CLINICAL CONTACT LENS PRACTICE

CLINICAL CONTACT LENS PRACTICE

Editors

EDWARD S. BENNETT, OD, MS, FAAO

Associate Professor of Optometry
Director of Student Services
University of Missouri-St. Louis College of Optometry
St. Louis, Missouri

BARRY A. WEISSMAN, OD, PHD, FAAO

Professor of Ophthalmology
Jules Stein Eye Institute
UCLA School of Medicine
Los Angeles, California

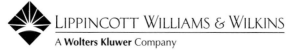

LIPPINCOTT WILLIAMS & WILKINS
A **Wolters Kluwer** Company
Philadelphia · Baltimore · New York · London
Buenos Aires · Hong Kong · Sydney · Tokyo

Acquisitions Editor: Jonathan Pine
Developmental Editor: Michael Standen
Manufacturing Manager: Ben Rivera
Cover Designer: Christine Jenny
Compositor: Maryland Composition
Printer: Maple Press

© 2005 by LIPPINCOTT WILLIAMS & WILKINS
530 Walnut Street
Philadelphia, PA 19106 USA
LWW.com

Library of Congress Cataloging-in-Publication Data

Clinical contact lens practice / editors, Edward S. Bennett, Barry A. Weissman.
    p. ; cm.
  Includes bibliographical references and index.
  ISBN 0-7817-3705-2
1. Contact lenses. I. Bennett, Edward S. II. Weissman, Barry A.
  [DNLM: 1. Contact Lenses. WW 355 C6408 2005].
RE977.C6C5225 2005
617.7′523—dc22

2004011055

Care has been taken to confirm the accuracy of the information presented and to describe generally accepted practices. However, the authors, editors, and publisher are not responsible for errors or omissions or for any consequences from application of the information in this book and make no warranty, expressed or implied, with respect to the currency, completeness, or accuracy of the contents of the publication. Application of this information in a particular situation remains the professional responsibility of the practitioner.

The authors, editors, and publisher have exerted every effort to ensure that drug selection and dosage set forth in this text are in accordance with current recommendations and practice at the time of publication. However, in view of ongoing research, changes in government regulations, and the constant flow of information relating to drug therapy and drug reactions, the reader is urged to check the package insert for each drug for any change in indications and dosage and for added warnings and precautions. This is particularly important when the recommended agent is a new or infrequently employed drug.

Some drugs and medical devices presented in this publication have Food and Drug Administration (FDA) clearance for limited use in restricted research settings. It is the responsibility of the health care provider to ascertain the FDA status of each drug or device planned for use in their clinical practice.

10 9 8 7 6 5 4 3 2 1

I would like to dedicate this book to the finest optometrist I know, my wife Jean, for allowing me the opportunity to do what I love. I would also like to acknowledge my children, Matt, Josh, and Emily, of whom I am very proud.

E.S.B.

I first dedicate my efforts on this text to my family: my wife Linda, and our children, Jeremy and Yardena, who have sacrificed time with me, not just for this text, but for many academic endeavors over the last several decades.

I also dedicate this book in appreciation to the Department of Ophthalmology of the David Geffen School of Medicine at UCLA and my colleagues: the many individual members of this department.

B.A.W.

CONTENTS

CONTRIBUTING AUTHORS

Dwight H. Akerman, OD   CIBA Vision Corporation, Duluth, Georgia

Anthony J. Aldave, MD   Assistant Professor of Ophthalmology, The Jules Stein Eye Institute, UCLA School of Medicine, Los Angeles, California

Keith Ames, OD   Chillicote, Ohio

Joseph T. Barr, OD, MS   Professor, Optometry and Vision Science, The Ohio State University, College of Optometry, Columbus, Ohio

Carolyn G. Begley, OD, MS   Professor, School of Optometry, Indiana University Bloomington, Indiana

William J. "Joe" Benjamin, OD, MS, PhD   Professor of Optometry and Physiological Optics, Director of Clinical Eye Research, School of Optometry, University of Alabama at Birmingham, Birmingham, Alabama

Peter D. Bergenske, OD   Chief, Contact Lens Service, College of Optometry, Pacific University, Forest Grove, Oregon

Cheryl Bergin, BA   University of Missouri-St. Louis College of Optometry, St. Louis, Missouri

Jan P.G. Bergmanson, OD, PhD   Professor/Director, Texas Eye Research and Technology Center, University of Houston, College of Optometry, Houston, Texas

James A. Bonafini, Jr., MS   Research Director, Research, Development & Engineering, Bausch & Lomb, Rochester, New York

Noel A. Brennan, OD, PhD   Brennan Consultants Pty Ltd, Kew, Australia

Urs Businger, OD   Josef Uoch Optiker AG, Luzern, Switzerland

Barbara Caffery OD, MS   Toronto, Ontario, Canada

Alexander Cannella, RN, FCLSA   Global Professional Services, Polymer Technology-A Bausch & Lomb Company, Wilmington, Massachusetts

Leo G. Carney, PhD, DSc   Professor, School of Optometry, Queensland University of Technology, Kelvin Grove, Australia

Nicole A. Carnt, BOptom   Senior Research Optometrist, Vision CRC, The University of New South Wales, Sydney, Australia

Patrick J. Caroline, COT   Associate Professor, Pacific University College of Optometry, Forest Grove, Oregon; Assistant Professor, Oregon Health Sciences University, Casey Eye Institute, Department of Ophthalmology, Portland, Oregon

Wing-Kwong Chan, FRCS (Edinburgh)   Clinical Senior Lecturer, Department of Ophthalmology, National University of Singapore; Senior Consultant, Refractive Surgery Service, Singapore National Eye Centre, Singapore

Melissa W. Chun, OD, FAAO   Assistant Clinical Professor of Ophthalmology, Department of Ophthalmology, Jules Stein Eye Institute, UCLA, Los Angeles, California

Brigitte Cowell, PhD   Research Associate, Cooperative Research Centre for Eye Research and Technology, University of New South Wales, Sydney, Australia

Anthony P. Cullen, OD, PhD   Professor, School of Optometry, University of Waterloo, Waterloo, Ontario, Canada

Larry J. Davis, OD   Dean, University of Missouri-St. Louis College of Optometry, St. Louis, Missouri

Robert L. Davis, OD, FAAO   Oak Lawn, Illinois

Paul N. De Land, PhD   Professor of Mathematics, Department of Mathematics, California State University, Fullerton, California

Michael D. Depaolis, OD   Clinical Associate, Department of Ophthalmology, University of Rochester School of Medicine, Rochester, New York; Adjunct Faculty, Pennsylvania School of Optometry, Philadelphia, Pennsylvania

Robert E. Dister, OD, JD, MS   Associate Clinical Professor, School of Optometry, UC Berkeley, Berkeley, California

Michael J. Doughty, PhD, FAAO   Research Professor, Department of Vision Science, Glasgow Caledonian University, Glasgow, Scotland

James P. Dunn, Jr., MD   Associate Professor of Ophthalmology, The Wilmer Eye Institute, The Johns Hopkins Hospital, Baltimore, Maryland

Rènée du Toit, Mphil, Optom   Manager Clinical Research, Vision CRC, The University of New South Wales, Sydney, Australia

Timothy B. Edrington, OD, MS   Professor, Cornea and Contact Lens Service, Southern California College of Optometry, Fullerton, California

Garold L. Edwards, OD   Felton, California

Nathan Efron, PhD, DSc   Professor of Clinical Optometry, Dean of Research, Department of Optometry and Neuroscience, University of Manchester Institute of Science and Technology, Manchester, United Kingdom

Arthur B. Epstein, OD, FAAO   Clinical Adjunct Assistant Professor, Northeastern State University, College of Optometry, Tahlequah, Oklahoma; Director of the Contact Lens Service, Ophthalmology, North Shore University Hospital, NYU School of Medicine, Manhasset, New York

Desmond Fonn, Dip Optom, M.Optom, FAAO   Professor, Centre for Contact Lens Research, School of Optometry, University of Waterloo, Waterloo, Ontario, Canada

Lisa Barnhart Fox, OD   Jules Stein Eye Institute, David Geffen School of Medicine at UCLA, Los Angeles, California

Rex Ghormley, OD   St. Louis, Missouri

Michael J. Giese, OD, PhD   Associate Professor of Clinical Optometry, College of Optometry, Ohio State University, Columbus, Ohio

Robert M. Grohe, OD, FAAO   Assistant Professor of Clinical Ophthalmology, Northwestern University, Department of Ophthalmology, Chicago, Illinois

David W. Hansen, OD, FAAO   Des Moines Eye Care, P.C., Des Moines, Iowa

Najat J. Harmis, Bachelor of Applied Science (Biomedical)   Laboratory Manager, Vision CRC, University of New South Wales, Kensington, Australia

Michael G. Harris, OD, JD, MS, FAAO   Director of Policy and Planning, Associate Dean Emeritus, School of Optometry, University of California; Clinical Professor, School of Optometry, Meredith W. Morgan Eye Center, University of California, Berkeley, California

Beth Henderson, OD   Assistant Clinical Professor, University of Missouri-St. Louis College of Optometry, St. Louis, Missouri

Vinita Allee Henry, OD   Clinical Associate Professor, University of Missouri-St. Louis College of Optometry, St. Louis, Missouri

Richard M. Hill, OD, PhD   Dean and Professor Emeritus, College of Optometry, The Ohio State University, Columbus, Ohio

Brien A. Holden, PhD, DSc, FAAO   The Cornea and Contact Lens Research Unit, School of Optometry and the Cooperative Research Centre for Eye Research and Technology, The University of New South Wales, Sydney, Australia

Milton M. Hom, OD, FAAO, (DipCL)   Azusa, California

John Mark Jackson, OD, MS   Assistant Professor, Optometry, Southern College of Optometry, Memphis, Tennessee

Jeffrey D. Johnson, OD   Refractive Surgery Service, Massachusetts Eye and Ear Infirmary; Instructor of Ophthalmology, Harvard Medical School, Boston, Massachusetts

Janice M. Jurkus, OD, MBA   Professor, Illinois College of Optometry; Staff Doctor, Cornea & Contact Lenses, Illinois Eye Institute, Chicago, Illinois

Lisa Keay, BOptom   Research Optometrist, Cornea and Contact Lens Research Unit, University of New South Wales, Sydney, Australia

Patricia Keech, OD   Shoreline, Washington

Harue J. Marsden, OD, MS   Associate Professor, Chief, Cornea and Contact Lens Department, Southern California College of Optometry, Fullerton, California

Timothy T. McMahon, OD, FAAO   Professor of Ophthalmology, Department of Ophthalmology and Visual Sciences, University of Illinois at Chicago, Chicago, Illinois; Director, Contact Lens Service, University of Illinois Medical Center, Chicago, Illinois

Bartly J. Mondino, OD   University of California, Los Angeles, Jules Stein Eye Institute, UCLA School of Medicine, Los Angeles, California

Bruce W. Morgan, OD, FAAO   Associate Professor, Chief of Cornea and Contact Lens Service, Michigan College of Optometry, Big Rapids, Michigan

Eric B. Papas, PhD   Executive Director Research and Development, Vision CRC, University of New South Wales, Sydney, Australia

Jerry R. Paugh, OD, PhD   Associate Professor and Director of Research, Basic and Visual Science, Southern California College of Optometry, Fullerton, California

Kenneth W. Pullum, OD   Senior Optometrist, Optometry, Moorfields Eye Hospital, London; Senior Optometrist, Optometry, Oxford Eye Hospital, Oxford, United Kingdom

Thomas Quinn, OD, MS   Athens, Ohio

Yaron S. Rabinowitz, MD   Clinical Professor, Ophthalmology, UCLA School of Medicine, Los Angeles, California; Director of Ophthalmology Research, Surgery, Cedars-Sinai Medical Center, Los Angeles, California

Marjorie J. Rah, OD, PhD　Assistant Professor of Optometry, The New England College of Optometry, Boston, Massachusetts

Melvin J. Remba, MOPT, OD　Chief, Optometry, Cedars Sinai Medical Center, Los Angeles, California

Cristina M. Schnider, OD　Manager, R & D Clinical Claims, Vistakon Global Franchise, Jacksonville, Florida

Julie A. Schornack, OD, MEd　Southern California College of Optometry, Fullerton, California

Ronald G. Seger　Mountain View, California

Manoj Sharma　University of California, Los Angeles, Jules Stein Eye Institute, UCLA School of Medicine, Los Angeles, California

Joseph P. Shovlin, OD, FAAO　Senior Optometrist, Northeastern Eye Institute, Scranton, Pennsylvania

Joel A. Silbert, OD, FAAO　Professor of Optometry, Pennsylvania College of Optometry, Elkins Park, Pennsylvania; Director, Cornea & Specialty Contact Lens Service, The Eye Institute, Philadelphia, Pennsylvania

Rajni Singh, OD　University of Missouri-St. Louis College of Optometry, St. Louis, Missouri

Cheryl Skotnitsky, BS, OD　Research Optometrist, Vision Cooperative Research Centre, The University of New South Wales, Sydney, Australia

Jennifer Smythe, OD, MS, FAAO　Assistant Professor of Optometry, Pacific University, Forest Grove, Oregon

Luigina Sorbara, OD, M.Sc　Lecturer, Head of Contact Lens Clinic, School of Optometry, University of Waterloo, Waterloo, Ontario, Canada

Fiona Stapleton, PhD, FAAO, McOPtom　Senior Lecturer, Cornea and Contact Lens Research Unit, School of Optometry and Vision Science and Vision CRC, University of New South Wales, Sydney, Australia

Judith Stern, BOptom　Program Director, Vision CRC, The University of New South Wales, New South Wales, Australia

Serina Stretton, PhD　Science Writer, Vision Co-operative Research Centre, The University of New South Wales, Sydney, Australia

Kai C. Su, PhD　President, Technology Resource International Corporation, Alpharetta, Georgia

Helen A. Swarbrick, PhD, FAAO　Senior Lecturer, School of Optometry and Vision Science, University of New South Wales, Sydney, Australia

Deborah F. Sweeney, PhD　CEO, Vision Co-operative Research Centre, The University of New South Wales, Sydney, Australia

Loretta B. Szczotka-Flynn, OD　Assistant Professor, Ophthalmology, Case Western Reserve University; Director, Contact Lens Service, Ophthalmology, University Hospitals of Cleveland, Cleveland, Ohio

Carol Tam, OD　Clinical Assistant Professor, University of Missouri-St. Louis College of Optometry, St. Louis, Missouri

Alan Tomlinson, PhD　Professor, Chairman of the Department, Glasgow Caledonian University, Department of Vision Science, Glasgow, Scotland

Heidi Wagner, OD　Assistant Professor, College of Optometry, Nova Southeastern University, College of Optometry, Ft. Lauderdale, Florida

Jeffrey Jay Walline, OD, PhD　Research Scientist, College of Optometry, Ohio State University, Columbus, Ohio

Richard E. Weisbarth, OD, FAAO　Vice President, Professional Services, Professional Services North America, CIBA Vision Corporation, Duluth, Georgia

Mark D.P. Willcox, PhD　Professor, Optometry and Vision Science, University of New South Wales, Sydney, Australia

Lynn C. Winterton, PhD　Distinguished Research Fellow, CIBA Vision Corporation, Duluth, Georgia

Jack J. Yager, OD　Orlando, Florida

Karen K. Yeung, OD　Director of Optometry, Arthur Ashe Student Health, University of California, Los Angeles, Los Angeles, California

Julie A. Yu, OD　Assistant Professor, Southern California College of Optometry, Fullerton, California

Alana J. Zhou, OD　Jules Stein Eye Institute, David Geffen School of Medicine at UCLA, Los Angeles, California

Hua Zhu, PhD　Senior Research Associate, School of Optometry and Vision Science, University of New South Wales, Sydney, Australia

PREFACE

Contact lenses remain an important component of eye care practice. As the contact lens field continues to progress at a rapid pace, textbooks such as *Clinical Contact Lens Practice* are necessary from time to time. We are therefore pleased to provide this book and hope you, our reader, will enjoy reading and using it as much as we have enjoyed preparing this material for you.

A number of very important new applications of contact lens care have developed during the past decade. Practitioners should appreciate the latest clinical paradigms used to approach challenging patients, such as postrefractive surgery and other forms of irregular cornea, utilizing the latest technology, research results, and lens designs. Several exciting new areas, such as corneal reshaping as a nonsurgical alternative to myopia reduction, are emphasized in this text. Other developing areas include the introduction of highly oxygen permeable silicone hydrogels and the new and improved multifocal lens designs that have been increasingly successful in contact lens management of the presbyopic patient.

On the one hand, we present a series of practical case grand round chapters on topics such as torics, bifocals, and irregular cornea to benefit the clinician interested in new methods of managing these challenging cases. On the other, we are very excited about presenting chapters pertaining to important but infrequently aired topics such as scleral lenses, contact lenses and the environment, legal issues, and clinical research applications.

Our goals are practical: to assist the clinician in his or her daily practice of contact lens care; to bring together many of the outstanding teachers, scholars, scientists, and clinicians to provide the best, most up-to-date information. We have attempted to provide a clear, concise, but also comprehensive text. It is certainly a text that does not necessitate reading from front to back, as a novel. Instead, one can customize study to reflect interests in specific areas (i.e., torics, bifocals, keratoconus, anterior segment disease, contact lens care, etc.).

Edward S. Bennett
Barry A. Weissman

ACKNOWLEDGMENTS

We would like to recognize a few individuals to whom we are especially indebted. The original idea for this text was proposed by Dr. Bob Grohe. This text is the result of the fine efforts of Michael Standen, Developmental Editor, and Jonathan Pine, Senior Executive Editor, for Lippincott Williams & Wilkins. Their ongoing assistance and support have been invaluable in making this project a reality. We would also like to acknowledge individuals who assisted in this effort by reviewing drafts, providing graphical assistance, inputting information, and assisting with literature reviews. These include Cheryl Bergin, Maria Taylor, and Janice White. The support of Dr. Jack Bennett, past Dean and Dr. Larry Davis, current Dean of the University of Missouri-St. Louis College of Optometry, was greatly appreciated by Ed Bennett. Bartly J. Mondino, MD, Director of the Jules Stein Eye Institute and Chairman of the Department of Ophthalmology and David Geffen School of Medicine at UCLA, should be similarly acknowledged for his continuing support of Barry Weissman.

Most of all, we thank the contributors, whose expertise and unselfish devotion toward enhancing and upgrading the contact lens education of interested contact lens practitioners, researchers, students, and assistants, has made this text possible.

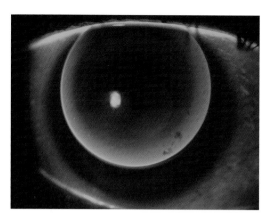

COLOR PLATE 7B.10. A static lid-attachment fit on a with-the-rule cornea showing horizontal alignment with pooling below (in the steep vertical meridian).

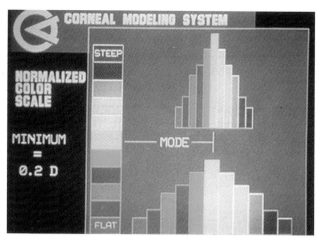

COLOR PLATE 9.6. Color scale used in a videokeratograph.

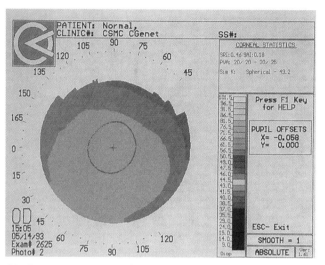

COLOR PLATE 9.10. Videokeratograph of a normal human cornea in the "absolute" scale.

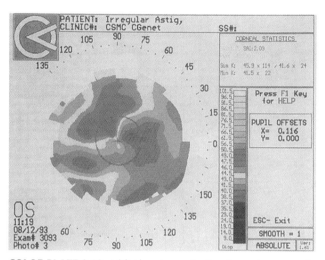

COLOR PLATE 9.12. Videokeratograph of an irregular cornea in the "absolute" scale.

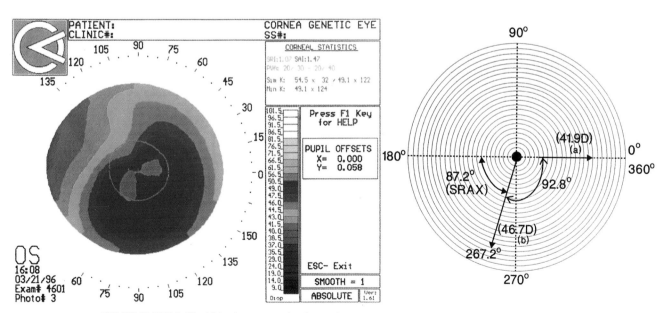

COLOR PLATE 9.13. Videokeratograph of a patient with keratoconus demonstrating the three topographic features of keratoconus and the calculation of the SRAX index.

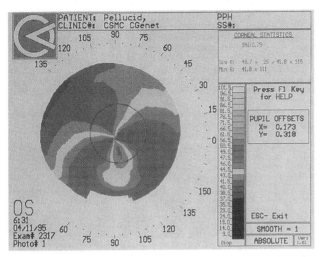

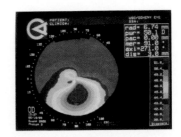

COLOR PLATE 9.14. Videokeratograph of a patient with pellucid marginal degeneration showing a typical butterfly pattern.

COLOR PLATE 9.15. Videokeratograph of a patient with keratoconus illustrating calculation of the I-S value.

Table 1
Calculation of I-S Value in Patient 5 (Right Eye)*

Inferior cornea							
degrees	330	300	270	240	210		
diopters	45.9	49.7	50.1	48.6	44.7	239 /5	= 47.8 (I) (average inferior corneal power)
Superior cornea							
degrees	150	120	90	60	30		
diopters	41.6	40.9	40.6	40.2	40.2	203.5/5	= 40.7 (S) (average superior corneal power)

I-S Value = 47.8 (I) − 40.7 (S) = 7.1 diopters

* Measurements taken 3 mm from center of cornea

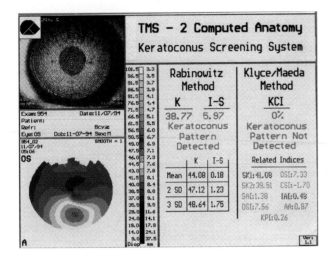

COLOR PLATE 9.16. Videokeratograph of a patient with "early" keratoconus and the Rabinowitz and Maeda-Klyce indices on the Tomey topographer.

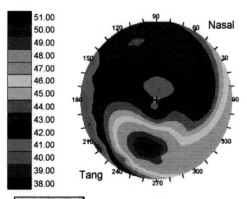

COLOR PLATE 9.17. Videokeratograph of the fellow eye of a patient with keratoconus. The eye appeared clinically normal, showing calculation of the KISA% index in both the sagittal and tangential views on the Alcon topographer.

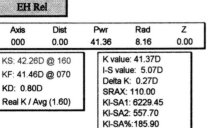

EH Rel

Axis	Dist	Pwr	Rad	Z
000	0.00	41.36	8.16	0.00

KS: 42.26D @ 160	K value: 41.37D
KF: 41.46D @ 070	I-S value: 5.07D
KD: 0.80D	Delta K: 0.27D
Real K / Avg (1.60)	SRAX: 110.00
	KI-SA1: 6229.45
	KI-SA2: 557.70
	KI-SA%:185.90

Axis	Dist	Pwr	Rad	Z
000	0.00	41.36	8.16	0.00

K value: 41.32D	KS: 41.96D @ 170
I-S value: 2.40D	KF: 40.97D @ 070
Delta K: 0.92D	KD: 0.99D
SRAX: 40.00	Real K / Avg (1.60)
KI-SA1: 3649.38	
KI-SA2: 96.00	
KI-SA%:32.00	**Tang. vs. Sag.**

Keratoconus: one or more of the following: Corneal thinning by slit-lamp evaluation, an iron ring, Vogt's striae

Early Keratoconus: no slit-lamp findings, with scissoring on retinoscopy

Keratoconus Suspect: clinically normal, with suspicious topography

COLOR PLATE 9.19. Classification scheme for keratoconus using videokeratography and clinical signs.

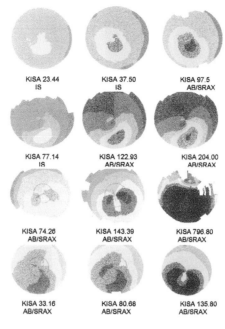

KISA 23.44 IS   KISA 37.50 IS   KISA 97.5 AB/SRAX

KISA 77.14 IS   KISA 122.93 AB/SRAX   KISA 204.00 AB/SRAX

KISA 74.26 AB/SRAX   KISA 143.39 AB/SRAX   KISA 796.80 AB/SRAX

KISA 33.16 AB/SRAX   KISA 80.68 AB/SRAX   KISA 135.80 AB/SRAX

COLOR PLATE 9.20. Videokeratographs with pattern and indices analysis showing progression of keratoconus from suspect to clinically affected over a 5-year period.

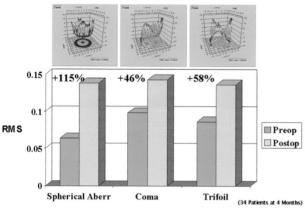

COLOR PLATE 9.21. Higher-order aberrations induced by LASIK surgery.

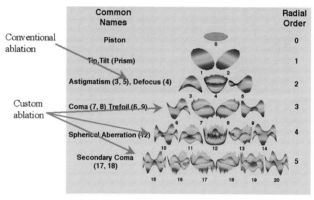

COLOR PLATE 9.25. Zernicke aberration components up to fifth-order aberrations also illustrating which aberrations are treated with conventional versus wavefront LASIK.

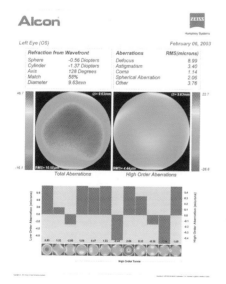

COLOR PLATE 9.26. Preoperative wavefront map output of the Alcon LADARWAVE Hartman-Shack sensor illustrating the total and the higher-order aberrations, as well as their decomposition.

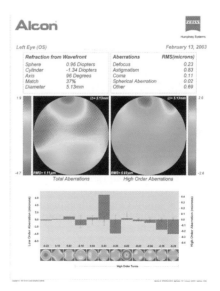

COLOR PLATE 9.27. Postoperative wavefront map 1 week after treatment with wavefront LASIK using the Alcon Custom Cornea system. The patient's night vision and quality of vision improved significantly, his total aberrations decreased to 1.1 (m, and higher-order aberrations decreased to 0.69 μm.)

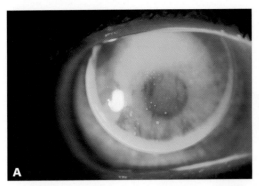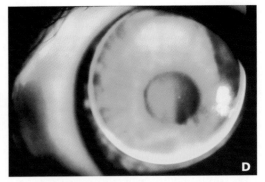

COLOR PLATE 10.11. A: Fluorescein appearance before yellow filter use (pseudo-steep). **D:** Fluorescein appearance after yellow filter use to show subtle pattern details.

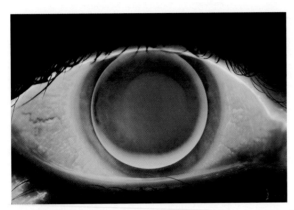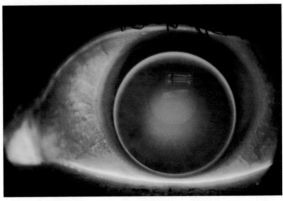

COLOR PLATE 16A.4. Alignment fluorescein pattern (posterior surface of the lens matching the corneal contour) with adequate edge clearance.

COLOR PLATE 16A.5. Lens with minimal edge clearance (tight periphery). This represents approximately 60 t of tear lens thickness at the edge.

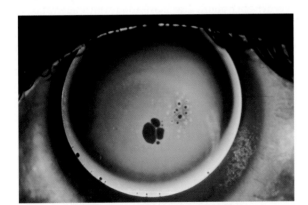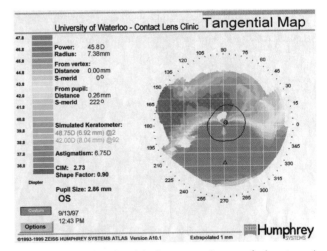

COLOR PLATE 16A.6. Lens fit demonstrating excessive edge clearance in depth and width characterized by the bubbles at the edge, as well as the bright fluorescein appearance. The inferior edge clearance is accentuated by the lid pressure imparted on the superior region of the lens.

COLOR PLATE 16A.13. Videokeratoscopic map of a keratoconic cornea depicting flatter (blue color) and steeper (red color) with inferior decentration of the steeper zone.

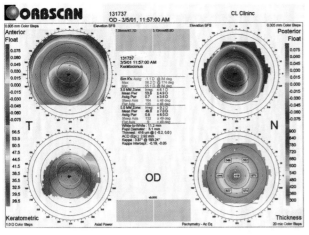

COLOR PLATE 16A.14. Printout from the Orbscan showing the anterior and posterior topography maps with a corneal thickness plot.

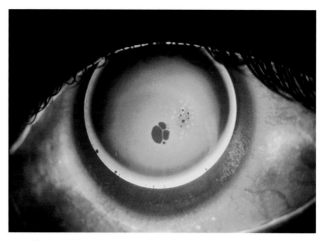

COLOR PLATE 16B.2. Excessive apical and peripheral clearance showing air bubbles at the edge and under center of the lens.

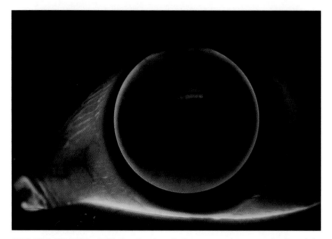

COLOR PLATE 16B.3. Optimal lens-to-cornea relationship showing alignment and adequate edge clearance.

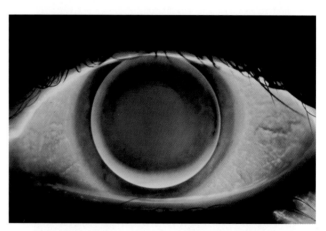

COLOR PLATE 16B.6. Optimal fluorescein pattern showing slightly more inferior edge clearance than lateral clearance.

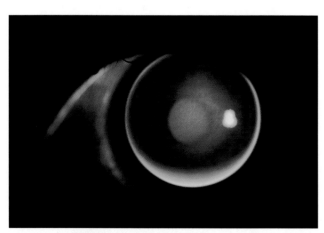

COLOR PLATE 16B.7. Aspheric design optimally fitted (spherical base curve) lens on a with-the-rule astigmatic cornea. The fluorescein pattern shows some apical clearance and relatively more inferior edge clearance consistent with this astigmatic cornea. This is a good example of gradual transition between touch and clearance consistent with an aspheric lens design.

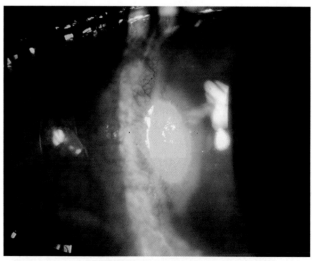

COLOR PLATE 16B.13. Large dellen (fluorescein staining in epithelial excavation) secondary to 3- and 9-o'clock corneal staining.

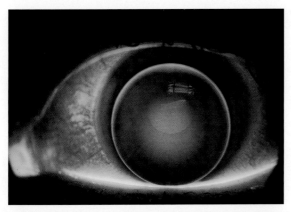

COLOR PLATE 16B.26. Steep lens showing apical clearance with minimal edge clearance in this inferiorly decentered gas permeable lens.

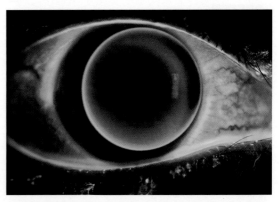

COLOR PLATE 16B.27. Flat (base curve) nasally decentered gas permeable lens.

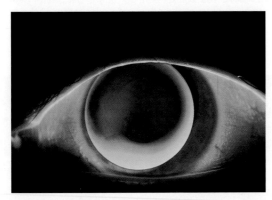

COLOR PLATE 16B.28. Flat base curve with excessive edge clearance causing nasal decentration of this aspheric gas permeable lens.

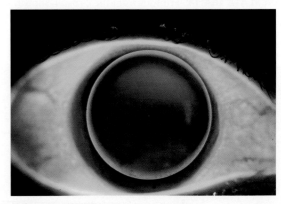

COLOR PLATE 16B.29. Alignment fit showing improved centration and acceptable fluorescein pattern. This is the same eye as shown in Color Plate 16B.27, which has been fitted with a steeper base curve lens.

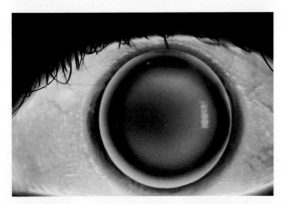

COLOR PLATE 16B.30. Large-diameter and large optic zone depicting excessive central clearance.

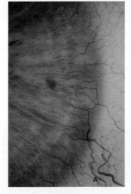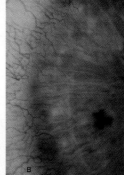

COLOR PLATE 22.10. Peripheral neovascularization **(A)** subsequent to long-term wear of low-Dk soft lens and **(B)** 30 days after refitting with high-Dk lens.

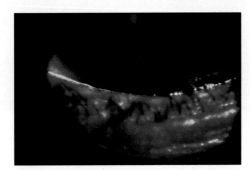

COLOR PLATE 23.4. Unsaturated tear meniscus. (Courtesy of J.E. Josephson.)

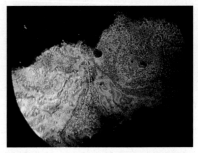

COLOR PLATE 23.7. "Colored fringe" interference pattern. (From Josephson JE. Appearance of the preocular tear film lipid layer. *Am J Optom Physiol Opt* 1983:60:885, with permission.)

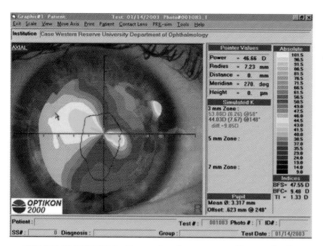

COLOR PLATE 28.1. Example of a steep-to-flat graft tilt.

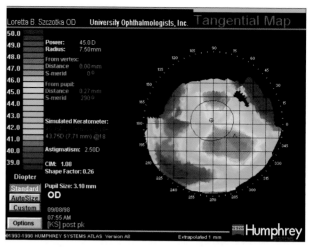

COLOR PLATE 28.2. Example of a prolate shape after corneal transplantation.

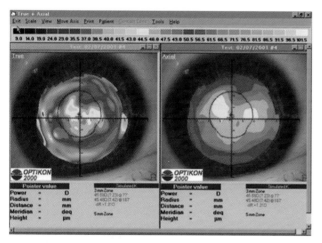

COLOR PLATE 28.3. Example of an oblate corneal shape after penetrating keratoplasty.

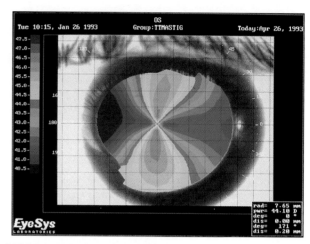

COLOR PLATE 28.7. Global astigmatism. With-the-rule astigmatism topographic pattern involving virtually the entire mappable surface.

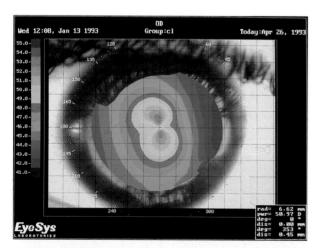

COLOR PLATE 28.8. Focal astigmatism. With-the-rule astigmatism topographic pattern primarily involving a 4-mm central zone. Note the lower amplitude oval-shaped global astigmatism pattern by observing just the green and blue colors.

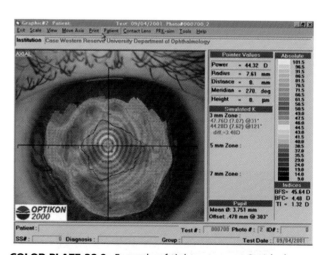

COLOR PLATE 28.9. Example of tight sutures at 8 o'clock causing localized steepening.

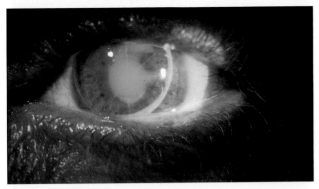

COLOR PLATE 28.10. Example of optically plus-powered lacrimal lens (formed beneath a rigid gas-permeable lens after radial keratotomy).

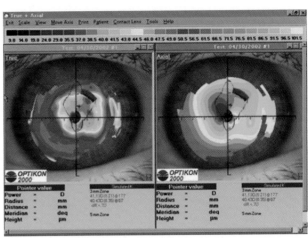

COLOR PLATE 28.11. Topographical differences noted on axial versus tangential maps after radial keratotomy.

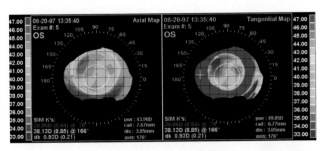

COLOR PLATE 28.12. Topographical differences noted on axial versus tangential maps on the same eye after automated lamellar keratoplasty. Note the cursor positioned over the same point on the two different maps results in very different corneal curvature readings.

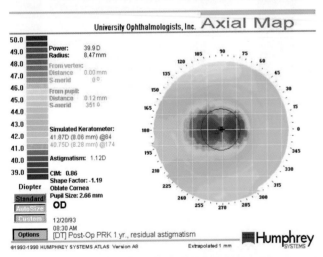

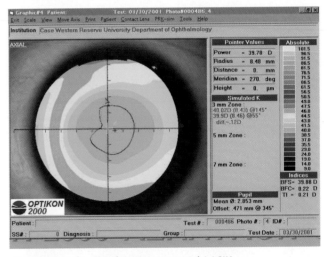

COLOR PLATE 28.13. Example of topography after photorefractive keratectomy and LASIK. **(Left)** This eye underwent photorefractive keratectomy and has a symmetrical peripheral cornea surrounding the ablation. **(Right)** This eye underwent laser-assisted in situ keratomileusis and has more asymmetry surrounding the ablation zone.

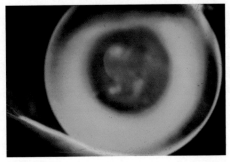

COLOR PLATE 28.14. Large, flat-fitted lens on an eye with keratoconus.

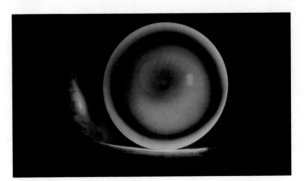

COLOR PLATE 28.15. "Three-point-touch" fluorescein pattern in keratoconus.

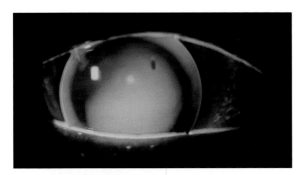

COLOR PLATE 28.16. Apical clearance fit.

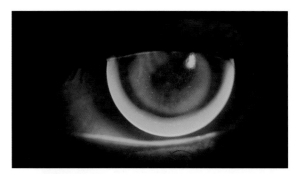

COLOR PLATE 28.17. Overall diameter/posterior optic zone: 8.6/7.6-mm gas-permeable lens shown on a keratoconus cornea.

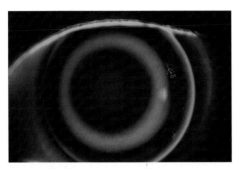

COLOR PLATE 29.3. Fluorescein pattern of an ideal fit of a reverse-geometry lens design.

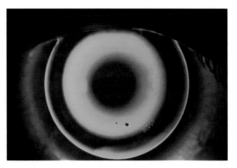

COLOR PLATE 29.5. Photo of a lens with sagittal depth that is too deep.

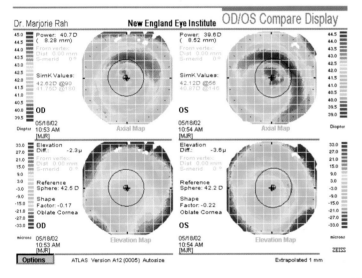

COLOR PLATE 29.6. Central island corneal topography caused by a lens with excess sagittal depth.

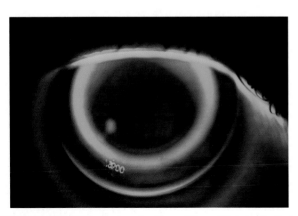

COLOR PLATE 29.8. Photo of a lens with sagittal depth that is too shallow.

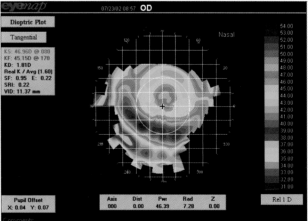

COLOR PLATE 29.9. Topography map from a lens with shallow sagittal depth.

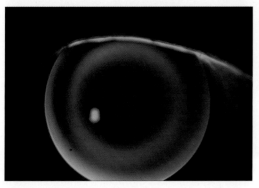

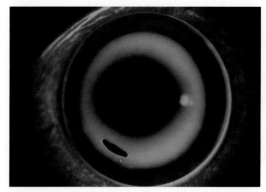

COLOR PLATE 29.11. Decentered lens due to a flat alignment zone.

COLOR PLATE 29.13. Photograph of a lens with a steep alignment zone.

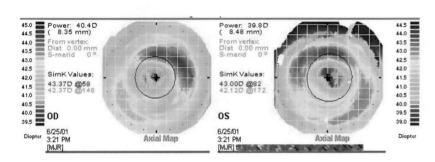

COLOR PLATE 29.14. Topography pattern for Case 1 depicting a small treatment zone from a lens with excessive sagittal depth.

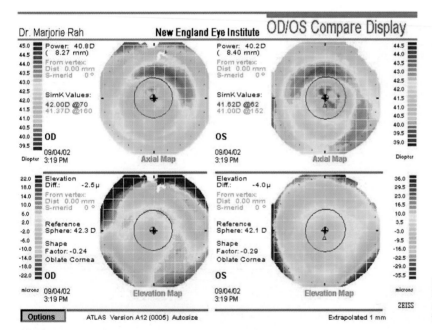

COLOR PLATE 29.15. Corneal topography for Case 1 following a change in contact lens parameters to increase the treatment zone diameter.

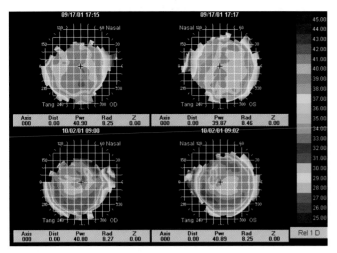

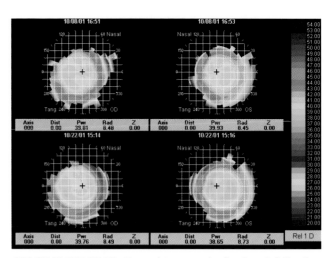

COLOR PLATE 29.16. Baseline corneal topography for Case 2.

COLOR PLATE 29.17. Corneal topography for Case 2 following 1 week of treatment.

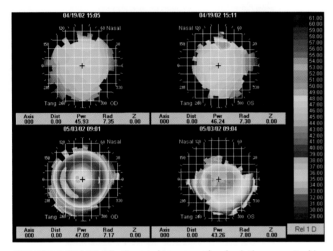

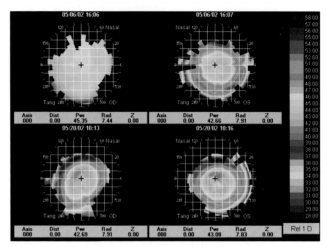

COLOR PLATE 29.18. Corneal topography depicting a central island in Case 3 following 1 day of treatment.

COLOR PLATE 29.19. Corneal topography showing the change in corneal curvature in Case 3 after 3 days of treatment. The central island has resolved, the right eye had returned to baseline values, and the left eye showed improved progress of the treatment.

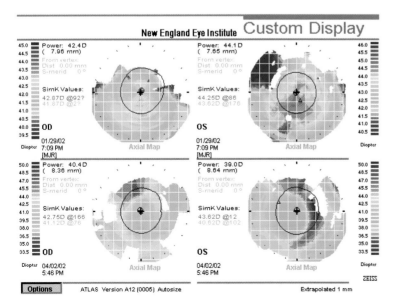

COLOR PLATE 29.20. Corneal topography maps following treatment with overnight corneal-reshaping contact lenses in Case 4.

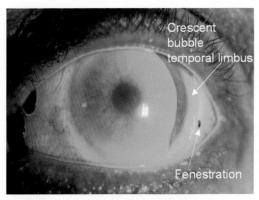

COLOR PLATE 33.4. Fenestrated scleral lens *in situ*. Note the crescent shaped bubble on the temporal side and reduced clearance on the nasal side.

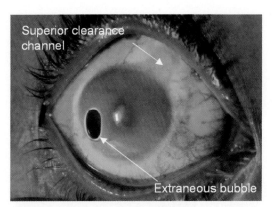

COLOR PLATE 33.7. Channeled scleral lens *in situ*.

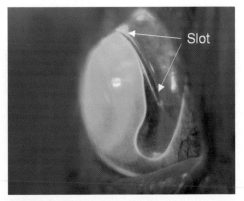

COLOR PLATE 33.10. Slotted scleral lens *in situ* fitted to a highly protrusive keratoglobus. Even a thinly cut slot, as shown here, enables excellent tear coverage.

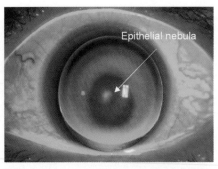

COLOR PLATE 33.40. A proud central nebula with corneal lens wear in keratoconus. Apical contact with the lens abrades the delicate surface.

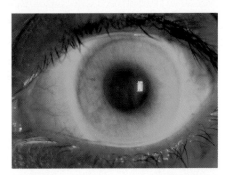

COLOR PLATE 33.42. The same eye as shown in Fig. 33.41 fitted with a scleral lens with central contact zone. There is good limbal clearance, but note that the contact zone extends more to the nasal side than to the temporal side.

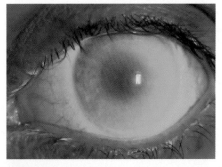

COLOR PLATE 33.43. One significant OZP increment of 0.24 mm gives minimum apical clearance. The upper nasal quadrant clearance is still noticeably less than the inferior temporal quadrant.

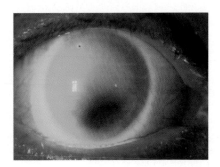

COLOR PLATE 33.45. Same eye as shown in Fig. 33.44 fitted with a rigid gas-permeable sealed scleral lens giving apical contact but clearance at the visual axis.

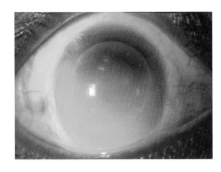

COLOR PLATE 33.47. Same eye as shown in Fig. 33.46 fitted with a sealed rigid gas-permeable scleral lens giving full clearance except at the upper limbus and just inside. Typically, nearly all the astigmatism is corrected by the precorneal fluid reservoir without a visual axis contact zone, as is often necessary with some forms of primary corneal ectasia fitted with scleral lenses prior to a transplant. Achieving visual axis clearance is not usually a problem because of the symmetry about the geometric axis. Superior contact may be difficult to avoid with such a protrusive profile because of the tendency for the lens to displace downwards and temporally.

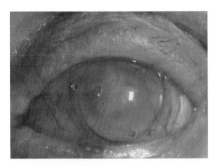

COLOR PLATE 33.49. A patient with Stevens-Johnson syndrome fitted with a fenestrated rigid gas-permeable scleral lens. In this example there is a fenestration at the nasal limbus, one just above the lid on the temporal side and a third (unseen) just under the upper lid in the upper temporal quadrant. The corneal surface is not distended, as is often the case with primary corneal ectasia or postoperative transplant, but the surface is still irregular. An area of clearance can be seen over the inferior half of the cornea, and a contact zone over the superior half. The small bubbles trapped under the optic zone are not a problem, but their presence suggests there could not be much more clearance if the lens is to retain a functional precorneal fluid reservoir. The corneal neovascularization is also clearly visible: this is part of the Stevens-Johnson syndrome disease process and was present before scleral lens fitting was undertaken.

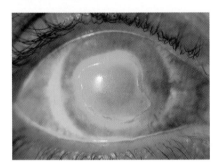

COLOR PLATE 33.50. A massive neurotrophic epithelial defect that was refractory to treatment.

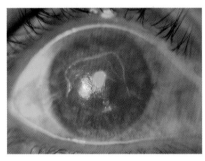

COLOR PLATE 33.51. The same lesion following 3 weeks day wear of a rigid gas-permeable scleral lens. The defect has almost resolved, although its original margin is still clearly visible.

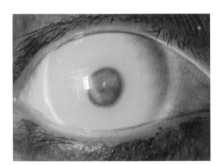

COLOR PLATE 33.54. A rigid gas-permeable scleral lens fitted for primary corneal ectasia with a central apex. Corneal stain is visible within the contact area.

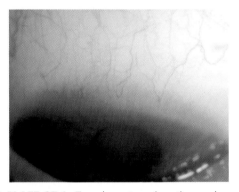

COLOR PLATE 37.1. Translucent conjunctiva and associated normal vessels encroaching onto the superior cornea.

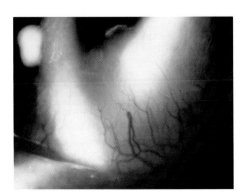

COLOR PLATE 37.2. Corneal vascularization.

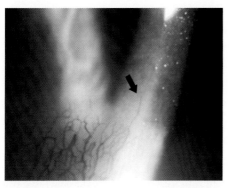

COLOR PLATE 37.3. A single straight superficial vessel (arrow) penetrating into the cornea of a 46-year-old woman who is a 38%-pHEMAi wearer.

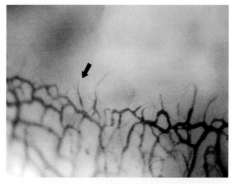

COLOR PLATE 37.4. High-magnification view of the limbus showing general hyperaemia and parallel tracked arterial and venous sections (arrow).

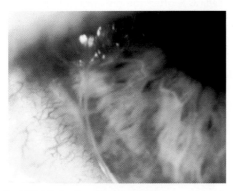

COLOR PLATE 37.5. Opacification and vascularization of peripheral cornea due to a poorly fitting rigid gas-permeable contact lens.

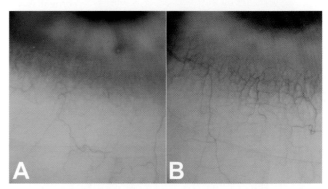

COLOR PLATE 37.6. Red-free image of right and left eyes of the same subject wearing a silicone hydrogel lens (A) and a 38% pHEMA lens (B). Note relative hyperaemia of the limbal vessels.

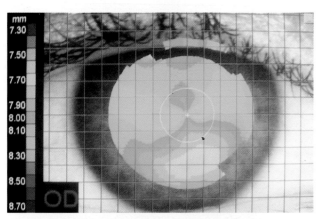

COLOR PLATE 40.9. Topography of the cornea shows inferior steepening, a sign that also can be seen in early keratoconic eyes. If no other classic signs of keratoconus can be found, then only time will tell if refitting was justified or if the finding was an indication of early keratoconus.

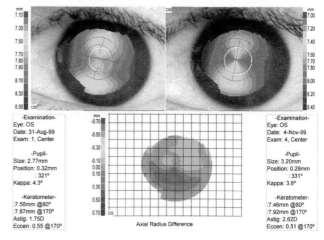

COLOR PLATE 40.10. Corneal topographies of a patient who complained that her vision decreased when wearing glasses instead of GP lenses for several days. **Left:** topography after wearing a spherical GP lens that gave 20/20 acuity; refraction was -7.25 -1.00 x 170 degrees. **Right:** topography after fitting the patient with a toric GP lens (20/20 acuity); refraction changed to -7.75 -3.00 x 170 degrees and the patient could switch between glasses and contact lenses without perceptible decrease in vision.

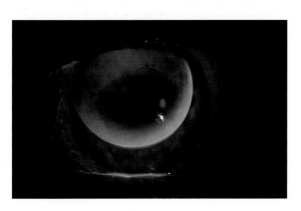

COLOR PLATE 40.11. Fluorescein pattern of a high-riding lens.

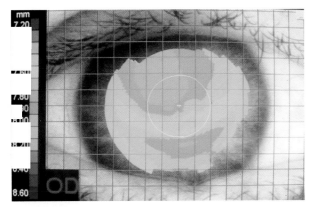

COLOR PLATE 40.12. Corneal topography after the lens was taken off the eye shown in Figure 40.11.

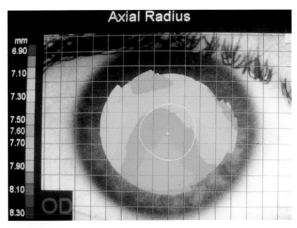

COLOR PLATE 40.13. Corneal topography after wearing a lens that rides constantly low.

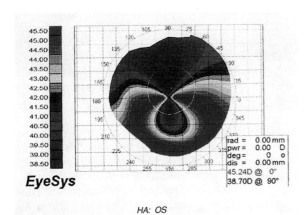

HA: OS

COLOR PLATE 49.5. Videokeratography map of pellucid marginal corneal degeneration.

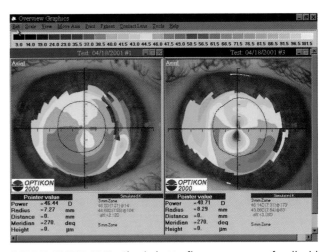

COLOR PLATE 49.7. Classic butterfly appearance of pellucid marginal degeneration showing inferior corneal steepening, superior corneal flattening, and high against-the-rule toricity.

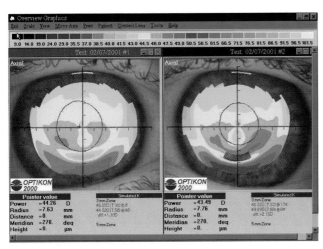

COLOR PLATE 49.8. Epithelial impression ring noted on topography of patient in this case and in Fig. 49.7, after wearing corneal gas-permeable lenses of diameter 9.9 mm OU. This explains the patient's spectacle blur upon lens removal.

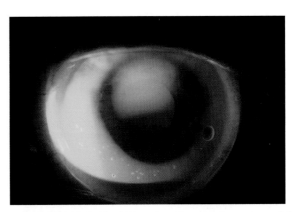

COLOR PLATE 49.9. Final Macrolens fluorescein pattern of the patient shown in Fig. 49.7.

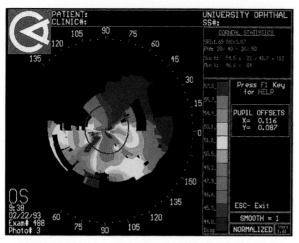

COLOR PLATE 49.11. Irregular corneal topography after penetrating keratoplasty.

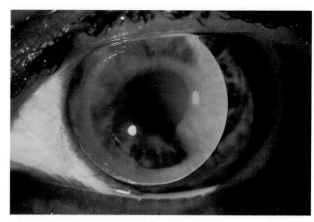

COLOR PLATE 49.12. Spherical rigid gas-permeable fluorescein pattern on cornea in Figure 49.11.

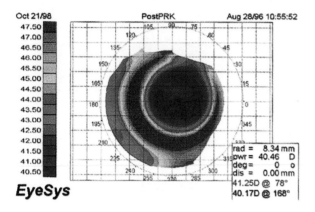

COLOR PLATE 49.16. Videokeratography map of post–photorefractive keratectomy.

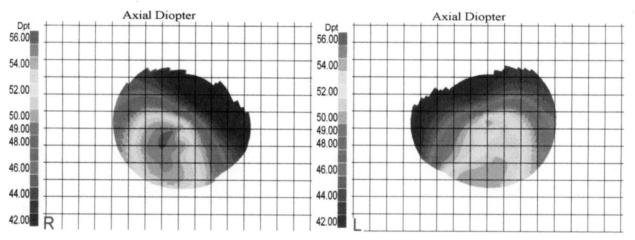

COLOR PLATE 49.17. Topography of a post-LASIK (laser *in situ* keratomileusis) patient revealing ectasia indicative of keratoconus.

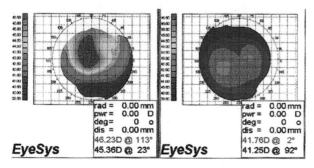

COLOR PLATE 49.19. Videokeratography maps of corneas after penetrating injury in the left eye.

BASIC TOPICS

HISTORY AND DEVELOPMENT OF CONTACT LENSES

JOSEPH T. BARR

INITIAL CONCEPTS

It was most likely Frederick A. Muller, a Weisbaden glass blower, who made the first scleral, nonoptical contact lens in 1887. His achievement was followed a year later by the optically useful scleral contact lenses designed independently by Adolph Eugen Fick, a Zurich physician, and Euegene Kalt, a French physician. It seems likely that each of these three pioneers was unaware of the work of his contemporaries. This is the history as we believed at the 100-year anniversary of the use of contact lenses.

Priority in the history of the principles and practice of contact lens design before 1887 is not easy to establish. da Vinci, Descartes, Young, and Herschel probably all deserve some credit for their experiments and theoretical efforts, which form the basis for the optical systems of contact lenses as we know them today (Table 1.1) (1).

In 1953, Hofstetter and Graham (2) discussed Leonardo da Vinci's contribution to the contact lens field. According to Hofstetter, da Vinci's real concept of a simple contact lens appears not in the body of the page of his notebook (in about 1508) but in the margin of the paper where da Vinci had penciled in some ideas and drawings on the nature of afterthoughts only remotely associated with his main text.

Leonardo da Vinci's large water-filled glass sphere with a face immersed in the water is generally interpreted as a contact lens only in the sense that the water in the glass bowl is in contact with the eye. However, his concept of a simple small contact lens is described and illustrated in the margin of the page. Four tiny drawings, each approximating

the size of ordinary contact lenses, are shown. One of these is the glass ampule from which the lens is to be cut. Hofstetter indicates that "Two (of the other) . . . may be interpreted as lenses in contact with the eye; the inside curve in each instance appearing to represent the cornea . . . it is clear that Leonardo described a small lens to be placed directly on the eye . . . " (Fig. 1.1).

Rene Descartes, in 1636 to 1637, used a hydrodiascope

TABLE 1.1. CONTACT LENS CHRONOLOGY

Material	Overall Diameter (mm)	Posterior Central Radius (mm)
Glass		
Fick (1888)	17–21 or 10–13	8–14
Kalt (1888)	16–22 or 11–13	7.9
PMMA		
Feinbloom (1936)	20	6.5–9.0
Tuohy (1948)	11–13	7.5–8.5
Microcorneals (1952)	9–10	Near corneal radius
Conforming contour corneals (1956)	7–9.4	Near corneal radius
Rigid gas permeable		
Polycon (1979)	9.5	0.2 flatter to on K
Soft		
Soft (1971)	12.0, later to 16.0	8.0–9.2
Silicone elastomer (1981)	10.5–12.5	7.5–8.3
Silicone hydrogel (1998)	14.0	8.5–8.8

PMMA, polymethyl methacrylate.

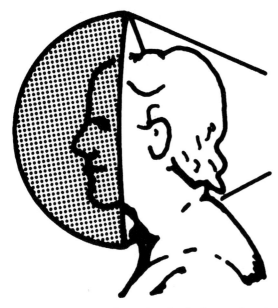

FIG. 1.1. Drawing illustrating da Vinci's experiment.

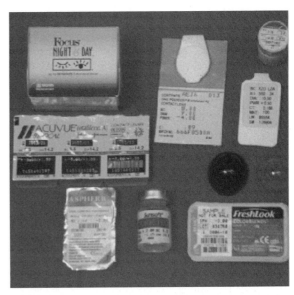

FIG. 1.2. Today's silicone hydrogel and disposable contact lenses **(top left).** Aspheric lens, toric soft lens, opaque cosmetic lens **(bottom row left to right).** Replicas of the Weisbaden lens (dark lens) and scleral lens (right of dark lens). Gas permeable lenses in **top right corner:** Polycon with brown label, Menicon Z in vial, and Corneal Refractive Therapy (Paragon Vision Sciences) in white flat pack.

(a water-filled tube with a glass lens at the distal end), which neutralized the refractive power of the cornea, as an aid in his study of corneal astigmatism. An apparatus similar to that of Descartes also was used by Thomas Young in 1801 to eliminate the refractive effect of the cornea during his investigation of accommodation. Enoch (3), in 1956, indicated that Descartes was not only the first to suggest applications of a contact lens but also was the first to apply such a lens to the eye and that Young apparently was first to correct an error of refraction with a contact lens plus an auxiliary lens.

Sir John F.W. Herschel, in 1827, precisely described the neutralization of a distorted cornea by a contact lens, and he also discussed the adaptation of this lens to the eye. Although Herschel did not make a contact lens, he described the practical optical principles perfectly. He suggested that fitting a contact lens would be delicate and that one could use a jelly substance between the eye and lens and perhaps take an actual mold of the cornea (3).

THE FIRST ATTEMPTS

F.A. Muller, a prosthetic eye manufacturer from Weisbaden, Germany, made a blown glass protective shell in 1887 for eyes with lagophthalmos and an eyelid deformed by cancer, as suggested by Saemisch, a physician (Fig. 1.2). A. Eugene Fick performed corneal contact lens experiments in 1888 and described the first contact lens worn beneath the eyelids with refractive power in his treatise *Eine Contactbrille,* a contact spectacle. Fick also experimented with a dextrose 2% solution between the small blown glass lens and the eye and later added a scleral flange to his corneal lens, resulting in improved comfort. Fick probably was the first to describe misting vision in his early contact lens work.

Prepared by Professor Abbe in Jena, Fick's glass hemispheres were 19 to 21 mm in diameter. Fick fitted animal eyes from animal eye molds and used molds from cadaver eyes to make lenses for himself and for other human subjects. Friedrich Muller of Wiesbaden describes some of Fick's lenses as "corneal lenses." These glass lenses weighed much more than present-day lenses, i.e., about 0.5 g. Fick used single curve blown glass lenses of 9.5- to 10.5-mm radius, concentric surfaced, and 17 to 19 mm in diameter, on animal eyes with good results. For human eyes, bicurve lenses of blown glass, 18 to 21 mm in diameter, were attempted for irregular astigmatism, aphakia, myopia, and keratoconus. Similar lenses were used on eyes suffering from opacities of the cornea. Some of Fick's earliest lenses for scarred corneas were made with the lens surface blackened except for a centrally placed stenopaic slit. Improved vision with contact lenses used by Fick on humans was due either to the lens itself or to an artificial pupil in the lens.

Eugene Kalt, in Paris, France, probably was second to Fick in describing a single curve blown glass corneal lens (11- to 12-mm diameter) in his early work with keratoconus in 1887 and 1888. Previously, keratoconus had been treated with silver nitrate cautery, pressure patches, and miotics. Kalt's lenses of 16 to 22 mm were worn by a keratoconic patient for a few hours; the results of this "experiment" were presented at a meeting.

However, it is possible that Kalt's work actually preceded Fick's (4,5). Early lenses made of blown glass usually were preferred to those made from grinding and polishing glass. Ground lenses had better optics but were less comfortable than blown glass lenses. Both Fick and August Muller used eye molds to make forms for contact lenses. Albert Carl Muller and Franciscus Albrecht Muller made blown glass scleral lenses until 1912, and another Kalt (Edouard) ground contact lenses for Dr. August Muller in 1889. These early lenses often induced significant amounts of residual astigmatic error.

August Muller (of Kiel, Germany, but no relation to Dr. F.A. Muller), a high myope, corrected his myopia with corneoscleral lenses in 1889 and is credited with an early understanding of lacrimal lens optics and the importance of lacrimal interchange behind the lens. He molded eyes of live humans and cadavers and used bicurve and tricurve lenses of 7- to 12-mm radius and 15- to 20-mm diameter. Curvature, thickness, and edge tolerance aspects of contact lens fitting were discussed by Muller. Muller also observed and explained overwear of the lens, or edema. He attempted to improve metabolism by improving the limbal fit of the lens.

Because glass is damaged by lacrimal fluid, these early glass lenses lasted only 6 to 18 months. Ground and polished glass lenses were made in the early 1900s by Karl Zeiss Optical Works in Jena and the Mueller Company in Wiesbaden. Some lenses even had ptosis crutches and drug delivery grooves, but these lenses suffered from poor surfaces.

FURTHER DEVELOPMENTS

Fluidless Glass Scleral Lenses

Josef Dallos, a physician in Budapest, refined the use of Negacol for making eye molds. From these molds he made 22- to 25-mm glass fluidless scleral lenses with ground corneal sections. It might take 20 hours of his time to make such a lens. Dallos understood the need for a slight mismatch between the shape of the contact lens and the eye as a physiologic fitting aid to lacrimal exchange. He also used fenestrations in the limbal area of the lens for the same purpose. Ida Mann, Senior Ophthalmologist from Moorfields Eye Hospital in London, reported that she persuaded Dallos to avoid the "menace of Hitler" and become a refugee when he moved to London and worked with her and Williamson-Noble's Rugg Gunn (6).

In London, Dallos and Adolf Mueller-Welt, who was in Stuttgart, both worked with "fluidless" glass scleral contact lenses. These minimum clearance lenses did not require use of the auxiliary contact lens solution so essential to the excessive corneal clearance lens, or "fluid" lens, fitted in the United States. A minimum clearance, or "fluidless," lens allowed lacrimal fluid to circulate between the lens and the cornea with varying degrees of freedom; this type of lens could be worn for much longer periods without corneal edema. However, lenses made of glass were a tedious chore for both the clinician and glass blower.

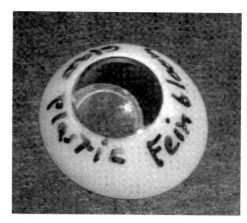

FIG. 1.3. Illustration of the polymethyl methacrylate (PMMA) scleral lens manufactured by Feinbloom in 1936.

George Nissel, Dallos' brother-in-law and an excellent contact lens technician, later made lenses with Dallos in London. Much success was needed with this new modality to minimize the risk of corneal transplantation (7).

Adolph W. Mueller-Welt, in Stuttgart, produced hand-blown glass scleral lenses as early as 1927. His laboratory, Mueller-Welt Contact-Linsen, produced many large trial sets of lenses. Joseph L. Breger brought the Mueller-Welt systems first to Canada in 1949 and then to the United States in 1950. Mueller-Welt made and distributed corneal polymethyl methacrylate (PMMA) lenses, including injection molded lenses and lathe cut lenses, in Detroit in the 1950s.

Scleral PMMA Lenses

William Feinbloom started working with contact lenses prior to 1932 and marketed a PMMA scleral portion and glass corneal portion lens in 1936 (Fig. 1.3). A variation of this same material combination lens was promoted without success in 1939. He also introduced bifocal and multifocal scleral lenses in a 1936 patent (Fig. 1.4). Feinbloom carefully described fitting plastic scleral lenses from an eye mold (8).

It may have been John Mullen, Theodore Obrig, or Istvan Gyorrfy who first made an all-PMMA lens between 1938 and 1940 (7). The lower specific gravity, inert, durable, machinable, transparent PMMA was far superior to

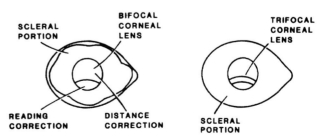

FIG. 1.4. Drawings of the bifocal lenses designed and introduced by Feinbloom in 1936.

glass and served as the primary rigid material for lenses from the late 1930s to the late 1970s (9).

Rhom and Hass introduced optically clear PMMA lenses in 1936, and both John Mullen and Theodore Obrig made scleral PMMA lenses in 1938. These lenses were reproduced more accurately by shaping and reshaping at temperatures that were not too high, lathing, and polishing. They also could be made much thinner than glass lenses, and fenestration was relatively simple. Dallos, Bier, and others improved the design and fitting of these plastic scleral lenses. Although few fitters exhibited expertise with scleral lenses, special attention to lens shape, fitting, bubble size, and position, as well as fenestration, made them more wearable.

Theodore Obrig and Philip L. Salvatori formed Obrig Laboratories in New York in 1938. During the 1940s and early 1950s, the books by these authors were the best source of information on contact lenses. In 1936 or 1937, Obrig accidentally developed the use of black light with fluorescein for evaluating lacrimal exchange behind the contact lens. Fluorescein had been used prior to this time, but only with white light. Black light added immeasurably to this observation technique. Obrig Laboratories and Precision-Cosmet were the major scleral lens makers in the 1940s (10).

Solon Braff was the first to use a nonirritating hydrocolloid that replaced Negacol, which required anesthesia, for eye molding. The use of molding material without anesthetic in 1945 helped allow more practitioners to learn to mold and fit scleral lenses (11,12).

Using sodium bicarbonate, saline, and methyl cellulose as part of the fluid in a "fluid" contact lens to prevent or delay the onset of Sattler's (or Fick's) veil met with failure. It was still not apparent to most clinicians and researchers that the edema that developed after a few hours of scleral lens wear was the result of hypoxia, which accompanied a stagnant tear layer under the "fluid" lens (13).

PMMA Corneal Designs

Kevin Tuohy, first a technician with Obrig Laboratories in New York and Montreal and later manager and part owner of Solon Braff's Solex laboratory, is credited by most with being the first inventor of the PMMA corneal lens (9). Early investigators, such as Edward Goodlaw, explained how the "sealed" chamber between the eye and a scleral lens did not allow carbon dioxide release with resultant lowering of the pH in the fluid trapped behind the lens. Prior to early 1949, fitters believed that Sattler's veil could be reduced by using the correct pH-balanced solution between the lens and the eye. This concept even had encouraged Harry Hind (Barnes-Hind) to develop a variety of contact lens solutions in an effort to combat corneal edema, which occurred with wearing of scleral lenses.

Goodlaw reports that in 1946 Villagran showed Tuohy and Braff the optical section of what was to have been a scleral lens. Xavier had unintentionally cut the corneal section off when he had made too deep a cut along the limbal groove of the scleral lens. With the realization that more oxygen could get to the eye with this smaller lens, Tuohy proceeded to develop the corneal lens. He used this accident to guide himself toward lenses that were smaller than the cornea. Corneal lenses were made for his wife and for himself (they both had myopia). Tuohy filed his flatter-than-the-cornea contact lens patents on February 28, 1948. Some of the patients on whose eyes he had used these monocurve lenses had already been wearing them daily for 10 months.

Tuohy's patent described a "contact lens applicable to the human eye comprising a concave-convex lens formed of light transmitting material having a marginal size smaller than the limbus portion of the eye for which it is applicable but larger than the maximum iris opening, said lens having a radius of curvature of the cornea to which it is applied so that radially from the center of the lens there will be a small but gradually increasing clearance for the natural entrance of eye fluids between the lens and the cornea, said lens to be ground for visual deficiency."

His monocurve (some had a narrow bevelled posterior surface) corneal lens eliminated many subjective symptoms of edema, which were common when scleral lenses were worn. These early lenses were about 0.3 mm thick.

The Tuohy patent was granted in June 1950. His early lenses were 11.5 to 12.5 mm in overall diameter, were fitted 1.50 or more diopters (D) flatter than the flattest corneal meridian, and exhibited a very high edge lift.

Dennis C. England filed his patent application on January 19, 1946. His corneal lens design was to conform exactly to the curvature of the cornea "to allow smooth passage of the eyelids over the lens." This patent was first denied in October 1946 and again in 1949. A third petition was not made, and the English patent was never granted (13).

George H. Butterfield's patent filed in August 1950 described a posterior surface that more nearly matched the corneal curvature than the flat-fitting Tuohy lenses. Butterfield's thinner contour, or alignment, lens, which was to approximate the shape of a paraboloid, was the thinner precursor of nearly all rigid lens designs from the early 1950s to the present (1).

Thus, PMMA haptics from the late 1930s and then flat Tuohy and contour PMMA corneal lenses dominated the contact lens field until hydrogel contact lenses became available in about 1971 (Table 1.1).

MODIFIED DESIGNS

A number of developments occurred in 1953. The Keraform lens, with four equally spaced, narrow, raised facets inside the edge of the posterior surface and designed to prevent rotation on the eye, was introduced by Noel O. Stimson, a California optician (10).

Of greater significance was the acceptance by many clinicians of the micro lens developed by Wilhelm Sohnges of Germany, Jack Neill of the United States, and Frank Dickinson of England. These micro lenses were approximately 9.5 mm in diameter, with 0.20 mm of center thickness, and were fitted 0.3 to 0.6 mm flatter than the corneal curvature.

The Vent Air lens, with semicircular grooves in the posterior surface, was introduced in the middle 1950s as a relatively successful franchised contact lens. Stanley Gordon filed a patent for the SpiroVent Lens in 1959 and received the patent in 1961. The posterior grooves were designed to ensure rotation and tear flow (10).

The Plastic Contact Lens Company was formed in 1946 in Chicago by Newton Wesley and George Jessen. In the early days, three pairs of lenses were provided for each patient to determine the best fit; one pair "on K," one flatter than "K," and one steeper than "K." Wesley and Jessen taught, promoted, and sold contact lenses throughout the world. In 1956, their laboratory introduced the extremely popular 9.2-mm diameter Sphercon lens, which had a 12.5-mm peripheral curve, or bevel, radius 0.4 mm wide. The Plastic Contact Lens Company sponsored the First Annual National Contact Lens Congress and formed the National Eye Research Foundation (NERF) in 1956. The Plastic Contact Lens Company also was responsible for the Aseptoplast lens, which incorporated hexachlorophene and corobex as germicides. Also, in the 1950s, Barnes-Hind, led by Harry Hind and John Petriciani, provided nearly all the contact lens solutions (10).

In 1960, Charles A. (Ted) Bayshore introduced his fitting technique with a lens, which was 7.0 to 8.6 mm in diameter, fitted 1.5 D steeper than "K," with an optical zone of 6.0 to 6.6 mm and a central fenestration of 0.009 inch. During the 1960s, lens diameters were reduced to 8.0 to 8.8 mm to provide more corneal exposure. At the time of his death in January 2002, Charles Neefe, Big Springs Texas, had 98 contact lens-related patents to his name.

Hydrogel Contact Lens Development

Otto Wichterle and Drahoslav Lim designed hydroxyethyl methacrylate (HEMA) at the Institute of Macromolecular Chemistry of the Czechoslovak Academy of Sciences to be used for a broad range of applications. In 1952, Professor Wichterle, a Czechoslovakian polymer chemist, met an ophthalmologist from Prague and, while observing the nature of the material of the orbital implants, which the ophthalmologist was reading about, considered designing a new material for this purpose. Wichterle's assistant, Lim, synthesized HEMA and glycol diester in 1954. This early HEMA was called *Hydron*. Wichterle and Lim worked together on the HEMA (lens) material patent application.

Wichterle adapted the spin casting method for lens manufacturing in 1951 using his sons' erector set (1,14). Table 1.2 lists Wichterle's and Lim's material design characteristics.

Wichterle later implanted HEMA material in animals,

TABLE 1.2. DEMANDS FOR A SUITABLE PLASTIC BY WICHTERLE AND LIM (15)

Structure permitting the desired water content
Intertness to normal biologic processes, including resistance to degradation of the polymer and to reactions unfavorable to the organism
Permeability for metabolites

with little reaction. Later he consulted with Maximillian Dreifus, an ophthalmologist, who was interested in implanting the material.

Thousands of lenses were made in Wichterle's home by polymerization in open rotating molds. These lenses were fitted first to Wichterle and then to others by M. Dreifus in 1956. This material was patented in 1963. Wichterle (Fig. 1.5) not only overcame the complication of incorporating his applied research into that of the Institute of Macromolecular Research, which emphasized basic research, but he also overcame the skepticism of the optical community.

Wichterle published his work in *Nature* in January 1960 after more than 4 years of testing. He stated that these materials now have passed through the stage of application, such as filling after enucleation of the eye. Promising results also have been obtained in experiments in other cases (e.g., in manufacturing contact lenses) and in arteries (15).

Martin M. Pollak (Fig. 1.6) and Jerome I. Feldman of National Patent Development Corp., via licensing the Wichterle technology to Bausch & Lomb, probably are most responsible for commercialization of hydrogel contact lenses in the world. Robert Morrison and Allan Isen also were instrumental in bringing soft lenses to the United States. Table 1.3 lists representative examples of other hydrogel lens polymer developments (16).

On March 18, 1971, Bausch & Lomb announced United States Food and Drug Administration (FDA) approval of their SofLens. Although there were numerous

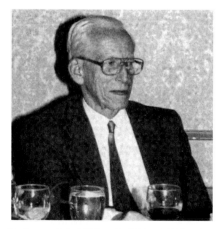

FIG. 1.5. Professor Otto Wichterle (1914–1998), who performed the initial research on the hydroxyethyl methacrylate (HEMA) lens.

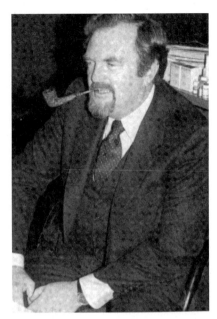

FIG. 1.6. Martin M. Pollak, who, with Jerome I. Feldman, was instrumental in the commercial success of hydrogel contact lenses worldwide.

problems with this and other early-generation lenses, including decentration, hypoxia, and "tight lens syndrome," improvements in design and material occurred frequently in the 1970s, resulting in the successful and popular lenses available today.

In 1981, soft lenses were approved by the FDA for over-

TABLE 1.3. DEVELOPMENTS OF SOFT LENS MATERIAL FROM THE 1950S THROUGH 1980

Material	Developer
Poly-HEMA	Wichterle and Lim
HEMA and vinyl pyrrolidine or PHP	Seiderman (Hydrocurve)
HEMA and PVP	Ewell, Griffen, Isen (Softcon)
HEMA, methacrylic acid, VP	Cordrey, Frankland, Highgate (Sauflon)
HEMA, methacrylic acid, VP	Union Corp. (Aquaflex), Stanley Gordon
Glycerol methacrylate	Corneal Sciences, Inc., Refojo (CSI), Korb
Polyvinyl alcohol	CIBA Vision Corp. (Atlafilcon A; Nelfilcon)
Etafilcon (disposable)	Vistakon (Johnson & Johnson) from Danalens (Bay)
Silicone hydrogels Trimethylsiloxy-silypropylvinyl Carbamate and fluoroether based	Bausch & Lomb and CIBA Vision
Tris-*N*, N-dimethyl acrylamide (16)	

HEMA, hydroxyethyl methacrylate; PVP, polyvinylpyrolidone; VP, vinyl pyrolidone.

night or extended wear. In the late 1980s, soft lenses, packaged and priced for disposability, were introduced by Johnson & Johnson (Acuvue), Bausch & Lomb (SeeQuence), and CIBA Vision Corp. (NewVues) (17).

Hydrogel Disposable Soft Contact Lenses

Johnson & Johnson (Vistakon) introduced the Acuvue lens for 1-week extended wear in six packs in 1987. Each lens was to be worn for 1 week and then disposed of. Disposable actually means a contact lens should be worn once and then discarded. Soon practitioners used the lenses for daily wear, with the direction to replace them every 2 weeks. According to Mertz, the concept that led the Danish Company Danalens to make disposable lenses was Scandinavian Klas Nilsson's idea that replacing high-water-content extended wear lenses every 6 months prompted Michael Bay to produce the multipack Danalens. Johnson & Johnson bought Danalens in 1984 (18). Later, Bausch & Lomb purchased the Scottish company Award PLC to make disposable lenses and launched a daily disposable lens in the United Kingdom in 1993. In 1993, Vistakon first introduced its 1-Day Acuvue lens for daily disposable use. CIBA Vision developed their own daily disposable lens made from and first distributed it in Norway in 1996. Mass production of quality lenses was not possible until the late 1980s. The new disposable lenses were more reproducible than previous soft lenses and led to improved contact lens safety, especially from inflammatory causes (19).

Many believe that disposable lenses led to the widespread sales of mail order and Internet order contact lenses. This may be true, but mail order sales began before disposable lenses and would have increased without their widespread use.

Rigid Gas Permeable Material Lenses

The first rigid gas permeable (RGP) lens (also termed *GP* lens) made of cellulose acetate butyrate (CAB) was approved by the FDA for use in the United States in 1978. Like many other contact lens materials, CAB had been in common use for years outside of the United States prior to this time.

In 1971, however, Norman G. Gaylord, a polymer chemist, had been commissioned by Polymer Optics Contact Lens Company to develop a GP contact lens material. Leonard Seidner, an optometrist, and his brother, Joseph Seidner, an engineer, assisted Gaylord in developing the Polycon lens material, commonly referred to as silicone/acrylate, but more correctly called a *copolymer of polysiloxanylalkyl acrylic ester and alkyl acrylic ester.* The material patent was awarded in 1974 (11). In 1977, Syntex purchased the Polycon lens system from Polymer Optics. In 1979, the Polycon lens was introduced initially in a thin, 9.5-mm diameter, 8.4-mm optic zone design. Later, 9.0- and 8.5-mm designs were added. The original material was more stable than CAB; therefore, Polycon lenses could be made much thinner than CAB lenses.

Pilkington brought suit against Paragon (Paraperm material) and Wilsa (Optacryl material) in 1984 and won in 1987. Paragon was sold to Pilkington in 1988, and Pilkington later acquired Optacryl's materials. Permeable Contact Lenses, owned by Leonard Seidner, and Polymer Technology Corporation, owned by Bausch & Lomb (20), were named in patent infringement suits by Pilkington in 1988, and a settlement in both cases occurred 1 year later.

Later, lenses made from other silicone/acrylates, fluoro silicone/acrylates, fluoropolymers, polystyrene (Wesley Jessen Airlens, Precision Cosmet OPUS III), polycarbonate, and polysulfone were developed. The butyl rubber Revlens, originally developed by BioContacts, was acquired by Cooper Laboratories but never was commercialized. Table 1.1 lists rigid lens developments from 1888 to the 1980s.

Menicon, founded by Japanese artist and businessman Kyoichi Tanaka, celebrated its fiftieth anniversary making rigid contact lenses in 2001 and obtained FDA approval for 30-day continuous wear of its Menicon Z lens in 2002. Prior to this, GP lenses had been approved for 7-day extended wear since the late 1980s in the United States.

Reverse geometry lenses for orthokeratology were used and FDA approved for daily wear in the late 1990s. In 2002, Paragon Vision Sciences obtained FDA approval for its Paragon Corneal Refractive Therapy (CRT), corneal refractive therapy, overnight corneal reshaping procedure. Rigid contact lens use continued to decline in the early part of the twenty first century due primarily to the many advances in disposable soft contact lenses, especially toric soft contact lenses (Fig. 1.7).

Aspheric Corneal Lenses

Daniel Elliot first described aspheric lenses in 1964. Later, Charles Neefe received a patent for a sine curve concave surface lens in 1965. David Volk's 1965 patent described an aspheric lens surface generation method, whereas William Feinbloom's 1966 patent describes a spherical optical zone, aspheric periphery lens. Volk and Eugen Hirst developed the Con-O-Coid lens in New Zealand in the 1960s. In the 1970s, the use of aspheric lenses was expanded for presbyopia by Goldberg. Further development of aspheric lenses was accomplished by Breger in 1983, Bronstein in 1985, and Volk in 1987 (multiple aspheric).

Special anterior designs include the Panofocal lens by Neefe, the RAU lens by Tabb in the 1970s, and the CALS lens by Carl Evans in 1980, which led to the Unilens and Dill's PS45 design (13). In addition, the Boston Envision, a bispheric design, was developed by Hanita in Israel, and marketed by the Polymer Technology Corporation (21). At the turn of the millennium, Cooper Vision and Specialty Ultravision (lens later acquired by CIBA Vision) produced aberration-reducing soft disposable lenses.

Silicone Elastomer Contact Lens

Silicone elastometer contact lenses have been plagued by reports of poor wetting, discomfort, and adherence of the lens to the cornea. Walter Becker, a Pittsburgh optician, began development of the silicone elastomer lens in 1956. He sold his patent in 1959 to Joe Breger, who further developed the silicone lens until it was sold to Dow Corning in 1972. Breger's Mueller-Welt elastometer lens was a 10.5-mm diameter, corneal lens that he called the *Silcon Lens*. Dow Corning altered the material, and a new lens called *Silsoft* (later Silsight in minus lenses) was produced. FDA approval for daily wear for cosmetic reasons and extended wear for aphakia followed in 1981. In 1983, the Silsight lens became the first 30-day extended wear lens for cosmetic use. These lenses were made in 11.3- and 12.5-mm diameters. Dow Corning removed itself from the contact lens arena in 1984, and Bausch & Lomb purchased the silicone lens from them in 1985.

Danker Labs, formerly Danker and Wohlk, developed silicone lenses in the 1970s. These lenses were later acquired by Bames-Hind. Wohlk's Silflex and Titmus' Tesicon lenses, both made of silicone material, were developed in Germany in the 1970s.

Silicone lenses have been made wettable on the eye by coating with hydrogel materials and by plasma surface treatment. Koziol, Gholam, Peyman, and Yasuda have developed a plasma treatment using methane gas (22).

Silicone Hydrogel Contact Lenses

In 1998, Bausch & Lomb introduced the PureVision lens. Lenses made from silicone hydrogel material have high oxygen permeability (Dk 100 or greater) and thus cause less corneal swelling. In 2001, CIBA Vision introduced the Focus Night & Day silicone hydrogel lens for up to 30 days

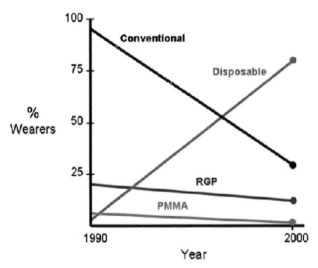

FIG. 1.7. Trends in wearers of conventional lenses (no planned replacement schedule), disposable, rigid gas permeable, and polymethyl methacrylate (PMMA) contact lenses.

TABLE 1.4. MAJOR UNITED STATES FOOD AND DRUG ADMINISTRATION APPROVALS AFTER 1988

Lens/Material	Type	Manufacturer	Year
Fluoroperm 60	RGP	Paragon Vision Sciences	1988[a]
Boston XO	RGP	Polymer Technolgy/Bausch & Lomb	2000
PureVision	Soft	Bausch & Lomb	1998
Night & Day	Soft	CIBA Vision	2001
Menicon Z	RGP	Menicon	2002

Note: The last three lenses eventually were approved for 30-day continuous wear.
[a]For daily wear; later approved in 1990 for extended wear. Later modified version, called Paragon HDS, was introduced in the 1990s.
RGP, rigid gas permeable.

TABLE 1.5. OUTLINE OF FOOD AND DRUG ADMINISTRATION APPROVALS FOR CONTACT LENSES IN THE UNITED STATES

Lens	Type	Manufacturer	Date (month/year)	Approval
SofLens	S	Bausch & Lomb	3/1971	DW
Softcon	S	American Optical	9/1973	T
Hydrocurve	S	Soft Lenses, later Barnes-Hind	4/1974	DW
Aquaflex	S	Union Corp., later Cooper and Wesley Jessen	6/1976	DW
Permalens	S	Cooper	6/1979	AEW
			1/1981	CEW
Hydrocurve	S	Soft Lenses, later Barnes-Hind	6/1979	AEW
			1/1981	CEW
SilSoft	Si	Dow Corning, later Bausch & Lomb	7/1981	DW
			9/1981	AEW
CS1	S	Syntex, later Sola and Barnes-Hind	2/1982	T
SilRX	Si	Danker, later Barnes-Hind	5/1982	AEW
BiSoft	S Bifocal	CIBA Vision Corp.	6/1982	DW
PA1	S Bifocal	Bausch & Lomb	11/1982	DW
Silsight	Si	Dow Corning	3/1983	CEW
CustomEyes	S Tinted	CTL, later Barnes-Hind	9/1983	DW
Softcolors	S Tinted	CIBA Vision Corp.	2/1984	DW
Meso	RGP	Danker	1/1978	DW
Polycon	RGP	Syntex, later CIBA Vision Corp.	1/1979	DW
Polycon 11	RGP	Barnes-Hind CIBA Vision	7/1982	DW
Silcon	Si, RGP	Dow Corning, later Conforma	10/1981	DW
Opus	RGP	Precision Cosmet	7/1983	DW
Boston 11	RGP	Polymer Technology	11/1983	DW
Paraperm 02	RGP	Paragon	11/1983	DW
Optacryl 60	RGP	Optacryl	11/1983	DW
Paraperm EW	RGP	Paragon	12/1986	EW
Equalens	RGP	Polymer Technology Corp.	11/1987	EW
Fluoroperm 90	RGP	Paragon	12/1987	EW
Advent	F	Allergan/3M Corp.	6/1988	EW
Saturn SoftPerm	S/RGP	Soft-RGP combination. Precision Cosmet, later Barnes-Hind, WJ, CIBA Vision Corp.	1/1985	DW

S, soft contact lens; Si, silicone; RGP, rigid gas permeable; F, fluoroether; DW, daily wear; T, therapeutic; AEW, aphakic extended wear; CEW, cosmetic extended wear.

of continuous wear (Table 1.4). At the time of the writing of this chapter, at least three other companies were developing these materials and the two manufacturers mentioned earlier were locked in a number of patent lawsuits. In 2002, due to the Harvey patent owned by CIBA Vision's subsidiary Wesley-Jessen, for the first time in contact lens history a company, Bausch & Lomb, was required to stop selling lenses in the United States due to a court decision that it was in violation of the patent. In early 2004 Vistacon introduced a silicone hydrogel contact lens as well.

Bifocal Contact Lenses

William Feinbloom patented, but did not manufacture, scleral bifocal and multifocal contact lenses in 1936. The Williamson-Noble scleral bifocal was developed in 1950 in England.

Both John DeCarle and Wesley-Jessen promoted bifocal contact lenses in 1957. DeCarle's design incorporated an inside surface segment and was designed around the simultaneous vision concept. The Wesley-Jessen alternating vision design had a bicurve anterior surface geometry. In 1970, Wesley-Jessen introduced the multirange design, which had multiple blackened pie-shaped portions centrally forming both a pinhole and stenopaic slit effect (7).

From 1981 through 1983, three new soft bifocal contact lens designs were introduced. The CIBA BiSoft lens, which has an anterior surface, bicurve (center distance portion) design, was the first to be FDA approved (Table 1.5). Bausch & Lomb's PA1, posterior aspheric multifocal lens (stated $+1.50$ D add power) was introduced in November 1982. Wesley-Jessen obtained FDA approval for its anterior surface, segmented, prism ballasted Trufocal in April 1983. Nevertheless, most presbyopes continue to be corrected with spectacles, distance vision contact lenses and reading glasses, or a monovision system.

Silcon VFL was the first FDA-approved GP multifocal design. The lens was approved in 1983 and later sold by Conforma Laboratories. Tangent Streak, a popular rigid contact lens bifocal made by Fused Kontacts of Chicago, was introduced in the mid 1980s. This truncated, prism ballast, alternating vision design has an anterior surface flat top segment.

Allen Cohen, an American optometrist, and Michael Freeman, an ophthalmic optician (optometrist) of Great Britain, simultaneously developed a diffraction grating (sometimes called *holographic*) bifocal for soft and rigid contact lenses. The central lens portion has posterior surface grooves or eschelettes, which cause interference of light due to diffraction at the eschelettes, thus providing a second focal length for near objects. Diffraction grating contact lenses function on the simultaneous vision principle. Allergan Optical (hydrogel) and Pilkington (GP) are currently manufacturing the diffraction grating bifocal contact lens.

Vistakon, CIBA Vision, and numerous other companies introduced disposable multifocal lenses in the late 1990s.

Until the late 1990s, bifocal contact lens wearers numbered in the hundreds of thousands in the United States. The introduction of disposable bifocal contact lenses at this time resulted in double-digit growth in the number of bifocal wearers. Indeed, near the turn of the millennium even toric-multifocal lenses were available (23).

SUMMARY

What is most fascinating about the contact lens industry is its dynamic nature (Fig. 1.7). It seems as though new developments occur every day. With the contact lens innovations of the past 100 years outlined in this chapter, it makes one wonder what will occur during the next 100 years. The field has expanded from small laboratories that often grew out of an optometrist's practice to where most lenses today are manufactured by large multinational corporations. Nearly 35 million persons in the United States and 85 million or more persons worldwide wear contact lenses.

Although the greatest risk of contact lens wear, corneal ulcer, occurs in 1 of 1/10,000 GP lens daily wearers, 3.5 of 10,000 soft daily wear patients, and 20 of 10,000 soft (hydrogel) extended wear patients (24), most wearers today are safer than ever and use contact lenses for many purposes (Table 1.6). In 1987, the FDA changed approval for soft contact lens extended wear from 30 days to only 7 days. Yet, in the past few years, 30-day approval with newer, highly oxygen transmissible lenses has recurred.

Manufacturing methods have ranged from blown glass scleral lenses to lathe cut and polished rigid and soft lenses to spin cast and cast molded soft lenses to stabilized soft molded and other injection molded processes. Once made by human hands with many tedious steps, modern lenses are made by computer-designed, computer-controlled, robotic assembly lines where humans simply oversee the computers. Manufacturers have evolved (Table 1.7), and consolidation of many manufacturers has been inevitable.

Contact lenses remain an important part of modern eye care and culture.

TABLE 1.6. INDICATIONS FOR CONTACT LENS WEAR

Optical correction of myopia, hyperopia, astigmatism, aphakia, presbyopia, and irregular astigmatism (postsurgical, posttrauma, postinfection)
Therapeutic bandage for corneal disease
Corneal reshaping for refractive error reduction
Prosthetic and cosmetic enhancement
Keratoconus

TABLE 1.7. CONTACT LENS MANUFACTURERS AND THEIR MAJOR ACQUISITIONS OVER THE YEARS

Bausch & Lomb
  Polymer Technology Corp.
  Custom Tint Labs, Inc. (CTL)
  Unilens
CIBA Vision Corp. (Novartis)
  Wesley Jessen
  Barnes-Hind/Hydrocurve (once owned by Revlon)
  Syntex (CSI and Polycon lenses)
  Precision Cosmet (Softperm lenses)
  American Optical lenses and solutions
Vistakon—Johnson & Johnson
  Frontier
  Danalens
XCEL
  Flexlens (from Paragon Vision Sciences)
CooperVision
  Union Corp. Aquaflex and Gordon RGP lenses
  Coast Vision
  Biocompatibles
Ocular Sciences
  American Hydron (once owned by Allergan[a])
  Essilor soft contact lenses/Sunsoft
Alcon (solutions)
  Burton Parsons

[a]Allergan once owned and marketed the Advent perfluoroether flexible GP lens developed by 3M Corp.
GP, rigid gas permeable.

ACKNOWLEDGMENT

The author thanks Neal Bailey for helping with the original version of this chapter.

REFERENCES

1. Mandell R. Historical development. In: Mandell R, ed. *Contact lens practice,* 4th ed. Springfield, IL: Charles C. Thomas Publisher, 1988:5.
2. Hofstetter HW, Graham R. Leonardo and contact lenses. *Am J Optom Arch Am Acad Optom* 1953;30:41.
3. Enoch JM. Descartes' contact lens. *Am J Optom Arch Am Acad Optom* 1956;33:77.
4. Pearson RM. Kalt, keratoconus, and the contact lens. *Optom Vis Sci* 1989;66:643–646.
5. Pearson RM, Efron N. Hundredth anniversary of August Muller's inaugural dissertation on contact lenses. *Surv Ophthalmol* 1989;34:133–141.
6. Ezekiel D. Personal communication, 2003.
7. Dallos J. Contact glasses, the invisible spectacles. *Arch Ophthalmol* 1956;15:617.
8. Feinbloom W. Contact lenses. *Am J Optom Arch Am Acad Optom* 1932;9:78.
9. Feinbloom W. A plastic contact lens chronicle. *Am J Optom Arch Am Acad Optom* 1937;14:41.
10. Bailey NJ. Neal Bailey's contact lens chronicle. *Contact Lens Spectrum* 1987;2:29.
11. Goodlaw EL. How corneal contacts were born. *Contact Lens Forum* 1978;2:31.
12. Graham R. The evolution of corneal contact lenses. *Am J Optom Arch Am Acad Optom* 1959;36:55.
13. Bailey NJ. The England lens. *Contact Lens Spectrum* 1986;1:56.
14. Heitz RF. History of contact lenses. In: *Contact lenses.* New York: Grune & Stratton, 1984:1.1.
15. Wichterle O, Lim D. Hydrophilic gels for biological use. *Nature* 1960;185:177.
16. Tighe B. Silicone hydrogels: how do they work? In: Sweeney DF, ed. *Silicone hydrogels.* Oxford: Butterworth-Heinemann, 2000:1-21.
17. McMahon TT, Zadnik K. Twenty-five years of contact lenses. *Cornea* 2000;19:730–740.
18. Mertz GW. Development of contact lenses. In: Hamano H, Kaufman HE, eds. *Corneal physiology and disposable contact lenses.* Boston: Butterworth-Heinemann, 1997:65–99.
19. Efron N. Historical perspective. In: *Contact lens practice.* Oxford: Butterworth-Heinemann, 2002:1–10.
20. Barr JT, Bailey NJ. 1988 annual report. *Contact Lens Spectrum* 1988;3:19.
21. Barr JT. A genealogy of aspheric lenses. *Contact Lens Spectrum* 1987;2:81.
22. Barr JT. Silicone elastomer: still a challenge. *Contact Lens Spectrum* 1987;2:29.
23. Barr J. Contact lenses 2001. *Contact Lens Spectrum* 2002;15:22–28.
24. Poggio EC, Glynn RJ, Schein O, et al. The incidence of ulcerative keratitis among users of daily-wear and extended-wear soft contact lenses. *N Engl J Med* 1989;321:779.

2

ANATOMY, MORPHOLOGY, AND ELECTRON MICROSCOPY OF THE CORNEA AND CONJUNCTIVA

JAN P.G. BERGMANSON AND MICHAEL J. DOUGHTY

Insight on corneal anatomy has evaded mankind for a long time. Perhaps this ignorance is due to the fact that the cornea is optically transparent. Subsequently, there is not much to see until something goes wrong and transparency is lost. In this respect, clinical slit-lamp biomicroscope evaluation (SLE) is of limited assistance in detecting or diagnosing changes in corneal structure and transparency. A reduction in central corneal transparency, however, can be devastating to vision, on a temporary or permanent basis, depending on its cause, location, and treatment outcome.

The primary goals of this chapter are to provide a balanced overview of anatomy, morphology, and ultrastructure of the mammalian cornea and conjunctiva, and to link these structural characteristics with current perspectives on physiology. Emphasis will generally be placed upon aspects of particular interest to the practicing clinician.

TERMINOLOGY

The International Anatomical Nomenclature Committee (IANC) has made an international effort to standardize anatomical terminology because it was recognized that eponyms are simply not descriptive and that uniformity is needed in the use of anatomical terms. The first effort to standardize anatomical language occurred in Basel in 1895 and resulted in a text in Latin. This *Nomina Anatomica* has been updated at intervals, and sections on embryology and histology have been added. The sixth edition was published in 1989 and involved the input of more than 100 senior academics from all over the world, so the accuracy and logic of the recommended nomenclature represent the synthesis of a range of ideas and perspectives.

From the perspective of the IANC, it has to be accepted that some ocular and corneal terms persist and are unlikely to be abandoned. It is our opinion, however, that attention should be given to this internationally accepted terminology in the interest of progress toward a uniform and appropri-

ately descriptive nomenclature in ocular anatomy. Therefore, the IANC-based nomenclature (1989) will be used here, with the older eponymous terms provided for completeness.

METHODS IN ANATOMY, MORPHOLOGY, AND ULTRASTRUCTURE OF THE CORNEA AND CONJUNCTIVA

Anatomical measurements made on living eyes or postmortem specimens in early studies of the cornea provided valuable insight on the condition of normal tissue (1). The conjunctiva and eyelids were similarly evaluated, but these can be easily observed in the living eye as well. Measures of corneal dimensions were therefore coarse and usually limited to a resolution of 0.5 or 1 mm. The human cornea and sclera are generally too thin to be measured with calipers, but it was possible to generate highly magnified images and use these to make measurements (2). Similarly, with histologic tissue sections, the thickness of the cornea (3) or its constituent cell layers (4,5) could be estimated from magnified images.

Biomicroscopy of transparent cornea, in optical section, at increased magnification and over localized areas is valuable; however, as mentioned earlier, only when the normal organization is disturbed will the elements of the cornea really be visible. Of interest, the single layer corneal endothelium is viewable in specular reflection, but usually at a resolution that does not allow one to make many conclusions.

A range of clinical instruments using optical or ultrasound principles were developed recently, and these instruments provide measurements of these tissues to within a few micrometers (6,7). Newer developments today even allow *in vivo* visualization and accurate measurement of corneal layers (8). Two different advanced forms of biomicroscopy, one based on specular reflection (the *specular microscope*) and the other on laser light sources (the *confocal microscope*), have been developed. Specular microscopes routinely allow imaging and objective assessment of the corneal endothelium (9–12), whereas confocal instruments allow one to see all the various types of cells in the cornea, including nerves (13,14). Ultrasound-based instruments, such as the Orbscan (15), not only measure corneal thickness at discrete locations but also provide maps of corneal curvature and thickness. Notwithstanding, it is the basic approach of using thin tissue sections of the cornea viewed with a laboratory light microscope or an electron microscope that likely will continue to provide the bulk of information on corneal structure and ultrastructure.

Light microscopes have allowed visualization of sections of corneal tissue for more than 100 years, but they have been largely used for qualitative purposes and rarely have been accompanied by significant dimensional measures of tissue sections (3). Perhaps a contributing reason for this has been the difficulty in reproducibly preparing the tissue for microscopy, with a resultant distorted and poorly preserved view of the corneal tissue. In retrospect, this outcome perhaps is hardly surprising because the general approach in such studies is to immerse either the whole eyeball or the isolated cornea in formalin, a diluted solution of formaldehyde (perhaps with some alcohol added) (16,17). That tissue contraction and distortion occur during the subsequent processing steps is a recognized problem (18), as can be objectively proven with comparative studies of fresh and processed tissues (19,20).

A much greater problem potentially arises when the interest is to examine the tissue at high resolution. It might well be argued that instruments that allow viewing of the corneal tissue at a resolution of 10 to 20 nm would be useless unless parallel advances were made in preserving the tissue in its natural shape and appearance without creating distracting artifacts. In this context, the cornea presents a unique problem to researchers who wish to achieve its optimal fixation. Perfusion of fixatives through the vascular system, which is the optimum procedure for fixation of most other organs and tissues, does not yield optimal results for the cornea. The problem is that the cornea lacks a blood supply; therefore, the only method by which the cornea may be successfully fixed is through some form of repeated application of a fixative, immersion, or, for isolated corneas, use of a special apparatus that provides superfusion of the two surfaces of the cornea with fixative. The cornea consists of a dense and relatively dehydrated collagenous stroma packed between two cellular layers that also function as fluid barriers; this anatomical fact does not make the task easier.

In the 1960s, the use of better aldehyde fixatives, namely glutaraldehyde (16) or a formaldehyde-glutaraldehyde mixture (21), was promoted. It must be noted, however, that scrutiny of numerous attempts over a 40-year period to use the newer glutaraldehyde-based fixatives indicates that it is still all too easy to produce substantial structural modifications to the corneal tissue if attention is not also given to the milieu under which the fixative is presented to the tissue (18,20). These conditions especially include consideration of the ionic strength (osmolality) of the fixative, because even a quality fixative can only preserve corneal tissue in something that approaches its natural condition if its ionic strength and pH are similar to that of the living eye. Formaldehyde-glutaraldehyde fixatives are likely to have an osmolality $3\times$ or $4\times$ greater than physiologic (20). It is not only possible, but reasonable, to consider by how much the chemical fixation of the cornea might change its curvature (22,23) or thickness (20), rather than selecting images from fixed tissue that appear to be conceptually pleasing. Based on systematic studies, it is possible to note that improved preservation of the corneal tissue organization can be realized with a 2% glutaraldehyde fixative in 80 mM buffer, which yields a solution with a reasonable osmolarity (of 330–340 mOsm/L) and a physiologic meaningful pH (of 7.2–7.4) (20). In the further processing of tissue for transmission electron microscopy (TEM), consideration needs to be given to the embedding medium (the plastic), especially if the area of interest is that of the collagen fibrils of the cornea (24). For scanning electron microscopy (SEM), even greater attention must be given to the impact of the extreme drying sustained by the tissue prior to metal coating, because such a process can induce cracking of cell surfaces (18). Overall, the goals of the contemporary microscopist desiring to study the cornea should be to achieve corneal cellular preservation with maintenance of a normal corneal shape and with minimal shrinkage or distortion of the tissue. Some changes are inevitable, but at least the gross artifacts should be recognized and such images discarded.

GROSS ANATOMY OF THE CORNEA

The cornea is part of the outer coat of the eye and continuous with the sclera, the conjunctiva and ultimately the skin. Its physiology is uniquely adapted to its functions because it is an avascular structure continuously bathed in fluid, by the tears anteriorly and the aqueous posteriorly. In the normal human eye, the cornea has been considered to extend over as much as 1/5 (25) or 1/6 (26) of the circumference of the eyeball, with sclera providing for the remaining surface. Alternatively, and as based on measures of area, corneal area is somewhere between 1/14 (27) and 1/10 of the surface area of the globe (2). Similarly, corneal area is small (approximately 1/15) compared to the surface area of the conjunctiva (28).

When viewed from the outside, the cornea has a certain diameter (Fig. 2.1). It appears round but actually has a slightly oval shape, with its vertical dimensions marginally smaller than the larger diameter along the horizontal meridian (29). It is likely that assessments of so-called corneal diameter are actually a measure of the visible iris diameter (29). In primary eye gaze, the superior edge of the cornea is covered by the upper eyelid.

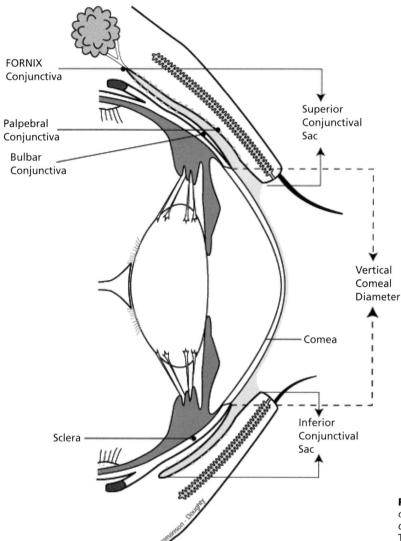

FORNIX
Conjunctiva

Palpebral
Conjunctiva

Bulbar
Conjunctiva

Superior
Conjunctival
Sac

Vertical
Corneal
Diameter

Cornea

Sclera

Inferior
Conjunctival
Sac

Bergmanson - Doughty

FIG. 2.1. Schematic diagram of the anterior aspects of the human eye. (From Bergmanson JPG. *Clinical ocular anatomy and physiology,* 11th ed. Houston, TX: Texas Eye Research and Technology Center, University of Houston College of Optometry, 2004, with permission.)

At its extreme periphery, the cornea gradually transforms into sclera (30,31). The transitional zone is known as the *corneoscleral junction* or *limbus.* A number of important structural modifications occur within the vicinity of the limbus but, with the exception of the epithelium, are considered outside the scope for this chapter.

The cornea undergoes rapid growth—as assessed by its increase in diameter—during the very early postnatal years and reaches adult values usually by age 2 or 3 years (Fig. 2.2) (32). Older texts give the horizontal diameter of the adult human cornea as around 11.7 mm in horizontal and 10.6 in vertical meridians, but it is unclear how these measurements were achieved (33). Evaluation of numerous values from the literature yield values of 11.1 mm for a 1-year-old (32), which indicates that the diameter is slightly smaller than the 11.6-mm value quoted for adults (29).

Although once regarded as a well-defined characteristic of the cornea, central corneal thickness (CCT) now must be recognized as a rather variable feature of the adult human cornea. Based on a comprehensive review of literature reports over a 30-year period, an average corneal thickness of 0.536 mm was calculated, for which a 95% confidence interval ([CI] based on $\pm 1.96 \times$ SD reported from 230 separate clinical studies) of between 0.473 and 0.595 mm was suggested (7). It should be noted, however, that different instruments and techniques appear to produce slightly different results (Fig. 2.3). In general, an historical review of published data indicates that slit-lamp–based techniques tend to yield slightly lower CCT values compared to ultrasound-based techniques, with specular microscopy techniques yielding values very similar to those with ultrasound (Table 2.1).

In human corneas, central regions are thinner than more peripheral regions. Numerous studies of these regional dif-

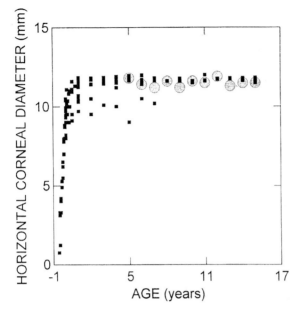

FIG. 2.2. Age-related changes in the human horizontal corneal diameter (visible iris diameter) in the early postnatal years and into childhood. (Modified from Muller A, Doughty MJ, [32], with permission.)

Physiologic Functions of the Cornea

In simple terms, several functions can be ascribed to the cornea:

1. Optical
   A. Transparency—to facilitate the transmission of light to the retina
   B. Refraction—to help focus the object viewed onto the retina. The cornea provides two thirds of the ocular refractive power that focuses images upon the retina.

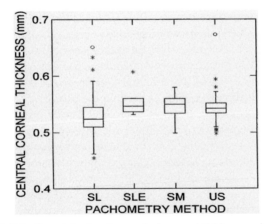

FIG. 2.3. Box plots showing central corneal thickness values in adult humans as assessed by optical slit-lamp (SL), slit lamp methods with extra electronic accessories (SLE), specular microscopy (SM), and ultrasound (US) pachometry. (From Doughty, Zaman, 2000, with permission.)

TABLE 2.1. PHYSICAL MEASUREMENTS OF THE HUMAN CORNEA

Characteristic	Infants (~ 1-year old)	Adults
Horizontal diameter (mm)	11.1	11.7
Anterior corneal curvature (mm)	7.56	7.8
Posterior corneal curvature (mm)	6.42[a]	6.5
Central thickness (mm)	0.571	0.536 (95% CI 0.473–0.595)
Water content	76%–78% (for bulk of cornea)	
Collagen protein (as percentage of wet mass)		15%
Proteoglycans (as percentage of wet mass)		5%–10%

[a]For children aged 6 to 17 years.
CI, confidence interval.

2. Protection—to protect the delicate intraocular structures from trauma. The cornea is a somewhat rigid fibrous structure with a renewable epithelial surface.

Measures of light transmission through the eyelid *in vivo* indicate that at least 90% of light in the visible portion of the spectrum should be transmitted, especially at the red end of the spectrum (34). For the normal cornea with lids open, light transmittance is even higher with at least 95% throughout in the visible range (35,36).

Corneal refractive characteristics result from a combination of the tissue composition and the character of the curved surfaces in contact with the tear film and aqueous humor. Recent estimates of the refractive indices of the corneal epithelium, anterior stroma, and posterior surface yield values of 1.401, 1.380, and 1.373, respectively (37). Using various methods, the refractive indices for the fibrils that make up the corneal stroma appear to have values higher than the corneal epithelium (i.e., >1.4), whereas the extracellular matrix (ground substance) within the stroma has lower values than the tissue as a whole (i.e., close to 1.35) (38).

Corneal Curvature

The anterior corneal surface is somewhat flatter than the posterior curvature. The anterior curvature generally is steep at birth, with average values for anterior curvature at age 1 year reported to be 7.58 mm (39); various contemporary studies yield similar values. The cornea flattens rapidly with aging so that, for adults, values at the central location are generally considered to be 7.8 and 6.5 mm for the anterior and posterior surfaces, respectively. Such estimates of curvature are rather simplistic because the actual geometric shape of the corneal surface is more complex (37,40). Based on central keratometry measures, the curved anterior corneal surface is capable of providing substantial refractive power, on the order of 43 D.

ferences have been reported, and, on average, the paracentral cornea (approximately 3 mm from the center) is likely to be at least 21% thicker than the central cornea (7).

Layers of the Cornea

The cornea traditionally is described as a five-layered structure (Fig. 2.4). This may seem inconsistent because we treat the endothelial basement membrane as a separate layer, but this distinction is not bestowed on the epithelium.

1. Epithelium (outermost cell layers)
2. Anterior limiting lamina ([ALL] Bowman membrane)
3. Stroma
4. Posterior limiting lamina ([PLL] Desçemet membrane)
5. Endothelium (innermost cell layer)

Although considered simply to be a five-layered structure, there is actually an anterior coating layer on the corneal surface. This mucus (mucin) coat is largely produced by the goblet cells (30,41,42) and can be considered to be functionally attached to the surface cells. It has been shown to be protective in that the penetration (and thus staining) of the ocular surface cells with dyes (such as rose bengal) depends on whether there is a mucous coat present (43). If a "toxic" agent strips off the mucous coating, then the surface cells will stain with a vital stain such as rose bengal, a result indicating that surface protection has been removed (see Chapter 23).

FIG. 2.4. Low-magnification transverse section through a monkey cornea as viewed by light microscopy. The cornea is bounded anteriorly by a stratified, nonkeratinized epithelium and posteriorly by a single layer of squamous endothelial cells. Stromal tissue occupies the space between these two boundary layers. Dense staining keratocytes are found within the stroma. These cells can be seen to be more numerous anteriorly. (Magnification approximately 100×.)

The coating is presumed to be primarily composed of mucous; therefore, it can be visualized if the ocular surface tissue is prepared for microscopy with a chemical agent (cetylpyridinium chloride) that "fixes" this mucin (44,45). When such special fixation is performed, all that is evident at the corneal or conjunctival surfaces is essentially an amorphous coat, that is, a gray, largely featureless image. This coat contains ultramicroscopic debris (Fig. 2.5A). TEM studies of the bulbar conjunctiva after such special preparations indicate an amorphous layer that is approximately 0.8 μm thick (45). At much higher magnification in SEM, a distinct texture can be observed in the precipitated and desiccated mucous layer (Fig. 2.5B). It still appears to be a largely amorphous matrix (i.e., it is not fibrous or globular), but there appear to be numerous small pores in the matrix (46).

Corneal Chemistry

The cornea also can be described in terms of both its water content and chemical composition. The percentage of the tissue composed of water (determined by heat drying) usually is quoted to be between 76% and 78%, although slight differences from these values can easily arise from methodologic errors or postmortem changes (47). Stated another way, the dry mass of the complete cornea is between 22% and 24% of the wet mass. The collagens of the cornea make up the bulk of this tissue dry mass, around 15% of the wet mass (or about 68% of the dry mass) (27,48). The corneal stroma also contains proteoglycans. These are large glycosylated protein molecules consisting of a protein core linked to a carbohydrate-like glycosaminoglycan (GAG) chain. These chains are polyanionic in nature and so can be detected both histochemically and biochemically with polycationic molecules such as Alcian blue. The relative amount of these proteoglycan molecules in the cornea usually is based on measures of the GAGs. Older literature values are between 1% and 5% of the dry mass (27), but more recent estimates are much higher at 9% (48). In absolute terms, the total quantity of proteoglycans in human corneas (based on an immunochemical detection method for the GAGs) has been reported at around 18 μg/mg wet mass in one study (49), whereas another study reported a value just 1/10 of this (50). In contrast, recent estimates of the total proteoglycan content (based on Alcian blue positive material) of bovine corneal stroma indicate values of 33 μg/mg wet mass (or 150 μg/mg dry mass) (51), higher than previous estimates (also based on Alcian blue staining) where the proteoglycan content was estimated to be around 40 μg/mg dry mass (52). These large differences likely reflect different extraction techniques and whether corrections are made for interfering polyanions (52). Further research clearly is needed to resolve these fundamental issues related to corneal composition. In addition to insoluble protein and readily solubilized proteoglycans, the cornea contains considerable quan-

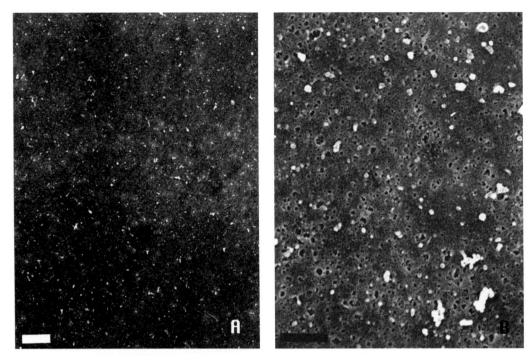

FIG. 2.5. Low-magnification **(A)** and high-magnification **(B)** scanning electron microscopic images of the mucin coat on the rabbit corneal surface precipitated with cetylpyridinium chloride-glutaral-dehyde. (From Doughty MJ, [46], with permission.)

tities of other proteins. Some of these make up the corneal epithelial and endothelial cell layers, but it should be recognized that substantial quantities of soluble protein can be extracted from the corneal stroma. These proteins, which presumably are largely derived from the keratocytes, have been recently estimated to be 20 μg/mg wet mass (51) or comprising some 18% of dry mass of the cornea (48).

EMBRYOLOGY OF THE CORNEA

The earliest corneal manifestation, a single layer of ectodermal cells, is noted after 5 weeks of gestation (31,53). This layer will become the corneal epithelium, which can be seen to show signs of stratification (i.e., into basal, wing and superficial cells) by mid gestation (54). It will acquire an almost adult appearance as the fetus opens its eyes, just over halfway through gestation (31). At about one fifth of the gestational period, mesoderm enters to form stromal tissue.

The ALL (Bowman membrane) and PLL (Desçemet membrane) also appear at mid gestation. The former appears to be formed by anterior keratocytes that later leave the area to create a cell-free zone (31,54,55). The collagenous secretion of stromal cells, later to become keratocytes, produces the corneal lamellae, which increase in number throughout gestation (31,54,55).

The corneal endothelium is thought to be of neural crest origin, but this has been a matter of debate (56). Immunohistochemical research indicates that both keratocytes and endothelial cells derive from neural crest cells that later differentiate into mesenchymal cells (57).

The secreted collagen network initially is loose, but continuous growth gradually creates denser and more parallel organized collagen bundles, termed *lamellae.* The cornea grows both in thickness, adding lamellae, and in width, from elongation of lamellae (31,54,55).

A double row of flattened mesenchymal cells appear relatively early in gestation, posterior to the basal lamina of two rows of epithelial cells (54,55). This will become the endothelium, which simultaneously will secrete its basement membrane, the PLL (Desçemet membrane). The PLL continues to grow throughout life, whereas the endothelium will have its adult configuration by birth (58).

The earliest signs of ciliary nerves form shortly after the appearance of the primitive endothelial cell layer. These can be observed initially at the edge of the optic cup, and within a few weeks fine neural twigs are present in the stroma (53).

As noted earlier, corneal dimensions in humans do not realize adult values until sometime after birth (Fig. 2.2). Similarly, substantial changes in corneal thickness occur. In early to mid stages of embryogenesis, the cornea has a relatively uniform thickness, but from mid gestation the peripheral cornea thickens (59). Rapid postnatal changes in the CCT can be expected (7). An analysis of literature studies over a 30-year period indicates that CCT values decline by about 10% over the first year or so of life and reach adult values in early childhood (Fig. 2.6) (60). As noted earlier, the peripheral corneal thickness is greater than the CCT in

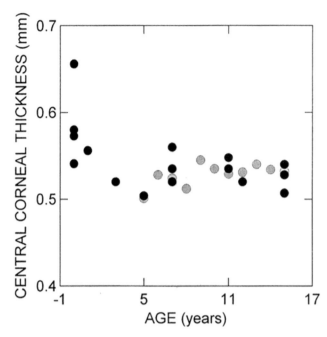

FIG. 2.6. Changes in human central corneal thickness in the postnatal period. (Modified from Doughty MJ, et al., [60], with permission.)

humans; limited data suggest that this difference lessens in the elderly (7).

MICROSCOPIC ANATOMY OF THE CORNEA

Epithelium

Various functions have been attributed to the corneal epithelial cell layer, namely, optical, protective, barrier, and shield properties, and as a stabilizer of the tear film. The optical roles obviously include transparency and refractive power (see earlier). The protective roles are related to the possible impact of external trauma on the ocular surface, with the corneal epithelium constituting a renewable protective layer over the corneal stroma. The corneal epithelium also serves as a fluid barrier with the surface layer of epithelial cells containing special cell–cell linking structures, the zonula occludentes. These serve as a barrier to limit fluid leakage into the cornea from the tear film. Similarly, the corneal epithelium can be considered a protective shield against microorganisms normally present in the tear fluid. Any significant perturbation of the integrity of the ocular surface is believed to compromise or even remove this shield and can result in microbial invasion of the cornea. Last, the corneal epithelial surface can be considered a tear film stabilizer, with the microplicae and microvilli along the epithelial surface promoting tear film interaction with the corneal surface and thus contributing to the stability of the tear film (see Chapter 23).

The corneal epithelium is classified as a stratified squamous epithelial layer. It is formed by five to six, or even seven, layers of tightly packed cells in humans and primates (Fig. 2.7) (4,5). No spaces are evident between the cells in the postnatal corneal epithelium; the paracellular space is very limited as a result of numerous connections (desmosomes) between the cells and a lack of edema. The corneal epithelium shows continuity with the conjunctival epithelium, which itself is continuous with the skin of the eyelid. In the healthy eye, the epithelium is not keratinized.

Older histologic studies report the thickness of the human corneal epithelium to be between 30 and 40 μm (4,5), but the thickness also has been quoted as being around 50 μm, presumably from histologic sections (25). A value of 54 + 4 μm has been obtained by through-focusing confocal microscopy in the living human eye (8). The epithelium conventionally is considered to be organized into three layers.

Three separate shapes of cells are recognized in the corneal epithelium: basal, wing, and squamous cells (Fig. 2.8). The cells that make up these layers are not generally considered to represent three different classes of cells but rather the same cell lineage at different stages between genesis and eventual loss from the corneal surface (see later).

Basal cells are sited at the innermost layer and are attached to the basement membrane, which itself is secreted by these cells. In human or monkey cornea, rather rounded nuclei are located close to the bases of the cells (Fig. 2.8). The arrangement sometimes is slightly different in that basal cells have slightly more elongated nuclei, oriented in the same anteroposterior direction as the cells (25,61). The same characteristic is generally found in rabbit corneal epithelium, where nuclei can be lobulated.

Above the basal cells are intermediate layers of cells often referred to as *wing* or *umbrella cells* because of their shape. These cells are found immediately above the single row of basal cells. Their nuclei are also usually relatively rounded

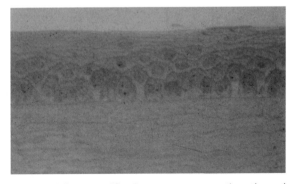

FIG. 2.7. Higher-magnification transverse section through a monkey corneal epithelium viewed by light microscopy. The epithelium is formed by 5 to 7 layers of tightly packed epithelial cells with no spaces present between them. A linear basement membrane facilitates the attachment of the epithelium to the remainder of the cornea. (Magnification approximately 250×.)

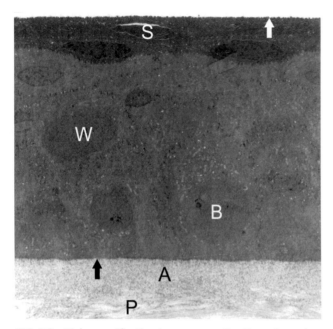

FIG. 2.8. High-magnification transverse section through monkey corneal epithelium as viewed by transmission electron microscopy. The epithelial surface is anteriorly lined by small projections (microplicae and microvilli, *white arrow*) and posteriorly by its basement membrane *(black arrow)*. The cells forming the epithelium are classified according to their shape and location as basal (B), wing (W), and squamous (S) cells. Internally, the basement membrane of the epithelium borders the anterior limiting lamina (A), which itself is facing the stroma posteriorly (P). (Magnification 5,300×.)

but have a tendency to be slightly oval in section, with the longest dimension oriented parallel to the epithelial surface.

External to two or three rows of intermediate cells are two to three rows of flattened *squamous cells*. The term *squamous* literally means flat but is generally used to also imply that these special cells routinely undergo a desquamation from the ocular surface (see later). Transverse section through the squamous cell nucleus reveals a notably elongated shape that is oriented parallel to the ocular surface. The corneal surface is formed by this most external layer of squamous cells.

The outline of the external squamous cells along the surface forms an irregular pattern, and the apical surfaces that are in contact with the tears are specially formed into very high numbers of special microprojections. For the normal corneal epithelium, these projections from the cell surfaces appear to principally be microscopic ridges (called *microplicae*) as opposed to individual features (called *microvilli*). As viewed in conventional sections, these projections are hard to distinguish (Fig. 2.8), but when viewed with SEM, a complex pattern of little ridges is clearly evident (Fig. 2.9A) (62). At extremely high magnification (50,000× at the microscope stage), the ridges can be seen to be decorated with small globular protrusions (Fig. 2.9B) that may be the glycocalyx (63) (see Chapter 23).

Epithelial renewal previously was believed to be accomplished through a simple process that involved mitotic cell division at the basal cell level, occurring across the entire cornea. Early histologic studies that used labeling of cells with [³H]-thymidine resulted in estimates of the life cycle of an epithelial cell of about 7 days (64), that is, a basal cell

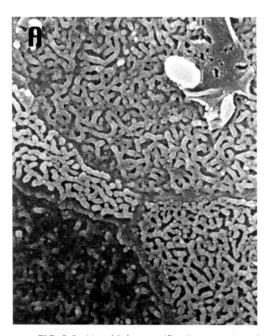

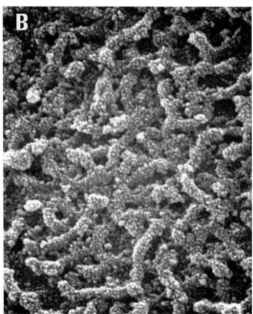

FIG. 2.9. Very-high-magnification scanning electron microscopic views of the surface of rabbit corneal epithelial cells show high density of microplicae on the lighter appearing cells **(A)** and the glycocalyx on the surfaces of the microplicae **(B)**. (From Doughty MJ, Fong WK, [62] and Doughty MJ, [63], respectively, with permission.)

would take this period of time to slowly migrate to the ocular surface. Following division, the cells would move toward the corneal surface and ultimately desquamate into the tears.

New evidence suggests a more complex cycle of epithelial renewal. It was observed some years ago that the destruction of limbal and conjunctival epithelium through trauma or disease leads to loss of epithelial integrity in central cornea. Thoft and Friend (65) suggested the X,Y,Z hypothesis: the proliferation of basal cells (in the X direction) together with a centripetal movement of peripherally located cells (Y direction) equals the desquamation rate (Z) at the surface. Thoft and Friend suggested that the central epithelium cannot solely depend on mitosis of corneal cells to remain healthy but requires a net flux of cells from the periphery. More recent studies using bromodeoxyuridine (BrdU) labeling to detect cell mitoses indicate that peripheral basal cells divide at a faster rate when challenged by overnight contact lens wear (66).

From a morphologic perspective, it is generally observed that the most superficial cells of the corneal epithelium have different sizes, shapes, and appearances. The best view of this is achieved with the SEM operated at lower magnifications (62). Such images (Fig. 2.10) show the cells to have light, medium, and dark appearances. In addition, there are topographical differences in the size, shape, and appearance of these surface cells (67). Some have argued that the different appearances reflect the period of time to which these cells were exposed at the tear film interface after having migrated from deeper levels of the corneal epithelium (68). In such a scheme, the largest and darkest appearing cells, with fewer surface projections (microplicae), are considered to be those that were at the surface for the longest period of time and are preparing to desquamate from the surface.

Desquamating cells have a very different appearance in that they can be "bright" cells with abundant surface projections (69). It has been argued (69) that the different character of desquamating cells indicates that there are several types of surface epithelial cells, with a subtly different lineage and differentiation. Such differences in the cells occur at some stage, during the course of their migration through the corneal epithelium, after differentiation from a precursor cell at the limbus, the stem cell. It now is recognized that some of the most superficial epithelial cells do not simply desquamate but undergo a special type of degeneration or cell death, called *apoptosis* (70), and perhaps this is the main mechanism by which cells are "deleted" from the corneal epithelium (71). The differences in SEM appearance of the superficial cells that are undergoing desquamation may be that some are apoptotic while others are not.

Although some cells populating the corneal epithelium are able to migrate from the basal layer to suprabasal location, those basal cells in contact with the basement membrane are extremely firmly attached. This adhesion is achieved through a large number of hemidesmosomes found along the internal plasmalemma of the basal cells, which adhere to the underlying cornea. There are also numerous desmosomes formed between neighboring cells throughout the epithelial layer, effecting substantial cell-to-cell adhesion and thus minimizing the paracellular space. Further enhancement of the cell-to-cell adhesion is achieved through interdigitations between neighboring cells. The combination of extensive intercellular interdigitations and numerous desmosomes acting as "spot weldings" results in a very resilient structure that will, for instance, permit very vigorous eye rubbing without secondary abrasion. The overall adhesion of corneal epithelial cells to the basement membrane is so strong that its weakest part is found in the tall columnar basal cells that fragment rather than loss of adhesion with the basement membrane or its attachment to overlying cells (72).

Other cell junctions in the epithelium are gap junctions and zonula occludentes (73). The gap and adherens junctions are found between cells in all layers and promote intercellular attachment and communication. The zonula occludentes are found only in the superficial squamous cell layer, where they provide an anterior fluid barrier. When this barrier is disturbed by some form of trauma, including any exposure to a hypotonic solution, fluid enters the epithelium and accumulates between cells. This is known as *epithelial edema*, clinically called *Sattler veil* because of the significant visual effects of this condition (74).

The name *corneal epithelium* implies that only epithelial

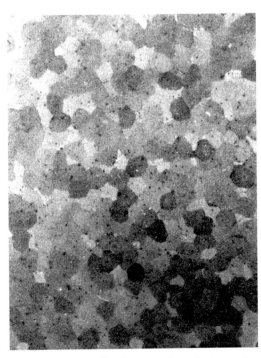

FIG. 2.10. Lower-magnification scanning electron microscopic view of the surface of the rabbit corneal epithelium showing the appearances of the polygonal cells, often referred to as light, medium, and dark cells. (From Doughty MJ, [62], with permission.)

cells are found in this layer, but this is not strictly true. It is well known that this layer has dense innervation (Fig. 2.11). Most epithelial nerves are located deep, in the basal cell layer. This also is the location of a third class of cells, Langerhans cells, which normally are resident in the epithelium. The Langerhans cell can be regarded as a special element of the immune system and can generally be found in the cornea (75), albeit at a much lower density than found in the skin. The small body of the Langerhans cell usually is found deep in the corneal epithelium among the basal cells, and long, rounded, processes project from its body to span significant corneal distances. Langerhans cells are antigen-processing cells, like macrophages (see Chapter 4). Extended wear of contact lenses can promote elevation of the number of Langerhans cells migrating into the cornea (76), whereas ultraviolet B (UVB) radiation causes a net reduction in the number of Langerhans cells (77). On occasion, white blood cells are observed within the epithelium. In all likelihood, these have been called upon in response to a challenge to the health of the cornea. Therefore, these cells should not be regarded as residents of the normal cornea but rather cells recruited when the integrity of the cornea is threatened.

Anterior Limiting Lamina

The ALL (also known as *Bowman membrane*) can be considered specially modified stromal tissue. It is substantial in

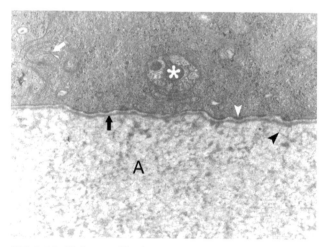

FIG. 2.11. High-magnification transmission electron microscopic view of a transverse section through primate corneal epithelium anterior limiting lamina interface at the basal cell level. The anterior limiting lamina (A) lies immediately posterior to the basement membrane *(black arrow)* of the epithelium, with which it is linked via a series of fine collagen type VII fibers (black arrowhead). The slightly interdigitated outline of the tightly packed epithelium has no spaces between the cells *(white arrow)*. Numerous hemidesmosomes *(white arrowhead)* are found along the basal side of basal cells and provide adhesion to the basement membrane. A small group of epithelial axons *(white asterisk)* is accommodated by an infolding of the basal plasmalemma. (Magnification 22,400×.)

human and primate corneas but is a mere vestige in corneas from animals such as rabbits. The ALL is strictly a corneal structure that does not extend beyond the corneal edge. In transverse section, the ALL narrows in width close to the corneal periphery as the limbus is approached (25,30,31, 78).

The ALL has been measured to be 8 to 14 μm in thickness using TEM in human and primate corneas (25). *In vivo* confocal microscopy ALL measurements of human corneas yield a value of 16.6 ± 1.1 μm (8). The ALL is acellular, except for occasional nerve fibers (neural ramus perforans) that are fine neural branches penetrating this layer on their way to the epithelium (see later). SEM observations of rabbit corneal surface after removal of the corneal epithelium shows "holes" through which nerve fibers are thought to emerge (79), but it should be noted that the ALL in rabbits is not a well-developed structure.

As viewed by TEM, the ALL is formed by a dense network of fine, randomly oriented collagen type I fibers, slightly finer in cross-section than the underlying stromal collagen (Fig. 2.11) (80). The ALL provides attachments for the epithelial basement membrane by means of type VII collagen fibers. These fibers originate from within the ALL and at their other end insert in the basement membrane. Thus, these fine fibrils are fused with the basement membrane anteriorly, whereas posteriorly they are located in anchoring plaques found within the ground substance of the ALL. There are additional structures or proteins that contribute to the complex arrangement involved in epithelial adhesion, including laminin and fibronectin.

Corneal Stroma

The corneal stroma (substantia propria) comprises around 90% of the corneal thickness in humans. Therefore, it often is considered to be approximately 0.5 mm thick, although in even a normal human cornea this stromal thickness could be between 0.42 and 0.54 mm based on CCT measures (7). The corneal stroma is a three-dimensional matrix of collagen fibers; an interstitial proteoglycan ground substance, which both coats the collagen fibrils and fills the space between them; and the overall matrix, which is populated by numerous keratocytes.

Collagen molecules make up some 68% of the corneal stromal dry mass (48), and the fibrils that make up the corneal stroma are principally type I collagen (considered to represent some 70% of the stromal collagen). The fully assembled adult corneal stroma also contains several other collagens, namely, types V, VI, XII, and XIV (48). Some of these are directly associated with the collagen fibrils, whereas others are found in the spaces between the flat bundles of the fibrils.

Type I collagen forms the basis of minute fibrils that, in turn, are arranged in a highly organized pattern in bundles called *lamellae*. The lamellae are visible as striations across lower-magnification transverse sections through the corneal stroma (Fig. 2.12) (81). In the more anterior stroma, the lamellae appear to be thinner and less organized (Fig. 2.12A), whereas in the posterior stroma collagen fibrils in each lamellae appear to be arranged more in uniform thickness sheets with parallel surfaces (Fig. 2.12B). It is not unusual for the posterior stromal lamellae to be slightly undulating; in the absence of any edema, this is a likely feature of corneas fixed without a perfusion method (81). It should be noted that although the lamellae apparently form parallel plates when viewed in transverse section by TEM, SEM studies clearly show that the lamellae cross each other at various angles (82–84). The cross-over of the lamellae at various angles also can be observed by interference light microscopy (85,86), through silver staining of the stroma, (87) and is implied from both polarized light transmission (88) and x-ray transmission studies (89).

A simplistic perspective of the corneal lamellae is that they are flat and very elongated bundles that stretch from one side of the cornea to the other. The extent of interlacing between the most anterior lamellae, however, is clearly more substantial than in the mid or posterior stroma (83,84, 90,91). In addition, lamellae can branch and even insert through one another (84). Lastly, it has yet to be well established exactly how the lamellae are organized at the periphery of the corneal stroma. Early light microscopy studies indicated that at least some of the lamellae adopt a circumcorneal (radial) orientation as they approach the limbus (85,86), and evidence for such an orientation has also been obtained from SEM (83) and x-ray studies (92). Some lamellae may well bridge the maximum diameter of the cor-

nea, but others can be arranged across much shorter distances (85). Regardless of what proportion of lamellae have circumcorneal orientation at the corneal periphery (84), an equally important issue is the nature of lamellae that cross the corneal periphery in a radial orientation from the episclera and sclera (86). Recent TEM studies on rabbits indicate that at least some of the anterior radial fibrils in the episclera are of the same dimensions as those in the corneal sclera, whereas most of the deeper-located fibrils in the anterior and posterior sclera are much larger (93). The nature of this interface between the various levels of the corneal stroma and the surrounding episclera and sclera surely must be a very important determinant of the shape and mechanical strength of the anterior segment of the eye. Similarly, the substantially interlaced nature of the most anterior lamellae play an important part in determining the shape of the anterior cornea and its resistance to change (90,91).

Stromal lamellae generally appear to have thickness values around 1 to 2 μm, but quality normative values remain to be established from TEM studies. There has been considerable interest in the gross organization of the lamellae, but relatively little attention has been given to quantitative analyses of the lamellae in terms of their thickness and whether there are any obvious age-related changes. Marshall and Grindle (53) reported that the lamellae in human corneas are 2 μm thick. In early studies, Schwartz and Keyserlingk (94) reported human stromal lamellae thicknesses between 0.75 and 5 μm, whereas an average thickness value of 1.15 μm, with a tendency to be thicker (average 1.29 μm) for the central cornea, was reported by Hamada et al. (95). In recent studies, the more anterior stromal lamellae from

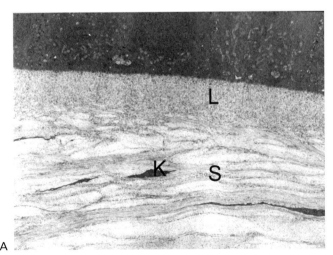
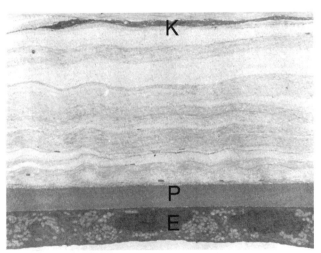

FIG. 2.12. Higher-magnification transmission electron microscopic images of transverse sections through monkey corneal stroma illustrating the arrangement of the collagen lamellae within **(A)** the most anterior location and **(B)** at the posterior aspect of the cornea. In the anterior location, the lamellae of the stroma (S) immediately under the anterior limiting lamina (L) are thinner and more interwoven compared to the thicker and flatter lamellae in the posterior stroma. The posterior stromas includes the posterior limiting lamina (P) and the corneal endothelium (E). Keratocytes (K) are present both anteriorly and posteriorly but are more numerous in anterior stroma than in the posterior stroma. (Magnification 4,000×.)

human corneas were reported to have average thickness values of 1.29 ± 0.23 μm, whereas the posterior lamellae were thicker, averaging 2.92 ± 1.54 μm. An overall average lamella thickness value of 1.66 ± 0.11 μm was calculated (96). In another study, it was noted simply that the more anterior lamellae varied in thickness from about 0.2 to 1.2 μm, whereas a range from 0.2 to 2.5 μm was found in the posterior stroma (82). Further work clearly is needed to assess the extent of differences in lamellae when comparing central versus peripheral locations or anterior versus posterior locations.

It remains to be established whether there are significant age-related differences in human stromal lamellae thickness. Data from rabbit corneas indicates that this may be the case. Hart et al. (97) implied that rabbit corneal stromal lamellae have an approximately uniform thickness of about 10 μm, yet a thickness of just 1 to 2 μm was noted by Gallager and Maurice (98). In recent detailed quantitative studies, the average thickness for posterior lamellae in corneas of adult rabbits (body weight around 2.5 kg) was found to be 2.45 ± 1.15 μm (99). More recent studies on younger 2-kg rabbits, however, indicates an average thickness closer to 2 μm for the posterior lamellae (Doughty, Bergmanson, and Gondo, *unpublished data*).

As noted earlier, the more anterior stromal lamellae are slightly thinner and appear to follow a more intertwined path (Fig. 2.12A), whereas posteriorly the lamellae appear to be more organized with respect to each other (Fig 2.12B). This anatomical variation between anterior and posterior lamellae may be part of the explanation to the substantial tendency for corneal stroma swelling to occur in the posterior direction (100) and for the anterior stroma to change relatively little even when there is substantial posterior swelling (91).

Collagen fibrils within stromal lamellae of a normal mammalian cornea are of very similar diameter and relatively uniformly spacing (Fig. 2.13A). Such very high magnification quality TEM images are easily procured from very recent postmortem corneal samples, especially if they are processed so as to minimize tissue distortion. With the type of material that might be obtained from an eye bank, unfortunately, it is more likely that images of the type shown in Figure 2.13B will be obtained. The observation of such generally well-organized arrays of fibrils is critically dependent on the hydration of the tissue, that is, the interfibril distance, and the apparent organization will change in a cornea that has developed edema (101). X-ray studies indicate that the interfibril distance will change substantially with even small deviations from the normal hydration values (102). Although the data are limited, both TEM (103) and x-ray studies (104) indicate that slightly smaller interfibril distances may be present in the corneal stroma of elderly humans compared to those from much younger patients.

Between the collagen fibrils is a complex inner matrix of proteoglycan molecules called the *extracellular matrix*

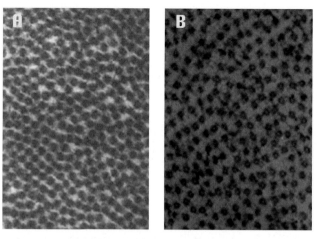

FIG. 2.13. Very-high-magnification transmission electron microscopic images of sections through rabbit **(A)** and human **(B)** lamellae within the posterior third of the corneal stroma. The organization in the freshly fixed rabbit sample is the result of the tissue being at normal hydration, whereas the human sample shows clear signs of postmortem edema.

(ECM). It is an ECM because it is external to the corneal cells (keratocytes; see later). TEM studies of both polycation-stained stroma (105) and freeze-etched stroma (106) clearly show the ECM is a complex array of microfilaments between adjacent collagen type I fibrils. Some of the filaments include some of the lesser collagen molecules as well. With some types of conventional TEM studies, some filaments also can be seen between the fibrils (24). Although it is possible to assign a certain index of refraction to the ECM (see corneal physiology section earlier), it should not be considered an amorphous ground substance without any structure.

Considerable attention has been given to the combination of small collagen type I fibrils, their relatively uniform spacing, and their relative refractive index compared to that of the ECM, to explain the optical transparency of the corneal stroma (107). The size (diameter) of individual collagen fibrils is considered too small to scatter significant light (108–110). It has generally been proposed that as long as the fibers remain of fairly uniform small size and are not spaced further apart than about λ/2n (where λ is the wavelength and n is the refractive index of the media), the requirements of corneal stromal transparency modeling would be satisfied (111).

The mammalian corneal stroma is populated with large numbers of keratocytes, but until relatively recently, these cells were all but ignored (Fig. 2.14) (112). More than a century ago, Claréus (113) observed that keratocytes appeared to form a closely linked network (in flat mounts of cornea stained with silver). Such a network has been readily demonstrated by this method in more recent assessments (114). As might be expected from flat mount or *en face* section views, the keratocytes are flattened because they are lodged between the lamellae of the corneal stroma. Evidence sup-

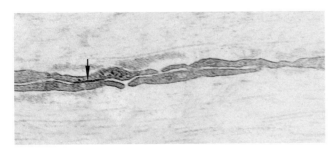

FIG. 2.14. High-magnification transmission electron micrograph of section through rabbit corneal stroma showing two keratocytes (a gap junction is seen at arrow). (Magnification 26,000×.)

porting the idea that the appearance of the keratocytes, as viewed in transverse section, is related to physical compression comes from comparative measures of keratocyte thickness and the thickness of adjacent lamellae (99); the thinner the lamellae, the thinner the keratocyte. As viewed in transverse section in TEM (Fig. 2.15), keratocytes are spindle shaped, with long processes that extend horizontally; these processes can reach 30 μm and sometimes even longer (99). TEM studies suggest that some keratocytes have vertical projections that actually cross the entire thickness of the lamellae (99). These have been termed *translamellar keratocytes* (TLKs) (99), and their presence has been confirmed by confocal microscopy (115). The long processes of the keratocytes make contact with each other via gap junctions (99,116–118), and it is via these gap junctions that the keratocytes communicate across the cornea, both horizontally and vertically (through the TLKs) (115,116). Normally keratocytes are in what has been termed a *quiescent* state, and their cell nuclei have smooth and oval profiles. In response to stress (including edema) and wounding, however, keratocytes can change to an activated phenotype in which the cell nucleus undergoes characteristic changes and rough endoplasmic reticulum becomes very prominent (119).

As viewed by light microscopy in transverse section (not shown) or TEM (Fig. 2.12), more keratocytes appear in anterior than posterior stroma. Serial section TEM studies indicate that the keratocytes are not randomly distributed but appear to be arranged in a regular, clockwise spiraling pattern throughout the full stromal thickness (118). It also is possible to view the keratocytes in the living stroma by confocal microscopy (Fig. 2.16). This technique principally allows the observer to see light reflected off the nuclei of the keratocytes *in vivo* (although high-resolution instruments and staining of the cells with fluorescent traces *ex vivo* have been used to show the cell processes as well) (115, 120). *In vivo* confocal microscopy confirms that the highest density of keratocytes is found in the more anterior stroma, with density declining by as much as 30% in a posterior direction (14,121,122).

Keratocytes produce the corneal stroma collagen fibrils during development and presumably maintain this function as a "housekeeping" activity throughout life. At the ultrastructural level, the newly assembled collagen fibrils can be seen to emanate from the keratocytes through what appear to be ultramicroscopic pores in the cell membrane (Fig. 2.17) (99,118). Newly assembled collagen fibrils are secreted from the keratocytes and, therefore, at least at some points in time, are attached to them.

The last ultrastructural feature of the keratocytes (Fig. 2.18) is very relevant to current interest in their role beyond the production of collagen for maintenance and repair of the corneal stroma (119). The corneal keratocytes contain contractile proteins [such as myosin and α-actinin (114)], which are considered important in both maintenance of cell shape and organization of connections between adjacent keratocytes. That these contractile proteins are functional

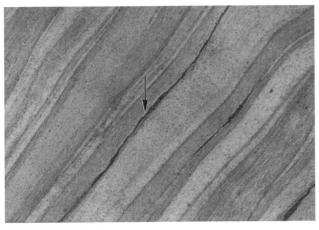

FIG. 2.15. High-magnification transmission electron micrographic image of transverse section through monkey corneal stroma showing the presence of a flattened keratocyte *(arrow)* between collagen lamellae. (Magnification 6,600×.)

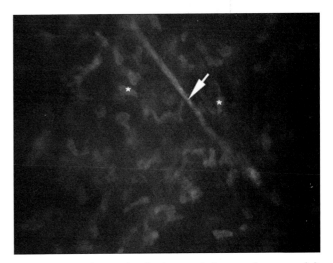

FIG. 2.16. *In vivo* confocal microscopic image of young adult human central corneal stroma. The anterior stroma has a high number of keratocytes, which are visualized here by their rounded, elongated nuclei *(asterisks).* An anterior stromal nerve *(arrow)* is traversing the field of view. (Micrograph courtesy of Dr. William Miller, University of Houston, College of Optometry.)

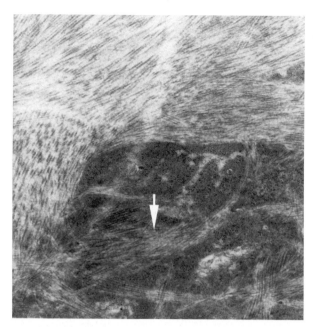

FIG. 2.17. High-magnification transmission electron micrographic view of coronal sections through a rabbit corneal stroma showing the cell body region of a keratocyte and the interface with surrounding collagen fibrils. The cell outline is very complex and extensively intermingled with collagen fibers *(arrow)*. (Magnification 20,000×.)

has been demonstrated *in vivo;* these cells change their characteristics in wound healing so as to draw together edges of corneal stroma incisions (123). They play a similar role in the organization of embryonic corneal stroma (124). Attachment of corneal keratocytes to collagen fibrils and their ability to exert traction on these fibrils also have been demonstrated *in vitro* (125). This close relationship between collagen fibers and keratocytes suggests that keratocytes also may be involved in supporting lamellar stability, that is, the keratocytes could help keep the different lamellae stable in their intended locations (82,99,118).

Although the keratocyte is the principal cell of the stroma, other cells have been observed in normal stromal tissue. For example, Kuwabara (126) reported small numbers of neutrophils, lymphocytes, plasma cells, and histocytes in the normal stroma. The anterior stroma also harbors a plexus of unmyelinated nerve fibers (Fig. 2.16); thus, the stroma also is inhabited by Schwann cells and neurons.

Posterior Limiting Lamina

The PLL (Descemet membrane) is a flat largely amorphous layer immediately adjacent to the corneal endothelium (Fig. 2.12). It may be 20 μm thick in the adult cornea (127). It is also a true corneal layer as it stops at the limbus (31). It is the basement membrane of the endothelium; it is also

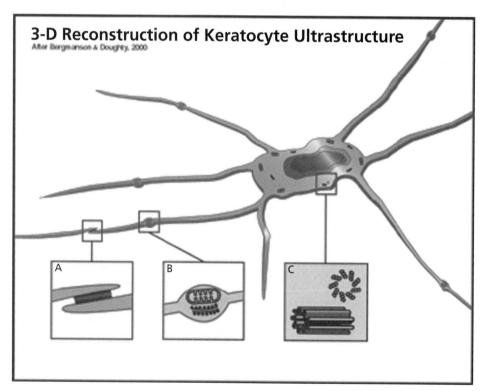

FIG. 2.18. Schematic three-dimensional reconstruction of a keratocyte showing its paper-thin proportions, peripheral displacement of organelles (except for the nucleus), and gap junction for intercellular communication. (From Bergmanson JPG. *Clinical ocular anatomy and physiology,* 11th ed. Houston, TX: Texas Eye Research and Technology Center, University of Houston College of Optometry, 2004, with permission.)

the thickest basement membrane in the body. The PLL is composed of a mixture of type IV and VIII collagen, with the former collagen type being very evident in histochemical analyses but likely the lesser component (48). Both collagens can be shown to be synthesized by corneal endothelial cells in culture, proving that the PLL is produced by these cells.

The PLL is approximately 3 μm thick at birth but thickens progressively throughout life (128). The most anterior portion is the oldest and least uniform. This is the fetal part of the membrane and is known as the *banded layer*, whereas the postnatal component of the membrane is uniform in texture and is the portion that thickens with age. Despite being a thin portion of the cornea, the PLL is a very resilient structure, with substantial capacity to resist deformation under applied hydrostatic pressure (129–131). The PLL often is the last corneal layer to disintegrate (descemetocele) in disease conditions such as corneal melting.

The adult peripheral PLL can show local thickenings known as Hassell-Henle warts (31). Similar irregularities in the PLL occasionally are noted in the central cornea and clinically termed *corneal guttae*. (Due to misuse of the Latin language, this condition has been referred to as *guttata* in some texts.) Corneal guttae usually are self-limiting, but occasionally this condition (due to an abnormal endothelial basement membrane synthesis) advances (132) to become known as Fuch endothelial corneal dystrophy. Subsequent loss of endothelial cell function may lead to stromal and epithelial edema and thus loss of corneal transparency. Fuchs endothelial corneal dystrophy is one of the most common reasons for keratoplasty (see Chapter 28).

Endothelium

A single layer of cells forms the corneal endothelium. The endothelial cells normally are relatively thin, with apical and basal sides strictly parallel to each other in the plane of the cornea (Fig. 2.12). With SEM, the cells are observed as a compact layer with rather prominent cell-to-cell borders and visible apical flaps between cells (Fig. 2.19). SEM also reveals the presence of scattered apical cell surface microvilli, and, at least under some circumstances, primary cilia are observed (133). As mentioned earlier, the cells have very flat, parallel, and linear apical and basal outlines, but their lateral walls show extensive interdigitations, of which the apical flap, the most posterior, is visible in the SEM (Fig. 2.20) (134). Junctional complexes between the cells can be found associated with these apical flaps (135), containing gap and intermediate junctions and zonula occludentes. The zonula occludens, as elsewhere in the body, function as a fluid barrier, but the endothelial zonular occludentes do not wrap entirely around each cell. Therefore, the corneal endothelium is a leaky membrane, allowing aqueous humor to pass from the anterior chamber into the relatively dehydrated corneal stroma. Gap junctions found within the junctional complexes provide intracellular communications,

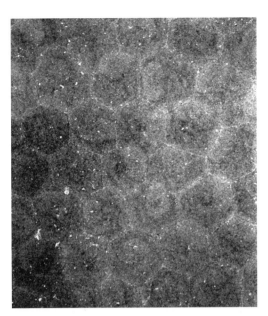

FIG. 2.19. Scanning electron microscopic image of the anterior (apical) surface of "normal" corneal endothelium from a young adult monkey. Note the interdigitated outline of cells.

whereas intermediate junctions (zonula adherentes) are responsible for cell-to-cell adhesion. These junctions are weaker than the desmosomes found in the epithelium, perhaps because the endothelium is not subject to the physical stresses of the anterior corneal surface.

When viewed clinically, as with a specular microscope, the posterior (aqueous chamber side) surfaces of the endothelial cells form a rather uniform, regular mosaic (Fig. 2.21). In either light microscopy of flat mounts or SEM (136) or specular microscopy (137), a relatively large proportion of the endothelial cells are seen as six sided. It is a common misnomer to refer to these cells as *hexagonal*; however many of the cells actually do not conform to this geometrical shape (134,138). Studies of the anterior surface of the corneal endothelium, facing the PLL, reveal that the cells here also are six sided and sometimes have a remarkable symmetry (136). Although one surface of these cells conforms to something resembling a hexagon, this does not mean that a similar configuration is present at the other surface (139). This observation is also not age related, as quantitative studies of the corneal endothelia of children clearly indicate that there are a large number of non–six-sided cells (140).

Corneal endothelial cells do not normally replicate after birth in either human or primate cornea (141). Any cells lost by stress, trauma, or damage will not be replaced, leading to an age-related decline in the number of corneal endothelial cells (readily observed by specular microscopy). At birth, the endothelial cell density is about 5,500 cells/mm^2 (32, 142). Cell density declines by about 1,000 to 2,000 cells to reach values close to 3,500 cells/mm^2 by childhood (32, 142). This initial apparent reduction is not all loss of cells,

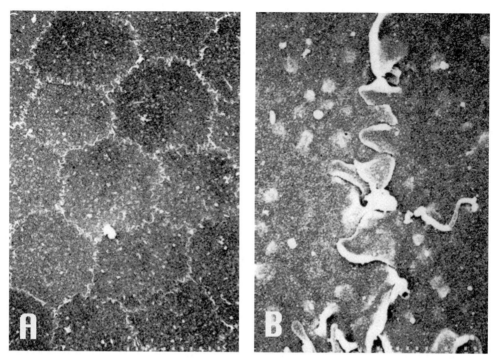

FIG. 2.20. Moderate **(A)** and high **(B)** scanning electron microscopic appearance of the apical surface of the rabbit corneal endothelium showing the interdigitation between cells **(A)** and these apical flaps at very high magnification **(B).** [Magnification 3,000× **(A)**, 10,000× **(B)**]. (From Doughty MJ, Sivak JG, [134], with permission.)

as it occurs during dramatic corneal growth (enlargement) (32). Although somewhat debatable, a further decline in cell density occurs slowly thereafter (as a result of cell loss) so that endothelial cell density values close to 2,000 cells/mm^2 are observed in the elderly (Fig. 2.22) (11,141–144). As cell density declines, some individual cells increase in

area. With age, the resultant endothelium contains a mixture of some smaller and some larger cells. The range of cell areas thus is greater than in a younger endothelium, and this appearance is generally referred to as *polymegethism* (145). Associated with the decline in cell density, the percentage of six-sided cells also declines with age (i.e., in-

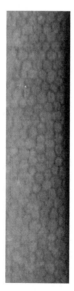

FIG. 2.21. Noncontact specular microscopic appearance of a "normal" corneal endothelium in a young adult. (From Doughty MJ, [137], with permission.)

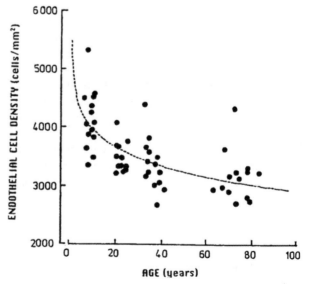

FIG. 2.22. Age-related changes in the density of human corneal endothelial cells as observed with the specular microscope. (From Doughty MJ, et al., 2000, with permission.)

creased proportions of non–six-sided cells). The range of cell shapes thus increases, and this type of change is generally referred to as *pleomorphism.* Neither polymegethism nor pleomorphism, *per se,* appears to result in abnormal microscopic morphology or lead to clinical complications (139, 146). However, substantial endothelial cell loss, above age-related normal changes, can compromise endothelial cell function and subsequent corneal edema could impair vision, necessitating a corneal transplant (141). It is believed that the functional limit of the corneal endothelium is approximately 700 to 1,000 cells/mm^2.

Endothelial function is believed to regulate fluid balance between the corneal stroma and the aqueous. It is generally accepted that the endothelium accomplishes this by acting both as a "leaky" fluid barrier and as a fluid pump (141). In the laboratory, with isolated corneal preparations, net fluid pump activity can be measured in the stroma-to-aqueous direction (147). Although this has been considered the *in vivo* corneal fluid pump fluid (141), a case can be made that keratocytes also serve to contract the collagen matrix of the corneal stroma to indirectly remove fluid from the stroma (148).

Corneal Nerves

The cornea is richly supplied with sensory nerve fibers, which are primarily derived from the ophthalmic division of cranial nerve V, but there may also be a minor maxillary contribution. Those nerves located within the corneal epithelium form an epithelial plexus and may be considered a first-line system. Conversely, stromal nerves form a stromal plexus, a separate second-line defense for detection of a range of stimuli. In the normal human cornea, no nerve fibers are of autonomic origin, as neither blood supply nor secretory organs are present.

Small corneal nerves, primarily from the long ciliary nerves but also from the short ciliary nerves, enter the cornea near the limbus at the mid stromal level. Some 1.5 mm from the limbus these fibers, if myelinated, lose their myelinated sheath (myelination is opaque and would obscure vision). Unmyelinated fibers divide and further subdivide into smaller branches that can cross two thirds of the cornea. These nerves may be seen clinically. Other nerve fibers of similar origin follow a similar route in the epithelium. These epithelial nerves lack the Schwann cell wrapping of fibers in the stroma. The close association between these axons and epithelial cells suggests that the epithelium has taken over the function of the Schwann cell. Single traversing neural ramus perforans moving from between stroma to the epithelium have been noted but are not common (149).

Nerve plexuses can be readily visualized in flat mounts of corneal tissue by nonspecific gold staining (150). Another partially specific histochemical staining method also can be applied, such as formaldehyde-induced fluorescence of catecholamine-containing nerves for associated with adrenergic (sympathetic) nerves and terminals, but they have only proved positive in lower animals (151,152). Alternatively, specific methods can be used, such as histochemical staining for the enzyme activities associated with neurotransmitter processing or immunochemical localization of antibodies specific for a type of neurotransmitter terminal. Examples include histochemical detection of acetylcholinesterase enzyme activity for a cholinergic innervation (152) or immunohistologic detection with anti-substance P antibodies for peptidergic nerve terminals (153,154).

Stromal nerve fibers terminate usually within 25 μm of the epithelium. Therefore, like the epithelial nerves, they are positioned to respond to external stimuli. Few axons will ascend to reach the surface cells of the cornea. This arrangement explains why the epithelial trauma threshold is lower than the corneal touch threshold (155). The epithelial nerve plexus is denser than the stromal plexus by a factor of 2:1 (156).

Corneal sensitivity most commonly is measured as its mechanical touch threshold with the use of the fine nylon filament of the Cochet-Bonnet esthesiometer (157). Recent alternatives include delivery of either a pulse of air to the cornea, which elicits a sensation by transiently cooling the corneal surface (158), or a pulse of CO_2, which results in transient local acidification of the tear film (159). All three instruments essentially measure different aspects of corneal sensitivity, although there may be some overlap.

Measurements of mechanical touch thresholds indicate that the central cornea is twice as sensitive as the peripheral cornea, and corneal sensitivity declines by about 50% during aging (adulthood to old age) (157,160,161).

GROSS ANATOMY OF THE LIMBUS AND CONJUNCTIVA

The cornea merges into the limbus at its periphery, and a further transition occurs to conjunctiva. The limbus is a circular (annular) strip of tissue, the *corneoscleral junction.* It is not a specific anatomical dividing mark but more a 0.5- to 1-mm wide zone. On the corneal side, the transition to the limbal epithelium is called the *corneolimbal junction,* whereas on the scleral side the transition is called the *limbo-scleral junction* (25).

The conjunctiva of the eye usually is divided into three main regions, namely, bulbar, fornix, and palpebral (Fig. 2.1). Bulbar conjunctiva covers the anterior part of the surface of the eye that is not included in the cornea and limbus and extends peripherally to the fornix. The fornix (Latin for arch or archlike structure or space) is the *cul-de-sac* at the inferior and superior extremes of the conjunctival sac that bridges the bulbar to palpebral conjunctiva. The palpebral conjunctiva covers the internal surface of the eyelid, from the fornix to the eyelid margin, where mucous-covered conjunctiva meets the skin (*oculomucocutaneous junction*).

The depth (extent) of the conjunctival sac is not symmetrical, with superior and inferior aspects dominant in both children and adults (Fig. 2.1). Commonly quoted values are 14 to 15 mm for the superior sac, 10 to 12 mm for the inferior sac, and 5 to 8 mm for the lateral (temporal) aspect. The medial (nasal) aspect of the conjunctival sac has no depth because it terminates at the plica semilunaris (25).

Both the limbus and the conjunctiva essentially have a two-layered structure consisting of an epithelial layer with underlying stroma. This stromal tissue is subdivided into a more superficial loose adenoid layer immediately under the epithelia and a deeper fibrous layer. Underlying the adenoid layer in both the limbal region and the proximal portions of the bulbar conjunctiva is the Tenon capsule, which itself merges into episcleral connective tissue. The Tenon capsule is a dense fibrous collagen sheath. When preparing blocks of tissue from this part of the eye, the tissue often separates at the plane of the capsule. Under the distal bulbar conjunctiva and, for the most part, under the rest of the palpebral conjunctiva, the loose adenoid tissue gives way to a deeper-lying fibrous layer that can be considered the conjunctival equivalent of the episclera.

Physiologic Functions of the Limbus and Conjunctiva

As discussed earlier, current thinking suggests that renewal of the corneal epithelium very much depends on a special population of cells, the stem cells, located deep in limbus (71,162,163). Stem cells are identified by specific biochemical markers and considered to be underdeveloped or primitive cell types genetically programmed for a long life. Their turnover rate (life cycle) is very slow. Providing they themselves are not damaged, stem cells are considered to have an unrestricted capability to produce identical daughter cells by mitosis that is either symmetric or asymmetric. Asymmetric division occurs when one daughter cell stays to provide replenishment to the stem cell pool (164,165). Stem cells have an unrestricted capacity for cell division. The daughter cells produced are known as *transient amplifying cells* (166) or *transitional cells* (167). These cells migrate into the cornea and upward through the corneal epithelial cell layers, divide a few times before they reach the corneal surface, and then desquamate. Although cell division (mitosis) is most commonly observed at the basal cell level, cells also may occasionally divide in the wing cell layers on their way to the corneal surface (168). It follows that the central cornea does not have resident stem cells.

Conjunctival tissue contains numerous sensory nerve endings. As with the cornea, various types of stimuli prompt reflex blinking to protect the ocular surface from trauma or damage. The conjunctiva is the most immunologically active tissue of the external eye (169,170). Even the normal conjunctival epithelium contains white blood cells (e.g., neutrophils and lymphocytes). Conjunctival allergic reactions are characterized by two gross structural changes (papillae and follicle formation), generalized vasodilation, and other aspects of the inflammatory response. Conjunctival papillae are areas of conjunctival hypertrophy, which contain mast cells and basophils, eosinophils, and neutrophils, and they are distinguished from follicles by the presence of blood vessels in their core. Papillae are most commonly found in the upper lid (everted for visualization) (171). Conjunctival follicles are similar to lymphoid follicles found elsewhere on the body: clear, fluid-filled pockets containing lymphocytes and macrophages. Blood vessels pass either above or below but not within them, and follicles can be found in both upper and lower conjunctival sacs. Eosinophils and basophils are not found in the normal conjunctival epithelium (169).

EMBRYOLOGY OF THE LIMBUS AND CONJUNCTIVA

The upper and lower eyelids are of ectodermal origin and fuse during the third month of pregnancy (172). Goblet cells first appear within the conjunctival epithelium about this time (173). Fusion of the eyelids serves to provide a barrier that seals the developing conjunctival sac from the amniotic fluid. It is believed that the period of eyelid fusion is important to protect both the corneal and conjunctival epithelium from trauma (173). The limbus is evident as a defined structure about one fourth of the way through gestation and is fully organized at about the sixth month (25).

MICROSCOPIC ANATOMY OF THE LIMBUS AND CONJUNCTIVA

Limbal Epithelium

At the limbus, where the conjunctival epithelium is continuous with the corneal epithelium, a local thickening occurs. The corneal epithelium (5–7 cell layers thick) shows signs of change at the location where the ALL of the cornea terminates (167). It is at this point that the basement membrane of the basal cells starts to become very irregular in profile (174) and has been described as serrated (25). Limbal epithelial cells at this location appear to be more compact than the corneal epithelial cells so that a slightly higher number of cell layers are evident (i.e., 6–9 layers) without noticeable thickening, and stratification of the cells is not so obvious. This is the *corneolimbal junction*. The immediately adjacent limbal epithelium is a stratified epithelium that may be 10 to 15 cell layers thick (25,167,175). The thickness of the limbal epithelium is not constant because of a unique feature, the palisades of Vogt (175).

In the slit lamp, these palisades are observed as fine, radial, whitish or gray lines, some 2 mm long and 0.1 to 1 mm apart (30,176). The same appearance can be seen in light microscopy at this location (175). The palisades may be substantially pigmented in some individuals. Although the limbal epithelial surface is smooth in this region, portions of the actual epithelium are thin (i.e., 6–9 cell layers thick) and other portions are thickened (i.e., 10–15 cell layers thick in an internal direction). Thicker and thinner portions are repeated at regular intervals to form the palisades, which result from the limbal epithelium following the contour of ridges on the loose adenoid layer (30,167). The thicker portions of the epithelium sometimes are referred to as *rete pegs* and serve to firmly anchor the limbal epithelium (25,31).

Stem cells, and their transient amplifying cells (also called *transitional cells*), are found in the basal layers of the most peripheral aspects of the corneal epithelium and within the limbal epithelium (167).

The ultrastructure of the limbal epithelial cells is not that different from corneal epithelium, except that the superficial cells are not as pronounced and the wing (intermediate) cells are more abundant. At the apical surface, it can be assumed that the cell-to-cell contacts are closed by zonula occludens similar to those in corneal epithelium (30,177). Limbal basal cells have slightly more prominent interdigitations compared to corneal epithelial basal cells, and their desmosomes are less numerous (25). A basement membrane, approximately 0.1 μm thick, is evident but is very irregular compared to the basement membrane of the corneal epithelium. Hemidesmosomes connect the basal cells to the basement membrane, and small arrays of anchoring filaments connect the basement membrane to the underlying loose connective tissue (25,30). As noted earlier, no ALL is found internal to the limbal epithelium.

The transition from corneal epithelium to limbal epithelium is evident in SEM for, at least in rabbits, a marked decrease in cell size occurs (Fig. 2.23). In the limbal region, the superficial epithelial cells have lighter and darker appearances, and the cell surfaces are predominantly decorated with microplicae. The limbal epithelium also is characterized by an almost complete lack of goblet cells (30).

Within the limbal epithelium, some lymphocytes and even some melanocytes can be found, especially between the deeper-lying cells (25,30).

Epithelium of the Bulbar Conjunctiva

As noted earlier, the limbal epithelium gives way to conjunctival epithelium at the sclerolimbal junction. As viewed in section with light microscopy or TEM, the bulbar conjunctiva right at the sclerolimbal junction may be six or more cell layers thick (177), but across the bulbar conjunctiva generally only two to four layers of stratified epithelial cells rest on an undulating basement membrane (Fig. 2.24) (25).

Apical surfaces of these cells are decorated with both microvilli and microplicae, and sparse tight junctions (zonula occludentes) are evident between the superficial cells

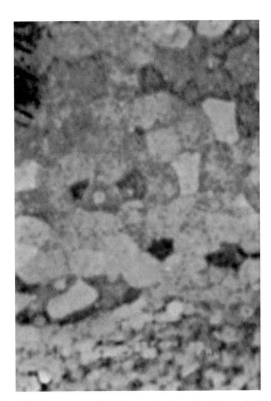

FIG. 2.23. Low-magnification scanning electron microscopic image of the transition zone in the rabbit between the peripheral corneal epithelium across the limbal epithelium to the bulbar conjunctiva. (From Doughty MJ, [63], with permission.)

(30). Although deeper-lying cells of the conjunctiva still make contact with each other, desmosomes are less common than between limbal or corneal epithelial cells. Part of the reason for fewer lesser cell-to-cell desmosomes between the bulbar conjunctival cells must be related to the large number of goblet cells (see later). The prominent spaces between the cells indicate a higher paracellular permeability for the conjunctival cell layers, at least based on measurements of drug permeation (178).

Viewed by SEM, the bulbar conjunctival surface can be seen to be made up of a layer of small polygonal cells that frequently are interrupted by orifices of goblet cells (Fig. 2.25) (179). Compared to the corneal epithelium, such SEM images clearly show the small size of these cells (compare Fig. 2.25 with Fig. 2.10). The average surface area for the bulbar conjunctival cells is approximately 125 μm^2, regardless of whether this value was obtained by SEM of rabbit material (e.g., Fig. 2.25) or from human conjunctival epithelial cells collected by impression cytology (180,181).

Goblet cells can be considered unicellular mucin-secreting glands (apocrine) within the conjunctival epithelium. Intact goblet cells are a normal feature of the conjunctival surface. They are interposed between superficial cells of both bulbar and palpebral conjunctiva and are present at relatively high density across both the bulbar and palpebral conjunctiva (44,182–184). The goblet cells are located be-

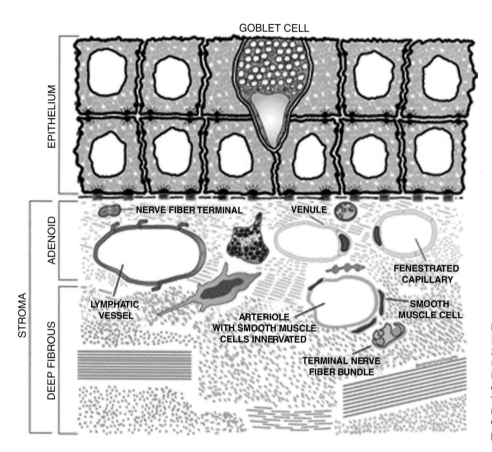

GOBLET CELL

EPITHELIUM

STROMA

ADENOID

DEEP FIBROUS

NERVE FIBER TERMINAL

VENULE

FENESTRATED
CAPILLARY

LYMPHATIC
VESSEL

ARTERIOLE
WITH SMOOTH MUSCLE
CELLS INNERVATED

SMOOTH
MUSCLE CELL

TERMINAL NERVE
FIBER BUNDLE

FIG. 2.24. Schematic diagram showing the overall structure and organization of the bulbar conjunctiva and underlying connective tissue. (From Bergmanson JPG. *Clinical ocular anatomy and physiology,* 11th ed. Houston, TX: Texas Eye Research and Technology Center, University of Houston College of Optometry, 2004, with permission.)

tween the cells of the bulbar conjunctiva (Fig. 2.26) (30, 41,177,184–186), although the "goblet" shape characteristic will very much depend on how the tissue was processed for microscopy (Fig. 2.26). Goblet cells are formed in the deeper epithelium and then migrate to the surface where they discharge their entire contents. Any stressful stimulus will likely result in goblet cell discharge (187), that is, the granulelike components that make up the goblet cell contents are released onto the ocular surface. This discharge, if substantial enough, can result in mucus strands being evident on the ocular surface. After the goblet cells expel their contents, TEM images suggest that a crater is left in the surface of the conjunctival epithelium, but this is an artifact. With discharge, the orifice changes and partly collapses. The stimuli that elicit goblet cell discharge can be allergic or toxic in origin, but the stimuli that result in this activity and the nature of the mucin "granules" remain to be characterized. Elevated secretion (hypersecretion) of goblet cells and epithelial mucin-producing cells may account for the mucoid characteristic of ocular inflammatory conditions.

The density of goblet cells in the bulbar conjunctiva is generally considered to be less than at the fornix or across the palpebral conjunctiva (30,183), but there is considerable diversity in estimates. For example, several estimates of gob-

let cell density across the bulbar conjunctiva in nominally healthy humans are 25 cells/mm^2 (188), 250 cells/mm^2 (189), 500 cells/mm^2 (41), and even close to 2000 cells/mm^2 (190). The method most commonly used to assess the presence of goblet cells is to stain an impression cytology sample with the periodic acid–Schiff stain so that the darkly staining round-to-ovoid goblets containing mucin can be visualized and counted. This impression cytology method relies on adherence of the goblet cell to the impression filter in a reproducible fashion. The marked differences in goblet cell density may simply reflect inconsistencies in this adherence (185). In addition, one must consider the way in which the goblet cells are counted, that is, whether one is trying to obtain an estimate of the total population of goblet cells or just the most superficial ones. In SEM (Fig. 2.25), obviously only those goblet cells within the most superficial cell layer of the conjunctiva will be observed. However, with impression cytology, those goblet cells in deeper-lying layers of the conjunctiva also will be visualized if, as so often appears to occur, multilayers of cells are removed onto the impression filter (i.e., the cell sample is not a monolayer) (189). If staining of whole-mount tissue is used to visualize goblet cells (183), then goblet cells at all depths of the conjunctival epithelial layer will be observed.

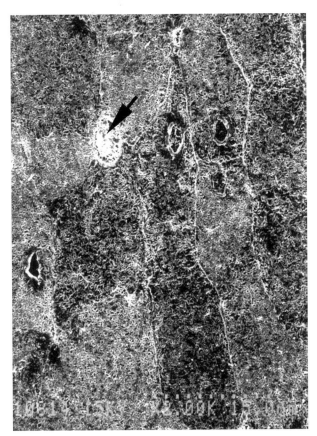

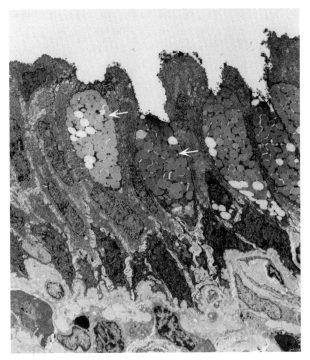

FIG. 2.26. Lower magnification transmission electron microscopic image of the palpebral conjunctiva of rabbit upper lid showing the presence of goblet cells *(arrows)*, which are elongated here. (Magnification 5,500×.) (From Doughty MJ, Bergmanson JPG, Optometry, 74: 485–500, with permission.)

FIG. 2.25. Lower-magnification scanning electron microscopic image of the rabbit bulbar conjunctiva. The mosaic of small polygonal cells is frequently punctuated by the round or oval orifices of the goblet cells *(arrow)*. (Magnification 3,000×.)

As noted earlier (corneal epithelium section), a mucin coat is present across the corneal and conjunctival surfaces; its origin is predominantly the goblet cells. The principal component of goblet cells mucin is the MUC5AC glycoprotein (191,192). In addition to goblet cells, there is some evidence that conjunctival epithelial cells also produce mucin because numerous small vesicles can be seen in the superficial conjunctival cells (193–195). It has been suggested that the conjunctival epithelial secretory contribution, a mucoprotein with long chemical chains, functions to anchor the goblet cell mucus to the epithelial cell surfaces.

There is one last aspect of the conjunctival epithelium that deserves more attention, not least because of the substantial confusion in the literature relating to it. This feature is the so-called crypts of Henle (30,31). The surface of the human bulbar conjunctiva usually is very smooth, but in some cases the bulbar conjunctiva and its underlying loose connective tissue can be irregular in that small undulations, wrinkles, or even microfolds are evident. During preparation of bulbar conjunctival tissue for tissue sections or SEM, it is extraordinarily difficult to prevent the tissue from being fixed with numerous wrinkles (Fig. 2.26). Notwithstanding, in some individuals, these folds are sufficiently prominent

to be observed with the slit lamp (196), especially highlighted by fluorescein. These have been referred to as *lid-parallel conjunctival folds* (LIPCOF) (196). It seems likely that infoldings of the conjunctival surface, seen across the bulbar or orbital conjunctival surface, are the same features referred to as the *crypts of Henle* or the *mucus gland of Henle* (30,197). Tissue sections of bulbar conjunctiva with conspicuous infoldings that are lined with goblet cells have been visualized by light microscopy (30). Such infoldings often are marked on schematic diagrams of the conjunctival epithelium (30,41). The confusion arises, in part, because an association has been made between such saccular invaginations of the bulbar (or palpebral) conjunctiva and the presence of other cryptlike openings seen in TEM of the palpebral conjunctiva (193,198). Thus, it has been stated that the crypts of Henle open onto the bulbar conjunctival surface with pores up to 60 μm in diameter (30) or very small pores in the conjunctiva labeled as Henle crypts (199). In our opinion, at least for normal adult rabbit bulbar conjunctiva (Doughty, unpublished data), no such "pores" exist, although infoldings containing goblet cells are commonplace (especially if the tissue is not stretched flat prior to fixation). In marked contrast, across the distal tarsal conjunctiva and proximal orbital conjunctiva, there are large numbers of such 60-μm-diameter pores that are thought to be the outlet not of the crypts of Henle but of the accessory lacrimal gland of Wolfring (44,195).

The epithelium of the bulbar conjunctiva is stratified but normally is nonsquamous, that is, it normally does not show the type of renewal pattern seen in the corneal epithelium and the cells do not normally desquamate. As just noted, these surface cells typically are small and, when viewed in coronal section, contain a nucleus that appears to fill most of the cell. In reality, the zone of cytoplasm around the nucleus occupies a similar area to the nucleus, that is, the nucleus-to-cytoplasmic fraction is close to 0.5 (or the nucleus-to-cytoplasmic ratio is around 1:1) (180). Under chronic stress, including that associated with immune reactions or exposure to toxic chemicals, however, nonsquamous cells of the bulbar conjunctiva can undergo a transformation to squamous-type cells (200). This new state of squamous metaplasia results in cell enlargement and decrease in the nucleus-to-cytoplasm ratio, or an increase in the cytoplasm-to-nucleus ratio (180). It has yet to be established if the nature of the cell-to-cell junctions changes as a result of the metaplasia. However, it is well established that the acute or chronic use of a range of pharmaceuticals can result in this cell transformation (180) and that this likely occurs concurrently with other changes to the ocular surface and eyelid margins. Part of the reason for the cell transformation likely is the result of reduction in the quantity or integrity of the mucus coating. There are two reasons for this. First, squamous metaplasia of the bulbar conjunctiva likely is associated with a reduction in mucus-secreting goblet cells (199). Second, ocular surface staining with rose bengal can be related to reduced goblet cell density (201).

Some migratory Langerhans cells also are found in the bulbar conjunctival cell layer (30).

Adenoid Layer of the Conjunctiva

The adenoid layer under the limbal and bulbar epithelia is a loose fibrous structure containing a number of melanocytes. A rich network of capillaries is found in this layer; some of them are nonfenestrated and others are fenestrated (25,30,31). As viewed in TEM at very high magnification, the fenestrations are locations in the endothelial lining of the blood vessels that are substantially attenuated and only the two membranes are evident (25). The same general features can be found under the palpebral conjunctiva (184).

Mast cells normally are found in the adenoid layer of the conjunctival stroma, just below the interface with the epithelium (78,201). The cytoplasm of mast cells are filled by numerous metachromatic round-to-oval shaped granules that can stain reddish purplish with the appropriate dyes and appear electron dense in TEM (78). As viewed by high-magnification TEM, all mast cells contain numerous granules that can have slightly different ultrastructural features (25,78,174,186) but are distinctly different from the ultrastructure of granules found in goblet cells, melanocytes, or various types of white blood cells. The mast cell granules contain both vasodilation-inducing substances (e.g., histamine) and other mediators of the inflammatory responses (prostaglandins, interleukins, and enzymes such as chymase and tryptase) (170,202,203).

Mast cells are numerous in the conjunctival stroma, but their presence, *per se,* does not mean that inflammation is present. In quiescent noninflamed normal tissue, these mast cells have certain characteristics and are referred to as *connective tissue-type mast cells.* Some mast cells, usually referred to as the *migratory mucosal phenotype,* can migrate toward the tissue surface when allergens are present (170,202–204). The mucosal-type mast cells presumably are activated in some way as a result of the presence of allergens. If the mast cell system is fully activated, their granules are released into the surrounding tissue and onto the ocular surface.

Deep Fibrous Layer of the Conjunctiva

The deep fibrous layer contains numerous small and large blood vessels and nerves (25,30,78,167). The layer is structurally organized into dense bundles of collagen fibers, as opposed to lamellae that are found in the cornea. In the sclerocorneal region, the diameters of the collagen fibrils in the most superficial bundles have been considered similar to those in the cornea (25), but deeper bundles contain ever increasing numbers of larger diameter fibrils (93).

A special case can be made for the deep fibrous layer underlying the tarsal conjunctiva. The collagen bundles under the tarsal portion of the palpebral conjunctiva, and which surround the main tarsal gland (the meibomian gland), are very densely packed to form a fibrous sheath. This is more developed in the upper than lower eyelid, and its development allows for eversion of the upper eyelid during clinical examination.

Conjunctival Nerves and Nerve Endings

The nerve supply to the limbus and conjunctiva is complex because it serves to support sensory and secretory functions as well as the vasculature.

Conjunctival sensory nerve branches and the nerve terminals are widely distributed within both epithelial layers and stroma. Epithelial and stromal distributions have sensory origin from both the ophthalmic and maxillary divisions of the trigeminal nerve. The ophthalmic division of the trigeminal nerve provides branches to the infratrochlear, supratrochlear, supraorbital, and lacrimal nerves. The maxillary division of the trigeminal nerve links to the infraorbital nerve. Neural distribution to the vasculature is dually autonomic, with a sympathetic supply from the superior cervical ganglion and a parasympathetic supply from the pterygopalatine ganglion (30).

Limbal and bulbar conjunctiva has complex sensory nerve endings called *corpuscles* (30,176). The corpuscular nerve endings are described as round or oval encapsulated structures served mostly by a single myelinated nerve fiber derived from nerve fiber bundles deeper in the conjunctiva or even within the episclera. The corpuscular nerve endings are most numerous in the limbal conjunctiva and are located immediately under the epithelium, often among the ridges of the palisade region (176).

In contrast (in very general terms), it can be stated that a large number of the conjunctival capillaries receive both sympathetic and parasympathetic innervation, which may help explain the remarkable local control of blood flow often seen in the irritated or inflamed eye.

Nerve ending corpuscles in the conjunctiva have a sensory role similar to that of nerves in the cornea (205). The touch sensitivity of the limbal conjunctiva is slightly less than that of the peripheral cornea, being about half that of the central cornea. Sensitivity to touch is slightly less across the exposed portion of the temporal bulbar conjunctiva and substantially less (by a factor of 100) both close to the plica and under the upper eyelid (157). As with corneal sensitivity, conjunctival sensitivity declines with age (161).

Recent research indicates that the relative sensitivity and the sensations to chemical and thermal stimulation experienced by the human conjunctiva are distinctly different from the cornea (205), with the stimuli to the conjunctiva being less irritating than to the cornea.

VASCULAR AND LYMPHATIC SYSTEM IN THE VICINITY OF THE LIMBUS AND BULBAR CONJUNCTIVA

Arterial Supply

Arterial supply has two principal sources, namely, the anterior ciliary arteries, which supply the bulbar region, and the palpebral branches of the dorsonasal and lacrimal arteries, which supply the palpebral region (25,30,31).

Venous Drainage

Conjunctival veins, which are more numerous than arteries, drain into the palpebral veins and superior and inferior ophthalmic veins. Three principal venous drainage routes exist. The anterior ciliary veins receive branches from the conjunctiva, the inferior ophthalmic vein receives tributaries from the conjunctiva, and the superior and posttarsal venous plexus receives contributions from both tarsal and bulbar vessels.

The blood vessels found in large numbers underlying the conjunctival epithelium, within the parenchyma, react to exposure to vasodilators such as histamine and prostaglandins (206). One result of these changes is the well-known dilation of the more superficial blood vessels. However, largely hidden from view is a complex process involving recruitment of white blood cells toward the site wherever an allergen is initially presented or encountered. Blood vessels dilate and the conjunctival appearance changes from a quiet "white" state to characteristic hyperemia and injection. A

not uncommon feature of even a quiet conjunctiva is the presence of some white blood cells. These often irregularly shaped cells can be found within both the conjunctival epithelial cell layer and the conjunctival parenchyma underlying the palpebral conjunctiva, where these cells will be very close to the superficial vasculature. These white blood cells largely originate from the blood vessels that routinely contain circulating white blood cells, principally eosinophils and granulocytes (170,207). As with the mast cells, these inflammatory cells contain secretory granules so that, in response to stimulation, a similar repertoire of inflammatory mediators are released into both the blood vessels and surrounding tissue. During chronic inflammation, specific types of T lymphocytes, with distinct immunocytochemical properties, emigrate out of the blood vessels and end up within the connective tissue of the conjunctiva (208,209). If the white blood cells are allowed to migrate into the conjunctival parenchyma for extended periods of time (weeks to months), some may form distinct dense aggregates. If these aggregates form in the vicinity of the limbus and palisades, they are referred to as *Herbert pits;* if they form underneath the bulbar or palpebral conjunctiva, they generally are known as *follicules* (30).

The blood vessels are supplied by nerves and display distinct pharmacologic characteristics, basically α_1-adrenoceptor for vasoconstriction and muscarinic cholinergic receptors for vasodilation. Substance P also is an effective vasodilator.

Lymphatic System of the Limbus and Conjunctiva

The lymphatic system is an essential element of all tissues supplied with blood and provides the natural mechanism by which the fluid balance within the tissues is maintained. This is especially important for the conjunctival tissues.

Overall, compared to our knowledge of the epithelial cells of the cornea and conjunctiva, the lymphatics of the limbus and conjunctiva are a poorly characterized system. They can be seen in tissue sections viewed by light microscopy, often partly collapsed, as vessels without any obvious contents and located immediately underneath the conjunctiva (30). They form a complex network of lymph-filled vessels or "channels" that are located both within the loose adenoid layer and, to a lesser extent, in the deeper fibrous layer (25,78,210,211), that is, there are both superficial and deeper-lying vessels. According to some researchers, these vessels form a distinct ring under limbus, sometimes referred to as the *circulus lymphaticus* or even the *lymphatic circle of Teichman* (210,211). The lymphatic vessels often follow the route of the blood vessels, principally the venous capillaries (25). This is especially true near the limbus where superficial lymph vessels are located between the palisades of Vogt, just as other capillaries often are, to reach the extreme periphery of the cornea (30,212). When neovascularization of the cornea develops, lymphatic vessels may extend into the cornea (213).

The lymphatic vessels are not well characterized from an ultrastructural perspective, probably because they collapse so readily postmortem. At the resolution available in light microscopy, it is possible to discern which vessels (capillaries) contain blood and which contain lymph. Vessels with very attenuated endothelia and no cells within the lumen are likely to be lymph vessels (30), but it is really only possible to identify these vessels in high-magnification TEM. A number of major ultrastructural features of the lymphatic vessels distinguish them from other capillaries: the nature of the contact between neighboring endothelial cells, the lack of an obvious or continuous basement membrane associated with the endothelial cells, and the lack of supportive structures (fibrocytes, pericytes, collagen) (25, 213–215). Cell-to-cell contacts are more in the form of overlap, without obvious cell-to-cell junctional complexes (78,186,213). In addition, there are special bundles of collagen fibrils that appear to anchor the lymph vessels to surrounding loose tissue (25).

There are no lymphatic nodes within the globe itself, that is, the lymphatic vessels only contact the globe at the limbus where fine branches follow the pattern of the limbal loop blood vessels, and there do not appear to be any lymphatic nodes within the globe itself. The deep plexus usually contains the larger vessels. The flow of lymph is generally in a temporal direction toward the lateral extremes of the lid, eventually connecting with the parotid node. There is also a medial route leading to the submandibular lymph nodes. Two principal lymphatic drainage sources are the superficial plexus, which drains the adenoid layer that drains into the parotid node, and the deep plexus, which drains the deep fibrous layer into the submandibular node.

In response to allergens, or mixtures of histamine and prostaglandins (206), the bulbar conjunctiva can become grossly dilated, resulting in the puffy (swollen) character of the bulbar and palpebral conjunctiva associated with an allergic reaction. The exact cause of this marked swelling reaction is unknown, but it presumably is a combination of the dilation of blood and lymphatic vessels and an increase in the interstitial fluid of the adenoid layer. This fluid must come from the blood vessels and eventually should drain back into the lymphatic system. The marked nature of an acute-onset chemosis that can develop in an allergic reaction may be related to the nature of the lymphatic drainage, which is more substantial at superotemporal sites compared to inferior sites (211). As a result, the interior aspect of the adenoid layer can become grossly distended. Such an effect might be the result of an abrupt change in the patency of the lymph drainage. The exact location of any valves within the conjunctival vessels that may influence the flow has yet to be established.

It should be noted that a slightly different effect of tissue edema may occur across the palpebral conjunctiva and involve the adenoid layer. Here, a generalized edema can develop that often leads to formation of discrete arrays forming rather than general distention of the tissue. Why these arrays form is not known, but they are generally referred to as *papillae*. These features reflect a combination of tissue edema, the presence of some aggregates of white blood cells, and the development of scar tissue within the papillae. They can be seen to form distinctive arrays when the surface is viewed by biomicroscopy, especially with fluorescein present. The size of these fluorescein-highlighted features is normally on the order of 0.025 mm^2 but can attain sizes in excess of 1 mm^2 in chronic conditions (171). Although the development of these arrays can be associated with an allergic reaction (and a follicular-papillary reaction is possible), there also seems to be an extramechanical component involved, such as rubbing of the palpebral surface against the cornea (or a contact lens surface, or suture).

ACKNOWLEDGMENT

The authors appreciate the skilled technical support of Ms. Margaret Gondo in the preparation of tissue and micrographs.

REFERENCES

1. Wilmer HA, Scammon RE: Growth of the components of the human eyeball. I. Diagrams, calculations, computation, and reference tables. *Arch Ophthalmol* 1950;43:599–637.
2. Olsen TW, Aaberg SY, Geroski DH, et al. Human sclera: thickness and surface area. *Am J Ophthalmol* 1998;125:237–241.
3. Stysznski A, Bruska M, Wozniak W. Morphometric study of the cornea in human embryos. *Folia Morphol (Warsz)* 2001;60: 57–59.
4. Ehlers N. Morphology and histochemistry of the corneal epithelium of mammals. *Acta Anat* 1970;75:161–198.
5. Calmettes L, Deodati F, Planel H, et al. Étude histologique et histochimique de L'épithélium antérieur de la cornée et de ses basales. *Arch d' Ophtalmol (Paris)* 1956;16:481–506.
6. Mishima S. Corneal thickness. *Surv Ophthalmol* 1968;13: 57–96.
7. Doughty MJ, Zaman ML. Human corneal thickness and its impact on intraocular pressure measures: a review and meta-analysis approach. *Surv Ophthalmol* 2000;44:367–408.
8. Li HF, Petroll WP, Møller-Pedersen T, et al. Epithelial and corneal thickness measurements by in vivo confocal microscopy through focusing (CMTF). *Curr Eye Res* 1997;16:214–221.
9. Bourne WM, McCarey BE, Kaufman HE. Clinical specular microscopy. *Trans Am Acad Ophthalmol Otolaryngol* 1976;81: OP743–OP753.
10. Binkhorst CD, Loones LH, Nygaard P. The clinical specular microscope. *Doc Ophthalmol* 1977;44:57–75.
11. Bigar F. Specular microscopy of the corneal endothelium. *Dev Ophthalmol* 1982;6:1–94.
12. Cotinat J. Microscopie spéculaire de l'endothélium cornéen. *J Fr Ophtalmol* 1999;22:255–261.
13. Cavanagh HD, Petroll WM, Jester JV. Confocal microscopy: uses in measurement of cellular structure and function. *Prog Retinal Eye Res* 1995;14:527–565.

14. Hollingsworth J, Perez-Gomez I, Mutalib HA, et al. A population study of the normal cornea using an in vivo, slit-scanning confocal microscope. *Optom Vis Sci* 2001;78:706–711.
15. Lattimore MR, Kaupp S, Schallhorn S, et al. Orbscan pachymetry. Implications of a repeated measures and diurnal variation analysis. *Ophthalmology* 1999;106:977–981.
16. Yanoff M, Zimmerman LE, Fine BS. Glutaraldehyde fixation of whole eyes. *Am J Clin Pathol* 1965;44:167–171.
17. Ko M-Y, Park WK, Lee JH, et al. A histomorphometric study of corneal endothelial cells in normal human fetuses. *Exp Eye Res* 2001;72:403–409.
18. Doughty MJ. Correcting cell density measures for tissue hydration changes in scanning electron microscopy: application to the rabbit corneal epithelium. *Tissue Cell* 1995;27:207–220.
19. Geroski DH, Edelhauser HF. Morphometric analysis of the corneal endothelium Specular microscopy vs. alizarin red staining. *Invest Ophthalmol Vis Sci* 1989;30:254–259.
20. Doughty MJ, Bergmanson JPG, Blocker Y. Shrinkage and distortion of the rabbit corneal endothelial cell mosaic caused by a high osmolarity glutaraldehyde-formaldehyde fixative compared to glutaraldehyde. *Tissue Cell* 1997;29:533–547.
21. Yanoff M. Formaldehyde-glutaraldehyde fixation. *Am J Ophthalmol* 1973;76:303–304.
22. Doughty MJ. A morphometric analysis of the surface cells of rabbit corneal epithelium by scanning electron microscopy. *Am J Anat* 1990;189:316–328.
23. Doughty MJ. Scanning electron microscopy study of cell dimensions of rabbit corneal epithelium surface. *Cornea* 1991;10:149–155.
24. Fullwood NJ, Meek KM. A synchrotron X-ray study of the changes occurring in the corneal stroma during processing for electron microscopy. *J Microsc* 1993;169:53–60.
25. Hogan MJ, Alvarado JA, Weddell JE. *Histology of the human eye.* Philadelphia: WB Saunders, 1971.
26. Bergmanson JPG. *Clinical ocular anatomy and physiology,* 11th ed. Houston, TX: Texas Eye Research and Technology Center, 2004.
27. Maurice DM. Cornea and sclera. In: Davson D, ed. *The eye, vol. 1B,* 3rd ed. London: Academic Press, 1984:1–158.
28. Watsky MA, Jablonski MM, Edelhauser HF. Comparison of conjunctival and corneal surface areas in rabbit and human. *Curr Eye Res* 1988;7:483–486.
29. Martin DK, Holden BA. A new method for measuring the diameter of the in vivo human cornea. *Am J Optom Physiol Opt* 1982;59:436–441.
30. Ruskell GL. The conjunctiva. In: Bennett ES, Weissman BA, eds. *Clinical contact lens practice.* Philadelphia: JB Lippincott, 1991:3-1–3-18.
31. Bron AJ, Tripathi FC, Tripathi BJ. Development of the human eye. In: *Wolff's anatomy of the eye & orbit,* 8th ed. London: Chapman & Hall, 1997:620–664.
32. Müller A, Doughty MJ. Assessments of corneal endothelial cell density in growing children, and its relationship to horizontal corneal diameter. *Optom Vis Sci* 2002;79:762–770.
33. Duke-Elder S, Wybar KC. *Cornea. System of ophthalmology, vol. 2: the anatomy of the visual system.* Henry Kimpton, 1961:95–131.
34. Ando K, Kripke DF. Light attenuation by the human eyelid. *Biol Psychiatry* 1996;39:22–25.
35. Beems EM, Van Best JA. Light transmission of the cornea in whole human eyes. *Exp Eye Res* 2000;50:393–395.
36. Ventura L, Sousa SJF, Messias AMV, et al. System for measuring the transmission spectrum of "in vitro" corneas. *Physiol Meas* 2000;21:197–207.
37. Patel S, Marshall J, Fitzke FW. Refractive index of the human corneal epithelium and stroma. *J Refract Surg* 1995;11:100–105.
38. Leonard DW, Meek KM. Refractive indices of the collagen fibrils and the extracellular material of the corneal stroma. *Biophys J* 1997;72:1382–1387.
39. Von Reuss A. Untersuchungen ueber den Einfluss der Lebenssalers auf die Kruemmung der Hornhaut nebst einigen Bemerkungen ueber die Dimensionen der Lidspalte. *Albrecht v Graefes Arch Ophthalmol* 1881l27:27–53.
40. Wichterle K, Vodaňsk J, Wichterle O. Shape of the cornea and conjunctiva. *Optom Vis Sci* 1991;68:232–235.
41. Rohen JW, Lütjen-Drecoll E. Functional morphology of the conjunctiva. In: Lemp MA, Marquardt R, eds. *The dry eye.* Berlin: Springer-Verlag, 1992:38–63.
42. Gipson IK, Inatomi T. Mucin genes expressed by the ocular surface epithelium. *Prog Retinal Eye Res* 1997;16:81–98.
43. Feenstra, Tseng. What is actually stained by rose bengal? *Arch Ophthalmol* 1992;110:984–993.
44. Doughty MJ. Scanning electron microscopy study of the tabal and orbital conjunctual surfaces compared to peripheral corneal epithelium in pigmented ral. *Doc Ofuthalmologing* 1997;13:345–371.
45. Nichols BA, Chiappino ML, Dawson CR. Demonstration of the mucus layer of the tear film by electron microscopy. *Invest Ophthalmol Vis Sci* 1985;26:464–473.
46. Doughty MJ. Impact of brief exposure to balanced salts solution or cetylpyridinium chloride on the surface appearance of the rabbit corneal epithelium: a scanning electron microscopy study. *Curr Eye Res* 2003;26:335–346.
47. Doughty MJ, Aakre BM, Patel S. Hydration (water binding) of the mammalian corneal stroma ex vivo and vitro: sample mass and error considerations. *Optom Vis Sci* 1996;73:666–675.
48. Panjwani N. In: Harding JJ, ed. *Cornea and sclera.* London: Chapman & Hall, 1997:15–51.
49. Quantock AJ, Meek KM, Brittain P, et al. Alteration of the stromal architecture and depletion of keratin sulphate proteoglycans in oedematous human cornea: histological immunochemical and x-ray diffraction evidence. *Tissue Cell* 1991;23:593–606.
50. Soriano ES, Campos MSQ, Michelacci YM. Effect of epithelial debridement on the glycosaminoglycan synthesis by human corneal explants. *Clin Chim Acta* 2000;295:41–62.
51. Doughty MJ. Changes in hydration, protein, and proteoglycan composition of the collagen-keratocyte matrix of the bovine corneal stroma ex vivo in a bicarbonate-mixed salts solution, compared to other solutions. *Biochim Biophys Acta* 2001;1525:97–107.
52. Scott JE, Bosworth TR. A comparative biochemical and ultrastructural study of proteoglycan-collagen interactions in corneal stroma. *Biochem J* 1990;270:491–497.
53. Marshall J, Grindle FJ. Fine structure of the cornea and its development. *Trans Ophthalmol Soc UK* 1978;98:320–328.
54. Ozanics V, Rayborn M, Sagun D. Observations on the morphology of the developing primate cornea: epithelium, its innervation and anterior stroma. *J Morphol* 1977;153:263–298.
55. Cook CS, Ozanics V, Jakobiec FA. Prenatal development of the eye and its adnexa. *Biomed Found Ophthalmol* 1999;2000:1–48.
56. Bahn CF, Falls HF, Varley GA, et al. Classification of corneal disorders based on neural crest origin. *Ophthalmology* 1984;91:558–563.
57. Hayashi K, Sueishi K, Tanaka K, et al. Immunohistochemical evidence of the origin of human corneal endothelial cells and keratocytes. *Graefes Arch Clin Exp Ophthalmol* 1986;224:452–466.
58. Ko M-K, Kim J-G, Chi JG. Cell density of the corneal endothe-

lium in human fetus by flat preparation. *Cornea* 2000;19: 80–83.

59. Styszynski A, Bruska M, Wozniak W. Morphometric study of the cornea in human embryos. *Folia Morphol (Warsz)* 2001;60: 57–59.

60. Doughty MJ, Laiquzzaman M, Müller A, et al. Central corneal thickness in European (white) individuals, especially children and the elderly, and assessment of its possible importance in clinical measures of intra-ocular pressure. *Ophthal Physiol Optics* 2002;22:491–504

61. Klyce SD, Beuerman RW. Structure and function of the cornea. In: Kaufman HE, et al., eds. *The cornea.* New York: Churchill Livingstone, 1988:3–54.

62. Doughty MJ. On the evaluation of the corneal epithelial surface by scanning electron microscopy. *Optom Vis Sci* 1990;67: 735–756.

63. Doughty MJ. Re-wetting, comfort, lubricant and moisturizing solutions for the contact lens wearer. *Contact Lens Anterior Eye* 1999;22:116–126.

64. Hanna C, O'Brien JE. Cell production and migration in the epithelial layer of the cornea. *Arch Ophthalmol* 1960;64:536.

65. Thoft RA, Friend J. The X, Y, Z hypothesis of corneal epithelial maintenance. *Invest Ophthalmol Vis Sci* 1983;24:1442–1443.

66. Ladage PM, Yamamoto K, Ren DH, et al. Proliferation rate of rabbit corneal epithelium in overnight contact lens wear. *Invest Ophthalmol Vis Sci* 2001;42:2804–2812.

67. Doughty MJ, Fong WK. Topographical differences in cell area at the surface of the corneal epithelium of the pigmented rabbit. *Curr Eye Res* 1992;11:1129–1136.

68. Hazlett LD, Wells P, Spann B, et al. Epithelial desquamation in the adult mouse cornea. A correlative TEM-SEM study. *Ophthal Res* 19809;12:315–323.

69. Doughty MJ. Evidence for heterogeneity in a small squamous cell type (light cells) in the rabbit corneal epithelium: a scanning electron microscope study. *Doc Ophthalmol* 1996;92:117–136.

70. Ren H, Wilson G. Apoptosis in the corneal epithelium. *Invest Ophthalmol Vis Sci* 1996;37:1017–1025.

71. Ladage PM, Yamamoto K, Li L, et al. Corneal epithelial homeostasis following daily and overnight contact lens wear. *Contact Lens Anterior Eye* 2002;25:11–21.

72. Bergmanson JPG, Chu LWF. Contact lens induced corneal epithelial injury. *Am J Optom Physiol Opt* 1982;59:500–506.

73. Sugrue SP, Zieske JD. Z01 in corneal epithelium: association to the zonula occludens and adherens junctions. *Exp Eye Res* 1997;64:11–20.

74. Krutsinger BD, Bergmanson JPG. Corneal epithelial response to hypotonic exposure. *Int Eye Care* 1985;1:440–443.

75. Gillette TE, Chandler JW, Greiner JV. Langerhans cells. A review of their nature with emphasis on their immunologic function. *Ophthalmology* 1982;89:700.

76. Hazlett LD, McClellan SM, Hume EB, et al. Extended wear contact lens usage induces Langerhans cell migration into cornea. *Exp Eye Res* 1999;69:575–577.

77. Hill JC, Sarvan J, Maske R, et al. Evidence that UV-B irradiation decreases corneal Langerhans cells and improves corneal graft survival in the rabbit. *Transplantation* 1994;57: 1281–1284.

78. Iwamoto T, Smelser GK. Electron microscopic studies on the mast cells and blood and lymphatic capillaries of the human corneal limbus. *Invest Ophthalmol* 1965;4:815–834.

79. Kaji Y, Obata H, Usui T, et al. Three-dimensional organization of collagen fibrils during corneal stromal wound healing after excimer laser keratectomy. *J Cataract Refract Surg* 1998;24: 1441–1446.

80. Kayes J, Holmberg A. The fine structure of Bowman's layer

and the basement membrane of the corneal epithelium. *Am J Ophthalmol* 1960;50[Pt 2]:1013–1021.

81. Gallagher B, Maurice D. Striations of light scattering in the corneal stroma. *J Ultrastruct Res* 1977;61:100–114.

82. Kamai Y, Ushiki T. The three-dimensional organization of collagen fibrils in the human cornea and sclera. *Invest Ophthalmol Vis Sci* 1991;32:2244–2258.

83. Radner W, Zehetmayer M, Mallinger R, et al. Zur dreidimensionalen Anordnung der kollagenen Lamellen im posterioren Stroma der menschlichen Hornhaut. *Spektrum Augenheilkd* 1993;7:77–80.

84. Radner W, Zehetmayer M, Aufreiter R, et al. Interlacing and cross-angle distribution of collagen lamellae in the human cornea. *Cornea* 1998;17:537–543.

85. Krauss R. Der konstruktive Bau der Cornea. *Z Mikrosk* 1937; 53:420–434.

86. Kokott W. Uber mechanisch-functionelle Strukturen des Auges. *Albrecht v Graefes Arch Ophthalmol* 1938;138:424–485.

87. Polack FM. Morphology of the cornea. I. Study with silver stains. *Am J Ophthalmol* 1961;51:1051–1056.

88. Christens-Barry WA, Green W, Conolly PJ, et al. Spatial mapping of polarized light transmission in the central rabbit cornea. *Exp Eye Res* 1996;62:651–662.

89. Daxter A, Fratzl P. Collagen fibril orientation in the human corneal stroma and its implications in keratoconus. *Invest Ophthalmol Vis Sci* 1997;38:121–129.

90. McTigue JW. The human cornea: a light and electron microscopic study of the normal cornea and its alterations in various dystrophies. *Trans Am Ophthalmol Soc* 1967;65:591–660.

91. Müller LJ, Pels E, Vrensen GFJM. The specific architecture of the anterior stroma accounts for maintenance of corneal curvature. *Br J Ophthalmol* 2001;85:437–443.

92. Newton RH, Meek KM. The integration of the corneal and limbal fibrils in the human eye. *Biophys J* 1998;75:2508–2512.

93. Doughty MJ, Bergmanson JPG. A further assessment of the collagen fibril characteristics at the corneo-scleral boundary and their role in determination of the swelling characteristics of the rabbit corneal stroma ex vivo. *Clin Exptl Optom* (in press).

94. Schwartz W, Keyserlingk DG. Uber die Feinstruktur der menschlichen Cornea, mit besonderer berucksichtigung des problems der transparenz. *Z Zellforsch* 1966;73:540–548.

95. Hamada R, Giraud J-P, Graf B, et al. Etude analytique et statistique des lamellas, des keratocytes, des fibrilles de collagene de la region centrale de la cornée humaine normale (microscopique optique et electronique). *Arch Ophtalmol (Paris)* 1972;32: 536–570.

96. Takahashi A, Nakayasu K, Okisaka S, et al. Quantitative analysis of collagen fiber in keratoconus [in Japanese]. *Acta Soc Ophthalmol Jpn* 1990;94:1068–1073.

97. Hart RW, Farrell RA, Langham MEL. Theory of corneal structure. *APL Digest* 1969;Jan-Feb:1–11.

98. Gallager B, Maurice D. Striations of light scattering in the corneal stroma. *J Ultrastruct Res* 1977;61:100–114.

99. Doughty MJ, Seabert W, Bergmanson JPG, et al. A descriptive and quantitative study of the keratocytes of the corneal stroma of albino rabbits using transmission electron microscopy. *Tissue Cell* 2001;33:408–422.

100. Cogan DG. Applied anatomy and physiology of the cornea. *Trans Am Acad Ophthalmol Otolaryngol* 1951;55:329–359.

101. Kanai A, Kaufman HE. Electron microscope studies of swollen corneal stroma. *Ann Ophthalmol (Chic)* 1973;5:178–190.

102. Sayers Z, Koch MH, Whitburn SB, et al. Synchrotron X-ray diffraction study of corneal stroma. *J Mol Biol* 1982;160: 593–607.

103. Kanai A, Kaufman HE. Electron microscopic studies of corneal

stroma: aging changes of collagen fibers. *Ann Ophthalmol (Chic)* 1973;5:285–292.

104. Malik NS, Moss SJ, Ahmed N, et al. Ageing of the human corneal stroma: structural and biochemical changes. *Biochim Biophys Acta* 1992;1138:222–228.

105. Meek KM, Elliott GF, Nave C. A synchrotron X-ray diffraction study of bovine cornea stained with Cupromeronic Blue. *Collagen Res Rel* 1986;6:203–218.

106. Hirsh M, Prenant G, Renard G. Three-dimensional supramolecular organization of the extracellular matrix in human and rabbit corneal stroma, as revealed by ultrarapid-freezing and deep-etching methods. *Exp Eye Res* 2001;72:123–135.

107. Maurice DM. The structure and transparency of the cornea. *J Physiol* 1957;136:263–286.

108. Smith JW. The transparency of the corneal stroma. *Vision Res* 1969;9:393–396.

109. Benedek GB. Theory of transparency of the eye. *Appl Optics* 1971;10:459–473.

110. Vaezey S, Clark JI. A quantitative analysis of transparency in the human sclera and cornea using Fourier methods. *J Microsc* 1991;163:85–94.

111. Farrell RA, Hart RW. On the theory of the spatial organization of macromolecules in connective tissue. *Bull Math Biophys* 1969; 31:727–760.

112. Snyder MC, Bergmanson JPG, Doughty MJ. Keratocytes: no more quiet cells. *J Am Optom Assoc* 1998;69:180–187.

113. Clarèus F. *Hornhinnans, Histologi.* Thesis, Uppsala University Medical School, E. Westrell, Stockholm, 1857.

114. Jester JV, Barry PA, Lind GJ, et al. Corneal keratocytes: in situ and in vitro organization of cytoskeletal contractile proteins. *Invest Ophthalmol Vis Sci* 1994;35:730–743.

115. Poole CA, Brookes N, Clover GM. Keratocyte networks visualized in the living cornea using vital dyes. *J Cell Sci* 1993;106: 685–692.

116. Watsky MA. Keratocyte gap junctional communication in normal and wounded rabbit corneas and human corneas. *Invest Ophthalmol Vis Sci* 1995;36:2568–2576.

117. Ueda A, Nishida T, Otori T, et al. Electron microscopic studies on the presence of gap junctions between corneal fibroblasts in rabbits. *Cell Tissue Res* 1987;249:473–475.

118. Müller LJ, Pels L, Vrensen GFJM. Novel aspects of the ultrastructural organization of human corneal keratocytes. *Invest Ophthalmol Vis Sci* 1995;36:2557–2567.

119. Fini ME. Keratocyte and fibroblast phenotypes in the repairing cornea. *Prog Retinal Eye Res* 1999;18:529–551.

120. Hahnel C, Somodi S, Weiss DG, et al. The keratocyte network of human cornea: a three-dimensional study using confocal laser scanning fluorescence microscopy. *Cornea* 2000;19:185–193.

121. Petroll WM, Boettcher K, Barry P, et al. Quantitative assessment of anteroposterior keratocyte density in the normal rabbit cornea. *Cornea* 1995;14:3–9.

122. Patel SV, McLaren JW, Hodge DO, et al. Normal human keratocyte density and corneal thickness measurement using confocal microscopy in vivo. *Invest Ophthalmol Vis Sci* 2001;42: 333–339.

123. Petroll WM, Cavanagh HD, Barry P, et al. Quantitative analysis of stress fiber orientation during corneal wound contraction. *J Cell Sci* 1993;104:353–363.

124. Tomasek JJ, Hay ED, Fujiwara K. Collagen modulates cell shape and cytoskeleton of embryonic corneal and fibroma fibroblasts: distribution of actin, α-actinin and myosin. *Dev Biol* 1982;92:107–122.

125. Roy P, Petroll WM, Cavanagh HD, Chuong CJ, et al. An in vitro force measurement assay to study the early mechanical interaction between corneal fibroblasts and collagen matrix. *Exp Cell Res* 1997;232:106–117.

126. Kuwabara T. Current concepts in anatomy and histology of the cornea. *Contact Intraocul Lens Med* J 1978;4:101–132.

127. Leuenberger PM. Morphologie functionnelle de la cornée. *Adv Ophthalmol* 1978;35:94–166.

128. Johnson DH, Bourne WM, Campbell RJ. The ultrastructure of Descemet's membrane: I. Changes with age in normal corneas. *Arch Ophthalmol* 1982;100:1942–1947.

129. Thiele H, Flasch R, Joraschky W. Histolyse der Cornea. Descemet-Membran. *Albrecht v Graefes Arch Klin Exp Ophthalmol* 1969;179:157–174.

130. Yue B, Maurice D. The mechanical properties of the rabbit and human cornea. *J Biomech* 1986;19:847–853.

131. Altman PA, Hoeltzel DA. Comments on "the mechanical properties of the rabbit and human cornea." *J Biomech* 1991;24: 869–872.

132. Bergmanson JPG, Sheldon TM, Goosey JD. Fuch's endothelial dystrophy: a fresh look at an aging disease. *Ophthal Physiol Opt* 1999;19:210–222.

133. Doughty MJ. Changes in cell surface primary cilia and macrovilli concurrent with measurements of fluid flow across the rabbit corneal endothelium ex vivo. *Tissue Cell* 1998;30: 634–643.

134. Doughty MJ, Sivak JG. Scanning electron microscope evaluation of the corneal endothelium in a case of unilateral microphthalmos with retrobulbar cyst in the pigmented rabbit. *Cornea* 1993;12:341–347.

135. Barry PA, Petroll WM, Andrews PM, et al. The spatial organization of corneal endothelial cytoskeletal problems and their relationship to the apical junctional complex. *Invest Ophthalmol Vis Sci* 1995;36:115–124.

136. Sherrard ES, Ng YL. The other side of the corneal endothelium. *Cornea* 1990;9:48–54.

137. Doughty MJ. Prevalence of "non-hexagonal" cells in the corneal endothelium of young Caucasian adults and their inter-relationships. *Ophthal Physiol Opt* 1998;18:415–422.

138. Doughty MJ. Concerning the symmetry of the "hexagonal" cells of the corneal endothelium. *Exp Eye Res* 1992;55:145–154.

139. Bergmanson JPG. Histopathological analysis of corneal endothelial polymegethism. *Cornea* 1992;11:133–142.

140. Müller A, Doughty MJ, Wright L. Reassessment of the corneal endothelial cell organization in children. *Br J Ophthalmol* 2000; 84:692–696.

141. Waring GO, Bourne WM, Delharser HF, et al. The corneal endothelium. Normal and pathologic structure and fraction. *Ophthalmology* 1982;89:531–559.

142. Doughty MJ, Müller A, Zaman ML. Assessment of the reliability of human corneal endothelial cell density estimate using a non-contact specular microscope. *Cornea* 2000;19:148–158.

143. Hollingsworth J, Perez-Gomez I, Mutalib HA, et al. A population study of the normal cornea using an in vivo, slit-scanning confocal microscope. *Optom Vis Sci* 2001;78:706–711.

144. Abib FC, Barreto J. Behavior of corneal endothelial density over a lifetime. *J Cataract Refract Surg* 2001;27:1574–1578.

145. Doughty MJ. Toward a quantitative analysis of corneal endothelial cell morphology: a review of techniques and their application. *Optom Vis Sci* 1989;66:626–642.

146. Bergmanson JPG. Endothelial complications. In: Silbert JA, ed. *Anterior segment complications of contact lens wear.* New York: Churchill Livingstone, 1994:91–121.

147. Doughty MJ, Maurice DM. Bicarbonate sensitivity of rabbit corneal epithelium fluid pump in vitro. *Invest Ophthalmol Vis Sci* 1988;29:216–223.

148. Doughty MJ. Evidence for a direct effect of bicarbonate on rabbit corneal stroma. *Optom Vis Sci* 1989;68:687–698.

149. Laties AM, Jacobwitz D. A comparative study of the autonomic

innervation of the eye in monkey, cat, and rabbit. *Anat Rec* 1967;156:383–396.

150. Chan-Ling T. Sensitivity and neural organization of the cat cornea. *Invest Ophthalmol Vis Sci* 1989;30:1075–1082.

151. Laties AM, Jacobowitz D. A comparative study of the autonomic innervation of the eye in monkey, cat, and rabbit. *Anat Rec* 1967;156:383–396.

152. Tervo T. Consecutive demonstration of nerves containing catecholamine and acetylcholinesterase in the rat cornea. *Histochemistry* 1977;50:291–299.

153. Colin S, Kruger L. Peptidergic nociceptive axon visualization in whole-mount preparations of cornea and tympanic membrane in rat. *Brain Res* 1986;398:199–203.

154. Muller LJ, Pels L, Vrensen GFJM. Ultrastructural organization of human corneal nerves. *Invest Ophthalmol Vis Sci* 1996;37:4.

155. Millodot M, O'Leary DJ. Corneal fragility and its relationship to sensitivity. *Acta Ophthalmol* 1981;59:820–826.

156. Bergmanson JPG. The central corneal innervation in primates. *Am J Optom Physiol Optics* 1988;65:56.

157. Draeger J. *Corneal sensitivity. Measurement and clinical importance.* New York: Springer-Verlag, 1984.

158. Murphy PJ, Patel S, Marshall J. A new non-contact corneal aesthesiometer (NCAA). *Ophthal Physiol Opt* 1996;16:101–107.

159. Belmonte C, Acosta MC, Schmelz M, et al. Measurement of corneal sensitivity to mechanical and chemical stimulation with a CO_2 esthesiometer. *Invest Ophthalmol Vis Sci* 1999;40:513–519.

160. Millodot M. The influence of age on the sensitivity of the cornea. *Invest Ophthalmol Vis Sci* 1977;16:240–242.

161. Norn MS. Conjunctival sensitivity in normal eyes. *Acta Ophthalmol* 1973;51:438–444.

162. Kruse FE. Stem cells and corneal epithelial regeneration. *Eye* 1994;8:170–183.

163. Zieske JD. Perpetuation of stem cells in the eye. *Eye* 1994;8:163–169.

164. Tseng SCG. Regulation and clinical implications of corneal epithelial stem cells. *Mol Biol Rep* 1996;23:47–58.

165. Dua HS, Azuara-Blanco A. Limbal stem cells of the corneal epithelium. *Surv Ophthalmol* 2000;44:415–425.

166. Cotsarelis GCS, Dong G, Sun T-T, et al. Existence of slow-cycling limbal epithelial basal cells that can be preferentially stimulated to proliferate: implications on epithelial stem cells. *Cell* 1989;57:201–209.

167. Lauweryns B, Vanden Oord JJ, Missotten L. The transitional zone between limbus and peripheral cornea. An immunohistochemical study. *Invest Ophthalmol Vis Sci* 1993;34:1991–1999.

168. Bergmanson JPG. Corneal epithelial mitosis. A possible explanation to corneal stippling. *Contacto* 1981;25:19–22.

169. Allansmith MR. Immunology of the external ocular tissues. *J Am Optom Assoc* 1990;61:S16–S22.

170. Bielory L. Allergic and immunologic disorders of the eye. Part 1: immunology of the eye. *J Allergy Clin Immunol* 2000;106:805–806.

171. Doughty MJ, Potvin R, Pritchard N, et al. Evaluation of the range of areas of the fluorescein staining patterns of the tarsal conjunctiva in man. *Doc Ophthalmol* 1995;89:355–371.

172. Barishak RY. *Embryology of the eye and its adnexa.* Basel: Karger, 2001.

173. Cook CS, Ozanics V, Jakobiec FA. Prenatal development of the eye and its adnexa. In: Tasman W, Jaeger EA, eds. *Biomedical foundations of ophthalmology, vol. 1.* Philadelphia: Lippincott Williams & Wilkins, 2000:1–93.

174. Gipson IK. The epithelial basement membrane zone of the limbus. *Eye* 1989;3[Pt 2]:132–140.

175. Busacca A. Étude de la structure et de la nature des palisades considérées jusu'ici comme un réseau de lymphatiques. *Arch d' Ophthal Mol (Paris)* 1939;3:593–705.

176. Lawrenson JG, Ruskell GL. The structure of corpuscular nerve endings in the limbal conjunctiva of the human eye. *J Anat* 1991;177:75–84.

177. Wanko T, Lloyd BJ, Mathews J. The fine structure of the human conjunctiva in the perilimbal zone. *Invest Ophthalmol* 1964;3:285–301.

178. Huang AJW, Tseng SCG, Kenyon KR. Paracellular permeability of corneal and conjunctival epithelial. *Invest Ophthalmol Vis Sci* 1989;30:684–689.

179. Steul K-P. Ultrastructure of the conjunctival epithelium. *Dev Ophthalmol Series.* Basel: Karger, 1989.

180. Blades K, Doughty MJ. Comparison of grading schemes to quantitative assessments of nucleus-to-cytoplasmic ratios for human bulbar conjunctival cells collected for impression cytology. *Curr Eye Res* 2000;20:335–340.

181. Doughty MJ, Blades K, Button NF, et al. Further analysis of the size and shape of cells obtained by impression cytology obtained from the exposed portion of the human bulbar conjunctiva. *Ophthal Physiol Opt* 2000;20:391–400.

182. Breitbach R, Spitznas M. Ultrastructure of the paralimbal and juxtacaruncular human conjunctiva. *Graefes Arch Clin Exp Ophthalmol* 1988;226:567–575.

183. Kessing SV. The mucus gland system of the conjunctiva. *Acta Ophthalmol (Copenh)* 1968;95[Suppl]:1–19.

184. Doughty MJ, Bergmanson JPG. New insights into the surface cells and glands of the conjunctiva and their relevance to the tear film. *Optometry* 2003:74:485–500.

185. Kruse FE, Jaeger W, Götz ML, et al. Conjunctival morphology in Sjögren's syndrome and other disorders of the anterior eye. A light and electron microscopic study based on impression cytology. *Scand J Rheumatol* 1986;61[Suppl]:206–214.

186. Nichols BA. Conjunctiva. *Microsc Res Techn* 1996;33:296–319.

187. Verges Roger C, Pita Salorio D, Refojo MF, et al. Cambios en la poblacion de celulas calciformes conjunctivales tras la aplicacion de una solucion hiperosmolar. *Arch Soc Esp Oftalmol* 1986;51:403–406.

188. Adar S, Kanpolat A, Sürücü S, et al. Conjunctival impression cytology in patients wearing contact lenses. *Cornea* 1997;16:289–294.

189. Rolando M, Terragna F, Giordano G, et al. Conjunctival surface damage distribution in keratoconjunctivitis sicca. An impression cytology study. *Ophthalmologica* 1990;200:170–176.

190. Dogru M, Katakami C, Miiyashita M, et al. Ocular surface changes after excimer laser phototherapeutic nerateitomy. *Ophthalmology* 2000;107:1144–1152.

191. Inatomi T, Spurr-Michaud S, Tisdale AS, et al. Expression of secretory mucin genes by human conjunctival epithelial. *Invest Ophthalmol Vis Sci* 1996;37:1684–1692.

192. Ellingham RB, Berry M, Stevenson D, et al. Secreted human conjunctival mucus contains MUC5AC glycoforms. *Glycobiol* 1999;9:1181–1189.

193. Takakusaki I. Fine structure of the human palpebral conjunctiva with special reference to the pathological changes in vernal conjunctivitis. *Arch Histol Jpn* 1969;30:247–282.

194. Dilly PN. On the nature and the role of the subsurface vesicles in the order epithelial cells of the conjunctiva. *Br J Ophthalmol* 1985;69:477–481.

195. Bergmanson JPG, et al. The acinar and ductal organization of the tarsal accessory lacrimal gland of Wolfing in rabbit eyelid. *Exp Eye Res* 1999;68:411–421.

196. Höh H, Schirra F, Kienecker C, et al. Lid-parallel conjunctival folds (LIPCOF) and dry eye: A diagnostic tool for the contactologist. *Contactologia* 1995;17:104–117.

197. Parsons JH. *The pathology of the eye, vol. 1.* London: Hodder and Stroughton, 1904.
198. Greiner JV, Covington HI, Allansmith MR. Surface morphology of the human upper tarsal conjunctiva. *Am J Ophthalmol* 1977;83:892–905.
199. Rohen JW, Lutjen-Drecoll E. Functional morphology of the conjunctiva. In: Lemp MA, Marquardt R, eds. *The dry eye.* Berlin: Springer-Verlag, 1992:35–63.
200. Rolando M, Brezzo V, Giordano G, et al. The effect of different benzalkonium chloride concentrations on human normal ocular surface. A controlled prospective impression cytology study. In: Van Bijster OP, Lemp MA, Spinelli D, eds. *The lacrimal system.* Amsterdam: Kugle & Ghedini Publ., 1991;87–91.
201. Paschides CA, Petroutsos G, Psilas K. Correlation of conjunctival impression cytology results with lacrimal function and age. *Acta Ophthalmol* 1991;69:422–425.
202. Yanni JM, Sharif NA, Gamache DA, et al. A current appreciation of sites for pharmacological intervention in allergic conjunctivitis: effects of new topical drugs. *Acta Ophthalmol Scand* 1999;77:33–37.
203. Welle M. Development, significance, and heterogeneity of mast cells with particular regard to the mast cell-specific proteases chymase and tryptase. *J Leukoc Biol* 1997;61:233–245.
204. Merayo-Lloves J, Calonge M, Foster CS. Experimental model of allergic conjunctivitis to ragweed in guinea pig. *Curr Eye Res* 1995;14:487–494.
205. Acosta MC, Tan ME, Belmonte C, et al. Sensations evoked by selective mechanical, chemical, and thermal stimulation of the conjunctiva and cornea. *Invest Ophthalmol Vis Sci* 2001;42:2063–2067.
206. Wirostko E, Bhattacherjee P, Eakins KE, et al. Cellular aspects of conjunctival inflammation induced by the synergistic action of histamine and prostaglandins. *Immunopharmacology* 1978;1:49–56.
207. Woodward DF, Spada CS, Hawley SB, et al. Conjunctival eosinophil infiltration evoked by histamine and immediate hypersensitivity. *Invest Ophthalmol Vis Sci* 1986;27:1495–1503.
208. MacLeod JDA, Anderson DF, Baddeley SM, et al. Immunolocalization of cytokines to mast cells in normal and allergic conjunctiva. *Clin Exp Allergy* 1997;27:1328–1334.
209. Abu El-Asrar Am, Struyf S, Al-Mosallam AA, et al. Expression of chemokine receptors in vernal keratoconjunctivitis. *Br J Ophthalmol* 2001;85:1357–1361.
210. Sugar HS, Riazi A, Schaffner R. The bulbar conjunctival lymphatics and their clinical significance. *Trans Am Acad Ophthalmol Otolaryngol* 1957;61:212–223.
211. Collin HB. Ocular lymphatics. *Am J Optom Am Acad Optom* 1966;43:96–106.
212. Gusev AM. Lymph vessels of human conjunctiva. *Arch Anat Gistologii Embriologii* 1963;45:T1099–T1102.
213. Cursiefen C, Schlötzer-Schrehardt U, Küchle M, et al. Lymphatic vessels in vascularized human corneas: immunohistochemical investigation using LYUE-1 and podoplanin. *Invest Ophthalmol Vis Sci* 2002;43:2127–2135.
214. Swartz MA. The physiology of the lymphatic system. *Adv Drug Delivery Rev* 2001;50:3–20.

CORNEAL OXYGEN CONSUMPTION AND HYPOXIA

NOEL A. BRENNAN AND
NATHAN EFRON

INTRODUCTION

The eyes of certain annelids and molluscs, and all vertebrates including humans, basically consist of a lens-pupil system that focuses the image of the visual field onto a light-sensitive retina in an arrangement that resembles a common camera. This scenario demands transparent living tissue to comprise the lens system, a requirement at odds with metabolic systems in other parts of the body.

The bioenergetic processes that sustain life for most eukaryotes depend on a continuous supply of oxygen. This substrate, while used in greater quantity than any other, is not stored by any body tissues. Species have developed elaborate systems, including lungs and an extensive vascular system, to ensure a supply that matches variable metabolic requirements. However, a vascularized system is not a transparent system, so the anterior-most layer of the eye has evolved a unique method of obtaining oxygen for respiration.

In the case of the crystalline lens, low metabolic demand in the absence of aerobic metabolism allows cells to survive by diffusion of metabolites from the bathing fluids. Corneal tissue demands are significantly higher, with the dual function of providing a refractive optical surface plus performing critical barrier functions. The cornea has therefore evolved to take advantage of a greater oxygen supply, derived by diffusion across the limiting membranes. When the eye is open, it derives the bulk of its oxygen supply from the atmosphere; during eye closure, oxygen diffuses from the blood vessels of the overlying palpebral conjunctiva. A constant limited supply is available from the aqueous humor, but the limbal capillaries provide little supplementation to these other supplies because of the long diffusion distances involved.

Wearing of contact lenses interferes with the normal flow of oxygen under both open- and closed-eye conditions, with a range of consequences. The study of this aspect of corneal physiology has therefore become a major focus of contact lens research. The development of silicone-hydrogel materials with oxygen permeability values substantially higher than those of traditional hydrogels has enabled clearer definition of the role of hypoxia in a number of contact lens related effects. In this chapter, we review corneal oxygenation, its quantification, the cellular and tissue adaptations to hypoxia, critical values of oxygen supply, and comparative performance of different types of contact lenses.

OXYGEN TENSION

Atmosphere

The atmosphere exerts a pressure of approximately 101 kPa (1 kPa = 7.501 mm Hg) at sea level, although this varies according to weather patterns and ambient humidity. Oxygen comprises some 21% of the total gases in the atmosphere in terms of pressure exerted, thus producing a partial pressure (pO_2) of 21 kPa at sea level. Partial pressure, but not oxygen concentration, falls with height above sea level; a useful rule of thumb for altitudes up to 10,000 m is that pO_2 falls by about 0.16 kPa (or 1.2 mm Hg) for every 100-m increase in altitude. Thus, the average pO_2 in Denver and Mexico City drops by more than 1/10 and nearly 1/5, respectively, compared to that at sea level. The Peruvian city of Cusco at an altitude of 3,200m has a pO_2 of about two thirds that at sea level, base camp at Mount Everest is at about one half, and the highest place on earth, the summit of Mount Everest, is at one third of what we consider to be a normal oxygen tension ("normoxia"). Many people live between 3,000 and 4,000 m above sea level and thus endure a relatively chronic hypoxia throughout life. We shall refer to these places later in our discussions about adaptation to hypoxia.

Body Tissues

Oxygen tension in body tissues has important connotations for contact lens wear. Oxygen is supplied to various bodily tissues by convective or bulk flow through the lungs and vascular system and then by diffusion from capillaries to cells to the target site, the mitochondria, wherein aerobic catabolism is accommodated. Partial pressure of oxygen continues to fall along this supply line. Arterial pO_2 is approximately 13 kPa, falling to 5 to 13 kPa in the capillaries. Average capillary pO_2 is around 7.5 to 8.0 kPa. Within cells, the partial pressure of oxygen is generally maintained at 1.3 to 2.7 kPa and falls to 0.1 to 1.3 kPa in mitochondria under conditions of normoxia. This level of oxygen clearly is sufficient to support most forms of life on the planet, a circumstance likely to be in teleologic accord with the laws of natural selection and evolution rather than mere coincidence. Various publications have shown that mitochondrial respiration remains constant down to very low levels (1) and is indeed more efficient at low pO_2. However, should the oxygen supply be interrupted, tissues such as brain cells will not survive more than a matter of minutes. Other body tissues can survive without oxygenation for minutes, hours, or even days (e.g., hair and nails continue to grow for several days after death).

The oxygen pressure of the highly vascular palpebral conjunctiva under the upper eyelid, and also at the anterior corneal surface during eye closure, approximately equals average pressure in the capillaries, that is, 7.5 to 8 kPa (2–6). Various estimates of aqueous humor partial pressure (mostly from animals) range from 3 to 7.5 kPa, depending upon the position within the aqueous (7–13).

CELLULAR METABOLISM

In general, eukaryotic cells make good use of aerobic metabolism because of efficiencies over anaerobic glycolysis. Aerobic metabolism requires mitochondria, subcellular organelles that house the enzymes of the Krebs tricarboxylic acid cycle and oxidative phosphorylation. (It is believed that mitochondria originally were bacteria that were incorporated into cells very early in the evolution of organisms.) A few human tissues, for example, red blood cells and the crystalline lens, do not have mitochondria and thus do not respire aerobically.

Energy Usage

As occurs in other tissues, energy derived from corneal cellular metabolic processes supports physiologic functions (maintenance of cellular and extracellular homeostasis and chemical balance). Specific examples include the active transport mechanisms of the epithelium and endothelium, which keep the cornea deturgescent; regulatory activities; cellular and tissue adhesions and junctional attachments; production of extracellular matrix; synthesis of proteins, deoxyribonucleic acid (DNA)/ribonucleic acid (RNA), lipids, and other essential components; programmed cell maturation; cellular division; tissue migration; and repair and resili-

ence to external threat. Although the exact breakdown of energy expenditure in the cornea has not been precisely expounded, there are guides from other tissues in the body.

Some 20% of whole-mammal oxygen usage is due to mitochondrial proton leak or nonmitochondrial respiration, although this may rise to much higher levels in individual tissues. Rolfe and Brown (14) summarize the breakdown of energy destinations as follows: 25% to 30% is used for protein, RNA, and DNA synthesis, 19% to 28% by Na^+/K^+-ATPase, 4% to 8% by Ca^{2+}-ATPase, 2% to 8% by actinomyosin-ATPase, 7% to 10% by gluconeogenesis, and 3% by ureagenesis (14). Protein synthesis and ionmotive ATPases are therefore the principal energy sinks in aerobically respiring cells and account for more than 90% of the oxidative adenosine triphosphate (ATP) production of rat skeletal muscle and as much as 66% of the ATP turnover in rat thymocytes. Given the functions of the cornea, it would be expected that these functions would similarly be its principal energy-consuming activities, especially in the limiting layers.

Metabolic Pathways

Corneal metabolic processes are similar to those found elsewhere in the body. Glucose, amino acids, vitamins, and minerals required for corneal metabolism appear to be derived from the aqueous; therefore, unlike oxygen, the supply of these metabolites is not interrupted by contact lenses. Aerobic catabolism involves stripping glucose of hydrogen in a series of redox reactions that release energy in the form of ATP, and the byproducts carbon dioxide and water. Figure 3.1 is an illustration of the pathways involved in the aerobic catabolism of glucose.

In summary, aerobic metabolism involves three main phases:

1. *Glycolysis* breaks down glucose into two pyruvate molecules, yielding two molecules of ATP. This process occurs in the cytoplasm and does not consume oxygen.
2. *The Krebs tricarboxylic acid (citric acid) cycle.* Pyruvate from glycolysis binds with coenzyme A, then is entirely decarboxylated in eight steps within the mitochondria. Coenzymes $NADH^+$ and $FADH^+$ capture most of the energy, with only 2 additional mole of ATP produced per mole of glucose.
3. *Oxidative phosphorylation* consists of two components: *electron transport chain* and *chemiosmosis*. The coenzymes accumulated from Krebs cycles are oxidized in the electron transport chain by a series of redox reactions using "electron acceptors" embedded in the mitochondrial cristae. As the electron is passed from one acceptor to the next, energy is captured temporarily in the form of pH and electrical potential gradients across the inner mitochondrial membrane by moving hydrogen ions into this space. The energy stored in this "proton gradient"

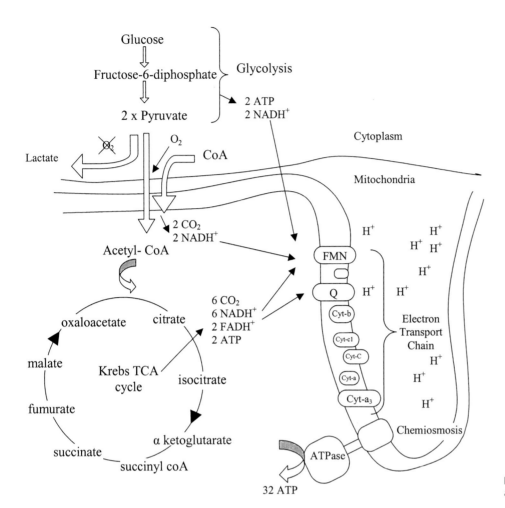

FIG. 3.1. Glucose catabolism via aerobic and nonaerobic pathways.

is later exploited to drive ATP synthase, a process known as *chemiosmosis.* Another 32 mole of ATP are derived per mole of glucose through this process. The eventual byproducts from these reactions are carbon dioxide and water.

In the absence of oxygen, glycolysis alone occurs with the production of lactate and yields relatively low amounts of energy. The pentose pathway (or hexose monophosphate shunt) is alternatively used for synthesis of nucleic acids and lipids, but it also yields 1 mole of ATP per mole of glucose. This pathway plays a significant role in corneal epithelium and endothelium, accounting for about 35%–65% of glucose metabolism in these layers. The rate of cellular respiration is controlled by feedback inhibition. The pacemaking step involves the enzyme phosphofructokinase, which can be inhibited by ATP and citric acid. Citric acid accumulation facilitates the conversion of acetyl-coenzyme A (acetyl-CoA) to fatty acid.

The aerobic pathway described earlier outlines the normal metabolic processes common to many cell types, including those of the cornea. When the oxygen supply is interrupted, there are a number of possible outcomes, ranging from cell damage and death to adaptive responses. In the

next section, we discuss cellular events before looking at the global response.

LOCAL RESPONSE TO HYPOXIA

The stark difference in energy yields from the aerobic and anaerobic pathways raises the question as to why species have maintained anaerobic glycolysis through their evolution when it is so inefficient. The answer lies in the fine balance between not having enough oxygen and having too much oxygen. To this end, cells are maintained virtually on the brink of asphyxiation. The oxygen supply to mitochondria in most cells matches consumption to a remarkable degree under a broad spectrum of challenges, and pO_2 consequently falls within very narrow physiologic constraints. Departure from this concentration can have dramatic consequences. High oxygen levels can lead to formation of reactive oxygen species and possibly toxic oxidative damage. Despite the remoteness of the intracellular microenvironment in most body tissues from air-level oxygen pressure, well-developed mechanisms exist to minimize the toxicity of oxidative damage. The corneal epithelium, in which cellular pO_2 may be as high as 20.1 kPa or fall to zero during closed-eye wear of contact lenses, dramatically contrasts with other body tissues. It is clear that the cornea shows outstanding resistance to the threat of oxidative damage.

Whereas high pO_2 may be toxic, low concentrations produce a range of well-known responses, including cellular, tissue, organ, and entire animal damage or death, and are a topic of great interest in contact lens research. Some tissues, such as the brain and heart, may only tolerate low oxygen for a matter of minutes before severe adverse cellular events arise. These include failure of energy-dependent membrane ion channels, breakdown of cellular calcium equilibrium, and disruption of cellular enzymes, ultimately leading to loss of cellular homeostasis. Traditionally, hypoxia-induced cell death was considered to be necrotic, but recently there has been overwhelming evidence that tissue damage is controlled by apoptosis. Moreover, it has become apparent that cells undergo an amazing array of adaptive responses due to the threat of low pO_2. Many of these responses to hypoxia are universal in aerobically respiring animals, occurring at both the local and global levels. The following discussion outlines the local molecular aspects of the general response to hypoxia, with reference to specific cell types of interest and the cornea where appropriate.

Critical Oxygen Levels

Critical oxygen supply to different cell types varies widely but is difficult to quantify because damage is dependent on the duration of exposure and preadaptation, as well as pO_2. Nonetheless, some indication of metabolic activity at low pO_2 can be extracted from microrespirometry studies of mitochondria. Respiration decreases by only about 10% as pO_2 falls from 20 to 1 kPa (1). Below 1 kPa, the relationship between oxygen flux (equivalent to oxygen usage and thus aerobic respiration rate) and pO_2 shows a hyperbolic relationship. Assuming saturation levels of adenosine diphosphate (ADP), respiration is about 80% of maximum at 0.27 kPa in rat heart mitochondria and is still maintained at about 50% of maximum activity at 0.035kPa. Critical pO_2 values for mitochondrial metabolism have been reported widely about this level by numerous authors (15–20). This partial pressure is 1/600 of atmospheric pressure, showing that respiration of cells is maintained despite great restriction to oxygen supply. It should be remembered that such a mitochondrial pO_2 may require a cytosolic pO_2 considerably greater than this, say 1.3 to 2.7 kPa as described earlier. Other cellular activities may be more sensitive to oxygen restriction, as indicated by the pO_2 for 50% activity of different cellular enzymes (21).

Cellular Responses

The range of cellular responses to hypoxic threat is quite dramatic. Despite this, the effect on local pO_2 may be minimal as both local and global mechanisms compensate for changed energy demands. For example, exercise induces increased oxygen consumption in muscle cells. Additional oxygen is supplied through greater inspiration and increased circulation and vasodilation, but the local pO_2 remains remarkably constant. Conversely, many body cells suppress metabolic rate during sustained hypoxia. For example, mammalian heart and liver cells will reduce metabolism by up to 50%. This occurs at levels well above the pO_2 at which diffusion of oxygen to the mitochondria should begin to limit oxidative phosphorylation. Harvitt and Bonanno (22) reported increased corneal oxygen consumption in response to acidosis induced by hypoxia. It is unclear what advantage this provides as increased surface layer consumption means additional hypoxia in deeper stromal layers.

In many cases, restricted oxygen supply does not mean tissue death or permanent damage, and adaptational changes are important. Preventing oxidative damage is a prime concern, and the body systems seem to have adapted to keep oxygen tension at the lowest level consistent with energy demands. The term *symmorphosis* refers to a functionality and efficiency of design in biologic tissues such that there is minimal surplus and wastage of energy resources. This theory envisages that greater metabolic efficiency should not be possible; however, it seems that there is a margin of redundancy and numerous functional gains to be extracted when times of plenty come to an end. In these circumstances, cells in the body make "tough" decisions and basically begin a programmed sequence of shutdown. Anoxia-tolerant species, such as some turtles, frogs, and fish, show the capacity to reduce membrane permeability, thereby greatly reducing oxygen demand. Carp, such as the common goldfish, are unique in that they produce ethanol as opposed to lactate as their bioenergetics switch to anaerobic metabolism. In anoxia-intolerant species, hypoxia may induce "hibernation" strategies in which high-energy functions such as ion transport and protein production are down-regulated to balance supply and demand, oxygen extraction from surrounding tissues is increased, and adaptations of enzymes allow metabolism at low partial pressures of oxygen. Anaerobic energy production is important to the survival of some tissues, despite its inefficiency. Skeletal muscle increases glucose uptake by 600% during hypoxia; bladder smooth muscle can generate up to 60% of the total energy requirement by anaerobic glycolysis. Anaerobic metabolism can maintain potassium channels in cardiac cells, protecting cell membrane integrity. These various adaptive processes begin at oxygen levels much higher than those necessary for basic metabolism. Despite taking advantage of the efficiencies of aerobic metabolism, the cells of the cornea seem to be particularly resilient to hypoxia, and this feature is discussed further later. In order to understand the adaptive mechanisms that occur in the cornea, it is pertinent to consider the features that characterize adaptation to hypoxia in most mammalian cells.

Molecular Oxygen Sensor

Oxygen sensors in prokaryotes and yeasts have been well known for many years. It has been evident that active oxygen control in higher organisms exists at the cellular, local, and systemic levels through a series of highly regulated and coordinated responses. Significant advances in our understanding of the molecular basis of this control were made in the 1990s (23,24). In the following discussion, the current understanding of the molecular basis for hypoxia-mediated gene expression is discussed [for more detail, refer to reviews by Semenza (25), Wenger (26), Hochachka and Rupert (27), Huang and Bunn (28), and Lando et al. (29)]. This process appears to have universal application in mammalian tissues, including the cornea.

Master transcriptional regulators in oxygen-regulated gene expression were first identified in novel investigations of erythropoiesis in the early 1990s. These proteins were dubbed hypoxia-inducible factors (HIFs). The following decade saw an explosion of research into oxygen-regulated gene expression, culminating with the sensational identification of the cellular oxygen sensing mechanism in 2001 (30–32).

HIFs are implicated in the expression of an impressive suite of target genes, totaling several dozen (more continue to be revealed). HIF transcriptional targets include those involved in iron metabolism (required for heme formation), angiogenesis (vascular endothelial growth factor [VEGF]), erythropoiesis, and modulators of vascular tone. Many are involved in glucose uptake, glycolysis, and pH buffering, as well as apoptotic and proliferative functions. HIF-1 has been linked to the pathogenesis of tumor vascularization, myocardial ischemia, and stroke through a localized regulatory control in response to the hypoxia prevailing under these conditions.

Figure 3.2 presents a schematic diagram of hypoxically induced molecular regulation. The HIF-1 DNA binding complex is a heterodimer of two basic helix-loop-helix PAS proteins, referred to as the α and β subunits. The β subunit, also known as aryl hydrocarbon receptor nuclear translator (ARNT), is stable across the commonly encountered range of pO_2. In mammalian transcription factors, ARNT serves primarily as a heterodimerization partner. Formation of the heterocomplex is necessary for DNA binding and *trans*-activation. However, despite the term *nuclear translocator*, ARNT is not required for HIF-1α translocation into the nucleus. HIF-1 protein is regulated mainly through the oxygen-dependent proteolysis of its α subunit. Under hypoxic conditions, the α subunit HIF-1α is stabilized to initiate a multistep pathway of activation. This includes nuclear translocation, dimerization with its partner ARNT to form HIF-1, recruitment of transcriptional coactivators, and subsequent specific binding to hypoxia response elements ([HRE] -ANACGTGC-) of DNA at a number of specific locations activating genetic expression as detailed earlier.

HIF-1α is unstable in oxygenated cells and is subject to rapid turnover. Its half-life is as few as 5 minutes, making detection in normoxic cells somewhat difficult. HIF-1α is degraded following binding of the von Hippel-Lindau tumor suppressor protein (pVHL), which recruits an E3 ubiquitin-protein ligase complex that targets HIF-1α for proteosomal degradation. In 2001, it was revealed that the interaction between pVHL and HIF-1α is regulated through hydroxylation of two proline residues, located within the carboxyl terminal transactivation domain (TAD-C), a process that is catalyzed by HIF-1α–proline hydroxylase requiring molecular oxygen as a substrate in the presence of Fe^{2+}. This finding constituted the discovery of the elusive hypoxia sensor in the body. Hydroxylation of an asparagine residue under normoxic conditions also prevents the interaction of the amino-terminal transactivation domain (TAD-N) with coactivator p300, which is necessary for transactivation of target genes by HIF-1. Although HIF-1 is regulated principally by oxygen tension, other factors also modulate its expression and consequent function. Extraordinarily, the rudimentary components of hypoxia-regulated gene expression may have been in place extremely early in evolution, prior to the appearance of the first eukaryotic organisms some 4 billion years ago (33). Certainly, the sophisticated regulation system described earlier exists in most, if not all, mammalian cells.

Corneal epithelium occupies a unique position in the study of hypoxia-induced gene expression. Makino et al. (34) identified an inhibitory PAS domain protein (IPAS) structurally related to the HIFs and intensely expressed in the corneal epithelium of mice. Predominantly localized in the nucleus, IPAS is present under normoxic conditions, but expression of its mRNA is up-regulated during hypoxia. It is found in lower concentrations in other tissues but is induced by hypoxia in mouse cerebrum, cerebellum, heart, and skeletal muscle, as in the cornea. IPAS lacks a *trans*-activation domain, thus serving as a natural HIF antagonist.

IPAS demonstrates dominant negative regulation over HIF-1α in the corneal epithelium. It does not affect hypoxia-induced protein stabilization of HIF-1α but provides a cell-type–specific or conditional negative regulatory strategy by the formation in the nucleus of an abortive complex with HIF-1α with regard to its ability to recognize the HRE motif. In particular, IPAS is important in negative regulation of both basal expression level and hypoxia-dependent activation of the VEGF gene in corneal epithelium. As noted earlier, hypoxic adaptive processes begin at partial pressures that are well above the critical level for normal mitochondrial function. Under normal conditions of eye closure, the corneal environment is sufficiently hypoxic to generate conditions that in other tissues would stimulate stabilization of HIF-1α. To maintain its avascularity, a consistent inhibitory action of IPAS over HIF-1 is necessary; indeed, inhibition of IPAS experimentally leads to corneal vascularization. Mechanisms investigated in the cornea also

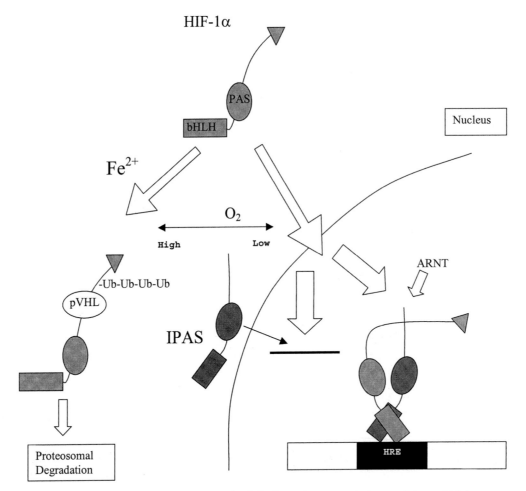

FIG. 3.2. Diagrammatic representation of cellular hypoxia sensor. Under conditions of high oxygen tensions, hypoxia-inducible factor 1α (HIF-1α) is quickly degraded by complexing with the von Hippel-Landau protein and ubiquitinization. When oxygen tension is low, HIF-1α is stabilized by binding with aryl hydrocarbon receptor nuclear translator (ARNT) and transactivates specific genetic loci. In cornea, retina, and to a lesser extent in most other tissues, the adaptive response to hypoxia may be blocked by inhibitory PAS domain protein (IPAS).

may inhibit hypoxically regulated gene expression in other tissues.

The corneal response to hypoxia is therefore a finely balanced act with a negative feedback loop rather than a disordered struggle for tissue survival. Despite inhibitory restraint on the adaptive response, aspects of altered gene expression in response to hypoxia are apparent in the cornea. For example, high corneal ATP levels observed during hypoxia most likely can be attributed to compensatory ATP generation by enhanced glycolysis (35). Consider also the response with regard to laminin 5, a key component of junctional complexes, during hypoxia. Production of laminin 5 is decreased overall, but extracellular processing of the laminin 5 γ2 chain is up-regulated, indicative of a finely tuned response to hypoxia by corneal cells (36). Moreover, it seems that regulation of the fellow eye will occur in some instances (37,38), implying that there is a central control or that regulatory signals can be transferred systemically from one eye

to the other. It will be interesting to reconcile the observed whole-tissue "adaptations" that the cornea makes to hypoxia with contact lens wear (see later) with changes at the molecular level over the next few years.

GLOBAL ADAPTIVE RESPONSES

We discussed earlier the cellular molecular response to hypoxia. The following discussion focuses more on tissue-, organ-, and whole-organism–based adaptations to the hypoxic state.

Tissue Variations

Each organ or tissue has its own unique sensitivity to hypoxia. At one end of the spectrum, as discussed earlier, hair and nails continue to grow for days after death. Vascular smooth muscle can survive a few days of hypoxia, skeletal muscle 60 to 90 minutes, and the kidney and liver no more than 20 minutes. At the other end of the spectrum, the brain and heart will not survive more than a few minutes without oxygen. The cornea, particularly its epithelium, is relatively resilient to hypoxia.

Animals

The animal kingdom provides a rich tapestry of adaptive mechanisms to hypoxia. The bar-headed goose, during its flight from southern India to breeding grounds in Tibet, ascends to over 9,500 m. It can ascend to 12,000 m, during which arterial pO_2 drops to 2.5 to 3 kPa. The only apparent adaptation is increased capillary density in the flight muscles, maximizing pO_2 to each cell. The freshwater turtle is able to survive brain anoxia for days by lowering energy consumption such that its needs can be fully met by anaerobic glycolysis. The mammals best adapted to hypoxia tolerance are seals; Weddell seals represent the elite in this group. They typically remain submerged during foraging dives up to 350 m deep for 15 to 20 minutes, with a maximum recorded duration of 82 minutes! Physiologic adaptations allowing these long periods of apnea seem to be a greater reliance on fatty acid catabolism based on increased β-hydroxyacyl CoA dehydrogenase activity, enhanced oxygen storage and diffusion capacity, decreased capillary density, and increased volume and density of mitochondria and citrate synthase activity.

Human Response to Altitude

Many people in Nepal, Tibet, Peru, and Kenya live at altitude (3,000–4,000m) and thus face a constantly reduced oxygen level. These highlanders show interesting adaptations to low oxygen tensions, some of which are adaptational while others are clearly programmed in individual races at the genetic level. Quechuas native to the high Andes show modest hypometabolism in regions of the brain, whereas Sherpas, native to the Himalayas and considered to show the greatest adaptation to high altitude, do not. In a study of marines adapting to high-altitude flying, Hochachka et al. (39) found that some areas of the brain showed depressed respiratory activity while others show enhanced activity, consistent with the concept of a highly regulated reaction to hypoxia. Acclimatized healthy highlanders living in mining towns at high altitude (4,000 m) with a resting arterial pO_2 of 6.5 to 7.5 kPa have a relatively normal life expectancy and suffer few medical problems despite the heavy manual work. Altitude acclimatization in lowlanders also has been well described. Experienced mountaineers can tolerate an arterial pO_2 of 4 to 5 kPa for several hours, whereas a lowlander who did not have altitude exposure would experience loss of breath, disorientation, and nausea, and finally would lose consciousness within a few minutes at such a partial pressure. Among other changes, increased red blood cell count is a primary feature of altitude adaptation. As for visual function, it is well known that relatively modest degrees of hypoxia can suppress aspects of color vision and dark adaptation (40,41).

Primed for Hypoxia?

Despite the research emphasis on aerobic corneal metabolism, the extent to which the cornea is predisposed to survive anaerobically is remarkable. The high concentration of the IPAS protein, which inhibits hypoxia-induced gene regulation (34) in corneal epithelium, is indicative of corneal evolution to tolerate closed lid hypoxia.

To illustrate the reliance on nonaerobic pathways, the following points should be noted:

- The cornea undergoes and withstands greater fluctuations in oxygen concentration than most body tissues.
- The cornea is avascular; thus, it derives nutrients and oxygen exogenously in lieu of an extensive vascular bed to provide these substrates at a consistent rate and constant level.
- It has been estimated that only 15% of corneal glucose substrate is metabolized aerobically (42).
- Corneal epithelium has an inhibitory protein to prevent vascularization in the absence of oxygen (34).
- Corneal epithelium does not show ultrastructural changes to prolonged systemic hypoxic threat, whereas both its stroma and endothelium do (43).
- Human corneal epithelial cells are resistant to apoptosis for 5 days of hypoxia (pO_2 of 2 kPa) in culture, and Poly (ADP-ribose) polymerases (PARP) cleavage (signaling initiation of the apoptotic pathway) is not evident for 7 days (36).
- *In vivo,* the cornea can withstand long periods (more than 8 hours) of zero oxygen tension at its anterior surface.
- During these periods of prolonged hypoxia, it does not lose either transparency or shape, and it maintains its barrier functions.
- A strong "Pasteur effect" has been noted in the endothelium (44).
- In keeping with a low organelle count to maintain transparency, corneal epithelial cells have a low count of mitochondria, the site of aerobic respiration.
- Its partner tissue, the lens, has no mitochondria. Although the sequence in which the metabolic systems in these tissues developed is a matter of some conjecture, it is evident that the transparent ocular tissues have evolved to be less dependent on aerobic respiration than most other body tissues.

Corneal resilience to hypoxia is illustrated by "safe" extended wear of oxygen-impermeable polymethyl methacrylate (PMMA) lenses in a cohort of 50 subjects for up to 7 years (45) and the widespread extended wear of low oxygen transmissibility (Dk/t*) soft lenses in the early 1980s, with approximately 99.8% of subjects not experiencing severe consequences. Curiously, it is the less than one in a million chance that an individual will lose vision if he or she chooses to sleep on a given night with contact lenses manufactured from these traditional hydrogel materials that has led to the widespread conviction that the cornea is susceptible to the effects of hypoxia. The probabilities manifest as an incidence of microbial keratitis (MK) in the population that is unacceptable to the community at large but represent what is a very modest reduction in the otherwise excellent robustness of this tissue.

CORNEAL RESPONSE TO HYPOXIA

Understanding the corneal response to hypoxia is a complicated task. The science of cellular metabolism teaches us that there are certain highly regulated responses to hypoxia in the cornea. Evolutionists and physiologists invoke different concepts when interpreting the term *adaptation*. To this end, it is difficult to decipher which corneal changes in response to hypoxia might be considered beneficial or compromising. A further group of observations made by corneal physiologists might simply be termed *side effects* to either hypoxia *per se* or the adaptive mechanism. Although speculative, we attempt here to identify observations into adaptations and side effects. Finally, when corneal hypoxia is marked and prolonged, the system may fail and adverse reactions may result; these circumstances are easily identified and fortunately rare.

Identifying the effects of hypoxia on the cornea is a complex task because corneal hypoxia is not a usual occurrence. Most information on the effects of corneal hypoxia has been derived from observations of corneas of contact lens wearers. Some short-term studies of hypoxia on the human cornea have been performed, enabling alteration of oxygen levels in isolation. Longer studies have been performed on animals with the potential to also restrict the influence of extraneous variables but with the limitation of cross-species application. Recently, the introduction of high Dk/t contact lenses has provided researchers with a persuasive tool for isolating hypoxic effects. Different properties of lens types, however, through modulus of elasticity and surface chemistry, complicate interpretation. Added to the complexity of studying the hypoxia response is the influence of time course; there are both short- and long-term effects.

We attempt to synthesize current thoughts linking the changes to hypoxic origin in the following discussion, rather than provide summaries of individual experiments. This discussion principally considers laboratory studies with emphasis on demonstrating ocular changes of hypoxic origin, with

more clinically biased considerations covered in the section on How Do Current Contact Lenses Measure Up?. Changes with contact lens wear thought to be due to other causes are not listed. More in-depth reviews on the entire spectrum of changes with contact lens wear are available (46–49).

Epithelial Respiration

The immediate and most studied corneal response to hypoxia is corneal swelling. The cornea will increase in thickness by approximately 8% over a 3-hour period of anoxia. This swelling appears to be caused by lactate production in the epithelium as a result of shutdown of aerobic metabolic pathways, which accumulates and leads to subsequent osmotic imbibition of water into the stroma (50,51). Both contact lens wear and eye closure exacerbate this swelling response so that a lens with low Dk/t may produce approximately 14% swelling if it is worn during eye closure (52). Despite its prominence as an index of corneal physiology, increased corneal thickness as a direct result of hypoxia has no known adverse effects. Therefore, it can be regarded as a side effect, although it is indicative of one of the adaptive mechanisms of the cornea—the conversion of metabolism from aerobic to anaerobic pathways. Activation of genetic loci to up-regulate anaerobic metabolism in the cornea is presumed rather than documented, but corneal ATP levels observed during hypoxia most likely can be attributed to compensatory ATP generation by enhanced glycolysis (35). Chemical analysis of the levels of various substrates, enzymes, and byproducts of metabolism show changes indicative of altered pathways during hypoxia (53–58).

The cornea demonstrates adaptation in its swelling response. Numerous studies found that prolonged exposure to low Dk/t contact lenses reduces the edema response by about 2% with daily wear lenses and 3% to 4% with extended wear lenses (59–64). This effect includes a reduction in overnight edema response without lens wear (64) and is directly related to hypoxia, as shown by the absence of such an effect with wear of high Dk/t lenses (65). The mechanism behind this adaptation is yet to be elucidated but may be related to altered oxygen consumption.

Harvitt and Bonanno (22) found a short-term increase in rabbit corneal oxygen consumption with decreasing corneal pH. During contact lens-induced hypoxia, corneal pH falls and the consumption rate is paradoxically predicted to rise. The authors used this effect to explain, in part, differences in anterior oxygen tension between measured and modeled values (see later for more details) (66). More information regarding control of corneal metabolic homeostasis is necessary to ascertain the role of the regulatory mechanism in promoting increased consumption in the short-term response to hypoxia.

Longer-term studies showed decreased corneal oxygen consumption as measured by a polarographic oxygen sensor (67–69). One can hypothesize that this would be based on a decreased volume of epithelial tissue or direct regulation

---

Throughout this chapter, Dk/t is presented in units of $\times 10^{-9}$ [cm/sec] [mLO$_2$/mL $\cdot$ mmHg.].

of respiratory activity. However, Bonanno et al. (70) recently were unable to show altered consumption in a sample of soft lens wearers using phosphorescence spectroscopy. One possible explanation for the difference in these studies may be the degree of hypoxic stress between wearing groups.

Epithelial Architecture

Basal epithelial cells may undergo mitosis several times before terminally differentiating, advancing toward the surface, undergoing apoptosis, and finally sloughing into the tears. The general population of corneal cells is renewed from stem cells, however, located at the limbus. As a result, there is both centripetal and forward movement of cells. Under normal conditions, an unknown control mechanism maintains an equilibrium in which cell division, size, movement, and exfoliation are coordinated to achieve a stable corneal epithelial volume and shape. Contact lens wear impacts proliferation in the basal layers of the corneal epithelium (55). All types of contact lens wear, soft or rigid, low Dk/t or high Dk/t, lead to decreased cellular division. Reduced mitosis with contact lens wear must be followed by, at minimum, one of the following three occurrences—increased cell life, cell enlargement, or epithelial thinning—and all appear to happen (38,68,71–82). The role of hypoxia in contact lens-related changes to epithelial homeostasis is confounded by other effects. Hypoxia reduces exfoliation rate but only in the short term (83). The effect of contact lens wear on epithelial cell size may be related to Dk/t, as silicone-hydrogel lenses produce no change in cell size (84). Low Dk/t lenses suppress proliferation more than do high Dk/t lenses, but there remains a one-third reduction with high Dk/t lenses (38). It seems that the mechanical presence of the lens or reduced post-lens tear flow plays a role. Similarly, there is a decrease in apoptotic figures (76,78) and an increase in the number of viable cells at the central cornea under a contact lens, regardless of soft lens Dk/t (80). All contact lenses decrease surface cell shedding rate, possibly as a result of reduced blink shear pressure, and this may signal the basal layer to reduce mitotic activity. The epithelial architectural equilibrium certainly is subject to mechanical forces, as the effect of orthokeratology is produced at least in part by redistribution of the epithelial volume (85). Control of epithelial architectural homeostasis is a complex phenomenon and is certain to be a topic of much research over the coming years.

Microcysts

Cellular production, lowered in rate during contact lens induced hypoxia, may be dysfunctional, disorganized, or incomplete, and epithelial appearances such as microcysts result (68,86–89). Although there may be microcysts in the normal cornea, numbers are limited usually to fewer than 10 per cornea. Formation of microcysts occurs over the first few months of extended wear of low Dk/t rigid or soft lenses. The microcyst response is therefore generally considered to be the classic clinical indicator of medium-term corneal hypoxia. They most typically appear in large numbers 2 to 3 months after initiating extended wear, but they are not of immediate pathologic significance (89). The role of hypoxia is confirmed by studies considering microcyst counts with lenses of different Dk/t. Most convincingly, wear of silicone-hydrogel lenses does not induce a microcyst response greater than that observed in the absence of lens wear (90–92). The microcyst response does not correlate with an individual's corneal edema response. suggesting that there may different mechanisms in play for these two classic indicators of hypoxia (93).

Epithelial Junctional Integrity

Another important effect of contact lens wear is loosening of tight junctions, separation of epithelial cells, and reduction in the number of hemidesmosomes (94–96). Laminin 5, a major adhesive ligand of basement membrane that participates in the complexes mediating cell–extracellular matrix attachment, is deposited in decreased amounts with hypoxia (36). However, in keeping with the concept of a controlled regulated response to hypoxia, up-regulation in the extracellular processing of laminin 5 $\gamma 2$ chain occurs for up to 5 days in low-oxygen tissue culture. The overall reduction in laminin 5 also may play a role in cellular apoptosis (36).

Clinically, junctional compromise is manifest as a more fragile epithelium (97), which is classically manifest as staining (62,95) or, in more severe cases, as abrasion (71,72,98). Intuitively, compromised junctional integrity should lead to an increase in epithelial permeability. Early research was unable to identify such a change (99,100), but more recently McNamara et al. (101,102) found a substantial increase without visible surface disruption. Increasing lens Dk/t reduces the effect of lens wear on epithelial barrier function, but it appears that factors other than hypoxia may be involved (103,104).

Corneal Sensitivity

Wear of contact lenses leads to reduced corneal sensitivity (105–108). Millodot and O'Leary (109) investigated the effects of oxygen deprivation on corneal sensitivity and found that loss of sensitivity is dependent upon both the degree and duration of hypoxia. It was observed that a significant loss of corneal sensitivity occurred in response to a range of hypoxic stresses, including the closed eyelid [supported recently by duToit et al (110)]. Decreased corneal sensitivity in contact lens wearers appears to be due to a functional change in nerves rather than a change in nerve density (111).

Stroma

Long-term extended wear of low Dk/t hydrogel lenses has been found to produce slight thinning (about 2%) of corneal stroma [monocular contact lens wearers compared to the contralateral non–lens-wearing eyes (68)]. Liu and Pflugfelder (112) replicated this finding in long-term contact lens wearers; however, they stated that the subjects had worn lenses "on a continuous basis for more than 5 years," and it is not clear whether this is meant to indicate extended wear or daily wear without discontinuation. Further, the role of mechanical effects of rigid lens wear on corneal thickness cannot be discounted in their study because most of the soft lens wearers also had rigid lens wearing experience. Patel et al. (111) were unable to find a difference in daily wearers of any type of lens with greater than 10 years' experience.

It may be conjectured that the basis for stromal thinning is related to the health of keratocytes. Keratocyte degeneration has been found after 24-hour wear of PMMA lenses, suggesting an effect of hypoxia on these cells (71). In longer-term extended wear of hydrogel lenses, there also is evidence of keratocyte loss (113,114) that was not found with long-term daily lens wear (111). However, Efron et al. (114) showed that the effect is not hypoxia related, as the posterior stromal keratocyte loss in their study occurred to a similar extent with both low Dk/t hydrogel and high Dk/t silicone-hydrogel lenses. A mechanical effect is hypothesized. Another theory for stromal thinning is through leaking of proteoglycans out of the stroma during episodes of edema (115).

Corneal pH

During contact lens-induced epithelial hypoxia, aerobic metabolism is supplanted by anaerobic metabolism, producing an increase in lactate as a byproduct (50). Elimination of lactate does not occur as easily as the byproducts of aerobic metabolism, and its accumulation has been found to account for the osmotic gradient down which water flows into the stroma (51). Lactic acid accumulation is responsible, in combination with carbon dioxide buildup under contact lenses (9), for acidosis of the stroma (116–118). Harvitt and Bonanno (22) reported increased oxygen consumption associated with corneal acidosis. Clinically, reduced pH may be responsible for some of the endothelial observations reported later. Acidity in the stroma correlates with decreased functional capacity of the endothelium (119).

Limbal Vasculature

The limbal vessels become injected during wear of low Dk/t hydrogel contact lenses (120,121). Papas (122) clearly demonstrated the inverse relationship between lens Dk/t and limbal redness, and moreover a link between hypoxia and limbal redness. Silicone-hydrogel lenses do not appear to induce significant limbal injection compared to low Dk/t hydrogel lens wear (92,123–125).

As opposed to the engorgement of the blood vessels at the limbus, encroachment of new vessels into corneal tissue represents a potential pathologic condition. Differences in neovascularization have been noted between low Dk/t hydrogel lenses and high Dk/t silicone-hydrogels, the latter causing no apparent change in the degree of vessel encroachment (125,126). Systemic hypoxia also has been found to produce stromal neovascularization in the absence of epithelial changes (43). As detailed earlier, an inhibitory protein that prevents HIF-1a binding to the VEGF HRE site serves to prevent neovascularization in the normal cornea (34). The features that overcome this inhibitory effect to stimulate corneal neovascularization remain unclear.

Endothelial Anatomy and Function

Short-term contact lens wear leads to transient endothelial edema, sometimes referred to as *blebs,* in inverse proportion to Dk/t (127). It has been theorized that accumulation of carbon dioxide to lower pH near the endothelium is the factor leading to this localized endothelial cell swelling (128). The relation between contact lens oxygen and carbon dioxide transmissibilities (129) may explain the association of blebs and Dk/t Adaptation effect of endothelial edema occurs; reintroduction of a contact lens to an eye produces a lesser effect over a period of days (128). Aside from indicating short-term insult, there does not appear to be any dysfunctional outcome associated with this sign.

Chronic hypoxia may have some important long-term consequences for corneal endothelial health. Whereas endothelial cell density does not change with long term contact lens wear, the shape and size of cells can be dramatically influenced (111,130–132). These effects, known as *pleomorphism* and *polymegethism,* respectively (see Chapter 2) may be associated with corneal exhaustion (133). Endothelial polymegethism correlates with hypoxic dose and may explain, in part, individual variation in corneal edema (134, 135). Recovery appears to be slow; polymegethism persists for many months following cessation of contact lens wear (68,136). Chronic hypoxia is etiologically implicated because low oxygen conditions, such as wear of lenses with low oxygen permeability (e.g., PMMA) and extended wear, are associated with greater degrees of polymegethism (68, 130,131,136). Polymegethism may be the most useful indicator of long-term hypoxia.

Another feature that has been considered separate to anatomical aspects is the functional capacity of the corneal endothelium to maintain corneal thickness or recover it after a stressful episode (137,138). Considerable work was performed recently in this area by Polse, Bonanno, and co-workers (119,134,139,140), although the suggestion that endothelial polymegethism is associated with reduced func-

tional capacity of the endothelium has been challenged by Bourne et al. (141). Acidity in the stroma correlates with decreased functional capacity (119). An interesting recent finding is that acidification of endothelium appears to occur almost exclusively due to carbon dioxide buildup (142).

Adverse Effects

The most feared adverse event linked with contact lens-induced hypoxia is MK. Clinical aspects of MK associated with contact lens wear are described in detail elsewhere (49, 143–145) (see Chapter 39). In brief, MK is a sight-threatening condition, and contact lens wear is a major risk factor for this condition. In particular, wear of contact lenses during sleep increases the risk of developing MK; however, the role of hypoxia in causing infection is controversial and remains to be resolved. At the time of this writing, indications are that high Dk/t lenses will significantly reduce the incidence of MK (146), but clinicians, patients, and the industry alike await results of epidemiologic studies confirming this hypothesis.

Demonstrating the role of hypoxia in the pathogenesis of contact lens-related infection remains difficult. In a rabbit model, a lens contaminated with *Pseudomonas aeruginosa* under a closed eye more effectively induced corneal infection than did corneal wounding, inoculation of bacteria, and closing the eye (147). Fleiszig et al. (148) demonstrated that extended wear of soft contact lenses led to an increased degree of binding of *P. aeruginosa* to human corneal epithelial cells gathered from the eye by gentle irrigation. Cavanagh and co-workers (149,150) demonstrated a relationship between Dk/t and bacterial binding to sloughed cells as well as to whole cornea. Other factors, however, including duration of wear and lens rigidity, show roles in bacterial binding (77,79). Furthermore, short-term hypoxia alone does not lead to increased bacterial binding to sloughed cells (151). Hypoxia is just one factor in the pathway to bacterial attachment to corneal cells; further research is required to elucidate the mechanisms of corneal infection with contact lens wear.

The role of hypoxia in noninfectious inflammatory conditions also is unclear. Hypoxia appears to regulate the degree and duration of inflammatory responses in other body tissues. Evidence is accumulating that inflammatory processes within the cornea also are mediated in part by hypoxia (152–154). However, the key noninfectious inflammatory processes involved with contact lens wear—contact lens-related acute red eye (CLARE) and contact lens-related peripheral ulcers (CLPU)—appear to occur in equal number with high Dk/t silicone-hydrogel lenses as low Dk/t hydrogel lenses (92,155), indicating that other factors predominate over hypoxia in producing these effects.

Perhaps the only other conditions of significance with an association to contact lens-induced hypoxia are corneal vascularization (see earlier) and the corneal exhaustion syndrome (CES). CES has been predominantly diagnosed following daily as opposed to extended wear, and it usually involves many years of PMMA or thick hydroxyethyl methacrylate (HEMA) contact lens wear (both of very low Dk/t and rarely used today). CES symptoms are lens intolerance, decreased visual acuity, photophobia, alterations to the spherical and cylindrical components of refraction, endothelial irregularity, and irregularity of anterior corneal shape (133). Vision decreases in the short term, but subjects who endure this condition show good recovery after some time without lenses or wearing contact lenses of higher Dk/t. Of current concern is the continued use of low Dk materials in thick toric lens designs, which may fail to deliver adequate oxygen to prevent CES. It is unclear why this condition principally arises in connection with daily wear, but MK is a more common endpoint with extended lens wear.

Assessment of Corneal Oxygenation

To determine whether a contact lens allows adequate oxygenation for normal corneal function, we require both valid methods for assessing corneal oxygenation and criteria for comparison. Fatt and Bieber (156) set out the concepts for estimating the steady-state, time-independent distribution of oxygen in the cornea. This model has been expanded, updated, and reworked in a variety of formats (2,66,157, 158). Analysis of the oxygen profile paradigm allows identification of the key parameters that can be used to describe corneal oxygenation.

The following indices or systems might be proposed.

1. *Corneal oxygen consumption profile.* Ultimately, the adequacy of oxygen supply under a given condition might be best judged by comparing the oxygen consumption at individual points within the cornea against the critical oxygen consumption required at each point to maintain normal physiology. The minimum oxygen consumption required for normal function within the various layers is not known, but any reduction to normal consumption might be regarded as unsatisfactory. Several authors have measured normal oxygen consumption by layer; these estimates assume constant consumption within each layer. Harvitt and Bonanno (159) tabulated these results. Measurement of oxygen consumption in comparative terms at a given point in the human cornea in response to an applied condition is not feasible to date, but techniques such as redox fluorometry and magnetic resonance imaging might be adapted for this purpose (13, 160,161).

2. *Corneal oxygen tension profile.* Because consumption at any point through the cornea should be dependent on oxygen tension at that point under steady-state conditions, one might alternatively compare the oxygen tension at individual positions within the cornea against the critical oxygen tension required at each point to maintain

normal consumption. Assuming equal consumption through a given corneal layer, this amounts to determining the point within each layer at which oxygen tension is at a minimum and to ascertain whether the supply at that point is adequate for normal consumption. Given the relation between oxygen usage and pO$_2$ by mitochondria (see section on Critical Oxygen Levels), it is reasonable to assume that this amounts to non-zero partial pressures of oxygen. Consequently, a reasonable criterion for adequacy of the corneal oxygen supply is the maintenance of non-zero pO$_2$ throughout the profile, the same criterion used by Harvitt and Bonanno (66). To date, measurement of oxygen tension at various points through the *in vivo* human cornea cannot be achieved. Diffusion models based on the principles of Fatt and Bieber (156), however, can be used to make theoretical approximations of the oxygen profile, based on data for the boundary conditions and the thickness, oxygen permeability, and consumption of the various layers.

3. *Total corneal oxygen consumption.* Total consumption can be modeled theoretically based on the oxygen diffusion models or its components and compared to a known critical value, but it would not provide details of where any shortfall might occur within the cornea. Alternatively, total consumption could be calculated from the difference between anterior and posterior fluxes (see later). Numerous authors produced data or models of consumption, but these do not have practical value in determining corneal oxygenation during contact lens wear (42,157,162–164). Bonanno et al. (165) have provided a technique for estimating corneal oxygen consumption by noninvasive measurement of post-lens tear film oxygen tension.

4. *Boundary layer oxygen flux.* It is reasonable to assume that oxygen tension and local consumption at any point in the cornea under steady-state conditions will be consistent for given boundary conditions at the limiting layers. Thus, details of the oxygen flux at both anterior and posterior surfaces should provide a unique solution to the oxygen tension profile, consumption at individual points through the cornea, and total corneal oxygen consumption, which might be calculated from the sum of the absolute values of flux at the front and back surfaces adjusted for corneal volume. Empirical estimation of posterior corneal oxygen flux cannot be made *in vivo*, however, with current techniques. Measurement of anterior flux has been problematic, but several estimates have been made (see later).

5. *Boundary layer oxygen tensions.* Individually, boundary layer oxygen tensions do not provide information about the corneal oxygen profile but, like boundary layer oxygen flux, will define a unique solution if other aspects of the consumption and diffusion of oxygen in the cornea are known. Indeed, either the boundary fluxes or

boundary oxygen tensions are sufficient information and so can be considered interchangeable in terms of value if the other parameters necessary for profile calculations are known.

6. *Anterior corneal oxygen flux.* In reality, flux across the posterior surface for closed-eye conditions is relatively constant regardless of anterior oxygen flux. Thus, anterior corneal oxygen flux alone should be reasonably adequate to define oxygen supply to the cornea. Because neither contact lens materials nor the tear film consumes oxygen and oxygen supplementation via tear exchange (with soft lenses) appears to be limited, the flux through the anterior surface of a contact lens on the eye provides a firm approximation of anterior corneal oxygen flux, without the need to measure post-lens oxygen tension. Estimates of the anterior corneal oxygen flux during normoxia are provided in Table 3.1 (156,157,166–173). Fatt and colleagues (168,174) attempted to make direct measurements with contact lenses *in situ*, with modest success.

7. *Anterior corneal oxygen tension.* Like anterior oxygen flux, anterior corneal oxygen tension can provide a substantial amount of the information required to define corneal oxygenation. Developing a system of measuring anterior corneal oxygen tension has been a popular research task. The commonly quoted equivalent oxygen percentage (EOP) is such an attempt; the oxygen flow from a membrane reservoir placed on the cornea after removal of a contact lens is matched to the depletion rate following exposure of the cornea to reservoirs of known gaseous environments. Various authors have described different aspects of the technique (9,175–178), but Benjamin (179) provided the most comprehensive set of EOP measures for different contact lenses. Harvitt and Bonanno (180) described a phosphorescence dye technique that involves oxygen quenching of Pd-meso-tetra (4-carboxyohenyl) porphine. By combining the dye

TABLE 3.1. ESTIMATES OF ANTERIOR CORNEAL OXYGEN FLUX WITH NORMOXIA

First Author	Year	Technique	Estimate (μL/cm^2/h)
Hill (166)	1963	Sealed haptic	4.8
Haberich (167)	1966	Volumetric	9.0
Fatt (156)	1968	Diffusion model	6.9
Jauregui (168)	1972	POS in goggle	2.8
Fatt (157)	1974	Diffusion model	5.5
Larke (169)	1981	POS	6.0
Quinn (170)	1984	POS	1.6
Fitzgerald (171)	1986	POS	6.2
Horton (172)	1989	POS	10.9
Brennan (173)	2001	EOP modeling	7.5

EOP, equivalent oxygen percentage; POS, polarographic oxygen sensor.

with bovine serum albumin onto the surface of contact lenses, the technique has been applied to human eyes to estimate the anterior corneal oxygen tension (165).

8. *Lens oxygen transmissibility (Dk/t).* If oxygen tension and local consumption at any point in the cornea under steady-state conditions are dependent on the boundary conditions at the limiting layers and the flux across the posterior surface is relatively constant regardless of anterior oxygen flux, it then stands to reason that for a given tear layer thickness, the Dk/t of the contact lens should be a good predictor of the other parameters of corneal oxygen usage. It is this assumption that has led to the widespread popularity of this paradigm among researchers, material scientists, and clinicians. Oxygen transmissibility is measured most commonly by either the polarographic or coulometric techniques (181,182). In 1996, however, Fatt (183) commented that the Dk/t term "used by itself as a measure of lens performance has been a disappointment." He pointed out that Dk/t does not by itself allow calculation of oxygen flux into the cornea, nor does it provide any indication of how closely oxygen flux into the cornea under a lens matches that without a lens is in place and specifically does not give an indication of the proportionate change in oxygen flux between lenses of different Dk/t values. The Dk/t figure is a bench-top measurement that affords only a modest link to on-eye performance.

The order in which the numbered points are listed gives a rough guide to the value and ease of measurement of each of these paradigms. The first few points on this list are more definitive in describing corneal oxygenation but are less easily measured. The last few points highlight parameters that are more easily quantified but are increasingly reliant on estimates of other corneal parameters to give a true picture of corneal oxygenation.

OXYGEN PROFILE MODELS

If the Dk/t paradigm has outlived its usefulness, what alternative index or indices might be preferred? Anterior corneal oxygen tension suffers from similar problems to Dk/t. Although it allows a comparison of the lens-wearing scenario to that without lenses, it does not by itself allow calculation of oxygen flux into the cornea, nor does it give an indication of the proportionate change in oxygen flux between lenses of different Dk/t values. Examination of the graph of oxygen flux versus anterior oxygen tension shows the nonlinearity of this relationship (184). We propose that the parameters of greater importance that should be considered are corneal oxygen flux and consumption. Oxygen flux provides an exact indication of the amount of oxygen entering the cornea per unit time, and oxygen consumption will give a direct indicator of metabolic activity. As noted earlier, in the late

1960s and early 1970s, Fatt and co-workers (2,157,185, 186) modeled the steady-state (time-independent) distribution of oxygen in the cornea. The parameters necessary to make these calculations include the permeability, thickness, and consumption rates of the various corneal layers and knowledge of the boundary conditions. A differential equation for the steady-state oxygen diffusion and consumption is written for each layer of the cornea. Because the flux values and partial pressure values at the interfaces of adjoining layers must be equal, a set of simultaneous equations can be constructed. The solution provides details of the oxygen tension across the cornea, which also can be used to assess all other parameters concerned in corneal oxygenation. Fatt and Ruben (158) used a simplified model in which the cornea was considered a single layer.

Harvitt and Bonanno (66) reevaluated oxygen diffusion using revised values for some of the parameters of the model and incorporating a correction for altered consumption rate that they measured with corneal acidosis. More recently, Brennan (2003, *unpublished data*) modified the Harvitt–Bonanno model. The Brennan model provides two important "upgrades." It first corrects for spurious consumption when the oxygen tension falls to zero at any position within the cornea. Harvitt and Bonanno (66) set predicted negative values of oxygen tension to zero. Closer examination reveals that the areas where pO_2 falls to zero within the cornea maintain consumption mathematically. The correction for the spurious consumption requires an eight-layer model but uses the same basic mathematical paradigm, in this case solving 15 simultaneous equations. Figure 3.3 illustrates the scenarios under which consumption within certain layers are set to zero. Figure 3.4 shows the curve (from Harvitt and Bonanno's Fig. 8) to avoid epithelial anoxia using their layer thickness parameters with a lens of Dk/t 89, a curve correcting for spurious consumption at a Dk/t 89, and a curve correcting for spurious consumption that shows a Dk/t 47 is needed to prevent epithelial anoxia. This demonstration reveals a substantial difference to the predicted minimum Dk/t by correcting for spurious consumption.

The second correction to Harvitt and Bonanno's model applies values for the thicknesses of the various layers that have been derived since publication of their model and are more representative of those for the average human cornea wearing a soft lens. Harvitt and Bonanno used a value of 45 μm for the post-lens tear layer thickness, whereas recent estimates suggest a value between 2.3 and 12 μm, most probably at the lower end (187–189). Although not explicitly stated, examination of the figures in Harvitt and Bonanno's paper suggest that they used a value for corneal epithelial thickness of 40 μm and a total corneal thickness of 495 μm. Estimates of epithelial thickness from various studies seem to dichotomize values at either approximately 50 (77,82,190) or 60 μm (68,191–193) but certainly greater than 40 μm. Perez et al. (82) criticize the larger

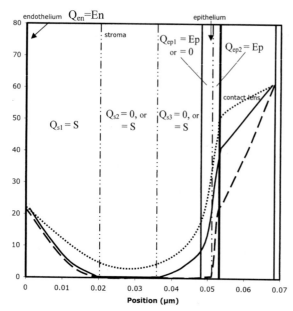

FIG. 3.3. Schematic diagram of the basis for the eight-layer oxygen diffusion model. Q_L denotes consumption of layer L, where L may be en, s1, s2, s3, ep1, or ep2 representing endothelium, stroma layer 1, stromal layer 2, stromal layer 3, epithelial layer 1 or epithelial layer 2, respectively. The value for consumption may be En S, Ep, or 0, representing the steady-state normal consumption of the endothelium, stroma, or epithelium with non-zero pO_2 or zero in cases where the pO_2 falls to zero, respectively.

formed a meta-analysis of some 600 data sets published from 1968 to 1999 and determined the mean result from these studies to be 534 μm, with optical pachymetry usually giving slightly lower values than ultrasound. Studies in our laboratories are in agreement with these findings. These differences in layer thicknesses produce substantial differences to the predicted pO_2 values from the diffusion model.

We plotted a range of curves for the thin and adjusted corneal thickness showing the minimum Dk/t levels theoretically required to avoid epithelial and stromal anoxia, using 3-μm tear layer thickness (Figs. 3.5–3.8).

Further research is needed to clarify the correction for altered consumption with corneal acidosis as proposed by Harvitt and Bonanno (66). Changes in corneal oxygen consumption with acidosis were investigated to account for low measured pO_2 values using the oxygen-dependent phosphorescent dye technique compared to diffusion modeled values (22,66,180). Part of the justification for reworking the models was that the EOP values quoted by Harvitt and Bonanno were more in keeping with empirical dye measures (180). These EOP values, however, derived from equations of Fatt and Chaston, seem to be low compared to the more extensively measured values of Benjamin (177,179). That the acidotic correction is linked to Dk/t also presents problems, because pO_2 may alter within the cornea through changes to tear layer thickness while Dk/t remains constant. Further, the effect is extrapolated to Dk/t values up to 126 despite the measures of acidosis being based on contact lenses of maximum Dk/t 56. It is noteworthy that the minimum Dk/t found to avoid corneal hypoxia is 125. A final concern is that increased oxygen consumption with hypoxic stress seems contrary to energy conservation strategies of

values measured by optical coherence tomography on the basis of including tear layer thickness, but it is not apparent how this would be eliminated with optical pachometry. Although there have been numerous studies of total corneal thickness undertaken, Doughty and Zaman (194) per-

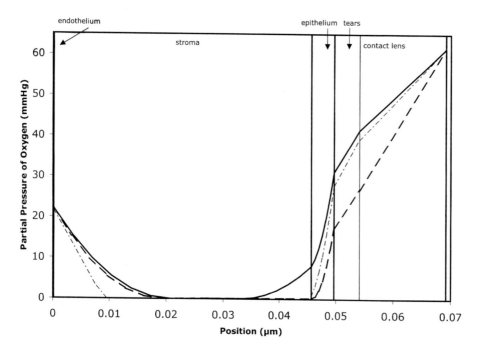

FIG. 3.4. Plots of oxygen tension distribution using the calculation and parameters of Harvitt and Bonanno (66) for avoiding epithelial edema (Dk/t = 89; *dash-dotted line*), with correction setting oxygen consumption to zero when oxygen tension equals zero *(dashed line)* for Dk/t of 89 *(solid line)* and to avoid epithelial anoxia *(broken line, Dk/t = 47)*.

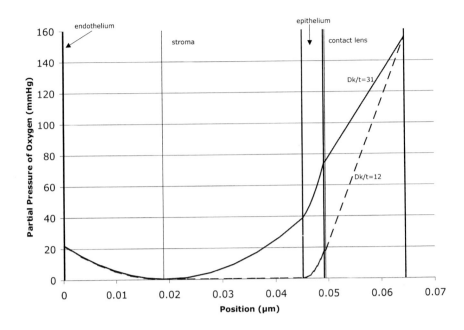

FIG. 3.5. Corneal oxygen tension profile for open eye with Dk/t = 31 and 12. The acidosis correction is switched on. Endothelial, stromal, epithelial, and tear layer thicknesses are 1.5, 450, 40, and 3 μm, respectively.

most tissues and, in the cornea, the apparent conversion to glycolytic pathways during hypoxia.

Models of steady-state oxygen distribution enable a comprehensive picture of corneal oxygenation, providing the model is truly representative and the parameter estimates accurate. Model performance can be assessed by comparison with empirical data where snapshots of the profiles are measured. Figure 3.9 plots anterior corneal oxygen tension versus lens Dk/t for open and closed eye as predicted by the oxygen diffusion model against some human and rabbit eye

empirical data (9,165,180). The model and EOP technique provide similar estimates for the open-eye condition. There is modest agreement between the profile model and EOP technique estimates for the closed eye (9). The phosphorescent dye technique yields values that are considerably smaller for both open- and closed-eye situations (165,180). The reason for the disparity between model predicted values and empirically derived phosphorescent technique values is not immediately apparent. It is unlikely that the difference can be explained by incorrect Dk/t measurements, as the

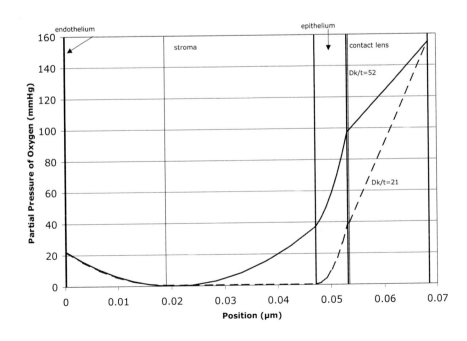

FIG. 3.6. Corneal oxygen tension profile for open eye with Dk/t = 52 and 21. The acidosis correction is switched on. Endothelial, stromal, epithelial, and tear layer thicknesses are 1.5, 470, 60, and 3 μm, respectively.

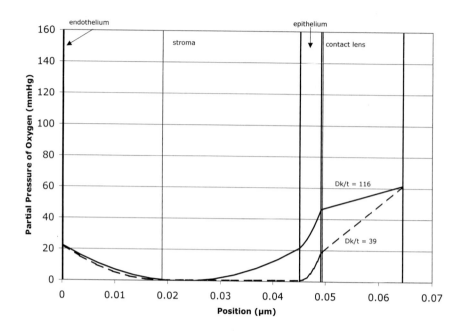

FIG. 3.7. Corneal oxygen tension profile for closed eye with Dk/t = 116 and 39. The acidosis correction is switched on. Endothelial, stromal, epithelial, and tear layer thicknesses are 1.5, 450, 40, and 3 μm, respectively.

results across a range of Dk/t values using both the rabbit and human eyes show consistency. Inaccuracies in boundary layer measures are a potential source of error, but the anterior oxygen tension under the closed lid has been measured many times using the polarographic technique with consistent findings, and error in the estimate of the posterior corneal oxygen tension would not have a dramatic effect on predicted values. If the dye technique values were correct, then the most obvious explanation would be an underesti-

mation in the consumption rate of the cornea. In order to generate oxygen tension values of the order of those presented here, we calculated that the consumption rate should be increased by 6.2 times for the closed eye and 3.6 times for the open eye. If oxygen consumption were truly this high, then a substantial part of the cornea would be anoxic when the eye is open in the absence of contact lens wear. Wear of any contact lenses under open- or closed-eye conditions would lead to predicted widespread anoxia within the

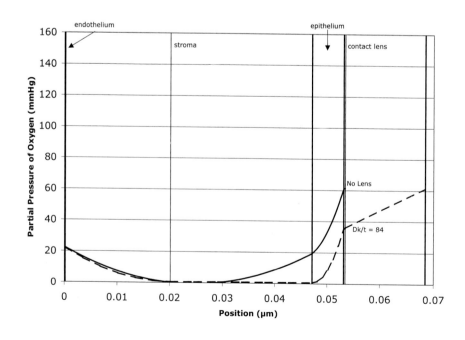

FIG. 3.8. Corneal oxygen tension profile for closed eye with no lens and Dk/t = 84. The acidosis correction is switched on. Endothelial, stromal, epithelial, and tear layer thicknesses are 1.5, 470, 60, and 3 μm, respectively.

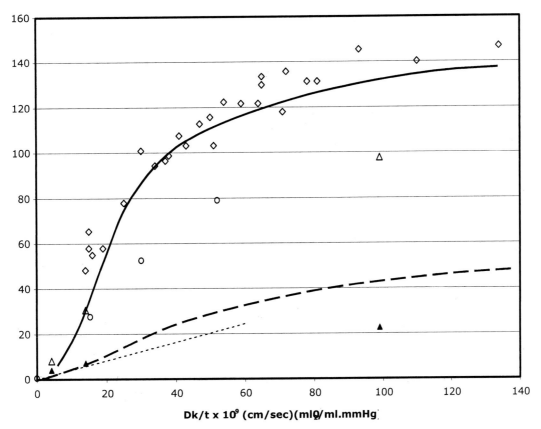

FIG. 3.9. Various estimates of anterior corneal oxygen tension versus contact lens Dk/t. Key to the studies: *diamonds,* Benjamin (179), open eye; *open triangles,* Bonanno (165), open eye; *closed triangles,* Bonanno et al. (165), closed eye: *circles,* Harvitt and Bonanno (180); *solid line,* Brennan (unpublished data), open eye; *broken line,* Brennan (unpublished data), closed eye; *dotted line,* Ang and Efron (9).

cornea. Further research is needed to elucidate the apparent discrepancy between model predictions and phosphorescent dye measurements.

CRITICAL VALUES

The section on cellular response to hypoxia discusses the difficulty of determining a critical oxygen value. There is a mismatch between what is capable of being measured versus what is functionally critical. And what constitutes compromise? Corneal researchers frequently have been restricted to measuring changes in structure; however, these changes may not directly bear on tissue function. For example, considerable attention has been devoted to the assessment of corneal edema, yet there is no direct evidence suggesting that small-to-moderate amounts of edema and related events compromise corneal integrity in the long term.

Conversely, changes in some aspect of corneal function that we are currently unable to detect may have serious consequences. An illustration of this is our inability to detect

a priori those patients who are at risk for developing corneal infection during contact lens wear. Despite strong circumstantial evidence linking hypoxia to susceptibility with infection, we currently do not have the techniques available to determine the point at which hypoxic stress renders the cornea vulnerable. With regard to corneal tissue, the problem of defining a critical oxygen requirement entails the additional feature of the level at which the criterion is defined, that is, should it be expressed as total consumption, anterior oxygen flux, anterior oxygen tension, or lens Dk/t? The most commonly used parameters for determining the critical oxygen requirement are the lens Dk/t and anterior corneal oxygen tension below which certain changes in structure or function may be measured. Tables 3.2 and 3.3 list some examples of criteria that have been determined using these parameters (118,128,156,195–209).

The Harvitt–Bonanno criterion of positive pO_2 values throughout the cornea represents an appealing standard, given the fact that-even if a tissue oxygen tension of 4 mm or so is needed—this will make modest difference to the oxygen diffusion model; however, further research is neces-

TABLE 3.2. ESTIMATES OF THE MINIMUM ANTERIOR CORNEAL OXYGEN TENSION REQUIRED TO PREVENT THE SPECIFIED CHANGES TO VARIOUS CORNEAL LAYERS

Author	Year	Criterion	pO_2 (mm Hg)
Epithelium			
Fatt and Bieber (156)	1968	Oxygen flux	20
Uniacke et al. (53)	1972	Thickness	37
Uniacke et al. (53)	1972	Glycogen depletion	37
Uniacke et al. (53)	1972	LDH concentration	37
Hill et al. (54)	1974	SDH reactivity	37
Millodot and O'Leary (109)	1980	Touch sensitivity	>57
Hamano et al. (55)	1983	Lactate	<98
Hamano et al. (55)	1983	Mitosis	<98
Masters (200)	1984	Mitochondria	>74
Benjamin and Hill (202)	1985	Oxygen flux	116
Mauger and Hill (206)	1992	Epithelial healing	77
Stroma			
Polse and Mandell (195)	1971	Corneal edema	11–19
Carney (196)	1974	Corneal edema	15
Mandell and Farrell (197)	1980	Corneal edema	23
Mizutani et al. (198)	1983	Corneal edema	111
Holden et al. (199)	1984	Corneal edema	75
Brennan et al. (204)	1987	Corneal edema (gas)	81
Brennan et al. (204)	1987	Corneal edema (EOP)	133
Endothelium			
Williams (128)	1986	Bleb response	123

EOP, equivalent oxygen percentage; LDH, lactate dehydrogenase; SDH, succinate dehydrogenase.

sary to refine the diffusion model to the extent that it will allow meaningful estimation of critical oxygen levels.

Recently, three separate investigations have reported a critical Dk/t of 125 to prevent hypoxic changes, and these deserve some discussion.

Papas (122) investigated the degree to which limbal in-jection is affected by lens Dk/t during open eye soft lens wear in 1998. The mean peripheral Dk/t required to prevent a change in limbal redness was determined to be 125, with 95% confidence intervals ranging from 56 to 274. The procedure to determine the critical Dk/t to prevent this vascular response can be approached from a number of angles. It is

TABLE 3.3. ESTIMATES OF CRITICAL OXYGEN TRANSMISSIBILITY TO AVOID CONTACT LENS-INDUCED CORNEAL CHANGES

Author	Year	Criterion	Dk/t
Holden et al. (199)	1984	Zero day-wear edema	24
Holden et al. (199)	1984	Zero residual O/N edema	34
Holden et al. (199)	1984	Closed-eye edema	87
O'Neal et al. (201)	1984	Closed-eye edema	75
Andrasko (203)	1986	Closed-eye edema	159
Ichijima et al. (205)	1992	Epithelial cells	64
Tsubota and Laing (207)	1992	PN/Fp ratio	59
Imayasu et al. (208)	1993	LDH, MDH	64
Giasson and Bonanno (118)	1994	Aqueous pH	18
Giasson and Bonanno (118)	1994	Epithelial pH	300
Ichijima et al. (209)	1994	LDH	84
Papas (122)	1998	Open-eye limbal injection	125
Harvitt and Bonanno (66)	1999	Oxygen profile modeling	125
Sweeney et al. (126)	2000	Closed-eye edema	125
Brennan and Coles (unpublished data)	2003	Closed-eye edema	300

Fp, flavoprotein; LDH, lactate dehydrogenase; MDH, malate dehydrogenase; O/N, overnight; PN, pyridine nucelotide.

noteworthy that the highest peripheral Dk/t value used by Papas was 71, meaning that extrapolation beyond the range of lenses tested was necessary to derive his result. There was no allowance for whether the mechanical presence of a lens *per se* might have an effect, although it is difficult to immediately foresee how such an allowance could be made. Papas used data for the inferior region of the cornea to estimate the critical Dk/t to prevent the vascular response. Although the inferior region may have shown the greatest response in his experiment, it is not clear whether this was a random event, how lower lid presence and associated lid problems might interact with lens wear in the induction of the limbal response, and how the selection of the worst case scenario interplays with the criterion. Despite these experimental challenges, this result has important consequences for negative power lenses. Dk/t values typically are quoted for central lens thickness. The periphery of myopic prescription lenses may be considerably thicker than central values, resulting in a high point-to-point loss of Dk/t (in the article by Papas, Dk/t in the periphery was reduced by as much as 80% in one lens). This result is significant because stem cells, which are the source of new corneal epithelial cells, are believed to exist only at the limbus. Hypoxic damage to stem cells may have serious long-term consequences for corneal health.

As previously discussed, Harvitt and Bonanno incorporated a correction for altered corneal oxygen consumption with varying degrees of corneal acidosis into an oxygen profile model in 1999. They concluded that Dk/t values of 84 and 125 were required to prevent epithelial and stromal anoxia, respectively. However, these results should be interpreted with caution. As detailed earlier, there are some deficiencies in their model, including use of nonrepresentative values for some of the layers. Figures 3.5 through 3.8 show the effect of alterations to their models on critical Dk/t values. To further illustrate the degree that errors in estimating layer thickness will have on critical Dk/t values, a simple resistors-in-series equation can be used for the estimate required to prevent stromal edema (210). A tear layer with Dk of 75×10^{-11} (cm^2/s) $(mL\ O_2/mL \bullet mm\ Hg)$ and thickness of 45 μm (as suggested by Harvitt and Bonanno) provides close to the same resistance to oxygen flow as would a lens with Dk/t of 125. In combination, a lens of this Dk/t, listed as their criterion to avoid corneal hypoxia, plus a tear layer thickness of 45 μm will provide the same resistance as a tear layer thickness of 3 μm plus a lens of Dk/t of 80. Thus, simply substituting a more appropriate tear layer thickness for a soft lens alters the minimum Dk/t estimate by a substantial amount, demonstrating further the vagaries involved in determining an oxygen criterion.

Sweeney et al. (126) reevaluated the famous Holden-Mertz criterion (178) in 2000. Holden and Mertz originally measured overnight corneal swelling of 10 subjects wearing lenses of differing Dk/t values. They calculated that a Dk/t of 87 was required to prevent overnight corneal swelling in

excess of 4%, which was the contemporaneous estimate of the amount of swelling that occurred overnight without a lens in place. Sweeney and co-workers argued that this estimate of overnight swelling may have been high and used data from La Hood et al. (211), who had found normal overnight swelling to be 3.2%. Using the original data of Holden and Mertz, Sweeney et al. calculated the minimum Dk/t to prevent edema beyond 3.2% was 125. However, deficiencies in the original Holden–Mertz methodology remain. The range of lenses was restricted with only one test lens having a Dk/t greater than 40, making interpretation outside of this range somewhat speculative. Standards for Dk/t measurement had not been written, leading to potential inaccuracy of the Dk/t estimates of lenses used in that study. The criterion then hinges to a large extent upon the mean swelling for the one lens with a Dk/t greater than 40 used in the study. These criticisms should not detract from the impact of the Holden–Mertz criteria on focusing the efforts of industry on the problem of hypoxia with contact lens wear.

Brennan and Coles (2003, *unpublished data*) repeated the Holden–Mertz experiment, extending the range of Dk/t values from which to estimate this critical oxygen requirement by using a hydrogel (Dk/t = 20), two silicone-hydrogels (Dk/t = 110 and 175), and a silicone elastomer (Dk/t = 265). Group mean overnight swelling in the absence of contact lens wear was 2.2%. The critical Dk/t to prevent overnight corneal edema in excess of that normally encountered without a worn contact lens was approximately 300.

The prediction of minimum oxygen criteria is prone to vagaries as demonstrated by the earlier discussion. The high degree of variation in estimates of the critical Dk/t adds weight to the Fatt notion that the Dk/t paradigm has limited utility, particularly when dealing with high Dk/t lenses such as silicone-hydrogels. We instead advocate an approach based on oxygen consumption similar to the theme of work by Bonanno and co-workers (66,70,165,212).

HOW DO CURRENT CONTACT LENSES MEASURE UP?

Although there are numerous laboratory and theoretical analyses of corneal physiology during contact lens wear, the ultimate proof of the role of hypoxia is in the clinical performance of contact lenses with high Dk/t. How do current contact lenses measure up in a clinical sense? Here we review reports of clinical experience with silicone-hydrogel lenses to assess the impact of hypoxia on corneal health.

Striae and Folds

As detailed earlier, increased corneal stromal thickness is the classic short-term physiologic response to hypoxia. Overnight corneal swelling is not, however, typically measured in practice because edema dissipates rapidly after awakening and pachymeters typically are not found in optometric practices. Slit-lamp examination of striae and folds can enable a rudimentary clinical assessment of edema levels (184). Silicone-hydrogel lenses produce significantly less evidence of striae than traditional hydrogels (92).

Microcysts

The microcyst response is the distinctive medium-term clinical indicator of corneal hypoxia (see earlier). High Dk/t lenses do not produce an appreciable microcyst response and produce significantly lower numbers of microcysts over a period of wear than do low Dk/t lenses (91,92).

Vascular Response

The relationship between Dk/t and limbal hyperemia was discussed in detail earlier. Numerous investigations demonstrate the manifestation of this effect in the clinical environment (92,123,125,213,214). In contralateral eye studies, where high Dk/t lenses are worn on one eye and low Dk/t lenses are worn on the other eye, differences in conjunctival injection are immediately apparent. In the only 3-year study of continuous wear of high Dk/t lenses to date, limbal injection was reduced compared to baseline levels with high Dk/t lenses (213). The likely scenario for the finding is a significant level of chronic limbal redness associated with daily wear of low Dk/t hydrogels prior to entering the study that subsided with wear of higher Dk/t lenses. There also are reports of lower levels of bulbar conjunctival hyperemia with wear of high Dk/t lenses compared to low Dk/t lenses (92, 124), although not all studies confirm this (126).

Vascularization of the cornea may be the most common change of pathologic significance during soft contact lens wear (215). Ordinarily it does not advance to an extent that compromises vision or further contact lens wear, but it has the potential to do so (121). Vascularization is more prominent in lower water content lenses for myopic correction (which have a lower peripheral oxygen transmissibility), during extended wear, with soft rather than rigid lens wear, and at the superior limbus, which is covered by the top lid, all implicating hypoxia as the vasogenic factor (121). Chan and Weissman found that hypoxia is a risk factor for corneal pannus, and this research is strongly supported by the finding of resolution of pannus following initiation of wear of high Dk/t silicone-hydrogel lenses (216,217). Clinical studies have found no evidence of vascularization with silicone-hydrogel lenses, whereas low Dk/t lenses induce measurable amounts in extended wear trials (125,126).

Refractive Error Changes

Nine months of extended wear of low-Dk/t lenses in adult myopes is associated with a small degree of myopic progres-

sion that appears to be reversible (218). The basis for this effect has not been clearly established but seems to be associated with small amounts of residual daytime edema. Wear of high Dk/t soft lenses generally has no impact on refractive error and may be associated with a small degree of central corneal flattening. There are anecdotal reports, however, of large refractive error changes when thicker silicone-hydrogel lenses, such as plus or higher minus powered lenses, are worn inside out.

Endothelial Effects

Wear of low Dk/t lenses has known long-term effects on corneal endothelial regularity (68,131,132,219,220). These effects can be discerned clinically. Endothelial morphologic changes may take years to develop, so it is not clear whether the use of silicone-hydrogel lenses will prevent changes in the endothelium. Bourne et al. (221) considered the impact of high Dk/t rigid lenses and found that endothelial changes still occurred. In studies where subjects wore silicone-hydrogel lenses for up to 9 months, Covey et al. (222) were unable to detect any clinical differences in endothelial morphology between these subjects and those who had not worn contact lenses.

Adverse Events

The performance criteria under examination showed that silicone-hydrogels, as expected, show superior performance from a corneal physiologic standpoint; however, it seems that noninfective complications, such as CLARE and CLPU, occur at about the same rate as with traditional hydrogel materials. The key to the success of silicone-hydrogels is to make an impact on the infection rate. Although anecdotal infections have been reported, in all of the clinical studies to date, there have been no cases of MK with silicone-hydrogel extended wear. Holden et al. (146) suggests that the incidence of MK with silicone-hydrogel lenses may be as much as 20 times less than with traditional hydrogels in extended wear (146); however, a full epidemiologic study is required to verify this claim.

CONCLUSION

The study of oxygen usage in the body was revolutionized in the past decade by molecular biology investigations, which led to the discovery of HIFs and the pathway for genetic regulation during hypoxia. Corneal epithelium has a strong presence of IPAS, a protein that inhibits the action of HIFs and inhibits vascularization. Together with other research findings, this indicates that the cornea is relatively resilient to hypoxia. Nonetheless, a range of corneal changes occur during hypoxia, and the genetic regulation suggests that these are adaptational in nature.

Describing the degree of corneal hypoxia during contact lens wear has become problematic with the advent of high Dk/t lenses and the concept that Dk/t has largely outlived its usefulness. We advocate exploring the concepts in oxygen diffusion models as methods for more adequately quantifying differences between contact lenses. To this end, critical oxygen criteria should be based around oxygen flux and total oxygen consumption rather than Dk/t. Regardless of these conceptual arguments, silicone-hydrogel lenses appear clinically to fulfill corneal oxygen requirements during closed-eye wear and seem to have solved the problem of corneal hypoxia during contact lens wear.

REFERENCES

1. Gnaiger E. Bioenergetics at low oxygen: dependence of respiration and phosphorylation on oxygen and adenosine diphosphate supply. *Respir Physiol* 2001;128:277–297.
2. Fatt I. Steady-state distribution of oxygen and carbon dioxide in the in vivo cornea II. The open eye in nitrogen and the covered eye. *Exp Eye Res* 1968;7:413–423.
3. Efron N, Carney LG. Oxygen levels beneath the closed eyelid. *Invest Ophthalmol Vis Sci* 1979;18:93–95.
4. Isenberg S, Green B. Changes in conjunctival oxygen tension and temperature with advancing age. *Crit Care Med* 1985;13:683–685.
5. Chapman KR, Liu FL, Watson RM, et al. Conjunctival oxygen tension and its relationship to arterial oxygen tension. *J Clin Monit* 1986;2:100–104.
6. Mader TH, Friedl KE, Mohr LC, et al. Conjunctival oxygen tension at high altitude. *Aviat Space Environ Med* 1987;58:76–79.
7. Hoper J, Funk R, Zagorski Z, et al. Oxygen delivery to the anterior chamber of the eye: a novel function of the anterior iris surface. *Curr Eye Res* 1989;8:649–659.
8. Stefansson E, Peterson JI, Wang YH. Intraocular oxygen tension measured with a fiber-optic sensor in normal and diabetic dogs. *Am J Physiol* 1989;256[4 Pt 2]:H1127–H1133.
9. Ang JH, Efron N. Corneal hypoxia and hypercapnia during contact lens wear. *Optom Vis Sci* 1990;67:512–521.
10. McLaren JW, Dinslage S, Dillon JP, et al. Measuring oxygen tension in the anterior chamber of rabbits. Invest *Ophthalmol Vis Sci* 1998;39:1899–1909.
11. Obata T, Saito K, Iwasawa T, et al. Dynamic MRI of transcorneal dispersion of oxygen into the anterior chamber of human eye. *J Magn Reson Imaging* 1998;8:508–510.
12. Fitch CL, Swedberg SH, Livesey JC. Measurement and manipulation of the partial pressure of oxygen in the rat anterior chamber. *Curr Eye Res* 2000;20:121–126.
13. Saito K, Obata T, Hirono K, et al. MR in vivo imaging of oxygen suppression effect of soft contact lens on the human cornea. *Magn Reson Imaging* 2000;18:357–360.
14. Rolfe DF, Brown GC. Cellular energy utilization and molecular origin of standard metabolic rate in mammals. *Physiol Rev* 1997;77:731–758.
15. Wilson DF, Erecinska M, Drown C, et al. Effect of oxygen tension on cellular energetics. *Am J Physiol* 1977;233:C135–C140.
16. Chance B, Quistorff B. Study of tissue oxygen gradients by single and multiple indicators. *Adv Exp Med Biol* 1978;94:331–338.
17. Wilson DF, Rumsey WL, Green TJ, et al. The oxygen dependence of mitochondrial oxidative phosphorylation measured by a new optical method for measuring oxygen concentration. *J Biol Chem* 1988;263:2712–2718.
18. Balaban RS. Regulation of oxidative phosphorylation in the mammalian cell. *Am J Physiol* 1990;258[3 Pt 1]: C377–C389.
19. Conley KE, Ordway GA, Richardson RS. Deciphering the mysteries of myoglobin in striated muscle. *Acta Physiol Scand* 2000;168:623–634.
20. Krumschnabel G, Schwarzbaum PJ, Lisch J, et al. Oxygen-dependent energetics of anoxia-tolerant and anoxia-intolerant hepatocytes. *J Exp Biol* 2000;203:951–959.
21. Leach RM, Treacher DF. The pulmonary physician in critical care c 2: oxygen delivery and consumption in the critically ill. *Thorax* 2002;57:170–177.
22. Harvitt DM, Bonanno JA. pH dependence of corneal oxygen consumption. *Invest Ophthalmol Vis Sci* 1998;39:2778–2781.
23. Semenza GL, Wang GL. A nuclear factor induced by hypoxia via de novo protein synthesis binds to the human erythropoietin gene enhancer at a site required for transcriptional activation. *Mol Cell Biol* 1992;12:5447–5454.
24. Wang GL, Semenza GL. Purification and characterization of hypoxia-inducible factor 1. *J Biol Chem* 1995;270:1230–1237.
25. Semenza GL. Physiology meets biophysics: visualizing the interaction of hypoxia-inducible factor 1 alpha with p300 and CBP. *Proc Natl Acad Sci U S A* 2002;99:11570–11572.
26. Wenger RH. Cellular adaptation to hypoxia: 02-sensing protein hydroxylases, hypoxia-inducible transcription factors, and 02-regulated gene expression. *FASEB J* 2002;16:1151–1162.
27. Hochachka PW, Rupert JL. Fine tuning the HIF-1 "global" O2 sensor for hypobaric hypoxia in Andean high-altitude natives. *Bioessays* 2003;25:515–519.
28. Huang LE, Bunn HF. Hypoxia-inducible factor and its biomedical relevance. *J Biol Chem* 2003;278:19575–19578.
29. Lando D, Gorman JJ, Whitelaw ML, et al. Oxygen-dependent regulation of hypoxia-inducible factors by prolyl and asparaginyl hydroxylation. *Eur J Biochem* 2003;270:781–790.
30. Ivan M, Kondo K, Yang H, et al. HIFalpha targeted for VHL-mediated destruction by proline hydroxylation: implications for O2 sensing. *Science* 2001;292:464–468.
31. Jaakkola P, Mole DR, Tian YM, et al. Targeting of HIF-alpha to the von Hippel-Lindau ubiquitylation complex by 02-regulated prolyl hydroxylation. *Science* 2001;292:468–472.
32. Lando D, Peet DJ, Whelan DA, et al. Asparagine hydroxylation of the HIF transactivation domain a hypoxic switch. *Science* 2002;295:858–861.
33. Webster KA. Evolution of the coordinate regulation of glycolytic enzyme genes by hypoxia. *J Exp Biol* 2003;206:2911–2922.
34. Makino Y, Cao R, Svensson K, et al. Inhibitory PAS domain protein is a negative regulator of hypoxia-inducible gene expression. *Nature* 2001;414:550–554.
35. Masters BR, Ghosh AK, Wilson J, et al. Pyridine nucleotides and phosphorylation potential of rabbit corneal epithelium and endothelium. *Invest Ophthalmol Vis Sci* 1989;30:861–868.
36. Esco MA, Wang Z, McDermott ML, et al. Potential role for laminin 5 in hypoxia-mediated apoptosis of human corneal epithelial cells. *J Cell Sci* 2001;114[Pt 22]:4033–4040.
37. Fonn D, du Toit R, Simpson TL, et al. Sympathetic swelling response of the control eye to soft lenses in the other eye. *Invest Ophthalmol Vis Sci* 1999;40:3116–3121.
38. Ladage PM, Ren DH, Petroll WM, et al. Effects of eyelid closure and disposable and silicone hydrogel extended contact lens wear on rabbit corneal epithelial proliferation. *Invest Ophthalmol Vis Sci* 2003;44:1843–1849.
39. Hochachka PW, Clark CM, Matheson GO, et al. Effects on regional brain metabolism of high-altitude hypoxia; a study of

six US marines. *Am J Physiol* 1999;277(Regul Integr Comp Physiol 46): R314-R319.

40. Kobrick JL, Zwick H, Witt CE, et al. Effects of extended hypoxia on night vision. *Aviat Space Environ Med* 1984;55: 191–195.

41. Vingrys AJ, Garner LF. The effect of a moderate level of hypoxia on human color vision. *Doc Ophthalmol* 1987;66:171–185.

42. Riley MV. Glucose and oxygen utilization by the rabbit cornea. *Exp Eye Res* 1969;8:193–200.

43. Mastropasqua L, Ciancaglini M, Di Tano G, et al. Ultrastructural changes in rat cornea after prolonged hypobaric hypoxia. *J Submicrosc Cytol Pathol* 1998;30:285–293.

44. Riley MV, Winkler BS. Strong Pasteur effect in rabbit corneal endothelium preserves fluid transport under anaerobic conditions. *J Physiol* 1990;426:81–93.

45. Sloan D. Another chapter in continuous contact lens wearing. *Contacto* 1965;9:19–22.

46. Bruce A, Brennan N. Corneal pathophysiology with contact lens wear. *Surv Ophthalmol* 1990;35:25–58.

47. Bruce A, Brennan N, Lindsay R. Diagnosis and management of ocular changes during contact lens wear, part 1. *Clin Signs Ophthalmol* 1995;16:2–11.

48. Bruce A, Brennan N, Lindsay R. Diagnosis and management of ocular changes during contact lens wear, part II. *Clin Signs Ophthalmol* 1995;17:2–11.

49. Efron N. *Contact lens complications,* 2nd ed. Oxford: Butterworth-Heinemann, 2004.

50. Smelser G, Chen D. Physiological changes in cornea induced by contact lenses. *Arch Ophthalmol* 1955;53:676–679.

51. Klyce S. Stromal lactate accumulation can account for corneal edema osmotically following epithelial hypoxia in the rabbit. *J Physiol* 1981;321:49–64.

52. Brennan NA, Efron N, Carney LG. Corneal oxygen availability during contact lens wear: a comparison of methodologies. *Am J Optom Physiol Opt* 1988;65:19–24.

53. Uniacke C, Hill R, Greenberg M, et al. Physiological tests for new contact lens materials. 1. Quantitative effects of selected oxygen atmospheres on glycogen storage, LDH concentration and thickness of the corneal epithelium. *Am J Optom Arch Am Acad Optom* 1972;49:329–336.

54. Hill R, Rengstorff R, Petrali J, et al. Critical oxygen requirement of the corneal epithelium as indicated by succinic dehydrogenase reactivity. *Am J Optom Physiol Opt* 1974;51:331–336.

55. Hamano H, Hori M, Hamano T, et al. Effects of contact lens wear on mitosis of corneal epithelium and lactate content in aqueous humor of rabbit. *Jpn J Ophthalmol* 1983;27:451–458.

56. Fullard RJ, Carney LG. Human tear enzyme changes as indicators of the corneal response to anterior hypoxia. *Acta Ophthalmol (Copenh)* 1985;63:678–683.

57. Ichijima H, Ohashi J, Cavanagh HD. Effect of contact-lens-induced hypoxia on lactate dehydrogenase activity and isozyme in rabbit cornea. *Cornea* 1992;11:108–113.

58. Bonazzi A, Mastyugin V, Mieyal P, et al. Regulation of cyclooxygenase-2 by hypoxia and peroxisome proliferators in the corneal epithelium. *J Biol Chem* 2000;275:2837–2844.

59. Bradley W, Schoessler JP. Corneal response to thick and thin hydrophilic lenses. *Am J Optom Physiol Opt* 1979;56:414–421.

60. Hirji NK, Larke JR. Corneal thickness in extended wear of soft contact lenses. *Br J Ophthalmol* 1979;63:274–276.

61. Lowther GE, Tomlinson A. Clinical study of corneal response to the wear of low water content soft lenses. *Am J Optom Physiol Opt* 1979;56:674–680.

62. Lebow K, Plishka K. Ocular changes associated with extended wear contact lenses. *Int Contact Lens Clin* 1980;7:49–55.

63. Schoessler JP, Barr JT. Corneal thickness changes with extended contact lens wear. *Am J Optom Physiol Opt* 1980;57:729–733.

64. Cox I, Zantos S, Orsborn G. The overnight corneal swelling response of non-wear, daily wear, and extended wear soft lens patients. *Int Contact Lens Clin* 1991;17:134–137.

65. Cornish R, Jaworski A, Brennan N. Overnight corneal swelling before and after 6 months of extended wear of high and low Dk hydrogel contact lenses. *Invest Ophthalmol Vis Sci ARVO Abstracts* 2001;42[Suppl]:Abstract 3168.

66. Harvitt DM, Bonanno JA. Re-evaluation of the oxygen diffusion model for predicting minimum contact lens Dk/t values needed to avoid corneal anoxia. *Optom Vis Sci* 1999;76: 712–719.

67. Farris R, Donn A. Corneal respiration with soft contact lenses. *J Am Optom Assoc* 1972;43:292–294.

68. Holden BA, Sweeney DF, Vannas A, et al. Effects of long-term extended contact lens wear on the human cornea. *Invest Ophthalmol Vis Sci* 1985;26:1489–1501.

69. Carney LG, Brennan NA. Time course of corneal oxygen uptake during contact lens wear. *CLAO J* 1988;14:151–154.

70. Bonanno JA, Nyguen T, Biehl T, et al. Can variability in corneal metabolism explain the variability in corneal swelling? *Eye Contact Lens* 2003;29[1 Suppl]: S7–S9.

71. Bergmanson J, Chu L. Corneal response to rigid contact lens wear. *Br J Ophthalmol* 1982;66:667–675.

72. Bergmanson J, Ruben C, Chu L. Epithelial morphological response to soft hydrogel contact lenses. *Br J Ophthalmol* 1985; 69:373–379.

73. Lemp MA, Gold JB. The effects of extended-wear hydrophilic contact lenses on the human corneal epithelium. *Am J Ophthalmol* 1986;101:274–277.

74. Tsubota K, Yamada M. Corneal epithelial alterations induced by disposable contact lens wear. *Ophthalmology* 1992;99: 1193–1196.

75. Tsubota K, Hata S, Toda I, et al. Increase in corneal epithelial cell size with extended wear soft contact lenses depends on continuous wearing time. *Br J Ophthalmol* 1996;80:144–147.

76. Yamamoto K, Ladage PM, Ren DH, et al. Effects of low and hyper Dk rigid gas permeable contact lenses on Bcl-2 expression and apoptosis in the rabbit corneal epithelium. *CLAO J* 2001; 27:137–143.

77. Cavanagh HD, Ladage PM, Li SL, et al. Effects of daily and overnight wear of a novel hyper oxygen-transmissible soft contact lens on bacterial binding and corneal epithelium: a 13-month clinical trial. *Ophthalmology* 2002;109:1957–1969.

78. Li L, Ren DH, Ladage PM, et al. Annexin V binding to rabbit corneal epithelial cells following overnight contact lens wear or eyelid closure. *CLAO J* 2002;28:48–54.

79. Ren DH, Yamamoto K, Ladage PM, et al. Adaptive effects of 30-night wear of hyper-O transmissible contact lenses on bacterial binding and corneal epithelium: a 1-year clinical trial. *Ophthalmology* 2002;109:27–39; discussion 40.

80. Yamamoto K, Ladage PM, Ren DH, et al. Effect of eyelid closure and overnight contact lens wear on viability of surface epithelial cells in rabbit cornea. *Cornea* 2002;21:85–90.

81. Ladage PM, Jester JV, Petroll WM, et al. Vertical movement of epithelial basal cells toward the corneal surface during use of extended-wear contact lenses. *Invest Ophthalmol Vis Sci* 2003; 44:1056–1063.

82. Perez JG, Meijome JM, Jalbert I, et al. Corneal epithelial thinning profile induced by long-term wear of hydrogel lenses. *Cornea* 2003;22:304–307.

83. Wilson G. The effect of hypoxia on the shedding rate of the corneal epithelium. *Curr Eye Res* 1994;13:409–413.

84. Stapleton F, Kasses S, Bolis S, et al. Short term wear of high Dk soft contact lenses does not alter corneal epithelial cell size or viability. *Br J Ophthalmol* 2001;85:143–146.

85. Alharbi A, Swarbrick HA. The effects of overnight orthokeratol-

ogy lens wear on corneal thickness. *Invest Ophthalmol Vis Sci* 2003;44:2518–2523.

86. Tripathi R, Bron A. Cystic disorders of the corneal epithelium. II. Pathogenesis. *Br J Ophthalmol* 1973;57:376–390.

87. Zantos S. Cystic formations in the corneal epithelium during extended wear of contact lenses. *Int Contact Lens Clin* 1983; 10:128–146.

88. Kenyon E, Polse KA, Seger RG. Influence of wearing schedule on extended-wear complications. *Ophthalmology* 1986;93: 231–236.

89. Holden BA, Sweeney DF. The significance of the microcyst response: a review. *Optom Vis Sci* 1991;68:703–707.

90. Holden BA, La Hood D, Sweeney DF. Prediction of extended wear microcyst response on the basis of mean overnight corneal response in an unrelated sample of non-wearers. *Am J Optom Physiol Opt* 1987;64[Suppl]:83.

91. Keay L, Sweeney DF, Jalbert I, et al. Microcyst response to high Dk/t silicone hydrogel contact lenses. *Optom Vis Sci* 2000;77: 582–585.

92. Brennan NA, Coles M-LC, Levy B, et al. One-year prospective clinical trial of balafilcon a (Purevision) silicone-hydrogel contact lenses used on a 30-day continuous wear schedule. *Ophthalmology* 2002;109:1172–1177.

93. Jaworski A, Cornish R, Brennan N. The relationship between an individual's overnight corneal swelling and the microcyst response for a low Dk contact lens worn in extended wear. *Optom Vis Sci* 2001;78[Suppl] S197.

94. Hamano H, Hori M, Hirayama K, et al. Influence of soft and hard contact lenses on the cornea. *Aust J Optom* 1975;58: 326–336.

95. Bergmanson J. Histopathological analysis of the corneal epithelium after contact lens wear. *J Am Optom Assoc* 1987;58: 812–818.

96. Madigan MC, Holden BA. Reduced epithelial adhesion after extended contact lens wear correlates with reduced hemidesmosome density in cat cornea. *Invest Ophthalmol Vis Sci* 1992;33: 314–323.

97. O'Leary D, Millodot M. Abnormal epithelial fragility in diabetes and in contact lens wear. *Acta Ophthalmol* 1981;59: 827–833.

98. Madigan M, Holden B, Kwok L. Extended wear of contact lenses can compromise corneal epithelial adhesion. *Curr Eye Res* 1987;6:1257–1260.

99. Boets E, van Best J, Boot J, et al. Corneal epithelial permeability and daily contact lens wear as determined by fluorophotometry. *Curr Eye Res* 1988;7:511–514.

100. Schurmans LR, Boets EP, van Best JA. Corneal epithelial permeability during extended wear of disposable contact lenses versus daily wear of soft contact lenses. *Br J Ophthalmol* 1995;79: 350–353.

101. McNamara NA, Fusaro RE, Brand RJ, et al. Epithelial permeability reflects subclinical effects of contact lens wear. *Br J Ophthalmol* 1998;82:376–381.

102. McNamara NA, Polse KA, Fukunaga SA, et al. Soft lens extended wear affects epithelial barrier function. *Ophthalmology* 1998;105:2330–2335.

103. McNamara NA, Chan JS, Han SC, et al. Effects of hypoxia on corneal epithelial permeability. *Am J Ophthalmol* 1999;127: 153–157.

104. Lin MC, Graham AD, Fusaro RE, et al. Impact of rigid gas-permeable contact lens extended wear on corneal epithelial barrier function. *Invest Ophthalmol Vis Sci* 2002;43:1019–1024.

105. Millodot M. Effect of soft lenses on corneal sensitivity. *Acta Ophthalmol* 1974;52:603–608.

106. Millodot M. Effect of hard contact lenses on corneal sensitivity and thickness. *Acta Ophthalmol* 1975;53:576–584.

107. Millodot M. Effect of length of wear of contact lenses on corneal sensitivity. *Acta Ophthalmol* 1976;54:721–730.

108. Millodot M. Effect of long term wear of hard contact lenses on corneal sensitivity. *Arch Ophthal* 1978;96:1225–1227.

109. Millodot M, O'Leary D. Effect of oxygen deprivation on corneal sensitivity. *Acta Ophthalmol* 1980;58:434–439.

110. du Toit R, Vega JA, Fonn D, et al. Diurnal variation of corneal sensitivity and thickness. *Cornea* 2003;22:205–209.

111. Patel SV, McLaren JW, Hodge DO, et al. Confocal microscopy in vivo in corneas of long-term contact lens wearers. *Invest Ophthalmol Vis Sci* 2002;43:995–1003.

112. Liu Z, Pflugfelder SC. The effects of long-term contact lens wear on corneal thickness, curvature, and surface regularity. Ophthalmology 2000;107:105–111.

113. Jalbert I, Stapleton F. Effect of lens wear on corneal stroma: preliminary findings. *Aust N Z J Ophthalmol* 1999;27:211–213.

114. Efron N, Perez-Gomez I, Morgan PB. Confocal microscopic observations of stromal keratocytes during extended contact lens wear. *Clin Exp Optom* 2002;85:156–160.

115. Kangas TA, Edelhauser HF, Twinning SS, et al. Loss of stromal proteoglycans during corneal edema. *Invest Ophthalmol Vis Sci ARVO Abstracts* 1988;29[Suppl]:215.

116. Bonanno J, Polse K. Effect of rigid contact lens oxygen transmissibility on stromal pH in the living human eye. *Ophthalmol* 1987;94:1305–1309.

117. Rivera R, Gan C, Polse K, et al. Contact lenses affect corneal stromal pH. *Optom Vis Sci* 1993;70:991–997.

118. Giasson C, Bonanno JA. Corneal epithelial and aqueous humor acidification during in vivo contact lens wear in rabbits. *Invest Ophthalmol Vis Sci* 1994;35:851–861.

119. Cohen SR, Polse KA, Brand RJ, et al. The association between pH level and corneal recovery from induced edema. *Curr Eye Res* 1995;14:349–355.

120. Tomlinson A, Haas DD. Changes in corneal thickness and circumcorneal vascularization with contact lens wear. *Int Contact Lens Clin* 1980;7:45–56.

121. McMonnies C. Contact lens-induced corneal vascularisation. *Int Contact Lens Clin* 1983;10:12–21.

122. Papas E. On the relationship between soft contact lens oxygen transmissibility and induced limbal hyperaemia. *Exp Eye Res* 1998;67:125–131.

123. Papas EB, Vajdic CM, Austen R, et al. High-oxygen-transmissibility soft contact lenses do not induce limbal hyperaemia. *Curr Eye Res* 1997;16:942–948.

124. Dumbleton K, Richter DB, Simpson T, et al. A comparison of the vascular response to extended wear of conventional lower Dk and experimental high Dk hydrogel contact lenses. *Optom Vis Sci* 1998;75[Suppl]:170.

125. Dumbleton KA, Chalmers RL, Richter DB, et al. Vascular response to extended wear of hydrogel lenses with high and low oxygen permeability. *Optom Vis Sci* 2001;78:147–151.

126. Sweeney DF, Keay L, Jalbert I, et al. *Clinical performance of silicone hydrogel lenses.* In: Sweeney DF, ed. *Silicone hydrogels: the rebirth of continuous wear contact lenses.* Oxford: Butterworth-Heinemann, 2000:90–149.

127. Holden BA, Williams L, Zantos S. The etiology of transient endothelial changes in the human cornea. *Invest Ophthalmol Vis Sci* 1985;26:1354–1359.

128. Williams L. *Transient endothelial changes in the in vivo human cornea.* PhD thesis University of New South Wales, 1986.

129. Ang JHB, Efron N. Carbon dioxide permeability of contact lens materials. *Int Contact Lens Clin* 1989;16:48–58.

130. Schoessler J, Woloshak M. Corneal endothelium in veteran PMMA contact lens wearers. *Int Contact Lens Clin* 1981;8: 19–25.

131. Schoessler J. Corneal endothelial polymegathism associated with extended wear. *Int Contact Lens Clin* 1983;10:148–156.

132. Carlson KH, Bourne WM. Endothelial morphologic features and function after long-term extended wear of contact lenses. *Arch Ophthalmol* 1988;106:1677–1679.

133. Sweeney DF. Corneal exhaustion syndrome with long-term wear of contact lenses. *Optom Vis Sci* 1992;69:601–608.

134. Polse KA, Brand RJ, Cohen SR, et al. Hypoxic effects on corneal morphology and function. *Invest Ophthalmol Vis Sci* 1990;31:1542–1554.

135. Erickson P, Doughty MJ, Comstock TL, et al. Endothelial cell density and contact lens-induced corneal swelling. *Cornea* 1998;17:152–157.

136. MacRae S, Matsuda M, Shelland S, et al. The effects of hard and soft contact lenses on the endothelium. *Am J Ophthalmol* 1986;102:50–57.

137. Sweeney D, Holden B, Vannas A. The clinical significance of corneal endothelial polymegathism. *Invest Ophthalmol Vis Sci ARVO Abstracts* 1985;26[Suppl]:53.

138. O'Neal MR, Polse KA. Decreased endothelial pump function with aging. *Invest Ophthalmol Vis Sci* 1986;27:457–463.

139. Cohen SR, Polse KA, Brand RJ, et al. Stromal acidosis affects corneal hydration control. *Invest Ophthalmol Vis Sci* 1992;33:134–142.

140. McNamara NA, Polse KA, Bonanno JA. Stromal acidosis modulates corneal swelling. *Invest Ophthalmol Vis Sci* 1994;35:846–850.

141. Bourne W, Hodge D, McLaren J. Estimation of corneal endothelial pump function in long-term contact lens wearers. *Invest Ophthalmol Vis Sci* 1999;40:603–611.

142. Giasson C, Bonanno JA. Acidification of rabbit corneal endothelium during contact lens wear in vitro. *Curr Eye Res* 1995;14:311–318.

143. Brennan NA, Coles ML. Extended wear in perspective. *Optom Vis Sci* 1997;74:609–623.

144. Willcox MD, Holden BA. Contact lens related corneal infections. *Biosci Rep* 2001;21:445–461.

145. Brennan NA. Is there a question of safety with continuous wear? *Clin Exp Optom* 2002;85:127–140.

146. Holden BA, Sweeney DF, Sankaridurg PR, et al. Microbial keratitis and vision loss with contact lenses. *Eye Contact Lens* 2003;29[1 Suppl]: S131–S134; discussion S43–S44, S92–S94.

147. Solomon O, Loff H, Perla B, et al. Testing hypotheses for risk factors for contact lens-associated infectious keratitis in an animal model. *CLAO J* 1994;20:109–113.

148. Fleiszig S, Efron N, Pier G. Extended contact lens wear enhances Pseudomonas aeruginosa adherence to human corneal epithelium. *Invest Ophthalmol Vis Sci* 1992;33:2908–2916.

149. Imayasu M, Petroll W, Jester J, et al. The relation between contact lens oxygen transmissibility and binding of *Pseudomonas aeruginosa* to the cornea after overnight wear. *Ophthalmology* 1994;101:371–388.

150. Ren H, Petroll WM, Jester JV, et al. Adherence of Pseudomonas aeruginosa to shed rabbit corneal epithelial cells after overnight wear of contact lenses. *CLAO J* 1997;23:63–68.

151. Ren DH, Petroll WM, Jester JV, et al. Short-term hypoxia down regulates epithelial cell desquamation in vivo, but does not increase Pseudomonas aeruginosa adherence to exfoliated human corneal epithelial cells. *CLAO J* 1999;25:73–79.

152. Stoltz RA, Conners MS, Dunn MW, et al. Effect of metabolic inhibitors on arachidonic acid metabolism in the corneal epithelium: evidence for cytochrome P450-mediated reactions. *J Ocul Pharmacol* 1994;10:307–317.

153. Conners M, Stoltz R, Webb S, et al. A closed eye contact lens model of corneal inflammation. Part 1: increased synthesis of cytochrome P450 arachidonic acid metabolites. *Invest Ophthalmol Vis Sci* 1995;36:828–840.

154. Vafeas C, Mieyal PA, Urbano F, et al. Hypoxia stimulates the synthesis of cytochrome P450-derived inflammatory eicosanoids in rabbit corneal epithelium. *J Pharmacol Exp Ther* 1998;287:903–910.

155. Dumbleton K, Fonn D, Jones L, et al. Severity and management of CL related complications with continuous wear of high Dk silicone hydrogel lenses. *Optom Vis Sci* 2000;77[Suppl]:216.

156. Fatt I, Bieber MT. The steady-state distribution of oxygen and carbon dioxide in the in vivo cornea. I. The open eye in air and the closed eye. *Exp Eye Res* 1968;7:103–112.

157. Fatt I, Freeman RD, Lin D. Oxygen tension distributions in the cornea: a re-examination. *Exp Eye Res* 1974;18:357–365.

158. Fatt I, Ruben C. New oxygen transmissibility concept for hydrogel contact lenses. *J Br Contact Lens Assoc* 1993;16:141–149.

159. Harvitt DM, Bonanno JA. Oxygen consumption of the rabbit cornea. *Invest Ophthalmol Vis Sci* 1998;39:444–448.

160. Masters B, Falks, Chance B. In vivo flavoprotein redox measurements of rabbit corneal normoxic-anoxic transitions. *Curr Eye Res* 1982;1:623–627.

161. Greiner J, Kopp S, Glonek T. Nondestructive metabolic analysis of a cornea with the use of phosphorus nuclear magnetic resonance. *Arch Ophthalmol* 1984;102:770–771.

162. Freeman RD. Oxygen consumption by the component layers of the cornea. *J Physiol* 1972;225:15–32.

163. Weissman BA. Oxygen consumption of whole human corneas. *Am J Optom Physiol Opt* 1984;61:291–292.

164. Holden BA, Sulonen J, Vannas A, et al. Direct in vivo measurement of corneal epithelial metabolic activity using a polarographic oxygen sensor. *Ophthalmic Res* 1985;17:168–173.

165. Bonanno JA, Stickel T, Nguyen T, et al. Estimation of human corneal oxygen consumption by noninvasive measurement of tear oxygen tension while wearing hydrogel lenses. *Invest Ophthalmol Vis Sci* 2002;43:371–376.

166. Hill R, Fatt I. Oxygen uptake from a reservoir of limited volume by the human cornea in vivo. *Science* 1963;142:1295.

167. Haberich F. Quelques aspects physiologiques de l'adaptation des verres de contact. *Cahiers Verres Cont* 1966;11:1–8.

168. Jauregui MJ, Fatt I. Estimation of the in vivo oxygen consumption rate of the human corneal epithelium. *Am J Optom Arch Am Acad Optom* 1972;49:507–511.

169. Larke JR, Parrish ST, Wigham CG. Apparent human corneal oxygen uptake rate. *Am J Optom Physiol Opt* 1981;58:803–805.

170. Quinn TG, Schoessler JP. Human corneal epithelial oxygen demand—population characteristics. *Am J Optom Physiol Opt* 1984;61:386–388.

171. Fitzgerald J, Efron N. Oxygen uptake profile of the human cornea. *Clin Exp Optom* 1986;69:149–152.

172. Horton P. *Changes in selected physiological parameters of the human cornea with age.* MScOptom thesis University of Melbourne, 1989.

173. Brennan NA. A model of oxygen flux through contact lenses. *Cornea* 2001;20:104–108.

174. Rasson JE, Fatt I. Oxygen flux through a soft contact lens on the eye. *Am J Optom Physiol Opt* 1982;59:203–212.

175. Efron N, Carney L. Oxygen performance of contact lenses: a human eye model. *Int Contact Lens Clin* 1981;8:17–21.

176. Novicky N, Hill R. Oxygen measurements: Dks and EOPs. *Int Contact Lens Clin* 1981;8:41–43.

177. Fatt I, Chaston J. Relation of oxygen transmissibility to oxygen tension or EOP under the lens. *Int Contact Lens Clin* 1982;9:119–120.

178. Holden B, Mertz G. Critical oxygen levels to avoid corneal edema for daily and extended wear contact lenses. *Invest Ophthalmol Vis Sci* 1984;25:1161–1167.

179. Benjamin WJ. EOP and Dk/L: the quest for hyper transmissibility. *J Am Optom Assoc* 1993;64:196–200.

180. Harvitt DM, Bonanno JA. Direct noninvasive measurement of tear oxygen tension beneath gas-permeable contact lenses in rabbits. *Invest Ophthalmol Vis Sci* 1996;37:1026–1036.

181. 9913-1, IIS. *Determination of oxygen permeability and transmissibility by the Fatt method.* Geneva, Switzerland: International Organization for Standardization, 1996.

182. 9913-2, I. *International Standard, Optics and Optical Instruments. Contact Lenses: Part 2: Determination of Oxygen Permeability and Transmissibility by the Coulometric Method.* Geneva, Switzerland: International Standards Organization, 2000:1–11.

183. Fatt I. New physiological paradigms to assess the effect of lens oxygen transmissibility on corneal health. *CLAO J* 1996;22:25–29.

184. Brennan NA, Coles M-LC. Continuous wear. In: Efron N, ed. *Contact lens practice.* Oxford: Butterworrth-Heinemann, 2002:275–294.

185. Fatt I. The oxygen electrode: some special applications. *Ann N Y Acad Sci* 1968;148:81–92.

186. Fatt I, St. Helen R. Oxygen tension under an oxygen permeable contact lens. *Am J Optom Arch Am Acad Optom* 1971;48:545–555.

187. Lin MC, Graham AD, Polse KA, et al. Measurement of post-lens tear thickness. *Invest Ophthalmol Vis Sci* 1999;40:2833–2839.

188. Nichols JJ, King-Smith PE. Thickness of the pre- and post-contact lens tear film interferometry. *Invest Ophthalmol Vis Sci* 2003;44:68–77.

189. Wang J, Fonn D, Simpson TL, et al. Precorneal and pre- and postlens tear film thickness measured indirectly with optical coherence tomography. *Invest Ophthalmol Vis Sci* 2003;44:2524–2528.

190. Ladage PM, Yamamoto K, Ren DH, et al. Effects of rigid and soft contact lens daily wear on corneal epithelium, tear lactate dehydrogenase, and bacterial binding to exfoliated epithelial cells. *Ophthalmology* 2001;108:1279–1288.

191. Feng Y, Varikooty J, Simpson TL. Diurnal variation of corneal and corneal epithelial thickness measured using optical coherence tomography. *Cornea* 2001;20:480–483.

192. Wang J, Fonn D, Simpson TL, et al. The measurement of corneal epithelial thickness in response to hypoxia using optical coherence tomography. *Am J Ophthalmol* 2002;133:315–319.

193. Wang J, Fonn D, Simpson TL. Topographical thickness of the epithelium and total cornea after hydrogel and PMMA contact lens wear with eye closure. *Invest Ophthalmol Vis Sci* 2003;44:1070–1074.

194. Doughty MJ, Zaman ML. Human corneal thickness and its impact on intraocular pressure measures: a review and meta-analysis approach. *Surv Ophthalmol* 2000;44:367–408.

195. Polse K, Mandell R. Critical oxygen tension at the corneal surface. *Arch Ophthalmol* 1971;84:505–508.

196. Carney L. Central and peripheral corneal thickness changes during contact lens wear. *Contact Lens J* 1974;5:3–10.

197. Mandell R, Farrell R. Corneal swelling at low atmospheric oxygen pressures. *Invest Ophthalmol Vis Sci* 1980;19:697–699.

198. Mizutani Y, Matsutakah H, Takemoto N, et al. The effect of anoxia on the human cornea. *Acta Soc Ophthalmol Jpn* 1983;87:644–650.

199. Holden B, Sweeney D, Sanderson G. The minimum precorneal oxygen tension to avoid corneal oedema. *Invest Ophthalmol Vis Sci* 1984;25:476–480.

200. Masters B. Oxygen tensions of rabbit corneal epithelium measured by non-invasive redox fluorometry. *Invest Ophthalmol Vis Sci ARVO Abstracts* 1984;25[Suppl]:102.

201. O'Neal MR, Polse KA, Sarver MD. Corneal response to rigid and hydrogel lenses during eye closure. *Invest Ophthalmol Vis Sci* 1984;25:837–842.

202. Benjamin WJ, Hill RM. Human cornea: oxygen uptake immediately following graded deprivation. *Graefes Arch Clin Exp Ophthalmol* 1985;223:47–49.

203. Andrasko GJ. Corneal deswelling response to hard and hydrogel extended wear lenses. *Invest Ophthalmol Vis Sci* 1986;27:20–23.

204. Brennan NA, Efron N, Carney LG. Corneal oxygen availability during contact lens wear: a comparison of methodologies. *Am J Optom Physiol Opt* 1988;65:19–24.

205. Ichijima H, Petroll WM, Jester JV, et al. Effects of increasing Dk with rigid contact lens extended wear on rabbit corneal epithelium using confocal microscopy. *Cornea* 1992;11:282–287.

206. Mauger TF, Hill RM. Corneal epithelial healing under contact lenses. Quantitative analysis in the rabbit. *Acta Ophthalmol (Copenh)* 1992;70:361–365.

207. Tsubota K, Laing RA. Metabolic changes in the corneal epithelium resulting from hard contact lens wear. *Cornea* 1992;11:121–126.

208. Imayasu M, Moriyama T, Ohashi J, et al. Effects of rigid gas permeable contact lens extended wear on rabbit cornea assessed by LDH activity, MDH activity, and albumin levels in tear fluid. *CLAO J* 1993;19:153–157.

209. Ichijima H, Cavanagh HD. Effects of rigid lens extended wear on lactate dehydrogenase activity and isozymes in rabbit tears. *Cornea* 1994;13:429–434.

210. Fatt I, Chaston J. Measurement of oxygen transmissibility and permeability of hydrogel lenses and materials. *Int Contact Lens Clin* 1982;9:76–88.

211. La Hood D, Sweeney D, Holden B. Overnight corneal edema with hydrogel, rigid gas-permeable and silicone elastomer contact lenses. *Int Contact Lens Clin* 1988;15:149–152.

212. Nguyen T, Soni PS, Brizendine E, et al. Variability in hypoxia-induced corneal swelling is associated with variability in corneal metabolism and endothelial function. *Eye Contact Lens* 2003;29:117–125.

213. Coles M, Brennan N, Jaworski A, et al. Ocular signs and symptom in patients completing 3 years with silicone-hydrogel contact lenses in 30-day continuous wear. *Optom Vis Sci* 2001;78[Suppl]S201.

214. Malet F, Pagot R, Peyre C, et al. Clinical results comparing high-oxygen and low-oxygen permeable soft contact lenses in France. *Eye Contact Lens* 2003;29:50–54.

215. Cunha M, Thomassen T, Cohen E, et al. Complications associated with soft contact lens use. *CLAO J* 1987;13:107–111.

216. Chan WK, Weissman BA. Corneal pannus associated with contact lens wear. *Am J Ophthalmol* 1996;121:540–546.

217. Chun MW, Kageyama JY. Corneal pannus resolved with silicone hydrogel contact lenses: a case series. *Int Contact Lens Clin* 2000;27:170–174.

218. Dumbleton KA, Chalmers RL, Richter DB, et al. Changes in myopic refractive error with nine months' extended wear of hydrogel lenses with high and low oxygen permeability. *Optom Vis Sci* 1999;76:845–849.

219. Carlson KH, Bourne WM, Brubaker RF. Effect of long-term contact lens wear on corneal endothelial cell morphology and function. *Invest Ophthalmol Vis Sci* 1988;29:185–193.

220. Bourne WM. The effect of long-term contact lens wear on the cells of the cornea. *CLAO J* 2001;27:225–230.

221. Bourne WM, Holtan SB, Hodge DO. Morphologic changes in corneal endothelial cells during 3 years of fluorocarbon contact lens wear. *Cornea* 1999;18:29–33.

222. Covey M, Sweeney DF, Terry R, et al. Hypoxic effects on the anterior eye of high-Dk soft contact lens wearers are negligible. *Optom Vis Sci* 2001;78:95–99.

IMMUNOLOGY AND INFLAMMATION

CAROLYN G. BEGLEY AND
MICHAEL J. GIESE

The human body constantly defends itself against invading microorganisms coming from an often threatening external environment. The active protective mechanisms of the body can be divided into two major responses: the immune response and inflammation. This chapter outlines the basic principles of immunology (the study of the immune response) and inflammation, and the application of these concepts to the eye.

ESTABLISHMENT OF INFECTIOUS DISEASE

There are quite a variety of microenvironments in just the anterior half of the eye and its adnexa. The ocular surface is a seemingly vulnerable mucous membrane bathed in warm tears, whereas the external surfaces of the lids are protected by thick, keratinized skin. The cornea is avascular; therefore, it lacks direct cellular defenses provided through blood vessels. Conversely, the conjunctiva is highly vascular and reacts quickly to external stimuli. All of these potential microhabitats must be protected from foreign invasion and injury.

Microorganisms interact with their potential hosts in many different ways. Some microorganisms are part of the normal flora and cause no disease. Opportunistic pathogens are those that cause disease only when the immune system is compromised. Other microorganisms may be pathogenic but are controlled by the normal flora. If the local environment changes, such pathogens can produce serious infections and host damage. Some microorganisms, however, are very pathogenic and able to defeat many of the defenses described later. A successful microbial pathogen by definition invades a host, survives and multiplies, and then conveys itself to a new and susceptible host.

The basic steps involved in the development of an infection include encounter, adherence and entry, local proliferation and spread, and production of tissue damage.

1. *Encounter.* The host and pathogen must interact.
2. *Adherence and entry.* The pathogen must possess a mechanism to adhere to or colonize host cells and tissue. At-

tachment is mediated by host and microbial cell-surface receptors known as *adhesin molecules* (1). Pinocytosis or membrane fusion (passive mechanism), and phagocytosis (active mechanism) bring the antigen (Ag) into the cell for processing.
3. *Local proliferation and spread (dissemination).* The pathogen multiplies (at the site of entry or another site) and spreads to other cells.
4. *Tissue damage.* Damage is caused by toxins produced by the pathogen, by the host's response to the pathogen, or by a combination of these activities (2).

HOST DEFENSE

The body's defense mechanisms can be divided into innate (nonspecific) and adaptive (specific) resistance. Innate resistance includes the mechanical protection afforded by the skin, secreted antimicrobial chemicals in the tears, and direct attack by inflammatory cells. The innate response is rapid and similar each time the individual is exposed to a given foreign invader. It relies on mechanisms present before infection starts. Conversely, adaptive resistance is stimulated by exposure to a foreign invader and operates by memory. Once the body has been exposed to a given microorganism, it becomes primed to specifically recognize that agent at the next encounter. At a second exposure, the reaction is much faster and of a greater intensity. Vaccinations manipulate this response by priming the immune system by exposure to a harmless form of a microorganism. With true exposure to the pathologic form, the body swiftly neutralizes the invader. These two types of responses, innate and adaptive, are not mutually exclusive. They often are intertwined, forming a complex meshwork of protection against foreign invaders.

Immunity involves a set of three disease-resistant processes.

Anatomic and Physiologic Barriers

The skin, with its tightly packed layers of epithelial cells (those on the surface are keratinized), provides an effective barrier to the entry of most microorganisms. Sebaceous glands in the skin produce sebum, which consists of lactic and fatty acids that maintain a relatively acidic pH to inhibit the growth of most microorganisms. Mucous membranes of the respiratory, digestive, and urogenital systems are major entry ports for microorganisms and contain lymphocytes and accessory cells that generate specific immune responses when challenged with Ag. These areas of tissue are called mucosa-associated lymphoid tissue (MALT) and include Peyer patches and pharyngeal tonsils. The primary ocular tissues involved in mucosal defenses are the lacrimal gland and conjunctiva. The lacrimal gland is important in host defense because of its ability to produce and secrete defense substances, both specific (e.g., immunoglobulin [Ig]) and nonspecific (such as hormones and growth factors). The conjunctiva is involved in the ocular mucosal immune system through "conjunctiva-associated lymphoid tissue" [CALT] (3). The following cells have been reported in the conjunctiva: plasma cells, T lymphocytes, major histocompatibility complex (MHC) class II expressing epithelial cells, stromal and Langerhans cells in the epithelium, and lymphatic channels. These findings suggest that the conjunctiva plays a role in Ag processing, lymphocyte migration, and defense mechanisms. CALT is composed of specialized cells that preferentially phagocytize Ags and bring them to lymphoid nodules. The multiple nodules are packed with small- and medium-sized lymphocytes that are activated by the processed Ag.

The eye provides an excellent example of physiologic defenses. The bony orbit, lids, and lashes and their blinking all provide protection. Tears, by their washing action and the ability of mucus to entrap pathogens, remove many microbes (4). A number of antimicrobial substances also are found in tears. These include IgA [which is an antibody (Ab) secreted into the tears by the lacrimal gland (5)] lactoferrin, lysozyme, and complement (6–8).

Phagocytic Barriers

Phagocytosis is a form of endocytosis that involves the cellular uptake of material found outside the cell. Specialized phagocytic white blood cells, also called *leukocytes,* such as blood monocytes, neutrophils, and tissue macrophages, comprise a group of warrior-like cells that rush to the site of infection, ingest bacteria and small foreign particles, and release extracellular chemicals that attack invaders.

Inflammatory Barriers

The acute inflammatory response is a series of events that act to contain and destroy invading microorganisms. In an affected area, blood vessels dilate and their cell walls become permeable (which allows a massive influx of inflammatory cells and chemical mediators into the area). Phagocytic cells attack and ingest microorganisms, and several plasma en-

zyme systems aid in the defense and cause clotting of the blood (9).

Both innate and adaptive immunity rely heavily on leukocytes for their actions. An overview of these cells and their functions is presented here.

LEUKOCYTES AND THEIR FUNCTIONS
Granulocytes

Granulocytes are the body's first line of cellular defense and therefore the first cells to appear at a site of injury or infection. These cells, composed of neutrophils, eosinophils and basophils, are characterized by multi-lobed, indented nuclei and numerous cytoplasmic granules. Their primary role is to release cytoplasmic granules at the site of inflammation; neutrophils, however, are also especially important in phagocytizing Ags.

Polymorphonuclear Neutrophils

Polymorphonuclear neutrophils (PMNs) are quiescent cells in the circulation that, when activated, become actively phagocytic. They accumulate early in bacterial infections, attracted to the site of infection by chemicals released from bacteria as well as damaged host cells. A smear of pus from a bacterial conjunctivitis (Fig. 4.1) contains many neutrophils and necrotic tissue. Granules in the cytoplasm of PMNs contain potent chemicals and enzymes that degrade bacteria and other foreign cells during phagocytosis. These cells also can accumulate in nonpathologic conditions, such as under the eyelids during sleep. Figure 4.2 shows a transmission electron micrograph of a neutrophil collected from human tears just after the individual awoke in the morning. This overnight accumulation of neutrophils in the closed-eye state is thought to protect the eye from infection (8). The neutrophil shown in Figure 4.2A is in the process of surrounding and in Figure 4.2b is phagocytizing a bacterium, presumably a Gram-positive *Staphylococcus* (10).

During phagocytosis, membrane protrusions called *pseudopodia* reach out and wrap around foreign particles, eventually enclosing them in a cellular vesicle (known as a *phagosome*) as they are pulled into the cell. As the phagosome moves through the cell, it fuses with intracellular granules and a lysosome to produce a phagolysosome, in which killing and breakdown of the entrapped microorganism occurs. This process involves two generalized antimicrobial mechanisms: oxygen independent and oxygen dependent. The oxygen-independent system includes intracellular granules that are filled with antimicrobial substances: hydrolytic enzymes and defensins (cytotoxic peptides that form ion-permeable channels in bacterial cell membranes) (11,12). Foreign substances also cause the neutrophil to undergo a "respiratory burst" in which oxygen is consumed (therefore oxygen dependent) and converted to reactive metabolites

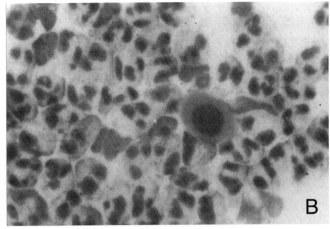
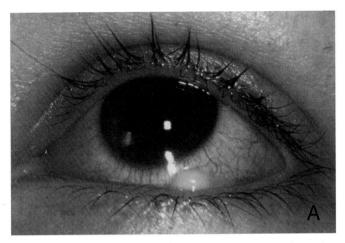

FIG. 4.1. **A:** Bacterial conjunctivitis with purulent discharge **B:** Smear of discharge using modified Wright stain. Note neutrophils with segmented nuclei. (Courtesy of Dr. Victor Malinovsky.)

(superoxide radical and hydroxide radicals). Superoxide can be converted to hydrogen peroxide, which reacts with other lysosomal chemicals in neutrophils to form very toxic compounds. All of these chemicals act to destroy the foreign particle, which is then "spit out" of the cell (exocytosed) along with the contents of the phagolysosome. The associated noxious chemicals can break down local tissue, forming the thick purulent exudate known as *pus.*

Polymorphonuclear Eosinophils

Polymorphonuclear eosinophils, like neutrophils, are phagocytic cells with granules in their cytoplasm. They are primarily tissue dwelling and, like neutrophils, are recruited to sites of inflammation.

One of their primary functions is to release their cellular contents into the extracellular environment when the foreign agent is too large for phagocytosis (such as parasitic worms) (13). The primary chemical released by eosinophils

during parasitic infections is called *major basic protein* (MBP), which binds to the parasite surface and disrupts cell membranes (leading to death) (14). Eosinophils are also active in allergic reactions, where Ag binding to IgE causes their activation and degranulation. Release of chemicals such as MBP can be toxic and may play a role in many allergic conditions. Shield ulcer formation in vernal conjunctivitis, for example, has been associated with eosinophil MBP (14). Eosinophils also release chemicals that inactivate compounds such as histamine and decrease granulocyte migration. Eosinophils therefore dampen the inflammatory response (15).

Polymorphonuclear Basophils and Mast Cells

This a heterogenous group of cells with many functions. Basophils and mast cells have large numbers of cytoplasmic granules that contain pharmacologically active substances.

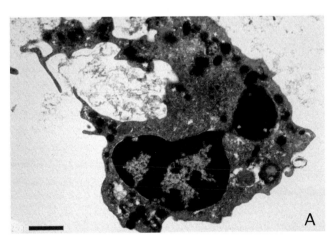
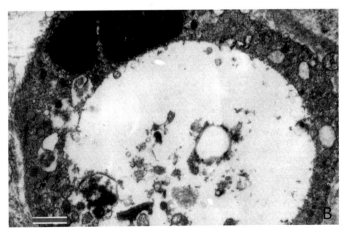

FIG. 4.2. Transmission electron micrograph of polymorphonuclear neutrophils (PMNs) collected from the eye upon awakening. **A:** PMN encircling debris. **B:** PMN phagocytizing a bacterium.

Blood basophils and tissue mast cells play an important role in allergies. Their degranulation causes the release of a number of inflammatory mediators, including histamine, prostaglandins, and leukotrienes (discussed later). Mast cells are found in a wide variety of tissues, including the skin, connective tissues, and mucosal surfaces such or the conjunctiva of the eye (16,17).

Mononuclear Cells

Highly specialized cells form the mononuclear phagocytic system that also functions in phagocytosis and intracellular degradation of foreign material. Monocytes circulate in the blood but differentiate into macrophages when they move into tissues.

Macrophages

Macrophages are morphologically large cells that are attracted to sites of acute inflammation after neutrophils. Their function is to phagocytize microorganisms and clean up necrotic tissue. Macrophages characteristic of various tissues are named according to the tissue. For example, histiocyte is another name for a macrophage that is permanently located in the connective tissue of many organs. Figure 4.3 illustrates a macrophage with phagocytosed debris in its cytoplasm. Phagocytosis by macrophages is similar to that of neutrophils, except that the lytic enzymes and antibacterial substances are not contained in cytoplasmic granules.

Macrophages are an important part of the overall immune response. They can wall off foreign Ags that cannot be managed by the immune system in any other way. When macrophages and dendritic cells phagocytize an Ag, it is broken down and products are expressed on their cell surfaces for recognition by lymphocytes. In this role, they function as Ag-presenting cells (APCs). This process is critical for initiation of the immune response (18). Macrophages also secrete biologically active substances such as complement proteins and other mediators of the inflammatory response, and they induce proliferation of T lymphocytes (19).

Lymphoid Cells

Lymphocytes (Fig. 4.4) are cells with large central nuclei; they comprise a population of cells that includes B, T, and null cells, all of which have different functions. B cells develop into plasma cells and secrete Abs. T cells have a variety of functions, which include recognition of foreign Ags, cytotoxicity, and stimulating B cells. The third class of lymphocytes are the natural killer (NK) cells, whose primary physiologic function is in host defense during viral infections. They also may be active in killing tumor and other foreign cells.

Lymphocyte subpopulations are morphologically identical but can be differentiated with the use of specific monoclonal Abs to characteristic cell surface protein markers. This classification system is called *c*luster of *d*ifferentiation and is denoted by the letters CD.

Lymphocytes circulate throughout the blood and lymphoid tissues, including lymph nodes and the spleen. Lymph nodes are bean-shaped structures packed with lymphocytes, macrophages, and dendritic cells. Other lymphoid tissues are more loosely aggregated, and many are components of MALT (previously discussed).

Plasma Cells

Plasma cells are terminally differentiated B cells that have been stimulated by Ag and other factors. When stimulated, B lymphocytes differentiate into effector cells, a subpopula-

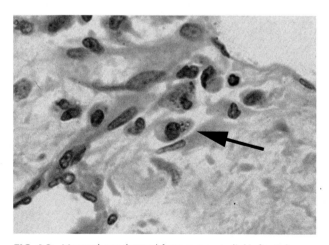

FIG. 4.3. Macrophage *(arrow)* from a myocardial infarct demonstrating phagocytosis of necrotic tissue.

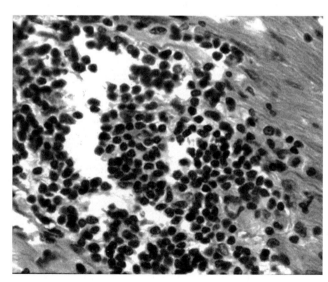

FIG. 4.4. Lymphocytes in a lymph node during acute appendicitis.

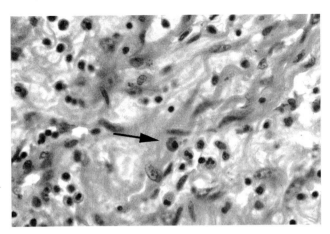

FIG. 4.5. Plasma cell *(arrow)* from a gastric ulcer.

tion of which mature into plasma cells. Plasma cells have eccentric nuclei that appear like wagonwheel spokes under light microscopy (Fig. 4.5). Plasma cells are generated at sites of an immune response and in lymphoid organs. They often migrate into the bone marrow where then can survive for long periods of time.

THE IMMUNE RESPONSE

As discussed earlier, the immune response is always present and adaptive in nature. Foreign molecules are recognized and the immune system stimulated to produce specific Abs or cells to mount an individual response. Production of Abs occurs due to the stimulation of B lymphocytes and is termed *humoral response* (alternatively, sensitization of T lymphocytes and macrophages produces *cell-mediated response*).

Antigens and Recognition of Self Versus Non-Self

In order for an immune response to occur, the body must first recognize a substance as foreign. A foreign substance is termed an *antigen* (Ag), and the degree to which an Ag can induce an immune response is referred to as its *antigenicity*. In general, large protein molecules are more antigenic, whereas small are less so. Small nonantigenic molecules may combine with a larger protein carrier (hapten-carrier complex), however, and become antigenic (e.g., thimerosal in contact lens solutions). Ags usually are foreign substances, but the body's own proteins may become antigenic with breakdown of the host ability to discriminate self from non-self. This leads to the generation of an immune response against self proteins and the development of an autoimmune disease.

How does the immune system of the human body recognize its own cells and keep them safe from internal attack? It does so through the recognition of specialized cell surface proteins, which are coded by genes in a large genetic locus called the *major histocompatibility complex* (MHC). In humans, these genes are located on the short arm of chromosome 6. Human leukocyte antigens (HLAs) are located within this gene locus and are subdivided divided into two basic gene groups known as *class I* and *class II*. Other MHC genes located within this locus code for complement components and are referred to as *class III* and *cytokines* (discussed later).

Class I MHC genes (HLA-A, HLA-B, HLA-C, HLA-E, HLA-F, HLA-G, HLA-H, and subclasses) code for proteins present on the surfaces of all nucleated cells in the body, including corneal epithelium, keratocytes, and endothelium. These genes are predominantly responsible for the recognition of self versus non-self. Graft rejection of foreign tissue occurs largely due to genes of the class I MHC, although both class I and II may be involved (20,21). Virally infected cells are recognized by T lymphocytes and later lysed because they express viral Ags in conjunction with class I proteins on their surfaces (22).

The class II region of the MHC (HLA-DP, HLA-DQ, HLA-DR) codes for proteins that modulate cell interactions during an immune response. Class II MHC molecules are expressed on APCs (such as dendritic cells, macrophages, and B cells). APCs first internalize Ags by phagocytosis or endocytosis, then display an Ag "piece" on the cell membrane bound to a class II MHC molecule. T cells then can "recognize" the foreign Ag to mount cell-mediated immune response (18,21). Because the MHC plays a central role in both humoral and cell-mediated immune responses, it has been used as a marker for a number of autoimmune diseases (e.g., HLA-B27 and uveitis) (23–25).

Antibodies

Five broad groups of Ig, have been identified in humans: IgG, IgA, IgM, IgD, and IgE. Igs consist of four polypeptide chains: two longer, "heavy" chains and two shorter, "light" chains, all covalently linked by disulfide bonds, and often schematically represented as a "Y." The top portion represents the variable region of the molecule and contains Ag binding sites. The remaining sequences are called the *constant region* and are essentially invariant. Cleavage of the Ig molecule with papain divides the Ab into two Fab fragments (Ag binding sites), the arms of the "Y," and the Fc fragment (crystallizable fragment), the stem of the "Y." The Fc fragment cannot bind with an Ag but contains effector sites that mediate functions common to a particular class of Ig.

Abs are produced by plasma cells that have differentiated in response to Ag activation. Each plasma cell is an "Ab factory," secreting a huge number of Ab. Abs in general function to bind Ags in all phases of the humoral immune response, but the five classes of Ig show different biologic functions determined by the structure of their Fc portion. Ig is distributed in biologic fluids throughout the body and on the surface of some cells. It is estimated that 10^8 or more different Ab molecules can be produced upon Ag stimulation (9).

Abs have a number of important functions in the inflammatory response. When Abs bind with an Ag at the site of infection, a cascade of protein evolution, known as the *complement pathway,* is initiated. Complement proteins attract inflammatory cells and may act directly to lyse bacterial cells. In addition, the presence of Abs and elements of the complement cascade on the surface of foreign cells makes them more readily phagocytized by macrophages (opsonization) or directly lysed by neutrophils or lymphocytes.

IgG comprises 80% of the total Ig in the body and is the principal Ab active against bacteria. It also passes through the placenta to the fetus and provides protective immunity to the newborn infant. About half of IgG is beneath epithelial surfaces and half in the serum. IgG enhances phagocytosis by coating foreign particles and binding to the Fc receptors of phagocytic cells, a process known as *opsonization.*

IgM accounts for approximately 5% to 10% of Ig in the serum. It is a large molecule composed of five "Y"s forming a pentamer linked by disulfide bonds. This increased size means that less IgM is needed to bind Ag compared to IgG. During the primary immune response (following initial Ag exposure), IgM is the first Ab class to be produced and the first Ab synthesized in neonates. IgM is very effective at "fixing" complement, greatly amplifying the immune response. IgM can be expressed on the surface of immature B lymphocytes (in conjunction with IgD) in addition to being actively secreted into the serum. When cells are activated, they develop into mature B lymphocytes (9).

IgD has a molecular weight slightly greater than IgA and is found in low concentrations in the serum. It functions as a receptor in B-cell development and in the activation of both B cells and lymphocytes.

IgA accounts for 10% to 15% of the total Ig in serum. It is known as the *secretory Ab* because it is found in mucous secretion and tears (5,26,27). Two IgA molecules bind to special receptors on mucosal epithelial cells and are transcytosed to the luminal cell surface. During this process, a secretory component is added, forming secretory IgA (sIgA). Secretory IgA inhibits viral adhesion and internalization; prevents bacterial adhesion and colonization; modulates the normal ocular flora; interferes with parasites; and reduces Ag-related damage to the conjunctiva and cornea. It prevents bacterial and viral adherence to the epithelia by binding to bacterial surface proteins (4) and may reinforce the mucus barrier by agglutinating pathogens to trap them in mucous threads and then flush them out of the system by either peristalsis or tear drainage.

IgE is both the "allergy Ab" and the primary Ab produced as a response to parasitic infections (9). It is present in very low concentrations in the serum and tears of normal individuals, but tear levels of IgE increase during atopic conjunctivitis (28). Most IgE in the body is bound to the surface of basophils and mast cells. When an allergic individual reencounters a specific Ag that binds to these molecules on mast cells, degranulation and subsequent release of vasoactive compounds (e.g., histamine) occurs. The consequences of this release include itching, coughing, lacrimation, and bronchoconstriction.

Ocular Immunoglobulins

The primary Ab involved in ocular protection is IgA (produced locally by lacrimal gland plasma cells). Secretory IgA, low levels of IgG (produced in lacrimal gland and derived from the serum), IgM (derived locally by lacrimal tissue), and IgE (origin unknown) all are found in the tears. IgA and IgG are found in similar concentrations in the central and peripheral zones of the cornea, whereas IgM is found only in the peripheral tissue. The ciliary body stroma contains all five Ab classes, whereas the pigmented and nonpigmented ciliary epithelium, iris, retina, and lens are Ab free (Table 4.1).

B Lymphocytes and Antibody Production

B cells mediate humoral immunity (the adaptive immune response mediated by Abs and the primary defense strategy against extracellular bacteria). These cells were so named because in birds they differentiate a cloacal pouch called the *bursa of Fabricius,* but B cells originate and mature in human bone marrow.

Each B cell is programmed to differentiate and produce specific Abs in response to exposure to a specific Ag. A large and constantly changing repertoire of appropriate Abs is necessary to adequately fight infection. What gives rise to this incredible Ab diversity and specificity?

The generation of Ab diversity is extremely complicated and beyond the scope of this chapter. In brief, however, the

TABLE 4.1. ESTIMATED LEVELS OF IMMUNOGLOBULINS IN THE EYE

Structure	Immunoglobulin (Protein Concentration [%] of Serum Level)	
	IgG	IgA
Sclera	10	5
Cornea	52	25
Conjunctiva	31	53
Choroid	38	30
Iris	1.0	—
Ciliary body	3	2
Retina	—	—
Aqueous	1.0	0.5
Vitreous	—	—
Muscles	12	10
Lens	—	—

process begins with the development of B cells in the bone marrow. During B-cell development, random rearrangements of Ig genes produce Ab specificity. Germline DNA contains multiple copies of variable region genes (V), joining region genes (J), and diversity genes (D). During B-cell maturation, deletion of intervening sequences between V and J, or V and D and J, causes "recombination" of genes (29,30), resulting in the transcription and translation of altered Abs and enhance diversity of possible Ab types. Following gene rearrangement, newly formed Igs are expressed on the B-cell surface as IgM or IgD, where they serve as Ag receptors. Although it is estimated that the bone marrow produces about 5×10^7 B cells per day in mice, only about 10% of these cells actually leave the bone marrow and enter the circulation. This is thought to be due to both negative selection and clonal deletion, which remove any B cells that express auto-Abs against self Ags in the bone marrow.

B cells circulate through the body after leaving the bone marrow, eventually entering lymph nodes and other secondary lymphoid tissues. Ags (e.g., viruses, bacteria) drain into or are carried to lymph nodes by APCs, where they stimulate specific B cells to differentiate and produce relatively low-affinity Abs of the IgM type. High-affinity Abs then are produced by hypermutation of B cells that bind to APCs in the lymph node. During a process called *affinity maturation,* a few B cells are preferentially selected for survival because they strongly bind to the Ag. Other lymph node cells that do not bind to the Ag eventually die. A miniature process of "natural selection" therefore occurs in the lymph node to produce Abs that provide a "best match" to the Ag (31–33).

Following production and selection of high-affinity Abs, a process of "class switching" from IgM and IgD to IgG, IgA, or IgE occurs (32,34) and Ab production moves into high gear. Some of the high-affinity cells will remain as long-lived memory cells following infection control. These cells activate quickly if the individual is reexposed to the same microorganism per Ag (35). This is why we do not suffer from the measles twice. A second encounter activates the memory cells to rapidly produce high-affinity, effective Abs.

The process of Ab generation requires "help" from activated T lymphocytes. Most protein Ags require this assistance by factors secreted by T lymphocytes, called *cytokines.* For example, interleukin (IL)-6 secretion by T helper cells promotes differentiation of B cells into plasma cells and thus stimulates further Ab production (Fig. 4.6).

T Lymphocytes: Cell-Mediated Immunity and Cytokines

Whereas B cells mediate humoral immunity, T cells form the basis of cell-mediated immunity. This form of immunity is an adaptive response that protects the host against intra-

cellular bacteria, viruses, and cancer, and it is important in graft rejection.

T lymphocytes comprise approximately 70% to 80% of the total lymphocyte population. Like B cells, T cells develop from stem cells in the bone marrow. T cells then circulate to the thymus where they mature and proliferate, hence their name.

All T cells possess membrane-bound receptors called *T-cell receptors* (TcR) that recognize Ag-bound MHC proteins to distinguish self proteins from foreign proteins. Developing T cells (thymocytes) acquire cell surface markers and become "educated" about self Ags by developing these receptors for self markers from the MHC.

"Naive" T cells (T cells that have not previously encountered Ag) circulate between the blood and lymphatics searching for their specific Ag. It is estimated that only 1 in 10^5 T cells "meets" its target Ag. Constant circulation increases the probability that a naïve T cell will encounter its specific Ag. The circulation time of naïve T cells throughout the blood and lymphatics is about 12 to 24 hours. During circulation, T cells reside in lymphoid tissues and lymph nodes, including ocular conjunctiva. T cells cannot recognize foreign Ags without the concurrent stimulation of accessory molecules. These include APC class I or II MHC molecules. In most cases, the APC is a macrophage. [As discussed earlier, macrophages phagocytize foreign proteins and present them in surface imbedded class I or II MHC molecules (9)].

T lymphocytes are subdivided into three functionally distinct populations: helper and suppressor (T_H), cytotoxic (also called *cytolytic;* T_c), and NK cells. All of these cells have different roles in the immune response.

Helper T Lymphocytes (T_H Cells)

T_H lymphocytes are restricted to recognizing Ags bound to class II receptors of the MHC. They are called T_H lymphocytes because they secrete cytokines that "help" other immune cells perform their functions (Fig. 4.6). These cells also express an accessory membrane glucoprotein molecule called *CD4* and are commonly referred to as *CD4⁺ cells.* The CD4⁺ subset of T cells comprises the majority of T cells in the thymus and 50% to 65% of peripheral T cells (9). T_H cells are activated by an Ag–class II MHC complex on an APC. Activation induces cell division giving rise to clones of T_H cells specific for the Ag. These cells then secrete cytokines (such as interleukins, interferon [IFN], and tumor necrosis factor), which increase the inflammatory response. The type of inflammatory response is based on the cytokines produced. Cells that produce IFN-γ, for example, produce a T_H1 response, and cells that produce IL-4 and IL-5 lead to a T_H2 response. Many cell types secrete cytokines, but those secreted by T_H cells influence or "help" all other types of immune and inflammatory cells, and promote Ab production.

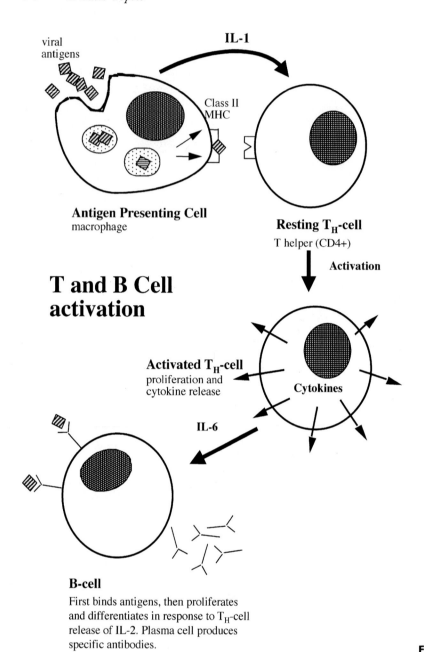

FIG. 4.6. T- and B-cell activation

Cytokines are low-molecular-weight glycoproteins that are not specific to any particular Ag, but they produce strong effects in minute quantities and can interact in a synergistic or antagonistic manner. They include ILs, tumor necrosis factors, IFNs, and a wide array of growth factors. Some cytokines attract PMNs and macrophages, and generally up-regulate the inflammatory response, whereas others act to dampen the response. Interleukins enhance macrophage function, increase expression of MHC molecules, promote B-cell maturation, and act as chemoattractants (Table 4.2). Interferons provide protection from viral infections by inactivating viral proteins and help to coordinate host defense mechanisms by influencing B lymphocytes. T_H lymphocytes secrete many cytokines, which gives them widespread chemical control over the immune system (9,36). They are very important in many ocular diseases because of their many inflammatory and antiinflammatory properties. Cytokines are involved in corneal would healing (growth factors), can induce corneal neovascularization, and are important in uveitis, keratitis, and corneal graft rejection. Cytokines also are involved in diabetic and other proliferative retinopathies, retinopathy of prematurity, in the formation of scar tissue after glaucoma surgery, and in the development of thyroid eye disease. It is likely that interactions between cytokines and inflammatory cells within the eye facilitate the development of many chronic ocular diseases.

The importance of T_H lymphocytes to the overall immune response is underscored by the devastating effects of

TABLE 4.2. SELECTED CYTOKINES AND THEIR BIOLOGIC ACTIVITY (9,36)

Cytokine	Secreted By	Major Biologic Functions
Interleukin-1 (IL-1α, IL-1β)	Monocytes, macrophages, dendritic cells, B cells, other body cells	Stimulates activation, maturation, and clonal expansion of B and T cells Increases expression of ICAMs
Interleukin-2 (IL-2)	T$_H$ cells	Stimulates proliferation of activated T cells Enhances activity of T$_C$ cells
Interleukin-3 (IL-3)	T$_H$ cells, NK cells, mast cells	Stimulates differentiation of bone marrow cells
Interleukin-4 (IL-4)	T$_H$ cells, NK cells, mast cells	Stimulates activation and proliferation of B cells Up-regulates class II MHC expression on B cells and macrophages Enhances phagocytic activity of macrophages Stimulates growth of mast cells
Interleukin-6 (IL-6)	Monocytes, macrophages, T$_H$ cells	Promotes B-cell differentiation into plasma cells Stimulates antibody secretion
Interleukin-8 (IL-8)	Macrophages, endothelial cells	Chemotactic attraction of PMNs Adherence to vascular endothelium and extravasation into tissue
Interleukin-10 (IL-10)	T$_H$ cells	Suppresses cytokine production by macrophages Down-regulates class II MHC expression
Interferon-γ (IFN-γ)	T$_H$ cells, T$_C$ cells, NK cells	Inhibits viral replication Enhances activity of macrophages Increases class I and II MHC expression Promotes cytotoxic functions by T$_C$ cells
Tumor necrosis factor (TNF–α, TNF–β)	T cells, macrophages, mast cells	Cytotoxic effect on tumor cells Induces cytokine secretion and phagocytic activity Causes cachexia (extensive weight loss) with chronic inflammation

ICAM, intracellular adhesion molecule; MHC, major histocompatibility complex; PMN, polymorphonuclear neutrophils.

the acquire immune deficiency syndrome (AIDS) epidemic. CD4+ T$_H$ lymphocytes are the main cell type infected by the human immunodeficiency virus. Loss or impairment of these cells leaves the patient severely immunocompromised and therefore highly susceptible to infection by a variety of bacteria, viruses, and fungi. This widespread chemical control over the immune system has led CD4$^+$ T$_H$ cells to be termed the "directors of the immunologic orchestra" (36).

Cytotoxic T Lymphocytes (T$_C$ Cells)

T cells that are positive for the cell surface molecule CD8$^+$ require activation by a class I MHC marker containing the appropriate Ag. These cells are termed *class I restricted*, as opposed to CD4$^+$ cells, which are *class II restricted*. They are important in fighting intracellular pathogens, and graft and tumor rejection (21). Because virtually all of the cells in the body express class I MHC molecules, T$_C$ lymphocytes can recognize and eliminate almost any altered body cell, but to perform this function, T$_C$ cells, like B cells, require cytokine "help" from T$_H$ cells (Fig. 4.7).

During viral infection, for example, effective defense is assisted by methods to recognize and eliminate infected cells. Subsequent attack of infected cells occurs via a "lethal hit," also known as the "kiss of death" (37). Virally infected cells express degraded viral Ags on their surfaces that act as a "red flag" to the immune system. T$_C$ cells recognize these viral Ags, along with class I MHC molecules. Upon binding, proteins (such as perforin) and several serine proteases (called *granzymes*) are released to lyse infected cells (the "lethal hit"). Some CD8$^+$ cells also suppress B-cell differentiation and Ab production, acting as a check to the overproduction of Abs (9).

Natural Killer Lymphocytes (NK Cells)

A third lymphocyte population can be defined by its lack of Ag receptors that distinguish other T or B lymphocytes. These cells are called *null cells*. Because null cells do not contain Ag-binding receptors on their cell surfaces, they are not specific for particular Ags. A subpopulation of this group of cells are granular lymphocytes that can nonspecifically kill or lyse virally infected or tumor cells. It is this population that are referred to as *NK cells*. NK cells do not need prior Ag interaction, although their killing mechanisms (granular exocytosis) are similar to those of T$_C$ lymphocytes. These cells are involved in the early response to infection (innate immunity) by viruses or intracellular bacteria while the Ag-specific T$_C$ lymphocyte response is developing. NK lymphocyte action is controlled by a balance of activating and inhibitory signals that allows the cells to distinguish healthy from infected or tumor cells. Normal levels of class I MHC expression on the cell surface override activation of NK cells to spare normal body cells (9).

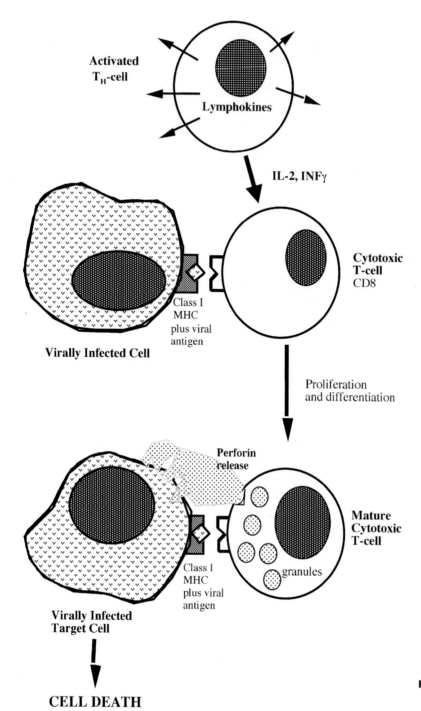

FIG. 4.7. Cytotoxic T-cell "kiss of death."

INFLAMMATION

With the immune response, the body first "learns" to recognize an invader or foreign Ag and then attacks it quickly on subsequent exposure. Conversely, inflammation is an innate response by which the body defends itself from infection and repairs damaged tissue. The inflammatory response does not require prior exposure to the offending organism to mount a fierce and effective counterattack. Although im-

mune and inflammatory responses are separated here for explanatory purposes, the two are infinitely interwoven *in vivo* to provide effective defense against invading microorganisms and tumors.

Inflammation can be divided into two main categories: acute and chronic. The acute inflammatory response is characterized by increased blood flow and vascular permeability in the affected area leading to infiltration by PMNs. Chronic inflammation often follows the acute phase and is typified by macrophages, lymphocytes, and scar formation.

Acute Inflammation

The primary purpose of acute inflammation is to increase blood flow in an affected area so that inflammatory cells, Abs, and chemical mediators of inflammation can attack, wall off, and destroy invading organisms. The clinical signs of inflammation were largely described by the ancient Greeks, who noted that inflammation was accompanied by *rubor* (redness), *tumor* (swelling), *calor* (heat), *dolor* (pain), and *functio laesa* (loss of function). Preseptal cellulitis (Fig. 4.8) demonstrates these signs, with redness, swelling, and ptosis due to loss of function. We also know from experience that the affected area feels warm to the touch, and that the patient experiences considerable discomfort.

Inflammatory signs of redness and heat are due to increased blood flow and vasodilation in the affected area. Blood vessels also become more leaky, and fluid moves into the extracellular space causing swelling and subsequent loss of function. Tissue swelling and chemical mediators act together to produce pain. The acute inflammatory response is of short duration and does not involve generation of a specific immune response.

Vascular Changes in Acute Inflammation

Under normal physiologic conditions, fluid flow across the blood vessel wall is regulated by Starling's Law, which describes fluid transport across the membrane as an interplay between two forces: i) intravascular hydrostatic pressure forcing fluid out of, and ii) osmotic pressure differential drawing fluid into, the vessel. Normally, hydrostatic forces are slightly greater so that there is a net movement of fluid out of the vessel, eventually drained by the lymphatics.

During acute inflammation, vascular changes alter this balance. First, a transient vasoconstriction of arterioles occurs at the site of injury, of seconds to minutes duration,

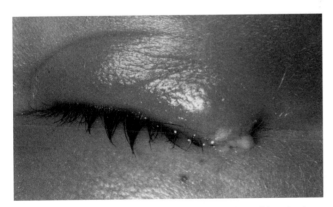

FIG. 4.8. Preseptal cellulitis secondary to infected hordeolum. (Courtesy of Dr. Victor Malinovsky.)

quickly followed by a profound vasodilation of the precapillary arterioles in the area. Vessels, especially postcapillary venules, become more permeable. Fluid, full of plasma proteins and ions, moves out of the vessel, shifting the direction of the osmotic pressure across the blood vessel wall. When this happens, both hydrostatic and osmotic pressure combine to force fluid out of the vessel, resulting in edema in the affected area.

Transient vasoconstriction is caused by both neurogenic and chemical mediators, but vasodilation and increase in permeability are due to vasoactive mediators. These chemicals cause actual gaps to form between vascular endothelial cells, allowing fluid and large molecules to escape into the intercellular space. Inflammatory cells, largely PMNs, also squeeze between vascular endothelial cells, a process mediated by adhesion molecules (discussed later) to escape into the tissue and attack Ag (e.g., foreign cells).

High protein content fluid escapes from the blood vessel through endothelial gaps during acute inflammation. This fluid can differ in appearance based on its specific content. For example, serous exudate, exemplified by a skin blister, is clear to yellowish and contains few inflammatory cells. Alternative purulent exudates are quite familiar to eye care practitioners (e.g., as in bacterial conjunctivitis). Large numbers of inflammatory cells (e.g., PMNs) impart a whitish color to the exudate. Pus from a bacterial conjunctivitis (Fig. 4.1) is composed of both necrotic debris and numerous PMNs. A fibrinous exudate usually occurs in more severe inflammation when the gaps between vascular endothelial cells are large enough to allow fibrin to escape (9).

Cellular Recruitment

Leukocytes are attracted to the site of inflammation by chemotactic factors, which are generated in high concentrations at sites of tissue injury or infection. Aided by slower blood flow in areas of inflammation, these factors cause circulating leukocytes, which normally flow along a central stream in blood vessels, to move peripherally toward the vessel wall (38). Leukocytes slow down, roll, and come to rest on the vascular endothelium. Cell rolling is mediated by repeated transient binding to adhesion molecules, called *selectins,* on vascular endothelial cells. These molecules briefly tether the leukocyte to the vascular endothelium and then "let go" as the force of the circulating blood breaks the bond, thus slowing the progress of the leukocytes. Adhesion molecules on the leukocyte surface, known as *integrins,* allow binding to corresponding adhesion molecules on the surface of on vascular endothelium, called *intracellular adhesion molecules* (ICAMs). Integrin association creates high-affinity (stronger and tighter) leukocyte binding, allowing leukocytes to stop and migrate into surrounding tissues. Adhesion molecules also can be expressed on other cells types during both inflammation and disease (13,39).

Leukocyte migration through the vessel wall and into

the surrounding tissue is called *emigration* or *transendothelial migration*. Neutrophils and few monocytes are observed in tissues in the first 3 to 6 hours during acute inflammation. After the initial neutrophil response, monocytes continue to infiltrate into the tissue and differentiate into macrophages, the predominant cell type in the later stages of inflammation. A chemotactic agent in tissues is the inducer of leukocyte migration. Chemotaxis is the process of directional movement of cells toward an increasing concentration of a stimulus called a *chemoattractant*. Chemoattractants are soluble molecules that diffuse away from their site of production into the surrounding tissue. They can be cytokines, bacterial and mitochondrial products, (e.g., *N*-formylated peptides), components of the complement system (e.g., C5a), or byproducts of arachidonic acid metabolism, such as leukotrienes, prostaglandins, and thromboxanes. Chemoattractants act broadly to control leukocyte traffic and are expressed in many infectious, autoimmune, and allergic conditions of the eye (40–43).

Cell-Derived Vasoactive Mediators

A number of inflammatory cell types are implicated in the release of chemical mediators of acute inflammation. Circulating platelets, tissue mast cells, basophils, PMNs, endothelial cells, macrophages, and the injured tissue are all sources of vasoactive mediators. These mediators may be stored in cytoplasmic granules, or they may require metabolism.

Arachidonic Acid Metabolites

Membrane phospholipids of several types of inflammatory cells, including mast cells, macrophages, and granulocytes, can be metabolized to form powerful chemical mediators of inflammation. Membrane phospholipids are broken down by the enzyme phospholipase A_2 to arachidonic acid and lyso-PAF, which subsequently is converted to platelet-activating factor (PAF) to cause both platelet activation and leukocyte chemotaxis (9). Arachidonic acid is metabolized by i) the cyclooxygenase pathway, which yields prostaglandins and thromboxanes; and ii) the lipoxygenase pathway, which produces leukotrienes (Fig. 4.9).

The cyclooxygenase pathway yields a number of clinically significant prostaglandins and thromboxanes. Thromboxanes cause vasoconstriction, bronchoconstriction, and platelet aggregation. The actions of prostaglandins include vasodilation, increased vascular permeability, and increased sensitivity to pain (with bradykinin). Prostaglandins also are involved in the production of fever, which is a clinical hallmark of inflammation. Bacteria, viruses, and injured cells stimulate macrophages to release IL-1, which stimulates prostaglandin synthesis in hypothalamic thermoregulatory centers in the brain to alter the body's "thermostat" producing fever. Nonsteroidal antiinflammatory drugs (NSAIDs) reduce fever by blocking the formation of prosta-

glandins. Leukotrienes, which are produced by the lipoxygenase pathway, are chemotactic (attractants) for PMNs, increasing vascular permeability (36).

A number of drugs interrupt arachidonic acid metabolite formation. Corticosteroids induce the synthesis of an inhibitor of phospholipase A_2, thereby inhibiting the synthesis of both prostaglandins and leukotrienes. The effectiveness of corticosteroids in the treatment of ocular inflammation is well documented, although numerous side effects make these drugs undesirable for use on a long-term basis (44). NSAIDs block specifically the cyclooxygenase pathway, inhibiting the synthesis of prostaglandins and thromboxanes. NSAIDs can be used topically in the eye to reduce inflammation and to treat symptoms of allergic conjunctivitis (45) as an alternative to steroids, and they have fewer side effects.

Histamine

The early events in inflammation, vasodilation, and increased vascular permeability are mediated largely by mast degranulation and the release of histamine. Mast cells are especially prevalent in mucosal surfaces, the dermis of the skin, and adjacent to small arterioles. Histamine release produces an almost immediate reaction in these tissues. Histamine is a preformed vasoactive mediator, stored within granules inside both mast cells and basophils. In classic anaphylactic reactions (see section of Type I Hypersensitivity), Ag binding with IgE causes degranulation of the mast cell and the release of histamine and other vasoactive substances. Because histamine is preformed and stored, its release results in rapid biologic effects, within minutes of mast cell degranulation. Histamine causes a variety of inflammatory effects, including vasodilation and increased vascular permeability through contraction of vascular endothelial cells. These effects result when histamine binds H1 receptors on the blood vessel wall. Histamine also causes bronchoconstriction and stimulates the production of prostaglandins. H2 and H3 receptors also have been identified, with different tissue distributions. Classic antihistamines specifically block H1 receptors so that histamine cannot bind and exert its effects (9).

The role of histamine in ocular allergy has been well documented (46,47). When histamine is applied topically to the rabbit eye, vascular injection occurs. When applied together with prostaglandins, vasodilation and increased vascular permeability are more marked.

Inflammatory Products Released from Neutrophils

Neutrophils are the main cell type participating in the acute inflammatory response. The cells are attracted to the site of inflammation by a number of factors, including products released from bacteria or damaged tissue, or by specific che-

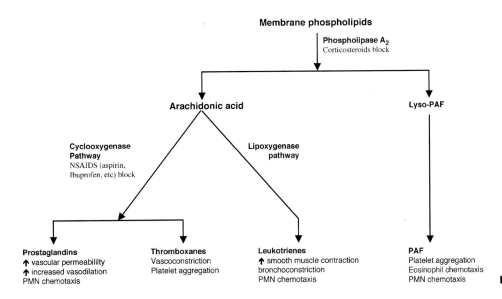

FIG. 4.9. Arachidonic acid pathway.

motactic factors. Once PMNs arrive at the site of inflammation, they attempt to phagocytize or "eat" foreign proteins or bacteria. During this process, PMNs release a number of lysosomal enzymes contained in cytoplasmic granules that break down or "digest" the foreign material inside the cell. During this process, lysosomal enzymes may leak into the surrounding tissue and cause collateral local tissue digestion and pus formation. Some of the substances released from PMNs also serve to attract macrophages to the site of inflammation, thereby further increasing the inflammatory response (9).

Plasma-Derived Inflammatory Mediators

The plasma contains three interrelated enzyme cascades that are active in acute inflammation. These enzyme cascades include the complement system (important in innate immune protection), coagulation cascade, and kinin generation.

Complement System

The complement cascade consists of more than 30 plasma and cell-bound proteins, many of which have vasoactive effects or otherwise interact with the immune system. Figure 4.10 diagrams the complement cascade with the factors that control its actions. Activation of the complement system can occur by either the "classic" or "alternate" pathways. A third pathway called the *lectin pathway* was described recently. This pathway induces activation of complement by glycoproteins or carbohydrates on the surface of microorganisms.

Activation of the classic pathway occurs in the presence of Ag–Ab complexes. Complement fragment C1 binds to the Fc region of an Ab molecule that has been previously altered by contact with Ag. Through a series of steps, C1 forms C3 convertase, which is a complex of C4b and C2a. C3 convertase binds and cleaves C3 into C3a and C3b. Complement fragment C3a is termed an *anaphylatoxin.* This means that, if systemically released, C3a is capable of causing anaphylactic shock through extensive peripheral vasodilation. C3a releases histamine and other vasoactive mediators from mast cells, which in turn causes increased vascular permeability and vasodilation. C3a also produces direct contraction of smooth muscle.

Complement fragment C3b coats foreign particles and is active in opsonization (literally, "to prepare for digestion"). When a phagocytic cell approaches a bacteria coated with C3b and Ab, it more readily phagocytizes the cell. A single molecule of C3 convertase can produce more than 200 molecules of C3b, thus amplifying this step of the sequence. Fragment C3b continues the complement cascade. In combination with other complement fragments, it forms the enzyme C5 convertase, which cleaves complement fragment C5 into C5a and C5b. Both C5a and C3a are potent anaphylatoxins. C5a causes a marked release of histamine and other vasoactive mediators from mast cells. C5a also serves as a strong chemotactic molecule for PMNs, thereby greatly increasing the acute inflammatory response. C5b continues the complement cascade to form the remaining complement fragments C6–C9. These fragments form a membrane-attack complex (MAC)m which can displace membrane phospholipids, resulting in a transmembrane channel leading to cell lysis (9). This process kills both target and "innocent bystander" or normal cells (48), so regulators (inhibitors) of the complement pathway are present in many tissues and fluids such as the tear film (49). Bacteria can produce some of these inhibitory factors, which greatly enhances their ability to infect (50).

The alternate pathway for complement activation does

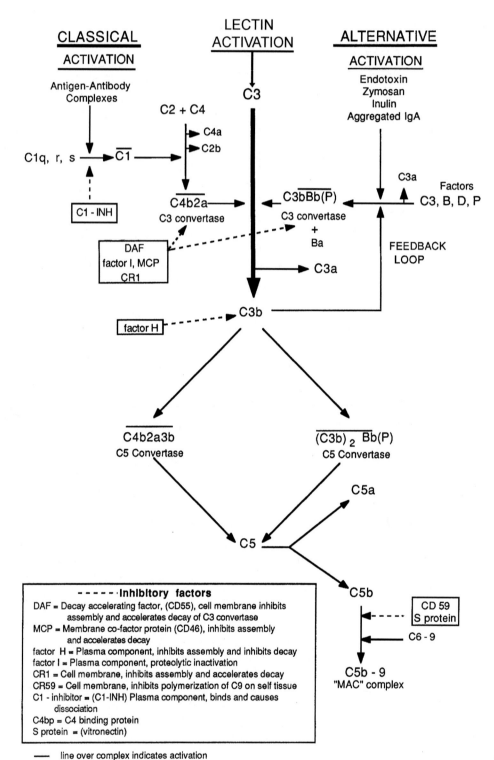

FIG. 4.10. Complement cascade.

not require Ag-Ab binding and is activated during contact with many strains of gram negative bacteria, yeasts, and some viruses, parasites, and tumor cells. As Figure 4.10 indicates, this pathway forms C3b by a different route. Following the point at which C3b combines with other comple-

ment fragments to form C5 convertase, the remainder of the pathway is similar.

Complement has been identified in tears, cornea, and aqueous humor. It has been shown to have protective roles in both corneal in intraocular infections.

Coagulation Cascade and Kinin Generation

Specific clotting factors are generated in the plasma and, in turn, produce vasoactive factors. The kinin system is an enzymatic cascade that begins with the Hageman factor, which is activated following tissue injury. Activated Hageman factor produces kallikrein, which cleaves kininogen to form bradykinin. Bradykinin causes increased vascular permeability, vasodilation, and contraction of smooth muscle. In combination with prostaglandins, it produces pain. Kallikrein also acts directly on the complement system to cleave C5 into C5a and C5b. The Hageman factor also acts on the fibrinolytic system to produce plasmin, which breaks down fibrin clots, and is chemotactic for leukocytes and activates the complement system. Another enzymatic pathway activated by the Hageman factor is the clotting cascade, which produces fibrin and fibrinopeptides. Fibrin produces clots and fibrinopeptides, both of which increase vascular permeability and cause PMN chemotaxis (9,36).

OVERVIEW OF ACUTE INFLAMMATION

Often acute inflammation begins with complement activation in response to Ab binding or other mechanisms. Complement fragments C3a and C5a cause the degranulation of mast cells, which release histamine and other vasoactive components, including prostaglandins and leukotrienes. These, along with plasmin and kinins, bring about increased vascular permeability, vasodilation, and increased blood flow to the area. Neutrophils then are chemotactically attracted to the site by a number of mediators, including C5a and leukotrienes. Neutrophils, macrophages, and other inflammatory cells move toward the vessel wall (margination), stick to the vascular endothelium (pavementing), and move through the wall into the surrounding tissue (emigration).

CHRONIC INFLAMMATION

Chronic inflammation often follows acute inflammation and serves to contain and remove infectious agents. It is associated with both immunologic and nonimmunologic mechanisms. Repair (scar formation) often begins during the chronic inflammatory phase. Cells typically involved in chronic inflammation are macrophages, lymphocytes, plasma cells, and eosinophils. Fibroblasts, cells that form scar tissue, are also often present.

Macrophages are the pivotal cells in the chronic inflammatory response (36). They are attracted to the site of inflammation by products derived from neutrophils, lymphocytes, and complement fragment C5a. Macrophages then become activated in the tissue by a number of factors, including lymphokines. Activated macrophages show in-creased phagocytosis and secrete chemicals to activate other cells. One of the most important mediators secreted by macrophages is IL-1, which has numerous effects, including activation of CD4$^+$ lymphocytes, production of fever, proliferation of many cell types, and production of prostaglandins.

Lymphocytes also are critical cells in the chronic inflammatory process. Lymphocytes regulate the activity of macrophages and other cells through lymphokine secretion. Plasma cells produce Abs that aid in neutralization of foreign cells.

However, chronic inflammation does not necessarily follow acute inflammation. Some Ags or foreign cells directly stimulate the chronic inflammatory response. Viral infections, for example, stimulate a lymphocytic response because T$_C$ lymphocytes (CD8$^+$ cells) lyse virally infected cells. Tumors, parasitic infections, and autoimmune responses also directly activate the chronic immune response.

When some T$_H$ lymphocytes encounter certain types of Ags, they produce a local inflammatory reaction known as the *delayed-type hypersensitivity response*. If the Ag is not removed easily, an intense response or granuloma develops. This type of inflammation is termed *granulomatous* and serves to wall off the offending substance or microorganism because it cannot be easily eliminated. This process is mediated by macrophages, which are very long-lived cells. Macrophages are called to the site of inflammation by cytokines from activated T lymphocytes, where they attempt to phagocytize the foreign substance. The macrophages lose their motility and begin to accumulate at the site. They change their basic shape and beginn to resemble epithelial cells. These epithelioid macrophages form ball-like clusters of cells around the indigestible foreign substance or cell. The clusters, termed *granulomas* (Fig. 4.11), may become

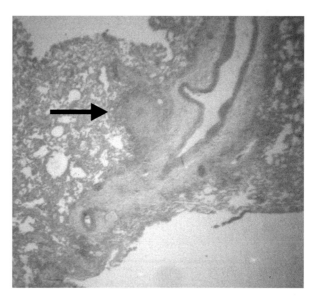

FIG. 4.11. Granuloma *(arrow)* formation in tuberculosis of the lung.

necrotic in the center and often show a rim of lymphocytes in the periphery. Large multinucleated giant cells, which result from a fusion of macrophages, also may be present.

Granulomatous inflammation occurs in a number of diseases, including tuberculosis, leprosy, parasitic infestations, sarcoid, and in response to foreign bodies such as asbestos or sutures (36,51). Figure 4.11 illustrates a pulmonary granuloma from a patient with tuberculosis. Tuberculosis an infectious disease caused by *Mycobacterium tuberculosis,* an acid-fast bacteria that can successfully survive and reproduce inside macrophages. In most cases, the initial pulmonary infection is contained by the granulomatous inflammation and immune response. If the patient is not immunologically competent or the number of infecting organisms is high, however, the initial granulomatous inflammation may not control the infection. The microorganism then spreads throughout the body inside macrophages, producing progressive primary tuberculosis.

HYPERSENSITIVITY REACTIONS

Immune reactions and the inflammatory response constitute an effective mechanism to protect the body against infection. This response can lead to host tissue damage and disease, however, and then is termed *hypersensitivity.* When the hypersensitivity reaction occurs in response to foreign Ags, it may produce a short-term allergic response or long-term disease. If self antigens or autoantigens activate the immune reaction, an autoimmune disease results. The etiology of autoimmune diseases is still unclear, but evidence suggests a loss of immune tolerance to self Ags (52). Hypersensitivity reactions involved different immune mechanisms, which historically have been divided into the four basic types presented later. Although these classification schemes outline basic immune mechanisms, actual hypersensitivity reactions and autoimmune diseases are much

more complex so that the boundaries between categories have become blurred (9).

Type I Hypersensitivity

Type I hypersensitivity (immediate or anaphylaxis) reactions occur immediately (within minutes) of exposure to an Ag to which the host has been presensitized by previous exposure. The reaction can be local and cause edema or hives, or it can be systemic. Systemic type I reactions are potentially lethal, resulting in bronchoconstriction, airway obstruction, and collapse if treatment is not immediately instituted. A bee sting in an allergic individual provides an excellent example of systemic anaphylaxis. Localized type I reactions (atopy) can lead to hay fever, asthma, food allergies, or atopic dermatitis.

As Figure 4.12 demonstrates, type I hypersensitivity reactions often are mediated by IgE, although complement fragments C5a and C3a and other substances can initiate the reaction. Atopic individuals form IgE in response to allergens, and the IgE Abs selectively bind to the membranes of mast cells by their Fc portions. Divalent binding to the Fab portion of the IgE molecule occurs with subsequent reexposure to the Ag. Once binding occurs, there is an influx of calcium into the cell, and the mast cell degranulates. Mast cell stabilizers block the calcium influx, thus preventing degranulation of the mast cell.

Mast cell degranulation releases preformed products, such as histamine, and synthesized products, such as prostaglandins, which participate in the early phase of the immediate response. The early phase develops within a few minutes of exposure to the Ag and persists for several hours. Late-phase reactions may develop, beginning anywhere from 3 to 12 hours after exposure to last for many hours. Eosinophils are present in late-phase reactions, apparently releasing inflammatory mediators that prolong inflammation (53). As late-phase reactions follow early-phase reactions, both

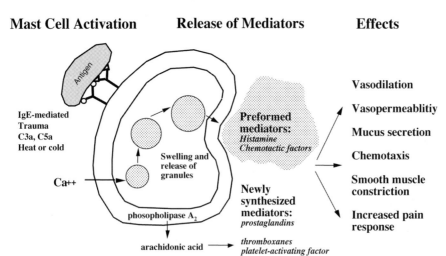

Mast Cell Activation   **Release of Mediators**   **Effects**

FIG. 4.12. Type I hypersensitivity: mast cell activation.

are likely to be mediated initially by mast cells. However, mast cell stabilizers do not always inhibit late phase reactions (54).

Allergic rhinitis and conjunctivitis provide excellent examples of localized IgE-mediated hypersensitivity reactions. Both are common in the United States, reaching a prevalence of 5% to 22% (55). Acute symptoms of sneezing, itchy eyes, nasal congestion, and rhinorrhea develop rapidly, suggesting that the reaction is mediated in large part by histamine. Antihistamines, mast cell stabilizers, and NSAIDs provide effective treatment of the early stages of either disease (56–58).

Type II Hypersensitivity

Type II hypersensitivity (cytotoxic) also is mediated by Abs, but, in this case, the Abs often are directed against fixed Ags on cell surfaces. IgM and IgG usually are involved and have the ability to fix complement through Fc receptors. Ab binding causes activation of the complement system that eventually destroys target cells, either by direct membrane lysis (C5–C9) or by enhancing phagocytosis. The classic example of this process is a transfusion reaction that occurs with blood type incompatibility; foreign red blood cells are lysed by complement fragments C5–C9 (36).

Other scenarios are possible in type II hypersensitivity reactions. Binding of Abs can promote functional changes rather than lysing targeted cells. In Graves disease (Fig. 4.13), for example, an auto-Ab forms against thyroid-stimulating hormone (TSH) receptors on thyroid cell surfaces. Ab binding acts to continuously stimulate the TSH receptor to produce thyroid hormone, thereby producing excess secretion. An overabundance of thyroid hormone causes the symptoms of hyperactivity, tremor, and cardiac arrhythmia noted in the disease. Exophthalmos is thought to be caused by some of the same auto-Abs that develop in response to Ags on thyroid follicular cells. Thyroid auto-Abs may

recognize epitopes on tissues contained in the orbital space, most likely preadipocytes and fibroblasts (59).

Type III Hypersensitivity

Type III hypersensitivity (immune complex diseases) reactions are characterized by the formation of immune complexes. IgM, IgG, or IgA binds to a circulating or fixed self Ag to initiate the complement cascade. Neutrophils and macrophages then are chemotactically attracted to the site and begin active phagocytosis of these immune complexes. During phagocytosis, these cells release lysosomal enzymes, which cause extensive tissue damage and scarring.

Rheumatoid arthritis exemplifies a type III hypersensitivity reaction. It is the most common autoimmune disease, affecting many more women more than men. Up to 80% of patients with rheumatoid arthritis are positive for rheumatoid factor, which consists of multiple Abs formed against the Fc portion of IgG. These Ab–Ab complexes can be found in the articular cartilage and synovium of the joints, where they participate in fixing complement to cause inflammation. The joint becomes swollen, hot, and painful. Leukocytes are attracted and release lysosomal enzymes and other inflammatory products to cause further tissue damage and eventual scarring of the joints (55).

Sjögren syndrome is another type III autoimmune condition. Multiple autoantibodies develop to nuclear proteins. As with other autoimmune conditions, the cause is unknown but may be related to a viral infection. The classic triad of clinical features in Sjögren syndrome is dry mouth, dry eyes, and a nondeforming arthritis. Both salivary and lacrimal glands are infiltrated by T lymphocytes that eventually destroy the acini and ducts, leaving nonfunctional scar tissue. Figure 4.14 shows a portion of a salivary gland from a Sjögren syndrome patient. Lymphocytes have invaded the

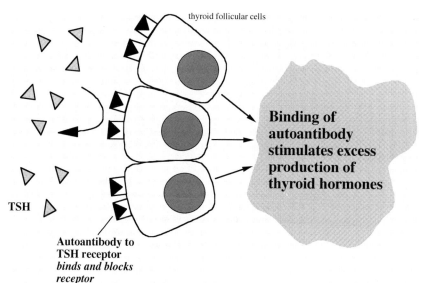

FIG. 4.13. Graves disease. Autoantibody formation to thyroid-stimulating hormone receptor stimulates overproduction of thyroid hormones.

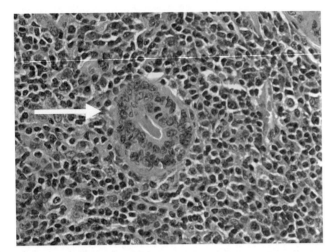

FIG. 4.14. Salivary gland in Sjögren syndrome. T lymphocytes have infiltrated the gland and destroyed all but a few "islands" of normal glandular tissue *(white arrow).*

gland, leaving only a small "island" of normal glandular tissue.

Type IV Hypersensitivity

Unlike the previous hypersensitivity reactions, type IV hypersensitivity (cell-mediated immunity) occurs independent of Abs. It is a delayed, cell-mediated reaction involving lymphocytes and macrophages. Type IV hypersensitivity reaches its greatest intensity 24 to 48 hours, or even later, after exposure to the Ag. During this reaction, Ags are phagocytosed by macrophages, processed, and presented to T lymphocytes. T "helper" lymphocytes then secrete lymphokines, which influence and attract a number of cell types and incite a vigorous inflammatory response. (This delayed-type hypersensitivity was discussed earlier in the section on Chronic Inflammation).

Contact dermatitis of the skin is an example of a type IV hypersensitivity response. When this occurs around the eye, it is likely to be due to cosmetics, topical ocular medications, or preservatives in contact lens solutions. Reactions to poison oak and poison ivy typify general skin contact dermatitis. These are small molecules that complex with skin proteins to elicit a delayed-type hypersensitivity reaction. Macrophages release lytic enzymes that result in the pustules characteristic of these allergic reactions (9).

SUMMARY

The eye functions as a window; therefore, ocular inflammatory responses are easily visualized (e.g., infiltrates in the cornea, cells and flare in the anterior chamber, vitreous snowballs in pars planitis) with our clinical techniques. Differences in presentation of primary ocular inflammation on the one hand and ocular inflammation from systemic disease on the other (both signs and symptoms), and their treatments, often can be better understood if the pathophysiology of the inflammatory reaction, discussed here in brief, is kept in mind. We note that the immune system must decide if an Ag is foreign (distinguish self from non-self) and then respond with cellular immune response, Ab (humoral) response, or tolerance. It also must regulate the magnitude and duration of these responses. Through this chapter we briefly reviewed aspects of how the body protects itself with these mechanisms and how they occasionally fail or act inappropriately. Aspects of ocular specific immunology and host defense mechanisms, and how they secondarily affect the eye, were discussed to emphasize how the ocular response is similar to systemic responses. The interested reader should importantly note that this short introduction is by no means a complete description of immunology. Many modern texts and journals are devoted to immunology, and they should be consulted to develop further appreciation and understanding of this very complex and evolving science.

REFERENCES

1. Rhem MN, Lech EM, Patti JM, et al. The collagen-binding adhesin is a virulence factor in *Staphylococcus aureus* keratitis. *Infect Immun* 2000;68:3776–3779.
2. Hoepelman AI, Tuomanen EI. Consequences of microbial attachment: directing host cell functions with adhesins. *Infect Immun* 1992;60:1729–1733.
3. Chodash J, Kennedy RC. The conjunctival lymphoid follicle in mucosal immunology. *DNA Cell Biol* 2002;21:421–433.
4. McNamara N, Fleizig SMJ: Human tear film components bind *Pseudomonas aeruginosa. Adv Exp Med Bio Lacrimal Gland, Tear film, and Dry Eye Syndromes* 1998;438:653–658.
5. Leher H, Zaragoza F, Taherzadeh S, et al. Monoclonal IgA antibodies protect against Acanthamoeba keratitis. *Exp Eye Res* 1999; 69:75–84.
6. Stuchell RN, Farris RL, Mandel ID. Basal and reflex human tear analysis part II: chemical analysis: lactoferrin and lysozyme. *Ophthalmology* 1981;88:858–861.
7. Lal H, Ahluwalia BK, Khurana AK, et al. Tear lysozyme levels in bacterial, fungal, and viral corneal ulcers. *Acta Ophthalmol (Copenh)* 1991;69:530–532.
8. Sack RA, Beaton AR, Sathe S, et al. Towards a closed eye model of the pre-ocular tear layer. *Prog Retinal Eye Res* 2000;19:649–668.
9. Goldsby RA, Kindt TJ, Osborne BA. In: *Kuby immunology.* New York: WH Freeman and Co., 2000.
10. Zhou J, Begley CG, Wright A, et al. Characterization of cells collected from the normal human ocular surface by contact lens cytology. *Cornea* 2000;19:824–832.
11. Haynes RJ, Tighe PJ, Dua HS. Antimicrobial defensin peptides of the human ocular surface. *Br J Ophthalmol* 1999;83:737–741.
12. Lehmann OJ, Hussain IR, Watt PJ. Investigation of beta defensin gene expression in the ocular anterior segment by semiquantitative RT-PCR. *Br J Ophthalmol* 2000;84:523–526.
13. Kaifi JT, Diaconu E, Pearlman E. Distinct roles for PECAM-1, ICAM-1, and VCAM-1 in recruitment of neutrophils and eosinophils to the cornea in ocular onchocerciasis (river blindness). *J Immunol* 2001;166:6795–6801.
14. Messmer EM, May CA, Stefani FH, et al. Toxic eosinophil granule protein deposition in corneal ulcerations and scars associated

with atopic keratoconjunctivitis. *Am J Ophthalmol* 2002;134: 816–821.

15. Popper H, Knipping G, Czarnetzki BM, et al. Activation and release of enzymes and major basic protein from guinea pig eosinophil granulocytes induced by different inflammatory stimuli and other substances. A histochemical, biochemical, and electron microscopic study. *Inflammation* 1989;13:147–162.

16. Buckley RJ. Allergic eye disease—a clinical challenge. *Clin Exp Allergy* 1998;28[Suppl 16]:39–43.

17. Church MK, McGill JI. Human ocular mast cells. *Curr Opin Allergy Clin Immunol* 2002;2:419–422.

18. Hamrah P, Liu Y, Zhang Q, et al. The corneal stroma is endowed with a significant number of resident dendritic cells. *Invest Ophthalmol Vis Sci* 2003;44:581–589.

19. Bauer D, Schmitz A, Van Rooijen N, et al. Conjunctival macrophage-mediated influence of the local and systemic immune response after corneal herpes simplex virus-1 infection. *Immunology* 2002;107:118–128.

20. She SC, Moticka EJ. Ability of intracamerally inoculated B- and T-cell enriched allogeneic lymphocytes to enhance corneal allograft survival. *Int Ophthalmol* 1993;17:1–7.

21. Reinhard T, Bohringer D, Enczmann J et al. HLA class I and II matching improves prognosis in penetrating normal-risk keratoplasty. *Dev Ophthalmol* 2003;36:42–49.

22. Carr DJ, Noisakran S. The antiviral efficacy of the murine alpha-1 interferon transgene against ocular herpes simplex virus type 1 requires the presence of CD4(+), alpha/beta T-cell receptor-positive T lymphocytes with the capacity to produce gamma interferon. *J Virol* 2002;76:9398–9406.

23. Schreiber K, Otura AB, Ryder LP, et al. Disease severity in Danish multiple sclerosis patients evaluated by MRI and three genetic markers (HLA-DRB1*1501, CCR5 deletion mutation, apolipoprotein E). *Mult Scler* 2002;8:295–298.

24. Grams SE, Moonsamy PV, Mano C, et al. Two new HLA-B alleles, B*4422 and B*4704, identified in a study of families with autoimmunity. *Tissue Antigens* 2002;59:338–340.

25. Haines JL, Bradford Y, Garcia ME, et al. Multiple susceptibility loci for multiple sclerosis. *Hum Mol Genet* 2002;11:2251–2256.

26. Pearce DJ, Demirci G, Willcox MD. Secretory IgA epitopes in basal tears of extended-wear soft contact lens wearers and in non-lens wearers. *Aust N Z J Ophthalmol* 1999;27:221–223.

27. Mestecky J, Fultz PN. Mucosal immune system of the human genital tract. *J Infect Dis* 1999;179[Suppl 13]:S470–S474.

28. Baudouin C, Bourcier T, Brignole F, et al. Correlation between tear IgE levels and HLA-DR expression by conjunctival cells in allergic and nonallergic chronic conjunctivitis. *Graefes Arch Clin Exp Ophthalmol* 2000;238:900–904.

29. Coffman R,L Weissman IL. Immunoglobulin gene rearrangement during pre-B cell differentiation. *J Mol Cell Immunol* 1983; 1:31–41.

30. Alt FW, Blackwell TK, DePinho RA, et al. Regulation of genome rearrangement events during lymphocyte differentiation. *Immunol Rev* 1986;89:5–30.

31. Leanderson T, Kallberg E, Gray D. Expansion, selection and mutation of antigen-specific B cells in germinal centers. *Immunol Rev* 1992;126:47–61.

32. Manser T. Evolution of antibody structure during the immune response. The differentiative potential of a single B lymphocyte. *J Exp Med* 1989;170:1211–1230.

33. Liu YJ, Joshua DE, Williams GT, et al. Mechanism of antigen-driven selection in germinal centers. *Nature* 1989;342:929–931.

34. Shan H, Shlomchik M, Weigert M. Heavy-chain class switch does not terminate somatic mutation. *J Exp Med* 1990;172: 531–536.

35. Picker L, Siegelman M. Lymphoid tissues and organs. In: Paul WE ed. *Fundamental immunology.* New York: Raven Press, 1993: 145–197.

36. Rubin E, Farber J. *Pathology.* Philadelphia: JB Lippincott, 1998.

37. Berke G. The functions and mechanisms of action of cytolytic lymphocytes. In: Paul WE ed. *Fundamental immunology.* New York: Raven Press, 1993:965–1014.

38. Carlos TM, Harlan JM. Leukocyte-endothelial adhesion molecules. *Blood* 1994;84:2068–2101.

39. Oh JW, Shin JC, Jang SJ, et al. Expression of ICAM-1 on conjunctival epithelium and ECP in tears and serum from children with allergic conjunctivitis. *Ann Allergy Asthma Immunol* 1999; 82:579–585.

40. Abu El-Asrar AM, Struyf S, Al-Kharashi SA. et al. Chemokines in the limbal form of vernal keratoconjunctivitis. *Br J Ophthalmol* 2000;84:1360–1366.

41. Adamus G, Manczak M, Machnicki M. Expression of CC chemokines and their receptors in the eye in autoimmune anterior uveitis associated with EAE. *Invest Ophthalmol Vis Sci* 2001;42: 2894–2903.

42. Hall LR, Pearlman E. Pathogenesis of onchocercal keratitis (river blindness). *Clin Microbiol Rev* 1999;12:445–453.

43. Verma MJ, Lloyd A, Rager H, et al. Chemokines in acute anterior uveitis. *Curr Eye Res* 1997;16:1202–1208.

44. Hammond R. General principles of corticosteroids. In: Onfrey BE, ed. *Clinical optometric pharmacology and therapeutics.* Philadelphia: JB Lippincott, 1993:43.

45. Schalnus R. Topical nonsteroidal anti-inflammatory therapy in ophthalmology. *Ophthalmologica* 2003;217:89–98.

46. Leonardi A. Role of histamine in allergic conjunctivitis. *Acta Ophthalmol Scand* 2000;Suppl 1230:18–21.

47. Leonardi A, Radice M, Fregona IA, et al. Histamine effects on conjunctival fibroblasts from patients with vernal conjunctivitis. *Exp Eye Res* 1999;68:739–746.

48. Bardenstein DS, Cheyer CJ, Lee C, et al. Blockage of complement regulators in the conjunctiva and within the eye leads to massive inflammation and iritis. *Immunology* 2001;104:423–430.

49. Cocuzzi E, Szczotka LB, Brodbeck WG, et al. Tears contain the complement regulator CD59 as well as decay-accelerating factor (DAF). *Clin Exp Immunol* 2001;123:188–195.

50. Cocuzzi E, Guidubaldi J, Bardenstein DS, et al. Release of complement regulatory proteins from ocular surface cells in infections. *Cur Eye Res* 2000;21:856–866.

51. Angi MR, Forattini F, Chilosi M, et al. Immunopathology of ocular sarcoidosis. *Int Ophthalmol* 1990;14:1–11.

52. Schwartz R. Autoimmunity and autoimmune diseases. In: Paul WE, ed. *Fundamental immunology.* New York: Raven Press, 1993:1033–1097.

53. Charlesworth EN, Hood AF, Soter NA, et al. Cutaneous late-phase response to allergen. Mediator release and inflammatory cell infiltration. *J Clin Invest* 1989;83:1519–1526.

54. Plaut M, Zimmerman E. Allergy and mechanisms of hypersensitivity. In: Paul WE, ed. *Fundamental immunology.* New York: Raven Press, 1993:1399–1425.

55. Smith J. Epidemiology and natural history of asthma, allergic rhinitis and atopic dermatitis (eczema). In: Middleton E, Reed CE, Ellis EF, et al., eds. *Allergy, principles and practice.* St Louis: Mosby, 1988:891–921.

56. Anderson DF, MacLeod JD, Baddeley SM, et al. Seasonal allergic conjunctivitis is accompanied by increased mast cell numbers in the absence of leucocyte infiltration. *Clin Exp Allergy* 1997;27: 1060–1066.

57. Howarth PH. Assessment of antihistamine efficacy and potency. *Clin Exp Allergy* 1999;29[Suppl 13]:87–97.

58. Arimura A, Yasui K, Kishino J, et al. Prevention of allergic inflammation by a novel prostaglandin receptor antagonist, S-5751. *J Pharmacol Exp Ther* 2001;298:411–419.

59. Heufelder AE, Joba W. Thyroid-associated eye disease. *Strabismus* 2000;8:101–111.

MICROBIOLOGY OF CONTACT LENSES

MARK D.P. WILLCOX
NAJAT J. HARMIS
HUA ZHU
BRIGITTE COWELL
AND FIONA STAPLETON

This chapter details the types and frequency of microorganisms that can colonize the ocular surfaces or contact lens during normal asymptomatic lens wear. Details of the effects of contact lens wear on the normal ocular microbiota and of the microbiota that can cause adverse responses during lens wear are provided. Sources of the normal and potentially pathogenic microbiota are outlined, as are the potential bacterial pathogenic traits involved in the induction of the adverse responses (particularly microbial keratitis [MK]). Finally, measures that are designed to limit the colonization of ocular surfaces and/or contact lenses are discussed.

The human eye is continually exposed to microorganisms, most of which are nonpathogenic. However, occasionally pathogenic microorganisms can contact the eye and produce adverse responses, such as MK and other noninfectious keratitis conditions associated with contact lens wear.

NORMAL OCULAR MICROBIOTA

The conjunctiva and lids have a normal microbiota, although the numbers of this microbiota are very low. This scarcity of colonization of the normal microbiota has led some researchers to question whether this is, in fact, a real and stable normal microbiota. A simple demonstration of the scarcity of the ocular microbiota can be seen by applying a swab to the conjunctiva and culturing under a number of atmospheric conditions (1). When compared to similarly swabbing and culturing a buccal (mouth) swab, the level of the normal conjunctival microbiota is at least two logs reduced. The lids have a slightly higher level of normal microbiota than the conjunctiva, but again the levels do not approach those seen in the mouth (Fig. 5.1). The cornea is considered to be sterile.

The main types of microorganisms that form the normal ocular (conjunctival or lid) microbiota are bacteria (Tables 5.1 and 5.2). In particular, Gram-positive cocci and rods, especially members of the coagulase negative staphylococci, *Corynebacterium* sp and *Propionibacterium* sp (2,3). For the coagulase-negative staphylococci, members of the capitis/warneri group (*S. capitis, S. warneri, S. cohnii, S. saprophyticus*) and members of the epidermidis group (*S. epidermidis, S. hominis*) have been shown to be the most common types (4). Approximately 50% of the population harbors one or more of these bacterial types on their conjunctiva at any given time (Table 5.1) (2,4,5). Other microorganisms may be isolated from the conjunctiva, but at much lower rates [e.g., *Staphylococcus aureus, Micrococcus* sp, *Bacillus* sp, certain Gram-negative bacteria (Table 5.1) (2,3)]. The lids are colonized more frequently (Table 5.2) and heavily (4,5) than is the conjunctiva. The number of bacteria colonizing the conjunctiva and lid increases during sleep (6).

Relatively few studies have examined the normal ocular microbiota for any differences between populations in differing geographic regions, and it is difficult to compare between different studies because differences in methodology of sample collection and bacterial enumeration and identification may confound interpretation. A study conducted by us and the LV Prasad Eye Institute, Hyderabad, India, examined the differences between a contact lens-wearing population in Sydney, Australia, and a similar population in Hyderabad. This study demonstrated that the type of microbiota did not differ between the two regions, but the frequency of isolation of the normal microbiota was significantly increased in Hyderabad compared to Sydney. This may reflect differences in climate.

There have been several investigations into the effects of contact lenses on the normal ocular microbiota. Elander et al. (7) demonstrated that for short wearing times (1 week) of contact lenses did not alter the conjunctiva microbiota. Other studies have examined lens wearers over a longer period of time or after a longer period of wear. In a mixed group of lens wearers, coagulase-negative staphylococci were the most common isolates from the conjunctiva. During lens wear there was an increased frequency of negative cul-

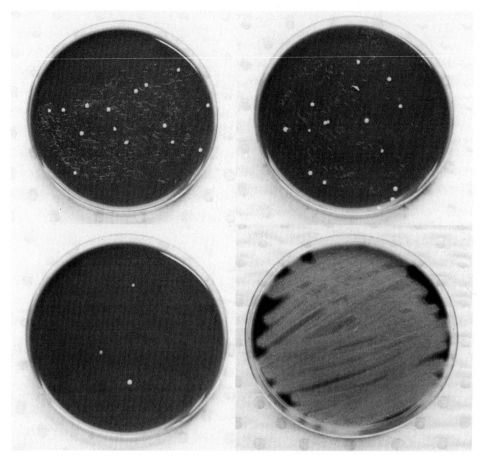

FIG. 5.1. Examples of the number of microorganisms that can be isolated from specific ocular sites and a buccal swab. **A:** Bacteria from a conjunctival swab. **B:** Bacteria from a lid swab. **C:** Bacteria from a tear sample. **D:** Bacteria from a buccal (mouth) swab. All photographs ×0.7 magnification. For isolation and culturing conditions of ocular samples, refer to Willcox et al. (2003). For the buccal swab, the swab was gently rotated on the inside of the cheek and placed in 400-μL phosphate-buffered saline, then 100 μL was plated onto a hemolyzed blood agar plate. The plate was incubated for 24 hours in normal atmospheric conditions at 35°C and photographed. The buccal swab has many more bacteria than all other swabs, so many bacteria that it is difficult to make out individual colonies. Tears have the least number of bacteria. Bacterial colonies appear, generally, as white spots on the agar plate.

tures in wearers (soft, hard, or silicone) compared with non-wearers, although Gram-negative bacteria occurred more frequently during wear (8). Table 5.3 (showing daily wear subjects) and Table 5.4 (showing extended wear subjects) show that in a controlled population of wearers in Sydney over a 2-year time period, there was a general significant decrease in the frequency of sterile cultures on their lids and on their conjunctiva, apart from the conjunctival microbiota of neophyte extended wear subjects (Table 5.1) whose frequency of sterile cultures increased with increasing years of wear. An increase in the number of bacteria isolated from the conjunctiva and lids during daily lens wear has been reported (5,9), although the types of microorganisms were not found to differ from non–lens-wearing eyes. An alteration in the types of microorganisms isolated from the conjunctiva or lids was seen with extended lens wear (isolation of more Gram-negative bacteria) along with an increase in the frequency of cultures growing no microorganisms (5, 8). This finding is significant because Gram-negative organisms are common ocular pathogens (10). Other studies, however, have reported no differences between wearers and non-lens wearers, although an increase in positive ocular cultures was found in former lens users and in association with certain modes of lens wear and types of disinfection

systems (3). A study comparing changes in the conjunctival microbiota during wear of soft hydrogel lenses, rigid gas permeable (GP) lenses and no lens wear demonstrated that there were similar rates of culture of Gram-positive bacteria (including coagulase-negative staphylococci), but for Gram-negative bacteria the average rate of colonization was 0% during soft lens wear, 2.5% with no lens wear, but 46% during wear of GP lenses (11). These differences may have been associated with the different lens care systems (11) (see later).

MICROBIOTA OF CONTACT LENSES DURING ASYMPTOMATIC WEAR

Small numbers of microorganisms infrequently colonize the contact lens during wear (12). Usually only an average of six colony-forming units per lens is cultured for the most common bacterial types (Table 5.5). The most common bacteria isolated are coagulase-negative staphylococci (Table 5.6) (3,8,12,13). Occasional isolation of *S. aureus, Corynebacterium* sp, micrococci, streptococci, a variety of Gram-negative bacteria, and fungi (either yeasts or molds) also has been noted (Table 5.6) (3,8). In a group of seamen, *S.*

TABLE 5.1. FREQUENCY OF ISOLATION OF NORMAL CONJUNCTIVAL MICROBIOTA

Visit	Microorganism	Daily Wear percent Isolation Frequency (No. of Sampling Occasions)	Extended Wear percent Isolation Frequency (No. of Sampling Occasions)	P Value[b]
Baseline				
	Coagulase-negative staphylococci	21 (53)	25 (132)	NS
	Corynebacterium sp	6 (53)	8 (132)	NS
	Fungi	0 (53)	1 (132)	NS
	No growth	74 (53)	30 (132)	<0.001
1-year visit				
	Coagulase-negative staphylococci	33 (54)	15 (65)	<0.05
	Staphylococcus aureus	0 (54)	3 (65)	NS
	Propionibacterium sp	7 (54)	15 (65)	NS
	Corynebacterium sp	4 (54)	2 (65)	NS
	Micrococcus sp	2 (54)	3 (65)	NS
	Streptococcus viridans	4 (54)	3 (65)	NS
	Nonhemolytic streptococci	2 (54)	0 (65)	NS
	Neisseria sp	0 (54)	2 (65)	NS
	Fungi	2 (54)	0 (65)	NS
	No growth	46 (54)	54 (65)	NS
2-year visit[a]				
	Staphylococcus saprophyticus	14 (58)	16 (76)	NS
	Staphylococcus epidermidis	12 (58)	13 (76)	NS
	Staphylococcus schleiferi	2 (58)	0 (76)	NS
	Propionibacterium sp	17 (58)	15 (76)	NS
	Corynebacterium sp	3 (58)	0 (76)	NS
	Micrococcus sp	2 (58)	0 (76)	NS
	Streptococcus viridans	0 (58)	1 (76)	NS
	Bacillus sp	7 (58)	3 (76)	NS
	Lactobacillus sp	2 (58)	0 (76)	NS
	Planococcus sp	2 (58)	1 (76)	NS
	Stomatococcus sp	2 (58)	0 (76)	NS
	Moraxella sp	2 (58)	0 (76)	NS
	Fungi	3 (58)	1 (76)	NS
	No growth	33 (58)	61 (76)	<0.01

Subjects were enrolled into a clinical study at the Cornea and Contact Lens Research Unit, School of Optometry and Vision Science, University of New South Wales. Subjects wore contralateral group IV and group I hydroxyethyl methacrylate (HEMA)-based hydrogel contact lenses. The extended wear schedule was 6 nights of continuous wear, with lens replacement on the seventh day. The daily wear schedule was 1 month of daily wear, with disinfection/cleaning in multipurpose solution overnight and monthly replacement of lenses.
Microorganisms were collected by swabbing the bulbar conjunctiva and cultured as described in Willcox et al. (2003).
[a]At the 2-year visit, the coagulase-negative staphylococci were differentiated into individual species.
[b]Statistical analysis for differences between daily wear and extended wear using Test of Proportion in CCSTAT—Quick Statistics for Optometrists (version 3.5).

epidermidis (coagulase-negative staphylococci) and *S. aureus* were most frequently isolated, followed by *Enterobacter* sp and *Pseudomonas* sp (14).

Other data from our laboratories have shown that contamination of lenses during wear is sporadic. Wearing lenses for increasing lengths of time did not result in increasing microbial contamination (15). Under certain circumstances, organisms may adhere to and form a glycocalyx on the posterior lens surface, thus prolonging the retention time of microorganisms at the ocular surface, and *Pseudomonas* sp encased within a biofilm on the posterior surface of the contact lens have been demonstrated during MK (16).

Table 5.6 presents data collected from a group of hydrogel lens wearers during 2 years of either daily wear or extended wear. The same types of bacteria were isolated at baseline as over the wear period, although there was a tendency for isolation of more different genera of bacteria during wear. Similar results for the frequency of isolation of bacteria from silicone hydrogel lenses have been reported (17). The apparent appearance of *Propionibacterium* sp during wear probably is due to better isolation conditions (this bacterium is obligatory anaerobic) rather than a real increase. However, we believe that the decrease in the frequency of sterile lenses during daily wear (which cannot alone be accounted for by better isolation/growth conditions) is real and indicates increasing colonization over time but not by any specific microbial type (Table 5.3).

Comparison of Tables 5.1, 5.2, and 5.6 demonstrates that

TABLE 5.2. FREQUENCY OF ISOLATION OF NORMAL LID MICROBIOTA

Visit	Microorganism	Daily Wear percent Isolation Frequency (No. of Sampling Occasions)	Extended Wear percent Isolation Frequency (No. of Sampling Occasions)	P Value[b]
Baseline				
	Coagulase-negative staphylococci	47 (58)	47 (137)	NS
	Staphylococcus aureus	0 (58)	1 (137)	NS
	Corynebacterium sp	10 (58)	16 (137)	NS
	No growth	40 (58)	36 (137)	NS
1-year wear				
	Coagulase-negative staphylococci	49 (69)	50 (64)	NS
	Staphylococcus aureus	1 (69)	0 (64)	NS
	Propionibacterium sp	16 (69)	23 (64)	NS
	Corynebacterium sp	4 (69)	2 (64)	NS
	Micrococcus sp	3 (69)	5 (64)	NS
	Streptococcus viridans	1 (69)	2 (64)	NS
	Acinetobacter sp	1 (69)	0 (64)	NS
	Pseudomonas fluorescens	1 (69)	0 (64)	NS
	Fungi	3 (69)	3 (64)	NS
	No growth	9 (69)	16 (64)	NS
2-year wear[a]				
	Staphylococcus saprophyticus	16 (73)	19 (86)	NS
	Staphylococcus epidermidis	22 (73)	20 (86)	NS
	Staphylococcus haemolyticus	4 (73)	1 (86)	NS
	Staphylococcus hyicus	1 (73)	2 (86)	NS
	Staphylococcus intermedius	0 (73)	1 (86)	NS
	Staphylococcus lugdunensis	1 (73)	0 (86)	NS
	Staphylococcus schleiferi	1 (73)	0 (86)	NS
	Propionibacterium sp	27 (73)	30 (86)	NS
	Corynebacterium sp	1 (73)	1 (86)	NS
	Micrococcus sp	3 (73)	4 (86)	NS
	Streptococcus viridans	0 (73)	2 (86)	NS
	Bacillus sp	3 (73)	1 (86)	NS
	Lactobacillus sp	0 (73)	1 (86)	NS
	Planococcus sp	3 (73)	1 (86)	NS
	Stomatococcus sp	1 (73)	0 (86)	NS
	Fungi	0 (73)	1 (86)	NS
	No growth	14 (73)	12 (86)	NS

Subjects were enrolled into a clinical study at the Cornea and Contact Lens Research Unit, School of Optometry and Vision Science, University of New South Wales. Subjects wore contralateral group IV and group I hydroxyethyl methacrylate (HEMA)-based hydrogel contact lenses. The extended wear schedule was 6 nights of continuous wear, with lens replacement on the seventh day. The daily wear schedule was 1 month of daily wear, with disinfection/cleaning in multipurpose solution overnight and monthly replacement of lenses. Microorganisms were collected by swabbing the lid margin and cultured as described in Willcox et al. (2003).
[a]at the 2-year visit, the coagulase-negative staphylococci were differentiated into individual species
[b]Statistical analysis for differences between daily wear and extended wear using Test of Proportion in CCSTAT—Quick Statistics for Optometrists (version 3.5).

there was a trend of increasing colonization frequency from the lowest for the conjunctiva, through contact lens contamination, to the highest for lids. This has been demonstrated previously for the coagulase-negative staphylococci (4).

DIFFERENCES WITH DIFFERENT LENS TYPES

Relatively few studies have compared differences in the colonization frequency between different lens types. A study by

Gopinathan et al. (13) examined the colonization of two groups of subjects wearing contralateral group IV or group I hydrogel lenses on an extended (6-night) or daily wear schedule in India or Australia. The same types and frequency of isolation were seen for the major bacterial types, whichever lens was worn. The contact lenses of the Indians were more commonly contaminated than those of the Australians. For individual bacterial species, streptococci and *Propionibacterium* sp were more commonly isolated from Australian lenses whereas fungi and *Bacillus* sp were more common on Indian lenses (13). Wearing silicone hydrogel

TABLE 5.3. EFFECT OF INCREASING YEARS OF DAILY WEAR ON NORMAL OCULAR MICROBIOTA

Sample Site	Significant Differences	Magnitude of Difference	p Value[a]
Conjunctiva	*Propionibacterium* sp baseline vs 2-year wear	Increase by 17×	<0.01
	No growth baseline vs 1-year wear	Decrease by 2×	<0.01
	No growth baseline vs 2-year wear	Decrease by 2×	<0.001
Contact lens	*Propionibacterium* sp baseline vs 1-year wear	Increase by 10×	<0.05
	Propionibacterium sp baseline vs 2-year wear	Increase by 21×	<0.001
	No growth baseline vs 1-year wear	Decrease by 21×	<0.001
	No growth baseline vs 2-year wear	Decrease by 16×	<0.001
Lid	*Propionibacterium* sp baseline vs 1-year wear	Increase by 16×	<0.01
	Propionibacterium sp baseline vs 2-year wear	Increase by 27×	<0.001
	No growth baseline vs 1-year wear	Decrease by 5×	<0.001
	No growth baseline vs 2-year wear	Decrease by 3×	<0.01

See Table 5.1 for more detailed description of the clinical trial and culture conditions.
For coagulase-negative staphylococci, comparisons could only be made between baseline and 1 year of lens wear.
[a]Statistical analysis for during the wear schedule using Test of Proportion in CCSTAT—Quick Statistics for Optometrists (version 3.5). No other comparisons were statistically significant.

TABLE 5.4. EFFECT OF INCREASING YEARS OF EXTENDED WEAR ON NORMAL OCULAR MICROBIOTA

Sample Site	Significant Differences	Magnitude of Difference	p Value[a]
Conjunctiva	*Propionibacterium* sp baseline vs 1-year wear	Increase by 15×	<0.001
	Propionibacterium sp baseline vs 2-year wear	Increase by 15×	<0.001
	No growth baseline vs 1-year wear	Increase by 2×	<0.01
	No growth baseline vs 2-year wear	Increase by 2×	<0.001
Contact lens	Coagulase-negative staphylococci baseline vs 1-year wear	Decrease by 2×	<0.05
	Propionibacterium sp baseline vs 1-year wear	Increase by 29×	<0.05
	Propionibacterium sp baseline vs 2-year wear	Increase by 31×	<0.05
Lid	*Corynebacterium* sp baseline vs 1-year wear	Decrease by 8×	<0.01
	Propionibacterium sp baseline vs 1-years wear	Increase by 23×	<0.001
	Propionibacterium sp baseline vs 2-year wear	Increase by 30×	<0.001
	No growth baseline vs 1-year wear	Decrease by 2×	<0.01
	No growth baseline vs 2-year wear	Decrease by 3×	<0.001

See Table 5.1 for more detailed description of the clinical trial and culture conditions.
For coagulase-negative staphylococci comparisons could only be made between baseline and 1 year of lens wear.
[a]Statistical analysis for during the wear schedule using Test of Proportion in CCSTAT—Quick Statistics for Optometrists (version 3.5). No other comparisons were statistically significant.

TABLE 5.5. NUMBER OF MICROBIAL COLONIES ON HYDROGEL CONTACT LENSES AFTER 12 MONTHS OF EXTENDED WEAR (6 NIGHTS)

Microorganism	Number of Times Isolated (No. of Times Sampled = 45)	Median Colony-Forming Units per Lens	Range
Coagulase-negative staphylococci	16	6	1–20
Propionibacterium sp	13	6	6–170
Corynebacterium sp	3	7	6–>300[a]
Streptococcus viridans	4	23	6–60

Other organisms were recovered but only on single occasions.
Details of clinical trial and microbial culture are described in Table 5.1 and Willcox et al. (1).
[a]>300 colony-forming units is the maximum number that is counted; equivalent to confluent growth.

TABLE 5.6. FREQUENCY OF ISOLATION OF NORMAL CONTACT LENS MICROBIOTA

Visit	Microorganism	Daily Wear percent Isolation Frequency (No. of Sampling Occasions)	Extended Wear percent Isolation Frequency (No. of Sampling Occasions)	P Value[b]
3-month visit				
	Coagulase-negative staphylococci	26 (62)	68 (19)	<0.01
	Staphylococcus aureus	0 (62)	5 (19)	NS
	Corynebacterium sp	2 (62)	0 (19)	NS
	Streptococcus viridans	0 (62)	5 (19)	NS
	Stomatococcus sp	0 (62)	5 (19)	NS
	Klebsiella sp	2 (62)	0 (19)	NS
	Stenotrophomonas maltophilia	3 (62)	0 (19)	NS
	Fungi	3 (62)	0 (19)	NS
	No growth	63 (62)	11 (19)	<0.001
1-year visit				
	Coagulase-negative staphylococci	24 (59)	36 (45)	NS
	Staphylococcus aureus	3 (59)	2 (45)	NS
	Corynebacterium sp	0 (59)	7 (45)	NS
	Propionibacterium sp	10 (59)	29 (45)	<0.05
	Micrococcus sp	2 (59)	0 (45)	NS
	Streptococcus viridans	2 (59)	9 (45)	NS
	Streptococcus pneumoniae	0 (59)	2 (45)	NS
	Nonhemolyitc streptococci	0 (59)	2 (45)	NS
	Neisseria sp	0 (59)	2 (45)	NS
	Pasteurella sp	0 (59)	2 (45)	NS
	Pseudomonas paucimobilis	0 (59)	2 (45)	NS
	Serratia marcescens	2 (59)	0 (45)	NS
	Fungi	0 (59)	2 (45)	NS
	No growth	3 (59)	4 (45)	NS
2 year visit[a]				
	Staphylococcus saprophyticus	21 (73)	19 (64)	NS
	Staphylococcus epidermidis	15 (73)	23 (64)	NS
	Staphylococcus haemolyticus	1 (73)	5 (64)	NS
	Staphylococcus lugdunensis	1 (73)	0 (64)	NS
	Propionibacterium sp	21 (73)	31 (64)	NS
	Corynebacterium sp	0 (73)	5 (64)	NS
	Micrococcus sp	3 (73)	2 (64)	NS
	Streptococcus viridans	0 (73)	2 (64)	NS
	Non-hemolytic streptococci	1 (73)	0 (64)	NS
	Bacillus sp	4 (73)	5 (64)	NS
	Planococcus sp	1 (73)	0 (64)	NS
	Stomatococcus sp	0 (73)	3 (64)	NS
	Listeria sp	0 (73)	2 (64)	NS
	Acinetobacter sp	1 (73)	0 (64)	NS
	Moraxella sp	1 (73)	0 (64)	NS
	Nocardia sp	3 (73)	0 (64)	NS
	Pseudomonas paucimobilis	1 (73)	0 (64)	NS
	Pseudomonas pickettii	1 (73)	0 (64)	NS
	Pseudomonas stutzeri	0 (73)	2 (64)	NS
	Serratia marcescens	1 (73)	0 (64)	NS
	Fungi	3 (73)	2 (64)	NS
	No growth	4 (73)	0 (64)	NS

Subjects were enrolled into a clinical study at the Cornea and Contact Lens Research Unit, School of Optometry and Vision Science, University of New South Wales. Subjects wore contralateral group IV and group I hydroxyethyl methacrylate (HEMA)-based hydrogel contact lenses. The extended wear schedule was 6 nights of continuous wear, with lens replacement on the seventh day. The daily wear schedule was 1 month of daily wear, with disinfection/cleaning in multipurpose solution overnight and monthly replacement of lenses.
Microorganisms were collected by sterilely removing the contact lens from the subjects eye and cultured as described in Willcox et al. (2003).
[a]At the 2-year visit, the coagulase-negative staphylococci were differentiated into individual species.
[b]Statistical analysis using Test of Proportion in CCSTAT—Quick Statistics for Optometrists (version 3.5).

lenses on a 30-night extended wear schedule does not greatly alter the types of bacteria that colonized the lids or conjunctiva (17) or the lenses worn on either a 6-night or 30-night schedule (18).

DIFFERENCES WITH DIFFERENT LENS WEAR REGIMENS

Several studies have examined changes to the contact lens microbiota during daily versus extended wear. The wear regimens for daily wear were usually monthly replacement and daily cleaning with a multipurpose hydrogel lens solution and for extended wear were usually 6 nights of wear with lens replacement on every seventh day. Willcox et al. (19) demonstrated no differences between bacteria colonization of hydrogel lenses worn on either a daily or extended wear schedule. Extended wear did not change the frequency or spectrum of bacteria isolated compared to daily wear (13) in Indian or Australian populations. Tables 5.1, 5.2, and 5.6 show the analysis of the conjunctival, lid, and contact lens microbiota over time (2 years of contact lens wear) in a population of daily lens wearers versus extended lens wearers (hydrogel lenses worn in both cases). Daily wearers were a group of previous daily wearers enrolled into a large scale clinical trial in Sydney. The extended wearers were a group of neophytes similarly enrolled and at approximately the same time. For the conjunctival microbiota, there was no significant difference in the frequency of isolation of microbial types at baseline, but there was a significant difference in the frequency of sterile cultures ($p < 0.001$), with an increased frequency of sterile cultures in the daily wearers (experienced wearers). After 1 year of wear, daily wearers had an increased colonization frequency of coagulase-negative staphylococci on their lenses. This may be related to increased handling of lenses during daily wear, as coagulase-negative staphylococci are commonly isolated from skin (20), although this did not reach significance for staphylococcal types at 2 years of wear. After 2 years of wear, the only differences between the wearers was the increased frequency of sterile cultures for the extended wear group. A similar finding has been reported for experienced extended wearers (5).

There were no significant differences in the frequency of isolation of any microbial type on the lids or the frequency of sterile cultures (Table 5.2). For the contact lens microbiota (Table 5.6), there was, initially at baseline, an increase in the frequency of isolation of coagulase-negative staphylococci ($p < 0.01$) and decreased frequency of sterile cultures ($p < 0.001$) in the extended wear group, but this had evened out at the 1-year visit. The only other change was an apparent increase in isolation frequency of *Propionibacterium* sp in the extended wear group at the 1-year visit ($p < 0.05$). Thus, there are remarkably few changes to the ocular or lens microbiota when daily and extended wear of

lenses are examined. A possible reason for this is the remarkably quick way that the eye can remove bacteria, at least from handled lenses (20).

MICROBIOTA DURING ADVERSE RESPONSES ASSOCIATED WITH CONTACT LENS WEAR

It is generally accepted that the microorganisms that cause adverse responses during contact lens wear are present on the contact lens surface and are not present on ocular tissues. The exception is MK, where the bacteria penetrate and infect the cornea. Contact lens-induced corneal adverse responses recently have been classified into serious sight-threatening responses, of which MK is the only one; significant adverse responses such as contact lens-induced acute red eye (CLARE), contact lens-induced peripheral ulcers (CLPU), and infiltrative keratitis (IK); and nonsignificant adverse responses such as asymptomatic infiltrative keratitis (AIK) and asymptomatic infiltrates (AI) (21). Of these adverse responses, bacterial colonization is one of the initiating factors in MK (22), CLARE (23,24), CLPU (25), and certain IK and AIK events (26). There are a wide variety of clinical signs and symptoms associated with MK. The common symptoms include moderate to severe pain of rapid onset, severe redness of the conjunctiva, blurred or hazy vision, photophobia, discharge, and puffy lids. Common signs include corneal infiltration (usually central or paracentral; large irregular infiltrate; diffuse infiltration surrounding epithelial lesion; infiltrate usually anterior to mid stromal), epithelial loss overlying the infiltrate (ulceration), and cells in the anterior chamber adhering to the endothelium. The clinical signs and symptoms associated with the noninfected adverse responses are more defined in nature (21). Gram-positive bacteria are commonly associated with CLPU (25, 26), whereas Gram-negative bacteria are commonly associated with CLARE (23,26,27). For CLARE, *Haemophilus influenzae* is the most commonly isolated bacterium (24). AI is associated with contamination of contact lens by Gram-positive bacteria, whereas IK is associated with contamination of lids of wearers with Gram-negative bacteria (1). In a study conducted in India using subjects in extended wear of disposable hydrogel lenses, the incidence of contamination of contact lenses by Gram-negative bacteria, Gram-positive bacteria, or fungi was greater during adverse responses (infiltrates in general) than during asymptomatic wear (28). *Streptococcus pneumoniae* ($>10\times$) or Gram-negatives ($6\times$) isolation was more frequent during adverse responses than asymptomatic lens wear (28).

Studies have examined the relative rate of adverse responses. In a study in Sweden examining the rates of adverse responses including MK from 1981 to 1982, the lowest level of complications occurred with hard lenses and the highest incidence of severe complications (including MK) occurred with the extended wear of hydrogels (29). In general, extended wear of lenses poses the highest risk of corneal infection, and use of hydrogel lenses appears to have a greater risk compared with use of rigid lenses (30). In the United States, 56% of MK has been associated with contact lens wear (31). In a review of published data by Liesegang (32), the risk of MK was estimated in various studies to be 2 per 10,000 during wear of GP lenses, 2.2 to 4.1 per 10,000 during daily wear of hydrogel lenses, 13.3 to 20.9 per 10,000 during extended wear of hydrogel lenses, and 52 per 10,000 for therapeutic lenses. The relative risk associated with contact lens wear has been estimated to be 1 for GP (referent), 0.5 to 2.74 for polymethyl methacrylate (PMMA) lenses, 1.0 to 4.2 for daily wear hydrogel lenses, 2.7 to 36.8 for extended wear hydrogel lenses, and 13.0 to 13.3 for wear of disposable hydrogels. Risk factors that have been identified include smoking, extended wear, male gender, and socioeconomic factors (32).

An interesting comparison can be made between the risks associated with MK in different lenses, with the lowest risk generally being daily wear of GP lenses and the apparent increased colonization of GP lenses of potentially pathogenic Gram-negative bacteria (11). This may reflect other changes to the cornea that occur during (especially extended) wear of hydrogel lenses that predispose the MK over and above an apparent increase in Gram-negative bacterial colonization.

Reasons for the increased risk of MK with lens wear have included failure to follow standard contact lens care, which was present in 88% of culture- or histology-proven MK (33). The spectrum of causative organisms in lens-related infections differs from that associated with non–lens-related infections, with up to 70% of culture-proven cases attributable to *Pseudomonas aeruginosa* (10), in contrast to non-contact lens wearers in whom *S. aureus* is the predominant bacterium. Other Gram-negative rods, such as *Serratia* sp, *Proteus* sp, and other *Pseudomonas* sp, have been reported to cause MK during lens wear. Of the Gram-positive species, *Staphylococcus* sp are the most prevalent. This is illustrated in a study by Tabbara et al. (34), where of a total of 11 MK cases, 7 were able to culture *P. aeruginosa*, 1 cultured *S. aureus,* and 3 cultured *S. epidermidis* (coagulase-negative staphylococci). Similarly, examining cases of MK over a 14-year period demonstrated that 40% of cases were attributed to *P. aeruginosa* and 31% to staphylococci; *S. pneumoniae, S. viridans,* and *Serratia marcescens* were the next most common (35). Bandage contact lens use was associated with quasi-commensal microbiota causing MK or polymicrobial MK (35). Fungi are uncommon causes on MK during contact lens wear, and no cases of fungal MK were found in a contact lens-wearing group compared to 17% of cases in a non-contact lens-wearing group (36). In a retrospective study from 1972 to 1987, 4% of 90 cosmetic or aphakic contact lens wearers had fungal MK and 27% of 15 therapeutic contact lens wearers had fungal MK. Filamentous

TABLE 5.7. SUMMARY OF BACTERIA ISOLATED FROM CASES OF MICROBIAL KERATITIS WITH HEMA-BASED HYDROGEL LENSES

Causative Bacteria (Total Culture Positive Cases)	HEMA-Based hydrogel 100[a] [Isolation Frequency (%)]
Gram-negative bacteria	73
Pseudomonas aeruginosa or sp	66
Serratia marcescens	4
Haemophilis influenzae	1
Morganella morgani	1
Escherichia coli	1
Gram-positive bacteria	25
Coagulase negative staphylococci	13
Staphylococcus aureus	6
Corynebacterium sp	3 (mixed)
Propionibacterium sp	3
Bacillus cereus	1
Unidentified	1

[a]Data from Patrinely et al. (107), Mondino et al. (108), Weissman et al. (109), Cohen et al. (110), Donnerfeld et al. (111), and Schein et al. (10).
HEMA, hydroxyethyl methacrylate.

fungi are more likely to be associated with cosmetic/aphakic lens wear (37).

Table 5.7 summarizes the isolation frequency of a series of studies on MK over a number of years. The types of microorganisms isolated has been remarkably similar, although in a study by Cohen et al. (38) there was an apparent steady decrease in the isolation frequency of *P. aeruginosa* from MK from 1993 to 1995, and the total number of contact lens related MK also decreased. This latter finding could have been the result of treating MK outside of a hospital environment (in which the study was carried out). Other microorganisms that have been reported to cause corneal infections during contact lens use include *Acanthamoeba* sp and viruses (although whether contact lens use increases the rate of viral keratitis remains uncertain).

For *Acanthamoeba* MK, the greatest risks include contact lens wear, with the incidence increasing in the 1980s (39, 40). Contact lens solutions for soaking/rinsing that were made with nonsterile water and salt tablets contributed to the increase (40). Another risk factor for developing *Acanthamoeba* MK includes the use of chlorine-based disinfection systems (41).

SOURCES OF OCULAR MICROBIOTA

The source of the normal and pathogenic microbiota in lens wearers is not always clear, although lens care material (42, 43), the hands (44), and ocular contamination (45) have been implicated. Contact lens contamination commonly occurs through lens handling (46), but it appears that during uncomplicated lens wear these organisms are readily cleared from the lens surface by the ocular defense mechanisms. Other sources of contamination of lenses by the normal microbiota include the eye lids of wearers (45). Colonization by Gram-negative bacteria, including potential agents of MK, is likely to be from environmental sources, such as the domestic water supply (45).

In a study of the source of bacteria found on the lenses of seamen, *Enterobacter* sp and *Pseudomonas* sp found on lenses were also found in the ships environment, whereas the normal ocular microbiota, e.g., coagulase-negative staphylococci, were found on lids as well as the lenses (14). Bottled water can contain potential ocular pathogens; 12 samples from eight brands contained microorganisms, with 37% of samples being contaminated (47).

The area that has received most attention is contact lens storage, and cleaning and disinfecting solutions. Five percent of contact lens storage solutions have been demonstrated to be contaminated with *P. aeruginosa* (48). In Turkey, medical personnel had 22% of solutions and contact lenses contaminated, whereas nonmedical personnel had only 2% solutions and contact lenses contaminated (49), which may reflect changes in the environment where solutions are kept affecting the type or frequency of contamination.

In a study examining preserved saline, patients used the saline for specified time periods (7–28 days), after which the saline underwent microbial analysis (43). The overall contamination rate was approximately 26%, and this rate remained similar for all periods of use. The coagulase-negative staphylococci were the most frequently isolated bacteria. Bacteria and fungi were isolated more frequently from bottle nozzles than from the saline contents. No *Acanthamoeba* were isolated. Saline preserved with ethylene-diamine-tetra-acetic acid in conjunction with sorbic acid showed the highest percentage sterility. A direct comparison between the 1999 study and a previous investigation into the contamination rate of unpreserved saline was possible (50). This comparison demonstrated that preserved saline became contaminated with Gram-positive bacteria rather than Gram-negative bacteria, and that the overall contamination rate was lower for preserved than unpreserved saline (43). A similar result was found in the study by Theng et al. (14).

Contact lens storage cases are another potentially important source of lens contamination, especially for daily wearers. For example, *Bacillus cereus* isolated from MK with daily wear of soft lenses also was isolated from the lens case of the patient (51). In a study in Scotland, 53% (n = 178) of cases were contaminated during normal wearer use and 4% in total were contaminated with amoeba (52). Up to 24% of cases can show contamination with *Stenotrophomonas* sp, *Pseudomonas* sp, and *Serratia* sp, but this study could find no *Acanthamoeba* in cases (53). Another study demonstrated that 13% of contact lens storage cases were contaminated with *P. aeruginosa* (48). A large study examining 101 asymptomatic daily wearers found that 81% of cases were contaminated: 77% grew bacteria, 24% fungi, 20% protozoa, and 8% *Acanthamoeba* (54). Interestingly, H_2O_2 was the most common method of disinfection, and all the bacteria that were isolated from the cases possessed catalase, an enzyme that breaks down H_2O_2. A study of 178 contact lens wearers in Scotland demonstrated that the method of disinfection, use of tap water, and age of the lens was associated significantly with case contamination (55).

Cold water (especially from tanks and with lime scale) has been associated with *Acanthamoeba* contamination of water (56). In this same study, 19 of 50 cases, 12 of 122 rinsing solutions, and 59 of 100 cold taps yield Gram-negative bacteria that could be used as food source by *Acanthamoeba* (56). *Acanthamoeba* is only commonly found in those cases with concomitant bacteria and/or fungal contamination (57), possibly because the amoeba can use the bacteria as a food source. For example, an *in vitro* study showed that *Acanthamoeba* growth was stimulated well by *Stenotrophomonas (Xanthomonas) maltophilia*, *Flavobacterium breve,* or *Pseudomonas paucimobilis* (58).

BACTERIAL PATHOGENIC TRAITS INVOLVED IN PRODUCTION OF ADVERSE RESPONSES DURING LENS WEAR

Because most bacterial-driven adverse responses that occur during lens wear are attributed initially to bacterial colonization of contact lenses, the ability of bacteria to adhere to lenses has been studied. This initial adhesion is followed, in cases of MK, by adhesion to the corneal epithelium, which may be mediated by specific proteins on the bacterial surface. Tissue penetration then occurs, which may be mediated by the production of bacterial toxins or proteases and subsequently by activation of host proteases. Activation of host defense mechanisms causes cytokine production and white blood cell recruitment. This leads to the characteristic clinical signs and symptoms of MK (21).

Adhesion to Contact Lenses

Studies have estimated the adhesion of various bacteria to contact lenses, including estimation of the strength of adhesion, the nonspecific factors involved in adhesion, the effect of lens wear on bacterial adhesion, and the role of possible specific bacterial–lens deposit interactions in mediating adhesion and colonization. For *S. epidermidis* adhesion to contact lenses, adhesion was greatest for the strain that produced slime (an adhesive extracellular polysaccharide substance). In general there was greater adhesion to low-water-content hydrogels than ionic lenses, and spin-cast lenses adhered less bacteria than lathe cut (perhaps because of differences in less surface roughness) (59). Figure 5.2 shows a similar trend for some strains of *P. aeruginosa* (6294, Paer1) but not all strains. Examination of nonspecific adhesion mechanisms demonstrated that *Pseudomonas* are more hydrophobic than *Staphylococcus* (and neither of the bacteria had a particularly charged surface). This difference in hydrophobicity was related to some extent to the greater numbers adhering to either a hydrophilic or hydrophobic lens surface (60). Stapleton et al. (61) observed *P. aeruginosa* adhered more to low-water-content nonionic hydrogels than to ionic hydrogels. Three strains of bacteria (two of *P. aeruginosa* and one of *Aeromonas hydrophila*) adhered in increased numbers to silicone hydrogel lenses compared to hydrogel lenses. This increase may have been due to the more hydrophobic nature of the underlying contact lens material in the silicone hydrogel lenses (19).

P. aeruginosa adhesion to unworn lenses is affected by changes in salt concentrations in the environment (62) and growth temperature (19). Figure 5.3 demonstrates the effect of environmental conditions on adhesion of *P. aeruginosa* to a group IV hydrogel. The bacteria were grown and simply exposed to various environmental conditions. Decreasing the temperature to which the bacteria were exposed to the lens surface from 37°C to 30°C resulted in less adhesion, as did decreasing the pH of the environment.

Effect of Adsorbed Tear Film Components on Bacterial Adhesion to Contact Lenses

Lens surface deposits have been shown to increase adhesion of *P. aeruginosa,* but enzyme cleaning (using papain, pancreatin, neuraminidase, mannosidase, or glucosidase) did not

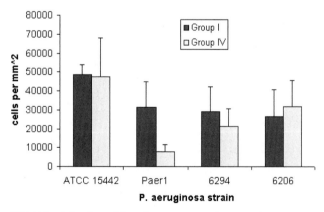

FIG. 5.2. Adhesion of *Pseudomonas aeruginosa* strains to group I and group IV hydrogel contact lenses. Bacteria were grown overnight in trypticase soy broth at 35°C, then washed and resuspended in phosphate-buffered saline to an optical density of 0.1 at 660 nm. Bacteria were allowed to adhere to washed contact lenses for 10 minutes at ambient temperature, nonadherent bacteria were removed, and the numbers of bacterial cells adhered to the lens surface were counted microscopically after staining with crystal violet. For further details see Taylor et al. (67).

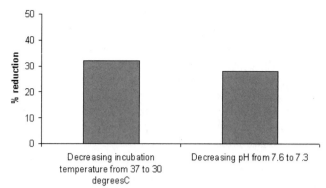

FIG. 5.3. The effect of changing environmental conditions on the adhesion of *Pseudomonas aeruginosa* to albumin-coated group IV hydrogel contact lenses. See Fig. 5.2 and Taylor et al. (67) for description of bacterial adhesion conditions and albumin adsorption to lenses.

reduce adhesion (63), and total protein did not correlate with adhesion of *P. aeruginosa* to lenses (64). Worn lenses usually increased the adhesion of bacteria (65). After wear of silicone hydrogel lenses, the adhesion of *P. aeruginosa, A. hydrophila, H. influenzae,* and *S. maltophilia* increased (19). Tear proteins lysozyme (on group IV lenses) and lipocalin or lactoferrin/secretory component of sIgA (on group I lenses) increased adhesion of *S. aureus* but also increased the ability to detach bacteria from the lens surface (60). Miller et al. (66) demonstrated that mucin, lactoferrin, lysozyme, IgA, BSA, and mixtures of these agents enhanced *P. aeruginosa* adhesion to hydrogels, but coating lenses in tears resulted in both increase and decrease, depending on underlying hydrogel polymer. Albumin coated onto the surface of contact lenses increased the adhesion of *P. aeruginosa* (60,67). Similarly, some strains of *S. marcescens* adhered better to lenses coated in an artificial tear fluid (68). Lysozyme adsorbed to a contact lens increases the adhesion of *S. aureus* to lenses (69), but it does not appear to affect the adhesion of *P. aeruginosa* (19).

Role of the Contact Lens in Promoting Adhesion of Bacteria to the Ocular Surface

After adhesion to the lens surface and probably bacterial growth, under the right conditions the bacteria adhere to and penetrate the cornea. A series of elegant experiments performed in the laboratories of H.D. Cavanagh aimed to understand the effects of the contact lens, especially low Dk versus high Dk lenses, on corneal epithelial cell turnover and bacterial binding to the cells. Rabbits wearing low Dk/t GP lenses or high Dk/t GP lenses or high Dk/t silicone hydrogel lenses have increased levels of viable epithelial cells on the corneal surface, and there was no difference between lens type (70). The conclusion drawn was that lenses acted like a bandage, protecting the cornea from the shear force of the lid and so protecting the cornea from this stimulator of epithelial cell death/sloughing. Previous experiments had shown that GP lens wear (regardless of Dk/t) prevented corneal epithelial cells apoptosis (a controlled method of cell death) but increased corneal stromal keratocyte apoptosis (71).

Do these effects translate to changes in the ability of bacteria to adhere to the cornea? It appears that there is not a direct relationship. There are differences in the levels of bacteria that can adhere to shed corneal epithelial cells, with more bacteria adhering to the shed epithelial cells during 3 months of extended wear hydrogel lens wear compared to extended wear silicone hydrogel lens wear (72). A hierarchy was noted in the adhesion of *P. aeruginosa* to epithelial cells of 6-night extended wear hydrogel wear > 6-night or 30-night extended wear silicone hydrogel wear > 30-night extended wear High Dk/t GP wear. High Dk/t GP wear did not increase bacterial binding to epithelial cells at all during the 1-year study. Interestingly, there appeared to be adaptation to lens wear during the study, with decreases in bacterial binding to shed epithelial cells over 12 months whether subjects wore hydrogel or silicone hydrogel lenses. Because this study and a previous study by the same group (73) using lenses worn on a daily wear basis had shown a correlation between bacterial binding to shed epithelial cells and the relative risk of lens wear schedules for MK (extended wear hydrogel > daily wear hydrogel > daily wear GP lens wear), it is tempting to speculate that the incidence of MK might be reduced with the silicone hydrogel lenses. However, definitive proof of this awaits the results of postmarket analysis and long-term clinical trials.

BACTERIAL PATHOGENIC TRAITS INVOLVED IN PRODUCTION OF MICROBIAL KERATITIS

Animal models have demonstrated the absolute requirement of a contact lens for the development of MK. Using tarsorrhaphy, contact lenses were inserted into rabbit eyes. Only those eyes with contact lenses produced MK (74). It is generally accepted that trauma of cornea is needed to develop MK (trauma may result from lens removal/insertion, hypoxia, deposits/debris, toxic reactions solutions). Animals with no trauma, even during contact lens wear, do not develop MK in the presence of a highly virulent *P. aeruginosa* isolate (27). Figures 5.4 and 5.5 demonstrate that growing bacteria cells at low temperature (25°C) increases the adhesion of *P. aeruginosa* strain Paer1 to a wounded epithelial surface, in a similar way to the increase on bacterial adhesion to contact lenses (19).

P. aeruginosa has four main strategies for adhering to ocular epithelial cells, namely, the production of pili (or fimbriae) on its cell surface, the production of exoenzyme S, cell surface lipopolysaccharide (LPS), and alginate synthesis (75,76), with pili probably being the dominant specific ad-

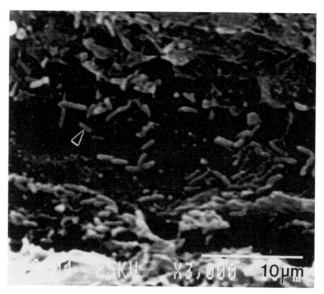

FIG. 5.4. Photomicrograph showing cells of *Pseudomonas aeruginosa* Paer1 adhering to scarified mouse cornea. Paer1 grown at 25°C in trypticase soy broth for 18 hours, then washed and resuspended in phosphate-buffered saline to an optical density of 1.0 at 660 nm. Cells then were allowed to adhere to scarified mouse corneas in organ culture. *Arrowhead* indicates *Pseudomonas* cells.

hesin. Pili are cell surface-associated protein structures that protrude from the cell. It is this protrusion of the pili and their specific protein confirmation/sequence that enables them to interact with receptors on the surface of the epithelial cells. Exoenzyme S is another cell surface protein that has been reported to mediate adhesion. Lipopolysaccharide is the main component of the cell-surface of all Gram-negative bacteria including *P. aeruginosa*. LPS is composed of both lipid and carbohydrate, with the carbohydrate component most likely being involved in adhesion. Alginate is an extracellular polysaccharide synthesized by *P. aeruginosa* after it has initially adhered to a surface and enables the adhered cells to remain firmly attached.

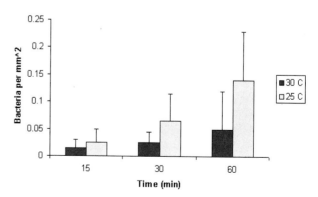

FIG. 5.5. Effect of changing the temperature of growth of *Pseudomonas aeruginosa* on the ability to adhere to scarified mouse corneas. Bacterial numbers were counted from micrographs similar to those shown in Fig. 5.4 and then numbers calculated to give bacterial cells per square millimeter of the whole cornea.

Adhesins of the bacterium appear to bind specifically to a 57-kDa sialylated protein of immature corneas, or asialo GM$_1$ glycolipid or cytokeratins exposed in wounded tissue (77,78). Mucin recently has been shown to inhibit *P. aeruginosa* binding to intact rabbit corneal epithelial cells (79), which implies that it also may act as an adhesin for the bacteria as all epithelial cells have cell surface-associated mucin. *P. aeruginosa* can bind to mucin (80) and to fibronectin, another epithelial cell surface protein (81). Strains isolated from MK have been compared with strains isolated from CLARE for their abilities to adhere to corneal epithelial cells. Interestingly, strains from MK and CLARE were equally able to adhere to epithelial cells (82). In a study examining potential virulence factors in *P. aeruginosa* isolated from MK, CLARE, or asymptomatic contact lens wearers, there was no clear distinction between clinical outcome and phenotype; strains that were able to kill corneal epithelial cells or to invade those cells were isolated from all three conditions (83). These results suggest that other factors are involved in the initiation of the respective conditions, possibly simply the presence of an epithelial break.

After adhesion to the cornea, the bacteria liberate powerful toxins that enable the bacteria to grow inside the cornea and result in a large-scale inflammatory response. *P. aeruginosa* and other Gram-negative bacteria can release LPS, or endotoxin, which is a potent inflammatory mediator. Intracorneal injection of *P. aeruginosa* endotoxin causes corneal "rings" seen clinically in human corneal infections due to *P. aeruginosa* (84). Exotoxins (exoproteins) produced by *P. aeruginosa* also may be involved in pathogenesis of corneal infection. Exotoxin A production has been shown to enable *P. aeruginosa* to infect and damage corneas (85). Extracellular proteases, elastase, and alkaline protease also may be involved in corneal ulceration, not only by their direct effect on corneal proteins but also by the activation of corneal proteases.

Epidemic clones of *P. aeruginosa* have been found among isolates from patients with MK. They were characterized by high activity of a size variant of the protease elastase, high alkaline protease activity, and possession of the *exoU* gene encoding exoenzyme U (86). Exoenzyme U appears to be associated with the ability to kill corneal epithelial cells. However, these virulence determinants were not exclusive traits in strains causing keratitis, as strains with other properties may cause keratitis in the presence of predisposing conditions. Indeed, another study has shown that *P. aeruginosa* strains that can invade inside corneal epithelial cells are more commonly isolated from MK (83). However, the finding related to cytotoxic strains is particularly interesting when compared with the finding that acute cytotoxic activity toward corneal epithelial cells correlates with resistance to contact lens disinfection systems, suggesting that chemical disinfection solutions may select for contamination with cytotoxic strains (87). A study examining the resistance of *P. aeruginosa* ocular isolates to commonly prescribed antibiotics has shown that a large number of isolates were resistant to the antibiotics. On average, 47% of isolates were resistant to β-lactam antibiotics, 10% were resistant to aminoglycosides, 4% were resistant to fluoroquinolones, and an additional 26% were resistant to ofloxacin. Approximately 22% of isolates showed multidrug resistance, and most of these were categorized as cytotoxic and serotype E (88). In another study, using the same strains of *P. aeruginosa*, serotype E strains were generally more adherent to contact lenses than most other serotypes (89).

MEASURES TO CONTROL PATHOGENIC MICROBIOTA ASSOCIATED WITH ADVERSE RESPONSES

Several measures have been put in place to try to control the exposure of contact lenses to potentially pathogenic bacteria and therefore avoid the production of adverse responses. Although contact lens disinfecting and cleaning solutions do become contaminated (see earlier), the presence of the disinfecting solutions probably helps reduce exposure to bacteria. In addition, good contact lens hygiene practices are important. In a study of 150 contact lens wearers in the United Kingdom, subjects instructed on best practice of lens/case use showed no isolation of *Acanthamoeba*, and bacteria were less frequently isolated from cases (90). In a study examining the ocular contamination of contact lens wearers, it appeared that the use of nonperoxide solutions was associated with a higher proportion of positive cultures of pathogenic microorganisms (3).

Various studies have examined the *in vitro* efficacy of contact lens solutions. For GP solutions, polyhexamethyl biguanide (PHMB)-containing solutions reduced the level of added bacteria and yeast but were less effective against molds unless PHMB plus chlorhexidine gluconate was used. Thimerosal-preserved solutions reduced the levels of all added bacteria and fungi tested. This held true even when "adapted" (preservative-resistant) bugs were used to challenge the solutions. A solution containing chlorhexidine by itself was not effective against "adapted" bacteria (*Serratia* or *Pseudomonas*). Benzalkonium chloride-containing solutions were less able to kill adapted *Serratia*. Polyquaternium-1 as the disinfecting agent was not effective against *Pseudomonas cepacia*. Some solutions required up to several days (> 14) to produce maximum effect (91). In another study, most solutions, particularly those containing phenylmercuric nitrate and polyaminopropyl biguanide, resulted in marked inhibition of bacterial cells in suspension (92). Solutions containing chlorhexidine and benzalkonium chloride showed survival of *S. marcescens* and *Candida albicans*, whereas cells of all tested microorganisms survived better in biofilm (cells adhered and encased in polysaccharide film) state (92). Drying of lens cases for 10 hours prior to testing reduced the survival of biofilm bacteria (92). For *Acantha-*

moeba, chlorhexidine may be more effective than polyhexamethylene biguanide (93).

For hydrogel lens care solutions, H_2O_2 systems are better able to kill *Candida* during recommended disinfection times than chemical (e.g., polyquat)-based systems, although after the H_2O_2 system was neutralized there could be significant regrowth (94). Two-step H_2O_2 systems (i.e., those that require an additive or step to neutralize the H_2O_2) are more effective at killing *Acanthamoeba* (95,96). One-step (neutralized) H_2O_2 and multipurpose solutions are similar to each other in controlling *Acanthamoeba* (97). Coculture with *P. aeruginosa* (a strain that can invade mammalian cells) increased *Acanthamoeba* survival (97,98). Interestingly, the presence of *Acanthamoeba* does not protect *P. aeruginosa* from contact lens solutions (99).

In other *in vitro* studies, H_2O_2 or chlorhexidine systems were effective against *Acanthamoeba* trophozoites and cysts, benzalkonium systems were only effective against trophozoites, and solutions containing polyaminopropyl biguanide or polyquaternium-1 were ineffective against trophozoites or cysts (100). Up to 9 hours was needed to kill cysts but only 30 minutes was required to kill trophozoites in H_2O_2 (100). When *Acanthamoeba* cysts were exposed to solutions *in vitro,* it was shown that saline solutions allowed the survival for 14 to 90 days and cleaning solutions allowed survival for 1 to 90 days, whereas disinfecting solutions allowed survival for 6 hours to 14 days (101). None of the solutions killed cysts in less than 6 hours of exposure (101). Multipurpose solutions may have the ability to dislodge adhered *Acanthamoeba* from contact lenses (102,103). Versions of multipurpose solutions that do not require any rubbing for apparent efficacy have antiamoebal activity (104) and activity against *S. aureus, S. marcescens, P. aeruginosa, C. albicans,* and *Fusarium solani* (105).

For control of contact lens storage case contamination, recommendations include regular scrubbing of lens cases to disrupt biofilm, exposure to hot (>70°C) water, allowing the case to dry between use, use of two-step H_2O_2 solutions, and regular replacement of cases (54). In an *in vitro* study, the most efficient treatment for removing *P. aeruginosa* from a case was the use of H_2O_2, the rinsing of the cases, and subsequent air drying (106).

CONCLUSIONS

Although new and better contact lens solutions to control bacteria are being produced and the best practice advise for their, and contact lens storage case, use is recommended and appropriate, we believe that until contact lenses that actively discourage bacteria from colonization are available, these measures will have only a small impact on the rate of MK. This belief is supported by the continued findings of increased risk of MK during extended wear of lenses, when the lenses do not come into contact with storage cases or

solutions. We look forward to the time when antimicrobial contact lenses are available on the market.

ACKNOWLEDGMENTS

This work was supported in part by the Australian Federal Government through the Cooperative Research Centres Scheme. The authors thank Professor Linda Hazlett for help with the adhesion of bacteria to mouse corneas in organ culture. The skilled help of Savtri Sharma, Usha Gopinathan, Patricia Munoz, S.K. Shynn, and the clinical staff of the Cornea and Contact Lens Research Unit, School of Optometry and Vision Science, and Cooperative Research Centre for Eye Research and Technology, University of New South Wales, Sydney, Australia, and the LV Prasad Eye Institute, Hyderabad, India, are gratefully acknowledged.

REFERENCES

1. Willcox MDP, Zhu H, Sharma S, et al. Microbiology of the external ocular surface. *Optician* 2001;211:5795–5799.
2. Perkins RE, Kundsin RB, Pratt MV, et al. Bacteriology of normal and infected conjunctiva. *J Clin Microbiol* 1975;1: 147–149.
3. Fleiszig SM, Efron N. Microbial flora in eyes of current and former contact lens wearers. *J Clin Microbiol* 1992;30: 1156–1161.
4. Leitch EC, Harmis NY, Corrigan KM, et al. Identification and enumeration of staphylococci from the eye during soft contact lens wear. *Optom Vis Sci* 1998;75:258–265.
5. Stapleton F, Willcox MD, Fleming CM, et al. Changes to the ocular biota with time in extended- and daily-wear disposable contact lens use. *Infect Immun* 1995;63:4501–4505.
6. Ramachandran L, Sharma S, Sankaridurg PR, et al. Examination of the conjunctival microbiota after 8 hours of eye closure. *CLAO J* 1995;21:195–199.
7. Elander TR, Goldberg MA, Salinger CL, et al. Microbial changes in the ocular environment with contact lens wear. *CLAO J* 1992;18:53–55.
8. Hovding G. The conjunctival and contact lens bacterial flora during lens wear. *Acta Ophthalmol* 1981;59:387–401.
9. Larkin DF, Leeming JP. Quantitative alterations of the commensal eye bacteria in contact lens wear. *Eye* 1991;5:70–74.
10. Schein OD, Ormerod LD, Barraquer E, et al. Microbiology of contact lens-related keratitis. *Cornea* 1989;8:281–285.
11. Izquierdo N, Diaz Mendoza S, Townsend W, et al. Prevalence of the microbiologic flora in contact lens wearers at the Puerto Rico Medical Center. *Bol Asoc Med Puerto Rico* 1991;83:96–68.
12. Hart DE, Reindel W, Proskin HM, et al. Microbial contamination of hydrophilic contact lenses: quantitation and identification of microorganisms associated with contact lenses while on the eye. *Optom Vis Sci* 1993;70:185–191.
13. Gopinathan U, Stapleton F, Sharma S, et al. Microbial contamination of hydrogel contact lenses. *J Appl Microbiol* 1997;82: 653–658.
14. Theng JT, Kiak LW, Lee BG, et al. Microbiological profile of a shipboard environment and the flora on contact lenses of seamen. *CLAO J* 2001;27:47–52.
15. Sweeney DF, Stapleton F, Leitch EC, et al. Microbial colonisa-

tion of soft contact lenses over time. *Optom Vis Sci* 2000;78:100–105.

16. Stapleton F, Dart J. *Pseudomonas* keratitis associated with biofilm formation on a disposable soft contact lens. *Br J Ophthalmol* 1995;79:864–865.

17. Willcox MDP, Harmis NY, Holden BA. Bacterial populations on high-Dk silicone hydrogel contact lenses: effect of length of wear in asymptomatic patients. *Clin Exp Optom* 2002;85:172–175.

18. Keay L, Willcox MDP, Sweeney DF, et al. Bacterial populations on 30N EW silicone hydrogel contact lenses. *CLAO J* 2001;27:30–34.

19. Willcox MDP, Harmis N, Cowell BA, et al. Bacterial interactions with contact lenses; effects of lens material, lens wear and microbial physiology. *Biomaterials* 2001;22:3235–3247.

20. Mowrey-McKee MF, Sampson HJ, Proskin HM. Microbial contamination of hydrophilic contact lenses. Part II: quantitation of microbes after patient handling and after aseptic removal from the eye. *CLAO J* 1992;18:240–244.

21. Holden BA, Sankaridurg P, Jalbert I. Adverse responses. Which ones and how many. In: Sweeney DF, ed. *Silicone hydrogels. The rebirth of continuous wear contact lenses.* Oxford: Butterworth Heinemann, 2000:150–213.

22. Solomon OD, Loff H, Perla B, et al. Testing hypotheses for risk factors for contact lens-associated infectious keratitis in an animal model. *CLAO J* 1994;20:109–113.

23. Holden BA, La Hood D, Grant T, et al. Gram-negative bacteria can induce contact lens related acute red eye (CLARE) responses. *CLAO J* 1996;22:47–52.

24. Sankaridurg PR, Willcox MD, Sharma S, et al. *Haemophilus influenzae* adherent to contact lenses associated with production of acute ocular inflammation. *J Clin Microbiol* 1996;34:2426–2431.

25. Jalbert I, Willcox MD, Sweeney DF. Isolation of *Staphylococcus aureus* from a contact lens at the time of a contact lens-induced peripheral ulcer: case report. *Cornea* 2000;19:116–120.

26. Sankaridurg PR, Sharma S, Willcox M, et al. Colonization of hydrogel lenses with Streptococcus pneumoniae: risk of development of corneal infiltrates. *Cornea* 1999;18:289–295.

27. Willcox MDP, Sankaridurg P, Lan J, et al. Inflammation and infection and effects of the closed eye. In: Sweeney DF, ed. *Silicone hydrogels. The rebirth of continuous wear contact lenses.* Oxford: Butterworth Heinemann, 2000:45–75.

28. Sankaridurg P, Sharma S, Willcox MDP, et al. Bacterial colonization of disposable soft contact lenses is greater during corneal infiltrative events than during asymptomatic extended lens wear. *J Clin Microbiol* 2000;38:4420–4424.

29. Chalupa E, Swarbrick HA, Holden BA, et al. Severe corneal infections associated with contact lens wear. *Ophthalmology* 1987;94:17–22.

30. Dart JK, Stapleton F, Minassian D. Contact lenses and other risk factors in microbial keratitis. *Lancet* 1991;338:650–653.

31. Zegans ME, Becker HI, Budzik J, et al. The role of bacterial biofilms in ocular infections. *DNA Cell Biol* 2002;21:415–420.

32. Liesegang TJ. Contact lens-related microbial keratitis: Part I: epidemiology. *Cornea* 1997;16:125–131.

33. Bowden FW 3rd, Cohen EJ, Arentsen JJ, et al. Patterns of lens care practices and lens product contamination in contact lens associated microbial keratitis. *CLAO J* 1989;15:49–54.

34. Tabbara KF, El-Sheikh HF, Aabed B. Extended wear contact lens related bacterial keratitis. *Br J Ophthalmol* 2000;84:327–328.

35. Ormerod LD, Smith RE. Contact lens-associated microbial keratitis. *Arch Ophthalmol* 1986;104:79–83.

36. Koidou-Tsiligianni A, Alfonso E, Forster RK. Ulcerative keratitis associated with contact lens wear. *Am J Ophthalmol* 1989;108:64–67.

37. Wilhelmus KR, Robinson NM, Font RA, et al. Fungal keratitis in contact lens wearers. *Am J Ophthalmol* 1988;106:708–714.

38. Cohen EJ, Fulton JC, Hoffman CJ, et al. Trends in contact lens-associated corneal ulcers. *Cornea* 1996;15;566–570.

39. Stehr-Green JK, Bailey TM, Visvesvara GS. The epidemiology of *Acanthamoeba* keratitis in the United States. *Am J Ophthalmol* 1989;107:331–336.

40. Illingworth CD, Cook SD. *Acanthamoeba* keratitis. *Surv Ophthalmol* 1998;42:493–508.

41. Illingworth CD, Cook SD, Karabatsas CH, et al. *Acanthamoeba* keratitis: risk factors and outcome. *Br J Ophthalmol* 1995;79:1078–1082.

42. Mayo MS, Schlitzer RL, Ward MA, et al. Association of *Pseudomonas* and *Serratia* corneal ulcers with use of contaminated solutions. *J Clin Microbiol* 1987;25:1398–1400.

43. Sweeney DF, Willcox MDP, Sansey N, et al. Incidence of contamination of preserved saline solutions during normal use. *CLAO J* 1999;25:167–175.

44. Hart DE, Shih KL. Surface interaction on hydrogel extended wear contact lenses: microflora and microfauna. *Am J Optom Physiol Optics* 1987;64:739–748.

45. Willcox MDP, Power KN, Stapleton F, et al. Potential sources of bacteria that are isolated from contact lenses during wear. *Optom Vis Sci* 1997;74:1030–1038.

46. Mowrey-McKee MF, Monnat K, Sampson HJ, et al. Microbial contamination of hydrophilic contact lenses. Part I: quantitation of microbes on patient worn-and-handled lenses. *CLAO J* 1992;18:87–91.

47. Penland RL, Wilhelmus KR. Microbiologic analysis of bottled water: is it safe for use with contact lenses? *Ophthalmology* 1999;106:1500–1503.

48. Micallef C, Cuschieri P, Bonnici MR. Contamination of contact-lens-related sources with *Pseudomonas aeruginosa*. *Ophthalmologica* 2000;214:324–331.

49. Kozer-Bilgin L, Demir N, Altan-Yaycioglu R. Microbiological evaluation of contact lenses and contact lens disinfection solutions in an asymptomatic population and in medical personnel. *CLAO J* 1999;25:228–232.

50. Sweeney DF, Taylor P, Holden BA, et al. Contamination of 500 ml bottles of unpreserved saline. *Clin Exp Optom* 1992;75:67–75.

51. Pinna A, Sechi LA, Zanetti S, et al. *Bacillus cereus* keratitis associated with contact lens wear. *Ophthalmology* 2001;108:1830–1834.

52. Devonshire P, Munro FA, Abernethy C, et al. Microbial contamination of contact lens cases in the west of Scotland. *Br J Ophthalmol* 1993;77:41–45.

53. Midelfart J, Midelfart A, Bevanger L. Microbial contamination of contact lens cases among medical students. *CLAO J* 1996;22:21–24.

54. Gray TB, Cursons RT, Sherwan JF, et al. *Acanthamoeba*, bacterial, and fungal contamination of contact lens storage cases. *Br J Ophthalmol* 1995;79:601–605.

55. Clark BJ, Harkins LS, Munro FA, et al. Microbial contamination of cases used for storing contact lenses. *J Infect* 1994;28:293–304.

56. Seal D, Stapleton F, Dart J. Possible environmental sources of *Acanthamoeba* spp in contact lens wearers. *Br J Ophthalmol* 1992;76:424–427.

57. Donzis PB, Mondino BJ, Weissman BA, et al. Microbial analysis of contact lens care systems contaminated with *Acanthamoeba*. *Am J Ophthalmol* 1989;108:53–56.

58. Bottone EJ, Madayag RM, Qureshi MN. *Acanthamoeba* keratitis: synergy between amebic and bacterial cocontaminants in

contact lens care systems as a prelude to infection. *J Clin Microbiol* 1992;30:2447–2450.

59. Garcia-Saenz MC, Arias-Puente A, Fresnadillo-Martinez MJ, et al. Adherence of two strains of *Staphylococcus epidermidis* to contact lenses. *Cornea* 2002;21:511–515.

60. Bruinsma GM, van der Mei HC, Busscher HJ. Bacterial adhesion to surface hydrophilic and hydrophobic contact lenses. *Biomaterials* 2001;22:3217–3224.

61. Stapleton F, Dart JK, Minassian D. Risk factors with contact lens related suppurative keratitis. *CLAO J* 1993;19:204–210.

62. Cowell B, Willcox MDP, Schneider R A relatively small change in sodium chloride concentration has a strong effect on adhesion of ocular bacteria to contact lenses. *J Appl Microbiol* 1998;84: 950–958.

63. Butrus SI, Klotz SA. Contact lens surface deposits increase the adhesion of *Pseudomonas aeruginosa*. *Curr Eye Res* 1990;9: 717–724.

64. Mowrey-McKee MF, Monnat K, Sampson HJ, et al. Microbial contamination of hydrophilic contact lenses. Part I: quantitation of microbes on patient worn-and-handled lenses. *CLAO J* 1992; 18:87–91.

65. Williams TJ, Willcox MDP, Schneider RP. The role of tear fluid in the growth of gram negative bacteria on contact lenses. *Aust N Z J Ophthalmol* 1997;25:s30–s32.

66. Miller MJ, Wilson LA, Ahern DG. Effects of protein, mucin and human tears on adherence of *Pseudomonas aeruginosa* to hydrophilic contact lenses. *J Clin Microbiol* 1988;26:513–517.

67. Taylor RL, Willcox MDP, Williams T, et al. Modulation of bacterial adhesion to hydrogel contact lenses by albumin. *Optom Vis Sci* 1997;75:23–29.

68. Hume EBH, Willcox MDP. Adhesion and growth of *Serratia marcescens* on artificial closed eye tears (ATF) soaked hydrogel contact lenses. *Aust N Z J Ophthalmol* 1997;25:s39–s41.

69. Thakur A, Chauhan A, Willcox MDP. Effect of lysozyme on adhesion of *Staphylococcus aureus* strains, isolated from contact lens induced peripheral ulcers, to contact lenses and toxin release. *Aust N Z J Ophthalmol* 1999;27:224–227.

70. Yamamoto K, Ladage PM, Ren DH, et al. Effect of eyelid closure and overnight contact lens wear on viability of surface epithelial cells in rabbit cornea. *Cornea* 2002;21:85–90.

71. Yamamoto K, Ladage PM, Ren DH, et al. Effect of low and hyper Dk rigid gas permeable contact lenses on Bcl-2 expression and apoptosis in the rabbit corneal epithelium. *CLAO J* 2001; 27:137–143.

72. Ren DH, Yamamoto K, Ladage PM, et al. Adaptive effects of 30-night wear of hyper-O_2 transmissible contact lenses on bacterial binding and corneal epithelium. A 1-year clinical trial. *Ophthalmology* 2002;109:27–40.

73. Ladage PM, Yamamoto K, Ren DH, et al. Effects of rigid and soft contact lens daily wear on corneal epithelium, tear lactate dehydrogenase, and bacterial binding to exfoliated epithelial cells. *Ophthalmology* 2001;108:1279–1288.

74. Koch JM, Refojo MF, Hanninen LA, et al. Experimental *Pseudomonas aeruginosa* keratitis from extended wear of soft contact lenses. *Arch Ophthalmol* 1990;108:1453–1459.

75. Gupta SK, Berk RS, Masinick S, et al. Pili and lipopolysaccharide of *Pseudomonas* aeruginosa bind to the glycolipid asialo GM1. *Infect Immun* 1994;62:1025–1035.

76. Fletcher EL, Fleiszig SMJ, Brennan NA. Lipopolysaccharide in adherence of *Pseudomonas aeruginosa* to the cornea and contact lens. *Invest Ophthalmol Vis Sci* 1993;34:1930–1936.

77. Hazlett LD, Rudner X, Masinick S, et al. In the immature mouse, *Pseudomonas aeruginosa* pili bind a 57-kd (α2-6) sialylated corneal epithelial cell surface protein: a first step in infection. *Invest Ophthalmol Vis Sci* 1995;36:634–644.

78. Wu X, Kurpakus M, Hazlett LD. Some *P. aeruginosa* pilus-

79. Fleiszig SMJ, Zaidi TS, Ramphal R, et al. Modulation of *Pseudomonas aeruginosa* adherence to the corneal surface by mucus. *Infect Immun* 1994;62:1799–1804.

80. Aristoteli LP, Willcox MDP. The adhesion of *P. aeruginosa* ocular isolates to mucin. *Clin Exp Ophthalmol* 2001;29: 143–146.

81. Baleriola-Lucas C, Willcox MDP. The ability of ocular bacteria to bind to fibronectin. *Clin Exp Optom* 1998;81:81–87.

82. Willcox MDP, Hume EBH. Differences in the pathogenesis of bacteria isolated from contact lens induced infiltrative conditions. *Aust N Z J Ophthalmol* 1999;27:231–233.

83. Zhu H, Thuruthyil S, Willcox MDP. Determination of quorum-sensing signal molecules and virulence factors of *P. aeruginosa* strains isolated from contact lens-induced microbial keratitis. *J Med Microbiol* 2002;51:1063–1070.

84. Belmont JB, Ostler B, Dawson CR, et al. Non-infectious ring shaped keratitis associated with *Pseudomonas aeruginosa*. *Am J Ophthalmol* 1982;93:338–341.

85. Pillar CM, Hobden JA. *Pseudomonas aeruginosa* exotoxin A and keratitis in mice. *Invest Ophthalmol Vis Sci* 2002;43: 1437–1444.

86. Lomholt JA, Poulsen K, Kilian M. Epidemic population structure of Pseudomonas aeruginosa: evidence for a clone that is pathogenic for the eye and that has a distinct combination of virulence factors. *Infect Immun* 2001;69:6284–6295.

87. Lakkis C. Fleiszig SM. Resistance of *Pseudomonas aeruginosa* isolates to hydrogel contact lens disinfection correlates with cytotoxic activity. *J Clin Microbiol* 2001;39:1477–1486.

88. Zhu H, Thuruthyil S, Willcox MDP. *Pseudomonas aeruginosa* ocular isolates: antibiotic resistance, phenotypes and serotypes. *Cornea* 2003 *(in press)*.

89. Thuruthyil S, Zhu H, Willcox MDP. Serotype and adhesion of *Pseudomonas aeruginosa* isolated from contact lens wearers. *Clin Exp Ophthalmol* 2001;29:147–149.

90. Seal DV, Dalton A, Doris D. Disinfection of contact lenses without tap water rinsing: is it effective? *Eye* 1999;13:226–230.

91. Keeven J, Wrobel S, Portoles M, et al. Evaluating the preservative effectiveness of RGP lens care solutions. *CLAO J* 1995;21: 238–241.

92. May LL, Gabriel MM, Simmons RB, et al. Resistance of adhered bacteria to rigid gas permeable contact lens solutions. *CLAO J* 1995;21:242–246.

93. Borazjani RN, May LL, Noble JA, et al. Flow cytometry for determination of the efficacy of contact lens disinfecting solutions against *Acanthamoeba* spp. *Appl Environ Microbiol* 2000; 66:1057–1061.

94. Rosenthal RA, Stein JM, McAnally CL, et al. A comparative study of the microbiologic effectiveness of chemical disinfectants and peroxide-neutralizer systems. *CLAO J* 1995;21:99–110.

95. Hiti K, Walochnik J, Haller-Schober EM, et al. Viability of Acanthamoeba after exposure to a multipurpose disinfecting contact lens solution and two hydrogen peroxide systems. *Br J Ophthalmol* 2002;86:144–146.

96. Hughes R, Kilvington S. Comparison of hydrogen peroxide contact lens disinfection systems and solutions against Acanthamoeba polyphaga. *Antimicrob Agents Chemother* 2001;45: 2038–2043.

97. Cengiz AM, Harmis N, Stapleton F. Co-incubation of Acanthamoeba castellanii with strains of *Pseudomonas aeruginosa* alters the survival of amoeba. *Clin Exp Ophthalmol* 2000;28:191–193.

98. Stapleton F, Harmis N, Deshpande R, et al. Preliminary studies on the amoebicidal efficacy of contact lens disinfection systems. *Aust N Z J Ophthalmol* 1998;26:s44–46.

99. Willcox MDP, Low R, Hon J, et al. Does *Acanthamoeba* protect

Pseudomonas aeruginosa from the bactericidal effects of contact lens disinfecting systems? *Aust N Z J Ophthalmol* 1998;26: s32–s35.

100. Zanetti S, Fiori PL, Pinna A, et al. Susceptibility of *Acanthamoeba castellanii* to contact lens disinfecting solutions. *Antimicrob Agents Chemother* 1995;39:1596–1598.

101. Brandt FH, Ware DA, Visvesvara GS. Viability of *Acanthamoeba* cysts in ophthalmic solutions. *Appl Environ Microbiol* 1989;55:1144–1146.

102. Raali E, Vaahtoranta-Lehtonen HH, Lehtonen OP. Detachment of trophozoites of *Acanthamoeba* species from soft contact lenses with BEN22 detergent, BioSoak, and Renu multi-purpose solutions. *CLAO J* 2001;27:155–158.

103. Kilvington S, Anger C. A comparison of cyst age and assay method of the efficacy of contact lens disinfectants against *Acanthamoeba*. *Br J Ophthalmol* 2001;85:336–340.

104. Rosenthal RA, McAnally CL, McNamee LS, et al. Broad spectrum antimicrobial activity of a new multi-purpose disinfecting solution. *CLAO J* 2000;26:120–126.

105. Lever AM, Miller MJ. Comparative antimicrobial efficacy of multi-purpose lens care solutions using the FDA's revised guidance document for industry: stand-alone primary criteria. *CLAO J* 1999;25:52–56.

106. Larragoiti ND, Diamos ME, Simmons PA, et al. A comparative study of techniques for decreasing contact lens storage case contamination. *J Am Optom Assoc* 1994;65:161–163.

107. Patrinely JR, Wilhelmus KR, Rubin JM, et al. Bacterial keratitis associated with extended wear soft contact lenses. *CLAO J* 1985; 11:234–236.

108. Mondino BJ, Weissman BA, Farb MD, et al. Corneal ulcers associated with daily-wear and extended-wear contact lenses. *Am J Ophthalmol* 1986;102:58–65.

109. Weissman BA, Mondino BJ, Pettit TH, et al. Corneal ulcers associated with extended-wear soft contact lenses. *Am J Ophthalmol* 1984;94:476–481.

110. Cohen EJ, Laibson PR, Arentsen JJ, et al. Corneal ulcers associated with cosmetic extended wear soft contact lenses. *Ophthalmology* 1987;94:109–114.

111. Donnerfeld ED, Cohen EJ, Arentsen JJ, et al. Changing trends in contact lens associated corneal ulcers: an overview of 116 cases. *CLAO J* 1986;12:145–149.

CHAPTER

6

CONTACT LENS DESIGN

BARRY A. WEISSMAN
EDWARD S. BENNETT
AND RONALD G. SEGER

The purpose of the study of contact lens design is to help the reader become a better contact lens fitter and problem solver. In this chapter we discuss the importance of (i) lens surface geometries, including base curve or back central optic radius (BCOR), and the variables that affect them; (ii) various lens diameters, including overall or total diameter (OAD); (iii) lens thicknesses and mass and their influence upon fitting; and (iv) lens edges. The basic principles discussed apply equally to both rigid and soft contact lens designs.

The goals of lens design are to achieve excellence in vision quality, minimum physical awareness of worn contact lenses, and minimal physiologic insult to the eye(s) and supporting structures.

A contact lens prescription consists of a number of elements. It has become popular (especially since the introduction of hydrogel contact lenses) to specify a contact lens by only several measurements: power, OAD, base curve radius, and perhaps brand name or material. Unfortunately, the selection of important parameters such as central thickness and edge design is left by default to the laboratory. Even if the practitioner elects to specify a lens by stock or preset measurements, knowledge of laboratory-supplied measurements is essential so that accurate modifications and duplication will be possible at a later time. This holds true for rigid gas permeable (GP) contact lenses and perhaps for some custom hydrogel contact lenses as well.

It should be noted that the material from which the lens is shaped is itself a variable. Rigid materials include polymethyl methacrylate (PMMA) and various oxygen permeable plastics, such as silicone/acrylates, fluorinated silicone/acrylates, polystyrenes, and fluoropolymers. Flexible lenses are made of various soft hydrogel materials with water contents ranging from about 40% to 80%, and two current silicone hydrogels with water content of 24% or 36%. There have been additional "hybrid" materials on the market from time to time, but none has yet achieved substantial popularity and many have been withdrawn.

These materials can differ in oxygen permeability (Dk) and other characteristics such as refractive index, specific gravity, and thermal conductivity (Table 6.1). All of these factors may have a role in contact lens design. For example, two lenses with identical posterior curves, OADs, and central thicknesses may have very different front curvatures if they are made of materials with different refractive indices

TABLE 6.1. EXAMPLE PROPERTIES OF RIGID CONTACT LENS MATERIALS[a]

Material	Optical Index	Specific Gravity	Dk in cm mL O$_2$ sec mL mm Hg ($\times$ 10–11) at 35°C (approximate values)
PMMA	1.49	1.18	—
CAB	1.48	1.20	8
Silicon/acrylates			
Polycon	1.49	1.15	5
Polycon II	1.48	1.14	10
Polycon HDK	1.47	1.12	45
Boston II	1.47	1.13	11
Boston IV	1.47	1.10	18
Paraperm O$_2$	1.47	1.11	14
Paraperm O$_2$+	1.47	1.07	31
Paraperm EW	1.46	1.10	39
SGP	1.47	1.11	15
SGP II	1.47	1.10	40
Polystyrene			
Airlens	1.54	0.99	20
Opus III	1.53	1.02	14
Fluoropolymers			
Advent	1.39	1.60	78
Boston RxD	1.435	1.27	45
Equalens	1.44	1.19	44
Fluoroperm 30	1.46	1.12	30
Fluoroperm 60	1.45	1.13	60
Fluoroperm 92	1.45	1.10	90
Quantum	1.43	1.25	45
Fluorex 700	1.46	1.10	70

[a]Data presented here have been collected by the authors from various sources, including manufacturers' reports, and rounded off to two decimal places where possible. Particularly helpful were Dr. Ronald Herskowitz (Polymer Technology Corporation) and Dr. Tracy K. Tsuetaki (Fused Contacts). Data also from Fatt I, Rosoon JE, Melpolder JB. Measuring oxygen permeability of gas permeable hard and hydrogel lenses and flat samples in air. *Int Contact Lens Clin* 1987;14:386–401.

and yet achieve identical optical power on an eye. All differences can affect *in situ* performance.

BASE CURVE RADIUS

The base curve radius of a contact lens is the radius of curvature of the central posterior optical portion in millimeters. This also is known as the back central optic radius (BCOR) (Fig. 6.1) or sometimes r_2. Tuohy's original corneal rigid (PMMA) contact lenses were selected with a base curve radius flatter than the patient's corneal curvature (1). In later years, hard contact lens base curve radius sometimes was prescribed relatively steeper than the patient's corneal curvature. Both to improve distribution of mass and to increase tear exchange, these original rigid corneal lens base curve "philosophies" eventually were compromised to produce a corneal contour concept in which the ideal fitting relationship was proposed to be corneal alignment (1). Rigid lenses of smaller OADs could vault the corneal apex slightly, as the small OAD allows for increased corneal exposure and demands decreased movement for optical performance. Larger OAD rigid lens usually are slightly flatter in BCOR than the apical corneal curvature to allow for tear exchange

and permit lens movement without sealing the tear pool (2). Modern GP lenses are less dependent on tear exchange for the supply of corneal oxygen needs, and they naturally fall into the latter category. These lenses usually are about 9.2 to 9.6 mm in OAD and are intended to be fitted slightly but definitely flatter than corneal curvature in base curve radius (discussed later). Hydrogel lenses originally were used without regard to the base curve radius/corneal curve relationship, but Sarver (3) showed that Bausch & Lomb aspheric lenses 12.5 mm in diameter worked best if they were about 0.5 mm flatter in their posterior apical radius (PAR)—which is a simulation of BCOR for these aspheric posterior surface lenses—than was the curvature of the central cornea. As the hydrogel contact lens OAD increases, this flattening factor should increase to maintain sagittal depth alignment. Therefore, modern low minus powered hydrogels (about 14.0 mm in diameter) usually are fitted about 1.0 mm flatter in the base curve radius than is corneal curvature. This usually results in alignment on the eye after flexure or wrapping (4).

This discussion illustrates that OAD and contact lens base curve radius are relatively linked; thus, the primary clinical goal is to match closely the front surface of the cornea with the back surface of the lens. This is a sagittal

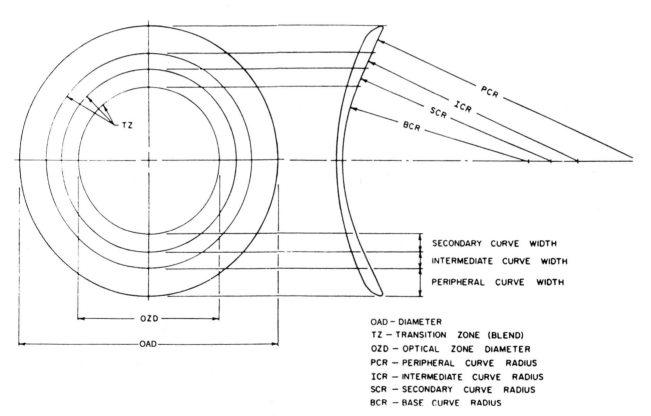

SECONDARY CURVE WIDTH
INTERMEDIATE CURVE WIDTH
PERIPHERAL CURVE WIDTH

OAD – DIAMETER
TZ – TRANSITION ZONE (BLEND)
OZD – OPTICAL ZONE DIAMETER
PCR – PERIPHERAL CURVE RADIUS
ICR – INTERMEDIATE CURVE RADIUS
SCR – SECONDARY CURVE RADIUS
BCR – BASE CURVE RADIUS

FIG. 6.1. Cross-section profile of a theoretical contact lens, rigid or hydrogel, showing overall or total diameter, base curve radius, central thickness (t_c), junction thickness (t_j), edge thickness, posterior peripheral curve system (radii and widths), anterior peripheral curve (radii and width), and anterior and posterior optic zone diameters. (From Bennett ES, Grohe RM. *Rigid gas permeable contact lenses.* New York: Professional Press Books, 1986, with permission.)

depth concept. Although there have been several efforts to unify contact lens base curve radius and OAD into a code for sagittal depth, none has been clinically accepted. It seems more flexible to maintain both overall diameter and base curve radius as independent variables. The clinician should recognize, however, that sagittal depth is being manipulated with changes in either the contact lens BCOR or OAD, or both.

POWER

Lens power (F) is the dioptric power of the contact lens, usually back vertex power. Contact lenses are considered thick lenses, and the standard formula is used:

$$F = (F_1/1 - \{t_{CL}F_1/n\}) + F_2,$$

where F_1 is the front surface power in diopters or $(n - 1)/r_1$ (r_1 is the radius of the front surface), F_2 is the back surface power $(1 - n)/r_2$, n is the refractive index of the lens material, and t_{cl} is lens central thickness (values of r and t_{cl} are in meters). Front vertex power often is preferable for in-office measurement of contact lenses; placement of the lens against the lensometer stop in back vertex position may allow the base curve to influence power determination as the lens central optics will vault away variably from the measurement position. This potential source of variability and error is minimized when the lens is measured in front vertex position and the central optical portion of the lens is directly placed in the stop location.

Optical power is considered a constant with rigid lenses but may be variable with hydrogel lenses. Weissman (5,6) noted that low minus powered hydrogel lenses do not change substantially in power with flexure, but that plus powered lenses should lose plus power slightly as they steepen in base curve radius.

OVERALL DIAMETER

The linear, chord, edge-to-edge measurement of the lens in millimeters is the OAD; truncated lenses have two diameters oriented at a 90° angle.

CENTER THICKNESS

Center thickness (t_c) influences contact lens flexibility, lens mass, and potential oxygen transmissibility (defined as Dk/t_{ave}, where t_{ave} is the average lens thickness), as well as other measurements. OAD, power, peripheral curve design, and edge thickness of the lens may all be affected. Central thickness is specified in millimeters.

Minus powered lenses usually are designed with specific functional goals with regard to central thickness. In an effort to minimize edge thickness, most PMMA lenses have been made with a central thickness between 0.12 and 0.14 mm. GP materials are more flexible and often are made with central thicknesses between 0.15 and 0.18 mm to minimize flexure (7,8). This should not substantially affect the oxygen available to the cornea under daily wear conditions in which some oxygen is supplied by tear exchange. Minus powered hydrogel lenses are commonly made with central thicknesses of 0.05 to 0.15 mm, depending upon the material, to allow for sufficient oxygen transmission. Tear exchange is minimal with soft contact lenses (9).

Plus powered lenses face the limitation that center thickness is a function of power; the greater the power for the same anterior optical zone diameter (OZD), the greater the central thickness. Thus, most manufacturers vary either center thickness or anterior optical zone (cap) diameter, or both, to arrive at what they consider a good compromise. Low plus powered (+0.25 to +1.50) contact lenses typically have central thicknesses of about 0.21 mm, and higher plus powered contact lenses are in the range from 0.25 to 0.60 mm.

EDGE THICKNESS

Traditionally, lens designers usually like to obtain unpolished edge thickness of about 0.10 to 0.12 mm for contact lenses, both rigid and flexible. After polishing, this decreases to about 0.08 mm immediately adjacent to the absolute edge and should have a specific shape that is slightly rounded toward the posterior surface (1). Peripheral curve systems on anterior or posterior surfaces, or both, are used to obtain the rough unpolished edge, and then lenses are given a final polish by hand or by machine. With the advent of disposable soft contact lenses, there has been a paradigm shift in lens edge shapes. Companies now produce contacts that are untouched by human hands and taper to thin pointed edges. Patients wear these lenses without complaint.

POSTERIOR PERIPHERAL CURVE SYSTEMS

Rigid contact lenses have posterior peripheral curve systems to (i) contour more closely the shape of the cornea and thereby prevent compression of the lens edge into the corneal epithelium and scleral conjunctiva; (ii) control lens excursion (movement) and tear exchange (for both reoxygenation and mechanical elimination of entrapped epithelial and tear debris); (iii) provide a tear meniscus to hydrate the cornea immediately peripheral to the lens edge; and (iv) reduce edge thickness (10).

GP lenses often are *tricurve* in design, which means that there is both a secondary curve (of specified width and radius) and a peripheral curve (width and radius specified) on the posterior surface in addition to the base curve radius.

Occasionally, especially when they are small in OAD (about 8.6 mm), rigid lenses usually are *bicurve* designs, with just a base curve radius and a single peripheral curve. Other rigid contact lenses can have four or more posterior peripheral curves.

When designing tricurve contact lenses, many laboratories suggest a secondary curve system about 0.8 to 1.0 mm flatter than the base curve radius and perhaps 0.2 mm wide, with a peripheral curve between 10.5 and 12.0 mm in its radius (depending on base curve) and 0.3 mm wide. Another system, modified from Dyer (11), suggests three peripheral curves, called a *tetracurve* design, with width of 0.2/0.2/0.3 mm for large-diameter lenses and 0.1/0.1/0.2 mm for smaller-diameter lenses (i.e., about 8.4 mm and less). Intermediate curve radii are each 0.7 to 0.9 mm flatter than the preceding curve, whereas the final curve is about 1.1 mm flatter than the intermediate one.

Edge lift is the distance between extension of the tangent of the base curve radius surface and the absolute edge after peripheral curves are added. *Radial edge lift* (REL) is measured normal to the base curve radius extension, and *axial edge lift* (AEL) is measured parallel to the lens optic axis (Fig. 6.2). As peripheral curves are either flattened in radius or widened, edge lift is increased. A greater lift increases the volume of fluid available for tear exchange and, potentially, the ability of the lens to move across the cornea. Alternatively, shorter radius and narrower peripheral curves decrease edge lift and usually result in less movement, but potentially better comfort. Most laboratories suggest edge lift values on the order of 0.10 mm. One should note, however, that the actual distance between the edge of the lens and the corneal surface is termed *edge clearance* (both radial and axial, respectively). Considering the aspheric and variable natures of the corneal topography, this quantity is not measurable but can be estimated.

Most laboratories have their own standard peripheral curve systems designed to standardize edge thickness and edge lift at certain value (i.e., AEL at 0.15 mm). It also would be theoretically possible to set a peripheral tear reservoir volume mathematically and then design or adjust peripheral curve systems to maintain this as a constant. This assumes that all corneas have the same peripheral topography. Unfortunately, it is well known that corneas vary greatly in peripheral topography.

It is common to design GP contact lenses somewhat differently from the designs used for the now-antiquated PMMA lenses. As tear exchange is less important from the perspective of oxygen resupply, GP lenses usually are larger in OAD, which enhances tolerance/comfort. Increased OAD often is accompanied by increased OZD, which decreases visual flare from lens edges. It is important, given the earlier discussion on base curve radius, to maintain slight central apical touch fit on the eye (central corneal alignment), which will maintain tear exchange and decrease the tendency for lens flexure and secondary optical astigmatism. Silicone-based copolymer materials tend to elicit corneal drying at the 3 o'clock/9 o'clock position; thus, it may be advantageous to decrease both the volume and edge lift of posterior peripheral curve systems by steepening the radii and narrowing widths of the peripheral curves. The secondary curve often is wider than the final peripheral curve. These lenses are less dependent on tear exchange for oxygen resupply; therefore, such changes are feasible. Bennett (8) has described a system for posterior peripheral curve design of RGP lenses to accomplish these goals. Increased total lens diameter and decreased edge lift tend to suppress lens movement and tear exchange, decreasing patient awareness of the lens and improving overall comfort as well. One must take care not to go too steep with the peripheral system or too large with the optical zone, however, because either or both may result in the lens "binding," or rubbing on the peripheral cornea, thus creating epithelial damage and discomfort.

Many modern hydrogel lenses have no posterior peripheral curve (i.e., they are *monocurve* in construction that may be spherical or aspherical in design). Some designs have one peripheral curve, which can be either routinely 0.8 to 1.0 mm flatter than the base curve radius or routinely 11.5 to 12 mm in radius, and about 0.5 mm wide. Each of these designs is intended to align the lens periphery with peripheral limbal or scleral topography.

We believe that it is not important which particular pe-

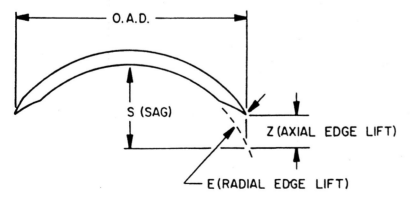

FIG. 6.2. Radial (REL) and axial (AEL) edge lifts are shown as distances between the edge of the contact lens and the extension of the base curve radius, measured along a line along a radial from the center of curvature of the base curve or parallel to the optic axis, respectively. (From Bennett ES: Silicone/acrylate lens design. *Int Contact Lens Clin* 1985;12:45, with permission.)

ripheral curve system is selected. It is important, however, to know which specific system is used on the lens, particularly with use of rigid lenses, so that *in situ* performance can be evaluated using the listed goals and any subsequent modification can be intelligently prescribed. For example, once a rigid lens originally designed with a peripheral curve of 11.0/0.3 mm (originally noted by fluorescein pattern evaluation to be inadequate) is modified to 12.0/0.4 mm to increase lens movement and tear exchange, the resultant prescription is changed. Subsequent orders for replacement lenses should reflect the modified rather than the original peripheral curve.

ANTERIOR PERIPHERAL CURVE SYSTEMS

With modern technology, lens front surface geometry is primarily determined by the interaction of center thickness, optical power, and edge thickness. The variable in the equation is the front peripheral, or carrier, curve that extends from the optical zone junction to the edge of the lens. With lower minus power lenses, the front peripheral curve is difficult to observe. With higher minus and plus powered lenses, one may easily observe the junction between the central optical radius and the anterior peripheral curve radius. The benefits of a geometrically defined radius for the peripheral curves include improve comfort/tolerance, controlled lens movement characteristics, and controlled lens centration. Front surface peripheral curves were sometimes applied using cone-shaped tools to thin the edges of minus lenses in the past (called a *Conlish* or CN bevel after its inventor, Calvin Nishimura).

Anterior peripheral curves are now mostly molded or lathed onto lens front surfaces. Both large OAD plus optically powered rigid contact lenses and hydrogel contact lenses (because their OADs are so much greater than smaller OAD rigid lenses) commonly have bicurve anterior surfaces. This means that there is a single peripheral curve with both a radius and a width in addition to the central "power" radius (within the optic zone) on the anterior lens surface. The lens designer first selects the desired values for the back central radius (r_2) and posterior peripheral curve(s). Optical power is the critical control variable for the front surface. Central thickness and size of the anterior optic zone are dependent variables that are selected to give the largest practical optical zone for any specific power without making the lens too thick or too thin both centrally and at the junction of the carrier curve. Formulas then are used to describe the spherical curve that will result in a specific unpolished edge thickness, generated from the junction of the anterior optical zone to the edge of the lens. This is termed *lenticular* construction (Fig. 6.3).

When considering hydrogel contact lenses, the thinner the overall profile of the lens, the greater the oxygen transmissibility of the contact lens and the greater the availability

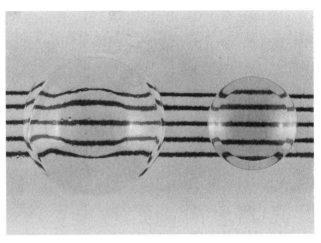

FIG. 6.3. Lenticular contact lenses: soft **(left)** and rigid **(right)**.

of oxygen for the underlying cornea. Because lenticular lenses are thinner and have increased flexure, a single lens design can be applied successfully to a variety of corneal shapes and sizes. Conversely, the thinner the lens profile, the more difficult lens handling becomes for a hydrogel contact lens wearer. Such concepts, therefore, lead to individual clinical tradeoffs and compromises, often dependent on other characteristics of the lens material, such as elasticity and breakage resistance.

Plus optically powered rigid contact lenses tend to ride inferiorly on the cornea because of increased weight, sharp edges, and movement of the center of gravity of the lens anterior to the corneal surface. Lenticular design improves this by decreasing lens mass, providing a better edge shape (12) and moving the center of gravity of the lens back toward the cornea. The smaller the anterior optical zone or optic cap for a specific overall diameter of a lenticular design, the better a lens will center. However, the structural quality of the lens may suffer and the patient may be more likely to observe flare from the nonoptical/carrier portion of the lens. Typically, the optic cap diameter of a rigid lens is 1.4 to 2.0 mm smaller than the overall contact lens diameter. Decreasing the optical cap diameter or flattening the anterior curve peripheral radius (usually 1.0–3.0 mm flatter than the base curve radius) will help to position a plus optically powered contact lens on a more superior portion of the cornea. It is easier to use optical cap diameter modifications to aid in lens positioning because verifying the curvature of an anterior surface peripheral curve is not clinically possible. The lenticular junction thickness is best maintained at about 0.13 mm to reduce breakage (12).

OPTICAL ZONE DIAMETER

The OZD is the usable optical portion of the lens. There is an OZD on both anterior and posterior surfaces, wherever there are peripheral curves. By convention, the lens OZD for rigid lenses usually is overall lens diameter minus twice the posterior peripheral curve width in millimeters, and the OZD for soft lenses is the overall lens diameter minus twice anterior peripheral curve width in millimeters.

MASS

Lens weight is the measurement that best reflects lens mass. Because many contact lens materials with very differing specific gravity values are now in clinical use (Table 6.1), lens weight has become another element subject to manipulation. Because the refractive index also is a variable, the front surface curvature needed to provide a specific lens power may differ from material to material for the same posterior surface, base and peripheral curve radii, and central thickness values, and calculations must be made on a lens-by-lens basis in order to assess changes in overall lens volume and weight (Fig. 6.4) (13). Contact lens weight may affect lens tolerance. Some patients may feel this difference; in other cases, decreasing lens weight or increasing the bearing area (for a better mass/unit area value) may result in less mechanically induced epithelial staining. Table 6.1 shows oxygen permeability values, refractive indices, and specific gravities for many popular rigid contact lens materials. A substantial reduction in lens weight can be made by the simple substitution of a polystyrene material for a silicone/acrylate (for example) when a contact lens of substantial refractive power and large diameter is manufactured. Changes in material weight with considering solely low minus powered contact lenses, however, may not be clinically important.

SUMMARY

A specific hydrogel or rigid contact lens performs mechanically and optically *in situ* as a result of how it was designed. This chapter presents an overview of important spherical lens design parameters and an introduction to their specific

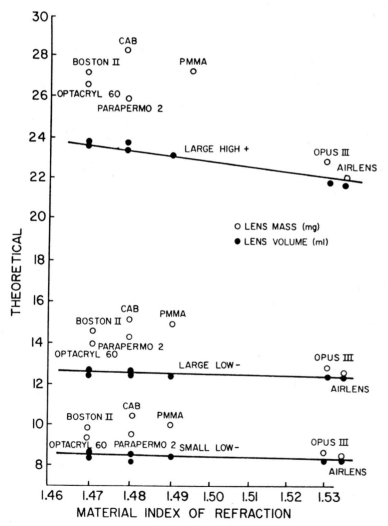

FIG. 6.4. Changes in theoretical rigid contact lens volume (in mL) and mass (in mg) compared to material optical index for three sample lens designs made from seven different common rigid gas permeable materials: Optacryl 60, Boston II, CAB, PMMA, Paraperm O₂, Opus III, and Airlens. *Solid lines* show relationship between volume–mass and index for each design. (From Weissman BA. Mass of rigid contact lenses. *Am J Optom Physiol Opt* 1985;62:322, with permission.)

application and modification. This discussion will be continued in specific detail in other chapters in this text.

REFERENCES

1. Mandell RB. *Contact lens practice,* 3rd ed. Springfield, IL: Charles C Thomas, 1981:13.
2. Korb DR, Korb JE. A new concept in contact lens design—parts I and II. *J Am Optom Assoc* 1970;41:1023.
3. Sarver MD. Fitting the Bausch & Lomb Softlens contact lens. *J Am Optom Assoc* 1973;44:258.
4. Weissman BA, Gardner KM. Power and radius changes induced in soft contact lens systems by flexure. *Am J Optom Physiol Opt* 1984;61:239.
5. Weissman BA. A general relation between changing surface radii of flexing soft contact lenses. *Am J Optom Physiol Opt* 1984;61:651.
6. Weissman BA. Loss of power with flexure of hydrogel plus lenses. *Am J Optom Physiol Opt* 1986;63:166.
7. Herman JP. Flexure of rigid contact lenses on toric corneas as a function of base curve fitting relationship. *J Am Optom Assoc* 1983;54:209.
8. Bennett ES. Silicone/acrylate lens design. *Int Cont Lens Clin* 1984;11:547.
9. Wagner L, Polse KA, Mandell RB. Tear pumping and edema with soft contact lenses. *Invest Ophthalmol Vis Sci* 1980;19:1397.
10. Bibby MM. Factors affecting peripheral curve design. *Am J Optom Physiol Opt* 1979;56:2.
11. Dyer JA. A practical nomogram for fitting contact lenses. *Contact Lens Med Bull* 1968;1:8.
12. Nelson G, Mandell RB. The relationship between minus carrier design and performance. *Int Contact Lens Clin* 1975;2:75.
13. Weissman BA. Mass of rigid contact lenses. *Am J Optom* 1985;62:322–328.

OPTICAL PHENOMENA OF CONTACT LENSES

WILLIAM J. "JOE" BENJAMIN

Much time and effort have been spent concentrating on the physiologic effects of contact lenses, so much so that the clinician is apt to forget that the basic reason for their existence is *optical* in nature. Contact lenses, first and foremost, fulfill the optical correction of ametropia in ways that allow the patient's vision to *exceed* that of other corrective modalities. The methods by which contact lenses are verified and their effects on the eye evaluated are based on optical principles. The goal of this chapter is to review visual optics in areas pertinent to contact lens practice and to outline how contact lenses fulfill the role of optical correction for the human binocular optical system. Along the way it will be specified how *contact lenses are unique* among the forms of correction available to the patient, and how *optimum vision* can be attained through the use of contact lenses. The Cartesian sign convention is used throughout this chapter, and a working knowledge of optical principles on the part of the reader is assumed.

OPTICS OF THE FIRST THREE MILLIMETERS

Corneal Reflex and Other Reflections

It may seem peculiar that a chapter on contact lens optics starts with the optics of reflection; however, many of the structures of the eye and especially the optical components observed by the clinician in everyday practice are transparent. As such, they must be viewed biomicroscopically with the use of *reflections.* Some reflections even hinder our observation of ocular structures by acting as glare sources. Thus, we angle the slit-lamp beam to change the position of reflections or to reduce their intensity so that we can see what we require. The intensities of reflections from interfaces of transparent media are minimized when the angle of incidence and angle of reflection are near zero, in other words, rays of light are incident perpendicular to the plane of the interface. As the angle of incidence increases, intensity of reflection also increases (Fig. 7A.1).

At small angles of incidence (less than 40 degrees), intensity of reflection is relatively constant but not zero (1). The relative intensity of reflection for light of near-normal incidence at a transparent interface can be calculated by *Fresnel's Formula for Reflection,* which shows that as refractive indices of the two interfacial media differ more greatly, intensity of reflection increases:

$$R = [n' - n/n' + n]^2 \quad \text{Equation 7A.1}$$
Fresnel's Formula for Reflection

where

R = Reflectance relative to 1.0 (all light reflected) and zero (no light reflected)
n = Refractive index of medium which contains incident and reflected ray
n' = Refractive index of medium which contains transmitted ray

Reflection from the precorneal tear film often is called the *corneal reflex* because it once was assumed to come from the air/corneal interface. To be sure, the tear/corneal interface does contribute some reflection to the corneal reflex; however, its contribution is very small compared to that of the air/tear film interface. Because the tear film is very thin, the two reflections appear even under the biomicroscope to be at the same position, in other words, superimposed. Using Fresnel's formula, intensities of reflection from each of these two "precorneal" interfaces can be calculated using refractive indices of the sodium "D" wavelength of light (587.6 nm) published by Gullstrand (2) for his schematic eyes (Table 7A.1):

$$R = [1.336 - 1.000/ 1.336 + 1.000]^2$$
Air/Tear Interface (R = 0.0207)
$$R = [1.376 - 1.336/1.376 + 1.336]^2$$
Tear/Cornea Interface (R = 0.0002)

The "corneal reflex," therefore, is made up of about 2.1% of the light incident upon the tear film. This, of course, is slightly greater when considering only blue light due to a slightly larger index of refraction and is lesser for red wavelengths. By wrongly assuming that the corneal reflex (the specular reflection called *Purkinje-Sanson image I*) was formed at an air/corneal interface, our calculations would

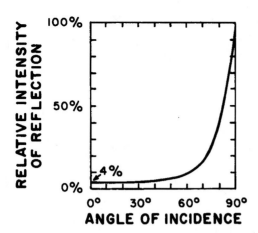

FIG. 7A.1. Plot of reflectance versus angle of incidence for light incident on a transparent refractive interface. Reflectance of light at near-normal incidence (<40 degrees) is described by Fresnel's Formula for Reflection (R = [(n′ − n)/(n′ + n)]²). (From Jenkins FA, White HE. Reflection. In: Jenkins FA, White HE, eds. *Fundamentals of optics,* 4th ed. New York: McGraw-Hill, 1976:523–543, with permission.)

have resulted in R = 0.025, or 2.5% reflectance. Therefore, the technicality over the surface or surfaces responsible for Purkinje-Sanson image I often is ignored.

When a contact lens is placed on the eye, the corneal reflex might be more aptly termed the "cornea and contact lens reflex." Again, however, this reflex is mostly derived from light reflected from the air/tear film interface. The higher refractive index of the contact lens material provides for a slightly larger contribution from the tear/contact lens interface than from a tear/cornea interface:

R = [1.490 − 1.336/1.490 + 1.336] ²
    Tear/ RIGID Contact Lens Interface (n = 1.49, R = 0.003)
R = [1.430 − 1.336/1.430 + 1.336]²
    Tear/ SOFT Contact Lens Interface (n = 1.43, R = 0.001)

The "corneal reflex," when wearing a contact lens, is a superimposition of reflections from the air/tear interface, the anterior and posterior tear/lens interfaces, and the tear/corneal interface. Because rigid lenses usually are of higher refractive index than soft lenses, the corneal reflection when

TABLE 7A.1. REFRACTIVE INDICES OF THE OPTICAL MEDIA BASED ON GULLSTRAND'S EXACT SCHEMATIC EYE (2)

Transparent Medium	Index of Refraction
Tear fluid	1.336
Cornea	1.376
Aqueous	1.336
Crystalline lens	1.386/1.406
Vitreous	1.336

wearing rigid lenses is brighter (refractive indices of contact lens materials are covered later in this chapter). In the examples just calculated, the corneal reflection composed of all four subcomponent reflexes for the rigid lens would total 2.5% of incident light and for the soft lens 2.3%. "Corneal reflections" when wearing rigid and soft contact lenses, therefore, can be 20% and 10% brighter, respectively, than the normal corneal reflex. This gives a noticeable extra *"sparkle" to the eyes of contact lens wearers* when observed by the untrained eye (especially rigid lens wearers) and can be a tell-tale sign of lens wear to the critical eye of the contact lens practitioner.

Several ocular structures are viewed with the use of *specular reflection* from the tear film. Smoothness of the tear fluid layer over the surface of the cornea, conjunctiva, and contact lens can be assessed with a biomicroscope. Reflections from the tear menisci along the tear prisms and around the edges of contact lenses may indicate whether the menisci are overfilled or underfilled with tear fluid (Fig. 7A.2). A special case of destructive interference involving reflection from the front and back surfaces of the thinnest portion of tear film next to a tear meniscus (about 0.25 of a light wavelength thick) results in a *"black line"* typical of any concave tear fluid meniscus (3,4).

Breakup times of tear fluid on top of the cornea, conjunctiva, and contact lenses can be analyzed by observing reflections off of the tear fluid layer. Special grids and lighted objects are reflected off of the cornea in order to assess corneal topography (keratometry, keratoscopy) and tear film thinning (xerometry, interference fringing) by reflection from the tear layer. Even binocular status can be assessed using reflections from the precorneal tear film (tests for angles Kappa and the Hirschberg test). Size and quantity of small reflections from the preconjunctival tear film are used to identify papillae and follicles for determination of severity of papillary hypertrophy and follicular conjunctivitis, respectively (Fig. 7A.3).

Total internal reflection from the anterior and posterior corneal surfaces is used in the well-known *"sclerotic scatter"* technique when screening for corneal opacities. Another internal reflection from the posterior corneal surface, at the interface of the endothelium and aqueous fluid of the anterior chamber, also is viewed and photographed with magnification for *in vivo* assessments of the endothelial mosaic (specular reflection). So dependent is the technique for viewing the endothelium on a proper angle of incidence and reflection that endothelial cells not in the same plane as the endothelial sheet, such as those overlying endothelial guttata (5), will not reflect light at the appropriate angle for viewing through the eyepiece of a biomicroscope (Fig. 7A.4). Thus, they may be misinterpreted as "holes" in the endothelial mosaic. Because the refractive index change between cornea (n = 1.376) and aqueous chamber fluid (n = 1.336) is small and similar to the change at the tear/corneal interface, the *endothelial reflex* is very dim (0.02% of light incident on the posterior cornea) compared to the

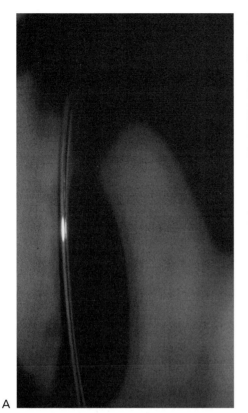

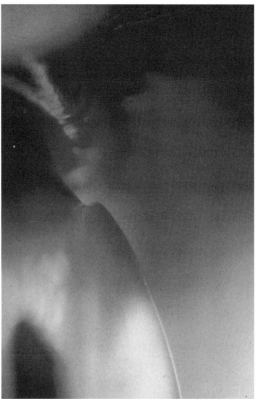

A

B

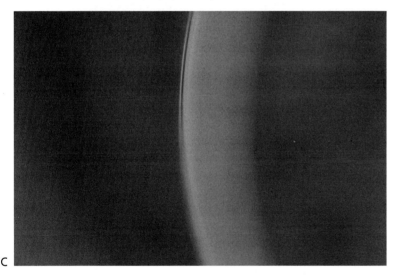

C

FIG. 7A.2. Specular reflection from a tear meniscus and the "black line" seen at the cornea immediately posterior to a meniscus (encircling a rigid lens) seen in a magnified slit-lamp view **(A)**. The black line is the result of destructive interference of reflected light at the thinnest area of the tear film adjacent to a meniscus **(B)** and can be accentuated with the use of fluorescein **(C)**. (From Benjamin WJ. Examination of the tear fluid meniscus. *Int Cont Lens Clin* 1988;15:390–391, with permission.)

bright anterior corneal reflex, which is greater than 100 times more intense and sometimes acts as a glare source to hide the endothelial reflex (Fig. 7A.4).

Purkinje-Sanson images I and II are formed by specular reflection at the anterior and posterior corneal surfaces (2). These images are the result of light that is initially diverging from objects *in front of the eye.* The images are positioned approximately 3.9 and 3.6 mm behind the anterior corneal surface, respectively, according to geometric optics of curved mirrors. Fresnel's Formula for Reflection remains the same when using a *biomicroscope,* and reflections from various

optical interfaces have the same relative intensities as would be calculated for the Purkinje-Sanson images from those surfaces, to include images III and IV from the anterior and posterior lenticular surfaces.

However, light from a biomicroscope originates from a filament that illuminates a slit aperture. The aperture is focused simultaneously with the binocular at the plane of regard. Light incident on the ocular surface (the object of regard) is *convergent.* When viewing the corneal reflex, the viewer moves the focus of the slit aperture to the tear film surface and effectively creates a conjugate source of light (a new object) at

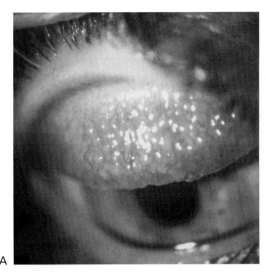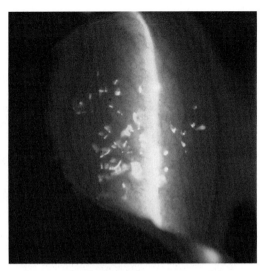

A   B

FIG. 7A.3. Small specular reflections occur at rounded conjunctival elevations, such as those seen on the palpebral conjunctiva during papillary hypertrophy **(A)** or follicular conjunctivitis **(B)**.

the surface with reflection at that surface. The "corneal reflex" in this case is positioned *at the surface of the tear film* and is different than the traditional first Purkinje-Sanson image. Likewise, when viewing the endothelial mosaic or reflections from anterior and posterior lens surfaces with a biomicroscope, the binocular is focused on the reflexes at those surfaces and not on traditional Purkinje-Sanson images. Therefore, corneal reflexes under normal circumstances are synonymous with "Purkinje-Sanson images I and II," but the surface reflections that are viewed with a biomicroscope are not normal Purkinje-Sanson images. However, with the biomicroscope focused at the crystalline lens and the slit aperture open, normal Purkinje-Sanson images I and II of the source filament can be seen in focus. When this occurs the corneal surfaces will not be in focus.

Transparency of the Cornea

The epithelial layer of the cornea, being *unkeratinized,* normally is transparent and approximately 50 to 60 μm thick with a refractive index of 1.41. The *roughened microvillous anterior cellular surface* of the epithelium is filled in by a *mucinaceous layer* of the tear film and so forms a *smooth optical surface.* The epithelium essentially adds no power to the optical system of the eye because it constitutes a thin lens with parallel anterior and posterior surfaces. Similarly, the anterior limiting lamina (Bowman's membrane), posterior limiting lamina (Descemet's membrane), and endothelial monolayer of the cornea are very thin (each <20 μm thick) and can be shown to be optically insignificant with regard to corneal refractive power.

The *air/tear film interface* is the refractive interface of the eye that has the most refractive power. The precorneal tear film, however, being less than 10 μm thick and formed by parallel optical interfaces, is (ironically) also optically

insignificant as far as refractive power of the normal eye is concerned. It is often remarked, therefore, that the *"cornea"* is the optical element of the eye making the greatest refractive contribution to the retinal image.

The refractive index of the *stroma* (n = 1.376, on average) is taken for that of the entire cornea due to the optical insignificance of the other corneal layers and tear film when considering refractive power. In previous examples using Fresnel's Formula for reflection, stromal refractive index was assumed for the tear/cornea interface instead of the higher epithelial index for a tear/epithelial interface. Light scatter from the epithelial surface and the adsorbed glycoproteinaceous tear layer probably act to negate any additional reflection from the cornea that would have been calculated for a tear/epithelial interface.

The corneal stroma is optically significant in terms of refractive power. The stroma is transparent to visible light in its normal state and consists of approximately 200 sheets, or *lamellae,* which are arranged parallel to the surface of the cornea. Relatively small numbers of *fibroblasts* and leukocytes are scattered sporadically through the stroma; they are *flattened* within the plane of the lamellae in which they are contained. The stroma, like the other layers of the cornea, is *avascular* such that transparency of the cornea is maintained.

Stromal lamellae are stacked one upon the other in an anteroposterior direction. Each consists of fibers or bundles of *collagen fibrils* running in the same direction and in parallel, although fibrils of a particular lamella run at various angles to those of other lamellae. Collagen fibrils are surrounded by a *ground substance* made of mucopolysaccharides and are regularly spaced 65 nm apart in a "lattice" arrangement (Fig. 7A.5). The diameters of fibrils range from 19 nm (anterior stroma) to 34 nm (posterior stroma); however, at any one depth within the cornea they are uniform in diameter and circular in cross-section (cylindrical). According to Maurice

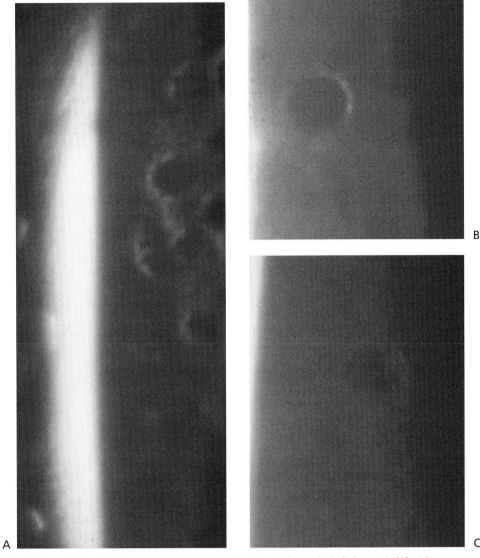

FIG. 7A.4. Endothelial guttata are seen as a "holes" in the endothelial mosaic **(A)**. A large guttatum also looks like a "hole" **(B)** but is actually lined by endothelial cells seen when the slit-lamp beam is oriented so as to also reflect light from those cells **(C)**. Note the wide bright (white) vertical stripe of the anterior corneal reflex, which can obscure the endothelial reflex or act as a glare source. (Panels B and C from Benjamin WJ. Endothelial guttatae: a type of corneal "drusen." *Int Cont Lens Clin* 1988;15:294, with permission.)

(6,7), collagen has a refractive index of 1.55 and the ground substance has a refractive index of 1.354. The refractive index of the stroma is by the *Principle of Gladstone and Dale,* an average of the refractive indices of its components:

$$n_s = n_c V_c + n_g V_g$$

   Equation 7A.2: Principle of Gladstone & Dale

where

n_s = Refractive index of corneal stroma
n_c = Refractive index of collagen (1.550)
n_g = Refractive index of ground substance (1.354)
V_c = Volume fraction of collagen within stroma (0.10)
V_g = Volume fraction of ground substance within stroma (0.90)

Maurice's *"Lattice Theory"* of corneal transparency holds that spacing between collagen fibrils (65 nm) is sufficiently small that light scattered by individual fibrils mutually interferes and scatter is, therefore, eliminated (6). Goldman and Benedek (8) believe that the interfibrillar spacing is small in comparison to wavelengths of light (400–630 nm) so that light traversing the stroma is not scattered. Perhaps both of these theories are true to some extent and explain why the cornea is transparent.

Loss of Corneal Transparency

When traumatized by various agents, including contact lenses, the corneal epithelium can become edematous, lose

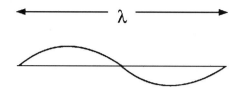

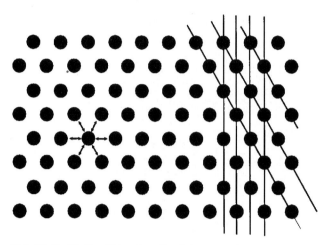

FIG. 7A.5. Fibrils within a lamella of the corneal stroma are regularly spaced and closely packed in a lattice arrangement. A wavelength of light is shown above for size comparison. (From Maurice DM. The structure and transparency of the cornea. *J Phys* 1957; 136:263–286, with permission.)

its normally tight adherences between cells and its basement membrane, and develop intercellular spaces filled with fluid that scatter light. Such hazing of the epithelium often is called *epithelial edema*. *Subepithelial infiltrates* may invade the epithelium and cause transparency to be lost at foci of infiltration. The epithelium also may keratinize in response

to chronic trauma and so lose its transparency. Certain keratopathies may cause *deposits* that are calcium or lipid in nature to form in or under the epithelium such that transparency is degraded. *Dry spots* appearing in the precorneal tear film or on top of contact lenses may scatter light and so reduce the transparency of the tear/cornea optical system.

Trauma affecting the stroma, whether it is direct or indirect by influence of the epithelium or endothelium, interrupts the uniform spacing and lattice structure of collagen fibrils. *Corneal scarring* is visible when the healing process fails to preserve the stroma's fibrillar organization (Fig. 7A.6). *Corneal vascularization* induces a reorganization of the normal stromal structure and so reduces stromal transparency. *Stromal edema* is thought to enlarge the spacing between fibrils, such that the "lattice" is not only irregular but is not packed as tightly, and scatter of light from fibrils is allowed to occur (following the hypothesis of Goldman and Benedek) and/or is no longer eliminated by interference (according to Maurice's Lattice Theory).

Many forms of trauma can result in corneal clouding (edema), for instance, mechanical, chemical, toxic, osmotic, and hypoxic trauma. All of these are present to some extent with contact lens wear, but the most well-known and recognized trauma during contact lens wear is hypoxic. Fig. 7A.7A shows *central circular corneal clouding* (ccc) of the stroma following wear of a rigid contact lens of low oxygen transmissibility. The peripheral cornea in this photo is not clouded because oxygenation was maintained there, so the demarcation between adequate and inadequate oxygenation to provide for corneal physiology is most obvious. *Stromal infiltrates* are collections of lymphocytes that form in the cornea around foci of infection or inflammation (Fig. 7A and 7B).

When the epithelium or stroma become edematous, patients begin to perceive *hazing* (called *Sattler's "veil"* or *Fick's phenomenon*) and *colored haloes* when gazing at lighted objects

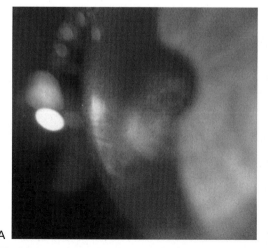

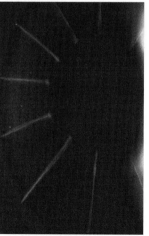

FIG. 7A.6. A: Corneal scarring is brought about by a healing process, in response to trauma, which does not preserve the original fibrillar spacing of the stroma. **B:** Radial scars were the result of radial keratotomy, the first refractive surgery technique to be widely used.

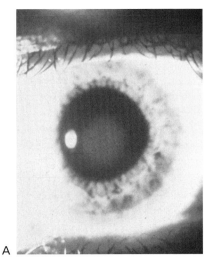 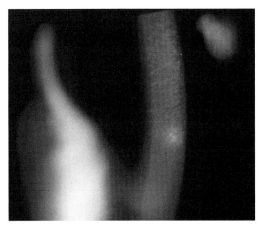

A   B

FIG. 7A.7. A: Central corneal clouding (ccc) is a result of abnormal fibrillar spacing within the stroma, brought about by a localized stromal edema. **B:** A stromal infiltrate is an opacity that often looks like a round scar with indistinct edges. (Courtesy of Dr. Chris Snyder.)

against a dark background (e.g., car headlights at night). It is thought that colored haloes are the result of diffraction of light by a rough grating formed by the basal cells of the epithelium, endothelium (which also can become edematous), and/or stromal collagen fibers (7). In extreme cases of stromal edema, the cornea can become opaque.

Polarized Biomicroscopy and Birefringence of the Stroma

When stress is placed on a transparent isotropic material, the material becomes "optically anisotropic," or *birefringent*. Birefringence induced by stress is called *stress birefringence,* or *photoelasticity.* Incident rays of light are polarized into ordinary and extra-ordinary rays of light that have different indices of refraction and whose planes of oscillation are at right angles. Photoelasticity is the phenomenon that causes a "polarization cross" and peripheral annular "compression ring" to be seen in a glass spectacle lens compressed by heat treatment when viewed against polarized light through a crossed polaroid.

The stroma is placed under stress by pull of extraocular muscles, intraocular pressure, and other forms of mechanical pressure. In addition, stromal lamellae are anisotropic and birefringent due to their "crystalline-like" lattice structures and inherent refractive properties of collagen fibrils. Stromal birefringence seems to be due mostly to lattice arrangement of fibrils rather than properties of the fibrils themselves (6), altered by the various constant and transient stresses noted earlier. The maximum difference of refractive index between the ordinary and extraordinary rays is 0.0028 for light passing through one stromal lamella. Birefringence of light passing through the entire cornea (index difference = 0.0014) is half of the birefringence occurring as a result of passing through

only one stromal lamella. This is because fibrils of different lamellae are arranged at angles to each other, with no consistent direction taken for all lamellae (9).

By establishing a source of partially polarized light behind the stroma and then viewing the cornea through a crossed polaroid, the effects of stromal anisotropy can be seen as a dark cross on a lighter background typical of photoelasticity and of crystals capable of uniaxial birefringence. White light in the beam of a biomicroscope can be sent through a polaroid filter prior to incidence on the eye. Reflected light from the posterior corneal surface and other structures is by then only partially polarized. The light passes back through the stroma and is viewed through a crossed polaroid at the binocular. Annular chromatic fringes seen at the corneal periphery are called *isochromes* and are seen in addition to a polarization cross (two crossed dark lines, called *isogyres* or *isoclinics*) in Fig. 7A.8. Such a scheme for analyzing birefringence of the cornea has been called *polarized biomicroscopy* by Mountford (10).

Isoclinics and isochromes alter their typical corneal pattern in response to various stresses placed on the cornea. Pull of the extraocular muscles, surgery, scarring, corneal edema, and other stresses, including those of contact lens wear, can change the anisotropic pattern of the cornea. At one time it was hoped that these patterns might someday be used as diagnostic tools to check the proper tightening of sutures during the healing process after ocular surgery and to follow fluctuations of intraocular pressure. However, alterations in the polarization stress pattern were too gross to accurately monitor those clinical parameters.

Inclusions Within the Corneal Epithelium

Transparent and translucent round refractile elements can be found in the corneal epithelium. These range up to 150

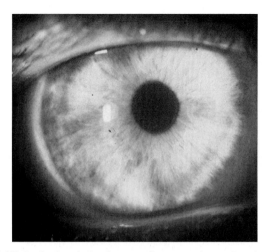

FIG. 7A.8. Dark polarization cross is seen at the cornea through a biomicroscope with a polaroid analyzer when using polarized incident light. The lines making up the cross are called *isogyres* or *isoclinics*. Annular chromatic rings also are seen in the periphery of the cornea and are called *isochromes*.

μm in diameter as seen through the biomicroscope and are sometimes difficult to perceive. They are best viewed in *"marginal retroillumination"* against either edge of a lighted section of iris or against the edge of the pupil (11). *Microcysts* are thought to be the result of chronic hypoxia during contact lens wear, are 15 to 50 μm in diameter, and usually do not stain with fluorescein because they are contained within the epithelium. Microcysts are irregularly shaped translucent bodies filled with a substance of higher refractive index than the surrounding epithelium. Therefore, under high magnification they produce "against" motion of light upon biomicroscopic examination, as they have essentially rounded optical surfaces forming lenses of plus power within the epithelium. Under low magnification they can appear like "dust particles" within the epithelium (12,13).

Motion of light within the aperture of a microcystic "lens" is achieved by altering the marginal position of lighted iris behind the "lens" (by moving the slit-lamp beam) from one side of the "lens" to the other (back and forth). This is analogous to hand neutralization of spectacle lenses (or retinoscopy of the eye), the performance of which results in "against" motion for plus lenses, or for eyes that are "plus" and thus require minus correction; and "with" motion for minus lenses, or for eyes that are "minus" and require plus correction.

Vacuoles are round and regular. They also are contained within the epithelium such that they do not stain with fluorescein. Vacuoles are about the same size as microcysts, about 20 to 50 μm in diameter, although they exhibit "with" motion as they are filled with fluid (or gas) of lesser refractive index than the surround. *Epithelial bullae* are larger than vacuoles (>40 μm), but they appear very similar, are subepithelial, and usually do not stain with fluorescein (12).

Pits or facets in the surface of the epithelium can occur. Being filled with tear fluid, they produce "with" orientation of light as would a minus lens (Fig. 7A.9) and stain with fluorescein. *Dimple veiling* results from large indentations in the corneal epithelium caused by trapped air bubbles between contact lenses and the corneal surface. Round surface pits 40 to 120 μm in diameter are left in the epithelium when *"microdeposits"* or *"mucin balls"* formed under extended wear gel lenses dislodge, leaving small pockets filled with tear fluid (14,15). Optical effects of these refractile elements within the cornea are, therefore, of diagnostic value for the practitioner monitoring contact lens wearers.

Corneal Topography: Front and Back Corneal Surface Power

The shape of the anterior corneal surface often is measured by *keratometry*. Keratometry results are in radii of curvature for a central annular zone of the cornea, approximately *3 mm in diameter,* surrounding the visual axis of the eye. The measurement assumes that the two primary meridians crossing the central corneal area are spherical. The method seems to be accurate enough for clinical work in the contact lens field, but it has significant drawbacks in describing the actual topography of the cornea due to assumptions of curvature sphericity, constancy of curvature across the corneal

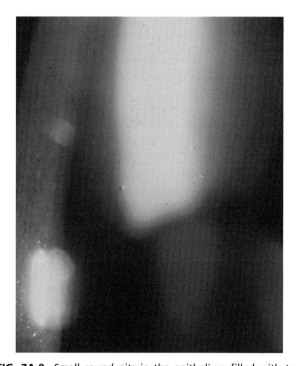

FIG. 7A.9. Small round pits in the epithelium filled with tear fluid exhibit "with" orientation of light shown in marginal retroillumination against a lighted strip of iris. (From Bourassa S, Benjamin WJ. Transient corneal surface "microdeposits" and associated epithelial surface pits occurring with gel contact lens extended wear. *Int Cont Lens Clin* 1988;15:338–340, with permission.)

surface, and regular surface toricity, which is limited to two primary meridians. Keratometry also assumes that the apex of the anterior corneal surface is coincident with the visual axis.

The keratometer uses a refractive index of 1.3375 to convert corneal radii of curvature to corneal refractive power. This number was chosen instead of the actual index of the corneal stroma (n = 1.376) in order to compensate for the negative refractive power of the posterior corneal surface (radius $\cong$ 8.00 mm, power $\cong$ -5.00 D). An important distinction needs to be made here between *corneal refractive power, anterior corneal surface power,* and *corneal curvature.* Let us say that the keratometer measures a radius of 7.50 mm. The dioptric value calculated by the keratometer with an index of 1.3375 is $+45.00$ D. This is essentially an estimate of the corneal refractive power with a "fudge factor" of -5 D thrown in for the posterior corneal surface. With a refractive index of 1.376, the actual power of the anterior corneal surface is $+50.13$. "Curvature," on the other hand, is an optical term for the reciprocal of the radius of curvature in meters and would work out to be $+133.33$ D. Confusion in terminology over the years has led the practitioner to call a dioptric K reading, actually an estimate of "corneal refractive power," by the name "corneal curvature." When radii of curvature are converted to refractive powers in air using n = 1.3375 in the manner of a keratometer, the units of power are often called *keratometric diopters.*

Conversion tables are commonly seen in contact lens practice and are used to convert radii of curvature to keratometric diopters and *vice versa.* These are remnants of the "precalculator" era; now conversions can be easily performed with hand calculators in seconds and often before the practitioner could have located a conversion table. A conversion to keratometric diopters can be quickly performed by *dividing 337.5 by the radius of curvature in millimeters;* likewise, a conversion to radius of curvature (in mm) can be done by *dividing 337.5 by the surface power in keratometric diopters.*

The *apex* of the cornea lies, on average, at the geometric center of the cornea along the optic axis of the eye, but the position is widely variable between subjects. It averages 0.5 mm temporal and superior to the visual axis such that light rays from a fixated point travel somewhat inferonasally to the corneal apex, fortunately through the center of that portion of the cornea measured by the keratometer. The *central cap* of the cornea contains the intersection of the visual axis and the cornea, an area over which the corneal refractive power is within 0.50 D for a given meridian (16). The central cap is approximately 2.4 mm^2 in size (16) and may or may not contain the corneal apex. In actuality the central cornea closely approximates an elliptical surface that flattens toward the periphery. In some patients the central ellipsoid is much different than a sphere. The *eccentricity* of the central corneal surface averages 0.45 and varies from -0.4 to 1.0 (see definition of ellipse in section on Radii of Curvature

and Sagittal Depths of Conic Sections). In the periphery the cornea becomes even flatter than an ellipsoid, and this area is not really described by any simple geometric relationship (17,18).

Keratometric measurements of the primary meridians average 7.8 mm, with a large range from 7.0 to 9.5 mm for "normal" corneas. Corneal toricity is generally *"with the rule."* Two perpendicular primary meridians have been assumed; however, most corneas have been shown to be slightly *irregular.* Toric corneas are better described as having four primary *semi-meridians* that range from 55 to 120 degrees apart instead of 90 degrees as assumed. The majority of semi-meridians are greater than 2.5 degrees away from normality with adjacent semi-meridians (19). However, assumption of two regular primary meridians suits the clinical situation, because optical devices are only reasonably available in regular astigmatic corrections. Rigid contact lenses are the only practical correction for significantly irregular corneas by virtue of the "lacrimal lens," a topic to be covered later.

Optical Aperture of the Eye

The *entrance pupil* of the eye is formed by refraction of the real pupil by the cornea and is just over 3 mm behind the anterior corneal surface. The entrance pupil is very important to contact lens wearers for several reasons. Illumination of the retina is proportional to the square of pupillary diameter. Depths of field and focus for clear vision are inversely proportional to pupil diameter. The lower limit of pupil size for optimum visual acuity is approximately 2 mm, below which effects of reduced retinal illuminance and diffraction outweigh beneficial aspects of an increase in depth of field and reduction of ocular spherical aberration. The entrance pupil also controls blur circle size on the retina for object rays not originating from the far point plane of the eye.

The entrance pupil averages 3.5 mm in diameter in adults under normal illumination and ranges from 1.3 to 10 mm. It often is centered on the optic axis of the eye but is displaced temporally away from the visual axis by an average of 5 degrees. The typical entrance pupil is decentered approximately 0.15 mm nasally and 0.10 mm inferior to the geometric center of the visible iris circumference (20). In general, the diameter of the pupil gradually becomes smaller during the lifetime of a patient after about age 12 to 18 years. This seems to be a linear relationship in which pupil sizes for light-adapted and dark-adapted eyes at age 20 (mean nearly 5 and 8 mm, respectively) both diminish to about 2 and 2.5 mm, respectively, at age 80 (21,22). The progressive change in pupil size is known as *senile miosis.* Pupil size is always changing in the normal eye due to small slow oscillations, convergence (near triad response), and pupillary responses to light. Pupil size can be influenced by drugs and medications and is slightly larger in persons with light irides compared to dark irides. Pupils become mydriatic in response to large sensory and psychological stimuli and become miotic in response to pain or irritation within the globe (oculopupillary reflex). Pupils are not larger for females (compared to males) and myopes (compared to hyperopes) when accommodation has been accounted for, although these relationships may be present under normal conditions when accommodation is uncontrolled (23).

It is apparent that the entrance pupil sets the limits of translation and centration of contact lenses on the eye, because the optic zone of a contact lens must be able to sufficiently cover the entrance pupil of the eye to obtain excellent vision. Flare seen by patients wearing rigid contact lenses occurs when the optic zone of the contact lens is smaller than the entrance pupil of the eye, or when the lens is positioned such that its optic zone does not cover the pupil. Optimal diameters of central clear zones of tinted gel lenses are dependent on pupil diameter of each wearer and can reduce field of view if improperly matched in size or if decentered before the pupil (24). The entrance pupil is of special importance when wearing bifocal contact lenses (20, 25,26). Pupillary diameter and position relative to the distance and near portions of the bifocal contact lens determine effective visual performance.

A good part of the difficulty of designing and fitting contact lenses, especially bifocal contact lenses, is caused by the fact that entrance pupils vary considerably between individuals and constantly change size in the same individual. Contact lens wear can dramatically enhance vision in a case of an abnormal pupil or iris, such as in aniridia or ocular albinism, for which contact lenses containing apertures can act in lieu of or in addition to the entrance pupil of the eye to perform its optical function. Cases of anisocoria, polycoria, and distorted pupils also can be managed by placing apertures within contact lenses (27). Positions and sizes of contact lens optic zones relative to the size and location of the pupillary reflex can be analyzed with the use of a retinoscope or ophthalmoscope, a technique recommended to contact lens practitioners by Josephson (28).

Transmittance of the Cornea to Electromagnetic Radiation

The spectrum of visible light (400–700 nm) is surrounded by infrared radiation ([IRR] from 700 to 10^6 nm) and ultraviolet radiation ([UVR] from 200–400 nm). The cornea absorbs nearly all radiation that enters it at wavelengths below 300 nm. Transmittance of the cornea climbs for wavelengths above 300 nm to about 80% at 400 nm, then more gradually increases to greater than 90% at 600 nm. UVR passing through the cornea is almost totally absorbed by the crystalline lens of the eye. In the infrared range above 700 nm the cornea absorbs radiation essentially the same as does water (29).

Of particular concern in recent years has been the protec-

tion of the eye from the effects of UVR. UVR can be subdivided into near UV (UV-A, from 315–400 nm), middle UV (UV-B, from 280–315 nm), and far UV (UV-C, from 200–280 nm). The ozone layer of the atmosphere is responsible for absorption of almost all of the most destructive UVR below 290 nm; therefore, UV-C is a consideration for the eye only when the ozone layer is thin or nonexistent, for instance, at the north or south poles of the earth. Small, transient thin areas in the ozone layer ("holes" in the layer) are thought to sometimes develop over other areas of the earth and may cause visual damage, especially in aphakes or pseudophakes without adequate retinal protection from UVR. Eyes of persons in space must be protected from harmful UVR (29,30).

The cornea and crystalline lens absorb most of UV-A and UV-B passing through the atmosphere. UV-B, in particular, is the portion of UVR that induces tanning of the skin and is suspected of having carcinogenic actions as well. All cells of the cornea are affected, even damaged, by sufficient quantities of UVR. Endothelial polymegethism during the aging process may be due in part to the destructive effects of UVR over a person's lifetime. In addition, UVR has been implicated as a causative factor in senile macular degeneration and senile cataract formation, and it may hasten onset of presbyopia.

Contact lenses normally transmit high levels of radiation from the lower end of UV-C far into the infrared. Some rigid and gel polymers have been developed, however, to specifically absorb UVR below 400 nm. Included in the contact lens standard from the American National Standards Institute (31) are criteria for UVR absorption when a manufacturer claims its contact lens to be a UVR absorber (Table 7A.2).

The "Phantom Fluorescein Effect"

Radiation from 365 to 470 nm must be used to stimulate *sodium fluorescein* when instilled in the eye. This can be done via a biomicroscope beam using a *cobalt filter* that illuminates the eye with blue light in the visible spectrum above 400 nm. It also can be performed by illumination with an *ultraviolet lamp* common to contact lens practitioners. Once excited, molecules of fluorescein emit light at 522 nm (32).

When a UVR-absorbing contact lens is placed on the eye, UVR from a UV lamp is not permitted to reach fluorescein in the post-lens tear pool. Thus, the lens/cornea fitting relationship cannot be properly assessed. A small amount of blue light emitted by the UV lamp might be used to view the fluorescein pattern, but the pattern is unacceptably dim even when contrast is enhanced by viewing through a *yellow (Wratten no. 12) filter*. Most radiation from a cobalt filter, transmission 300 to 550 nm, peaking at 440 nm (32), is not blocked by the contact lens and is allowed to stimulate post-lens fluorescein so that the lens/cornea relationship can

TABLE 7A.2. ALLOWABLE TRANSMITTANCE OF ULTRAVIOLET RADIATION FOR ULTRAVIOLET RADIATION ABSORBERS ACCORDING TO ANSI Z80.20:1998

Ultraviolet Radiation	UV–A 316–380 nm	UV–B 280–315 nm
Transmittance[a]		
Class 1 absorber	τUVR <0.10	τUVR <0.01
Class 2 absorber	τUVR <0.30	τUVR <0.05

[a] τUVR = ultraviolet radiation (UVR) transmittance of the contact lens; multiply by 100 to obtain UVR transmittance in percent (%). An average transmittance summed over the range of wavelengths is indicated.

be evaluated. The practitioner might be advised to have *both* types of illumination available. A UV lamp can be used to identify UVR-absorbing lenses on the eye; a cobalt filter then can be used to evaluate the lens fit (33). Spectral composition of "blue light" emitted by biomicroscopes may vary; therefore, amounts of fluorescence behind normal and UVR-blocking contact lenses may vary between instruments.

Alteration of the Eye's Optical Parameters

The wear of contact lenses can induce several changes in addition to loss of transparency that affect the optical performance of the eye. By far the most significant refractive change is that of the anterior corneal surface curvature, both during and after contact lens wear. These effects on the eye are outside the scope of this chapter, but suffice to say here that corneal curvature and toricity alterations with rigid contact lens wear and to a lesser extent with soft lens wear are mostly responsible for *"spectacle blur"* and longer-term changes in the spectacle refraction.

Myopic creep is a gradual increase in myopia associated with young adult patients during extended wear of contact lenses. Corneal curvature in these cases does not alter enough to explain the additional myopia evident in overrefraction (OR). The physiologic/anatomical basis of this optical effect has not been adequately investigated and, therefore, is not yet known.

The wear of rigid lenses can produce centralized edema (Fig. 7A.7) that creates a steeper corneal surface, thus increasing the eye's spectacle refraction into the minus and flattening the contact lens/cornea fitting relationship. Alterations of spectacle correction and spectacle blur are the result, but rigid lenses *"mask"* most of these refractive changes when the lenses are actually being worn. For soft lenses, corneal edema is more evenly distributed across the cornea. The anterior corneal surface radius of curvature is only slightly elongated, and this creates only a small subclinical deviation of the refractive error. Corneal thickness is increased during episodes of edema, but its influence on corneal refractive power is sufficiently small as to be subclinical. Stromal refractive index is lowered subclinically due to in-

flux of water and tends to counteract the increase in myopia caused by rigid lens-associated hypoxia but adds to an elongation of corneal radius of curvature created by soft lens wear. Further effects of corneal surface curvature changes on the lens/cornea fitting relationship and the masking of these power changes by rigid contact lenses are discussed in the section on "Exploding" the Lacrimal Lens Concept.

REFRACTIVE CORRECTION WITH CONTACT LENSES

Nuances of Contact Lens Refractive Power

A contact lens is treated, in terms of geometrical optics, as a "thick lens," in spite of the fact that contact lenses are actually quite thin. Refractive power is the result of the curvatures of both surfaces as well as the index of refraction and center thickness of the contact lens material. The "thick lens" formula for computing refractive power of lenses is shown in Equation 7A.3 and is necessary in comparison to treatment as a "thin lens" because the *sagittal depth* (sagitta, or sag of surface curvature) of a contact lens is short in comparison to chord diameter:

$$F_T = F_1 + F_2 - (t/n)F_1F_2 \qquad \text{Equation 7A.3}$$
$$\text{Equivalent Refractive Power}$$

where

F_T = equivalent, or true, lens refractive power in diopters
F_1 = $(n' - n)/r_1$ = refractive power of the anterior lens surface
F_2 = $(n - n')/r_2$ = refractive power of the posterior lens surface
t = center thickness of lens in meters
n' = refractive index of the lens material
n' = refractive index of medium surrounding lens
r_1 = radius of curvature of anterior surface, in meters
r_2 = radius of curvature of posterior surface, in meters

By Cartesian convention, a typical contact lens might be illustrated as in Fig. 7A.10, with light traveling from left to right in a positive (+) direction. The meniscus design

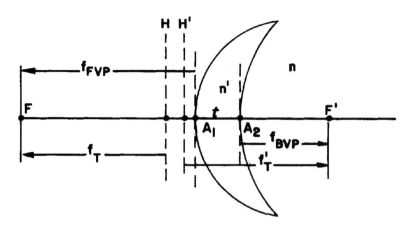

FIG. 7A.10. A typical contact lens is a "thick lens," optically speaking. It has a meniscus design, such that the principal planes (H,H') lie anterior to a plus lens, as shown, but posterior to a minus lens. Made of material having a refractive index (n') greater than air (n), the front (convex) lens surface has a plus power (F_1) and the back (concave) lens surface a minus power (F_2). The front-surface vertex (A_1) and back-surface vertex (A_2) are separated by center thickness (t). The refractive power of the lens is a function of F_1, F_2, t, and n', but it depends on the reference points from which focal lengths are measured. The diagram indicates three possible reference points, principal planes (F_T); front vertex (FVP); and back vertex (BVP), from which focal lengths can be measured (f_T, f_{FVP}, and f_{BVP}, respectively).

of a contact lens produces a front surface with a positive refractive power and a posterior surface with a negative refractive power. The resultant true or equivalent power (F_T), therefore, is the sum of the surface powers and a correction factor due to lens thickness. The true focal lengths of a contact lens are measured from the principal planes:

$$f'_T = -f_T = 1/F_T \qquad \text{Equation 7A.4}$$

in air, where

f_T = anterior focal length, in meters
f'_T = posterior focal length, in meters

It is impractical to use the true, or equivalent, power of a contact lens as a definition of refractive power because the positions of the principal planes vary with the design of the lens and its two surface powers. A fixed position from which to measure refractive power can be found by adopting the measurement of either *front vertex power* (FVP) or *back vertex power* (BVP). The equations for these powers are as follows:

$$FVP = F_1 + (F_2/ [1 - (t/n')F_2]) \qquad \text{Equation 7A.5}$$
$$BVP = (F_1/[1 - (t/n')F_1]) + F_2 \qquad \text{Equation 7A.6}$$

Front and back vertex powers are useful in that their points of reference (front-surface vertex and back-surface vertex, respectively) are easily localized in order to position a lens for measurement. Vertex focal lengths in meters are reciprocals of the vertex powers in diopters. When measuring refractive power, the contact lens can be placed on top of the lens stop of a projection lensometer as shown Fig. 7A.11. Hence, the front-surface vertex is located at the site of the lens stop when the convex surface is against the lens stop

in order to assess front vertex power in air. The opposite is true for measurement of back vertex power, in which the back-surface vertex is located at the lens stop when the concave surface is placed against the lens stop. When lens center thickness and/or surface powers are small, the differences between front and back vertex powers usually are clinically insignificant. However, as center thickness increases the two power measurements become progressively disparate according to Equations 7A.5 and 7A.6.

Because lenses of minus power usually have small center thicknesses and lenses of plus power have large center thicknesses, the disparity between front and back vertex power grows as lens power goes into the plus and especially into aphakic powers. Table 7A.3 lists disparities between the two vertex powers for back vertex powers ranging from −10 to +20 D. The front vertex powers have been calculated for rigid lenses in a typical design and center thickness for the particular power involved, having a refractive index of 1.49, base curve of 7.8 mm, and center thickness as indicated. The exact disparities would differ depending on lens design and surface powers, such that Table 7A.2 is representative within those constraints. Note that for a plus lenticular design, the disparity between vertex powers reaches a difference of 0.25 D just below +10 D of power. The disparity increases above that point, to 0.50 D just below +15 D of power and approaches 100 D at a back vertex power of +20 D.

Front vertex power is always of lesser magnitude than back vertex power when considering lenses designed in a meniscus fashion, as are contact lenses. Lens materials or designs that necessitate an increase in lens center thickness, therefore, induce higher disparities between the two vertex powers.

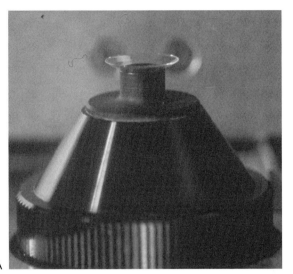
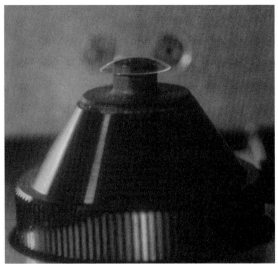

A   B

FIG. 7A.11. A contact lens has been placed on the stop of a projection lensometer, in order to measure front vertex power with convex surface toward the stop **(A)** and back vertex power with concave surface toward the stop **(B).**

Measurement of the appropriate front or back vertex power is predicated on the correct placement of either the front or back-surface vertex of a contact lens at the site of measurement on a lensometer. Unfortunately for contact lens practitioners, the typical lensometer has been made with measurement of spectacle lenses in mind, such that the vertex of the posterior spectacle lens surface is correctly positioned for accurate measurement when the concave surface of the lens contacts the lens stop. Because contact lenses have steep curvatures in comparison to spectacle lenses, the sagittal depth of a concave contact lens surface does not allow for correct placement of the back-surface vertex relative to the lens stop of the lensometer (Fig. 7A.12). The resultant measurement of back vertex power for contact lenses can be misleading, especially for lenses of higher minus or plus powers, because the contact lens power may in reality be more minus/less plus than determined. Most lensometers can be fitted with a different (smaller) lens stop for use with contact lenses so as to minimize the effects of

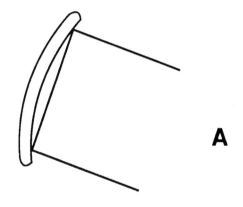

A

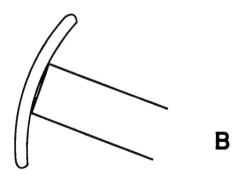

B

FIG. 7A.12. A: When measuring back vertex power on a lensometer, the large sagittal depth of a contact lens may not permit proper placement of the back-surface vertex at the middle of the stop aperture. **B:** Special stop attachments can be used for contact lenses to eliminate this problem. (From Fannin TE, Grosvenor TG. Optics of contact lenses. In: Fannin TE, Grosvenor TG, eds. *Clinical optics.* Stoneham, MA: Butterworth Publishers, 1987:415–453, with permission.)

TABLE 7A.3. DIFFERENCES BETWEEN FRONT VERTEX POWER AND BACK VERTEX POWER IN AIR FOR RIGID CONTACT LENSES

Back Vertex Power (D)	Front Vertex Power (D)	Center Thickness (mm)	Power Disparity (D)
−10	−9.92	0.10	−0.08
−5	−4.95	0.12	−0.05
0	0.00	0.15	0.00
+5	+4.90	0.23	+0.10
+10	+9.71	0.32	+0.29
+15	+14.44	0.41	+0.56
+20	+19.06	0.50	+0.94

sagittal depth on measurement of back vertex power. This stop is called a *"contact lens stop."*

Nearly all contact lenses now are specified by their back vertex powers in air, using the same convention as for spectacle lenses. However, the "sagittal depth" effect on power measurement probably is less, and positioning of rigid contact lenses easier when front vertex power is measured, making for more consistent and accurate front vertex power readings. Practitioners, therefore, often measure front vertex power at the office as a routine, but they must realize the technique's significant difference from back vertex power for high lens powers. In the past, some rigid lens manufacturers have marked their lenses according to front vertex power and, for higher plus and minus powers, a practitioner measuring the back vertex power should note values that are of higher magnitude than those of the manufacturer. In addition, should the lens be spherocylindrical or prismatic, the axis of cylinder or prism will appear rotated around a vertical meridian when front vertex power is assessed on the lensometer.

Indices of Refraction

Although the effects of surface curvature on lens refractive power are routinely considered by practitioners, changes in the *index of refraction* from one lens to another, and during the wear of the same hydrophilic lens, are increasingly becoming important. Table 7A.4 reveals various indices of refraction for rigid lens materials, ranging from 1.44 to 1.53. The index of polymethyl methacrylate (PMMA) at 1.49 was the index typically remembered by students of contact lenses, but with development of new materials has come some deviation from that earlier index "standard." Lens curvatures and thicknesses must be adjusted according to these indices in order to obtain appropriate refractive powers by rigid and other nonhydrogel lenses.

Table 7A.4 also shows that indices of refraction of conventional hydrophilic (soft) materials range from 1.38 to 1.44. In Fig. 7A.13 it is shown that the index is negatively correlated with the water content of their polymer matrices. *Water content* is the ratio of water mass within a gel lens to the mass of the hydrated lens, and it is the primary determi-

TABLE 7A.4. INDICES OF REFRACTION OF SOME CURRENT AND FORMER RIGID, NONHYDROGEL FLEXIBLE, AND SOFT CONTACT LENS MATERIALS

	Material Class	Index of Refraction
Rigid Lenses		
Airlens	Styrene	1.53
Opus III	Styrene	1.53
Silcon	Silicone resin	1.52
PMMA	Polymethyl methacrylate	1.49
CAB	Cellulose acetate butyrate	1.48
Polycon II	Silicone-acrylate	1.48
Paraperm O₂	Silicone-acrylate	1.48
Paraperm EW	Silicone-acrylate	1.475
Optacryl 60	Silicone-acrylate	1.47
Boston II	Silicone-acrylate	1.47
Boston IV	Silicone-acrylate	1.47
Fluoroperm 30–90	Fluoro/silicone-acrylate	1.47
Equalens	Fluoro/silicone-acrylate	1.44
Nonhydrogel Flexible Lenses		
SilSoft	Flexible silicone elastomer	1.44
Advent	Flexible fluoropolymer	1.39
Hydrogel Lenses		
CSI	Low water content gel	1.44
Durasoft 2	Low water content gel	1.44
Optima FW	Low water content gel	1.43
Cibasoft	Low water content gel	1.43
Optima Toric	Mid water content gel	1.42
Tresoft	Mid water content gel	1.42
Gold Medalist	Mid water content gel	1.41
Frequency 55	Mid water content gel	1.41
Acuvue	Mid water content gel	1.40
Proclear	Mid water content gel	1.40
SofLens 66	High water content gel	1.39
Compatibles	High water content gel	1.387
Permalens	High water content gel	1.38
Precision UV	High water content gel	1.38
Pure Vision	Silicone-hydrogel	1.426
Focus Night & Day	Silicone-hydrogel	1.43

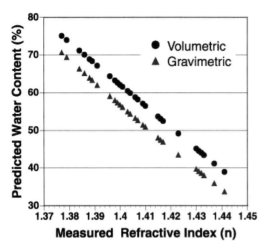

FIG. 7A.13. Relationship between refractive index of a conventional hydrogel contact lens and its water content. Note that the volumetric water content (%v/v) is 5% to 7% higher than gravimetric water content (%w/w). (From Young MD, Benjamin WJ. Calibrated oxygen permeability of 35 conventional hydrogel materials and correlation with water content. *Eye Contact Lens* 2003; 29:126–133, with permission.)

nant of the oxygen permeability of conventional hydrophilic contact lens materials. Water content is correlated to refractive index of hydrated gel lenses by a relationship derived from the principle of Gladstone and Dale (34):

$$\text{Water Content} = \frac{n_{\text{dehydrated}} - n_{\text{hydrated}}}{n_{\text{dehydrated}} - n_{\text{saline}}} \quad \text{Equation 7A.7}$$

where

$n_{\text{dehydrated}}$ = Refractive index of dry contact lens material (~1.51)

n_{hydrated} = Refractive index of hydrated contact lens material, measured

n_{saline} = Refractive index of medium in which lens has hydrated (1.333)

Water contents determined in this way are in terms of percent volume (%v/v), or approximately 5% to 7% higher than water contents calculated as a percentage of weight (%w/w). Percent volume can be translated to percent weight knowing the specific density of saline (1.000) and of the dry hydrogel (~1.25). It is as a percentage of weight (%w/w) that water contents are typically published. This is the result of the *gravimetric method* with which water content usually is assessed. Measurement of refractive index involves finding of the angle of critical reflection, for example, with an Abbe refractometer. The *refractometer* assesses only the few micrometers of material near the surface of contact lenses. The material deeper within the lens matrix is assumed to be of the same refractive index. However, water content and refractive index at the surface of a hydrogel contact lens are not always representative of those deeper within the lens matrix (35,36).

Thus, when measuring the refractive power of gel lenses in air, level of hydration ideally should be kept constant and near that encountered when the lens is on the eye. This typically has been done by *blotting* (with a lint-free cloth or filter paper) or *wiping* (with a "squeegee" technique) excess water from the lens surface prior to measurement; however, gel lens surfaces after such treatment are generally not optically excellent. The degree of surface degradation due to the lens preparation procedure is highly dependent on the operator or technician. Therefore, optical quality, measurement consistency, and accuracy are relatively low when lensometers are used to measure refractive power of most gel lenses in air. Power determination becomes even more difficult for gel lenses of high water content. One exception may be measurement of the CSI contact lens manufactured by Ciba Vision Corporation, which has a low water content for a hydrogel and more rigidlike surface optics than other hydrophilic lenses. Examples of the target images seen when measuring the CSI lens in air by projection lensometry compared to another gel lens of similar water content and a rigid lens are shown in Fig. 7A.14.

Blotting of hydrogel lenses should be performed with *lint-free filter paper or cloth* to remove excess water from their surfaces immediately before measurement of vertex powers. The accuracy of this method is limited by the difficulty of reliably blotting the test specimen to remove excess saline from the surfaces before determination of the hydrated refractive power. Care must be taken to remove all surface water; however, the specimens must not be overblotted so as to remove water from within the material. Blotting must be performed as quickly as possible to prevent loss of water from the test specimen by evaporation. The test specimens may be "dry blotted" or "wet blotted" at room temperature.

In *dry blotting,* the specimen is placed on a dry, clean, lint-free, absorbent cotton or linen cloth. The cloth is folded over the specimen, and the specimen is blotted lightly with a fingertip. The probability of overblotting is increased with the dry blotting technique, which can lead to an overestimation of the refractive power. In *wet blotting,* the specimen is placed on a clean, lint-free portion of Whatman no. 1 filter paper that has been barely dampened with saline. The filter paper is folded over the specimen, and the specimen is blotted lightly with a fingertip. The probability of leaving surface water on the lens is increased with the wet blotting technique, which can lead to an underestimation of the refractive power. Perhaps a better technique is to hold the soft lens up vertically with a pair of soft lens tweezers and to *drain off excess saline at the bottom of the lens* with an absorbent cloth or tissue. This leaves the central optical area untouched with theoretically smoother optical surfaces.

The Wet Cell

An often-quoted technique for measurement of gel lens refractive power involves a *"wet cell"* filled with saline, into

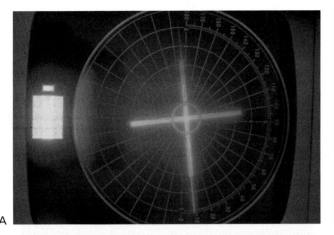

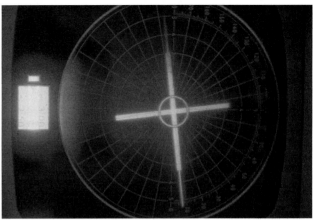

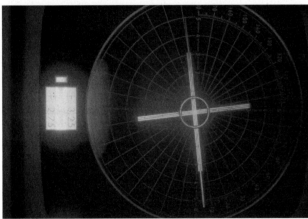

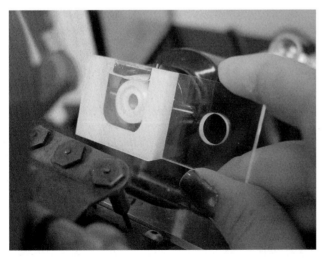

FIG. 7A.14. Views of the projection screen of a projection lensometer, when measuring a typical 38% water hydrogel contact lens **(A)**, when measuring the CSI gel contact lens **(B, also 38% water)**, and when measuring a rigid contact lens **(C)**. Note that the image formed through the CSI lens is clearer and more defined than that of the other low-water soft lens, but both have less definition than the image projected through the rigid lens.

which the lens is submerged prior to and during power measurement with a lensometer (Fig. 7A.15). Using this method, optical quality of the lensometer target images is excellent; however, correction factors based on the refractive index of the material are required in order to convert the

FIG. 7A.15. Soft contact lens immersed in a wet cell filled with saline, held against the lens stop of a lensometer for measurement of refractive power.

refractive power measured in saline to that which would be encountered in air. The correction factor results in a power in air that is 4 to 4.5 times that measured in saline, depending on the index of refraction and surface curvatures of the gel material. Two major deficiencies found with the wet cell method limit its usefulness: (i) correction for index of refraction can be elaborate (37) and *multiplies measurement error by 4 or more times;* and (ii) index of refraction is so dependent on water content, which for the specific lens at the time of measurement usually is unknown and not accurately obtainable, that wet cell measurement of refractive power is imprecise. More manageable deficiencies of the technique involve the importance of consistent lens hydration with isotonic (to tear fluid) buffered saline within the wet cell to maintain proper lens surface geometry and refractive index. Appropriate positioning of gel lenses directly against the lens stop of a lensometer is not possible; therefore, errors in measurement due to "sagittal effects" for lenses of high refractive power should be evident.

One of the problems in contact lens practice is the inability of the manufacturer and the practitioner to accurately assess optical quality of hydrogel lenses prior to insertion on the patient's eye. Without the tight production controls available for optical quality of rigid lenses, practitioners likely receive a higher proportion of gel lenses that are optically deficient, but additionally, they are unable to properly assess gel lenses before those lenses are dispensed. Rigid lenses with defective optics can be screened out with the use of a lensometer; however, this is not generally true of gel lenses. The practitioner may conclude with help of an OR that the refractive power of a gel lens is incorrect, but diagnosis of inferior vision due to gel lenses with defective surface optics must await analysis of all other possible causative factors until the practitioner finally defines the problem by "process of elimination." Fortunately, most hydrogel lenses are now easily replaced at low or no cost when their powers or surface optics are found to be insufficient.

Wet Cell Measurement of the Bifocal Add Power

An interesting feature of *diffractive* bifocal contact lenses and all *rigid back-surface* bifocals (including one-piece and fused-segment back-surface rigid designs), is that the near "add" power may be determined directly on the lensometer with the use of a "wet cell." Verification of add power for *rigid* back-surface bifocals has been practical for many years. Distance and near powers were easily determined in air, and other parameters of rigid lenses were easily assessed in order to verify lens design. Therefore, the refractive power of the back-surface bifocal "add" was verified although its power was measured in air. Use of a wet cell to verify adds of rigid back-surface bifocal contact lenses was possible but not necessary.

Wet cells assumed special importance with the introduction of the diffractive *Echelon* soft lens (38,39), now still available from Ocular Sciences, Inc. A photograph of a diffractive bifocal is shown in Fig. 7A.16. The optic zone of this lens is composed of multiple annular concentric zones of equal area, whose widths become progressively thinner into the periphery of the optic zone. Clinically speaking, accurate assessment of gel lens power in air and design parameters necessary for add verification are beyond the capabilities of normal office instrumentation. However, with the wet cell, add power was verified directly and accurately without the need for correction factors notorious for otherwise reducing the wet cell's practical value. The wet cell is useful because the thin annular optical curves of the soft Echelon lens, like those of rigid back-surface bifocals, do not conform to the cornea when the lenses are on the eye. The back surface adds of *rigid* diffractive bifocals (e.g., the discontinued Diffrax rigid lens) also was verified with the wet cell (40).

These *back-surface* bifocals are designed to produce the correct "add" powers when their posterior surfaces are immersed in tear fluid. The index of refraction (n = 1.336) of tears is similar to that of water (saline) bathing the posterior surface of the lens in a wet cell (n = 1.333). Therefore, the refractive power of the add of these back-surface bifocal contact lenses (the difference between the distance and near

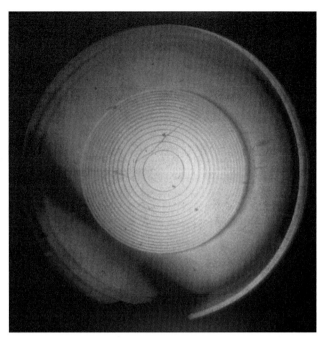

FIG. 7A.16. Diffractive bifocal showing the many concentric zones of equal area on the back surface. (From Benjamin WJ, Borish IM. Presbyopia and the influence of aging on prescription of contact lenses. In: Ruben, CM, Guillon M, eds. *Textbook of contact lens practice.* London: Chapman & Hall, 1994:763–830, with permission.)

powers) is correct when read through a lensometer (focimeter) with the use of a wet cell, although the distance power must be corrected (by a factor of 4 or more).

For instance, let us assume that the refractive index of an Echelon back-surface soft bifocal lens is such that a 4× correction factor should be used to convert power in saline to power in air. If the practitioner reads −0.87 DS and +0.87 DS with a focimeter for the distance and near images through a wet cell, then the add is +1.75 DS (−0.87 to +0.87 DS). However, the distance power is −0.87 DS multiplied by 4, the correction factor, or −3.50 DS. The lens is −3.50 DS with +1.75 DS add on the eye. Had the distance and near powers been obtained in air, the add (in air) would have measured +7.00 DS.

The adds of most back-surface hydrogel bifocal lenses cannot be measured directly using the wet cell. This includes back-surface concentric bifocal lenses and back-surface hydrogel progressive lenses. Although technically of back-surface design, the back curvatures are thought to conform to the cornea such that the adds are produced by front-surface curvatures when on the eye. The lenses are back-surface bifocals off of the eye but essentially function as front-surface bifocals on the eye (41). As a result, the wet cell does not give the equivalent of an "in eye" add measurement for these lenses. Hence, the add powers of most hydrogel presbyopic lenses should be estimated on the lensometer in air.

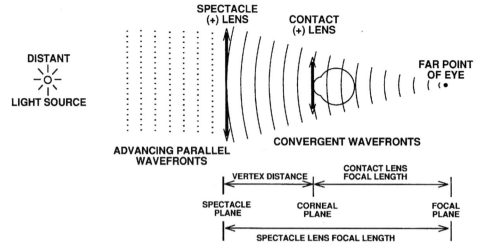

FIG. 7A.17. Refractive power of the correcting lens depends on vertex distance. For a *plus* lens, correction at the corneal plane will require a shorter focal distance than at the spectacle plane by an amount equal to the vertex distance.

Effective Power and Vertex Distance

Optical corrections for ametropia are situated in front of the eye at a distance from the anterior corneal apex called the *vertex distance.* When of appropriate back vertex power, the secondary focal point of the correcting lens coincides with the far point *(punctum remotum)* of the ametropic eye. Figures 7A.17 and 7A.18 show the placements of two commonly prescribed lenses—a spectacle lens and a contact lens—each on a myopic and a hyperopic eye. Spectacle lenses can be placed at vertex distances of 8 to 18 mm in front of the corneal apex. Contact lenses are worn at a vertex

distance of zero. Intraocular lenses have a negative vertex distance, in that they are implanted behind the cornea within the eye itself.

Because each correcting lens must place its focal point at the far point of the eye in order to optimally correct ametropia, variations in vertex distance between corrections produce corresponding deviations in the necessary power of the correcting lens. The reader can see in Fig. 7A.17 that, when correcting a hyperope, a contact lens will require a smaller focal length (a higher plus refractive power) than will a spectacle lens. An intraocular lens will require a smaller focal length than even a contact lens. On the other

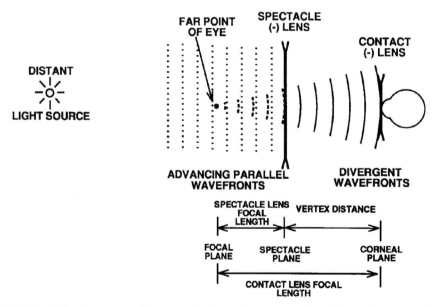

FIG. 7A.18. Refractive power of the correcting lens depends on vertex distance. For a *minus* lens, correction at the corneal plane will require a longer focal distance than at the spectacle plane by an amount equal to the vertex distance.

hand, a contact lens will require a longer focal length (lesser magnitude of minus power) than a spectacle lens for a myope, and the focal length of an intraocular lens should be even longer (Fig. 7A.18).

Stated simply, as a minus lens is brought closer to the eye its *effective power* increases, such that its refractive power must be decreased in order to maintain a constant amount of power relative to the eye. As a plus lens is brought closer to the eye its effective power decreases, such that its refractive power must be increased in order to maintain a constant amount of power relative to the eye. Effective power differences between contact lenses and spectacle corrections become clinically significant at about ± 4.00 D. Hence, vertex distance changes should be taken into account for spectacle corrections with back vertex powers greater than 4 D. The process by which the power change is calculated can be called *referring power to the cornea* and must be performed for each primary meridian of the correction. The refractive error at the spectacle plane, called the *spectacle plane refraction,* must be converted to the refractive error at the corneal plane, called the *corneal plane refraction,* in order to properly determine the appropriate contact lens power.

In order to "refer power to the cornea," it is necessary to remember that the difference in power between corrections placed at two vertex distances is related to the difference in focal lengths required by altering the vertex distance. Let us assume an eye with spectacle plane refraction of $+7.00 - 2.00 \times 0.90$ at a vertex distance of 12 mm is to be fitted with contact lenses. The focal lengths of the two primary meridians are as follows:

Horizontal Meridian:

$$f_{180} = \frac{1}{F_{180}} = \frac{1}{+5\ D} = 0.200\ m = 200\ mm$$

Vertical Meridian:

$$f_{090} = \frac{1}{F_{090}} = \frac{1}{+7\ D} = 0.143\ m = 143\ mm.$$

The focal lengths of the necessary contact lens are 12 mm shorter and, therefore, are 188 and 131 mm, respectively. The powers for the two meridians referred to the corneal plane are as follows:

Horizontal Meridian: $F_{180} = \dfrac{1}{+0.188\ m} = +5.32\ D$

Vertical Meridian: $F_{090} = \dfrac{1}{+0.131\ m} = +7.63\ D.$

The corneal plane refraction is, therefore, $+7.63 - 2.31 \times 090$. Note that for *compound hyperopic astigmatism,* both *sphere* and *cylinder* components are *larger* when referred to the corneal plane. Had the spectacle plane refraction been $-5.00 - 2.00 \times 180$, the vertex distance change would have increased the magnitudes of the focal lengths to -212 and -155 mm for the horizontal and vertical meridians, respectively:

Horizontal Meridian: $F_{180} = \dfrac{1}{-0.212\ m} = -4.72\ D$

Vertical Meridian: $F_{090} = \dfrac{1}{-0.155\ m} = -6.45\ D$

The corneal plane refraction in this case is $-4.72 - 1.73 \times 180$. Note that for *compound myopic astigmatism,* both *sphere* and *cylinder* components are *smaller in magnitude* when referred to the corneal plane. Table 7A.5 relates those spectacle lens powers that, when placed at a vertex distance of 15 mm, will result in powers referred to the corneal plane that are different by 0.25, 0.50, 0.75, and 1.00 D.

Contact Lenses on the Eye

Refractive effects of contact lenses when they are placed on the eye are largely dependent on whether those lenses do or do not conform to the topography of the cornea, or the degree to which the lenses conform (flex) to the cornea. A cross section of a contact lens/cornea optical system is shown in Fig. 7A.19. Taking the reader through layer by layer, the pre-lens tear film covers the contact lens, which sits on top of the post-lens tear pool. Underneath all of these optical media, then, is the cornea and the rest of the optical system of the eye. Each optical component from pre-lens tear film to the anterior corneal surface will be considered here and can be viewed as individual refractive components through which incident light must pass.

A *common misconception* is that the refractive power of a contact lens in air does not translate the same amount of power to the lens/cornea optical system when on the eye, supposedly because the lens is then immersed in a medium (tear fluid) with a lesser index of refraction (1.336) than air (1.000). Let us say, for purposes of argument, that a gel contact lens with BVP = -10.00 DS in air was placed on

TABLE 7A.5. SPECTACLE PLANE REFRACTION COMPARED TO CORNEAL PLANE REFRACTION AT A VERTEX DISTANCE OF 15 MM

Hyperopic (+) Correction at Spectacle Plane	Amount of Effective Change When Referred to Cornea	Myopic (−) Correction at Spectacle Plane
+4.00	±0.25 D	−4.25
+5.50	±0.50 D	−6.00
+6.75	±0.75 D	−7.50
+7.75	±1.00 D	−8.75
+9.25	±1.50 D	−10.75
+10.50	±2.00 D	−12.50
+12.75	±3.00 D	−15.75
+14.50	±4.00 D	−18.50
+16.00	±5.00 D	−21.00

Referral of (+) refractive power to the cornea requires a net increase of (+) power, whereas referral of (−) refractive power requires a net decrease of (−) power.

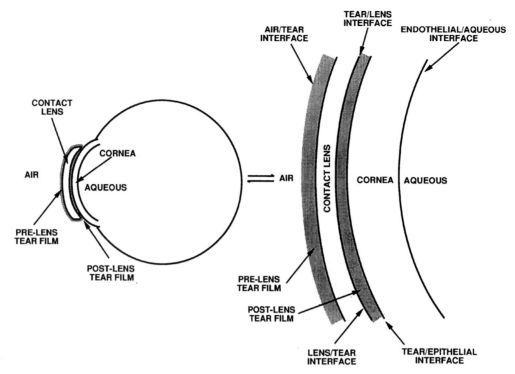

FIG. 7A.19. Cross-sectional diagram of the contact lens/cornea optical system, showing the various optical interfaces involved.

the eye and conformed to the shape of a spherical cornea (in this instance, "spherical" means *nontoroidal* or that both central primary meridians are of the same surface power). The critical optical parameters are given as follows:

Radii of Curvature	(mm)
Anterior cornea	7.80
Anterior contact lens	9.56
Posterior contact lens	7.80
Indices of refraction	
Cornea	1.376
Tears	1.336
Contact lens	1.430
Center Thicknesses	*(mm)*
Precorneal tear film	0.001
Pre-lens tear film	0.001
Contact lens	0.10
Post-lens tear pool	0.004

The precorneal and pre-lens tear films are composed of fluid with an index of 1.336 formed into refractive components of zero power, because the films have parallel anterior and posterior surfaces and are very thin. For purposes of determining refractive power, then, the tear films can be ignored and light can be assumed to first enter the visual system at an air/cornea interface. The vergence of light from a distant object encountered just after penetrating the anterior corneal surface, assuming no contact lens in place, would be $+48.20$ D:

$$F_c = (n' - n)/r_c = +48.20 \text{ D}$$

where

F_c = refractive power of air-cornea interface
r_c = 0.0078m = corneal radius of curvature, in meters
n' = 1.376 = refractive index of cornea
n = 1.000 = refractive index of air.

When the gel lens is placed on the eye, assuming the refractive effects of the pre-lens tear film to be negligible due to its zero refractive power and thinness, vergence of light penetrating the anterior corneal surface will be the result of vergence alterations at the "air/lens interface," lens/tear pool interface, and tear pool/corneal interface. Again, however, because the post-lens tear pool is very thin and is of zero refractive power (the gel lens conformed to the corneal surface curvature, such that the interfaces of the tear pool are parallel), its existence is negligible with regard to vergence of light. We can assume that a contact lens/cornea interface exists instead of a post-lens tear pool. After penetrating the anterior contact lens surface ($F_1 = +44.98$ D) and traversing through the contact lens, light originally from a distant object would have a vergence of $+45.12$ D immediately before exiting the lens. The vergence change induced by then next penetrating the lens/cornea interface would be as follows:

$$F_{L\text{-}C} = (n' - n)/r_c = -6.92 \text{ D}$$

where in this case:

$F_{L\text{-}C}$ = refractive power of lens-cornea interface
r_c = 0.0078m = corneal radius of curvature, in meters

n' = 1.376 = refractive index of cornea
n = 1.43 = refractive index of contact lens.

The vergence of light just after it penetrates the anterior corneal surface is $+45.12 - 6.92 = +38.20$ D, which is exactly 10 D less than calculated when the -10.00 D contact lens was not in place. Therefore, a contact lens on the eye will effect a change in vergence of light equal to the power of the contact lens in air. This analysis can be confirmed using an "exploded" view of the lens/cornea optical system (Fig. 7A.20), in which each optical component can be individually inspected as if in air using principles of geometric optics.

The "Lacrimal Lens Theory" and an "Exploded" View

When an *inflexible* contact lens is placed on the eye, the surfaces of the contact lens do not conform to the cornea. Under such circumstances, the post-lens tear pool does not assume parallel surfaces as in the case of the hydrophilic lens discussed earlier, unless by design the back surface of the rigid contact lens matches that of the anterior central cornea. Such a lens/cornea fitting relationship is called an *"on K"* fit, and the power of the post-lens tear pool, now called the *"lacrimal lens,"* is zero. Other names for the "lacrimal lens" are *"tear lens"* and *"fluid lens."* The *"Lacrimal Lens Theory"* is a clever mental device that was invented to explain certain optical effects of lens/cornea fitting relation-

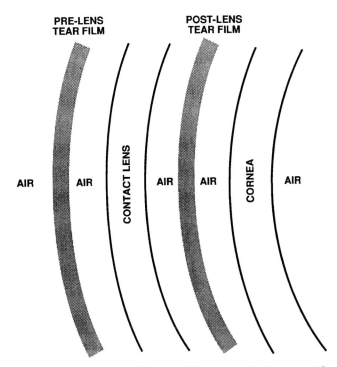

FIG. 7A.20. "Exploded" diagram of the contact lens/cornea optical system, showing each optical component as if in air.

ships (42). Refractive power calculations involving the lacrimal lens are performed as if the lacrimal lens was in air, viewed as in the "exploded" diagram shown in Fig. 7A.20.

In many situations the base curve of a rigid contact lens is not the same as the radius of curvature of the central cornea, and the lacrimal lens takes on shapes indicative of the power change that is attributed to it. Figure 7A.21 shows the shapes of the post-lens tear pool (panel A) when a lens has been fitted steeper than the cornea *("steeper than K"),* imparting a plus power to the overall lens/cornea optical system by creation of a "plus" lacrimal lens, and (panel B) when a lens has been fitted flatter than the cornea (*"flatter than K"*), imparting a minus power to the optical system by creation of a "minus" lacrimal lens. The reader should note, however, that in reality the contact lens/tear pool interface is always of minus power. Perception of plus or minus refractive power for the "lacrimal lens" depends on an "exploded" view in which the lacrimal lens is surrounded by air.

For argument's sake, let us say that the rigid lens shown in Fig. 7A.21A was fitted with a base curve of 7.62 mm and in Fig. 7A.21B was fitted with a base curve of 7.98 mm. The lenses are made of a material having a refractive index of 1.49 with back vertex powers of -5.00 D and center thicknesses of 0.10 mm. The cornea has a central radius of 7.80 mm, and by using a refractive index of 1.3375 as does a keratometer to compute refractive powers, we can see that lens A has been fitted approximately "1 D steeper than K" and that lens B has been fitted about "1 D flatter than K" (Table 7A.6). Such an analysis of the contact lens/cornea fitting relationship ignores the true refractive indices of the lens, tear fluid, and cornea, but the following paragraphs will show this use of Lacrimal Lens Theory to give correct analyses of the fitting relationship for most clinical applications.

The actual differences in refractive power between the various optical components of the two contact lens/cornea systems shown in Fig. 7A.21 can be found at two interfaces. The first, and most obvious, is the contact lens/tear pool interface, which has a smaller radius of curvature in Fig. 7A.21A and a larger radius in 7A.21B than would an "on K" (parallel) fit. The second is the air/contact lens interface (remember, the pre-lens tear film is optically inconsequential in terms of refractive power), because in order to have two contact lenses in Fig. 7A.21A and 7A.21B with the same refractive power in air (-5.00 D) but with different base curves, the front-surface curvature of the lens in A must be steeper and in B must be flatter. Table 7A.6 lists the refractive powers of the two optical interfaces with reference to an "on K" fit on the same cornea.

Note that in Table 7A.6, alterations of front-surface power from those of an "on K" fit (values in parentheses in column 1) are about *three times* the magnitude of power alterations at the lens/tear pool interface induced by changing the base curve of the rigid lens (values in parentheses

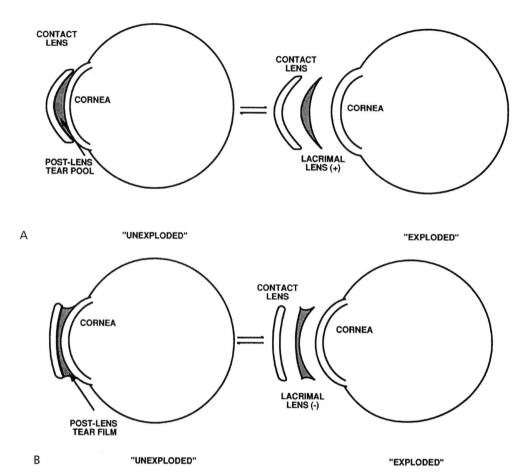

FIG. 7A.21. A: Post-lens tear pool of a *steeply* fitting rigid contact lens can be viewed "unexploded" or "exploded." The shape of the lacrimal lens is like that of a plus lens. **B:** Tear pool of a *flat* fit takes on a shape like that of a minus lens.

in column 2). The overall power changes of the system away from that of an "on K" fit (values in parentheses in column 3) match those predicted by the Lacrimal Lens Theory (within parentheses in column 4).

The Lacrimal Lens Theory uses a refractive index of 1.3375 to predict power changes relative to an alignment ("on K") fit resulting from base curve selections by the practitioner. Although originally derived for the keratometer to compensate for the average power of the posterior corneal surface when measuring corneal refractive power (K readings), by coincidence, 1.3375 is very close to the refractive index of tear fluid (n = 1.336 according to Gullstrand). As it happens, the use of a fictitious refractive index for the contact lens and cornea allows the practitioner to easily

TABLE 7A.6. REFRACTIVE POWERS DERIVED FOR INFLEXIBLE (RIGID) CONTACT LENSES OF −5.00 D IN AIR, WITH DEVIATIONS FROM "ON K" FIT IN PARENTHESES

	Power of Air–Lens Interface (D)	Power of Lens–Tear Pool Interface (D)	Back Vertex Power of (−5 D) Rigid Lens on Eye (D)	Lacrimal Lens Theory (D)
Steep Fit (A)	+59.07 (+1.47)	−20.21 (−0.47)	+39.10 (+1.02)	+44.29 (+1.02)
"On K" Fit	+57.60 (0)	−19.74 (0)	+38.08 (0)	+43.27 (0)
Flat Fit (B)	+56.19 (−1.41)	−19.30 (+0.44)	+37.10 (−0.98)	+42.29 (−0.98)

predict refractive power changes in the contact lens/cornea optical system due to lens/cornea fitting relationships affecting the power of the "lacrimal lens." This is done by visualizing an "exploded" view of the lacrimal lens (Fig. 7A.20) without having to compute the actual power alterations that are induced at both surfaces of a contact lens *in vivo* such as reported in Table 7A.6.

The practitioner then may compensate for refractive power alterations attributed to the lens/cornea fitting relationship by selecting a contact lens with a back vertex power to optimally correct the ametropic eye. Equations relating the refractive power of the "lacrimal lens" to the lens/cornea optical system are contained in the next few paragraphs, and clinical examples are included to help additionally explain the use of the Lacrimal Lens Theory in everyday contact lens practice.

Residual Astigmatism: Definition and Utility

Residual astigmatism is the refractive astigmatism left uncorrected when an optical correction is placed in front of the eye. It is the cylindrical component of *residual ametropia*. In terms of contact lenses, residual astigmatism appears in the OR determined when a contact lens is being worn. When a spherical *hydrogel contact lens* is worn, its back surface is assumed to conform to the corneal surface because the lens is highly flexible. The lacrimal lens is of zero power in all meridians and does not contribute to the correction of ametropia. Thus, "LLP" and "ΔLLP" are zero in Equations 7A.9, 7A.10, 7A.11, and 7A.12. The amount of residual astigmatism showing through the spherical soft lens will be equal to the *refractive astigmatism* found in the corneal plane refraction.

When an *inflexible rigid lens* is worn, on the other hand, the component of refractive astigmatism due to corneal toricity is masked, and only the *internal astigmatism* of the eye contributes to the cylinder in the OR. Internal astigmatism is also sometimes referred to as *"lenticular astigmatism"* because it is thought primarily to be the result of the ocular crystalline lens. The residual astigmatism is equal to the internal astigmatism when an inflexible rigid lens is worn.

$$CPA = CA + IA \qquad \text{Equation 7A.8}$$

where

CPA = Corneal Plane Astigmatism (DC), also called "Refractive Astigmatism"
 CA = Corneal Astigmatism (DC), or "Corneal Toricity"; the component of refractive astigmatism due to the toricity of the anterior corneal surface in keratometric diopters.
 IA = Internal Astigmatism (DC); the component of refractive astigmatism due to ocular optical elements behind the anterior corneal surface (i.e., posterior corneal surface and crystalline lens). Sometimes also called merely "lenticular astigmatism."

The *predicted* residual astigmatism is an important factor when considering the type of contact lens to be prescribed for a particular patient. If the refractive astigmatism is low, 0.75 DC or less, the eye may be able to wear a spherical hydrogel contact lens. This lens will allow most, or all, of the refractive astigmatism to show through the lens, because little, if any, corneal astigmatism will be masked by the soft lens. If the refractive astigmatism and corneal astigmatism are roughly equal in magnitude (± 0.50 DC) and direction (± 10 degrees) but less than 2.00 DC, a spherical rigid lens would likely correct nearly all of the refractive cylinder as it masks the corneal toricity. Similarly, a bitoric rigid lens exhibiting the "spherical power effect" (SPE), discussed in a subsequent chapter, could be a viable mode of contact lens correction when the corneal toricity and refractive cylinder are simultaneously greater than 2.00 DC. In these instances the residual astigmatism through the spherical or SPE rigid contact lens is predictably zero or nearly so (± 0.50 DC).

When refractive cylinder and corneal cylinder are not equal, such that 1.00 DC or more of internal cylinder is predicted to show through an inflexible spherical rigid contact lens, the front toric rigid lens and toric soft contact lens become viable options. Finally, in cases of large corneal toricity (>2.00 DC) when refractive cylinder and corneal cylinder are not equal, bitoric lenses exhibiting the "cylindrical power effect" (CPE) can be prescribed. Toric soft contact lenses of high cylinder have a lower probability of success, yet they also may be occasionally prescribed in these latter instances. A flow chart is shown in Table 7A.7, which may help the practitioner in the initial determination of the type of contact lens to be recommended to the patient. The various contact lens methods for correction of astigmatism is discussed further in Chapter 7B.

Lacrimal Lens and Masking of Corneal Shape: Example 1

The practitioner has several optical measures from which to assess the optical status of the eye, such as the refraction providing maximum visual acuity *(spectacle plane refraction)* and keratometry readings of the central cornea *(K readings)*. These techniques also can be performed with a contact lens in place, in which case they are called *overrefraction* and *over-K readings,* respectively. The following equations relate these measures for use by the clinician with respect to each primary meridian of correction:

$$CPR = CLP + OR + LLP$$

$$\text{Equation 7A.9}$$

where

CPR = Corneal Plane Refraction (D)
CLP = Contact Lens Power, in air (D)
 OR = Over-Refraction, referred to the corneal plane (D)
LLP = Lacrimal Lens Power, in air (D)

TABLE 7A.7. CONTACT LENS CORRECTION OF ASTIGMATISM

Condition	Contact Lens Options
Refractive Cylinder ≤ 0.75 DC	
Corneal toricity = Refractive cylinder	Spherical rigid lens[a]
	Spherical or aspheric soft lens
Corneal toricity ≠ Refractive cylinder	Spherical or aspheric soft lens[a]
	Spherical rigid lens
Refractive Cylinder = Corneal Toricity (within ± 0.50 DC)	
Low astigmatism (0.75–2.00 DC)	Spherical rigid lens[a]
	Toric soft lens
High astigmatism (>2.00 DC)	Bitoric "SPE" rigid lens[a]
	Spherical rigid lens
	Custom toric soft lens
Refractive Cylinder ≠ Corneal Toricity (difference > 0.50 DC)	
Low corneal toricity (≤2.00 DC)	Toric soft lens[a]
	Front toric rigid lens
High corneal toricity (>2.00 DC)	Bitoric "CPE" rigid lens[a]
	Custom toric soft lens

[a] Optimal option, on average, considering optical quality of correction, comfort, and fit of contact lenses.
CPE, cylindrical power effect.

When the OR is zero and no alterations of base curve radius (ΔLLP) are made when the final contact lens is specified, the diagnostic contact lens power becomes the final contact lens power when ordering the contact lens prescription (Rx):

$$FCLP = DCLP + OR - \Delta LLP$$
Equation 7A.10

where

$FCLP$ = Final Contact Lens Power to be ordered (D)
$DCLP$ = Diagnostic Contact Lens Power (D)
OR = Over-Refraction, referred to the corneal plane (D)
ΔLLP = Change in Lacrimal Lens Power, in air (D), when altering from the diagnostic contact lens to the final contact lens

The base curve radius of the contact lens and the K reading of the primary meridian must be known to derive the appropriate power of the "lacrimal lens." Using 1.3375 as the refractive index in order to compute refractive power of the front surface of the lacrimal lens, a comparison between the front lacrimal surface power and rear lacrimal surface power (derived from the corneal K reading) will ascertain the "power" of the lacrimal lens:

$$LLP = F_1 LL + F_2 LL \quad \text{Equation 7A.11}$$

where

LLP = Lacrimal Lens Power, in air (D)
$F_1 LL$ = Front Surface Power of the Lacrimal Lens, in air (D, based on n = 1.3375 and the base curve radius of the contact lens)
$F_2 LL$ = Back Surface Power of the Lacrimal Lens, in air

(D, based on n = 1.3375 and the keratometry reading of the cornea)

If the dioptric power of the posterior contact lens surface is treated as a positive value, Equation 7A.11 can be rewritten for clinical use:

$$LLP = BC - K \quad \text{Equation 7A.12}$$

where

LLP = Lacrimal Lens Power, in air (D)
BC = Base Curve (D), based on n = 1.3375 (keratometric diopters) and the base curve radius of the contact lens (treated as + value)
K = Keratometry Reading (D), based on n = 1.3375 (keratometric diopters) and the corneal radius of curvature

As can be noted from Fig. 7A.21 and Equation 7A.12, a contact lens fitted "1 D steeper than K" when using n = 1.3375 to judge the lens/cornea relationship will result in a lacrimal lens with +1 keratometric diopter of power. Although we know that, technically, the Lacrimal Lens Theory is a simplified version of the truth, it is clinically much easier to use the Lacrimal Lens Theory and to visualize an "exploded" view of the contact lens/cornea optical system when determining the proper contact lens power for a patient.

Let us suppose that the practitioner has attempted to fit a −2.50 DS rigid diagnostic lens with a base curve radius of 7.90 mm on an eye for which he or she earlier measured K readings of 42.25 DC @ 180 and 45.00 DC @ 090. The patient's spectacle refraction was −1.00 −2.75 × 180. What should be the expected OR for this eye? If we were to fit a lens having an equivalent lens/cornea relationship, what would be the ideal contact lens power to prescribe?

Example 1: Pertinent parameters
Spectacle Rx: $-1.00 -2.75 \times 180$
K readings: 42.25/45.00 @ 090
Diagnostic contact lens
    Base curve radius: 7.90 mm (42.75 D)
    Power: -2.50 DS

Using Equations 7A.9 and 7A.12, we can calculate the expected OR, initially for each primary meridian and then combine the two to form a spherocylindrical result. First, the lacrimal lens powers must be calculated from Equation 7A.12:

* Horizontal Meridian: Lacrimal Lens Power =
            (0.3375/.0079) − 42.25 = *+0.47* D
* Vertical Meridian: Lacrimal Lens Power =
            (0.3375/.0079) − 45.00 = *−2.28* D

These values can be rounded to the nearest quarter diopter and next substituted into Equation 7A.9. The expected OR in each meridian then is resolved:

* Horizontal Meridian: $-1.00 =$
            $-2.50 + OR + (+0.50)$
* Horizontal OR = *+1.00* D
* Vertical Meridian: $-3.75 =$
            $-2.50 + OR + (-2.25)$
* Vertical OR = *+1.00* D

The OR for this eye should be $+1.00$ DS as calculated. The ideal contact lens Rx could be obtained using Equation 7A.10, assuming that the practitioner would not alter the base curve of the lens when ordered from the laboratory (the alteration of lacrimal lens power for the final contact lens would then be zero from that of the diagnostic lens). It also could be computed by using Equation 7A.9 and assuming an OR of zero:

* Horizontal Meridian: $-1.00 =$
            CL Rx + OR + (+0.50), where OR = 0
* Horizontal FCLP = *−1.50* D
* Vertical Meridian: $-3.75 =$
            CL Rx + OR + (−2.25), where OR = 0
* Vertical FCLP = *−1.50* D

The result shows a convenient situation in which a spherical OR is obtained over a spherical inflexible contact lens (a rigid lens without toric surfaces), such that the rigid contact lens ideally suited for this eye's refractive status would have a back vertex power of -1.50 DS in air. A rigid lens of -1.50 DS would result in an OR of zero and would become the best rigid lens Rx assuming that the fit of the lens was appropriate. For eyes that have *corneal toricity (as*

measured by the keratometer) equal to the cylindrical component of the corneal plane refraction, an inflexible contact lens is predicted to require only spherical front and back surfaces for best optical correction. This type of rigid lens is the least complicated of all lens designs to prescribe for a patient. Note that internal astigmatism for this eye is zero and that the residual astigmatism seen through the inflexible rigid lens also was zero.

Corneal toricity is said to be *"masked"* by rigid lenses, because the difference in refractive power between the two primary corneal meridians (2.75 DC with-the-rule toricity in Example 1) is offset exactly by the difference in power between the lacrimal lens powers of those two meridians when an inflexible rigid lens of spherical base curve is placed on the cornea (2.75 D in the earlier case, more minus in the vertical meridian). Should the patient's corneal toricity change over time after initiating wear of a rigid lens, these toricity alterations also would be masked by equal, but opposite in sign, power alterations of the lacrimal lens. Therefore, rigid lenses are sometimes said, *incorrectly,* to lessen the incidence of refractive changes of the eye. However, rigid lenses mask corneal shape changes so that power changes requiring *replacement or modification of rigid contact lenses are not as frequent as found with spectacle correction or by correction with flexible soft lenses.*

Masking of corneal shape is perhaps the most striking advantage of rigid contact lenses over all other forms of ametropic correction. Not only can rigid lenses mask regular corneal astigmatism and astigmatic changes in time, but *irregular corneal astigmatism* and other corneal topographical abnormalities or *distortions* can be masked as well. For instance, in *keratoconus* where highly irregular astigmatic and distorted corneas are encountered, rigid contact lenses are most often a necessity because no other form of correction can provide excellent vision. In cases of *keratoplasty, keratorefractive surgery,* and *corneal trauma,* rigid contact lenses are often the best form of correction, due to the ability of the lacrimal lens to compensate for refractive corneal surface abnormalities.

Front Toric Rigid Contact Lenses: Example 2

In Example 1, corneal toricity and refractive astigmatism were both with-the-rule and of equal magnitude. The result was that, when fitted with an inflexible rigid lens of spherical base curve radius, the lacrimal lens masked corneal astigmatism such that no astigmatic component was necessary in the contact lens Rx. What if all of the patient's refractive astigmatism was *not* the result of corneal toricity? For instance, let us say that the eye described earlier had a spectacle Rx of $-1.00 -1.75 \times 180$ and all other critical parameters remained the same. What would be the best rigid lens Rx in this case? The answer might be tied to which type of rigid lens design best fit the cornea: a front toric design or a bitoric design.

> Example 2: Pertinent parameters
> Spectacle Rx: $-1.00 -1.75 \times 180$
> K readings: 42.25/45.00 @ 090
> Diagnostic contact lens
> Base curve radius: 7.90 mm (42.75 D)
> Power: -2.50 DS

If the practitioner deems that a spherical base curve of 7.90 mm radius of curvature properly fits the cornea, as in our earlier example, a front toric design may be appropriate. The optical calculations to ascertain the appropriate contact lens Rx closely resemble those previously shown, with the exception that the OR over a -2.50 DS diagnostic contact lens and the final contact lens power will have identical cylindrical components. The lens/cornea fitting relationship remains the same as in Example 1, therefore, again using Equation 7A.9:

* Horizontal Meridian: $-1.00 =$
  $$-2.50 + OR + (+0.50)$$
* Horizontal OR $= +1.00$ D
* Vertical Meridian: $-2.75 =$
  $$-2.50 + OR + (-2.25)$$
* Vertical OR $= +2.00$ D

The OR is predicted to be $+2.00 -1.00 \times 090$. Residual astigmatism through the inflexible diagnostic lens was -1.00 DC $\times$ 090, which is the internal astigmatism of the eye. When an OR of zero is substituted in Equation 7A.9 in order to ascertain the front toric rigid contact lens power (or, this can be done using Equation 7A.10), the calculations areas follows:

* Horizontal Meridian: $-1.00 =$
  $$CLP + OR + (+0.50), \text{ where } OR = 0$$
* Horizontal CLP $= -1.50$ D
* Vertical Meridian: $-2.75 =$
  $$CLP + OR + (-2.25), \text{ where } OR = 0$$
* Vertical CLP $= -0.50$ D

The final front toric rigid contact lens power with a 7.90-mm spherical base curve radius is, therefore, $-0.50 -1.00 \times 090$. The amount of toricity in the final contact lens is equal to the internal astigmatism, which is also the amount of astigmatism that was residual when the inflexible rigid diagnostic contact lens was worn.

Bitoric Rigid Lenses: Example 3, Spherical Power Effect

Let us assume in our earlier case in which a spectacle refraction of $-1.00 -2.75 \times 180$ was found (Example 1) that a rigid lens with a toric back surface was required to obtain an acceptable corneal fit, such that one primary meridian had a radius of curvature of 7.90 mm and the other meridian had a radius of 7.63 mm. This lens would be expected to fit with its steep meridian aligned vertically with the steep corneal meridian. The bitoric diagnostic rigid lens has a back vertex power of $-2.50 -1.50 \times 180$, and all other parameters remain the same as in our earlier examples. What is the expected OR for the bitoric diagnostic lens, and what should be the final bitoric lens refractive power?

> Example 3: Pertinent parameters
> Spectacle Rx: $-1.00 -2.75 \times 180$
> K readings: 42.25/45.00 @ 090
> Diagnostic contact lens
> Base curve: 7.90/7.63 mm (42.75/44.25 D)
> Power: $-2.50 -1.50 \times 180$

The calculations closely resemble our earlier examples. However, in this case the lacrimal lens power has been altered due to the fitting relationship in the vertical meridian. Because we have steepened the lens fit from 7.90 to 7.63 mm in that meridian, the lacrimal lens in the vertical meridian has a power of -0.75 D (computed from Equation 7A.12), whereas the lacrimal lens power in the horizontal meridian remains at $+0.50$ D. Using Equation 7A.9 to estimate the OR:

* Horizontal Meridian: $-1.00 =$
  $$-2.50 + OR + (+0.50)$$
* Horizontal OR $= +1.00$ D
* Vertical Meridian: $-3.75 =$
  $$-4.00 + OR + (-0.75)$$
* Vertical OR $= +1.00$ D

The OR is predicted to be $+1.00$ DS. When an OR of zero is substituted in order to ascertain the rigid bitoric final contact lens power, the calculations areas as follows:

* Horizontal Meridian: $-1.00 =$
  $$CLP + OR + (+0.50), \text{ where } OR = 0$$
* Horizontal CL Rx $= -1.50$ D
* Vertical Meridian: $-3.75 =$
  $$CLP + OR + (-0.75), \text{ where } OR = 0$$
* Vertical CL Rx $= -3.00$ D

The bitoric rigid contact lens Rx with a 7.90 mm/7.63 mm back surface is, therefore, $-1.50 -1.50 \times 180$ as measured by a lensometer in air.

Example 3 is a special case where the patient's ametropia could have been excellently corrected by an inflexible spherical rigid lens, as *corneal toricity matched the cylindrical component of the eye's spectacle refraction*. Yet, a lens of bitoric design was required in order that the lens fit the cornea properly. The final bitoric lens design and refractive power achieved an optical correction in which front-surface toricity of the lens was required to make up for the lack of power of the lacrimal lens (induced by steepening the posterior contact lens surface in the vertical meridian). An interesting aspect of this rigid lens is that it has a spherical refractive power when placed on the eye (Table 7A.8), thus illustrating *SPE*. Rigid SPE lenses can rotate on the eye without inducing astigmatism and can be used when back-surface toricity in keratometric diopters (n = 1.3375) equals the eye's refractive cylinder. Note that the SPE diagnostic lens provided a residual astigmatism of zero, as did the spherical lens in Example 1. An SPE lens can easily be identified because its *cylinder power in air (by lensometry) equals its back-surface toricity in keratometric diopters* (43). The fitting of bitoric lenses specifically for "spherical power effect" is covered more fully in Chapter 7B.

Bitoric Rigid Lenses: Examples 4 to 6, Cylindrical Power Effect

When corneal toricity does not match corneal plane refractive cylinder, bitoric lenses that optimally correct the eye's ametropia create cylinder when placed on the eye. Let us suppose that the eye's spectacle correction in Example 3 was actually −1.00 DS. The diagnostic bitoric lens was the same as that in Example 3, with a back vertex power of −2.50 −1.50 × 180 and back-surface radii of 7.90 and 7.63 mm. All other parameters of the eye and contact lens were the same as in our earlier examples. Note that internal astigmatism is −2.75 DC × 090, and that this amount of cylinder should be residual through an inflexible spherical or SPE rigid lens.

Example 4: Pertinent parameters
Spectacle Rx: −1.00 DS
K readings: 42.25/45.00 @ 090
Diagnostic contact lens:
    Base curve: 7.90/7.63 mm (42.75/44.25 D)
    Power: −2.50 −1.50 × 180

Using Equations 7A.9, 7A.10, and 7A.12, it can be determined that the expected OR is +3.75 −2.75 × 090 and the final contact lens power should be −0.25 −1.25 ×

090. Table 7A.9 reveals that the back vertex power of the final rigid lens Rx is spherocylindrical when placed on the eye. The Rx in this case is, therefore, representative of *CPE*.

CPE lenses induce astigmatism when they rotate away from correct axis orientation. The amount of cylinder that rotates with a CPE lens on the eye is the difference of refractive cylinder between the CPE lens and an SPE lens that has the same base curve radii. With 1.50 DC of back-surface toricity, an SPE lens would have −1.50 DC of refractive cylinder oriented axis 180. Therefore, with −1.25 DC oriented axis 090, this CPE lens creates −2.75 DC × 090 when it is on the eye. Because we refracted over an SPE diagnostic lens, this is the amount of cylinder found in the OR. The reader might note that, when refracting over an SPE lens, the residual cylinder is equal to the eye's internal astigmatism. The fitting of bitoric lenses specifically for CPE is covered more fully in Chapter 7B.

It is not necessary that a rigid lens be bitoric to produce the CPE. Should the patient's corneal topography and spectacle Rx be appropriate, on rare occasion, the CPE can be produced by a *back toric lens* with a spherical front surface that optimally corrects for the eye's ametropia.

As can be seen in Table 7A.6, the actual refractive alteration at the lens/tear pool interface induced by a change in the base curve radius of a rigid lens is slightly less than *half* of the keratometric diopter value (n = 1.3375) of the base curve radius change. The front surface of the contact lens must undergo a change in power of *almost three times* that of the lens/tear pool interface, in other words, nearly *1.5 times* that of the dioptric base curve change (n = 1.3375), when back vertex power is held constant. These relationships are often called the *"1:2:3 rule,"* because the refractive alterations due to base curve changes at the (i) posterior lens/tear pool interface, (ii) posterior lens surface in air in keratometric diopters (n = 1.3375), and (iii) posterior lens surfaces in air according to a refractive index of 1.49 are in ratios of 1:2:3, respectively. The reader will note that the values in Table 7A.6 (in parentheses) represent refractive alterations computed due to base curve radius changes and that these values approximate the ratios of 1:2:3.

Suppose, then, that the spectacle refraction called for

TABLE 7A.8. REFRACTIVE POWER OF THE BITORIC CONTACT LENS COMPUTED IN EXAMPLE 3 CALCULATED FOR THAT LENS WHEN PLACED ON THE EYE

	Front Surface Power in Air (D)	Back Surface Power in Tears (D)	Back Vertex Power on the Eye (D)
Horizontal meridian	+60.28	−19.49	+41.04
Vertical meridian	+60.97	−20.18	+41.04

The back vertex powers for the two primary meridians are the same when the lens is on the eye, even though the lens had a spherocylindrical power when both surfaces were surrounded by air. Such lenses contribute no cylinder to the overall optical system of the eye and are representative of the spherical power effect.

TABLE 7A.9. REFRACTIVE POWER OF THE BITORIC CONTACT LENS COMPUTED IN EXAMPLE 4 CALCULATED FOR THAT LENS WHEN PLACED ON THE EYE

	Front Surface Power in Air (D)	Back Surface Power in Tears (D)	Back Vertex Power on the Eye (D)
Horizontal meridian	+60.28	−19.49	+41.04
Vertical meridian	+63.70	−20.18	+43.52

The back vertex powers for the two primary meridians are not the same when the lens is on the eye, even though the lens had a spherocylindrical power when both surfaces were surrounded by air. Such lenses contribute cylinder to the overall optical system of the eye and are representative of the cylindrical power effect.

cylinder power at 1.5 times the dioptric difference (n = 1.3375) between base curves of a back toric rigid contact lens. Suppose, also, that the base curves were fitted "on K" to both primary corneal meridians, such that spectacle cylinder is 1.5 times the corneal cylinder as well:

Example 5: Pertinent parameters
Spectacle Rx: −1.00 −4.00 × 180
K readings: 42.25/45.00 @ 090
Diagnostic contact lens
    Base curve: 7.99/7.50 mm (42.25/45.00 D)
    Power: −2.50 −2.75 × 180

The diagnostic lens in Example 5 is an SPE lens (refractive cylinder is equal to back-surface keratometric toricity). The OR should be +1.50 −1.25 × 180, and the final contact lens power −1.00 −4.00 × 180. In this case, all refractive astigmatism is corrected by the toric back surface; therefore, the front surface must be spherical. The final contact lens Rx is a *back toric/front surface sphere,* technically not a bitoric lens but nevertheless representative of the CPE. The amount of cylinder that rotates with the final CPE lens on the eye is −1.25 DC × 180.

Another peculiar circumstance occurs when a bitoric rigid lens is designed such that back-surface toricity in keratometric diopters (n = 1.3375) is only slightly greater than refractive astigmatism. Consider Example 6:

Example 6: Pertinent parameters
Spectacle Rx: −1.00 −1.25 × 180
K readings: 42.25/45.00 @ 090
Diagnostic contact lens
    Base curve: 7.90/7.63 mm (42.75/44.25 D)
    Power: −2.50 −1.50 × 180

The OR should be +2.50 −1.50 × 090 and the final contact lens power −1.50 DS. In this case, a bitoric lens exhibits CPE on the eye but actually has a spherical refractive power in air as measured with the lensometer. This lens would be difficult to distinguish from a warped spherical rigid lens, because both lenses have spherical refractive powers when measured by lensometry (see section on Lens Flexure and Warpage). One difference would be that back-surface toricity of the CPE lens should be much greater than back-surface toricity of the warped spherical lens. The amount of cylinder that would rotate with the CPE lens in Example 6 is −1.50 DC × 090, which is the internal astigmatism of the eye.

Lacrimal Lens Theory and Refractive Index

The ability of the lacrimal lens to fully compensate for optical power effects of the base curve/cornea relationship has been based on the wear of PMMA lenses with a refractive index of 1.49. Could the "lacrimal lens theory" break down when rigid lenses having refractive indices other than 1.49 are prescribed? Extreme indices for currently available rigid lenses listed in Table 7A.4 were 1.53 on the high side and 1.44 on the low side of PMMA. Perhaps future rigid lenses could be made to attain the very high index of 1.82 (possible now with some types of glass) or a very low index of 1.33, like that of water.

Table 7A.10 lists the actual refractive changes encountered in a lens/cornea optical system when altering base curves of rigid lenses having various refractive indices. It can be seen that predicted power alterations based on the Lacrimal Lens Theory are very accurate for all real and hypothetical index extremes for lenses fitted even 5 D steep or flat. The only way to marginally improve the Lacrimal Lens Theory is to accept the index of tear fluid (1.336) instead of that used by the keratometer (1.3375) for the calculation of lacrimal lens power! The Lacrimal Lens Theory is, therefore, insensitive to refractive index differences between contact lens materials and is only marginally improved by assuming the actual index of tear fluid for calculations involving the post-lens tear pool.

Interestingly enough, the index of 1.336 was used to calculate "corneal curvature" by the old Ophthalmometer manufactured by American Optical Corporation. This device did not survive in the marketplace as did the Bausch & Lomb Keratometer, for reasons other than assumption of a different refractive index. The proper use of 1.336, therefore, fell into disfavor in comparison to 1.3375 because it was associated with an otherwise unsuccessful instrument.

TABLE 7A.10. CALCULATED POWER ALTERATIONS OF THE CONTACT LENS/CORNEA OPTICAL SYSTEM INDUCED BY RIGID LENSES OF THREE DIFFERENT BASE CURVES

Base Curve (mm)	Lacrimal Lens Power (n = 1.3375)	Lacrimal Lens Power (n = 1.3360)	Induced Refractive Power Alteration for Lenses of Several Indices				
			n = 1.82	1.53	1.49	1.44	1.33
6.99	+5.01 D	+4.99 D	+4.99	+4.99	+4.99	+4.99	+4.99D
7.80	0.0 D	0.0 D	0	0	0	0	0 D
8.82	−5.00 D	−4.98 D	−4.98	−4.98	−4.98	−4.98	−4.98 D

Len fits were "5 diopters steeper than K," "on K," and "5 diopters flatter than K" according to the Lacrimal Lens Theory. All calculations assumed a rigid lens power of −5.00 D and that the central corneal radius of curvature was 7.80 mm. Note that the Lacrimal Lens Theory using an index of 1.3375 accurately predicted the actual power alterations and was made only slightly more accurate by assuming a refractive index of 1.336. The refractive index of the lens material had no impact on power alterations induced by the lens/cornea fitting relationship.

Base Curve Radius Changes and a "Rule of Thumb"

A practitioner often makes changes in the base curve radius of a lens when a new lens is ordered for the patient. Perhaps the lens on the patient's eye is a diagnostic lens for which the parameters and OR are known, but the practitioner believes that a better fitting relationship can be obtained by altering the base curve radius of the lens. Or perhaps the patient's eye has changed curvature over time such that the patient's present lens, although it has "masked" refractive changes of the cornea such that the OR is zero, requires an alteration of the lens/cornea fitting relationship. In these cases, Equation 7A.10 can be invoked to calculate the appropriate refractive powers to be ordered. The equation should be solved for each of the primary meridians.

Assume that the eye and lens in Example 1 did not provide an excellent fitting relationship and that the practitioner wished to fit the lens with a spherical base curve of 7.80 mm instead of 7.90 mm. This would result in a lacrimal lens that is approximately 0.50 DS steeper (ΔLLD = +0.50 DS) than the original fit in keratometric diopters. As stated in Example 1, the diagnostic rigid lens power was −2.50 DS and the OR was +1.00 DS. With a base curve radius of 7.90 mm, a final contact lens power of −*1.50 DS* was to be ordered. In this case, calculations from Equation 7A.10 are the same in both primary meridians; however, base curve radius alterations might require consideration in only one meridian (in fitting a bitoric lens, for instance):

Final Contact Lens Power =
$$-2.50 + (+1.00) - (+0.50) = -2.00 \text{ DS}$$

Note that by steepening the base curve radius by +0.50 keratometric diopter, a net addition of −0.50 DS of power to the final lens Rx was necessary. For every base curve radius change that is made, there is an *equal but opposite* change of power necessary in the rigid contact lens Rx. Had the practitioner flattened the base curve radius by, say, 0.15 mm and ordered a base curve radius of 8.05 mm, the necessary contact lens Rx would have been −0.75 DS, reflecting

a +0.75 D back vertex power modification for a −0.75 power alteration of the lacrimal lens.

A good rule to remember is that *0.05 mm ≅ 0.25 D* of lacrimal lens power in keratometric diopters for small base curve alterations (<0.20 mm, or 1.0 D). This "rule of thumb," as is typical of rules of thumb, accurately describes effects of base curve radius alterations on lacrimal lens power for a limited range of base curve values (from 7.85–8.65 mm, or 43.00–39.00 D in terms of keratometry readings). Table 7A.11 shows that a 0.25 D change in power of the lacrimal lens can be achieved with as little as 0.03-mm alteration of base curve should the base curve be very steep or as much as 0.06 mm should it be very flat. The practitioner, therefore, should be wary when making mental calculations based on this "rule of thumb," especially for large base curve radius changes on steep lenses.

Lens Flexure and Warpage

Previous equations and calculations involving the lacrimal lens were derived assuming that the rigid contact lens was *inflexible* to forces acting on it *in vivo*. In many situations, however, contact lenses flex on the eye to either partially or fully conform to the shape of the cornea. The amount of flexure is a function of flexural strength of the lens material (e.g., highly oxygen-permeable polymers generally flex more than polymers having low permeability), design of the lens (e.g., thin lenses flex more than thick lenses), corneal topography, and lens/cornea fitting relationship. Concerns about the effects of lens flexure have mounted in recent years because of emphasis placed on oxygen transmissibility of contact lenses (44). Highly flexible "rigid" oxygen-permeable materials made in designs as thin as tolerable to meet corneal oxygen demands have made rigid lens flexure a common problem for today's practitioners.

Soft Lens Flexure

The most extreme example of lens flexure is, of course, a hydrophilic lens that conforms to the topography of the cornea. The match between back-surface curvature of a typi-

TABLE 7A.11. BASE CURVE RADIUS COMPARED TO BASE CURVE IN KERATOMETRIC DIOPTERS

Keratometric Diopters	Base Curve (mm)	Base Curve Radius Alteration To Change 0.25 D (mm)	Base Curve Radius Alteration To Change 1.00 D (mm)
53.00	6.37	0.03	0.12
51.00	6.62	0.0325	0.13
49.00	6.89	0.035	0.14
47.00	7.18	0.04	0.16
45.00	7.50	0.04	0.16
43.00	7.85	0.045	0.18
41.00	8.23	0.05	0.20
39.00	8.65	0.055	0.22
37.00	9.12	0.06	0.24

Values have been computed for a range of base curve radii from 6.37 mm (53.00 D) to 9.12 mm (37.00 D). Note that the rule of thumb specifying that 0.05 mm = 0.25 D is correct only for a limited range.

cal thin minus hydrogel *in vivo* and corneal toricity is assumed to be parallel, and the lacrimal lens contributes no power to the lens/cornea optical system. Technically, as contact lenses are treated as "thick" lenses according to geometric optics, lens flexure should result in an alteration of back vertex power (45–48). Let us assume that a hydrogel lens of −5.00 back vertex power in air (n = 1.43), having a base curve of 8.50 mm and center thickness of 0.10 mm, was placed on a cornea measuring 43.00 D (7.85 mm) by keratometry (n = 1.3375). What is the actual back vertex power in air when the contact lens conforms to the topography of the cornea?

Early theorists thought that the front surface of the soft contact lens must alter its radius equal to, or at some constant ratio with (called a *wrap factor*), alteration of the posterior lens surface in order for flexure to occur (45,46). By using the back vertex power formula (Equation 7A.6), one can compute the front-surface radius of curvature for the contact lens in its unflexed state:

$$BVP = -5.00 \text{ D} = \frac{F_1}{1 - (0.0001/1.43)F_1} + (-50.59 \text{ D}).$$

Therefore,

$$F_1 = 45.45 \text{ D, and } r_1 = 9.46 \text{ mm}$$

When the soft lens conforms to the corneal radius, the posterior lens surface will alter from 8.50 to 7.85 mm and the anterior lens surface was proposed to undergo an equal transition, from 9.46 to 8.81 mm. The front and back surfaces of the contact lens then will be +48.81 D and −54.78 D, respectively, such that the recalculated back vertex power would be −5.80 D. This proposed "on the eye" power is significantly different than that encountered "off of the eye."

Table 7A.12 shows how "on the eye" back vertex power for −5.00 D and +5.00 D hydrophilic lenses alter with central corneal radius of curvature, assuming equal alterations of front- and back-surface radii [Sarver's *"Equal Change Hypothesis,"* cited by Picker et al. (45)]. Contact lens powers have been calculated as if the lens was in air but conforming exactly to the shape of the cornea. Note

TABLE 7A.12. BACK VERTEX POWERS OF HYDROPHILIC LENSES WITH POWERS OF −5.00 D AND +5.00 D IN AIR, BASE CURVE = 8.50 MM, AND CENTER THICKNESSES OF 0.10 MM AND 0.20 MM, RESPECTIVELY

Keratometry Readings (D)	Back Vertex Power in Air of −5 Gel Lens Conformed to Cornea (D)	Back Vertex Power in Air of +5 Gel Lens Conformed to Cornea (D)
Model: Front and Back Surfaces Flex Equally		
40.00	−5.06	+5.05
42.50	−5.67	+5.73
45.00	−6.32	+6.47
47.50	−7.00	+7.25
50.00	−7.71	+8.08
Model: Flexed Lenses Maintain Same Volume		
40.00	−5.01	+4.98
42.50	−5.06	+4.88
45.00	−5.12	+4.76
47.50	−5.18	+4.64
50.00	−5.24	+4.52

Calculations were made for lenses after they conformed to corneas with several different radii of curvature. According to Sarver's model, the back vertex powers increase in magnitude as the lenses flex to corneas of steeper and steeper curvature. Bennett's model predicts equal power changes into the minus for all lens powers, but of much less magnitude than the earlier model. Refractive index of the contact lenses was 1.43.

that as the cornea steepens, the magnitude of back vertex power is predicted to increase for minus and plus lenses. Exact conformation to the cornea may not be entirely realistic especially for plus lenses (49). Therefore, soft lens flexure might not be as great in some cases as assumed here.

Clinical experiences of early investigators showed that high-plus gel contact lenses seemed to *lose power* when on the eye even after vertex distance effectivity was taken into account. Also, the power changes that were encountered were not as large as predicted by calculations based on the Equal Change Hypothesis (50). Actual power changes upon gel lens insertion also did not agree with predictions of Strachan (46), whose model assumed a "wrap factor" in order to predict flexure of front and back lens surfaces. Bennett (47) proposed a model for gel lenses of refractive index 1.43, in which the front lens surface maintained *constant lens volume and thickness* when the back surface flexed. This model seemed to better predict the clinical situation especially for plus lenses:

$$F_{ch} = -300(t)[(1/r_k^2) - (1/r_2^2)]$$

$$\text{Equation (7A.12)}$$

where

F_{ch} = Change in back vertex power induced by flexure, in diopters

t = Center thickness of contact lens, in mm

r_k = Radius of curvature of cornea, determined by keratometry, in mm

r_2 = Radius of curvature of posterior contact lens surface, in mm

Also in Table 7A.12 are shown refractive powers induced by flexure based on Equation 7A.12. Bennett's model predicts that conformation of a flatter gel lens to the cornea will always result in *net addition of minus power,* even for plus lenses. The power alterations are nearly unaffected by the original power of the lens, plus or minus, and are most significantly proportional to lens *center thickness.* This model was very nearly the same as that proposed by Wichterle (48).

For practical reasons, then, soft contact lenses cannot be assumed to provide the labeled lens power on the eye, and the practitioner might not obtain the expected OR. Even if labeled with a more applicable power (say, -5.25 D instead of -5.00 D for the minus lens shown in Table 7A.12), soft lenses will assume various "on the eye" powers depending on the amount of flexure incurred by each lens when on the cornea. This effect is clinically significant for thick, high-plus gel lenses and can account for up to 0.75 D less plus than indicated on the packaging of those lenses.

Dehydration of gel lenses brought about by evaporation and ocular temperature also influences refractive power on the eye. Dehydration raises the refractive index of the lens, the net effect of which is to increase the magnitude of plus and minus corrections. In addition, gel lens surfaces steepen during dehydration, again causing back vertex powers to increase in magnitude. A thick (high-plus) gel lens can create a negative "lacrimal lens" when it does not completely conform to the curvature of the cornea (49). There are several factors, therefore, that alter the refractive power of a soft lens when it is placed on the cornea.

Hydrogel lens powers are difficult to confirm in the office, because back vertex power evaluated by the lensometer has only limited ability to estimate the power of a gel lens. Contact lenses also may vary by a few quarters of a diopter from the indicated value when placed on the eye. Therefore, ORs may not confirm that a given lens power in air is appropriate for the particular eye involved. Many practitioners attribute variations in ORs ($\pm$ 0.75 D from that expected) to poor control of refractive parameters by the manufacturer. It may just be, on the other hand, that quality control is not the entire problem, as the lenses themselves take on various powers when placed on different eyes. Indeed, various environmental (heat, humidity) and physiologic influences (tear fluid tonicity, pH, temperature) on gel lens hydration probably are responsible for fluctuations of refractive power when lenses are worn on any eye.

Thick hydrogels have been said to offer some masking of corneal astigmatism on the order of 0.25 to 1.00 D due to flexural strength gained with increased lens thickness (49). Increased gel lens flexure in the steeper corneal meridian also may "mask" some corneal astigmatism by slightly increasing minus power in the steep meridian over that in the flat meridian, particularly for thick gel lenses. Sarver (51) and Wechsler et al. (52) analyzed the masking of corneal toricity by hydrogels and concluded that the effect was small, but significant, and highly variable between patients and contact lens materials.

Rigid Lens Flexure

When a *rigid contact lens* flexes, in contrast, its posterior surface only conforms slightly to corneal surface topography. Rigid lenses are assumed to flex to the meridian of steepest corneal curvature. That is, on a with-the-rule cornea, a spherical rigid lens is assumed to steepen in the vertical meridian and only slightly flatten in the horizontal meridian. Fatt (53) indicated, however, that the two meridians actually flex by equal and opposite amounts. The lacrimal lens power in both primary meridians will be affected accordingly, and the power difference between the two meridians caused by flexure will be measured as toricity with over-Ks. Over-keratometry readings (over-Ks) can be used to evaluate the amount of lens flexure *in vivo* by measurement of toricity from the anterior contact lens surface.

The amount of lens *flexure* is applied clinically to only the steep corneal meridian because the amount of flattening in the other primary meridian is assumed traditionally (and, falsely) to be subclinical. The calculated effect of flexure is to lessen the minus power of the lacrimal lens in the steeper corneal meridian (decrease minus/increase plus), thus requiring the OR to make up the lost minus according to Equation 7A.9.

Interestingly enough, a *regularly warped* spherical lens will most likely orient on the eye with its steep curve aligned at the steep corneal meridian. *Warpage and flexure*, therefore, may have the same optical effects on the eye (spherical lenses become bitoric lenses on the eye), although bitoricity will be maintained *off* of the eye only by the regularly warped lens. *Irregular warpage* does not imitate flexure. A regularly warped spherical rigid lens can be distinguished from nearly all bitoric lenses because its refractive power is spherical by lensometry and its back-surface toricity is small, generally less than 1.50 DC. This is in contrast to the bitoric lens, which will be spherocylindrical by lensometry (nearly always, but note previous Example 6) and will have a large back-surface toricity, generally greater than 1.50 DC.

In Example 1, a rigid lens of −2.50 DS with a base curve radius of 7.90 mm was placed on a cornea measuring 42.25 @ 180 and 45.00 @ 090. The eye's spectacle refraction was −1.00 −2.75 × 180. We assumed at the time that the lens was inflexible, but let us say now that over-Ks were 39.75 @ 180 and 40.50 @ 090. What would be the expected OR?

The over-Ks show that 0.75 DC of flexure has occurred compared to the spherical base curve when off of the eye. We will attribute the toricity to steepening of the vertical base curve, from 42.75 D (7.90 mm) to 43.50 D (7.76 mm). Calculation of lacrimal lens power will, therefore, not be altered by flexure in the horizontal (flat) corneal meridian (42.75 − 42.25 = *+0.50* D according to Equation 7A.12). However, lacrimal lens power is different from that calculated in Example 1 by the amount of steepening of the vertical meridian (43.50 − 45.00 = *−1.50* D, instead of −2.25 D) and the expected OR is now +1.00 −0.75 ×

180 instead of +1.00 DS. The amount of flexure in diopters (n = 1.3375, measured by keratometer) attributed to the steep corneal meridian resulted in an *equal* amount of additional minus overcorrection for that meridian and *created residual astigmatism* found in the OR. The practitioner will now need to assess the patient's contact lens options for elimination of flexure or correction of its visual effects. Because flexure for rigid lenses is usually of small magnitude (unlike soft lenses), alterations of back vertex power due to flexure are subclinical in nature.

"Exploding" the Lacrimal Lens Concept

Fannin and Grosvenor (54) developed a unique approach to illustrate why the Lacrimal Lens Theory must be used with care. The approach involves a one-piece concentric back-surface bifocal of *distance-center* design (Fig. 7A.22). The central portion of the lens is to be used for distance vision and the periphery is to be more plus for near vision. A question is asked: Should the back-surface periphery be made flatter or steeper than the central area in order to provide plus power for near vision?

The answer to this question has been known for many years. However, many clinicians who use the lacrimal lens concept for fitting rigid lenses will reply to this question that the back peripheral curve should be steeper to induce plus power. Their rationale is that the lacrimal lens (viewed "exploded" as if in air) will be more plus and, therefore, will add plus to the overall lens/cornea optical system. However, as noted earlier in this chapter, the refractive powers of contact lenses must be held the same in order to compare optical effects of back-surface curvatures with the lacrimal lens concept. When back-surface curvature is steepened, it actually imparts more negative power to the optical system (viewed "unexploded" at the lens/tear pool interface) that

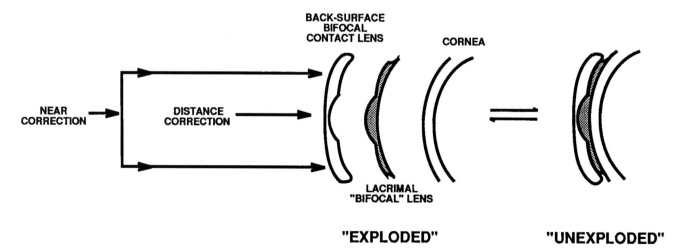

FIG. 7A.22. "Back-surface" rigid one-piece bifocal contact lens, in which the distance correction is in the center of the lens. The posterior peripheral curve must be flatter than the central curvature in order to impart a plus power to the overall optical system in the periphery.

is counteracted by a simultaneous alteration of the front-surface power into the plus by three times that magnitude. Like the aspheric back-surface bifocal described later, however, back-surface concentric bifocals have the same front surface for central and peripheral lens areas. Increased front-surface curvature to overcome increase in minus by steepening of the back surface is not present; therefore, the lacrimal lens theory has been thought not to apply. The correct answer to the question posed by Fannin and Grosvenor (54) is that the peripheral curvature of the posterior lens surface should be *flattened!* The contact lens/tear pool interface will then impart less minus (more plus) to the overall optical system, given that the front-surface curvature of the periphery remains the same as that at the center of the lens. The peripheral back surface curvature for a concentric *near-center* bifocal will, of course, need to be steeper than the central curvature in order to provide the appropriate add power.

The example provided by Fannin and Grosvenor (54) also may be ameliorated using an "exploded" view. The refractive power difference, in air, between the back-surface bifocal lens center and periphery will be nearly 1.5 times the magnitude and of opposite sign than the power difference between the center and periphery of the lacrimal lens in air. Even though the lacrimal lens in air induces minus power for the flatter periphery compared to the center, the contact lens in air is even more plus in the periphery. Thus, the bifocal add will be the sum of these two differences, and we see that the problem can be correctly solved using the Lacrimal Lens Theory.

The Lacrimal Lens Theory also assumes that the post-lens tear pool is a "thin lens," such that its thickness does not affect the refractive power of the lacrimal lens. An estimate of tear pool center thickness can be performed by calculation according to the equations for sagittal depth listed in Table 7A.13 (see section on Radii of Curvature

and Sagittal Depths of Conic Sections). For flat, "on K," or slightly steep fits, the tear pool may be assumed to have minimal thickness and be a "thin lens." However, for very steeply fitting lenses and especially for *haptic (scleral) contact lenses,* tear pool thickness becomes significant such that even the lacrimal lens must be considered a "thick lens." Fortunately for advocates of lacrimal lens theory, most practitioners do not have to worry about lacrimal lens thickness, as very steep lenses and haptic lenses are not often prescribed.

Corneal curvature alteration during the wear of rigid lenses is a more common instance in which the Lacrimal Lens Theory does not quite predict the actual situation. Let us assume that a cornea has steepened by 2.00 D in the vertical meridian as measured by keratometry, and that this occurred while a patient wore a lens that was originally fit "on K" with respect to that meridian at 45.00 D. By the Lacrimal Lens Theory, again looking at an "exploded" view of the lens/cornea optical system, a -2.00 D change in the lacrimal lens should effectively mask the corneal surface alteration. The net change in OR should be zero, and the patient's contact lens should require no power modification by the practitioner in order to maintain optimum vision.

Once again, however, the front-surface curvature of the rigid contact lens has not been changed as is necessary to meet the requirements of the Lacrimal Lens Theory! Another complicating factor is that it is not the front surface of the lacrimal lens that has been altered, but the back surface. The net change in power is really at the tear/cornea interface, and the cornea has altered curvature from 7.50 mm (45.00 D) to 7.18 mm (47.00 D). The actual refractive powers of the tear/cornea interface, both before and after the keratometric alteration, are as follows:

$$\text{Before} \qquad\qquad \text{After}$$
$$\frac{1.376 - 1.336}{0.00750 \text{ m}} = +5.33 \qquad \frac{1.376 - 1.336}{0.00718 \text{ m}} = +5.57.$$

TABLE 7A.13. SAGITTAL DEPTHS GIVEN FOR A SPHERICAL SURFACE HAVING A RADIUS OF CURVATURE OF 7.80 MM, COMPARED TO CONOIDAL SURFACES HAVING THAT SAME APICAL RADIUS OF CURVATURE, THOUGH WITH DIFFERENT ECCENTRICITIES

Chord Diameter (mm) 2h	Oblate Elliptical Sagitta (mm) e = −0.45	Spherical Sagitta (mm) e = 0	Prolate Elliptical Sagitta (mm) e = 0.45	Parabolic Sagitta (mm) e = 1	Hyperbolic Sagitta (mm) e = 2
1.0	0.016	0.016	0.016	0.016	0.016
2.0	0.064	0.064	0.064	0.064	0.063
3.0	0.146	0.146	0.145	0.144	0.140
4.0	0.262	0.261	0.260	0.256	0.245
5.0	0.414	0.412	0.409	0.401	0.374
6.0	0.606	0.600	0.595	0.577	0.524
7.0	0.842	0.829	0.820	0.785	0.693
8.0	1.128	1.104	1.086	1.026	0.878
9.0	1.472	1.429	1.340	1.298	1.076
10.0	1.890	1.813	1.761	1.603	1.285
11.0	2.403	2.269	2.183	1.939	1.504
12.0	3.061	2.816	2.673	2.308	1.731

Sagittal depth increases with chord diameter and decreases with eccentricity.

The net change in power for the entire optical system is +0.24 D, not zero as predicted by the Lacrimal Lens Theory, and the patient's contact lens should require about a quarter diopter of minus added in order to maintain optimum correction (OR should be about −0.25 D in the vertical meridian). Overall, the Lacrimal Lens Theory *underestimates* the OR by −0.12 D per full keratometric diopter of corneal steepening (+0.12 D per diopter of flattening). Fortunately, this is a small error that is subclinical for most cases in which corneal curvature has changed and may become of importance only for very large K differences such as those associated with keratoconus or refractive surgery.

Misorientation of Spherocylinders: Crossed Cylinder Effect

The practitioner often is confronted with spherocylindrical contact lenses, whether they are rigid front toric, CPE bitoric, or hydrogel toric lenses, with axes of cylinder that do not align with the axis of spectacle correction. Such misalignment, or misorientation, is actually a condition of *"crossed cylinders."* Briefly stated, when the axis of cylinder of a correcting contact lens does not align with that of best optical correction, an OR will show cylinder at an axis oblique to that of the axis of best correction. The eye, therefore, will not be optimally corrected by the misaligned lens, and the patient's visual acuity will be decreased from its maximal corrected level. Residual cylinder will show through the contact lens on the eye and be present in the OR.

Crossed cylinder effects are minimized for cylinders of low refractive power and for small amounts of misorientation. The practitioner should attempt to reduce misorientation as much as possible and keep contact lens refractive cylinder as low as possible in order to lessen the impact of crossed cylinders on the patient's vision (55). Crossed cylinder effects resulting from the fitting of highly astigmatic contact lenses probably are a limiting factor for success with toric soft lenses in many such cases, because even a small misorientation can produce large visual acuity deficits. A common crossed cylinder effect is covered in Chapter 7B, in which the correcting cylinder and refractive astigmatism are of the same power.

Radii of Curvature and Sagittal Depths of Conic Sections

New instrumentation has brought about an increased understanding of the topography of the ocular surface, and recent technologic improvements in manufacturing have led to an enhanced ability to produce contact lens surfaces of various aspheric forms. Such forms are generally the result of surfaces produced by rotation of a *conic section* around its axis. Though potentially confusing to practitioners who wish to tailor the design of contact lenses to the individual patient, *conoidal aspheric surfaces* can be described in a way that is consistent with the practitioner's prior knowledge of design characteristics involving spherical surfaces (56).

A circle is a geometric form that can be produced by sectioning a cone with a plane parallel to the base of the cone, hence the term *conic section*. Rotation of a circle around an axis containing any two points on the circle produces a sphere. Aspheric surfaces are usually also the result of conic sections in directions other than parallel with the base of the cone. Figures 7A.23 and 7A.24 show the various conic sections, from *sphere* (circle), to *ellipse, parabola,* and *hyperbola.* A spherical surface has only 1 radius of curvature, whereas surface curvatures of the aspheric surfaces continuously vary with distance from an apex. An ellipse has a *prolate apex,* from which curvature continuously flattens toward the periphery, and an *oblate apex,* from which curvature continuously steepens toward the periphery. Parabolas and hyperbolas have only prolate apices.

The anterior central corneal surface is considered to be elliptically prolate, and most aspheric contact lenses have an elliptical surface. An *ellipse* has two foci, a major axis of length "2a" and a minor axis of length "2b." The combined distance from any point on the ellipse to the two foci equals the length of the major axis (2a). A *hyperbola* also has two foci, a transverse axis between apices of length "2a" and a

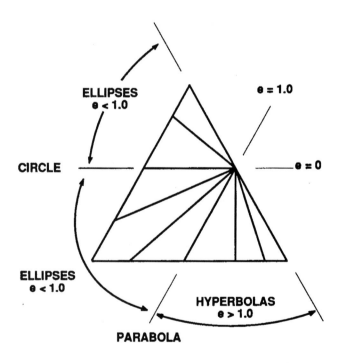

SECTIONS OF A CONE

FIG. 7A.23. Sections of a cone. Eccentricity (e) of an ellipse is less than 1.0 (e < 1). Spheres (circles) are a subset of ellipses having eccentricity of zero (e = 0). Eccentricity of a parabola is equal to 1.0 (e = 1) and for a hyperbola is greater than 1.0 (e > 1).

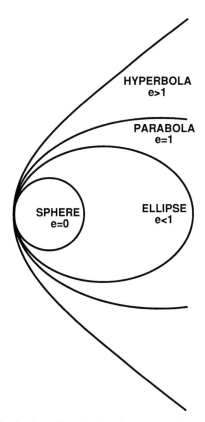

FIG. 7A.24. Conic sections having the same prolate apical radius of curvature and apex position, but differing with respect to eccentricity (e). Prolate surfaces are steepest at the apex and flatten toward the periphery. Note that the ellipse has two prolate apices and two oblate apices. The oblate surfaces are flattest at the apex and steepen toward the periphery. When referring to the oblate surface of an ellipse, e is often given a negative sign that is not used in computations.

conjugate axis of length "2b." The *difference* between distances from any point on a hyperbola to its two foci equals the length of the transverse axis (2a).

Eccentricity of ellipses and hyperbolas is related to lengths of their axes. Eccentricity (e) is zero (0) for a sphere (circle), which is actually an ellipse for which major and minor axes are the same length (a = b in Equation 7A.13); e < 1.0 for an ellipse; e = 1.0 for a parabola (b = 0 in Equations 7A.13 and 7A.14); and e > 1.0 for a hyperbola. The value of "e" is positive or zero, but when referring to oblate elliptical surfaces, e is sometimes given a negative sign, which is not used in computations. *Eccentricity of the central cornea averages 0.45 (elliptically prolate), with a range from − 0.4 (elliptically oblate) to 1.0 (parabolic).* The corneal periphery is even flatter than an ellipsoid and may be hyperbolic. Therefore, the entire corneal surface cannot be simply described by any single geometric relationship.

$$e = \frac{(a^2 - b^2)^{1/2}}{a} \qquad \text{Equation 7A.13}$$

Eccentricity for Ellipse

where

2a = Major axis of ellipse

2b = Minor axis of ellipse

and

$$e = \frac{(a^2 + b^2)^{1/2}}{a} \qquad \text{Equation 7A.14}$$

Eccentricity for Hyperbola

where

2a = Transverse axis of hyperbola

2b = Conjugate axis of hyperbola

The square of eccentricity (e^2) and also ($1 - e^2$) are each sometimes referred to as a *shape factor,* not to be confused with the "shape factor" related to spectacle magnification.

Local Radius of Curvature for Conic Sections

Schroeder (57) derived a method to estimate curvature surrounding any point on a conic section, in terms of a *"local" radius of spherical curvature,* which best approximated the curvatures surrounding the point. Basically, the local radius of curvature was computed knowing the two basic parameters of a conic section (eccentricity, e, and prolate apical radius, r_{a-p}) and the chord diameter of the surface (2h). This relationship is reproduced here as Equation 7A.15:

$$r_L = r_{a-p}[1 + e^2(h^2/r_{a-p}^2)]^{3/2} \qquad \text{Equation 7A.15}$$

Local Radius of Conic Section

where

r_L = Local radius of curvature

r_{a-p} = Apical radius of prolate curvature

e = Eccentricity of conic section

2h = Chord diameter at point on conic section.

When the point in question is any point on a spherical surface, e = 0 and the "local radius" becomes the apical radius of prolate curvature, which in fact is the radius of spherical curvature. When the point in question is the prolate apex of an aspheric conic section (ellipse, parabola, or hyperbola), h = 0 and the local radius in Equation 7A.15 again becomes the apical radius of prolate curvature. Bennett (58) defined the prolate apical radius of an ellipse in terms of the major and minor axes, and the equation also holds true for a hyperbola:

$$r_{a-p} = \frac{b^2}{a} \qquad \text{Equation 7A.16}$$

Prolate Apical Radius For Ellipse or Hyperbola

where

r_{a-p} = Apical radius of prolate surface

2a = Length of major axis of ellipse or transverse axis of hyperbola

2b = Length of minor axis of ellipse or conjugate axis of hyperbola.

Thus, the base parameters of an ellipse or hyperbola (e, $r_{a\text{-}p}$) can be computed from their axes. When the point in question is the oblate apex of an ellipse, h = b. Because $r_{a\text{-}p} = b^2/a$ and it is known from Equation 7A.13 that $(1 - e^2) = b^2/a^2$, algebraic manipulation of Equation 7A.15 leads to the apical radius of oblate curvature in terms of the major and minor elliptical axes:

$$r_{a\text{-}o} = \frac{a^2}{b} \qquad \text{Equation 7A.17}$$

Oblate Apical Radius for Ellipse

where

$r_{a\text{-}o}$ = Apical radius of oblate elliptical curvature
2a = Length of major axis of ellipse
2b = Length of minor axis of ellipse

For spherical surfaces, Equations 7A.16 and 7A.17 reduce to b or a, which in fact are both equal to the radius of spherical curvature, which could refer to the back central optic radius (base curve radius) of a contact lens. For parabolic and hyperbolic surfaces, only the prolate apical radius need be considered. Parabolic apical radii are equal to "2a" (see Equation 7A.23).

Sagittal Depths of Conic Sections

Sphere (Circle)

By use of the Pythagorean Theorem, assuming that an arc of spherical curvature forms one side of a right triangle (h), whose hypotenuse is the spherical radius of curvature (r) and other side is (r − s):

$$(r - s)^2 + h^2 = r^2 \text{ by Pythagorean Theorem.}$$

Therefore, by selection of the correct sign (−) of the square root:

$$s = r - (r^2 - h^2)^{1/2}, \quad \text{Equation 7A.18}$$

Sagittal Depth of a Spherical Surface

where

s = Sagitta of spherical surface
r = Radius of surface curvature
2h = Chord diameter.

From the Pythagorean Theorem, it is also true that

$$r^2 - 2rs + s^2 = r^2 - h^2$$

When the sagittal depth (s) is much smaller than the radius of curvature (r), s^2 is negligible, thus:

$$s = \frac{h^2}{2r}$$

Approximated Sagittal Depth of Sphere when r >> s

"Approximated Sagittal Depth" is often used when dealing with spectacle lenses because radii of surface curvature are much greater than sagittal depths of spectacle lenses. For contact lenses, however, this condition is not met, and Equation 7A.18 is most appropriate.

Prolate Ellipse

We have denoted the apical radius of curvature "$r_{a\text{-}p}$" for prolate surfaces and "$r_{a\text{-}o}$" for oblate surfaces. The equation for the ellipse shown in Fig. 7A.25, with prolate apex at the origin (0,0), is as follows:

$$\frac{(X - k)^2}{a^2} + \frac{Y^2}{b^2} = 1 \quad \text{Equation 7A.19}$$

where

X = Horizontal component of distance from origin to where vertical chord of diameter 2h intersects ellipse in Fig. 7A.25 ($= s_p$)
Y = Vertical component of distance from origin to where vertical chord of diameter 2h intersects ellipse in Fig. 7A.25 ($= h$)
k = Displacement of elliptical center from origin ($= a$)
2a = Length of major axis of ellipse
2b = Length of minor axis of ellipse

The center of the ellipse in Fig. 7A.25 is at point "E." The distance "a" extends from the prolate apex at the origin to the elliptical center. The distance from the apex to the center of curvature of the apex is the apical radius of prolate curvature ($r_{a\text{-}p}$). It can be shown that the sagittal depth is as follows(56,59):

$$s_p = \left(\frac{r_{a\text{-}p}}{1 - e^2}\right) - \sqrt{\left(\frac{r_{a\text{-}p}}{1 - e^2}\right)^2 - \left(\frac{h^2}{1 - e^2}\right)}$$

Equation 7A.20: Sagittal Depth of a Prolate Elliptical Surface

where

s_p = Sagittal depth of prolate elliptical surface
e = Eccentricity of elliptical surface
2h = Diameter of contact lens surface
$r_{a\text{-}p}$ = Apical radius of curvature at prolate end of ellipse

Sagittal depth of an elliptical surface not only depends on a radius of curvature and chord diameter as it does for a spherical surface, but also on eccentricity of the surface. For a spherical surface, e = 0 and Equation 7A.20 reduces to Equation 7A.18. The reader will note that, for a given apical radius of curvature in Table 7A.13, the sagitta for a prolate elliptical surface will be less (flatter) than for a spherical

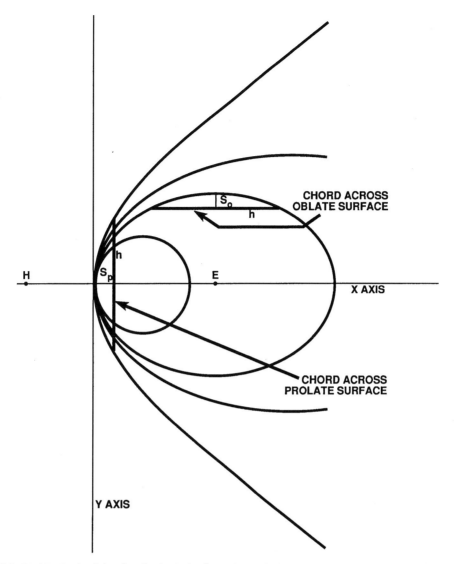

FIG. 7A.25. Sagittal depths of spherical, elliptical, parabolic, and hyperbolic surfaces having the same prolate apical radius of curvature, with prolate aspheric apices coincident at the origin (0, 0). Holding sagittal depth constant, chord diameter (2h) increases with eccentricity (e). Sagittal depth at the prolate apex, sagittal depth at the oblate apex, and semi-diameters of the chords are labeled s_p, s_o, and h, respectively. The magnitude of (a) is measured from the prolate apex to the center of an ellipse or hyperbola. As shown here, the elliptical center (point "E") is located to the right of the origin and the hyperbolic center (point "H") is left of the origin.

surface. As eccentricity increases, the surface flattens more rapidly in the periphery.

Oblate Ellipse

There are occasions when an elliptical surface must be oblate in order to fulfill its refractive function, that is, the surface must become progressively steeper in the periphery than the apical curvature. For instance, a front-surface distance-center *or* back-surface near-center progressive aspheric contact lens intended for correction of presbyopia must have an oblate surface (60). Fig. 7A.25 shows a horizontal chord (2h) across the oblate surface of the ellipse. Hence, Equation

7A.19 is modified here as Equation 7A.21 with respect to the oblate apex of the ellipse:

$$\frac{(X - k)^2}{a^2} + \frac{Y^2}{b^2} = 1, \quad \text{Equation 7A.21}$$

where

Y = Vertical component of distance from origin to where horizontal chord of diameter 2h intersects ellipse in Fig. 7A.25

X = Horizontal component of distance from origin to where horizontal chord of diameter 2h intersects ellipse in Fig. 7A.25

k = Displacement of elliptical center from origin
2a = Length of major axis of ellipse
2b = Length of minor axis of ellipse

It can be shown that the sagittal depth is as follows (56):

$$s_o = r_{a\text{-}o}(1 - e^2) - \sqrt{[r_{a\text{-}o}(1 - e^2)]^2 - h^2(1 - e^2)}$$

Equation 7A.22:
Sagittal Depth of an Oblate Elliptical Surface

where

s_o = Sagittal depth of oblate elliptical surface
e = Eccentricity of elliptical surface
2h = Diameter of contact lens surface
$r_{a\text{-}o}$ = Apical radius of curvature at oblate end of ellipse

Note the symmetry between the sagittal equations for prolate and oblate elliptical surfaces by comparing Equations 7A.20 and 7A.22. For every term in the prolate equation having $(1 - e^2)$ in the denominator, $(1 - e^2)$ is in the numerator for oblate curvatures. When e = 0, Equation 7A.22 (like Equation 7A.20) also reduces to Equation 7A.18. For a given apical radius of curvature in Table 7A.1, the sagitta for an oblate elliptical surface will be greater (steeper) than for a spherical surface. As eccentricity increases, the surface steepens more rapidly in the periphery.

Parabola
A parabola has a single focus and a single axis (a) equal to the distance between the apex and the focus. A chord running parallel to the Y axis and through the focus has a diameter (4a). The curve is prolate, and the radii of curvature of the asymptotic ends of the parabola approach infinity (i.e., they are nearly flat in the far periphery). The general formula for the parabola shown in Fig. 7A.25, with apex at the origin (0,0), is as follows:

$$Y^2 = 4aX = 2Xr_{a\text{-}p} \quad \text{Equation 7A.23}$$

where

X = Horizontal component of distance from apex of parabola to where chord of diameter 2h intersects parabola in Fig. 7A.25 (= s_p)
Y = Vertical component of distance from apex of parabola to where chord of diameter 2h intersects parabola in Fig. 7A.25 (= h)
a = Length of parabolic axis (e = 1)
$r_{a\text{-}p}$ = Apical radius of prolate curvature = 2a

It can be shown the sagittal depth is as follows (56,59):

$$s_p = \frac{h^2}{2r_{a\text{-}p}} \quad \text{Equation 7A.24:}$$

Sagittal Depth of a Parabolic Surface

Equation 7A.24 is identical to that of "approximated sagittal depth" of spherical surfaces, derived earlier, when r =

$r_{a\text{-}p}$. Hence, the equation is also known as the *parabolic approximation* for sagittal depth of a spherical surface.

Hyperbola
At least one contact lens manufacturer has claimed to produce hyperbolic lens surfaces. The general equation for the hyperbola depicted in Fig. 7A.25, with apex at the origin (0,0), is as follows:

$$\frac{(X - k)^2}{a^2} - \frac{Y^2}{b^2} = 1 \quad \text{Equation 7A.25}$$

where

X = Horizontal component of distance from origin to where chord of diameter 2h intersects hyperbola in Fig. 7A.25 (= s_p)
Y = Vertical component of distance from origin to where chord of diameter 2h intersects hyperbola in Fig. 7A.25 (= h)
k = Displacement of hyperbolic center from origin (= −a)
2a = Length of transverse axis of hyperbola
2b = Length of conjugate axis of hyperbola

The center of the hyperbola in Fig. 7A.25 is at point "H" and the distance "a" extends from the prolate apex at the origin to the hyperbolic center. In actuality, the hyperbola has a second prolate surface at a distance "a" to the left of its center, which has been omitted from Fig. 7A.25 to simplify the diagram. It can be shown that the sagittal depth is as follows (56):

$$s_p = \left(\frac{r_{a\text{-}p}}{1 - e^2}\right) + \sqrt{\left(\frac{r_{a\text{-}p}}{1 - e^2}\right)^2 - \left(\frac{h^2}{1 - e^2}\right)}$$

Equation 7A.26:
Sagittal Depth of a Hyperbolic Surface

where

s_p = Sagittal depth of hyperbolic surface
e = Eccentricity of hyperbolic surface
2h = Diameter of contact lens surface
$r_{a\text{-}p}$ = Apical radius of prolate curvature

Summary

The ability to map corneal surface topography and to manufacture contact lens surfaces in various geometries has become more sophisticated in recent years. Optical design of rigid and soft contact lenses may now take into account enhanced knowledge of corneal topography, correction for presbyopia, and reduction of optical aberrations inherent in contact lenses and the eye. The entire range of prolate conic sections (sphere, ellipse, parabola, and hyperbola) and the oblate surface of the ellipse can now be used in the form of a contact lens. A summary of the sagittal depth equations for these surfaces is given in Table 7A.14.

TABLE 7A.14. SUMMARY OF THE CONIC SECTION, THEIR APICAL RADII OF CURVATURE, ECCENTRICITIES, AND SAGITTAL DEPTHS

Conic Section	Apical Radius/Eccentricity	Sagittal Depth Equation
Sphere	$e = \dfrac{r}{0}$	$s = r - \sqrt{r^2 - h^2}$
Ellipse (prolate)	r_{a-p} $\quad e < 1$	$s_p = \left(\dfrac{r_{a-p}}{1-e^2}\right) - \sqrt{\left(\dfrac{r_{a-p}}{1-e^2}\right)^2 - \left(\dfrac{h^2}{1-e^2}\right)}$
Ellipse (oblate)	r_{a-p} $\quad e < 1^a$	$s_o = r_{a-o}(1-e^2) - \sqrt{[r_{a-o}(1-e^2)]^2 - h^2(1-e^2)}$
Parabola	r_{a-p} $\quad e = 1$	$s_p = \dfrac{h^2}{2r_{a-p}}$
Hyperbola	r_{a-p} $\quad e > 1$	$s_p = \left(\dfrac{r_{a-p}}{1-e^2}\right) + \sqrt{\left(\dfrac{r_{a-p}}{1-e^2}\right)^2 - \left(\dfrac{h^2}{1-e^2}\right)}$

^{a} For the oblate surface, e is given a negative value that is not used in computations. From Benjamin WJ, Rosenblum WM. Radii of curvature and sagittal depths of conic sections. *Int Contact Lens Clin* 1992; 1963: 76–82.

Sagittas of spherical surfaces have been useful for calculation of contact lens thicknesses and, therefore, the appropriate front-surface design for attaining prescribed back vertex power. The "base curve radius" of a back-surface aspheric bifocal lens is not an applicable term, for *apical radius of curvature* and *eccentricity* are necessary to define the surface if it is a conic section. Regardless of the surface geometry, however, sagittal depths of all types of surfaces may still be used in these computations. Minimum contact lens thickness is achieved at some point on a lens (the center of a minus lens, or the edge of a plus lens) critical for stability of lens shape. The minimum thickness is related to physical factors of the lens material (flexibility, hardness, durability, tear resistance) as well as to lens design. Such a point on the lens is called a *"point of critical thickness."* Lens shape and thicknesses at all other points are functions of sagittas of both the front and back contact lens surfaces relative to the point of critical thickness:

$$CT + s_2 = ET + s_1$$

Equation 7A.27 for a Meniscus Lens

where

CT = Center thickness of contact lens
ET = Thickness of contact lens at distance h away from center, or Edge Thickness for lens of diameter 2h
s_1 = Sagittal depth of front lens surface
s_2 = Sagitta depth of back lens surface

For example, in a given rigid *minus lens,* thinnest at the center, it is assumed that at least 0.08 mm is required to maintain lens stability. Let us further assume that the prescribed posterior lens surface has a parabolic apical radius of 7.80 mm (e = 1); central back vertex power has been prescribed at −5.00 D; refractive index of the prescribed rigid contact lens is 1.47; the prescribed optic zone diameter is 8.0 mm; and the front surface is to be elliptically oblate (e = −0.45). Apical radius of the front surface depends on center thickness of a contact lens and can be calculated to be 8.53 mm using refractive power formulas for optically "thick" lenses. The sagittas of the front and back curves (from Equations 7A.22 and 7A.24) are 1.013 and 1.026 mm, respectively. The thickness of the lens at the edge of the optic zone then can be calculated from Equation 7A.27: ET = 0.093 mm.

Given a *plus lens,* thinnest at the edges, it is assumed that at least 0.08 mm is required to maintain lens stability. Again, let us further assume that the prescribed posterior lens surface has a parabolic apical radius of 7.80 mm (e = 1); refractive index of the prescribed rigid contact lens is 1.47; the prescribed optic zone diameter is 8.0 mm; and the front surface is to be elliptically oblate (e = −0.45). The prescribed central back vertex power shall be +5.00 D. The minimum center thickness (CT) possible for this lens could be calculated from Equation 7A.27; however, there is another unknown value in the equation that cannot be determined without knowledge of center thickness: apical radius of front-surface curvature.

Faced with solving an equation with two unknowns, we can resort to trial and error, by inserting several thicknesses first into a "thick lens" refractive power formula, then Equations 7A.22 and 7A.24, until we arrive at a center thickness that will produce the appropriate back vertex power yet give a front-surface sagitta that will comply with Equation 7A.27. For instance, a center thickness of 0.28 mm will require that the front-surface radius be 7.29 mm, whose sagitta of 1.226 mm then complies with Equation 7A.27.

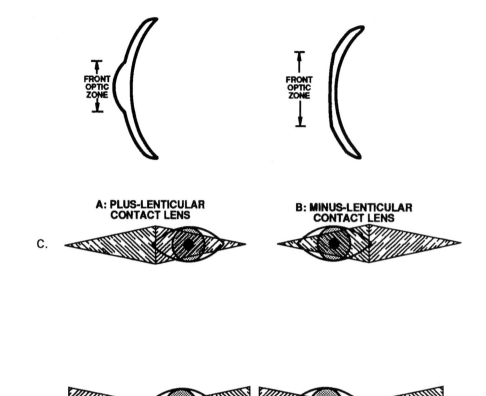

FIG. 7A.26. A: Front-surface plus lenticular and minus lenticular contact lenses **(B)**. "Base out" effect of plus spectacle correction **(C)** and "base in" effect of minus spectacle correction **(D)**. When a person converges to a near object, the eyes deviate from the optic axes of his spectacle lenses and generate prism according to Prentice's Rule (Equation 7A.29).

Creighton's contact lens fabrication tables (61) give excellent examples of the effects of various lens parameters on lens shape with respect to spherical surfaces and are recommended by the author for those readers more interested in applying sagittal depths of conic sections to clinical manipulation of contact lens design. The important aspect of the last few paragraphs is to realize that the refractive power of a lens, its critical thickness, diameter, and the base curve chosen for the patient, all will have their impacts on shape of a *conventional* contact lens, its mass, and thickness at any point. Practitioners versed in the art of *contact lens design* are able to manipulate parameters of the lens in order to achieve the appropriate lens shape, size, thickness, and mass for their patient.

Unconventional contact lens designs limit the effects of refractive power on thickness and shape of lenses by reducing the diameter (2h) of the front optic zone. A *plus-lenticular lens* and a *minus-lenticular lens* (Fig. 7A.26A) both have small front optic zones in comparison to their conventional design counterparts. Sagittal depth of the front surface is reduced for the plus-lenticular lens such that center thickness can be reduced. Sagittal depth of the front surface is increased for the minus-lenticular lens so that edge thickness

can be reduced. The well-known "CN bevel" placed on high-minus contact lenses at the practitioner's office to reduce edge thickness is actually a way of creating a minus-lenticular design from a conventional minus lens. New optical designs may free practitioners to design lenses specific to the patient's eye without consideration for design alterations now necessary to incorporate optical correction into lenses as well.

CONTACT LENS OPTICS: BINOCULAR VISION AND PERCEPTION

Prism and Prismatic Effects of Contact Lenses

A prismatic component in a contact lens Rx is produced by varying the thickness of the contact lens while maintaining the same front- and back-surface curvatures required for proper refractive power. Most prisms in contact lenses are *base down* in orientation and are used to *stabilize lens rotation* in toric and bifocal lens Rxs. The back surface of the prismatic contact lens on the eye is at the same angle with respect to incoming rays of light that would be encountered by the same lens if produced without prism. Therefore, the angle of incidence of light upon the *front surface* of the prismatic lens determines the amount of prismatic power when the lens is on the eye. This can be simplistically viewed as placing a right angle prism on the eye with its flat face against the cornea. The apical angle (a) of the prism is related to prismatic thickness and prismatic power (P) in prism diopters:

$$\tan a = \frac{BT - AT}{BAL} \text{ and } P = 100(n' - 1)\tan a$$

therefore,

$$P = \frac{100(n' - 1)(BT - AT)}{BAL}$$

Equation 7A.28

where

P = Prismatic power in prism diopters (cm/m, or $^\Delta$)
n′ = Refractive index of prismatic lens
BT = Base thickness of prismatic component of lens
AT = Apex thickness of prismatic component of lens
BAL = Length of base-apex line, usually the *diameter of contact lens* along base-apex line of prism

The fact that a prism is technically bathed in tear fluid does not lessen the amount of effective prismatic power when a prismatic lens is on the eye. Therefore, the prismatic component measured in air will impart an equal prismatic power on the eye (62).

However, because lens thickness is increased toward the base with no alteration in surface curvature to maintain consistent refractive power, refractive power of a prismatic lens varies along the base-apex line according to the thick lens formula for back vertex power (Equation 7A.6). Back vertex power becomes *more plus/less minus* as thickness increases toward the base of prism.

$$P = h(BVP)$$

Equation 7A.29: Prentice's Rule

where

P = Prismatic power in prism diopters (cm/m. or $^\Delta$)
h = Distance ray of light penetrates lens away from optic center of refractive component, in cm
BVP = Back vertex power of contact lens in diopters

Due to Prentice's Rule, variation of refractive power along the base-apex line generates a variation of net prismatic power across the surface of the prismatic contact lens. Prismatic power then *decreases* as the lens thickens toward the base. Fortunately, variations of back vertex power and prismatic power along the base-apex line of contact lenses are small for lenses of low refractive power and usually are clinically inconsequential even for patients with high amounts of

anisometropia. Perhaps these variations could assume some infrequent significance in the wear of bifocal prism-ballasted contact lenses when anisometropic patients are forced to view through the thicker portions of the lenses in order to attain near correction.

Contact lenses slide around on the cornea during and just after the blink, when the patient's eyes assume various gaze positions, and during ocular vergence movements. In addition, the lenses may not center on the eye even in straight-ahead gaze. Small prismatic fluctuations are, therefore, occurring as a result of Prentice's Rule for all contact lenses and for all eyes at nearly any time during open-eye contact lens wear. Prismatic fluctuations occur, for the most part, equally in each eye of the patient, assuming that the lens powers are approximately the same for each eye. However, contact lens practitioners should be aware that, in high anisometropia or high ametropia, these fluctuations can be fairly large (up to 2 or 3 prism diopters) and disconcerting to some patients, particularly just after the blink.

Vergence Demands with Contact Lenses

Contact lenses move with the cornea as the eyes rotate into different positions of gaze, in contrast to spectacle lenses, which remain fixed in orientation to the head while the eyes move. Prismatic effects of spectacle lenses, which are incurred as a result of movement of the lines of sight away from *major reference points* of the lenses, do not significantly occur when contact lenses are worn. Wear of contact lenses, therefore, eliminates or substantially reduces a host of prismatic effects common to spectacle lens wear:

1. Base right prism and base left prism for bilateral myopes, and base left prism and base right prism for bilateral hyperopes, in right and left gaze, respectively
2. Vergence demand alterations in anisometropia or antimetropia, required for right and left gaze
3. Vertical prismatic effects in up and down gaze, and imbalances in downgaze resulting from anisometropia or antimetropia
4. Increased near convergence demand for bilateral hyperopes and decreased near convergence demand for bilateral myopes (63) shown in Fig. 7A.26.

Because minus spectacle lenses create a ''base in'' effect in near vision (Fig. 7A.26B), a binocular myopic patient who switches to contact lenses may undergo adaptation problems, outright diplopia, or otherwise begin having symptoms suggestive of binocular vision problems. This might occur especially if the patient was initially an exophore on the borderline of fusional convergence ability with spectacles at near. A similar situation might exist for an esophoric hyperope on the border of fusional divergence capability at near when wearing spectacles. Contact lens correction would decrease convergence demand at near, perhaps pushing this esophoric patient over the limit of binocular ability (63,64).

Fortunately for the contact lens patient and practitioner, as will be pointed out in the next section of text, accommodative demands are different with contact lenses in comparison to spectacles. Accommodative vergence is biased in the direction of compensating for differences in vergence demands between the two modes of correction *via* the near triad response.

It is important to note that although contact lenses eliminate or reduce many undesirable prismatic effects of spectacle lenses, beneficial prismatic aspects of spectacle lenses are eliminated as well. For instance, the ability to correct for lateral prismatic deviations is lost when wearing only contact lenses. Vertical deviations requiring small amounts of base down prism in one eye (<2.5 prism diopters) can be handled with contact lenses; however, significant corneal physiologic compromise due to lens thickness and altered fit may be endured to do so in comparison with the eye not wearing the prismatic correction. Unilateral prescription of a prism-ballasted lens may induce a significant vertical imbalance in some patients, for instance, if a ballasted toric soft lens is prescribed unilaterally.

Accommodative Demand at the Corneal Plane

As we noted with respect to effective power, the vertex distance at which a correcting lens is placed influences the magnitude of refractive power required for optimum refractive correction of an eye for *distance vision*. In a similar manner but in a differing amount, vertex distance also influences the amount of correction required for an object *at near*. Vertex distance has a lesser impact on optimal refractive correction for near vision (compared to its impact at distance) when considering a plus lens and a larger impact for a minus lens. The difference between distance and near refractive corrections is actually *accommodative demand* when only the distance correction is worn by a patient, but it must be referenced to the vertex plane in which correction was determined. Therefore, accommodative demand at the corneal plane is less for a myopic eye corrected by a spectacle lens than for an emmetropic eye. A spectacle-corrected hyperopic eye has a higher accommodative demand at near than does an emmetropic eye (63–66).

Consider correction of a +6.00 D hyperopic eye measured at a spectacle plane 15 mm in front of the cornea (Fig. 7A.27). Light from a *distant object* would have a vergence of zero just before passing through the +6.00 D correction. Following the change in vergence to +6.00 D at the back surface of the lens, the light would travel 15 mm to the corneal plane, thus lessening the radius of curvature of the wavefront immediately exiting the lens from +166.7 mm (+6 D) to 151.7 mm just before entering the cornea. Vergence of light at the corneal plane from a distant source

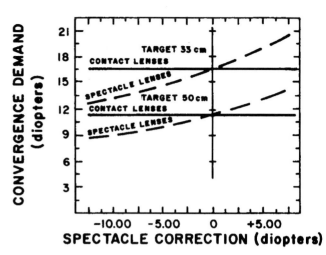

FIG. 7A.27. Amount of convergence demand for ametropic patients with interpupillary distances of 65 mm, when wearing spectacles having a vertex distance of 14 mm *(dashed lines)* or contact lenses *(solid lines)* and viewing objects 50.0 and 33.3 cm in front of the spectacle plane. (From Westheimer G. The visual world of the new contact lens wearer. *J Am Optom Assoc* 1962;34:135–138, with permission.)

would, therefore, be 1/0.1517 m or +6.59 D. This value has been listed in Table 7A.15 and would be the optimum distance contact lens correction for the hyperopic eye considering a vertex distance of zero for the contact lens. Note that for an emmetrope who has no lens in front of the eye, the vergence of light at the cornea is zero.

Light from a *near object* 40 cm in front of the spectacle plane in Fig. 7A.28 would have a vergence of −2.50 D before entering the +6 lens; therefore, vergence of light

TABLE 7A.15. VERGENCES OF LIGHT COMPUTED FOR CORNEAL AND LENTICULAR PLANES ORIGINATING FROM DISTANT AND NEAR OBJECTS FOR A +6 HYPEROPIC EYE, EMMETROPIC EYE, AND −6 MYOPIC EYE CORRECTED AT THE SPECTACLE PLANE

	Vergence of Light at Cornea		Corneal Plane Accommodative Demand (D)
	Near (D)	Distance (D)	
+6 D hyperope	+6.59	+3.69	+2.90
Emmetrope	0.00	−2.41	+2.41
−6 D myope	−5.50	−7.54	+2.04

	Vergence of Light at Anterior Lens		Ocular Accommodative Demand (D)
	Distance (D)	Near (D)	
+6 D hyperope	+59.97	+55.74	+4.23
Emmetrope	+50.50	+47.17	+3.33
−6 D myope	+43.00	+40.30	+2.70

Parameters of Gullstrand's Simplified Schematic Eye have been assumed, as well as a near object distance 40 cm in front of a spectacle plane with a 15-mm vertex distance.

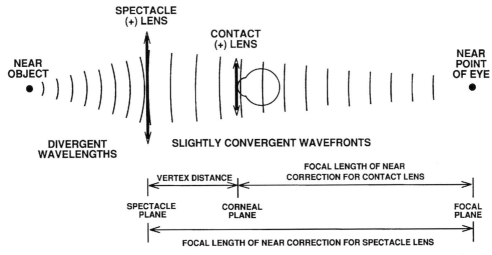

FIG. 7A.28. Vergence of light at the cornea of a *hyperopic* eye from a near source 40 cm in front of the spectacle plane with a vertex distance of 15 mm. The equivalent diagram for a distant object is shown in Fig. 7A.17.

just exiting the posterior lens surface would be $-2.50 + 6 = +3.50$ D. This wavefront would begin traversing the spectacle vertex distance with a radius of curvature of $+285.7$ mm ($+3.50$ D) and at the corneal plane would have a radius of $+270.7$ mm. Vergence of light at the cornea from the near object would be $1/0.2707$ m or $+3.69$ D. For the emmetrope, the wavefront at the spectacle plane has a radius of curvature of -400 mm (-2.50 D), which increases by 15 mm upon reaching the corneal plane. Vergence of light at the emmetropic cornea (from the near object) would be $1/(-0.415$ m$) = -2.41$ D.

The difference between vergences of light at the cornea for near and distant objects is the *accommodative demand at the corneal plane* shown for the $+6.00$ D hyperope and the emmetrope in Table 7A.15. Note that the hyperopic eye requires more accommodation effective at the corneal plane than does an emmetropic eye to clear a near object when wearing spectacles. The case of a -6.00 myope corrected at the spectacle plane is diagrammed in Fig. 7A.29. Light from a *distant object* (Fig. 7A.18) exits the spectacle lens with a radius of curvature of -166.7 mm (-6 D), which lengthens to -181.7 mm (-5.50 D) by the time the wavefront traverses the vertex distance to the cornea. For a *near object* at 40 cm (Fig. 7A.29), light exiting the lens at -8.50 D has a radius of curvature of -117.6 mm that becomes -132.6 mm at the cornea (-7.54 D). The *accommodative demand at the corneal plane* for the myope is $+2.04$ D (Table 7A.15). Note that the myopic eye requires less accommodative demand effective at the corneal plane than does the hyperopic eye or even the emmetropic eye to clear a near object when corrected at the spectacle plane.

As one might guess, accommodative demand differences between ametropes and emmetropes are further magnified

as distance to near objects is reduced (Fig. 7A.30) (63,64). For the clinician, however, it might be advantageous to refer to Table 7A.16 in which hyperopic and myopic spectacle corrections at 15 mm are listed that induce differences in corneal accommodative demand of $\pm$ 0.25, 0.50, 0.75, and 1.00 D from that necessary for the emmetropic eye viewing a near object at 40 cm. Differences of accommodative demand at the corneal plane become clinically significant at $+3.25$ D and -3.87 D (0.25D change of demand per emmetropia).

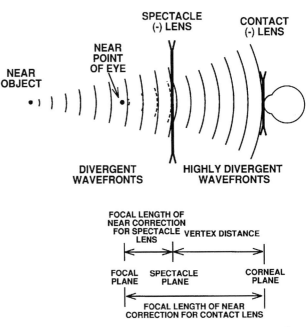

FIG. 7A.29. Vergence of light at the cornea of a *myopic* eye from a near source 40 cm in front of the spectacle plane with a vertex distance of 15 mm. The equivalent diagram for a distant object is shown in Fig. 7A.18.

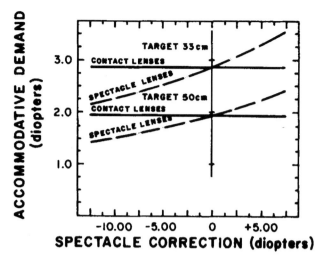

FIG. 7A.30. Accommodative demand at the corneal plane for ametropic patients wearing spectacles having a vertex distance of 14 mm *(dashed lines)* or contact lenses *(solid lines)* and viewing objects 50.0 and 33.3 cm in front of the spectacle plane. (From Westheimer G. The visual world of the new contact lens wearer. *J Am Optom Assoc* 1962;34:135–138, with permission.)

The term *ocular accommodation* has often been used to signify accommodative demands at the corneal plane listed in Tables 7A.15 and 7A.16. However, with the advent of intraocular lenses for which accommodative demand should be calculated at the position of the anterior crystalline lens (3.6 mm behind the cornea), a further distinction between accommodative demands at the *spectacle, corneal,* and *anterior lenticular* planes should be made in order to compare corrections placed at those planes. Using ocular constants taken from Gullstrand's Simplified Schematic Eye (2), calculations show that the crystalline lens itself must contribute even more accommodation than that effective at the corneal plane for the hyperopic eye corrected with spectacles, whereas the opposite is true for the spectacle-corrected myopic eye (Table 7A.15). The distinction between "corneal plane" and "lenticular plane" accommodation might be additionally important for correction of aphakia with intraocular lenses when compared to contact lenses.

TABLE 7A.16. ACCOMMODATIVE DEMANDS AT THE CORNEAL PLANE WHEN WEARING SPECTACLE LENSES, ASSUMING A VERTEX DISTANCE OF 15 MM AND NEAR OBJECT DISTANCE OF 40 CM

Difference in Corneal Plane Accommodative Demand Compared to Emmetropia (D)	Back Vertex Power of Hyperopic Spectacle Lens (D)	Back Vertex Power of Myopic Spectacle Lens (D)
±0.25	+3.25	−3.87
±0.50	+6.00	−8.37
±0.75	+8.62	−13.75
±1.00	+10.87	−20.87

Because contact lenses are placed at the corneal plane, contact lenses correcting for ametropia induce corneal plane accommodative demands *equivalent to that of emmetropia.* Clinical manifestations of accommodative problems for patients wearing spectacles can be either helped or hindered. For instance, the age of presbyopic onset, when refractive correction is by spectacles, is slightly less for hyperopes and slightly more for myopes than found in emmetropia (40–45 years of age). Contact lenses, therefore, eliminate the accommodative benefits of wearing spectacles in myopia and the detriments of wearing spectacles in hyperopia. The practitioner should be wary of correcting *pre-presbyopic myopes* with contact lenses because the accommodative demand will be increased, thus possibly precipitating presbyopia. On the other hand, pre-presbyopic hyperopes may benefit from lessening of accommodative demand with contact lenses. Most first-time contact lens wearers are young myopes who have become accustomed to decreased accommodative demand when wearing spectacles. Therefore, *postfitting near vision problems* related to an increase in accommodative demand with contact lenses can be encountered even with young patients.

Accommodative imbalances in anisometropia can be effectively managed with contact lenses, because corneal plane accommodative demands are equalized between the two eyes. Similarly, astigmatic accommodative imbalances (monocular conditions in which spectacle correction induces different accommodative demands for the two primary meridians of one eye) can be effectively managed with contact lenses.

A misconception commonly heard in clinical circles is that a hyperopic eye may require a more powerful near add in a spectacle correction than does a myopic eye. However, this is true only if a low-power add is prescribed. The rationale for this misconception is based on corneal accommodative demands as outlined earlier and is sometimes used to mistakenly justify the prescription of different spectacle add powers for the two eyes of an anisometrope or antimetrope (more plus add for the more hyperopic eye) when full near correction is required. In aphakia, higher spectacle adds are generally prescribed to obtain acceptable near vision, presumably because of increased accommodative demand at the corneal plane incurred as a result of high-plus spectacle lenses. Contact lenses are sometimes said, in error, to eliminate the need for different adds (for the anisometrope, antimetrope) or a more powerful add (for the patient with aphakia) when worn in conjunction with a spectacle overcorrection used for near vision.

Upon closer scrutiny, however, the accommodative rationale for these claims is proven false when full near adds are prescribed at the spectacle plane. The addition of +2.50 DS (a full add for a 40-cm working distance) eliminates any differences of corneal plane accommodative demand between hyperopic, myopic, and emmetropic eyes. With +2.50 DS adds, the hyperope, myope, and emmetrope all have accommodative demands of zero when viewing a near object at 40 cm with spectacles. Full near correction in the form of an add at the spectacle plane alters vergence of light from the near object such that it equals that of a distant object without an add. This occurs before light traverses the space between correcting lens and cornea, thus negating any effective power difference between near and far vision.

Accommodative demand imbalances between anisometropic eyes may exist at low add powers, for instance, in early presbyopia when the visual system is expected to partially accommodate to a near target. Corneal plane accommodative imbalances have been calculated as increasing amounts of near spectacle correction have been applied to an anisometrope in Table 7A.17. Note that corneal accommodative imbalance approaches zero as the bifocal add is increased to full near correction at the patient's working distance.

Most first-time contact lens wearers are young myopes who have become accustomed to decreased accommodative demand when wearing spectacles. Therefore, postfitting near vision problems related to an increase in accommodative demand with contact lenses can be encountered. When prescribing *bifocal* contact lenses for the early presbyope, bifocal adds may be strengthened for myopic patients whose eyes will be required to accommodate more than they did with spectacles. Contact lens adds may be less than that prescribed for spectacles of early hyperopic presbyopes. As adds approach full near correction of complete presbyopia (the patient has lost all accommodative ability), the difference between adds required for myopes and hyperopes approaches zero. Therefore, *full* correction at near (i.e., +2.50 adds at a 40-cm working distance or +4.00 adds at a 25-cm working distance) can provide optimum correction for contact lenses *and* spectacles irrespective of the degree of ametropia.

TABLE 7A.17. ACCOMMODATIVE DEMANDS AT THE CORNEAL PLANE FOR A NEAR TARGET 40 CM IN FRONT OF THE SPECTACLE PLANE, FOR THREE DIFFERENT EYES WEARING SPECTACLE BIFOCAL ADDS RANGING FROM 0 TO +2.50 D

Spectacle Add	Emmetropic Eye	+6 D Right Eye	−6 D Left Eye	Accommodative Demand Imbalance
No add	2.42	2.81	2.12	0.69 D
+1.00 D	1.47	1.71	1.29	0.42 D
+1.50 D	0.99	1.15	0.86	0.29 D
+2.00 D	0.50	0.58	0.43	0.15 D
+2.50 D	0	0	0	0 D

Spectacle refractions of the three eyes were plano (emmetropia), +6 D, and −6 D, respectively, at a vertex distance of 12 mm. The right column shows corneal plane accommodative demand imbalances of an antimetrope with distance spectacle refraction right +6 D, left −6 D. The accommodative demand imbalance decreases to zero as the bifocal add is increased to full correction for the 40-cm target distance.

Spectacle Magnification, or Magnification of Correction

Spectacle magnification (SM) is the ratio of retinal image size of the *corrected ametropic eye* to the retinal image size of the *same eye uncorrected* and has been used as an index of how corrective lenses alter retinal image size as compared by the patient before and after corrective lenses are placed on the eye. Formulas for spectacle magnification (64,67–69) include a *power factor* and a *shape factor*:

$$SM = \underbrace{[1/\,1 - h(BVP)]}_{\text{Power FActor}} \times \underbrace{[1/1 - (t/n')F_1]}_{\text{Shape Factor}}$$

Equation 7A.30

where

SM = Spectacle Magnification, or Magnification of Correction
BVP = Back vertex power of correcting lens (D)
h = Stop distance, from plane of correcting lens to ocular entrance pupil in meters = vertex distance + 3mm
t = Center thickness of correcting lens (m)
n' = Refractive index of correcting lens
F_1 = Front surface power of correcting lens (D)

The "shape factor" is nearly always greater than 1.0, indicating magnification, because ophthalmic spectacle lenses rarely have anything but convex anterior surfaces (F_1 is a positive number in Equation 7A.30). F_1 is also a positive number for contact lenses so that the "shape effect" induces magnification for these lenses as well. However, if one assumes an exploded view of the contact lens/cornea system, the presence of the "lacrimal lens" confuses calculation of the shape factor. One might conclude that there are two lenses placed at the cornea in the case of a contact lens: (i) the correcting lens itself, and (ii) the associated lacrimal lens. By combining shape factors designated for the correcting contact lens and its associated lacrimal lens (by multiplying them together), the overall shape factor for a contact lens can be derived:

$$\text{Shape Factor} = [1/1 - (t/n')F_1] \times [1/1 - (t_L/n_L)F_L]$$

Equation 7A.31
(Contact Lens)

where

t = Center thickness of correcting lens in meters
n' = Refractive index of correcting lens
F_1 = Front surface power of correcting lens in diopters
t_L = Center thickness of lacrimal lens in meters
n_L = Refractive index of lacrimal lens (1.3375)
F_L = Front surface power of lacrimal lens in keratometric diopters

The reader might note in Equation 7A.31 that increased

shape magnification due to higher front-surface powers of a contact lens and lacrimal lens in comparison to a spectacle lens is offset by comparative minification due to lower center thicknesses of both shape factor components when contact lenses are worn. Scleral (haptic) lenses, which vault over the cornea, have much thicker "lacrimal lenses" and so create more shape magnification than do other types of contact lenses, on the order of 1% to 3%.

The "power factor" for contact lenses is essentially the same as that for spectacle lenses, except that with a vertex distance of zero, stop distance is 3 mm (h = 0.003 m). This stop distance is also approximated by refractive surgery, stromal implants, and corneal onlays. For purposes of magnification computations, back vertex power is the corneal plane refraction (which is equal to the contact lens power plus the contribution of the lacrimal lens when the OR is zero: see Equation 7A.9). Fig. 7A.31 shows spectacle magnifications for a range of back vertex powers determined at the spectacle plane 15 mm in front of the cornea, calculated for both spectacle lenses (standard "corrected-curve" design in CR-39 polymer) and contact lenses (base curve radius 7.80 mm, "on K"). Indices of refraction of both types of correction were assumed to be 1.49, and standard lenticular designs for each lens were adopted where appropriate. The broken line in Fig. 7A.31 indicates the net change in spectacle magnification occurring when the eye is switched from spectacles to contact lenses.

Note that for high myopes, a significant minification (SM < 1.0) of the retinal image occurs with spectacle correction, which is substantially alleviated when contact lenses are worn. The net change in spectacle magnification, therefore, is to increase retinal image size when myopic patients opt to wear contact lenses. High myopes often remind the practitioner that their *vision is much "clearer" with contact lenses than with spectacles,* even for soft lenses that do not usually distort the cornea or cause "spectacle blur." Part of

the reason for this beneficial patient symptom is due to the larger retinal image supplied by the contact lens in comparison to spectacles, and highly myopic patients often have slightly *enhanced acuities* when contact lenses are worn. For high hyperopes and aphakes, on the other hand, contact lens correction results in a much smaller retinal image than does spectacle correction, and a corresponding slight reduction of visual acuity with contact lenses can be the result. The majority of contact lens wearers are myopes for which acuity benefits from spectacle magnification.

A rough predictor of the change in spectacle magnification when an eye switches from spectacle to contact lens correction can be made with the use of Equation 7A.32. This equation is essentially a simplification of division of power factors derived for contact and spectacle lenses. Contributions of shape factors have been ignored due to the complexity of shape factors for contact lenses:

$$\frac{\text{Contact Lens Power Factor}}{\text{Spectacle Lens Power Factor}} = 1 - h(BVP)$$

Equation 7A.32

where

h = Stop distance of spectacle lens in meters = vertex distance + 3 mm

BVP = Back vertex power of spectacle lens in diopters

Though spectacle magnification is much reduced in magnitude when wearing contact lenses in comparison to spectacles, significant magnification (for hyperopes) and minification (for myopes) still occur, especially when the eye is highly ametropic. This is a result of the much lower stop distance for contact lenses (h = 0.003 m), which is not quite negligible as it is for intraocular lenses (h = 0). In unilateral aphakia, for instance, spectacle correction can result in upwards of 25% to 30% magnification for the aphakic eye (SM = 1.25 and higher), thus helping to induce

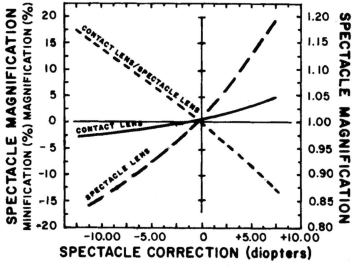

FIG. 7A.31. Spectacle magnification, for correction by spectacles *(dashed line)* and by contact lenses *(solid line)*. Contact lenses have been fitted "on K" to a 43.50 D cornea, with assumed thicknesses appropriate for conventional rigid lenses. Spectacle lens designs are according to the Orthagon Series, with a vertex distance of 14 mm. The net change in magnification going from spectacle to contact lens correction is also shown *(dotted line)*. (From Westheimer G. The visual world of the new contact lens wearer. *J Am Optom Assoc* 1962;34:135–138, with permission.)

diplopia and aniseikonia. Even when corrected with a contact lens, however, a difference of 5% to 8% (SM = 1.05–1.08) may be apparent between the patient's two eyes, and binocular vision problems, even diplopia, may prevent otherwise successful contact lens wear. The optimum correction for aphakia, using spectacle magnification as the only criterion, is with intraocular lenses for which the power factor theoretically contributes little or no magnification or minification of the retinal image.

Relative Spectacle Magnification

Another method of estimating retinal image size is to compare the *corrected ametropic* retinal image to that of a standard *emmetropic schematic eye*. A ratio called *relative spectacle magnification* (RSM) was derived for spectacle lenses (64, 67–69). In purely *axial ametropia,* for which ametropia is a result of axial elongation of the globe (Fig. 7A.32):

$$RSM = \frac{1}{1 + g(BVP)}$$

Equation 7A.33: Axial Ametropia

where

RSM = Relative Spectacle Magnification for axial ametrope

g = Distance in meters from anterior focal point of eye to correcting lens; g = 0 if lens is 15.7mm in front of the eye

BVP = Back Vertex Power of refractive correction (D)

Note that because "g" is a distance that is zero or close to zero for most spectacle lenses, relative spectacle magnification is zero or close to it. In other words, the retinal image of an axially ametropic eye corrected with a spectacle lens is the same as that of an emmetropic schematic eye. This

TABLE 7A.18. RELATIVE SPECTACLE MAGNIFICATIONS COMPARED TO THE EMMETROPIC SCHEMATIC EYE (E = EMMETROPIA) FOR AMETROPIC CORRECTIONS PLACED AT THE SPECTACLE PLANE (VERTEX DISTANCE = 15.7 MM), THE CORNEAL PLANE, AND THE PLANE OF THE ANTERIOR CRYSTALLINE LENS

	Correction Placed at		
	Spectacle	**Corneal**	**Lenticular**
Axial myopia	= E	>> E	>> E
Axial hyperopia	= E	>> E	>> E
Refractive myopia	<< E	< E	= E
Refractive hyperopia	>> E	> E	= E

is the essence of *Knapp's Law* (69). As "g" becomes larger, for instance, with a contact lens, the retinal image becomes significantly larger for myopes (RSM > 1.0) and smaller for hyperopes (RSM < 1.0) in comparison to the standard schematic eye. The optical position of a contact lens will be imitated when corneal refractive surgery is performed, or for stromal implants and corneal onlays. When an axially ametropic eye is corrected with an intraocular lens, "g" is at a maximum and the largest clinically relevant relative spectacle magnification for axial ametropia is apparent. This last hypothesis could occur, for instance, when the crystalline lens of a very high myope (usually of axial origin) is removed and replaced with an intraocular lens. A summary of relative spectacle magnification is given in Table 7A.18.

The theory of relative spectacle magnification predicts that anisometropia of axial origin is best corrected with spectacles. It also predicts that problems related to aniseikonia may develop if axial anisometropes are corrected with contact lenses or some other form of correction not placed at the spectacle plane (e.g., refractive surgery or ocular implants).

In purely *refractive ametropia* (Fig. 7A.33), in which ame-

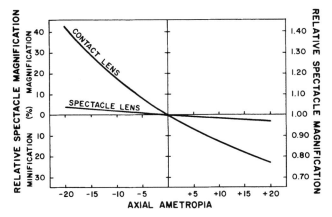

FIG. 7A.32. Relative spectacle magnification for *axial* ametropia when corrected by spectacles and contact lenses). (From Mandell RB. Corneal topography. In: Mandell RB. *Contact lens practice,* 4th ed. Springfield, IL: Charles C. Thomas, 1988:107–135, with permission.)

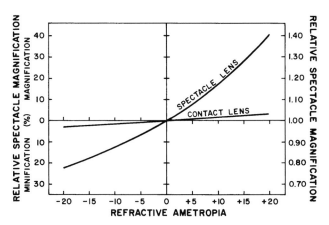

FIG. 7A.33. Relative spectacle magnification for *refractive* ametropia when corrected by spectacles and contact lenses. (From Mandell RB. Corneal topography. In: Mandell RB. *Contact lens practice,* 4th ed. Springfield, IL: Charles C. Thomas, 1988:107–135, with permission.)

tropia is a result of an abnormal refractive component or components of the eye, the equation for relative spectacle magnification (64,67–69) is the same as that of the *power factor* for spectacle magnification:

$$RSM = \frac{1}{1 - d(BVP)}$$

Equation 7A.34: Refractive Ametropia

where

RSM = Relative Spectacle Magnification for refractive ametrope

d = Stop distance in meters from correcting lens to entrance pupil = vertex distance + 3mm

BVP = Back Vertex Power of refractive correction (D)

Note that because "d" is a distance that is zero or close to zero for intraocular lenses, relative spectacle magnification is then zero or close to it. In other words, the retinal image of a refractively ametropic eye (an aphakic eye, for instance) corrected with an intraocular lens is the same as that of an emmetropic schematic eye. As "d" becomes larger, for instance, with a contact lens, corneal refractive surgery, stromal implants, or corneal onlays, the retinal image becomes slightly smaller for myopes (RSM < 1.0) and larger for hyperopes (RSM > 1.0) in comparison to the standard schematic eye. When a refractively ametropic eye is corrected with a spectacle lens, "d" is at a maximum and relative spectacle magnification becomes much more significant for both refractive myopes and hyperopes (Table 7A.18).

The theory of relative spectacle magnification predicts that anisometropia of refractive origin is best corrected with intraocular lenses (e.g., unilateral aphakia). It also predicts that problems related to aniseikonia may develop if high axial anisometropes are corrected with contact lenses or other forms of correction placed at the corneal plane (e.g., refractive surgery, stromal implants, or corneal onlays). It further predicts greater aniseikonic problems with refractive anisometropes when corrected with spectacles.

Spectacle magnification (magnification of correction) was used primarily to compare optical image sizes of a corrected ametropic eye to that of itself uncorrected, but optical image sizes for *relative spectacle magnification* have been referenced to a standard eye. Therefore, *relative spectacle magnification* is more specific and appropriately used to compare corrected image sizes of a patient's two eyes theoretically *if* the difference in ametropia between the two eyes is known to be of axial or refractive origin. The origin of anisometropia may be clinically determined with the use of the spectacle refraction, keratometry readings, and, if the practitioner's office is so equipped, ultrasonic measurement of an eye's axial length. Clinically speaking, however, anisometropias are seldom found to be purely results of axial or refractive anomalies, and this confuses clinical application of *relative spectacle magnification*. Many practitioners rely on *spectacle magnification* (power and shape factors) to deal with individual

patients because application of relative spectacle magnification theory is so difficult in many cases.

One might wonder why aniseikonic symptoms with axial anisometropia are *rarely encountered* in contact lens practice. The majority of contact lens wearers are young myopes, and many of them should have anisometropia of primarily axial origin. However, magnification of the retinal image is an optical phenomenon that has been presented here as if various ametropic retinas and related neurologic systems are identical. Such is probably not the case, given that axial myopia likely occurs in conjunction with retinal "stretching" to cover the posterior pole of the eye. Thus, the retina of an axial myope may have greater separation between receptors and receptive fields that effectively reduce the "neurological image" of the larger optical image predicted on the basis of optical principles alone (70).

Fields of View and Fixation

"Field of view" is the angular separation of those limiting rays of light at the edges of a correcting lens aperture that become directed to the entrance pupil of the eye after refraction by the correcting lens and are viewed by the peripheral retina (Figs. 7A.34 and 7A.35). Simply stated, it is the angle through which light entering the spectacle lens aperture can be viewed by the patient *during one fixation.* *"Field of fixation"* is the angular separation of the peripheral limiting rays of light that become directed after refraction toward the center of curvature of the globe and are able to be viewed by the fovea as the eye rotates to fixate the limiting rays (Figs. 7A.34 and 7A.35). Again, more simply, field of fixation is the angle through which light entering the correcting lens aperture can be viewed by the patient using central vision and by *rotating the eyes.*

Fields of view and fixation are brought about by *prismatic deviation of the limiting rays* of light at the edges of the spectacle lens aperture. Rays of light that are directed toward the entrance pupil and center of curvature, respectively, but pass just outside the lens aperture are undeviated (Figs. 7A.34 and 7A.35) and help to define *"ring scotoma"* (for hyperopic spectacle corrections) and *"ring diplopia"* (for myopic spectacle corrections). These prismatic effects are especially severe in cases of high ametropia and can influence testing of visual fields in the office as well as visual performance of the patient related to sports and safety in driving automobiles or negotiating stairways.

Because contact lenses follow the eye's angular movements, *fields of fixation* are not limited by the relatively small apertures of contact lenses. Practically speaking, *fields of view* are not much limited, either, by apertures of contact lenses. Contact lenses are located 3 mm in front of the entrance pupil, however, and small limitations on the field of view may exist if a contact lens and/or its central optical zone are small. *Flare and glare,* in the case of rigid corneal contact lenses, may be partly due to slightly reduced fields of view

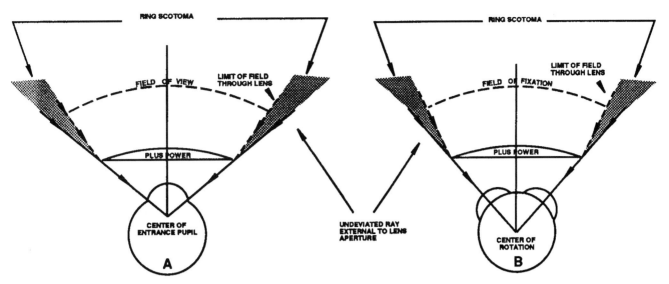

FIG. 7A.34. Fields of view **(A)** and fixation **(B)** of a *plus* correction at the spectacle plane. Note the "ring scotoma."

and glinting of light off of rigid lens edges and edges of central optic zones during lens wear.

Optical Aberrations with Contact Lenses

It is beyond the scope of this chapter to review optical aberrations of the eye and of correcting lenses in great detail. However, suffice it to say that vision using any form of ametropic correction is influenced by all optical aberrations. During contact lens wear, because the lens follows the line of sight during eye movements, the impacts of aberrations inherent in objects *off of the optic axis* of the correcting contact lens

on the *central vision* of patients are minimized. For spectacle correction, these "off axis" aberrations can influence central vision when the eyes are rotated away from the optical centers of the spectacle lenses. Table 7A.19 lists chromatic and various monochromatic aberrations and indicates which aberrations are alleviated by contact lens correction.

The retinal image of the eye corrected with contact lenses, similar to that of the eye corrected with spectacles, suffers from *"off-axis"* aberrations affecting *peripheral vision.* Spectacles and contact lenses also allow *"on-axis"* aberrations to influence *central vision.* The cornea's flattened periphery tends to reduce spherical aberration; however, increased

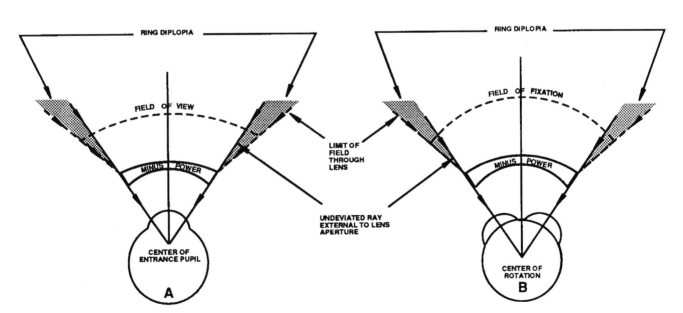

FIG. 7A.35. Fields of view **(A)** and fixation **(B)** of a *minus* correction at the spectacle plane. Note the "ring diplopia."

TABLE 7A.19. OPTICAL ABERRATIONS OF CORRECTING LENSES AND VISUAL DEFICITS PRODUCED WHEN WEARING CONTACT LENSES COMPARED TO SPECTACLES

Aberration	Object Position	Visual Deficit with	
		Spectacles	Contact Lenses
Spherical aberration	On axis	Central	Central
Coma	Off axis	Central and peripheral	Peripheral
Radial astigmatism	Off axis	Central and peripheral	Peripheral
Curvature of field	Off axis	Central and peripheral	Peripheral
Distortion	Off axis	Central and peripheral	Peripheral
Chromatic aberration	On and off Axis	Central and peripheral	Central and peripheral
Prismatic dispersion	Off axis	Central and peripheral	Peripheral

positive spherical aberration is the result when the corneal surface is covered with a contact lens made of spherical surfaces (peripheral light rays encounter more refractive power than do paraxial rays). Front-surface aspheric contact lenses may be better in this regard because their peripheries can be made to flatten and to lessen spherical aberration. It may be possible in the future to design contact lenses such that their surfaces further correct for optical aberrations and even those aberrations present in optical elements of the eye. Lenses with elliptical front surfaces may, for instance, reduce or eliminate spherical aberration. Efforts are underway with the Shack-Hartmann Aberrometer Sensor to be able to measure residual aberrations of eyes wearing contact lenses (71). The hope is to design contact lenses for the reduction of residual optical aberrations in each eye and to correspondingly increase visual performance for the individual patient.

Optics of a Spectacle–Contact Lens Telescope

The last special optical phenomenon to be covered in this chapter is that of the spectacle–contact lens telescope. The magnification of a telescopic system is the negative ratio of the refractive power of the eyepiece (F_e) to that of the objective lens (F_o), or the inverted ratio of their primary or secondary focal lengths (f_e and f_o, or f'_e and f'_o, respectively):

Magnification of Spectacle − Contact Lens Telescope =

$$\frac{-F_e}{F_o} = \frac{f_o}{-f_e} = \frac{f'_o}{-f'_e}$$

Equation 7A.35

In cases of low vision, a *contact lens of high-minus* refractive power can be used as the *"eyepiece"* of a Galilean telescopic system. A *high-plus spectacle lens* is used as the *"objective."* The secondary focal point of the objective and the primary focal point of the eyepiece are coincident (Fig. 7A.36), such that the difference in focal lengths must be the vertex distance (v.d. = $f'_o - f_e$).

Potential for high magnification exists; however, practi-

cal limits on magnification have been found in application to ophthalmic use. A reasonable vertex distance must be maintained, requiring differences between eyepiece and objective focal lengths to be from 8 to 24 mm. This necessitates the use of very high powers for the contact lens, on the order of −20 to −40 D and limits magnification to at most 2.0× in clinical situations (72). For most applications, magnification may vary from 1.3× to 1.7×. Accurate placement of the objective spectacle lens (powers ranging from +13.5 to +30 D) at the appropriate vertex distance is of importance, because even small deviations from the proper vertex distance produce large alterations in refractive power effective at the corneal plane.

Use of the spectacle–contact lens telescope is further complicated for near vision, because accommodative demand is generally above that which the eye can reasonably produce. Let us assume for a moderate case that a −25.00 D contact lens has been overcorrected with a +18.25 spectacle lens at a vertex distance of 14.8 mm. The magnification for this telescopic system is +1.37×. Light incident on the cornea from a distant object is parallel, with a vergence of zero. Light from a near object 40 cm in front of the spectacle plane has a vergence of −4.46 D when entering the cornea. The accommodative demand is +4.46 D, much higher than an eye can be expected to produce on a regular basis. A plus add of higher power than normal must be used in order to obtain clear near vision.

Magnification at near is also introduced for the eye by the near add (F_{add}) and is similar to that calculated for a simple microscope (Magn. = $F_{add}/4$). Magnification at near for the spectacle–contact lens telescope with an add is, therefore:

Magnification of Spectacle − Contact Lens Telescope with Add =

$$\frac{-F_e}{F_o} \times \frac{F_{add}}{4}$$

Equation 7A.36

Other optical difficulties with the spectacle–contact lens telescope are (i) decreased fields of view and fixation due

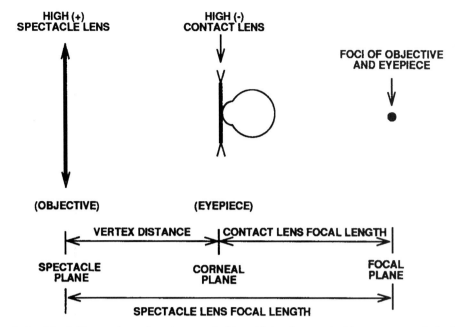

FIG. 7A.36. Galilean telescopic system created by a high-minus contact lens overcorrected with a high-plus spectacle lens. Focal points of the objective (+) lens and the ocular (−) lens are coincident. The lenses are separated by the vertex distance.

to the high-plus nature of the objective spectacle lens, (ii) "ring scotoma," and (iii) prismatic effects of high-plus spectacle lenses (72,73). These optical effects were covered earlier in this chapter.

SUMMARY: OPTICAL CORRECTION WITH CONTACT LENSES

The availability of contact lens materials and designs has grown extensively over time as contact lens wear expanded into the population. One reason contact lenses became so popular could be the desire of most wearers to eliminate the need for spectacles. Patients and practitioners tend to ignore the beneficial optical effects of contact lenses as they strive to improve cosmesis. Other modes of correction now are available, such as various forms of refractive surgery, which also promise to eliminate the need for glasses. The contact lens is being moved into more intimate association with the eye in the form of corneal onlays, stromal implant lenses, and anterior chamber intraocular lenses. These ophthalmic optical devices are experimental at this time, but eventually they may emerge to compete with traditional contact lenses. However, traditional contact lenses meet the optical requirements of correction in ways that no other form of correction has yet accomplished, when materials and designs are prescribed for individual eyes and patients under the appropriate circumstances. One can point only to small special groups of people for whom certain of the alternative modes of correction might provide excellent vi-

sion. It is the contact lens that will continue to provide the best vision, most of the time, for the majority of people who do not wear spectacles. Vision most often is superior to that of even spectacles, too, for those who wear contact lenses.

The exceptional quality of vision associated with contact lens wear is the result of a combination of factors. As discussed in this chapter, retinal image sizes, fields of view and fixation, and prismatic effects when wearing contact lenses are very close to those encountered in emmetropia. Convergence and accommodative demands also are virtually the same as in emmetropia. Central and peripheral residual aberrations resemble those encountered in emmetropia. Rigid contact lenses, in particular, have excellent surface optics and are able to mask corneal topographical irregularities and toricity. The overwhelming majority of contact lens wearers achieve clarity of vision *better* than 20/20 in each eye when properly prescribed, and they then live in an almost natural visual world. These are the benefits of contact lenses that professionals should be making their patients aware of in addition to the cosmetic advantage.

Wear of contact lenses is accompanied by rather minimal disruption of the ocular tissues in comparison to the current and emerging alternatives to spectacles noted above. Nearly all of the adverse effects are reversible when contact lens wear is temporarily arrested or discontinued. Contact lenses are relatively easily replaced with others of the same or different powers, materials, and/or designs, in order to arrive at the optimum correction for each eye of every patient. Contact lenses are similarly replaced if they become damaged or if the patient changes over time in terms of ocular refraction, corneal curvature, or otherwise. Replacement is performed without the need for additional surgery or further interruption of ocular tissues. The optical correction achieved with contact lenses is more exacting in that the visual result does not depend on healing of the eye, a factor known to induce variability into the optical correction, and that the optical correction can be "fine tuned" to the requirements of each eye. Specified changes in contact lens power, material, and design can correspond to changes in the patient's eyes and needs throughout a lifetime. Every advance in the contact lens field increases the benefit-to-risk ratio, as has most recently occurred with the advent of silicone-hydrogel soft lens materials. Hence, contact lenses will remain the most versatile, capable, accurate, and least invasive of the alternatives to spectacles in the foreseeable future. There is no doubt that now is the best time in all of history to be an ametrope!

REFERENCES

1. Jenkins FA, White HE. Reflection. In: Jenkins FA, White HE, eds. *Fundamentals of optics,* 4th ed. New York: McGraw-Hill, 1976:523–543.
2. Emsley HH. Visual optics. In: Emsley HH, ed. *Visual optics, volume 1: optics of vision,* 5th ed. London: Butterworth & Co., 1976:336–403.
3. Holly FJ. Tear film physiology and contact lens wear. I. Pertinent aspects of tear film physiology, and II. Contact lens-tear film interaction. *Am J Optom Physiol Opt* 1981;58:324–341.
4. Benjamin WJ. Examination of the tear fluid meniscus. *Int Cont Lens Clin* 1988;15:390–391.
5. Benjamin WJ. Endothelial guttatae: a type of corneal "drusen." *Int Cont Lens Clin* 1988;15:294.
6. Maurice DM. The structure and transparency of the cornea. *J Phys* 1957;136:263–286.
7. Maurice DM. The cornea and sclera. In: Davson H, ed. *The eye, volume 1: vegetative physiology and biochemistry,* 2nd ed. New York: Academic Press, 1969:489–600.
8. Goldman JN, Benedek GB. The relationship between morphology and transparency in the non-swelling corneal stroma of the shark. *Invest Ophthalmol Vis Sci* 1968;6:574–600.
9. Naylor EJ. Polarized light studies of corneal structure. *Br J Ophthalmol* 1953;37:77–84.
10. Mountford J. Polarized biomicroscopy. *Int Cont Lens Clin* 1982;9:373–384.
11. Brown N. Visibility of transparent objects in the eye by retroillumination. *Br J Ophthalmol* 1971;55:517–524.
12. Zantos SG. Cystic formations in the corneal epithelium. *Int Cont Lens Clin* 1983;10:128–146.
13. Zantos SG. Corneal infiltrates, debris, and microcysts. *J Am Optom Assoc* 1984;55:196–198.
14. Bourassa S, Benjamin WJ. Transient corneal surface "microdeposits" and associated epithelial surface pits occurring with gel contact lens extended wear. *Int Cont Lens Clin* 1988;15:338–340.
15. Tan J, Keay L, Jaobert I, et al. Mucin balls with wear of conventional and silicone hydrogel contact lenses. *Optom Vis Sci* 2003;80:291–297.
16. Edmund C. Location of the corneal apex and its influence on the stability of central corneal curvature. A photokeratoscopy study. *Am J Optom Physiol Opt* 1987;64:846–852.
17. Lowther GE. Preliminary investigation and initial examination. In: Bier N, Lowther GE, eds. *Contact lens correction.* London: Butterworth & Co., 1977:113–121.
18. Mandell RB. Corneal topography. In: Mandell RB, eds. *Contact lens practice,* 4th ed. Springfield, IL: Charles C. Thomas, 1988:107–135.
19. Schultz DN. Asymmetry of central and peripheral corneal astigmatism measured by photokeratoscopy. *Am J Optom Physiol Opt* 1976;54:776–781.
20. Erickson P, Robboy M. Performance characteristics of a concentric hydrophilic bifocal contact lens. *Am J Optom Physiol Opt* 1985;62:702–708.
21. Loewenfeld IE. Pupillary changes related to age. In: Thompson MS, ed. *Topics in neuro-ophthalmology.* Baltimore: Williams & Wilkins, 1979.
22. Pitts DG. The effects of aging on selected visual functions: dark adaptation, visual acuity, stereopsis, and brightness contrast. In: Sekular R, Kline D, Dismukes K, eds. *Aging and human visual function.* New York: Alan R. Liss, 1982:131–159.
23. Jones R. Do women and myopes have larger pupils? *Invest Ophthalmol Vis Sci* 1990;31:1413–1415.
24. Josephson JE, Caffery BE. Visual field loss with colored hydrogel lenses. *Am J Optom Physiol Opt* 1987;64:38–40.
25. Borish IM. Pupil dependency of bifocal contact lenses. *Am J Optom Physiol Opt* 1988;65:417–423.
26. Erickson P, Robboy M, Apollonio A, et al. Optical design considerations for contact lens bifocals. *J Am Optom Assoc* 1988;59:198–202.
27. Bier N. Albinism. *Int Cont Lens Clin* 1981;8:10–15.
28. Josephson JE. Locating the central bifocal zone. *Int Eyecare* 1986;2:441.
29. Pitts DG. Threat of ultraviolet radiation to the eye—how to protect against it. *J Am Optom Assoc* 1981;52:949–957.
30. Pitts DG. Comments made for Benjamin WJ: Protection against ozone layer "donut holes." *Int Cont Lens Clin* 1987;14:333–334.
31. ANSI Z80.20-1998. *American National Standard for Ophthalmics—Contact lenses—Standard terminology, measurements and physicochemical properties.* Merrifield, VA: Optical Laboratories Association, 1998.
32. Refojo MF, Korb DR, Silverman HI. Clinical evaluation of a new fluorescent dye for hydrogel lenses. *J Am Optom Assoc* 1972;43:321–326.
33. Benjamin WJ. Ultraviolet-absorbing contact lenses: fluorescent analysis. *Int Eyecare* 2:442.
34. Teuerle W. Refractive index calculation of hydrogel lenses. *Int Cont Lens Clin* 1984;11:625–628.
35. Galas SL, Enns JB. Humidity-conditioned gravimetric method to measure the water content of hydrogel materials. *Optom Vis Sci* 1993;70:577–586.
36. Young MD, Benjamin WJ. Calibrated oxygen permeability of 35 conventional hydrogel materials and correlation with water content. *Eye Contact Lens* 2003;29:126–133.
37. Campbell CE. Converting wet cell measured soft lens power to vertex power in air. *Int Cont Lens Clin* 1984;11:168–171.
38. Loshin DS. The holographic/diffractive bifocal contact lens. *Int Cont Lens Clin* 1989;16:77–86.
39. Benjamin WJ. Back-surface hydrogel bifocals: part I, featuring the Echelon diffractive bifocal. *Int Cont Lens Clin* 1994;21:151–153.
40. Benjamin WJ. Wet cells, back-surface bifocals, and the "lacrimal lens theory." *Int Cont Lens Clin* 1990;17:157–158.
41. Benjamin WJ. Back-surface hydrogel bifocals: part II, featuring the Spectrum bifocal. *Int Cont Lens Clin* 1994;21:199–201.
42. Sarver MD. The fluid lens power effect with contact lenses. *Am J Optom* 1962;39:434–437.
43. Weissman BA, Chun MW. The use of spherical power effect

rigid bitoric contact lenses in hospital practice. *J Am Optom Assoc* 1987;58:626–630.

44. Harris MG, Gale B, Gansel K, et al. Flexure and residual astigmatism with Paraperm O$_2$ and Boston II lenses on toric corneas. *Am J Optom Physiol Opt* 1987;64:269–273.

45. Picker DM, Egan DJ, Bennett ES. Theories on the flexure of "hard" and "soft" contact lenses. *Cont Lens J* 1984;12:5–11.

46. Strachan JPF. Some principles of the optics of hydrophilic lenses and geometrical optics applied to flexible lenses. *Austr J Optom* 1973;56:25–33.

47. Bennett AG. Power changes in soft contact lenses due to bending. *Ophthal Optician* 1976;16:939–945.

48. Wichterle O. Changes of refracting power of a soft lens caused by its flattening. In: Girard LJ, ed. *Corneal and scleral contact lenses, The Proceedings of the International Congress, March 1966.* St. Louis: CV Mosby, 1967:247–256.

49. Weissman BA. Loss of power with flexure of hydrogel plus lenses. *Am J Optom Physiol Opt* 1986;63:166–169.

50. Weissman BA. A general relationship between changing surface radii of flexing soft contact lenses. *Am J Optom Physiol Opt* 1984; 61:651–653.

51. Sarver MD. Vision with hydrophilic contact lenses. *J Am Optom Assoc* 1972;43:316–320.

52. Wechsler S, Ingraham TE, Sherrill DD. Masking astigmatism with spherical soft lenses. *Cont Lens Forum* 1986;11:42–45.

53. Fatt I. Hard contact lens flexing—a preliminary study of a new experimental procedure. *Int Cont Lens Clin* 1987;14:360–367.

54. Fannin TE, Grosvenor TG. Optics of contact lenses. In: Fannin TE, Grosvenor TG, eds. *Clinical optics.* Stoneham, MA: Butterworth Publishers, 1987:415–453.

55. Weissman BA. Theoretical optics of toric hydrogel contact lenses. *Am J Optom Physiol Opt* 1986;63:536–538.

56. Benjamin WJ, Rosenblum WM. Radii of curvature and sagittal depths of conic sections. *Int Cont Lens Clin* 1992;19:76–83.

57. Schroeder DJ. *Astronomical optics.* San Diego, CA: Academic Press, 1987:33–38.

58. Bennett AG. Personal letter to Dr. W.J. Benjamin, dated August 31, 1989.

59. Bennett AG. Aspherical contact lens surfaces, parts I, II, III. *Ophthal Optician* 1966;8:1037–1040, 8:1297–1311, 9: 222–230.

60. Benjamin WJ, Borish IM. Presbyopia and the influence of aging on prescription of contact lenses. In: Ruben, CM, Guillon M, eds. *Textbook of contact lens practice.* London: Chapman & Hall, 1994:763–830.

61. Creighton CP. *Contact lens fabrication tables.* Alden, NY: Alden Laboratories, Inc., 1976.

62. Mandell RB. Prism power in contact lenses. *Am J Optom* 1967; 44:573–580.

63. Alpern M. Accommodation and convergence with contact lenses. *Am J Optom* 1949;26:379–387.

64. Westheimer G. The visual world of the new contact lens wearer. *J Am Optom Assoc* 1962;34:135–138.

65. Neumueller J. The effect of the ametropic distance correction upon the accommodation and reading addition. *Am J Optom* 1938;15:120–128.

66. Hermann JS, Johnson R. The accommodation requirement in myopia. *Arch Ophthalmol* 1966;76:47–51.

67. Bennett AG. *Optics of contact lenses,* 4th ed. London: Association of Dispensing Opticians, 1966.

68. Neumueller JF. The optics of contact lenses. *Am J Optom Arch Am Acad Optom* 1968;45:786–796.

69. Duke-Elder S, Abrams D. Optics, section I. In: Duke-Elder S, Abrams D, eds. *Ophthalmic optics and refraction,* volume V of Duke-Elder S, ed. *System of ophthalmology.* St. Louis: CV Mosby, 1970:25–204.

70. Douthwaite WA. *Contact lens optics.* London: Butterworth & Co., 1987:23.

71. Hong X, Himebaugh N, Thibos LN. One-eye evaluation of optical performance of rigid and soft contact lenses. *Optom Vis Sci* 2001;78:872–880.

72. Byer A. Magnification limitations of a contact lens telescope. *Am J Optom Physiol Opt* 1986;63:71–75.

73. Lewis HT. Parameters of contact lens-spectacle telescopic systems and considerations in prescribing. *Am J Optom Physiol Opt* 1986; 63:387–391.

PRACTICAL OPTICS OF CONTACT LENS PRESCRIPTION

WILLIAM J. "JOE" BENJAMIN

Now that the reader is well versed in the optical phenomena of contact lens wear, which were discussed in Chapter 7A, a practical approach to the derivation of the *optical parameters of a contact lens prescription* will be discussed. It is the object of the author to also note other interesting practical considerations that are optical in nature and to leave nonoptical contact lens matters to other chapters. This approach stems from Table 7A.7 and expands upon some earlier publications (1–3). A *worksheet* from Benjamin (1) is reproduced for use in computing refractive powers of rigid contact lenses, especially those that are bitoric. If desired, it can be of help in the prescription of soft contact lenses (SCLs). Several examples show how the worksheet is used to determine the refractive powers of contact lens prescriptions. A collection of *58 optical problems,* accompanied by their answers, is reproduced from Benjamin (4) so that the busy practitioner or student of contact lens optics can relatively quickly prove his or her knowledge in this detailed and critical area.

SPHERICAL AND TORIC HYDROGEL (SOFT) CONTACT LENSES

If the patient's *refractive astigmatism is 0.75 DC or less,* a spherical soft lens may be prescribed because it will generally provide acceptable vision unless the patient is visually critical or otherwise susceptible to small amounts of residual cylinder. The spherical refractive power of the final SCL prescription (CLP in Equation 7A.9, with lacrimal lens power [LLP] = 0 and overrefraction [OR] = 0) will be equal to the *spherical equivalent* of the corneal plane refraction, or slightly less minus/more plus if the refractive cylinder is with the rule. Many patients with 0.25 or 0.50 DC of residual cylinder will not notice any difference between their acuities with spherical equivalent soft lenses and spherocylindrical spectacle refractions. Indeed, the patients will likely feel that his or her vision with contact lenses is better for the following reasons. (i) The fields of view and fixation through spectacles no longer hinder peripheral vision and

vision in extreme gaze positions, respectively. (ii) The adverse prismatic effects of spectacles are nearly eliminated. (iii) Because most contact lens candidates are myopic, the greater spectacle magnification with contact lenses may enhance visual acuity so positively that the small negative effect of residual cylinder is offset (in low myopia) or even superseded (in moderate and high myopia). Simple myopes in the low-to-moderate ranges will often find that their visual acuities are better with contact lenses than with spectacles by approximately half of a Snellen acuity line. Simple high myopes may find their visual acuities to be higher by a line or more.

Some patients having 0.75 DC of refractive astigmatism, typically hyperopes and low myopes, will find their vision with the residual cylinder unacceptable, unless they are moderate or high myopes for which the influence of spectacle magnification is large. Others will learn to accept the blur rather than to wear soft toric contact lenses or rigid lenses, or to remain wearing spectacles. Aspheric SCLs, such as the Cooper Frequency 55 Aspheric, are now often used for correction of an eye having astigmatism of 0.25 or 0.50 DC. This is attempted if the patient has a visual decrement with a spherical soft lens, yet toric soft lenses are not available with astigmatic powers below 0.75 DC. At 0.75 DC, a toric soft lens like the *double-thin-zone* Vistakon Acuvue Toric is often prescribed. These options work well in *unilateral astigmatism* by avoiding the imposition of vertical prism before only one eye and by providing comfort equivalent to that of the spherical lens worn in the patient's other eye. Prismatically ballasted toric soft lenses are generally not as comfortable as the double-thin-zone variety or spherical soft lenses, and the thick prismatic base intensifies inferior corneal hypoxia (5). Should the patient have 0.50 DC or 0.75 DC of refractive cylinder that is matched by corneal toricity, a common finding, a decision will be required between the *immediate comfort associated with SCLs* and *the clarity of vision associated with spherical rigid contact lenses.*

If the patient's *refractive astigmatism is 1.00 DC or more,* a toric soft lens may be prescribed because it will generally provide acceptable vision for cases of astigmatism at the corneal plane of *up to 2.00 DC.* The selection of powers and fitting parameters of toric soft lenses often is somewhat limited, and the quality control of SCL refractive powers is such that vision with replacement toric lenses might not match that of the original lens. Toric soft lenses are fitted and designed to *remain as rotationally stable on the eye as possible.* Even so, the lenses can *rotate significantly* in different gaze positions, with varying blinking habits, and with changing environmental conditions that affect the hydration of the lenses on the eye. Thus, the axis of cylinder fluctuates from its ideal position during wear. As a result, vision with soft toric lenses is more variable than vision with other forms of contact lens correction, and this is especially so for some patients. The *amount of cylinder correction possible with toric soft lenses is limited by the variable rotation* of these lenses on the eye. Although toric soft lenses can be obtained with cylinder powers much greater than 2.00 DC, successful toric SCL wear becomes progressively less probable as the cylinder power is increased. Cylinder powers greater than 2.00 DC may sometimes be prescribed successfully for *highly compound myopes* because these individuals are tolerant of blur, including variable blur induced by wear of highly astigmatic toric soft lenses. Even so, a back-toric rigid lens becomes the preferred option when the major component of high refractive astigmatism is corneal toricity.

Refractive cylinder is often *undercorrected* with soft toric lenses so as to reduce the visual influences of *variable lens rotation* on the eye. Indeed, should the patient have 1.00 to 2.00 DC of refractive cylinder that is nearly matched by corneal toricity, as is a common finding, a decision will again be required between the relative comfort associated with toric SCLs and the clarity of vision associated with spherical rigid contact lenses.

Adjustment of the Prescribed Axis of Astigmatism

The axis of astigmatism for a toric soft lens is specified relative to the prismatic portion(s) of the lens with the base-apex line (BAL in Equation 7A.28) in the vertical meridian. There are scribe (etch) marks on the peripheral front surfaces of toric soft lenses that indicate either the 090 (vertical) meridian or the 180 (horizontal) meridian of the lens. Four such lenses are shown in Fig. 7B.1 (6), three with markings in the 270 position to specify the vertical meridian of the lens (A, B, and D) and the other with markings at the 000 and 180 positions to specify the horizontal meridian of the lens (C). When prescribing these lenses it is important to assess the initial rotational stability of the lenses on the eyes in the office, by observing the rotational orientation of the markings. If the lenses appear to be rotationally stable enough to justify the ordering of toric soft lenses, the axes of cylinder must be adjusted according to the degree of rotation of the lenses on the eyes.

The direction of rotation of a toric lens is specified according to the movement of the bottom of the lens on the eye, *from the vantage point of the practitioner.* This is in apparent contradiction to the specification of "right" and

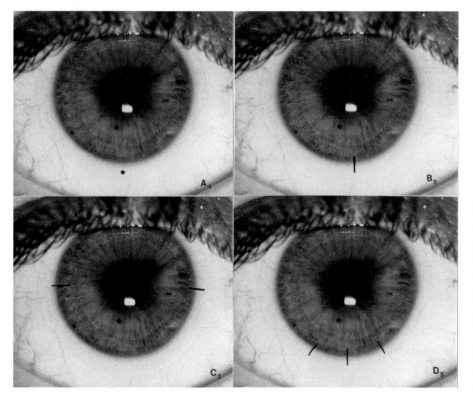

FIG. 7B.1. Toric soft contact lenses with reference (scribe) markings. The scribe marks are enhanced with a black pigment for easy visibility by the reader but would normally appear as light etch marks. **A:** Single dot marking base of prism. **B:** Single line marking base of prism. **C:** Horizontal scribe marks typical of "double thin zone" toric soft lenses. **D:** Three lines marking base of prism and 30 degrees to either side. (From Snyder C, Daum KM. Rotational position of toric soft contact lenses on the eye—clinical judgments. *Int Contact Lens Clin* 1989;16:146–151, with permission.)

"left" eyes, which are designated from the point of view of the patient. If the bottom of the lens rotates nasally, the rotation is "nasal rotation." *Nasal rotation* is counterclockwise in the patient's right eye and clockwise in the patient's left eye, as viewed by the practitioner. If the bottom of the lens rotates temporally, the rotation is "temporal rotation." *Temporal rotation* is clockwise in the right eye and counterclockwise in the left eye. The magnitude of the rotation can be measured using the protractor scale of the slit-lamp beam supplied on most biomicroscopes. Relatively stable toric soft lenses usually average *0 to 10 degrees of nasal rotation.*

The cylinder axis to be prescribed in the toric SCL must take into account the *direction and magnitude of stable lens rotation* (Fig. 7B.2). Let us assume that a right eye's refractive cylinder axis is 015 and that the toric soft lens assumes a stable orientation of 5 degrees nasal rotation (counterclockwise) on the eye. The prescribed cylinder axis will need to be 010 such that the lens rotation will move the cylinder axis into the 015 meridian on the eye (Fig. 7B.2A). Suppose that the refractive cylinder axis is 015 and that the lens rotated 5 degrees tempo-

rally on the right eye. The prescribed cylinder axis should then be 020. For the left eye, let us assume a refractive cylinder axis of 110. If the lens rotates 10 degrees nasally (clockwise), the prescribed axis should be 120 (Fig. 7B.2B). If temporal rotation is 10 degrees, the prescribed axis becomes 100. Hence, it is a simple matter to predict the required axis of cylinder in the prescribed lens conceptually.

Although adjustment of the prescribed cylinder axis is easily performed conceptually, a widely accepted pneumonic device is that of the *LARS (left add, right subtract) Principle.* Regardless of which eye is being fitted with a toric soft lens, if the bottom of the lens rotates to the *left,* the magnitude of rotation is to be *added* to that of the actual refractive cylinder axis in order to arrive at the axis of cylinder to be prescribed in the toric lens. The direction of rotation is expressed from the vantage point of the practitioner. If the bottom of the lens rotates to the *right,* the magnitude of rotation is to be *subtracted* to that of the actual refractive cylinder axis in order to arrive at the axis of cylinder to be prescribed in the toric lens.

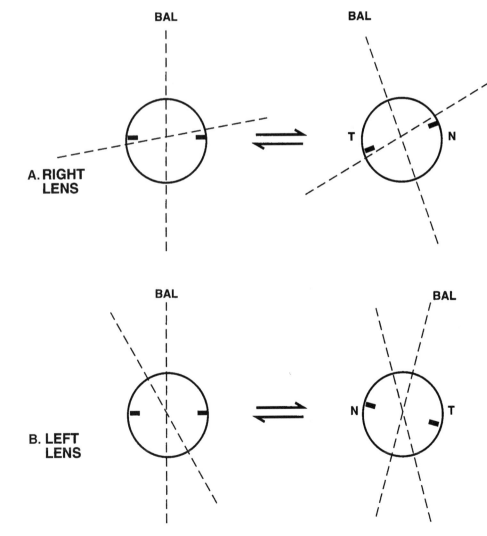

FIG. 7B.2. Rotational orientation of cylinder axis to compensate for nasal rotation of toric soft lenses, shown for right and left lenses on the *left.* Note the cylinder axis should be off-set clockwise from the base–apex line (BAL) on a right lens that will rotate nasally, whereas the cylinder axis on the left lens should be rotated counterclockwise. When the segs rotate into position, shown "on the eye" at the *right,* they are positioned in the appropriate meridians. (From Benjamin WJ. Contact lenses: clinical function and practical optics. In: Benjamin WJ, ed. *Borish's clinical refraction.* Philadelphia: WB Saunders, 1998: 956–1021, with permission.)

Upside Down, Inside Out, and Axis Location by Prism or Markings

Many toric SCLs are designed with *base-down vertical prism,* such that there is only a single proper orientation of the lens on the eye: the base of the prism is inserted down so as to stabilize near the 270 position. These lenses are rotationally stabilized by this design according to the "watermelon seed effect" of the superior eyelid and the "nasal kick" of the lower eyelid. However, an increasing number of toric soft lenses are available in a *"double-thin-zone"* design, exemplified by the original Torisoft lens from Ciba Vision Corporation, in which the lens is prismatically slabbed off in the superior and inferior areas in order to achieve orientation through the "watermelon seed effect" using both eyelids. "Double-slab-off" designs can be inserted in two stable rotational orientations, one *"upside down"* from the other. It should be noted that, *if a toric lens is inserted upside down, the cylinder axis is also rotated through 180 degrees and should achieve the correct axis orientation on the eye.*

Patients occasionally will insert an SCL on the eye *"inside out."* When a spherical thin soft lens is inserted in this manner, the patient often will report that his or her vision is surprisingly excellent. The patient may know that "something is wrong" with the lens but will not be able to define the cause. The comfort and refractive power of a thin spherical soft lens will not be drastically altered when inserted inside out as long as the back surface conforms sufficiently to the corneal surface. The intended refractive power of thick soft lenses (plus lenses) may be altered significantly and vision will be correspondingly affected adversely. The cylinder axis of a toric SCL will be *rotated around the vertical meridian* when inserted inside out. Thus, the intended cylinder axis of a toric lens at 005 will be located at 175 when inserted. Similarly, lenses having axes at 045 and 085 will be inserted at axes 135 and 095. Only for toric lenses having cylinder axes at 090 or 180 will the axes remain the same upon insertion inside out. The amount of visual degradation upon insertion will be commensurate with the magnitude of the cylinder and the degree of rotation from the intended cylinder axis.

It is common for contact lens practitioners or technicians to measure the refractive powers of contact lenses with a lensometer of the projection type. *Projection lensometers* are handy devices in contact lens practice because lens stops for contact lenses are available and are easily removed and replaced. Contact lenses can be situated on the lens stop for measurement using gravity as an aid to stable positioning (as in Fig. 7A.11). The stop can be removed before centration and rotational orientation of the lens on the stop are achieved, then replaced in concert with the lens on the lensometer prior to measurement. Lens stops of projection lensometers for contact lenses can be interchanged easily and rapidly with those for spectacle lenses when the need arises.

The optical design of a projection lensometer is such that the *bottoms of spectacle lenses are inserted away from the*

operator and *vertical prism* is signified by deflection of the target in a manner opposite that of traditional lensometers: base down is signified by an upward deflection of the target on the screen of a projection lensometer. Unaware of these facts, many contact lens practitioners and technicians insert a toric contact lens on the lens stop with the bottom of the lens toward the operator. In this rotational orientation, *upside down* from that for which the projection lensometer was designed, the cylinder axis is rotated through 180 degrees. Therefore, the appropriate cylinder axis should be indicated by the lensometer. Any base down prism in the contact lens results in a deflection of the target downward on the screen of the projection lensometer, which is interpreted by the clinician as being "base down" even though the projection lensometer is actually signifying "base up." Hence, the contact lens practitioner can get away with an "alternative" measurement technique with the projection lensometer as long as he or she does not attempt to measure prism in spectacles!

Situation of a contact lens on the lens stop is easier when the front surface is against the stop as compared to location of the back surface against the stop. As a result, practitioners and technicians often measure front vertex power (FVP) routinely rather than back vertex power (BVP) at the office. Clinicians should note that their FVP values will be different for contact lenses of high refractive power (Table 7A.3) than those BVP values indicated by the manufacturer. In addition, the axis of cylinder of a toric contact lens will appear *rotated around the vertical meridian* when front vertex power is assessed on the lensometer.

A question arises as to how to localize the cylinder axis of a toric soft lens that is stabilized on the eye by means of prism. Is the lens to be initially aligned on the lens stop of the lensometer with the *etch markings* in the appropriate vertical or horizontal positions, or is the lens to be rotated until the *base down prism* is properly located at 270 in the reticle of the lensometer? In "double-thin-zone" designs this is of no consequence because prism is not located in the optic zone of these lenses and the etch markings must be used to rotationally orient the lenses on the lens stop. For lenses that are "prism ballasted," on the other hand, there may be some error involved in the marking of the designated meridian relative to the vertical prismatic component. The clinician probably should measure the cylinder axis of prismatically ballasted toric lenses *according to the etch markings,* because these markings will be used to assess rotation and rotational stability when the toric lenses are on the eye. The clinician may simultaneously evaluate the axis of the prism relative to the etch markings by observing the direction in which the lensometer target has been deflected when the etch markings have been properly aligned.

Use of the Retinoscope

As noted in the earlier discussion on the optics of hydrogel contact lenses, the *optical quality* of soft lenses is difficult to assess. Whether lensometer mires are observed with the lens power measured in the dry state or the wet state, variations of optical quality seen in the mires are difficult to discern. Major imperfections in the optic zone of a soft lens sometimes are detectable; therefore, the reason for a patient's reduced vision can be deduced. A new soft lens with a central front-surface imperfection is shown in Fig. 7B.3A. This blemish reduced the patient's vision to Snellen 20/30 (6/9) when the lens was inserted as a replacement, in comparison to the expected 20/20 (6/6). When the blemish was discovered biomicroscopically, the lens was itself replaced and 20/20 (6/6) was achieved. The patient had evidently scratched the central front surface of a soft lens (Fig. 7B.3B), reducing visual acuity to 20/60 (6/18). The eye cosmetics of another patient had deposited on the front surface (Fig. 7B.3C), lessening visual acuity to 20/40 (6/12). Replacement of these lenses alleviated the problems.

Reduced optical quality of the optic zone of SCLs often can be the result of imperfections that are not easily recognized upon simple inspection or biomicroscopic evaluation.

A technique (originally recommended to the author by Dr. Jan Bergmanson of the University of Houston and reinforced by Dr. Christopher Snyder of the University of Alabama at Birmingham) is the use of *retinoscopy* for the detection of central optical defects in soft lenses. The procedure involves examination of the fundus reflexes with a streak retinoscope while the patient is wearing soft lenses. It also can be performed with a direct ophthalmoscope used as a "spot retinoscope." This method allows the practitioner to detect otherwise unobservable optical deformities in SCLs and explain visual deficits that patients may have with certain lenses. The technique becomes of even greater importance in the evaluation of toric SCLs and multifocal contact lenses, which are more difficult to manufacture, verify, and prescribe than spherical lenses. Josephson (7) found this technique especially useful for identification and location of the central optical zones and near segments of *bifocal contact lenses* relative to the entrance pupil of the eye. Retinoscopes also are used without contact lenses in place to assess the degree and location of optical distortion of the cornea relative to the pupil in cases of keratoconus.

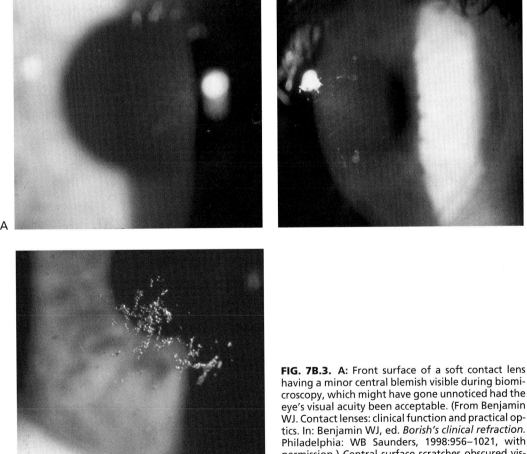

A

B

C

FIG. 7B.3. A: Front surface of a soft contact lens having a minor central blemish visible during biomicroscopy, which might have gone unnoticed had the eye's visual acuity been acceptable. (From Benjamin WJ. Contact lenses: clinical function and practical optics. In: Benjamin WJ, ed. *Borish's clinical refraction.* Philadelphia: WB Saunders, 1998:956–1021, with permission.) Central surface scratches obscured visual acuity **(B)**, as did central deposition from eye makeup **(C).**

Cylinder Axis and Power in Refractions Over Toric Soft Lenses

A typical finding in a refraction over a toric SCL is a seemingly inexplicable axis of residual astigmatism that is oblique to the axis of the eye's astigmatism and the axis of the correcting cylinder. Basically, the obliquity and magnitude of the residual cylindrical error are the result of an optical combination of two crossed cylinders by vector addition (8). The ocular astigmatism can be considered to be a plus cylinder that requires correction by an overlying minus cylinder. This calculation can be performed using a properly programmed hand-held calculator/computer, but the time, effort, and optical expertise required for an *exact* numerical result often are prohibitive. This is especially true considering that the vector addition can be approximated mentally in the most common clinical scenarios, for instance, when the refraction is over a toric SCL having a cylinder power equal to, or nearly equal to, the actual cylindrical component of the eye's refractive error (2,3).

A typical scenario occurs during the fitting of a toric SCL when a trial or diagnostic contact lens is chosen for the patient's eye. Ideally, the trial contact lens should have the correct spherocylindrical powers and axis, but the limitations of a trial lens set most likely preclude immediate availability of the most appropriate powers and axis in a single toric lens. Most clinicians will attempt to locate a diagnostic lens that has the correct cylinder power with an axis and sphere power that are as close to the patient's refractive error as possible from those selections available in the fitting set. The result is a diagnostic lens that incorporates a cylinder component equal to, or nearly equal to, the eye's astigmatic correction in terms of power. On the eye, however, the correcting cylinder of the diagnostic lens most likely will be crossed with respect to the eye's astigmatic axis. This will be due to the concurrent effects of the rotational orientation that the lens assumes on the eye and the fact that the desired cylinder axis was not available in the trial lens set. We will ignore here the possible influence of a potential "lacrimal lens," which is thought to be small and unpredictable by those who theorize the effect.

The typical scenario also occurs when the refraction is performed over a toric soft lens during progress visits during the adaptation period to toric SCLs or during later checkup visits after adaptation. In these situations, the cylinder power of the toric SCL is that required, or very nearly so, but the cylinder axis may be crossed due to lens rotation stemming from soft lens degradation and coatings. Perhaps the eye's astigmatic axis has changed somewhat from that apparent when the lens was first prescribed. As a result, the contact lens practitioner often is confronted with a correcting minus cylinder in the toric SCL being somewhat crossed with respect to the axis of the eye's astigmatism. Hence, the spherocylindrical overrefraction corrects for the *combination of two cylinders (ocular and correcting) having powers of opposite sign and roughly equal magnitude* (2,3).

Underlying Optics: The Short Version

When two cylinders are combined so that their axes are coincident, a resultant cylinder will be formed with its axis in the original position. The resultant refractive power is equal to a simple numerical addition of the dioptric strengths of the two original cylinders. If the minus correcting cylinder is of the same magnitude and is at the same axis as the plus cylinder ocular astigmatism, the minus cylinder refractive error is neutralized by the minus cylinder lens. The residual astigmatic error, in this case zero, is the cylinder error left uncorrected by the lens that has been placed in front of the eye (Fig. 7B.4).

If two cylinders of opposite sign and equal magnitude are combined so that their axes are not coincident, the result is a spherocylinder having a cylinder axis oblique to those of the original two cylinders. Pascal (9) calculated the extent of the shift in position of the resultant plus cylinder axis for two cylinders of equal power but opposite sign from the formula (90 + a)/2, where a is the angular discrepancy between the two combined cylinders. This relationship states, essentially, that *the resultant plus cylinder axis is 45 degrees from the midpoint between the axes of the two combined*

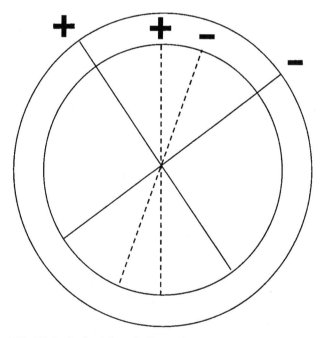

FIG. 7B.4. *Dashed lines* indicate the axes of a plus cylinder (×090, representing ocular astigmatism) and a correcting minus cylinder (×070), each power having the same magnitude but being opposite in sign. *Solid lines* represent the plus and minus cylinder axes of the resultant combination of the two original cylinders. The resultant plus cylinder axis of the combination (×125) is located 45 degrees away from the midpoint between the two (×080) and on the side of the original plus cylinder opposite to that of the original minus cylinder. A minus cylinder will need to be placed at the axis of 125 in order to neutralize the residual refractive error. (From Benjamin WJ. The "explicability" of cylinder axis and power in refractions over toric soft lenses. *Int Contact Lens Clin* 1998;25:89–92, with permission.)

cylinders. The axis of the resultant plus cylinder of the crossed cylinder combination will appear on the side of the axis of the original plus cylinder opposite to that of the original minus cylinder. For example (Fig. 7B.4), if the axis of ocular astigmatism is 090 and a minus cylinder of equal power is placed at axis 070, 20 degrees away, the resultant plus cylinder axis will appear (90 + 20)/2 = 55 degrees from 070 on the opposite side, or "×125." The resultant plus cylinder will require a minus cylinder correction. Thus, the residual astigmatic *error* left by the correcting lens is minus cylinder axis 125, which is 45 degrees from the midpoint between the axes of the correcting cylinder and ocular astigmatism (10). Figure 7B.2 shows the *axis* of the residual astigmatic error in graphical form with respect to the angular difference between axes of ocular astigmatism and correcting cylinder having powers of equal magnitude and opposite sign.

The clinician attempts to reduce, as much as possible, the discrepancy between the axes of ocular astigmatism and the correcting cylinder in a toric SCL. Hence, the clinician rarely refracts over these two cylinders when crossed by more than 30 degrees. Linksz (11) calculated that, when cylinders

of equal but opposite power are crossed by 30 degrees, the resultant cylinder power is equal in magnitude to the original (100%). If crossed by 15 degrees, the resultant power is equal to 50% of the original; if crossed by 5 degrees, the resultant is equal to 17% of the original. The power of the resultant cylinder closes to zero as the angular separation between the plus and minus cylinders reduces to zero. One way to estimate the power of the residual cylinder is to realize that the magnitude of the residual cylinder error shown in Fig. 7B.4, where the cylinders are crossed by 20 degrees, should be greater than 50% yet less than 100%, perhaps around *70%* of the original magnitude.

Figure 7B.5 also reveals the relative *power* of the residual astigmatic error with respect to the angular difference between axes of ocular astigmatism and correcting cylinder having powers of equal magnitude and opposite sign. Another way of estimating the residual astigmatism is to note that it increases roughly 10% of the refractive/correcting cylinder for every 3 degrees of crossing between the two (12). In the earlier example in which the cylinders were crossed by 20 degrees, the residual cylinder power should

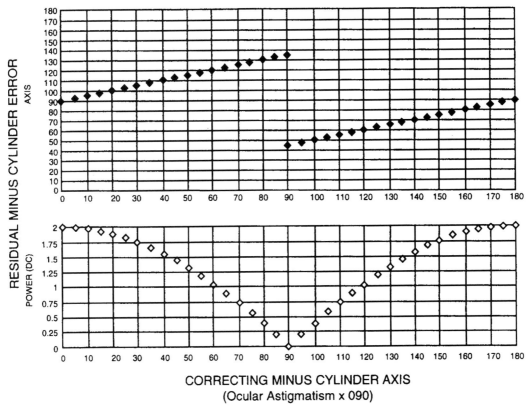

FIG. 7B.5. Graph showing the refractive power and axis of the residual astigmatic error with respect to the meridian in which a correcting cylinder of − 1.00 DC is placed. The ocular astigmatism is +1.00 DC × 090, resulting in an astigmatic error of − 1.00 DC × 090. This is a case where the ocular astigmatism and the correcting cylinder have powers of equal magnitude and opposite sign, typically encountered during examinations of wearers of toric soft contact lenses. Note that the magnitude of the residual cylinder power is approximately 10% for every 3 degrees of cross. (From Benjamin WJ. The "explicability" of cylinder axis and power in refractions over toric soft lenses. *Int Contact Lens Clin* 1998;25:89–92, with permission.)

have been 20/3 = 6⅔ times 10%, or *67%* of the refractive/correcting cylinders. Hence, these two methods of estimating the residual cylinder produce similar results.

It can be noted in Fig. 7B.5 that the closer the axis of the correcting minus cylinder comes to matching the eye's astigmatic axis, the farther the axis of the residual astigmatic error moves from the eye's axis of astigmatism and the smaller the cylinder power of the residual error becomes. The influence of the angular separation is *intuitive* with respect to the *refractive power* of the residual minus cylinder in the overrefraction, because the power of the residual cylinder decreases to zero with the separation. However, the effect of the angular separation on the *axis* of the residual cylinder is *counterintuitive,* because the residual cylinder becomes more oblique as the angular separation between the two original cylinders is closed! As a result, *clinicians often believe something to be "wrong,"* or that the correcting cylinder axis is far removed from the eye's actual cylinder axis, when the overrefraction reveals the residual cylinder axis to be significantly oblique. Instead, however, the oblique residual axis indicates that the correcting minus cylinder is really close to, or even nearly coincident with, the axis of the eye's minus cylinder error!

When the axes of the ocular astigmatism and the correcting minus cylinder coincide, the computed residual astigmatic axis is 45 degrees away and the computed magnitude of the cylinder error is zero. A correcting cylinder only slightly misplaced results in a small residual error nearly 45 degrees from the midpoint between the ocular and correcting cylinders. As the axis of the correcting cylinder is moved away from the axis of ocular astigmatism, the axis of the residual error moves toward the axis of ocular astigmatism by half that amount and becomes greater in terms of power, as noted earlier (11). The largest residual error is twice that of the original refractive error when the correcting minus cylinder is moved 90 degrees from the axis of ocular astigmatism. At this point, the axis of the residual error coincides with that of the original cylinder error.

Application to Specific Cases

To reiterate, because the correcting minus cylinder is often of roughly equal magnitude to that of the eye's astigmatic error, *the refraction over a toric SCL is merely the result of combination of two cylinders having nearly equal magnitude but being opposite in sign.* The plus cylinder is the eye's astigmatism and the minus cylinder is the correcting cylinder. *The outcome of the cylindrical combination is that the residual minus cylinder error in the overrefraction is 45 degrees from the midpoint between the two original cylinders, on the side of the eye's astigmatic axis.* When crossed by 30 degrees, the residual minus cylinder power is equal in magnitude to the original (100%). If crossed by 15 degrees, the residual power is equal to 50% of the original; if crossed by 5 degrees, the residual is equal to 17% of the original. The power of

the residual minus cylinder error closes to zero as the angular separation between the original plus and minus cylinders reduces to zero. Another way of estimating the residual error is to add *10% of the original cylinder power for every 3 degrees of crossing.*

The reader now can realize that a right eye with refractive error − 2.00 − 1.25 × 180, corrected with a toric SCL of the same power that is rotating nasally by 10 degrees (×010), will be properly overrefracted with a minus cylinder component at axis 140. The power of the residual cylinder will be approximately − 0.25 DC or more likely − 0.50 DC when assessed using a refractor capable of 0.25 DC steps. Similarly, for a left eye with refractive error + 1.00 − 1.75 × 160, corrected with a toric SCL of the same power that is rotating nasally by 20 degrees (×140), the residual minus cylinder error will lie at an axis of 015. The residual cylinder power in the overrefraction should come out − 1.00 to − 1.25 DC. If the eye has a refractive error of − 1.75 − 1.50 × 020 and the overrefraction shows a residual minus cylinder at axis 060, the minus cylinder of the correcting SCL must be located near axis 010. Hence, the oblique residual cylinder axes and the powers in the refraction over a toric SCL are actually explicable, to the point that the magnitude and direction of the rotation of toric SCLs can be approximated in practice!

SPHERICAL AND FRONT-TORIC RIGID CONTACT LENSES

If the patient's corneal plane astigmatism (refractive cylinder) and corneal toricity in keratometric diopters are *similar* (± 0.50 DC), spherical rigid contact lenses may be prescribed because they will generally provide acceptable vision for cases of corneal astigmatism *up to 2.00 DC.* Above 2.00 DC of corneal toricity the ability of spherical rigid lenses to provide an acceptable fit is progressively reduced. Thus, back-toric rigid lenses become the preferred option when the major component of high refractive astigmatism is corneal toricity. The selection of powers and fitting parameters of spherical rigid lenses is excellent because they are customized devices. In addition, the quality of rigid lens refractive power and optical surface quality are excellent. Rigid lenses now are made of materials of various permeabilities to oxygen and are called *gas permeable* (GP) contact lenses.

Front-toric rigid lenses are rarely prescribed today and are somewhat of a curiosity to younger contact lens practitioners. They were originally designed with a spherical back surface and base down prism to rotationally stabilize the correcting cylinder ground into the front surface. Front-toric rigid lenses were fitted when significant residual cylinder was revealed in the refraction over a spherical rigid lens, i.e., when refractive cylinder did not match corneal toricity. Corneal toricity was less than 2.00 DC such that a spherical base curve provided an acceptable fit, and back-surface toric lenses were recommended above this amount of corneal to-ricity. The advent of toric SCLs has all but eliminated the prescription of front-toric rigid lenses, for toric soft lenses are applicable to the same population as were front-toric rigid lenses. In addition, soft toric lenses are more comfortable, they fit the cornea better, and the orientations of cylinder axes are more stable. Hence, the prescription of front-toric rigid lenses is now only a minimal specialty within contact lens practice.

In a *lid-attachment fit,* a spherical GP lens is desired that is close to central alignment ("on K"), and the lens must be large enough to facilitate lid attachment. Most corneas are at least slightly "with the rule," and the flat corneal meridian is fitted "on K" or a little "steeper than K." This means that the steep corneal meridian is fitted "flatter than K." The static base curve/corneal surface fitting relationship ideally should be one of alignment or slight central clearance ("slightly steep") in the flattest meridian. The static *base curve/cornea relationship* should be "flatter than K" in the steepest corneal meridian and will allow some rocking of the lens during the blink to promote tear fluid exchange underneath the GP lens. The overall "flat" nature of the *static fit* permits lid attachment of the lenses for those patients whose upper eyelids are able to control the vertical centration of the lenses.

Dynamic lens centration of a spherical GP lens is brought about by steepening the overall base curve/cornea relationship when an *interpalpebral fit* is required. Interpalpebral fits may be necessary when corneas are *spherical, against the rule, or obliquely toric,* and especially when the superior eyelid will not control the position of rigid lenses. In these instances, a shorter base curve radius may be prescribed in the posterior surface of a lens having small optic zone and overall diameters so as to effect vertical lens centration over the apex of the cornea in the absence of lid attachment. The eyelid should more easily slide over the upper edge of the steeper lens so as to enhance comfort, reduce vertical movement of the lens on the blink, and/or avoid pushing the lens inferiorly on the cornea. The necessity for an interpalpebral fit will incur the costs of incomplete tear flushing during the blink and less comfort due to blinking over the exposed upper edge of the contact lens. Prescription of a steeper lens will require slightly more minus power in the lens to compensate for the increased plus power in the lacrimal lens.

Diagnostic Session for Spherical Gas Permeable Lenses

It is wise to prescribe GP lenses only after having first performed a diagnostic session so as to arrive at the back-surface design necessary for optimal lens performance. The cornea is steepest centrally and usually flattens peripherally, but the degree of flattening varies from meridian to meridian and from eye to eye. The central cornea is an irregularly astig-matic surface, although we assume regularity for purposes of optical correction, and the degree of irregularity increases into the periphery. Thus, the appropriate back surface of the GP contact lens prescription should be determined by assessment of *the static and dynamic fluorescein patterns* of at least one diagnostic rigid contact lens. It is important that the parameters of the diagnostic lens be verified before proceeding with the diagnostic session.

The *static fluorescein pattern* is that seen with the GP contact lens centered over the apex of the cornea with eyelids removed from contact with the front surface of the lens. The practitioner may observe this pattern with a cobalt filter on the biomicroscope or with an ultraviolet lamp, while holding the eyelids away from the lens. The lens may be propped on top of the margin of the lower eyelid such that it is centered in the cornea. The *dynamic fluorescein pattern* is that seen when the lens is allowed full contact with the eyelids and reaches a location on the cornea determined by a competition between the "watermelon seed effect" and the "minus carrier effect" to be fully discussed in another chapter. The lens may or may not be centered over the corneal apex when the dynamic pattern is observed, and this position is where the lens would ride if it were to be worn by the patient.

A diagnostic lens could be selected using the following "rule of thumb": The *initial base curve radius should be approximately equal, in keratometric diopters, to the flat K reading plus 20% of the corneal toricity.* The overall diameter (OAD) and optic zone diameter (OZD) of the diagnostic lens should be large enough to attach to the upper lid. A lens with OAD = 9.5 mm and OZD = 8.1 mm would likely be appropriate, but a smaller OAD (e.g., 9.0 mm, with OZD = 7.8 mm) might be appropriate in some cases depending on the corneal diameter, pupil diameter, and upper lid anatomy. If fitting interpalpebrally, a steeper base curve with the 9.0 overall diameter or even smaller might be optimal. Ideally, the refractive power of the diagnostic lens should approximate that of the final prescription. In the case where the diagnostic lens is of significantly different power than that which will be later worn by the patient, the lens design will need to be adjusted according to what the practitioner believes the incorporation of the final lens power will do to the performance of the final lens. This will be covered later in this section.

The basic idea here is to obtain a representative spherical lens on the eye close to the appropriate diameter and base curve of the spherical lens that will be prescribed. The next step is to assess the *static* base curve/cornea fitting relationship in the flat (horizontal) and steep (vertical) meridians so that an estimate can be made of how much flatter or steeper the base curve radius must be fitted in order to obtain the concept of how a well-fitted GP lens should perform. The clinician must make an "educated guess" as to the degree the final lens should be steepened or flattened according to the fit of the diagnostic trial lens that was evaluated. The *static and dynamic fluorescein patterns* of the final lens should be evaluated when it is first placed on the patient's eye to see if the base curve radii of the spherical GP lens prescription will require alteration the next time a lens is ordered for that eye.

A spherocylindrical overrefraction should be done before taking the spherical diagnostic lens off of the eye. If the patient has been appropriately preselected on the basis of K readings and refractive astigmatism, the overrefraction should yield only a small cylindrical component (≤1.00 DC).

The cylindrical correction in the overrefraction (residual astigmatism) should be equal to the internal astigmatism of the eye, but this concept is confused by the fact that "rigid" spherical GP lenses actually *flex* on toric corneas. The optics of rigid lens *flexure* was covered in detail in Chapter 7A, but in practical terms flexure is considered to lessen the correction of corneal astigmatism by decreasing the minus power of the "lacrimal lens" in the steep meridian. The result of flexure can be to overestimate the amount of with-the-rule cylinder that shows through an assumed "inflexible" spherical GP lens. If the residual astigmatism in the overrefraction does not match the predicted internal astigmatism, over-keratometry (over-K) can be performed to see how much flexure is occurring.

The overall diameter and/or the optic zone diameter of the final contact lens prescription may require alteration according to the fit and centration of the diagnostic lens. To a large extent, selection of these parameters will be influenced by the corneal diameter, pupil diameter, and eyelid anatomy of the individual eye.

Selecting the Peripheral Curves of Spherical Gas Permeable Lenses

Another empirically derived rule of thumb for peripheral curves is applied here to a tricurve back-surface design having an axial edge lift of 0.08 to 0.10 mm. If a computer program is not available, the axial edge lift may be approximated by producing the secondary and peripheral curves according to the guidelines in Table 7B.1.

If, when the diagnostic spherical GP lens fit on the individual cornea is assessed, the peripheral edge clearance is less or more than what might be expected for the average cornea, the peripheral curves of the final lens can be either flattened (axial edge lift and clearance increased) or steepened (axial edge lift and clearance decreased) accordingly. Upon dispensing of the initial GP lens prescription, the peripheral curve selection may be further assessed and modified appropriately the next time that a lens is ordered for the patient's eye. An order form showing the data for two lenses prescribed in Example 7 (right eye) and Example 8 (left eye) is included in Fig. 7B.6.

Ordering the Final Refractive Powers

The basic optical principles concerning the refractive properties of spherical GP lenses were described in Equations 7A.9, 7A.10, and 7A.11 in Chapter 7A. In Fig. 7B.7 is shown the *Rigid Lens "Form 1040,"* which can be used to predict the refractive power of the final lens (1). Already known should be the keratometry measurements of the eye being fitted, the pertinent parameters of the diagnostic contact lens, the central back-surface parameters of the contact lens to be ordered, and the spectacle refraction of the eye referred to the corneal plane so that the *basic information* section of the form can be filled out. What is done next is to make *two estimates of the final contact lens power* (final CLP) in both primary meridians. The *first estimate* is based on the spherocylindrical overrefraction that was performed over the diagnostic contact lens power (Diag. CLP) and the change in the power of the "lacrimal lens" in the final base curve radius compared to the base curve radius of the diagnostic lens (ΔLLP). Remember that a base curve change of 0.05 mm is roughly equivalent to a power change of 0.25 D. The *second estimate* is based on the spectacle refraction referred to the corneal plane (corneal plane refraction [CPR]) and the lacrimal lens power (LLP) of the final lens as computed from the K readings and final base curve radius. The last evaluation of refractive power is a *comparison of the first and second estimates* and prescription of the final CLP based on an evaluation of the *credibility* of those two initial estimates.

Example 7: Spherical Gas Permeable Lens Without Flexure

The numbering of the examples in this chapter continues from the six examples covered in Chapter 7A. Let us now look at Example 7 shown in Fig. 7B.8, with the basic infor-

TABLE 7B.1. TYPICAL TRICURVE GP BACK SURFACE DESIGN

Lens Diameters (OAD/OZD, in mm)	Secondary Curve Radius (SCR)	Peripheral Curve Radius/ Width (PCR/PCW)
9.5/8.1	1.0 mm flatter than BCR	2.0 mm flatter than BCR/0.2 mm
9.0/7.8	1.5 mm flatter than BCR	2.5 mm flatter than BCR/0.2 mm
8.5/7.5	2.0 mm flatter than BCR	3.0 mm flatter than BCR/0.2 mm

BCR, base curve radius, OAD, overall diameter; OZD, optical zone diameter.

CONTACT LENS ORDER FORM

| TYPE OF LENS: | SPHERICAL RGP LENS |
| MATERIAL: | BOSTON RXD |

	BC	SCR/W	PCR/W	OAD	OZD	POWER	CT
R	8.00	9.00/.5	10.00/.2	9.5	8.1	−3.50 DS	.14
L	7.70	9.20/.4	10.20/.2	9.0	7.8	−4.75 DS	.17

NOTES: Blue #1 Tint ; Dot R Lens

FIG. 7B.6. Contact lens order form filled out for the spherical rigid lenses prescribed in Example 7 (right eye) and Example 8 (left eye). (From Benjamin WJ. Contact lenses: clinical function and practical optics. In: Benjamin WJ, ed. *Borish's clinical refraction.* Philadelphia: WB Saunders, 1998:956–1021, with permission.)

mation as listed in the upper section of the document. The corneal cylinder was equal to refractive cylinder, so we expect no internal (residual) cylinder to show up in a refraction over the diagnostic lens, which was a − 3.00 DS spherical GP lens with a base curve radius of 7.90 mm. In fact, an overrefraction of − 1.00 − 0.25 × 180 DS was obtained, which is within acceptable error of the expected zero residual astigmatism. The base curve radius selected on the basis of the diagnostic lens fit was 8.00 mm.

The practitioner would proceed to compute the first and second final CLP estimates from the data accumulated and according to the established equations shown on the Rigid Lens "Form 1040." The two estimates are within 0.25 D of each other in both primary meridians, such that the practitioner can be relatively sure that the final CLP is an accurate value.

Example 8: Spherical Gas Permeable Lens with Flexure

Let us look at Example 8 shown in Fig. 7B.9, with the basic information as listed in the upper section of that document. The corneal cylinder was again equal to refractive cylinder, so we expect no internal (residual) cylinder to show up in a refraction over the diagnostic lens, which was the − 3.00 DS spherical GP lens with a base curve radius of 7.80 mm. An overrefraction of − 1.00 − 1.00 × 180 was obtained. The base curve radius selected for the final prescription on the basis of the static and dynamic fluorescein patterns of the diagnostic lens was 7.70 mm for an interpalpebral fit in which the base curve radius was slightly steeper than the central corneal curvature in the flat meridian.

The practitioner would proceed to compute the first and second final CLP estimates from the data accumulated and

according to the established equations shown on the Rigid Lens "Form 1040." Perhaps the practitioner would identify that some flexure of the spherical diagnostic lens could account for the discrepancy between the two final power estimates in the vertical meridian and measure over-K readings to see if flexure did, indeed, exist. Sure enough, the over-K readings indicated that the spherical diagnostic lens was flexing by 1.00 D! The lens design could be altered by increasing lens thickness in order to lessen the degree of flexure and/or a stiffer material could be used in the contact lens. Should these steps be taken, the appropriate final CLP could be biased in the direction of the second estimate.

Front-Surface Design: Adjusting for Incorporation of Refractive Power

The final CLP in Example 7 was in the low minus range and would not greatly influence the fitting and rotation of the final lenses in comparison to the diagnostic lens, which was of similar power. However, when the refractive powers of the final contact lens will be different than those of the diagnostic lens, the practitioner should make some educated guesses as to the manner in which the final lens may fit differently and try to compensate for any adverse differences by adjusting the design of the spherical GP lens. This is especially important with respect to vertical lens centration.

With a *lid-attachment fit,* minus lenses that are less minus than about − 2.00 DS (and especially lenses having plus power) likely will require a plus lenticular construction in which a minus carrier is used to obtain greater lid attachment. The more pronounced the minus carrier prescribed, the more eyelid attachment will be obtained in order to vertically center the lens. The lens also can be fit slightly flatter than normal in order to enhance lid attachment.

RIGID LENS "FORM 1040"

PATIENT NAME: _____   DATE: _____

1. EYE: R or L   CPR = [   ] – [   ] X [   ]

BASIC INFORMATION   sphere   minus cylinder   axis

	FLAT MERIDIAN			STEEP MERIDIAN	

2. K's [   ] = [   ] @ [   ]   [   ] = [   ] @ [   ]
         mm   D   mm   D

3. DIAG. CL   [   ] = [   ]   Verified?   [   ] = [   ]
   BASE CURVE   mm   D   Y or N   mm   D

4. FINAL CL   [   ] = [   ]   [   ] = [   ]
   BASE CURVE   mm   D   mm   D

Rx POWER ESTIMATE #1:   FINAL CLP = DIAG. CLP + OR – ΔLLP

	FLAT MERIDIAN		STEEP MERIDIAN

5. DIAG. CLP [+ or –   D]   Verified?   [+ or –   D]
                                     Y or N

6. OR   + [+ or –   D]   + [+ or –   D]

7. ΔLLP   – [+ or –   D]   Line 4 – Line 3 – [+ or –   D]

8. FINAL CLP [+ or –   D] Line 5 + Line 6 – Line 7 [+ or –   D]
   EST. # 1

Rx POWER ESTIMATE #2:   FINAL CLP = CPR – LLP

	FLAT MERIDIAN		STEEP MERIDIAN

9. CPR   [+ or –   D]   From Line 1   [+ or –   D]

10. LLP   – [+ or –   D]   Line 4 – Line 2 – [+ or –   D]

11. FINAL CLP [+ or –   D]   Line 9 – Line 10   [+ or –   D]
    EST. #2

CL REFRACTIVE POWER ADJUSTMENT WEIGHING ESTIMATES #1 and #2

	FLAT MERIDIAN		STEEP MERIDIAN

12. FINAL CLP [+ or –   D]   From Lines 8 & 11   [+ or –   D]

FIG. 7B.7. Form worksheet for derivation of the refractive correction for rigid contact lenses. (From Benjamin WJ. Bitoric rigid gas permeable lenses. In: Schwartz CA, ed. *Specialty contact lenses: a fitter's guide.* Philadelphia: WB Saunders, 1995:21–41, with permission.) *(Figure continues.)*

NOTES:
GENERALLY FIT ABOUT 2/3 OR 3/4 OF THE CORNEAL TORICITY
JUDGE CREDIBILITY OF ESTIMATE #1 vs. CREDIBILITY OF ESTIMATE #2, BEFORE
ADJUSTING POWER TO THAT WHICH WILL BE ORDERED (FINAL CLP)
BIAS TOWARD "SPHERICAL POWER EFFECT" WHEN APPROPRIATE, WHERE BACK-
SURFACE TORICITY IN DIOPTERS (Line 4) = CLP REFRACTIVE CYLINDER (Line 12)

DEFINITIONS:
CPR = CORNEAL PLANE REFRACTION
DIAG. CL = DIAGNOSTIC CONTACT LENS
DIAG. CLP = DIAG. CL (REFRACTIVE) POWER
FINAL CL = THE CONTACT LENS THAT WILL BE ORDERED
FINAL CLP = FINAL CL (REFRACTIVE) POWER
LLP = LACRIMAL LENS (REFRACTIVE) POWER
ΔLLP = CHANGE OF LLP TO THAT OF THE FINAL CL BASE CURVE
FROM THAT OF THE DIAG. CL BASE CURVE
OR = OVER-REFRACTION AT THE CORNEAL PLANE

FIG. 7B.7. (Continued)

In the case of an *interpalpebral fit,* plus lenticular designs with a plano carrier or minus carrier may be prescribed to decrease lens mass and thickness of lenses having powers greater than +2.00 DS. In this case, lenticularization could help compensate for inferior lens centration as a result of excessive mass of full-cut plus lenses. As the interpalpebral design may have already been steepened slightly to obtain centration of the diagnostic lens, perhaps due to against-the-rule or oblique corneal toricity, further steepening of the fit could result in tear fluid stagnation and poor central corneal physiology. Plus lenticularization has the added advantage of thinning the central optic cap, allowing greater oxygenation to the cornea under the center of the GP lens where tear fluid exchange is least efficient.

More often, however, contact lens practitioners run into the problem of prescribing significantly more minus power than was in the diagnostic lens, such that the upper lid is expected to attach too aggressively to the final lens. In these instances, a minus lenticular design is used. Starting at −5.00 DS of power, a "CN bevel" may be prescribed, which is a form of minus lenticular that is easy for the laboratory to manufacture using cone tools. In Fig. 7B.6, the order for the left lens calls for a CN bevel. Laboratories, however, will determine the actual parameters of the CN bevel, and the practitioner will have to accept the consequences of not defining the front surface more specifically. The author is willing to accept those consequences with lens powers in the −5 to −7 DS range but gets increasingly uneasy with the use of CN bevels as the refractive power mounts above this range. Therefore, above 8 DS of minus power it is best to specify the exact front-surface design that is needed, to include the front optic zone diameter, junction thickness, and uncut edge thickness. These parameters can be found easily with the use of a computerized lens design program.

For the interpalpebral fit, the edges of nonlenticularized high-minus lenses are uncomfortable because they are thick. These lenses tend to move excessively during the blink and can be driven inferiorly on the cornea by the upper eyelid margin. A CN bevel or other minus lenticular design may be prescribed to allow the lid to more easily slide over the upper lens edge so as to enhance comfort, reduce vertical movement of the lens on the blink, and/or avoid pushing the lens inferiorly on the cornea.

SUMMARY

Spherical GP lenses can give a *quality of vision* unequaled by any other form of correction for most compound myopic astigmats, who comprise the overwhelming majority of contact lens candidates. These lenses have excellent surface optics and are able to mask corneal topographical irregularities and toricity. Spectacle magnification, fields of view and fixation, and prismatic effects are close to those encountered in emmetropia. Thus, the "clarity of vision" associated with rigid contact lenses is the result of a confluence of beneficial factors. The primary detraction of rigid lenses is relative discomfort, especially during the adaptation period. Hence, patients who are wearing rigid lenses successfully often inquire of the practitioner about their ability to wear soft lenses. Based on the patients' K readings and refraction, it may appear that little or no residual cylinder will result from the wear of soft lenses. Even in these cases, however, the *patient and practitioner must be forewarned that "vision with soft lenses is just not the same as vision with rigid lenses."*

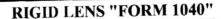

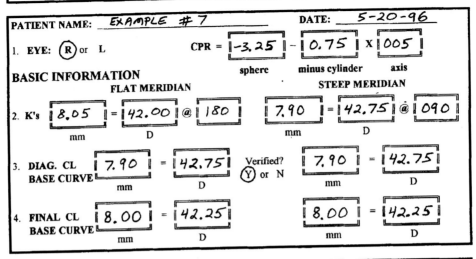

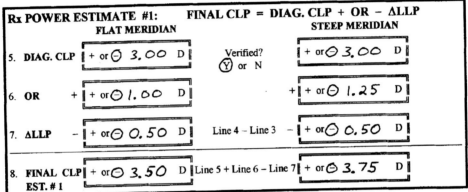

FIG. 7B.8. Worksheet filled out for Example 7. (From Benjamin WJ. Contact lenses: clinical function and practical optics. In: Benjamin WJ, ed. *Borish's clinical refraction.* Philadelphia: WB Saunders, 1998:956–1021, with permission.)

RIGID LENS "FORM 1040"

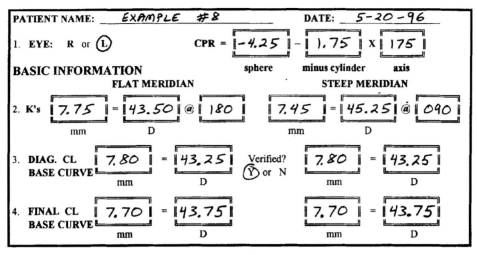

PATIENT NAME: _EXAMPLE #8_   DATE: _5-20-96_

1. EYE: R or Ⓛ   CPR = | -4.25 | – | 1.75 | X | 175 |
                        sphere   minus cylinder   axis

BASIC INFORMATION
     FLAT MERIDIAN   **STEEP MERIDIAN**

2. K's | 7.75 | = | 43.50 | @ | 180 | | 7.45 | = | 45.25 | @ | 090 |
      mm   D   mm   D

3. DIAG. CL BASE CURVE | 7.80 | = | 43.25 | Verified? Ⓨ or N | 7.80 | = | 43.25 |
       mm   D   mm   D

4. FINAL CL BASE CURVE | 7.70 | = | 43.75 | | 7.70 | = | 43.75 |
       mm   D   mm   D

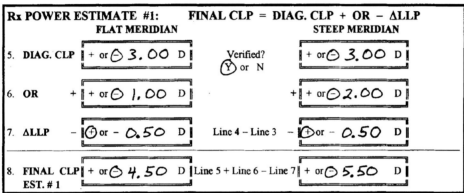

Rx POWER ESTIMATE #1:   **FINAL CLP = DIAG. CLP + OR – ΔLLP**
     FLAT MERIDIAN   **STEEP MERIDIAN**

5. DIAG. CLP | + or ⊖ 3.00 D | Verified? Ⓨ or N | + or ⊖ 3.00 D |

6. OR   + | + or ⊖ 1.00 D | + | + or ⊖ 2.00 D |

7. ΔLLP   – | ⊕ or – 0.50 D | Line 4 – Line 3   – | ⊕ or – 0.50 D |

8. FINAL CLP EST. #1 | + or ⊖ 4.50 D | Line 5 + Line 6 – Line 7 | + or ⊖ 5.50 D |

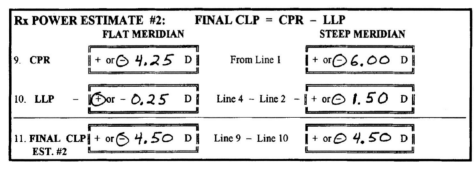

Rx POWER ESTIMATE #2:   **FINAL CLP = CPR – LLP**
     FLAT MERIDIAN   **STEEP MERIDIAN**

9. CPR | + or ⊖ 4.25 D | From Line 1 | + or ⊖ 6.00 D |

10. LLP   – | ⊕ or – 0.25 D | Line 4 – Line 2   – | + or ⊖ 1.50 D |

11. FINAL CLP EST. #2 | + or ⊖ 4.50 D | Line 9 – Line 10 | + or ⊖ 4.50 D |

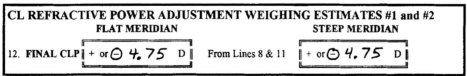

CL REFRACTIVE POWER ADJUSTMENT WEIGHING ESTIMATES #1 and #2
     FLAT MERIDIAN   **STEEP MERIDIAN**

12. FINAL CLP | + or ⊖ 4.75 D | From Lines 8 & 11 | + or ⊖ 4.75 D |

FIG. 7B.9. Worksheet filled out for Example 8. (From Benjamin WJ. Contact lenses: clinical function and practical optics. In: Benjamin WJ, ed. *Borish's clinical refraction.* Philadelphia: WB Saunders, 1998:956–1021, with permission.)

BACK-TORIC RIGID CONTACT LENSES

In the past, considerable mystique has surrounded the prescription of back-surface toric rigid lenses. Yet, the basic principles surrounding the fitting of spherical rigid lenses to slightly toric corneas (<2.00 D of corneal toricity) are merely applied to both primary meridians of back-toric lenses in the fitting of corneas having greater toricity (=2.00 D of corneal toricity). More emphasis should be placed on adherence to these basic principles in the case of back-surface torics because there is less room for error than with spherical lenses. The manufacture of back-surface torics is more difficult and exacting, such that inaccuracies in the prescription are compounded by heightened financial and other consequences. Meticulous verification of back-surface toric lenses is a necessary requirement for successful prescription. Even so, the required greater level of attention to detail can supply a sense of accomplishment to the practitioner who becomes successful with patients for whom optical correction is best undertaken with back-surface toric GP corneal lenses.

Back-surface toric lenses are prescribed in cases of high corneal toricity when a spherical GP lens will not ride appropriately on the toric corneal surface. Most corneas and especially highly toric corneas are "with the rule," being steeper vertically than horizontally, and the initial discussion will be concerned with fitting *"with-the-rule"* corneas. Management of "against-the-rule" and "oblique" corneas will be covered later. The same rules of thumb apply to "back torics" that apply to spherical rigid lenses in a *lid-attachment fit.* The lens should be close to central alignment ("on K"), *in an overall sense,* and the lens must be large enough to facilitate lid attachment. The stated goal of an "overall alignment" fit, however, is difficult to achieve with a significantly toric cornea (13). As when fitting a spherical lens to a slightly toric cornea, the flat corneal meridian is fitted "on K" or a little "steeper than K" and the steep corneal meridian is fitted somewhat "flatter than K." The static base curve/corneal surface fitting relationship ideally should be one of alignment or slight central clearance ("slightly steep") in the flattest meridian. The static base curve/cornea relationship should be "flatter than K" in the steepest corneal meridian by an amount that allows some rocking of the lens during the blink to promote tear fluid exchange underneath the GP lens (14). The overall "flat" nature of the static fit permits lid attachment of the lenses for those patients whose upper eyelids are able to control the vertical centration of the lenses. Care should be taken to avoid an overly flat fit in the vertical meridian, because this creates excessive dynamic rocking, discomfort, and inadequate vertical lens centration due to aggressive lid attachment. If the vertical meridian is fitted too steeply, dynamic lid attachment will generally be less effective and tear fluid flushing will be limited.

In general, back-toric lenses are prescribed to fit about two thirds to three fourths of the corneal toricity and slightly steeper than K in the flatter horizontal meridian. It is necessary that at least 2.00 DC of corneal toricity be present so that the toric back surface can rotationally match the cornea to align the optical power meridians in the correct axis and to allow the additional effort and cost of back-toric GP lenses to be justified over spherical GP lenses in terms of enhanced vision and comfort. The static fluorescein pattern of such a lens will appear with slight central clearance horizontally (slight fluorescence) and will have two zones of slight "touch" (minimum fluorescence) on the cornea in the horizontal periphery of the optic zone. There will be some tear fluid pooling (significant fluorescence) underneath the static lens superiorly and especially inferiorly in the midperiphery and periphery of the optic zone (Fig. 7B.10; see Color Plate 7B.10). It is important to ensure that the horizontal pattern has, in fact, slight central clearance when that is desired. In the presence of significant tear fluid pooling above and below, the relative lack of fluorescence horizontally may induce the practitioner to falsely recognize the horizontal pattern as being in "alignment" or, perhaps, even "slightly flat." In some cases the practitioner may actually wish the horizontal pattern to be in alignment or slightly flat across the entire optic zone in order to obtain greater lid attachment.

As in the case of a spherical GP lens, dynamic lens centration of a back-surface toric lens is brought about by steepening the overall base curve/cornea relationship when an *interpalpebral fit* is required. In these instances the full corneal toricity may be prescribed in the posterior surface of a lens having small optic zone and overall diameters so as to effect vertical lens centration over the apex of the cornea in the absence of lid attachment. Prescription of the full corneal cylinder on a with-the-rule cornea will allow the eyelid to more easily slide over the upper lens edge so as to enhance comfort, reduce vertical movement of the lens on the blink, and/or avoid pushing the lens inferiorly on the cornea. The necessity for an interpalpebral fit will incur the costs of

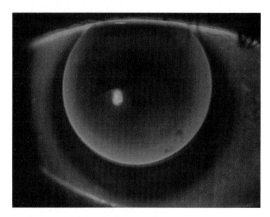

FIG. 7B.10. Static lid-attachment fit on a with-the-rule cornea showing horizontal alignment with pooling below (in the steep vertical meridian). (See Color Plate 7B.10.)

incomplete tear flushing during the blink and less comfort due to blinking over the exposed upper edge of the contact lens. Prescription of full corneal toricity will require more minus power in the steep meridian, thus reducing the supply of oxygen through the higher-minus periphery to the cornea. Fortunately, the oxygen capabilities of GP materials have greatly increased over the last 15 years, such that incorporation of refractive power should have less adverse impact on corneal physiology than in the past (15,16). The cornea is now more forgiving when optimum tear fluid exchange is not attained.

Diagnostic Session for Back-Surface Toric Gas Permeable Lenses

The first order of business when prescribing a back-toric GP lens is to perform a diagnostic session so as to arrive at the back-surface design necessary for optimal lens performance. It is of even more importance in comparison to the fitting of spherical GP lenses that the evaluation be performed with diagnostic GP lenses on the eye so that a best "educated guess" of the proper lens geometry can be ascertained. The cornea is steepest centrally and usually flattens peripherally, but the degree of flattening varies from meridian to meridian and from eye to eye. The amount and axis of corneal toricity change from the center to the periphery of the cornea. There is no guarantee, for instance, that a cornea having 3 DC of "with-the-rule" astigmatism according to keratometry will be 3 DC in the periphery, or even "with the rule" for that matter! The central cornea is an irregular surface, although we assume regularity for purposes of optical correction, and the degree of irregularity increases into the periphery. Therefore, the amount of back-surface toricity that an eye will require must be determined by assessment of the static and dynamic fluorescein patterns of at least one diagnostic rigid contact lens. It is very important that the parameters of the diagnostic lens be accurately verified before proceeding with the diagnostic session.

If Only a Spherical Gas Permeable Lens Fitting Set is Available

With a set of spherical trial lenses, an initial diagnostic lens would be selected in the same manner that a diagnostic lens for a spherical GP lens fitting would be selected: The initial base curve radius (BC) should be approximately equal, in keratometric diopters, to the flat K reading plus 20% of the corneal toricity. The overall diameter (OAD) and optic zone diameter (OZD) of the diagnostic lens should be large enough to attach to the upper lid. A lens with OAD = 9.5 mm and OZD = 8.1 mm would likely be appropriate, but a smaller lens could be selected having OAD = 9.0 mm and OZD = 7.8 mm in some cases, depending on the corneal diameter, pupil diameter, and upper lid anatomy. If the fit was to be interpalpebral, a steeper base curve could

be used with the 9.0 diameter lens or generally smaller, perhaps with OAD = 8.5 mm and OZD = 7.5 mm. Ideally, the refractive power of the diagnostic lens should approximate that of the final prescription, but the fitting set that is available might not allow for a wide range of powers. In the case where the diagnostic lens is of significantly different power than that which will be later worn by the patient, the lens design will require adjustment according to what the clinician believes will be the effect of incorporation of the final lens power on the performance of the final lens (to be covered later).

The basic idea is to obtain a representative spherical lens on the eye similar to the appropriate overall diameter and base curve radius of the spherical lens that might be prescribed if toric GP lenses were not available. The next step is to assess the static base curve/cornea fitting relationship in the flat (horizontal) and steep (vertical) meridians. An estimate of how much flatter or steeper these two meridians must be fitted is performed in order to obtain the concept of how a well-fitted GP lens should perform. It usually is true that the fitting relationship of the horizontal (flattest) meridian is not difficult to judge because the base curve of the lens is not far from the horizontal corneal curvature. Because the diagnostic fit here has been chosen to be *"20% of the corneal toricity steeper than the flat K,"* the horizontal base curve for the final back-toric lens will generally require flattening by a small amount, approximately 0.50 D depending on the amount of corneal toricity. The diagnostic fit in the vertical (steepest) meridian is going to be significantly flat; therefore, the base curve selection for the final back-toric lens will be much steeper than that of the diagnostic lens. In general, this curve will be steepened by a dioptric value about 45% to 55% (half) of the corneal toricity. An "educated guess" as to the degree to which this meridian will be steepened according to the spherical lens fit that you evaluated will be the factor that has the least accuracy concerning the back-surface design of the final lens. The static and dynamic fluorescein patterns of the final lens should be evaluated when it is first placed on the patient's eye. This is especially true for the steep meridian, in order to see if it will require further steepening, or even flattening, of the base curves of the back-toric prescription the next time a lens is ordered for that eye.

Of course, a spherocylindrical overrefraction must be performed before taking the spherical diagnostic lens off the eye. In cases of highly toric corneas, the cylinder within the spectacle refraction is substantially the result of corneal astigmatism and only a minor astigmatic contribution comes from internal astigmatism. In many instances, the overrefraction will yield only a small cylindrical component.

The cylindrical correction in the overrefraction (residual astigmatism) should be equal to the internal astigmatism of the eye, but this concept is confused by the fact that "rigid" spherical GP trial lenses actually flex on toric corneas. The optics of rigid lens flexure was covered in detail earlier, but in practical terms flexure is considered to lessen the correction of corneal astigmatism by decreasing the minus power of the "lacrimal lens" in the steep meridian. The result of flexure can be to overestimate the amount of with-the-rule cylinder showing through an assumed "inflexible" spherical GP trial lens. If the cylinder in the overrefraction does not match the predicted residual astigmatism, over-K can be performed to see how much flexure is occurring. Because the back-toric lenses to be ordered will match corneal toricity more closely, they will not flex as much as spherical trial lenses on the eye. In fact, usually, back-toric lenses do not flex much. The front surfaces of back-surface toric lenses are toric in nearly all instances, hence, the term *bitoric* and the implication that over-K cannot be as practically used to verify the degree of on-eye bitoric lens flexure.

The overall diameter and/or the optic zone diameter of the final contact lens prescription may require alteration according to the fit and centration of the diagnostic lens. To a large extent, selection of these parameters will be influenced by the corneal diameter, pupil diameter, and eyelid anatomy of the individual eye. Normally, a good job of determining the toric base curves and powers of the final lens can be achieved with a spherical GP diagnostic lens if the corneal toricity is less than 4 DC. Sometimes a second lens will need to be ordered when the evaluation of lens fit and overrefraction are updated after the original ordered lens is dispensed. If the corneal toricity is greater than 4 DC, the original order may be treated as a diagnostic lens or the fitting may be performed from a set of bitoric trial lenses as mentioned later. A theoretical maximum limit is the ability to manufacture toric GP lenses, at about 10 DC of back-surface toricity. Below 6 DC of toricity can be easily produced, but above 6 DC the laboratory will have a harder time of it. Therefore, about 12 to 15 DC of corneal toricity is all that may be corrected with GP contact lenses, unless the toricity is concentrated centrally so that in the periphery the lenses ride on portions of the cornea that are of considerably less toricity.

"Spherical Power Effect" Bitoric Trial Lenses

"Connoisseurs" of back-toric GP lenses will have one or two fitting sets of special *"spherical power effect"* (SPE) bitoric lenses available. The optics of these lenses were covered in detail in Chapter 7A, but suffice it to say here that the front surfaces of these lenses are made so as to produce the same optical effect on the eye as would an inflexible spherical lens. If a refraction is performed over an SPE bitoric, the same answer is obtained as if the refraction were performed over an inflexible spherical lens having the same overall parameters as the flat meridian of the bitoric. SPE trial sets will have back-surface toricities of 2 D, 3 D, or 4 D, and they make great diagnostic lenses because an accurate overrefraction can be achieved without worrying about how the lenses rotate on the eye. When an SPE bitoric rotates on

the eye, there is no "in-eye" cylinder power to rotate with it! A more accurate estimate of the fluorescein pattern (compared to a spherical trial lens) can be made and the base curves more accurately prescribed in the vertical and horizontal meridians in order to achieve the final lens performance that is desired. SPE lenses can easily be identified because the back-surface toricity, in keratometric diopters, is equal to the refractive cylinder of the lens measured in air with the lensometer.

Using SPE trial lenses for a lid-attachment fit, a diagnostic lens would be selected that has two-thirds or three fourths of the corneal toricity and a base curve in the flat meridian that is in alignment with or slightly steeper than that of the cornea. For an interpalpebral fit, a lens would be selected that essentially matches the central K readings or, perhaps, is slightly steeper. Basically, a lens is selected from the fitting set that is as close as possible to the predicted best fit. Because the SPE lens fits better than a spherical lens on the highly toric cornea and because the SPE lens fits in a manner more representative of the final lens to be ordered, the clinician's estimate about how much flatter or steeper the two major meridians must be fitted in order to obtain the best final lens performance will be more accurate. This will be of even more importance in the fitting of corneas having toricity greater than 4 D. Before taking the lens off the cornea, a spherocylindrical overrefraction must be performed. Comfort of the SPE bitoric lens will be better than that of a spherical lens, and as a result the refraction over an SPE lens should be more accurate due to reduced reflex tearing. As with spherical trial lenses, in many instances, the spherocylindrical refraction over an SPE bitoric lens will yield only a small cylindrical component equivalent to the internal astigmatism of the eye.

Selecting the Peripheral Curves for Back-Toric Gas Permeable Lenses

Much has been said about the benefits of rigid lenses with spherical base curve and toric peripheral curves versus rigid lenses with toric base curves and spherical peripheral curve versus rigid lenses having toric central and peripheral surfaces. From a practical point of view, it is a rare cornea that is best fitted with a spherical optic zone but needs a toric back peripheral zone. This cornea would have little toricity centrally and a lot of toricity peripherally. Likewise, it would be a rare cornea that is best fitted with a toric central back surface but not also a toric back peripheral zone. Perhaps this cornea would be very toric centrally but have only minor toricity peripherally. All other highly toric corneas will require a toric back optic zone and a toric back peripheral zone for best fit.

The author follows the same empirically derived rule of thumb for toric peripheral curves as was described for spherical peripheral curves, keeping the same difference between radii of curvature of the two primary meridians in the periphery as in the optic zone. In this way the junctions between the optic zone, secondary curve, and peripheral curve are concentric and circular. Back lens surfaces are tricurve designs in which each primary meridian has an axial edge lift of 0.08 to 0.10 mm

If, when the diagnostic spherical or SPE lens fit on the individual cornea is assessed, it is seen that the peripheral edge clearance is less or more than what might be expected for the average cornea, the peripheral curves may be flattened or steepened accordingly. Upon dispensing of the initial back-toric prescription, the peripheral curve selection may be further assessed and modified appropriately the next time a lens is ordered for the eye. An order form showing the data for two lenses prescribed in Example 9 (right eye) and Example 10 (left eye) is included in Fig. 7B.11.

Ordering the Final Refractive Powers

Back-toric GP lenses obey all of the optical principles that were expressed for spherical GP lenses. All that is necessary is to pay a little more attention to refractive power in each primary meridian. The keratometry measurements of the eye being fitted, the pertinent parameters of the diagnostic contact lens, the central back-surface parameters of the contact lens to be ordered, and the spectacle refraction of the eye referred to the corneal plane should already be known so that the *basic information* section of the *Rigid Lens "Form 1040"* can be filled out. Then, *two* estimates of the final CLP in both meridians are made, as described previously for spherical rigid lenses. The last evaluation of refractive power is a comparison of the first and second estimates and prescription of the final CLP based on an evaluation of the credibility of those two initial estimates.

Example 9: Spherical Power Effect

Let us look at Example 9 shown in Fig. 7B.12, with the basic information as listed in the upper section of the document. The corneal cylinder was equal to refractive cylinder, so we expect no internal (residual) cylinder to show up in a refraction over the diagnostic lens, which was a -3.00 spherical GP lens with a base curve of 7.90 mm. However, an overrefraction of $+1.50 - 1.00 \times 180$ was obtained. The toric base curves that were selected on the basis of the diagnostic lens fit were 7.90 and 7.63 mm.

The practitioner would proceed to compute the first and second final CLP estimates from the data accumulated and according to the established equations shown on the Rigid Lens "Form 1040." Perhaps he or she would identify the fact that some flexure of the spherical diagnostic lens could account for the discrepancy between the two final power estimates in the vertical meridian and measure over-K readings to see if flexure did, indeed, exist. Let us assume that the over-K readings indicated that the spherical diagnostic lens was flexing by 1.00 D. This would not be expected for a final back toric lens that would be more closely aligned with the toric central corneal curvature. Thus, the final CLP was selected to be closer to the second estimate in the hopes that the back-toric rigid contact lens would not flex nearly as much as the diagnostic lens.

The reader will note that the final contact lens found in this example is very nearly a bitoric lens having the SPE on the eye. The final lens power is only 0.25 DC away from being equal to the back-surface toricity in diopters. When this lens rotates on the eye, only 0.25 DC of cylinder will rotate with the lens, a negligible amount that will go unnoticed by the patient.

CONTACT LENS ORDER FORM

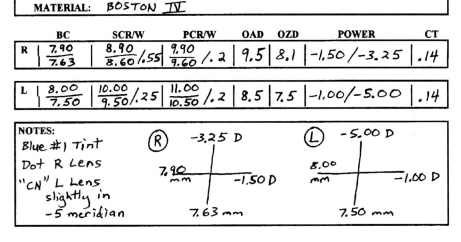

FIG. 7B.11. Contact lens order form filled out for the lenses prescribed in Example 9 (right eye) and Example 10 (left eye). The meridional refractive powers and radii of curvature have been spelled out (*bottom*) in case the laboratory encounters some confusion concerning the parameters listed in the boxes (*top*). The prescription in the left eye calls for a slight "CN bevel" to be applied to the periphery of the most minus meridian. (From Benjamin WJ. Contact lenses: clinical function and practical optics. In: Benjamin WJ, ed. *Borish's clinical refraction.* Philadelphia: WB Saunders, 1998: 956–1021, with permission.)

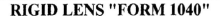

RIGID LENS "FORM 1040"

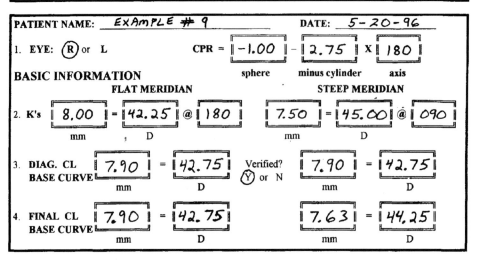

PATIENT NAME: *EXAMPLE # 9*   **DATE:** *5-20-96*

1. **EYE:** Ⓡ or L   CPR = | -1.00 | - | 2.75 | X | 180 |

BASIC INFORMATION   sphere   minus cylinder   axis

FLAT MERIDIAN   STEEP MERIDIAN

2. **K's** | 8.00 | = | 42.25 | @ | 180 | | 7.50 | = | 45.00 | @ | 090 |
    mm   D   mm   D

3. **DIAG. CL BASE CURVE** | 7.90 | = | 42.75 | Verified? Ⓨ or N | 7.90 | = | 42.75 |
    mm   D   mm   D

4. **FINAL CL BASE CURVE** | 7.90 | = | 42.75 | | 7.63 | = | 44.25 |
    mm   D   mm   D

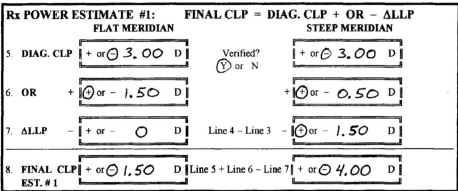

Rx POWER ESTIMATE #1:   **FINAL CLP = DIAG. CLP + OR − ΔLLP**

FLAT MERIDIAN   STEEP MERIDIAN

5. **DIAG. CLP** | + or ⊖ 3.00 D | Verified? Ⓨ or N | + or ⊖ 3.00 D |

6. **OR** + | ⊕ or - 1.50 D | + | ⊕ or - 0.50 D |

7. **ΔLLP** − | + or - 0 D | Line 4 − Line 3 − | ⊕ or - 1.50 D |

8. **FINAL CLP EST. # 1** | + or ⊖ 1.50 D | Line 5 + Line 6 − Line 7 | + or ⊖ 4.00 D |

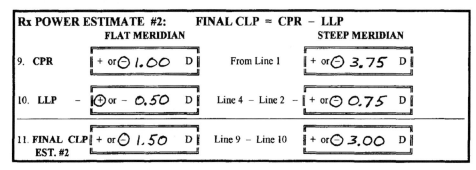

Rx POWER ESTIMATE #2:   **FINAL CLP = CPR − LLP**

FLAT MERIDIAN   STEEP MERIDIAN

9. **CPR** | + or ⊖ 1.00 D | From Line 1 | + or ⊖ 3.75 D |

10. **LLP** − | ⊕ or - 0.50 D | Line 4 − Line 2 − | + or ⊖ 0.75 D |

11. **FINAL CLP EST. #2** | + or ⊖ 1.50 D | Line 9 − Line 10 | + or ⊖ 3.00 D |

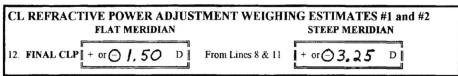

CL REFRACTIVE POWER ADJUSTMENT WEIGHING ESTIMATES #1 and #2

FLAT MERIDIAN   STEEP MERIDIAN

12. **FINAL CLP** | + or ⊖ 1.50 D | From Lines 8 & 11 | + or ⊖ 3.25 D |

FIG. 7B.12. Worksheet filled out for Example 9, a lid-attachment fitting on the right eye of a 2.75 DC with-the-rule toric cornea. Note that between two thirds and three fourths of the corneal toricity has been prescribed in the back surface of the contact lens. (From Benjamin WJ. Contact lenses: clinical function and practical optics. In: Benjamin WJ, ed. *Borish's clinical refraction.* Philadelphia: WB Saunders, 1998:956–1021, with permission.)

Example 10: Cylindrical Power Effect

Let us look at Example 10 shown in Fig. 7B.13, with the basic information as listed in the upper section of that document. The corneal cylinder was not equal to refractive cylinder, so we expect some internal (residual) cylinder to show up in a refraction over the diagnostic lens, which was an SPE bitoric with power of ± 2.75 D and base curves of 8.00 and 7.50 mm. An overrefraction of $-1.00 -1.25 \times$ 180 was obtained. The toric base curves that were selected for the final prescription on the basis of the static and dynamic fluorescein patterns of the diagnostic lens were 8.00 and 7.50 mm for an interpalpebral fit in which the base curves matched the central corneal curvatures.

The practitioner would proceed to compute the first and second final CLP estimates from the data accumulated and according to the established equations shown on the Rigid Lens "Form 1040." In this case, an uncommon instance occurred: both estimates came out the same! Thus, the final CLP would be -1.00 DS with -4.00 DC of cylinder in the steep meridian.

The reader will note that the final contact lens found in this example is a back toric lens having a *"cylindrical power effect"* (CPE) on the eye. The final lens power is 1.25 DC away from being equal to back-surface toricity in diopters. When this lens rotates on the eye, 1.25 DC of the cylinder will rotate with the lens, a significant amount that could be noticed by the patient. More attention must be paid to lenses that have 1.00 DC or more effective cylindrical power so that stable lens rotation is achieved in a manner to obtain the correct axis orientation for the effective cylinder. Fortunately, *corneal astigmatism accounts for the majority of refractive astigmatism in cases where back-toric lenses are needed,* so internal cylinder rotating with the CPE lens usually is small and relatively insignificant. In cases where significant effective cylinder power could be prescribed, one technique suggested is to bias the spherocylindrical contact lens power in the direction of the SPE, thus reducing the amount of effective "on-eye" cylinder.

It turns out that there is a peculiarity about the final contact lens in Example 10; the back surface of this lens corrects for all of the refractive cylinder in this case. Thus, the front surface of the lens must be spherical. The final contact lens is a back-toric/front-surface sphere, technically not a bitoric lens but nevertheless representative of CPE. It often is unrecognized that the term *back-surface toric,* rather than *bitoric,* is a more accurate descriptor of the kind of rigid contact lens covered in this section.

Front-Surface Design: Adjusting for Incorporation of Refractive Power

The final CLP in Example 9 was in the low minus range and would not greatly influence the fitting and rotation of the final lenses in comparison to the diagnostic lens, which

was of similar power. Because the lens was nearly an "SPE" bitoric anyway, an amount of unexpected lens rotation would have little effect on the optical correction of the ametropia. However, when the refractive powers of the final contact lens will be different than those of the diagnostic lens, it is necessary to make an educated guess as to the manner in which the final lens may fit differently and try to compensate for any adverse differences by adjusting the design of the back-toric lens. With respect to vertical lens centration, this process of compensating for expected problems created by incorporation of the final power is similar to that used in prescribing spherical GP lenses!

There are no great mysteries about the adjustments and compensations for final refractive power in the vertical centration of back-toric lenses that have not been covered in more detail elsewhere with respect to spherical lenses. In the past, however, manufacturers were not prepared to add a lenticular flange to the front surface of a bitoric GP lens, although a flange could be produced for the rare case in which a back-toric/front-surface sphere (Example 10) was necessary. Today, on the other hand, lenses with front-surface toricity can be manufactured in plus lenticular designs due to improvements in computer control and precision of lathing. For a lid-attachment fit, minus lenses that are less minus than about -2.00 D and especially lenses having plus power will likely require a plus lenticular construction in which a minus carrier is used to obtain greater lid attachment. The more pronounced the minus carrier prescribed, the more eyelid attachment will be obtained in order to vertically center the lens. The lens also can be fitted slightly flatter than normal in order to enhance lid attachment.

In the case of an interpalpebral fit, plus lenticular designs with a plano carrier or minus carrier may be prescribed to decrease lens mass and thickness of lenses having powers greater than $+2.00$ D. In this case, lenticularization could help compensate for inferior lens centration as a result of excessive mass of full-cut plus lenses. As the interpalpebral design may have already been steepened slightly to obtain centration of the diagnostic lens, further steepening of the fit could result in tear fluid stagnation and poor central corneal physiology. A difference in the design of back-toric lenses, compared to spherical lenses, is that the clinician has the powers of two primary meridians to worry about instead of only a single power for the entire lens. Thus, lenticularization may be required even though the final refractive power of only one of the meridians may have a predictably adverse impact on the manner in which the lens centers on the eye. Plus lenticularization has the added advantage of thinning the central optic cap, allowing greater oxygenation to the cornea under the center of the GP lens where tear fluid exchange is least efficient.

More often, however, contact lens practitioners run into the problem of prescribing significantly more minus power than was in the diagnostic lens, such that the upper lid is expected to attach too aggressively to the final lens. In these

RIGID LENS "FORM 1040"

PATIENT NAME: EXAMPLE # 10   **DATE:** 5-20-96

1. **EYE:** R or Ⓛ   CPR = | -1.00 | - | 4.00 | X | 180 |

                             sphere   minus cylinder   axis

BASIC INFORMATION

          FLAT MERIDIAN   **STEEP MERIDIAN**

2. **K's** | 8.00 | = | 42.25 | @ | 180 | | 7.50 | = | 45.00 | @ | 090 |

           mm   D   mm   D

3. **DIAG. CL** | 8.00 | = | 42.25 | Verified? | 7.50 | = | 45.00 |
BASE CURVE   Ⓨ or N

           mm   D   mm   D

4. **FINAL CL** | 8.00 | = | 42.25 | | 7.50 | = | 45.00 |
BASE CURVE

           mm   D   mm   D

Rx POWER ESTIMATE #1:   **FINAL CLP = DIAG. CLP + OR – ΔLLP**

          FLAT MERIDIAN   **STEEP MERIDIAN**

5. **DIAG. CLP** | + or –   0   D | Verified? | + or ⊖ 2.75 D |
                                   Ⓨ or N

6. **OR**   + | + or ⊖ 1.00 D | + | + or ⊖ 2.25 D |

7. **ΔLLP**   – | + or –   0   D | Line 4 – Line 3   – | + or –   0   D |

8. **FINAL CLP** | + or ⊖ 1.00   D | Line 5 + Line 6 – Line 7 | + or ⊖ 5.00 D |
EST. # 1

Rx POWER ESTIMATE #2:   **FINAL CLP = CPR – LLP**

          FLAT MERIDIAN   **STEEP MERIDIAN**

9. **CPR** | + or ⊖ 1.00   D | From Line 1 | + or ⊖ 5.00 D |

10. **LLP**   – | + or –   D | Line 4 – Line 2 – | + or –   D |

11. **FINAL CLP** | + or ⊖ 1.00   D | Line 9 – Line 10 | + or ⊖ 5.00 D |
EST. #2

CL REFRACTIVE POWER ADJUSTMENT WEIGHING ESTIMATES #1 and #2

          FLAT MERIDIAN   **STEEP MERIDIAN**

12. **FINAL CLP** | + or ⊖ 1.00   D | From Lines 8 & 11 | + or ⊖ 5.00 D |

FIG. 7B.13. Worksheet filled out for Example 10, an interpalpebral fitting on the left eye of a 2.75 DC with-the-rule toric cornea. Note that the full corneal toricity has been prescribed in the back surface of the contact lens. (From Benjamin WJ. Contact lenses: clinical function and practical optics. In: Benjamin WJ, ed. *Borish's clinical refraction*. Philadelphia: WB Saunders, 1998:956–1021, with permission.)

instances, a minus lenticular design is used, with special emphasis on the most minus meridian. Starting at about −5.00 D of power, the clinician may prescribe a CN bevel, which is a form of minus lenticular that is easy for the laboratory to manufacture using cone tools. In Fig. 7B.11, the order for the left lens calls for a CN bevel. Laboratories, however, will determine the actual parameters of the CN bevel, and the practitioner will have to accept the consequences of not defining the front surface more specifically. The practitioner may be willing to accept those consequences with lens powers in the −5 to −7 D range, but the author gets increasingly uneasy with the use of CN bevels as the refractive power mounts above this range, especially when dealing with back-toric lenses. Therefore, above 8 D of minus power the exact front-surface design should be specified in the most minus meridian, to include the front optic zone diameter, junction thickness, and uncut edge thickness that are derived using a computerized lens design program. One caveat here is that the specified uncut edge thickness of the lenticularized most minus meridian must be the same or less than the predicted uncut edge thickness of the least minus meridian before lenticularization. An example of a back-toric lens order having these ingredients is shown in Fig. 7B.14. The uncut edge thicknesses listed for the lenticularized most minus meridians are equivalent to the uncut edge thicknesses of the unlenticularized least minus meridians. Were the edge thicknesses specified to be lower than those of the unlenticularized least minus meridians, the least minus meridians would become lenticularized as well.

For the interpalpebral fit, the edges of nonlenticularized high-minus lenses are uncomfortable because they are thick. These lenses tend to move excessively during the blink and can be driven inferiorly on the cornea by the upper eyelid margin. A CN bevel or minus lenticular design may be prescribed to allow the lid to more easily slide over the upper lens edge so as to enhance comfort, reduce vertical movement of the lens on the blink, and/or avoid pushing the lens inferiorly on the cornea. It is worth noting, again, that lenticularization may be required even though the final refractive power of only one of the meridians may have a predictably adverse impact on lens centration and/or comfort. Minus lenticularization has the added advantage of thinning the periphery of a high-minus lens, allowing greater oxygenation to the cornea under the periphery of the GP lens, which is of special importance in the meridian of most minus power.

The edge of an unlenticularized back-toric GP lens is of varying thickness around its circumference, which presents a situation that is greatly different than that of a spherical GP lens. Unfortunately, back-toric rigid lenses will rotate on the eye in response to eyelid forces invoking the "watermelon seed effect" or the "minus carrier effect." *Back-toric lens rotation* on the eye as a result of the equilibrium between these two competing effects can be *seemingly inexplicable* and may not be adequately predictable during the diagnostic fitting session. Although the optical correction will not be significantly affected by rotation of SPE or "near-SPE" bitoric lenses for the majority of bitoric GP lens wearers, as noted earlier in Example 9, visual performance will suffer in those fewer patients wearing misoriented back-toric lenses having significant effective on-eye CPE.

These rotations may be minimized by alteration of the periphery of the contact lens: plus lenticular or minus lenticular designs may be used. Still, when the final lens is dispensed to the patient, lid forces often can rotate the CPE prescription enough to significantly disturb vision. An in-office modification procedure has been recommended for

CONTACT LENS ORDER FORM

TYPE OF LENS:	BITORIC RGP LENSES						
MATERIAL:	FLUOROPERM 60						

	BC	SCR/W	PCR/W	OAD	OZD	POWER	CT
R	7.75 / 7.20	9.00 / 8.40 /.45	10.00 / 9.40 /.2	9.2	7.9	−5.00/−9.00	.15
L	7.80 / 7.40	9.00 / 8.60 /.45	10.00 / 9.60 /.2	9.2	7.9	−4.50/−8.25	.15

NOTES: Blue #1 Tint ; Dot R Lens
MINUS LENTICULAR IN MOST ⊖ MERIDIAN

	Junction Thickness	Uncut Edge Thickness	Front OZD	
R	.35	.22	8.0	mm
L	.33	.21	8.0	mm

FIG. 7B.14. Contact lens order form filled out for lenses prescribed with a minus lenticular design in the most minus (steeper) meridian. In addition to the usual bitoric figures, the exact parameters related to the front-surface design are detailed in the notes (*bottom*). In this case, the uncut edge thicknesses of the lenticularized most minus meridians are the same as the calculated uncut edge thicknesses of the unlenticularized least minus meridians. (From Benjamin WJ. Contact lenses: clinical function and practical optics. In: Benjamin WJ, ed. *Borish's clinical refraction.* Philadelphia: WB Saunders, 1998:956–1021, with permission.)

correction of the rotation of GP lenses from that initially seen on the eye (17). By polishing off peripheral thicknesses at the peripheral points on minus lenses that have been grasped by the upper eyelid, one of the authors (IMB) over many years was able to overcome lens rotation so that the correct CPE axis orientations were achieved. Another method of lessening the visual influence of off-axis effective cylinder is to bias the cylinder power of the final GP lens in the direction of SPE.

Highly Against-the-Rule and Obliquely Toric Corneas

The thickest portion of the minus-powered back-toric lens edge is situated superiorly such that the "minus-carrier effect" most often results when the upper eyelid overhangs onto a *"with-the-rule"* cornea by at least 2 mm. The lens usually is fitted flat in the vertical meridian, which facilitates lid attachment and tear fluid flushing induced by rocking of the lens during the blink. If the refractive power of the lens does not allow lid attachment, we have discussed ways to increase the attachment. If the lens attaches too aggressively, we have discussed ways to decrease the degree of lid attachment. However, the situation is somewhat different when prescribing for *"against-the-rule"* or *"oblique"* corneas.

Prescribing for the Against-the-Rule Cornea

If the base curves of a conventional back-toric lens align with the appropriate *against-the-rule* corneal meridians, the thick portions of the minus lens periphery will be positioned horizontally in the interpalpebral space, and the thin portions of the periphery will be located superiorly and inferiorly. This will likely be excellent for an *interpalpebral fit*, as the upper eyelid should easily slide over the top edge of the lens with minimal effect on lens centration. Because in an interpalpebral fit we have prescribed the full corneal toricity often in a slightly steep manner, the lens should not significantly decenter right or left of the flat (vertical) corneal meridian. The upper lid in a *lid-attachment* fit, which is far more prevalent than the interpalpebral fit, may do one of two things to the conventional minus back-toric lens: (i) the lid could force the lens inferiorly as in the "watermelon seed" effect, such that the opposite of lid attachment occurs; or (ii) with blinking, the upper eyelid could attach strongly to the nasal or temporal portion of the thicker lens edge and rotate the lens considerably off axis. In addition, the lens will have a tendency to decenter right or left away from the flatter vertical corneal meridian.

It is important, accordingly, to alter our fitting philosophy for *lid attachment* of back-toric lenses in cases of against-the-rule corneas. An alignment fit in the vertical (flat) meridian and prescription of the full corneal toricity in the horizontal (steep) meridian should increase the chances of lateral centration, but we will have to forego the beneficial

rocking motion necessary for optimum tear fluid exchange. The fit will be steeper in the vertical meridian than for the equivalent with-the-rule corneal fit, so we will have to concentrate on lid attachment with plus and low-minus lenses by using the minus carrier in a plus lenticular design. The plus lenticular design should also decrease the variation of peripheral thickness around the edge circumference of the lens so that the lens is less prone to off-axis rotation and can be oriented primarily by the match between the toric back surface and the cornea. If our lens is to be of high-minus power, we will not have as much lid attachment to worry about when fitting the against-the-rule cornea, if the least minus meridian orients vertically. We can decrease off-axis rotation by prescribing a minus lenticular design emphasizing its use in the horizontal (more minus) meridian to decrease lid grasp of the otherwise thick lateral edges. Fortunately, back-toric lenses requiring significant CPE are not as prevalent as those nearly exhibiting SPE. As a result, corrections for off-axis lens rotation by prescription of special lens designs and by in-office modification (noted earlier) are not often necessary.

Prescribing for the Obliquely Toric Cornea

Let us assume that the base curves of a conventional back-toric lens align with a flat meridian at 045 and a steep meridian at 135 on the *obliquely toric* right cornea of a patient. The thick portions of the minus lens periphery will be positioned superotemporally and inferonasally, and the thin portions of the periphery will be located superonasally and inferotemporally. In the case of an *interpalpebral fit*, it is likely that the upper eyelid would slide over the superonasal edge of the lens but not as adequately the superotemporal edge. As a result, the lens may rotate and/or decenter inferonasally. The upper lid in a *lid-attachment* fit may do one of two things to the conventional minus back-toric lens. (i) The lid could force the thick superotemporal lens edge inferiorly as in the "watermelon seed" effect, such that counterclockwise lens rotation occurs. In addition, the lens would have a tendency to decenter inferonasally below the flat oblique corneal meridian. (ii) With blinking, the upper eyelid could attach strongly to the thick superotemporal lens edge and rotate the lens in a clockwise fashion. The lens then will have a tendency to decenter superotemporally above the flat oblique corneal meridian.

Again, it is important to alter our fitting philosophy for back-toric lenses in cases of obliquely toric corneas. An alignment fit in the flat meridian and prescription of the full corneal toricity in the steep meridian should increase the chances of lateral and vertical centration. The overall fit will be steeper than for the equivalent with-the-rule lid-attachment fit, so we will have to concentrate on lid attachment with plus and low-minus lenses by using the minus carrier in a plus lenticular design. As with against-the-rule corneas, the plus lenticular design should decrease the variation of peripheral thickness around the edge circumference of the lens so that the lens is less prone to off-axis rotation and can be oriented primarily by the match between the toric back surface and the cornea. If our lens is to be of high-minus power, we can decrease rotation by prescribing a minus lenticular design emphasizing its use in the meridian of most minus power. It may be reiterated that back-toric lenses requiring significant CPE are not as prevalent as those nearly exhibiting SPE. Corrections for off-axis lens rotation by prescription of special lens designs and by in-office modification are not often necessary.

Prescription of Bitoric "Crossed Cylinder" GP Lenses

Up to this point we have been assuming that corneal astigmatism, internal astigmatism, and refractive astigmatism were of the same or similar axis orientation. This is usually a safe assumption to make because corneal astigmatism and refractive astigmatism are often within 10 degrees of each other. A crossed alignment within this range would lead only to a small (less than 0.50 DC) discrepancy in our calculations for refractive correction in the contact lens prescription. It should be remembered that in most cases of high corneal toricity, corneal cylinder is the largest contributor to refractive cylinder, and the influence of internal astigmatism is minor. Even if the internal astigmatism was aligned at an oblique angle with the corneal cylinder, the visual effect of the internal astigmatism could be small. The cylinder axes of corneal and refractive cylinder would still be similar. We proceed with our back-surface toric lens prescription, ignoring the fact that a situation of "crossed cylinders" existed, knowing that a small bit of uncorrected astigmatism would probably not be visually significant. As a general rule, therefore, contact lens practitioners ignore the effect of crossed cylinders when corneal astigmatic correction and refractive astigmatism are *crossed less than 10 degrees*. It is a good idea to always compare the corneal and refractive cylinder axes at the beginning of a back-toric contact lens fitting, in order to screen for more pronounced cases of crossed astigmatic components that could influence your prescription of refractive power.

As the magnitude of internal astigmatism increases, the alignment of corneal cylinder axis and internal cylinder axis becomes more critical. This will be noted by the practitioner when corneal astigmatic correction and refractive astigmatism differ by more than 10 degrees. To the extent that these differ by more than 10 degrees, internal astigmatism will be of greater magnitude relative to corneal astigmatism and/or its axis of cylinder more obliquely oriented with that of corneal astigmatism. When the spherical or SPE bitoric diagnostic lens is placed on the cornea, significant residual astigmatism should be revealed in the overrefraction at an axis oblique to that of corneal cylinder. If you were to add the corneal astigmatic correction calculated from the K readings and the residual cylinder from the overrefraction in the well-known, though complicated manner necessary for crossed cylinders, the resultant should equal the refractive cylinder. A good lens design computer program should have the capability of determining the resultants of crossed cylinders.

As in any other CPE back-toric lens fit, the effective on-eye (residual) cylinder must be added to the front surface of the correction for corneal astigmatism, which is essentially equivalent to an SPE bitoric lens. After all, if there were no residual cylinder, the optimum correction would be an SPE bitoric lens correcting only for corneal astigmatism. The problem is that the axis of residual cylinder is oblique to the astigmatic axis of the toric front surface of the SPE equivalent. The proper front surface of the final CPE prescription must be derived by adding these two crossed cylinder powers together. The primary meridians of the final toric front surface of the CPE lens will not be in alignment with the meridians of the toric back surface, hence the term *crossed cylinder bitoric lens.* Providing the practitioner has the ingenuity to formulate a prescription in the form of a bitoric lens having toric front and back surfaces of different axes, modern lathing processes are able to manufacture bitoric crossed cylinder lenses according to the prescription.

SUMMARY

Prescription of back-toric GP corneal lenses should be done with the knowledge that a second or occasionally even a third lens will be necessary before the eye is optimally fitted. The practitioner must be a little more fanatical about the details of the fitting, be more fastidious about verification of the contact lenses used for diagnosis and prior to dispensing, and make a more extensive educated guess about final lens powers and parameters in comparison to the equivalent spherical GP lens fitting. In addition, if the back-toric lens power deviates slightly from that desired, the practitioner cannot practically alter lens power in the office as with spherical GP lenses. As we discussed earlier, edge thicknesses sometimes can induce seemingly inexplicable lens rotations on the eye in response to eyelid forces, rotations that may not be adequately predictable during the diagnostic fitting session. For these reasons, it reduces the potential for practitioner and patient frustration, on occasion, to order back-surface toric lenses on a "per case" basis. It is a simple matter to avoid undue expectations by more completely educating the patient in the more difficult back-toric cases, for instance, when against-the-rule or obliquely toric corneas also require significant effective on-eye cylinder (CPE). One of the toughest prescriptions in the area of contact lens practice is the bitoric crossed cylinder lens, especially if corneal toricity is oblique or against the rule!

Fortunately, several positive factors work in favor of excellent vision with back-surface toric GP lenses. The overwhelming majority of highly toric corneas are "with the rule," having the most minus optical correction oriented near the vertical meridian. This allows a fitting method that captures the beneficial aspects of lid attachment and allows plenty of tear fluid exchange under the lens. In most cases the bitoric correction approximates SPE. Thus, lens rotations on the cornea usually do not result in visual decrements. Even in cases where significant effective cylinder is present to rotate with the lens, as in CPE, the visual result usually is acceptable until a second lens with adjustments made on the basis of the initial lens fit is received. The magnitude of internal astigmatism usually is minor in comparison to refractive astigmatism in cases of highly toric corneas, and it is the internal cylinder of the eye that composes the effective cylinder of a correcting CPE lens. Today more than in the past, it is possible to adjust the centration and rotation of back-surface toric lenses with plus lenticular and minus lenticular designs, because lenses with toric front surfaces now can be lenticularized. The oxygen permeabilities of GP materials have risen so greatly that lens parameters promoting tear fluid exchange are not as critical as they once were, and the deleterious impacts of lens design and refractive power on corneal oxygenation have been significantly alleviated. Indeed, the potential for success with "bitoric" GP lenses has never been greater! To take advantage of this updated technology, practitioners must be versed in the art and science of rigid lens prescription, and simultaneously they must be eager to take on challenges that entice them to break away from the "soft lens mentality."

CONTACT LENS OPTICS PROBLEMS AND ANSWERS

General Optical Concepts

1. A patient has a spectacle Rx of -11.00 DS at a vertex distance of 11 mm. What is the refractive error referred to the cornea?

Answer: -9.81 DS

2. If the spectacle correction is $+15.00 -5.00 \times 180$ at a vertex distance of 12 mm, what correction is required at the cornea?

Answer: $+18.29 -6.93 \times 180$

3. The following spectacle prescriptions for two ametropic eyes were obtained at a vertex distance of 12 mm: (A) $-5.25 -3.50 \times 010$; (B) $+15.50 -2.25 \times 165$. What are the powers referred to the cornea and rounded to the nearest eighth of a diopter?

Answer: (A) $-5.00 -3.00 \times 010$. (B) $+19.00 -3.25 \times 165$

4. A contact lens has a back-surface radius of 7.80 mm. (A) What is the refractive power of the surface in air if its refractive index is 1.49? (B) What would be the refractive power of the front surface of the tear film in air if it had the same radius of curvature as did the back surface of the

contact lens (7.80 mm)? (C) How do these two values compare to the power of the posterior lens/tear film interface formed at the back surface of this lens?

Answer: (A) -62.82 D. (B) $+43.08$ D. (C) -19.74 D. Their sum is the same as actual power calculated for the interface.

5. A polymethyl methacrylate (PMMA) contact lens has a back vertex power of -3.00 DS, a back-surface radius of 8.00 mm, and a center thickness of 0.15 mm. What is the front-surface radius of this lens?

Answer: 8.46 mm

6. A contact lens has a back-surface radius of 7.50 mm, a center thickness of 0.18 mm, front optic radius of 7.95 mm, and a refractive index of 1.47. What are the vertex powers of this lens?

Answer: BVP = -3.12 D, FVP = -3.07 D

7. You have measured a back-surface bifocal contact lens in a wet cell and know that for this particular lens material the refractive power in air is four times that in water. The lensometer measured -0.37 D when the distance image was in focus and measured $+1.12$ D when the near image was in focus. (A) What is the distance power in air? (B) What is the near "add" *in air?* (C) What is the true add that this lens will correct?

Answer: (A) -1.50 DS. (B) $+6.00$ DS. (C) $+1.50$ DS

8. A back-surface concentric bifocal contact lens is to have a $+2.25$ DS peripheral addition. What posterior peripheral radius is required if the base curve is 7.60 mm, center thickness is 0.21 mm, refractive index is 1.49, and central power is -1.00 DS?

Answer: 8.55 mm

9. If a front-surface concentric bifocal contact lens is to have a $+2.25$ D peripheral add, what anterior peripheral radius is required if the base curve is 7.60 mm, center thickness is 0.21 mm, refractive index is 1.49, and central power is -1.00 DS?

Answer: 7.55 mm if "add" is generated by front vertex power, 7.59 mm if "add" is generated by back vertex power.

10. A patient has a -9.00 DS spectacle correction at a vertex distance of 13 mm. (A) When fitted with contact lenses, will the patient require more or less accommodation for a 40-cm viewing distance than with spectacles? What dioptric amount of accommodation would this patient require (B) with spectacles and (C) with contact lenses when viewing a target 40 cm in front of the spectacle plane?

Answer: (A) More accommodation required with contact lens. (B) Corneal plane accommodation = $+1.95$ D. (C) Corneal plane accommodation = $+2.42$ D

11. A spectacle–contact lens telescope was designed by adding -27.00 DS to a contact lens Rx in order to serve as an eyepiece. This now requires a $+19.25$ DS spectacle lens to serve as the objective lens for distance viewing. Calculate (A) the magnification of the telescope and (B) the vertex distance required by the spectacle lenses.

Answer: (A) $1.4\times$. (B) 14.9 mm

12. A patient being fitted with a gel contact lens has the following Rx: $-6.00 -0.62 \times 165$ at a vertex distance of 15 mm. What is (A) the corneal plane refraction and (B) the expected equivalent sphere power required for the contact lens?

Answer: (A) $-5.50 -0.50 \times 165$. (B) -5.75 DS

13. In the problem above, the spectacle Rx was made of resin (n = 1.50), $+3.75$ base curve, and 2.0-mm center thickness. The contact lens has a 0.08-mm center thickness, n = 1.45, and the base curve is 8.60 mm on the eye. Using equivalent spherical correction, calculate the spectacle magnification (A) when wearing spectacles and (B) when wearing contact lenses. (C) What is the net change in magnification when this eye switches from spectacles to contact lenses? (D) What is the net change in magnification attributable only to the power factors when switching from spectacles to contact lenses?

Answer: (A) 0.902, or -9.8% (minification). (B) 0.986, or -1.4% (minification). Note: Use power factor only. (C) $+8.4\%$ (magnification). (D) 1.1035, or $+10.35\%$ (magnification)

14. Gullstrand's exact schematic eye has been fitted with a contact lens made of a material having a refractive index of 1.53. (A) What is the increase of relative intensity (in percent) for the "corneal reflex" visible when the contact lens is worn in comparison to when it is not?

Answer: 43% increase (3.0% vs 2.1%.) Hint: Use Fresnel's Formula for Reflection.

15. In its rigid form, unhydrated, a hydrophilic material has a refractive index of 1.49. The contact lens to be made of the material requires a water content of 37.5%. What will be the refractive index of the hydrated contact lens material?

Answer: $n' = 1.43$

16. A patient's cornea has become swollen to the point that visual acuity has decreased. A biopsy of the stroma and resultant analysis shows the ground substance to have a refractive index of 1.348. Assuming that all other refractive indices and proportional contributions of stromal components remain the same as in a transparent cornea, what is the refractive index of the swollen stroma?

Answer: $n' = 1.368$ Hint: Use Principle of Gladstone and Dale.

17. K readings for an eye are 41.50/46.75 @ 180. (A) What is the actual refractive astigmatism at the cornea that is a result of the difference between primary meridians? (B) What is the estimated refractive astigmatism encountered at the *posterior* corneal surface?

Answer: (A) -5.85 DC $\times$ 090. (B) $+0.60$ DC $\times$ 090. Hint: n = 1.3375 was used for the keratometer instead of n = 1.376 to account for the power of the posterior cornea.

18. A rigid gas permeable contact lens has a base curve of 7.90 mm, center thickness of 0.15 mm, back vertex power of -4.00 D, and refractive index of 1.47. (A) What are the vertex focal lengths of this lens? (B) What would the front-surface radius have to be in order for the lens be of zero back vertex power?

Answer: (A) $f_{BVP} = -250$ mm, $f_{FVP} = +253$ mm. (B) 7.95 mm

19. The refractive index of a dry button of gel material is 1.49. It is to be made into a finished hydrophilic contact lens that, when hydrated, will have a center thickness of 0.07 mm, back vertex power of -8.50 D, and base curve of 8.80 mm. (A) If the water content of hydrated material is 38.6%, what is the refractive index of the hydrated lens? (B) What is the radius of curvature of the front surface (hydrated)? (C) What is the front vertex power of the hydrated lens? (D) What would be the back vertex power of the lens (as if in air) when placed on a cornea having a K reading of 43.00 D? Assume that the front surface flexes an amount equal to that of the back surface and that the lens completely conforms to the cornea. (E) What would be the back vertex power of the lens (as if in air) when placed on the same cornea, but assuming flexure maintains equal center thickness and lens volume?

Answer: (A) n = 1.43. (B) 10.67 mm. (C) -8.45 D. (D) -10.44 D This is not representative of the real power of the lens on the eye. (E) -8.57 D. This is a small change, into the minus, which is more representative of the change that actually occurs.

20. A patient has a spectacle prescription of R $+7.50 -4.00 \times 180$ and L -5.00 DS at a vertex distance of 13 mm and views an object 40 cm in front of the spectacle plane. (A) What is the monocular accommodative imbalance at the corneal plane between primary meridians of the right eye? (B) What are the binocular accommodative imbalances at the corneal plane between eyes for the horizontal and vertical meridians? (C) If rigid contact lenses were fitted that excellently corrected the patient's ametropias, what accommodative imbalances would remain at the corneal plane between meridians and between eyes?

Answer: (A) 0.30 D (horizontal meridian greater). (B) 0.82 D and 0.52 D, respectively (R eye greater). (C) None would exist; however, slight accommodative imbalances would remain at the lenticular plane.

21. The same patient as in problem 20 has presented to your office. K readings are R 44.50/49.12 @ 090 and L 44.50 DS. (A) What are the differences of relative spectacle magnification between the two eyes in the horizontal and vertical meridians when corrected with spectacles? (B) Spectacle base curves are R $+13.00$ DS, L $+4.00$ DS, and center thicknesses are R 5.5 mm, L 2.0 mm. The refractive index of these lenses is 1.49. What are the differences of spectacle magnification between the two eyes in the horizontal and vertical meridians? (C) If contact lenses are fitted that optimally correct the patient's ametropia, what are the differences of relative spectacle magnification between the two eyes in the horizontal and vertical meridians? (D) Considering only the power factor, what will be the differences of spectacle magnification between the two eyes in the hori-

zontal and vertical meridians when corrected with contact lenses?

Answer: (A) 3.35% (R eye smaller) horizontally and 13.3% (R eye larger) vertically. Hint: K readings indicate anisometropia to be of axial origin in horizontal meridian but refractive in the vertical meridian. Note that vertex distance is not 15.7 mm; thus, slight aniseikonia exists even for axial anisometropia corrected with spectacles. (B) 26.3% (R larger) horizontally and 18.2% (R larger) vertically. Hint: Use shape and power factors. Note that the origin of anisometropia does not enter into calculations. (C) 19.5% (R eye smaller) horizontally and 2.5% (R eye larger) vertically. Hint: Refer power to the cornea. Note that contact lenses reduce aniseikonia for refractive anisometropes but do the opposite for axial problems. (D) 3.9% (R larger) horizontally and 2.5% (R larger) vertically. Hint: Refer to cornea, and remember that d = 0.003 m.

22. A conventional monocurve rigid contact lens has a front-surface sagitta of 1.80 mm and a diameter of 9.5 mm. Two prism diopters ($^\Delta$) of prism are to be added to the Rx (base down). The thickness of the lens edge at the prism apex is to be 0.10 mm, refractive index is 1.49, and base curve is 7.80 mm. (A) What are the center thickness, thickness of the lens at the base of prism, and front-surface radius? (B) What is the back vertex power at the apex, center, and base of the lens? (C) What is the prismatic power at the apex and base of the lens compared to the center?

Answer: (A) 0.49 mm, 0.49 mm, and 7.17 mm, respectively. Hint: Thicknesses are result of contributions from prism and sagittas. (B) +5.83 D, +7.09 D, and +7.09 D, respectively. Note: BVP alters vertically across lens due to thickness. (C) 4.8$^\Delta$ BD, 2.0$^\Delta$ BD, and 1.4$^\Delta$ BU, respectively. Hint: Total prism is 2.0$^\Delta$ BD plus that added by Prentice's Rule at each point. Note: Prismatic power varies vertically across lens.

23. An emmetropic low-vision patient requires the use of a spectacle–contact lens telescope. You believe that 1.5× is an excellent magnification to obtain for this patient and have the availability of prescribing up to a −40 D contact lens. (A) The patient's spectacle frame allows only a 15-mm vertex distance. What is the maximum magnification that you can obtain and with what power of spectacle lens? (B) If you fit the patient with a frame that has adjustable pads, in which a vertex distance of 20 mm is attainable, what is the lowest power of spectacle lens that you can use and still obtain 1.5× magnification?

Answer: (A) 1.6×, with +25.00 D spectacle lens and −40.00 D contact lens. (B) +16.67 D, with contact lens of −25.00 D.

Lacrimal Lens Problems

24. A patient who wears a rigid lens on one eye has come in for a check-up after 7 years without otherwise visiting your office. The lens was fit over a central corneal graft that originally had an average K reading of 47.00 DS and now has a K reading of 43.00 DS, yet the patient still wears the same lens. For smaller amounts of corneal shape alteration, the lacrimal lens should "mask" nearly all refractive changes as long as the rigid lens is worn. However, for very large K changes the lacrimal lens theory may not completely predict changes in the overrefraction and the optimum rigid lens Rx. In this case, what overrefraction could have resulted from the K change noted?

Answer: +0.47 DS

25. If a patient has a K reading of 43.00 @ 180, 43.00 @ 090, a spectacle Rx of −3.00 DS, and is fitted with a lens with a base curve of 7.60 mm, what power is needed in the contact lens?

Answer: −4.37 DS

26. If a patient has a K reading of 44.00 @ 180, 44.00 @ 090, a spectacle Rx of −4.00 DS, and is fitted with a lens with a base curve of 7.60 mm, what power is needed in the contact lens?

Answer: −4.37 DS

27. A patient has on his eye a diagnostic lens with a 7.50-mm base curve and power of −1.50 DS. A refraction over the lens indicates the need for an additional −1.25 DS, and the practitioner's analysis of the fit indicates that a base curve of 7.40 mm would be better. (A) What refractive power is required if the 7.40-mm base curve is ordered? (B) If the patient required a lens with a base curve of 7.55 mm, what refractive power would be needed?

Answer: (A) −3.36 DS. (B) −2.47 DS

28. A patient has K readings of 45.00 @ 180, 47.00 @ 090, a spectacle Rx of −1.00 −2.00 × 180, and is fitted with a lens with a base curve of 7.50 mm. (A) What power is needed in the contact lens? (B) Did corneal toricity match refractive cylinder in this case?

Answer: (A) −1.00 DS. (B) Yes

29. A patient has K readings of 46.00 @ 180, 47.50 @ 090, a spectacle Rx of −2.00 −1.50 × 180, and is fitted with a lens with a base curve of 7.18 mm. What power is needed in the contact lens?

Answer: −3.00 DS

30. A patient has K readings of 44.00 @ 180, 45.50 @ 090, a spectacle Rx of +2.00 −2.00 × 180, and is fitted with a base curve of 7.50 mm. (A) What spherical power is needed in the contact lens, and (B) what is the amount of residual astigmatism? (C) Did corneal toricity match refractive cylinder in this case?

Answer: (A) +0.75 DS, equivalent sphere. (B) −0.50 DC × 180. (C) No

31. A patient has a K reading of 45.00 DS, a spectacle prescription of −2.00 DS, and is to be fitted with a rigid lens (n = 1.49) with a base curve of 7.40 mm. What power would be required in the contact lens?

Answer: −2.61 DS

32. A patient has a spectacle prescription of −2.25 −0.50 × 180 and K readings of 45.00 @ 180, 45.50 @

090. If a 7.40-mm base curve contact lens is fitted to this eye, (A) what power should be ordered, and (B) how much residual astigmatism is expected? (C) Did corneal toricity match refractive cylinder?

Answer: (A) − 2.86 DS. (B) None. (C) Yes.

33. The spectacle prescription of a patient is + 12.00 DS measured at a vertex distance of 14 mm, and his K reading is 42.00 DS. He is to be fitted with a contact lens with base curve 7.89 mm. What power should be ordered in the contact lens?

Answer: + 13.65 DS

34. If a patient is wearing a 7.85-mm base curve, − 4.00 DS corneal lens and the overrefraction is − 1.25 DS, what power should be ordered in a new lens with a 7.71-mm base curve?

Answer: − 6.03 DS

35. If a patient is wearing a 7.42-mm base curve, − 2.50 DS lens and the refraction over the lens is − 0.75 DS, what power should be ordered in the new lens with a 7.50-mm base curve?

Answer: − 2.76 DS

36. A patient's K readings are 42.00 @ 180, 44.00 @ 090, and the spectacle Rx is − 2.00 − 1.00 × 180. What is the predicted residual astigmatism with a spherical (A) rigid contact lens and with a spherical (B) soft contact lens?

Answer: (A) − 1.00 DC × 090. (B) − 1.00 DC × 180

37. Find the predicted overrefraction when a diagnostic rigid contact lens having a base curve of 42.00 D and power of − 2.00 D is used on a patient with a spectacle Rx of − 3.00 − 0.50 × 175 and K readings of 41.75 @ 180, 43.00 @ 090.

Answer: − 0.50−0.75 × 095 or 090

38. A patient's eye has K readings of 43.00 @ 180, 45.00 @ 090, a spectacle Rx of − 1.00 − 2.00 × 180, and is being fitted with a lens with a base curve of 7.76 mm. Your over-K readings are 42.50 @ 180, 43.50 @ 090. (A) What is your expected refraction over a − 1.50 DS diagnostic lens? (B) Did corneal toricity match refractive cylinder in this case?

Answer: (A) pl − 1.00 × 180. (B) Yes

39. An eye has been fitted with a rigid contact lens having a base curve of 7.94 mm and of − 3.00 DS power. The K readings are 42.50 @ 180, 44.00 @ 090, and the spectacle Rx is − 2.00 − 0.75 × 180. (A) Assuming that this lens is inflexible, what is the expected overrefraction for the lens? (B) What would be your recommended refractive power if you were to correct the ametropia with (B) a front-toric rigid lens or (C) a toric soft lens, ignoring rotational and orientation effects on the eye?

Answer: (A) + 1.75 − 0.75 × 090. (B) − 1.25 − 0.75 × 090. (C) − 2.00 − 0.75 × 180

40. Surprise! You ordered a spherical rigid lens with a power of − 1.62 DS according to the spherical equivalent of your overrefraction at the fitting session for the patient in problem 39, and your over-K readings now show at dis-

pensing that the lens is flexing on the eye with the rule by 0.75 D! (A) What is your expected overrefraction? (B) Given that you could order a lens of similar parameters that would flex in an identical manner, what spherical refractive power would you now order?

Answer: (A) − 0.37 DS. (B) − 2.00 DS

41. A patient has a spectacle prescription of − 3.50 − 1.00 × 180. While wearing a rigid contact lens with a base curve of 7.70 mm and of − 2.00 DS, the obtained overrefraction was − 2.00 DS. What are this person's K readings?

Answer: 43.33 @ 180, 44.33 @ 090

42. A soft contact lens is fitted to a patient with K readings of 43.00 @ 180, 44.25 @ 090, and a spectacle Rx of − 3.00 − 0.75 × 180. What residual astigmatism would be expected with the soft lens on the eye?

Answer: − 0.75 DC × 180

43. A 1.00 DS myope with K readings of 45.00 DS is fit with a plano-powered rigid contact lens. What base curve must be used to optimally correct this person's ametropia?

Answer: 7.67 mm

44. A patient initially was fitted with a rigid contact lens having a base curve of 44.00 D and a power of − 3.50 D. It later was necessary to change the base curve to 43.00 D. What power must now be ordered?

Answer: − 2.50 DS

45. Calculate the corneal curvatures using the following:
Spec Rx: − 2.50 − 0.75 × 180
Diagnostic rigid lens: 43.00 BC, − 3.00 Power
Overrefraction: + 0.50 − 1.75 × 090
Answer: 41.25 @ 180, 43.75 @ 090

46. Find the predicted overrefraction when a rigid contact lens with a 42.25 BC and − 3.00 D power is fitted on an eye having the following parameters:
Spec Rx: − 4.50 − 1.00 × 172
Vertex distance: 13 mm
K readings: 44.50 @ 180, 46.25 @ 090
Answer: + 1.87 − 0.87 × 090

47. Suppose that on the eye in problem 46, the overrefraction was − 1.25 − 1.50 × 180. What are the calculated K readings?

Answer: 42.25 @ 180, 41.63 @ 090

48. You have placed an inflexible rigid lens on a 43.50/ 44.00 @ 090 cornea from your fitting set of − 3.00 DS lenses. You meant to place a lens with 7.90-mm base curve on the eye but found out just after the lens was on the patient that your set of trial lenses had been mixed up. (A) If the spectacle Rx was − 2.00 − 1.25 × 180 and the overrefraction was + 1.75 − 0.75 × 180, what was the base curve of the lens that you placed on the eye? (B) Suppose that you thought that the lens looked too "flat," and upon subsequent testing you found that a lens with a 7.70-mm base curve fitted the best. What should be your expected overrefraction with your 7.70-mm base curve trial lens, rounded to the nearest eighth of a diopter? (C) You

could prescribe the "equivalent sphere" Rx and forget about the cylinder in the overrefraction, but you have the ability to increase flexure of the lens by making it thinner. If you could place a lens of the appropriate thickness on the eye such that it would flex to correct for the residual cylinder found with your inflexible trial lens, what amount of cylinder in the over-K readings would be ideal? Is this realistically achievable?

Answer: (A) 7.90 mm. Hint: Use lacrimal lens theory applied to both meridians. Note: Lucky! The correct lens was on the cornea. (B) $+0.62 -0.75 \times 180$. (C) 0.75 DC, steeper in horizontal meridian. No. This cannot be reasonably expected. Hint: Flexure is attributed to meridian of steepest corneal curvature. Lens power does not alter. Flexure can only correct for refractive astigmatism that is not the result of corneal toricity. Had the overrefraction been $+0.62 -0.75 \times 090$ and corneal curvature remained the same, flexure could correct for the refractive cylinder.

49. A patient's eye is $+8.50 -4.50 \times 010$ at a vertex distance of 14 mm and has K readings of 43.50/48.00 @ 100. (A) A $+5.00$ D diagnostic rigid lens with 7.50-mm base curve seems to fit in a reasonable manner, for a spherical lens. What amount of residual astigmatism should show through the overrefraction? (B) The lens flexes on the eye such that 0.50 D of flexure is revealed in the over-K readings. What is the expected overrefraction? (C) To obtain a better fit, you wish to order a bitoric rigid lens. Not having a bitoric diagnostic lens available, you estimate that about 2.50 D of back-surface toricity should be correct and order a lens with back-surface radii of 7.60 and 7.20 mm. What refractive power should you order, assuming that this lens will not flex?

Answer: (A) -0.90 DC $\times 010$. Hint: Refer power to cornea before using lacrimal lens theory. Note: Although it appears that corneal toricity and refractive astigmatism are equal, once referred to the cornea they are not. Astigmatism is not completely masked. (B) $+3.14 -1.40 \times 010$. Hint: Flexure increases power of lacrimal lens into the plus/less minus in the steeper corneal meridian. Flexure in this case, as in most cases, worsens residual astigmatism. (C) $+8.75 -3.37 \times 010$. Note that in most bitoric fits, increasing back toricity necessitates an increase of refractive astigmatic correction in the lens.

Back-Toric Contact Lens Problems

50. A patient has a spectacle prescription of $-0.50 -3.50 \times 180$ and K readings of 42.00 @ 180, 45.00 @ 090. If fitted with a toric base curve of 7.94/7.58 mm, what power must be ordered in the contact lens?

Answer: $-1.00 -2.50 \times 180$, or -1.00 D @ 180/-3.50 D @ 090

51. A refraction over a 7.70-mm base curve rigid diagnostic lens of -3.00 DS power is $-1.75 -1.00 \times 090$. The lens ordered has a toric back surface with radii of 7.50 and 7.90 mm (on a with-the-rule cornea). What lens power should be specified for this lens to correct the patient's refractive error?

Answer: $-4.64 -1.27 \times 180$, or -4.64 D @ 180/-5.91 D @ 090

52. A patient has K readings of 42.00 @ 180, 46.00 @ 090, a spectacle Rx of $-2.00 -5.00 \times 180$ at a vertex distance of 12 mm, and is fitted with a contact lens with base curve radii 7.95 and 7.50 mm. What power is needed in the contact lens?

Answer: $-2.45 -3.00 \times 180$, or -2.45 D @ 180/-5.45 D @ 090

53. A diagnostic lens with a base curve of 7.50 mm and -3.00 DS is placed on a patient's eye, and a refraction over the lens indicates a need for the following additional power: $-0.50 -0.75 \times 090$. The lens to be ordered for this patient is to have a base curve of 7.35/7.70 mm (toric). What power is needed in the contact lens, assuming with-the-rule corneal toricity?

Answer: $-3.08 -1.34 \times 180$, or -3.08 D @ 180/-4.42 D @ 090

54. A patient has K readings of 43.00 @ 180, 46.25 @ 090, a spectacle Rx of $-8.00 -3.50 \times 180$ at a vertex distance of 12 mm, and is fitted with a lens with base curve radii of 7.45 and 7.85 mm. The lens has a diameter of 9.50 mm, optic zone of 7.50 mm, secondary curve radii of 8.45 and 8.85 mm, and center thickness of 0.12 mm. The refractive index of the rigid lens is 1.52. (A) What power should be ordered in the lens, and (B) what front radii are needed?

Answer: (A) $-7.30 -1.86 \times 180$, or -7.30 D @ 180/-9.16 D @ 090. (B) 8.86 mm @ 180, 8.62 mm @ 090

55. A patient has a spectacle prescription of $-10.00 -5.00 \times 180$ at a vertex distance of 12 mm, and K readings of 44.00 @ 180, 49.00 @ 090. If the patient is fitted with spherical rigid lens with a radius of 7.30 mm, (A) what spherical power would be required in the contact lens? (B) What residual astigmatism would be expected? (C) Does corneal toricity match refractive cylinder in this case? (D) Would lens flexure help or hinder in this case?

Answer: (A) -10.55 DS, equivalent sphere. (B) -1.22 DC $\times 090$. (C) Actually, it does not. Once the refractive cylinder is referred to the cornea, it amounts to -3.78 DC $\times 180$, which is less than corneal toricity. (D) Up to 1.25 DC of flexure would help correct the refractive astigmatism

56. If the eye in problem 55 is fitted with a toric base curve lens with radii of 7.55 and 6.96 mm, (A) what power would be required in each meridian to correct the patient's refractive error? (B) This lens is representative of what optical fitting effect? (C) How much cylinder rotates with this lens on the eye?

Answer: (A) -9.63 D @ 180, -12.20 D @ 090. (B) Cylindrical power effect. (C) Approximately 1.25 DC

57. A patient's corneal toricity matches that of the refractive cylinder, yet the toricity does not allow a rigid con-

tact lens with a spherical base curve to fit correctly. K readings are 40.00 @ 180, 44.50 @ 090, and the spectacle refraction is $+1.00 -4.50 \times 180$. With your office fitting set, you estimate that a bitoric lens having base curves of 8.33/7.76 would provide the best fit. (A) What would be the refractive power of the ordered lens (n = 1.47) in air? (B) What would be the power of the lens on the eye, its posterior surface immersed in tear fluid? (C) This lens is an example of what type of optical fitting effect? (D) How much cylinder rotates with this lens on the eye?

Answer: (A) $+0.50 -3.00 \times 180$, or $+0.50$ D @ 180/-2.50 D @ 090. (B) $+40.79$ @ 180, $+40.83$ @ 090 (essentially spherical). (C) Spherical power effect. (D) Almost none; zero

58. A bitoric rigid contact lens has base curve radii of 8.03 and 7.67 mm, and back vertex powers of -1.00 D and -4.00 D in those meridians, respectively. What amount of cylinder power rotates with this lens as it varies rotational orientation on the eye?

Answer: 1.00 DC

REFERENCES

1. Benjamin WJ. Bitoric rigid gas permeable lenses. In: Schwartz CA, ed. *Specialty contact lenses: a fitter's guide.* Philadelphia: WB Saunders, 1995:21–41.
2. Benjamin WJ. Contact lenses: clinical function and practical optics. In: Benjamin WJ, ed. *Borish's clinical refraction.* Philadelphia: WB Saunders, 1998:956–1021.
3. Benjamin WJ. The "explicability" of cylinder axis and power in refractions over toric soft lenses. *Int Contact Lens Clin* 1998;25:89–92.
4. Benjamin WJ. Companion for contact lens optics. In: Bennett ES, Henry VA, eds. *Clinical manual of contact lenses,* 2nd ed. Philadelphia: Lippincott Williams & Wilkins, 2000:34–56.
5. Westin EJ, McDaid K, Benjamin WJ. Inferior corneal vascularization associated with extended wear of prism-ballasted toric hydrogel lenses. *Int Contact Lens Clin* 1989;16:20–23.
6. Snyder C, Daum KM. Rotational position of toric soft contact lenses on the eye—clinical judgments. *Int Contact Lens Clin* 1989;16:146–151.
7. Josephson JE. Locating the central bifocal zone. *Int Eyecare* 1986;2:441.
8. Stephens GL. Correction with single vision lenses. In: Benjamin WJ, ed. *Borish's clinical refraction.* Philadelphia: WB Saunders, 1998:823–887.
9. Pascal JI. Cross cylinder tests—meridional balance technique. *Opt J Rev Optom* 1950;87:31–35.
10. Borish IM, Benjamin WJ. Monocular and binocular subjective refraction. In: Benjamin WJ, ed. *Borish's clinical refraction.* Philadelphia: WB Saunders, 1998:629–723.
11. Linksz A. Determination of axis and amount of astigmatic error by rotation of trial cylinder. *Arch Ophthalmol* 1942;28:632–651.
12. Heiby JC, personal phone communication, fall 1998. Dr. John C. Heiby of St. Clairsville, Ohio, had read the Benjamin reference (3) and astutely noted that the residual cylinder was approximately the addition of 10% of the original cylinder for every 3 degrees of crossed cylinders.
13. Silbert JA. Rigid lens correction of astigmatism. In: Bennett ES, Weissman BA, eds. *Clinical contact lens practice.* Philadelphia: JB Lippincott, , Philadelphia, PA, pp. 1991:1–42.
14. Mandell RB. Toric lenses. In: Mandell RB, ed: *Contact lens practice.* Springfield, IL: Charles C. Thomas Publisher, 1988:284–309.
15. Richardson SS, Benjamin WJ. Oxygen profiles and contact lens design. *Cont Lens Spectrum* 1993;8:57–58.
16. Benjamin WJ, Cappelli QA. Oxygen permeability (Dk) of thirty-seven rigid contact lens materials. *Optom Vis Sci* 2002;79:103–111.
17. Benjamin WJ, Borish IM. Presbyopia and the influence of aging on prescription of contact lenses. In: Ruben CM, Guillon M, eds. *Textbook of contact lens practice.* London, UK: Chapman & Hall, 1994:763–830.

PRELIMINARIES

INITIAL EVALUATION

TIMOTHY B. EDRINGTON AND JULIE A. SCHORNACK

When you begin to evaluate a potential contact lens patient, it is important to consider the major indications and contraindications to contact lens wear. Performing an appropriate screening of contact lens candidates at the front end of the evaluation process is vital in assuring long-term patient success. Providing adequate consultation to patients who have a guarded prognosis or a distinct contraindication to contact lens wear is also an important part of contact lens practice.

INDICATIONS FOR CONTACT LENS WEAR

Refractive Error

Most patients who require a refractive error correction desiring freedom from spectacles or rejecting refractive surgery options can benefit from contact lens wear. Gas permeable (GP) and soft contact lens designs may be prescribed to correct myopia, hyperopia, astigmatism, and presbyopia. GP lenses are available in more design choices and in expanded parameters. A comprehensive case history, corneal curvature assessment, manifest refraction, assessment of binocular vision status, and evaluation of the cornea will determine the appropriateness of prescribing contact lenses for an individual patient. Patients with high amounts of myopia, hyperopia, and astigmatism benefit from reduced visual distortion and enhanced peripheral vision when wearing contact lenses.

Cosmesis

Patients seek contact lenses as a choice for a variety of reasons, including cosmesis. Contact lenses may be prescribed to enhance or change the appearance of the eye. Handling, enhancement, and opaque tints are available. Prosthetic lenses may be prescribed to mask corneas or irides disfigured by trauma or disease. Most prosthetic contact lenses use opaque tints to match the fellow eye's iris color. These lenses can be dispensed to the patient with corrective power or with a blackened central occluder pupil area.

Presbyopia

There are countless soft and GP contact lens prescribing options for presbyopic patients who request a multifocal correction. Patients may wear their distance contact lens correction with a pair of part-time reading glasses for near or intermediate tasks. Or the patient may wear near or intermediate contact lenses with a pair of overcorrection spectacles for distance tasks. Monovision correction, where one eye is prescribed for distance correction and the fellow eye is designated for near correction, is the most commonly applied contact lens option for presbyopia (1). Multifocal correction also is available in both soft and GP materials. Most multifocal contact lenses are either prescribed for simultaneous vision (where both distance and near images are focused on the retina at the same time) or alternating vision (where the distance and near corrections are viewed independently). Many practitioners prescribe modified monovision in which one eye wears a single vision or multifocal design that optimizes distance vision and a single vision or multifocal design that optimizes near vision that is worn in the fellow eye (2).

Irregular Astigmatism

Irregular astigmatism may be induced by corneal conditions such as keratoconus, postrefractory surgery, corneal scarring, and postpenetrating keratoplasty (post-RK). Spherical, aspheric, bitoric, and reverse geometry GP lens designs are prescribed to optimize vision for patients with irregular corneal surfaces (3). The front surface of the GP contact lens creates a smooth refracting surface. The tear lens between the lens base curve and the cornea minimizes the optical distortion caused by the corneal surface irregularity.

Corneal Dystrophies

Some corneal dystrophies (such as Cogan's map-dot-fingerprint dystrophy) may lead to recurrent corneal erosions. Eyelid interaction with the fragile corneal epithelium and the mechanical effects of contact lens application and removal tend to disrupt the epithelium, delaying healing. A soft contact lens prescribed as a "bandage" lens and worn on an extended wear basis often is the best treatment for chronic and recurrent corneal erosions (4).

Amblyopia

An opaque contact lens with a solid black base tint may be used as an occluder contact lens for patients undergoing occlusion therapy for amblyopia (5). The use of a high-plus contact lens can serve the same purpose by blurring the retinal image to a significant degree.

Nystagmus

Patients with nystagmus might benefit from the wear of GP contact lenses to reduce the amplitude of nystagmus. The theory to explain this phenomenon is that the eyelids interact with the lens edge and provide biofeedback to the patient on the movement of the lens. This sensation may enable the patient to reduce the amplitude and frequency of the nystagmus (6). It is not unusual for the effect to diminish as the patient adapts to the feel of the lens over time.

Prism Correction

Prism may be prescribed in contact lenses to correct or reduce a vertical hyperphoria. Base down corrections up to four prism diopters may be achieved in either soft or GP lens designs. Lid interaction with the prism profile and gravity allow for only base down prism corrections in contact lenses. On average, patients accept approximately 0.75

diopters less prism on associated vertical phoria testing through contact lenses compared to spectacles (7,8).

PROCEED WITH CAUTION IN CONTACT LENS WEAR

Pinguecula and Pterygium

The presence of pinguecula and pterygia presents special concerns to contact lens fitting. Prediger and Edmondson surveyed diplomates in the Cornea and Contact Lens Section of the American Academy of Optometry regarding their prescribing habits for patients presenting with pingueculae or pterygia. Ninety-six percent of the respondents had prescribed contact lenses to patients with pingueculae within the previous year. Slightly over half of the practitioners who prescribed contact lenses for patients with pingueculae had no preference between fitting soft or GP contact lenses on these patients. Twenty-nine percent preferred prescribing soft contact lenses, and 19% preferred prescribing GP lenses on patients with pingueculae.

Sixty-four percent of the respondents had prescribed contact lenses for a patient presenting with a pterygium in the previous year. Forty-eight percent of the practitioners who prescribed contact lenses for pterygia patients preferred soft contact lenses, whereas 26% were more likely to prescribe GP lenses (9). In patients with pterygia, care should be taken to monitor changes in corneal topography and keratometry distortion that may be related to progression.

Efforts to minimize the level of conjunctival injection, corneal staining adjacent to the leading edge of the pterygium, and peripheral corneal desiccation will increase the success rate of contact lens wear for these patients.

Dexterity

Contact lens patients should be capable of applying and removing their lenses. Patients with decreased manual dexterity due to physical limitations or restrictions need to make compensations or contact lens wear should be limited. Continuous wear lenses or an available and willing assistant in lens application and removal, as well as lens care, may be needed for lens wear to be possible. These issues are most prevalent in the geriatric and pediatric populations.

Hygiene

Contact lens wear may be ill advised when patients present with poor hygiene or report a clear history of noncompliance with contact lens wear or lens care recommendations. Although patient education can be helpful in correcting many of these issues, the best choice for some patients is to advise against contact lens wear.

Environmental

During the course of taking a case history, information about a patient's work and leisure activities should include environmental details. It is important to educate and make recommendations to patients concerning environments hazardous to contact lens wear. Jobs that have dusty or dirty workplaces may contaminate lenses or decrease lens comfort. Circumstances where noxious fumes are present can produce ocular irritation with or without contact lens wear.

Severe Allergies

Allergies may be present with many degrees of severity. Contact lens wear has a guarded prognosis for patients who report severe ocular allergic reactions on either a continual or seasonal basis. In addition to the overall ocular irritation, the itching, and redness that accompany most severe ocular allergies, and mucus discharge may limit successful lens wear. The alterations that occur to the palpebral conjunctiva associated with allergies can diminish contact lens comfort and cause excessive lens movement. If allergies cannot be controlled with systemic and ocular medications to ease patient symptoms to a significant degree, contact lens wear probably should not be pursued.

Dermatologic Problems

Certain dermatologic conditions may have secondary ocular complications that hinder contact lens success. As an example, acne rosacea patients often have staphylococcal lid disease that produces exotoxins that can deteriorate the integrity of the cornea so that contact lenses are contraindicated. Other dermatologic conditions such as psoriasis and eczema may produce similar complications.

Glaucoma

Patients who are taking ocular medications for glaucoma should be warned about alteration of drug delivery caused by the presence of a soft contact lens. Any soft lens may imbibe medication and prolong the contact time of the medication to the anterior chamber or completely hinder delivery of the medication to the eye (10,11). Removal of lenses prior to medication instillation is the safest recommendation in these situations. If the glaucoma patient has a filtering bleb, the presence of a contact lens is risky because the incidence of intraocular infection and endophthalmitis may be increased under these conditions.

Dry Eye

Although dry eye is a common complaint among contact lens patients on a continual or episodic basis, some patients fall into severe dry eye categories where cosmetic contact lens wear would be contraindicated. Many complaints associated with dry eye fall along a continuum that only contraindicates contact lenses in their most advanced states. Dry eye conditions that exhibit corneal staining and significant epithelial disruption do not bode well for contact lens success. Breaks in the natural defenses of the epithelium may lead these eyes to secondary infection (12). Treatment options to increase success may include altering the water content or thickness of the selected contact lenses, changing the lens, materials or changing the contact lens care system.

Many other treatment options to improve dry eye complaints in contact lens patients are aimed at applying supplemental lubrication in rewetting drops, artificial tears, and ointments. Punctal plugs to decrease the natural drainage of tears also have been identified as a treatment to improve contact lens comfort. Dietary supplements and therapies related to the inflammatory theory of dry eye symptomology have been proposed.

Thyroid Dysfunction

Either an overactive or underactive thyroid gland can cause complications in contact lens practice. A hyperactive thyroid can cause degrees of exophthalmia that could lead to incomplete closure of the eyelids during a blink. Secondary drying of the ocular environment could contraindicate contact lens wear. On the other hand, a hypothyroid condition also can cause dry eye symptoms. Either of these situations is typically well controlled with medication that may alleviate symptoms making successful contact lens wear possible.

Diabetes

Diabetic patients can exhibit corneal basement membrane disorders that make them more prone to erosions. In addition, corneal sensitivity may be diminished, and corneal healing often is slower in these patients. This cluster of corneal conditions should cause the eye care practitioner to proceed with caution in fitting diabetic patients. Clear patient education concerning the potential complications and warning signs should occur before prescribing contact lenses.

March et al. (13) demonstrated no statistical difference in overall rates of corneal complications when comparing diabetic (22% incidence of complications) to nondiabetic (17% incidence of complications) soft contact lens patients.

Past research has shown increased rates of corneal complications in diabetic patients wearing extended-wear soft contact lenses. Caution and regular follow-up care are advised when prescribing contact lenses for diabetic patients.

Immunocompromised Patients

Patients who have compromised immune systems can be at increased risk for ocular infections secondary to contact lens wear. Patients typically fall into two major categories of immunocompromise: (i) human immunodeficiency virus (HIV), or (ii) medication related. Patients who test positive for HIV are not necessarily at risk from contact lens wear unless it has progressed to autoimmune deficiency syndrome (AIDS). Medication-related immunocompromised patients should be carefully evaluated for ocular complications prior to commencing with any type of contact lens wear because their susceptibility to infection may be increased.

Use of specific categories of medications has been implicated in compromised immunity. Drugs that diminish immunity include topical and systemic steroids, many drugs used in the treatment of cancer, and drugs used for treatment of rheumatoid arthritis.

CASE HISTORY

Chief Complaint

It is vitally important to elicit the primary reason for the patient's office visit. The patient might offer a general reason for the visit, such as responding to your recall letter, or the patient might reveal a specific concern, such as acute onset of red eye. There may be more than one reason for the visit. Additional elements of the patient history should continue to be elicited throughout the examination based on findings.

Closed-ended questions often are used in patient intake history forms in eye care practitioners' offices. These data can be obtained with a mailed questionnaire or administered in the waiting room just prior to the examination. In the examination room, the eye care practitioner generally starts with open-ended questions and then uses a more focused strategy to ask follow-up questions (Table 8.1) (14).

The words used in the case history should be concise and should be at a level of understanding that is comfortable for each individual patient (Table 8.2) (14). Care should be taken to minimize the use of professional terms and eye care jargon. For example, use a word like "focus" instead of "accommodate."

It is important to describe in detail to the patient your findings and recommendations regarding his or her chief complaint(s) at the end of the visit. Assuring that the chief complaint is resolved is central to patient satisfaction.

Personal Medical History

As health care providers, eye care practitioners modify their recommendations regarding contact lenses based on systemic conditions and medications. Eye care practitioners also may be the health care provider initially responsible for observing changes in the eye that could lead to a systemic diagnosis such as hypertension or diabetes.

As an example of the impact of systemic disease on contact lens wear, diabetics may experience reduced corneal sensitivity and a poor corneal healing response (15,16). They also are more likely to experience corneal ulceration from contact lens wear. Diabetics may experience refractive error fluctuations due to variations in blood sugar levels. Extra patient education discussing these potential side effects should be provided. Many eye care practitioners view moderate and severe diabetes as a contraindication to contact lens wear. Exceptions are made for patients with corneal conditions, such as keratoconus, which necessitate contact lens wear. Most eye care practitioners believe that extended wear is contraindicated for diabetic patients.

Current demographics indicate that the largest group of contact lens patients are females between the ages of 15 and 45 years. Because these ages encompass the prime ages for child bearing, contact lens issues associated with pregnancy will be significant issues for this population. Pregnancy has been shown to contribute to a less stable tear film resulting in generalized contact lens intolerance (17). The patient may complain of decreased wearing time or a change in the comfort associated with contact lens wear. Studies also have suggested that the corneal curvature may steepen during pregnancy (18). This potentially could alter the fit of the patient's contact lenses or lead you to believe that the changes are contact lens related rather than of systemic origin. Changes in the eye and the contact lens environment often continue after pregnancy and persist if the patient chooses to breast feed her child.

Medications for acute and chronic conditions have the potential to cause ocular side effects (Table 8.3). Many side effects of medications may impact the success of contact lens wear. Over-the-counter, as well as prescription, medications need to be documented. Patients often forget to include birth control medications or nutritional and herbal supplements when listing their current medications.

Medications that exacerbate dry eye symptoms may diminish contact lens wearing time and lead to decreased overall lens comfort. This is an important issue to address as decreased comfort is the number one reason for discontinuation of contact lens wear (19). Patient education regarding potential side effects and palliative therapy with lubricating drops may enhance patient tolerance to contact lens wear.

Even subtle refractive changes may be missed as a side effect of systemic medications. Small-to-moderate increases in myopia may be observed with some systemically administered medications. Changes in refractive error can be as small as 0.25 D of minus, but increases as dramatic as 7.00 D have been reported (20–23). Discontinuation of the medication usually results in a change in refractive error back toward baseline within several days to weeks. Distinguishing between a medication side effect and contact lens-related problem often can be difficult in these circumstances.

Some drugs taken at high therapeutic doses to achieve systemic effects will cause ocular irritation because they are excreted in the tears. Salicylates prescribed for arthritic con-

TABLE 8.1. DEFINITION AND PURPOSES OF FOUR TYPES OF QUESTIONS

Type of Response	Definition	Purpose in Interview
Open-ended question	A question beginning with "what," "how," "when," or "who," which asks for information without specifying the content and requires more elaboration than a one-word response	1. To invite the patient to talk at the beginning of an interview 2. To encourage patient elaboration during early stages of an interview 3. To obtain specific examples of a patient problem 4. To inform patients of their illness and to determine the kind and amount of information they need 5. To assess type and level of vocabulary used by the patient
Closed question	A question beginning with words like "are," "do," "did," "is," or "can," which asks for a specific fact or piece of information and can be answered with one word or short phrase	1. To obtain a specific fact or piece of information; or when a one-word answer is desired, as in "review of systems" in a health history 2. To narrow rather than broaden an area of discussion, as in introducing a specific area of history taking, such as social or family history 3. To stop a patient who is rambling from overtalking
Focused question	A question often beginning with "have you," "can you," or "do you," which narrows or defines the topic by asking for a specific response	1. To define a topic and request for a response in a more definitive manner than the open-ended question 2. To characterize a symptom or obtain descriptive information about a clinical sign or event
"Laundry-list" question	A question that provides the patient with a list of adjectives or descriptive phrases from which to choose	1. To obtain specific information about a symptom or illness by providing a series of choices 2. To obtain patient identification of a piece of information that has not been obtained from open-ended or focused questions.

Excerpted from Cormier LS, Cormier WH, Weissner RJ. *Interviewing and helping skills for health professionals.* Boston: Jones and Bartlett Publishers, 1986.

ditions often result in superficial punctuate keratitis and generalized ocular irritation.

Drugs that cause mydriatic effects may lead to patient complaints of flare and glare associated with contact lens wear as the pupil size exceeds the workable optic zone of the contact lens. Although this complaint is more common among GP contact lens wearers, soft contact lens patients also may experience this side effect. The mydriatic or miotic effect associated with some drugs may adversely affect the performance of any patient wearing a contact lens design that is dependent on pupil size, such as soft and GP multifocal lenses.

Allergies may affect contact lens wear. A thorough investigation of a contact lens patient's allergies, reactions, and medications is important in managing and sustaining successful contact lens wear. Patients with mild or seasonal allergies generally succeed with contact lens wear. They may benefit from reducing their hours of lens wear during times when their allergies are most bothersome. Systemic medica-

TABLE 8.2. GUIDELINES FOR WORDING QUESTIONS

1. Phrase questions simply. Avoid medical jargon.
2. Phrase questions concisely. Avoid long windedness.
3. Ask only one question at a time. Avoid "stacking" questions.
4. Phrase questions in a nonaccusatory way, using "what" or "how." Avoid using "why" questions.
5. Phrase questions so that they do not suggest or influence patient answers. Avoid parenthetical phrases or sequences of words that suggest a particular symptom, illness, or diagnosis.

Excerpted from Cormier LS, Cormier WH, Weissner RJ. *Interviewing and helping skills for health professionals.* Boston: Jones and Bartlett Publishers, 1986.

TABLE 8.3. OCULAR SIDE EFFECTS AND PATIENT SYMPTOMS WITH COMMONLY PRESCRIBED SYSTEMIC MEDICATIONS

Symptom	Drug Category
Dry eye	Decongestants, antihistamines, antihypertensives, oral contraceptives, antiacne medications, muscle relaxants, anticholinergics, phenothiazines
Mydriasis	Stimulants, anticholinergics, antihistamines, antipsychotics
Miosis	Codeine
Ocular irritation	Gold salts, salicylates
Refractive changes	Acetazolamide, oral contraceptives, sulfamethizole, sulfamethoxalate, sulfisoxazole

tions taken for allergies, such as antihistamines, may lead to dry eye symptoms. Symptoms may become exacerbated by contact lens wear. A small percentage of patients are allergic to preservatives and other components in eye drops and contact lens care solutions. Thimerosal, a mercury-based preservative, has been implicated in the past for causing both immediate and delayed sensitivity reactions. Preservative-free drops should be prescribed when possible for patients with a history of allergic responses to solutions. Daily disposable soft contact lenses may benefit patients exhibiting solution sensitivities.

The lifestyle history of potential contact lens patients should be investigated. Dietary supplements and overall hydration of the patient can impact on contact lens comfort and success. Issues of alcohol consumption are important to elicit because alcohol can contribute to dry eye complaints. Smoking has been shown to increase the risk of microbial keratitis with contact lens wear (24,25). McNally et al. (26) reported that silicone hydrogel patients who smoked cigarettes were 1.7 times more likely to develop corneal infiltrative events than were nonsmokers. If the smoker was younger than 30 years, infiltrative events were 2.7 times more likely to occur than in an age-matched nonsmoking population (26). Documentation of these key aspects of a case history should not be overlooked.

Personal Ocular History

Past eye history including diseases, injuries, and eye care and eyewear should be elicited. If the patient's most recent primary care eye examination is not current (within the past year) or was not thorough, a complete primary care eye examination should be performed. The patient should be questioned regarding his or her perception of vision during work and leisure activities. If the patient states that his or her vision has steadily become worse, this could be the result of progressive myopia or cataract formation. Further case history and clinical testing will determine the correct diagnosis and therapy.

Recent use of prescribed and over-the-counter (OTC) eye drops and the reason for their use should be determined. Eye drops can be absorbed by soft contact lenses, thereby increasing their contact time in the eye and potentially altering their desired effect (11). Also, the preservatives, especially benzalkonium chloride, used in many eye drop formulations may be absorbed by a soft contact lens and lead to a hypersensitivity reaction (27). Ointments may coat a lens and cause blurred vision or contaminate the lens, rendering it useless.

Family Medical and Ocular History

Heredity does not generally play a significant role in contact lens success. However, a family history of systemic conditions, such as diabetes, should be investigated. Eye conditions with a hereditary basis, such as glaucoma, should be ruled out by examination. Parents who are significantly myopic may be concerned about their children's refractive status and prognosis. GP lens wear or orthokeratology often are requested to stabilize or reduce the progression of myopia.

Contact Lens Experience and Expectations

Determine the reasons the patient desires contact lenses, as well as his or her expectations regarding contact lens wear. Even though the patient might desire a certain type of correction, it might not be appropriate for the planned use. Patient education on the front end can increase the ultimate success of the patient in contact lens wear.

The fact that a patient previously was unsuccessful with contact lenses does not mean that he or she is not now a good candidate. Careful investigation of the circumstances of the patient's previous contact lens experience will be extremely useful to plan future contact lens strategies. Determine the type of contact lenses he or she wore previously and the reason lens wear was not successful. Did the patient stop wearing contact lenses because of cost, inconvenience, unacceptable vision, or poor comfort? Be sure to address how the new contact lens modality will alleviate or decrease the past problems. More frequent lens replacement, new lens materials, advanced lens designs, and improved care systems allow many patients who failed contact lens wear to successfully wear lenses. Often patients discontinue contact lens wear due to poor motivation. Circumstances regarding motivation may have changed. Many contact lens patients drop in and out of contact lenses several times over their lifetime. Providing the best contact lens choices, tailor made for their needs, may help to break the cycle.

When discussing the contact lens history of any patient, a record of previously used solutions and care systems is an important aspect of the conversation. Sometimes sensitivities to previously used solutions, incorrectly used solutions, or noncompliance with care systems can sabotage success. Obtaining these details in the patient's case history can uncover aspects of lens care to remediate and ensure future contact lens satisfaction.

Many factors contribute to the overall acceptance of contact lens wear. Both signs and symptoms are considered when an eye care practitioner determines contact lens performance. Terry et al. (28) reported proposed standards to provide a framework to judge "success" with contact lens wear. These guidelines are summarized in Table 8.4.

Vocations and Avocations

It is imperative to understand patients' work and avocational vision needs and the environments in which they perform these activities. Without carefully listening to the way patients use their vision and the specific visual demands

TABLE 8.4. STANDARDS FOR SUCCESS FOR DAILY AND EXTENDED CONTACT LENS WEAR

Wearing time	Daily wear	12 hours per day, 6 days per week
	Extended wear	6 or more consecutive nights
Comfort	Subjective rating	Grade 3 (comfortable) or better
Vision	Subjective rating	Grade 3 (good) or better
	Visual acuity	Within 1 line of best spectacle visual acuity, under high and low illumination
		$\leq$1 line reduction from optimum contact lens visual acuity
Ocular tissue changes	Hypoxic effects	$\leq$10 microcysts or vacuoles
		No striae in daily wear
		No striae after 1 hour of open eye in extended wear
		No endothelial folds in daily or extended wear
	Corneal vascularization	$\leq$0.5 mm vessel penetration beyond translucent limbal transition zone
	Endothelial polymegathism	$\leq$1 grade increase (Cornea and Contact Lens Research Unit [CCLRU] grading scale)
	Changes in corneal curvature and refractive error	No irregular corneal distortion or warpage $\leq \pm 0.50$ D change in flatter K, and/or ± 0.75 D change in steeper K
		$\leq \pm 0.50$ D sphere, and/or ± 0.75D cylinder change in spectacle refraction
	Corneal staining	$\leq$ Grade 2 type of staining (macropunctate)
		$\leq$ Grade 1 depth of staining (superficial epithelial involvement)
		$\leq$ Grade 1 extent of staining (1%–15% surface involvement)
	Lens adherence	No signs during daily wear, or after 1 hour of open eye during extended wear
	Eyelid changes	$\leq$1 grade increase in papillae or redness of superior palpebral conjunctiva
	General appearance	No unacceptable change
Patient appearance	Bulbar redness	$\leq$1 grade increase

Excerpted from Terry RL, Schnider CM, Holden BA, et al (28), with permission.

of particular tasks in their job or avocation, you cannot adequately address their needs. Contact lenses offer an additional option for refractive error correction for many of your spectacle-wearing patients.

Contact lenses can provide a benefit to patients who complain of spectacle lenses that fog associated with changes in temperatures in their environment. Contact lenses do not become fogged in cold environs.

Contact lenses offer minimal ocular protection when performing tasks where small wood or metal objects may enter the ocular surface, so safety eyewear still needs to be prescribed to wear over the contact lenses.

Athletes benefit from the use of contact lenses over spectacle wear due to the increased field of view offered by contact lenses. Spectacles also may be dislodged or broken during contact sports. In sports where balls that travel at high-velocity are used (e.g. handball, racquetball), protective goggles over the contact lenses are required for ocular safety.

Patients who are frequent travelers or go camping on a regular basis may benefit from the advantages of single-use contact lenses. This modality can significantly minimize care system use and simplify packing and care of the contact lenses. Even having single-use lenses in addition to other contact lens modalities is a great way to satisfy the changing needs of your patients.

Even though patients who participate in water sports benefit from contact lens wear, patient education regarding

lenses becoming contaminated with organisms such as *Acanthamoeba* must be conveyed (29). Prescription diving masks or watertight goggles should be worn whenever possible. In situations where this is not feasible, such as water polo, patients must be advised and medical records need to reflect that contact lens wear is not recommended. Some patients wear daily disposable lenses for water-related sports and activities. Under these circumstances, it is important that the lens move freely on the eye before lens removal is attempted.

Many patients would enjoy or benefit from part-time wear of contact lenses. Explore the possibility of part-time contact lens wear with your spectacle-wearing patients. Part-time wear may be desired due to vocational, hobby, sports, or social reasons. Also keep in mind that contact lens patients should possess a "backup" pair of spectacles with their current prescription. In addition, the eye care practitioner's recommendation about appropriate sun wear for their contact lens patients will assist in eye protection and visual comfort.

TESTING PROCEDURES

It is important that your prefitting data are precise, because these data will serve as baseline to monitor and compare changes over time.

Visual Acuity

Entrance visual acuity through the patient's habitual vision correction is desired before any measurements or testing is performed to establish baseline findings for medical-legal purposes. Monocular and binocular visual acuities at distance and near need to be recorded.

Preliminary Measurements

Several preliminary measurements are performed to assist the practitioner in determining the most appropriate contact lens modality and design.

Horizontal Visible Iris Diameter

The horizontal visible iris diameter (HVID) can be used to determine the overall diameter (OAD) of the GP lens. For example, some GP-prescribing philosophies set the OAD at 2 mm smaller than the HVID.

HVID may be considered in soft contact lens base curve determination. Corneal diameter plays a significant part in base curve determination due to the sagittal height factors that impact on soft contact lens fitting relationships (30).

Pupil Size

Pupil size can be measured to determine the optic zone diameter (OZD) for GP contact lenses. Pupil size is also an important variable to evaluate in specialty lens designs such as multifocal contact lenses. Many practitioners use moderate-to-low room illumination to measure the pupil size with a millimeter rule. Another method is to view the pupil through an ultraviolet (UV) lamp to measure pupil size. Generally, the OZD will be prescribed 1 to 2 mm larger than the measured pupil size.

Palpebral Fissure

The palpebral aperture or fissure (PF) can be used to determine OAD; the wider the PF in straight-ahead gaze, the larger the OAD prescribed. Overall GP lens diameters based on palpebral fissure size and/or pupil size recommended by Bennett (31) are listed in Table 8.5.

TABLE 8.5. RELATIONSHIP BETWEEN OVERALL DIAMETER AND PALPEBRAL FISSURE/PUPIL SIZE

Overall Diameter (mm)	Palpebral Fissure Size (mm)	Pupil Size in Dim Illumination (mm)
8.8–9.0	<9.0	<6
9.2–9.4	9.0–10.5	6–8
9.6–9.8	>10.5	>8

Excerpted from Bennett (31).

Young et al. (32) found that smaller palpebral fissure size was related to enhanced soft toric lens rotational stability. This implies that patients with smaller palpebral apertures may obtain increased visual performance and consistency of vision while wearing soft toric contact lenses. Young et al. also determined that lid anatomy, especially the angles of the lids, plays a role in toric soft contact lens orientation and stability.

Eyelid Position

Eyelid position and tension are important factors in contact lens centration and lens rotation. If the upper eyelid covers the superior limbus in straight ahead gaze, a lid-attachment GP contact lens fit may be considered (33). If the upper eyelid does not cover a portion of the superior cornea, an interpalpebral GP lens design is generally indicated (34). Larger OADs (>9.5 mm) are generally prescribed when fitting lid-attachment GP lenses; smaller OADs (<9.2 mm) are generally used in fitting interpalpebral designs.

Lower eyelid position is important in prescribing translating design multifocal GP contact lenses. Many translating multifocal designs are dependent on the bottom of the contact lens resting on the lower eyelid or the inferior edge of the lens being stopped by the lower lid on downgaze. The lens may be truncated to achieve this goal. Success with translating multifocal contact lenses is therefore improved if the lower lid is tangent to or slightly above the inferior limbus. If the position of the lower lid is greater than 1 mm higher or lower than the inferior limbus, the success of many translating design multifocals may be in question.

Eyelid Tension

Eyelid tension is important for multifocal GP fitting. Eyelid tension may be assessed during lid eversion. If the tension of the lids is exceedingly lax in patients being considered for translating vision multifocal contact lenses, the lid may not provide adequate resistance for translation. Upon downgaze, the lens may slip under the lower eyelid, rendering the design unworkable. Additionally, a flaccid upper lid could pose problems when trying to remove GP lenses. Sufficient tension must be achieved for successful GP lens removal. On the other hand, patients who have undergone blepharoplasty procedures for cosmetic or therapeutic reasons may experience difficulties in contact lens wear because their lids may be excessively taut. Achieving a lens position that does not tuck under the upper lid is often a problem.

Blink

The frequency of the patient's blink, as well as the completeness of the blink, should be evaluated. If the patient partially blinks, consider fitting the patient with either soft or lid-attachment GP contact lenses in order to optimize the stability of the tear film (35). Partial blinkers also may show evidence of corneal staining with fluorescein on slit-lamp examination. This classic pattern of staining appears in the lower third of the cornea. If the staining is severe, contact lens success may be questionable.

Iris Color

Iris color assists the practitioner in recommending cosmetic or therapeutic tints. Tinted soft contact lenses allow the patient to enhance or change the natural color of the eyes. Enhancement tints do little to alter the appearance of patients with dark irides. Opaque tinted lenses are necessary for these patients to alter their eye color. Patients with corneal scarring or iris colobomas may benefit from being prescribed opaque or custom prosthetic tinted contact lenses, which will mask the appearance and improve cosmesis. GP lenses also are tinted, but generally for handling purposes. Because GP lenses usually are prescribed smaller in diameter than the cornea and tend to move significantly on a blink, they are not widely used for cosmetic tints. Some practitioners prescribe a g(R)een lens for the right eye and a b(L)ue lens for the left eye to aid their patients in maintaining the correct lens for each eye.

Keratometry

Keratometry should be performed prior to applying diagnostic contact lenses. Keratometry remains a staple for prescribing GP contact lens base curves. The amount of corneal toricity assists the practitioner in deciding the most appropriate lens design. Patients with corneal toricity of less than 1.50 diopters are generally prescribed spherical or aspheric base curve GP lenses. Base curve torics and biotrics are often prescribed when corneal toricity exceeds 2.50 diopters.

Many fitting philosophies have been proposed for GP lenses. A popular fitting philosophy recommends prescribing the base curve equal to the flat keratometry value. This is referred to as fitting "on K." Other philosophies recommend prescribing the base curve based on the flat K value and adjusting for the amount of corneal toricity. An example of a fitting philosophy using corneal toricity to determine the base curve is given in Table 8.6.

Note that the base curve is generally prescribed flatter when a larger overall diameter is used. This maintains a similar central fitting relationship.

Although keratometry values are not as critical in prescribing soft contact lenses, they may be used as general guidelines to select the initial diagnostic base curve. Soft contact lens manufacturers often recommend flat base curves for corneas flatter than 43.00 diopters and steep base curves for corneas steeper than 43.00 diopters.

TABLE 8.6. BASE CURVE SELECTION AS A FUNCTION OF LENS DIAMETER AND CORNEAL CYLINDER

Corneal Toricity (D)	Lens Overall Diameter		
	8.9 mm	9.3 mm	9.7 mm
0.00–0.50	0.25 D steep	On K	0.25 D flat
0.62–1.25	0.50 D steep	0.25 D steep	On K
1.37–2.00	0.75 D steep	0.50 D steep	0.25 D steep
2.12–2.75	1.00 D steep	0.75 D steep	0.50 D steep
2.87–3.50	1.25 D steep	1.00 D steep	0.75 D steep

When performing keratometry, mire quality should be evaluated. Tear film insufficiencies or corneal distortion may result in poor mire quality. If mire distortion is due to poor tear film integrity, it should improve immediately following a blink. If the mires remain significantly distorted after a blink, the patient's corneal surface is irregular, or he or she may suffer from tear film deficiency. An irregular corneal surface may be due to injury, corneal surgery, or disease. Keratometric mire distortion should be crudely graded (on a 4 point clinical scale).

Most keratometers provide curvature readings from 36 to 52 diopters. It is common for postrefractive surgery patients to have keratometry readings flatter than 36 diopters. A -1.00 D spectacle trial lens may be attached to the objective (patient) side of the keratometer to expand the range by approximately 6 diopters. For example, if the extended range drum reading is 40.00 D, subtract approximately 6 diopters for an adjusted K value of 34.00 diopters. On the other hand, if the patient's corneal curvature is steeper than 52 diopters, such as for a keratoconus patient, attach a $+1.25$ D spectacle trial lens to the objective side of the keratometer and add approximately 8 diopters to the drum reading. For example, if the extended range value is 50.00 D, add approximately 8 diopters for an adjusted K value of 58.00 diopters (36).

Over-keratometry (keratometry performed on the front surface of a GP contact lens on the eye) can be used to determine the amount of on-eye lens flexure or warp. If the front surface of the GP lens is spherical in design, the difference between keratometry findings indicates the amount of lens flexure. Over-keratometry also can be performed with soft contact lenses on the eye. If mire quality improves immediately following a blink, the lens may be too steep or the tear film inadequate. If mire quality improves as the patient stares, the lens may be fit too flat. Over-keratometry is not a routine clinical procedure but can be performed to help solve problems.

Corneal curvature has been used to determine the initial OAD for GP contact lens fitting. Mandell (36) recommends a 9.6-mm OAD for corneas flatter than 42.00 diopters, a 9.2-mm diameter for corneas between 42.00 and 44.00

diopters in curvature, and an 8.8-mm diameter for corneas steeper than 44.00 diopters.

Corneal Topography

Corneal topography is beneficial for understanding the corneal contour and curvature across the central and midperipheral cornea (see Chapters 9 and 28). Central curvature readings are reported as simulated keratometry values (sim K), and corneal contour regularity may be described by a surface regularity index (SRI) or surface asymmetry index (SAI). Baseline topography is helpful for monitoring corneal change subsequent to contact lens wear, especially GP contact lens wear. Topography is widely used in cases where the corneal contour is unique or irregular in shape, such as after corneal injury or surgery. Orthokeratology and corneal refractive therapy are GP contact lens applications where monitoring the treatment by corneal topography is essential. Obtaining centration of the treatment zone and avoiding induced corneal distortion are crucial to achieving the desired effect.

Corneal topography should be performed at regular intervals following corneal refractive surgery. Topography also is helpful in determining the initial lens design and lens parameters following PK. The post-PK corneal contour will dictate whether to prescribe a sphere, toric, or reverse-geometry lens design. Fluorescein pattern evaluation will allow fine tuning of the fit.

Many corneal topography instruments offer software that enables the practitioner to vary GP lens parameters and to view a simulated fluorescein pattern prior to applying a diagnostic lens or ordering an initial lens. Direct ordering via e-mail is another option with some software packages.

Refractive Error Determination

Objective and subjective determination of a patient's refractive error should be performed for baseline purposes. Retinoscopy and/or autorefraction are objective and supportive measurements of refractive error. Retinoscopy generally provides the practitioner with a full plus determination of the patient's refractive error. This is especially helpful when prescribing for a hyperopic patient. If a patient is a slow or poor responder during the subjective refraction, the retinoscopy finding will serve as an efficient and accurate assessment of the patient's refractive error. Verify the retinoscopy finding by using a trial frame with the patient's tentative prescription. An added advantage of retinoscopy is that the regularity of the reflex provides the clinician with an assessment of the regularity of the corneal surface. Scissors motion retinoscopy reflex, for example, may lead the eye care practitioner to suspect keratoconus.

Manifest refraction determines the amount of the refractive error and the resulting visual acuity. If the best-corrected visual acuity is reduced, pinhole visual acuity may be performed to estimate the best potential vision. The amount of the sphere and cylinder, as well as the axis of the cylinder, is important in determining the best contact lens correction. Spherical refractions alone do not reveal the optimal prescription for patients who could benefit from an astigmatic correction. Some eye care practitioners theorize that only a spherical refraction is needed if a spherical soft contact lens is to be prescribed. Ignoring astigmatic corrections, even if they are small, could significantly diminish the patient's vision and subsequent satisfaction with the prescribed contact lenses.

The thickness of the contact lens profile for patients who are high hyperopes or myopes (>6 diopters) may encourage the practitioner to prescribe high Dk GP or silicone hydrogel materials to minimize localized areas of corneal edema (37). For example, high-minus conventional soft contact lenses may contribute to neovascularization, whereas silicone hydrogels probably will not.

Manifest refractive errors of 4 diopters or more need to be adjusted for vertex distance to obtain the power at the corneal plane. Powers less than this do not result in a clinically significant difference. An overrefraction (OR) through a trial contact lens generally provides a more precise method for determining contact lens power by combining the power of the trial lens with the equivalent sphere of the OR. Any OR greater than ± 4 diopters also must be adjusted for vertex distance to determine the appropriate contact lens power.

The following formula is used to adjust the effective power of a manifest or spectacle refraction to the corneal plane:

$$Fc = \frac{Fs}{1 - dFs}$$

where

Fc = power at the corneal plane (in diopters)
Fs = power at the spectacle plane (in diopters)
d = vertex distance (in meters).

Example: Manifest refraction = $-5.00 - 4.00 \times 180$
Vertex distance = 12 mm

In the 180th meridian: $Fc = \dfrac{-5.00}{1 - (0.012)(-5.00)}$

$$Fc = -4.717 = -4.75 \text{ D}$$

In the 90th meridian: $Fc = \dfrac{-9.00}{1 - (0.012)(-9.00)}$

$$Fc = -8.123 = -8.12 \text{ D}$$

Power at the corneal plane = $-4.75 - 3.37 \times 180$.

Another consideration when prescribing contact lenses is that myopes have to converge and accommodate more through contact lenses than when they are wearing spectacles (38). Therefore, myopic contact lens patients may develop symptoms of presbyopia sooner while wearing contact lenses than with spectacles. Conversely, contact lens wear might delay the need for additional help at near for hyperopic patients. These effects are amplified in higher prescriptions.

A comparison of corneal curvature (keratometry or simulated K readings) and manifest refraction findings assists the practitioner in determining the most appropriate GP contact lens design. Other factors, such as the patient's tolerance to uncorrected astigmatism, also are considered when selecting lens materials and designs. If the amounts of corneal toricity and refractive cylinder are similar, a spherical base curve GP lens design should provide the patient with excellent vision. If the corneal toricity exceeds 2.50 diopters, a bitoric GP lens design is generally indicated. If the cornea has 1.00 diopter or less of corneal toricity and the refractive cylinder exceeds the corneal toricity by more than 0.75 diopter, a front-surface toric, spherical base curve, GP lens design is indicated (Table 8.7) (39).

Many practitioners fit a back-surface toric soft contact lens to enhance rotational stability if the refractive cylinder is primarily corneal and a front-surface toric soft contact lens if the cornea is nearly spherical and the refractive cylinder is primarily internal. Both front- and back-surface toric soft contact lenses may be acceptable choices, however, regardless of the corneal toricity.

Soft contact lens design choices are generally determined by the amount of refractive cylinder. If the refractive cylinder is 0.75 diopter or less, a spherical soft contact lens will generally be prescribed. If the refractive cylinder is more than 0.75 diopter, a toric soft contact lens will usually be indicated.

Because of Knapp's Law, anisometropic patients (especially if refractive) have fewer problems with image size differences when wearing contact lenses compared to spectacles (38). Patients with unequal refractive errors between the two eyes may experience symptoms of visual discomfort or diplopia when not viewing through the optical centers of their spectacles. This is due to the unequal amount of prism induced through each lens. The effect is larger for greater amounts of anisometropia. Contact lenses minimize this effect because the patient tends to view through the optical centers of the contact lenses even in different positions of gaze.

TABLE 8.7. GAS PERMEABLE TORIC LENS DESIGN CONSIDERATIONS

Rigid Gas Permeable Lens Design	Residual Cylinder in Over refraction (D)	Corneal Toricity (D)
Sphere	≤0.75	≤2.50
Base curve toric	≥0.75 at same axis as corneal toricity	≥1.50
Spherical power effect (SPE) bitoric	<0.75	≥1.50
Cylinder power effect (CPE) bitoric	≥0.75	≥1.50
Front surface toric	≥1.00	≤1.00

Excerpted from Edrington TB. Rigid gas permeable lenses for astigmatism. In: Hom MM, ed. *Manual of contact lens prescribing and fitting with CD-ROM.* Washburn, MA: Butterworth Heinemann, 2000:144.

Binocular Status

An evaluation of binocular vision should be included as part of the initial contact lens examination. Decisions on lens types and modes of correction may be influenced by findings in this portion of the examination. The optical differences between spectacle correction and contact lens correction could work to the patient's advantage or disadvantage based on binocular findings.

Many approaches have been used to determine the eye to select for near viewing when prescribing monovision. The most prevalent practice is to fit the dominant eye for distance and the nondominant eye for near. Eye dominancy may be determined by performing a sighting test or by assuming eye dominancy is the same as hand dominancy. Another technique is to have the patient wear his or her distance prescription over both eyes and then place a loose spectacle trial lens with the needed add power alternately over each eye to determine which is more visually comfortable for both distance and near viewing. Refractive error sometimes helps to determine which eye is initially selected for distance or near. If the patient is emmetropic in one eye, initially select that eye for distance viewing. If the patient is myopic by an amount that is similar to his or her near or intermediate add requirement, select that eye for near. Some patients prefer an eye for distance due to the location of their rear view mirror when driving or where they place their reading material during computer work.

Slit-Lamp Evaluation

A thorough slit-lamp biomicroscopy examination should be completed prior to fitting a patient with contact lenses. This should include examination of the cornea, bulbar conjunctivae, tear film, eyelids, eyelashes, and palpebral conjunctivae. Practitioners should develop a routine examination procedure for using the slit lamp.

The slit lamp is composed of two systems: (i) a binocular microscope for viewing the patient's eye and ocular adnexa; and (ii) an illumination system where the light can be varied in height, width, and intensity. Filters are available to enhance the practitioner's observations.

Commonly used illumination and observation combinations are described in Table 8.8 (40,41) Performing slit-lamp biomicroscopy is a dynamic process. Illumination and viewing angles are regularly adjusted during the procedure (Table 8.8.)

Filters can be used to enhance slit-lamp observations. A cobalt (blue) filter is used in front of the illumination source to excite the wavelength of sodium fluorescein, thereby enhancing the view of corneal staining or fluorescein pattern evaluation. The blue filter also is used in performing Goldmann tonometry. A red-free (green) filter can be used in front of the illumination source to enhance the view of blood vessels or other observed blood elements. A yellow

TABLE 8.8. BIOMICROSCOPY TECHNIQUES AND THEIR PURPOSE

Method of Illumination	Name of Procedure	Character of Aperture	Typical Magnification	Angle of Illumination	Purpose
Diffuse	Diffuse	Wide open	5–15×	~ 45°	1. Extent of corneal scars 2. Presence of folds in Descemet's membrane 3. Presence of invading blood vessels 4. Edema of epithelium 5. Gross observation of anterior segment
Direct	Optic section (narrow beam)	Narrow beam	5–45×	~ 450	1. Thinning or thickening of corneal contour 2. Localize depth of corneal foreign bodies 3. Angle estimation 4. View crystalline lens
	Parallelepiped (broad beam)	Medium–broad beam	5–45×	~ 450	1. Broad view of anterior and posterior corneal surfaces and stroma 2. General survey of cornea 3. View crystalline lens 4. Sodium fluorescein evaluation
	Conical beam	Small, circular	30–45×	~ 450	1. Evaluation for cells and flare in the anterior chamber
Retro illumination	Direct and indirect	Medium beam; light is focused on deeper structures while scope is focused anteriorly	30–45×	Wide angle (>450)	1. Studying deposits on Descemet's membrane 2. Examination of epithelial vacuoles, edema, delicate scars, microcysts, precipitates
Specular reflection		Parellepiped	30–45×	Angle of incidence = angle of reflection	1. Elevations and depressions of anterior surface 2. Details of precorneal tear film 3. Examination of endothelium
Sclerotic scatter		Parellepiped	5–30×	Light focused at limbus, view in central cornea	1. Observation of a disturbance of normal corneal transparency

filter can be used on the objective side of the microscope (in conjunction with a cobalt blue illumination source) to enhance viewing of corneal staining and fluorescein pattern evaluation. Yellow filters are particularly helpful when photographing the fluorescein pattern or corneal staining. It is necessary to use a yellow filter to evaluate fluorescein patterns of GP contact lens materials containing a UV inhibitor.

Eversion of the upper and lower eyelids should be performed for baseline purposes and regularly on follow-up examinations. Evaluation of the tarsal area on upper eyelid eversion is of increased importance for patients who wear contact lenses on an extended or continuous wear basis. Allansmith (42) documented increased formation of giant papillary conjunctivitis (GPC) in patients who wore soft contact lenses for extended periods without frequently replacing their lenses.

Contact lens-induced papillary conjunctivitis (CLIPC)

observed with silicone hydrogel wear is more localized in appearance and is proposed to be mechanical in nature (43). Other mechanical etiologies of papillary conjunctivitis can be observed with exposed corneal sutures following PK and in patients with ocular prosthetics.

The crystalline lens should be evaluated for cloudiness or opacities to aid the practitioner in explaining any reduction in visual acuity and educating the patient about future expectations. If the patient has had cataract surgery without an intraocular lens implant, consider prescribing a contact lens material with a UV inhibitor, as well as spectacles with UV-blocking lenses.

VITAL DYES AND STAINS

When using the slit lamp to evaluate the anterior segment prior to contact lens application in the initial examination, several vital stains and dyes are often used. These stains and dyes provide additional information to the practitioner about whether or not the patient is a good candidate for contact lens wear.

Sodium Fluorescein

Sodium fluorescein is a water-soluble dye with very low toxicity to ocular tissues. Sodium fluorescein does not penetrate intact epithelial cells; rather, it stains intercellular spaces and damaged epithelial cells. It has the ability to fluoresce under cobalt blue lighting conditions. Common uses for sodium fluorescein are (i) to evaluate corneal epithelial integrity, and (ii) to determine the fitting characteristics of GP contact lenses. The most common administration of sodium fluorescein is by impregnated sterile strips that are wet with saline and then applied to the conjunctiva. A yellow filter may be used to enhance viewing.

Rose Bengal

Rose Bengal stains dead or devitalized cellular tissue on the anterior segment. No filter is needed to view this reddish-brown stain because white light illumination is used. Rose Bengal can be applied in much the same way as fluorescein with the use of impregnated sterile strips that should be wet with a few drops of saline prior to instillation. Rose Bengal also is available in liquid unit doses.

Lissamine Green

Lissamine green may be used as an alternative to Rose Bengal stain. This vital stain also identifies dead and devitalized cells and mucus. It has an advantage over Rose Bengal in that it does not cause the same degree of ocular irritation upon instillation (44). With white light illumination, lissamine green will stain the cornea blue in areas of devitalized tissue.

TEAR FILM OBSERVATIONS AND ASSESSMENT (SEE ALSO CHAPTER 23)

Gross observation of the tear film quality should be conducted upon slit-lamp examination. Debris and mucus often can be viewed as major components of the tear film environment. Patients with blepharitis often show increased cellular debris present in the tear film. The presence of makeup and oils in the tear film can be observed on casual slit-lamp examination. Determination of the cause of excessive tear film debris and an attempt to clean up the ocular environment may lead to increased patient comfort and success with contact lenses.

Dry Eye Questionnaires

Several questionnaires have been developed and tested to assess dry eye symptoms for contact lens wearing and non–contact lens wearing patients. Questionnaires for both patient care and research purposes are available (45–48).

Tear Film Breakup Time and Noninvasive Breakup Times

Tear film break-up time (TBUT) provides a measure of tear film quality. A theory is that short TBUTs (<10 s) may identify patients with dry eye. TBUT may be determined by instilling sodium fluorescein in the eye and measuring the time until a dry area within the tear film is observed with the slit lamp. A problem with this method is that instillation of the fluorescein disrupts the normal quality of the tear film. Several "noninvasive" breakup time (NIBUT) methods (in which the tear film is not disturbed by the testing procedure) have been developed and investigated (49). One method readily available to eye care practitioners is observing the amount of time until the image of the reflected keratometry mires distorts following a blink to determine tear breakup time by noninvasive means.

Schirmer Tear Testing

This test attempts to quantify the tear production capability of a patient. A thin paper strip with a tab is placed inside the lower au de sac for 5 minutes, and the length of the wetting observed on the paper strip is measured from the notch of the paper tab. A value of 15 mm of wetting in 5 minutes is considered normal. Values less than 15 mm are suggestive of dry eye. The presence of the strip can have an irritating effect, which may produce increased reflex tearing that clouds the significance of the results of this test. It has been theorized that basal tear production can be assessed independent of reflex tearing by measuring with a Schirmer strip after the instillation of anesthetic, although this contention is somewhat controversial.

Phenol Red Thread

The Phenol red thread test also measures the tear production capability of the patient. In a similar fashion to Schirmer tear testing, a 70-mm thread impregnated with phenol red dye is bent on one end and placed in the lower au de sac. Measurements are taken of the length of wetting on the thread, shown by a color change from red to yellow, after a 15-second period of time. Because the thread that is introduced into the lower eyelid is smaller and not as irritating, the test may have the advantage of causing less reflex tearing reaction than the Schirmer test. Normal values for this test are between 9 and 20 mm of wetting in 15 seconds. Recently, the significance of this test adequately measuring tear production also has been brought into question (50).

Tear Meniscus Height

Using the slit lamp to evaluate the height of the tear meniscus at the lower lid margin may provide insight into overall tear volume. In addition to the height of the meniscus, the regularity of the volume across the span of the lower lid can be assessed. A normal value for tear meniscus height is 0.22 mm (51).

ADDITIONAL INITIAL EVALUATION TESTING
Ophthalmoscopy

Ophthalmoscopy should be performed as a routine portion of the patient's general eye care examination. Ophthalmoscopy may reveal the reason for reduced vision or visual function loss. Ophthalmoscopy may be useful in determining the extent of cataract formation or confirming an irregular corneal surface by viewing the red reflex.

Intraocular Pressure

As with all patients, intraocular pressure measurements should be routinely performed on contact lens patients. Intraocular pressure readings tend to be low (<10 mm) for post–laser-assisted *in situ* keratomileusis (post-LASIK) and keratoconus patients due to the decreased ocular rigidity from thinned central corneas (52). The appearance of the optic nerve head and visual field findings warrant close monitoring to assess for any evidence of glaucomatous changes because the intraocular pressure measurements may be misleading in patients with thin corneas.

Visual Fields

Contact lenses may be used rather than spectacles to correct refractive error when conducting visual field testing. This will reduce false-positive "ring scotoma" findings caused by the rim of the spectacles. The experience also might encourage a patient to try contact lenses for cosmetic reasons.

OPAQUE CONTACT LENS CONSIDERATIONS
Contact Lens Selection

Case history and testing results help the practitioner determine the optimal contact lens option for the patient. Past contact lens experiences, lifestyle needs, expectations, and refractive data all contribute to the decision.

Trial Lens Fitting

Many practitioners prefer to empirically order the patient's initial contact lenses. Advantages include (i) increased efficiency and decreased chair time for both the practitioner and the patient; and (ii) the patient's initial experience may be more favorable because the specifications of the lens have been custom ordered, often resulting in better initial vision and comfort. To order GP contact lenses empirically, keratometry (or corneal topography) and manifest refraction data are used to design the initial base curve and lens power. A popular fitting philosophy referred to as fitting "on K" is to prescribe the base curve equal to the flat K value. The contact lens power is the most plus (after adjustment when prescribing "on K" for vertex distance to the corneal plane) meridian of the manifest refraction. Empirically ordering lenses also is common for lens designs that the practitioner infrequently uses, such as toric GP and soft lens designs.

Diagnostic fitting with trial lenses allows the practitioner to fine-tune lens parameters prior to ordering the patient's first pair of lenses. Before empirically ordering or trial fitting a patient, determine if the patient is interested in tinted or opaque lenses and if the patient is interested in flexible or continuous wear. When fitting soft contact lenses, first verify that the brand of trial lens you select is available in the parameters, such as lens power, required by your patient. This is particularly important in selecting toric soft contact lenses, which often have limited parameter availability.

If you are applying a GP lens to a patient's eye for the first time, consider using an anesthetic to minimize the initial lens discomfort and resulting tearing (53).

Overrefractions

ORs are performed to fine-tune and check the contact lens power. Sphere-only ORs may be used to efficiently determine contact lens power and resulting visual acuity. Spherocylinder ORs offer the added advantage of determining the optimal vision through the optics of the contact lens. The equivalent sphere may be used to determine the sphere power of the contact lens.

Autorefractors may be used to perform contact lens ORs to increase patient care efficiency.

Fluorescein Pattern Interpretation

To evaluate the GP lens-to-cornea fitting relationship, apply sodium fluorescein to the conjunctiva and view the pattern with either a Burton UV lamp or a slit lamp. If observing by slit lamp, use the cobalt filter over the illumination source and a yellow filter over the objective portion of the microscope to enhance viewing.

After the initial diagnostic GP lens is applied, fluorescein pattern interpretation and an OR should be performed. Fluorescein patterns allow the practitioner to fine-tune the lens-to-cornea fitting relationship. The apical or central fitting relationship (alignment, touch, or clearance), peripheral edge lift, and lens position and movement should be assessed. The quality of the tear film and lens wetting characteristics can be observed at the same time.

In evaluating a fluorescein pattern, the practitioner should carefully determine where the lens bears on the cornea. If only the fluoresced areas are interpreted, the practitioner may misjudge the fitting relationship due to excessive fluorescein or fluorescein coating the front surface of the lens.

PRESCRIBING CONSIDERATIONS

Refractive Error

Myopia

The effects of prescribing minus power contact lenses with thicker midperipheral lens profiles to correct myopia should be considered. The edge profile of high-minus-power GP contact lenses may lead to discomfort as the upper eyelid interacts with the thick lens edge during a blink. Edge thinning, such as lenticulation, reduces this lens–lid interaction. A thicker edge profile may cause the eyelids to vault the cornea beyond the edge of the lens, possibly inducing 3-o'clock to 9-o'clock peripheral corneal desiccation (54).

The edge thickness of a high-minus-power soft contact lens may lead to peripheral corneal neovascularization. Contact lens-induced neovascularization tended to be more pronounced with extended wear using nonsilicone hydrogel lenses (55), probably due to hypoxia leading to decreased compactness of the corneal tissue. Prescribing high Dk silicone hydrogel lenses tends to stabilize or reduce existing neovascularization (37).

Hyperopia

High-plus-power GP contact lenses should be lenticulated to reduce the center thickness, thereby placing the lens' center of gravity closer to the corneal surface. This encourages the lens to position centrally or superiorly. A lenticular design when compared to a single-cut lens reduces the center thickness by approximately 25%.

Consider higher Dk lenses for your hyperopic patients. Patients wearing high-plus-power soft contact lenses need to be monitored regularly to determine if excessive corneal swelling is occurring. This swelling is due to limited oxygen transmissibility through the thicker profile of the contact lens center (56). If striae or other signs of corneal edema occur, reduce the wearing time or refit the patient into a silicone hydrogel or high Dk GP lens material. Increasing soft lens water content alone probably will not sufficiently alter the available oxygen to acceptable levels (57).

Astigmatism

The amount of refractive cylinder is used to determine whether a soft sphere or a soft toric is indicated for an astigmatic patient. Many practitioners prescribe soft toric lenses when the cylinder is 0.75 D or more. The reproducibility of today's soft toric lenses encourages practitioners to prescribe the toric option more often and for smaller amounts of astigmatism. Practitioners also factor in variables such as the patient's vision needs and the magnitude of the spherical portion of the refraction (58).

The majority of today's soft toric contact lenses use prism ballasting or dual thin zones to achieve rotational stability. Eghbali et al. (59) found that oxygen transmissibility (Dk/t) was approximately half the amount through the inferior portion of a prism ballasted toric soft contact lens when compared to the available oxygen through similar superior lens locations. Prism ballasted soft toric lenses may be designed using eccentric lenticulation to minimize central lens thickness.

Contact Lens Replacement Options

Improvements in manufacturing in terms of cost of production and increase in soft lens reproducibility have enabled more frequent lens replacement. Patients enjoy the improved comfort and vision with new lenses. Also, there are fewer corneal and lid complications when patients replace their lenses more frequently. Traditional or conventional lenses were generally replaced annually. (Currently lenses can be prescribed for frequent replacement schedules of 1 to 3 months, or for *disposable* daily or after 1 to 2 weeks of wear.) Michaud and Giasson (60) found that lenses replaced after a longer interval than recommended by the manufacturer led to increased bound protein deposits, which contributed to increased upper eyelid papillae and hyperemia. Solomon et al. (61) reported fewer adverse patient symptoms with daily disposable versus 1- to 3-month replacement cycles. They also found that patients reported greater overall satisfaction with daily disposable lenses. There were fewer complications and fewer unscheduled office visits with daily disposables (61).

The practitioner should tailor the lens replacement schedule to meet the eye care needs (and budget) of each individual patient. Modify the replacement schedule by prescribing a different lens based on clinical findings and patient compliance.

Patients desiring part-time soft contact lens wear should consider daily or 2-week replacement soft lenses. If 2-week replacement lenses are dispensed, recommend lens replacement intervals based upon the number of days of lens wear. For example, if the patient wears the lenses 3 days a week to play tennis, recommend monthly replacement. If a lens is going to be reused, it must be disinfected again within 24 hours prior to wear.

PATIENT CONSIDERATIONS

Patient Compliance

The more emphasis is placed on patient education, the more likely the patient will comply with wearing schedules, lens care instructions, lens replacement schedules, and follow-up care. A relationship has been shown between patient compliance and contact lens complications, including microbial contamination (62).

Patient Education

At the end of the examination, the eye care practitioner should inform the patient of the examination results and how the findings relate to the patient's chief complaint and other symptoms. It is important for the practitioner to convey all vision correction options, including spectacles, contact lenses, and surgery, to their patients. The advantages, disadvantages, and expectations of each option should be explained, and the practitioner should provide recommendations. Patient education regarding the necessary visits and the rationale for those visits should be conveyed. All contact lens-wearing patients should have functional spectacles to allow for breaks within their wearing schedule and to wear in case of eye infections or injuries.

SUMMARY

Prescribing contact lenses is both an art and a science. The practitioner will not be able to fit every patient using textbook or nomogram philosophies. Preliminary data assist the practitioner in determining and recommending initial contact lens options for their patients and establishes baseline information. Changes to the patient's refraction, visual acuity, and corneal health, curvature, or shape are more easily noted and monitored over time. To succeed at and enjoy contact lens fitting and patient care, it is necessary to apply the artistic side of the equation and to be both resourceful and creative.

REFERENCES

1. Josephson JE, Erickson P, Back A, et al. Monovision. *J Am Optom Assoc* 1990;61:820–825.
2. Pence NA. Strategies for success with presbyopes. *CL Spectrum* 1994;9:30–39.
3. Edrington TB. Diagnosing and fitting irregular corneas. *CL Spectrum*. 1998;13[Suppl]:3s–5s.
4. Hayworth NAS, Asbell PA. Therapeutic contact lenses. *CLAO J* 1990;16:137–142.
5. Moore BD. Contact lens therapy for amblyopia. In: Rutstein RP, ed. *Problems in optometry*. Philadelphia: JB Lippincott, 1991: 355–368.
6. Allen ED, Davies PD. Role of contact lenses in the management of congenital nystagmus. *Br J Ophthalmol* 1983;67:834–836.
7. Cotter SA. *Clinical uses of prism: a spectrum of applications,* 1st ed. St. Louis: Mosby, 1995:170.
8. Mandell RB. The prism controversy. *J Am Optom Assoc* 1967; 38:190.
9. Prediger JP, Edmondson LL. Management of contact lens patients with pingueculae or pterygia. *Optom Vis Sci* 1993;70:9–14.
10. Waltman SR, Kaufman HE. Use of hydrophilic contact lenses to increase ocular penetration of topical drugs. *Invest Ophthalmol* 1970;9:250–255.
11. Karlgard CC, Wong NS, Jones LW, et al. In vitro uptake and release studies of ocular pharmaceutical agents by silicon-containing and p-HEMA hydrogel contact lens materials. *Int J Pharm* 2003;257:141–151.
12. Seal DV, McGill JI, Mackie IA, et al. Bacteriology and tear protein profiles of dry eyes. *Br J Ophthalmol* 1986;70:122–125.
13. March W, Long B, Hofman W, et al. Retrospective trial of daily wear contact lenses in diabetic patients. *Optom Vis Sci* 2002; 79[12s]:249.
14. Cormier LS, Cormier WH, Weisser RJ. *Interviewing and helping skills for health professionals.* Boston: Jones and Bartlett Publishers, 1986.
15. Inoue K, Katos S, Ohara C, et al. Ocular and systemic factors relevant to diabetic keratoepitheliopathy. *Cornea* 2001;20: 798–801.
16. O'Donnell C, Efron N, Boulton AJ. A prospective study of CL wear in diabetes mellitus. *Ophthal Physiol Opt* 2001;21:127–138.
17. Imafidon CO, Imafidon JE, Akingbade OA, et al. Symptomatology of contact lens wear in pregnancy. *Optom Vis Sci* 1991; 68[Suppl 12]:111.
18. Blackstone D. Wearing difficulties during pregnancy. *Optician* 1965;149:12.
19. Young G, Veys J, Pritchard N, et al. A multi-centre study of lapsed contact lens wearers. *Ophthal Physiol Opt* 2002;22: 516–527.
20. Hook SR, Holladay JT, Prager TC, et al. Transient myopia induced by sulfonamides. *Am J Ophthalmol* 1986;113:1231–1232.
21. Chirls IA, Norris JW. Transient myopia associated with vaginal sulfanilamide suppositories. *Am J Ophthalmol* 1984;98:120–121.
22. Bovino JA, Marcus DF. The mechanism of transient myopia induced by sulfonamide therapy. *Am J Ophthalmol* 1982;94:99.
23. Grinbaum A, Ashkenazi I, Gutman I, et al. Suggested mechanism for acute transient myopia after sulfonamide treatment. *Ann Ophthalmol* 1993;25:224–226.
24. Schein OD, Glynn RJ, Seddon JM, et al. The microbial keratitis study group. The relative risk of ulcerative keratitis among users of daily-wear and extended-wear soft contact lenses. *N Engl J Med* 1989;321:773–778.
25. Cutter G, Chalmers R, Roseman M. The clinical presentation, prevalence, and risk factors of focal corneal infiltrates in contact lens wearers. *CLAO* 1996;22:30–36.
26. McNally JJ, Chalmers RL, McKenney CD, et al. Risk factors for corneal infiltrative events with 30-night continuous wear of silicone hydrogel lenses. *CLAO* 2003;29[1s]:153–156.
27. Peyton SM, Joyce RG, Edrington TB. Soft contact lens and corneal changes associated with Visine use. *J Am Optom Assoc* 1989;60:207–210.
28. Terry RL, Schnider CM, Holden BA, et al. CCLRU standards for success of daily and extended wear contact lenses. *Optom Vis Sci* 1993;70:234–243.
29. Available at *http://www.siliconehydrogels.org*
30. Caroline PJ, Andre MP. The effect of corneal diameter on soft lens fitting, part 2. *CL Spectrum* 2002; May:56.
31. Bennett ES. Master the art of rigid lens design. *Rev Optom* 1994; 131[Suppl]:15A.
32. Young G, Hunt C, Covey M. Clinical evaluation of factors influencing toric soft contact lens fit. *Optom Vis Sci* 2002;79:11–19.

33. Korb DR, Korb JE. A new concept in contact lens design—part I and II. *J Am Optom Assoc* 1970;41:1023–1032.
34. Bruce, AS. Rigid gas permeable lens fitting and eyelid geometry. In: Hom MM ed. *Manual of contact lens prescribing and fitting with CD-ROM,* 2nd ed. Woburn, MA: Butterworth-Heinemann, 2000.
35. Josephson JE. Examination of the anterior ocular surface and tear film. In: Stein H, Slatt B, Stein R, eds. *Fitting guide for rigid and soft contact lenses,* 3rd ed. St. Louis: Mosby, 1990:39–50.
36. Mandell RB. *Contact lens practice,* 4th ed. Springfield, IL: Charles C. Thomas, 1988:998–999.
37. Dumbleton KA, Chalmers RL, Richter DB, et al. Vascular response to extended wear of hydrogel lenses with high and low oxygen permeability. *Optom Vis Sci* 2001;78:141–151.
38. Benjamin WJ. *Borish's clinical refraction.* Philadelphia: WB Saunders, 1998:990–997.
39. Edrington TB. Rigid gas permeable lenses for astigmatism. In: Hom MM, ed. *Manual of contact lens prescribing and fitting with CD-ROM.* Washburn, MA: Butterworth Heinemann 2000:144.
40. Brandreth RH. Biomicroscopic techniques for hydrogel lenses. *Int Contact Lens Clin* 1975;2:33–41.
41. Goldberg JB. *Biomicroscopy for contact lens practice: clinical procedures,* 2nd ed. Chicago: The Professional Press, 1984.
42. Allansmith MR. Giant papillary conjunctivitis. *J Am Optom Assoc* 1990;61:42–46.
43. Skotnitsky C, Sankaridurg PR, Sweeney DF, et al. General and local contact lens induced papillary conjunctivitis (CLPC). *Clin Exp Optom* 2002;85:193–197.
44. Manning FJ, Wehrly SR, Foulks GN. Patient tolerance and ocular surface staining characteristics of lissamine green versus rose Bengal. *Ophthalmology* 1995;102:1953–1957.
45. McMonnies CW. Key questions in a dry eye history. *J Am Optom Assoc* 1986;57:512–517.
46. Doughty MJ, Fonn D, Richter D, et al. A patient questionnaire approach to estimating the prevalence of dry eye symptoms in patients presenting to optometric practices across Canada. *Optom Vis Sci* 1997;74:624–631.
47. Begley CG, Caffery B, Nichols KK, et al. Responses of contact lens wearers to a dry eye survey. *Optom Vis Sci* 2000;77:40–46.
48. Nichols JJ, Mitchell GL, Nichols KK, et al. The performance of the contact lens dry eye questionnaire as a screening survey for contact lens-related dry eye. *Cornea* 2002;21:469–475.
49. Guillon M, Ho A. Photokeratoscopy and corneal topography. In: Reuben, Guillon, eds. *Contact lens practice.* Chapman and Hall Medical, 1997:313–357.
50. Tomlinson A, Thai LC, Doane MG, et al. Reliability of measurements of tear physiology. *Adv Exp Med Biol* 2002;506[Pt B]:1097–1105.
51. Guillon JP, Guillon M. Tear film examination of the contact lens patient. *Optician* 1993;206:21–29.
52. Brooks AMV, Robertson IF, Mahoney AM. Ocular rigidity and intraocular pressure in keratoconus. *Aust J Ophthal* 1984;12:317–324.
53. Bennett ES, Smythe J, Henry VA, et al. The effect of topical anesthetic use on initial patient satisfaction and overall success with rigid gas permeable contact lenses. *Optom Vis Sci* 1998;75:800–805.
54. Holden T, Bahr K, Koers D, et al. The effect of secondary curve lift-off on peripheral corneal desiccation. *Am J Optom Physiol Optics* 1987;64:108P.
55. Holden BA, Sweeney DF, Swarbrick HA, et al. The vascular response to long-term extended contact lens wear. *Clin Exp Optom* 1986;69:112–119.
56. Holden BA, Mertz GW. Critical oxygen levels to avoid corneal edema for daily and extended wear contact lenses. *Invest Ophthal Vis Sci* 1984;25:1161–1167.
57. Morgan PB, Efron N. The oxygen performance of contemporary hydrogel contact lenses. *Contact Lens Ant Eye* 1998;21:3–6.
58. Dabkowski JA, Roach MP, Begley CG. Soft toric versus spherical contact lenses in myopes with low astigmatism. *Int Contact Lens Clin* 1992;19:252–255.
59. Eghbali F, Hsu EH, Eghbali K, et al. Oxygen transmissibility at various locations in hydrogel toric prism-ballasted contact lenses. *Optom Vis Sci* 1996;73:164–168.
60. Michaud L, Giasson CJ. Overwear of contact lenses: increased severity of clinical signs as a function of protein absorption. *Optom Vis Sci* 2002;79:184–192.
61. Solomon OD, Freeman MI, Boshnick EL, et al. A 3-year prospective study of the clinical performance of daily disposable contact lenses compared with frequent replacement and conventional daily wear contact lenses. *CLAO J* 1996;22:250–257.
62. Bowden FW, Cohen EJ, Arentsen JJ, et al. Patterns of lens care practices and lens product contamination in contact lens microbial keratitis. *CLAO J* 1989;15:49–54.

CORNEAL TOPOGRAPHY: CORNEAL CURVATURE AND OPTICS, CLINICAL APPLICATIONS, AND WAVEFRONT ANALYSIS

YARON S. RABINOWITZ

CORNEAL CURVATURE AND OPTICS

The ocular anterior surface (with its tear film) is the major refractive element of the eye. Even minute surface disruptions can result in decreased vision. Such minor distortions often are not appreciated on slit-lamp evaluation and are best evaluated by methods that measure corneal topography. Topography is the science of describing or representing features of a particular surface (1). The most widely used technique to assess corneal shape utilizes the reflection of a target object from the anterior corneal surface with convex mirror optical principles (1). The ophthalmometer (Keratometer, Bausch & Lomb, Rochester, NY) is one such device. Ophthalmometers define the anterior cornea's radius of curvature by measuring four sites of reflected mires approximately 3 mm apart. Ophthalmometers are limited in that they provide no meaningful information regarding corneal shape central or peripheral to these points. Photokeratoscopes, which use optical principles similar to those of the ophthalmometer, measure larger surfaces and provide more complete appreciation of corneal shape.

The first known keratoscope target was a window pane. In 1619, Scheiner estimated corneal curvature by comparing the size of an image of a window pane seen in a human cornea to those seen in a series of marbles; his goal was to find that marble that duplicated the size of the corneal image (1). Alignment of the natural light, the target, and observer with the patient's visual axis was a major problem. This was overcome in 1882 by Placido, who placed an observation hole in the center of the target (2). Placido's target of alternating black and white rings (the Placido disk) still is used in many current corneal topography devices, hence the term *Placido disk keratoscopy.*

A modern version of the original Placido disk is the Klein hand-held keratoscope (Fig. 9.1), which is useful for detecting irregular astigmatism such as that induced by contact lens warpage, dry eye, or keratoconus. Its mire pattern has an outer diameter of 5.5mm, however, which limits its utility for evaluating peripheral corneal topography.

Photokeratoscopes project a series of concentric circular mires to form a virtual image located within the anterior chamber of the eye (Fig. 9.2). Information regarding the power of the anterior corneal surface is derived from visual inspection of the size and shape of the mires. Information regarding the radius of curvature of a localized area of the cornea is simultaneously obtained by the separation between the mires reflected from that area of the cornea. In areas of steep cornea, the mire images are smaller and the rings appear closer together. In flat areas of the cornea, the mire images are larger, so the rings appear further apart. In patients with regular astigmatism, the mires appear elliptic, with the short axis of the ellipse corresponding to the meridian corneal steepening and highest power (3). Photokeratoscopes are clinically useful in that they provide qualitative information about the peripheral cornea. Limitations include the lack of information about the central 3 mm of the cornea and the fact that up to 3 D of cylinder may go undetected by visual inspection of photokeratographs alone.

Computer-Assisted Videokeratoscopy

Quantitative analysis of photokeratograms became practical when Gullstrand applied photography to keratoscopy (photokeratoscopy) in 1896 (3). This allowed the clinician to fix the image and measure the size of the rings; however, this analysis is slow and subject to major errors (3). Computer power was adapted to the task of automated high-resolution corneal topography analysis in the 1980s, most popularly implemented in commercially available computer-assisted videokeratoscopes.

These devices overcome the deficiencies of the previous photokeratoscopes, both in speed and in gathering quantitative information about the anterior corneal surface (4). Most

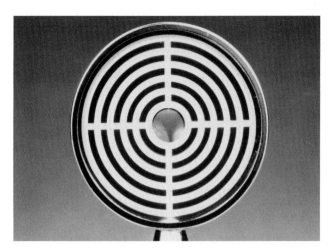

FIG. 9.1. Klein hand-held keratoscope.

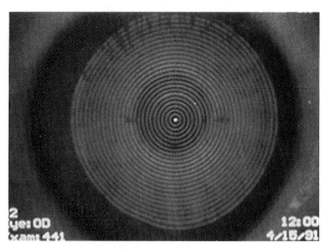

FIG. 9.3. Placido disk reflection of videokeratoscope showing 32 rings.

systems use illuminated Placido-type mires with nose cones that provide a broad area of corneal coverage, from the apex to the limbus of the cornea (Fig. 9.3).

These novel conical mire targets provide very high radial resolution; details are separated by 0.17 mm when reflected on normal corneal surfaces. Additionally, the central fixation light and the first mire of the standard cone provide excellent central corneal coverage, ensuring that corneal topographic details important to visual function are not obscured as they are with keratometers and traditional photokeratoscopic targets. Because direct measurements are made from the centrally visually important area as well as from the periphery, a clinically complete dataset derived from between 6 and 13,000 datapoints on the cornea, depending on the device, is available for clinical interpretation.

Other advantages of videokeratoscopy over photokeratoscopy are speed in gathering quantitative information and

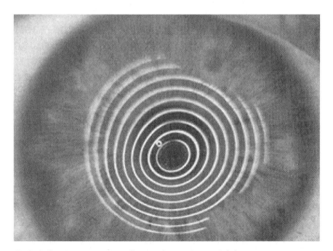

FIG. 9.2. Corneascope photo of a patient with keratoconus. Note the mires are closer together inferotemporally where the cornea is steepest.

ability to display data in a clinically useful format that is both accurate and reproducible (5–7).

Computer-assisted videokeratoscopes consist of a Placido disk on a slit-lamp–type platform and a video camera linked to a computer (8,9). In the topographic modeling system, the patient views a fixation target within the nose cone (Figs. 9.4 and 9.5). The operator, viewing a video display of the Placido disk mire images, brings them into focus while aligning a central target in the pupil with a joystick. Two peripheral targets also aid in focusing.

When the three targets overlap, maximum focus has been reached and an electronic snapshot of the video picture of the reflection of the Placido mires is acquired. The computer analyzes this image (to determine the size and the shape of the mires), reconstructs the patient's corneal surface, and presents a graphic picture of the topography in a suitable form.

The most useful form of data presentation is a color-coded corneal contour map in which steep areas are depicted as "hot colors" such as reds and browns and shallow areas as "cool colors" such as blues and greens (Fig. 9.6). Two scales are commonly used: absolute and normalized. In the absolute scale, each color represents 1.5 diopter intervals between 35 and 50 diopters, whereas above and below this range colors represent 5 diopter intervals. This scale is useful in routine practice (e.g., preoperative screening). In the normalized scale, the cornea is divided into 11 equal colors spanning the eye's total dioptric power. In this scale, more minute topographic details within an individual cornea can be appreciated. As part of the topographic display, quantitative indices are generated, including the following: predicted visual acuity based on corneal shape, simulated keratometry readings, minimum keratometry reading, surface regularity index, and surface asymmetry index (10).

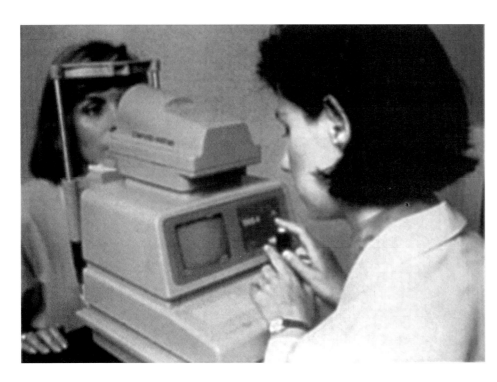

FIG. 9.4. Topographic modeling system showing video capturing of a patient's anterior corneal surface.

OPTICS: CALCULATION OF CORNEAL SURFACE POWER

Videokeratoscopic analysis of corneal shape relies on the optical principle that the tear film on the anterior corneal surface acts as a convex mirror. A light (mire) directed toward the cornea gives rise to a virtual erect image located approximately 4 mm posterior to the anterior surface of the cornea, at the level of the anterior capsule. This is the corneal light reflex, or the first Purkinje-Sanson image, which is viewed during both keratoscopy and keratometry. The size of this image can be used to quantify the curvature of the cornea: the steeper the cornea (i.e., the smaller the radius of curvature), the more powerful the convex mirror and thus the smaller the image. By the same principles, any

toricity (different radii of curvature in different meridians) or irregularity of the corneal surface will cause regular or irregular distortion of the image (2). The image of a convex mirror can be constructed in two rays: (i) a ray parallel to the principal axis, which reflected away from the principal focus; and (ii) a ray from the top of the object traveling toward the center of curvature and reflecting back along the same path (Fig. 9.7).

The magnification produced by a curved mirror is the ratio of image (I) to object size (O). This in turn is proportional to the ratio of the distance of the image (v) and the object (u) from the mirror as follows:

$$\text{Magnification} = I/O = v/u.$$

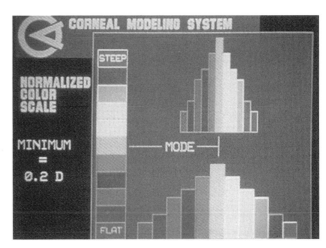

FIG. 9.6. Color scale used in a videokeratograph. (See Color Plate 9.6.)

FIG. 9.5. Nose cone of the topographic modeling system.

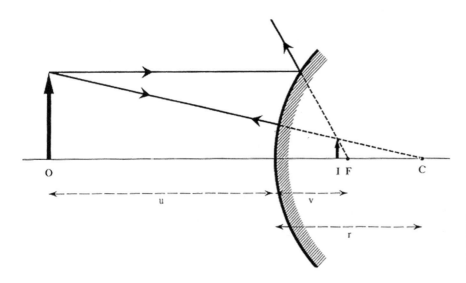

FIG. 9.7. Ray diagram depicting ray tracing in convex mirrors. (From Corbett MC, Obart DPS, Saunders DC, et al. The assessment of corneal topography. *Eur J Implant Refract Surg* 1994;6:98, with permission.)

In practice, the image (I) is located close to the focal point (F), which is halfway between the center of curvature of the mirror (C, at the principal focus) and the mirror itself. Therefore, v may be taken to equal half the radius of curvature of the mirror (r/2). Upon substituting r/2 for v in the preceding equation (I = O × r/2u), it can be seen that as the cornea becomes steeper and its radius of curvature (r) becomes smaller, so the image (I) becomes smaller and the topography mires appear closer together.

In a given keratometer, u, the focal distance of the viewing telescope, is constant. Rearrangement of the equation (r = 2u × I/O) shows that the radius of curvature is proportional to image size if the object remains constant (2). The geometrics optics equation that relates corneal power in diopters (D) to the radius of corneal curvature (R, measured in millimeters) is adapted from Snell's Law of Refraction, with differences of refractive index combined with corneal thickness and corneal back surface, to give the following equation:

$$D = K1/R2,$$

where K1 is the keratometric index usually assigned a numeric value of 337.5. For example, a cornea with a radius of curvature (R2) of 7.8 mm equates with this convention to a corneal power of 43.25 diopters (i.e., 337.5/7.8). The keratometric index differs from the corneal refractive index (1.376) in that it takes into account both the anterior and posterior corneal surfaces; however, it fails to recognize the different refractive properties of the epithelium and the stroma (1).

Corneal Contour Display

Corneal contour usually is described in one of three ways: qualitative, mathematical, or point to point. In the qualitative method, the cornea is said to consist of two zones: (i) a central zone or corneal cap of nearly constant corneal curvature surrounded by (ii) a peripheral zone with an increasingly longer radius of curvature. The corneal cap is an artifact of measurement methods and continues to be used only because it provides a convenient clinical construct. The cornea actually has a radius of curvature that changes immediately as one moves away from the apex. Near the apex the rate change is slow, but it increases rapidly toward the periphery. Cap diameter therefore depends on an arbitrary criterion for the amount of radius change that can occur before it is considered significant: 1 diopter of change has typically been adopted as a criterion, which yields a corneal cap of approximately 4 mm (11,12).

The second method of describing corneal contour is the mathematical method, using expressions such as an ellipse or polynomials. This method is favored by most authorities because it has a number of applications to ocular optics, such as in analysis of aberrations. Of the various simple mathematical expressions that can be used to describe the cornea, the ellipse is arguably the best. It usually is possible to describe an elliptic curve very closely to radius data from any single meridian or hemi-meridian of the cornea, except in the periphery where the rate of flattening exceeds that of an ellipse. Thus, for the optic portion of the cornea, the ellipse is an adequate model (2,11).

The third approach is the point-to-point method, which simply consists of an array of corneal radius or power values found at various corneal positions. Although this method seems simple and straightforward, it is difficult to assimilate an overall impression of the corneal contour merely by looking at an array of numbers. If all adjacent numbers with the same values are connected as in contour mapping, however, the display is transformed into a comprehensive pattern that provides an overall impression of corneal shape. Currently the preferred method of displaying the corneal topography by videokeratoscopy is the topographic map.

This method provides a large amount of information about the corneal contour in a single display. The corneal topographic map applies the principles of a geographic topographic map, except that instead of providing equal elevations, the isometric zones represent different radii of curvature. The topographic map is derived from the radius measurements at several thousand corneal positions, which can be displayed in either millimeters of curvature or dioptric power values. The diopters that are used for corneal power, however, have only a relative relationship to the true corneal power in the optical sense.

For example, if a cornea has power of 42 diopters at its apex and 40 diopters at some peripheral point, we would expect the peripheral point to be about 2 diopters out of focus. With current videokeratoscopy, however, the radius of curvature is actually measured and power displayed simply represents a conversion from radius to power using the following keratometric formula: $P = (n - 1)/r$, where $n = 1.3375$.

This formula is not applicable to the peripheral cornea because the keratometric formula is valid only for paraxial rays and becomes increasingly inaccurate as one moves further peripherally. The power used in the calculation of the corneal topographic map is based on the keratometric formula and uses the radius of curvature (AC) ending at the optic axis (Fig. 9.8) (11).

Alignment

Videokeratoscopes are aligned along an axis that is neither in the line of sight nor in the visual axis, both of which could be practical reference points. The subject looks at a fixation point on the optic axis of the instrument. The videokeratoscopic axis is aligned perpendicular to the cornea and thus is directed toward the center of curvature of the cornea for some unknown peripheral position (Fig. 9.9) (11).

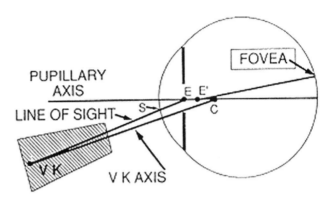

FIG. 9.9. Alignment of videokeratoscope axis relative to the cornea, pupillary axis, and line of sight. (From Mandell RB. The enigma of corneal contour. *CLAO J* 1992;18:267, with permission.)

Image Processing

From an optical standpoint, the videokeratoscope has no advantage over the photokeratoscope; however, it is superior to the photokeratoscope in terms of image processing. What previously required hours to days for hand analysis now can be completed in minutes. Not only are the measurements faster, they are more accurate. For example, using manual digitization a resolution of 500 lines per frame gives an accuracy of 1.2 diopters. Automated digitization statistical procedures can produce subpixel resolution and accuracy of less than 0.25 diopters. Formerly it required great skill to construct a photokeratoscope with target rings that were perfectly round so that the object size would be the same in all meridians. With the videokeratoscope, the target roundness is immaterial because every meridian can be calibrated separately. The ability of the instrument to measure the curvature of any small area depends largely on the instrument algorithm, which is a series of calculations involved in converting videokeratoscope image sizes into radius of curvature values for the cornea (2).

Software

A reference point is established from which the position of each other point can be identified mathematically. Ideally, the reference point should be related to an ocular feature such as the visual axis or corneal apex. Because the area of the cornea forming the sharpest retinal image frequently is not centered on any of these landmarks, it often is more appropriate to select the most convenient reproducible reference point. Most systems use the center of the innermost mire, the position of which can be determined in one of three ways. If the first mire is relatively large, computational techniques must be used to calculate either the centroid of its corneal surface area or its geometrically averaged center. These techniques have been obviated since the development of collimated devices, which can reduce the diameter of the innermost mire to 0.7 mm and use the reflection of the

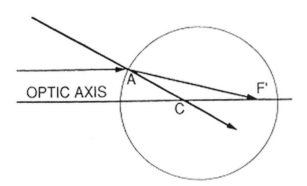

FIG. 9.8. Ray diagram illustrating radius of curvature AC used in the corneal power calculations of topographic maps. (From Mandell RB. The enigma of corneal contour. *CLAO J* 1992;18:267, with permission.)

fixation light as a central reference point. The accuracy of the reference center depends on patient fixation and proper alignment of the instrument. Once a central reference point is established, rectangular coordinates are given to each datapoint where a semi-meridian intersects a mire. Most commercial systems have 15 to 38 circular mires and 256 to 360 equally spaced semi-meridians, theoretically providing between 6,000 and 11,000 datapoints.

The accuracy of the final construction does not depend on the total number of datapoints but on their density, provided the same video pixel is not sampled multiple times. Rectangular coordinates locating the datapoints are converted to polar coordinates on the keratoscope mires to facilitate corneal reconstruction. A reconstruction algorithm is applied to the location of each point on the two-dimensional reflection to give a three-dimensional position of the cornea from which the reflection originated. The algorithm consists of a mathematical formula from which the curvature of the anterior corneal surface is calculated. This is converted to total corneal power by the standard keratometric index (2). Because there is no mathematical formula that describes the shape of the normal cornea, the algorithm gives only an approximation of corneal shape, which is most accurate centrally where the cornea is most spheric. For each point on mire reflection to correspond to a unique position on the cornea, the following assumptions about the cornea are made: the surface is spherical within the small area being measured, the surface is of uniform refractive index, and the centers of curvature for all reflecting points are on the optic axis. Algorithms are derived in several ways. In the one-step curve-fitting method, the geometry of reflected mires is globally fitted to a polynomial. A refinement fits the global geometric model to the cornea at each meridian individually, with the allowance of local nonconformance. The one-step profile method normalizes the central radius of curvature to a standard 7.8 mm and then uses a successive approximation method to calculate the corneal shape in the periphery in a given meridian.

A more accurate reconstruction of the central cornea is obtained by a two-step profile method, which compares the diameters of individual keratoscope mires reflected from the cornea with those from calibration spheres (2).

Accuracy and Reproducibility

The accuracy of any instrument depends on the resolution it achieves at each stage between the generation of mire pattern and presentation of the data. The final transverse spatial resolution ideally should be sufficient to detect surface irregularities just large enough to degrade visual function. This precise level has yet to be determined and may vary from the center to the periphery of the cornea. Videokeratoscopy measures corneal power with a sensitivity of 0.25 diopters or better within the central 6 mm of the cornea. Sensitivity is reduced toward the periphery for very

steep (>46 diopters) or very flat (<38 diopters) corneas, as well as in the presence of marked surface irregularity (13–17).

CLINICAL APPLICATIONS OF CORNEAL TOPOGRAPHY

Normal Cornea

Prior to detecting the shape of diseased cornea, it is imperative to develop an understanding of how the normal cornea is depicted by videokeratography.

The normal cornea is aspheric, steeper centrally while flattening toward the periphery. Flattening may vary from 1 to 4 diopters (Fig. 9.10). There is significant variability in the shape of videokeratographs of normal human corneas, with 10 classifiable shapes if a single consistent scale such as the absolute scale is used (Fig. 9.11). A normal cornea will not look the same when displayed in normalized as opposed to absolute scale. To develop an appreciation of normal shape, it is recommended that the clinician only use the absolute scale initially for diagnostic purposes. Red colors (range 49–50.5 diopters) are seen only very rarely in normal corneas (18–21) in the absolute scale. Although there are interindividual differences in corneal shape, the corneal surface shapes of the companion eye in a single patient often are strikingly similar.

Astigmatism

Regular Astigmatism

Regular astigmatism is either congenital or surgically induced and is depicted as a figure-of-eight pattern (Fig. 9.11.6), with the two lobes being almost equal in size. Regu-

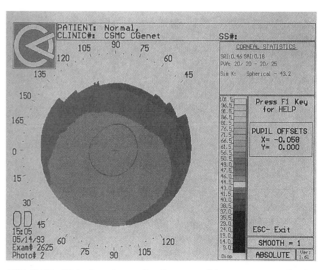

FIG. 9.10. Videokeratograph of a normal human cornea in the "absolute" scale. (See Color Plate 9.10.)

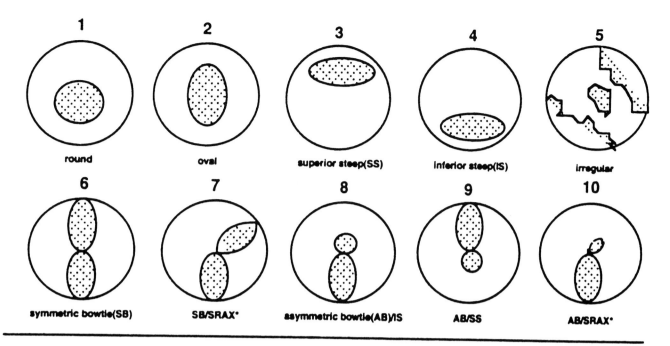

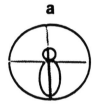
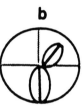

Explanation of how to interpret SRAX*(skewed radial axes):
this pattern suggests that there is skewing of the steepest radial axes above and below the horizontal meridian. To interpret this as such, an imaginary line is drawn to bisect the upper and lower lobes of asymmetric bowtie(see solid line). If there is no deviation from the vertical meridian, there is no skewing and the pattern is labelled AB(figure a). However if the lines bisecting the two lobes appear skewed by more than 30 degrees from the vertical meridian, it is called skewed(as in figure b), and this pattern is labelled AB/SRAX.

FIG. 9.11. Classification scheme for normal human corneas showing the variation in normal shape using the "absolute" scale.

lar astigmatism may be with the rule (figure-of-eight at 90 degrees), against the rule (figure-of-eight at 180 degrees), or oblique (figure-of-eight at an oblique axis) (1).

Irregular Astigmatism

In irregular astigmatism, the major steep axes above and below the visual axis are not separated by 180 degrees, and there may be multiple zones of increased or decreased surface corneal power depending on the cause of the astigmatism (Fig. 9.12).

Causes of irregular astigmatism are multiple and may include tear film abnormalities as seen with keratitis sicca or severe meibomitis. The latter is depicted on videokeratography as absent areas of digitization or irregular or defocused keratoscopic rings. Topographic alterations are commonly the result of focal elevations of the epithelium over dystrophic tissue or subepithelial scarring from previous epithelial erosions. If irregular astigmatism is the sole source of the patient's decreased vision, acuity should improve with rigid contact lens overrefraction (as the lens' smooth ante-

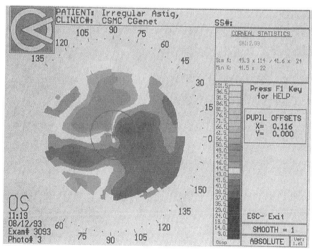

FIG. 9.12. Videokeratograph of an irregular cornea in the "absolute" scale. (See Color Plate 9.12.)

rior refracting surface optically neutralizes surface irregularities).

Other causes of irregular astigmatism include inflammatory processes affecting the stroma, trauma, peripheral limbal masses, and pterygia, all of which may cause significant reduction in visual acuity. In these instances, the cornea may appear normal on clinical examination, whereas videokeratography reveals typical and obvious topographic alterations (1).

Keratoconus

Corneal topography of keratoconus is highly complex and extremely variable. The cone can assume many different shapes, and its apex can be located at variable points relative to the center of the cornea. Prior to the introduction of videokeratography, cones were described as having two basic shapes, oval and nipple, which could be differentiated by slit-lamp microscopy and corneoscopy. Videokeratography has demonstrated that the corneal shape in keratoconus is more complex (22–24). Classically, keratoconus is depicted as a localized area of increased surface power surrounded by concentric zones of decreasing surface power (Fig. 9.13). The area of steepening may occur anywhere on the cornea. Inferior steepening, more prominent temporally, is the most common pattern seen. Other complex patterns, such as central steepening with a superimposed asymmetric bowtie pattern, have been noted.

Videokeratography is useful for distinguishing keratoconus from other thinning disorders such as pellucid marginal degeneration and Terrien's marginal degeneration. Pellucid marginal degeneration patients have videokeratographs of butterfly-shaped patterns that demonstrate low corneal power along the central vertical axis, increased power as the peripheral cornea is approached, and high corneal power in the midperipheral cornea along the inferior oblique meridians (Fig. 9.14) (25). Terrien's marginal degeneration causes a variety of patterns, depending on areas of involvement. Most common superior corneal thinning will show an inverted butterfly-shaped appearance in the videokeratograph, that is the wings of the "butterfly" point upward and superiorly (26).

"Early Detection" of Keratoconus

One of the most useful applications of computer-assisted videokeratography is the detection of keratoconus before the onset of slit-lamp or retroillumination signs. Even in the presence of regular keratoscopy mires, there may be subtle signs of keratoconus as displayed by the color-coded videokeratographs (27,28).

Marc Amsler used a photographic Placido disk to first describe early corneal topographic changes in keratoconus patients (prior to the detection of clinical or biomicroscopic signs). His classic studies on the natural history of keratoconus documented its progression from minor corneal surface distortions to clinically detectable keratoconus. He classified keratoconus into clinically recognizable stages and an earlier latent stage recognizable only by Placido disk examination of corneal topography. These early stages were subdivided into two categories: "keratoconus fruste" (1- to 4-degree deviation of the horizontal axis of the Placido disk), and "early or mild keratoconus" (4- to 8-degree deviation of the

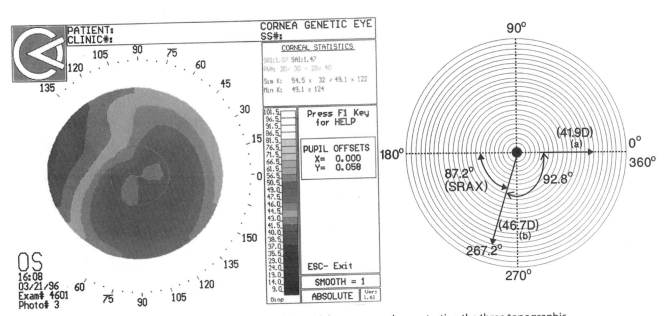

FIG. 9.13. Videokeratograph of a patient with keratoconus demonstrating the three topographic features of keratoconus and illustrating the calculation of the SRAX index. (See Color Plate 9.13.)

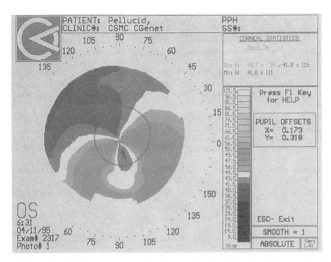

FIG. 9.14. Videokeratograph of a patient with pellucid marginal degeneration showing a typical butterfly pattern. (See Color Plate 9.14.)

horizontal axis). Only slight degrees of asymmetric oblique astigmatism could be detected in these early forms of keratoconus. Similar findings were absent in patients with regular astigmatism (29,30).

In Amsler's study of 600 patients 22% had clinically obvious keratoconus in both eyes, 26% had clinical keratoconus in one eye and latent keratoconus in the other, and 52% had latent keratoconus bilaterally. Progression was highly variable and most often asymmetric. The cone could remain stationary, progress rapidly over 3 to 5 years, and arrest or progress intermittently over an extended period of time. When Amsler reexamined 286 eyes 3 to 8 years after the diagnosis, only 20% of the entire group, including 66% of the latent cases, had progressed. Progression was most likely to occur in patients between 10 and 20 years of age, decreased slightly between ages 20 and 30 years, and was less likely to increase after age 30 years (29,30).

Modern videokeratoscopes detect subtle changes in corneal topography prior to the onset of clinical disease. This has assumed even greater importance with the increasing popularity of refractive surgery because it is important to detect abnormal topography prior to embarking on any refractive surgical procedure. Videokeratography is therefore used routinely to screen patients for these procedures (31, 32). As previously described, keratoconus sagittal videokeratography has three characteristics that are not present in normal videokeratographs: an increased area of corneal power surrounded by concentric areas of decreasing power, inferior–superior power asymmetry, and skewing of the steepest radial axes above and below the horizontal meridian (Fig. 9.13).

Similar patterns have been noted in clinically normal family members of keratoconus patients and in the clinically "normal" fellow eye of patients with clinically unilateral keratoconus (28,33,34). These patterns are milder (as mea-

sured by dioptric power) than the patterns noted in clinically obvious keratoconus. Because it may be difficult to interpret subtle changes resembling keratoconus on the videokeratograph, two methods have been suggested to differentiate subtle keratoconus from normal videokeratographs: pattern recognition and differentiation through quantitative descriptors (35–37).

Videokeratography Pattern Recognition

Pattern recognition with color-coded maps becomes easier as a practitioner gains experience. Diagnosing keratoconus based on videokeratograph pattern recognition alone appears difficult for inexperienced clinicians. Maps suspicious for keratoconus in the presence of an otherwise clinically normal eye should be labeled "keratoconus suspect" until progression to keratoconus is documented (38). Proficiency in distinguishing normal from subtle pathology is gained by use of the absolute scale (in the Topographic Modeling System [TMS-1] this scale divides the cornea into 1.5 D intervals between 35 and 50 D and 5 D intervals outside of this range) (39). The normalized scale in this device (which divides the cornea into 11 equal colors) is confusing, and many clinically normal patients with slight inferior steepening might inadvertently be labeled as "suspect." For the purposes of our research in trying to define an "early keratoconus" phenotype by videokeratography, we compiled a database of normal videokeratography patterns of 195 normal individuals using this absolute scale (Fig. 9.11). This baseline database of videokeratography patterns (sagittal topography) will be used as a reference for our longitudinal topographic studies of keratoconus family members and can determine subtle deviations in corneal topography at any point in time. Although the ultimate determination as to which patterns ultimately progress to keratoconus has yet to be finalized, our database of videokeratography patterns suggests that only 1 (0.5%) of 195 normal patients have mild topographic features similar to, but milder than, those seen in clinically detectable keratoconus asymmetric bowtie with skewed radical axes (ab/srax) (19,40,41).

"Pseudokeratoconus"

Videokeratography patterns simulating keratoconus (videokeratographic pseudokeratoconus) confound the minimal topographic criteria for keratoconus (42,43). The most common culprit is wear of contact lenses, both hard and soft, that induces patterns of inferior steepening almost indistinguishable from keratoconus (42). These patterns, however, disappear with time after contact lens wear is discontinued. Videokeratographic pseudokeratoconus also may occur when either inferior eyeball compression or misalignment of the eye (inferior or superior rotation) occurs during video capture. Inferior corneal steepening also is simulated from dry spot formation with incomplete digitization of mires. Early pellucid marginal degeneration, inflammatory corneal thinning, and previous ocular surgery all can induce videokeratography patterns that simulate keratoconus (43). Awareness of these pitfalls allows for better appreciation of the true topographic changes occurring in the earliest stages of keratoconus. Analyses of videokeratography data described thus far are based on data generated by sagittal algorithms, which are spherically biased. Recent preliminary studies suggest that tangential algorithms may have more promise for identifying the "early" topographic features of keratoconus. Studies are underway to determine whether such algorithms might be the preferred method for studying keratoconus (44).

Quantitative Descriptors

Accurate quantitative descriptors of videokeratography patterns in keratoconus would enhance pattern recognition and might assist determination of minimal topographic criteria for diagnosing keratoconus. The use of quantitative videokeratography-derived indices potentially represents a more reproducible way of quantifying keratoconus, especially its early phenotypes (41).

This has particular application in screening patients for refractive surgery, because unpredictable results and patient dissatisfaction have been attributed to refractive surgery performed on myopic patients with undiagnosed "early" keratoconus (45–47). The many topographic forms of keratoconus may make recognition of early or forme fruste keratoconus videokeratographs difficult. Software programs with quantitative indices have been developed to alert the clinician to the presence of keratoconus or "suspect" topography during the refractive surgery screening process.

Three such software programs exist: (i) the Rabinowitz K and I-S indices on the Tomey topography; (ii) the Maeda-Klyce system, also on the Tomey system; and (iii) the most recent KISA% system, currently available on the Alcon topographer and being developed as broad cross-platform software to be used on all topographic devices (22,36,37).

The Rabinowitz K and I-S indices (Figs. 9.15 and 9.16) quantify the central steepening found in nipple cones and the superior inferior dioptric asymmetry found in oval cones. Advantages of these indices were simplicity and extreme sensitivity. Disadvantages were a relatively high false-positive rate and inability to quantify irregular astigmatism occurring in keratoconus. It should be noted that false-posi-

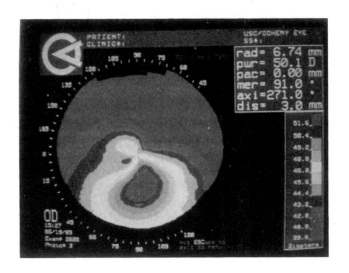

Calculation of I-S Value in Patient 5 (Right Eye)*

Inferior cornea							
degrees	330	300	270	240	210		
diopters	45.9	49.7	50.1	48.6	44.7	239 /5	= 47.8 (I) (average inferior corneal power)
Superior cornea							
degrees	150	120	90	60	30		
diopters	41.6	40.9	40.6	40.2	40.2	203.5/5	= 40.7 (S) (average superior corneal power)

I-S Value = 47.8 (I) – 40.7 (S) = 7.1 diopters

---

* *Measurements taken 3 mm from center of cornea*

FIG. 9.15. Videokeratograph of a patient with keratoconus illustrating calculation of the I-S value. (See Color Plate 9.15.)

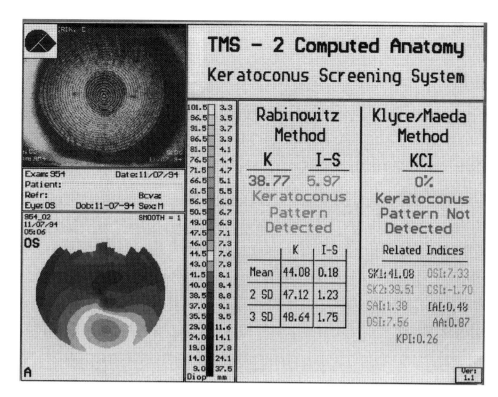

FIG. 9.16. Videokeratograph of a patient with "early" keratoconus and the Rabinowitz and Maeda-Klyce indices on the Tomey topographer. (See Color Plate 9.16.)

tive results alert the clinician to other conditions to be ruled out prior to refractive surgery (35).

The Maeda-Klyce system (available only on the Tomey topographer) was developed to be more specific, decrease the false-positive rate, and differentiate keratoconus from a wide range of other corneal pathologies. A series of neural network systems perform this function in its current version (36). Disadvantages of this system include its complexity, that it is specific only to the Tomey topographer, and that its keratoconus prediction index (KPI; expressed as percent keratoconus) bears no correlation to the clinical degree of keratoconus because it was derived in the laboratory from videokeratographs only, not clinical data (36).

The KISA% index is a product of the previously developed K and I-S values and a new index, the SRAX index (Fig. 9.13), which was developed to quantify the irregular astigmatism that occurs in keratoconus (37). It was devised using both sagittal and tangential algorithms. and is a most useful index for videokeratography screening in refractive surgery because it is a single index with excellent clinical correlation to disease status. It clearly differentiates keratoconus from normal and provides a range for potential "suspects" with minimal overlap with the normal population. Additionally, the KISA% index is more accurate and specific than any of the previously described keratoconus detection systems (37).

When the KISA% has a value of 100 or more, the patient always has clinically detectable keratoconus. As disease severity increases, so does the numerical value of the index.

Normal patients and those with keratoconus are clearly separated, with almost no overlap. Values ranging from 60% to 100% are used to designate or label patients as "suspects" with minimal fear of significant overlap with the normal population (<0.5%) (Figs. 9.17 and 9.18). These patients can be followed for development of keratoconus.

Because this index has excellent clinical correlation, it is highly likely that any topographic map with a KISA% index over 100% represents keratoconus and that patient should be excluded from undergoing laser-assisted *in situ* keratomileusis (LASIK) (45–47). If no clinical signs were detected prior to the patient undergoing topography, a value over 100% should alert the clinician to the possibility of keratoconus, to carefully look for "scissoring of the red reflex" on dilated retinoscopy, or to perform pachymetry and look for corneal thinning to verify the presence of "early" keratoconus. If eventually verified by independent observers using different sets of normal controls and keratoconus patients, the simplicity of this index allows it to be universally used on many different videokeratoscopes. Although currently available only on the Alcon topographer, this system should soon be available on all topographic devices to diagnose and quantify keratoconus.

Classification Scheme and Progression

Using a combination of videokeratography and clinical signs, keratoconus can be classified into three distinct categories, each of which has its own unique corneal topogra-

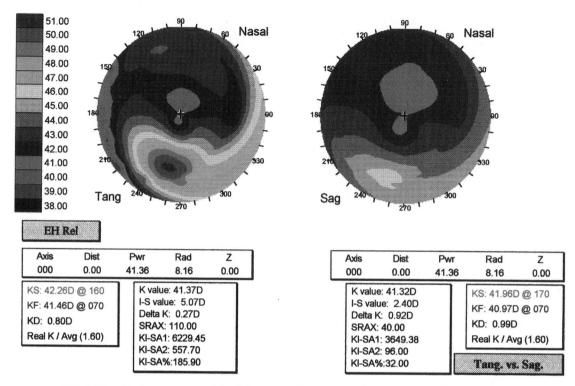

Axis	Dist	Pwr	Rad	Z
000	0.00	41.36	8.16	0.00

KS: 42.26D @ 160	K value: 41.37D
KF: 41.46D @ 070	I-S value: 5.07D
KD: 0.80D	Delta K: 0.27D
Real K / Avg (1.60)	SRAX: 110.00
	KI-SA1: 6229.45
	KI-SA2: 557.70
	KI-SA%: 185.90

Axis	Dist	Pwr	Rad	Z
000	0.00	41.36	8.16	0.00

K value: 41.32D	KS: 41.96D @ 170
I-S value: 2.40D	KF: 40.97D @ 070
Delta K: 0.92D	KD: 0.99D
SRAX: 40.00	Real K / Avg (1.60)
KI-SA1: 3649.38	
KI-SA2: 96.00	**Tang. vs. Sag.**
KI-SA%: 32.00	

FIG. 9.17. Videokeratograph of the fellow eye of a patient with keratoconus. The eye appeared clinically normal, showing calculation of the KISA% index in both the sagittal and tangential views on the Alcon topographer. (See Color Plate 9.17.)

phy. The three categories, in decreasing order of severity, are as follows (Fig. 9.19). (i) *Keratoconus.* Disease is detected by slit-lamp evaluation. Patient may have one or more of the following clinical signs: stromal corneal thinning, Vogt striae, Fleischer ring, and a typical ab/srax pattern with videokeratography. (ii) *"Early" keratoconus.* No slit-lamp findings of disease but scissoring or a "Charleaux" oil droplet sign on retroillumination and a typical ab/srax pattern with videokeratography. (iii). *Keratoconus "suspect."* No clinical signs of keratoconus on either slit-lamp evaluation or retroillumination but a typical ab/srax pattern (Fig. 9.13).

Classifying keratoconus into shapes and quantifying these shapes with indices allows quantification of disease progression (Fig. 9.20). Subsequent analysis allows definition of early phenotypes, which are used both in screening prior to refractive surgery and for genetic analyses in keratoconus pedigrees and genetic studies. Genetic analyses using these methods to quantify 'early' disease phenotypes dem-

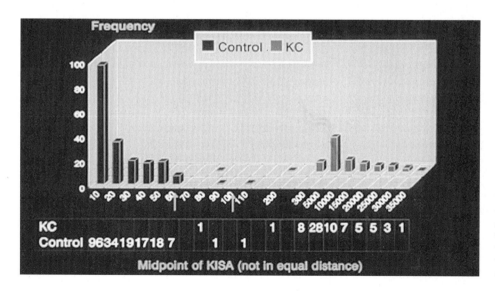

FIG. 9.18. Histogram of the KISA% index calculated in 195 normal patients and 60 patients with keratoconus. Note the clean separation of the two groups. Most normal patients have a value less than 60, whereas the majority of keratoconus patients have a value over 100.

onstrate that genes play a major role in the pathogenesis of keratoconus (48,49).

Contact Lenses

Before evaluating a videokeratograph, it is critical to determine whether a patient is a contact lens wearer, what type of lenses he or she wears, and how long the lens had been off the eye when the videokeratograph was acquired. Normal contact lens wear is likely the most common cause of alterations of corneal topography. Topographic changes are more common with rigid gas permeable contact lenses, but they occur with daily and extended wear soft contact lenses as well. Topographic alterations induced by contact lens wear are frequently characterized by a reversal of the normal topographic pattern, evident as progressive flattening of the corneal surface from the center to the periphery, loss of radial symmetry, and central irregular astigmatism.

Following wear of decentered rigid contact lenses, there is frequently a correlation between the most common resting position of the contact lens and corneal topography distortions. A relative flattening zone occurs beneath the decentered contact lens, and relative steepening of the corneal contour is observed outside the area of contact with the decentered contact lens, called *corneal warpage.* Symptoms include decreased visual acuity with eyeglass wear and intolerance to contact lenses (infrequent). The time for resolution of corneal warpage after discontinuation of contact lens wear varies among patients.

Contact lens-induced alterations of corneal contour should be excluded before refractive surgical procedures are considered. Before surgery is undertaken in these patients, contact lens wear should be discontinued and topography monitored until results are normal and stable (50). Topographic changes frequently resolve within 6 weeks in soft lens wearers. Rigid contact lens wearers may require longer

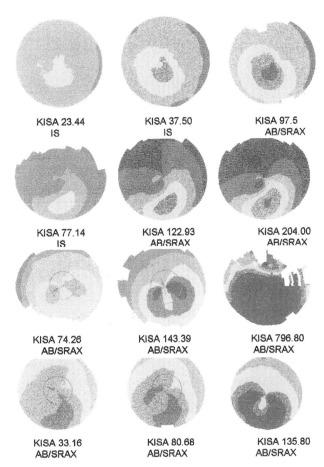

FIG. 9.20. Videokeratographs with pattern and indices analysis showing progression of keratoconus from suspect to clinically affected over a 5-year period. (See Color Plate 9.20.)

Keratoconus: one or more of the following: Corneal thinning by slit-lamp evaluation, an iron ring, Vogt's striae

Early Keratoconus: no slit-lamp findings, with scissoring on retinoscopy

Keratoconus Suspect: clinically normal, with suspicious topography

FIG. 9.19. Classification scheme for keratoconus using videokeratography and clinical signs. (See Color Plate 9.19.)

times, ranging from 8 weeks to 8 months. Corneal topography should be monitored on a regular basis until results are stable 2 weeks apart prior to initiating any refractive procedure.

Because videokeratography provides important information about corneal curvature in the periphery of the cornea, it also shows promise as an aid to contact lens fitting in patients with complex corneal topographies, such as keratoconus and after corneal transplant, radial keratotomy, and LASIK (51,52).

WAVEFRONT ANALYSIS

An exciting new method for determining the true refractive state of the eye and measurements of associated aberrations has recently become popular. Wavefront analysis is an objective and quantifiable measure of visual performance. Prior to the introduction of refractive surgery, wavefront aberration played a small role in clinical ophthalmic optics. Even at relatively large apertures, wavefront aberrations do not degrade image quality below 20/20 in normal eyes (53).

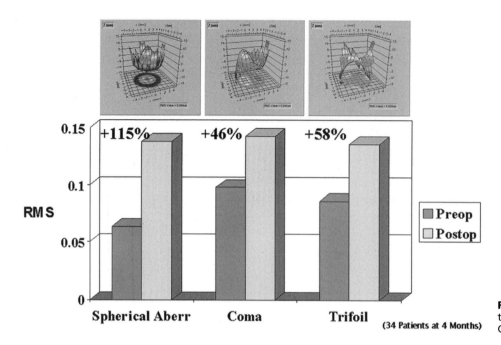

RMS

0.15 +115% +46% +58%

0.1

0.05

0

Spherical Aberr **Coma** **Trifoil**

(34 Patients at 4 Months)

■ **Preop**
□ **Postop**

FIG. 9.21. Higher-order aberrations induced by LASIK surgery, (See Color Plate 9.21.).

Refractive surgery-induced aberrations, however, become important under low levels of illumination and with large pupil apertures.

Spherical aberration and coma, particularly, are both induced in eyes treated with excimer laser procedures (Fig. 9.21). Fig. 9.22 illustrates this point. After LASIK, wavefront measurements illustrate why this patient is unhappy when his eye achieves 20/20 vision. This has spurred interest in both the measurements of high-order chromatic aberrations and techniques for their elimination among refractive surgeons.

Refraction and visual acuity measurements suggest which letters on the vision chart are correctly identified, but there is a wide variability in perceived image quality for the same level of illumination (54). Consider the optics of the Kodak Instamatic camera compared to the sophisticated Canon

EOS Élan 7. Both cameras focus an image on a film plane, but one produces a much better quality picture.

Wavefront aberration detection and reconstruction are based on either interferometry or ray tracing. The interferometric method has not found much application in physiologic optics, primarily due to difficulties in stabilizing the eye and constructing appropriate reference surfaces (54). All other methods have been based on ray tracing and reconstruction of the wavefront aberration by integrating the slopes of an array of beams intersecting the eye's entrance pupil. Several current commercial devices measure wavefront error, including the Tracey system, the Tschering method used by Wavelight, and the Hartman-Shack wavefront sensor by Alcon's Autonomous Technologies, called the LADARWAVE system. The Hartman-Shack wavefront sensor (Fig. 9.23) is based on an astronomy method that uses a deformable mirror to analyze atmospheric aberrations above a telescope. This device has been adapted to detect aberrations of the eye (54). The measurement is made by

Visual Acuity

- Identifies which letters on a chart can be correctly identified.
- Limitation: Wide variability in perceived image quality for the same level of visual acuity.

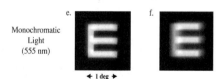

Monochromatic Light (555 nm)

e. f.

◄ 1 deg ►

FIG. 9.22. Difference in quality of vision of two patients who can see the same letter E on the acuity chart. One is unhappy because of poorer image quality induced by higher-order aberrations.

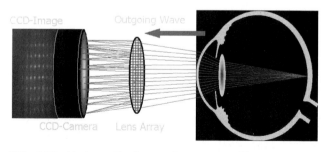

CCD-Image   Outgoing Wave

CCD-Camera   Lens Array

FIG. 9.23. Hartman-Shack wavefront sensor illustrating how light rays are captured on the CCD camera after being reflected from the retina back through the lens and cornea.

focusing a bright spot of light on the retina and projecting the exiting quasi-planar wave onto a matrix of lenslets that focus spots of light on a CCD video array. The displacement of spots from their unaberrated positions yields the average slopes of wavefront at each lenslet's position (55).

The wavefront sensor includes an input laser, a wavefront sensor that measures the slope of the exiting wavefront, and software that determines aberration characteristics. A visual fixation target assists the patient in maintaining view, direction, and accommodation during wavefront measurement. While the patient fixates, the laser beam generates a point light source on the retina. When the laser beam enters the eye, it has a flat wavefront. The light is reflected from the retina back through the pupil. In theory, a perfect human eye would reflect back a beam with its wavefront still flat. However, after the beam of light has traveled through homogeneities in the refractive media (an imperfect crystalline lens, an irregular cornea, or other ocular media), the flat wavefront has become irregular (Fig. 9.24). Analysis of the wavefront reveals the aberrations of the human optical system through which it has just traveled.

The wavefront errors of the eye's optical system are registered by the wavefront sensor, and the software analyzes the results. The wavefront sensor measures the slopes of the wavefront across the pupil of the eye. Zernicke decomposition is one of the methods used to convert the measurements. The software reconstructs a wavefront map using a least squares fit with the Zernicke polynomials.

Conventional LASIK corrects two types of corneal optical error: spherical and cylindrical. Wavefront-guided refractive surgery promises to create treatments tailored to the individual eye based on the total wavefront error rather than the conventional manifest refraction. Zernicke polynomials are used as mathematical blueprints of ocular aberrations. Each Zernicke polynomial, called a *mode,* describes a certain type of shape, a certain three-dimensional surface. The second-order Zernicke terms represent the conventional aberrations: defocus (spherical aberration) and astigmatism. Zernicke aberrations above the second order are called *high-order aberrations.* The third-order Zernicke terms are *coma* and *trefoil* (a wavefront shape with threefold symmetry).

Fourth-order Zernicke terms include spherical aberrations, four other terms, and so on. The Zernicke polynomials are an infinite set, but ophthalmic discussion has generally been limited to the first 15 or so (Fig. 9.25) (55).

The particulars of Zernicke decomposition are integral to the measurement capabilities of the sensor. By using this information, aberrometer software plots ocular aberrations on a graph, creating a wavefront map, similar to a topography map, for clinical interpretation. Evaluation is essentially the same. Clinicians are given information in two additional ways: through conventional refraction (in diopters) and in Zernicke form. Once the aberrations are described, the image blur of a point object, like a star, called the *point-spread function,* is quantified. The point-spread function is the energy distribution of light associated with the image of a perfect point (infinitesimal) object. This added information helps determine the quality of visual performance, that is, how well the patient's eyes are imaging objects.

The wavefront map generated by the Alcon LADAR-WAVE provides information useful in planning customized excimer laser treatment: a pictorial map of the total number of aberrations of the eye and second a pictorial map of the higher-order aberrations only. These maps can be displayed as three-dimensional pictures to create a better understanding of these aberrations (Figs. 9.26 and 9.27). Next to each map, a number abbreviated as "the RMS" appears. The RMS is the root mean square, the integrated root mean square of the differences between the wavefront surface and the mean value of the surface (Fig. 9.28). A perfectly normal eye with a perfect optical system and no aberrations would have an RMS of 1. The higher the RMS, the more the eye is aberrated. A plot map for each Zernicke describing each higher-order aberration is provided so that the clinician will understand which aberrations have most effect on each particular eye and appropriately plan treatment (Figs. 9.26 and 9.27). An additional refractive output is provided assuming a 3-mm pupil, although wavefront measurements are computed all the way out to 9 mm because all wavefront treatments are done at a 6.5-mm pupil with a 1.25 blend, that is, treatment out to 9 mm. Next to the refraction, a percent match also is provided; the smaller the percent match, the greater the effect of higher-order aberrations on visual function.

Wavefront technology has tremendous potential. Undoubtedly, this new way of looking at optics will increasingly be used to customize laser ablations and reduce the higher-order aberrations induced by LASIK. The power of this revolutionary new technology is beautifully illustrated in a clinical case illustrated in Figs. 9.26 and 9.27.

A 49-year-old man reported previous radial keratotomy and LASIK, both in his left eye. Although his distance vision was reasonable during daylight hours, it decreased to 20/80 vision at night, and he suffered from distortion, massive haloes, and glare, to the point he could neither drive nor see street signs. Neither spectacles nor contact lenses im-

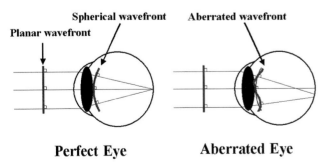

FIG. 9.24. Wavefront of a potentially perfect eye and wavefront of an aberrated eye.

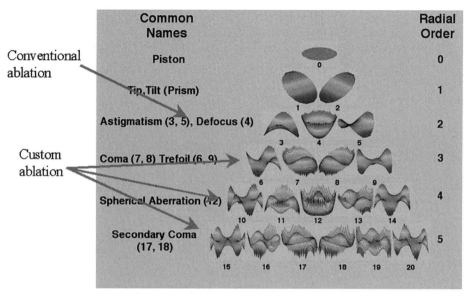

Conventional ablation

Custom ablation

FIG. 9.25. Zernicke aberration components up to fifth-order aberrations also illustrating which aberrations are treated with conventional versus wavefront LASIK. (See Color Plate 9.25.)

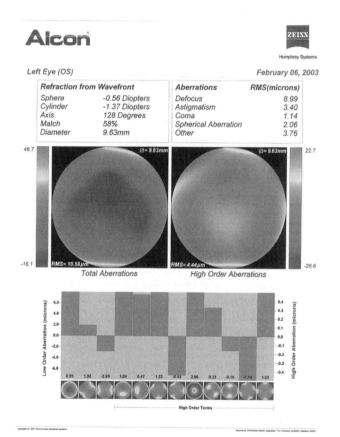

FIG. 9.26. Preoperative wavefront map output of the Alcon LADARWAVE Hartman-Shack sensor illustrating both the total and the higher-order aberrations, as well as their decomposition. This patient had massive high-order aberrations, root mean square (RMS) of 4.4 μm, and total aberrations of 10.5 μm. Note the pupil is dilated to 9 mm, which exaggerates the aberrations. (See Color Plate 9.26.)

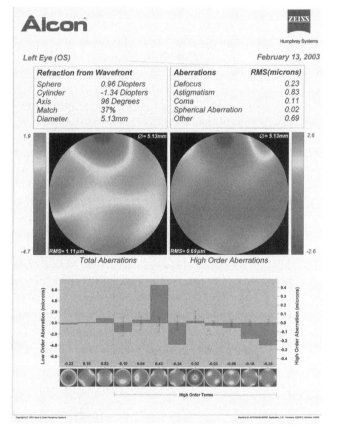

FIG. 9.27. Postoperative wavefront map 1 week after treatment with wavefront LASIK using the Alcon Custom Cornea system. The patient's night vision and quality of vision improved significantly, and his total aberrations have decreased to 1.1 μm and higher-order aberrations have been reduced to 0.69 μm. (See Color Plate 9.27.)

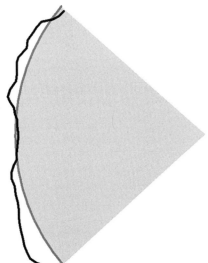

The difference between the actual wavefront (black) and
the ideal wavefront (dark grey)
in the plane of the eye's exit pupil defines the optical
aberrations of the eye = r m s (root mean squared) error

(RMS takes wavefront elevations above and below reference plane, squares them and takes the root mean) RMS value indicates the quality of the retinal image)

Slide courtesy of Ray Applegate, OD,PhD

FIG. 9.28. How the root mean square (RMS) for wavefront aberrations is calculated.

proved his vision. The preoperative wavefront map (Fig. 9.26) suggests massive aberrations (Alcon LADARWAVE Hartman-Shack device). Total aberrations were on the order of 10 μm and higher-order aberrations in the order of 4.4 μm. Each Zernicke component is displayed by the red bar graphs beneath the wavefront map.

Our patient underwent custom cornea ablation with the newly FDA (US Food and Drug Administration)-approved Custom Cornea LASIK with the Alcon autonomous LADARWAVE laser. One week later, his acuity had improved to 20/30, but dramatically his night vision and quality of vision improved significantly. The postoperative map (Fig. 9.27) beautifully illustrates this subjective improvement objectively. Total aberrations were reduced to 1.1 μm and higher-order aberrations were reduced to 0.69 μm.

Wavefront technology therefore has tremendous potential for treating irregular corneas with distortion-inducing aberrations and particularly in the management of keratoconus. Keratoconus patients whose corneas are highly aberrated have significant higher-order aberrations. Wavefront technology has the potential to reduce their aberrations through improved rigid contact lens fitting, guiding surgical implantation of INTACS in select patients who are contact lens intolerant, and even possibly customized excimer photorefractive keratectomy (PRK) or laser epithelial keratomileusis (LASEK) in select keratoconus patients over age 40 years with early and stable disease whose corneas are sufficiently thick.

CONCLUSION

This chapter has guided the reader through the many technologies available to qualitatively and quantitatively measure corneal surface shape, from matching reflected images in marble templates through keratometry and then modern videokeratography and wavefront analysis.

ACKNOWLEDGMENT

Supported in part by the Eye Birth Defects Research Foundation Inc. and grant NEI RO1 09052 from the National Eye Institutes of Health.

REFERENCES

1. Rabinowitz YS, Wilson SE, Klyce SD, eds. *A color atlas of corneal topography: interpreting videokeratography.* Tokyo: Igaku Shoin Medical Publishers, 1993.
2. Corbett MC, O'Bart DPS, Saunders DC, et al. The assessment of corneal topography. *Eur J Implant Refract Surg* 1994;6:98–105.
3. Rowsey JJ, Reynolds AE, Brow R. Corneal topography: corneascope. *Arch Ophthalmol* 1981;99:1093–1100.
4. Klyce SD. Computer-assisted corneal topography: high-resolution graphic presentation and analysis of keratoscopy. *Invest Ophthalmol Vis Sci* 1984;25:1426–1435.
5. Dingeldein SA, Klyce SD. Imaging of the cornea. *Cornea* 1988; 7:170–182.
6. Gormley DJ, Gersten M, Koplin RS, et al. Corneal modeling. *Cornea* 1988;7:30–35.
7. Koch DD, Foulks GN, Moran CT, et al. The corneal EyeSys system: accuracy analysis and reproducibility of first-generation prototype. *Refract Corneal Surg* 1989;5:424–429.
8. Klyce SD, Wilson SE. Methods of analysis of corneal topography. *Refract Corneal Surg* 1989;5:368–371.
9. McDonnell PJ. Current applications of the corneal modeling system. *Refract Corneal Surg* 1991;7:87–91.
10. Wilson SE, Klyce SD. Quantitative descriptors of corneal topography: a clinical study. *Arch Ophthalmol* 1991;109:349–353.
11. Mandell RB. The enigma of corneal contour. *CLAO J* 1992;18: 267–273.
12. Mandell RB, St. Helen R. Mathematical model of the corneal contour. *Br J Physiol Opt* 1971;26:183–197.
13. Hannush SB, Crawford SL, Waring GO III, et al. Reproducibility of normal corneal power measurements with a keratometer, photokeratoscope, and video imaging system. *Arch Ophthalmol* 1990;108:539–544.

14. Hannush SB, Crawford SL, Waring GO III, et al. Accuracy and precision of keratometry, photokeratoscopy, and corneal modeling on calibrated steel balls. *Arch Ophthalmol* 1989;107:1235–1239.

15. Koch DD, Wakil JS, Samuelson SW, et al. Comparison of the accuracy and reproducibility of the keratometer and the EyeSys corneal analysis system model I. *J Cataract Refract Surg* 1992;18:342–347.

16. Maguire LJ, Wilson SE, Camp JJ, et al. Evaluating the reproducibility of topography systems on spherical surfaces. *Arch Ophthalmol* 1993;111:259–262.

17. Wilson SE, Verity Sm, Conger DL. Accuracy and precision of the corneal analysis system and the topographic modeling system. *Cornea* 1992;11:28–35.

18. Bogan SJ, Waring GO III, Ibrahim O, et al. Classification of normal corneal topography based on computer-assisted videokeratography. *Arch Ophthalmol* 1990;108:945–949.

19. Rabinowitz YS, Yang H, Akkina J, et al. Videokeratography of normal human corneas. *Br J Ophthalmol* 1996;80:610–616.

20. Wilson SE, Klyce SD, Husseini ZM. Standardized color-coded maps for corneal topography. *Ophthalmology* 1993;100:1723–1727.

21. Dingeldein SA, Klyce SD. The topography of normal corneas. *Arch Ophthalmol* 1989;107:512–518.

22. Rabinowitz YS, McDonnell PJ. Computer-assisted corneal topography in keratoconus. *Refract Corneal Surg* 1989;5:400–408.

23. Wilson SE, Klyce SD. Corneal topography of keratoconus. *Cornea* 1991;10:2–8.

24. McMahon TT, Robin JB, Scarpulla KM, et al. The spectrum of topography found in keratoconus. *CLAO J* 1991;17:198–204.

25. Maguire LJ, Klyce SD, McDonald MB, et al. Corneal topography of pellucid marginal degeneration. *Ophthalmology* 1987.94:519–524.

26. Wilson SE, Klyce SD, Insler MS. Terrien's marginal degeneration: corneal topography. *Refract Corneal Surg* 1990;6:21–25.

27. Maguire LJ, Bourne W. Corneal topography of early keratoconus. *Am J Ophthalmol* 1989;108:107–112.

28. Rabinowitz YS, Garbus J, McDonnell PJ. Computer-assisted corneal topography in family members of keratoconus. *Arch Ophthalmol* 1990;108:365–371.

29. Amsler M. Le keratocone fruste au javal. *Ophthalmologica* 1938;96:77–83.

30. Amsler M. Keratocone classique et keratocone fruste, arguments unitaires. *Ophthalmologica* 1946;111:96–101.

31. Wilson SE, Klyce SD. Screening for corneal topographic abnormalities before refractive surgery. *Ophthalmology* 1994;101:147–152.

32. Rabinowitz YS, Klyce SD, Krachmer JH, et al. Videokeratography, keratoconus, and refractive surgery. *Opin Refract Corneal Surg* 1992;5:403–407.

33. Rabinowitz YS, Nesburn AB, McDonnell PJ. Videokeratography of the fellow eye in unilateral keratoconus. *Ophthalmology* 1993;100:181–186.

34. Lee LR, Hirst LW, Readshaw G. Clinical detection of unilateral keratoconus. *Aust N Z J Ophthalmol* 1995;23:129–33.

35. Rabinowitz YS. Videokeratographic indices to aid in screening for keratoconus. *J Refract Surg* 1995;11:371–379.

36. Maeda N, Klyce SD, Smolek MK, et al. Automated keratoconus screening with corneal topographic analysis. *Invest Ophthalmol Vis Sci* 1994;35:2749–2757.

37. Rabinowitz YS, Rasheed K. KISA% index: a quantitative videokeratography algorithm embodying minimal topographic criteria for diagnosing keratoconus. *J Cataract Refract Surg* 1999;25:1327–1335.

38. Waring GO, Rabinowitz YS, Sugar J, et al. Nomenclature for keratoconus suspects. *Opin Refract Corneal Surg* 1993;9:219–221.

39. Rasheed K, Rabinowitz YS, Remba M, et al. Interobserver and intraobserver reliability of a classification scheme for corneal topographic patterns. *Br J Ophthalmol* 1998;82:1401–1406.

40. Rabinowitz YS. Keratoconus: update and new advances. *Surv Ophthalmol* 1998:42:297–319.

41. Szczotka L, Rabinowitz YS, Yang H. The influence of contact lens wear on the topography of keratoconus. *CLAO J* 1996;22:270–273.

42. Wilson SE, Lin DTC, Klyce SD, et al. Topographic changes in contact lens-induced corneal warpage. *Ophthalmology* 1990;97:734–44.

43. Wilson SE, Lin DTC, Klyce SD, et al. Rigid contact lens decentration: a risk factor for corneal warpage. *CLAO J* 1990;16:177–182.

44. Rabinowitz YS. Tangential vs sagittal videokeratographs in the "early" detection of keratoconus. *Am J Ophthalmol* 1996:122:888–889.

45. Argento C, Cosentino MJ, Tytiun A, et al. Corneal ectasia after laser in situ keratomileusis. *J Cataract Refract Surg* 2001;27:1440–1448.

46. Jabbur NS, Stark WJ, Green WR. Corneal ectasia after laser-assisted in situ keratomileusis. *Arch Ophthalmol* 2001;119:1714–1716.

47. McLeod SD, Kisla TA, Caro NC, et al. Iatrogenic keratoconus: corneal ectasia following laser in situ keratomileusis for myopia. *Arch Ophthalmol* 2000;118:282–284.

48. Wang Y, Rabinowitz YS, Rotter JI, et al. Genetic epidemiological study of keratoconus: evidence for major gene determination. *Am J Med Genet* 2000;93:403–409.

49. Rabinowitz YS, Maumenee IH, Lundergan MK, et al. Molecular genetic analysis in autosomal dominant keratoconus. *Cornea* 1992;11:302–308.

50. Ruiz-Montenegro J, Mafra CH, Wilson SE, et al. Corneal topographic alterations in normal contact lens wearers. *Ophthalmology* 1993;100:128–134.

51. Rabinowitz YS, Garbus JJ, Garbus C, et al. Contact lens selection for keratoconus using a computer-assisted videophotokeratoscope. *CLAO J* 1991;17:88–93.

52. McDonnell PJ, Garbus JJ, Caroline P, et al. Computerized analysis of corneal topography as an aid in fitting contact lenses after radial keratotomy. *Ophthalmic Surg* 1992;23:55–59.

53. Howland HC. Ophthalmic wavefront sensing. History and methods. In: Macrae SM, Kruger RR, Applegate RA, eds. *Customized corneal ablations. The quest for supervision.* Thorafore, NJ: SLACK Inc., 2001.

54. Miller DT, Williams DR, Morris G, et al. Images of cone photoreceptors in the living human eye. *Vision Res* 1996;36:1067–1079.

55. Macrae SM, Kruger RR, Applegate RA, eds. *Customized corneal ablations. The quest for supervision.* Thorofare, NJ: SLACK Inc., 2001.

RIGID CONTACT LENS APPLICATION, CARE, AND EVALUATION

C H A P T E R

10

POLYMER CHEMISTRY

ALEXANDER CANNELLA AND
JAMES A. BONAFINI, JR.

BACKGROUND

The first contact lenses were rigid made out of glass in Europe in the 1880s by Adolf Fick (Zurich, Switzerland), Friederich Müller (Wiesbaden, Germany), August Müller (Kiel, Germany) (Fig. 10.1; see also Chapter 1). The 1930s saw the introduction of plastics for use as contact lens materials in both Europe and the United States (1,2).

The plastic polymethyl methacrylate (PMMA) proved to have extremely good physical properties for use as a contact lens. This material

1. has excellent optical properties
2. is extremely durable
3. is easy to manufacture using a multitude of methods (lathing, molding)
4. has excellent surface wetting and good deposit resistance, and is easy to clean with relatively weak surfactants
5. is not rejected by the body

Despite the excellent physical properties offered by PMMA, the glaring deficiency is that this material is not oxygen permeable. PMMA lenses depend solely on a "tear pump" to deliver oxygen to the central cornea following each blink. Rigid lens tear pumps unfortunately supply only minimal oxygen to the underlying tear layer.

Resultant corneal hypoxia and edema were managed by fitting these lenses as small as possible in order to cover as little of the cornea as possible. If this failed to relieve corneal

clouding, minute openings were made through the lens (fenestrations) in an attempt to increase tear flow under the lens (Fig. 10.2).

The first gas permeable (GP) material, cellulose acetate butyrate (CAB), was introduced for use in contact lenses in the early 1970s. This material proved to be variable in terms of parameter stability, and its oxygen permeability (Dk) was very low (4 Dk units, see later for units; see also Chapter 3). It was not until the late 1970s that a stable GP rigid contact material of sufficient permeability (12 Dk units), known as Polycon™ silicone/acrylate (S/A), was introduced by Leonard Seidner, OD.

KEY GAS PERMEABLE PHYSICAL PROPERTIES

Permeability and Transmissibility

Dk is the term used to denote the *permeability* of rigid and soft contact lens materials. "D" stands for the inherent ability of the material to allow gas through; "k" represents the degree to which oxygen is solubilized within the material (often related to water content in hydrogels because water plays a role in absorbing and assisting in the transport of oxygen).

Several methods are used to measure permeability. As the world becomes a global market, the necessity for standardization of measurements has become apparent in order to ensure uniformity and avoid confusion. The International

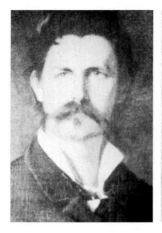 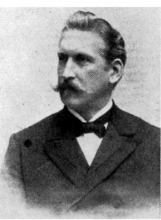 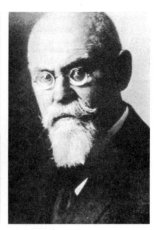

FIG. 10.1. Contact lens pioneers Adolf Fick, Friederich Müller, and August Müller (shown from **left** to **right**).

Organization for Standardization (ISO)/Fatt method has been chosen as the international standard for all contact lens material manufacturers to state the permeability of their materials for ISO and CE marking. The European Community (EU) and other countries use the ISO/Fatt standard (ISO 9913.1). The United States alternately uses the ISO/American National Standards Institute (ANSI) standard (2). Both the ISO/Fatt and ISO/ANSI standards use the same formula for stating contact lens material Dk or permeability units (see earlier). It is stated as $\times 10^{-11} (\text{cm}^2/\text{s})([\text{mL O}_2]/[\text{mL} \cdot \text{mm Hg}])$ @ 35°C (Table 10.1) (3,4).

Because newer permeability standard figures are approximately 25% less than those obtained using previous measurement methods, the key for the practitioner is understanding that all contact lens material companies have not universally adopted standards as of this time. New measurement standards may cause confusion if materials are compared using a mixture of methods.

Dk/L incorporates the Dk measurement and is *transmissibility* of a material when it is made into either a lens of a given thickness (*L*). Internationally, this measurement is being standardized into a new designation, *Dk/t*, where *t* has replaced *L* for lens thickness. The significance of this

parameter is that the amount of oxygen that is able to diffuse through any lens to the underlying tears and cornea is governed by the thickness of the lens as well as the inherent permeability of the material.

TABLE 10.1. ISO/ANSI, ISO/FATT OXYGEN PERMEABILITY STANDARDS

Lens Name	Corrected, Calibrated Dk in ANSI Units	95% Confidence Limits[a]
Alberta 45	28.0	23.8–34.0
Boston II	16.3	13.5–21.0
Boston IV	20.8	18.5–23.8
Boston Equalens I	67.9	62.7–73.9
Boston Equalens II	85	82.8–87.9
Boston ES	27.3	22.9–34.1
Boston EO	57.6	53.7–62.1
Boston XO	101	94.2–109.6
Fluorex 300	23.9	22.1–26.0
Fluorex500	29.6	28.3–31.0
FluoroPerm 30	30.3	28.8–31.9
FluoroPerm 60	42.7	41.4–44.0
FluoroPerm 92	61	59.7–62.5
FluoroPerm 151	99.3	—
Flurocon	44.0	40.4–48.3
OP-2	17.5	15.5–20.3
OP-3	27.1	24.2–30.9
OP-6	57.0	51.9–63.2
Optacryl 60	13.8	12.1–16.4
Paragon HDS*	39.3	37.3–41.5
Paragon Thin	23.0	21.9–24.2
Paraperm EW	49.5	46.6–52.8
Paraperm 02	15.7	13.9–18.3
Polycon II	14.1	11.7–18.5
SGP I	14.9	13.4–17.0
SGP II	31.9	30.1–33.8
SGP III	33.5	31.8–35.4
Trans-Aire	19.7	19.1–20.5

[a] 95% confidence limits derived from + 2 standard errors (N = 6) surrounding the edge-corrected slope of the linear resistance (t/Dk) vs thickness (t) equation used to correct for boundary layer effect for each material.
*Paragon HDS 100 was not tested in recent studies but manufacturer lists ISC/ANSI DK as 100.

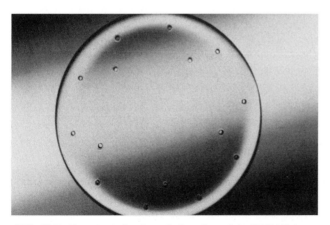

FIG. 10.2. Fenestrated polymethyl methacrylate (PMMA) lens.

EOP (equivalent oxygen percentage) is another clinically relevant value, which represents the effect of oxygen passing through a lens to the cornea. This *in vivo* measurement takes into account contact lens oxygen delivery (permeability and lens thickness) compared to various benchmarks based on available oxygen to the open eye and predicts the amount of oxygen required to avoid certain clinical events, such as corneal hypoxia, edema, and endothelial cell changes (Fig 10.3).

Mechanical Properties

Hardness is measured in two ways. One method measures the hardness of GP materials while they are in the button form. This is known as *Rockwell R hardness.* Using this method, a round-head probe is used to apply steady pressure to determine the amount of compression the GP button will withstand to measure its hardness and resilience. The second test method is called *Shore D hardness* for finished GP lenses. This test method indicates surface resistance to penetration from pressure by a sharp probe and is used to predict the scratch resistance of a GP lens material. These tests are not definitive indicators for predicting the dimensional stability and the life of a GP lens. More accurate tests for predicting durability are modulus and toughness measurements.

Modulus or *slope* of the stress–strain curve is a term that refers to the stiffness of a plastic and can be stated in *megapascals (MPa)* (5). This quality is a critical property of GP materials. Clinically, this property relates to the stiffness of the material (also resistance to flexure) and relates to the ability of a GP lens to "mask" corneal astigmatism. GP materials that have good stiffness properties will mask astigmatism better than those with less stiffness. Modulus is measured by applying force (stress) to a lens until it begins to

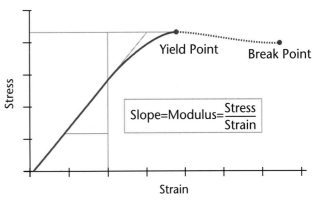

FIG. 10.4. Stress–strain testing to determine slope (modulus). (From *Contact Lens Spectrum,* April 1993, with permission.)

deform (strain). The application of force is continued until lens breakage occurs (Fig. 10.4).

Modulus ratings may approximate a range as high as 2,250 MPa in the case of PMMA and as low as 1,200 MPa for high-Dk, softer lens materials (Table 10.2).

Toughness (MPa mm/mm) testing determines lens fracture resistance by simply flexing the lens sample until it breaks. This property is quantified by measuring the "area under the curve." In a GP lens, this quality relates to lens durability and handling characteristics (Fig. 10.5).

These material stiffness and toughness characteristics are determined by the chemistry of each material, particularly by the type, amount, and manner in which cross-linking agents are used to stabilize the polymer chains. If cross-linking agents are used extensively, material hardness can be very high; however, material permeability will be subsequently decreased. These materials may be able to mask corneal astigmatism well because they have characteristics

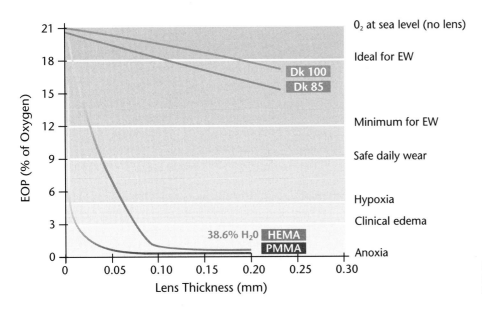

FIG. 10.3. Equivalent oxygen percentage (EOP) chart. (For this figure, all values are estimates only.)

TABLE 10.2. EXAMPLE OF AVERAGE RESIDUAL CYLINDER RELATED TO MODULUS (5)

Sample	Stress–Strain Technique Flexural Modulus (MPa)	Clinical Average Residual Cylinder (D)
PMMA	2,250	0.83
Dk = 45	1,800	1.18
Dk = 75	1,400	1.33
Dk = 30	1,300	1.34
Dk = 65	1,200	1.41

PMMA, polymethyl methacrylate.

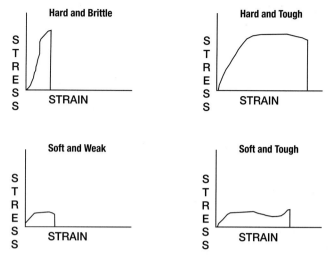

FIG. 10.6. Fracture characteristics of glassy materials. (From *Contact Lens Spectrum*, April 1993, with permission.)

that give the polymer a hard and glassy characteristic (Fig. 10.6).

Materials that use less cross-linking can be categorized as rubbery (soft and weak, or soft and tough) with a very poor ability to resist flexure, thus masking corneal astigmatism.

Wettability or *wetting angle* measurements are meant to be clinical predictors of how well a contact lens will wet and stay wet when placed and worn on the eye. In theory, a low wetting angle will equate to good on-eye lens wetting. These measurements historically have been performed using several methods: Wilhelmy plate method, sessile drop method, and captive bubble method (Fig. 10.7).

The Wilhelmy plate method is a dynamic test performed by dipping a GP material in and out of a test solution to measure the contact angle (meniscus) between the lens material and the solution as the GP test material advances and is withdrawn (receding).

The sessile drop method uses a drop of saline placed on a lens material in order to measure the contact point between the drop of solution and the test lens material. This method is deemed to be one of the oldest but least accurate of all the methods used.

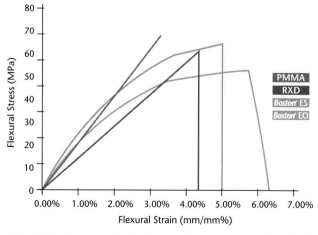

FIG. 10.5. Stress–strain fracture testing examples. (Modified from original artwork provided by Polymer Technology Corporation, a Bausch & Lomb company.)

In 1978, the captive bubble technique for wetting angle measurement (developed by Maurice Poster, OD, of New York) (6) was adopted as both the US Food and Drug Administration (FDA)- and ANSI-approved method for measuring lens wetting angle in the United States. This method uses a bubble of air trapped against the surface of the GP test material to determine the contact angle (similar to the sessile drop method).

It is important to note that, although wetting angle measurements are a requirement for GP lens testing and approval, these tests have proven *not* to have a correlation with on-eye lens wetting and comfort. The human tear film contains many components, which include lipids, mucin, lactoferrin, and lysozyme. These components form a *biofilm* that acts as a natural wetting agent to coat the lens within a few blinks. This lowers the lens wetting angle, contributing significantly to creating and maintaining on-eye contact lens wettability for periods of time determined by the individual chemistry of each patient's tear film (7). Given this fact, in-laboratory wetting angle measurements usually are not indicative of on-eye performance.

In recent years, other more dynamic and therefore seemingly more realistic methods of testing lens wetting have been proposed (8).

The method known as *dynamic contact angle (DCA)* uses the Wilhelmy plate method of dipping a test plastic in solution to test both the advancing and receding contact angles, obtaining the *contact angle hysteresis* by subtracting the receding angle from the advancing angle to determine the DCA (Fig. 10.8). A wide gap between the *advancing* and *receding* contact angles indicates a poorly wetting GP material surface. This may be due to hydrophobicity or lack of soaking the lens material prior to testing.

Specific gravity is the ratio of the mass of solid or liquid to an equal volume of distilled water at 4°C (9). This is used as a standard and is given a nominal of 1.00 (Table 10.3).

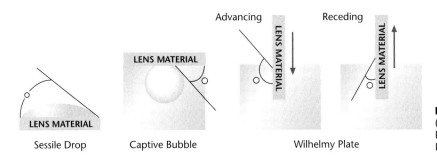

FIG. 10.7. Contact angle testing methods. (Modified from original artwork provided by Polymer Technology Corporation, a Bausch & Lomb company.)

Specific gravity is normally of no concern when fitting GP lenses of conventional designs and powers. However, high-plus lens powers have increased lens mass due to increased center thickness. Lens position on single-cut (non-lenticulated) plus lenses also is adversely affected because the center of gravity of the lens is displaced forward. For this reason, all plus lenses should be ordered with a lenticular edge design to avoid the "watermelon seed" effect.

Lens mass is also increased in high-minus lenses where edge thickness becomes an issue in terms of both lens weight and comfort. Lenses above -4.00 D or -4.50 D power

should be made with a lenticular edge that will reduce edge thickness and lens mass, thereby increasing lens comfort and improving lens position and centration (Fig. 10.9).

The only other area where specific gravity may play some role is if a front-toric-design GP lens, requiring prism ballast, is being fitted. In this case, use of a higher specific gravity (heavier) GP material may assist in positioning the lens and may also require less edge thickness (prism diopters) to stabilize the lens.

Ultraviolet Blockers

Ultraviolet radiation (UVR) is emitted in a range of wavelengths and is found adjacent to visible light on the electro-

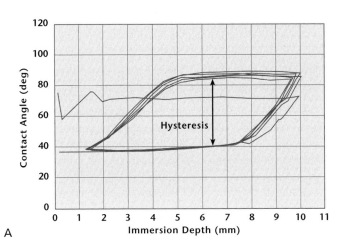

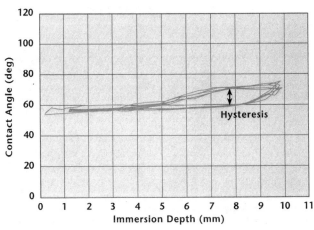

FIG. 10.8. A: Poorly wetting gas permeable material as demonstrated by wide hysteresis angle. **B:** Good wetting gas permeable material as shown by narrow hysteresis angle.

TABLE 10.3. SPECIFIC GRAVITY OF VARIOUS GAS PERMEABLE MATERIALS

Material	Type	Specific Gravity
Boston II	S/A	1.13
Boston IV	S/A	1.10
Boston Equalens I	F-S/A	1.19
Boston Equalens II	F-S/A	1.24
Boston ES	F-S/A	1.22
Boston EO	F-S/A	1.23
Boston XO	F-S/A	1.27
FLOSI	F-S/A	1.27
Fluorex 300	F-S/A	1.11
Fluorex 500	F-S/A	1.10
FluoroPerm 30	F-S/A	1.14
FluoroPerm 60	F-S/A	1.15
FluoroPerm 92	F-S/A	1.10
Hybrid FS	F-S/A	1.18
Hydro 02	F-S/A	1.15
Menicon Z	F-S/A	1.20
Optacryl 60	S/A	1.13
Paragon HDS	F-S/A	1.16
Paragon HDS 100	F-S/A	1.10
Paraperm 02	S/A	1.13
Paraperm EW	S/A	1.07
Polycon II	S/A	1.13
SGP I	S/A	1.13
SGP II	S/A	1.13
SGP III	F-S/A	1.13
Trans-Aire	F-S/A	1.08
PMMA	—	1.20

FS/A, fluoro-silicone acrylate; S/A, silicone acrylate.

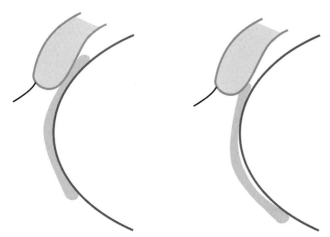

FIG. 10.9. Lens centration with **(left)** and without **(right)** lenticulation.

magnetic spectrum. Shorter wavelengths are more energetic and more harmful to living cells.

Energy wavelengths are measured in nanometers (nm), which are billionths of meters. UVR begins at approximately 100 nm and extends to 400 nm and is split into three bands: UVC, UVB, UVA. UVC rays (100–200 nm) are absorbed by the earth's atmosphere.

UVB (200–300 nm) are the rays that pass through cloud cover and cause sunburns. UVA rays are nearest to the visible light spectrum and are the least dangerous of the UV wavelengths. Significant evidence exists that there is a correlation between UVR exposure and ocular conditions such as conjunctival pterygium, photokeratitis, cataracts, and retinal degenerative changes. Use of UVR absorbers in contact lenses can help to protect the underlying structures of the

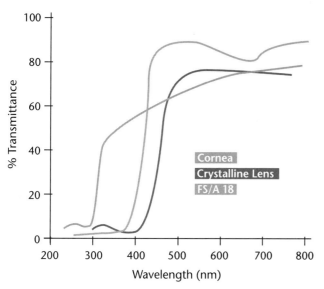

FIG. 10.10. Ultraviolet light transmittance through eye structures and lens material.

eye to some degree, but it does not offer total protection. Protective eyewear (sunglasses, goggles) is still recommended for maximum protection (Fig. 10.10).

The presence of UV absorbers in GP contact lenses may cause fluorescein pattern detail to be very difficult to determine when viewed with UV light, such as that used in a normal clinical Burton lamp. Slit-lamp viewing is possible, but the fluorescein pattern may appear "washed out."

The adjunctive use of a yellow Wratten filter helps to bring out greater details and subtle differences in tear film thickness. Most laboratories have these kits available for a very low cost (Fig. 10.11).

TYPES OF GAS PERMEABLE MATERIALS AND SURFACE CHARACTERISTICS

The basic elements in a GP contact lens material consists of the following:

- Methacrylic acid
- Hydrophilic monomers
- Silicone/fluorine
- Cross-linking agents

Silicone/Acrylate Chemistry: The First Generation of Gas Permeable Lenses

The addition of silicone to the hard lens chemistry provided for permeability and the exchange of gases beneath the lens, reducing or eliminating the problems encountered with PMMA. PMMA lenses, however, are very wettable, deposit resistant, and easily cleaned, due to the relatively neutral surface properties of PMMA (Fig. 10.12).

The surface of PMMA is polar (hydrophilic) but contains no surface charge. This may explain why the surface attracts little surface deposits and maintains its high level of wetting. This type of surface interacts favorably with tear fluid components.

The introduction of S/A lenses in the 1970s brought new issues to the management of rigid contact lens wearers, namely, an increase in hard-to-remove protein deposition. The S/A lenses had surfaces with negative ionic charges that dried faster, attracted protein more, and bound deposits more tightly to the surfaces (Fig. 10.13).

The surface of an S/A material contains a relatively large amount of both charged groups (negative, hydrophilic) and silicone groups (hydrophobic). This type of surface can attract both protein and lipid deposits (Fig. 10.14).

S/A lens deposits bind to dry spots on the lens surface and begin to form plaque layers that typically appear as a dull-appearing, nonelevated coating that is difficult to remove using solutions that contain weak surfactants, such as solutions designed for PMMA hard lenses (Fig. 10.15). The

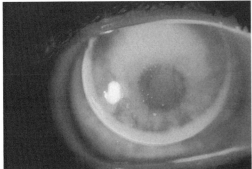

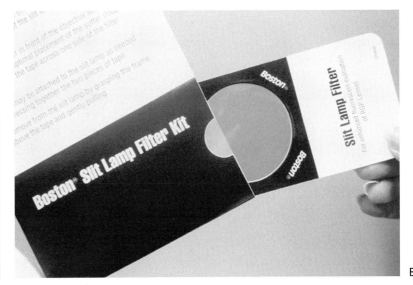

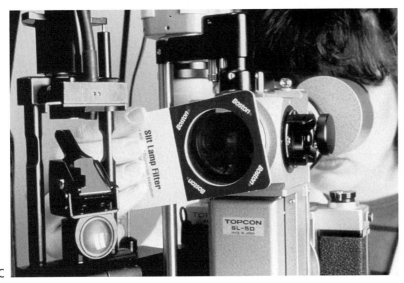

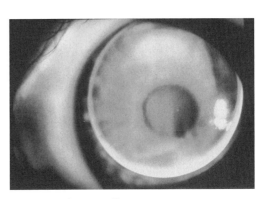

FIG. 10.11. **A:** Fluorescein appearance before yellow filter use (pseudo-steep). **B, C:** Yellow Wratten filter kit. **D:** Fluorescein appearance after yellow filter use to show subtle pattern details. (See Color Plate 10.11)

predominant and fastest forming type of deposit found on contact lenses is protein. Protein deposits are reported to begin forming on contact lenses in as few as 30 minutes (10,11).

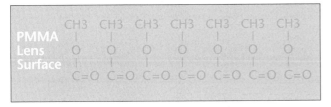

FIG. 10.12. Chemical surface of a polymethyl methacrylate (PMMA) lens.

This property of silicone causes lens drying that leads to patient complaints of dryness, scratchiness, and red eyes. More aggressive cleaners that contain friction agents and improved wetting and soaking solutions were required and eventually introduced by the contact lens industry to help patients keep their lenses clean, wet, and comfortable longer. Use of adjunct proteolytic weekly enzymatic cleaners also helped patients keep their lenses clean and comfortable (12).

As additional materials with increasingly higher Dk values were introduced, material surface wettability and deposit resistance decreased. This increase in silicone caused an increase in lens material instability that ultimately led to lens warpage, crazing, and breakage (Fig. 10.16).

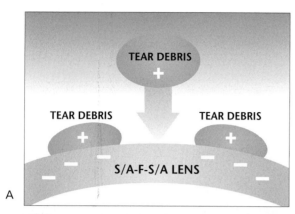

A

B

FIG. 10.13. Tear debris attraction and binding to gas permeable lens surfaces.

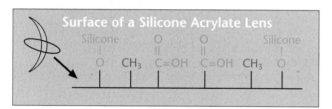

FIG. 10.14. Silicone/acrylate surface chemistry.

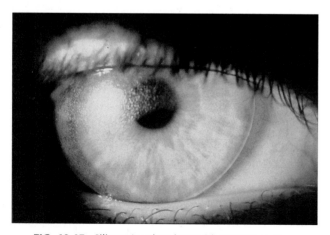

FIG. 10.15. Silicone/acrylate lens with protein coating.

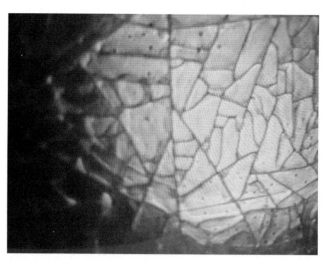

FIG. 10.16. Crazed gas permeable lens. Image taken directly from inspection monitor. (Courtesy of Polymer Technology Corporation.)

Fluoro-Silicone/Acrylate Materials: The Second Generation of Gas Permeable Lenses

The custom of adding more silicone to increase permeability created a concept known as the *silicone/acrylate barrier*. This is the point at which the addition of more silicone to a lens only serves to compromise other critical lens properties in favor of higher oxygen permeability. The introduction of fluoro-silicone/acrylate (F-S/A) GP materials (such as Boston® Equalens™ by Polymer Technology Corporation) in the late 1980s helped to solve this problem. F-S/A materials differed from earlier S/A materials by the addition of fluorine whereby permeability was increased (through increased oxygen solubility in fluorine) and silicone was reduced.

GP materials now could have permeabilities that surpassed 20 or 30 Dk units, rising to the range from 50 to 70 units while still containing significant amounts of silicone (11%–13%). This level may still cause lenses to flex and exhibit wetting and deposit problems related to their composition. Generally, the higher the Dk, the more flexibility the lens might exhibit.

However, these new material formulations positively affect lens stability and make the material more wettable and more deposit resistant because of the Teflon™-like nonstick characteristic that is imparted by fluorine to the polymer (Fig. 10.17).

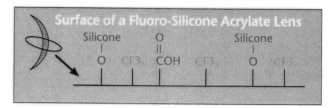

FIG. 10.17. Chemical surface of a fluoro-silicone/acrylate lens.

In F-S/A materials, the negative charge and hydrophobic properties observed in S/A lens surfaces are masked because of the presence of fluorine (hydrophobic, resists surface deposits) at the surface. When the proper balance of fluorine, charged groups, and silicone is achieved, positive surface wetting and deposit resistance properties result. With the addition of fluorine, some of the silicone composition can be reduced. The key is to maintain a wettable nondrying surface that is not disturbed by the presence of deposits.

These materials assist in alleviating symptoms of dryness commonly experienced by S/A lens wearers. Because of the addition of fluorine, lenses stay wet longer, deposits adhere less tightly, and the lenses are easier to keep clean.

As with any gain, there is also a downside. F-S/A materials resist protein deposits very well. In terms of surface characteristics related to fluorine content, these lenses attract and bind lipid rather than protein deposits to their surfaces. F-S/A lenses deposited with lipids present a much different clinical picture than lenses with protein deposits. Lipid deposits are elevated, clear conglomerations of fatty, oily substance, similar to the jelly bumps observed on conventional soft contact lenses (Fig. 10.18).

F-S/A lenses are more prone not only to lipid depositing but also to attracting and binding lipid-like deposits, such as those from lotions, shampoos, soaps, and other personal care products that contain lanolin, palm oil, cocoa butter, and other moisturizing agents. This includes perfumes, deodorants, and emollients (Fig. 10.19). Patients and office staff need to be aware that these products can adsorb to F-S/A lens surfaces, and this will affect GP lens clinical performance. These deposits may be difficult to remove and *should not* be polished. Polishing will spread the oily material over a larger surface of the lens, making vision, wettability, and comfort worse. Instead, a professional cleaner containing a mild solvent can be used in the office to remove these deposits.

Fluoro-Silicone/Acrylate Materials: The Third Generation of Gas Permeable Lenses

Improvements and refinements to the F-S/A chemistry took place in the late 1990s and early 2000s. Companies such as Polymer Technology Corporation and Paragon Vision Sciences developed polymer refinement systems that maximized permeability, lens stability, and wetting. Polymer Technology Corporation introduced the Boston® AER-COR® low-silicone chemistry with materials such as Boston EO, and Boston ES, and super-Dk materials such as Boston XO. Paragon Vision Sciences introduced the Hyperpurified Delivery System (HDS)™, which maximized the silicone in the lens to derive maximum permeability. This third generation of GP materials now moves the permeability bar up into the range from 60 to 100, with little negative affect on lens wetting, deposit resistance, and lens stability.

As the result of these developments, a reclassification of GP materials was necessary in order to help practitioners look at GP materials based on the modality for which they are used. Although there are more materials to choose from, there also are more options as to which materials would be best suited for toric designs, orthokeratology, thin lens designs, daily wear, and extended wear (Table 10.4) (13).

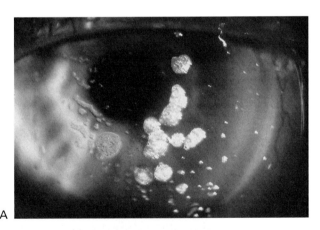

A

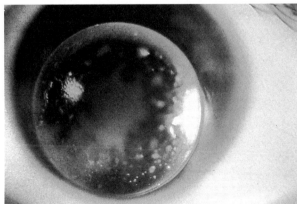

B

FIG. 10.18. Nonwetting lipid deposits on lens.

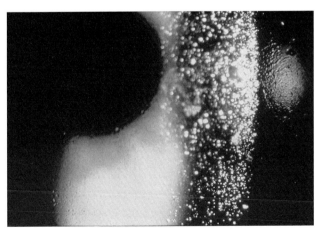

FIG. 10.19. Gas permeable lens surface contaminated with skin care lotion.

TABLE 10.4. CLASSIFICATION OF Dk RANGES FOR GAS PERMEABLE MATERIALS (NOT LENSES)

Name	Dk Range[a]	Description
Low Dk	<15	Materials with low Dk/L at 0.12-mm thickness
Medium Dk	15–30	Materials with medium Dk/L at 0.12-mm thickness
High Dk	31–60	Materials with high Dk/L at 0.12-mm thickness
Super Dk	61–100	Materials with super Dk/L at 0.12-mm thickness
Hyper Dk	>100	Materials with hyper Dk/L at 0.12-mm thickness

[a] Dk units = 10^{-11} $(cm^2/s)(mLO_2/[mL\text{-}mm\ Hg])$ or equivalently: 10^{-11} $(cm^3[O_2].cm)/(cm^2.s.mm\ Hg)$ as determined by gas-to-gas method.

Other Materials

Hyper-Dk materials such as Menicon Z have pushed the envelope of oxygen permeability, offering an F-S/A material that has a permeability of 163 using ISO 9913.1. This is accomplished using higher amounts of silicone.

Surface biocompatibility is achieved by putting lenses through a plasma treatment that effectively "hides" any hydrophobic elements on the lens surface from attracting deposits. However, care must be taken not to compromise the surface integrity of the material by using abrasive cleaners on these lenses or by accumulating scratches. Newly introduced GP materials, such as FLOSI (Lagado Corp.), Hydro O_2 (Innovision), and Hybrid FS (Contamac Ltd.), propose better wetting GP materials in low- to mid-Dk GP materials.

SUMMARY

It is important that practitioners understand and consider the bulk properties (Dk, wetting, specific gravity, modulus, refractive index) of GP contact lenses. It is equally important that the surface properties of these lens materials and how they interact with the ocular environment, as well as with all substances with which they come into contact, are considered when deciding which GP material to use when designing a lens for various modalities and indications.

REFERENCES

1. DeCarle J. Who fitted the first contact lens? *The Optician Supplement—100 Years of the Contact Lens,* May 1988.
2. Sabell T. The early years. *The Optician Supplement—100 Years of the Contact Lens,* May 1988.
3. Benjamin WJ, Cappelli QA. Oxygen permeability (Dk) of thirty-seven rigid contact lens materials. *Optom Vis Sci* 2002;79:103–111.
4. Bonafini JA. Finally . . . an international standard for Dk measurement. *Global Contact* 1998;19.
5. Raheja MK, Huang H. Mechanical property testing of RGP materials. *Contact Lens Spectrum* 1993;8:45.
6. Poster MG, Gelfer DM, Fermamdez NM. Wetting angles of rigid contact lens plastics: the effect of contact lens wear. *J Am Optom Assoc* 1986;57:452–454.
7. Benjamin WJ. Pellicle, biofilm, mucin layer, surface coating, or contact lens camouflage. *Int Contact Lens Clin* 1989;16:183–184.
8. Zhang J, Herskowitz R. Is there more than one angle to wetting characteristics of contact lenses? *Contact Lens Spectrum* 1992;7:26–30.
9. *The American Heritage Desk Dictionary.* Boston: Houghton Mifflin Company, 1981:893.
10. Jones LWJ. Contact lens deposits: their causes and control. *Contact Lens J* 1992;20:6–15.
11. Leahy CD, Mandell RB, Lin ST. Initial in vivo tear protein deposition on individual hydrogel contact lenses. *Optom Vis Sci* 1990;67:504–511.
12. Lippman JI. Surface properties of a contact lens. *Contact Lens Spectrum* 1988;3:47–49.
13. Benjamin WJ. EOP and Dk/L: the quest for hyper transmissibility. *J Am Optom Assoc* 1993;64:196–200.

MATERIAL SELECTION

EDWARD S. BENNETT AND
JEFFREY D. JOHNSON

Before fitting evaluation and patient education procedures, it is important to select the most appropriate rigid lens material for a given patient. An understanding of the benefits, applications, material properties, and composition is important in assisting in this decision. In addition, factors such as the patient's ocular health and general health, occupation, hobbies, and motivation are extremely important to consider.

GAS PERMEABLE LENSES: BENEFITS, APPLICATIONS, AND LIMITATIONS

Benefits

In large contact lens specialty practices and medical clinics, the percentage of gas permeable (GP) lens wearers has increased from 30% to 50% (1–3). The latter values can be attributed to the numerous benefits and applications of GP lenses, including quality of vision, ocular health, stability/durability, and patient retention.

Quality of Vision

Studies comparing hydrogel and GP lenses have found significantly better visual performance with GP lenses. This includes both subjective patient preference (4,5) and contrast sensitivity function (6,7). The superior optical quality provided by a stable refractive surface accounts for much of this difference. GP lenses also maintain surface wettability better than hydrogel lenses. This can lead to improved long-term comfort and less deposit formation. They may slow down the progression of myopia in young people and, in fact, reduce existing myopia via lenses designed specifically for corneal reshaping. Finally, GP lenses are the lenses of choice for correcting high astigmatic, presbyopic, and irregular cornea patients (discussed later).

Ocular Health

GP lenses have been reported to be less compromising to ocular health than hydrogel lenses (8). They have resulted in less corneal staining (7,9) and ocular infection (8). In addition, because GP lenses have a comparatively smaller surface area and deposits are removed more easily, giant papillae conjunctivitis is an uncommon complication (10). *Acanthamoeba* adherence to the lens surface is also greatly reduced with rigid lenses (11). Another important ocular health benefit results from the increased oxygen transmission potential of GP lens materials (discussed later). Finally, the smaller overall diameter of rigid lenses does not allow for many of the peripheral corneal complications resulting from hydrogel lens limbal compression (12,13).

Stability/Durability

Unlike hydrogel lenses, rigid lenses do not tear or easily change shape or coloration; therefore, frequent lens replacement is not necessary.

Patient Retention/Profitability

One of the most important advantages of rigid lenses in the 1990s was increased patient retention. With mail-order and Internet sites offering replacement lenses, many patients feel that they can bypass the professional care provided by eye care practitioners. As a custom device, GP lenses are much more difficult to obtain through these unconventional channels; in fact, only approximately 1% of mail-order lenses are GP lenses. Also, an increasing number of patients are asking for their contact lens prescriptions to be released. The variety of parameters specified in a GP lens prescription (including base curve, overall diameter, optic zone diameter, peripheral curve radii and widths, and power) helps to demonstrate the specialty nature of the device to patients. Further, studies have shown that greater revenue is generated from GP lens patients than from soft lens patients. This can be attributed to several factors, including the fact that GP lens patients return more frequently for eye examinations and purchase eyeglasses more often than soft lens patients.

APPLICATIONS

Myopia Reduction

Clinical research by Perrigin et al. (14) concluded that GP lens wear in children ages 8 to 13 years resulted in a total increase in myopia of 0.48 D over a 3-year interval, compared to an increase of 1.53 D for a matched spectacle-wearing control group. In addition, once rigid lens wear was discontinued, very little residual increase in myopia occurred (15). These results are similar to those from a study by Khoo et al. (16) but were not found by Katz et al. (17). Because the latter study was compromised by a high dropout rate, the definitive study on the effect of GP lenses on myopia progression in young people, as well as the possible mechanisms, is the Contact Lenses and Myopia Progression (CLAMP) study by Jeff Walline. The results of this study are expected to be published as this text goes to press. GP lenses also are used in corneal reshaping (orthokeratology), a nonsurgical approach to reducing myopia. Although orthokeratology has been available for many years, it recently has enjoyed a renewed popularity. The widespread use of corneal topography and the advent or reverse-geometry GP lenses have been important factors in this resurgence. A more comprehensive discussion of corneal reshaping is provided in Chapter 30.

Hydrogel Lens Refits

It has been reported that patients who failed with hydrogel lens wear due to factors such as poor vision or giant papillary conjunctivitis have been successfully refitted with GP lenses (18–20). Connelly (19) reported on a retrospective study of 200 consecutive patients refit from one contact lens material to another; Ninety percent of these patients were refit from either polymethyl methacrylate (PMMA) or hydrogel lenses into GP lenses. It is apparent that if a patient is unhappy with his or her vision or has experienced ocular compromise, GP lenses are a viable option. The use of a topical anesthetic prior to the initial application of GP lenses in addition to providing—via inventory or empirical fitting—lenses in the patient's correct power will optimize the initial experience and likely result in successful lens wear (21).

Postsurgical/Irregular Cornea

GP lenses also are the material of choice when fitting postsurgical and irregular corneas. Patients who have undergone refractive surgery and still require an optical correction benefit from the increased oxygen delivery of GP lenses versus hydrogel lenses. Post-RK radial keratotomy eyes often have an unusual topographic pattern in which the central cornea is flatter than the peripheral cornea. This topographic pattern—although often less radical—is present in the eyes of patients after laser-assisted *in situ* keratomileusis (LASIK)

as well. Reverse-geometry GP lenses have been developed in which secondary curves are steeper than the base curve, thus improving the fitting relationship of these lenses to the postsurgical cornea. Patients who have undergone penetrating keratoplasty are also good candidates for GP lenses, not only because of the increased oxygen delivery but also because of the spherical anterior refracting surface provided by these lenses. Finally, patients with keratoconus (and other irregular corneal disease) also benefit from GP lenses due to the spherical refracting surface of these lenses, which can allow better-quality vision than hydrogel lenses. These topics are covered more thoroughly in chapters throughout this volume.

Astigmatism

GP lenses correct corneal astigmatism by allowing the tear layer to compensate for the corneal curvature changes. Therefore, GP lens rotation does not affect quality of vision as does hydrogel toric contact lens rotation.

Presbyopia

Presbyopes also benefit from any one of several rigid bifocal designs. These lenses depend on either simultaneous vision or translation to produce the necessary near add power. Translating GP bifocal lenses produce excellent success rates, reported to be as high as 85% (22–24). These lenses typically use prism ballasting and truncation to position properly on the lower lid. Simultaneous vision lenses require precise centration as the near power increases from the center to the edge of the lens. However, as a result of improvements in manufacturing technology, higher-add aspheric multifocal and translating segmented designs with an intermediate correction have been introduced.

LIMITATIONS

Initial Comfort

The most commonly reported cause of discontinuation of rigid lens wear is discomfort (7,19,25). The initial sensation experienced by new rigid lens wearers varies from mild awareness to much discomfort and tearing. Conversely, hydrogel lenses are more comfortable initially, primarily as a result of their much larger diameter. Andrasko and Billings (26) evaluated numerous factors in new rigid lens wearers after 20 to 30 minutes of wear. Poor comfort and itching were associated on the basis of this study (Fig. 11.1). Whether discomfort is going to be problematic can sometimes be determined during the prefitting evaluation. If the patient exhibits apprehension such as lid eversion, fluorescein application, or tonometry during tests, then hydrogel lenses should be considered. Initial lens awareness can result in increased chair time for the patient and practitioner. It

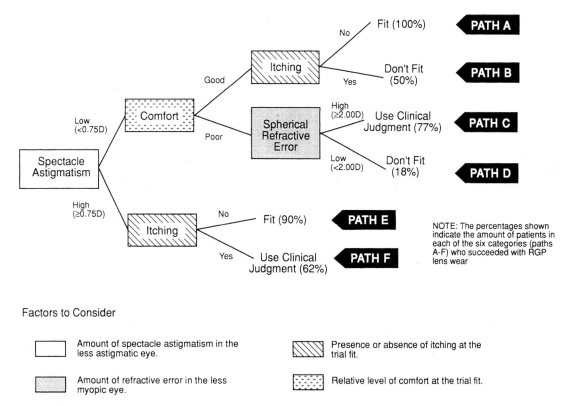

Factors to Consider

☐ Amount of spectacle astigmatism in the less astigmatic eye.

▨ Presence or absence of itching at the trial fit.

▨ Amount of refractive error in the less myopic eye.

▨ Relative level of comfort at the trial fit.

FIG. 11.1. Patient selection model. (From Andrasko GJ, Billings R. A simple nomogram for RGP fitting success. *Contact Lens Spectrum* 1993;8:28, with permission.)

also can affect the lens-to-cornea fitting relationship. Therefore, the use of a topical anesthetic often is recommended for the diagnostic fitting visit to ease patient apprehension. Clinical studies have demonstrated that the use of a topical anesthetic at the fitting visit, when compared to placebo use on new GP wearers, resulted in improved patient perception of GP lenses and greater overall satisfaction success (27,28). In one study, 80% of the patients who discontinued lens wear had not received a topical anesthetic at the fitting visit.

Another important factor integral to initial comfort is how GP lenses are communicated to a patient. The initial application of GP lenses often arouse fear, and the practitioner should almost assume that the patient has heard that "hard lenses are uncomfortable." Therefore, it is important to avoid fear-arousing words such as discomfort or pain when describing adaptation to GP lenses. In fact, it was found that when new GP patients are provided with a doctor–patient scenario in which the doctor presents GP lenses using fear-arousing terms, 6 of 19 patients were not able to adapt successfully to the GP lenses (29). Conversely, when a more realistic doctor–patient scenario was provided, all patients in this group were able to adapt to GP lenses. The use of terms such as "lens awareness" or "lid sensation" are preferable when describing adaptation to a new GP patient. Likewise, avoiding the word "rigid" will lessen any initial

apprehension the patient may have. This presentation can be supplemented by showing video tapes such as "Building Your Practice with GPs" and "GP Lens Care and Handling," which are available from the RGP Lens Institute.

Inventory

As a result of their custom nature, GP lenses are more difficult to inventory than hydrogel lenses. Therefore, the immediate availability of lenses for new patients or those requiring replacement lenses is much less common. Some large rigid lens manufacturers are providing inventories of rigid lenses in commonly used base curve radii and powers.

Occasional/Cosmetic Wear

Hydrogel lenses have the benefit of allowing occasional or intermittent wear with relatively little effect on comfort. Hydrogel lenses also can be used to change or enhance eye color, whereas the small diameter of GP lenses precludes iris color changes.

Environmental Limitations

Another limitation of rigid lenses includes increased susceptibility for dust and debris to become trapped underneath the lens. Patients who work exclusively outdoors in a dusty, windy environment may be better served by hydrogel lenses. Further, participation in contact sports may limit the use of rigid lenses. Although many athletes can successfully wear large-diameter, low-edge-lift rigid lenses, hydrogel lenses may be a necessary alternative (30).

MATERIAL PROPERTIES

Oxygen Permeability

Many properties are deemed desirable for successful long-term contact lens wear. GP lenses have many of these qualities, including meeting the corneal oxygen requirements, good on-eye surface wettability, stability, and crisp visual acuity (31).

Oxygen permeability (Dk) is a property of the lens material independent of the size, shape, or surface condition of a lens. Oxygen transmissibility (Dk/L), a measure of the amount of oxygen transmitted through the lens, depends on the Dk value of the material and on lens thickness (typically center thickness for rigid lenses). Lenses manufactured with identical materials and Dk values but with different thicknesses have different oxygen transmissions; the greater the lens thickness, the lower the oxygen transmission. For example, if a lens has a Dk value of 40 and a center thickness of 0.10 mm, the Dk/L is equal to 40; if the center thickness of this material is 0.20 mm, the Dk/L is decreased by half to a value of 20 Fatt units, that is, $(10^{-11} \text{ cm}^2 \times \text{mL O}_2)$ (sec $\times$ mL $\times$ mm Hg) for Dk and $10^{-9} \times$ cm mL O$_2$/s mL mm Hg for Dk/L. Another method of evaluating oxygen transfer through a rigid lens is equivalent oxygen percentage (EOP). EOP is a measure of the amount of oxygen in the tears between the lens and the cornea and is determined *in vivo*. Essentially, EOP is a predictor of how much oxygen will reach the anterior corneal surface with a particular lens material and design, with a maximum value of 21%. A method of oxygen permeability recently reported by Benjamin and Cappelli (32) has been adopted by the Contact Lens Manufacturers Association (CLMA).

How much oxygen is necessary for corneal physiologic success? Certainly there are advantages in potential oxygen transmission with GP lenses versus hydrogel lenses. As a rule, GP lenses can deliver two to three times more oxygen to the cornea than hydrogen lenses of equal thickness (33). This is a result of both the availability of higher-Dk materials and the fact that these lenses exchange up to 20% of the tear volume per blink (34,35). Conversely, hydrogel lenses can exchange only approximately 1% of the tears per blink (36). GP lenses with Dk values in the range from 18 to 25 have exhibited an amount of overnight corneal swelling (10%–12%) similar to that of many hydrogel extended wear lenses (37,38). However, on awakening, the cornea deswells much faster with a rigid lens and, unlike with hydrogel lenses, typically returns to the zero swelling level.

Research has shown that a Dk/L of 24 (10% EOP) should satisfy the daily wear oxygen requirements of every patient, whereas a Dk/L of 34 should satisfy the extended wear requirements of no residual swelling approximately 4 hours after awakening (39). Further, a Dk/L of 75 to 100 would be required for there to be no corneal physiologic changes noted at any time with lens wear (40). When the oxygen transmission values of several commonly used hydrogel and rigid minus- and plus-power daily wear and disposable lenses were compared, rigid lenses were much more likely to meet this Holden-Mertz criteria (Fig. 11.2) (41).

For daily wear, a 30-Dk lens with a center thickness of 0.12 mm would meet this requirement, as would a 60-Dk material with a center thickness of 0.24 mm. Some newer materials, with Dk of approximately 120 and an average thickness of 0.15, are approaching the range of producing no corneal physiologic changes at any time during wear.

With these newer materials in mind, the classification system for GP lenses has expanded from the earlier low-Dk and high-Dk categories. Benjamin (42) has divided GP lenses into five categories based on Dk (and using a standard thickness of 0.12 mm): low Dk (<15), medium Dk (15–30), high Dk (31–60), super-Dk (61–100), and hyper-Dk (>100). However, the bottom line is that oxygen transmission, although important to successful lens wear, should not be viewed apart from other lens performance factors, such as adequate movement, comfortable edge design, resistance to deposit buildup, flexural resistance, and dimensional stability (43).

Surface Wettability

Lens surface wettability is of major importance to polymer chemists, manufacturers, and clinicians. In fact, better wetting materials was the number one request for desired rigid lens improvements in the 1990s in a nationwide survey of optometrists (44). It has been hypothesized that lenses that dry between blinks are more prone to deposits (45). When this occurs, the mucin layer remaining on the surface could undergo chemical changes that reduce the mucin's wettability; a similar result would be expected on the contact lens surface. Surface wettability problems are many and varied and include reduced comfort and vision. Management of these problems is discussed elsewhere in this volume.

Flexural Resistance

Flexural resistance pertains to the ability of a rigid lens to resist the bending or flexing forces when it is on a toric cornea. A lens with poor flexural resistance will tend to flex during the blinking process and therefore inadequately correct the patient's corneal astigmatism. Flexure is more commonly experienced with high-Dk materials and thin center thicknesses, steep base curve radii, and large optical zone diameter lens designs (46–48).

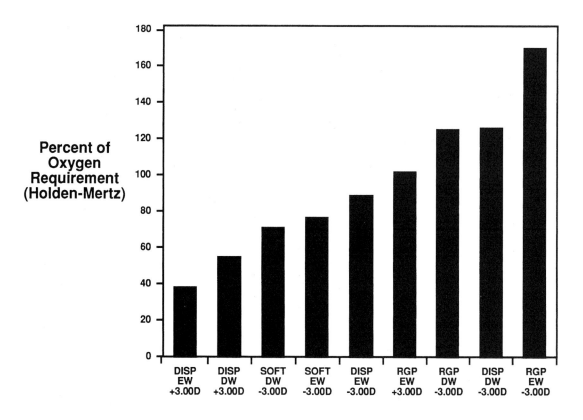

FIG. 11.2. Comparison of the oxygen transmission values of hydrogel and gas permeable minus- and plus-power daily wear, extended wear, and disposable lenses. (From Gordon JM, Bennett ES. Dk revisited: the hypoxic corneal environment. Presented at the Annual Meeting of the American Academy of Ophthalmology, Chicago, Illinois, November 1993, with permission.)

Specific Gravity

Specific gravity refers to the weight of an GP lens at a given temperature divided by the weight of an equal volume of water at the same temperature. It often is compared to water, which has a specific gravity of 1.00. Specific gravity values for rigid lens materials can be divided into low (=1.10), medium (1.11–1.20), and high (>1.20). These values can play an important role in the success of rigid lenses. If all other parameters are held constant, changing to a different lens material (and hence different specific gravity) can produce as much as a 20% change in lens mass, therefore greatly affecting lens positioning (49). It is possible that the higher specific gravity (i.e., heavier) lens materials may have more of a tendency to position inferiorly on the cornea because of the forces of gravity (50,51).

Other Properties

Other properties pertain to the so-called "softness" of a given material. Factors such as hardness value, scratch resistance, and optical quality have been described and compared.

MATERIAL TYPES AND COMPOSITION

Silicone/Acrylate

The first successful GP lens materials were of silicone/acrylate (S/A; also termed siloxane/methacrylate) composition. Also referred to as silicone-based, these copolymers actually contained the element silicon as siloxane bonds in side branches of the main carbon–carbon polymer chain. The introduction of silicone-based copolymers in 1979 was a major breakthrough because silicone has excellent oxygen permeability characteristics. Unlike homogeneous PMMA lens materials, S/A materials are polymers with silicone, methacrylate, wetting agents, and cross-linking agents. The latter two ingredients are important because of the dryness (hydrophobicity) and flexibility of silicone. Wetting agents, including hydroxyethyl methacrylate and methacrylic acid (the most common), achieve their effect through their strong affinity with water molecules. Cross-linking agents have the ability to strengthen the material; therefore, the flexibility is decreased, matching characteristics are improved, and the material is less sensitive to the effect of solvents. S/A materials, notably high-Dk polymers, have a greater tendency for lipid accumulation (52).

Currently available S/A lens materials are listed in Table 11.1. (53) As it became apparent that higher-Dk lens materials would be necessary to meet the cornea's daily wear oxygen requirements and to allow for flexible/extended wear schedules, higher-Dk lens materials were introduced. However, increasing the siloxane bonding to increase oxygen permeability increases both the hydrophobic properties and the flexibility of the lens, possibly resulting in problems such as corneal desiccation, surface deposits, warpage, and flexure, with subjective symptoms such as dryness and reduced vision (47,54). Increasing the amount of wetting agent to offset these problems typically results in excessive material hydration, causing poor contact lens stability. An excess of cross-linking agents to enhance stability could result in a brittle material (55).

Modified silicone-based materials designed to offset these problems have been introduced. These lenses include the Trans-Aire lens (Bentec), a 45-Dk silicone copolymer, and the Novalens (Ocu-Tec Corp.), a 44-Dk GP core with a hydrophilic surface. Due to their surface chemistry, these lens materials purportedly have excellent surface wettability and initial comfort (56,57). A tedious care system, however, has resulted in limited use of the Novalens (58,59).

Fluoro-Silicone/Acrylate

Fluoro-silicone/acrylate (F-S/A) lens materials are similar to S/A materials, with the notable exception of the addition of fluorine. Fluorine, known for its nonstick properties in Teflon-coated cooking materials, increases the deposit resistance of the lens materials by promoting tear film interaction with the lens surface. In addition, low surface tension (energy) is present; that is, there is a reduced affinity of polarized tear components to become adherent to the contact lens surface (45). Therefore, the primary problem experienced with S/A lens material—dryness—should be reduced with F-S/A materials. This has, in fact, been the case;

several comparison studies have concluded that F-S/A lenses are more wettable and are perceived as more comfortable (47,60,61) and less prone to surface deposits (62) compared with S/A lenses. It has been found that the tear film stays in contact with the lens surface for about twice as long with the F-S/A materials than with S/A materials. In addition, the rate of tear film breakup is slower over the fluorinated lens material (63).

The fluorinated component also aids oxygen transmission through the lens material. This is accomplished by oxygen's increased ability to dissolve into fluorinated materials (i.e., oxygen transmission is achieved by solubility, not diffusion, in fluorine) (55,64). It is apparent that although the ability of silicone to promote diffusion of oxygen through the lens material is important, the additional permeability provided by fluorine will reduce the need to use excessive amounts of silicone. Therefore, it has been found that the F-S/A materials are more dimensionally stable than S/A materials (47,55).

F-S/A lenses can be divided into five categories, as discussed earlier. The authors prefer to combine these categories into low Dk (25–50), high Dk (51–99), and hyper-Dk (= 100). Lens materials in these categories are listed in Tables 11.2, 11.3, and 11.4. Low-Dk materials are the lenses of choice for most daily wear patients (i.e., myopes) due to the benefits of surface wettability and dimensional stability (65–67). High-Dk F-S/A materials have been the lenses of choice for patients needing higher oxygen transmission levels (i.e., daily wear hyperopes and patients desiring a flexible wear schedule). Hyper-Dk lenses can be worn by all patients but are definitely indicated for patients desiring an extended wear schedule. High-Dk and hyper-Dk lens materials, although more stable than previous generation

TABLE 11.1. SILICONE/ACRYLATE LENS MATERIALS (53)

Name	Dk	Manufacturer
Boston II	12	Polymer Technology
Paraperm 02	15.6	Paragon Vision Sciences
SA-18	18	Lagado Corporation
Optacryl 60	18	Paragon Vision Sciences
Boston IV	19	Polymer Technology
SGP I	22	Life-Style Co.
SA-32	32	Lagado Corp.
SGP II	43.5	Life-Style Co.
Trans-Aire	45	Rand Scientific Research
Paraperm EW	56	Paragon Vision Sciences

Manufacturer Dk values listed; method may vary among manufacturers.

TABLE 11.2. LOW DK FLUORO-SILICONE/ACRYLATE LENS MATERIALS (53)

Name	Dk	Manufacturer
Boston ES UV[a]	18	Polymer Technology
Boston RXD[a]	24	Polymer Technology
Accucon	25	Innovision
Flosi	26	Lagado Corp.
Paraperm Thin	29	Paragon Vision Sciences
FluoroPerm 30	30	Paragon Vision Sciences
Sportsight GP	30	Paragon Vision Sciences
Fluorex 300	30	GT Laboratories
Hybrid FS	31	Contamac U.S.
SGP III	43.5	Life-Style Co.
Equalens	47	Polymer Technology
Boston 7 UV	49	Polymer Technology
Fluorex 500	50	GT Labs
Hydr02	50	Innovision

Manufacturer Dk values listed; method may vary among manufacturers.
[a] Has been listed with a Dk >25 with other methods of measurement.

TABLE 11.3. HIGH DK FLUORO-SILICONE/ACRYLATE LENS MATERIALS (53)

Name	Dk	Manufacturer
Boston EO UV	58	Polymer Technology
Boston EO Envision UV	58	Polymer Technology
Paragon HDS	58	Paragon Vision Sciences
FluoroPerm 60	60	Paragon Vision Sciences
Fluorex 700	70	GT Laboratories
Equalens II	85	Polymer Technology
FluoroPerm 92	92	Paragon Vision Sciences

Manufacturer Dk values listed; method may vary among manufacturers.

TABLE 11.5. GAS PERMEABLE MATERIAL SELECTION (IN GENERAL)

Low Dk	High Dk	Hyper Dk
Myopia	Hyperopia	Hyperopia
Daily wear	Flexible wear (hyperopia)	Extended wear (myopia and hyperopia)
Optimum wettability	Extended wear (myopia)	
Optimum stability	Prism ballasted lens designs	

materials, are more likely to experience compromises in dimensional stability and surface wettability. These applications are summarized in Table 11.5.

Improved material composition and manufacturing processes have resulted in the production of higher-Dk lenses that are durable and flexure resistant and maintain good wettability. For example, the Boston XO (Polymer Technology) GP lens has a Dk of 100 but is promoted as having increased durability and wettability. Polymer Technology has developed the Boston XO (and ES and EO) lens using a unique chemistry termed AERCOR O technology. The lens contains an oxygen-permeable backbone and AERCOR O cross-linking agents, allowing more free volume within the lens and thus allowing more oxygen to reach the cornea. This also allows the lens to be manufactured with a low level of silicon, thus improving wettability. The Menicon SF-P and Z lenses (Menicon, Con-Cise) also offer extremely high levels of oxygen transmission with improved comfort and wettability (68–70). The Menicon Z, in particular, is a hyper-Dk lens material that can be manufactured in an ultrathin design. It is also the only GP lens material approved by the United States Food and Drug Administration (FDA) for continuous wear.

Even with improved material composition and manufacturing techniques, these super-Dk and hyper-Dk lenses often have shorter lifespans than the lower-Dk lenses (71–73). Because of this, several manufacturers offer a fre-

quent replacement program with their lenses. Fluoroperm 151 (Paragon Vision Sciences) and Menicon SF-P (Menicon USA) are two examples of GP lens materials that can be purchased under a planned replacement schedule. Some practitioners suggest dispensing both pairs of lenses at one time, with the second pair used initially as a backup if needed. Others suggest dispensing only the first pair and then dispensing the new pair of lenses at 6-month follow-up (74).

Super-Dk and hyper-DK patients are not the only patients who may benefit from a planned replacement schedule. Patients with dry eye or meibomian gland dysfunction in whom deposits form quickly on their lenses, as well as patients who work under deposit-forming environmental conditions (e.g., hairdressers), also would benefit from a frequent replacement program.

Oxygen transmission is not the only factor that should be considered when using an F-S/A lens. Some materials have an ultraviolet absorber within the lens material, and this can be a potentially significant benefit as we learn more about the harmful effects of sunlight on the eye and particularly on the crystalline lens. Also, several lens materials are available in a biaspheric lens design (i.e., aspheric both centrally and peripherally, in contrast to a peripheral-only aspheric design). There are fewer parameters with this type of lens design (i.e., base curve radii and overall diameters); therefore, the design is less complicated to fit, and an in-office inventory of this design could be maintained.

It is apparent that this and similar designs will become popular in the United States as a result of their popularity (and the high percentage of GP lenses fitted) in many parts of Europe, particularly in technologically advanced countries such as Germany, Switzerland, and Holland (1,75). This popularity appears to be the result of European fitters' knowledge in areas such as contact lens optics and corneal topography, in combination with the available aspheric manufacturing technology. The result is what has been termed "design compatibility," or the matching of a material's fitting characteristics with a posterior surface design that optimizes initial comfort and "forgiveness" of fit (76).

TABLE 11.4. HYPER Dk FLUORO-SILICONE/ACRYLATE LENS MATERIALS (53)

Name	Dk	Manufacturer
Boston XO UV	100	Polymer Technology
Paragon HDS 100	100	Paragon Vision Sciences
FluoroPerm 151	151	Paragon Vision Sciences
Menicon Z	163	Menicon America, Inc./Con-Cise

Manufacturer Dk values listed; method may vary among manufacturers.

Polystyrene

Styrene-based materials were introduced in the 1980s as a result of benefits such as low specific gravity and good flexural resistance (38). This material has been incorporated into the center of a material that cross-links or molecularly bonds an outer hydrophilic skirt with the GP center material (77). The final result, the SoftPerm lens (Ciba Vision), has a rigid center (8.0 mm with a 7-mm optical zone and one peripheral curve) composed of tertiary butyl styrene, silicon/methacrylate, and a wetting agent. The surface wettability also is enhanced by the surface neutralization of silicone when in contact with the tear film. This material can be manufactured to a minimal thickness of 0.08 mm at −4.50 D and 0.08 mm at plano. The outer skirt portion of the SoftPerm is a hydroxyethyl methacrylate-based hydrogel with an approximate water content of 25%. The overall diameter of this lens material is 14.3 mm.

This lens should be fitted 0.1 to 0.2 mm steeper than "K." Essentially it can be thought of as an 8-mm diameter rigid lens; therefore, a steeper than "K" base curve radius should promote more of an alignment fitting relationship while allowing adequate movement and good comfort (77). Fluoresoft (Holles Laboratories), a macromolecular fluorescein solution, not fluorescein, should be used to evaluate the fit. At minimum, a 0.25-mm lag in upgaze is recommended.

The primary benefits of the SoftPerm lens are good initial comfort, astigmatic correction, and centration (78). The latter benefit is especially important for patients with irregular corneas as a result of keratoconus, trauma, or other causes, because a rigid lens may not center properly and a hydrogel lens most likely will not provide adequate vision. Borderline dry eye and corneal exhaustion syndrome patients also have benefited from being refit with the SoftPerm lens (79).

Problems with the SoftPerm lens include the cost, edema, and neovascularization resulting from a tight-fitting relationship, tearing at the junction between the rigid and hydrogel portions (although the latter two problems are less in the SoftPerm than in its predecessor, the Saturn II, because of an improved design that increases the probability of lens movement with the blink), limited parameters, flexure, and difficulty in lens removal. Currently, the SoftPerm can be ordered in base curves of 6.5, 6.7, 6.9, and 7.1 to 8.1 (in 0.1-mm steps) and with powers of +6.00 to −16.00 D. Difficulty with lens removal can be addressed by educating patients to apply a few drops of saline in the eye before removing the lens. The lens can then be removed, either by gently pinching the lower section and removing it like a hydrogel lens or moving it onto the sclera and pinching it off. The SoftPerm can be cleaned with any Allergan cleaning solution, although UltraCare or Consept is recommended.

In summary, the SoftPerm lens is not the lens of choice for most patients. However, it is a niche lens that should be considered for use in contact lens practices that specialize in fitting patients with irregular corneas.

Silicone Elastomer

The silicone elastomer lenses, introduced by Dow Corning in the 1980s, have the definite advantages of outstanding oxygen permeability (DK = 340) and intermediate lens diameters (11.3 and 12.5 mm), which are beneficial to children. The greatest problem with silicone elastomer lenses has been their hydrophobic nature. The hydrophobic surface is treated by ionic bombardment near the end of the manufacturing process, thus making the surface more hydrophilic (80). Mucous adhesion is still a problem, however, as are dryness and corneal adhesion. Because of these problems, the silicone rubber lens is rarely used in a clinical setting. Pediatric aphakic patients are an exception to this rule, and the lenses currently are available in aphakic powers from Bausch & Lomb (Silsoft). The selection of base curve radii varies from 7.5 to 8.3 mm (i.e., between characteristic GP and hydrogel radii) in the standard aphakic power range. Although these lenses may last only 6 months when worn on an extended wear basis, their excellent oxygen transmission, ease of handling (vs a larger hydrogel lens), and better initial comfort (than that of a rigid lens) make them a viable option for the pediatric aphakic patient.

MATERIAL SELECTION

The availability of all these different rigid (or semirigid) lens materials presents a myriad of choices to the practitioner. What GP material is preferable for our patients? The answer depends on the particular patient to be fitted. In other words, it is recommended to use diagnostic lens sets of several different materials. Fig. 11.3 shows the authors' recommendations for material selection (81–83). They can be divided into five categories: (i) refractive error, (ii) corneal topography, (iii) refits, (iv) occupation/hobbies, and (v) age.

REFRACTIVE ERROR

Because of the thin center thicknesses typically available in minus-power lenses, most myopic patients would benefit from the dimensional stability provided by low-Dk to medium-Dk F-S/A lenses while still meeting (or approximating) the cornea's daily wear oxygen requirements. However, if corneal edema is present with a low-Dk or medium-Dk lens material, which often results from either a high corneal oxygen need (which varies between individual patients) or a tight-fitting lens, the patient should be refit into a higher-Dk material. Hyperopic patients will benefit most from a super-Dk or hyper-Dk lens material because of the greater center thickness present in these lens powers.

CORNEAL TOPOGRAPHY

Patients with moderate astigmatism (i.e., >1.50 D) benefit from the flexural resistance provided by low-Dk F-S/A lens

GP Material Selection

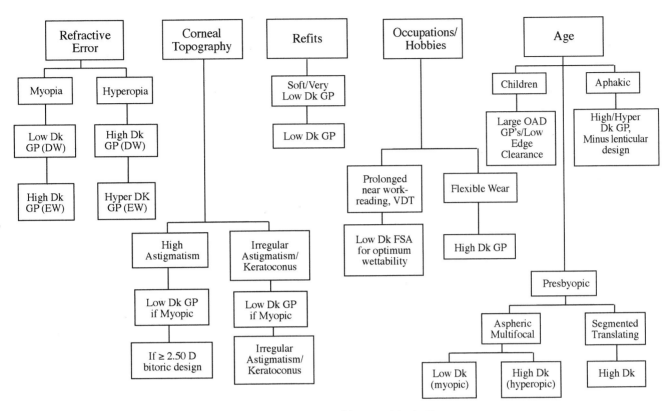

FIG. 11.3. Gas permeable material selection.

materials. Patients with high astigmatism (i.e., ≥2.50 D) often benefit from spherical power effect or cylinder power effect bitoric designs. It is preferable, however, to use these same designs in a higher-Dk material than the currently available Polycon II (Ciba Vision) material (Dk = 10). As mentioned previously, patients with irregular corneas from keratoconus, trauma, or another cause may benefit from the SoftPerm lens, although it is recommended that the clinician initially diagnostically fit a low-Dk F-S/A lens material and evaluate the fitting relationship and centration.

If inferior decentration is a problem (often a result of the rate of flattening of the cornea and/or the location of the corneal apex), a lid-attachment lens design is recommended. For a laterally decentered lens, common in against-the-rule astigmatism, an aspheric design may be of value. Managing GP lens decentration is discussed in greater detail in another chapter.

REFITS

Former PMMA and first-generation GP lens wearers should be refit into low-Dk rigid lenses. Typically, these patients have established care habits that could be damaging to the higher-Dk lens materials. Surface scratches and warpage could occur (see Chapter 13), especially if these patients are not properly educated.

Previous hydrogel wearers who have experienced deposit-related problems (i.e., redness, itching, decrease in wearing time) resulting in papillary hypertrophy would benefit from being refit into essentially any GP material, preferably the most wettable available material. These materials also would be recommended for all borderline dry eye patients and mild allergy sufferers.

OCCUPATION

Individuals who perform much near work would benefit from the most wettable materials available (similar to those for papillary hypertrophy patients), supplemented by frequent application of rewetting/reconditioning drops. Athletes benefit most from hydrogel lenses. If this option is not satisfactory, a large-diameter, low-edge-lift GP may be considered, as may a semirigid lens such as the SoftPerm. This larger-diameter may help limit less displacement. Individuals who desire (or need) to wear their lenses on a flexible schedule or on an extended wear basis (e.g., nurses, police, firefighters) would benefit from a super-Dk or hyper-Dk F-S/A material. Likewise, pilots and flight attendants, who often are exposed to less-than-optimal oxygen levels, would benefit from the higher-Dk materials.

AGE

As mentioned previously, aphakic children often benefit from being fitted with a silicone elastomer lens or a high-Dk F-S/A lens with an ultraviolet filter. Phakic children would benefit from larger-diameter GP lenses with an ultraviolet filter, which should be less likely to dislodge. Initial comfort could be optimized by achieving an underneath the upper lid fitting relationship and by using a rolled, tapered-edge design. Adult aphakic patients would benefit from a super-Dk or hyper-Dk F-S/A lens with an ultraviolet filter material in a minus lenticular design and large (9.2–9.6 mm) overall diameter.

SUMMARY

GP lenses have numerous benefits and applications and, in fact, can differentiate the novice contact lens practitioner from the practitioner who considers all of the available options, including GP lenses, before fitting the patient. It is important to determine the patient's level of motivation, sensitivity to something approaching the eyes, and factors such as desired wearing time, occupation, and refractive error. Once it is decided that a given patient will be fitted into GP lenses, it is important to remember that no one rigid lens material should be used for all such patients.

REFERENCES

1. Ames K. Rethink your approach to RGP lenses. *Contact Lens Spectrum* 1993;8:24.
2. Connelly S. Who really decides which material to fit, the patient or the practitioner? *Contact Lens Spectrum* 1992;7:45.
3. Bennett I. *State of the ophthalmic industry address.* Advisory Enterprises, 1989.
4. Ziel CJ, Gussler JR, Van Meter WS, et al. Contrast sensitivity in extended wear of the Boston IV lens. *CLAO J* 1990;16:276.
5. Fonn D, Gauthier CA, Pritchard N. Patient preferences and comparative ocular responses to rigid and soft contact lenses. *Optom Vis Sci* 1995;72:857.
6. Timberlake GT, Doane MG, Bertera JH. Short-term low contrast visual acuity reduction associated with in vivo contact lens drying. *Optom Vis Sci* 1992;69:755.
7. Johnson TJ, Schnider C. Clinical performance and patient preference for hydrogel versus RGP lenses. *Int Contact Lens Clin* 1991;18:130.
8. Contact lenses: what to consider. *Consumer Reports* 1989;54:411.
9. Goldberg EP, Bhatia S, Enns JB. Hydrogel contact lens-corneal interactions: a new mechanism for deposit formation and corneal injury. *CLAO J* 1997;23:243.
10. Poggio EC, Glynn RJ, Schein OD, et al. The incidence of ulcera-

tive keratitis among users of daily-wear and extended-wear contact lenses. *N Engl J Med* 1989;321:779.
11. Seal DV, Bennett ES, McFayden AK, et al. Differential adherence of *Acanthamoeba* to contact lenses: effects of material characteristics. *Optom Vis Sci* 1995;72:23.
12. Suchecki JK, Ehlers WH, Donshik PC. Peripheral corneal infiltrates associated with contact lens wear. *CLAO J* 1996;22:41.
13. Dart JK. The epidemiology of contact lens-related diseases in the United Kingdom. *CLAO J* 1993;19:241.
14. Perrigin J, Perrigin D, Quinteros S, et al. Silicone-acrylate contact lenses for myopia control: 3-year old results. *Optom Vis Sci* 1990;67:764.
15. Grosvenor T, Perrigin D, Perrigin J, et al. Rigid gas-permeable contact lenses for myopia control: the effects of discontinuation of wear. *Optom Vis Sci* 1991;68:385.
16. Khoo CY, Chong J, Rajan U. A 3-year study on the effect of RGP contact lenses on myopic children. *Singapore Med J* 1999;40:230–237.
17. Katz J, Schein OD, Levy B, et al. A randomized trial of rigid gas permeable contact lenses to reduce progression of children's myopia. *Am J Ophthalmol* 2003;136:82–89.
18. Ames K. Clinical experiences with Boston Envision. *Contact Lens Spectrum* 1991;6:21.
19. Connelly S. Why do patients want to be refit? *Contact Lens Spectrum* 1992;7:39.
20. Andrasko G, Smiley T, Nichold L, et al. Clinical recommendations for the management of symptomatic soft contact lens wearers. *Contact Lens Spectrum* 1993;8:24.
21. Davis R, Bennett ES. Refitting soft lens wearers into GPs. *Contact Lens Spectrum* 2003;18:48–49.
22. Remba MJ. The Tangent Streak rigid gas-permeable bifocal contact lens. *J Am Optom Assoc* 1988;59:212.
23. Kirman ST, Kiman GS. The Tangent Streak bifocal contact lens. *Contact Lens Forum* 1988;13:38.
24. Gussler JR, Lin ES, Litteral G, et al. Clinical evaluation of the Anterior Constant Focus (ACF) annular bifocal contact lens. *CLAO J* 1993;19:222.
25. Hewett TT. A survey of contact lens wearers, part II: behaviors, experiences, attitudes and expectations. *Am J Optom Physiol Opt* 1984;61:73.
26. Andrasko GJ, Billings R. A simple nomogram for RGP fitting success. *Contact Lens Spectrum* 1993;8:28.
27. Bennett ES, Smythe J, Henry VA, et al. The effect of topical anesthetic use on initial patient satisfaction and overall success with rigid gas-permeable contact lenses. *Optom Vis Sci* 1998;75:800–805.
28. Schnider DM. Anesthetics and RGPs: crossing the controversial line. *Rev Optom* 1996;33:41.
29. Bennett ES, Stulc S, Bassi CJ, et al. The effect of patient personality profile and verbal presentation on successful adaptation, satisfaction and compliance. *Optom Vis Sci* 1998;75:500–505.
30. Schwartz CA. New strategies for screening RGPs. *Rev Optom* 1994;131:29.
31. Jones L. Modern contact lens materials: clinical performance update. *Contact Lens Spectrum* 2002;17:24–35.
32. Benjamin WJ, Cappelli QA. Oxygen permeability of thirty-seven rigid contact lens materials. *Optom Vis Sci* 2002;79:103–111.
33. Mandell RB, Lieberman GL, Fatt I. Corneal oxygen supply: RGP versus soft lenses. *Contact Lens Spectrum* 1987;2:37.
34. Bennett ES, Ghormley NR. Rigid extended wear; an overview. *Int Contact Lens Clin* 1987;14:319.
35. Maehara JR, Kastl PR. Rigid gas-permeable extended wear. *CLAO J* 1994;20:139.
36. Polse KA. Tear flow under hydrogel contact lenses. *Invest Ophthalmol Vis Sci* 1979;18:409.
37. O'Neal MR, Polse KA, Sarver MD. Corneal response to rigid

and hydrogel lenses during eye closure. *Invest Ophthalmol Vis Sci* 1986;27:837.

38. Tomlinson A, Armitage B. Closed-eye corneal response to a tertiary butyl styrene gas-permeable lens. *Int Eyecare* 1985;1:320.
39. Holden BA, Mertz GW. Critical oxygen levels to avoid corneal edema for daily- and extended-wear contact lenses. *Invest Ophthalmol Vis Sci* 1984;24:1161.
40. Sigband DJ, Bridgewater BA. Fluoroperm 151 extended wear: a clinical study. *CLAO J* 1994;20:37.
41. Gordon JM, Bennett ES. Dk revisited: the hypoxic corneal environment. Presented at the Annual Meeting of the American Academy of Ophthalmology, Chicago, Illinois, November 1993.
42. Benjamin WJ. EOP and Dk/L: the quest for hypertransmissibility. *J Am Optom Assoc* 1993;64;196.
43. Bennett ES. How important are lens oxygen ratings? *Cornea* 1990;9[Suppl 1]:4.
44. Maruna C, Yoder M, Andrasko GJ. Attitudes toward RGPs among optometrists. *Contact Lens Spectrum* 1989;4:25.
45. Feldman G, Yamane SJ, Herskowitz R. Fluorinated materials and the Boston Equalens. *Contact Lens Forum* 1987;12:57.
46. Herman JP. Flexure of rigid contact lenses on toric corneas as a function of base curve fitting relationship. *J Am Optom Assoc* 1983;54:209.
47. Bennett ES, Tomlinson A, Mirowitz MC, et al. Comparison of overnight corneal swelling and lens performance in RGP extended wear. *CLAO J* 1988;14:94.
48. Egan DJ, Bennett ES. Trouble shooting rigid contact lenses flexure—a case report. *Int Contact Lens Clin* 1985;12:147.
49. Levitt AO. Specific gravity and RGP lens performance. *Contact Lens Spectrum* 1996;11:43.
50. Bennett ES. Problem-solving with rigid gas-permeable lenses. *Practical Optom* 1991;2:9.
51. Ghormley NR. Specific gravity—does it contribute to RGP lens adherence? *Int Contact Lens Clin* 1991;18:125.
52. Quinn TG. Material solutions for gas permeable questions. *Contact Lens Spectrum* 2000;15:19.
53. Thompson T. *Tyler's quarterly soft contact lens parameter guide.* 2003;20:52–53.
54. Henry VA, Bennett ES, Forrest JF. Clinical investigation of the Paraperm EW rigid gas-permeable contact lens. *Am J Optom Physiol Opt* 1987;64:313.
55. Weinschenk JI. A look at the components of fluoro-silicone acrylates. *Contact Lens Spectrum* 1989;4:61.
56. Baker MA. Clinical results from 6 months with the Novalens H_2OGP. *Optical Prism* 1990;Sept–Oct:30.
57. LaFerla J. Novalens: clinical views. *Contact Lens Forum* 1991;16:371991.
58. Clark SA, Bennett ES, Henry VA, et al. The effect of contact lens cleaners on lens parameters and surface quality of the Novalens. *J Am Optom Assoc* 1993;64:169.
59. Hatfield RO, Jordan DR, Bennett ES, et al. Initial comfort and surface wettability: a comparison between different contact lens materials. *J Am Optom Assoc* 1993;64:271.
60. Gelnar PV, Behnken BH. Paraperm EW vs. Fluoroperm 90 gas-permeable contact lens study. *Contact Lens J* 1989;17:15.
61. Andrasko GJ. Comfort comparison between silicon acrylates and the Boston Equalens. *Contact Lens Spectrum* 1988;3:61.
62. Bark M, Hanson D, Grant R. A guide to rigid gas-permeable contact lens materials. *Optician* 1994;207:17.
63. Doane M, Gleason W. Tear film interaction with RGP contact lenses. Presented at the First International Material Science Symposium, St. Louis, Missouri, March 1988.
64. Caroline PJ, Ellis EJ. Review of the mechanisms of oxygen transport through rigid gas-permeable lenses. *Int Eyecare* 1986;2:210.
65. Quinn TQ. Clinical experience with Fluoroperm 30 lenses. *Contact Lens Spectrum* 1989;4:63.
66. Quinn TQ. Base curve stability of a fluoro-silicone-acrylate material of moderate permeability. *Contact Lens Spectrum* 1989;4:52.
67. Bennett ES. Basic fitting. In: Bennett ES, Weissman BA, eds. *Clinical contact lens practice.* Philadelphia: JB Lippincott, 1991.
68. Mackeen DL, Sachdev M. Ballou V, et al. A prospective multicenter clinical trial to assess safety and efficacy of Menicon SF-P RGP lenses for extended wear. *CLAO J* 1992;18:183.
69. Ichikawa H, Kozai A, Mackeen DL, et al. Corneal swelling responses with extended wear in naïve and adapted subjects with Menicon RGP contact lens. *Contact Lens Spectrum* 1992;7:23.
70. Hayashida J, Kame RT. Correction of hyperopia with a novel high-Dk RGP contact lens. *Contact Lens Spectrum* 1992;7:23.
71. Jones L, Woods CA, Efron N. Life expectancy of rigid gas-permeable and high water content contact lenses. *CLAO J* 1996;22:258.
72. Woods CA, Efron N. Regular replacement of rigid contact lenses alleviates binding to the cornea. *Int Contact Lens Clin* 1996;23:13.
73. Woods CA, Efron N. Regular replacement of extended-wear rigid gas-permeable contact lenses. *CLAO J* 1996;22:172.
74. Bridgewater BA. Why you should consider a planned replacement program for RGP lenses. *Contact Lens Spectrum* 1997;13[Suppl]:5.
75. Herskowitz R. Boston Equacurve: a new concept in design compatibility. *Contact Lens Forum* 1990;15:49.
76. Kok JH. A European fitting philosophy for aspheric, high-Dk RGP contact lenses. *CLAO J* 1992;18:232.
77. Dubow BW, Vrchota, LR. SoftPerm: the "quintessential" lens design for practice-building professionals. *Contact Lens Forum* 1990;15:17.
78. Morgan P. Practical experience with a new soft/RGP combination lens. *Optician* 1992;204:16.
79. Tucker IS. Insights on using the SoftPerm lens. *Contact Lens Spectrum* 1993;8:53.
80. Huppertz HL. Observations on the fitting of silicone rubber lenses. *J Br Contact Lens Assoc* 1980;3:87.
81. Bennett ES. Matching the patient with the gas permeable material. *Rev Optom* 2002;139:45–46.
82. Bennett ES, Levy B. Material selection. In: Bennett ES, Henry VA, eds: *Clinical manual of contact lenses,* 2nd ed. Philadelphia: Lippincott Williams & Wilkins, 2000:59–74.
83. Bennett ES. Choose the right RGP lens material for your patient. *Contact Lens Spectrum* 2001;16:19.

One of the most important indicators of a practitioner's skill is the ability to successfully design and apply a gas permeable (GP) contact lens. The art of fitting a rigid lens demands a considerable degree of skill and knowledge, much more so than with hydrogel lenses. However, the effort associated with developing this expertise can be well rewarded. The high quality of vision, ocular health, durability, and surface wettability associated with GP lenses are advantages that cannot be overemphasized. Successful GP lens fitting begins with proper material selection and continues with careful application of diagnostic lenses and identification of appropriate lens design parameters.

OPTIMIZING INITIAL COMFORT

For GP lenses to be successfully fit, the initial experience has to be optimized. The perception of initial comfort often is negative, and it represents the most common reason why patients discontinue GP lens wear (1). Although in a recent study 70% of new GP lens wearers were able to wear their lenses 14 hours per day, 60% of those who could not achieve all-day wear were unable to do so as the result of either unacceptable comfort or vision, often the former. It is evident that if the patient has a poor initial experience with GP lenses, he or she will influence others away from considering this option. One of the primary problems is a poorly motivated practitioner. If the clinician—via his or her educational background (or lack thereof) or current employment environment—is not motivated to fit GP lenses, it is likely that, despite the many benefits of GP lenses, patients will not be fit into the mode of correction that would be indicated due to quality of vision, eye health, or some other reason.

The author has presented a threefold approach to optimizing the initial comfort (2). This includes proper presentation, use of a topical anesthetic, and optimizing lens design and fitting. As described in Chapter 11, it begins with the initial approach in presenting this modality to patients. New contact lens wearers often are hesitant to place a foreign object on their eyes. Male patients, in particular, are apprehensive because they are not accustomed to applying cosmetics around their eyes. The method used by the practitioner and staff member to present GP lenses can have a dramatic effect on the patient's perception of these lenses (3). If tentativeness is exhibited in recommending GP lenses, the patient will understandably be hesitant in accepting this option (4). In fact, if it is evident via verbal or nonverbal communication that the practitioner prefers soft lenses, the patient can be easily influenced toward this option. It is preferable to present GP lenses in a favorable but realistic manner. The benefits of eye health, quality of vision, ease of handling, durability, and possible myopia control should be presented (5,6). It is apparent that patients can tolerate the initial lens awareness if these benefits are explained and they are told what to expect during adaptation and how improvement in comfort will gradually occur.

The initial lens sensation should be explained in a calm, matter-of-fact manner. Using strong terms such as "discomfort" or "pain" has been found to result in increased discontinuation from lens wear as opposed to when terms such as "lens awareness" and "lid adaptation to the edge" were used (3). Likewise, omitting the word "rigid" and using "oxygen permeable," "gas permeable," or "GP" to describe this lens modality is more reassuring to the patient (7). If the patient is told that discomfort or even pain can result when wearing GP lenses, it makes it an easy decision for the patient to select soft contact lenses as the preferred mode of correction. Numerous aids available from the RGP Lens Institute *(www.rgpli.org)* will be beneficial in assisting the patient through the adaptation process, including the GP Benefits/Applications laminated pocket card and the video entitled "Have You Considered Oxygen Permeables." It is apparent that if GP lenses are explained properly to the patient, it is very likely that the percentage of patients adapting to GP lenses will be higher than otherwise. In addition, as practitioners acquire more experience in fitting GP lenses, they will acquire a greater level of confidence and will be comfortable in presenting this option in a positive but realistic manner.

A second important component to optimizing initial comfort is the use of a topical anesthetic immediately prior to the initial application of a GP lens on a new wearer. This has been considered controversial due to concerns pertaining to its potential for softening the epithelium, resulting in a greater incidence of corneal staining (8,9). In addition, there is always the potential for misleading the patient who will ultimately experience the typical lens awareness with GP lenses. Fortunately, although these are legitimate considerations, they have not been confirmed by clinical research (10,11). In an 80-subject multicenter study, half of the subjects received a placebo at dispensing while the other half received a topical anesthetic immediately prior to application of GP lenses (10). At the completion of 1 month of lens wear, anesthetized subjects perceived their fit experience, long-term wear, adaptation time, and overall satisfaction to be significantly higher than subjects who had a placebo. Seventy of 80 subjects completed the study, and only 2 of the 10 who discontinued the study were in the anesthetic group. In addition, no significant difference in corneal staining between these two groups was found at consecutive visits. For apprehensive patients such as children, patients with keratoconus, and those with soft lens refits, topical anesthetic use is beneficial. However, it is especially beneficial for all first-time GP lens wearers because it allows practitioners the ability to quickly assess the fluorescein pattern, as opposed to waiting until the patient has reduced the awareness symptoms. This allows rapid lens changes, if necessary; therefore, efficiency is increased, which is important when competing with soft lenses.

The most critical factor for GP lens success, however, is the first few minutes of lens wear. If lens wear is not unpleasant during this period, patient satisfaction and the potential for long-term successful wear should be good. It could be theorized that if the patient's first experience with lens wear is also with lenses in his or her correction, the resulting visual benefit would contribute to a positive first impression. It is also important to note, however, that the effect of the topical anesthetic should be allowed to wear off, with the patient gradually experiencing lens awareness during this initial fitting session. Likewise, frequent anesthetic application is unnecessary and could result in the aforementioned side effects. Likewise, providing patients with topical anesthetic—even in a diluted concentration—to take home is contraindicated.

Nonsteroidal anti-inflammatory drugs (NSAIDs) also have been used to reduce awareness during adaptation (12, 13). Because NSAIDs reduce production of prostaglandins, which are mediators of pain, reducing their production reduces pain. The most effective drug within this class at inhibiting prostaglandin synthesis appears to be Voltaren. A recommended NSAID dosage for GP lens adaptation is as follows (13):

- Instill one drop of Voltaren in each eye 30 minutes and then 15 minutes prior to lens insertion.
- Instill a third drop just prior to lens insertion.
- A fourth drop can be instilled 1 hour after insertion.

- This regimen can be maintained for 3 to 5 days or until adaptation is completed.

Although it is apparent that initial presentation, topical anesthetic use, and lens design (to be discussed) are important factors for successful adaptation to GP lenses, there is no substitute for experience in fitting this modality. It is evident that experienced GP lens fitters do not perceive comfort as an important concern with their patients; in fact, they exhibit great pride in fitting this modality to their patients.

LENS DESIGN AND FITTING

Once the appropriate material has been selected, a decision has to be made regarding which method to use for fitting: empirical design or application of diagnostic lenses. Both methods are commonly used, and both have certain advantages. I recommend diagnostic fitting if an inventory is available or for patients benefitting from a special design (i.e., bifocal, keratoconus). However, with the manufacturing methods in use today, empirical fitting can result in a more user-friendly and efficient method that allows patients to experience good vision on the initial application.

Empirical Fitting

Empirical fitting refers specifically to designing lenses empirically or without using diagnostic lenses. Practitioners who use empirical fitting methodologies claim that manufacturers' recommendations (supplying the laboratory with such minimal prefitting information as keratometry values and refraction) and fitting guides provide effective means to obtain maximum lens performance and fit. Empirical fitting also means that a new, unworn, lens will be fitted to one patient only. Finally, empirical fitting has the attraction of eliminating a fitting visit and, consequently, enabling a simplistic fitting approach (14). Whereas it is important for the novice GP lens fitter to gain experience in the diagnostic fitting and evaluation of spherical GP lenses, empirical fitting ultimately allows the fitter to save time and to provide the patient with good vision on the initial application. It could be argued that the initial comfort may be improved in the mind of a patient if he or she experiences good vision. Diagnostic fitting of a −3.00 D lens on a 6 D myope denies the patient the opportunity to initially experience this important benefit of GP lenses. In addition, the combination of a standard lens design (i.e., practitioner specifies diameter, base curve, and power only) using modern lathing methods and an empirical approach allows the practitioner to compete more effectively with soft lenses as they pertains to chair time and simplicity. Most laboratories have such a design; representative examples include Achievement (Art Optical), E-lens (Conforma), and Visions

Ultrathin (X-Cel). This last example is available in a two-pack, which allows the practitioner to send back both the opened pair and the unopened pair for a full exchange and ultimately provides the patient with a spare pair (15). Likewise, the use of corneal topography software programs has allowed the ability to utilize comprehensive corneal topography information in recommending a specific design while also allowing the practitioner to view a simulated lens-to-cornea fitting relationship. Topography-based empirical fits have rivaled diagnostic fitting in their success rates (16–19).

Empirical fitting has a few limitations. One study in which a group of patients fitted empirically (using the manufacturer's fitting guide) was compared with another group of patients who obtained the best diagnostic fit with the same lens material found a higher success rate with the diagnostically fitted patients (84% vs 71%) (20). The results of this study suggested that diagnostic lens fitting results in both fewer lens reorders and greater patient compliance to the visit schedule. In addition, if diagnostic lenses are not used, factors such as lens centration and residual astigmatism cannot be evaluated. In addition, with more challenging cases such as patients exhibiting irregular corneas or presbyopia, diagnostic fitting is important to ensure an optimum fitting relationship.

Diagnostic Fitting

Although diagnostic fitting requires a fitting visit and the use of several diagnostic lenses, practitioners can evaluate the lens-to-cornea fitting relationship to provide the best fit and acceptable vision for the patient. The confidence of both the patient and the practitioner in the eventual success of the lenses is enhanced if a good fit is achieved during the diagnostic fitting process. Fewer reorders will be necessary to improve fit or visual acuity, which minimizes interruptions in the patient's wearing schedule. In addition, many observations beyond lens diameter and base curve radius (BCR)—depending upon the design—often are necessitated. Factors such as pupil size, tear quality, lid tension, movement, lateral decentration, peripheral curve relationship, lens movement, lens position, and wetting characteristics of the lens material need to be evaluated to achieve an optimal fitting relationship (21).

The primary limitation, as noted earlier, pertains to the inability of the patient to experience the benefit of excellent vision upon initial application if the diagnostic lens power differs greatly from the predicted contact lens power. In addition, the process could be more time consuming compared to the current generation of commonly used, empirically based lens designs. For maximum success, it is recommended to diagnostically fit the same GP material and design that eventually will be ordered from the manufacturer to ensure a similar lens-to-cornea fitting relationship.

Diagnostic Fitting Sets

Having several diagnostic fitting sets is strongly recommended. For example, 20-lens diagnostic sets in a –3.00 D power would be beneficial in both low-Dk (<50) and high-Dk (≥50) materials. It is recommended that the low-Dk diagnostic set be in an ultrathin design. An example of such a diagnostic set is given in Table 12.1. In addition, similar diagnostic sets in low plus (e.g., +3.00 D in the same parameters with a minus lenticular edge in a high-Dk material) and high minus (e.g., −8.00 D in the same parameters with a plus lenticular edge in lower-Dk material powers) will be beneficial. Keratoconic, bitoric, aphakic, and bifocal diagnostic sets are recommended and discussed in other chapters of this text. A good average overall diameter is 9.4 mm with a 8.0-mm optical zone diameter in BCRs ranging from 40.75 D (8.28 mm) to 45.50 D (7.42 mm) in steps of 0.25 D. A relatively constant edge lift design also is recommended for the diagnostic lenses. Finally, the appropriate center thickness should be ordered (e.g., a −3.00 D lens in a low-Dk material should have a center thickness of approximately 0.11 mm; a −3.00 D lens in a high-Dk material would be about 0.15 mm). All of the diagnostic lenses of the same power would have equal and appropriate center thickness.

The use of a large (100- to 200-lens) inventory system, which has been popular with hydrogel lenses, is also an option with GP lenses. Due to their custom design, notably in BCR, GP lenses require an inventory of at least 200 lenses if the majority of patients are to be fitted directly without having to order the lenses from a laboratory. A 200-lens inventory is given in Table 12.2.

Because of the labor and expense involved, not all rigid lens manufacturers are willing to supply such large inventories. However, they often are available to practitioners who fit a large number of rigid lenses. As with hydrogel lenses, the initial expense to the practitioner is minimal. The laboratory usually requires the practitioner to meet the following conditions: (i) maintain an inventory of lenses equal to the original consignment; (ii) fit a certain number of lenses within a specified period; and (iii) use the manufacturer's lens design parameters. The advantages of using an inventory are many and include the following: (i) some patients can be fitted out of stock; (ii) replacement lenses can be provided without delay, thereby enhancing patient satisfaction; and (iii) lens parameters can be changed in the office without delay (22).

Storage of Diagnostic Lenses

Although storing diagnostic lenses in the hydrated state provides good initial wettability while maintaining the lenses in a somewhat sterile condition, depending on the frequency with which the solution is changed, there are many advantages to keeping the lenses in the dry state. It is both efficient

TABLE 12.1. RECOMMENDED PARAMETERS FOR A 20-LENS DIAGNOSTIC SET, LOW DK GAS PERMEABLE MATERIAL

Overall diameter:	9.4 mm
Optical zone diameter:	8.0 mm
Center thickness:	0.11 mm
Power:	−3.00 D

	BCR (mm)	SCR/W (mm)	ICR/W (mm)	PCR/W (mm)
1.	7.42	8.00/.2	8.80/.2	10.0/.3
2.	7.46	8.10/.2	8.90/.2	10.1/.3
3.	7.50	8.20/.2	9.00/.2	10.2/.3
4.	7.54	8.20/.2	9.00/.2	10.2/.3
5.	7.58	8.30/.2	9.10/.2	10.3/.3
6.	7.63	8.30/.2	9.20/.2	10.4/.3
7.	7.67	8.40/.2	9.30/.2	10.5/.3
8.	7.71	8.50/.2	9.40/.2	10.6/.3
9.	7.76	8.50/.2	9.50/.2	10.7/.3
10.	7.81	8.60/.2	9.60/.2	10.8/.3
11.	7.85	8.60/.2	9.60/.2	10.9/.3
12.	7.89	8.70/.2	9.70/.2	11.0/.3
13.	7.94	8.70/.2	9.70/.2	11.1/.3
14.	7.99	8.80/.2	9.80/.2	11.2/.3
15.	8.04	8.80/.2	9.90/.2	11.3/.3
16.	8.08	8.90/.2	10.0/.2	11.4/.3
17.	8.13	8.90/.2	10.1/.2	11.5/.3
18.	8.18	9.00/.2	10.2/.2	11.6/.3
19.	8.23	9.10/.2	10.3/.2	11.7/.3
20.	8.28	9.20/.2	10.4/.2	11.8/.3

BCR, base curve radius; ICR/W, intermediate curve radius/width; PCR/W, peripheral curve radius/width; SCR/W, secondary curve radius/width.

TABLE 12.2. GAS PERMEABLE LENS INVENTORY

Power (D)	Base Curve Radius (mm)														
	7.46	7.50	7.54	7.58	7.63	7.67	7.71	7.76	7.80	7.85	7.89	7.94	7.99	8.04	8.08
−1.25								94	110	123	136	149	162	175	188
−1.50							79	95	111	124	137	150	163	176	189
−1.75							80	96	112	125	138	151	164	177	190
−2.00	1	14	27	40	53	66	81	97	113	126	139	152	165	178	191
−2.25	2	15	28	41	54	67	82	98	114	127	140	153	166	179	192
−2.50	3	16	29	42	55	68	83	99	115	128	141	154	167	180	193
−2.75	4	17	30	43	56	69	84	100	116	129	142	155	168	181	194
−3.00	5	18	31	44	57	70	85	101	117	130	143	156	169	182	195
−3.25	6	19	32	45	58	71	86	102	118	131	144	157	170	183	196
−3.50	7	20	33	46	59	72	87	103	119	132	145	158	171	184	197
−3.75	8	21	34	47	60	73	88	104	120	133	146	159	172	185	198
−4.00	9	22	35	48	61	74	89	105	121	134	147	160	173	186	199
−4.25	10	23	36	49	62	75	90	106	122	135	148	161	174	187	200
−4.50	11	24	37	50	63	76	91	107							
−4.75	12	25	38	51	64	77	92	108							
−5.00	13	26	39	52	65	78	93	109							

Other parameters: Low Dk fluoro-silicone/acrylate (F-S/A) lens material
9.4-mm overall diameter/ 8.0-mm optical zone diameter
Secondary curve radius (SCR) = Base curve radius + 1 mm
Peripheral curve radius (PCR) = Secondary curve radius + 2 mm
Secondary curve width = 0.3 mm; Peripheral curve width = 0.4 mm.

and convenient to store the lenses dry because they can be kept in flat-pack cases and occupy very little space in the office. If lenses are stored in the hydrated state, the solution can either dry up in the case or leak out; both possibilities result in a lens that may adhere to the case or even change in BCR because of variation between the hydrated and the dry state. The dried solution also may be difficult to remove from the lens surface. Whenever a diagnostic lens has been applied, however, it should be carefully cleaned and blotted dry with a soft tissue prior to disinfection and placement into the appropriate diagnostic lens set. The Centers for Disease Control and Prevention (CDC) recommends ophthalmic-grade hydrogen peroxide for GP lenses; therefore, AOSept Clear Care (Ciba Vision) for a 5- to 10-minute soak has been recommended (23). GP lenses that are going to be dispensed to a patient should be hydrated for a minimum of 24 hours prior to application to enhance surface wettability and maintain the BCR in the hydrated state (i.e., similar to the "on-eye" condition).

FLUORESCEIN APPLICATION

Sodium fluorescein is an organic compound that is inert and harmless to tissue (24). Its initial application in 1938 to rigid lens fitting has been credited to Obrig (25). When applied to the upper bulbar conjunctiva, fluorescein causes the tears to fluoresce a yellow-green color when viewed with a cobalt blue light source. This enables the practitioner to evaluate the lens-to-cornea fitting relationship. Fluorescein is invaluable, if not essential, in the assessment of GP lens fit. The application of fluorescein to the tear film is essential for proper evaluation of the lens-to-cornea fitting relationship. However, its omission represents a common shortcut taken by practitioners in an effort to increase efficiency. This error of omission could result in practitioner failure to observe (i) peripheral sealoff and the resulting absence of tear exchange, thereby eliminating debris removal and additional oxygen supply; (ii) areas of bearing or contact of lens against cornea, which could result in corneal distortion with time; (iii) regions of excessive edge clearance, which could result in greater lid awareness, corneal dryness or desiccation, and lens decentration; and (iv) areas of coalesced corneal staining (26).

The technique of fluorescein application is as follows. The fluorescein strip is wetted with an ophthalmic irrigating solution—exhibiting care to avoid contact between the tip of the solution bottle and the fluorescein strip—and is gently applied against the superior bulbar conjunctiva, with the patient viewing inferiorly. It is important to reassure the patient that this procedure is painless. The thumb should carefully pin back the upper lid to prevent the lid from pushing the strip into contact with the superior cornea, causing both discomfort and corneal staining.

Use of an ophthalmic irrigating solution is advantageous because it is sterile and its slightly alkaline pH enhances fluorescein (24). It has been shown that a solution having a pH less than 6.0 will fluoresce at less than half of the intensity of a solution with a pH of 7.0 (27). Thus, if an unbuffered (acidic) saline is used to wet the strip, the fluorescein pattern is not as easy to evaluate as when buffered saline is used (28). A buffered saline also reduces the chances of burning or stinging upon application of the strip. A rigid lens wetting solution is not as advantageous to use as an irrigating solution because it is more viscous and results in an abnormally thick tear layer.

Methods of Observation

Burton Lamp

The traditional method of evaluating the fluorescein pattern is by use of an ultraviolet fluorescent lamp that utilizes a +5.00 D magnification lens to assist in viewing (Fig. 12.1). This method has the advantages of being inexpensive and simple, and it allows a good overall view of the fluorescein pattern. In fact, it allows the practitioner to easily view and compare the patterns between the two eyes. However, the Burton lamp is limited in its abilities. It does not allow for variable magnification or illumination, and it is an ineffective method of observing the fluorescein pattern of GP materials with ultraviolet-absorbing properties. This is a result of the decreased fluorescence that occurs when short-wavelength blue light is attenuated by the lens material, because the Burton lamp has its highest emission in the 300- to 400-nm range. Thus, it is not appropriate to use this as the only method of evaluating a fluorescein pattern. However, it is a useful adjunct to the biomicroscope because of the overall field of view and is especially beneficial in observing

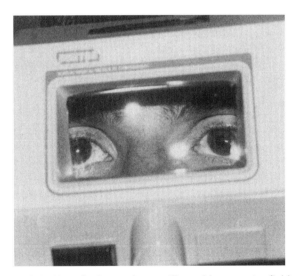

FIG. 12.1. Use of a Burton lamp will provide a greater field of view and allow simultaneous bilateral observation of the fluorescein pattern.

some of the more distinctive patterns, such as those pertaining to high corneal toricity and keratoconus.

Biomicroscope

The most popular and effective method of evaluating the fluorescein pattern of a GP lens is with the biomicroscope. The primary advantage of this over other observation methods is flexibility. It allows the practitioner to vary the magnification, illumination, and slit-beam width while observing the fluorescein pattern. Proper use of a biomicroscope is essential for successful GP lens fitting and evaluation.

Biomicroscopes vary considerably among manufacturers: a good illumination source and variable magnification must be present to evaluate the fluorescein pattern effectively. Variable magnification is important because the field of view decreases rapidly as the magnification is increased (24). It has been determined that with many biomicroscopes it is not possible to use greater than 10× magnification and still retain an adequate field of view (29).

The fluorescein pattern is viewed with the assistance of a cobalt blue filter placed over the illumination system, which transmits blue light, activating the fluorescein dye. It also has become standard practice to use a yellow barrier filter (i.e., Wratten no. 12 or equivalent) over the observation system. Application of this filter will enhance the fluorescence of the pattern evaluation (Color Plate 2, Color Fig. 23.1A and B), especially with GP materials that have ultraviolet-blocking agents (26). This filter is available from many ,sources including many contact lens companies, notably Polymer Technology Corporation (Rochester, New York) and photographic supply companies. In addition, biomicroscope manufacturers are currently incorporating this type of yellow filter into their instruments.

Pattern Evaluation

Once fluorescein has been properly instilled, the patient should be instructed to blink several times to distribute the fluorescein adequately on the eye. The fluorescein pattern should be observed initially using low magnification, a wide (diffuse) slit beam, and high-intensity illumination. The central and peripheral fluorescein pattern should be relatively easy to determine after several blinks. This pattern assumes a variety of forms. Areas of fluorescein pooling appear green, whereas areas in which fluorescein is absent or where the tear layer is too thin to detect appear dark or black. Between these extremes, the varying thicknesses of the tear layer are observed as varying shades of green. An optic section, with the angle of illumination 45 to 60 degrees, also can be used to observe the pooling of tears in relation to the contact lens. It will appear as a green layer representing the outer layer of tears on the lens, then a wider dark layer that is the contact lens, next another green layer representing tears between the lens and cornea, and finally

a bright grayish layer, the cornea (24). The lens-to-cornea fitting relationship can be evaluated by viewing the thickness of the tear layer along the optic section.

An *alignment* fit is observed when the lens evenly contours the cornea with a light, even tear pooling (Color Plate 2, Fig. 23.1B). *Apical clearance* exists when a steep central fit with excessive fluorescence or central tear pooling is present (Color Plate 2, Color Fig. 23.1.C). This can result in midperipheral bearing and sealoff, with a reduced ability to remove cellular debris and mucus, which may be an important precursor to rigid lens adherence to the cornea. *Apical bearing* exists when the lens is in direct contact with the central cornea or the tear pool is too shallow to detect with fluorescein (Color Plate 2, Color Fig. 23.1D). Excessive apical bearing can result in corneal molding with distortion or warpage. It also may lead to gradual formation of a central corneal abrasion. A description of the various fluorescein patterns behind different regions of the lens is given in Table 12.3.(30)

With corneal astigmatism greater than 1 D, a dumbbell-shaped fluorescein pattern is observed (Color Pate 2, Color Fig. 23.1E). Typically, along the steeper meridian of the cornea, the tear layer thickness gradually increases toward the edge and the lens does not touch the cornea. Along the flatter meridian, however, the tear layer thickness decreases toward the periphery, and the lens comes in contact with the cornea at the edge of the optical zone. As corneal astigmatism increases, the difference in tear layer thickness between the two major meridians becomes greater, the area of alignment becomes smaller, and the astigmatic or dumbbell-shaped fluorescein pattern becomes exaggerated (28). If the cornea exhibits with-the-rule corneal astigmatism, the pooling is in the vertical meridian, with alignment or bearing in the horizontal meridian. If the cornea exhibits against-the-rule astigmatism, the opposite is true: the pooling is in the horizontal meridian, with alignment or bearing in the vertical meridian. In high corneal astigmatism (typically > 2 D), use of a high-Dk material with a steeper-than-K BCR will result in excessive flexure and reduced visual acuity. The "rocking" of the lens during the blink process may result in discomfort, mechanical corneal staining, and possibly lens adherence. A material with lower oxygen permeability and perhaps a flatter BCR should be selected. Another option would be a bitoric design, especially if the high amount of corneal toricity results in inferior decentration of the lens.

It is important to evaluate the fluorescein pattern after the blink because the amount of pooling and bearing will vary during the blinking process. If the lens is decentered, the position of the lens relative to the cornea must be considered before the fluorescein pattern is evaluated. For example, an inferior decentering lens typically will exhibit excessive superior pooling because the flatter peripheral bevel is adjacent to the steeper central cornea.

Evaluation of the fluorescein pattern at the lens periphery

TABLE 12.3. HOW TO INTERPRET FLUORESCEIN PATTERNS

Parameter	Appearance	Management
Base curve radius	Too flat: black appearance centrally	Steepen base curve
	Too steep: green appearance centrally	Flatten base curve
Optical zone	Too small: black appearance centrally	Increase optical zone/Steepen base curve
	Too large: green appearance centrally	Reduce optical zone/flatten base curve
Intermediate	Too flat/wide: green appearance in mid-periphery	Steepen/narrow curves
	Too steep/narrow: black appearance signifies insufficient edge clearance	Flatten/widen curves
Peripheral curves	Too flat/wide: green appearance in periphery	Steepen/narrow curves
	Too steep/narrow: black appearance signifies insufficient edge clearance	Flatten/widen curves

Modified from Bennett (2a).

is beneficial. There should be enough peripheral clearance (typically it should be greater than apical clearance) to allow sufficient tear exchange and debris removal while avoiding mechanical irritation from the lens movement on the cornea. If fluorescein pooling is minimal or absent peripherally and sealoff exists, the peripheral curve(s) should be flattened.

Fluorescein pattern evaluation of the GP lens-to-cornea fitting relationship should be performed at the fitting visit and on all follow-up visits. A practitioner's ability to assess fluorescein patterns develops with experience and frequent evaluation. The lens material is only as good as the practitioner's ability to evaluate it, and a poor lens-to-cornea fitting relationship can result in numerous problems, including corneal desiccation, adherence, and abrasion. In particular, the fluorescein pattern evaluation is invaluable in the more challenging cases, such as high corneal toricity and irregular or distorted corneas, including keratoconus, corneal trauma, and postsurgical. Another important reason to assess fluorescein patterns pertains to the fact that GP lens laboratories tend to vary considerably in the design parameters that that they recommend (31). These factors, in combination with individual corneal topographic differences, make evaluating the fitting relationship of a GP lens to the cornea with fluorescein critical to long-term patient success with these lenses. An extremely beneficial teaching aid is the videotape "GP Fitting and Evaluation," available from the Contact Lens Manufacturers Association (1-800-346–5367) and its member laboratories. This and related instructional resources are given in Table 12.4.

False Fluorescein Patterns

On many occasions, unexpected fluorescein patterns are observed. This phenomenon can have a variety of causes, including the following. (i) Unusual corneal topography. The corneal "cap," defined as the area within 0.50 D of the steep apex, varies considerably between individuals (32,33). For example, a patient with a small corneal cap will exhibit a somewhat steeper fluorescein pattern than a patient with

a larger-than-average cap, all other factors being equal. (ii) The selection of a steep BCR may result in poor tear exchange and a misleadingly small amount of fluorescein pooling behind the center of the lens, especially if lens adherence is present. (iii) If the peripheral curve is too steep, peripheral sealoff can occur, and the fluorescein pattern will exhibit apical clearance regardless of the BCR. (iv) In certain individuals, the fluorescein will dissipate quickly and may mislead the practitioner into the belief that excessive apical bearing is present. In such cases, care must be taken to ensure that sufficient fluorescein has been applied and that the pattern is evaluated soon after application. (v) The existence of a "pseudo-steep" fluorescein pattern has been reported in high-minus lenses made from a fluoro-silicone/acrylate lens material (34,35). It is theorized that the thickness of the edge blocks the fluorescence of the tears, giving the appearance of central pooling from the more brilliant fluorescent appearance in the center (Color Plate 2, Color Fig. 23.1F). One would expect that a high-plus lens may demonstrate a flatter-than-actual base curve fitting relationship because the thick center would attenuate the light more.

AUTHOR'S FITTING PHILOSOPHY

Several methods for determining the GP lens design parameters in diagnostic fitting are available. In this section, my own philosophy is presented; several other philosophies are discussed later in this chapter.

Overall Diameter and Optical Zone Diameter

The overall diameter (OAD) of a GP lens should be large enough to allow for a sufficient optical zone while providing good lag with the blink. The optical zone diameter (OZD) typically encompasses anywhere from 65% to 80% of the lens diameter.

The size of both the OAD and OZD depends on several factors, including the following.

TABLE 12.4. GAS PERMEABLE LENS EDUCATIONAL RESOURCES

Resource	Source	Contact No./Web Site
GP Fitting and Evaluation	RGP Lens Institute	800–344–9060; *rgpli.org*
GP Lens Management Guide	RGP Lens Institute	800–344–9060; *rgpli.org*
GP Fitting	Polymer Technology	800–847–0127; *polymer.com*
Fit Today's RGP (modules 1–5)	Paragon Vision Sciences	800–340–5129; *paragonvision.com*
Fluorescein Pattern Identification/Benefits and Applications	RGP Lens Institute Laminated Card	800–344–9060; *rgpli.org*
Contact Lens Fitting	International Association of Contact Lens Educators	*iacle.org*

Palpebral Aperture Size and Lid Position

The palpebral aperture size refers to the vertical separation of the lids in the normal state. An average amount of separation is 9.0 to 10.5 mm. More important, however, is the position of the lids, which varies between patients. A fitting relationship in which the upper edge of the lens rides underneath the upper lid on straight-ahead gaze has been found to be more comfortable than an interpalpebral fitting relationship (36,37). However, if the upper lid is positioned at or above the superior limbus, this position is not easily obtainable. It may be preferable to select a smaller-diameter lens (i.e., =9.0 mm), fit steeper than K, and obtain a well-centered lens that positions at least 1 mm below the upper lid (i.e., "interpalpebral").

Pupil Size

The diameter of the pupil should be measured in high and low illumination. These findings will be important in determining the OZD of the lens. Assuming a good lens-to-cornea fitting relationship, the OZD should be greater than the pupil size in dim illumination to minimize the risk of flare symptoms at night.

Refractive Power

Often it is necessary to select a larger OAD/OZD with hyperopic lens powers to provide adequate pupil coverage with a thicker, higher-mass lens.

Corneal Curvature

To maintain optimal centering, a larger-than-average OAD should be used with flat corneal curvatures (e.g., flatter than 41.00 D), and a smaller-than-average OAD should be used with steep curvatures (e.g., steeper than 45.00 D).

Lid Tension

The lens diameter to be used varies with the amount of lid tension, which can be determined by everting the lid. Because this should be performed at the prefitting evaluation

and at all subsequent follow-up visits, one can determine which patients have loose lids (i.e., upper lid everts very easily) or tight lids (i.e., upper lid everts with much effort, if at all). Because a loose upper lid will provide little assistance in raising a lens during the blink process, a larger than average OAD/OZD is recommended in this case.

What are good average OAD/OZD values? Average values are typically in the range from 9.2 to 9.6 mm for OAD and from 7.6 to 8.2 mm for OZD. I use a 9.4/8.0-mm design in approximately 65% to 70% of my custom-designed lenses. When a larger OAD/OZD is indicated, a 9.8/8.4-mm design is recommended; when a smaller OAD/OZD is indicated, a 9.0/7.6-mm design is recommended. When changing a lens design parameter such as diameter, one rule of thumb prevails: *Make the design change a significant one.* Merely increasing the OAD/OZD by 0.1 to 0.2 mm usually has no effect on lens performance.

The current trend with new GP materials is for manufacturers to recommend larger OADs (i.e., >10 mm) to increase initial comfort. These have included the ComfortFlow (Aculens), Macrolens (C & H), and Epicon (Specialty Ultravision) (38–40). It would not be surprising to see the introduction of such "comfort" designs increase in the near future. However, the fitting relationship becomes more critical with these designs. A larger lens tends to exert more of an effect on the cornea, possibly resulting in molding and distortion. In addition, highly flexible materials have the potential to cause limited lens lag and adherence. A large OZD may result in limited lens movement laterally with the blink and may encourage corneal desiccation because the lens does not move over the peripheral cornea (37). Some practitioners prefer to use a large OAD (e.g., 9.8 mm) with a small OZD (e.g., 7.4 mm) to create good midperipheral and peripheral alignment. This design is acceptable if there is both sufficient lens lag and sufficient pupil coverage. OAD/OZD of 9.4/8.0 mm should be successful in most cases, particularly when a lid-attachment fitting relationship is desired. A smaller-than-average OAD/OZD of 9.0/7.6 mm is recommended in cases where an interpalpebral fitting relationship is desired, as well as steeper-than-average corneal curvatures. A larger-than-average OAD/OZD is indicated for patients exhibiting a larger-than-average pupil size, as well as athletes.

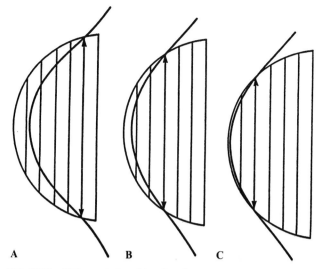

FIG. 12.2. Fitting relationship of various optical zone diameters. If optical zone diameter "a" or "b" is chosen, an apical clearance fitting relationship will result. The smaller optical zone "c" will provide an alignment fitting relationship. (From Caroline PJ, Norman CW. A blueprint for rigid lens design: part I. *Contact Lens Spectrum* 1988;3:39, with permission.)

Base Curve Radius

The primary function of the BCR is to optimize the fitting relationship of the lens to the central and midperipheral cornea. Selection of the BCR depends on several factors, including corneal curvatures, the observed fluorescein pattern, and the desired lens-to-cornea fitting relationship. It can be specified in diopters or millimeters (see Appendix 1).

The selection of a given BCR (e.g., "on K") in several patients will result in differences in the observed fluorescein patterns due to differences in corneal topography (apical area, rate of flattening) and lens design. A lens fitted "on K" often will provide an apical clearance fitting relationship because the optical zone typically is much larger than the corneal cap or apex (41). This steep pattern will be even more apparent as the optical zone increases (Fig. 12.2). (42) To maintain an alignment fitting relationship it is necessary, in most cases, to select a BCR flatter than K. A flatter BCR

will minimize lens-induced flexure and potential for sealoff of tear exchange that can occur with an "on K" fit on a spherical cornea (43). My criteria for BCR selection are given in Table 12.5.

It is important to note that if the OZD is smaller than normal, a slightly steeper BCR is necessary. For example, with corneal curvatures of more than 45 D, a smaller OZD is necessary to maintain alignment. Conversely, if the OZD is larger than normal, a slightly flatter BCR than recommended in Table 12.3 may be indicated. For example, with corneal curvatures flatter than 41 D, a larger OZD is necessary to maintain alignment. In addition, patients with large pupil diameters will need a larger OZD to minimize flare. A simple rule is to flatten the BCR by 0.25 D for each increase in OZD of 0.5 mm and steepen it by 0.25 D for every decrease in OZD of 0.5 mm (42). The specific BCR to be selected will depend primarily upon the fluorescein pattern, especially if an instrument to measure the eccentricity or shape factor of the cornea (i.e., from central to, at minimum, midperipheral cornea) is not available.

High astigmatic patients may require a steeper BCR than lower astigmatic patients for several reasons, the most important of which is to increase the probability of obtaining a good lens-to-cornea fit. With high astigmatic patients (i.e., corneal astigmatism >2 D), the BCR has to be steepened or a bitoric design must be used to determine the best distribution of lens alignment over the largest area (24). An "on K" BCR on high corneal astigmatism will not only provide very little corneal alignment and subsequent decentration, but the resulting areas of bearing and excessive clearance may cause lens "rocking" on the cornea with the blink, discomfort due to an increase in edge contact with the upper lid, and corneal desiccation.

A steeper-than-K BCR is also often necessary with hyperopic patients. In such patients the center thickness is greater and the center of gravity is located more anteriorly; therefore, the lens has a greater tendency to drop inferiorly after the blink (Fig. 12.3). A steeper-than-K BCR is more likely to provide well-centered lens positioning.

The geometric center of the lens should coincide with

TABLE 12.5. GAS PERMEABLE LENS DIAMETER AND BASE CURVE SELECTION[a]

Corneal Cylinder (D)	OAD/OZD		
	9.0/7.6 mm (Interpalpebral and Steep Corneas)	9.4/8.0 mm (Lid Attachment)	9.8/8.4 mm (Large Pupils and Athletes)
0–0.75	0.25D flatter than K	0.50D flatter than K	0.75D flatter than K
1.00–1.25	"On K"	0.25D flatter than K	0.50D flatter than K
1.50–1.75	0.25D steeper than K	"On K"	0.25D flatter than K
2.00–2.25	0.50D steeper than K	0.25D steeper than K	"On K"
≥2.50	Bitoric lens design is recommended		

[a] For minus lenses only; for plus lenses select base curve radius 0.50 D steeper than this philosophy.
OAD, overall diameter; OZD, optical zone diameter.

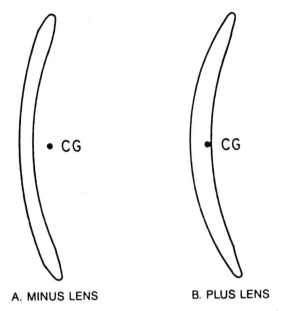

A. MINUS LENS   **B. PLUS LENS**

FIG. 12.3. Center of gravity for plus versus minus power lens designs.

or be positioned slightly above the patient's line of sight. A slightly superior lens-to-cornea fitting relationship in which the lens is "tucked underneath the lid" or "lid attachment" should maximize patient comfort by minimizing the interaction of the lens edge with the upper lid. This fitting relationship also has been found to result in less corneal desiccation than interpalpebral and inferior positioning lenses (44). The amount of lens lag or downward movement after the blink should be at least 1 mm and at most 3 mm. A larger lens may cause fluctuations in vision due to flare and awareness of the lens, whereas a smaller lag could cause adherence with resultant trapped debris and edema. The OZD should provide good papillary coverage throughout the blink process. Once again, no single selection philosophy for BCR can accurately predict lens positioning on a given patient; therefore, trial and error supplemented by fluorescein pattern evaluation is important in determining the appropriate BCR.

Peripheral Curve Radii and Width

Surrounding the OZD of the lens are the peripheral curve radii, which typically encompass the outer 20% to 35% of the lens. Designs in common use have either one (bicurve), two (tricurve with a secondary curve radius [SCR] and a peripheral curve radius [PCR]), or three (tetracurve with an SCR, intermediate curve radius [ICR], and PCR) peripheral curves. Some lens designs use an aspheric periphery with a continuous flattening of the peripheral region of the lens. Each curve must be progressively flatter than the adjacent, more centrally positioned curve to provide proper lens clearance from the cornea. The peripheral curve, in particular, serves the following three functions (45):

1. It prevents the edge of the lens from digging into the corneal surface during lens movement.

2. It permits proper circulation of the tears beneath the lens in order to maintain the metabolism of the cornea.

3. It supports a meniscus at the edge of the lens to provide forces that cause the lens to center.

The peripheral curves serve no optical purpose. If the contact lens is decentered such that the peripheral curves are directly in front of the visual axis, flare will result (46).

The distance from the lens edge perpendicular to the peripheral cornea is termed *edge clearance*. Closely related to *edge clearance* and more easily quantifiable is *edge lift*, a geometric term that pertains to the distance between the lens edge and an extension of the BCR of the lens. *Radial edge lift* is defined as the extension of the lens edge perpendicular to the extension of the BCR. *Axial edge lift*, which is more commonly used, refers to the vertical distance from the lens edge to an extension of the BCR of the lens (Fig. 12.4) (47,48). If the PCR is flattened or the peripheral curve width (PCW) is increased, edge clearance will increase, all other lens parameters held constant.

To provide good tear circulation and debris removal, a flat, wide peripheral curve customarily has been used in traditional polymethyl methacrylate (PMMA) lens designs. Such a design enhances oxygen flow to the cornea. These philosophies used a bicurve or tricurve design with an SCR approximately 1.0 to 1.5 mm flatter than the BCR and a PCR of 12.00 to 12.25 mm. For example, a lens design of BCR 7.8 mm, SCR/SCW (secondary curve width) 9.2/0.3 mm, and PCR/PCW 12.25/0.4 mm was not uncommon. However, excessive edge clearance may result in lens decentration, lens awareness, and corneal desiccation. (41, 48–50) The desiccation may result from a combination of a receding tear meniscus as it is pulled underneath the lens edge from the adjacent peripheral cornea and a possible alteration in the blink pattern due to the upper lid's contacting the anteriorly positioned edge (45,47,51). In addition, inferior decentration may result when a flat base curve–anterior apex lens design is used in an effort to achieve lid attachment due to the resulting increase in edge clearance (52).

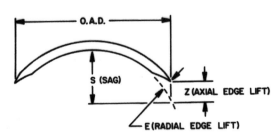

FIG. 12.4. Axial versus sagittal edge lift. (From Bennett ES. Silicone/acrylate lens design. *Int Contact Lens Clin* 1985;12:45, with permission.)

GP lenses, however, are not as dependent on the tear pump as PMMA lenses, and because many of these materials are silicone based, presenting the possibility of a short over-the-lens tear breakup time (53) and evaporation of the peripheral tear pool (47), a design incorporating lower edge clearance should be advantageous. The peripheral curve system I prefer is the following tetracurve design (Table 12.6):

SCR/W = BCR + 0.8/0.2 mm
ICR/W = SCR + 1.0/0.2 mm
PCR/W = ICR + 1.4/0.3 mm

where ICR is intermediate curve width.

For example, if the BCR = 7.8 mm:

SCR/W = 7.8 + 0.8 = 8.6/0.2 mm
ICR/W = 8.6 + 1.0 = 9.6/0.2 mm
PCR/W = 9/6 + 1.4 = 11.0/0.3 mm

To maintain a constant edge lift, the peripheral curve system must be flattened at a greater rate with flat BCRs and at a lesser rate for steep BCRs. Therefore, the aforementioned peripheral curve design philosophy can be used for average BCRs (i.e., 7.5–8.2 mm), but slightly flatter values should be used with flatter BCRs and slightly steeper values with steeper BCRs.

Lenses with edge lift values less than 0.08 mm may be more difficult to remove, and they may trap debris (54). In addition, increased lens adherence (55,56) and vascularized limbal keratitis (57) have been associated with the use of low edge lift designs. Therefore, it is always important to assess the peripheral lens-to-cornea fitting relationship with fluorescein to determine if design changes are necessary to result in the preferable slightly increased clearance (relative to center) relationship (Fig. 12.5).

Many aspheric lens designs are able to provide a uniform edge clearance resulting in the potential for better initial

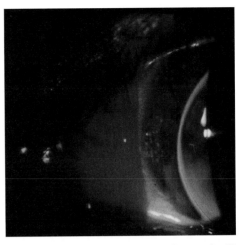

FIG. 12.5. Low edge clearance design that has resulted in sealoff and corneal desiccation.

comfort. These designs are the result of improved manufacturing technology resulting in a well-polished posterior surface with a standard rate of flattening (58,59). This is complemented by the introduction of many standard lens design with aspheric or pseudo-aspheric peripheries that have used advanced corneal topography software.

The application of peripheral curves during the manufacturing process creates a sharp ridge between peripheral curves. This ridge can prevent adequate circulation of tears to the central cornea and can impair the removal of metabolic debris from under the lens (Fig. 12.6). Therefore, the application of a blend will result in more even tear flow.

The blend, which is performed with a radius tool midway between the PCR values, can be light, medium, or heavy. At minimum, a medium blend should be performed to enhance debris removal. Blending the PCR junctions also may increase lens lag by creating a smoother posterior surface. It has been theorized that a blended lens is more comfortable initially to a new GP wearer than an unblended lens; however, confirmation of this concept is still needed.

Center Thickness

Many lens parameters affect center thickness, but the primary factors are lens power and OAD. The center thickness is greater and the center of gravity more anterior for plus

TABLE 12.6. AUTHOR'S RECOMMENDED PERIPHERAL CURVE PHILOSOPHY

> 9.0 mm OAD: tetracurve design

Secondary curve radius (SCR)/width = BCR + 0.8 mm/0.2 mm
Intermediate curve radius (ICR)/width = SCR + 1.0 mm/0.2 mm
Peripheral curve radius (PCR)/width = ICR + 1.4 mm/0.3 mm
  Example: BCR = 7.80 mm OAD/OZD = 9.4/8.0 mm
SCR/W = 7.80 + 0.8 = 8.60 mm/0.2 mm
ICR/W = 8.60 + 1.0 = 9.60 mm/0.2 mm
PCR/W = 9.60 + 1.4 = 11.00 mm/0.3 mm

≤9.0 mm OAD: tricurve design

Secondary curve radius (SCR)/width = BCR + 1.0 mm/0.3 mm
Peripheral curve radius (PCR)/width = SCR + 2.0 mm/0.4 mm
  Example: BCR = 7.80 mm OAD/OZD = 8.8/7.4 mm
SCR/W = 7.80 + 1.0 = 8.80 mm/0.3 mm
PCR/W = 8.80 + 2.0 = 10.80 mm/0.4 mm

OAD, overall diameter; OZD, optical zone diameter.

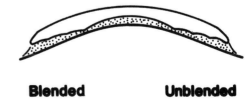

FIG. 12.6. Blended versus unblended peripheral curve junctions.

lenses, whereas the edge thickness is greater and the center of gravity more posterior for minus lenses.

In lens design there is a fine line between too thin and too thick. A lens that is too thin will likely be unstable, flex significantly on the eye, and be prone to warpage. A lens that is too thick may position inferiorly and cause fluctuating vision. Two rules of thumb are important:

1. Increase center thickness by 0.02 mm for lens materials with Dk values greater than 50.

2. Increase center thickness an additional 0.02 mm for each diopter of corneal astigmatism.

The recommended center thickness values vary among materials and manufacturers.

It is extremely important to verify center thickness because an inaccurate value may affect lens performance. A decision on center thickness should not be made on the basis of oxygen permeability but on factors such as vision, lens stability, and positioning. For example, increasing center thickness by 0.04 mm will increase mass by 24% but only decrease equivalent oxygen percentage by less than 1% (60). One of the many benefits of more advanced manufacturing processes has been the introduction of numerous ultrathin lens designs. Essentially, every laboratory has one or more such designs that can produce lenses as thin as 50% less than standard (61–63). For example, a 0.10- to 0.11-mm center thickness is possible for a −3.00 D power as compared to 0.14 to 0.15 mm. Therefore, the likelihood of inferior decentration should be reduced and initial comfort optimized. In fact, an ultrathin design should be the lens of choice whenever possible. A notable exception would be moderate-to-high corneal astigmatic patients (i.e., >1.50 D) in whom a steeper-than-K BCR often is selected, optimizing induced residual astigmatism via flexure (64,65).

Edge Thickness and Design

Edge design is an extremely important and often underestimated parameter that can be the primary variable affecting comfort and lens positioning (66). A thin, tapered, rolled-edge design simulating the gap between the bulbar and palpebral conjunctiva is desirable. The edge can be divided into three zones (67). The anterior zone interacts with the upper lid during blinking. The posterior zone is often a narrow reverse curve that is placed onto the posterior lens surface to flare the edge away from the cornea. This assists in lens removal but primarily has the role of permitting free movement of the lens across the cornea during the blink. The junction between the anterior and posterior zones is the lens apex, which must be well rounded to minimize lens awareness during the blink (Fig. 12.7). Korb and Korb (36) recommend an edge design that has its apex located anteriorly to assist the upper lid in lifting and attaching to the upper edge of the lens. Lenses with well-rounded anterior edge profiles have been found to be significantly more com-

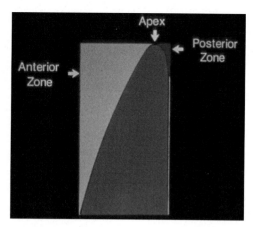

FIG. 12.7. Optimum edge design. (Courtesy of Craig Norman.)

fortable than lenses with square anterior edges; however, there was no significant difference between rounded and square posterior edge profiles (68). Thus, it was concluded that interaction of the edge with the eyelid is more important in determining comfort than edge effects on the cornea.

Several studies have found inconsistency of edge design with GP materials (68–70). Using four different materials, one study found that not only was there much inconsistency between materials, but there were large differences within lenses of the same material from the same manufacturer with identical parameters (70). Although edge quality has improved due to increasing use of sophisticated automated lathes, verification with a comparator or similar method still is important, both in the frontal position and in profile. However, a survey of contact lens practitioners found that approximately half do not verify the edge, in part a result of few sources of edge verification equipment (71). As a material increases in Dk value, it also increases in softness and potential for chipping and breakage. If an unverified lens is defective because an edge is too sharp, too blunt, or chipped but nevertheless is dispensed to the patient, the result may be a dissatisfied patient who may never again desire to wear GP lenses.

Both center thickness and edge thickness change with changes in OAD and with different lens powers. Edge thickness increases with increasing minus power while the center thickness decreases. If the center thickness is greater than average, as with low-minus and plus-power lenses, the edge thickness will be minimal as with spectacles. The edge and center thicknesses are equal, not at plano but at approximately −2.00 D power (41,72).

As a result of the variance in edge thickness with lens power and OAD, use of a lenticular design sometimes is indicated. In a lenticulated lens, the front surface consists of a central optical portion surrounded by a peripheral carrier portion that is thinner and flatter (73). The thickness of the lens at the junction of the optic cap and carrier portion should be 0.12 to 0.14 mm (74,75). If it is thicker, lens

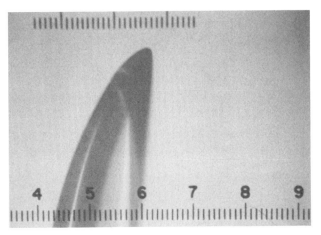

FIG. 12.8. High-minus-power gas permeable lens with an anterior tapered edge design via a CN bevel.

mass is unnecessarily added to the lens; if thinner, the lens can break at this junction.

Either an anterior (CN) bevel (Fig. 12.8) or plus lenticular design (Fig. 12.9) can be used to reduce edge thickness in high-minus-power lens designs; the latter option is used most often. Plus lenticular designs often are used because they minimize problems associated with thick edges, such as lens awareness, inferior positioning due to lid–lens interaction, and corneal desiccation resulting from compromise in the normal blinking process. Plus lenticular designs also reduce center thickness and overall lens mass. Typically, lens powers of −5.00 D and greater are lenticulated, because the edge thickness is 0.20 mm or greater without this modification (41).

A minus lenticular design to increase edge thickness is very important to enhance lid interaction with the edge and

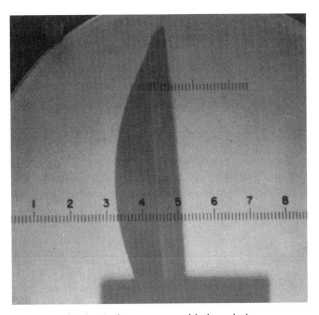

FIG. 12.9. Plus lenticular gas permeable lens design.

TABLE 12.7. CLINICALLY SIGNIFICANT PARAMETER CHANGES (53)

Parameter	Change for Clinical Significance
Base curve radius	0.50 D ($\sim$ 0.1 mm)
Overall diameter/optical zone	0.4 mm/0.3 mm
Peripheral curve radius	0.5 mm
Center thickness (for high DK gas permeable lenses)	0.02 mm

to minimize inferior decentration. A minus lenticular design is recommended with minus powers of −1.50 D or less and with all plus power lenses.

When making a change in any of the aforementioned parameters (BCR, diameter, PCR/PCW, center thickness), it is important to make a significant change when an improvement in the lens-to-cornea fitting relationship is desired. The magnitude of such design parameter changes are given in Table 12.7 (76).

POWER DETERMINATION AND LENS ORDER

Once the proper design and an optimum lens-to-cornea relationship has been achieved, the final lens power can be determined. This is obtained via a comprehensive overrefraction and an understanding of tear layer optics and vertex distance.

TEAR LAYER POWER

Tear layer effects are important when a rigid contact lens is fitted flatter or steeper than K. If a rigid lens is fitted flatter than K, a minus tear lens power is created; therefore, a corresponding plus power is necessary. If the lens if fitted steeper than K, a plus tear lens power is created; therefore, a corresponding minus power correction is indicated. For example, if a lens is fitted 0.75 D flat on a cornea with a flatter keratometry reading of 42.75 D and a spherical refractive value of −3.00 D, the tear layer power is equal to −0.75 D; therefore, +0.75 D is necessary to correct for the tear layer. The final predicted lens power is −2.25 D (Fig. 12.10). If a lens is fitted 0.50 D steeper than the flatter keratometry reading on this patient, a +0.50 D tear layer power is created; therefore, −0.50 D is necessary and the final predicted lens power is −3.50 D (Fig. 12.10). If a rigid lens is fitted "on K," or equal to the keratometry reading, the predicted lens power is equal to the spherical refractive value if the latter is less than 4 D. It is incorrect to assume that the final predicted lens power will be equal to the spherical equivalent (as is often true with hydrogel

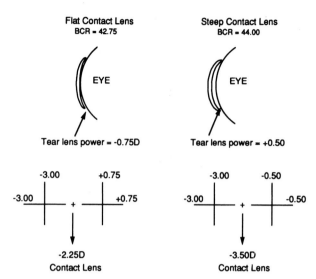

Refraction: -3.00 - 1.50 x 180

Keratometry Readings: 43.50 @ 180, 44.00 @ 90

FIG. 12.10. Example of the effect of tear lens on the power of a gas permeable lens.

lenses), unless the lens is being fitted to be half the difference steeper than K.

Vertex Distance

The effective power at the corneal plane is an important consideration when fitting patients exhibiting high myopia or hyperopia; specifically, the effective power difference becomes significant at 4 D or greater of ametropia. The effective power at the corneal plane is always increased in plus relative to the spectacle plane.

Appendix 2 presents the difference in effective power from the spectacle to the corneal plane, assuming a 12-mm vertex distance. The formula for determining the effective power is:

$$Fc = \frac{Fs}{1 - FS}$$

where Fc is the contact lens power
Fs is the spectacle lens power
d is the distance between the spectacle lens and the contact lens (in meters).

For example, if a 12-mm vertex distance is present and the patient's refractive error is $-6.50 - 1.00 \times 180$, at the corneal plane this will equal:

$$\frac{-6.50}{1 - (0.012 \times -6.50)} = -6.03 \text{ D}$$

$$\frac{-7.50}{1 - (0.012 \times -7,50)} = -6.88 \text{ D}$$

Rx spectacles $= +14.50 - 3.00 \times 010$

$$\frac{+14.50}{d1 - (0.012 \times +14.50)} = +17.55 \text{ D}$$

$$\frac{+11.50}{1 - (0.012 \times +11.50)} = +13.34 \text{ D}$$

$$= +17.55 - 4.21 \times 010 \text{ or}$$

$$+17.50 - 4.25 \times 010$$

It is important to measure vertex distance because it can vary among patients, and this factor increases in importance as the ametropia increases.

Ordering

Prior to fitting rigid diagnostic contact lenses, it is desirable to indicate the predicted vertexed lens powers on the fitting form. In addition, information pertaining to the diagnostic lens parameters, lens-to-cornea fitting relationship, and overrefraction should be provided. Figs. 12.11A and 12.11B are illustrations of a high-myopic patient using the vertexed refraction and a hyperopic patient who would benefit from a minus lenticular design. The predicted lens power can be obtained simply by adding the best sphere overrefraction value to the contact lens power. For example:

Keratometry: 42.50 @ 180, 42.75 @ 090
Spectacle refraction: $-6.50 - 0.25 \times 180$
Effective power: $-6.00 - 0.25 \times 180$
BCR (using aforementioned philosophy): 41.75 D or 0.75 D flatter than K
Predicted lens power: Spherical refractive value at the corneal plane minus tear lens power $= -6.00 - (-0.75) = -5.25$ D

In Fig. 12.11A and 12.11B and in the above example, the overrefraction values equal the predicted values. In many cases, this does not occur because of inaccuracies in refraction, keratometry values, BCR, or lens power, or because of flexure or lens decentration. If the discrepancy is 0.25 D, it probably is not significant; if it is higher, the other factors should be ruled out before the lenses are ordered. This is one of many important reasons for using diagnostic lenses as opposed to fitting empirically. The final power derived from adding the overrefraction and the diagnostic lens power usually will be more successful than selecting the lens power on the basis of predicted values. In addition, in some cases in which a high degree of residual astigmatism is predicted (implying that spherical rigid lenses may not be desirable), little or not cylinder is found on overrefraction, and the patient obtains satisfactory vision with a spherical overrefraction.

University of Missouri St.Louis

University of Missouri-Saint Louis

Contact Lens Fitting Data

School of Optometry

Patient ___Doe___ , ___Jane___   M.I. ___   File # ___2910___   Date ___11/19/90___

Keratometry
Average (Low K)   Average (High K)

Current Subjective Refraction

R 43.25 ⊃ 175, 44.50 ⊃ 085   R −8.25 −1.25 × 175   20/20 +2

L 42.75 ⊃ 010, 43.50 ⊃ 100   L −7.00 − 0.50 × 010 20/ 20

Predicted Lenses: Rigid ☑ Soft ☐   Special Design (specify) _____

	B.C.R.	S.C.R./W	P.C.R./W	Dia.	O.Z.D.	Power	C.T.
(43) R	7.85			9.2		− 7.25	.13
(42.25)	7.99			9.2		− 6.00	.13

	#1	#2	#3
Diagnostic Lens	_____	_____	_____
B.C./Dia./Power/C.T.	R 7.85 9.2 / −6.00 .13	R / / /	R / / /
	L 7.99/ 9.2 / −6.00 .13	L / / /	L / / /
Fluorescein Pattern (H.C.L.) or Over-K readings (S.C.L.)	R ◯ slight "astigmatic" pattern	R ◯	R ◯
	L ◯ alignment	L ◯	L ◯
Appearance of Mires (S.C.L.)	R	R	R
	L	L	L
Position and Lag	R ◯ good	R ◯	R ◯
	L ◯ centration OU	L ◯	L ◯
Retinoscopy (sphero-cyl)	R −1.00 −0.25 × 180 20/20	R 20/	R 20/
	L plano 20/20 +2	L 20/	L 20/
Subjective (best sphere)	R − 1.25 20/15 +2	R 20/	R 20/
	L plano 20/20 +2	L 20/	L 20/

Final Lens Design: Rigid ✓ Soft _____   Laboratory: Mid-South

	B.C.R.	S.C.R./W	P.C.R./W	Dia.	O.Z.D.	Power	C.T.	Tint
R	7.85	8.70/.3	11.20/.2	9.2	7.8	− 7.25	.13	blue
L	7.99	8.80/.3	11.20/.2	9.2	7.8	− 6.00	.13	blue

Blend ___Med___   Additional information ___Fluoroperm 30   ICR/W = 9.80/.2 OU___

Student Intern_____   Supervising Clinician_____

A   Comments:

FIG. 12.11. Examples of gas permeable lens diagnostic fits. **A:** Highly myopic patient. *(Figure continues.)*

University of Missouri St. Louis

University of Missouri-Saint Louis

Contact Lens Fitting Data

School of Optometry

Patient _Doe_, _John_   File # _3118_   Date _12/11/90_

Keratometry

	Average (Low K)	Average (High K)	Current Subjective Refraction
R	41.50 ⊃ 180	41.75 ⊃ 090	R +3.25 −0.25 × 170 20/15⁻²
L	41.75 ⊃ 180	42.50 ⊃ 090	L +3.00 −0.75 × 180 20/20⁺¹

Predicted Lenses: Rigid ☐ Soft ☐ Special Design (specify) _____

	B.C.R.	S.C.R./W	P.C.R./W	Dia.	O.Z.D.	Power	C.T.
(41) R	8.23			9.4		+3.75	
(41.50) L	8.13			9.4		+3.25	

	#1	#2	#3
Diagnostic Lens			
B.C./Dia./Power/C.T.	R 8.23 / 9.4 / +3.00	R / / /	R / / /
	L 8.13 / 9.4 / +3.06	L / / /	L / / /
Fluorescein Pattern (H.C.L.) or Over-K readings (S.C.L.)	R ◯ alignment	R ◯	R ◯
	L ◯ alignment	L ◯	L ◯
Appearance of Mires (S.C.L.)	R	R	R
	L	L	L
Position and Lag	R ◯ slightly superior	R ◯	R ◯
	L ◯ tucked under 1.0 OU	L ◯	L ◯
Retinoscopy (sphero-cyl)	R +0.50 DS 20/15⁻²	R 20/	R 20/
	L +0.25 DS 20/15⁻³	L 20/	L 20/
Subjective (best sphere)	R +0.75 DS 20/15⁻²	R 20/	R 20/
	L +0.25 DS 20/15⁻³	L 20/	L 20/

Final Lens Design: Rigid __✓__ Soft _____ Laboratory: _Mo-Con_

	B.C.R.	S.C.R./W	P.C.R./W	Dia.	O.Z.D.	Power	C.T.	Tint
R	8.23	9.0/.3	11.4/.2	9.4	8.0	+3.75	Min	blue
L	8.13	8.9/.3	11.4/.2	9.4	8.0	+3.25	Min	blue

Blend _Med_ Additional information _Boston RxD   ICR/w .10.00/2 OU_
Minus lenticular edge OU

Student Intern _____   Supervising Clinician _____

B   Comments:

FIG. 12.11. Continued. B: Hyperopic patient.

STANDARD DESIGN

Many practitioners order lenses using a standard design. BCR, OAD, and power are specified. The manufacturers use their own design to determine thicknesses, peripheral curves, optical zone, and other parameters. This method has the advantage of being less time consuming, and, if the practitioner has difficulty in determining what other parameter specifications to provide, an experienced laboratory should be able to assist in developing an effective design for a given GP material. In fact, many laboratories use one of many successful computer-assisted lens design programs. The disadvantages of this option versus custom lens designs are that it takes some control away from the practitioner, and no one diameter, OZD, center thickness, or peripheral curve system will be successful in every patient.

DESIGN PHILOSOPHIES

Korb

The "lid-attachment" fitting philosophy originated by Korb and Korb (36) is intended to optimize the interaction between the upper lid and the lens. This is accomplished via the edge contour and the shape of the anterior peripheral lens surface. Five variables are considered in this design:

1. Peripheral lens contour
2. Edge contour
3. Edge thickness
4. Lens mass
5. Secondary radii and edge curvatures

The goal of this philosophy is to use a lens design that will effectively simulate the actions and movements of the tear layer. Because most of the tear layer movement is the result of upper lid actions, this lens should, in effect, be attached to the upper lid. The normal act of blinking should not be compromised with this design.

The peripheral lens contour, or outer 1.00 mm, is considered the most important factor in lens–lid attachment. This lens design provides a broad area of lid–lens contact, with the peripheral lens and edge contour sloping toward the lid and not away from it, as with many standard designs. The edge contour should provide an adequate ski effect on the inner lens surface to enable the lens to move freely over the cornea or onto the sclera during blinking. An average edge thickness of 0.08 mm measured 0.2 mm from the apex of the edge is used in the +6.00 D to −6.00 D power range; larger edge thicknesses are commonly used for minus lenses. To reduce mass, Korb design lenses have minimal center thickness compared to lenses designed using other philosophies.

The average BCR is fitted 0.25 mm (approximately 1.5 D) flatter than K, varying from a minimum of 0.15 mm to as much as 0.70 mm. OAD ranges from 8.6 to 9.4 mm. The lens must maintain a superior-central lens-to-cornea fitting relationship and must remain attached to the upper lid. If the lens drops inferiorly as a result of partial blinking, the patient is given blinking exercises in an effort to concentrate on making complete blinks. Often it may be necessary to use diagnostic lenses 2 D to 4 D flatter than K to obtain the desired fit. If proper blinking and flattening the BCR do not result in a lid-attachment fit, a lenticular diagnostic set should be used to provide this relationship. The fluorescein pattern will demonstrate even bearing throughout the inferior 3 to 4 mm. If the lens decenters to an intrapalpebral position, the fluorescein pattern will reveal excessive central bearing.

An advantage of this philosophy includes the reduction of desiccation staining by a lid-attachment fitting relationship with a thin edge design. In addition, comfort should be enhanced because the lens edge is no longer in direct contact with the lid on the blink. Fewer lens deposits should be formed than with other lens design philosophies. The only possible complication is from corneal distortion, which may occur from long-term wear of a flat-fitting rigid lens. This could be a problem if the lens tends to drop and center in an intrapalpebral fitting relationship.

CALCULATING CORNEAL CURVATURE

Keratometry measurements are assumed to be a valid predictor of the BCR that should be selected for a given rigid lens patient. However, because they measure only approximately the central 3 mm of an aspheric, gradually flattening cornea, this may not be true (77,78). Keratometry has been found to be both invalid as a predictor of residual astigmatism (79) and unreliable when tested on different days (80). Because of these possible errors, a method of calculating keratometry values was developed by Brungardt (80,81) and later modified by Edrington (T. Edrington, *personal communication*). The corneal curvatures are calculated from the refractions with and without a rigid contact lens on the eye. An example is provided here.:

Calculating K Values

Solving for Tear Lens

Assume a vertexed spectacle refraction is equal in power to a contact lens refraction. The contact lens refraction is equal to the power of the contact lens plus the overrefraction plus the power of the tear lens, or:

SRv (subjective refraction vertexed) +
CLR (contact lens refraction)
OR (overrefraction)
SRv = *CLR* = *CLP* (contact lens power) + *OR* + *TL* (tear lens).

Rewrite the above formula to solve for the tear lens:

TL = *SRv* − *CLP* − *OR*.

Example:

$$SRv = -3.00{-}1.00 \times 180$$
$$(-)\ CLP\ (-){-}3.00\ (43.00\ \text{Base Curve})$$
$$\underline{(-)\ OR\ (-)\ +0.25{-}0.50 \times 180}$$
$$TL = -0.25{-}0.50 \times 180$$

This tear lens will be viewed when interpreting the fluorescein pattern.

Calculating Corneal Curvature

If you know the curvature of the contact lens BCR and the value of power of the tear lens, you can solve for the calculated corneal curvature.

TABLE 12.8. COMPARISON OF MEASURED AND CALCULATED CORNEAL CURVATURES (N = 84)

	Keratometry		Calculated		Difference in Means
	Mean	SD	Mean	SD	
Steep	44.150	1.48	43.959	1.54	+0.191
Flat	43.342	1.34	43.301	1.40	+0.041
Mean	43.746	1.38	43.630	1.45	+0.116
Toricity	0.808	0.57	0.658	0.54	+0.150

Means and standard deviations of each variable in corneal curvatures as measured and calculated. In every variable, the keratometer measurement is greater by the amount shown in the last column. From Brungardt TF. Corneal curvature determination by keratometry and refraction. *Int Contact Lens Clin* 1984;11:629.

$$Kc = BC\text{--}TL$$

For this example:

$$Kc @ 180 = 43.00\text{--}(\text{-})0.25 = 43.25 \text{ D}$$
$$Kc @ 090 = 43.00\text{--}(\text{-})0.75 = 43.75 \text{ D}$$

Generally, the mean calculated corneal curvatures are approximately 0.25 D flatter than the mean measured keratometry values. This is true because the resultant calculated curvatures depend upon all of the refractive light rays that enter through the pupil of the eye and the optical zone of the lens. Brungardt compared the two methods of determining corneal curvatures (i.e., via keratometry and calculated by refraction) (76). The results are given in Table 12.8. A high correlation was found between the two methods, with the keratometric readings on average slightly steeper and more toric than the values calculated from the two refractive findings.

This method is intended to be used as an adjunct to, and not *in lieu* of, keratometry plus fluorescein pattern interpretation in determining BCR. It also can be used to monitor changes due to corneal adaptation.

"INSIDE-OUT" DESIGN

The "inside-out" design is based on providing an aligned lens-to-cornea fitting relationship by designing the lens from the "inside out" (i.e., beginning with BCR, continuing with OZD, and later adding the secondary and peripheral curves to achieve the overall lens diameter) (42).

Step 1: Anatomic Features

When fitting a rigid lens, the ideal upper lid position is below the superior limbus, covering the superior third or fourth of the cornea. Therefore, a lens can be designed with apical alignment or apical bearing, and no posterior curve will be steeper than the adjacent cornea. Corneal astigma-tism also must be considered. According to this philosophy, it is the location, not the amount of astigmatism, that determines overall lens dynamics and design. Ideal fitting dynamics are created with a 2 D, with-the-rule cornea fitted with alignment along the horizontal meridian. A fulcrum effect exists along the horizontal meridian, and the lens will naturally follow the path of least mechanical resistance along the steep meridian. With an against-the-rule astigmat, however, the same principle typically will cause the lens to shift laterally, and another lens option may be necessary.

Step 2: Base Curve (Optical Zone) Radius

With regard to the first lens parameter to be selected, it is postulated that to obtain a true alignment fitting, a BCR 0.50 D flatter than K must be selected, regardless of corneal toricity (i.e., if keratometry = 45.00 @ 180, 46.50 @ 090; BCR/OZD = 44.50). This BCR is necessary to ensure that alignment is achieved, because a lens fit "on K" will result in apical clearance and midperipheral bearing.

Fig. 12.8 shows the relationship of OZD to lens-to-cornea fitting with this design philosophy. In this example, a lens of BCR 44.50 D is placed on a cornea with a central curvature of 45.00 D. Of the three OZDs shown, only the last shows an alignment fit; the first two exhibit a steep pattern. The OZD should decrease as BCR becomes steeper. OZD should never be greater than BCR in millimeters (i.e., if BCR = 44.50 D [7.58 mm], the maximum OZD = 7.6 mm).

Step 3: Secondary Curve Radius and Width

SCR should be 1.0 mm flatter than BCR to ensure adequate corneal clearance, compensating both for corneal flattening and for the inward tilting of the lens with the blink. If BCR is 7.60 mm, the SCR will be 8.60 mm. To maintain this relationship, SCR width will be dictated by OAD; it will increase for larger lenses and decrease for smaller lenses.

Step 4: Peripheral Curve Radius and Width

This will vary depending on the lens-to-cornea fitting relationship. A steeper curve is necessary with an interpalpebral fitting than with a superior fit (Fig. 12.12). The peripheral curve should typically have a radius of 12.25 mm or flatter with a width of 0.4 mm to ensure peripheral clearance.

Step 5: Lens Diameter

The diameter of a rigid lens is best determined by measuring the visible iris diameter and subtracting 2.3 mm (i.e., if visible iris diameter = 11.5 mm, OAD = 9.2 mm).

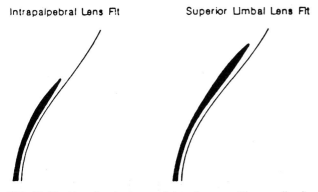

Intrapalpebral Lens Fit   Superior Limbal Lens Fit

FIG. 12.12. Use of a steeper peripheral curve with a smaller (intrapalpebral) lens design to maintain similar edge clearance with a larger-diameter lens. (From Caroline PJ, Norman CW. A blueprint for rigid lens design: part I. *Contact Lens Spectrum* 1988;3:39, with permission.)

Step 6: Blend Curve

This is determined in the same manner as with other methods (i.e., radius between the two curves). The blend should be heavy enough to remove any junction between the curves.

Step 7: Edge Profile

For minus lenses greater than 2 D, sufficient edge mass should be present for adequate lid support. Low minus and all plus lenses may require lenticulation to create the necessary edge thickness in the lens periphery. The edge profile can be changed dramatically to increase or decrease lid interaction by varying the radius of the lenticular flange.

Step 8: Center Thickness

This parameter depends on the dimensional stability of the lens material. Assuming the material has good stability, the center thickness values given in Table 12.9 are recommended.

TABLE 12.9. RECOMMENDED CENTER THICKNESS VALUES, "INSIDE-OUT" DESIGN PHILOSOPHY

Power (D)	Center Thickness (mm)
Plano	0.18
−1.00	0.17
−2.00	0.16
−3.00	0.15
−4.00	0.14
−5.00	0.13
−6.00	0.13
−7.00	0.13
−8.00	0.13

From Caroline PJ, Norman CW. A blueprint for rigid lens design: Part I. *Contact Lens Spectrum* 1988;3:39.

TABLE 12.10. SUMMARY OF "INSIDE-OUT" DESIGN PHILOSOPHY

Parameter	Design
Base curve radius	0.50 D flatter than K
Optical zone diameter	Never greater than the BCR in mm
Secondary curve	1.0 mm flatter than BCR; width increases as OAD increases
Peripheral curve	Typically 12.25/0.4 mm
Lens diameter	Visible iris diameter minus 2.3 mm
Edge profile	Low minus and all plus require lenticulation; proper lid interaction achieved by varying radius of lenticular flange
Center thickness	Depends on dimensional stability of material (values given in Table 12.9)

BCR, base curve radius; OAD, overall diameter.
From Caroline PJ, Norman CW. A blueprint for rigid lens design: Part I. *Contact Lens Spectrum* 1988;3:39.

Step 9: Lens Power

Power is determined as with other design philosophies, taking into consideration tear lens power. A summary of the Caroline-Norman "inside-out" design philosophy is given in Table 12.10.

SUMMARY

Selection of the most appropriate GP lens material for a given patient in combination with good judgment in lens design and fitting should result in both a high rate of use and a favorable success rate. In particular, application of diagnostic lenses to optimize the lens-to-cornea fitting relationship, custom design of the lenses, and comprehensive fluorescein evaluation of lens position and fit are important ingredients for long-term success with GP contact lenses.

ACKNOWLEDGMENT

The author thanks Dr. Tim Edrington for contributing information pertaining to the "calculating Ks GP fitting approach."

REFERENCES

1. Polse KA, Graham AD, Fusaro RE, et al. Predicting RGP daily wear success. *CLAO J* 1999;25:152–158.
2. Bennett ES. RGP fitting: how to increase comfort. *Practical Optom* 1997;8:148–152.
3. Bennett ES, Stulc S, Bassi CJ, et al. Effect of patient personality profile and verbal presentation on successful rigid contact lens adaptation, satisfaction and compliance. *Optom Vis Sci* 1998;75:500–505.

4. Bennett ES. How to present rigid lenses more effectively. *Rev Optom (Suppl)* 1995;132:8a–10a.

5. Davis R, Keech P, Dubow B, et al. Making RGP fitting efficient and successful. *Contact Lens Spectrum* 2000;15:40–47.

6. Benoit DP. Try RGPs for fun & profit. *Contact Lens Spectrum* 1996;11:47–48.

7. Quinn TG. Maximizing comfort with RGPs. *Contact Lens Spectrum* 1997;12:21.

8. Jervey JW. Topical anesthetic for the eye: a comparative study. *South J Med* 1989;48:770–774.

9. Lyle WM, Page C. Possible adverse effects from local anesthetics and the treatment of these reactions. *Am J Optom Physiol Opt* 1975;52:736–744.

10. Bennett ES, Smythe J, Henry VA, et al. The effect of topical anesthetic use on initial patient satisfaction and overall success with rigid gas permeable contact lenses. *Optom Vis Sci* 1998;75:800–805.

11. Schnider CM. Anesthetics and RGPs: crossing the controversial line. *Rev Optom* 1996;133:41–43.

12. Gordon A, Bartlett JD, Lin M. The effect of diclofenac sodium on the initial comfort of RGP contact lenses: a pilot study. *J Am Optom Assoc* 1999;70:509–512.

13. Caroline PJ, Andre MP. NSAIDs in RGP adaptation. *Contact Lens Spectrum* 2001;16.

14. Ames K. Rethink your approach to RGP lenses. *Contact Lens Spectrum* 1993;8:24–27.

15. Achiron LR. Custom-designed ultra-thin RGP lenses. *Contact Lens Spectrum* 2001;16.

16. Lebow KA. Fitting accuracy of an arc step-based contact lens module. *Contact Lens Spectrum* 1997;12:25–30.

17. Soper B, Shovlin J, Bennett ES. Evaluating a topography software based program for fitting RGPs. *Contact Lens Spectrum* 1996;11:37–40.

18. Szczotka LB. Clinical evaluation of a topographically based contact lens fitting software. *Optom Vis Sci* 1997;74:14–19.

19. Evardson WT, Douthwaite WA. Contact lens back surface specification from the EyeSys videokeratoscope. *Contact Lens Ant Eye* 1999;22:76–82.

20. Bennett ES, Henry VA, Davis LJ, et al. Comparing empirical and diagnostic fitting of daily wear fluoro-silicone/acrylate contact lenses. *Contact Lens Forum* 1989;14:38–44.

21. Davis R, Keech P, Dubow B, et al. Making RGP fitting efficient and successful. *Contact Lens Spectrum* 2000;15:40–47.

22. Keech P. The top 10 reasons to inventory RGPs. *Contact Lens Spectrum* 1996;11:32–36.

23. Szczotka LB. In-office RGP lens disinfection. *Contact Lens Spectrum* 2001;16:17.

24. Mandell RB. Trial lens method. In: Mandell RB, ed. *Contact lens practice*, 4th ed. Springfield, IL: Charles C. Thomas, 1988:243–264.

25. Obrig TE, Salvatori PL. *Contact lenses.* New York: Obrig Laboratories, 1957.

26. Bennett ES, Barr JT, Johnson J. Unmasking the RGP fit with fluorescein. *Contact Lens Spectrum* 1998;13:31–42.

27. Maurice DM. The use of fluorescein in ophthalmological research. *Invest Ophthalmol Vis Sci* 1967;6:464.

28. Young G. Fluorescein in rigid lens fit evaluation. *Int Contact Lens Clin* 1988;15:95.

29. Korb DR. Recent development in the observation of the cornea-lens relationship. In: *Encyclopedia of contact lens practice, vol. 3.* South Bend, IN: International Optics, 1959–1963:Appendix B:98–101.

30. Bennett ES. Easy ways to improve your RGP lens fitting. *Rev Optom (Suppl)* 1995;132:15A–17A.

31. Schwartz CA, Bennett ES, Moore C. Setting standards: what is a peripheral curve? *Contact Lens Spectrum* 1997;12:19–22.

32. Edmund C. Location of the corneal apex and its influence on the stability of the central corneal curvature: a photokeratoscopy study. *Am J Optom Physiol Opt* 1987;64:846.

33. Rowsey JJ, Reynolds AE, Brown R. Corneal topography: cornea scope. *Arch Ophthalmol* 1981;99:1093.

34. Grohe RM. RGP lens update. Presented at the Heart of America Contact Lens Congress, Kansas City, Missouri, February 1988.

35. Davis LJ, Bennett ES. Fluorescein patterns in UV-absorbing rigid contact lenses. *Contact Lens Spectrum* 1989;4:49.

36. Korb DR, Korb JE. A new concept in contact lens design. Parts I and II. *J Am Optom Assoc* 1970;4:1023.

37. Bier N, Lowther GE. Lens design. In: Bier N, Lowther GE, eds. *Contact lens correction.* Stoneham, MA: Butterworths, 1977.

38. Winkler TD. Case report of a corneo-scleral RGP lens. *Contact Lens Spectrum* 1999;14:41–43.

39. Cutler SI, Szczotka LB, Maynard R, et al. Managing irregular corneas with gas permeable lenses. *Contact Lens Spectrum* 2002;17:25–31.

40. Eisenberg JS. Safer, healthier, longer. *Rev Optom* 2001;138:71–76.

41. Lowther GE. Review of rigid contact lens design: part I. *Contact Lens Spectrum* 1988;3:39.

42. Caroline PJ, Norman CW. A blueprint for rigid lens design: part I. *Contact Lens Spectrum* 1988;3:39.

43. Herman JP. Flexure of rigid contact lenses on toric corneas as a function of base curve fitting relationship. *J Am Optom Assoc* 1983;54:209.

44. Henry VA, Bennett ES, Forrest JF. A clinical investigation of the Paraperm EW rigid gas permeable contact lens. *Am J Optom Physiol Opt* 1987;64:313.

45. Bibby MM. Factors affecting peripheral curve design. *Am J Optom Physiol Opt* 1979;56:2.

46. Honan PR, Morgan JF, Dabezies OH. Nomenclature, lens design, and fitting parameter. In: Dabezies OH, ed: *CLAO guide to contact lenses.* Orlando, FL: Grune & Stratton, 1984.

47. Stone J. Designing hard lenses in the 1980's. *J Br Contact Lens Assoc* 1982;4:130.

48. Bennett ES. Silicone/acrylate lens design. *Int Contact Lens Clin* 1985;12:45.

49. Atkinson TCO. The design of the back surface of gas permeable lenses. *J Br Contact Lens Assoc* 1982;5:16.

50. Holden T, Bahr K, Koers D, et al. The effect of secondary curve liftoff on peripheral corneal desiccation. Poster presented at the Annual Meeting of the American Academy of Optometry, Denver, Colorado, December 1987.

51. Schnider CM, Terry RL, Holden BA. Effect of patient and lens performance characteristics on peripheral corneal desiccation. *J Am Optom Assoc* 1996;67:144–150.

52. Sorbara L, Fonn D, Holden BA, et al. Centrally fitted versus lid-attached rigid gas permeable lenses. Part II. A comparison of the clinical performance. *Int Contact Lens Clin* 1996;23:121–126.

53. Doane M, Gleason W. Tear film interaction with RGP contact lenses. Presented at the First International Material Science Symposium, St. Louis, Missouri, March 1988.

54. Williams CE. New design concepts for permeable rigid contact lenses. *J Am Optom Assoc* 1979;50:331.

55. Zabkiewicz KR, Terry R, Holden BA, et al. The frequency of rigid lens binding in extended wear increases with time. *Am J Optom Physiol Opt* 1987;64:110.

56. Swarbrick HA, Holden BA. Rigid gas permeable lens binding: significant and contributing factors. *Am J Optom Physiol Opt* 1987;64:815.

57. Grohe RM, Lebow KA. Vascularized limbal keratitis. *Int Contact Lens Clin* 1989;16:197.

58. Bennett ES, Henry VA, Seibel DB, et al. Clinical evaluation of the Boston Equacurve. *Contact Lens Forum* 1990;15:49–52.

59. Andrasko GJ. A comfort comparison. *Contact Lens Spectrum* 1989;4:49–52.
60. Hill RM, Brezinski SD. The center thickness factor. *Contact Lens Spectrum* 1987;2:52.
61. Choatt C, Wing E. An RGP lens with a soft lens fit. *Contact Lens Spectrum* 2000;15:49–52.
62. Norman C. Today's RGPs: better performance through innovative technology. *Contact Lens Spectrum* 1996;11.:
63. Achiron LR. Custom-designed ultra-thin RGP lenses. *Contact Lens Spectrum* 2001;16.
64. Pole JJ, Kochanny L. The comparative flexure of Polycon II, Silcon and Boston II contact lenses on toric corneas. *Optom Monthly* 1984;75:151–155.
65. Corzine JC, Klein SA. Factors determining contact lens flexure. *Optom Vis Sci* 1997;74:639–645.
66. Edwards K. Rigid gas-permeable contact lens problem solving. *Optician* 2000;219:18–24.
67. Campbell R, Caroline P. Don't take RGP edge design for granted. *Contact Lens Spectrum* 1997;12.
68. La Hood D. The edge shape and comfort of RGP lenses. *Am J Optom Physiol Opt* 1988;65:613.
69. Picciano S, Andrasko GA. Which factors influence RGP lens comfort? *Contact Lens Spectrum* 1989;4:31.
70. Morris DS, Lowther GE. A comparison of different rigid contact lenses: edge thickness and contours. *J Am Optom Assoc* 1981;52:247.
71. Bennett ES, Grohe RM. RGP quality control: the results of a national survey. *J Am Optom Assoc* 1995;66:147–153.
72. Andrasko GJ, Stahl B. Hard choices made easy. *Rev Optom* 1986; 123:85.
73. Honan PR, Morgan JF, Dabezies OH. Nomenclature, lens design, and fitting parameter. In: Dabezies OH, ed: *CLAO guide to contact lenses.* Orlando, FL: Grune & Stratton, 1984.
74. Bier N, Lowther GE. Lens design. In: Bier N, Lowther GE, eds: *Contact lens correction.* Stoneham, MA: Butterworths, 1977.
75. Snyder C. Designing minus carrier RGP lenses. *Contact Lens Spectrum* 1998;13:20.
76. Szczotka LB. RGP parameter changes: how much change is significant? *Contact Lens Spectrum* 2001;16:18.
77. Brungardt TF. Corneal curvature determination by keratometry and refraction. *Int Contact Lens Clin* 1984;11:629.
78. Schultz DN. On asymmetry of central and peripheral corneal astigmatism measured by photokeratoscopy. *Am J Optom Physiol Opt* 1977;54:776.
79. Sarver MD. A study of residual astigmatism. *Am J Optom Arch Am Acad Optom* 1969;46:578.
80. Brungardt TF. Reliability of keratometry readings. *Am J Optom Arch Am Acad Optom* 1969;46:686.
81. Brundardt TF. *K* readings versus valid corneal curvature values. *J Am Optom Assoc* 1975;46;230.

RIGID LENS CARE AND PATIENT EDUCATION

**EDWARD S. BENNETT AND
HEIDI WAGNER**

INTRODUCTION

The ability to properly care for and handle gas permeable (GP) contact lenses depends upon several factors. First, the patient must be taught a primary method for insertion and removal, and proficiency in these methods must be demonstrated prior to leaving the office. Second, the patient must be aware of the function of each solution in the recommended care regimen; the importance of performing each function properly, in the correct order, and regularly; and why other solutions are not compatible with the particular material. Third, the patient must know the "dos and don'ts" relating to GP lenses; in other words, the patient must recognize the limitations of the lenses and the problems that can occur through noncompliance. The purpose of this chapter is to provide an overview of the ways in which these important factors can be satisfactorily addressed, thereby enhancing the probability of patient success.

CARE REGIMEN

Wetting and Soaking

The majority of solutions used for wetting and soaking of GP lenses combine several functions into one solution. These solutions have four major functions (1):

1. To temporarily enhance the lens surface wettability
2. To maintain the lens in a hydrated state similar to that achieved on the eye
3. To disinfect the lens
4. To act as a mechanical buffer between lens and cornea

The specific formulation of the ingredients in these solutions, especially the preservatives and wetting agents, is very important.

Disinfection

Prudent management by a contact lens-wearing patient includes the use of a lens care system that will minimize micro-

bial challenge to the eye and guard against problems such as microbial keratitis and conjunctivitis. Microbial contamination may be presented to the eye with the contact lens by way of the patient's hands, contaminated lens care products, lens care packaging, or a contaminated lens case.

GP lens care products accomplish lens disinfection by use of chemicals that act, first, as the lens care product preservative and, second, as the lens disinfecting agent. The choice and concentration of the chemical(s) are carefully selected in combination with wetting/soaking solutions so that, when in contact with living cells of the eye for a short duration (minutes), no toxicity or sensitivity reactions occur. The solution must, however, kill living cells (i.e., microorganisms) after a predetermined duration in a lens case (usually 4-hour minimum contact/soak time).

Preservatives

Preservatives are capable of either killing microorganisms (bactericidal agents) or inhibiting their growth (bacteriostatic agents) (2). They are the active ingredients in these solutions (and all other GP lens care solutions), which should perform the following functions (3):

1. Effectively provide the necessary degree of disinfection in the environment in which it is to be used
2. Not cause toxic reactions
3. Be compatible with the lens materials, avoiding adverse effects on surface wettability and lens parameters
4. Be compatible with the tear film

Numerous preservatives currently are in common use, all differing in their mode of action and effectiveness. The most common preservatives include benzalkonium chloride (BAK), chlorhexidine, thimerosal, ethylenediamine tetraacetate (EDTA), benzyl alcohol, polyaminopropyl biguanide (PAPB), polyquaternium-1 (polyquad), and polyhexanide hydrochloride (Tables 13.1 and 13.2).

Benzalkonium Chloride

BAK is a quaternary ammonium compound that is bactericidal against a wide spectrum of bacteria and fungi and

TABLE 13.1. STORAGE AND DISINFECTION SOLUTIONS

Manufacturer	Name	Preservative
Allergan	Barnes-Hind Comfort Care GP Wetting & Soaking Solution	Chlorhexidine
Bausch & Lomb	Wetting & Soaking Solution	Chlorhexidine
Optikem International	Sereine Wetting & Soaking Solution	
Polymer Technology	Boston Advance Conditioning Solution	Chlorhexidine and polyaminopropyl biguanide
Polymer Technology	Boston Conditioning Solution	Chlorhexidine

normally is used at a concentration of 0.004%. It is used in the majority of ophthalmic preparations and was first introduced as a preservative for hard contact lens solutions in the late 1940s (4). The effectiveness of BAK is enhanced when it is used in combination with EDTA, allowing a lower concentration than otherwise necessary (4). It is not used as a preservative with hydrogel lens solutions because the hydrogel material will bind the preservative and actually concentrate it, thereby allowing it potentially to reach toxic levels and cause ocular injury (5).

There has been some controversy as to the appropriateness of BAK as a preservative in GP lens solutions based on the fact that BAK is a cationic detergent with positively charged (hydrophilic) nitrogen head and a negative hydrocarbon chain (hydrophobic) tail. The theoretical binding mechanisms are complex. Practitioners have appeared to resolve this contradictory view of BAK efficacy by maintaining a clinical "wait and see" attitude. If a patient uses BAK successfully, no change is needed. However, the appearance of complications concurrent with the use of BAK prompts a temporary discontinuation of BAK to assess any clinical effect of lingering BAK on the lens surface or a permanent discontinuance of BAK by changing to a care product with a different preservative (6,7).

Chlorhexidine Gluconate
Chlorhexidine gluconate is bactericidal in action and traditionally has been used in a concentration of 0.005% in hydrogel lens chemical disinfection solutions. However, a primary reason for the gradual elimination of chlorhexidine-preserved hydrogel lens solutions from the marketplace has been the result of its tendency to bind to the lens surface and to concentrate by way of mucoprotein on the lens surface. However, the binding capacity of chlorhexidine to GP

lenses appears to be limited (8). Although chlorhexidine has been reported to have an excellent spectrum of antimicrobial activity, it has limited effectiveness against yeast and fungi; therefore, it often has been combined with EDTA or thimerosal for greater effectiveness. In addition, chlorhexidine has been found to be relatively ineffective against *Serratia marcescens* (9).

Thimerosal
Thimerosal is a bactericidal organic mercurial compound that at one time was a commonly used hydrogel lens solution preservative. However, some patients are sensitive to organic mercurial compounds and experience a burning sensation and associated clinical signs of redness and superficial punctate keratitis (10–12). In addition, it is both slow acting in nature and, in low concentrations (0.04%), may be ineffective against *Pseudomonas* (2,13). When compared with BAK, thimerosal was much less effective against a variety of Gram-positive and Gram-negative microorganisms (14). In addition, it has been found to be incompatible with EDTA (15). Although thimerosal has been found to be compatible with GP lenses (16,17) exhibiting only rare sensitivity reactions, for optimal antimicrobial effectiveness it should be used in combination with another preservative such as chlorhexidine.

Ethylenediamine Tetraacetate
EDTA is a chelating agent and not a true preservative. However, it is commonly used in combination with BAK and other preservatives in rigid contact lens solutions because of its synergistic ability to enhance bacterial action of pure preservatives against *Pseudomonas* (18).

Benzyl Alcohol
Benzyl alcohol originally was considered for use as a solvent for contact lens materials; however, it was also found to have

TABLE 13.2. COMBINATION SOLUTIONS

Manufacturer	Name	Preservative
Alcon	Unique pH Multipurpose Solution	Polyquaternium-1
CIBA Vision	Solo-Care Multipurpose Solution	Polyhexanide hydrochloride
Lobob	Optimum by Lobob	Benzyl alcohol
Menicon	Claris Cleaning & Soaking Solutions	Benzyl alcohol
Polymer Technology	Boston Simplicity Multi-Action Solution	Chlorhexidine and polyaminopropyl biguanide

good disinfection capabilities. Pure benzyl alcohol possesses certain physicochemical characteristics that are regarded as ideal for an ophthalmic preservative, including the following (19). First, it has a low molecular weight, and the molecules are capable of permeating small intermolecular spaces of tissues and lens polymers. Second, it has a bipolar molecule with a low order of polarity; therefore, benzyl alcohol would be expected to exhibit very little physical interaction or attraction with the polarized surface of the lens. Third, it is water soluble. Benzyl alcohol appears to show promise because it has been reported to exhibit negligible binding to the surface of GP lenses, especially fluoro-silicone/acrylate lens materials (19). In addition to its properties as a disinfectant, benzyl alcohol is effective in lipid removal (20).

Polyaminopropyl Biguanide

PAPB is similar in molecular structure to chlorhexidine and exhibits a lower sensitivity rate and greater antimicrobial effectiveness than chlorhexidine (8,21). PAPB has been used as a preservative/disinfectant agent in hydrogel lens disinfection regimens because of this low sensitivity rate, and recently it has supplemented chlorhexidine as a preservative/disinfectant agent in GP lens care systems. Polymer Technology Corporation has incorporated it into its GP lens care products.

Polyquaternium-1

Polyquaternium-1 is a large cationic (+) polymer that also is similar in molecular structure to chlorhexidine. The quaternary ammonium group has a lower cationic (+) charge than polyhexamethylene biguanide and, as a result, is used at higher concentrations (22). It is less likely to produce toxic or allergic reactions than previously developed preservatives such as benzalkonium chloride and thimerosal (23). It is unique to Alcon products.

Polyhexanide Hydrochloride

Polyhexanide hydrochloride, a relatively recent addition to contact lens disinfecting solutions, is also a chlorhexidine derivative (24). It appears to be well tolerated as a contact lens disinfectant. It is unique to Ciba Vision products.

Wetting Agents

Wetting/soaking solutions typically contain either polyvinyl alcohol or a methylcellulose derivative as a wetting agent.

Polyvinyl alcohol (PVA) has several properties that make it a beneficial additive to GP lens solutions (2). It is water soluble and is relatively nonviscous and nontoxic to ocular tissues. It has good viscosity-building properties and exhibits good spreading and wettability on the eye and lens surfaces (25). Also, unlike methylcellulose, PVA does not retard regeneration of corneal epithelium (26). Methylcellulose derivatives have been used successfully as wetting agents in more viscous rigid GP lens solutions.

Available wetting/soaking solutions are listed in Appendices 1 and 3 (27).

Cleaning

Several types of cleaners are available for use by GP lens wearers, including nonabrasive surfactant, abrasive surfactant, surfactant soaking, enzymatic, and laboratory cleaners.

Nonabrasive Surfactants

GP cleaners and traditional hard lens cleaners may contain nonabrasive surfactant (detergent) cleaning agents to remove contaminants (e.g., mucoproteins, lipids, debris) from the lens surface. These surfactants typically are formulated in one of three forms: (i) amphoteric, with either a positive or negative charge; (ii) cationic, with a positive charge; or (iii) anionic, with negative charge. The use of digital pressure or friction during the cleaning process is important in removing deposits from rigid lenses. Examples of such cleaners currently available include Resolve/GP and LC-65 (Allergan).

Abrasive Surfactants

Abrasive particulate matter has been used in cleaners as an effective adjunct in removing adherent substances or cleaning off mucoproteinaceous deposits from the lens that may be resistant to use of the surfactant alone. Examples of such cleaners currently available include Boston Cleaner and Boston Advance Cleaner (Polymer Technology Corporation) and Opti-Clean II Daily Cleaner (Alcon). Daily use of abrasive cleaning regimens has been demonstrated to be more effective than the use of nonabrasive cleaners (28). However, two potential problems have been described with abrasive cleaners. First, small surface scratches have been seen under high magnification (29). Second, reports of inducing minus lens power have been documented (30–32). Nevertheless, these cleaners have become a popular and effective option for GP lens patients.

Surfactant Soaking and Multipurpose Lens Care Products

GP lens care systems have traditionally embraced two-bottle regimens composed of separate cleaning and soaking solutions. One-bottle GP lens care systems combining these procedures recently have entered the marketplace. These solutions use surfactant soaking and are intended to dissolve deposits during the overnight soaking cycle; therefore, little digital pressure is necessary and warpage is less likely (33).

Claris (Menicon) and Optimum (Lobob) are variations of the former DE-STAT products by Sherman Pharmaceuticals (34). Both cleaners contain nonabrasive surfactants and are used for both disinfection and cleaning. Both products should be rinsed prior to insertion, to remove the benzyl alcohol and facilitate the mechanical removal of lens debris. Boston Simplicity (Polymer Technology Corporation), Unique pH (Alcon), and Solocare (CIBA Vision) are examples of multipurpose lens care products that do not require rinsing prior to insertion. Solocare is unique in that it is approved as a lens care system for both rigid and soft lenses. It also is distinctive in that it is significantly less viscous than other GP lens care products. Although the low viscosity may be a detriment to lens wettability, this product offers convenience to patients wearing hybrid or piggyback lens corrections (35).

Manufacturers have recently obtained approval from the United States Food and Drug Administration (FDA) to market "no rub" versions of multipurpose solutions approved for hydrogel lens disinfection. It remains to be seen whether this trend will follow in GP lens care practices. Patients welcome the added convenience while practitioners remain skeptical. Although the manufacturers have data documenting the efficacy of these regimens, it is important to note the importance of following the manufacturers' instructions for products that do not require digital rubbing because the efficacy may be based on a rinsing step. Patients who omit the rubbing and/or rinsing step or who are heavy depositors may experience deposit buildup or microbial contamination (35–37). Practitioners must educate themselves about the available lens care systems and then educate their patients about the systems they prescribe (38).

The lens care system should be prescribed for the needs of the patient. For example, Boston Original was formulated specifically for silicone/acrylate lenses that tend to deposit protein, whereas Boston Advance Comfort Care was designed for fluoro-silicone/acrylate lenses that are more likely to attract lipids (39). Multipurpose lens care systems may be most appropriate for patients who do not tend to deposit lenses or who are not compliant with two-bottle lens care regimens. Patients who exhibit sensitivity to one formulation may be better served by a system using a different preservative.

Enzymatic Cleaning

The use of a weekly enzymatic cleaning regimen for GP lens wearers has been proven to be a beneficial adjunct in protein removal from the lens surface (40). In addition, enzyme use has not been reported to cause any adverse effects for GP lens wearers (41). Newly developed lens care products are in liquid, rather than tablet, form and may be used with the manufacturer's accompanying storage solution. Boston One-Step Liquid Enzymatic Cleaner (Polymer Technology) is added to the storage solution weekly, whereas SupraClens (Alcon) is added daily. Both products should be rinsed prior to lens insertion. Boston One-Step is composed of subtilisin; SupraClens is a pancreatin deriva-

tive (34). Both products are designed to promote patient compliance and meet the patients' desire for convenience.

Special Techniques

Occasionally, patients may need to supplement the regular surfactant cleaning step because of a buildup of a lens coating across the back surface of the lens. Plaque may deposit centrally or peripherally on the front or back surface (42). Rigid lenses with steep base curve radii are especially prone to buildup because of the physical limitations of digital cleaning of the steep posterior lens surface. Use of a cotton-tipped applicator and a few drops of an abrasive surfactant cleaner to swab the inside bowl of the lens held in the palm of the hand is recommended to be performed by the patient, at minimum, a few times each week in addition to the regular lens care routine. Enzymatic soaking often is recommended as an adjunct to this special step. The evidence of the need to prescribe this extra step may present as centralized superficial epithelial fluorescein staining or as lens adherence with daily or extended wear.

In-Office Cleaning

Laboratory Cleaners and Solvents

Use of laboratory-approved, extra-strength cleaners such as the Boston Laboratory Cleaner (Polymer Technology Corporation) or Fluoro-Solve (Paragon Optical, Inc.) can be beneficial. The Boston Laboratory Cleaner, a solution consisting of several surfactants, can be beneficial for in-office cleaning of lenses that either exhibit poor initial wettability or have acquired a heavy film over time. Surface debris that is more tenacious and difficult to remove, such as pitch or wax, can be better removed with Fluoro-Solve, which is a mild solvent. Miraflow and Quick-Care Starting Solution (CIBA Vision), although not approved for routine GP lens use, can be excellent restorers of lens surface wetting. Available GP lens cleaners are listed in Table 13.3 (27).

TABLE 13.3. DAILY CLEANERS

Manufacturer	Name
Alcon	Opti-Clean II Daily Cleaner
Allergan	Resolve/GP
Allergan	LC-65
Allergan	Barnes-Hind GP Daily Cleaner
Bausch & Lomb	Concentrated Cleaner
Lobob	Optimum by Lobob Extra Strength Cleaner
Optikem International	Sereine Cleaner
Polymer Technology	BOSTON Cleaner
Polymer Technology	BOSTON Advance Cleaner

Deposit Removal (Cleaning) and Polishing

Cleaning and polishing of GP lenses in the office can be easily performed using a contact lens polish, such as X-Pal, Sil-02-Care, or Boston Lens Polish, in conjunction with a foam tool on a rotating spindle of a lens modification unit. Spindle speed should be about 1,000 rpm, and generous amounts of lens polish should be used to minimize friction and the buildup of heat, which can damage the lens surfaces. A foam cone is recommended as the tool to use because it allows the lens front surface to be polished on the cone's side surface and the lens back surface at the cone apex. In addition, this tool is soft enough so as to be "forgiving," that is, the possibility of changing the lens power or warping the lens is negligible. A hand-held suction cup typically holds the lens. Many patients, even with appropriate and diligent execution of care and handling procedures throughout the year, will still develop a buildup of lens filming and coatings, especially on the back surface of the lens. This in-office cleaning and polishing done annually will rejuvenate lens surfaces and renew the lenses for another year of comfortable wear. Of course, regularly prescribed daily and weekly lens care and maintenance by the patient still is necessary!

Solution Controversies

Much controversy has surrounded the performance of BAK-preserved wetting/soaking solutions versus those preserved with chlorhexidine. Although early reports showed BAK to be compatible with polymethyl methacrylate (PMMA) and cellulose acetate butyrate (CAB) lens materials (43–46), more recent reports show dewetting of the lens surface, corneal dry spots, and patient intolerance with more recently marketed GP lens materials (7,46). This may explain why BAK-preserved solutions are not as prevalent as in the past.

Use of tap water with GP lenses remains contentious because of its association with *Acanthamoeba* keratitis. The effectiveness of several types of preserved solutions against two common *Acanthamoeba* species, *A. polyphaga* and *A. castellanii,* has been evaluated (47–49). The results of these studies have demonstrated that *Acanthamoeba* adherence is less to GP than to hydrogel lenses. It also is apparent that a lens care system that is more effective against bacteria will be more effective against *Acanthamoeba* because *Acanthamoeba* feed on bacteria. Without an available "meal" of bacteria, *Acanthamoeba* will have difficulty flourishing. The literature also illustrates the preventable nature of *Acanthamoeba* keratitis (50). Numerous studies have demonstrated that the preservatives in most contact lens solutions are not effective or are slow in killing *Acanthamoeba* (51–55). Therefore, it is beneficial to avoid the potential for contamination through daily lens disinfection, adequate contact lens storage case hygiene, and avoidance of swimming while wearing contact lenses.

Some debate exists over whether the Boston Advance Conditioning (wetting and soaking) Solution (Polymer Technology), which is preserved with PAPB (0.0015%), is truly an "advance" over the original Boston Conditioning Solution, which is preserved with chlorhexidine (0.006%). An animal study comparing Boston Advance Conditioning Solution, Boston Conditioning Solution, and the Allergan Wet-N-Soak Plus Solution (preserved with 0.006% benzalkonium chloride) showed that the Boston Advance Conditioning Solution was toxic to the rabbit corneal epithelium, causing extensive disruption of the superficial layer of cells (56). A parallel of that study performed on human eyes demonstrated significantly more corneal fluorescein staining with the Boston Advance Conditioning Solution (57). Practitioners were warned to educate their patients about the differences between the Boston Original Conditioning Solution and the Boston Advance Conditioning Solution. This controversy has been all but ended with the replacement of Boston Advance Conditioning Solution with the Boston Advance Comfort Formula, which has a significantly lower concentration of preservatives.

Although the preservative controversy continues, all commonly used preservatives in GP lens solutions appear to be safe and exhibit far fewer sensitivity reactions than do hydrogel lens disinfecting solutions. Additionally, modern preservatives, some of which are large-molecular-weight derivatives of older preservatives, tend not to bind to lens surfaces as readily (58). As a result, they are generally well tolerated. Although studies primarily have focused on silicone/acrylate materials, clinical experience suggests a similar preservative response to fluoro-silicone/acrylate lenses. It has been our clinical experience that a patient occasionally can exhibit a sensitivity reaction to any one of the aforementioned preservatives. This is manifested, as with allergic reaction, in the form of itching, burning, or redness. If this occurs, switching to a care regimen using a different preservative almost always eliminates the adverse response.

Wet Versus Dry Storage

Patients should store their GP lenses in the hydrated state upon removal. There are many reasons for this, including the following:

1. To disinfect the lenses
2. To maintain the lenses in the hydrated state (the lens is in contact with the tear film when on the eye)
3. To enhance wettability by soaking in the wetting/soaking solution
4. To minimize surface scratches that can occur when the lens is taken in and out of a dry, dirty case well
5. To decrease the intermittent tendency of rigid GP lenses to form areas of nonwetting

Because of minimal microbial recovery from dry stored GP lenses, coupled with the fact that rubbing (cleaning) and rinsing removes a significant amount (>99%) of microorganisms (58), dry storage of diagnostic lenses may be recommended. Prior to dry storage, current American Optometric Association Clinical Practice Guidelines (59) state that disinfection of diagnostic contact lenses should be performed by methods approved by the Centers for Disease Control and Prevention (CDC) (60,61). The CDC recommends a 5- to 10-minute soak in a commercially available hydrogen peroxide contact lens disinfecting system currently approved for soft contact lenses. The cleaning and rinsing of a dry-stored GP lens, followed by wetting with wetting/soaking solution prior to application, should leave little risk for microbial contamination of a healthy eye. Dry storage of diagnostic GP lenses seems to be standard practice.

Patient's own spare lens(es) should be treated differently. Patients may be instructed to store a spare GP lens or lenses in a clean and dry lens case for long-term storage. The lenses should, by package insert instructions, be cleaned and soaked for an appropriate period of time, usually 4 hours, in a GP lens soaking solution designed for lens disinfection before wearing the lenses.

The introduction of Visions (X-Cel), a lens manufactured in Paragon Vision Science's HDS material, may mark the advent of new lens storage practices for inventoried GP lenses. The lenses are shipped in glass vials, fully hydrated, and presumably ready for lens wear. Shipping lenses in the wet state rather than the traditional dry state is intended to prevent the initial poor wetting that occasionally results from residual pitch (62). The lens package also includes an identical lens, which some practitioners present to the patient as a spare lens while others prescribe the second lens for planned replacement. Planned replacement is suggestive of the trend in hydrogel lens care whereby lenses that are replaced more frequently are paired with more streamlined lens care systems.

Compliance

Ocular complications associated with noncompliance are more common with hydrogel lens wearers (63,64). However, GP lens wearers who do not comply with the recommended care guidelines may experience problems as well. Some of the more frequent causes of noncompliance problems with GP lens wearers include the following:

1. Patient does not clean the lenses as often or as comprehensively as desired (if at all)
2. Patient does not adhere to the prescribed wearing schedule
3. Patient does not use disinfection solution or, if used, does not replace it regularly
4. Patient does not wash hands before handling the lenses
5. An inappropriate wetting solution such as saliva or tap water is used

6. Expired solutions are used
7. Case is not cleaned and replaced regularly
8. Patient substitutes originally recommended solution with another brand

One study found that approximately 50% of rigid lens care solutions were contaminated (63). In addition, a much higher percentage of patients who admitted noncompliance were found to have contaminated care regimens than compliant patients. It is important to note that all solutions that were less than 21 days old were uncontaminated. Ghormley (65) has recommended a three-tier approach to noncompliance by emphasizing ongoing education of the practitioner, the staff, and the patient. Meichenbaum and Turk (66) have identified five variables that may affect patient compliance: (i) characteristics of the patient, (ii) characteristics of the treatment regimen, (iii) features of the disease, (iv) relationship with the clinician, and (v) the clinical setting (66). Podell and Gary (67) have suggested that one third of patients follow instructions, another third do sometimes, and the remaining third never do.

Tap Water

Use of tap water with GP lenses is very controversial. It is apparent that the use of tap water or homemade saline may result in serious ocular complication, especially when used as a wetting or rewetting solution. One reported case of *Acanthamoeba* was associated with a GP lens wearer who occasionally used municipal or well water or saliva to wet the lenses (68). Therefore, patients must be educated not only to avoid tap water as a wetting agent but also as to the consequences if they do not comply. Another issue is whether it is acceptable to use tap water as a rinsing agent. Obviously, hard lens patients are accustomed to using tap water for this purpose, and it certainly is inexpensive. If the patient uses tap water *only* to rinse off the cleaning solution before placing the lenses into the disinfecting solution, it most likely would be acceptable, and this has been recommended by several practitioners (69,70). A tap water rinse of the GP lens cleaner from the lens before the use of wetting solution and insertion of the lens onto the eye is common clinical practice. However, to totally avoid the possibility of ocular infections induced by tap water use, aerosol saline has been recommended as a rinse for GP lenses (69). Presumably, other saline or multipurpose hydrogel lens care solutions could serve the same purpose. This issue is further complicated by the fact that the manufacturers' instructions may recommend the use of tap water.

Solution Confusion

The large number of currently available GP and hydrogel lens care products makes patient compliance more challenging. Frequently, patients cannot recall the name of the product(s) and may inadvertently select a similar-appearing but incorrect (and possibly ill-advised) solution. This may be further confused by competitive contact lens solution marketing, which may result in companies' adopting similar-appearing label colors, print styles, and bottle sizes and shapes (71). Finally, solution substitution may simply be a result of pricing; the patient may purchase the solution just because it is less expensive.

The following steps can minimize solution confusion:

1. Thoroughly educate the patient as to what solutions they can use, including alternatives.
2. Emphasize *why* you are recommending specific solutions to discourage price shopping.
3. Inquire as to what solutions are being used at progress evaluation visits to ensure that solution switching has not occurred. To obtain an honest response, it is important that the doctor or assistant use neutral questioning, such as "What is the name of the solution you are using?" Otherwise, if patients are asked if they are still using the recommended solution, they will frequently and sheepishly answer "yes."
4. Stock lens care products for sale in your practice setting allows patients to buy their bundled, long-term supplies from you. This may prevent product purchase "noncompliance."

Rewetting and Relubricating

A solution that is used to rewet a GP lens surface while it is still on the eye should perform the following functions (72,73):

1. Rewet the lens surface
2. Stabilize (or at least not destabilize) the tear film
3. Rinse away trapped debris
4. Break up loosely attached deposits

Ideally, this solution should clean the lenses of any debris while rewetting them for an extended period of time (73). Because the key to rewetting a GP lens is contact time, PVA often is added to increase the length of contact time. In theory, the PVA molecule contains both lipophilic and hydrophilic groups. When applied to a GP lens, the lipophilic group binds to the plastic lens surface, forming a complex that exposes the hydrophilic portion of PVA. The new surface attracts and binds water. Other wetting agents are used as well. In fact, research has shown that the number of possible combinations in a relubricating solution potentially is unlimited (74). Some solutions contain hydroxyethyl cellulose, methylcellulose, or other cellulose derivatives to aid surface wetting by increasing viscosity. Several rewetting solutions also contain a mild nonionic detergent to loosen and solubilize mucus and debris and keep it from adhering tenaciously to the lens surface (73). Preservative-free rewetting drops are a useful adjunct for patients with a previous

TABLE 13.4. WETTING AND LUBRICATION SOLUTIONS

Manufacturer	Name
Alcon	Clerz Plus Lens Drops
Allergan	Refresh Contacts
CIBA Vision	CIBA Vision Lens Drops
Lobob	Optimum by Lobob Wetting and Rewetting
Polymer Technology	BOSTON Rewetting Drops

history of preservative sensitivity and/or frequent use of relubricating solutions.

Available rewetting/relubricating solutions are listed in Table 13.4 (27).

DISPENSING VISIT

Procedures

Knowledge about the available care regimens and their respective functions, applications, and benefits becomes especially important at the dispensing visit. Before dispensing new lenses to a patient, it may be beneficial to apply fluorescein dye to the tear film to rule out any baseline staining with the biomicroscope. Once the rigid lenses have been applied and the patient has stopped tearing and is able to gaze in the straight-ahead position with minimal difficulty (a variable period of time; typically 11–45 min), visual acuity and lens evaluation can be performed.

Visual Acuity

The patient's quality of vision should be assessed first, either by Snellen's test or with a contrast sensitivity or similar chart. In addition, a useful method is a reduced-contrast (Bailey-Lovie) acuity chart. If a reduction in visual acuity compared with baseline is found, biomicroscopy should be performed to evaluate lens position and surface wettability. If both good lens centration and surface wettability are present, an overrefraction can be performed to determine the necessary additional correction.

Overrefraction

If the visual acuity is equal to the expected value, typically a spherical overrefraction only is indicated. Monocular assessment of subjective response to +0.50 and −0.50 diopter trial lenses held over the eye (while viewing the distant eye chart) is a quick and easy way to grossly check the appropriateness of the contact lens prescription. If the overrefraction is 0.50 D or greater (equivalent sphere), resulting in a reduction in visual acuity, the lenses should not be dispensed because an adverse effect on the patient's perception of contact lenses may result. Just as the diagnostic fitting is imperative both for obtaining a proper fit and for enhancing patient motivation (by the knowledge that contact lenses can be tolerated), the dispensing visit is important in continuing this momentum toward eventual patient success by the ability to see, wear, handle, and care for the new GP lenses.

If a spherical overrefraction is present, in-office repowering of the lens surface is the quickest method of providing the appropriate correction. If uncorrected cylinder that is not residual in nature is causing reduced visual acuity, overkeratometry should be performed to determine if the lens is flexing. If the keratometry readings are not spherical, flexure is present. This induced flexure can be minimized by selecting a flatter base curve radius (i.e., 0.50 D minimum) or increasing center thickness by a minimum of 0.02 mm (75,76).

Slit-Lamp Biomicroscopy

Use of a biomicroscope is essential for evaluating lens centration, lag, fluorescein pattern, and surface wettability. The lens-to-cornea fitting relationship initially should be evaluated using a wide beam with low-intensity white light and low magnification to scan the lens surface. In addition, it can be evaluated for regions of poor wettability or hazing. If the patient experiences variable visual acuity in combination with poor initial wettability, this problem can be minimized by presoaking the lenses for a minimum of 24 hours to precondition the surface before insertion (77).

If poor wettability is present after presoaking the lenses, an in-office cleaner such as the Boston Laboratory Cleaner (Polymer Technology Corporation) can be used; approved laboratory solvents such as the Boston Solvent (Polymer Technology Corporation) or Fluoro-Solve (Paragon Vision Sciences) should eliminate the problem. Although some clinicians have used Quick-Care Starting Solution or Miraflow (CIBA Vision) for GP lenses, it should be noted that this is an "off-label" use of these cleaners, which are not intended for routine use with GP lenses. Because prolonged and repeated exposure to alcohol-based products, such as Miraflow, may cause permanent damage because of parameter changes (78) and brittleness and cracking due to isopropyl alcohol, (79) such products should be used for no more than 30 seconds and then thoroughly rinsed off. Polishing the front surface of the lens also may be beneficial. However, this should be performed after the lens is initially cleaned with an in-office cleaner.

Comprehensive evaluation of the fluorescein pattern is important. Is the pattern similar to that observed at the diagnostic fitting visit? The use of high illumination, low magnification, and a moderate-to-wide beam width should be beneficial when observation is by biomicroscope. If there is difficulty in observing the pattern, a Wratten no. 12 or similar filter can be used, especially if the lens material contains an ultraviolet inhibitor. In addition, if lower magnification is necessary to evaluate the pattern accurately, a common problem in cases of irregular cornea, a Burton lamp can be used.

Handling

The key to handling rigid lenses successfully is *reassurance.* No matter how frustrating it is to the person performing the instruction, that feeling of frustration must not be conveyed to the patient. The instructions must be provided slowly and one at a time. Performing group instruction is distracting and denies the patient the necessary one-on-one instruction. Your patient should not have the perception that you or your assistant has lost confidence in his or her ability to learn how to handle the lenses properly; otherwise, feelings of failure and surrender may result, possibly leading to the attitude that contact lenses will never be worn again. Conversely, if the patient feels confident about handling the lenses, a perception of satisfaction and success often is present. Patients frequently feel anxiety about being able "to put those things in my eyes." A minimum of three successful insertions and removals is recommended, although the number depends upon how confident the patient feels. If it takes two or three visits (closely spaced to maximize memory of techniques and to minimize further anxiety) for the patient to master lens handling, it often is worth the effort. This is more often a problem with presbyopic patients, who not only are experiencing blurred vision at near but also may have lived 40 or more years without having a foreign body placed on their eye, thereby increasing anxiety.

Patients should be instructed to insert and remove the lenses over a cloth or paper towel spread on a table (not over a sink drain). In addition, patients should be reminded to avoid oily substances such as hand creams, lotions, or cosmetics, and their hands should be washed and rinsed thoroughly before handling the lenses.

Insertion

Insertion by the Patient
Insertion of lenses by the patient is a three-step procedure.

1. Positioning. The patient should be encouraged to use an adjustable mirror when inserting the lenses. This will help to ensure that the lens is positioned properly on the finger and to view the position of the lens. The latter is especially important because patients may consistently bring the lens in contact with the upper or lower lid.

2. Lid retraction. For the right eye, the lens should be placed on the right index finger. The middle finger of the left hand should be placed *underneath* the upper lashes to lift up the upper lid. The middle finger of the right hand should be placed directly *over* the lower lashes to depress the lower lid (Fig. 13.1). The ability to retract the lashes successfully is essential.

3. Placement. The patient should be viewing inferiorly and can be instructed to view directly through the lens as it is brought toward the eye. Typically, the new rigid lens patient will experience difficulty maintaining proper fixation as the lens approaches the eye; therefore, encouragement should be provided that the lens will not damage the eye. Finally, once the lens has made contact with the eye, the patient should be instructed first to release the finger holding the lens, then the lower lid, and finally the upper lid. This procedure then can be performed in reverse for the other eye (i.e., use the index finger of left hand for holding the lens, the middle finger of right hand for holding the upper lid, and the middle finger of left hand for holding the lower lid).

Insertion by the Practitioner or Assistant

The procedure is similar if performed by an office member. If the lens is to be placed on the right eye, the lens will be placed on the index finger of the right hand, with the left middle finger holding the upper lid and the right middle finger holding the lower lid. Because the patient may become especially apprehensive with someone else inserting the lens, it is very important to apply pressure underneath the lashes to ensure that he or she will not move during this process (Fig. 13.2). Anchoring the heels of the hands on the patient's forehead and cheek, as well as positioning the patient's head with a head rest, are recommended to stabilize the patient's head and to have a controlled situation for insertion as well as removal of the lens.

Removal

Removal by the Patient

There are at least three methods for removing a rigid lens. Which method is used depends on factors such as lid tension, lens design, and personal preference.

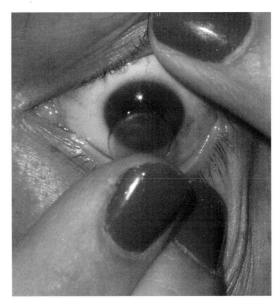

FIG. 13.2. Proper insertion of a gas permeable lens by an assistant.

The easiest method is to use the index finger of the same hand as the eye in which the lens is to be removed to eject the lens. The finger is placed at the junction of the lateral edge of the lids (Fig. 13.3). With the eye opened wide, the lids are pulled laterally; at the same time, the patient blinks and the lens is ejected. This procedure can be performed with both the middle and index fingers of the same hand to enhance the possibility of lens ejection. The other hand can be positioned underneath the eye to catch the lens if it fails to adhere to the lower eyelashes.

For patients who experience difficulty with the first method because of factors such as loose lid tension, low

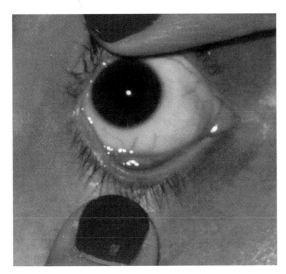

FIG. 13.1. Proper lid retraction for insertion of a rigid lens.

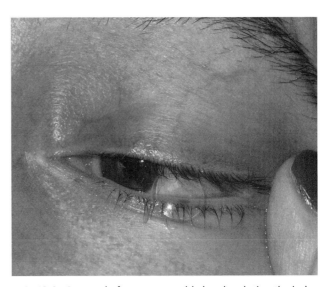

FIG. 13.3. Removal of a gas permeable lens by placing the index finger at the lateral edge of the lids.

edge lift, and large overall lens diameter, a more forceful method to remove the lens is to use both hands. The middle and index fingers of the same hand are positioned over the lower lid; the middle and index fingers of the opposite hand hold up the upper lid (Fig. 13.4A). As with the first method, the lids are pulled laterally and, while the patient blinks, the lens is ejected (Fig. 13.4B and 13.4C). As with all methods of removal, the most important factor is allowing the lid margins to eject the lens. Fig. 13.5 shows that if the lids are not retracted properly (i.e., if the finger is not placed *over* the lashes), the lid can evert and, therefore, apply very little pressure toward ejecting the lens.

Another method of removing the lens is to eject the lens with a vertical (not lateral) motion. The fingers are positioned as in the second method (i.e., fingers on the opposite hand holding the upper lid, fingers on the same hand positioned on the lower lid). The lower lid is pushed superiorly and the lens is ejected (Fig. 13.6).

Removal by the Practitioner

The same methods for removal by the patient can be used by the practitioner. The second and third methods are preferable because they minimize the amount of time necessary to eject the lens.

The fear of being unable to remove a rigid lens is perhaps the greatest cause of panic with a new wearer. Every patient should be able to remove his or her lenses easily, before

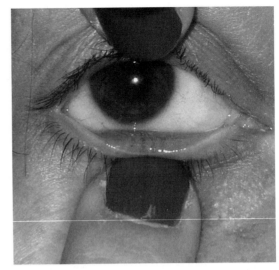

FIG. 13.5. Improper placement of the fingers can result in lid eversion and inability to remove the lens.

leaving the office. Although the temptation exists to allow the patient to practice at home, this may eventually result in a frustrated and dissatisfied patient. Both practitioners and assistants should be skilled at all of these removal methods.

A suction cup should not be used as a crutch for patients who experience difficulty with removal unless it is deemed

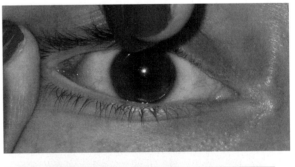

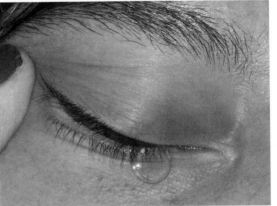

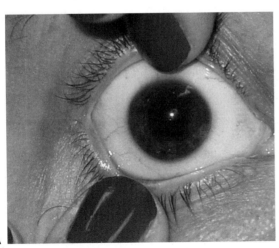

FIG. 13.4. Removal of a gas permeable lens is easily accomplished using both hands. The upper lid is held by the opposite hand; the lower lid is held by the same hand **(A).** As the lids are pulled laterally, the lens is ejected **(B, C).**

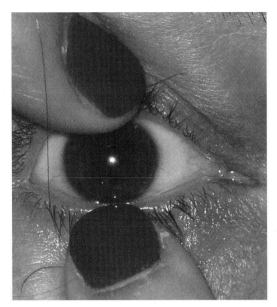

FIG. 13.6. Another effective method of gas permeable lens removal is to push the lids in a vertical motion with the fingers positioned the same as in Fig. 13.2.

absolutely essential. However, in an emergency situation in which a suction cup is unavailable, the patient's head can be placed in a sink filled with water and his or her eyes opened, allowing the lenses to wash off of the eye.

Recentration

It is extremely important to demonstrate to new rigid lens wearers how to recognize when a lens has decentered off of the cornea and how to reposition it. This often occurs dur-

ing adaptation, when lenses tend to drop further on the cornea after the blink.

If the patient notices a unilateral blurring of vision, the eye should be evaluated for the possibility of a decentered lens. Location can be determined by the use of a mirror or, if this is not possible, a finger can be placed gently over different regions of the lids to feel any region that may be overlying the lens. Once the lens has been located, it can be manipulated through the lids. The patient should look away from the lens and, after placing a finger on the opposite side of the lens, should look toward the direction of the lens, repositioning it on the cornea (Fig. 13.7).

Often, the patient will develop the confidence to reposition the lens gently without the benefit of the lids. If it is difficult for the patient to locate, it most likely is superior. The lens should be applied to the patient's eye in a decentered position to allow the patient an opportunity to practice recentering the lens under instruction in the office.

Cleaning

Patients should be told which specific brand cleaning solution(s) to use, when to use them, and how to clean the lens properly. Cleaning with a surfactant cleaner should be performed *immediately* upon removal at the end of the day, not before insertion the next morning. This is important in maintaining good surface wettability, both because the lens is inserted directly from the wetting/soaking solution and because debris is removed more easily given that the lens has been in contact with the tear film.

Cleaning should be performed carefully in the palm of the hand (not between the fingers). Excessive digital pressure can result in lens warpage or lens fracture, especially with the more flexible super permeable lens materials.

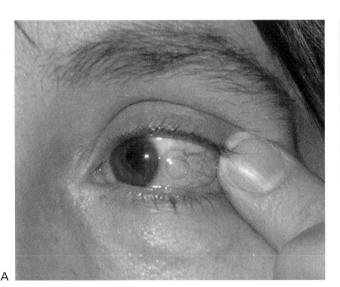
A

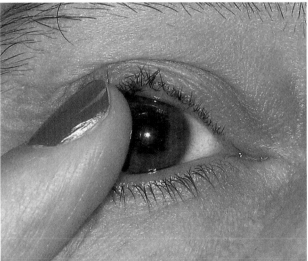
B

FIG. 13.7. To properly recenter a gas permeable lens, the patient must first look in the opposite direction of the lens **(A)**. The lens is gently nudged onto the cornea as the patient shifts gaze toward the lens **(B)**.

This has been shown to be a much greater problem in former PMMA wearers (80). These patients may be accustomed to lens care habits (i.e., cleaning between the fingers, storing in a dry state, carelessness in handling) for which little or no penalty results with PMMA. Because GP lenses appear similar to PMMA lenses, it is easy to understand why patients may mistakenly assume that the GP lenses can be cared for and handled in the same way as PMMA lenses. Patients should be warned about what can occur with noncompliance, and the proper cleaning techniques should be demonstrated at follow-up visits.

It is important to note that patients should be told what *not* to use in cleaning the lenses and why. Former PMMA wearers may have used products such as baking soda, toothpaste, baby shampoo, or dishwashing liquid to clean their lenses. It should be emphasized that these products are not approved for use with GP lenses and may be irritating and harmful to surface wettability.

Patients should be warned of the so-called "left lens syndrome." This pertains to the problem of patients who clean the right lens first and more thoroughly than the left. Eventually, the left lens becomes more deposit bound and problematic to the patient. Simply bringing this potential problem to the patient's attention should be sufficient to prevent its eventual occurrence.

In addition to a surfactant cleaner, use of an enzymatic cleaner should be recommended with some patients. Both extended wear and borderline dry eye patients should be started with enzyme cleaner. Other patients also may benefit from enzymatic cleaning, which can be provided once it has been established that surface deposits have been problematic.

Care Regimen

Every patient should know what solutions they can and cannot use with their lenses and why. For example, it should be emphasized that although other solutions (i.e., rigid and hydrogel) may cost less and appear to have similar functions, changing to such solutions may cause redness, burning, and reduced surface wettability. The specific recommended solutions and any acceptable alternative solutions should be provided as part of the patient instruction materials. In addition, progress evaluation visit forms should have a space for solutions such that patients can be asked to provide brand names of their care regimens at each visit.

Every product in the care kit provided to a new GP patient should be explained to the patient. What the assistant and practitioner believe is common sense may be confusing to the patient. It cannot be assumed that every patient will carefully read and understand product labels and care instructions. It is not uncommon for patients to believe that their wetting/soaking solution also cleans the lenses or that their wetting/soaking solution is used for wetting and soaking. In addition, there may be products in the kit that are

not desired by the practitioner (i.e., enzyme or lubricant); therefore, these should be omitted and, if desired, other products substituted. If each product is explained and the patient still appears to be confused, the specific care instructions for each care product can be provided in written form.

Rewetting or relubricating drops, although more important as an adjunct for rehydrating hydrogel lenses, do provide some important functions with GP lenses. Specifically, these solutions can rewet the lens surface while rinsing loosely adherent debris off of the lens surfaces. They can be used on an as-needed basis.

Patients should be advised *always* to soak the lenses in the recommended disinfecting solution, not in the dry state. Soaking the lenses overnight has numerous benefits as listed earlier in the section on wet versus dry storage issues.

In addition, the patient should be advised against "topping off" their disinfecting solution, which involves adding a small amount to top off what is already in the case instead of replacing the solution every night. The resulting solution is less efficacious and may cause potential sight-threatening ocular complications.

The lens case should have several important features to be effective for GP lens storage. It should easily differentiate left from right lenses. Many cases have an "L" and an "R" in the lens well or on the cap cover to serve as a reminder (Fig. 13.8). In addition, use of a hard plastic, ribbed, and deep-welled case is recommended, both to allow sufficient solution in the wells and to minimize leakage. The more flexible super permeable lens materials can adhere to a smooth-welled case if placed improperly (e.g., convex side up) in the case, possibly resulting in warpage due to the

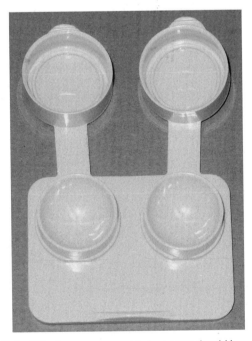

FIG. 13.8. Effective gas permeable lens cases should have ridges or holes in the well to minimize adhesion.

force required to remove the lens from the case. Also, lenses adhered to the bottom of a smooth-surface case may experience edge chipping from the excessive digital pressure needed to dislodge the lens. Using a case that has ridges or holes in the wells can eliminate both of these problems.

The moist environment of the contact lens storage case is a favorable environment for microbial growth. Biofilm, excreted by the bacteria, forms a "bathtub ring" film, which protects the microorganisms from the soaking solution and renders the disinfecting solution less effective. Bacterial biofilm formation on contact lens storage cases may be a risk factor for contact lens-associated corneal infection (81). Consequently, lens case care is an important component of patient education. Daily rinsing, allowing the case to air dry, and weekly cleaning with lens cleaner and a toothbrush exemplify good lens storage case hygiene (82). Patients also should be educated to replace the lens storage case on a frequent basis.

Scratches

Every patient should be warned about the softness of the lens materials, especially the super permeable materials. Lenses should be handled over a towel or soft tissue. If the concave surface of the lens comes in contact with a hard surface, a drop of wetting solution can be placed on a finger and the lens gently lifted off the surface.

Foreign-Body Particles

Patients wearing GP lenses should be informed about the possibility of dust or debris becoming trapped underneath the lens and irritating the cornea. If this trapping results in greater than momentary discomfort, the patient should be told to remove the lens and clean it. If the discomfort persists after lens removal or upon lens reinsertion, the patient should call the practitioner's office.

Cosmetics

Every contact lens patient should be thoroughly educated about the proper use of cosmetics. Cosmetics can cause lens discoloration, damage, and surface deposition. Because many popular cosmetics contain ingredients such as preservatives, pigments, oils, and cleaners, subjective discomfort and eye infection can result from their use (83). Cosmetics should be applied after lenses have been inserted. Mascara that contains "lash builders" can cause severe problems. These nylon or rayon fibers can flake off into the tear film, resulting in corneal abrasion. This is especially problematic with rigid extended wear lens patients in whom these flakes are trapped underneath an adherent lens during sleep (84). Bacterial infection is also a problem (85). A patient may transfer infectious organisms from the lashes to the mascara wand and then to the mascara tube, where they colonize.

In addition, eyeliner should not be applied to the inner lid margin because it may clog the meibomian glands, possibly resulting in blepharitis, hordeolum, or chalazion.

Numerous cosmetic products on the market are recommended for contact lens wearers. They are water soluble and contain little, if any, fragrances of fillers. Some practitioners carry such a line of cosmetic products in their office and include samples in the patient's initial care regimen. It is important to note again that cosmetics should be applied after lenses have been inserted. Any cream or oil that is used on the face or hands can be transferred to the contact lenses, resulting in discomfort and blurred vision; therefore, these substances should be applied after the lenses have been inserted. Any contaminant or residual oils on the hands can be transferred to the lens and possibly absorbed into the lens matrix. Hand soaps contain additives such as oils, perfumes, dyes, deodorants, and abrasives that can complicate the problem (86). The addition of a compatible hand cleaner developed specifically for contact lens wearers to the care regimen will minimize discoloration and deposit buildup on contact lenses. Two such cleaners are Optisoap (Optikem International, P.O. Box 27319, Denver, CO 80227) and Eye-care Special Hand Soap (Channel Laboratories, Ltd., 1215 Boissevain Avenue, Norfolk, VA 23507) (87).

Swimming

Rigid lens patients should be advised not to swim with their contact lenses unless watertight swimmer's goggles or a diving mask is worn (88). If a patient swims with the GP lenses but without goggles, he or she should know about the strong likelihood of lens loss, as well as the potential risk for ocular infection.

Adaptation

Patients should be told that adaptation varies from person to person, with an average of 10 to 14 days before the achievement of no lens awareness. This period can be estimated by how much tearing and discomfort is experienced at the dispensing visit. However, the patient also should know that it could last as long as 4 weeks in some people. The patient should be reassured that comfort typically will improve on a daily basis. Avoiding the use of sensitizing words such as pain and discomfort is helpful in reassuring the patient. Normal and abnormal adaptation symptoms are listed in Table 13.5. In addition, the patient should be told that, if lens wear must temporarily be discontinued (i.e., because of irritation or a lost lens), wearing time will need to be rebuilt gradually. A typical wearing schedule is as follows:

Day 1: 4 hours
Day 2: 4 hours
Day 3: 6 hours

TABLE 13.5. NORMAL AND ABNORMAL RIGID LENS ADAPTATION SYMPTOMS

Normal Adaptation Symptoms (Diminish Gradually)

1. Tearing. This is the natural response by eyelids that are not accustomed to having foreign objects on them. It will subside rapidly as wearing time increases.
2. Minor irritation. This tickling or awareness sensation gradually disappears with wear. It may cause mild discomfort on upward gaze due to the lens coming in contact with the upper lid.
3. Intermittent blurry vision. This usually is due to excess tears.
4. Light sensitivity as well as extra sensitivity to wind, smoke, and dust
5. Mild redness. This is common in patients with allergies or chronic sinus problems.

Abnormal Symptoms (Occur Suddenly)

1. Sudden pain or burning (greater than minor irritation). If a sudden sharp pain is felt, it probably is due to a dust particle or a lash under the lens. Remove, clean, and reinsert the lens.
2. Severe or persistent haze halo seen around lights
3. Severe redness or irritation
4. Blurry vision through spectacles for >1 hour
5. Increasing eye discharge or mattering
6. Lens adhering to the eye

Day 4: 6 hours
Day 5: 8 hours
Day 6: 8 hours
Day 7: 10 hours
Day 8: 10 hours

Current all-day rigid lens wearers should be able to go immediately into a full 12-hour wearing schedule after receiving their new GP lenses. All daily wear patients should be told to wear their lenses a minimum of 4 hours before their scheduled progress evaluation; therefore, it is important to schedule these visits in the afternoon or evening. Exceptions to this are GP extended wear patients, who should be seen in the morning. Progress visits for a daily wear patient should be scheduled as follows:

Visit 1: 1 week after dispensing
Visit 2: 1 month after visit 1
Visit 3: 3 months after visit 2
Visit 4: 6 months after visit 3

After the 6-month visit, patients should be scheduled at regular 6-month intervals.

For the extended wear patient, visits should be scheduled as follows:

Visit 1: 1 week after dispensing (daily wear)
Visit 2: 24 hours after initiating extended wear
Visit 3: 1 week after initiating extended wear
Visit 4: 2 weeks after visit 3
Visit 5: 1 month after visit 4
Visit 6: 3 months after visit 5

After the initial six visits, progress evaluations should be scheduled every 3 months for the extended wear patient.

Educational Materials

A four-step education process is recommended. This includes written information, verbal instruction, video demonstration, and ongoing reinforcement.

Written Information

A patient instructional manual is beneficial in the education process. It should be comprehensive and contain the information listed in Table 13.6. In addition, it should be written in layman's language, with a print quality that makes it easy for a patient to read, understand, and comply with the information presented. This manual can include customized inserts on information such as a fee or compliance agreement, cosmetic use, and extended wear. In some communities it may be beneficial to have inserts in multiple languages. It also can have a patient agreement that has important information such as the refund policy and care regimen (Fig. 13.9).

The instruction manuals preferably should be printed professionally or by a desktop publishing system. Small typewritten or poor-quality print will discourage the patient from reading the manual. Graphics showing how to handle the lenses also are beneficial. A graphic artist can provide these, or a manual complete with graphics can be obtained from Anadem Publications, Inc. (P.O. Box 14385, Columbus, OH 43214). The standard booklet from Anadem includes information with accompanying illustrations about rigid lenses, specialty lenses, proper blinking, insertion, re-

TABLE 13.6. CHECKLIST FOR GAS PERMEABLE LENS PATIENT INSTRUCTION MANUAL

1. Composition, benefits, and applications of a rigid gas permeable lens
2. Insertion, removal, and decentration
3. Cleaning techniques
4. Normal and abnormal adaptation symptoms (see Table 13.1)
5. Importance of adhering to prescribed wearing schedule
6. Causes of reduced wear (e.g., colds, hay fever, medications)
7. Importance of using the recommended care regimen (not saliva or nonrecommended brands); alternative acceptable solutions
8. How to minimize loss and surface damage
9. Benefits of a spare pair of lenses or spectacles
10. Swimming and showering
11. Cosmetic use
12. Caring for the lens case
13. Visit schedule
14. Fee and refund policy
15. Service agreement
16. Office telephone number
17. Doctor's after-hours emergency telephone number

Contact Lens Service

IN CASE OF EMERGENCY:

1. **During normal business hours**: please **remove** the contact lenses and call for an appointment at the Contact Lens Service, 516-5609 or Center for Eye Care, 516-5131 during clinic hours. You may leave a message at 516-5609 after clinic hours or if the phone is in use. We will return your call as soon as possible. If you have lost or damaged a contact lens, and need a replacement lens, please call the Contact Lens Service (516-5609).

2. **After hours**: if you remove the contact lens and the problem persists even after contact lens wear is discontinued, please contact us at 407-5375 or go to the nearest emergency service. This number is for <u>eye emergencies only</u> and is **not** for contact lens replacements. No one at this number will be able to provide you with a contact lens replacement.

REFUND POLICY:

It is our belief that most patients can be successfully fit with contact lenses. If we determine that a patient can not be successfully fit at the fitting examination, we inform the patient at that time and do not fit contact lenses. After a patient receives lenses, we try our best to work with a patient experiencing difficulty with lens wear, lens handling or vision, so that they may be successful. This may require ordering new or different lenses. If a patient is not happy with their contact lenses and wants to return their lenses within 60 days of the dispensing, we will refund a portion of their lens fees. Fitting fees are non-refundable. Please return for recommended follow-up visits so that potential lens wear difficulties may be addressed as early as possible. If you are experiencing any contact lens problems and do not have an appointment scheduled, please call to make a follow-up appointment as soon as possible.

REPLACEMENT POLICY:
Rigid Contact Lenses:
DW/EW Rigid lens*......................
*Keratoconic & High minus lenses
Toric Rigid lens...........................
Bifocal ....
Soft Contact Lenses:
DW SCL......................................
EW/Tinted SCL............................
Toric...
Bifocal ....
Prosthetic ....
FRP/Disposable........................

The fitting fee includes contact lenses, starter kit of solutions and 4 months of contact lens follow-up visits. Follow-up visits are suggested every 6 months after the initial period. The standard fee for a follow-up visit is $ A comprehensive eye examination should be performed every year.

Please be advised that a contact lens is a FDA regulated medical device used in direct contact with the eye, and has potential to cause damage to the eye. Ongoing professional care is essential in maintaining the safe use of contact lenses. Missouri State law does not require the release of a contact lens prescription to an individual; therefore, the release of your contact lens prescription is conditional upon your identification of either a licensed optometrist or ophthalmologist that will monitor and be responsible for your eye health while wearing contact lenses. Your contact lens prescription is not final until the contact lenses have been dispensed and followed for a period of time to ensure that the lens fit and prescription is accurate. Your contact lens prescription expires one year from your fitting examination.

FEES AND COSTS ARE SUBJECT TO PERIODIC REVISIONS

STATEMENT BY PATIENT
This is to certify that I received instructions in the proper methods of insertion, removal, use and care of my contact lenses; and have reviewed the information on this page. Having proven myself to be competent enough to carry out these instructions, the contact lenses were given to me. I realize that success with contact lenses cannot be guaranteed and that any refund will be subject to the policy outlined on this page.

_____   _____
Patient's Signature   Student Intern's Signature

_____   _____
Date   Clinical Instructor's Signature

FIG. 13.9. Representative patient agreement and education form.

moval, and care. If the office has an Apple or IBM-compatible computer, a floppy diskette that allows the practitioner to customize the information provided to GP lens patients can be ordered.

It should be noted that from a medical-legal point of view, an informed consent document listing wearing schedule and solution brands should be signed and dated by the patient (89). In a court of law two rules apply: (i) records are witnesses that never lie, and (ii) work not written is work not done. These records should be signed in duplicate; for example, the second form can be attached by perforation and easily removed for the patient's permanent record.

Verbal Instruction

The assistant can discuss the most important information with the patient and encourage the patient to ask questions. It should be emphasized that the *verbal* educational process is much more important than the written process because patients cannot be expected to understand all the information provided, and, on occasion, the manual may not be read at all.

Video Demonstration

An innovative and effective method of patient education is the use of video tapes. Rigid lens instructional videos produced by the Contact Lens Manufacturers Association (CLMA) and the RGP Lens Institute (RGPLI; *www.rgpli.org*) are available from the CLMA (1-800-344-9060) (90). If there are any reservations as to a patient's ability to handle or care for contact lenses, a video reviewed together in the office or for viewing at home is an excellent supplement to the instruction manual. Additional educational materials related to GP lens wear are available on the Internet. For example, the Rigid Gas Permeable Lens Institute, the educational division of the CLMA, maintains a web site targeted at consumers *(www.contactlenses.org)* (91).

Reinforcement

An invaluable method of patient education is reinforcement of important care instructions at follow-up visits. In one study, approximately 50% of the care samples were contaminated when instructions were not reinforced, whereas only 6% were contaminated when the manufacturers' care instructions were reinforced at every follow-up visit (8). The practitioner should inquire if the patient has any problems handling lenses, confirm that he or she is still using the recommended solutions, monitor the wearing time, and verify that the lenses are being cleaned properly upon removal at night. Any noncompliance should be noted in the patient's record.

SUMMARY

Rigid lenses provide easier care and a less expensive solution regimen than traditional hydrogel lenses. In addition, there is less risk of surface contamination and preservative sensitivity with GP lenses. Nevertheless, comprehensive and effective patient education is extremely important for the eventual success of the patient. If a GP wearer does not feel confident in handling lenses or is not properly educated about lens care and cleaning, failure most likely will result, with a loss in motivation for future contact lens wear.

REFERENCES

1. Bennett ES, Grohe RM. Lens care and solutions. In Bennett ES, Grohe RM, eds: *Rigid gas permeable contact lenses.* New York: Professional Press. 1986:225–246.
2. Mandell RB. Lens care and storage. In Mandell RB, ed: *Contact lens practice,* 4th ed. Springfield, IL: Charles C. Thomas, 1988: 326–351.
3. Hopkins GA. The formulation of rigid lens care systems. *Optician* 1986;191:18.
4. Brown MRW, Richards RME. Effect of ethylenediaminetetraacetate on the resistance of *Pseudomonas aeruginosa* to antibacterial agents. *Nature* 1965;207:1391.
5. MacKeen GD, Bulle K. Buffers and preservatives in contact lens solutions. *Contacto* 1977;21:33.
6. Herskowitz R. Solution interaction and gas-permeable lens performance. *Contact Lens J* 1987;15:3.
7. Rosenthal P, Chou MH, Salamone JC, et al. Preservation interaction with GP lenses. *Optician* 1986;192:33.
8. Lieblein JS. Overview of soft contact lens hygiene. *Rev Optom* 1978;115:29.
9. McLaughlin R, Barr JT, Rosenthal P, et al. The new generation of RGP solutions meets increasing demands. *Contact Lens Spectrum* 1990;5:45.
10. Mondino BJ, Groden LR. Conjunctival hyperemia and corneal infiltrates with chemically disinfected soft contact lenses. *Arch Ophthalmol* 1980;98:1767.
11. Binder PS, Rasmussen DM, Gordon M. Keratoconjunctivitis and soft contact lens solutions. *Arch Ophthalmol* 1981;99:87.
12. Witten EM, Molinari JF. Allergic keratoconjunctivitis from thimerosal in soft contact lens solutions. *South J Optom* 1981;23: 12.
13. Erikson S, et al. Suitability of thimerosal as a preservative in soft lens soaking solutions. In: Bitonte JL, Keates RH, eds. *Symposium on the flexible lens.* St Louis: CV Mosby, 1972.
14. Bach FC, Hansard JD. The germicidal action of contact lens soaking tablets. *Contacto* 1971;5:21.
15. Richards RME, McBride RJ. The preservation of ophthalmic solutions with antibacterial combinations. *J Pharm Pharmacol* 1972;24:145.
16. Huth S, Cohn L, Eriksen S. Care products for silicone-copolymer lens materials. *Optician* 1986;181:16.
17. Petricciani R, Krezanoski J. Preservative interaction with contact lenses. *Contacto* 1977;21:6.
18. Macaregor DR, Elliker PR. A comparison of some properties of strains of *Pseudomonas aeruginosa* sensitive and resistant to quaternary ammonium compounds. *Can J Microbiol* 1968;4:449.
19. Feldman GL. Benzyl alcohol. New life as an ophthalmic preservative. *Contact Lens Spectrum* 1989;4:41.
20. Weisbarth RE. Hydrogel lens care regimens and patient educa-

tion. In: Bennett ES, Weissman BA, eds. *Clinical contact lens practice.* Philadelphia: Lippincott, 1993:1–27.

21. McLaughlin R, Barr JT. Contact lens solutions update. *Contact Lens Spectrum* 1989;4:21.
22. Hom MM. Current multi-purpose solutions concepts. *Contact Lens Spectrum* 2001;9:33–39.
23. Gasson A, Morris J. Care systems. In: Gasson A, Morris J, eds: *The contact lens manual.* Oxford, England: Butterworth-Heinemann, 1992:234–244.
24. Olivieri J, Eigenmann PA, Hauser C. Severe anaphylaxis to a new disinfectant: polyhexanide, a chlorhexidine polymer. *Schweiz Med Wochenschr* 1998;128:1508–1511.
25. Hill RM, Terry JE. Ophthalmic solutions: viscosity builders. *Am J Optom Physiol Opt* 1974;51:847.
26. Krishna N, Brow F. Polyvinyl alcohol as an ophthalmic vehicle. *Am J Ophthalmol* 1964;57:99.
27. *Tyler's quarterly soft contact lens parameter guide.* 2003;20:52–53.
28. Chou MH, Rosenthal P, Salamone JC. Which cleaning solution works best? *Contact Lens Forum* 1985;10:41.
29. Doell GB, Palombi DL, Egan DJ. Contact lens surface changes after exposure to surfactant and abrasive cleaning procedures. *Am J Optom Physiol Opt* 1986;63:399.
30. Carrell BA, Bennett ES, Henry VA, et al. The effect of rigid gas permeable lens cleaners on lens parameter stability. J *Am Optom Assoc* 1992;63:193.
31. Bennett ES, Henry VA. Rigid lens power change with abrasive cleaner use. *Int Contact Lens Clin* 1990;17:152.
32. Caroline PJ, Andre MP. Inadvertent patient modification of RGP lenses. *Contact Lens Spectrum* 1999;14:56.
33. Feldman G. Manufacturer's report: a new system for RGP lens care. *Contact Lens Forum* 1989;14:48.
34. Pederson K. Exploring the differences in today's lens care options. *Contact Lens Spectrum* 1999;5:29–32.
35. Watanabe RK, Rah MJ. Preventative contact lens care: part III. *Contact Lens Spectrum* 2001;8:26–32.
36. Barr JT. Contact lens solutions and lens care update. *Contact Lens Spectrum* 2001;6:26–33.
37. McLaughlin R. Rub vs. no rub: skipping the rub leads to dirty lenses and complications. *Contact Lens Spectrum* 2001;9:40.
38. Edrington TB, Barr JT. Keep up-to-date with changes in soft lens solutions. *Contact Lens Spectrum* 2002;4:46.
39. Norman C. Solutions for keeping RGPs in top form. *Contact Lens Spectrum* 1998;10:165–185.
40. Lasswell LA, Tarantino N, Kono D. Enzymatic cleaning of extended-wear lenses: papain vs. pancreatin. *Int Eyecare* 1986;2:101.
41. Lowther GE. Caring for hard GP lenses. *Int Contact Lens Clin* 1984;11:75.
42. Caffery B, Cotter J, White P. Dry eye: a common and complicated problem. *Contact Lens Spectrum* 1997;5:41–48.
43. Walters KA, et al. The interaction of benzalkonium chloride with Boston contact lens materials. I. Basic interaction studies. *J Br Contact Lens Assoc* 1982;6:42.
44. Walters KA, et al. The interaction of benzalkonium chloride with Boston contact lens materials. II. *J Br Contact Lens Assoc* 1983;6:42.
45. Richardson NE, et al. The compatibility of benzalkonium chloride with a CAB lens material. *J Br Contact Lens Assoc* 1980;3:120.
46. Rosenthal P. Absorption of BAK. A differing view. Heard at the forum. *Contact Lens Forum* 1986;11:56.
47. John T, Desai D, Sahm D. Adherence of Acanthamoeba castellanii to new daily wear, extended wear, and disposable soft contact lenses. *CLAO J* 1991;17:109.
48. Kilvington S, Larkin DF, White DG, et al. Laboratory investigation of Acanthamoeba keratitis. *J Clin Microbiol* 1990;28:2722.

49. Seal DV, Bennett ES, McFadyen AK, et al. Differential adherence of Acanthamoeba to contact lenses: Effects of material characteristics. *Optom Vis Sci* 1995;72:23–28.
50. Radford CF, Lehmann OJ, Dart JK, for the National Acanthamoeba Keratitis Study Group. Acanthamoeba keratitis: multi-centre survey in England 1992–6. *Br J Ophthalmol* 1998;82:1387–1392.
51. Niszl IA. Markus MB. Anti-Acanthamoeba activity of contact lens solutions. *Br J Ophthalmol* 1988;2:1033–1038.
52. Buck SL, Rosenthal RA, Schlech BA. Methods used to evaluate the effectiveness of contact lens care solutions and other compounds against Acanthamoeba: a review of the literature. *CLAO J* 2000;26:72–84.
53. Rosenthal RA, McAnally CL, McNamee LS, et al. Broad spectrum antimicrobial activity of a new multi-purpose disinfecting solution. *CLAO J* 2000;26:120–126.
54. Kilvington S, Anger C. A comparison of cyst age and assay method of the efficacy of contact lens disinfectants against Acanthamoeba. *Br J Ophthalmol* 2001;85:336–340.
55. Hiti K, Walochnik J, Haller-Schober EM, et al. Viability of Acanthamoeba after exposure to a multipurpose disinfecting contact lens solution and two hydrogen peroxide systems. *Br J Ophthalmol* 2002;86:144–146.
56. Begley CG, Waggoner PJ, Hafner GS, et al. Effect of rigid gas permeable contact lens wetting solutions on the rabbit corneal epithelium. *Optom Vis Sci* 1991;68:189.
57. Begley CG, Weirich B, Benak J, et al. Effects of rigid gas permeable contact lens solutions on the human corneal epithelium. *Optom Vis Sci* 1992;69:347.
58. Shih KL, Hu J, Sibley MJ. The microbiological benefit of cleaning and rinsing contact lenses. *Int Contact Lens Clin* 1985;12:235.
59. *Clinical practice guidelines for optometry. Care of the contact lens patient.* American Optometric Association, 2000:23.
60. U.S. Food and Drug Administration, National Institutes of Health, Centers for Disease Control. Current trends: recommendations for preventing possible transmission of human T-lymphotropic virus type III/ Lymphadenopathy-associated virus from tears. *MMWR Morb Mortal Wkly Rep* 1998;34:533–534.
61. Szczotka LB. In-office RGP lens disinfection. *Contact Lens Spectrum* 2001;11:17.
62. Barr JT. Contact Lenses 2000. *Contact Lens Spectrum* 2001;23–31.
63. Donzis PB, Mondino BJ, Weissman BA, et al. Microbial contamination of contact lens care systems. *Am J Ophthalmol* 1987;104:325.
64. Smith RE, MacRae SM. Contact lenses: convenience and complications. *N Engl J Med* 1989;321:824.
65. Ghormley NR. Contact lens compliance: a solution? *Int Contact Lens Clin* 1989;16:250.
66. Meichenbaum D, Turk DC: *Facilitating treatment adherence.* New York: Plenum Press, 1987.
67. Podell RN, Gary LR. Compliance. A problem in medical management. *Am Fam Physician* 1976;13:74–80.
68. Koenig SB, Solomon JM, Hyndiuk RA, et al. *Acanthamoeba* keratitis associated with gas-permeable contact lens wear. *Am J Ophthalmol* 1987;103:832.
69. Bennett ES. Should tap water be used with RGP lenses? Presented at Contact '92, Anaheim, California, July 1992.
70. Shovlin JP. Acanthamoeba keratitis in rigid lens wearers: the issue of tap water rinses. *Int Contact Lens Clin* 1990;17:47.
71. Berenblatt AJ. Lens care systems: a practitioner's wish list. *Contact Lens Forum* 1988;13:37.
72. Sibley MJ, Barr JT, et al. Lubricating and rewetting solutions: a roundtable discussion—part 1. *Contact Lens Spectrum* 1989;4:41.

73. Greco A. Lubricating drops for hard and soft contact lenses. *Int Contact Lens Clin* 1985;12:205.

74. Carney LG, Hill RM, Barr JT, et al. Rigid lens care solutions: how different are they? *Contact Lens Spectrum* 1988;3:78.

75. Herman JP. Flexure of rigid contact lenses on toric corneas as a function of base curve fitting relationship. *J Am Optom Assoc* 1983;54:209.

76. Egan DJ, Bennett ES. Trouble-shooting rigid contact lens flexure: a case report. *Int Contact Lens Clin* 1985;12:147.

77. Grohe RM, Caroline PJ. RGP non-wetting lens syndrome. *Contact Lens Spectrum* 1989;4:32.

78. Lowther GE. Effect of some solutions on HGP contact lens parameters. *J Am Optom Assoc* 1987;58:188.

79. Rakow PL. Solution incompatibilities and confusion: observations and caveats. *Contact Lens Forum* 1989;14:60.

80. Henry VA, Bennett ES, Forrest J. Clinical investigation of the Paraperm EW rigid gas-permeable contact lens. *Am J Optom Physiol Opt* 1987;4:313.

81. McLaughlin-Borlace L, Stapleton F, Matheson M, et al. Bacterial biofilm on contact lenses and lens storage cases in wearers with microbial keratitis. *J Appl Microbiol* 1998;84:827–838.

82. Caroline PJ, André MP. Combatting the dreaded contact lens case. Contact lens case reports. *Contact Lens Spectrum* 2000;4:57.

83. Baldwin JS. Cosmetics: too long concealed as culprit in eye problems. *Contact Lens Forum* 1986;11:38.

84. Bennett ES, Ghormley NR. Rigid extended wear: an overview. *Int Contact Lens Clin* 1987;14:319.

85. Ng A, Mostardi B, Mandell RB. Adherence of mascara to soft contact lenses. *Int Contact Lens Clin* 1988;15:64.

86. Hoffman WC, Cook SA. Reducing lens spoilage via CL wearers' hand soap. *Contact Lens Forum* 1986;11:44.

87. Ghormley NR. Contact lens care. Hand soap? *Int Contact Lens Clin* 1984;11:318.

88. Barr JT. Swimming while wearing contact lenses. *Contact Lens Spectrum* 2002;8:15.

89. Harris MG. Is your CL practice vulnerable to legal action? *Contact Lens Spectrum* 1990;5:51.

90. *RGPLI Online,* the official site of the RGP Lens Institute. Available at: *http://www.rgpli.org*

91. *Contact lenses: a guide from the Contact Lens Manufacturers Association.* Available at: *http://www.contactlenses.org.*

INSPECTION AND VERIFICATION OF GAS-PERMEABLE CONTACT LENSES

**VINITA ALLEE HENRY AND
EDWARD S. BENNETT**

Inspection and verification of the contact lens is an important step in the successful fit of a gas permeable (GP) contact lens that often is regarded as unnecessary; yet it may be the most crucial step of all. This includes verifying the diagnostic lenses, previous lenses worn by the patient, and the lenses to be dispensed. The fit may not be satisfactory if the lenses are not manufactured to within tolerance of the practitioner's specifications, and patient comfort will be unsatisfactory if the edges are poor. This task of inspection and verification, although time consuming, is not difficult.

LENS PARAMETER VERIFICATION

Contact Lens Power

Contact lens power is determined by a lensometer in much the same way as is spectacle lens power. However, because a spectacle lens has a much flatter base curve, the sagittal depth of a contact lens over the lens stop of the lensometer is much greater than that of a spectacle lens (Fig. 14.1) (1, 2). This difference results in an error in the power measurement that increases the back vertex power of minus lenses. The error is most significant in high prescriptions (2,3). Most lensometers correct for this by a special accessory device that compensates for the difference (Fig. 14.2). This device positions a lens with its vertex point against the lens stop, assuring precise power measurements.

Back vertex power can be determined by placing the concave side of the contact lens against the proper lens stop. Likewise, front vertex power can be determined by placing the convex surface against the lens stop. Practitioners generally use back vertex power as phoropters, corrected curve trial lenses and spectacle lenses are measured in terms of back vertex power. However, it would be best to determine which method is used by the specific laboratory. Very little difference will be found between front and back vertex powers, except in high-plus prescriptions where as much as 1 D difference can be found between front and back vertex measurements (2,3). For example, a lens with a +15.00 D

back vertex power, base curve radius (BCR) of 43 D, and center thickness of 0.70 mm will have a front vertex power of +16.00 D (4).

In preparing to measure contact lens power, the eyepiece of the lensometer should be adjusted for the individual user by rotating the eyepiece counterclockwise to blur the lines on the reticule. Then it should be slowly rotated clockwise until the lines are sharply in focus (Fig. 14.3). With no lens in the lensometer, the target should be in focus when the power drum is set at zero.

After adjusting the lensometer, the clean, dry contact lens should be placed concave side against the lens stop. It can be gently held in this position with the thumb and index finger, or the lensometer can be set in a vertical position, allowing the lens to rest on the lens stop. If the lens is held on the lens stop, caution must be taken not to flex the lens by applying too much pressure, which may distort the mires or give an incorrect measurement. The power can be determined by turning the power drum toward the user until the target comes into sharp focus (2,5). The power should be within ±0.12 D for lens powers of ±10.00 D and within ±0.25 D for powers greater than ±10.00 D.

In order to measure prism on the contact lens, the contact lens must be centered carefully on the lens stop. A decentered lens provides an incorrect prism reading. With the target in focus, the amount of prism power can be determined by the amount of target decentration in relation to the center of the reticule. The reticule is designed with dark concentric rings corresponding to powers of 1.00 to 5.00 prism diopters (Fig. 14.4). For example, when the center of the target is on the first dark concentric ring of the reticule, it corresponds to one prism diopter.

Prism is used in front-toric contact lenses to prevent excessive lens rotation. When verifying a front-toric lens, it is placed on the lens stop with the center of the mires directly below the center of the reticule, which is the base down position of the prism (2). The sphere, cylinder, and axis are determined in minus cylinder form by positioning the power drum at the most plus reading. The cylinder axis

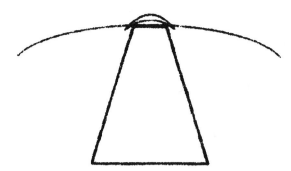

FIG. 14.1. Diagram demonstrating sagittal depth difference of a contact lens versus a spectacle lens on the lensometer stop without the use of a contact lens accessory device.

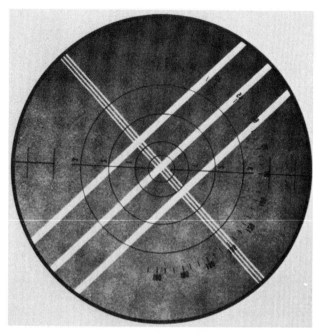

FIG. 14.3. Lensometer mire image in sharp focus.

should be rotated until the sphere target (three closely spaced lines) is in sharp focus. The power drum then is rotated to focus sharply the cylinder target (three lines spaced further apart). The sphere is the power found when the sphere target is in sharp focus. The cylinder power, in minus cylinder form, is the difference between the sphere power and the cylinder target focus point. The axis location is given on the cylinder axis drum (5).

In lenses with toric curves and no prism, the power is not recorded in cylindrical form but as the power found in each meridian, for example, BCRs 7.94/7.46 mm and Rx −3.75 D/ −6.75 D.

Base Curve Radius

The BCR of a GP contact lens can be determined using a radiuscope or keratometer; however, the radiuscope is the most commonly used and most accurate method. The ra-

diuscope uses the Drysdale principle to determine the radius of curvature by measuring the difference between the lens surface and the center of curvature (Fig. 14.5) (6).

GP lenses absorb some solution when they are soaked in an aqueous solution. This, in turn, can cause the BCR to flatten (3). Low myopic and hyperopic prescriptions have been found to be quite stable; however, as the center thick-

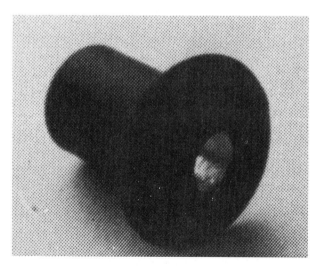

FIG. 14.2. Example of a contact lens accessory device for the lensometer.

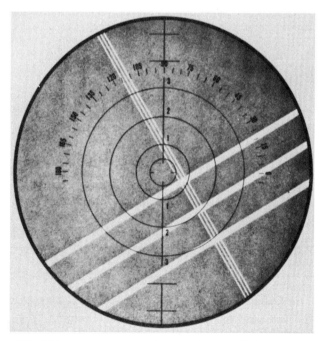

FIG. 14.4. Lensometer mire image of a prism-ballasted lens.

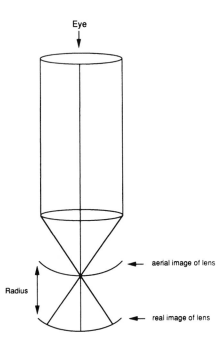

FIG. 14.5. Diagram demonstrating the Drysdale principle of the radiuscope.

ness of the lens decreases, as in high myopic prescriptions, the variation in BCR increases. This change in BCR of GP lenses may change the lens-to-cornea fitting relationship. As a result, it is extremely important to verify the BCR in both the dry and wet states to determine if BCR flattening is present. Likewise, a lens stored dry and then placed in contact with the tear film may exhibit a similar change in BCR. Therefore, it is important to maintain the lens in the hydrated state. Minimum recommended soaking times vary, but a soaking time of 12 to 24 hours should be adequate for determining base curve variations (3,7,8).

The steps for measuring the concave surface of BCR of a contact lens using the American Optical radiuscope are as follows (Courtesy of American Optical, Buffalo, NY):

1. Be certain that the contact lens is clean and dry.

2. Put a drop of water in the depression on the concave lens mount. Place the contact lens in the depression with the concave surface to be measured facing upward.

3. Position the lens mount in its support on the stage of the instrument. The mount should be reasonably level in its support and the lens level in its mount so that the center of the lens surface is normal to the optical axis of the microscope (Figs. 14.6 and 14.7).

4. Set the illumination control knob to your preferred position.

5. Check the aperture selector of the illuminator to be certain that the large aperture is in "working" position. (When facing the instrument, push the selector to your left to position the large aperture properly.)

6. Fully lower the objective of the microscope using a coarse adjustment knob.

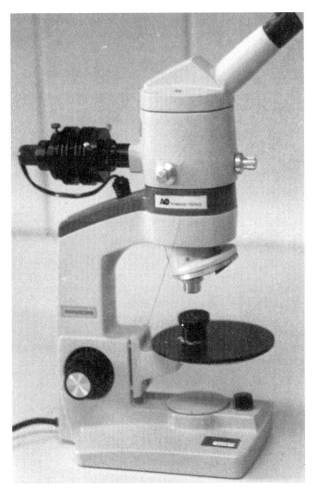

FIG. 14.6. Radiuscope.

7. Observe the beam of light coming from the objective and move the stage until the beam appears to be centered on the contact lens. The state can be rotated on its axis and moved in any horizontal direction by applying gentle pressure.

8. After visually centering the beam of light, fully raise the objective using a coarse adjustment knob. Note: If using a binocular model, adjust the interpupillary distance of the eyepiece(s).

9. Look into the eyepiece(s) and observe the scale on the right side of the field of view (Fig. 14.8). Bring this scale into sharpest focus using the scale focusing knob. If the same individual always uses the instrument, it is not necessary to make this focusing adjustment each time the radiuscope is used; however, it is important to occasionally reconfirm.

10. While viewing through the eyepiece(s), lower the objective slowly, using a coarse adjustment knob, until you see light come into focus forming part or all of a spoke pattern target (Fig. 14.9).

11. Move the stage horizontally until the target is centered in the field of view.

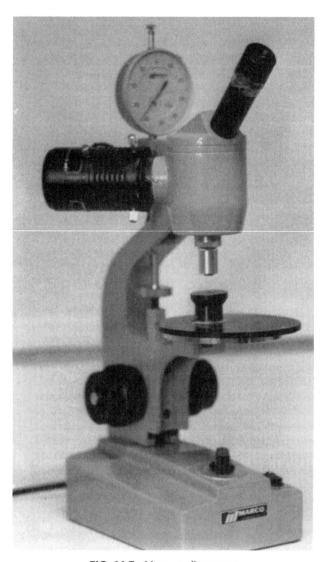

FIG. 14.7. Marco radiusgauge.

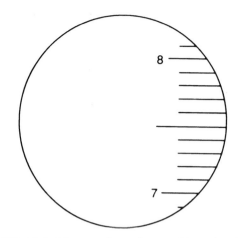

FIG. 14.8. Diagram of a radiuscope internal scale.

16. Bring the image of the target into sharp, clear focus using a fine adjustment knob.

17. If your original index line setting was at zero, read the radius of curvature directly from the scale at the position of the index line. If the original index line setting was at a plus whole number in the area on the scale below zero, add that whole number to the value shown by the index line at the aerial images.

To measure the convex radius, the procedure is generally the same as for the concave radius with one important exception: the positions of the aerial and real images are reversed. When measuring a convex radius, the "upper" image is the real image and the "lower" image is the aerial image. The steps are as follows:

12. Continue to lower the objective. At one point the filament of the lamp will come into focus. Disregard this image and continue lowering the objective with a coarse adjustment knob.

13. The target will again come into view. This is the "real" image of the target at the surface of the lens. As the focus begins to become sharper, change to a fine adjustment knob to bring the target into a clear, sharp focus.

14. When you have the target in clear focus, use the index adjustment knob to move the index line to zero. On occasion, you may not be able to move the index line to zero. In this case, set the index line to the nearest whole number.

15. Raise the objective until the upper (aerial) image of the target again comes into view. Raise the objective slightly beyond the point at which the image appears sharpest, then lower it. By focusing downward for final setting, more accurate readings are achieved.

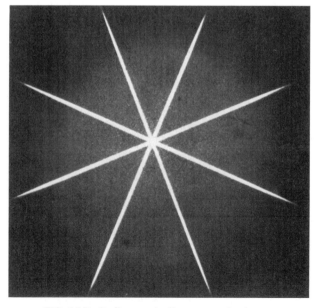

FIG. 14.9. Radiuscope/radiusgauge mire image.

1. Follow steps 1 through 5 used for concave measurement with the exception that in the convex lens mount the convex lens surface is facing upward (Fig. 14.10).

2. To center the beam of light on the convex lens surface (as described in step 7), the objective should be in the fully raised position. While in the raised position, bring the scale into sharpest focus using the scale focusing knob.

3. Fully lower the objective, then raise it until a spoke pattern target (the aerial image) comes into focus and center the target in the field of view.

4. Fully raise the objective, then lower it until the other target (the real image) comes into focus. Move the index line to the nearest whole number and note this number.

5. Continue lowering the objective to the lower target. Bring this into sharp focus, using the fine adjustment knob. Read the scale at the index line. Subtract this reading from the previously noted whole number. The difference is the radius of curvature of the convex lens surface measured.

The steps for measuring a toric base contact lens are as follows:

1. Follow steps 1 through 11 as before.

2. To orient the lens and mount properly, bring the target into the sharpest possible focus using a fine adjustment knob. Slowly turn the mount in a horizontal circular direction until one of the "spokes" of the target becomes clearer than the remaining spokes (Fig. 14.11). When turning, keep the whole target pattern centered in the field of view. It may be necessary to adjust the focus with a fine adjustment knob until this one spoke is in sharp focus. When this has been achieved, the lens is properly oriented for measurements

3. Lower the objective until the target (the real image) comes into view. Bring this into focus using a fine adjustment knob.

4. When you have the target in clear, sharp focus, use the index adjustment knob to move the index line to zero.

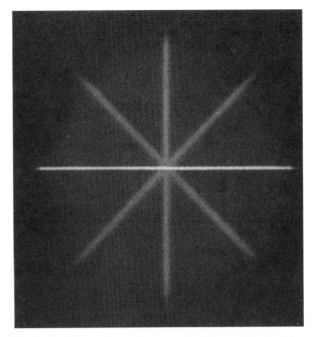

FIG. 14.11. Mire pattern of a warped or back-surface toric lens.

On occasion, you may not be able to move the index line to zero. In this case, set the index line to the nearest whole number.

5. Raise the objective until the upper (aerial) image of the target again comes into view. Bring the image of the same spoke, described in step 2, sharply into focus using a fine adjustment knob.

6. If your original index line setting was at zero, read the radius of curvature directly from the scale at the position of the index line. If the original index line setting was at a plus whole number in the area on the scale below zero, add that whole number to the value shown by the index line at the aerial image.

7. Using a fine adjustment knob, focus sharply on the spoke 90 degrees away from the spoke previously in focus.

8. Repeat procedure in step 6.

The lowest reading (smallest figure) is the meridian on the contact lens with the steeper curve. The highest reading represents the meridian on the contact lens with the flatter curve.

A person who experiences a reduction in visual acuity that is correctable with a spherocylindrical overrefraction most likely is experiencing either lens flexure or warpage. A warped lens can be determined by checking the BCR on the radiuscope. The mire pattern will have two separate foci as with a back surface toric lens (Fig. 14.11); however, verification of lens power on the lensometer will remain spherical. A lens that is flexing, as diagnosed by toricity exhibited with over-keratometry, may appear to be warped immediately on removal; however, typically within a matter

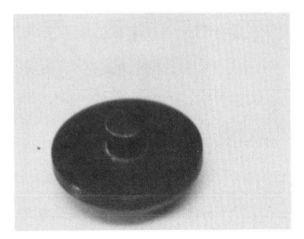

FIG. 14.10. Lens mounting device for convex surface measurement.

of seconds, the lens will return to its original spherical state and will appear as such with the radiuscope.

Peripheral Curve Radius

The peripheral curve radii of the contact lens can be measured using the radiuscope in the same manner as for measurement of the BCR. However, it is difficult to verify and is only possible if the curve width is, at minimum, 1 mm or wider and sufficiently polished to reflect a good image. The convex lens mount is tilted on the radiuscope in order to achieve this measurement (Fig. 14.12). After locating the curve mire, it may be desirable to use the small aperture of the radiuscope as it restricts the field of view to an area similar to that of the peripheral curve (9).

A variety of keratometer attachments can be used to measure the BCR of a rigid lens (2,3). Similar to measuring the convex surface of the cornea, the keratometer can measure the concave surface of the lens. The keratometer should be calibrated with a steel ball of known radius prior to determining BCR. After calibration, the contact lens is placed on the holder with a drop of saline and attached to the keratometer (Fig. 14.13A and 14.13B). A spherical contact lens should result in a spherical reading that can be converted from diopters to millimeters. It should be noted that although a keratometer can measure the BCR, the radiuscope is simpler and more precise because it is a separate instrument that can be used without interrupting an examination. In addition, the lens is held in a stable horizontal position with saline; conversely, some keratometer attach-

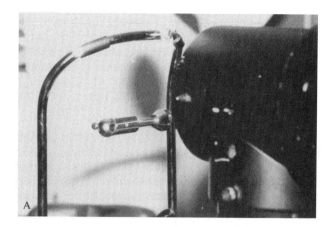

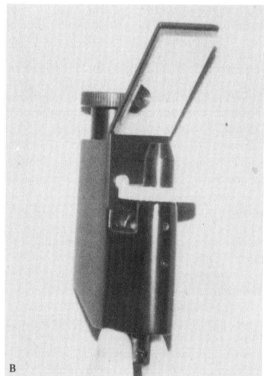

FIG. 14.13. Keratometer attachments for measuring the base curve radius of a gas permeable lens.

ments use clay or tape to hold the lens in the vertical position. The BCR should be with in ± 0.024 mm of the radius ordered.

Overall Diameter

The overall diameter of a lens is easily determined using a 7× or 10× measuring magnifier (reticule). The lens is held concave side down on the back of the measuring magnifier by the index finger with a window or fluorescent light source in the background. A scale of 0 to 20 mm can be found on the back lens of the magnifier (Fig. 14.14). This scale is divided into 0.1-mm increments. The lens and scale are

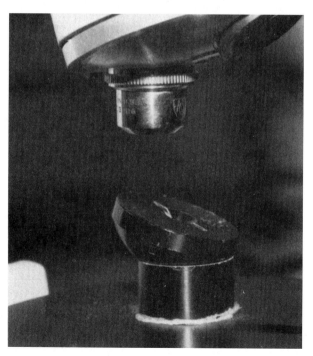

FIG. 14.12. Lens positioning for measurement of peripheral curve radius.

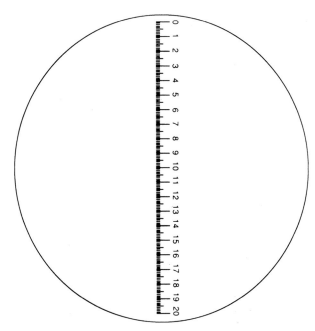

FIG. 14.14. Measuring magnifier scale.

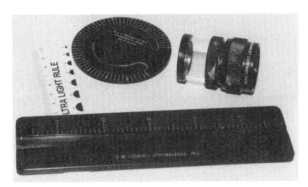

FIG. 14.15. Devices for measuring the overall diameter of a gas permeable lens.

magnified for the viewer by a plus lens with adjustable focus. The lens should be lined up against the zero edge of the scale, with the diameter read as the distance between the zero and the opposite edge of the lens. The lens should be rotated to verify the diameter is spherical, not oval. The lens and measuring magnifier should be clean and dry during this procedure.

The V-channel gauge is another method of determining overall diameter. The V-channel gauge consists of a plastic or metal plate with a channel down the center that becomes progressively smaller. The lens is placed in the slot and the gauge is tilted, allowing gravity to slide the lens down to the position where the lens diameter and the width of the channel are equal. The diameter is simply read off the gauge. Care should be taken not to force the lens down the channel because the edges might be damaged or the diameter read incorrectly because of lens flexure. The V-channel gauge is limited to overall lens diameter, whereas the measuring magnifier can be used in additional lens inspection.

Other techniques that are used infrequently are a dial gauge, a projection magnifier, and a PD stick (Fig. 14.15). A tolerance of ±0.05 mm difference between diameter ordered and diameter received is acceptable.

Optical Zone Diameter

The optical zone diameter is determined most easily by the use of a measuring magnifier (reticule). The lens is placed concave side down, similar to measuring overall diameter. By varying the light source with movement of the reticule, the optical zone diameter can be determined (Fig. 14.16). The lens should be rotated to check for an oval optical

zone. The optical zone will be oval if the lens has been manufactured with (i) a spherical BCR and a toric peripheral curve system, (ii) a toric base curve and a spherical peripheral curve system, or (iii) a toric base curve and toric secondary curve where the differences in curvature of the major meridians are not equal (2). If none of these conditions exists, an oval optical zone diameter is a result of poor manufacturing and the lens should be returned to the manufacturer.

The projection magnifier also can be used to determine

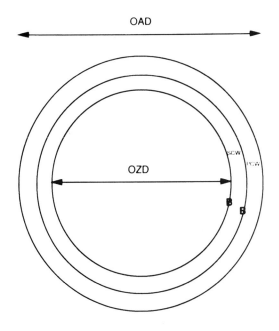

OAD = Overall Diameter
OZD = Optical Zone Diameter
SCW = Secondary Curve
PCW = Peripheral Curve Width
B = Blend or Transition Zone

FIG. 14.16. Diagram of lens measurements.

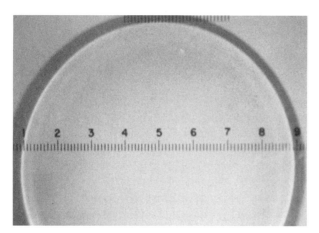

FIG. 14.17. Projection magnifier can be used to measure overall diameter, optical zone diameter, and peripheral curve widths.

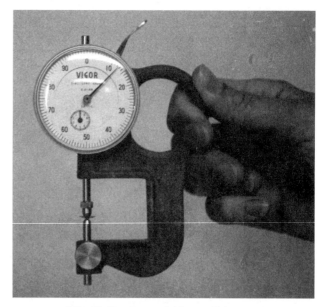

FIG. 14.19. Center thickness dial gauge.

optical zone diameter and peripheral curve widths. The lens is projected on the screen, and the optical zone diameter and peripheral curve widths can be determined by the scale on the screen (Fig. 14.17). The tolerance on the optical zone diameter should be within ±0.2 mm for medium-to-heavy blends and ±0.1 mm for light blends.

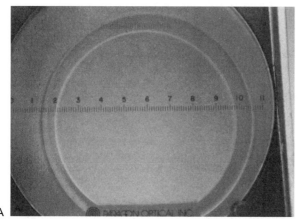

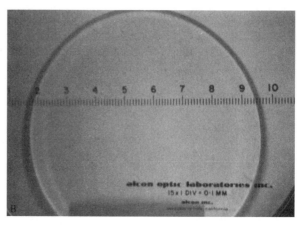

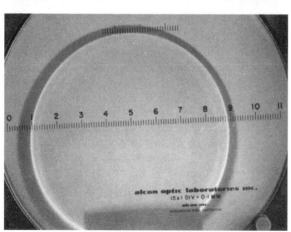

FIG. 14.18. As blend time increases from light blend **(A)**, to medium blend **(B)**, to heavy blend **(C)**, the specific peripheral curve width(s) is more difficult to verify.

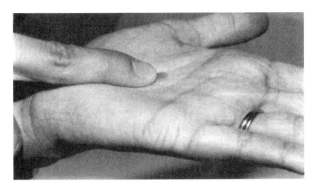

FIG. 14.20. Palm test for determining smoothness of edge.

Peripheral Curve Widths

A measuring magnifier, used in the same method as when determining optical zone diameter, will give an accurate reading of peripheral curve widths. The difficulty in determining these widths will be dependent on the blend of the lens. As the blend time is increased, the specific peripheral curve width becomes more difficult to verify (Fig. 14.18A–14.18C).

Center/Edge Thickness

The most frequently used method to measure lens thickness is a dial gauge. The lens is placed on the base of the gauge concave side up, and a plunger is carefully lowered onto the lens using a lever controlled by the thumb (Fig. 14.19) (10). The lens can be placed in a position to measure either center or edge thickness. The thickness is read off the gauge. If the needle is set on 20, the thickness reads 0.20 mm, as it can be determined to the hundredth thousandth. The Marco radiusgauge incorporates a center thickness gauge that allows the instrument to be used for measuring both lens radius and thickness. Proper thickness of the lens is important in providing comfort, preventing flexure, contributing to proper position, and obtaining needed oxygen

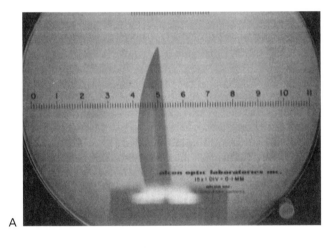

A

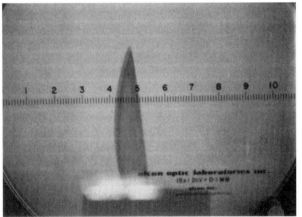

B

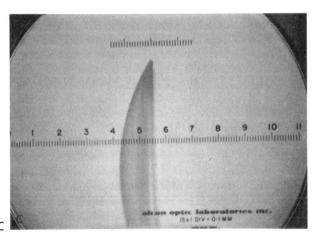

C

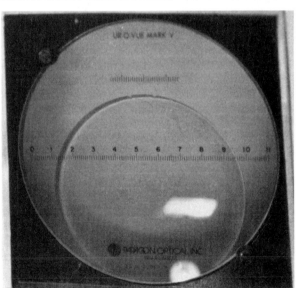

D

FIG. 14.21. Results showing round smooth edge **(A)**, sharp edge **(B)**, blunt edge **(C)**, and microchips at edge **(D)** when using a projection magnifier.

transmission. The tolerance factor is no more than ±0.02 mm.

Edge Shape

Careful examination of the edges on each lens dispensed is important because edge thickness and shape vary, not only among manufacturers but with the same manufacturer (11). The softness of the lens material makes it difficult to produce a consistent edge. A quick check of the edges may prevent the possibility of a dissatisfied GP lens wearer because of discomfort.

Methods of checking the edge of the lens include the "palm test" and the use of the projection magnifier. The two techniques work best in combination. Initially, the lens can be placed on the palm of the hand, concave side down, and pushed across the palm. If the lens is resistant to movement or an audible sound occurs, the edge is faulty (Fig. 14.20).

Placing the lens on the projection magnifier will confirm if the edge is sharp or blunt, or perhaps has microchips (Fig. 14.21A–14.21D).

Patient acceptance and comfort with GP lenses are dependent on the edge as it interacts with the lids and cornea. A poor edge will lead to lens intolerance, and even the best fit can result in failure if the edge is defective. Similarly, a satisfied patient with a damaged lens edge may return and complain of discomfort. The edge should be smooth and rounded on both the anterior and posterior surfaces; however, patients appear to be less tolerant of a blunt anterior surface because of its contact with the lids (12). Fortunately, with the introduction of higher-quality lathes and polishing methods, edge-related comfort problems are much less common than they were 10 to 20 years ago.

Surface Quality

The surface of a new lens should be free of scratches or tool marks. Scratches and deposits on a patient's lenses will be evident when the lens is viewed with the projection magnifier (Fig. 14.22). A measuring magnifier can be used to

TABLE 14.1. PRESCRIPTION REQUIREMENTS FOR CONTACT LENSES (ANSI Z80.20-1998)

Parameter	Tolerance
Diameter	±0.05 mm
Optical zone diameters	±0.1 mm
Base curve radius	±0.05 mm
Peripheral curve radius	±0.1 mm
Power	
0.00 to ±5.00 D	±0.12 D
5.12 to ±10.00 D	±0.18 D
10.12 to ±15.00 D	±0.25 D
15.12 to ±20.00 D	±0.37 D
>20D	±0.50 D
Prism power	
0–10 s	±0.25 s
>10 s	±0.50 s
Cylinder power	
<2.00 D	±0.25 D
2.00–4.00 D	±0.37 D
>4.00 D	±0.50 D
Cylinder axis	
0–1.50 DC	±5×
>1.50 DC	±3×
Toric base curve radii	
Back surface cylinder	
0–0.20 mm	±0.05 mm
0.21–0.40 mm	±0.06 mm
0.41–0.60 mm	±0.07 mm
>0.06 mm	±0.09 mm
Bifocal add power	±0.25 D
Center thickness	<±0.02 mm

evaluate the surface; however, the magnification is much greater and the defects more easily detectable with the projection magnifier.

Tint

The tint of the lens should be uniform throughout. The pair of lenses should be very similar in tint; however, small variations will be difficult to confirm *in vivo*. Differences in power between the two lenses may result in variations between the tint of the two lenses.

Summary

In conclusion, the measurements of a GP contact lens discussed in this chapter are important in obtaining a successful fit (Table 14.1) (13). Verification of these parameters is a simple step in assuring that the lenses received are as ordered and will aid the practitioner in the fitting of GP contact lenses.

REFERENCES

1. Henry VA. Verification of rigid lenses. In: Bennett ES, Henry VA, eds. *Clinical manual of contact lenses,* 2nd ed. Philadelphia: Lippincott Williams & Wilkins, 2000:160–180.

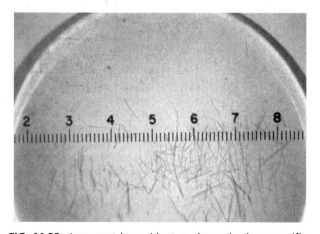

FIG. 14.22. Lens scratches evident on the projection magnifier.

2. Lowther GE. Contact lenses: procedures and techniques. In: *Inspection and verification.* Boston: Butterworth & Co., 1982: 153–192.

3. Mandell RB. Contact lens practice. In: *Inspection and verification,* 4th ed. Springfield, IL: Charles C. Thomas, 1988:352–387

4. Sarver MD. Verification of contact lens power. *J Am Optom Assoc* 1983;34:1304–1306.

5. Lensometer Instruction Manual. Buffalo, NY: Reichert Ophthalmic Instruments, 1998.

6. Lowther GE. Inspection and verification. In: Bier N, Lowther GE, eds: *Contact lens correction,* 3rd ed. Boston: Butterworth & Co., 1977:226–252.

7. Bennett ES. Lens care and solutions. In: Bennett ES, Grohe RM, eds. *Rigid gas-permeable contact lenses.* New York: Professional Press, Fairchild Publishers, 1986:225–240.

8. Barr, JT, Hettler DH. Boston II base curve changes with hydration. *Contact Lens Forum* 1984;9:65–67.

9. *AO radiuscope instructions.* Buffalo, New York: Reichert Ophthalmic Instruments, 1987.

10. Bennett ES. Lens design, fitting and troubleshooting. In: Bennett ES, Grohe RM, eds: *Rigid gas-permeable contact lenses.* New York: Professional Press, Fairchild Publishers, 1986:189–220.

11. Morris SD, Lowther GE. A comparison of different rigid contact lenses. Edge thickness and contours. *J Am Optom Assoc* 1981;52: 247–249.

12. LaHood D. Edge shape and comfort of rigid lenses. *Am J Optom Physiol Opt* 1988;65:613–618.

13. *Contact lenses—standard terminology, tolerances, measurements, and physicochemical properties.* ANSI Z80.20-1998:15-16. Optical Laboratories Association, 1998.

MODIFICATION

BRUCE W. MORGAN AND
EDWARD S. BENNETT

The ongoing development of shorter soft lens replacement schedules has been accompanied by a growing interest in placing gas permeable (GP) lenses on a planned replacement schedule. At least two manufacturers have developed such programs for their lens materials, and numerous practitioners have initiated planned replacement GP lens programs in their offices. These programs are especially important for materials with the so-called hyper-DK lens materials (i.e., DK [measure for oxygen permeability] >100). However, what about the so-called low-Dk (25–50 Dk) and medium-Dk (51–100) lens materials? It is apparent that these lens materials can perform well for up to several years. The keys to this longevity are proper lens care and in-office modification. The purpose of this chapter is to describe how to modify GP lenses and how these procedures can help increase patient satisfaction. Before discussing modification procedures, it is first important to describe the manufacturing process.

MANUFACTURING PROCESS

Not many practitioners are involved directly with the manufacturing of contact lenses, but a general knowledge of the basic techniques in manufacturing can help the practitioner understand the type of modifications that may need to be made on a lens in the office. It also is important to know what techniques are being used by particular local laboratories so that an educated choice can be made by the practitioner. Many times, the laboratory can make the difference between a successful and an unsuccessful fit of a GP lens.

As in other areas of the contact lens field, manufacturing of GP lenses is undergoing constant change. The addition of silicone, fluorine, and other materials to obtain ever-increasing oxygen transmissibility has created an environment in which the laboratories must make minor adjustments to maintain optical quality, wettability, and stability for each new polymer.

Cutting and Preparation of the Polymer

The first stage in GP lens manufacturing is preparation of the polymer. This process consists of essentially four steps

(1). The first is to evaluate the purity and quality of the raw materials. This is important for maintaining the stability and durability of the final product. Second, the material is refrigerated with minimal exposure to heat and light, both of which could cause a breakdown of components in the material, adversely affecting polymerization. Third, the raw materials are tested for impurities using distillation under stringent temperature and pressure controls. Once these three steps have been completed, the fourth step, polymerization, can begin. The proper combination of monomers and other additives, including tints, inhibitors (added to prevent breakdown of the monomer), and stabilizing and wetting agents, must be prepared. After the polymerization is completed, the first three steps are repeated on the new material to ensure the quality of the final product.

The material can be polymerized into rods, sheets, or buttons. It then must be put through an annealing process to eliminate areas of stress that could induce warpage in the final product. This process involves heating the material to an extremely high temperature in an oven and then cooling it very slowly (2). Annealing, as with all the aforementioned procedures, usually is performed by the laboratory supplying materials to the manufacturer.

The advantage of good oxygen transmission properties can be affected during the polymerization process. Manufacturers must be careful not to compromise one property when trying to improve another. The challenge of each manufacturer is to find the optimal combination of monomers to obtain a material with good wettability and stability, along with fairly high oxygen transmissibility.

Machining

The most common technique in machining GP lenses is lathe cutting. However, the heat generated by this procedure is the natural enemy of GP lens materials. Excessive heat can be produced by friction to the extent that a coolant often is necessary. Machining materials with heat distortion temperatures only slightly above room temperature requires extra care and attention to the cooling process (3).

Mechanical stress during machining eventually can lead

to undesirable changes in the lens measurements. It is recommended that the GP blank be mounted with a low-melting-point wax onto a steel button that is held in the spindle (4). This eliminates stress on the blank and decreases the possibility of radical flattening on the base curve radius, unwanted prism, and unwanted toricity. GP lens materials should be produced using very slow and shallow cuts with constant application of a liquid or air coolant to eliminate excessive heat production. It also is important that the polishing procedure be timed carefully so that the lens surface will not be polished excessively (5).

Lathe cutting the rigid button with the use of a natural diamond is preferred, although synthetic diamonds can be used. The advantage of using a diamond tool is that other tools tend to dull rapidly. The diamond requires relapping when small pits occur on the lens surface, which can affect wettability. Replacement of the cutting diamond is advised after every 800 to 1,000 lenses (6).

In recent years, advances have been made toward automatic lathes that use a DC servomotor that is vibration free and controlled by electro-optics for accuracy (5). The spindle rides on a cushion of air that results in production of a smoother surface requiring less polishing time. In contrast, the more conventional manual lathes use a drive belt from the motor to the spindle that, in turn, rests on a bearing. This configuration lends itself to vibrations that ultimately may cause ridges on the contact lens surface.

A few rigid lenses are being manufactured using a molding procedure similar to that used in producing hydrogel lenses. This technique has great potential because it eliminates many of the inconsistencies inherent in the lathing process. However, improvements in curing techniques must be made to increase the stability of a molded lens.

Each GP lens material has its own unique properties that may affect manufacturing and modification. Generally, the higher the DK of the material, the more difficult it is to manufacture, and more care must be taken when using slower lathe speeds and slower polishing techniques to reduce heat production. Certain GP lens materials, such as silicone resin, polystyrene, and surface-treated lenses, cannot be modified in any way after manufacturing.

Cutting and Polishing Base Curves

The base curve is cut by using any lathe specifically made for cutting a concave radius onto a contact lens blank (Fig. 15.1) (3). Care should be taken to ensure that the lathe is aligned precisely so that the cutting tool passes exactly through the axis of the spindle, because any displacement could result in a small bump in the center of the lens or in an unwanted prism. It is important that shavings be removed with compressed air or a vacuum during machining. The buildup of material at the cutting edge can generate heat that, in turn, will burn the lens surface.

Polishing the base curve after lathing requires the use of

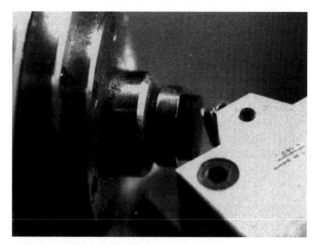

FIG. 15.1. Lathe cutting a base curve on a gas permeable lens.

pitch, soft waxes, or Pellon pads. Pitch can be heated gently while the lens blank is allowed to rotate over the surface. The pitch will then form to the blank and produce an excellent optical surface after approximately 2 minutes of polishing time. The use of a lap tool with Pellon pads also is effective, and polishing time again is approximately 2 minutes.

The lens surface must be kept moist with polish at all times during the polishing process. If the spindle speed exceeds 1,500 rpm, too much heat may be generated. Variable-speed machines should have spindle speeds set at 900 rpm with an oscillation rate of 25 strokes per minute. Many automatic polishing machines allow several lenses to be polished at the same time (Fig. 15.2).

Once the lens is polished, the surface should be inspected for lathe marks, scratches, and other abnormalities. If any are present, additional polishing is necessary. The optics and radius are verified for accuracy with the use of a radiuscope, and center thickness is checked with a gauge.

Front Curve Cutting and Polishing

The front surface power required for a lens is calculated using a computer or a programmable calculator. The same

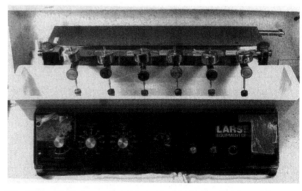

FIG. 15.2. Base curve polishing process for multiple gas permeable lenses.

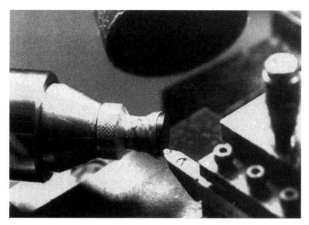

FIG. 15.3. Lathe cutting front or power curve on a gas permeable lens.

general procedures used for cutting the base curve are used for cutting the front curve, except for the use of a convex curve lathe-cutting device rather than a concave device (Fig. 15.3). At this stage, the blank is reduced to its final thickness and power. In addition, any necessary lenticulation is performed at this time.

The polishing for the front surface is very similar to the polishing of the back surface. Again, pitch or Pellon pads may be used, and the polishing time is approximately 2 minutes.

Finishing

Once the front and back surfaces are made to satisfaction, the lens can be cut down to the desired diameter. The overall diameter of the lens should be reduced to within 0.1 to 0.2 mm of the desired amount to allow for edge shaping and polishing (3). Peripheral curve radii then can be applied using a diamond-impregnated radius tool, progressing consecutively to flatter tools until the final design has been obtained. Minimal pressure should be used during these procedures, with special care being taken with the new softer materials. The use of a soft pad, such as velveteen, for polishing and blending the peripheral curve radii is recommended.

Initial edge shaping occurs during overall diameter reduction procedures. To do this, a cone-shaped tool with polishing compound should be used. To polish the edge, a drum tool with a soft sponge soaked in polishing compound is recommended because of its softness. Edge polishing is the final procedure and is discussed in more detail later in this chapter. After edge polishing, the lens is ready for final inspection.

MODIFICATION

Why Modify?

The ability to modify GP lenses is a powerful in-office problem solver. GP lens quality is improving due to technologic advancements in manufacturing. Nevertheless, there will be that occasional defective edge of a poorly wettable lens. Solving this problem in the office will not only result in a much more satisfied patient but also will minimize the resulting negative effects of a dissatisfied patient who may communicate his or her feelings to other people and, as a result of frustration, may give up on contact lens wear in general. Likewise, to compete with soft lens patients, it is important to have available as many in-office services as possible to keep the patient from discontinuing lens wear.

The problems that can occur often can be solved quickly by in-office modification. A patient with symptoms of lens awareness often can be managed by a simple edge polish. Dryness and/or fluctuating vision can be managed by surface polishing. A lens that feels dry and exhibits very little movement with the blink can be managed by blending and/or flattening the peripheral curves. If the addition of a slight amount of power will provide the patient with better vision while eliminating the need for reordering the lens, this can be performed in the office as well.

Patients in today's society do not want to be inconvenienced. If a problem can be solved without having to order an additional lens and risk forcing the patient to have to discontinue lens wear until the new lens arrives from the laboratory, it makes sense to solve it immediately, if possible. Patients place a high value on their time and appreciate receiving personalized custom services. It also reduces practice expenditures incurred by purchasing additional lenses. Any practice that is fitting GP lenses also should be verifying and, when indicated, modifying rigid lenses as well. It is a valuable service for both patient and practice. Just as obtaining a consistently excellent lens-to-cornea fitting relationship is difficult, so is receiving consistently perfect lenses from the manufacturing laboratory.

Modifying rigid lenses is simple and requires little time. The procedures discussed in this chapter all take no more than a few minutes to perform. As will be discussed, there are several ways for practitioners to gain proficiency in performing common modification procedures. In addition, technicians in the office can easily be trained to perform these procedures. The expense for equipment is, at most, a few hundred dollars; this is not much to ask to keep patients satisfied while enhancing lens performance. Some modifications, such as a clean and polish, can be provided as an annual service to patients who have a service agreement.

Instrumentation and Supplies

Modification equipment is not difficult to purchase; in fact, numerous Contact Lens Manufacturer's Association (CLMA) member laboratories either sell or distribute this equipment (Table 15.1) (7). Although a wide range of modification units, tools, and accessories are available, this chapter will focus on the basic equipment necessary for performing common in-office procedures.

TABLE 15.1. WHERE TO OBTAIN MODIFICATION EQUIPMENT

Laboratory	Location	Phone Number	E-mail
ABBA Optical	Stone Mountain, GA	770–498–8545	*lee@abbaoptical.com*
Acculens Inc.	Lakewood, CO	303–232–6244	*kdpcl@aol.com*
Aero Contact Lens	Carrollton, OH	937–866–1963	*aeroclohio@cs.com*
Conforma Contact Lenses	Norfolk, VA	800–426–1700	*info@conforma.com*
Contour Fine Tooling	Marlborough, NH	603–876–4908	*contour@top.monad.net*
G.P. Specialists	Phoenix, AZ	800–366–2522	*gp@gp2c.com*
Larsen Equipment Design	Seattle, WA	800–789–5121	*larseneq@aol.com*
Polychem, Inc.	Gaithersburg, MD	800–778–7206	*PolychmUSA@aol.com*
Precision Optics	Omaha, NE	800–584–9110	
Valley Contax	Springfield, OR	541–744–9393	*contax@valleycontax.com*
X-Cel Contacts	Duluth, GA	770–622–9235	*mparker@walman.com*

A Walman Co.: locations also in Baltimore, MD; Minneapolis, MN; Orlando, FL; Vista, CA; Pittsburgh, PA; and Redmond, WA.

Recommended Equipment

Modification Unit

Numerous types of units are available, and almost all units are compatible with GP lens materials. A box unit with a deep-set splash pan to minimize splash of the polish outside of the bowl is important (Fig. 15.4). If purchasing a modification unit for the first time, the accessory tools available for that same unit also should be purchased because spindle size can vary between units. Likewise, when purchasing a new unit, do not assume that the spindle size of this unit is identical to the previous one. This should be confirmed before purchasing the modification unit if a desire exists to continue to use the same modification tools. Because taper sizes vary for both units and tools, it is important to keep in mind that tapers must match exactly. Incorrect taper size can result in tool wobble and improper modification. In addition, the modification unit should have a spindle speed no greater than 1,200 rpm to minimize heat generation, which can be especially problematic for the softer high-Dk and hyper-Dk materials (8). Some manufacturers sell variable-speed units, which have the benefit of allowing the practitioner to use a higher spindle speed for lower-Dk materials as well as for procedures that carry a very low risk for compromising optical quality, such as edge polishing.

Lens Attachment Devices

Many options are available for holding or mounting lenses for modification. The most common include suction cup holders, concave and convex tools incorporating the use of double-sided tape, and spinners.

The most inexpensive tool may be the most important, and that is the two-piece green suction cup. Beneficial for many modification procedures, it is interchangeable, allowing the suction cup to be adhered to either the convex or concave side, depending on the procedure being performed. Most suction cup holders, such as the R&F stronghold, have interchangeable ends so that both the concave and convex surfaces of the lens can be attached. It is very important to center the lens on the cup to ensure proper modification results (Fig. 15.5). Failure to do this will result in an oval optical zone diameter or uneven edge or surface polishing, and may compromise the lens optics. Care also must be taken to use minimal pressure when applying the lens to the cup, or warpage may occur. Conforma Laboratories (Norfolk, VA) has developed a suction cup insert for the R&F stronghold that uses a larger surface area and a small flange to distribute the pressure more evenly and decrease

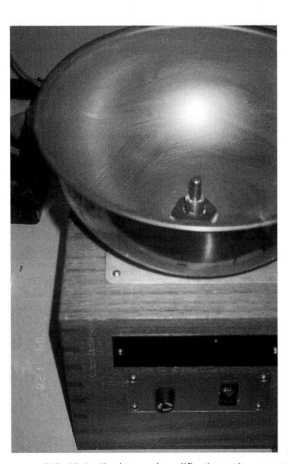

FIG. 15.4. Single-speed modification unit.

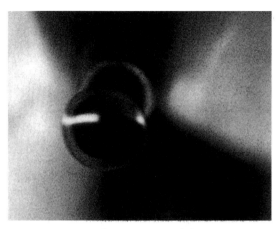

FIG. 15.5. Centration of a gas permeable lens on a suction cup.

the possibility of warpage (Fig. 15.6). The suction cup should be held by the operator as close as possible to the lens to impart maximal control during the modification process.

The use of double-sided tape is beneficial for several modification procedures, such as polishing and repowering. Again, centering the lens on the tool is vital. The disadvantage of using double-sided tape is that the tape will leave a residue on the surface of the lens that must be removed with a compatible solvent, such as Fluoro-Solve (Paragon Vision Sciences) or The Boston Solvent (Polymer Technology Corporation, Rochester, NY). In addition, adhesion of the tape is affected by time and moisture, so it must be replaced frequently.

Spinner tools are very beneficial for certain procedures requiring care in maintaining optical quality, such as power changes and front surface polishing. Several types of spinners are available, but all work similarly. They use either a suction cup or double-sided tape for lens attachment, and the lens is able to spin freely along with the spindle while the handle is held stationary. The end of the spinner is cushioned with a ball bearing so that it will spin along with the spindle. Because several spinner tools are commercially available, it is most important to confirm that this tool rotates freely with little resistance. With the spinner rotating

the lens during the modification procedure, it is likely that the change to the lens will be made very evenly or symmetrically, with little risk of optical compromise.

Sponge Tools

A flat sponge tool for polishing the front surface, a flat sponge tool with a central aperture for polishing the edge, and a cone-shaped sponge tool for polishing the back surface are commonly used. The sponge is presoaked with water before modifying, and polish is added frequently throughout the procedure. These tools are only mildly abrasive and, if kept moist, rarely cause optical compromise to the lens.

Radius Tools

Brass, Delrin (acetal resin), or plastic radius tools are used for performing peripheral curve modification procedures such as blending, flattening, and optical zone diameter reduction (Fig. 15.7). In addition, diamond-dusted or diamond-coated radius tools are available, although at a much higher cost. These tools are covered typically with velveteen. Precut velveteen pads are available from most laboratories. If using velveteen, it is advisable to stay with 100% cotton, because some of the polyester blends heat the lens too quickly, which can cause warpage or other distortion (9). A minimum radius tool set could consist of the following tools: 7.60, 7.80, 8.0, 8.2, 8.4, 8.6, 8.8, 9.0, 9.4, 9.8, 10.4, 11, and 12 mm.

Polish

To speed up the modification procedure while keeping the lens cool during the procedure, a liquid polish is required. These polishes have a grit aluminum oxide base and typically are applied every 3 to 5 seconds during the procedure.

Several polishes are available. A study by Reeder et al. (10) compared the performance of seven such polishes: five premixed polishes (Boston White Finishing Polish [Polymer Technology Corp.], Evergreen [R&F Products, Denver, CO], Mirapolish [ABBA Optical, Stone Mountain, GA], Nu-Care 2000 [Polychem, Gaithersburg, MD], and Sil-O-

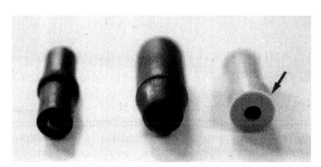

FIG. 15.6. Custom-made wide-flange suction cup insert (Conforma Laboratories).

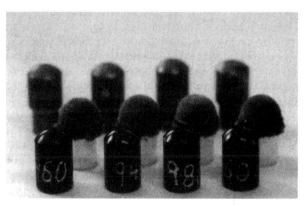

FIG. 15.7. Radius tools made of brass **(background)**, Delrin with velveteen cover **(center)**, and plastic **(foreground)**.

Care [Polychem, Gaithersburg, MD]) and two powder polishes (mixed one part powder and two parts saline; Al-Ox 721 [Transelco Ferro, Cleveland, OH] and X-Pal [Davison Chemical, Chattanooga, TN]). These polishes were compared when changing lens power on a 92-Dk GP lens material. The results showed that to add 0.50 D of minus power, it took anywhere from about 30 seconds to 2.5 minutes to achieve this change, with the powder polishes resulting in a shorter modification time. In addition, 60 of 70 lenses had good or very good optical quality after the procedure was performed, a very good result when changing the power of a hyper-Dk lens material. Obviously, an ammonia- and alcohol-based compound such as Silvo is contraindicated for use with GP lens materials.

Other Tools

Other tools that are commonly available, although perhaps not used as often as those discussed previously, include a velveteen-covered drum tool and a 90-degree anterior bevel tool. The drum tool is used much like the flat sponge tool in performing edge and surface polish procedures. It also can be used for repowering. The anterior bevel tool is used for thinning a blunt or thick edge. Common tools used for modification are shown in Fig. 15.8 (11).

Packages

The cost of modification equipment varies, depending on the number of procedures performed. For basic edge and surface polish procedures, many laboratories have economical packages ranging from $225 to $350. This typically includes a single-speed modification unit in addition to sponge and/or velveteen tools for polishing procedures (7). Suction cups and polish also are typically provided. This type of modification unit is acceptable, although a variable-speed unit would be preferable, especially if the spindle speed of the single-speed unit exceeds 1,000 rpm.

A deluxe package (often $300–$500) allows the practitioner and/or staff to perform peripheral curve procedures such as blending and flattening, in addition to changing the power of the lens. This package typically includes a suction cup spinner for polishing and repowering, radius tools for peripheral curve procedures, a 90-degree anterior based cone tool for thinning the edge, and possibly a 7× magnifying loupe and/or a diameter gauge. Because many laboratories either manufacture or distribute modification equipment, it is advisable to contact a local CLMA member laboratory to determine if it provides modification equipment and, if so, what type of packages are available.

Verification Equipment

Edge and surface verification equipment is strongly recommended, although such equipment is not as readily available today as in the past. The Contact Lens Edge Profile Analyzer (CLEPA [SGY Enterprises, Eugene, OR]) is quite valuable for using the optics of the radiuscope to verify the edge profile under high magnification. A list of required, strongly recommended, and recommended equipment is given in Table 15.2 (11).

Modification Procedures

Before performing any modification procedure, it is important to obtain some baseline data on the lenses, especially if the patient is new to the office. An educated decision as to how to modify a lens can be made only after knowing the initial specifications. All the optical and structural qualities of the lens should be verified and recorded before beginning any procedure, because modification of one measurement often can affect another measurement.

It would be beneficial to obtain the original specifications of the lens, if possible. It is, therefore, a good habit to verify all new lenses from the laboratory before dispensing them to patients. This is well worth the time if the lens should need modifying in the future. It also is important to know

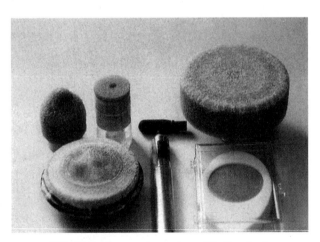

FIG. 15.8. Commonly used modification tools.

TABLE 15.2. IN-OFFICE MODIFICATION EQUIPMENT

Required
    Modification unit (variable speed or low single speed)
    Edge and surface sponge polishing tools
    Suction cups
    Polish
    7× or 10× magnifying loupe
Strongly Recommended
    Suction cup spinner
    CLEPA or projection magnifying device
Recommended
    Radius tools
    90° anterior bevel cone tool

CLEPA, Contact Lens Edge Profile Analyzer.

whether the laboratory measures the lens using the back vertex power or the front vertex power. This is critical for contact lenses for aphakia, where the power can vary 1 to 2 D depending on which vertex is used.

Peripheral Curve Fabrication/Blending

In-office blending and/or flattening of the peripheral curve radii allows the practitioner to adjust the fit of the lens and immediately observe an improved lens-to-cornea fitting relationship and, more than likely, an improvement in lens performance (12). If limited lens movement is present with the blink and is accompanied by tear stagnation, blending the junctions between peripheral curve radii should result in increased movement and better tear exchange. In addition, blending the peripheral curve junctions can increase patient comfort (13). If peripheral and/or midperipheral bearing is present, seal-off and possibly lens adherence can result. Once again, only limited—if any—tear exchange will result. Flattening the peripheral curve radius should resolve the problem and result in greater clearance peripherally. If these problems are not promptly managed, edema and dryness-related problems can result (14). Because these procedures typically take only a matter of seconds to perform in the office, there should be no reason to inconvenience the patient by returning the lens to the laboratory or ordering a new lens.

For peripheral curve blending and flattening procedures, all that typically is needed is a suction cup and a series of radius tools, as described previously. When blending the junction between two peripheral curves, it is important to determine the specific tool to be used. The first step is to add the two radii to be blended and then divide by two. For example, the following lens design to be modified is presented: base curve radius 7.8 mm, secondary curve radius 9.4 mm/0.4 mm width, and peripheral curve radius 11.0 mm/0.2 mm width. The first junction to be blended would be obtained by adding $7.8 + 9.4 = 17.2$. Because $17.2 \div 2 = 8.6$, the desired blend tool would be -8.6 mm. Because the velveteen used on the radius tool adds 0.4 mm to the radius, an 8.2-mm radius tool should be selected for blending these curves. To blend the junction between the secondary curve and peripheral curve radii, the desired radius (after compensation with velveteen) would be $9.4 + 11.0 = 20.4$. Because $20.4 \div 2 = 10.2$, the desired blend tool would be 10.2 mm (requiring a 9.8-mm radius tool). It is important not to attempt to blend with a velveteen-compensated tool less than 0.5 mm flatter than the base curve radius of the lens. A tool any steeper than this can flatten or warp the base curve radius quite rapidly while reducing the optical zone diameter, possibly resulting in compromised vision.

The degree of blend is related to the relative ease of being able to observe the optical zone and peripheral curve junctions (Fig. 15.9). Blending typically is differentiated into light, medium, and heavy, as follows (2):

- Light blend: 5 seconds on tool; junction easily observable
- Medium blend: 10 seconds on tool; junction still observable but shadows are beginning to form
- Heavy blend: 15 to 20 seconds on tool; junction is very difficult to read and can appear as one continuous shadow

When flattening and/or widening of the peripheral curve is desired, a flatter tool is selected. For example, in the earlier case, if peripheral bearing is observed with fluorescein application, because the peripheral curve radius is 11.0 mm and the width is 0.3 mm, a 12-mm tool can be used and the procedure can be performed until a slightly wider peripheral curve (i.e., 0.4 or 0.5) has been established. This should take only 10 to 30 seconds.

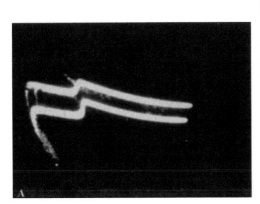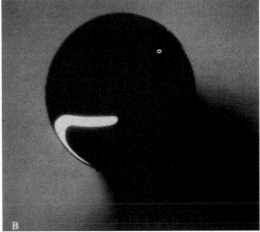

FIG. 15.9. A: Light reflex shows the distinct junctions between peripheral curves of an unblended lens. **B:** Light reflex shows the smooth transition between the peripheral curves of a heavily blended lens.

To perform blending or flattening, velveteen or a similar form of covering is properly placed over the appropriate radius tool, ensuring that no wrinkles or contaminants are present. The lens is attached to the suction cup, concave side out. It is important that good suction is obtained and that the lens is well centered on the suction cup. If the lens is not well centered or the lens shifts during the procedure because of inadequate suction, a decentered optical zone can result. The radius tool is then placed on the spindle of the unit, the motor is turned on, and polish is applied to the tool surface. Once the spindle is spinning, the lens is placed gently against the center of the tool in a perpendicular orientation (Fig. 15.10). For maximal control, the suction cup should be held as close as possible to the lens to minimize any wobble. The lens then is rotated in a figure-of-eight motion in small sweeps across the top of the radius tool (Fig. 15.11).

The lens should be lifted from the tool and polish added every 3 to 5 seconds (if not continuously) during this procedure to keep the lens cool. The importance of preventing heat buildup during peripheral curve modification procedures cannot be overemphasized. Insufficient polish, as well as excessive pressure, can lead to heat buildup and damage to the posterior surface of the lens, especially with the softer high-Dk lens materials (Fig. 15.12). For this same purpose, if a variable-speed modification unit is being used, a low spindle speed should be selected. In addition, posterior surface scratches can result if the surface of the modification tool is not kept clean. It is important to ensure that the velveteen covering is free of debris, dried polish, and other material at all times during the procedure. The lens then can be inspected with a $7\times$ or $10\times$ hand magnifier to view changes in junction quality, optical zone diameter, and peripheral curve width.

A second method for blending and/or flattening the pe-

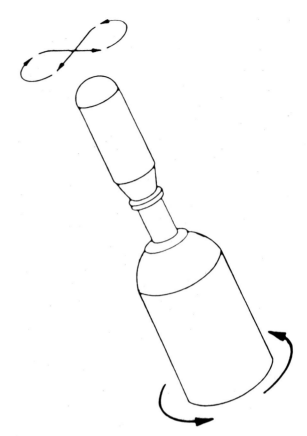

FIG. 15.11. Figure-of-eight design used to apply a peripheral curve.

ripheral curve radii is to place the suction cup at a 30-degree angle to the vertical, with the entire outer edge of the lens in contact with the covered tool at all times. The suction cup is rotated smoothly and evenly with the fingers in the opposite direction of the spindle rotation (i.e., typically counterclockwise). Both of these procedures require practice for proficiency but, when used properly, can produce the required result in a matter of seconds.

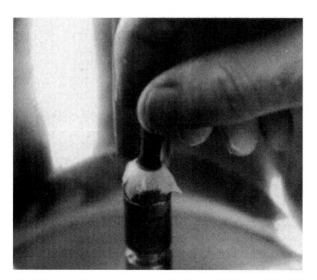

FIG. 15.10. Peripheral curve application with lens and suction cup.

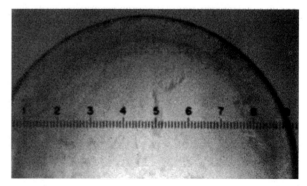

FIG. 15.12. Bull's-eye effect from scratches on the posterior surface due to excessive pressure from an unclean surface of the tool.

Edge Polishing/Shaping

This is the most important modification procedure to perform. In fact, some offices routinely polish the lens edge of every new lens to ensure optimal initial comfort for the lens wearer (12). It cannot be assumed that a replacement lens will have the same edge as the original or that the left lens will have the same edge as the right. Whenever a patient has symptoms of lens awareness or discomfort after insertion of a new lens, poor edge quality should be suspected. The lens edge then should be inspected for confirmation of a less-than-desirable lens shape or quality.

Because a defective edge that is not promptly managed can result in a very dissatisfied patient, edge inspection is a very important but much underused procedure. One simple initial method of determining if a lens edge is defective is the palm test (15). The lens, concave side down, is placed in the palm of the hand and then pushed across the palm by the forefinger of the other hand. If it fails to glide easily across the palm (i.e., does not tend to more or, if movement is present, the lens feels rough), the edge is defective. One of the projection edge inspection devices mentioned earlier should be used to determine the type of edge defect present. Both the anterior and posterior edges should be rolled and tapered, as the posterior edge is near alignment with the cornea and the anterior edge is often in contact with the upper lid. A defective edge will be too sharp or too blunt, have small microchips, or simply be somewhat abraded or rough in appearance. The latter two defective edges often can be diagnosed by having an inspection device that allows both frontal and profile views.

Edge Polishing Procedures

Edge Sponge Tool

Use of a flat sponge tool with an aperture in the center for edge polishing is a very common procedure for polishing the edge. In this procedure, the lens is first mounted on a suction cup. As with any procedure using a suction cup, proper mounting of the lens onto the suction cup is important. The lens should be clean before the procedure is performed to enhance the suction effect. The suction cup should be moistened with water before use; once water has been squeezed into the suction cup, it should be placed against the convex side of the device. When proper alignment is achieved, the pressure exerted on the top of the suction cup should be released and the lens will adhere to the suction cup. Minimal pressure should be used during lens application to prevent lens warpage. The importance of proper centration of the lens on the suction cup via visual inspection cannot be overemphasized. If the lens is decentered, an uneven edge design can result.

To perform this procedure, the sponge should be thoroughly moistened with water. As the sponge rotates, polish is applied every few seconds and the suction cup is held

vertically to the tool. The lens is then pushed into the central hole of the sponge and moved in an up-and-down manner (Fig. 15.13). The lens edge can be inspected every 30 seconds until the desired amount of polishing has been achieved.

Velveteen-Covered Tool

An often-used technique for polishing the lens edge involves a velveteen-covered pad tool. This tool consists of a large 3- to 4-inch flat sponge covered with velveteen or moleskin (16). The lens is attached to a spinner or suction cup with the convex side out and with the end of the tool pointing toward the center of the pad. The edge of the lens is lowered gently onto the pad about two thirds of the way out from the center. When the edge of the lens touches the rotating flat pad, the lens is moved across the pad, with the angle of the spinner of the suction cup to the pad varying from 45 degrees to parallel (Fig. 15.14). If a spinner is used, it should be allowed to rotate with the drum for about 15 seconds at a time. When using the suction cup, the lens should be rotated with the fingers in a counterclockwise direction as it is moved across the surface of the pad. The entire procedure may take anywhere from a few seconds to 2 to 3 minutes, depending on the bluntness or roughness of the original edge and the edge design desired. It is recommended that the pad be rotated against the lens edge from the concave, not the convex, side of the lens to obtain a more tapered and contoured edge.

A similar method would be simply to guide the lens across the sponge tool for about 30 to 60 seconds (17). Regardless of the procedure, it is extremely important that

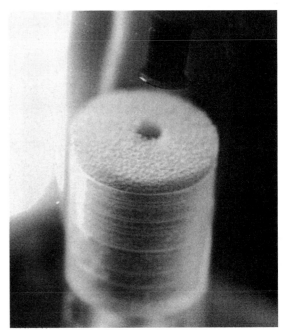

FIG. 15.13. Sponge tool with central hole used for edge polishing.

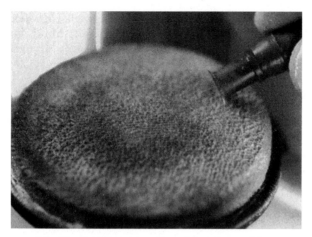

FIG. 15.14. Velveteen pad used for edge polishing.

the final position of the edge against the sponge tool be on the right side; otherwise, the plastic may be pushed or rolled toward the inner lens surface. Polish should be applied frequently, and the lens should be spinning at all times.

Finger Polishing

The edge can be polished by using the fingers as polishing pads. Using either a brass tool that holds the lens concave side out with double-sided tape or a tool that holds a suction cup with the lens in this position, the lens can be polished by using the thumb and forefinger (wetted with polish) to glide up and down the edge while the lens is rotating (Fig. 15.15). A suction cup tool or "fingerlishing" tool is available from SGY Enterprises/Valley Contax (Springfield, OR) (10).

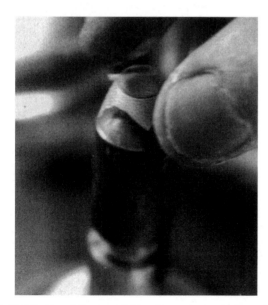

FIG. 15.15. Use of finger polishing to create a smooth, polished edge.

Edge Shaping Procedures

Moleskin-Covered Strip

The use of a moleskin-covered wood strip is effective in shaping the lens edge. The moistened moleskin-covered strip is held such that it is continually rolled over the edge of the rotating lens, from position A to position C and then back again (Fig. 15.16). Because the wood strip provides a solid support to the moleskin, pressure can be applied to the lens edge at its concave side, if desired. The wood strip should be held almost parallel to the rim of the lens (position 1) for a longer period of time (18). If more anterior bevel on the convex side of the lens is desired, the wood strip should be held at a considerable angle past the vertical (position C) for a longer period of time. Again, excessive pressure should be avoided with flexible GP lens materials that can easily chip or fracture.

Anterior Bevel

When the edge is too thick or blunt, an anterior bevel must be performed before edge polishing. This procedure also is beneficial in lowering a superiorly decentered lens. To thin the edge or create an anterior bevel, a cone tool is needed. A 90-degree cone tool usually is used to add an anterior (also termed "CN") bevel to the lens edge. Alternatively, a 120-degree tool can be used for a wider bevel or a 60-degree tool for a narrower bevel (11,13). This procedure is performed most often with the lens attached to a suction cup, convex side out. A velveteen (or similar material) pad with a one-quarter section cut out is placed within the tool so that it conforms to the cone surface. The lens is then placed within the cone and, with polish added frequently, the lens is gently rocked forward and backward and left and right (Fig. 15.17). This rocking motion allows application of a bevel with a smooth transition zone. It is important to avoid excessive rocking because peripheral anterior surface quality can be affected. The lens should be examined every 10 to 15 seconds until the desired edge thickness is obtained (Fig. 15.18). Once obtained, an edge polish should be performed.

Surface Polishing

Another common procedure, surface polishing, is indicated if the lens has an adherent mucoprotein film or surface

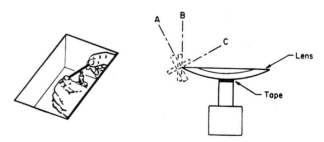

FIG. 15.16. **Left:** Use of a moleskin-covered strip in edge shaping. **Right:** Proper rotation of the strip in edge shaping.

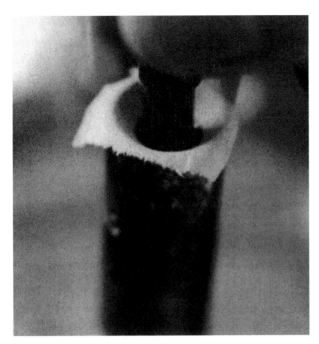

FIG. 15.17. A 90-degree tool used on the anterior bevel or thinner edge.

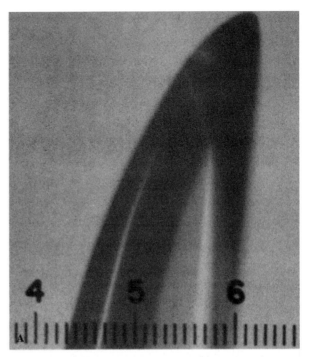

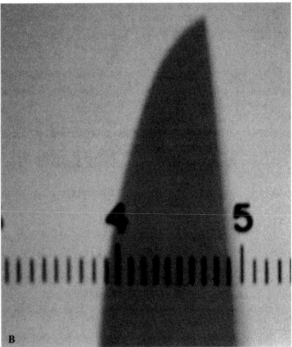

FIG. 15.18. A: Thick edge shown by magnifying comparator. **B:** Lens edge after being thinned by a 90-degree bevel tool.

scratches are present on the lens surface. Patients typically report transient blurry vision acquired over time, typically accompanied by redness and/or reduced wearing time. The specific problem can be diagnosed via biomicroscopic evaluation of the lens surface.

If a lens exhibits poor initial wettability, it is important first to use a laboratory cleaner or solvent to clean the lens, followed by rubbing/wetting solution to help condition the lens before it is reinserted (12). Polishing the front surface should be a last resort because of the possibility that the poor initial wettability is caused by residual pitch polish left on the lens during the manufacturing process. If so, the pitch may simply be distributed further on the lens surface, and the problem is not alleviated. If the problem is an acquired mucoprotein film that has become plaquelike and resistant to normal cleaning, once again a laboratory cleaner or solvent approved for use with GP lens materials should be used initially. If the deposits are not totally removed, a mild front surface polish should be considered. Only occasionally does the posterior surface attract sufficient debris or deposits to warrant polishing. In addition, the patient should be educated to clean the lenses every night on removal, supplemented by, at minimum, weekly enzymatic cleaning. The use of a liquid enzyme, if approved for that specific material, is another option.

If the problem is the result of surface scratches, a surface polish is indicated. In almost every case the scratches are limited to the front surface. In these cases, patients need to be educated about proper lens handling, especially with high-Dk and hyper-Dk lens materials. GP lenses should be handled over a soft cloth to minimize the possibility of the

lens displacing onto a hard surface. If the lens is dragged across a hard surface, such as a sink or floor, scratches invariably result. If the lens displaces onto a hard surface, a drop of wetting solution can be placed onto one finger and the lens gently lifted off the surface. Another source of scratches is a dirty case. Any particulate matter in a lens well can scratch a lens, especially if the lens is dragged out of the well. It is important that the lens case be maintained in good condition and replaced on a frequent basis. The patient should be advised always to be gentle when lifting the lens out of a case well.

Surface Polishing Procedures

Flat Sponge Tool

A common method of polishing the front surface of the lens is via the use of a large (3-inch) flat sponge tool in combination with a suction cup. The sponge is wetted with water and then polish, and the lens is attached to the suction cup, convex side out. Once the tool is rotating, the lens is placed halfway between the center and the edge of the sponge (8). The lens should be held at a 45-degree angle and rotated in a direction opposite the rotation of the tool (Fig. 15.19). The lens is depressed about one eighth into the sponge during the procedure, and polishing is continued for about 20 to 30 seconds before reevaluating the surface. In addition, the lens power should be verified to ensure that optical quality is unchanged and that no minus power has been added. This procedure may take up to 2 to 4 minutes. Fig. 15.20 shows the gradual improvement in lens surface quality after 30 seconds and 1 minute of polishing.

An alternative method would be to use a spinner, either in contact with the flat sponge, in a similar manner as with the suction cup, or in combination with a rounded sponge tool. In the latter method, the spinner rolls the lens from edge to center and back until the desired surface quality has been obtained (Fig. 15.21). As long as the spinner continues to rotate, the optical quality should not change.

In all of these procedures, frequent application of polish in combination with minimal pressure is very important. In addition, it is not advisable to attempt to polish out deep scratches totally, because optical quality could be compromised by frequent polishing.

Drum Tool

Another method is to use a 3-inch velveteen-covered drum tool with a suction cup. Similar to the first method de-

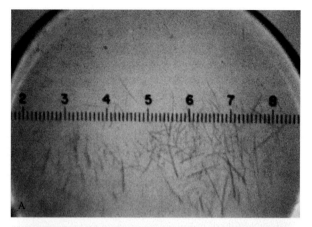
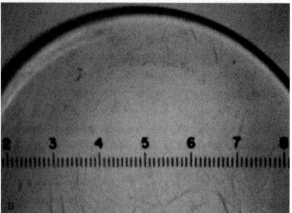
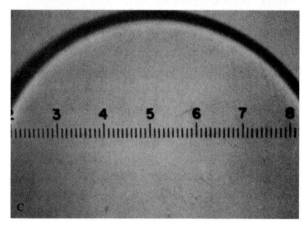

FIG. 15.20. **A:** Excessive front surface scratches on a gas permeable lens. **B:** Thinned scratches after initial front surface polishing. **C:** Remnant deep scratches after final surface polishing.

scribed, the lens is attached convex side out. The convex side of the lens should be positioned vertically over the center of the drum tool and the lens brought into light contact with the drum (16). The suction cup should be slowly rocked back and forth about 10 degrees for 1 to 3 seconds. This rocking motion minimizes the risk of adding plus power to the lens while polishing the front surface. It is not necessary to turn or rotate the suction cup between the fingers.

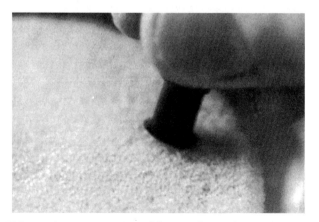

FIG. 15.19. Demonstration of front surface polish with the use of a flat sponge tool.

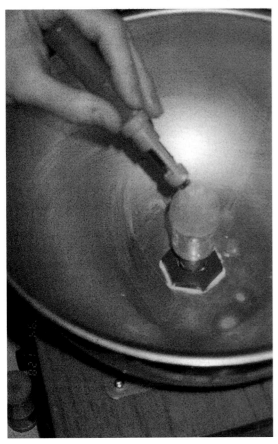

FIG. 15.21. Use of a spinner and rounded sponge tool for surface polishing.

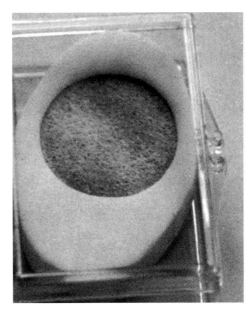

FIG. 15.22. Polishing pad used for manual front surface polishing (Eaton Medical Corp.).

Polishing Pad

For removing thick adherent mucoprotein deposits and very light scratches, a hand polishing pad such as The Cleaner Accessory Pad (Eaton Medical Corp.) can be used (Fig. 15.22) (19). The pad is wetted with preservative-free saline, followed by six to eight drops of a rigid daily cleaning solution. The lens is placed on the tip of the thumb or index finger and rubbed into the pad for approximately 20 seconds.

Cone-Shaped Sponge

Although rare, if adherent deposits and/or scratches are present on the back surface of the lens, a cone-shaped sponge in combination with a suction cup can be used. The sponge is moistened, first with water and then polish, and the lens is mounted onto the suction cup, concave side out. While the spindle is rotating, polishing compound is added and the suction cup is tilted slightly, with the lens placed just off the center of the sponge (Fig. 15.23) (8). The lens is depressed about one eighth into the sponge and rotated opposite of the spindle rotation for about 15 seconds before inspection. It can be repeated if necessary.

Repowering

For patients with consistently blurred vision through their GP lenses as a result of overcorrection or undercorrection, an overrefraction typically results in the need for more minus or plus power. A common solution to this problem is simply to order another lens (or lenses). However, in the interim the patient is inconvenienced, either by having to discontinue lens wear or to wear lenses that do not provide

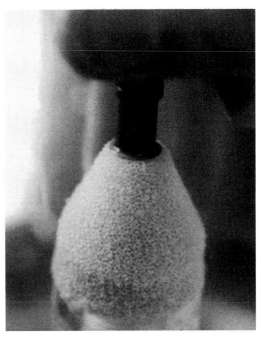

FIG. 15.23. Polishing the concave surface of a gas permeable lens with a cone-shaped sponge.

optimal vision. The ability to change the power, or repower, the lens in the office is an important benefit because the problem is solved immediately without patient inconvenience.

Repowering Procedures

Spinner/Rounded Sponge Tool

Use of a spinner with a rounded sponge tool is an excellent method of adding minus power. This sponge can be a cone sponge tool or any rounded sponge tool. The sponge tool is mounted vertically on the spindle and wetted thoroughly with water and polish. The lens is mounted convex side out and well centered on the spinner tool. It is particularly important in this procedure that the particular spinner tool being used rotates quite easily and freely. As the sponge tool rotates, the lens is first held with the edge adjacent to the side of the pad to initiate the spinning action (Fig. 15.24) (8). Once the lens is spinning freely, the spinner is rotated so that the lens is perpendicular to the sponge tool, approximately 1 to 1.5 cm from the apex (Fig. 15.25). It is important for this position to remain constant because this allows the center of the lens to be in direct contact with the pad while the periphery receives less friction. This creates a flatter front surface curvature and a resultant increase in minus power. As long as the lens is spinning during this procedure, lens optical quality should remain unchanged, and as much as 1 D of minus power can be added (8). The power should be monitored every 15 seconds; the actual amount of minus power added depends on the amount of pressure, time, and polishing compound used. This procedure should not take more than 1 to 2 minutes to perform.

Adding plus power with this procedure is very similar. The primary difference is that once the lens is spinning, instead of moving it such that the center is perpendicular to the center, the lens periphery remains in alignment with the sponge tool (Fig. 15.26). Plus power is being added as the front surface curvature increases by removal of material from the periphery of the lens and not the center. Only about 0.50 D of plus power can be added because the rate of power change is much slower with plus than with minus power.

Drum Tool/Suction Cup

An alternative method of adding plus power is to use a flat drum tool in combination with a suction cup. The drum tool typically is covered with velveteen or suede cloth (9). With the monitor running, a small amount of polish is added to the tool. The lens, convex side out on the suction cup, is brought in contact with the center of the drum tool with a perpendicular orientation (Fig. 15.27). With mild pressure, the lens is rotated both clockwise and counterclockwise. As with all other methods, polish should be applied liberally. Only about 0.50 D of plus power can be added with this method.

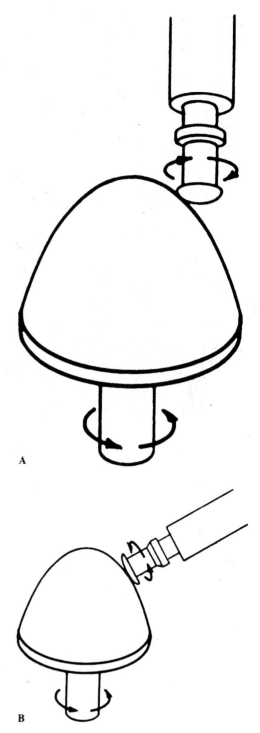

FIG. 15.24. **A:** Spinner and lens position for initiating lens movement against a rounded sponge. **B:** Position of lens against rounded sponge for the addition of minus power.

Flat Sponge Tool/Suction Cup

An alternative method of adding minus power is to use a flat sponge tool in combination with a suction cup (9). For adding minus power, the lens is mounted on the suction cup, convex side out. With the flat sponge spinning on the

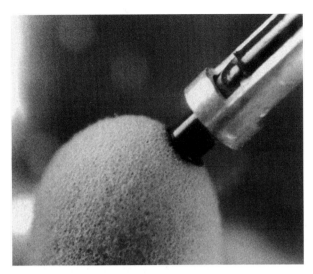

FIG. 15.25. Use of a rounded sponge and spinner for the addition of minus power.

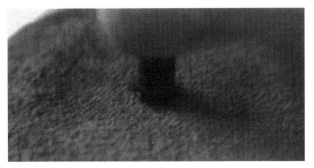

FIG. 15.27. Use of a drum tool for the addition of plus power.

spindle and thoroughly wetted with water and polish, the lens is placed approximately 0.5 inch from the edge of the tool. With the lens held perpendicular to the sponge, only mild pressure is exerted as the lens is revolved counterclockwise around the tool. Only through practice will the modifier be able to determine the number of revolutions needed for the desired amount of added minus power. Once again,

it is important to check power and optical quality with the lensometer approximately every 15 seconds. A maximum of 0.75 D of minus power can be added with this method.

Special Considerations

Obviously, there is a risk of compromising the optics of GP lenses, especially the high-Dk and hyper-Dk materials. Some procedures are not recommended for certain materials, whereas other procedures are recommended but only if certain precautions are taken.

Important Precautions

Several precautions are important to consider when modifying GP materials, particularly the high-Dk and hyper-Dk materials. Obviously, the use of a low-speed modification unit is desirable. In addition, not applying too much pressure will minimize the risk of distorting optics. Polish should be applied frequently, if not constantly, to minimize heat buildup. Likewise, it is beneficial to take frequent breaks so as not to burn or scorch the lenses. For the same reason, it is advisable to dip the lens in water before performing the modification procedure (and after each break). If a polishing sponge is used, it should be thoroughly soaked with water. It also is advisable to condition the lens in the palm of the hand with a wetting solution and then to soak the lens for a few minutes after performing the modification procedure.

Indicated Procedures

With low-Dk and high-Dk lens materials, it is apparent that edge polishing, surface polishing, blending and flattening the peripheral curves, and repowering should be performed with little risk of error, especially if the aforementioned precautions are taken into consideration. With hyper-Dk materials, edge polishing should not be a problem; however, when surface polishing to remove scratches and deposits, only very light pressure should be used to avoid heat-induced optical distortion or even breakage.

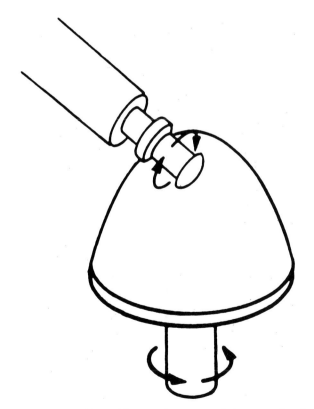

FIG. 15.26. Position of lens against a rounded sponge for the addition of plus power.

FIG. 15.28. Scanning electron microscopy of lens surface after the addition of minus lens power with a spinner and rounded sponge.

FIG. 15.30. Scanning electron microscopy of lens surface after the addition of minus power with velveteen pad.

Procedures to Either Avoid or Use with Extreme Caution

One procedure that should not be performed on contemporary GP lens materials is diameter reduction. Because these materials are softer and more likely to chip or break, it is not worth the time and effort to reduce the diameter and then reshape the edge and reapply peripheral curves. Likewise, prolonged surface polishing (i.e., several minutes) is not recommended, especially with high-Dk and hyper-Dk

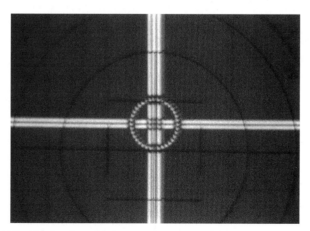

FIG. 15.29. Blurred lensometer image resulting from distortion of lens optics during attempted power change.

TABLE 15.3. MODIFICATION DO'S AND DON'TS

Do	Don't
Procedures	
Edge polish	Diameter reduction
Surface polish	Prolonged surface polish
Peripheral curve blending/flattening (low-high Dk)	Blending/flattening (hyper Dk)
Repowering	Repowering (velveteen pad/suction cup with higher/hyper Dk); infrequent polish
Techniques	
Keep lens cool	Allow heat to build
• Add polish frequently	
• Dip lens in water	
• Keep sponge tools saturated with water	
• Use a low spindle speed	
Optimize surface wettability	Dispense lens immediately after procedure
• Clean lens after procedure	
• Condition surface before dispensing	

lens materials. Some of the defects that result are not evident with biomicroscopy. Grohe et al. (20) evaluated the effect of front surface polishing on 20 GP lenses. The modified lenses were evaluated by high-magnification (100–500×) scanning electron microscopy. Several microscopic surface abnormalities were observed, including microcracks, splitting, scorching, and bleaching. It was concluded that prolonged polishing, diameter reduction, and repowering would be unacceptable in-office modification procedures for high-Dk GP lens materials. Walker (21) found similar results. If fluoro-silicone/acrylate lenses were surface polished for longer than 2 minutes, poor surface wettability, resulting in patient awareness of the lens over time, often resulted.

Repowering appears to be controversial. Whereas Grohe et al. (20) found it to be contraindicated with high-Dk lens materials, the studies by Reeder et al. (10) and Morgan et al. (22) appear to support it, although some precautions may be necessary, depending on the polish used and the specific procedure. The latter study found that repowering, even at a high (1,600 rpm) spindle speed with a high-Dk lens material, did not result in optical distortion or reduced quality of vision if a spinner tool was used in combination with a rounded sponge tool. Likewise, under scanning electron microscopy, the lens surface was free of defects (Fig. 15.28). However, use of a velveteen-covered tool resulted in significant optical distortion and reduced vision with the high-Dk lens material, even with the use of a low (550 rpm) spindle speed (Fig. 15.29). Numerous surface defects typically were present under scanning electron microscopy (Fig. 15.30).

An overview of recommended and not recommended modification procedures and techniques is given in Table 15.3.

Modification of Special Designs

It is apparent that modification procedures can be the difference between success and failure in bifocal/multifocal patients, as well as with keratoconic lens designs (11). In keratoconus, it is not uncommon to need to reduce the optic zone diameter and/or flatten the peripheral curve radii to reduce adherence and increase tear flow. Blending the peripheral curves can likewise have a dramatic effect (Fig. 15.31). As a result of the high minus powers often required for keratoconus correction, edge polishing and thinning are not uncommon procedures. The application of an anterior bevel, followed by an edge polish, is very beneficial in thinning a high minus edge (8).

Because many bifocal designs are prism ballasted and truncated and are designed to rest on the lower lid, thinning the upper edge to minimize the lifting effects of the upper lid is a beneficial procedure. To accomplish this, all but the upper edge can be covered by velveteen or a similar material. The edge can be rolled against a sponge using a suction cup spinner (Fig. 15.32). Polishing the occasional sharp thin

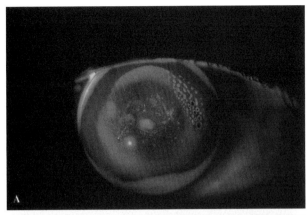

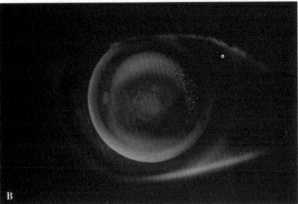

FIG. 15.31. A: Keratoconus lens design exhibiting harsh central bearing and peripheral sealoff. **B:** Same lens after reducing optic zone diameter and blending the peripheral curve radii. Note the increased fluorescein present peripherally and centrally. (Courtesy of Dr. Larry Davis.)

edge of a plus-powered bifocal/multifocal design can be beneficial. Although we have not done so, some practitioners have found it useful to modify the truncation angle of translating bifocal designs.

SUMMARY

Anyone can modify, and staff members can be of tremendous assistance in performing these procedures. Numerous organizations provide modification workshops, as do many members of the CLMA. The RGP Lens Institute also has an instructional videotape available (1-800-344-9060). Lenses to practice with should not be difficult to obtain, and rigid contact lens laboratories are excellent about assisting in these activities.

Modification of GP contact lenses is an invaluable asset to any practitioner. Although precautions must be taken with the newer high-Dk materials, most rigid contact lenses can be modified safely. Use of proper techniques and equipment, along with practice and experience, will greatly decrease the uncertainty and apprehension of in-office modification.

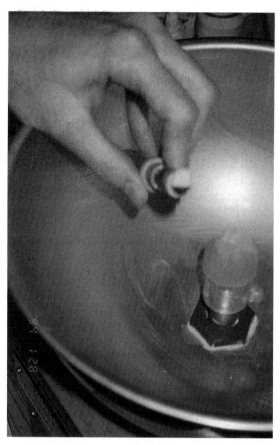

FIG. 15.32. Use of a velveteen pad to cover all but the superior edge of a prism-ballasted truncated lens. With the lens attached to the spinner, the edge is thinned when rotated into a sponge tool.

ACKNOWLEDGMENT

The authors thank Cheryl Bergin for assistance with this chapter.

REFERENCES

1. Hoffman WC. Mechanical and viscoelastic properties as they relate to machine and optical properties. *Optom Monthly* 1982; 73:340.
2. Fitzgerald JK. A comparison of selected rigid gas permeable contact lens material properties. *CLAO J* 1983;9:245.
3. Ratkowski D. The manufacture of rigid gas-permeable lens materials. In: Bennett ES, Grohe RM, eds. *Rigid gas-permeable contact lenses.* New York: Professional Press, 1986:99–114.
4. Schwartz CA. Radical flattening and RGP lenses. *Contact Lens Forum* 1986;11:49.
5. Mandell RB. Modification procedures. In: Mandell RB, ed. *Contact lens practice,* 4th ed. Springfield, IL: Charles C. Thomas, 1988:475–501.
6. *General manufacturing inspection procedure for the Boston lens.* Contact lens document no. OP2100, pp. 41–45, Polymer Technology Corporation, Rochester, New York.
7. Bennett ES. Offer-added value with in-office RGP modification. *Contact Lens Spectrum* 1996;11:18.
8. Morgan BW, Bennett ES. Modification. In: Bennett ES, Henry VA, eds. *Clinical manual of contact lenses,* 2nd ed. Philadelphia: Lippincott Williams & Wilkins, 2000:211–236.
9. Tracy D, Sanford M. Modification procedures, guidelines and tips. Conforma Laboratories, Norfolk, VA.
10. Reeder RE, Pate JR, Snyder C. Effectiveness and efficiency of rigid gas-permeable lens power modification with various polishes. *Int Contact Lens Clin* 1996;23:67.
11. Bennett ES. Successfully modifying contemporary RGP materials. *Optom Today* 1997;5:27.
12. Bennett ES, Clompus RJ, Hansen DW. A hands-on approach to RGP modification. *Rev Optom* 1998;135:88.
13. Picciano S, Andrasko GJ. Which factors influence RGP lens comfort? *Contact Lens Spectrum* 1989;4:31.
14. Meszaros GK. Simplifying lens modification. *Contact Lens Forum* 1986;11:42.
15. Morgan BW, Bennett ES. Modification of RGP lenses. *Contact Lens Forum* 1990;15:33.
16. Clompus R. How to polish and modify rigid lenses. *Rev Optom* 1987;124:106.
17. Jurkus JM. Modifying RGPs: a straightforward approach. *Optom Management* 1996;31:54.
18. *Gordon contact lens adjusting manual.* Division of UCO Optics, Rochester, NY.
19. Campbell R, Caroline P. New cleaning system for heavy depositors. *Contact Lens Spectrum* 1997;12:56.
20. Grohe RM, Caroline PJ, Norman C. The role of in-office modification for RGP surface defects. *Contact Lens Spectrum* 1988;3:52.
21. Walker J. Overpolishing fluoro-silicone/acrylates: the consequence and the cure. Transactions of the British Contact Lens Association Annual Clinical Conference, Birmingham, United Kingdom, 1989;6:29.
22. Morgan BW, Henry VA, Bennett ES, et al. The effect of modification procedures on rigid gas-permeable contact lenses: the UM-St. Louis study. *J Am Optom Assoc* 1992;63:201–206.

16A

PROGRESS EVALUATION PROCEDURES

DESMOND FONN AND
LUIGINA SORBARA

Aftercare is essential to ensure that the patient is comfortable and has adequate wearing time, has good vision, and is free of contact lens-induced complications. The practitioner and the patient share the responsibility of post-lens fitting follow-up. In order to confirm that a contact lens wearer is free from complications induced by contact lenses, whether it is soon after initiating lens wear or many years later, a detailed history should be obtained and a careful examination of eye and lenses must be conducted. It is not unusual for patients to develop chronic ocular changes (which are mostly subtle) without being symptomatic.

The contact lens wearer should be reexamined periodically, and each visit's evaluation procedures should follow a specific sequence. There is a consensus that patients should be reexamined more frequently during the first few months after initiating gas permeable (GP) lens wear. After dispensing GP lenses, we recommend a follow-up schedule with the following frequency: after 1 week, 3 weeks, 1 month, 3 months, and 6 months. Thereafter, patients are recommended to return every 6 months for as long as they wear contact lenses.

Most patients who successfully wear GP lenses will attain full-day wearing time, which may be anywhere between 8 and 16 hours per day (1). These patients should be examined toward the end of the day during their follow-up visits because some of the ocular manifestations may not be obvious after only a few hours of wear. During the adaptation period, which can range from days to months (2,3) for GP lens wearers, the daily wearing time invariably will be less than during postadaptation.

Patients who experience symptoms of discomfort or inability to wear the lenses should be instructed to discontinue lens wear prior to the consultation. The patient and lenses should be examined in order to establish the cause. However, if the diagnosis remains uncertain but the doctor is satisfied that there is no risk, lens wear may be resumed (even though the patient is uncomfortable) in the hope of eliciting the disorder and thus facilitating the diagnosis.

In the case of extended wear of GP lenses, it is preferable to examine these patients in the early morning when complications, such as corneal edema and lens binding from overnight wear, are more likely to manifest (4–10). This is especially true during the early stages of lens wear. When these complications have been determined to be either absent or insignificant, regular progress evaluation times may be considered.

Photodocumentation at the progress evaluation is a useful and sometimes essential method of recording obvious ocular signs. Following the progress of a condition, where one relies on written notes and drawings or grading from slit-lamp examinations, is a requirement but may be more precise with a series of photographs (11). Conventional photography requires a certain level of expertise to ensure the correct exposure, has high ongoing development costs, and cannot be viewed in real time. Image capture of the anterior segment has become much easier through the application of digital photography. To create a digital image, a system for recording the image, one for converting the image data into a digital file, and one for storage are required. The image can be captured by a still or video camera. The quality of the digital image captured will depend on the quality of the image capture board, video camera, and optics of the slit-lamp biomicroscope. Alternately, digital cameras can be attached directly to the slit lamp, and no image conversion is needed (12), The introduction of both illustrative and photographic grading scale systems (13) has resulted in a more structured and repeatable way of measuring and assessing ocular appearance; however, both time and skill are required in order to maximize their use.

ORDER OF THE PROCEDURES

The progress evaluation should be conducted efficiently and expediently so that the information yielded may result in an accurate diagnosis. This can best be achieved if the sequence of tests in the routine is structured (Table 16A.1) (14). Examples of data recording forms are given in Figures 16A.1 and 16A.2.

The sequence of procedures outlined in Table 16A.1 is a universal procedure that is applicable to all GP lens wearers

TABLE 16A.1. SEQUENCE OF PROCEDURES FOR A PROGRESS EVALUATION

With Lenses On
  History
    Posture and blinking
    Visual acuity
    Retinoscopy
    Overrefraction
    Overkeratometry
  Assessment of lens performance
    Fluorescein pattern
    Centration
    Movement
  Assessment of lens surface
    Wettability
    Deposits
With Lenses Off
  Biomicroscopy
  Keratometry/corneal topography
  Retinoscopy
  Refraction
  Visual acuity
  Examination of lenses
    Deposits
    Surface and edge inspection
    Parameter measurements

(15–18). To ensure that the patient's problem is lens related, other routine tests should be conducted, such as ophthalmoscopy, tonometry, and binocular evaluation, to rule out the possibility of ocular complications dissociated from lens wear. Patients seek aftercare for different reasons, such as emergency visits or routine 6-month consultations; therefore, all or part of the examination is conducted at the discretion of the doctor.

HISTORY

Occasionally, it is possible to extract sufficient information from a case history to diagnose the patient's problem, in which case only a few specific tests may be needed to confirm the diagnosis. However, it is imperative to establish whether the complaint or symptoms are serious enough to warrant resolution. Just as the examination routine is organized, so should the case history questions, in order to learn all relevant information.

Regardless of the condition or reason for the progress evaluation, all patients should be questioned about lens wearing time, comfort, vision, and compliance. They should be encouraged to state specifically what symptoms, if any, are experienced. Decreased wearing time or an inability to achieve sufficient wearing time is an indication of discomfort or intolerance. Excessive wearing time may cause complications often manifested as a delayed reaction. Comfort of GP lenses is relative and has been shown to improve with time (5). This phenomenon is interpreted as adaptation,

although there are measurable physiologic conditions that partially explain adaptation, such as decreases in corneal (19–23) and lid (24) desensitization.

The question regarding vision should be directed toward comparison between the two eyes and whether there has been a change in vision over time. It is always useful to question patients about compliance to ensure that they remember the necessities of cleaning, disinfecting, wetting, and using the appropriate solutions (25).

PROCEDURES WITH LENSES ON THE EYE

Posture and Blinking

During the case history it is important to observe the patient's posture and blinking habits at a time when the patient is unaware of the doctor's observations. Frequently GP lens wearers develop the contact lens "salute" (26). Backward head tilt, narrowing of the palpebral aperture, and restricted eye movement are characteristics of adaptation and usually are manifestations of discomfort.

Narrowing of the palpebral fissure has been observed with GP extended wear (5,27) and daily wear, particularly when the GP lenses are worn unilaterally (Fig. 16A.3). This pseudoptosis is observed more easily when it occurs in only one eye, but patients may become conscious of a bilateral change if the interpalpebral apertures decrease significantly. The precise repeated measurement of palpebral aperture height is difficult; therefore, practitioners and patients may remain unaware of subtle lid position changes. A photographic recording of the baseline may be helpful in this instance.

Some patients develop unnatural blinking habits with rigid lens wear, and it has been demonstrated that their blink rates increase (28–31). Of greater concern, however, is the partial blink that may occur during adaptation. The partial blink probably is in response to discomfort resulting from the lens edge causing a foreign body sensation.

Visual Acuity

Monocular and binocular acuity should be recorded at each visit. The measurement of visual acuity should correlate with the patient's symptoms related to vision. Visual acuity should be measured prior to examination of the eyes with bright white light, which produces after images and causes lacrimation, thus disturbing the lens, and could lead to an erroneous finding. In patients with symptoms related to reduced visual performance yet indicating normal visual acuity from standard letter charts, use of low-contrast acuity charts and measurement of contrast sensitivity also should be used.

Retinoscopy

There are at least three reasons for conducting retinoscopy. The first is to determine if a residual refractive error is pres-

University of Waterloo
School of Optometry
☐ Scheduled   **Progress Check/Delivery Visit No. _____**
☐ Unscheduled   **Frequent Replacement/Disposable**

Patient _____ Date _____ Health No. _____

History   W.T. Today _____ Usual W.T. _____ hours   **Summary of Visit**

Lens Name   OD _____ OS _____   Assessment (problems)

Care System _____ Compliance _____

Enzyme _____ How often? _____ Last used? _____

Vision ☐   Comfort ☐   Insertion/Removal ☐   Other ☐

Lens Age   OD _____ mos./yr   OS _____ mos./yr

CC

Change in health?/Meds?/Allergies? _____

With Old Lenses On	**OD**	**OS**	Plan
Visual Acuity 6/ Near	6/ Near		
Retinoscopy	6/	6/	
Balanced Best Sphere Subjective	6/	6/	

Mire Appearance (SCL)

before blink _____   before blink _____

after blink _____   after blink _____

RGP Position	RGP Position
Lag _____ ◯	Lag _____ ◯
SCL	SCL
Lag Str. Ahead _____	Lag Str. Ahead _____
Sup. Gaze _____ Cornea	Sup. Gaze _____ Cornea

Photos taken?   ☐ Yes   ☐ No

Next appointment date:

_____

Biomicroscopy indicate nicks, tears, scratches transient films   ◯ Lens   ◯ Lens

Recall factor: 3 months / 6 months / yearly

Modifications	**OD**	**OS**

With Lenses Off	**OD**	**OS**	Name	_____	_____
Biomicroscopy – See reverse for details			B.C.	_____	_____
Pachometry	mm	mm	S.C.R./W	_____	_____
Keratometry ____ / ____ X ____	____ / ____ X ____		P.C.R./W	_____	_____
mm ____ / ____	mm ____ / ____		O.Z.D.	_____	_____
Retinoscopy	6/	6/	Dia.	_____	_____
Subjective	6/	6/	Power	_____	_____

With New Lenses On	**OD**	**OS**	C.T.	_____	_____
Visual Acuity 6/ Near	6/ Near		Other	_____
Retinoscopy	6/	6/		
Balanced Best Sphere Subjective	6/	6/		

Mire Appearance (SCL)

before blink _____   before blink _____

after blink _____   after blink _____

RGP Position	RGP Position
Lag _____ ◯	Lag _____ ◯
SCL	SCL
Lag Str. Ahead _____	Lag Str. Ahead _____
Sup. Gaze _____ Cornea	Sup. Gaze _____ Cornea

Change of Address/Tele. No./Health No.

_____

_____

_____

Biomicroscopy indicate nicks, tears, scratches transient films   ◯ Lens   ◯ Lens

Intern

_____

Supervising Clinician

FIG. 16A.1. Progress evaluation form currently used at the Contact Lens Clinic, School of Optometry, University of Waterloo, Ontario, Canada.

Quantification of Slit Lamp Observations

SECTION A: Slit Lamp Examination

OD ☐ All Negative   ☐ All Negative OS

	OD						OS			
Absent ☐	Present ☐				**Corneal Striae**	Absent ☐	Present ☐			
Grade	0	1	2	3	**Corneal Edema**	Grade	0	1	2	3
Grade	0	1	2	3	**Corneal Neovascularization**	Grade	0	1	2	3
Grade	0	1	2	3	**3 and/or 9 o'clock Corneal Staining**	Grade	0	1	2	3
Grade	0	1	2	3	**Other Corneal Staining**	Grade	0	1	2	3
Grade	0	1	2	3	**Epithelial Microcysts**	Grade	0	1	2	3
Grade	0	1	2	3	**Limbal Injection**	Grade	0	1	2	3
Grade	0	1	2	3	**Bulbar Injection**	Grade	0	1	2	3
Grade	0	1	2	3	**Bulbar Edema**	Grade	0	1	2	3
Type	0	1	2	3	**Tarsal Conjunctival Abnormalities**	Type	0	1	2	3

SECTION B: Other Anterior Segment Abnormalities

OD ☐ All Absent   ☐ All Absent OS

Instructions: If abnormalities are present, indicate cause(s) by checking appropriate box(es) and note location in diagram below.

(1) Lens Related	(2) Solution Related	(3) Result of Other Factors (explain)		(1) Lens Related	(2) Solution Related	(3) Result of Other Factors (explain)
☐	☐	☐ _____	1. Blepharitis	☐	☐	☐ _____
☐	☐	☐ _____	2. Corneal Infiltrates	☐	☐	☐ _____
☐	☐	☐ _____	3. Iritis	☐	☐	☐ _____
☐	☐	☐ _____	4. Corneal Ulceration Confirmed By Microbiological Culture	☐	☐	☐ _____
☐	☐	☐ _____	5. Other (Explain)	☐	☐	☐ _____

SECTION C: Comments and Additional Tests (eg. photography)

FEB. 97   5109-1

FIG. 16A.2. Biomicroscopy form used in association with the progress evaluation form (Fig. 16A.1) from the same institution.

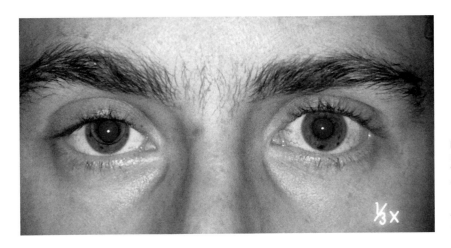

FIG. 16A.3. Unilateral ocular ptosis in the right eye 4 weeks after commencing extended wear. This subject is wearing a rigid gas permeable lens in the right eye and a soft lens in the left eye. (From Fonn D, Holden BA. Rigid gas-permeable vs hydrogel contact lenses for extended wear. *Am J Optom Physiol Opt* 1988; 65:536–544, with permission.)

ent while the patient is wearing the contact lens; therefore, retinoscopy would provide the starting point for the subjective overrefraction. Small amounts of residual astigmatism are common with spherical rigid lens wear, but this astigmatism is often considered clinically insignificant and tolerable (32–34). The second reason is that the optics of the system (lens + eye) can be viewed objectively to determine if any aberrations or distortions have occurred within the pupillary zone. The normal clear orange circular light reflex that is expected from this corrected system may contain blemishes, such as dark shadows in arcuate or linear form. These effects might be produced by either decentered lenses or small optical zone diameters, both of which would place the secondary curves within the pupil area. Warped, damaged, or badly scratched lenses can result in apparent opacities or multiple images within the reflex. The third reason to perform retinoscopy would be to use information gained from the previous two procedures to substantiate the symptomatology in cases where inadequate, reduced, or fluctuating vision has been reported.

Overrefraction

In some instances, monocular subjective overrefraction should be preceded by autorefraction. These instruments are simple to use, and their efficiency is especially evident when overrefractions are performed on patients wearing toric lenses. Unfortunately, these instruments also have certain limitations. For example, the end result of this procedure is always a spherocylindrical prescription, and often the instrument will signal error when the contact lens does not center perfectly.

One of the purposes of GP lens application is to neutralize corneal astigmatism. If residual astigmatism is present, it is often ignored, unless it is significant enough to reduce acuity and produce symptoms. It is for this reason that the first approach to overrefraction is spherical only. In the case of the undercorrected or overcorrected ametropia, if the visual acuity or symptoms are not predictably remedied by

spherical overrefraction, then a spherocylindrical overrefraction should follow.

Finally, the monocular overrefraction and then binocular balance should provide a clear endpoint result and should closely correlate with the retinoscopy result. If entering visual acuity is substantially lower due to incorrect refractive correction, the overrefraction should improve acuity proportionately. The relationship among visual acuity, overrefraction, and subjective symptoms should always be considered.

Overkeratometry

When made too thin, highly permeable GP lenses will flex on the cornea of patients with moderate-to-high corneal astigmatism. This results in lens flexure (toricity of the front surface of the lens *in situ*) and is measured clinically by manual or automated keratometry. The degree of lens flexure is influenced by material properties, lens design (thickness), lens fit (base curve radius), corneal toricity, lid tension, and tear film dynamics (35–43).

GP lenses neutralize corneal astigmatism through the tear lens and spherical surfaces of the contact lens. However, residual astigmatism will result if the GP lens flexes on the eye and a decrement in visual acuity can be expected (44). Lens flexure might be advantageous in cases where corneal astigmatism is greater than spectacle astigmatism (45).

ASSESSMENT OF LENS PERFORMANCE
Fluorescein Pattern

Assessment of the fluorescein pattern is considered mandatory in the progress evaluation sequence, regardless of the reason for the consultation. The fluorescein pattern should be examined carefully, particularly in patients who are not exhibiting satisfactory progress or who have symptoms of discomfort and are unable to achieve an acceptable wearing time. Reference has been made to the static and dynamic patterns (46). It would be appropriate to appraise the static lens-to-cornea relationship and then to examine the fluorescein pattern in the context of lens movement and centration.

Fluorescent hand-held lamps, such as the Burton lamp, can be used to view the fluorescein pattern but would be inappropriate if the lens contained an ultraviolet block. Our preference is to use a slit-lamp biomicroscope incorporating a cobalt blue filter to study the fluorescent tear film and contact lens. The slit lamp is advantageous because of the bright light source and variable magnification. A yellow barrier filter, for example, the Kodak Wratten filter no. 12, placed before the slit lamp-objective to enhance the contrast of the tear film is essential. Many new biomicroscopes now conveniently incorporate yellow barrier filters.

The GP lens fluorescein pattern can be subdivided into three components: the central apical area, the midperipheral zone, and the peripheral zone. There is general theoretic agreement that most of the back surface of the lens should parallel the central corneal curvature, and the balance of the posterior surface should gradually flatten at a greater rate than the corneal midperiphery, creating space for a reservoir of tears. If this principle were followed, then the fluorescein pattern observed in Fig. 16A.4 (see Color Plate 16A.4) would fulfill these criteria. It can be observed that there is central alignment (a dark central zone indicating minimal tear lens thickness), an apparent absence of midperipheral bearing, and minimal edge clearance. An apical clearance fit shows excessive pooling in the center and marked localized midperipheral bearing, which effectively seals the optical zone. A lens that is too flat exhibits localized central touch and excessive edge clearance. Figs. 16A.5 (see Color Plate 16A.5) and 16A.6 (see Color Plate 16A.6) depict edge lift only and demonstrate too little edge clearance (a tight periphery) and excessive edge clearance, respectively. Note the air bubbles at the inferior edge of the lens in Fig. 16A.6. It may be beneficial to grade the central and edge clearance

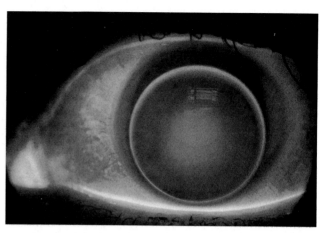

FIG. 16A.5. Lens with minimal edge clearance (tight periphery). This represents approximately 60 μm of tear lens thickness at the edge. (See Color Plate 16A.5.)

characteristics of the lens fit on an arbitrary scale (-2, -1, 0, $+1$, $+2$) for purposes of record keeping. This five-tier rating system, when used for central classification, would rate a very flat lens as -2 and a very steep lens as $+2$. Using these two examples of edge lift, the lens shown in Fig. 16A.5 would be rated as $+2$ edge clearance and in Fig. 16A.6 as -2.

Centration

GP lenses should center symmetrically within the corneal diameter to provide adequate coverage of the pupil. Centration is dependent on many variables, such as corneal astigmatism, shape and apex location, aperture size, lid force, and the many lens variables that affect the center of gravity of the lens (24). When lenses locate eccentrically (Fig.

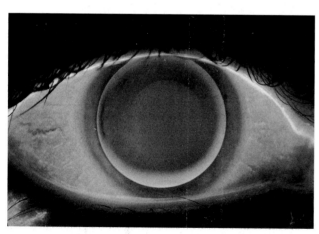

FIG. 16A.4. Alignment fluorescein pattern (posterior surface of the lens matching the corneal contour) with adequate edge clearance. (See Color Plate 16A.4.)

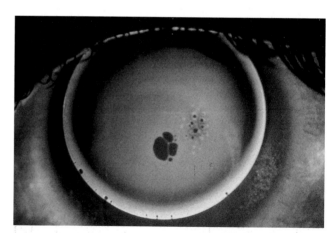

FIG. 16A.6. Lens fit demonstrating excessive edge clearance in depth and width characterized by the bubbles at the edge, as well as the bright fluorescein appearance. The inferior edge clearance is accentuated by the lid pressure imparted on the superior region of the lens. (See Color Plate 16A.6.)

16A.7), the lens-to-cornea fitting relationship alters as the lens tends to lodge on a flatter region of the cornea. In cases where lenses are manufactured with a traditional tricurve design without blending the transitions, corneal indentation and insult could occur and movement might be hampered.

It is fairly easy to determine if lenses are decentered, but again distinction should be made between the static and dynamic positions of the lens (24). The lens should always be viewed immediately after the blink within the confines of the corneal diameter and in relation to the pupil. The intensity of light entering the eye will determine the pupil size, so it may be preferable to evaluate the lens position using blue light with fluorescein. Rather than assessing the decentration and recording the relative position of the lens using a diagram, it is preferable to measure the amount of decentration. This can be accomplished by incorporating a graticule in the eyepiece of a biomicroscope. The millimeter scale is superimposed over the cornea. With the appropriate magnification, the geometric center of the cornea is located and the decentration of the lens is recorded for both principal meridians (47). These x and y values, denoting horizontal and vertical measurements, respectively, are recorded as either positive (+) or negative (−) values from standard graphic notations. It is important that the patient be comfortably positioned in the chin rest of the slit lamp, because the lens may appear decentered if an abnormal posture is adopted.

Movement

Lens movement is an essential element of the lens fit (48, 49). Movement encourages tear exchange, which, in turn, is responsible for supplying a limited amount of oxygen and for removing metabolic waste products (50–52). Movement also is a useful indicator of the lens-to-cornea relationship.

Steep fitting lenses or lenses that conform too closely to

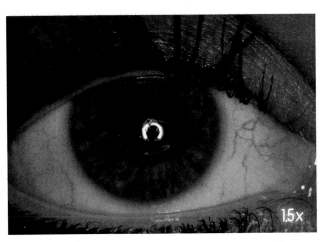

FIG. 16A.7. Typical superior decentration of high minus (−10.50 D) rigid gas permeable lens fitted slightly flatter than low K on a near spherical cornea.

the cornea (alignment) with very little edge lift can be termed *tight* and invariably will have restricted movement. Conversely, lenses that have apical touch and excessive edge lift usually will be looser and thus exhibit too much movement unless the lens decenters to a flatter region of the cornea or is partially covered by the superior lid.

Lens movement is measured most effectively using a graticule in the eyepiece of a biomicroscope. The amount of movement is observed most easily if the zero position of the scale is placed at the inferior edge of the lens. The patient is requested to blink and, immediately following the upward excursion of the lid, the position of rest of the lens is noted before it moves down again. The magnitude is generally 1 to 2 mm (53,54).

The clinician also should be aware of the downward excursion of the lens. The gradual and straight lag toward the inferior limbus is the expected motion. However, if the lens drops very quickly or an arcuate movement is observed, the lens fit can be classified as loose or the lens fit might be too flat. Other factors, such as lacrimation, excessive lens thickness, and the location of the center of gravity of the lens, also may be responsible for this movement.

ASSESSMENT OF LENS SURFACE

Wettability

In vitro wettability (wetting or contact angle) of GP lens surfaces has been described in detail elsewhere in this book. Although these measurements have been shown to be consistent for a given technique comparing different materials (55,56), there is skepticism about the relationship between this measurement and the *in situ* wetting performance of the lens (57–59).

It is clinically difficult to quantify or assess the in-eye wettability of contact lenses. Reports of techniques that describe slit-lamp and photographic procedures using tear film interference patterns and conventional illumination have been published (60–63).

Many factors can influence the integrity of the tear film on the GP lens, such as lacrimation produced by ocular irritation, lens thickness and design, excessive mucus or lipid contamination of the tear film, the condition of the lens surface, lens material, and the light source being used to examine the pre-lens tear film.

One method for evaluating the stability of the tear film on the lens surface is the tear lens breakup time (TBUT). The conventional procedure for measuring corneal surface TBUT using fluorescein has been challenged because it is an invasive technique. By using the slit lamp and low levels of white light illumination without fluorescein, it is possible to measure TBUT on the lens surface (64); however, the validity of this method has yet to be established.

What is perhaps more beneficial is to observe the characteristics of the tear film and appearance of the lens surface

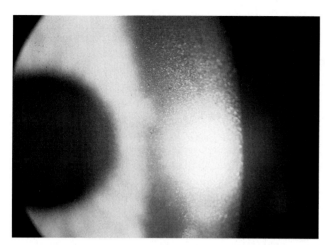

FIG. 16A.8. Tear film appearance photographed approximately 2 seconds after the normal transparent film transforms by the eyes being kept open. This *film* appearance is frequently observed on rigid lenses.

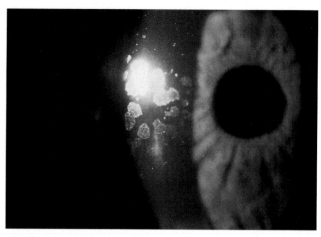

FIG. 16A.10. Dry patches or nonwetting areas on a rigid lens surface.

immediately following the break or interruption of the prelens tear film when the eye is purposefully held open for 10 seconds or longer. The appearance of the tear film–lens surface can be subdivided into three categories. The first is the normal film appearance (Fig. 16A.8), which is seen to consist of minute droplets or beads of lipid and probably is the most common. The second category of lens surface appearance is described as *hazing* (Fig. 16A.9). The haze seems to have a dry or powdery appearance and appears to occur with a faster TBUT on the lens surface, although there is no conclusive proof of this. It occurs much less frequently than the "film." The third category consists of what appear to be obvious dry patches (Fig. 16A.10) and is less common than the other two. These dry patches appear when the lens does not wet completely and are fairly com-

mon with new lenses during the first few days and are very common at dispensing.

Deposits

GP lens surfaces are likely to attract tear components, such as mucus, lipoprotein, and exogenous substances. These coatings, or deposits, are easily observed with a biomicroscope and white light. The precise composition of the material on the lens, however, can only be identified by elaborate laboratory techniques.

Deposits convey the connotation of tenaciously bound substances. Often, the coatings or concretions will remain persistently on the lens during blinking, but when the lens is removed for cleaning by rubbing, rinsing, and drying with tissue paper, the material that is removed is called *loosely bound deposits*. These tear solutes and other exogenous sub-

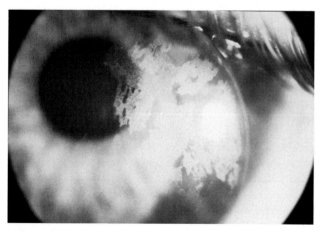

FIG. 16A.9. Appearance of *haze* on the lens surface displaying the powdery appearance as the tear film breaks. Tear film breakup time on the lens surface usually is faster when the haze appearance occurs.

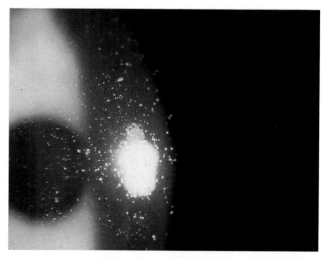

FIG. 16A.11. Appearance of pearlescent spots on a rigid lens surface. This is a deposit that is persistent only while the lens is on the eye.

stances, such as eye makeup that remains on the lens while in the eye, can cause irritation and interfere with vision.

One fairly common example (Fig. 16A.11) of a loosely bound deposit on a GP lens observed while in the eye has been termed *pearlescent spots* (65). The chemical composition of these spots has not yet been classified adequately, but they probably consist of lipoprotein and mucus.

PROCEDURES WITH LENSES OFF THE EYE

After all the preceding tests have been conducted, there is every likelihood that any existing complications would be identified. The manifestations of physical and physiologic stress imparted by a GP lens can be detected fairly easily if the patient has worn the lenses for as long as possible. The bulbar and tarsal conjunctiva, the tear film, and the lids should be examined as carefully as the cornea.

Biomicroscopy

Biomicroscopy should be the first procedure to be performed after lenses are removed. Clinical entities are difficult to quantify, such as 3- and 9-o'clock staining (Fig. 16A.12); therefore, a system to record and monitor slit-lamp signs (Fig. 16A.2) is essential (66,67). Most biomicroscopes include the fundamental elements needed for a full examination: sufficient light intensity (preferably quartz halogen); magnification up to at least 40×; cobalt blue and red-free filters in addition to white light and neutral density filters, with some slit lamps now incorporating yellow barrier filters; graticule options for the eyepiece; and a mechanism to offset the illumination and observation synchronization (breaking the linkage).

Using the techniques of direct focal and indirect illumination, direct and marginal retroillumination, and specular reflection, it should be possible to identify any corneal and conjunctival surface or refractile defects. The use of rose bengal, lissamine green, and fluorescein stains with a yellow barrier filter will highlight any surface defects and assist in the differential diagnosis.

One of the challenges that clinicians face after conducting a biomicroscopic examination is characterizing the condition and assessing the severity. To simplify matters, magnitude estimation scales (0–3) are used (Fig. 16A.2). Although these scales serve the purpose of being able to define whether or not a condition is serious, they do not offer sufficient variability to make judgments of more subtle changes. Alternative photographic (Cornea and Contact Lens Research Unit [CCLRU]) scales (68) or artist's rendition scales (11) offer the advantage of having a constant reference so that clinical judgment may be easier and more accurate.

Guillon and Guillon (69) have suggested that the Tearscope™ (Keeler Instruments) may be a useful instrument to observe the lipid layer of the tear film. Prior to instillation of any dyes, the Tearscope is held in front of the objective of the slit lamp and is the only magnification that is used to view the tear film. This diffuse cold light source illumination system allows noninvasive measurement of lipid coverage of the cornea (or over a contact lens) and patterns of lipid mixing, which are classified in order of increasing thickness. Patterns can be described from the thinnest open meshwork, tight meshwork, wave pattern, amorphous pattern to finally the thickest lipid pattern, a color pattern.

The methods of biomicroscopy and contact lens-induced complications have been comprehensively described (70–73). A convenient method is to operate from low magnification with diffuse light to highest magnification with maximum localized focal light, working from anterior to posterior surfaces of the cornea and then the anterior chamber, applying fluorescein, and finally examining the tarsal conjunctiva.

Keratometry and Corneal Topography

The shape of the cornea may alter as a result of the mechanical and physiologic influences of the GP contact lens (74, 75). Physiologic changes are less common now because present-day materials are sufficiently oxygen permeable for daily wear. Studies on extended wear GP lenses have demonstrated the mechanical influence of lenses as a sphericalization effect (the steeper meridian of the cornea flattening more than the flatter meridian) (8,76,77). Keratometric changes are observed as numerical quantitative alterations that either increase or decrease in value or as distortion of the mires, which should be recorded as a qualitative change or surface irregularity. Some of the newer autokeratometers also produce images and numeric values for central and midperipheral corneal areas. The limitation of keratometry is that it only measures a small area of the cornea (approxi-

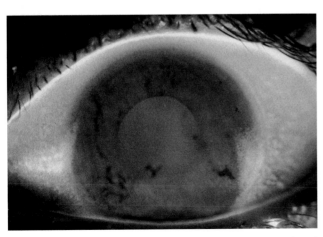

FIG. 16A.12. Severe 3- and 9-o'clock corneal staining produced by desiccation while wearing a rigid corneal contact lens.

mately 3 mm) unless eccentric fixation targets are used to offset the reflected mires, in which case multiple serial measurements across the surface are necessary to represent a larger area of the cornea.

The advent of corneal topography with videokeratoscopes has superseded keratometry for the purpose of capturing the shape of a much larger area of the cornea (approximately 8 mm) and, for some instruments, the entire cornea surface. A good example where corneal topography is so much more useful than keratometry is inferior corneal steepening due to warpage induced by a contact lens or the development of keratoconus (Fig. 16A.13; see Color Plate 16A.13).

The aim of corneal topography (or keratoscopy) is to accurately describe the shape of the corneal surface in all meridians (78–80). In most cases, the technique uses a principle similar to keratometry, in that the size of the image is determined from a target that is reflected from the corneal surface. The primary difference is that, in keratoscopy, a series of targets, usually circular (black and white rings), is used. This arrangement allows both central and peripheral curvature to be determined. Modern-generation topographers capture the corneal reflected image electronically on a computer and use sophisticated image processing software to provide immediate analysis of the image (videokeratoscopy).

Reflective devices measure topography based on the reflection of mires from the anterior surface tear film rather than from the corneal surface. Once the images are

recorded, then a computational approach is used to derive the corneal shape. The images (or "maps") produced by reflective keratoscopes characterize corneal surface power distribution using color-coded displays, in which greens and yellows represent powers characteristic of those found in normal corneas, blue represents flatter areas (low powers), and reds represent steep areas (high powers) (81). These maps permit recognition of corneal shape through pattern recognition and swiftly reveal the presence of abnormal powers (Fig. 16A.13; see Color Plate 16A.14). All devices display simulated keratometry (SimK) values, which are analogous to standard keratometry values and simultaneously display the power and axis of the flattest and steepest meridians. Topographers also can generate difference maps, which are useful for detecting subtle changes over time.

Pachymetry

Measurement of corneal thickness should be an essential element in the battery of tests used to monitor corneal status in response to contact lens wear. It is important to measure corneal thickness in refractive surgery, keratoconics, and patients with peripheral corneal thinning diseases. Serial thickness measurement should be conducted on orthokeratology patients. This proved to be difficult in the past because of the instruments available at the time. Off-the-shelf optical pachymeters and hand-held ultrasound instruments suffered from a lack of repeatability. With the development of newer ultrasound pachymeters and the Orbscan (Orbtek,

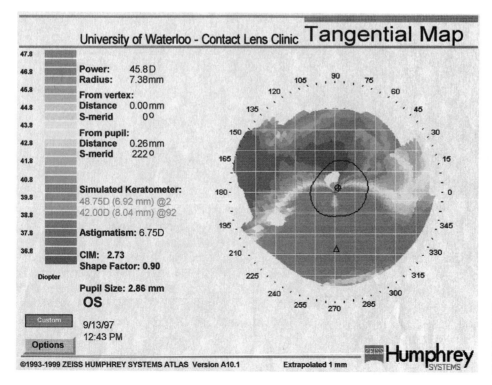

FIG. 16A.13. Videokeratoscopic map of a keratoconic cornea depicting flatter (blue color) and steeper (red color) with inferior decentration of the steeper zone. (See Color Plate 16A.13.)

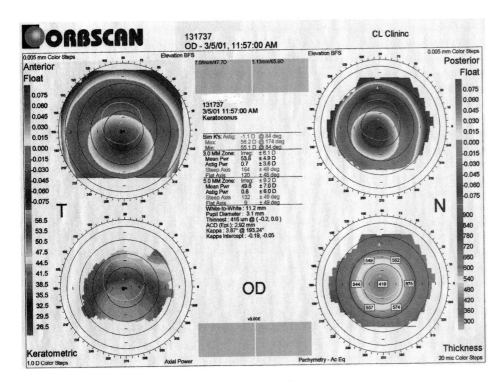

FIG. 16A.14. Printout from the Orbscan showing the anterior and posterior topography maps with a corneal thickness plot. (See Color Plate 16A.14.)

Bausch and Lomb Surgical), corneal thickness measurements can be performed with ease. The Orbscan automatically generates a thickness profile map of the cornea (approximately 8 mm) with maps of surface topography (Fig. 16A.14).

Corneal thickness changes can reflect alterations in hydration and metabolism. Most contact lenses will induce corneal swelling through hypoxia and osmotic fluid changes. Central corneal thickness has been shown to increase by about 10% to 15% during contact lens wear with eye closure, and this is predominantly a function of oxygen transmissibility for both GP and soft lenses (82,83). Corneal thickness also can be altered by mechanical pressure from GP lens designs or intentionally and specifically from orthokeratology reversed geometry design lenses.

Topographic corneal swelling has been measured, but it has been very difficult to determine with certainty whether the changes occur anteriorly or posteriorly. Less is known about the changes to the corneal epithelium, presumably due to the relative difficulty in measuring and imaging this thin layer. Epithelial thickness appears to be resistant to change from the hypoxic effects of contact lens wear but not to the mechanical effects of GP lenses (84–88). Erickson and Comstock (89) used mathematical models to describe corneal swelling after 4 hours of patched eye contact lens wear and concluded that swelling affected the posterior area of the cornea.

The Orbscan 2™, which is an optical based topographic imaging system, uses anterior and posterior corneal surface elevation data to calculate corneal thickness across a large corneal area (Fig. 16A.14) and would be a definitive instrument for characterizing corneal thickness changes (90). Orbscan corneal topography system is a noninvasive and noncontact computerized corneal mapping instrument that uses optical scanning slit to provide topographic analysis of both the front and back surfaces of the cornea, as well as pachymetric measurements. Lattimore et al. (90) used the Orbscan in a repeatability experiment and showed high repeatability with a standard deviation of 9.08 μm for 750 data points across the central 7 mm of the cornea.

Optical coherence tomography (OCT) is a noncontact imaging technique that can measure tissue thickness with the highest nominal resolution among current noncontact diagnostic instruments (91). Previous work has suggested that corneal and particularly corneal epithelial thickness can be measured using the OCT. Wang et al. (84) measured central and peripheral corneal thickness by mounting a fixation device on the OCT system.

Retinoscopy, Refraction, and Visual Acuity

Wearing a GP contact lens can alter the refractive error and corneal curvature of an eye. Increases or decreases in myopia or hyperopia and changes in astigmatism become apparent when corneas steepen or flatten or become more or less toroidal. There is usually a commensurate change in visual acuity. Retinoscopy is a sensitive procedure for determining the optical quality of the eye. If previously unobserved aberrations or distortions occur in the retinoscopic reflex, they can be attributed directly to the influence of the contact lens, but they also may be due to a corneal condition such as keratoconus.

Refractive error should remain constant with lens wear, but if an alteration in refraction occurs, then the corrected visual acuity should be identical to the baseline measurement. A clear endpoint of this procedure is indicative of little or no corneal deformation. A reduction in visual acuity with the best possible refractive error correction is indicative of corneal distortion, and if lens wear is discontinued, this phenomenon will invariably be found to be reversible.

EXAMINATION OF LENSES

Examination of the lenses is the final part of the progress evaluation. Although these issues have been discussed in detail elsewhere, each of the following subsections should be applied to aid in the diagnosis and care of the patient.

Deposits

Lenses that have been removed from the eye should be rinsed and dried clean with a Kimwipe or soft tissue paper. Tear solutes, debris, lipid coatings, and unbound protein layers usually will be removed with this action. The objective now is to determine whether any resistant deposits have remained on the lens. Such residues invariably will be bound or denatured protein sometimes described as plaque (Fig. 16A.15) (92). Lenses can be inspected with simple instruments as a magnification loupe or binocular magnifiers or more sophisticated instruments such as a stereomicroscope with dark-field illumination (Fig. 16A.16).

Surface and Edge Inspections

GP lenses have proved to be less durable than polymethyl methacrylate (PMMA) lenses. Frequent inspection (at each

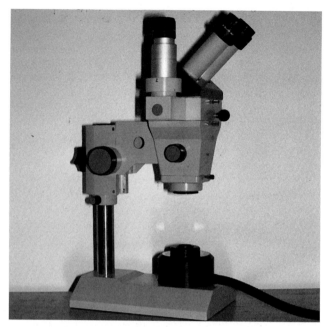

FIG. 16A.16. Zeiss "dark-field" stereomicroscope, which can be used to inspect rigid gas permeable and soft contact lenses.

progress evaluation) of the surfaces and edges of GP lenses is advised because they scratch and chip more easily. It is easy to inspect the lenses with a hand-held 7× or 10× loupe, but because this is a monocular instrument, it is preferable to use a stereomicroscope with dark-field illumination for identifying any surface irregularities. Alternatively, a high-magnification profile projector can be used for detailed inspection and measurement (Fig. 16A.17). Occasionally it has been observed that GP lens base curve radii alter appreciably with time (flatten or steepen), especially thinner lenses and lenses made of higher-permeability materials. In addition, these lenses are more susceptible to warpage, and in certain cases the measurement stability may be affected by solutions (93).

CONCLUSIONS

All currently available GP materials will, to some degree, attract deposits. Generally the extent of the deposits is proportional to the age of the lens and the wearing time. If lenses become deposited, the risk of trauma increases; therefore, patients must be encouraged to undergo periodic progress evaluations. A perplexing problem of GP lenses relates to lens surfaces. Compliance cannot be overemphasized. Careful and thorough cleaning, disinfection, and wetting preparation prior to insertion will, in most cases, limit the severity of contamination and enhance the wettability of the lenses.

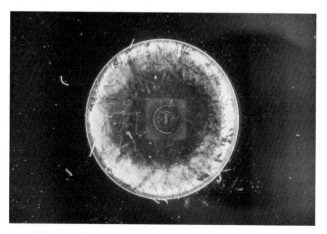

FIG. 16A.15. Rigid gas permeable lens showing protein deposit (plaque) surrounding a fairly clear central area, which is typical of a patient cleaning/rubbing only the central area of the lens.

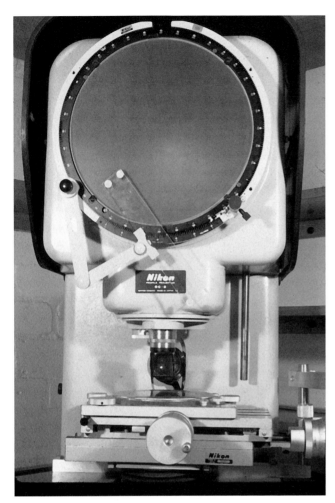

FIG. 16A.17. Nikon profile projector with interchangeable lenses providing variable magnification.

REFERENCES

1. Gasson A. Aspects of hard lens aftercare. *Contact Lens J* 1979;8:4–11.
2. Mandell RB, Harris MG. Theory of the contact lens adaptation process. *J Am Optom Assoc* 1968;46:296–302.
3. Harris MG, Mandell RB. Contact lens adaptation: osmotic theory. *Am J Optom Arch Am Acad Optom* 1969;46:196–202.
4. Fonn D, Holden BA. Extended wear of hard gas permeable contact lenses can induce ptosis. *CLAO J* 1986;12:93–94.
5. Fonn D, Holden BA. Rigid gas-permeable vs. hydrogel contact lenses for extended wear. *Am J Optom Physiol Opt* 1988;65:536–544.
6. Lattood, D. Edge shape and comfort of rigid lenses. *Am J Optom Physiol Opt* 1988;65:613–618.
7. Kenyon E, Polse KA, Mandell RB. Rigid contact lens adherence: incidence, severity and recovery. *J Am Optom Assoc* 1988;59:168–174.
8. Polse KA, Sarver MD, Kenyon E, et al. Gas permeable hard contact lens extended wear: ocular and visual responses to a 6-month period of wear. *CLAO J* 1987;13:31–38.
9. Swarbrick HA, Holden BA. Rigid gas permeable lens binding: significance and contributing factors. *Am J Optom Physiol Opt* 1987;64:815–823.
10. Swarbrick HA. A possible etiology for RGP lens binding (adherence). *Int Contact Lens Clin* 1988;15:13–19.
11. Efron N. Grading scales for contact lens complications. *Ophthal Physiol Opt* 1998;18:182–186.
12. Cox I. Digital imaging in the contact lens practice. *Int Contact Lens Clin* 1995;22:62–66.
13. Terry RL, Schnider CM, Holden BA, et al. CCLRU standards for success of daily and extended wear contact lenses. *Optom Vis Sci* 1993;70:234–243.
14. Jurkus J, Stein PD. An organized approach to solving problems of hard contact lens wearers. *Contacto* 1982;26:5–7.
15. Bennett ES. How to manage the rigid lens wearer. *Rev Optom* 1986;123:102–110.
16. Burnett Hodd FA. Aftercare and symptomatology. In: Stone J, Phillips AJ, eds. *Contact lenses.* London: Barrie and Jenkins, 1981;496–526.
17. Catania LJ. A categorical approach to the diagnosis and management of pre- and post-fit contact lens conditions. *J Am Optom Assoc* 1987;58:819–830.
18. McMonnies CW. Contact lens aftercare: a detailed analysis. *Clin Exp Optom* 1987;70.4:121–127.
19. Bergenske PD, Polse KA. The effect of rigid gas permeable lenses on corneal sensitivity. *J Am Optom Assoc* 1987;58:212–215.
20. Millodot M. Effect of the length of wear of contact lens on corneal sensitivity. *Acta Ophthalmol* 1976;54:721–730.
21. Millodot M. Effect of long-term wear of hard contact lenses on corneal sensitivity. *Arch Ophthalmol* 1978;96:1225–1227.
22. Millodot M, O'Leary DJ. Effect of oxygen deprivation on corneal sensitivity. *Acta Ophthalmol* 1980;58:434–439.
23. Polse KA. Etiology of corneal sensitivity changes accompanying contact lens wear. *Invest Ophthalmol Vis Sci* 1978;17:1202–1206.
24. Mandell RB. Basic principals of rigid lenses. In: Mandell RB, ed. *Contact lens practice,* 4th ed. Springfield, IL: Charles C. Thomas, 1988;173–202.
25. Chun MW, Weissman BA. Compliance in contact lens care. *Am J Optom Physiol Opt* 1987;64:274–276.
26. Mandell TB. Symptomatology and refitting. In: Mandell RB, ed. *Contact lens practice,* 4th ed. Springfield, IL: Charles C. Thomas, 1988;388–439.
27. Fonn D, Pritchard N, Garnett B, et al. Palpebral aperture sizes of rigid and soft contact lens wearers compared with nonwearers. *Optom Vis Sci* 1996;73:211–214.
28. Brown M, Chinn S, Fatt I, et al. The effect of soft and hard contact lenses on blink rate, amplitude and length. *J Am Optom Assoc* 1973;44:254.
29. Carney LG, Hill RM. Contact lenses and the blink. *Contact Lens J* 1986;14:3–6.
30. Hill RM, Carney LG. The effects of hard lens wear on blinking behavior. *Int Contact Lens Clin* 1984;11:242–248.
31. Korb DR. The role of blinking in successful contact lens wear. *Int Contact Lens Clin* 1974;1:59–71.
32. Bailey NJ. Residual astigmatism with contact lenses. *Arch Soc Am Ophthalmol* 1959;11:37–41.
33. Bailey NJ. Residual astigmatism with contact lenses: part 1. *Opt J Rev Optom* 1961;98:30–31.
34. Sarver MD. A study of residual astigmatism. *Am J Optom Physiol Opt* 1969;48:578–582.
35. Harris MG. The effect of contact lens thickness and diameter on residual astigmatism: a preliminary study. *Am J Optom Physiol Opt* 1970;47:442–444.
36. Harris MG, Chu CS. The effect of contact lens thickness and corneal toricity on flexure and residual astigmatism. *Am J Optom Arch Am Acad Optom* 1972;49:304–307.
37. Harris MG, Appelquist TD. The effect of contact lens diameter and power on flexure and residual astigmatism. *Am J Optom Physiol Opt* 1974;51:266–270.

38. Harris MG, Sweeney KE, Rocchi S, et al. Flexure and residual astigmatism with cellulose acetate butyrate (CAB) contact lenses on toric corneas. *Am J Optom Physiol Opt* 1982;59:858–862.

39. Harris MG, Kadoya J, Nomura J, et al. Flexure and residual astigmatism with Polycon and polymethyl methacrylate lenses on toric corneas. *Am J Optom Physiol Opt* 1982;59:263–266.

40. Harris MG, Gale B, Gansel K, et al. Flexure and residual astigmatism with Paraperm O_2 and Boston II lenses on toric corneas. *Am J Optom Physiol Opt* 1987;64:269–273.

41. Herman JP. Flexure of rigid contact lenses on toric corneas as a function of base curve fitting relationship. *J Am Optom Assoc* 1983;54:209–213.

42. Holden BA. Predicting contact lens flexure from in vitro testing. *J Am Optom Assoc* 1984;55:171.

43. Pole JJ, Kochanny L. The comparative flexure of Polycon II, Silicon and Boston II contact lenses on toric corneas. *Optom Monthly* 1984;75:151–155.

44. Sorbara L, Fonn D, MacNeil K. Effect of rigid gas permeable lens flexure on vision. *Optom Vis Sci* 1992;69:953–958.

45. Bennett ES. Astigmatic correction. In: Bennett ES, Grohe RM, eds. *Rigid gas permeable contact lenses*. Chicago: Professional Press, 1986;348–384.

46. Mandell RB. Trial lens method. In: Mandell RB, ed. *Contact lens practice*, 4th ed. Springfield, IL: Charles C. Thomas, 1988; 243–264.

47. Holden BA. Grading system, Personal Communication, 1986.

48. Korb DR, Korb JE. A new concept in contact lens design: parts 1 and II. *J Am Optom Assoc* 1970;40:1–12.

49. Korb DR. Fitting to achieve normal blinking and lid action. *Int Contact Lens Clin* 1974;1:57–70.

50. Efron N, Carney LG. Effect of blinking on the level of oxygen beneath hard and soft gas-permeable contact lenses. *J Am Optom Assoc* 1983;54:229–234.

51. Mandell RB. Gas-permeable contact lenses and corneal edema. *Contemp Optom* 1982;1:15–17.

52. Polse KA. Tear flow under hydrogel contact lenses. *Invest Ophthalmol Vis Sci* 1979;18:409–413.

53. Fonn D, Holden BA, Roth P, et al. Comparative physiologic performance of polymethyl methacrylate and gas-permeable contact lenses. *Arch Ophthalmol* 1984;102:760–764.

54. Knoll HA, Conway HD. Analysis of blink-induced vertical motion of contact lenses. *Am J Optom Physiol Opt* 1987;64:153–155.

55. Benjamin WJ, Ghormley NR. Wettability of silicone and silicon-acrylate contact lens materials. *Int Contact Lens Clin* 1983;10: 94–99.

56. Madigan M, Holden BA, Fong D. A new method for wetting angle measurement. *Int Eye Care* 1984;2:45–48.

57. Madigan M, Holden BA. Preliminary report: lens wear and its effect on wetting angle. *Int Eye Care* 1986;2:44.

58. Mandell RB. Is there an angle to wetting. *Contact Lens Forum* 1984;9:45–51.

59. Mandell RB. Lens design and function. In: Mandell RB, ed. *Contact lens practice*, 4th ed. Springfield, IL: Charles C. Thomas, 1988;883–912.

60. Doane MG, Korb D, Miller D. Diagnostic high-speed photography in ophthalmology. *Invest Ophthalmol Vis Sci* 1984;25[Suppl]: 192.

61. Doane MG, Gleason W. The marginal meniscus: a major factor in contact lens wetting. *Invest Ophthalmol Vis Sci* 1987; 25[Suppl]:372.

62. Guillon M, Guillon JP, Mapstone V, et al. Rigid gas permeable lenses in vivo wettability. *Trans Br Contact Lens Assoc* 1989; 24–26.

63. Shiobara M, Schnider CM, Back A, et al. Guide to the clinical assessment of on-eye wettability of rigid gas permeable lenses. *Optom Vis Sci* 1989;66:202–206.

64. Pole J, Lowther GE, Hammack GG. Clinical evaluation of RGP contact lens surface qualities and subjective lens comfort. *Int Contact Lens Clin* 1987;14:185–200.

65. Holden BA, Schnider C. Personal communication, 1986.

66. Allansmith MR, Korb D, Greiner J, et al. Giant papillary conjunctivitis in contact lens wearers. *Am J Ophthalmol* 1977;83: 697–708.

67. Mandell RB. Slit lamp classification system. *J Am Optom Assoc* 1987;58:198–201.

68. Cornea and Contact Lens Research Unit, UNSW. CCLRU grading scales. In: Phillips AJ, Speedwell L, Stone J, eds. *Contact lenses*, 4th ed. Oxford, England: Boston: Butterworth-Heinemann, 1997:Appendix;863–867.

69. Guillon JP, Guillon M. Tear film examination of the contact lens patient. *Optician* 1993;206:21–29.

70. Brown N. Visibility of transparent objects in the eye by retroillumination. *Br J Ophthalmol* 1971;55:517–524.

71. Goldberg J. *Biomicroscopy for contact lens practice: clinical procedures*, 2nd ed. Chicago: Professional Press, 1984:153–192.

72. Holden BA. High magnification examination and photography with the slit lamp. In: Brandeth RH, ed. *Clinical slit lamp biomicroscopy*. Berkley, CA: Multi Media Center, 1978;329–341.

73. Zantos S. *Slit lamp examination of contact lens wearers*. Bausch & Lomb Educational Pamphlet, Bausch & Lomb, Rochester, New York, 1984.

74. Carney LG. The basis for corneal shape change during contact lens wear. *Am J Optom Physiol Opt* 1975;52:445–454.

75. Rengstorff RH. Variations in corneal curvature measurements: an after-effect observed with habitual wearers of contact lenses. *Am J Optom Physiol Opt* 1969;46:45–51.

76. Fonn D. The clinical performance of high DK rigid gas permeable (RGP) lenses used for extended wear. *Am J Optom Physiol Opt* 1987;46:45–51.

77. Polse KA, Sarver MD, Kenyon E, et al. Gas permeable hard contact lens extended wear: ocular and visual responses to a 6-month period of wear. *CLAO J* 1987;13:31–38.

78. Guillon M, Lydon DPM, Wilson C. Corneal topography: a clinical model. *Ophthalmic Physiol Opt* 1986;6:47–56.

79. Mandell RB. The enigma of the corneal contour. *CLAO J* 1992; 18:267–272.

80. Mandell RB. A guide to videokeratography. *Int Contact Lens Clin* 1996;23:205–228.

81. Klyce SD. Developments in corneal topographic analysis following contact lens wear and refractive surgery. *Contact Lens Anterior Eye* 2001;24:168–174.

82. Fonn D, du Toit R, Simpson TL, et al. Sympathetic swelling response of the control eye to soft lenses in the other eye. *Invest Ophthalmol Vis Sci* 1999;40:3116–3121.

83. La Hood D, Sweeney DF, Holden B. Overnight corneal edema with hydrogel, rigid gas-permeable and silicone elastomer contact lenses. *Int Contact Lens Clin* 1988;15:149–153.

84. Wang J, Fonn D, Simpson TL, et al. The measurement of corneal epithelial thickness in response to hypoxia using optical coherence tomography. *Am J Ophthalmol* 2002;133:315–319.

85. Wang J, Fonn D, Simpson TL. Topographical thickness of the epithelium and total cornea after hydrogel and PMMA contact lens wear with eye closure. *Invest Ophthalmol Vis Sci* 2003;44: 1070–1074.

86. Wilson G, Fatt I. Thickness of the corneal epithelium during anoxia. *Am J Optom Physiol Opt* 1980;57:409–412.

87. Swarbrick HA, Wong G, O'Leary DJ. Corneal response to ortho-keratology. *Optom Vis Sci* 1998;75:791–799.

88. O'Leary DJ, Wilson G, Henson DB. The effect of anoxia on the

human corneal epithelium. *Am J Optom Physiol Opt* 1981;58: 472–476.

89. Erickson P, Comstock T. An improved technique for patched eye corneal swelling studies. *Int Contact Lens Clin* 1996;22:191–197.
90. Lattimore MRJ, Kaupp S, Schallhorn S, et al. Orbscan pachymetry: implications of a repeated measures and diurnal variation analysis. *Ophthalmology* 1999;106:977–981.
91. Hrynchak P, Simpson T. Optical coherence tomography: an introduction to the technique and its use. *Optom Vis Sci* 2000;77: 347–356.
92. Caroline PJ. Laboratory and clinical analysis of the surface characteristics of high oxygen flux RGP lenses. Fourteenth National Research Symposium on Contact Lenses, Washington, DC, Conference Proceeding, 1987.
93. Lowther GE. Effect of some solutions on HGP contact lens parameters. *J Am Optom Assoc* 1987;58:188–192.

16 B

RIGID GAS-PERMEABLE LENS PROBLEM SOLVING

DESMOND FONN AND LUIGINA SORBARA

The development of high-oxygen gas permeable (GP) materials has resolved the hypoxia-related complications of daily wear. Some of these lenses even exceed the Holden and Mertz extended wear Dk/t criteria of 87×10^{-9} (1). Subjective, visual, mechanical, surface, lens design, fitting, and tear film-related problems, however, continue to plague GP lens wearers. The objective of this chapter is to characterize these problems, describe their etiologies, and, most importantly, offer suggestions on management of the complications.

LENS DISCOMFORT

Discontinuation of contact lens wear continues to be a fairly common occurrence. It is estimated that there are about 10 million dropouts in the United States. The accuracy of this estimate is questionable because it is based on sampling, and some patients who abandon contact lenses return to wear after years of abstinence. The percentage of discontinuations may be higher in the United Kingdom (UK), leading Morgan (2) to suggest that this is the reason for the decline in the numbers of contact lens wearers in the UK.

Causes of contact lens discontinuation have been described previously (3–5). The primary reasons are discomfort and ocular dryness, redness, and handling/inconvenience difficulties. Other reasons, considered less significant, include decreased vision, expense, and, more recently, the attraction of permanent refractive correction through refractive surgery. Studies by Weed et al. (3) and Pritchard et al. (4) compared the reasons for rigid and soft lens discontinuation, and their results were remarkably similar. Table 16B.1 lists the top four reasons for discontinuation noted in the Weed survey study.

The most common symptom, and reason for discontinuation, among rigid GP lens wearers is discomfort. GP lens discomfort can be divided into acute and chronic. The acute cause is more obvious and usually mechanical, such as lens defects, foreign body entrapment, denatured deposits on the posterior surface, or very poor design and fitting characteristics.

Foreign body "tracking" of the cornea produces marked discomfort and responsive lacrimation. These particles, usually from extraneous sources such as environmental dust, permeate the tear film. As tear exchange occurs, with lens movement from blinking, the particles flow under the lens to abrade the cornea, causing discomfort. Biomicroscopic examination of the ocular surface exhibits corneal staining, such as the linear tracking shown in Fig. 16B.1. It has been shown that lens design may facilitate these incidents (6). The greater the edge clearance, the more likely debris will collect under the edge (Fig. 16B.2; see Color Plate 16B.2) and then traverse the cornea with lens movement. If there is central clearance (Fig. 16B.2), the foreign body can be trapped behind the lens. The discomfort in this case usually is unilateral. A more appropriate fitting relationship, that is, one that is aligned with the corneal surface centrally with less peripheral tear clearance (Fig. 16B.3; see Color Plate 16B.3), would likely alleviate this problem.

Acute discomfort may be due to a damaged lens (usually unilateral): the lens is chipped or has a poorly finished edge or unpolished secondary curves. All of these problems can be rectified by polishing the curves, rolling the edge, or replacing the lens. Edge thickness and profile is another controlling factor of lens discomfort. Fig. 16B.4 compares a poor and thick edge profile with a corresponding thinner and perfectly designed edge shape.

TABLE 16B.1. REASONS AND FREQUENCY (%) OF DISCONTINUATION FROM RIGID AND SOFT CONTACT LENS WEAR

	Rigid Lenses	Soft Lenses
Discomfort	30	25
Handling/inconvenience	15	20
Dryness	17	16
Red eyes	15	10

Data from Weed K, Fonn D, Potvin R. Discontinuation of contact lens wear. Optom Vis Sci 1993; 70 [125]:140.

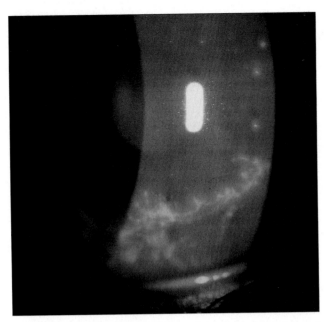

FIG. 16B.1. Foreign body tracking staining from debris trapped under a gas permeable lens.

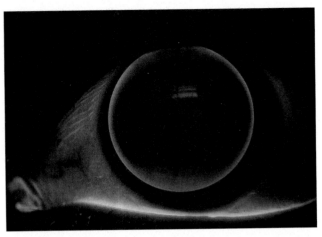

FIG. 16B.3. Optimal lens-to-cornea relationship showing alignment and adequate edge clearance. (See Color Plate 16B.3.)

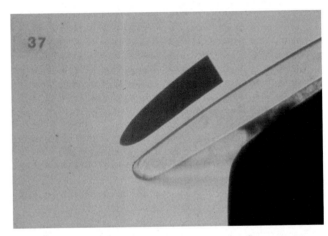

FIG. 16B.4. Thick poorly formed rigid lens edge **(lower transparent image)** compared to a thinner perfectly formed edge **(upper dark image).** (Courtesy of International Association of Contact Lens Educators [IACLE].)

Acute discomfort (burning and stinging) on lens insertion most likely is due to solution toxicity. The most common cause is when patients use lens cleaning solution prior to lens insertion in the morning, forget to rinse the lens, and then apply the lens, perhaps with a thin coat of wetting or conditioning solution. The signs are a dense circular patch of corneal staining approximately equal to the diameter of the lens (Fig. 16B.5), excessive lacrimation, and conjunctival hyperemia. All preservatives used for antimicrobial activity are potentially toxic; some patients specifically react to chlorhexidine digluconate, benzalkonium chloride, or polyaminopropyl biguanide. Tissue damage is dependent on exposure time and concentration. These preservatives

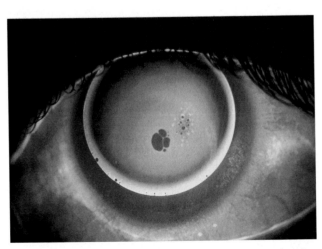

FIG. 16B.2. Excessive apical and peripheral clearance showing air bubbles at the edge and under center of the lens. (See Color Plate 16B.2.)

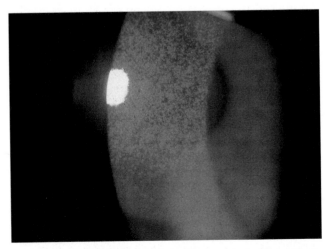

FIG. 16B.5. Dense severe toxic-induced corneal staining in response to use of a contact lens cleaner. The patient forgot to rinse the cleaner off the lens prior to lens insertion.

can bind to proteins, mucin, and the silicone components of the lens surface, but it is more likely that the direct presence of the preservative in the tear film causes the reaction.

Peripheral corneal ulcers associated with GP lens wear are rare events and are more likely to occur during extended than daily wear. Poggio et al. (7) found that the incidence of microbial keratitis with rigid lenses was 1 in 10,000, but the number of noninfectious cases is unknown. These lesions will invariably cause acute discomfort. After discontinuing lens wear, antibiotic therapy is invariably the appropriate treatment: ciprofloxacin 0.3% (Ciloxan) or fortified tobramycin 15 mg/mL with 5% homatropine or scopolamine 0.25%. Although this has been termed an *acute reaction*, the underlying etiology may be chronic (e.g., peripheral desiccation and/or lens adherence), in which case lens design may need alteration.

Chronic discomfort is much more difficult to alleviate because the symptom is often less specific. Discomfort is invariably accompanied by dryness. We have found a strong correlation between these two symptoms when they are graded independently by subjects using visual analogue scales, although this was in the context of soft lens wear (8).

Chronic rigid lens discomfort may result in failure to adapt to rigid lens sensation, but we do not know why some patients are able to adapt and others not. It probably is linked to the proprioception of the cornea, perhaps the conjunctiva, and to a lesser extent the interaction of the eyelid. Although the mechanisms of discomfort remain a mystery, here are some ideas on how to optimize rigid lens comfort:

Oxygen permeability should not be critical even though patients have different oxygen demands; as the vast majority of patients will be using these lenses on a daily wear basis, lens materials exceeding 50 Barrer (Dk units) should be physiologically sufficient. With regard to comfort, ensuring that the surfaces are wettable probably is more important than is the material oxygen permeability.

Lens design and mechanical fit are critical elements for optimizing comfort. Small overall diameter (OAD), decentered lenses with poor edge design, and excessive lens movement contribute to discomfort. Studies have shown that lenses with moderate edge clearance and fitted in an alignment pattern are more comfortable than high edge clearance, high riding lenses with minus lenticular carriers (9). Fig. 16B.6 (see Color Plate 16B.6) shows an optimal fluorescein pattern. Note that the lens is fairly large in diameter, positions centrally, and has some coverage by the superior lid. Williams-Lyn et al. (10) found that larger lenses (9.5–10.0 mm OAD) are generally more comfortable than smaller-diameter lenses. Achieving complete alignment across the majority of the posterior lens surface is not always possible because of the inevitable corneal astigmatism (usually "with the rule") that is corrected with spherical base curves. Fitting the lens slightly steeper than the flattest corneal meridian should create minimal central clearance,

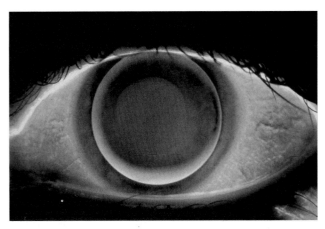

FIG. 16B.6. Optimal fluorescein pattern showing slightly more inferior edge clearance than lateral clearance. (See Color Plate 16B.6.)

midperipheral bearing, and sufficient edge clearance with a gradual transition between each (Fig. 16B.7; see Color Plate 16B.7). This particular example displays more than optimal inferior edge clearance. Any more than this can lead to excessive debris collection in the deep/wide peripheral zone.

The lens design should include an aspheric or a well-blended multicurve posterior surface with an optic zone diameter approaching 8.5 mm and a total diameter of 9.7 to 10.0 mm. Although center thickness is less critical for comfort (11), our recommendation would be to minimize this parameter; for minus power lenses, a range from 0.10 to 0.15 mm should be optimum.

Although excessive edge thickness and poor edge design were mentioned as causes of acute discomfort, either can also cause chronic discomfort. La Hood (12) showed comfort can be improved by optimizing edge design. The front

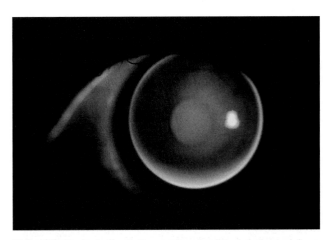

FIG. 16B.7. Aspheric design optimally fitted (spherical base curve) lens on a with-the-rule astigmatic cornea. The fluorescein pattern shows some apical clearance and relatively more inferior edge clearance consistent with this astigmatic cornea. This is a good example of gradual transition between touch and clearance consistent with an aspheric lens design. (See Color Plate 16B.7.)

surface should be continuous with the edge, and the edge should be thin and rounded with the apex centered between the front and the back surfaces, as in the optimal form shown in Fig. 16B.4.

Fitting back toric lenses on corneas with high amounts of corneal astigmatism will enhance comfort by achieving alignment relationships. Chronic discomfort also may be related to poor wettability, which can either facilitate or result from lens surface deposits. For further information, see the section on Surface Deposits.

CORNEAL STAINING

Three and nine o'clock corneal staining (see Chapter 40) (Figs. 16B.8 and 16B.9) affects an estimated 40% to 90% of rigid contact lens wearers (13,14). This complication can be classified as moderate/severe in about 15% of patients and thus requires intervention. It is more prevalent during GP extended than daily wear (15). The staining appears within the palpebral aperture on the corneal area that is not covered by the lens; therefore, it sometimes is referred to as *exposure staining*. Contact lens wearers have been shown to blink both less frequently and partially (16,17). Peripheral desiccation almost certainly results from blinking inhibition, and the partial blink pattern that develops most likely is due to lens discomfort. In those cases, the cause of the staining may be the inability of the eyelid to completely wet the corneal surface around the lens. The contact that the tarsal conjunctiva should make with the cornea during blinking is disturbed by the presence of a rigid lens, causing "bridging" between the tarsal conjunctiva and the cornea. Rigid lens wear causes accelerated tear film evaporation and decreased tear breakup time (BUT) (18). In addition, it has been demonstrated that tear film thinning occurs in the zone just beyond the edge of the tear menisci (19) because tear fluid is drawn toward the meniscus created by the peripheral curve edge clearance. All of these factors, which are

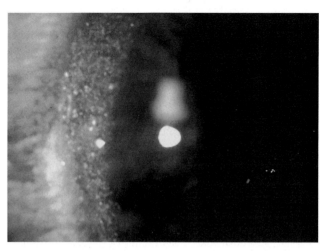

FIG. 16B.9. High magnification of severe coalesced temporal peripheral exposure staining from gas permeable lens wear.

listed in Fig. 16B.10, represent the etiology of 3- and 9-o'clock staining. The condition may be exacerbated by the presence of a pinguecula close to the limbus that accentuates the bridging (lid gap) effect.

Chronic irritation to the 3- and 9-o'clock areas can lead to hyperplasia of the peripheral corneal epithelium, followed by inflammation and infiltration of the affected area, peripheral corneal vascularization, and eventually erosion (20). This chronic form of inflammation and desiccation is called vascularized limbal keratitis (VLK). Chronic 3- and 9-o'clock staining also can lead to neovascularization (Fig. 16B.11) and scarring of corneal tissue (Fig. 16B.12). Another severe and very rare sequela of chronic 3- and 9-o'clock staining is dellen (21), where peripheral superficial punctate keratitis becomes very dense. It appears as if the epithelium has been denuded (Fig. 16B.13; see Color Plate 16B.13) because of a well-circumscribed vertically oval area of epithelial cell loss. If this area is examined with a slit lamp using an optical section, the thinning is obvious. Patients with dry eye (e.g., as a result of chronic use of Accutane™ for acne) or patients who have considerably

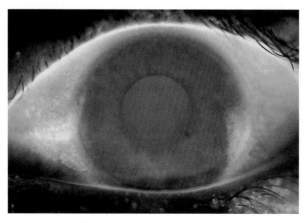

FIG. 16B.8. Marked 3- and 9-o'clock corneal staining induced by gas permeable lens wear.

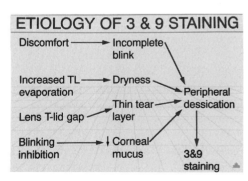

FIG. 16B.10. Etiology and development of 3- and 9-o'clock corneal staining.

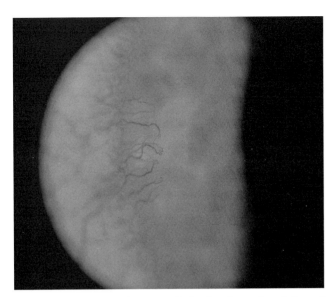

FIG. 16B.11. Temporal neovascularization from chronic 3- and 9-o'clock corneal staining.

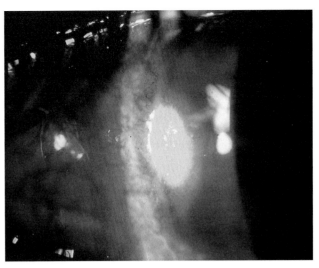

FIG. 16B.13. Large dellen (fluorescein staining in epithelial excavation) secondary to 3- and 9-o'clock corneal staining. (See Color Plate 16B.13.)

reduced blink frequency (as with a new nonadapted wearer) may be predisposed to dellen.

Management of 3- and 9-o'clock staining can be challenging. The strategy for all patients with this condition is to improve the comfort of the lens through lens design changes in order to improve and naturalize the patient's blinking pattern. We and others (22) advocate increasing lens OAD as a first modification. A larger lens will cover more area of the cornea, leaving less area exposed (13) and larger lenses are more comfortable (10). The lens should be as thin as possible, and this applies especially to edge thickness. Optimizing the edge profile has already been de-

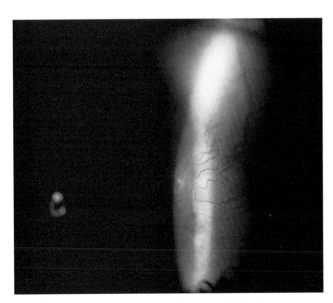

FIG. 16B.12. Corneal scarring and neovascularization as a consequence of chronic 3- and 9-o'clock corneal staining.

scribed. Edge clearance should be structured to minimize the effect of the meniscus. Adequate edge clearance should be ensured, and lens movement should be unrestricted but not excessive.

In many cases, patients' tear films will appear abnormal, but this may be in response to wearing "uncomfortable" lenses and the secondary partial and/or reduced frequency of blinking. Tear supplements (rewetting drops) help these cases. It has been suggested that blinking exercises may help patients who exhibit obvious partial blinking habits (23,24). Discontinuation of lens wear will depend on the severity of staining and the sequelae. Reduced wearing time is unsatisfactory in most cases, but it is an option as the condition generally worsens toward the end of the wearing period. If all else fails, refitting patients with hydrogel lenses will eliminate 3- and 9-o'clock staining (13).

Corneal staining due to the tracking of a foreign body trapped between the lens and the cornea was described. It usually is inconsequential and easily resolved by lens removal. The corneal staining usually will resolve within hours.

Corneal erosions due to GP lens wear are rare. Erosions usually are accompanied by discomfort, but patients who are asymptomatic may have compromised corneal sensitivity. These individuals include keratoconics and postsurgical patients, i.e., after penetrating keratoplasty, aphakia, and corneal refractive surgery. Previous polymethyl methacrylate (PMMA) wearers, diabetics, and immunosuppressed patients also have reduced corneal sensitivity. If patients are asymptomatic, making them aware of the possible complications of untreated corneal erosions is difficult. Associated conjunctival hyperemia and visual changes should prompt them to seek care. Management should include a prophylactic antibiotic and temporary discontinuation of contact lens wear until the epithelium heals.

Solution toxicity (described earlier) can manifest as a coalesced patch of corneal staining. Patients may have symptoms of discomfort and burning, especially upon lens insertion. Immediate discontinuation of the care regimen and temporary discontinuation of lens wear until the corneal staining has resolved are recommended. Ocular lubricants will help to alleviate acute discomfort. Prescribing an alternative care regimen, with a lower percentage of the preservative or a different preservative, is recommended.

Corneal ulcers are extremely rare in daily wear. They are characterized by full-thickness epithelial lesions with underlying infiltration and fluorescein staining that leaks into the stroma. Corneal ulcers can be distinguished from dellen and erosions by the absence of infiltrates in the latter two. The treatment was discussed previously.

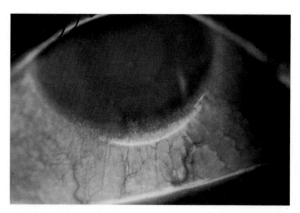

FIG. 16B.15. Edge-induced arcuate conjunctival staining with hyperemia induced by movement and edge of a gas permeable lens.

CONJUNCTIVAL HYPEREMIA

Conjunctival hyperemia typically involves the nasal and temporal quadrants of the bulbar conjunctiva, including the limbus and the area in apposition with the inferior limbus (Fig. 16B.14). The etiology is multifactorial (25). All of the foregoing complications would cause hyperemia. Conjunctival hyperemia almost always is secondary to some other form of ocular disturbance, such as peripheral corneal desiccation, toxicity reaction, edema, and trauma. The hyperemic response to mechanical trauma of the conjunctiva would be a primary reaction. An example where the edge of the lens has caused mechanical damage of the inferior conjunctival zone is shown in Fig. 16B.15. Management of this condition is preventing the lens from traversing the cornea by minimizing lens movement and designing the lens so that superior lid attachment is achieved. An imperfect lens edge also may contribute to the trauma.

Patients who have a pinguecula or pterygium invariably

exhibit hyperemia of this tissue, either through mechanical irritation of the lens or indirectly from desiccation. Fig. 16B.16 shows an example of marked inflammation of a pinguecula in association with GP lens wear. Managing the complications described earlier should alleviate the primary or secondary conjunctival injection (26). Unfortunately, conjunctival hyperemia also can be due to idiopathic causes, and the best that can be done is to minimize the injection by using tear supplements.

LENS ADHERENCE

Adherence was one of the first signs reported with GP lenses (27) and is the most common complication during extended wear (28–30). According to Swarbrick and Holden (31), 100% of patients have an adhered lens at some point in time, but only 22% have a persistent problem. The sign of lens adherence is an immobile lens with thick mucous

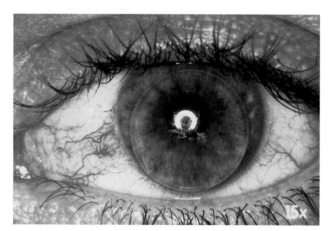

FIG. 16B.14. Marked nasal and temporal limbal and bulbar conjunctival hyperemia with some inferior limbal injection secondary to 3- and 9-o'clock corneal staining and inferior lens edge mechanical irritation.

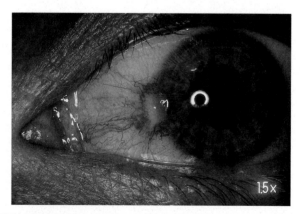

FIG. 16B.16. Severe pinguecula inflammation and nasal conjunctival hyperemia in response to wearing a gas permeable lens. This probably was induced by mechanical irritation and dryness from the rigid gas permeable lens.

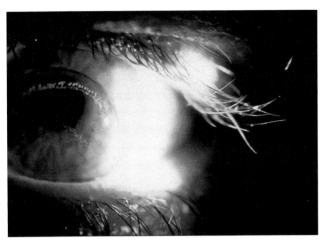

FIG. 16B.17. Lens adhesion depicting arcuate mucous/lipid deposits under the lens.

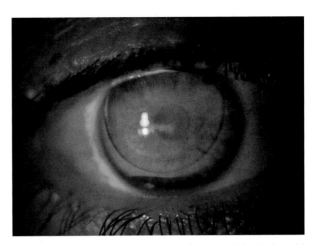

FIG. 16B.19. Imprint and central confluent staining induced by lens adhesion.

(ferning) beneath the lens (Fig. 16B.17). The adhesion can be broken with digital manipulation. If fluorescein is instilled prior to digital manipulation, the fluorescein can be observed seeping under the lens, which indicates an absence of tear film during the adhesion. If the lens is removed, an arcuate indentation of the cornea is apparent, due to fluorescein pooling (Fig. 16B.18), as well as both central punctate (Fig. 16B.19) and peripheral arcuate staining. Corneal distortion from the arcuate indentation of a decentered lens is easily observed with videokeratoscopy. Few symptoms usually accompany lens binding. In fact, some patients report lenses are more comfortable than usual because lens movement is absent.

Lens adherence has been attributed to a number of factors. For example, lid pressure on the lens during sleep squeezes out the tear film (aqueous layer) between the lens and the cornea, trapping mucous and debris and thus increasing the tear viscosity. Another contributing factor could be reduced aqueous production during sleep. The

lens invariably decenters during sleep because of lid pressure. If lens diameter is relatively large, with a large optic zone and little edge clearance, the risk of binding increases. GP lens adherence from overnight wear appears to be independent of lens design and fit, as authors disagree on a design recommended to minimize adherence (32–38). Although 22% of patients have repeated episodes of adherence (27), if the patient is asymptomatic and binding does not cause secondary complications, changes to lens design or wearing style are not considered essential unless the lens-to-cornea fitting relationship requires obvious modification.

Lens adherence during daily wear is rare, and the etiology may be different than extended wear. If a patient reports repeated episodes of adherence and examination of the lens indicates that it is indeed decentered, then it is essential to modify the design and fit to improve centration. When the lens decenters, peripheral and secondary curve junctions will contact flatter regions of the cornea, and the pressure induced by the lid will create an indentation of the cornea that facilitates lens binding. Lenses that decenter, especially laterally, usually are too flat (and the lens will exhibit excessive edge clearance if it is positioned centrally). Management here would be to optimize lens centration by steepening the base curve and maintaining a moderate amount of edge clearance, but ensure that the junctions between the curves are well blended, or use an aspheric back-surface design. Dry eye (aqueous deficient) should be considered another risk factor for lens adherence even if the condition is clinically marginal. Frequent use of rewetting preparations may prevent adherence. Management is important in either extended or daily wear situations to prevent severe secondary complications such as corneal distortion, dellen formation, and ulceration (39).

VISION PROBLEMS

Unilateral or bilateral reduced vision as a presenting symptom or a measured reduction of visual acuity during evalua-

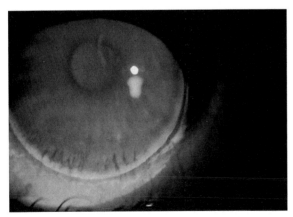

FIG. 16B.18. Imprint from a bound gas permeable lens after removal. Fluorescein has collected within the corneal imprint that was induced by the bound lens.

tion often can be rectified with a simple change in refractive optical power. Another common cause is lens reversal, that is, lenses accidentally switched, left for right or *vice versa.* Instability of refractive error can be more challenging, for example, with keratoconics or following refractive surgery complications, or while refitting long-term PMMA lens wearers. High-oxygen permeable GP lenses rehabilitate such corneas and provide required refractive correction. If the corneal shape alters significantly, the lens and tear lens should still provide the same net corrective power during the period of change. A change in the prescription of the GP lens would only be necessary if the base curve had to change after the corneal topography had stabilized to a different curvature.

Lens warpage may cause reduction in vision. Lens verification (radiuscope and focimeter) with an overrefraction should establish the cause of vision reduction. Excessive pressure with an abrasive cleaner also may cause the lens to increase in minus power over time, along with a decrease in center thickness (40). A less aggressive method of cleaning should be suggested.

Most patients who are fitted with GP lenses have corneal astigmatism. Spherical lenses are designed to neutralize corneal astigmatism by maintaining their shape, and if the lens flexes while on the eye, residual astigmatism will result. Flexure-induced residual astigmatism invariably will cause reduced or fluctuating vision. Flexure is due to a combination of factors that include pressure from the eyelid on the lens, which may be too thin and made from a flexible material, corneal astigmatism, the fluid force under the lens, and influence by lens parameters and designs (41–46). Flexure is detected by measuring the front surface of the lens *in situ* with a keratometer or corneal topographer. If visual acuity is affected, an overrefraction should be performed to establish if there is residual astigmatism, and this value should closely agree with the amount of flexure.

Flexure can easily be corrected. Increasing lens center thickness by 0.03 mm usually will suffice. As this will decrease the oxygen transmissibility, it may be prudent to use a material with a higher permeability because flexure will not necessarily increase with an increase in permeability (47). Herman (48) has suggested that flatter than K fitting relationships will reduce flexure regardless of lens position. However, flatter lenses will tend to decenter and be less stable. If vision and comfort are affected because the lens is too flat, then other choices should be considered for reducing flexure. If corneal astigmatism is greater than 2.00 D, the best alternative may be a back-surface toric design.

Lens decentration (Fig. 16B.20) may result in flare (haloes or ghosting) and variable vision with blinking (49). Flare is exacerbated with optical zones that are smaller than the patient's pupil. Decentration may be due to a number of lens design and patient factors but most likely is due to flat fitting lens designs, particularly if the lens is laterally and/or superiorly decentered. Flare worsens under scotopic

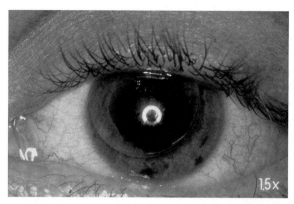

FIG. 16B.20. Decentered gas permeable lens on a fairly large pupil as an example of why patients may report flare or ghosting.

conditions because of pupil dilation. This complication should be relatively easy to correct. The optic zone diameter should be increased (so that it is larger than the pupil under scotopic conditions) and/or the base curve should be steepened to center the lens and tighten it if the edge clearance is reduced.

Poor surface wettability (particularly with new lenses) immediately after lens insertion will result in poor and inconsistent vision (50). The same visual response would be true of deposited and scratched lens surfaces. The following section on surface deposits describes how to manage wetting and deposit problems.

SURFACE DEPOSITS

Most GP lenses contain silicone, fluorine, and polymethyl methacrylate. Although these materials perform well in many ways, these lenses are inherently hydrophobic and it is necessary to wet or condition the lens surface with wetting agents. The introduction of fluorine appears to have improved wettability of the material and increased the permeability. Deposition also appears to have decreased.

New lenses frequently do not exhibit good wetting properties. The suggested reasons are residual blocking pitch on the lens or the fact that the surface is highly polished. Upon insertion and inspection with a slit lamp, dry patches are often observed, even though the lenses have been soaked for a few days in conditioning solution and then rubbed with the same solution prior to insertion. A typical example of a nonwetting lens is shown in Fig. 16B.21. After a few days of lens use, the surface wettability tends to improve. The dry patches on the surface naturally attract lipid, which appears as shiny, transparent, greasy spots over the lens surface known as *pearlescence.* Pearlescence (Fig. 16B.22) is a loosely bound deposit that can be removed easily with alcohol-based surfactant cleaners such as Miraflow® or Aoflow®.

Protein (primarily lysozyme) deposits develop as either

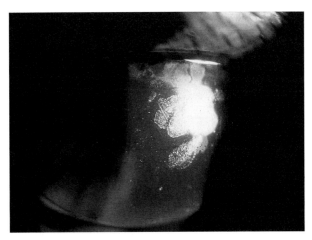

FIG. 16B.21. Nonwetting "dry patch" indicated on the front surface of a gas permeable lens.

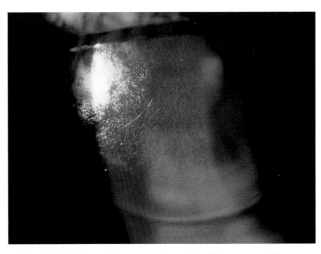

FIG. 16B.23. Bound denatured protein with poor wetting on a gas permeable lens surface.

transient and transparent films, become hazy areas when combined with lipid, and, finally, if untreated, protein becomes denatured, multilayered, and translucent (51). Fig. 16B.23 is an example of denatured protein deposits. In this particular case, the lens back surface also was severely deposited, as evidenced by the significant punctate corneal staining (Fig. 16B.24) associated with use of this lens. Irregular protein film on the front surface of a lens caused the somewhat localized papillary conjunctivitis observed in Fig. 16B.25. This lens might be salvageable by polishing its surfaces with an abrasive laboratory compound. If this is unsuccessful, the lens must be replaced. The use of surfactant cleaners and friction along with passive protein removal with enzymatic cleaners will help to prevent deposition and dislodge the loosely bound protein and thus prevent denaturation of the protein (52). Failure to prevent excessive deposit accumulation will result in decreased vision, dis-

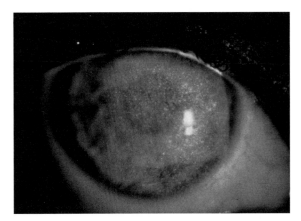

FIG. 16B.24. Diffuse punctuate corneal staining resulting from mechanical irritation from the bound protein on the gas permeable lens shown in Fig. 16B.23.

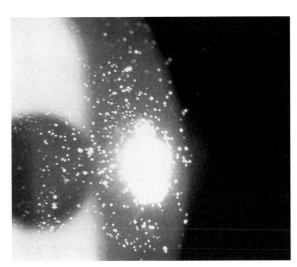

FIG. 16B.22. Pearlescent lipomucoid loosely bound deposits on a gas permeable lens surface. (Courtesy of International Association of Contact Lens Educators [IACLE].)

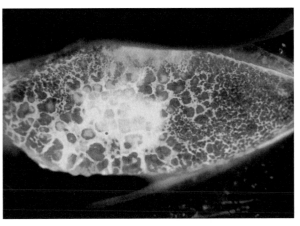

FIG. 16B.25. Papillary conjunctivitis (somewhat localized) induced by the bound protein on the gas permeable lens shown in Fig. 16B.23.

comfort, decreased wetting of the lens surface, increased corneal staining, and an increased upper tarsal papillary response (52).

PHYSIOLOGIC RESPONSES

As mentioned earlier, hypoxic edema with contact lens daily wear has virtually been eliminated by lenses that have exceeded the oxygen transmissibility criteria of Holden and Mertz (1) (this also is true for some instances of extended wear). Previously, choices of the material were based on rigidity to prevent flexure and wettability (53). Today, newer high Dk fluoro-silicone/acrylate materials have equal wettability, durability, and rigidity. For example, the Aercor™ materials (Polymer Technology Corporation, Wilmington, MA, USA) and Menicon™ super-Dk materials (Nagoya, Japan) (54) have Dk values ranging from 82 to 120.

Use of corneal topographers enhances our abilities to detect corneal distortion, sphericalization, or any other irregular shapes that contact lenses may induce. Corneal topographers also aid us in contact lens fitting, as most of the corneal surface can be considered when designing lens peripheries (55). The Orbscan™ topographer assesses both the front and back surfaces of the cornea using slit-scan photography; thus, changes due to edema with overnight wear can be monitored more easily simultaneously with topography (56).

LENS DECENTRATION

There are three essential reasons for optimizing the lens mechanical fit: making the lens as comfortable as possible, avoiding ocular tissue insult, and providing excellent vision. To accomplish this, the lens diameter should be as large as possible so that a portion of the lens is tucked under the superior lid. It should align the cornea with sufficient and gradually increasing edge clearance from the midperiphery to the edge of the lens. The lens should be centered over the pupil with an optic zone diameter larger than the pupil. Finally, the lens should move smoothly and vertically with the top lid during blinking to provide some tear exchange and avoid lens adherence. If a lens decenters, it is likely to affect each of the three essential elements, although it is unknown whether decentration will directly affect comfort[6].

Current high-oxygen transmission lenses will provide more than sufficient oxygen for daily wear, and it has been demonstrated that tear exchange provides an insignificant amount of oxygen compared to the amount that diffuses through high-Dk lenses (57). However, lenses with excessive apical clearance and little edge clearance will hinder tear exchange, are more likely to bind, and, if decentered, will

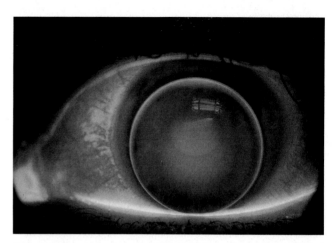

FIG. 16B.26. Steep lens showing apical clearance with minimal edge clearance in this inferiorly decentered gas permeable lens. (See Color Plate 16B.26.)

usually position inferiorly (Fig. 16B.26; see Color Plate 16B.26).

Flat fitting (base curve) lenses, or lenses with excessive edge clearance, are more likely to decenter than are aligned or steep fitted lenses. Decentration usually is laterally and/or superiorly, especially if there is accompanying excessive edge clearance (Figs. 16B.27 and 16B.28; see Color Plates 16B.27 and 16B.28). The GP lens shown in Fig. 16B.27 will cause flare and fluctuating vision because of decentration and an optical zone that does not cover the pupil. Flat fitting lenses will generally be looser (particularly plus power lenses), with quicker movement. In one instance (Fig. 16B.27), the mechanical fit was easily improved by a steeper base curve (Fig. 16B.29; see Color Plate 16B.29) where the centration and alignment are both observed to be improved. This is a preferred result compared with Fig. 16B.30 (see Color Plate 16B.30), where a larger optic zone diameter and steeper base curve were chosen, resulting in too much central clearance. Although this fit would not have caused

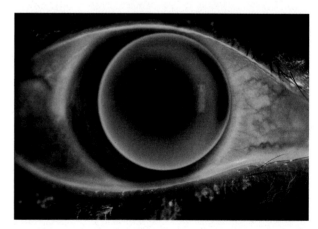

FIG. 16B.27. Flat (base curve) nasally decentered gas permeable lens. (See Color Plate 16B.27.)

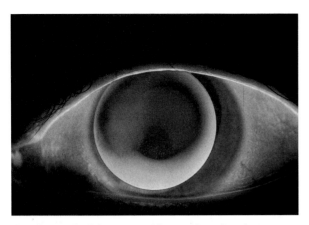

FIG. 16B.28. Flat base curve with excessive edge clearance causing nasal decentration of this aspheric gas permeable lens. (See Color Plate 16B.28.)

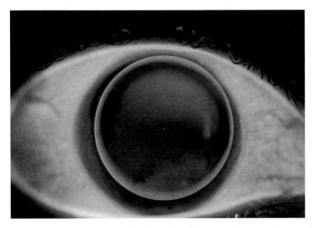

FIG. 16B.29. Alignment fit showing improved centration and acceptable fluorescein pattern. This is the same eye as shown in Fig. 16B.27, which has been fitted with a steeper base curve lens. (See Color Plate 16B.29.)

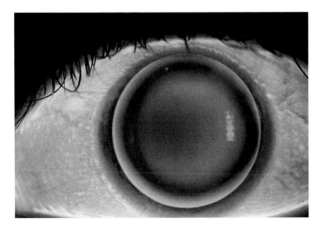

FIG. 16B.30. Large-diameter and large optic zone depicting excessive central clearance. (See Color Plate 16B.30.)

physiologic compromise, the patient's vision may have decreased (58).

PTOSIS

Some patients who have worn GP lenses for many years notice that their palpebral aperture sizes (PAS) have decreased, and patients are particularly concerned when there are unequal aperture sizes. Fortunately, it appears that only 10% of wearers are so affected.

A number of studies have established that PAS decreases with GP contact lens wear (59–65). An example of subsequent unilateral ptosis is shown in Fig. 16B.31. Both Fonn et al. (59) and Van den Bosch and Lemij (64) found that GP lens wear decreases PAS by approximately 0.50 mm. This decrease, resulting from blepharoptosis or drooping of the upper eyelid, is particularly noticeable when compared to the PAS of eyes wearing soft contact lenses or none at all. In fact, this condition rarely appears with soft contact lens wear, except with the development of severe papillary conjunctivitis, in which drooping is caused by edema and inflammation of the lid.

The causes of contact lens-induced blepharoptosis are unclear. Common explanations include vernal conjunctivitis, papillary conjunctivitis, and trauma resulting from a rigid lens becoming embedded in the superior lid. It also could be the result of edema or inflammation of the eyelid due to irritation caused by the lens edge or surface imperfections, or epithelial hyperplasia of the tarsal conjunctiva (59). Some investigators have suggested that this condition is a result of stretching of the superior eyelid that facilitates lens removal, which can lead to disinsertion of the levator aponeurosis and dehiscence (a tear or split) of the muscle of the superior lid (63,64). However, Fonn et al. (59) suggest that there are causes other than dehiscence, particularly when ptosis develops after a short time of wearing lenses. Studies have demonstrated that if lens wear is terminated, PAS increases in size, thus appearing to recover spontaneously (60–62).

Although it is possible to observe blepharoptosis with bilateral lens wear (Fig. 16B.32), it tends to be more obvious when the condition is asymmetric (one PAS is smaller than the other, as shown in Fig. 16B.31). Fig. 16B.33 illustrates the results of a study by Fonn and Holden (61), showing changes in PAS over 13 weeks of extended wear with a GP lens in one eye and a soft lens in the other eye, in addition to 7 weeks of recovery time.

To detect this condition bilaterally, it is necessary to take baseline measurements of the palpebral aperture, in order to notice if any changes have occurred (59,66). The clinical appearance of this condition includes narrowing of the palpebral aperture and a large space between the upper lid margin and skin fold at the top of the eyelid (66).

Management of this condition includes three options.

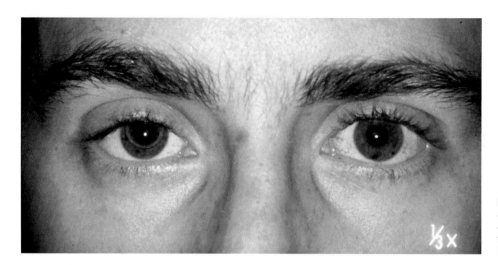

FIG. 16B.31. Unilateral ptosis induced by a gas permeable lens after 4 weeks of extended lens wear with the contralateral eye wearing a soft lens.

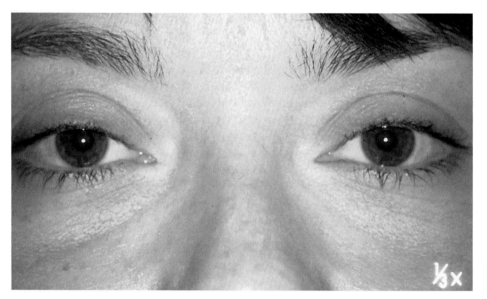

FIG. 16B.32. Bilateral reduction of palpebral aperture sizes in a long-term gas permeable lens wearer.

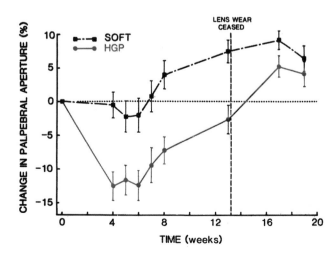

FIG. 16B.33. Comparative palpebral aperture size changes after 13 weeks of extended wear and recovery. (Adapted from Fonn D, Holden BA. Rigid gas permeable versus hydrogel contact lenses for extended wear. *Am J Optom Physiol Opt* 1988;65:536–544.)

The first option is to discontinue GP lens wear and wait for recovery. Patients may be refitted with soft lenses, and PAS usually will recover. If the condition does not resolve with time, indicating that muscular dehiscence has occurred, surgery may be necessary as a last resort.

REFERENCES

1. Holden BA, Mertz GW. Critical oxygen levels to avoid corneal edema for daily and extended wear contact lenses. *Invest Ophthalmol Vis Sci* 1984;25:1161–1167.
2. Morgan P. Is the UK contact lens market healthy. *Optician* 2001;221:22–26.
3. Weed K, Fonn D, Potvin R. Discontinuation of contact lens wear. *Optom Vis Sci* 1993;70[12s]:140.
4. Pritchard N, Fonn D, Brazeau D. Discontinuation of contact lens wear: a survey. *Int Contact Lens Clin* 1999;26:157–162.
5. Pritchard N. How can I avoid CL drop-outs? *Optician* 2001;222:14–18.
6. Sorbara L, Fonn D, Holden BA, et al. Centrally fitted versus upper-lid attached rigid gas permeable lenses. Part II: a comparison of the clinical performance. *Int Contact Lens Clin* 1996;23:121–127.
7. Poggio EC, Glynn RJ, Schein OD, et al. The incidence of ulcerative keratitis among users of daily-wear and extended-wear soft contact lenses. *N Engl J Med* 1989;321:779–783.
8. Fonn D, Situ P, Simpson TL. Hydrogel lens dehydration and subjective comfort and dryness ratings in symptomatic and asymptomatic contact lens wearers. *Optom Vis Sci* 1999;76:700–704.
9. Sorbara L, Fonn D, Holden BA, et al. Centrally fitted versus upper lid-attached rigid gas permeable lenses. Part I. Design parameters affecting vertical decentration. *Int Contact Lens Clin* 1996;23:99–104.
10. Williams-Lyn D, MacNeill K, Fonn D. The effect of rigid lens back optic zone radius and diameter changes on comfort. *Int Contact Lens Clin* 1993;20:223–229.
11. Cornish R, Sulaiman S. Do thinner rigid gas permeable contact lenses provide superior initial comfort? *Optom Vis Sci* 1996;73:139–143.
12. La Hood D. Edge shape and comfort of rigid lenses. *Am J Optom Physiol Opt* 1988;65:613–618.
13. Edrington TB, Barr JT. Peripheral corneal desiccation. *Contact Lens Spectrum* 2002;17:46.
14. Bennett ES. Lens design and trouble shooting. In: Bennett ES, Grohe RM, eds. *Rigid gas permeable contact lenses*. New York: Professional Press,1986:189–224.
15. Henry VA, Bennett ES, Sevigny J. Rigid extended wear problem solving. *Int Contact Lens Clin* 1990;17:121–133.
16. Hill R M. The quantitative blink. *Int Contact Lens Clin* 1984;11:366-368.
17. Holly FJ. Tear film physiology and contact lens wear: contact lens tear film interaction. *Am J Optom Physiol Opt* 1981;58:331–341.
18. Tomlinson A, Cedarstaff TH. Tear evaporation from the human eye. The effects of contact lens wear. *J Br Contact Lens Assoc* 1982;5:141–150.
19. McDonald JE, Brubraker S. Meniscus-induced thinning of tear films. *Am J Ophthalmol* 1971;72:139–146.
20. Grohe RM, Lebow KA. Vascularized limbal keratitis. *Int Contact Lens Clin* 1989;16:197–208.
21. Fonn D, Gauthier C. Aftercare of RGP lens wearers. *Contact Lens Spectrum* 1990;5:71–81.
22. Schnider CM, Terry RL, Holden BA. Effect of lens design on peripheral corneal desiccation. *J Am Optom Assoc* 1997;68:163–170.
23. Kerr C. 3 and 9 O'clock staining—a simple solution. *Optician* 1988;195:25.
24. Mackie IA. Localised corneal drying in association with dellen, pterygia and related lesions. *Trans Ophthalmol Soc UK* 1971;91:129–145.
25. Efron N. Contact lens-induced conjunctival hyperaemia. *Optician* 1997;213:22–27.
26. Catania LJ. A categorical approach to the diagnosis and management of pre- and post-fit contact lens conditions. *J Am Optom Assoc* 1987;58:819–830.
27. Zantos SG, Zantos PO. Extended wear feasibility of gas-permeable hard contact lenses for myopes. *Int Eyecare* 1985;1:66–75.
28. Kenyon E, Polse KA, Mandell RB. Rigid contact lens adherence: incidence, severity and recovery. *J Am Optom Assoc* 1988;59:168–174.
29. Benjamin WJ, Boltz RL. RGP lens adhesion is not a benign phenomenon. *Int Contact Lens Clin* 1989;16:60–62.
30. Levy B. Rigid gas-permeable lenses for extended wear—a 1-year clinical evaluation. *Am J Optom Physiol Opt* 1985;62:889–894.
31. Swarbrick HA, Holden BA. Rigid gas-permeable lens adherence. *Optom Vis Sci* 1996;73:473–481.
32. Kenyon E, Mandell RB, Polse KA. Lens design effects on rigid lens adherence. *Br Contact Lens Assoc J* 1989;12:32–36.
33. Jones L, Jones D. Effects of lens parameter variation on rigid gas-permeable lens adherence. *Optician* 1995;210:28–29.
34. Ghormley NR. Specific gravity: does it contribute to RGP lens adherence? Part six: RGP lens adherence (binding). *Int Contact Lens Clin* 1991;18:125–126.
35. Lin ST, Leahy CD, Mandell RB. The effect of time, patching, and lens flexibility on RGP lens adherence. *J Am Optom Assoc* 1989;60:182–187.
36. Kenyon E, Mandell RB, Polse KA. Lens design effects on rigid lens adherence. *Br Contact Lens Assoc J* 1989;12:32–36.
37. Swarbrick HA. A possible etiology for RGP lens binding (adherence). *Int Contact Lens Clin* 1988;15:13–19.
38. Swarbrick HA, Holden BA. Rigid gas permeable lens binding: significance and contributing factors. *Am J Optom Physiol Opt* 1987;64:815–823.
39. Terry R, Schnider CM, Holden BA. Maximizing success with rigid gas permeable extended wear lenses. *Int Contact Lens Clin* 1989;16:169–175.
40. Henry VA, Bennett ES. Explanation for parameter changes on RGP patients. *Contact Lens Forum* 1989;14:21.
41. Harris MG, Chu CS. The effect of contact lens thickness and corneal toricity on flexure and residual astigmatism. *Am J Optom Arch Am Acad Optom* 1972;49:304–307.
42. Harris MG. The effect of contact lens thickness and diameter on residual astigmatism: a preliminary study. *Am J Optom Physiol Opt* 1970;47:442–444.
43. Harris MG, Appelquist TD. The effect of contact lens diameter and power on flexure and residual astigmatism. *Am J Optom Physiol Opt* 1974;51:266–270.
44. Harris MG, Sweeney KE, Rocchi S, et al. Flexure and residual astigmatism with cellulose acetate butyrate (CAB) contact lenses on toric corneas. *Am J Optom Physiol Opt* 1982;59:858–862.
45. Harris MG, Kadoya J, Nomura J, et al. Flexure and residual astigmatism with Polycon and polymethyl methacrylate lenses on toric corneas. *Am J Optom Physiol Opt* 1982;59:263–266.
46. Harris MG, Gale B, Gansel K, et al. Flexure and residual astigmatism with Paraperm 02 and Boston II lenses on toric corneas. *Am J Optom Physiol Opt* 1987;64:269–273.
47. Sorbara L, Fonn D, MacNeil K. Effect of rigid gas permeable lens flexure on vision. *Optom Vis Sci* 1992;69:953–958.

48. Herman J P. Flexure. In: Bennett ES, Grohe RM, eds. *Rigid gas permeable contact lenses.* New York: Professional Press, 1986: 145.

49. Theodoroff CD, Lowther G. Quantitative effect of optic zone diameter changes on rigid gas permeable lens movement and centration. *Int Contact Lens Clin* 1990;17:92–94.

50. Guillon M, Guillon JP, Mapstone V, et al. Rigid gas permeable lenses in vivo wettability. *Trans Br Contact Lens Assoc* 1989; 24–26.

51. Grohe RM, Caroline PJ. RGP non-wetting lens syndrome. *Contact Lens Spectrum* 1989;4:32–44.

52. Tripathi TC, Tripathi BJ. Lens spoilage. In: Debezies O Jr., ed. *Contact lenses: the CLAO guide to basic science and clinical practices.* New York: Grune and Stratton, 1984;45.1–45.36.

53. Henry VA, Bennett ES, Forrest JF. Clinical investigation of the Paraperm EW rigid gas-permeable contact lens. *Am J Optom Physiol Opt* 1987;64:313–320.

54. Ghormley NR. New guy on the block. *Int Contact Lens Clin* 1995;22(Pt1):139–140.

55. Soper BA, Shovlin JP, Bennett E. Evaluating a topography software program for fitting RGPs. *Contact Lens Spectrum* 1996;11: 37.

56. Liu Z, Pflugfelder SC. The effects of long-term contact lens wear on corneal thickness, curvature, and surface regularity. *Ophthalmology* 2000;107:105–111.

57. Mandell RB. Oxygen supply and corneal needs. In: *Contact lens practice,* 4th ed. Springfield, IL: Charles C. Thomas, 1988;93: 81–106.

58. Sorbara L, Chong T, Fonn D. Visual acuity, lens flexure, and residual astigmatism of keratoconic eyes as a function of back optic zone radius of rigid lenses. *Contact Lens Anterior Eye* 2000; 23:48–52.

59. Fonn D, Pritchard N, Garnett B, et al. Palpebral aperture sizes of rigid and soft contact lens wearers compared with nonwearers. *Optom Vis Sci* 1996;73:211–214.

60. Fonn D, Gauthier CA, Pritchard N. Patient preferences and comparative ocular responses to rigid and soft contact lenses. *Optom Vis Sci* 1995;72:857–863.

61. Fonn D, Holden BA. Rigid gas permeable versus hydrogel contact lenses for extended wear. *Am J Optom Physiol Opt* 1988;65: 536–544.

62. Fonn D, Holden BA. Extended wear of hard gas permeable contact lenses induce ptosis. *CLAO J* 1986;12:93–94.

63. Epstein G, Putterman AM. Acquired blepharoptosis secondary to contact lens wear. *Am J Ophthalmol* 1981;91:634–639.

64. Van den Bosch WA, Lemij HG. Blepharoptosis induced by prolonged hard contact lens wear. *Ophthalmology* 1992;99: 1759–1765.

65. Levy B, Stamper RL. Acute ptosis secondary to contact lens wear. *Optom Vis Sci* 1992;69:565–566.

66. Efron N. Ptosis. In: BH/Optician, ed.: *Contact lens complications.* Oxford, UK: Butterworth Heinemann, 1999:10–14.

HYDROGEL CONTACT LENS APPLICATION, CARE, AND EVALUATION

CHEMISTRY AND PROCESSING OF CONTACT LENS MATERIALS

LYNN C. WINTERTON AND KAI C. SU

Today, the majority of materials used for commercialized soft contact lenses are hydrogel polymers. These hydrogels are cross-linked hydrophilic (water-loving) polymers that are made by polymerizing suitable monomers with a cross-linking agent. This same process can be achieved, less commonly, by the posttreatment of non–cross-linked hydrophilic polymers in which the cross-linking (also known as *vulcanization*) occurs through postthermal treatment or, even less commonly, by gamma irradiation. Cross-linking of the polymeric chains is necessary to make the entire lens matrix physically stable and nonsoluble in an aqueous environment.

The monomer is the fundamental building block for these polymers. A polymer is many of these "mer" units linked together in a chain, hence the name poly "mer," or *polymer*. In general, a monomer unit contains a polymerizable double bond, or vinyl group, i.e., C=C. The following are a few examples of monomers that are commonly used in contact lens materials. Because there are many derivations of monomer units, this listing is not intended to be all inclusive but only representative of the most common monomers used in contact lens applications.

1. *2-Hydroxyethyl methacrylate (HEMA)* monomer and its non–cross-linked low-molecular weight-polymer are water soluble. It is the primary monomer from which the first commercial soft contact lens was made. HEMA polymerization occurs through the double-carbon bond, which results in long, acrylate side-chains protruding from a carbon backbone. The chemical structure of the HEMA monomer is as follows:

2. *Ethylene glycol dimethacrylate (EGDMA).* This monomer contains two methacrylate groups in one molecule. Therefore, it is used primarily as a cross-linking agent, which is known as a vulcanizing agent used in rubber chemistry. Its main function is to increase the dimensional stability of the polymer. Excessive use of cross-linking agents tends to make the hydrogel stiff, lowers the water content, and renders the polymer less elastic (stretchable). The chemical structure of EGDMA can be written as follows:

3. *Methacrylic acid (MAA).* This unit is used to increase the water content in a hydrogel. The monomer is always charged at physiologic pH. Therefore, incorporating this monomer unit will result in the polymer being negatively charged. Depending on the resultant water content, the polymer will be an FDA type 2 or type 3 polymer. This monomer unit can be written as follows:

$$H_2C = \overset{\overset{\displaystyle CH_3}{|}}{C} - \overset{\overset{\displaystyle}{}}{\underset{\underset{\displaystyle O}{\|}}{C}} - OH$$

4. *Methyl methacrylate (MMA)* is the monomer unit that makes up the polymethyl methacrylate (PMMA) hard lens. It is sometimes used to lower water content or to improve durability and strength in some soft contact lenses. MMA can be illustrated as follows:

$$H_2C = \overset{\overset{\displaystyle CH_3}{|}}{C} - \underset{\underset{\displaystyle O}{\|}}{C} - O - CH_3$$

5. *Vinyl pyrrolidone,* or *n-vinyl-pyrrolidone (NVP),* can be an important monomer that is copolymerized with the vinyl functional copolymers. Due to its hydrophilicity, it has commonly been used to increase water content of traditionally hydrogel materials. It now is also used with silicone moieties to improve the wetting characteristics and water content of silicone hydrogels. Vinyl pyrrolidone is written as follows:

6. *Vinyl alcohol* is a monomer that has been used in medical devices for years. It can be made soluble in water. It is depicted as follows:

$$H_2C = CH - OH$$

7. *Styrene* is another monomer that is often used in contact lenses. It typically is brittle, hydrophobic, and water insoluble. When it is used in a hydrogel, it tends to increase the refractive index and lower the water content of the material. Increasing the refractive index of the resultant polymer allows the lens to be manufactured in a much thinner design to achieve the desired power target. Styrene is written as follows:

8. *Divinylbenzene* contains two polymerizable vinyl groups; therefore, it typically is used as a cross-linking agent. Divinylbenzene is written as follows:

9. *Polydimethylsiloxane (PDMS),* or *silicone rubber,* typically is used to increase the oxygen permeability of contact lenses. It is the principal component of both rigid gas permeable (GP) contact lenses as well as the new generation of silicone hydrogel materials that allows these lenses to transmit oxygen in higher quantities compared to traditional hydrogel materials, thus rendering them suitable for continuous wear without causing corneal swelling. Cross-linked PDMS lenses have been used successfully in the treatment of pediatric aphakia and as intraocular lenses. PDMS is depicted as follows:

10. *Tris-(trimethyl-silyl-propyl-methacrylate),* also simply referred to as *TRIS,* is a less expensive alternative to silicone monomer used to increase oxygen permeability in contact lenses. It is a very "bulky" monomer that allows significant oxygen to permeate the resultant polymer. It also has the advantage of making the resultant materials typically softer than ordinary pure PDMS materials. This monomer typically is copolymerized with silicone-containing moieties and not considered viable as a contact lens material when homopolymerized because it lacks strength. TRIS has the following structure:

11. *Dimethylacrylamide (DMA)* is a monomer that now is being used to copolymerize with acrylate moieties to increase the water content and hydrophilic character of the resultant copolymer. It is often used in silicone hydrogel chemistry. DMA is depicted as follows:

$$H_3C-N(CH_3)-C(=O)-CH=CH_2$$

Vinyl monomers can be polymerized by either free radical polymerization or via either cationic or anionic polymerization. Within the contact lens industry, ionic polymerization processes are rarely used; therefore, for this discussion, the focus is limited to free radical polymerization. The free radical polymerization scheme is typically represented by the following:

$$(C = C) + Rad^* \Rightarrow (Rad - C - C^*)$$

where *Rad** represents a reactive free radical chemical group that can attach itself covalently to a vinyl group (double bond between two carbons, i.e., $C = C$). Free radical polymerizations usually are initiated by decomposing a catalyst or initiator into a free radical. Free radicals can be generated either photochemically (i.e., sun lamp or ultraviolet [UV] light) or thermally (applying heat). Free radical formation is followed by the addition of other monomer units, in rapid succession, until a polymer is formed. This may be illustrated in the following scheme:

Initiator + *(UV/ heat)* $\rightarrow$ *Rad **
Rad * + *M* $\rightarrow$ *M ** *(RadM*)*
M * + *M* $\rightarrow$ *MM **
MM * + *M* $\rightarrow$ *MMM ** + *M* $\rightarrow$ *MMMM ** + *M* $\rightarrow$
etc. $\rightarrow$ *Polymer*

An example of this entire process can be shown through the polymerization of HEMA. First we have the generation of a free radical via the initiator: *Initiator* $\rightarrow$ *Rad **. Then the remaining process is depicted in Fig. 17.1. The "n" of the polymer refers to the average number of repeating HEMA monomer units in the polymer chain or backbone. The resultant polymer may not have dimensional stability and may partially dissolve in water (low-molecular-weight polyHEMA is water soluble). Adding a small amount of a cross-linking monomer, such as EGDMA, to the HEMA monomer increases the dimensional stability and renders the resultant polymer matrix insoluble in water. When placed in water, the resulting new polymer matrix will swell to a cross-linked three-dimensional hydrogel, not unlike a clear sponge (Fig. 17.2).

When a higher water content material is desired, monomers, such as MAA or vinyl pyrrolidone, are blended into the formulation. In this type of situation, a blend of more than one kind of monomer is used. Technically speaking,

when the polymer contains more than one kind of monomer, it is called a *copolymer,* and the process of making it is called *copolymerization.* Most of the commercially available high-water contact lenses are copolymers with one monomer adding water content and the other imparting the desired physical properties. The copolymerization process is schematically outlined in the following:.

Initiator $\rightarrow$ *Rad **
Rad * + M_1 $\rightarrow$ *RadM$_1$ **
Rad * + M_2 $\rightarrow$ *RadM$_2$ **

where M_1 and M_2 denote different kinds of monomers. Statistically, both *RadM$_1$** and *RadM$_2$** can react with remaining M_1 or M_2 monomers. However, in reality, the generated radicals react preferentially toward one or the other as driven by thermodynamic preference, depending on the nature of the M_1 and M_2 monomers, as well as the given reaction conditions. Therefore, all possible reactions are as follows:

RadM$_1$ * + M_1 $\rightarrow$ *RadM$_1$M$_1$ **
RadM$_1$ * + M_2 $\rightarrow$ *RadM$_1$M$_2$ **
RadM$_2$ * + M_1 $\rightarrow$ *RadM$_2$M$_1$ **
RadM$_2$ * + M_2 $\rightarrow$ *RadM$_2$M$_2$ **

Given the four possible reactions, the resulting copolymer may have monomers M_1 and M_2 in a random, an alternating, and/or a block configuration. These three configurations can be schematically represented as follows:

$M_1M_1M_2M_1M_2M_2M_1$	Random copolymer
$M_1M_2M_1M_2M_1M_2M_1$	Alternating copolymer
$M_1M_1M_1M_1M_1M_1M_2M_2M_2M_2$	Block copolymer

As a rule of thumb, monomers with similar chemical structures tend to copolymerize to form random copolymers. For example, due to the similarity in chemical structure, MMA (monomer 4) and ethyl methacrylate can be copolymerized to form a random copolymer.

$$H_2C=C(CH_3)-C(=O)-O-CH_2-CH_3$$

Ethyl Methacrylate

Copolymers of monomers with different chemical configurations may have significant differences in the final polymer physical properties, even when they start with the same comonomer mix. For example, MMA (monomer 4) and vinyl pyrrolidone (monomer 5) cannot be copolymerized to a random copolymer at all. When combined, these monomers will homopolymerize in the same vessel but will not react with each other to any significant extent. The result is two homopolymers and no copolymer. This is an extreme example, yet other comonomer blends may exhibit graded

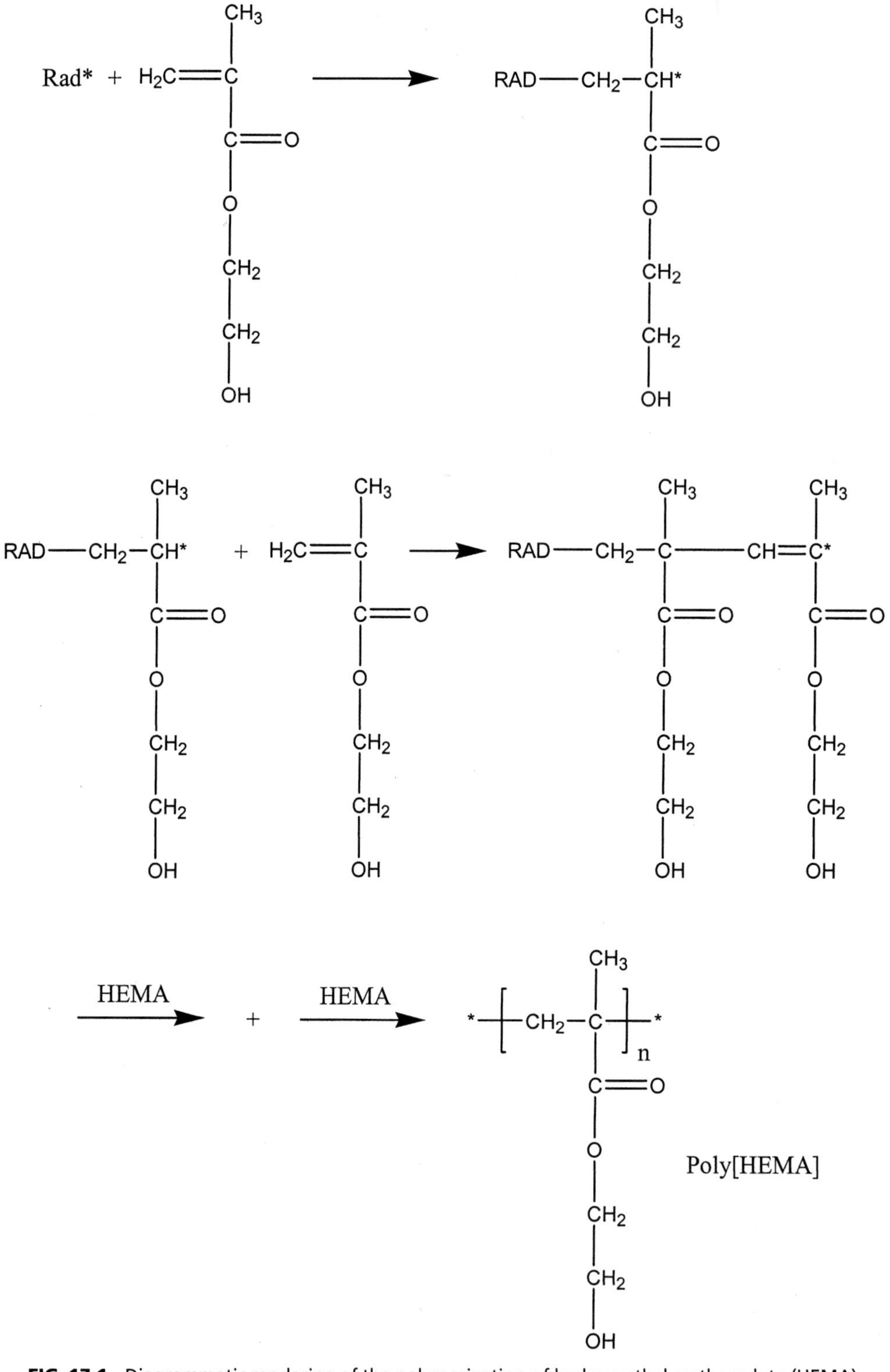

FIG. 17.1. Diagrammatic rendering of the polymerization of hydroxyethyl methacrylate (HEMA).

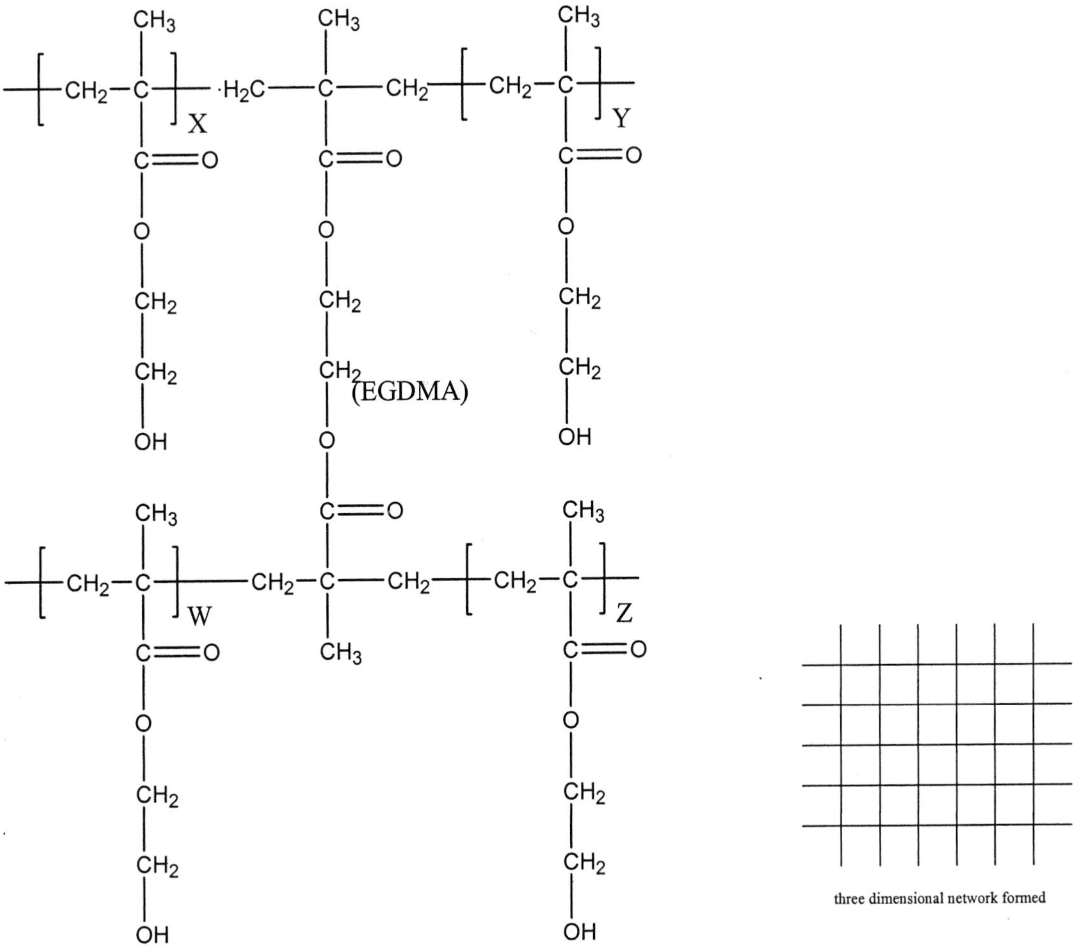

FIG. 17.2. The polymer becomes an insoluble three-dimensional polymer when cross-linking agents are added to the hydroxyethyl methacrylate (HEMA) monomer mixture and copolymerized together.

polymer properties as one monomer is incorporated into the final copolymer at the expense of the other.

In the contact lens industry, copolymerization is very important for both hydrogel and GP lens materials. Virtually all lens materials are copolymers. By polymerizing the proper combinations of different monomers, one can modify or determine the desired physical and chemical properties of a lens material. By varying the ratios of the same two monomers, one can create materials with various water contents, refractive indices, variable hardness, mechanical strengths, and oxygen permeabilities.

Depending on the compositional nature of the hydrogel copolymer, the temperature and pH (acidity) can have a great influence on the clinical performance of some hydrogel lenses. When the temperature rises, some low-water contact lens materials tend to swell and their diameter becomes larger. Conversely, many high-water contact lens materials tend to shrink when the temperature is raised from ambient to the patient's eye temperature (34°C).

Acidity has little effect on the dimensional stability of

the uncharged neutral hydrogel lens. Conversely, acidity can influence greatly the dimensions of a hydrogel material that contains MAA as a comonomer. At lower pH levels, the MAA units in the hydrogel mostly reside in the uncharged, neutral state. This enables the polymer to stabilize in the most compact conformation possible (Fig. 17.3).

However, in isotonic buffered saline solutions, the MMA residues in the polymer are charged (Fig. 17.4). In order to minimize the electrostatic repulsion between the negative charges of the carboxylate groups, the lens material expands

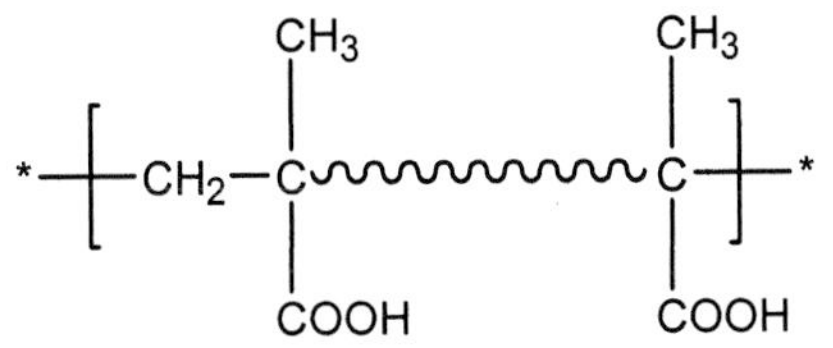

FIG. 17.3. Compact conformation of a methacrylic acid (MMA)-containing hydrogel polymer in acidic medium.

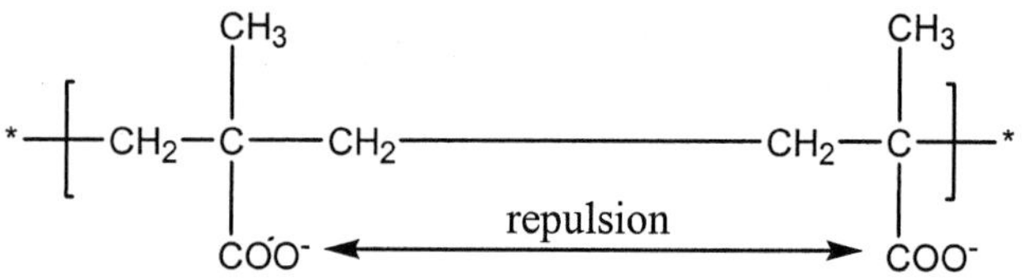

FIG. 17.4. Repulsion of like ionic charges causes the polymer chain to move apart, resulting in an increase in water content.

significantly, changing the dimensional characteristics of the lenses by essentially pushing the charges apart with water spacers. This raises the water content. In the eye, carbon dioxide generation by natural metabolism lowers the pH. Therefore, this type of lens tends to gradually tighten on the eye as the pH drops.

CHEMISTRY OF TINTED AND COLORED HYDROGEL CONTACT LENSES

Almost all GP lenses and hard lenses are tinted for easier handling. These tints are added by either dissolving dyes in the monomer or dispersing pigment into the monomer mixture. The resulting monomer mix is polymerized into tinted contact lens blanks, or *buttons.* This technology may not work for hydrogel soft contact lenses if the lens material swells too much in aqueous solutions. The dye or pigment may not be retained in the expanded lens matrix. However, if the cross-linked density (concentration) is sufficiently high, then the polymer chains and cross-links, together, may sufficiently cage the dispersed pigment so that it cannot be removed from the lens matrix. This technology must be applied with care so that the resultant polymer is not too stiff. Another option to disperse pigment into such a cage matrix is to incorporate larger pigment particles, which are trapped by a more open caged network. This technology also must be applied with care so that light does not scatter from the larger pigment particles, thus inducing visual defects in the wearer's visual field. Such visual defects may manifest themselves as rings about lights, also known as *halos* at night.

For both handling and cosmetic reasons, several tinting technologies have been developed for hydrogel lenses during the past two decades. However, the majority of tinted hydrogel soft lenses sold today are tinted by either the chemical bond process or the vat dye process.

In the chemical bond process, the dye molecules are fastened to the lens material by stable, chemical covalent bonds. Dyes used for this process are selected from various reactive dyes that were developed in the textile industry for dyeing cotton and silk. They are known for their color fastness. The chemical reaction is between the reactive dye and hydroxyl groups (–OH) in the lens material. This reaction can be expressed as follows:

$$dye - X + (HO - Lens) \rightarrow dye - X - O - Lens$$

where X is the reactive group.

The tinted lenses made from this process have clear and bright color. They are stable in both chemical, including hydrogen peroxide, and heat lens care regimens, but they can be bleached by chlorine and chlorine-containing disinfecting agents, as well as other halogen-containing systems. Therefore, this type of tinted lens should not come into contact with chlorinated tap water, swimming pool water, or household bleach. Before using novel disinfection systems, the user needs to verify that they are safe for tinted and colored contact lenses.

The application of such reactive dyes may be (i) after the lens is manufactured or (ii) before the lens is made. Both systems have their advantages and disadvantages.

Tinting After Lens Formation

If the tint is applied after the lens is formed, this requires a separate step in the process and, therefore, more costly. However, using appropriate masking techniques, this type of tint application can result in clear edges so that the handling tint or applied color is restricted only to the iris area of the wearer's eye. Because the color does not extend beyond the sclera, the white appearance of the sclera is not affected and, therefore, remains white. Because the sclera appearance is not affected by the tint color and remains clear, this type of color application is appropriate for handling tints, color-enhancing tints, and opaque color tints, which are used to change the appearance of the wearer's eye. After tinting, the lenses are extracted to remove any unreacted or unbonded dyes.

Tinting Before Lens Formation

The reactive dye may be applied to the monomer mixture before the lens is made. If we consider HEMA, which is rich in available hydroxyl groups, as an example, one can imagine a scheme in which reactive dye is added to monomeric HEMA and then reacted. This scheme can be depicted as follows:

$$dye - X + (HEMA) \rightarrow dye - X - HEMA$$

The resultant HEMA monomer is tinted before the HEMA polymerization reaction occurs. Therefore, this tinted HEMA monomer is be added back to the comonomer mixture and the polymerization reaction carried out normally. This results in an edge-to-edge tinted final lens. The cost is less than application of tint after the lens is formed. The drawback is that the color intensity is limited to light handling tints, so the sclera does not appear colored to the observer. A darker tint would make the sclera appear colored. This process does not require an additional extraction step solely for the tint, as all contact lenses are extracted after production to remove any unreacted monomers and solvents.

Another important tinting method is to let a water-soluble vat dye (reduced form) permeate into swollen lens material. Through an oxidation step, these dyes in the lens matrix are made insoluble in water and, therefore, become locked into the lens matrix. This tinting scheme is depicted in Fig. 17.5.

Lenses tinted with vat dye are somewhat dull in color because of the heterogeneity of the vat dye aggregates produced in this process. However, they are stable in both chemical and older heat lens care regimens.

Opaque Colored Lenses

Many contact lens wearers, particularly young wearers, would like to change the color of their natural eyes. To do this, they may wear a tinted lens that can add to or enhance the color of the natural eye or choose to mask the eye color using a lens that uses opaque colors.

To enhance a color, the lens wearer may choose a tinted lens without any apparent color pattern to the colored area. The wearer's iris color comes through the lens and is added to the enhancing tint of the lens. The result is a color blend of the two initial colors. The color chemistry of this type of lens was discussed previously.

To mask the natural eye color, such as changing a brown iris to appear blue, wearers must use opaque tints and pigments that mostly reflect only the color applied to the outside of the contact lens and block much of the natural color of the iris from dominating the viewer's perception. It is undesirable to mask all of the natural iris color, as this makes the appearance two dimensional, without depth, and very unnatural. To achieve this masking of the underlying iris color, there are two dominant techniques. One is *sandwich-*

ing color in the lens and the other is *printing* color to the outside of the front surface of the lens.

Sandwiching color involves manufacturing to produce a clear lens that has an annular trench cut around the iris area, leaving the optic zone unaffected. Into the trench is laid or stamped a very thin layer of reflective white, opaque material, using an irislike pattern. The colored material may be an off-white or colored mixture. The trench is then re-filled with monomer mixture and cured a second time. This additional cure step creates a patch that holds the patterned opaque material within the lens matrix. After cure, the lens is tinted using a reactive dye process (see earlier discussion). This process has the advantage that, after a common opaque process, any color can be applied to the surface to create any color of lens desired. In addition, because the color is on and in the lens, the appearance is three dimensional and very natural. The disadvantage is the cost involved with this process.

Printing color uses normal, clear, finished, contact lenses as stock material. No special trenching or handling is required. The lens is stamped with a mixture of monomer and opaque pigments on the front surface of the contact lens. The color is applied in an iris pattern using a soft, rubber stamp. The process can be repeated with other colors or patterns to enhance the pattern or color desired to make it look more natural or wild. After the color and monomer are applied, a heat or UV cure is performed to cure the monomer on the surface. The resultant lenses are colorfast and natural appearing. The majority of eye color-changing lenses are produced using this type of processing because of the ease of printing compared to the sandwiching process.

CHEMISTRY OF SILICONE HYDROGELS

It was shown in the late 1970s that the addition of silicone moieties to contact lenses can improve the oxygen and carbon dioxide transmission properties of the resultant lenses. However, since that time, the patent literature is filled with all types of soft, silicone contact lens materials that were never commercialized. During the past 25 years, researchers have been trying to blend the hydrophilic desired character of soft lenses with the hydrophobic character of silicone moieties. This has been likened to mixing oil and water to form a stable, optically clear mixture.

The key to mixing silicones with hydrogels is to incorporate monomers that compatibilize the two separate phases of organo-silicone and water. The monomeric means to accomplish this task could cover volumes within this text, alone. Good reviews and text books have been written that specifically address this novel chemistry and processing breakthrough (1,2). However, the polymerization of these materials occurs in the same fashion as does the polymerization techniques described previously.

The incorporation of silicone moieties renders these

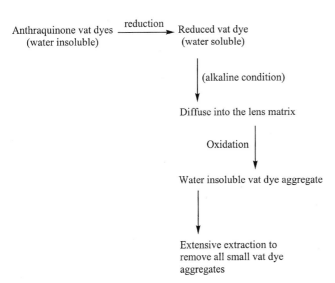

FIG. 17.5. Tinting method using vat dyes.

types of materials inherently nonwetting. As such, they will adsorb lipid and protein from the eye. To prevent this from occurring during wear, these materials need to mask the undesired hydrophobic (lipophilic) character of the silicone chemistry. To accomplish this, one can apply one of two surface modification techniques:

1. *Surface modify the contact lens.* This either applies a coating to the lens or modifies the surface chemistry of the lens to render it hydrophilic. Typically this can be accomplished by several means:

A. *Plasma reaction.* This is a vacuum system process in which molecules are energized so as to react in a fashion that normally would not occur. This may either modify the surface chemistry or coat the lens, depending on the gas used in the plasma chamber. A typical plasma reaction would be to use oxygen gas as an oxidizing agent to the lens surface. This would etch the surface and cause oxygen to react with the outermost lens molecules. Typically this produces hydroxyl moieties, such as those found on HEMA monomer. As such, this can render the surface wettable. However, due to the inherent chain mobility of polymers, such nominal oxidation of the surface is transient and not robust over time. Higher oxidation energies may overcome this problem by oxidizing the surface of the silicone to silicate (glass). However, plasma reactions are not limited to oxygen. One also can use alkyl carbon, which produces diamondlike thin films that are wettable and inert. Other possible reactions are nitrogen (amino)-containing systems, as well as other more elaborate chemicals.

B. *Surface grafting.* This is a wet, solution process that uses solution monomers that can react with the surface to graft a new polymer onto the outermost surfaces of the contact lens. For example, one could use HEMA monomers to graft onto the outermost surface and create a sandwich of silicone lens inside a thin HEMA shell. Of course, other hydrophilic monomers could be used to accomplish the de-

sired affect. However, the monomers do not have to be directly applied to the lens itself. The monomers also can be applied to the mold surface and cured into a thin sandwich half. The lens monomers then are cast into the coated molds and the outer coating releases during cure, resulting in a sandwich lens.

C. *Other means.* Any attached or adsorbed chemical that will create new surface properties and render the old surface masked to its undesired hydrophobic properties.

2. *Incorporate wetting agents that leach onto the surface with time.* In this process, one incorporates water-soluble, low-molecular-weight polymer chains into the monomer mixture during cure. These water-soluble agents are not functionalized, so they cannot participate in the polymerization process. They are left in the midst of the polymer matrix so as to leach slowly with time, much like sustained medications that release over a day or two. These leaching agents, such as polyvinylpyrrolidone or polyvinyl alcohol, can, to some extent, temporarily stick to the surface of the hydrophobic lens as they are released. However, such modifications are limited by time and are not optimal in that they rely on a sustained release; which cannot occur with regularity over time. The surface eventually will become depleted of release agent, and the time for replenishing will become increasingly longer. The resultant lenses will become increasingly hydrophobic with time. One way to attempt this scenario is to incorporate more wetting agent as a copolymer with the silicone moieties, yet this results in higher water content and lower oxygen permeability. This becomes a rather defeating purpose, because silicone was added to enhance the oxygen permeability in the first place.

REFERENCES

1. Sweeney D, ed. *Silicone hydrogels, the rebirth of continuous wear contact lenses.* Boston: Butterworth Heinemann, 2000.
2. Nicolson PC, Vogt J. Soft contact lens polymers: an evolution. *Biomaterials* 2001;22:3273–3283.

SOFT CONTACT LENS APPLICATION

KAREN K. YEUNG AND
BARRY A. WEISSMAN

Invented before 1960 by Otto Wichterle, hydrogels were developed during the creation of water-absorbing plastics for medical applications (1,2). Hydrogels are defined as a subclassification of "flexible" or "soft" contact lenses: contact lenses that can fold until opposite ends meet, return without damage into their original shape, and wrap toward the corneal surface upon application (3–5). Wichterle's promotion of hydrogel lenses began the global proliferation of hydrogel materials and designs as we know them today (2).

MATERIAL PROPERTIES

Chemistry

Both hydrogel and rigid gas permeable (GP) contact lens plastics are composed of *polymers,* which are monomers linked together to form large repetitive chains. A large monomer with preassembled structural units is a *macromer.* Its structural and functional group interactions affect its linkage to other polymers. Use of multiple types of monomers creates *copoylmers* (6). Polymer chains are then chemically bonded via cross-linking.

Hydrogels differ from GP lenses in their ability to bind substantial amounts of water (1). Differences in hydrogel cross-linking affect this ability to bond with water and thereby control many of the hydrated lens' physical properties, especially water content, elasticity, and tear resistance. Loose cross-linking allows the plastic to swell to several times its original dry volume; tight cross-linking may preclude swelling. Loose cross-linking also weakens the lens' ability to recover from mechanical deformation (modulus of elasticity) and resist breakage, whereas tight cross-linking decreases elasticity (6).

Water content is the primary factor, but other ingredients and cross-linking will affect the final plastic's effective "pore" size, which is estimated to be about 8 Angstroms (Å) for low-water-content materials and 20 to 30 Å for high-water-content materials (7), and affect the lenses' elasticity, tensile strength, optical index, adsorption of deposits, and oxygen transmissibility (8).

Wichterle made his first hydrogel contact lenses with poly-2-hydroxyethyl methacrylate (p-HEMA) cross-linked with ethylene glycol dimethacrylate (EDMA). Additional hydrogels were later created by the use of other monomers (such as n-vinyl-pyrrolidone) with p-HEMA to increase water content. Relatively small percentages of acrylic or vinyl monomers can be added to modify the final hydrogel properties, for example, both isobutyl methacrylate and pentyl methacrylate decrease the final plastic's equilibrium water content because of their hydrophobic properties (6). In addition, non–p-HEMA–based hydrogels (e.g., Focus Dailies nelfilcon A: polyvinyl alcohol) have become available.

More recently, monomers containing silicone as siloxane, fluorine, or carbon/carbon triple bonds have been added to produce higher oxygen permeable flexible lenses. Lotrafilcon A combines silicone with a polar fluorinated side-chain and hydrophilic monomers. Alternatively, balafilcon A has macromers with a biphasic hydrophilic polyethylene oxide segment and oxygen permeable polysiloxane units (9,10). The newest addition to the silicone hydrogels is Galyfilcon A with Hydraclear® integrated into the matrix of the lens. These silicone materials dramatically increase oxygen permeability (compared to traditional hydrogel materials) while hopefully maintaining many of the standard hydrogel mechanical fitting and comfort characteristics (11).

Water Content

Water content of a hydrogel contact lens is expressed by the following equation (12):

$$\text{Water content} = \left(\frac{\text{Weight of lens water}}{\text{Total weight of hydrated lens}} \right) \times 100$$

Hydrogel contact lens materials range in water content from about 25% to 80% when equilibrated in normal (0.9%) saline (6). Hydrogel contact lenses may be arbitrarily grouped into low (<45%), medium (45%–60%), and high (>60%) water content lens materials. The US Food and Drug Administration (FDA) has alternatively recommended that hydrogel lenses be divided into four groups

TABLE 18.1. FDA* HYDROGEL LENS GROUPS WITH A SAMPLE OF LENS MATERIALS AND BRANDS[a]

Group 1 (<50% H₂O nonionic)		Group 2 (>50% H₂O nonionic)		Group 3 (<50% H₂O ionic)		Group 4 (>50% H₂O ionic)	
Crofilcon A	*CSI EW*	Alphafilcon A	*Soflen66*	Balafilcon A	*Purevision*	Etafilcon A	*Acuvue*
Hefilcon B	*Optima Toric*	Hilafilcon B	*Resolution*	Bufilcon A	*Soft Mate B*	Focofilcon A	*Fre-flex*
Hioxifilcon B	*Alden HP*	Hioxifilcon A	*Satureyes*	Ocufilcon A	*Tresoft*	Methafilcon A	*Frequency 55*
Lotrafilcon A	*Night & Day*	Nelfilcon A	*Focus Dailies*	Phemfilcon A	*Fresh Look*	Ocufilcon F	*Hydrogenics 60*
Galyfilcon A	*Acuvue Advance*	Omafilcon A	*Proclear*			Perfilcon A	*Permalens*
Tetrafilcon A	*Preference*	Vasurfilcon A	*Precision UV*			Vifilcon A	*Focus 1–2 week*

[a] This list is not complete; more than one brand may use the same lens materials.
*FDA, U.S. Food and Drug Administration.

according to material water content and chemical (ionic or nonionic) properties (Table 18.1) (13). High-water-content ionic materials tend to be more easily and quickly soiled and chemically reactive during use. Low-water-content nonionic materials, however, tend to be relatively soilage and chemistry resistant. The other two groups fall in between. It is possible that the silicone hydrogels eventually may be considered a fifth group.

The oxygen permeabilities (Dk) of traditional hydrogel materials are directly related to their water contents (6,8, 14) (see later). Contrary to traditional hydrogel materials, the oxygen permeability of silicone hydrogel materials increases as water content decreases because oxygen is transported faster through the silicone polymer phase than through the bound water. Water content, however, is a relative parameter (15). First, there is some variation in water content among batches of hydrogel material. Conditions such as humidity and temperature of the wearer's surrounding environment may change the water content of any hydrogel lens while it is on the eye. Wearer-specific tear film conditions, such as tear pH and osmolarity, also contribute to the *in vivo* hydration of a hydrogel lens (16). High-water-content hydrogel lenses generally show a greater reduction in water content than low-water-content lenses (17). Off the eye, a hydrogel lens will begin to dry immediately in air. Drying begins rapidly and then slows to approach the dehydrated state (18). Some water may remain at equilibrium with the air, depending on air humidity, but further drying may be accomplished in a vacuum oven. Finally, different methods of measurement technique and expression of water content has led to confusion when comparing various studies of hydrogel lens water content changes (Fig. 18.1) (19,20).

Reduction in water content, on or off the eye, will decrease both overall diameter (OAD) and thickness, steepen the base curve to tighten the lens fit (21), change optical power (22), and reduce the Dk of the material (23).

Several presumably "dehydration-resistant" hydrogel materials have been recently developed: ocufilcon A, Benz-G 55, and omafilcon A. Compared to hydrogel materials of similar water contents, these materials are intended to

dehydrate less *in situ*, hence providing greater comfort (especially for dry eye patients). The polymers in these lenses (phosphorylcholine in omafilcon A and poly-HEMA/glycerol methacrylate (GMA) copolymer in Benz-G 55) have strong affinities for water and are claimed to be slow to dehydrate but rehydrate quickly (24–27). Lemp et al. (24) found that patients wearing omafilcon A reported improvement in subjective symptoms, such as burning, dryness, and eye irritations. Objectively the lenses also caused less fluorescein corneal staining.

Lens Rigidity

The "stiffness" of a hydrogel contact lens is thought to be a component of its thickness profile as well as the "integrity" (modulus of elasticity) of the hydrogel material. More rigid lenses tend to have lower water contents and thicker profiles. In myopia-correcting lenses, the most rigid part of a contact lens is in its midperiphery (where it is thickest), whereas

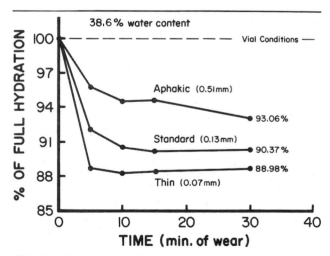

FIG. 18.1. Percentage of hydration at various time intervals of wear with different-thickness hydrogel contact lenses. Poly-2-hydroxyethyl methacrylate (p-HEMA) hydrogels had initial water content of 38.5%. (From Andrasko G. The amount and time course of soft contact lens dehydration. *J Am Optom Assoc* 1982; 53:207, with permission.)

hyperopia-correcting lenses are thickest centrally. Certain materials are known to have a lower or higher modulus of elasticity.

Temperature

An increase in temperature lowers the water content of a hydrogel, similar to drying (28). Low-water-content hydrogel lenses were found to change little in base curve, but high-water-content lenses were found to steepen in base curve (29). Additionally, high-water-content high-plus optically powered lenses were found to decrease in plus power (22,30) with increased temperature.

Refractive Index

The refractive index provided in the technical literature usually refers to that of a material's fully hydrated state. The refractive index of a hydrogel material is a property of the polymer and its cross-linking. It varies linearly with water content from about 1.37 at water content 80% to 1.44 at water content 42% (28). The silicone hydrogel contact lenses (both lotrafilcon A and balafilcon A) have refractive indexes of 1.43 (Package inserts: Bausch & Lomb, Rochester, NY, USA; CIBA Vision Care, Duluth, GA, USA).

Tonicity and pH

The stability of hydrogel lens parameters is promoted by packaging in solutions with pH and tonicity similar to that of human tears. Storing lenses in different solutions, however, can change the lens performance *in vivo*. For example, p-HEMA (38% water content) lenses were found to be stable in diameter through the pH range from 2.7 to 10.6, but vifilcon A (55% water content) lenses were stable only in basic solutions. Exposing lenses of this hydrogel to pH 3.7 resulted in permanently smaller diameters and warped edges. Similarly, the OADs of vifilcon lenses were found to be susceptible to changes in tonicity (0%–1.5% NaCl), being larger in hypotonic solutions and smaller in hypertonic solutions. p-HEMA lenses, however, were relatively insensitive to these tonicity changes (31). The tonicity of the storage solution also may influence subsequent *in vivo* performance. Lens movement decreases as storage solution salinity is reduced. A lens presoaked in 0.6% NaCl will typically show poor movement on the eye for several minutes, and a lens presoaked in a solution of less than 0.6% NaCl will adhere tenaciously to the eye for about 15 minutes (32). (Irrigation with 0.9% NaCl will eventually allow lens movement.)

Biocompatibility

Although hydrogel materials are extensively tested for biocompatibility prior to use in contact lenses, there remains a potential for various contaminants that are not compatible with human tissues (e.g., residual catalysts and monomers from manufacture, colorants, stabilizers). Concentrations capable of causing toxic effects should not be present if careful manufacturing techniques are followed (33,34).

Oxygen Permeability and Transmissibility

Corneal metabolism is dependent on oxygen supply to its anterior surface (35–37). A contact lens covering the ocular surface will form a potential barrier to oxygen, related directly to both the oxygen transmissibility of the lens itself (termed *Dk/t*, where *Dk* is the oxygen permeability of the material in units of cm^2 mL O_2/s mL mm Hg and *t* is lens thickness in cm) (8,14) and the exchange of tears (which carry diffused oxygen) around the edge of the lens. Whereas rigid lenses have been found to exchange about 10% to 20% of the underlying tear layer per blink, hydrogel lenses promote only minimal, if any, tear exchange (38). Oxygen supply to the hydrogel lens-wearing cornea is therefore almost totally dependent on the Dk/t of the lens.

The Dks of contact lens materials have been measured by the single-chamber polarographic method of Fatt and St. Helen (8) since the 1960s. There has been some controversy regarding alternative methodology and results (39–41), particularly with regard to GP materials, but recent work has resulted in general agreement for hydrogels (42). It is important that measurements be made at, or corrected for, ocular temperature (35°C) (8). Corrections for both boundary and edge effects also are necessary (1992, standard no. 9913, International Standards Organization, Westliche, Germany) (43–47). The single-chamber polarographic technique may not be appropriate for materials of Dk substantially higher than the highest water content hydrogel (47), so alternative methods are being developed (48).

The "boundary" effect will result in underestimation of Dk/t and therefore Dk. This effect was not initially important because the Dk/t values of early hydrogel lens designs (with water content approximately 40% and t values approximately 0.2 cm) were relatively low (8). As hydrogel lenses increased in Dk/t (with increased water content and decreased t) to approach the Dk and t values of any associated tear, saline, or water layers, the boundary effect became a concern. Fatt and Chaston (47) provided a technical solution to this problem: several samples (a minimum of four is recommended) of the same material but of varying t values are measured and the slope of the linear regression of the reciprocal of measured Dk/t (i.e., t/Dk) versus t is the reciprocal of Dk of the material without the effects of any boundary layers.

The "edge" effect, described by both Fatt et al. (44) and Brennan et al. (45), occurs because the polarographic electrode collects diffusing oxygen from an area in an overlying sample somewhat greater than its own diameter. The edge effect causes overestimation of first Dk/t and therefore Dk, and increases with increasing Dk/t. The edge effect can be removed from data by mathematical correction or through improved electrode design (46).

Dk is a characteristic of the plastic from which a lens is manufactured, increasing with the increasing fraction of oxygen permeable moiety in the material (e.g., water or silicone). Traditional hydrogel materials range in Dk from 5 to 35 × 10^{-11} cm^2 mL O$_2$/s mL mm Hg (or *Barrer*) (14). The Dks of these traditional hydrogel materials are directly related to their water contents in a logarithmic relationship (14,49); therefore, measurement of water content (50) can be used to estimate Dk (51) at ocular temperature and corrected for both edge and boundary effects for the whole spectrum of nonsilicone hydrogels (52):

Dk = 1.61 × 10^{-11} e$^{0.0411 \text{ water content}}$ (Fig. 18.2).

In silicone-containing hydrogels, however, Dk is dependent on first silicone content and then water content because oxygen is even more soluble in silicone than water. Hence, the permeability of oxygen increases as silicone content increases and water content decreases. The three current commercially available silicone hydrogel lenses have Dks of 60, 100, and 170 cm^2 mL O$_2$/s mL mm Hg, respectively.

On the eye, however, the contact lens specific value of Dk/t will be important. A lens manufactured from a low Dk hydrogel could be so much thinner (decreased t) than a similarly optically powered but very thick lens of a high Dk material, that the Dk/t and resultant oxygen flux to the underlying cornea would be relatively greater. Dk/t values of traditional hydrogel lenses range from about 10 to 30 × 10^{-9} cm mL O$_2$/s mL mm Hg (or *"Barrer/*cm"*") (49)

but silicone hydrogel Dk/ts are probably 85 × 10^{-9} Barrer/cm or greater, varying with thickness profiles.

Calculations often simply assume that the lenses are made of a uniform t. Optically powered lenses, however, only have uniform thickness at low minus (about −0.75 D) powers (53). Morris and Fatt (54) suggested that the central value of t for optical powers between ±1.50 D was close enough to average t that this value could be used. Fatt and others proposed mathematical techniques to provide an average t value (55–57). Holden and Mertz (58) and later Tomlinson and Bibby (59) suggested that t should only be averaged over a central zone about 6 mm in diameter (rather than the entire diameter) of each lens.

Fatt and Neumann (60) alternatively argued that average thickness is not appropriate for predicting lens physiologic performance in the absence of tear exchange or mixing, as in the case of hydrogel lens wear. They suggested that the thickest portion of the lens is most important because it is the Dk/t at that site which will produce the greatest hypoxic stress to the underlying corneal tissues. Later evidence was supportive of this concept (61,62).

Polse and Mandell (63) were the first to propose that there was a "critical tension" for the anterior corneal surface below which corneal metabolism would be compromised. "Critical" contact lens Dk/t values have been similarly quantified below which, for daily and extended wear, respectively, abnormal corneal metabolism—identified by measurable corneal swelling—can be anticipated; the open eye requires a contact lens of Dk/t 25 to 35 × 10^{-9} or greater and the closed eye requires a contact lens of Dk/t 90 to 125 × 10^{-9} cm mL O$_2$/s mL mm Hg or greater to preclude corneal edema (58,64,65). This difference is due to a decrease in oxygen tension, which is the driving force

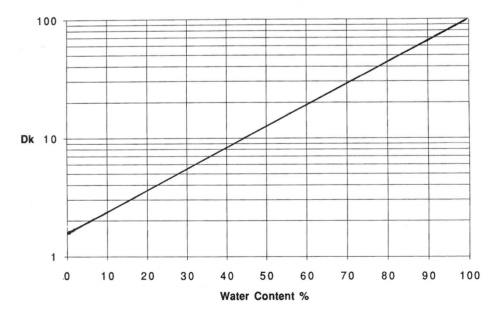

FIG. 18.2. Fatt-Chaston relationship of Dk (×10^{-11} cm^2 mL O$_2$/s mL mm Hg) versus water content (%) of hydrogel materials, modified to account for the edge effect. (From Brennan NA, Efron N, Weissman BA, et al. Clinical application of oxygen transmissibility of powered contact lenses. *CLAO J* 1991;17:169, with permission.)

for diffusion through the lens, from 155 mm Hg (open eye) to about 50 mm Hg (closed eye) (66,67) at the anterior surface of the lens.

Some corneal swelling during contact lens daily wear is clearly physiologically tolerated, because few, if any, traditional hydrogel contact lenses have Dk/t values (49,65) of 25×10^{-9} or greater (Fig. 18.3). Corneal edema may be observed clinically using the biomicroscope and can be measured with ultrasound or optical pachometers, but minimal amounts are difficult to detect clinically (58,68,69).

Silicone hydrogels (e.g., lotrafilcon A and balafilcon A) approach the theoretical minimum Dk/t criteria for pre-

cluding overnight contact lens-induced corneal swelling. Lin et al. (70) found corneal swelling after wearing CIBA Night & Day lenses for 1 hour in a closed-eye state to be equal to not wearing a contact lens at all. Both lotrafilcon A and balafilcon A have now achieved FDA approval for 30-day extended wear (71,72).

Ultraviolet Protection

Increasing numbers of contact lens materials incorporate ultraviolet (UV)-absorbing moieties, providing some protection from the damaging effects of UV radiation to the

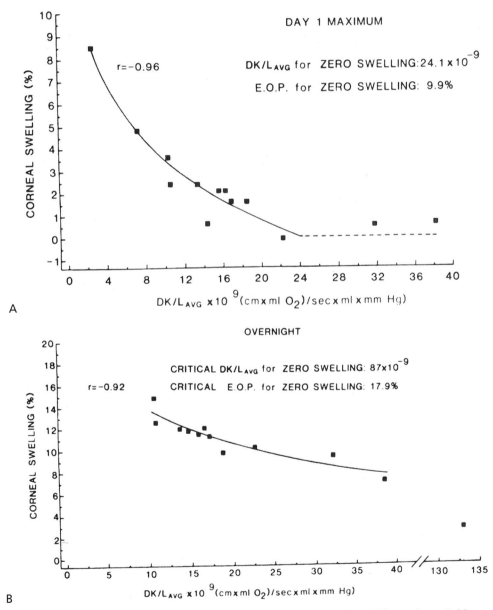

FIG. 18.3. Corneal swelling versus contact lens Dk/L for open **(A)** and closed **(B)** eyes. (From Holden BA, Mertz GW. Critical oxygen levels to avoid corneal edema for daily and extended-wear contact lenses. *Invest Ophthal Vis Sci* 1984;25:1161, with permission.)

wearer's eyes. The spectral absorption of UV varies among contact lens materials (73), and none appears to block all UV radiation less than 400 nm (74).

DESIGN

Hydrogel contact lenses are available in a wide variety of parameters. Each parameter ultimately affects the contact lens fit on the patient's eye. Elements of lens design include the following categories.

Base Curve Radius

The base curve radius (also known as the *back central optic radius*) is the spherical radius of curvature of the posterior surface central (optical) zone, measured in millimeters. Spherical surfaced hydrogel lenses have been produced in base curves ranging from 7.5 to 9.5 mm in steps of 0.2 to 0.4 mm (75–77). Many current lenses are available in only a limited number of base curves, more commonly about 8.4 for average to steeper corneas and about 8.7 for average to flatter corneas.

Some hydrogel lenses have been manufactured with aspheric surfaces. The "base curve" of aspheric spin-cast lenses, for example, has been defined as "posterior apical radius" (78,79). Lenses with elliptical posterior central curvatures have been specified by both apical radius and eccentricity factor (80–82).

Overall Diameter

The total or overall diameter of a hydrogel contact lens is the linear chord edge-to-edge measurement of the lens in millimeters and typically ranges from 12.0 to 16.0 mm. Current lenses usually are limited to one or two OADs, often close to 14.0 mm. Multiple OADs, if available, usually are obtained in 0.5- to 1.0-mm steps; intermediate values have not proved helpful (75,77,83,84). Early clinical hydrogel lens practice suggested that lenses that were too small would decenter, resulting in subsequent corneal exposure (85), whereas lenses that were too large could lead to poor tear mixing (86), limbal compression, erosion, and subsequent vascular congestion (84).

Posterior Peripheral Curve System

Unlike rigid contact lenses, which often have posterior peripheries with multiple curves, the posterior surfaces of hydrogel lenses usually are either *monocurve* with no posterior peripheral curve or *bicurve* with one peripheral curve, 11 to 13 mm in radius and 0.5 to 0.9 mm in width, or of a standardized edge lift, intended to promote alignment with scleral curvature (75,76,87).

Anterior Peripheral Curve System

The larger hydrogel lens OAD (compared to GP lenses) necessitates the use of anterior peripheral curve systems to produce reasonable edge thickness values (0.10–0.08 mm). In practice, the lens designer selects the desired values for the base and posterior peripheral curve(s). Lens optical power, central thickness, and anterior optical zone diameter are selected as a group to give the largest practical optical zone for any specific power without making the final hydrated lens too thick or thin (centrally and at the junction between the optical zone and the peripheral curve systems). Computerized calculations are used to define a curve from the anterior surface optical/periphery junction to the edge of the lens, which will result in the desired unpolished lens edge thickness. Occasionally, multiple anterior peripheral curves are used in the design of hydrogel lenses. The final edge should be rounded, smooth, and polished (75).

Spin-cast lenses posses a characteristic front surface bevel about 1 mm wide (88). One of the advantages of spin-cast production is that this bevel produces a very fine edge in a very reproducible shape.

Optical Power

Hydrogel contact lenses can be manufactured in a wide variety of optical powers. Although many lens designs are provided in limited optical powers (i.e., plano to ±20.00 D), custom lathe-cut lenses may be available from +60.00 DS to −40.00 DS. Steps of 0.25 D are common in optical powers up to ±6.00 DS; thereafter, availability often is in steps of 0.50 D. Toric hydrogel lenses are available in spherical power of −20.00 to +10.00 and commonly of astigmatic power of −0.75 to −2.00 DC; custom toric lenses can have up to −10.00 DC.

Optical power varies with hydration, which is related to changes in environmental temperature, pH, and osmolarity (22,28). Flexure on an eye also will play a role (3,89). Low minus powered hydrogel lenses do not change substantially with flexure, but plus optically powered lenses decrease in optical power as the base curve steepens (Fig. 18.4) (90, 91).

Central Thickness

Minus optically powered hydrogel contact lenses are commonly available with central thickness ranging from 0.04 to 0.18 mm; thinner lenses can lead to central corneal desiccation (92), whereas thicker traditional hydrogel lenses may induce physiologic complications through hypoxia (58) [e.g., peripheral corneal vascularization (93)]. Plus optically powered lenses usually range in central thickness from about 0.20 to 0.70 mm. These values vary with the edge and central thickness, size of the anterior surface optical zone, water content of the plastic, and optical power elected.

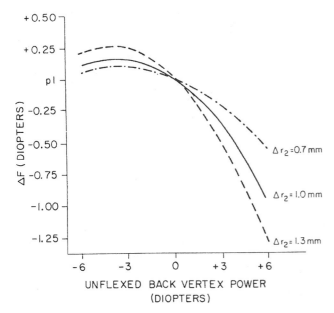

FIG. 18.4. Change in hydrogel contact lens back-vertex optical power versus original unflexed back-vertex power for various changes in base curve radius (Δr_2). (From Weissman BA. Clinical soft lens power changes. *Int Contact Lens Clin* 1984;11:342, with permission.)

Optical Zone Diameter

The optical zone diameter is the usable optical portion of the lens measured in millimeters. There is an optical zone diameter on both the anterior and posterior surfaces whenever there are peripheral curves.

MANUFACTURE

There currently are three manufacturing methodologies: spin casting, lathe cutting, and cast molding. Combinations of these processes have been used by several manufacturers, for example, one side of a lens is cast molded and then the other is lathed or spin cast. Hydrogel contact lenses are commonly manufactured in large batches at preselected parameters. The flexibility of the hydrated material allows a reduced set of specifications to be applicable to a multitude of ocular topographies. Finished lenses, which have been sterilized and are soaking in 0.9% saline solution in containers (glass vials or boxes of blister packs), are stocked in a central locale to be dispatched upon request.

Upon drying subsequent to initial hydration, lenses will both shrink and deform. In the dry state, a hydrogel contact lens is quite brittle and easily broken. However, if the lens is rehydrated intact, it will again assume the parameters of the proper flexible lens (75,94).

Spin Casting

Hydrogel contact lens designs have been produced by the original Wichterle method of spin casting for about 40 years

(2). Spin casting offers the advantage of consistent manufacture and low lens cost, but it is limited in optical powers as confined by the physical design of the lens.

During manufacture, a measured portion of a mixture of liquid monomers and a catalyst is injected onto a concave spinning mold. The front surface of the final lens is determined by the curvature of this mold and therefore is an independent variable. As the mold spins, the material spreads to the edges of the mold. Equilibrium is accomplished with surface tension, gravity, and centrifugal force. The posterior surface of the lens will assume a shape determined by the interaction of these forces; hence, no single spherical radius defines this curvature. Spinning the mold at different speeds causes different posterior surfaces (different posterior apical radii) and thereby different optical powers. In any given series of lenses made from the same mold, the posterior surface may vary from the polar section of an ellipse, a prolate spheroid, to the side of an ellipse, an oblate spheroid; within each series one posterior curve may even approach a spherical surface (99).

Polymerization is initiated by UV radiation and is completed while the mold is spinning. The lens is then hydrated, which frees it from the mold, and impurities are extracted by boiling the lens in saline (96).

Minus optically powered spin-cast lenses of the same series are available in standard central thickness, although the posterior apical radius decreases (curvature increases) with optical power (88). Plus optically powered lenses have central thickness ranging from 0.17 to about 0.60 mm, and the posterior apical radius increases with increasing optical power (88). (Note that some series have been discontinued.)

Lathe Cutting

Hydrogel contact lenses can be manufactured by machining on a lathe, similar to the manufacture of GP lenses. This method of production is relatively expensive and can be inconsistent, but it offers great latitude in possible parameters. Lathe cutting requires the use of dry plastic "buttons" that resemble the same initial material from which rigid lenses are produced. Every aspect of this form of hydrogel lens manufacture must be designed to prevent water from prematurely contacting the material. The manufacturing room has controlled humidity and lens buttons are stored in special containers to prevent their absorption of moisture from the atmosphere. Polishing is performed with compounds suspended in an oil base, and various inorganic rather than water-soluble solvents are used for cleaning. Correction factors are applied to determine the parameters at which a lens manufactured in the dry state will expand to produce the desired wet state values. The index of refraction is greater, front optic and base curves shorter, OAD smaller, and optical power greater than in the final hydrated lens. After manufacture, the final dry lens is placed in a saline bath and heated to undergo dimensional expansion

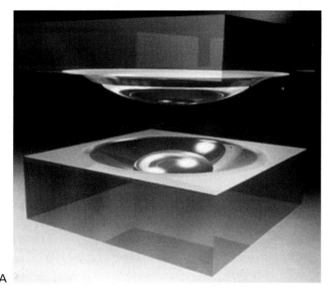
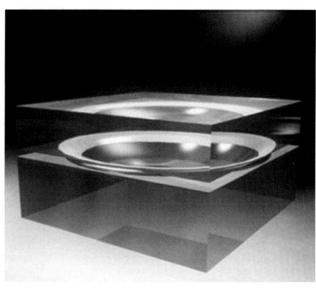

FIG. 18.5. **A:** CIBA Vision's patented cast-mold "Light Stream Technology" used to manufacture "1-day" lenses. Nelfilcon A is poured into a quartz mold. **B:** Cast molds are lowered within micrometers of each other. (Courtesy of CIBA Vision, a Novartis company.)

while being transformed from a hard to a flexible lens (12, 75,99–101).

Cast Molding

Cast molding is manufacture of lenses by injecting a monomer plastic between two molds, one concave and one convex. Similar to spin casting, some monomers are polymerized with UV radiation and then hydrated; others are molded with an already hydrated polymer. The lens is completed by removal of the mold shells. Multiple molds produce large numbers of lenses simultaneously; hence, cast molding can produce large quantities of inexpensive hydrogel lenses (102). With strict controls, quality can be excellent, but parameters are limited by the molds available (Fig. 18.5).

INDICATIONS AND CONTRAINDICATIONS

The primary clinical advantage of hydrogel contact lenses is enhanced *initial* patient comfort and tolerance compared to that achieved with rigid contact lenses. Clinicians rarely encounter patients who demonstrate contact lens adaptation problems with hydrogel lenses similar to those often encountered during rigid contact lens fitting. Hydrogel lens wearers also tolerate intermittent wearing periods well (103).

Overall, rigid contact lenses usually offer improved quality of vision, especially when astigmatism is considered (103), although several excellent designs of astigmatic ("toric") hydrogel lenses are now available (see Chapter 26).

Rigid lenses are easier and less expensive in terms of care, and they usually last longer than hydrogels (Table 18.2).

Despite rigid lens advantages, however, approximately 75% of patients currently dispensed contact lenses receive hydrogel lenses (104). This is due in part to the impression on the part of both patients and practitioners that hydrogel lenses are much more comfortable to wear than are rigid lenses (105). Previous rigid lens failure because of poor comfort is therefore a primary indication for hydrogel lens consideration. The comfort attained with hydrogel lenses may be so rewarding that negative attributes may be overlooked. It is only fair that a thorough discussion of the disadvantages, as well as the advantages, occur prior to prescription.

It often is assumed that comfort is related to the softness or water content of a hydrogel lens, but these factors probably play only minor roles. A hydrogel lens is comfortable when it has a large diameter, thin edges, smooth surfaces, and limited movement with the blink (106).

Relatively spherical refractive errors, particularly the extreme refractive errors (either very low myopia or very high myopia, or hypermetropia and aphakia) are indications for use of hydrogel lenses. Patients with minimal corrections often find adaptation to rigid lenses difficult, as they do not appreciate visual improvement enough to overcome initial discomfort. Alternatively, eyes of higher refractive errors (>3 D of hypermetropia or >7 D of myopia, although there is no absolute demarcation) often prove difficult to fit with rigid contact lenses because of problems with decentration and edging, some of which are more easily overcome with the larger OAD and improved tolerance offered by hydrogels. High myopes, in particular, do well optically with spherical hydrogel lenses; magnification often allows even patients with greater than 1 D of astigmatism to obtain

TABLE 18.2. ADVANTAGES AND DISADVANTAGES OF HYDROGEL COMPARED TO RIGID GAS PERMEABLE CONTACT LENSES

	Hydrogel Lenses	Rigid Gas-Permeable Lenses
Adaptation	Quick adaptation	Some patients may not adapt
Cleaning	One-day disposables eliminate cleaning	Traditionally easier to clean than daily wear hydrogels
Comfort	Initial comfort	Offer long-term comfort to patients who adapt
Cost	Traditionally more expensive than GPs (including solutions)	Less expensive than hydrogels
Durability	More fragile, especially disposables	More durable
Fit	Easy to fit by clinician	Require more chair time and expertise
Ocular health	Traditionally provides less oxygen to cornea than higher-Dk GPs	Can provide more oxygen to cornea
Sports	Good for sports because of larger diameters	Dislodge/pop out more easily while playing sports
Vision	Good vision if spherical power	Better vision, especially with astigmatism or corneal irregularities

RGPs, rigid gas-permeable lenses.

acceptable vision (Fig. 18.6) (107). Hyperopes or aphakes with substantial astigmatism, however, probably will obtain better optical results with rigid (or toric hydrogel) lenses, as the loss of acuity through minification compared to spectacles makes the need for astigmatic correction more apparent.

Both corneal distortion and subsequent spectacle blur are minimized (compared to rigid lens use) with hydrogel lenses (69). Because their optical zones are so much larger than those of most rigid lenses, hydrogel lenses rarely produce flare. Dislocation of contact lenses onto the sclera or ejection from the eye, and foreign body problems, are rare

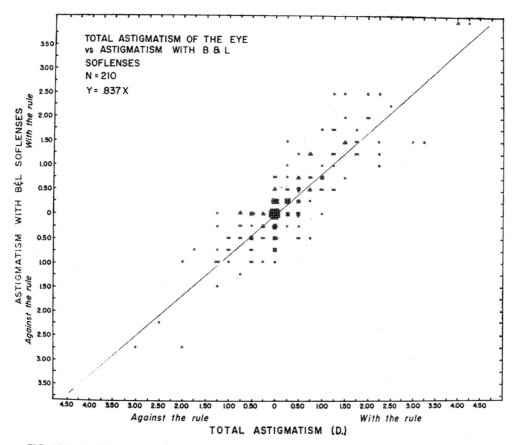

FIG. 18.6. Residual astigmatism with spin-cast hydrogel lenses on a large population (n = 210) of eyes compared with refractive interpretation, showing that nontoric hydrogel lenses do not neutralize refractive astigmatism. (From Sarver MD. Vision with hydrophilic contact lenses. *J Am Optom Assoc* 1972;43:316, with permission.)

with hydrogel lenses but common with rigid lenses, making hydrogels particularly advantageous for patients wishing correction for participation in sports.

The signs and symptoms of a poor tear layer and either a history or evidence of atopy and/or lid margin disease are relative contraindications for use of hydrogel lenses. Poor qualitative or quantitative tear layers result in unstable hydrogel lens parameters through dehydration, and both fit and optics can be variable (see earlier). Lenses soil more rapidly, and the optical quality of the lens surface may be seen to deteriorate with even short periods of wear. Dry eye and atopic patients also are believed to be more prone to infections and allergic reactions such as giant papillary conjunctivitis and solution sensitivities.

Relative contraindications include any active inflammation or disease of the anterior segment of the eye, corneal hypoesthesia, or any systemic/ocular disease that may affect the eye or be exaggerated by contact lens wear. Specific autoimmune diseases such as rheumatoid arthritis, systemic lupus erythematosus (both of which lead to dry eye problems), diabetes, or other immune compromise, acne rosacea, and atopic dermatitis (which leads to ocular surface problems including poor healing, risk of infection, and neovascularization) may cause concerns in patients wearing hydrogel contact lenses. Another relative contraindication is severe and/or irregular astigmatism (e.g., keratoconus or following corneal injury) for optical reasons.

The previous hydrogel lens problems of expense and limited durability, both from deposits as well as mechanical cracking or splitting, have been overcome for the most part by the introduction of inexpensive "disposable" hydrogel lens designs (108).

Driven by improved and more cost-effective manufacturing technologies, as well as a drive for patient convenience and competition with refractive surgery, a great variety of hydrogel contact lens designs now is available. One-day disposable contact lenses have developed a niche with either occasional contact lens wearers or those patients who prefer minimal contact lens care. They also work well for patients for whom soilage/deposits are a continuing problem with wear of traditional hydrogel lenses.

Driven by the increasing number of aging "baby boomers," disposable presbyopic contact lens designs (bifocal) now are available.

Disposable tinted contact lenses, such as Wild Eyes and Crazy Lens, have popularized effects that once were common only in the movie industry. With fixed pupils, however, they may limit contrast sensitivity and visual fields (109,110).

CLINICAL APPLICATION

The practitioner may elect to fit hydrogel contact lenses empirically, can use small "diagnostic" sets of hydrogel lenses, or (now more commonly) may have a large "inventory" of lenses of one or more brands to directly dispense to patients. All methods have advantages and disadvantages.

Ordering contact lenses empirically eliminates the need for the inventory and space for diagnostic lenses. Refraction and corneal topography measurements has been shown to allow successful empirical fits in corneas with low-to-moderate central and peripheral toricity, but success is limited with irregular and/or high-toricity corneas (111). Selecting from a small set of "diagnostic" lenses minimizes the space a clinician devotes for storage of contact lenses and makes the task appear customized and precise to the patients. Lenses dispensed to patients are new unworn lenses, but unfortunately they may vary in performance compared to the diagnostic lenses. Another lens will then be ordered, involving additional expense to the clinician and time delay to the patient. Additionally, the diagnostic set must be continuously maintained and sterilized (112). Alternatively, a large inventory allows for instantaneous changes, refinements and corrections, and rapid replacement of lost or damaged lenses. The deployment of a multitude of inexpensive frequent replacement and disposable hydrogel lenses in myopic, hyperopic, astigmatic, and presbyopic designs has revolutionized this practice.

The physical application of modern hydrogel contact lenses for correction of refractive error is rather direct. The clinician first performs a full ophthalmic evaluation, including balanced distance refraction, tonometry, visual field evaluation, keratometry, and examination of both anterior and posterior segments. The lids and tears should be carefully evaluated. All prefitting abnormalities should be documented and addressed before contact lens fitting. The clinician then attempts to provide hydrogel lenses that will be physically comfortable and cosmetically acceptable, will be physiologically tolerable under the intended *in vivo* conditions, and will provide the proper optical power to neutralize refractive error and allow for maximum visual acuity. This means that the clinician must select a hydrogel lens that will (i) fully cover the corneal surface, (ii) show relatively concentric positioning with the corneal limbus with slight scleral overlap, and (iii) move slightly from its primary position easily with a blink or when nudged gently by digital pressure through the lower lid, usually 0.5 to 1.0 mm (suggesting that the lens is not "gripping" the eye) (75,79,83, 84,87). The ideal fit hydrogel lens should move more rather than less easily, and it can show a slight inferior lag (87, 101). Optical correction should then be prescribed to optimize vision.

A hydrogel lens will undergo flexure when it is removed from its shipping vial and placed on an eye. It will flex or "wrap" so that its base curve radius changes from the original curvature (while floating in saline) toward duplicating the anterior ocular surface curvature (3,4). This probably is due to surface tension and thin film forces of the tears in combination with the action of the lids (113). Making a hydrogel lens design thinner—or increasing the water content of its material—allows the lens to be more flexible, increasing this mechanical applicability (and increasing both Dk/t and fragility). It appears that proper selection of lens material characteristics, thickness (central, peripheral, and edge), and base curve radius/diameter combinations may result in a few lens designs that will be applicable to most of the many possible corneal topographies found in the population. Additional sources will provide custom hydrogel lenses, which can extend this range to almost the entire population.

Modern hydrogel lenses usually are available with OADs of about 14.0 mm (101) with primary base curve radius about 8.6 mm. There may be additional base curves both 0.3 mm steeper or flatter. Central thickness of a low minus powered lens is approximately 0.08 mm at a power of −3.00 DS. Less minus powered lenses usually are thicker (central thickness 0.11 mm), and higher minus powered lenses often are somewhat thinner (central thickness 0.05 mm). Plus optically powered lenses are thicker. A thicker lens design may prove advantageous for patients who find lens manipulation difficult and for dryer-eyed patients (V. Finnemore, *unpublished data,* 1987). Thicker lenses are available in steeper base curve radii, as should be lenses made of lower water content or stiffer plastics (as these appear clinically less flexible). Higher-water-content and thinner lenses are available in flatter base curve radii designs with fewer (or larger) steps, as these appear to be more flexible.

The clinician could start the fitting process from a baseline measurement of corneal curvature and select a diagnostic lens with a base curve radius about 1 mm flatter than the mean corneal curvature (84,114–116). Hydrogel lenses of different water content, elasticity, and OADs may, however, achieve optimum mechanical fit at different base/ocular curve relationships. Cast molded lenses with OAD of 12.5 mm, were found to perform best when "base curve," i.e., posterior apical radius, was about 0.5 mm flatter than mean corneal curvature (72,99,100) [OAD of 13.6 suggested posterior apical radius 0.85–1.15 mm flat and OAD of 14.5 suggested posterior apical radius 1.2 mm flat (84)].

Alternatively, the "normal" manufacturer-suggested design may be applied if corneal curvature is not excessively steep (>46.00 D) or flat (<41.00 D). Some hydrogel lens designs have been identified as performing anomalously; however, one study suggests initial use of the "steeper" base curve (8.4 mm) in one particular design (55% water content) will result in the optimum fit for a majority of eyes (117).

Centration

If the OAD of a hydrogel lens is too small for an eye or if it decenters excessively for any other reason, a portion of the corneal surface may be left exposed beyond the edge of the lens (84,85,87). This may eventually result in corneal staining (85) and discomfort from desiccation analogous to the "3/9 stain" encountered with rigid lens fitting. Optics, especially with aspheric (i.e., spin-cast) lenses (100), may be adversely affected as well. It is not necessary that a lens position itself totally concentric with the limbus, but it is recommended that a lens overlap the limbus by about 1 to 2 mm all around its circumference (75,83,84,87,101,116). Decentration of hydrogel lenses, when it occurs, is generally in an upwards/temporal direction (101,116). Initial lathe-cut hydrogel lens designs were 14 to 16 mm in OAD to achieve this good centration, but as lenses became thinner it was found that smaller OADs could still achieve good centration (75). Kikkawa (118) proposed that centration of hydrogel lenses was governed by elastic forces generated by stretching of the lens periphery.

Movement

Poorly fitting hydrogel lenses are termed either "too tight" or "too loose." Lenses that are too tight will move poorly, if at all, following a blink or eye movement. They may cause indentation of the underlying sclera at their edge or constriction of the scleral vasculature from the mechanical pressure of the edge or posterior bevel just inward from the lens edge. Conjunctival vessels may be displaced with lens movement, called *conjunctival drag,* especially during use of lenses with thicker edges (87). Bubbles of air may be seen in the entrapped tear film between the posterior surface of the contact lens and the cornea. "Mucin balls" can appear under silicone hydrogel contact lenses, perhaps as a result of poor tear exchange due to lens rigidity (119,120). Initially "tight" hydrogel lenses are very comfortable, but with wearing time they can induce irritation and injection of the conjunctiva (Fig. 18.7) (75,84).

Vision may be slightly blurred just before, and temporarily improved just following, a blink. Retinoscopy shows a dark shadowy area in the central portion of the pupil, similar to the shadow reflex often seen with keratoconus. Immediately following a blink the shadow will disappear only to reappear a moment later. Similarly, a keratometry image of the lens anterior surface on the eye will be distorted but will temporarily clear somewhat just following a blink. It is thought that the tight hydrogel lens conforms to the peripheral corneal surface but deviates to vault the central cornea in an aspheric manner. A blink squeezes the central portion down momentarily, resulting in the changes noted (75).

Hydrogel lenses that are too "loose," on the other hand, commonly lag downward on the eye 2 to 4 mm and move excessively with a blink or eye movement, perhaps show a curling or lifting of the contact lens edge at some position within the palpebral aperture (87). They are less than optimally comfortable on the eye. Recentration occurs slowly, if at all. As opposed to the tight lens situation, vision will be best immediately prior and worst immediately following

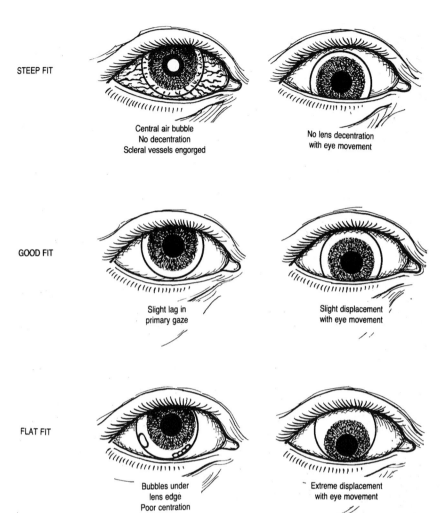

STEEP FIT

Central air bubble
No decentration
Scleral vessels engorged

No lens decentration
with eye movement

GOOD FIT

Slight lag in
primary gaze

Slight displacement
with eye movement

FLAT FIT

Bubbles under
lens edge
Poor centration

Extreme displacement
with eye movement

FIG. 18.7. Diagrammatic rendering of tight (steep), optimal, and flat (loose) fitting hydrogel contact lenses. All signs may not be observed at the same time in a real clinical situation. (From Weissman BA. *Contact lens primer.* Philadelphia: Lea & Febiger, 1984:35, with permission)

a blink. Retinoscopy may show a dark shadow in the inferior pupil that worsens immediately following a blink. The keratometric image of the *in situ* anterior lens surface may show increasing distortion just following the blink. All of these observations are explained by the inferior positioning (i.e., lag) of the lens.

Hydrogel lenses often act tighter with wear; the plastic dehydrates, debris may become entrapped in the thinning post-lens tear film, and movement of the lens slows (16,21, 122,123). The surface of the lens may be seen to become dry as well, losing its optical luster and becoming coated with tear layer constituents. Occasionally, however, a dried (dehydrated) hydrogel lens may become loose, displaying both edge lift and excessive motion.

Sagittal Relationship

Central corneal curvature as measured by keratometry is not universally a good indication of peripheral corneal to-

pography. Occasionally, the "normal" design hydrogel lens will fit poorly on a cornea measured at an "average" K of 44.00 D. The clinician should then select another hydrogel lens with a steeper/flatter base curve radius or larger/smaller OAD as appropriate to achieve the previously identified criteria of a "good fit." It is advantageous to have several base curve radius choices and at least one larger OAD (14.5 or 15.0 mm) available, in addition to the most commonly used 14.0-mm OAD. This will be helpful when caring for patients with (i) large corneal diameters, (ii) peculiar anterior segment topography (i.e., decentered corneal apex), or (iii) lid structures or other peculiarities that suggest the need for lens designs with improved centering abilities. These concepts suggest that the occasional patient requires a contact lens with a different sagittal depth than the standard to achieve proper contact lens positioning and movement (123,124).

The term *sagittal depth* refers to the distance defined by a line measured from the apex/optical axis of the contact

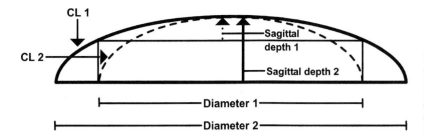

FIG. 18.8. Changing of sagittal depth relationship of contact lenses on the cornea by modifying contact lens diameters and base curves. The sagittal depth (sagittal depth 1) of contact lens 1 (CL1, diameter 1) can be modified to a greater sagittal depth (sagittal depth 2) by increasing diameter 1 or 2 or by decreasing the base curve such as that of contact lens 2 (CL2).

lens to the plane of the lens edge. This value is clearly dependent on both the base curve radius and OAD. Contact lenses with greater sagittal depths act steeper-tighter on the eye and *vice versa*. Sagittal depth may be increased by steepening (i.e., shortening) the base curve radius or alternatively increasing the lens diameter. Sagittal depth may be reduced by the reverse procedures, making a lens act physically looser. These same principles apply to both spherical and aspheric (and rigid as well as hydrogel) designs (Fig. 18.8).

Visual Correction

Visual correction through early hydrogel contact lenses was variable because manufacturers were unable to consistently manufacture or measure contact lenses (99) and vial labels often did not correspond to actual lens parameters (125), especially lens powers (126). Several studies found decrements in contrast sensitivity during hydrogel lens wear (compared to rigid contact lens or spectacle correction) despite acceptable visual acuity during clinical evaluation with standard high-contrast (Snellen) letter charts (127,128). Residual astigmatism (129), spherical aberration (130), deposits (131), optical (99,126) and material imperfections, and hypoxic-driven corneal edema (132–135) all were considered possible but nonexclusive etiologies.

Modern hydrogel lens designs, however, provide excellent vision for patients with relatively spherical refractive errors (<0.75 D refractive astigmatism) (135). Optical powers of initial (diagnostic) hydrogel contact lenses should be selected similar to the expected spherical equivalent refractive error after vertex distance correction.

Refractive astigmatism of 1 D or greater usually requires toric (astigmatic) hydrogel lens designs to optimize visual correction (78,99,103,136–138), although this rule is not always precise. High myopes often do well even if uncorrected astigmatism is greater than 1 D (because magnification works in their favor) (107). For the majority of patients, however, the clinician should consider that even small amounts of uncorrected residual astigmatism may decrease visual performance (129,139). Decreased visual acuity may be caused by misalignment of the axis and power of astigmatism, the polymer and exact nature of the hydrogel contact lens design, and patient visual sensitivity. Whereas one patient might be subjectively unaware of the difference between 20/25 − and 20/20 + vision, another patient might not be able to tolerate any visual compromise.

Although hydrogel contact lens flexure changes both the front and back optical radii, only minimal optical power change is induced with use of thin low minus-powered spherical hydrogel lenses (90,140) (Fig. 18.9). It has been clinically noted (141) and quantitatively verified (91) that plus-powered hydrogel lenses, however, decrease in effective power when they flex toward alignment with the underlying corneal curvature. Although most thin lenses align well with the corneal surface, a thicker lens [such as some astigmatic lenses (142)] or one with unusual curvatures may not come into perfect alignment with the anterior ocular surface, thus effectively creating a tear lens to complicate the optical effect of the lens on the eye (89). Diagnostic fittings and verification should be used whenever base curve radius changes are attempted with unusual designs, and thick and/or plus optically powered hydrogel lenses.

Once a diagnostic lens is on the eye and has equilibrated for tear temperature, pH, and osmolarity (see earlier) for a few minutes, its fit can be evaluated. Any changes suggested by movement, centration, and patient reactions should be explored. If the fit is found acceptable, then patient comfort, retinoscopy and subjective refraction by standard techniques, and balance of accommodation, when applicable, will suggest the optimum contact lens optical power. The level of visual acuity attained compared to that possible with best spectacle correction will alert the clinician to the success of the optical correction.

DISPENSING HYDROGEL CONTACT LENSES

At the dispensing visit, the clinician observes that the prescribed hydrogel lenses are properly inserted onto the eyes. Once the lenses have again been allowed to equilibrate with the ocular environment, they should be evaluated to verify proper mechanical fit, physical comfort, and optical correction of refractive error as anticipated. Instructions as to contact lens maintenance and handling should be conveyed to the patient. Guardians should sign consent forms if the patient is not capable of taking care of his or her own lenses.

Additional evaluations are suggested and scheduled. At

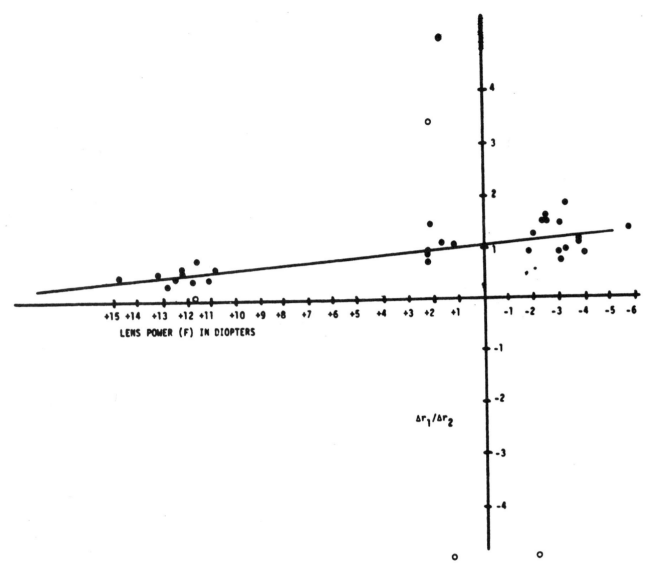

FIG. 18.9. Relationship between the covariance in front and back surface radii of curvature of hydrogel lenses versus optical back-vertex power. (From Weissman BA. A general relationship between changing surface radii or flexing soft contact lenses. *Am J Optom Physiol Opt* 1984;60: 651, with permission.)

these follow-up sessions, both patient vision and comfort, as well as lens fit and physiologic response, are evaluated by standard techniques, including history, refraction, and biomicroscope evaluation. After the patient has fully adapted, progress evaluations should be scheduled routinely at 6-month to 1-year intervals for patients who are not at risk, and at 3- to 6-month intervals for those whom the clinician feels may have some additional risk factors, such as extended wear schedules or presence of neovascularization or giant papillary conjunctivitis. Reinforcing proper contact lens care procedures, improving contact lens hygiene, providing appropriate routine general ophthalmic evaluations, and informing patients as to new contact lens options should be an ongoing process for all contact lens patients.

In conclusion, after an exhaustive period of both scientific research and trial-and-error clinical application during the past 50 years (much of which was described here), initial prescribing of hydrogel contact lenses has now become fairly straightforward. The review of historical considerations should be viewed as background to a now simplified procedure, but it may prove particularly valuable when (rarely) clinical care does not follow normal expectations.

REFERENCES

1. Wichterle O, Lim D. Hydrophilic gels for biological use. *Nature (Lond)* 1960;185:117–118.
2. Sposato P. The soft lens story. *Contact Lens Spectrum* 1987;2: 65–77.

3. Strachan JPF. Some principles of the optics of hydrophilic lenses and geometrical optics applied to flexible lenses. *Aust J Optom* 1973;56:25–33.

4. Holden BA, Zantos SG. On the conformity of soft lenses to the shape of the cornea. *Am J Optom Physiol Opt* 1981;58:139–143.

5. Mandell RB. What should we call gel lenses? *Int Cont Lens Clin* 1974;1:25.

6. Refojo MF. The chemistry of soft hydrogel lens materials. In: Ruben M, ed. *Soft contact lenses.* New York: John Wiley & Sons, 1978:19–39.

7. Fatt I. Water flow and pore diameter in extended wear gel materials. *Am J Optom Physiol Opt* 1978;55:294–301.

8. Fatt I, St Helen R. Oxygen tension under an oxygen permeable contact lens. *Am J Optom Arch Am Acad Optom* 1971;48:545–555.

9. Bambury RE, Seelye D. Vinyl carbonate and vinyl carbamate contact lens monomers. US Patent 5610252, 1997.

10. Kunzler J. Ozark R. Fluorosilicone hydrogels. US Patent 5321108, 1994.

11. Alvord L, Court J, Davis T, et al. Oxygen permeability of a new type of high Dk soft contact lens material. *J Am Acad Optom* 1998;75:30–36.

12. Refojo M. The relationship of linear expansion to hydration of hydrogel contact lenses. *Contact Intraoc Lens Med J* 1976;1:153–162.

13. Lowther GE. Updated lens classification tables. *Int Contact Lens Clin* 1988;15:205.

14. Fatt I. Gas transmission properties of soft contact lenses. In: Ruben M, ed. *Soft contact lenses.* New York: John Wiley & Sons, 1978:83–110.

15. Andrasko G. Hydrogel dehydration in various environments. *Int Contact Lens Clin* 1983;10:22–28.

16. Brennan NA, Efron N, Bruce AS, et al. Dehydration of hydrogel lenses: environmental influences during normal wear. *Am J Optom Physiol Opt* 1988;65:277–281.

17. Efron N, Brennan NA, Bruce AS, et al. Dehydration of hydrogel lenses under normal wearing conditions. *CLAO J* 1987;13:152–156.

18. Hill RM, Lindner DE. The two lives of a gel lens. *Int Contact Lens Clin* 1975;2:79-82.

19. Snyder AC, Koers DM. Water content measurement of hydrogel lenses—does technique make a difference? *Int Contact Lens Clin* 1983;10:344–347.

20. Brennan NA, Lowe R. The effects of hypotonic solutions on the fluid content of hydrophilic contact lenses. *Am J Ophthalmol* 1986;101:501–502.

21. Martin DK, Holden BA. Variations in tear film osmolarity, chord diameter and movement during wear of high water content hydrogel contact lenses. *Int Contact Lens Clin* 1983;10:323–342.

22. Fatt I, Chaston J. Swelling factors of hydrogels and the effect of deswelling (drying) in the eye on power of a soft contact lens. *Int Contact Lens Clin* 1982;9:146–153.

23. Hill RM, Andrasko G. Oxygen and water. *J Am Optom Assoc* 1981;52:225–226.

24. Lemp MA, Caffrey B, Lebow K, et al. Omafilcon A (Proclear) soft contact lenses in a dry eye population. *CLAO J* 1999;25:40–47.

25. Young G, Bower R, Hall B, et al. Clinical comparison of Omafilcon A with four control materials. *CLAO J* 1997;23:249–258.

26. Hall B, Jones S, Young G, et al. The on-eye dehydration of Proclear compatibles lenses. *CLAO J* 1999;25:233–237.

27. Quesnel N, Giasson C. On-eye dehydration of Proclear, Resolution 55G and Acuvue contact lenses. *CLAO J* 2001;24:88–93.

28. Fatt I, Chaston J. The effect of temperature on refractive index, water content and central thickness of hydrogel contact lenses. *Int Contact Lens Clin* 1980;7:37–42.

29. Janoff LE. The consequence of temperature change on hydrophilic lens base curve in hydrogels of varying water content. *Int Contact Lens Clin* 1982;9:228–231.

30. Fatt I, Chaston J. The response of vertex power to changes in dimensions of hydrogel contact lenses. *Int Contact Lens Clin* 1981;8:22–28.

31. Eriksen S, Randeri K, Ster J. Behavior of hydrophilic soft contact lenses under stress conditions of pH and tonicities. In: Bionite JL, Keates RH, eds. *Symposium on the flexible lens.* St Louis: CV Mosby, 1972:213–217.

32. Mandell RB. Sticking of gel contact lenses. *Int Contact Lens Clin* 1975;2:28–29.

33. Refojo MF. On the chemical stability of Softcon (Vifilcon A) lenses. *Cont Intraoc Lens Med J* 1975;1:36–39.

34. Marcus R, Hunt C, Windhorst R, et al. Acute systemic toxicological test of soft contact lens extractives. *Am J Optom Physiol Opt* 1980;57:360–362.

35. Smelser G, Ozanics V. Importance of atmospheric oxygen for maintenance of optical properties of the human cornea. *Science* 1952;115:140.

36. Klyce SD. Stromal lactate accumulation can account for corneal edema osmotically following epithelial hypoxia in the rabbit. *J Physiol* 1981;321:49–64.

37. Bonnano JA, Polse KA. Corneal acidosis during contact lens wear: effects of hypoxia and CO_2. *Invest Ophthalmol Vis Sci* 1987;28:1514–1520.

38. Polse KA. Tear flow under hydrogel contact lenses. *Invest Ophthalmol Vis Sci* 1979;18:409–413.

39. Holden BA, La Hood D, Sweeney D. Does Dk/L measurement accurately predict overnight edema response? *Am J Optom Physiol Opt* 1985;65:95.

40. Hamano H, Kawabe H, Mitsunaga S. Reproducible measurement of oxygen permeability (Dk) of contact lens materials. *CLAO J* 1985;11:221–226.

41. Winterton LC, White JC, Su KC. Coulometrically determined oxygen flux and resultant Dk of commercially available contact lenses. *Int Contact Lens Clin* 1988;15:117–123.

42. Holden BA, Newton-Howes J, Winterton L, et al. The Dk project: an interlaboratory comparison of Dk/L measurements. *Optom Vis Sci* 1990;67:476–481.

43. Weissman BA, Fatt I, Pham C. Polarographic oxygen permeability measurement of silicone elastomer contact lens material. *J Am Optom Assoc* 1992;63:187–190.

44. Fatt I, Rasson JE, Melpolder JB. Measuring oxygen permeability of gas permeable hard and hydrogel lenses and flat samples. *Int Contact Lens Clin* 1987;14:389–401.

45. Brennan NA, Efron N, Newman SD. An examination of the "edge effect" in the measurement of contact lens oxygen transmissibility. *Int Contact Lens Clin* 1987;14:407-411.

46. Fatt I, Mueller TD. Application of guard ring technology to measurement of oxygen permeability of contact lens materials by the polarographic method. *Int Contact Lens Clin* 1994;21:96–104.

47. Fatt I, Chaston J. Measurement of oxygen transmissibility and permeability of hydrogel lenses and materials. *Int Contact Lens Clin* 1982;9:76–88.

48. Fatt I. Gas-to-gas oxygen permeability measurements on RGP and silicone rubber lens materials. *Int Contact Lens Clin* 1991;18:192–198.

49. Sarver MD, Baggett DA, Harris MG, et al. Corneal edema with hydrogel lenses and eye closure: effect of oxygen transmissibility. *Am J Optom Physiol Opt* 1981;58:386–392.

50. Brennan NA. A simple instrument for measuring the water content of hydrogel lenses. *Int Contact Lens Clin* 1983;10:357–361.

51. Efron N, Brennan NA. Simple measurement of oxygen transmissibility. *Aust J Optom* 1985;68:27–35.

52. Brennan NA, Efron N, Weissman BA, et al. Clinical application of oxygen transmissibility of powered contact lenses. *CLAO J* 1991;17:169–172.

53. Weissman BA. Designing uniform-thickness contact lens shells. *Am J Optom Physiol Opt* 1982;59:902–903.

54. Morris JA, Fatt I. A survey of gas permeable contact lenses. *Optician* 1977;174:27–36.

55. Fatt I. The definition for thickness of a lens. *Am J Optom Physiol Opt* 1979;56:324-337.

56. Brennan NA. Average thickness of a hydrogel lens for gas transmissibility calculations. *Am J Optom Physiol Opt* 1984;61:627–635.

57. Weissman BA. Calculating area average thickness of rigid gas permeable contact lenses. *Am J Optom Physiol Opt* 1986;63:922–926.

58. Holden BA, Mertz GW. Critical oxygen levels to avoid corneal edema for daily and extended wear contact lenses. *Invest Ophthalmol Vis Sci* 1984;25:1161–1167.

59. Tomlinson A, Bibby MM. Determination of the effective diameter for the calculation of the equivalent thickness of soft contact lenses. *Am J Optom Physiol Opt* 1985;62:398–401.

60. Fatt I, Neumann S. The average oxygen transmissibility of contact lenses: application of the concept to laboratory measurements, clinical performance and marketing. *Neue Otickerjournal* 1989;31:55–58.

61. Weissman BA, Phan C. The L in Dk/L. *Optom Vis Sci* 1992;69:639–644.

62. Fatt I, Ruben CM. The point to point variation of oxygen delivery to a cornea covered by a hydrogel contact lens in the open eye. *Int Contact Lens Clin* 1994;21:50–56.

63. Polse KA, Mandell RB. Critical oxygen tension at the corneal surface. *Arch Ophthalmol* 1970;84:505–508.

64. Harvitt DM, Bonanno JA. Re-evaluation of the oxygen diffusion model for predicting minimum contact lens Dk/t values needed to avoid corneal anoxia. *Optom Vis Sci* 1999;76:712–719.

65. O'Neal MR, Polse KA, Sarver MD. Corneal response to rigid and hydrogel lenses during eye closure. *Invest Ophthalmol Vis Sci* 1984;25:837–842.

66. Fatt I, Bieber MT. The steady state distribution of oxygen and carbon dioxide in the in vivo cornea: the open eye in air and the closed eye. *Exp Eye Res* 1968;7:103–112.

67. Isenberg SJ, Green BF. Changes in conjunctival oxygen tension and temperature with advancing age. *Crit Care Med* 1985;13:683–685.

68. Mandell RB, Polse KA, Fatt I. Corneal swelling caused by contact lens wear. *Arch Ophthalmol* 1970;83:3–9.

69. Mandell RB. Corneal edema and curvature changes from gel lenses. *Int Contact Lens Clin* 1975;29:88–98.

70. Lin MC, Graham AD, Polse KA, et al. The effects of one-hour wear of high-Dk soft contact lenses on corneal pH and epithelial permeability. *CLAO J* 2000;26:130–133.

71. Levy B, Comstock T, Cresciullo T, et al. Randomized controlled clinical trial of silicone hydrogel contact lens for 30 days of continuous wear. *Invest Ophthalmol Vis Sci* 2000;41:74.

72. Nilsson SE. Seven-day extended wear and 30-day continuous wear of high oxygen transmissibility soft silicone hydrogel contact lenses: a randomized 1-year study of 504 patients. *CLAO J* 2001;27:125–133.

73. Quesnel NM, Fares F, Verret E, et al. Evaluation of the spectral transmittance of UV-absorbing disposable contact lenses. *CLAO J* 2001;27:23–9.

74. Anstey, A, Taylor, D, Chalmers I, et al. Ultraviolet radiation-blocking characteristics of contact lenses: relevance to eye protection for psoralen-sensitised patients. *Photodermatol Photoimmunol Photomed* 1999;15:193–197.

75. Mandell RB. Lathe-cut hydrogel lenses. *Int Contact Lens Clin* 1974;1:54–62.

76. Tomlinson A, Bibby MM. Movement and rotation of soft contact lenses. Effect of fit and lens design. *Am J Optom Physiol Opt* 1980;57:275–279.

77. Lowther GE, Tomlinson A. Critical base curve and diameter interval in the fitting of spherical soft contact lenses. *Am J Optom Physiol Opt* 1981;58:355–360.

78. Sarver MD. Fitting the Bausch & Lomb Soflens contact lens. *J Am Optom Assoc* 1973;44:258–262.

79. Touch AJ, Mertz GW, Seger RG. The best fit band theory—two years later. *Int Contact Lens Clin* 1976;3:32–36.

80. Bennett AG. Aspheric contact lens surfaces (part 1). *Ophthalmic Optician* 1968;8:1037–1040.

81. Bennett AG. Aspheric contact lens surfaces (part 2). *Ophthalmic Optician* 1968;8:1297–1311.

82. Bennett AG. Aspheric contact lens surfaces (part 3). *Ophthalmic Optician* 1969;9:222–224, 229–230.

83. Brucker D. The new hydrocurve contact lens. *Int Contact Lens Clin* 1974;1:33–42.

84. Touch AJ, Mertz GW. A research rationale for the multi-diameter philosophy of Bausch & Lomb Soflens (polymacon) contact lens fitting. *Int Contact Lens Clin* 1977;4:49–63.

85. Kline LN, DeLuca TJ. An analysis of arcuate staining with the Bausch & Lomb Soflens. *J Am Optom Assoc* 1975;46:1126–1132.

86. McNamara NA, Polse KA, Brand RJ, et al. Tear mixing under a soft contact lens: effects of lens diameter. *Am J Ophthalmol* 1999;127:659–665.

87. Dupont GZ, Remba MJ. Fitting evaluation tests for Tresoft and other lathe-cut semiscleral soft lenses. *Int Contact Lens Clin* 1979;6:263–267.

88. Gruber E. The Soflens contact lens; six years later. *Contact Lens Intraoc Lens Med J* 1975;1:70–82.

89. Sarver MD, Ashley D, Van Every J. Supplemental power effect of Bausch & Lomb Soflens contact lenses. *Int Contact Lens Clin* 1974;1:3–9.

90. Weissman BA. Clinical soft lens power changes. *Int Contact Lens Clin* 1984;11:342—346.

91. Weissman BA. Loss of power with flexure of hydrogel plus lenses. *Am J Optom Physiol Opt* 1986;63:166–169.

92. Orsborn GN, Zantos SG. Corneal desiccation staining with thin high water content contact lenses. *CLAO J* 1988;14:81–85.

93. Chan WK, Weissman BA. Corneal pannus associated with contact lens wear. *Am J Ophthalmol* 1996;121:540–546.

94. Brucker D, Malin AH. Fitting soft corneo-scleral lenses. *J Am Optom Assoc* 1972;43:287–290.

95. Wichterle K, Wichterle O. Surface shapes of fluids in rotating vessels. *Appl Sci Res* 1970;22:150–158.

96. Clements LD. Spincasting Bausch & Lomb Soflens (Polymacon) contact lenses. In: Ruben M, ed. *Soft contact lenses*. New York: John Wiley, 1978:435–442.

97. Coombs WF. Spin casting of HEMA lenses. *Int Contact Lens Clin* 1982;9:169–172.

98. Poster MG. A rationale for fitting the Bausch & Lomb Soflens. *J Am Optom Assoc* 1975;46:223–227.

99. Sarver MD. Vision with hydrophilic contact lenses. *J Am Optom Assoc* 1972;43:316–320.

100. Charman WN. Optical characteristics of Bausch & Lomb Soflens (PA1) bifocals. *Int Contact Lens Clin* 1984;11:564–575.

101. Grosvenor T. Lathe-cut soft contact lens fitting—part 1: materials and manufacturing process. *Optom Weekly* 1977;68:109–112.

102. Ruben M. *Color atlas of contact lenses and prosthetics,* 2nd ed. St Louis: CV Mosby, 1989.

103. Grosvenor T. Lathe-cut soft contact lens fitting—part 2: comparison with conventional hard lenses. *Optom Weekly* 1977;67: 38–40.

104. Health Products Research data, quoted in *Optom Manage* 1995; 30:3.

105. Sarver MD. The visual Rx. *J Am Optom Assoc* 1976;47:335.

106. Mandell RB. Why are gel lenses comfortable? *Int Contact Lens Clin* 1974;1:30–31.

107. Westheimer G. The visual world of the new contact lens wearer. *J Am Optom Assoc* 1962;34:135–138.

108. Donshik P, Weinstock FJ, Wechsler S, et al. Disposable hydrogel contact lenses for extended wear. *CLAO J* 1988;14: 191–194.

109. Spraul CW, Roth HJ, Gackle H, et al. Influence of special effect contact lenses (Crazy Lenses) on visual function. *CLAO J* 1998; 24:29–32.

110. Josephson JE, Caffery BE. Clinical performance of two opaque, tinted soft contact lenses. *J Am Optom Assoc* 1993;64:462.

111. Reddy T, Szczotka LB, Roberts C. Peripheral corneal contour measured by topography influences soft toric contact lens fitting success. *CLAO J* 2000;26:180–185.

112. Callender MG, Charles AM, Chalmers RL. Effect of storage time with different hydrogel trial lens disinfection efficacy: a multi-center study. *Optom Vis Sci* 1992;69:678–684.

113. Touch AJ. The lens-cornea relationship in Soflens (polymacon) contact lens fitting continued report. *Contacto* 1975;19: 33–34.

114. Campbell C. The fit of soft contact lenses. *Int Contact Lens Clin* 1984;11:219–240.

115. Kolom BM, Remba MJ. Some problems, some solutions, with Tresoft lenses. *Contact Lens Forum* 1978;3:46–51.

116. Olson M, Sarver MD. Apical bearing and success with the Bausch & Lomb Soflens (polymacon) contact lens. *Am J Optom Physiol Opt* 1976;53:173–176.

117. Roseman MJ, Frost A, Lawley ME. Effects of base curve on the fit of thin, mid water contact lenses. *Int Contact Lens Clin* 1993; 20:95–101.

118. Kikkawa Y. Kinetics of soft contact lens fitting. *Contacto* 1979; 23:10–17.

119. Dumbleton K, Jones L, Chalmers R, et al. Clinical characterization of spherical post-lens debris associated with lotrafilcon high-Dk silicone lenses. *CLAO J* 2000;26:186–192.

120. Pritchard N, Jones L, Dumbleton K, et al. Epithelial inclusions in association with mucin ball development in high-oxygen permeability hydrogel lenses. *Optom Vis Sci* 2000;77:68–72.

121. Refojo MF, Miller D, Fiore AS. A new fluorescent stain for soft hydrophilic lens fitting. *Arch Ophthalmol* 1972;87: 275–277.

122. Little SA, Bruce AS. Hydrogel (Acuvue) lens movement is influenced by the post lens tear film. *Optom Vis Sci* 1994;71: 364–370.

123. Bibby MM. Sagittal depth considerations in the selection of the base curve radius of a soft contact lens. *Am J Optom Physiol Opt* 1979;56:407–413.

124. Burnett-Hodd NFP. Soft lenses: fitting philosophies. *Ophthalmic Optician* 1984;24:817–826.

125. Davis H E, Anderson DJ. An investigation of the reliability of hydrogel lens parameters. *Int Contact Lens Clin* 1979;6: 136–142.

126. Sarver MD, Harris M, Mandell RB, et al. Power of a Bausch & Lomb Soflens contact lens. *Am J Optom Physiol Opt* 1973;50: 195–199.

127. Applegate RA, Massof RW. Changes in the contrast sensitivity function induced by contact lens wear. *Am J Optom Physiol Opt* 1975;52:840–846.

128. Wechsler S. Visual acuity in hard and soft contact lens wearers: a comparison. *J Am Optom Assoc* 1978;49:251–256.

129. Gundel RE, Kirshen SA, DiVergilio D. Changes in contrast sensitivity induced by spherical hydrogel lenses on low astigmats. *J Am Optom Assoc* 1988;59:636–640.

130. Cox I, Holden BA. Soft contact lens induced longitudinal spherical aberration and its effect on contrast sensitivity. *Optom Vis Sci* 1990;67:679–683.

131. Gellatly KW, Brennan NA, Efron N. Visual decrement with deposit accumulation on HEMA contact lenses. *Am J Optom Physiol Opt* 1998;65:937–941.

132. Kirkpatrick DL, Roggenkamp JR. Effects of soft contact lenses on contrast sensitivity. *Am J Optom Physiol Opt* 1985;62: 407–412.

133. Grey CP. Changes in contrast sensitivity during the first hour of soft lens wear. *Am J Optom Physiol Opt* 1986;63:702–707.

134. Grey CP. Changes in contrast sensitivity during the first six months of soft lens wear. *Am J Optom Physiol Opt* 1987;64: 768–774.

135. Nowozychyj A, Carney LG, Efron N. Effect of hydrogel lens wear on contrast sensitivity. *Am J Optom Physiol Opt* 1988;65: 263–271.

136. Harris MG, Goldberg T, McBride D, et al. Residual astigmatism and visual acuity with hydrogel contact lenses: a comparative study. *J Am Optom Assoc* 1979;50:303–306.

137. Lee AN, Sarver DS. The gel lens—transferred corneal toricity as a function of lens thickness. *Am J Optom Physiol Opt* 1972; 49:35–40.

138. Bernstein PR, Gundel RE, Rosen JS. Masking corneal toricity with hydrogels; does it work? *Int Contact Lens Clin* 1991;18: 67–70.

139. Dabkowski JA, Roach MP, Begley CG. Soft toric versus spherical contact lenses in myopes with low astigmatism. *Int Contact Lens Clin* 1992;19:252–255.

140. Weissman BA. A general relationship between changing surface radii of flexing soft contact lenses. *Am J Optom Physiol Opt* 1984;60651–60653.

141. Janoff L, Dabezies OH. Power change induced by soft contact lens flexure. *CLAO J* 1983;9:32–38.

142. Weissman BA. Theoretical optics of toric hydrogel contact lenses. *Am J Optom Physiol Opt* 1986;63:536–538.

CHAPTER 19

HYDROGEL LENS CARE REGIMENS AND PATIENT EDUCATION

RICHARD E. WEISBARTH AND BETH HENDERSON

Although it is an essential step, a good lens-to-cornea fitting relationship is only the first of many factors involved in successful contact lens wear. There are many potential problems with the contact lens cleaning, disinfection, and handling process, including patient noncompliance, solution misuse, concurrent use of incompatible products, preservative sensitivities or allergies, and contamination of solutions. Because a single clinical sign or symptom may result from a combination of closely interrelated causes, determining the etiology of and managing such complications can often be quite challenging. In addition, the rapidly expanding market of lens care products may become overwhelming for patients and contact lens practitioners alike. As the multitude of available products grows, it will become even more necessary for lens wearers to rely on the expertise of the contact lens professional for quality lens care information.

By their very nature, hydrogel lenses are affected greatly by contact lens solutions. These lens care products can often be an important factor in determining the success or failure of the patient as a contact lens wearer. Therefore, this chapter is intended to provide a comprehensive review of the varied aspects of hydrogel lens care, ranging from the clinical aspects of cleaning and disinfection to ways of enhancing patient compliance through proper patient education.

CLEANERS

The composition of the tears is complex, as they contain more than 60 different kinds of protein (1). Significant amounts of both protein and lipid deposits build up on lenses after only 1 day of wear (2). Therefore, proper cleaning is the essential first step in caring for hydrogel lenses. Cleaning removes deposits that can interfere with the disinfection procedure (3,4) and ultimately lead to reduced vision, shortened lens life, physiologic compromise, ocular infection, and discomfort (5–15).

The two primary types of cleaners for hydrogel lenses are surfactant (daily) cleaners, which remove lipids, mucin, cosmetics, and environmental pollutants, and enzymatic cleaners, which break down and remove protein deposits. Combining surfactant cleaning with regular enzyme cleaning minimizes the total amount of deposits and debris on the lens surface (5,16,17).

Daily Surfactant Cleaners

Surfactant cleaners have traditionally been used each time contact lenses were removed from the eyes. The purpose of a surfactant is to remove loosely adherent deposits and debris, including microorganisms. They act to break up the deposits through the formation of micelles (18). Most cleaners contain nonionic or ionic detergents, wetting agents, chelating agents, buffers, and preservatives (19,20).

The most common method of cleaning lenses uses digital rubbing of each lens surface with the cleaning solution. This is best accomplished in the palm of the hand. The lens should first be rinsed to increase hydration. The surfactant is then applied to both surfaces of the lens. The cleaning action is accomplished by means of the surfactant (surface active agent) attaching itself to the debris on the surface of the lens (19,21). Next, mechanical action emulsifies and loosens the debris. Thorough rinsing of the lens then allows for removal of the debris.

An alternative in lens cleaning is the Clensatron 700CL, an automatic device that agitates at 300 cycles per minute. This device produces turbulent movement that is claimed to be effective in removing deposits on lenses. One study has shown it is more effective after 2 minutes of cleaning in removing *Pseudomonas* and *Candida* than the digital cleaning method (22). However, more clinical studies are needed to determine the efficacy of this device.

Manufacturers have developed specialty type cleaners in recent years. Lens Plus Daily Cleaner (Advanced Medical Optics, formerly Allergan Optical) has several different surfactant agents in its formulation. The product is preservative-free and is packaged in a bottle that is available for multidose use. This is advantageous for the patient who has exhibited sensitivity to cleaning solutions with more traditional preservatives.

Opti-Clean Daily Cleaner (Alcon) has a unique formulation with special polymeric beads that provide an abrasive cleaning action. This particulate matter increases the mechanical cleaning action and may permit removal of deposits, as well as the normal debris on the surface of the lens (23,24). This product is in a suspension; therefore, every time it is used, it is imperative that the bottle be well shaken before dispensing the cleaner, otherwise it will not be of the proper consistency. The original formulation of Opti-Clean used thimerosal as the preservative, but it has been reformulated as Opti-Clean II Daily Cleaner (Alcon) and Opti-Free Daily Cleaner (Alcon), both of which are preserved with Polyquad. Opti-Free Daily Cleaner has been specifically formulated to be compatible with the Opti-Free disinfection system, while providing easy rinsing ability from the lens surface (25).

MiraFlow Extra-Strength Daily Cleaner (CIBA Vision), originally formulated for use with polymethyl methacrylate lenses, also is approved for use with all hydrogel lenses. MiraFlow carries the distinction of being an extra-strength cleaner because it contains the largest percentage of cleaning agents of any cleaner currently available. Cleaning ingredients include isopropyl alcohol (20%), poloxamer-407 (15%), and amphoteric-10 (10%). The primary advantage of MiraFlow appears to be the isopropyl alcohol ingredient, which is capable of dissolving lipids (26), making this an excellent cleaner for patients who have a propensity for lipid deposits (27). The alcohol component is also believed to be of benefit in removing mucin (28). Isopropyl alcohol imparts broad-spectrum microbicidal activity to the cleaner and at the same time eliminates the need for preservatives (29,30). Table 19.1 lists the daily cleaners presently available from major manufacturers.

Although digital cleaning is an important step in removing unbound protein deposits from hydrophilic contact lenses, it has been found that only one third to one half of protein deposits are removed with cleaning (31,32). In one study, never-worn soft lenses were incubated in an artificial tear solution, and only lysozyme was removed; albumin, lactoferrin, and glycoprotein remained on the lenses (31). Furthermore, decreasing the cleaning time with a surfactant has been shown to increase protein accumulation on lenses (32). Adherence to the full recommended cleaning time should, therefore, be emphasized to prevent excess deposit accumulation.

Cleaning plays more than just a debris-removal role in a contact lens care regimen. Studies have shown that the cleaning process itself is beneficial in eliminating some of the microorganisms that may be present on a lens before undergoing the disinfection procedure (33–38). It also has been shown that minor amounts of detergents can stimulate the detachment of *Pseudomonas aeruginosa* from contact lens surfaces (39).

According to United States Food and Drug Administration (FDA) regulations, manufacturers are required to inoculate lenses with 1 million (10^6) microorganisms to study the efficacy of a lens care system (40,41). The cleaning step alone reduces the number of microorganisms that may be present on a lens by approximately 1 log unit (90%). If the cleaner is rinsed from the lens, the number of microorganisms can be further reduced by an additional 2 log units (Fig. 19.1) (34,42,43). By the time a lens reaches the disinfection procedure, a substantial reduction in the number of microorganisms has already occurred. If a patient's lenses are contaminated, the cleaning step is very important to ensure that the care regimen works properly and that it provides lenses that are safe to wear.

TABLE 19.1. DAILY SURFACTANT CLEANERS

Product (Manufacturer)	Preservatives	Other Ingredients
CIBA Vision Cleaner (CIBA Vision)	Sorbic acid 0.1%, edetate disodium 0.2%	Cocoamphocarboxyglycinate, sodium lauryl sulfate, hexylene glycol
Lens Plus Daily Cleaner (Advanced Medical Optics)	—	Sodium lauryl sulfate, hexylene glycol, sodium chloride, sodium phosphate, cocoamphocarboxyglycinate
MiraFlow Extra-Strength Daily Cleaner (CIBA Vision)	—	Isopropyl alcohol (20%), poloxamer 407 (15%), amphoteric 10 (10%)
Opti-Clean II Daily Cleaner (Alcon)	Polyquad 0.001%, edetate disodium 0.1%	Tween 21, MICROCLENS special polymeric cleaning agents
Opti-Free Daily Cleaner (Alcon)	Polyquad 0.001%, edetate disodium 0.1%	Tween 21, MICROCLENS special polymeric cleaning agents
Pliagel Cleaning solution (Alcon)	Sorbic acid 0.25%, edetate disodium 0.5%	Sodium chloride, potassium chloride, poloxamer 407 (15%)
POLYCLENS II Daily Cleaner (Alcon)	Polyquad 0.001%, edetate disodium 0.1%	Special polymeric and surfactant cleaning agents
Sensitive Eyes brand Daily Cleaner (Bausch & Lomb)	Sorbic acid 0.25%, edetate disodium 0.5%	Hydroxypropyl methylcellulose, poloxamine, sodium borate, sodium chloride
Sof/Pro-Clean SA (Lobob)	Edetate trisodium 0.25%, sorbic acid 0.1%	Nontionic detergents

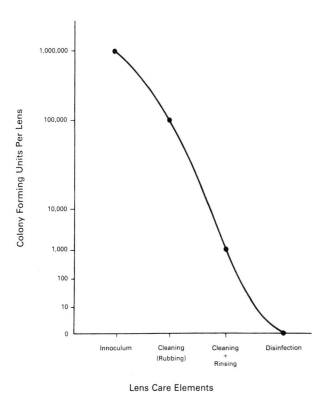

FIG. 19.1. Contribution of elements test.

Value of Rinsing

Regardless of the cleaner used, it is important for the patient to thoroughly rinse the cleaning solution from the lens. This has been well established (4,6,43–45), and most practitioners have observed patients who experience difficulties as a result of residual cleaner acting on the corneal epithelium. Also, any cleaner remaining on the lens may induce foaming when the lens is placed in enzymatic cleaner (6,43).

Experience with hydrogen peroxide disinfection systems further illustrates the value of rinsing. Some practitioners have found that if a patient does not thoroughly rinse the cleaner from a lens before the hydrogen peroxide disinfection process, foaming or sudsing may occur as a result of the bubbling action created when the hydrogen peroxide is neutralized (43). This has been responsible for the disinfection solution bubbling out of the lens case in some situations. The patient may later find the lenses in a dehydrated state, soaking in little, if any, disinfection solution. Thoroughly rinsing the cleaner from the lens before disinfection will solve this problem.

Enzymatic Cleaners

Enzymatic cleaners contain proteolytic enzymes that specifically cause hydrolysis of tear proteins to polypeptides and amino acids, causing them to release from the lens surface. Therefore, these products are far more effective for remov-

ing protein deposits than are surfactant cleaners (46–53). Up to 75% protein removal can be achieved using enzymatic cleaners, but the frequency of use, the tear proteins involved, and the state of the protein deposits all affect the efficiency of these cleaners (54). They are generally used on a weekly basis, but the frequency may vary depending on a person's rate of deposit formation (53,55,56). Because the enzymatic cleaning step is relatively costly and time consuming, it often is subject to noncompliance (18). With the growing popularity of 1- to 2-week "disposable" and frequent replacement lenses (57) and the introduction of multipurpose solutions (MPSs) that remove protein, the need for a separate enzymatic cleaner has decreased (57).

It has been estimated that 80% of all clinical complications related to contact lens wear can be attributed to lens deposits (54). Reduced acuity, decreased comfort and wettability, and increased inflammatory complications such as giant papillary conjunctivitis and contact lens acute red eye have been documented (54). The level of protein deposition has been reported to be dependent upon the water content and ionic nature of the lens material (58,59). Other sources state that water content is not a primary factor in determining protein absorption, rather the monomer constituents such as methacrylic acid or n-vinyl pyrrolidone control the adsorption of certain types of protein, with changes in water content being a byproduct of these monomers (60).

The earliest enzymatic cleaners available contained papain (Allergan Optical) or pancreatin (Alcon). These products have been successful in eliminating and preventing major protein deposits on contact lenses (46,61–69). When enzymatic cleaners were originally marketed in tablet form, distilled water was one of the vehicles in which the tablets were dissolved. In light of the high probability of microbial contamination (70–72), distilled water is now contraindicated. In addition, experience has shown that distilled water is not necessarily chlorine free (some distilled water bottlers actually add chlorine to the water after the process to ensure sterility at the time of shipment.) It has been shown that chlorine acts like a bleach on certain tinted lenses (73–75), and if patients are using such distilled water, either to mix salt tablet saline or to dissolve enzyme tablets, there can actually be fading or bleaching of the lens tint. Therefore, for papain- and pancreatin-containing enzyme products, it is important to verify that sterile saline solution is being used as the diluent.

A liquid enzyme daily protein remover called Opti-Free SupraCLENS Daily Protein Remover (Alcon) also is available. It is a pancreatin-based enzyme formulated to be used on a daily basis in conjunction with Opti-Free Express Multi-Purpose Solution, Opti-Free Rinsing, Disinfecting and Storage Solution, or Opti-One Multi-Purpose Solution (Alcon) (76). One study provided evidence that daily use is well tolerated and provides a more convenient method of achieving simultaneous disinfection and protein cleaning compared with enzyme tablets (77).

Another group of enzymatic cleaners uses subtilisin, an enzyme derived from the bacterial fermentation of *Bacillus licheniformis* (6,78). One of the cleaners is ReNu Enzymatic tablets (Bausch & Lomb), which have been available in several different forms. A thermal formulation was used in a heat disinfection case, which allowed simultaneous disinfection and enzymatic cleaning of the lens. The thermal version was not recommended for use with CSI lenses, because it could make this particular material stiff and brittle (79), resulting in patients tearing or damaging lenses. ReNu Effervescent Enzymatic Cleaner tablets (Bausch & Lomb) are formulated to accompany nonperoxide chemical disinfection systems. The most recent additions are ReNu 1 Step Enzymatic Cleaner (Bausch & Lomb) and the ReNu 1 Step Daily Protein Remover Liquid (Bausch & Lomb), which simultaneously disinfect and enzymatically clean the lens. These enzymatic tablets should be dissolved only in the ReNu Multi-Purpose Disinfection Solution.

Unizyme Enzymatic Cleaner (CIBA Vision) and Complete Weekly Enzymatic Cleaner (Advanced Medical Optics) are other enzymatic cleaners that contain subtilisin A. Ultrazyme Enzymatic Cleaner (Advanced Medical Optics, formerly Allergan Optical) also contains subtilisin, but this is specifically formulated to be dissolved in hydrogen peroxide disinfection solution and, therefore, achieves simultaneous lens disinfection and enzymatic cleaning of the lens (80,81). Lenses must be rinsed thoroughly with saline, however, after the procedure is completed. As with any enzymatic cleaner, if a patient does not completely rinse the lens, complications may ensue (10,82,83). The Ultrazyme tablet is specifically formulated to work at an alkaline pH (84). From a clinical standpoint, if Ultrazyme is used with a one-step peroxide system, the patient should rinse the lens thoroughly with a buffered sterile saline before lens application to reequilibrate the lens to physiologic pH. Failure to complete this step could result in varying degrees of burning and stinging, depending on the buffer capacity of a person's tears.

Compatibility of other enzymatic tablets in hydrogen peroxide has not been reported in the literature. No other enzymatic products are currently FDA-approved for use directly with hydrogen peroxide systems. It has been established, however, that enzymatic tablets derived from papain are not compatible with hydrogen peroxide (6,85,86). Hydrogen peroxide will deactivate papain before it has a chance to provide any significant enzymatic cleaning action.

Competitive evaluations of various products have been reported. A comparison of four marketed enzymatic cleaners, including Allergan Enzymatic (papain), Alcon Opti-Zyme (pancreatin), Bausch & Lomb ReNu Effervescent (subtilisin), and Advanced Medical Optics Ultrazyme (subtilisin A) was conducted (87). Lenses were examined using a scanning electron microscope, and the amount of deposition was quantified by digital analysis. All of the enzymatic cleaners tested were effective in removing deposits, but there was no significant difference in cleaning efficacy among the

TABLE 19.2. ENZYMATIC AND WEEKLY CLEANERS

Product (Manufacturer) Preservatives	Other Ingredients
Complete Weekly Enzymatic Cleaner (Advanced Medical Optics)	Subtilisin A
Ultrazyme Enzymatic Cleaner (Advanced Medical Optics)	Subtilisin A
Opti-Free Enzymatic Cleaner (Alcon)	Purified pork pancreatin
Opti-Free SupraCLENS Daily Protein Remover (Alcon)	Propylene glycol, sodium borate, purified pork pancreatin
Opti-Zyme Enzymatic Cleaner (Alcon)	Purified pork pancreatin
Polyzyme Enzymatic Cleaner (Alcon)	Purified pork pancreatin
ReNu 1 Step Daily Protein Remover Liquid (Bausch & Lomb)	Subtilisin, glycerin, borate
ReNu 1 Step Enzymatic Cleaner (Bausch & Lomb)	Subtilisin, sodium carbonate, sodium chloride, boric acid
ReNu Effervescent Enzymatic Cleaner (Bausch & Lomb)	Subtilisin, polyethylene glycol, sodium carbonate, sodium chloride, tartaric acid
Sensitive Eyes brand Enzymatic Cleaner (Bausch & Lomb)	Subtilisin
Unizyme Enzymatic Cleaner (CIBA Vision)	Subtilisin A, potassium carbonate, citric acid, polyethylene glycol, sodium benzoate

four cleaners tested. Another study used the Rudko classification for categorizing protein deposits and phase contrast microscopy for photodocumentation (88). Results showed that Allergan Enzymatic Cleaner and Ultrazyme were comparably effective in decreasing deposits. Ultrazyme was found to be slightly more effective at removing the light, type II protein deposits, whereas Allergan Enzymatic Cleaner was effective in cleaning medium- and heavy-bound protein deposits.

Lens materials react differently to the various enzymatic cleaners. *In vitro* lens studies have shown that pancreatin uptake is less than with papain (89). Even with short soaking times, 20% of group IV (high-water, ionic) lens wearers reported irritation from the use of papain (89). Therefore, cycle times may need to be altered, depending on the chemical composition of the lens materials involved (90). It also has been suggested that a cocktail of different enzymatic cleaners is not recommended, because enzyme products derived from different sources are likely to digest one another as opposed to being effective on the absorbed tear proteins (54).

Another approach to protein removal involves using strong surfactant cleaners (91,92). Table 19.2 lists the enzymatic and weekly cleaners currently available.

SALINE

Saline is used for rinsing and storing hydrogel lenses. Most products are formulated with a neutral pH (7.0–7.4) and are isotonic (0.9% NaCl) with human tears. Saline is available in a variety of forms, ranging from self-prepared, made-with-salt tablets to the many premixed brands packaged in either unit-dose or multidose containers. Preservatives are added to many saline preparations to prevent microorganisms from growing in them. An alternative method to minimize the risk of solution contamination involves packaging the saline in aerosol containers or unit-dose vials. This packaging eliminates the need for preservative agents. The types of saline solutions currently available are listed in Table 19.3.

Salt tablet-formulated saline can be used safely only for rinsing or storing lenses before heat disinfection. Contamination is likely if patients fail to follow labeling directions properly (3,10,44,45,56,72,93). Common errors include handling the tablets with unclean hands; not cleaning or rinsing the mixing bottle as directed; dissolving the tablet in nonsterile water; and using the product for a final rinse or directly in the eye. It is well documented that salt tablet-prepared saline carries a high risk of contributing to serious eye infections, including *Acanthamoeba* keratitis (72,83,91, 94–112). Therefore, it is important for the contact lens practitioner to identify those patients who still may be using these products and educate them on the risks involved. If indicated, patients should be switched to a more appropriate product. From a medical-legal standpoint, it is always im-

portant to document any recommendations regarding the discontinuation of salt tablet-prepared saline in the patient's record.

Patients tend not to be brand-loyal when it comes to purchasing saline. Manufacturers formulate their products similarly, but sometimes there can be slight differences in the chemical formulation of the different salines, which ultimately can determine their success. A wide variation in pH values has been shown to exist in different saline solutions (113–118). If a patient begins with a particular brand of saline that has a pH of 7.00 and then switches to a saline with a pH of 7.40 or 6.05, a burning or stinging sensation may be experienced, depending on the buffer capacity of the tears. Therefore, if a patient complains of burning or stinging, one of the first factors that should be investigated is the brand of saline being used. One cannot assume that the brand in use is the one that was originally recommended. Complaints of discomfort or lens parameter changes also may be due to using outdated or long-opened solution containers (119). A routine evaluation of solution bottles during patient follow-up visits may heighten patient awareness of the risks associated with old products and prevent such problems from occurring.

Aerosol saline products are preservative-free, resulting from the use of a one-way valve that does not allow contamination to enter the can (45). Aerosol salines initially were offered only in a nonbuffered version (118). As with any nonbuffered solution, the pH of the solution often decreased into the acidic range, causing some patients to experience a burning and stinging sensation (71,118,120). Also,

TABLE 19.3. SALINE SOLUTIONS

Product (Manufacturer)	Preservatives	Other Ingredients
Preserved Saline		
Good Sense Saline Solution (Amcon, Inc.)	Sorbic acid 0.1%, edetate disodium	Sodium chloride
Sensitive Eyes brand Plus (Bausch & Lomb)	Polyaminopropyl biguanide 0.00003%, edetate disodium 0.025%	Boric acid, sodium borate, potassium chloride, sodium chloride
Sensitive Eyes brand Saline Solution (Bausch & Lomb)	Sorbic acid 0.1%, edetate disodium 0.025%	Boric acid, sodium borate, sodium chloride
Soft Wear Saline (CIBA Vision)	Antimicrobial buffer system generating up to 0.006% hydrogen peroxide	Sodium borate, boric acid, sodium perborate, phosphonic acid
Nonpreserved Saline		
Blairex Sterile Saline Solution (Blairex)	—	Sorbic acid 0.1%, edetate disodium
CIBA Vision Saline (CIBA Vision)	—	Sodium chloride, borate buffer
Clear Conscience Saline Solution (Clear Conscience)	—	Sodium chloride, boric acid, sodium borate
Lens Plus Sterile Saline Solution (Advanced Medical Optics)	—	Sodium chloride, boric acid
Sensitive Eyes brand Sterile Saline Spray (Bausch & Lomb)	—	Sodium chloride 0.4%, boric acid, sodium borate
Unisol 4 (Alcon)	—	Sodium chloride, boric acid, sodium borate

high-water-content, ionic lenses (group IV) could react to the acid environment and change in parameters (83,121, 122). One study found the mean pH of buffered aerosol saline products averaged 7.30 pH units, whereas the mean pH of unbuffered aerosol saline was 5.79 pH units (123).

Most major manufacturers currently include buffering ingredients in their aerosol saline formulations. One can always tell if a saline is buffered simply by looking at the ingredients (113,124). The presence of any type of borate or phosphate is an indication that the saline has some buffer capacity. With the introduction of buffered aerosol saline products, problems due to pH level are minimized. When replacing saline, however, an individual may obtain a brand of the nonbuffered variety. If a patient reports burning and stinging on lens application, the brand of saline being used (buffered or nonbuffered) should be investigated.

There are some disadvantages to aerosol saline. One difficulty is that in some situations, the nitrogen propellant becomes spent before the saline is completely expelled (125). To minimize the occurrence of this situation, the nozzle should be lined up with the imprinted dot on the rim of the can. This ensures that the dipstick lines up properly to maximize the use of the propellant in the bottom of the can (Fig. 19.2). Additionally, when rinsing a lens, the can should not be tipped past the horizontal, or this may expel

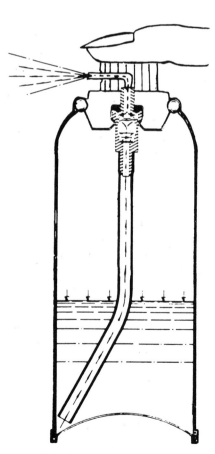

FIG. 19.2. Proper use of aerosol saline.

the propellant at a more rapid rate than was intended for the contents of the can. Proper patient education can minimize difficulties. Finally, a short spurt of saline should be directed into the sink to clear the nozzle of the aerosol saline can before its use to eliminate the possibility of contamination (from the nozzle tip) reaching the patient's lenses.

SoftWear Saline (CIBA Vision) is a unique saline that uses a borate buffering system, rather than a standard preservative, as an antimicrobial agent (126). A 6-month clinical study of 159 patients (318 eyes) was conducted to evaluate the safety and efficacy of SoftWear Saline (127). The results revealed no attributable slit-lamp findings and no adverse reactions. In addition, a study conducted on 21 patients with a history of sensitivity reactions demonstrated that SoftWear Saline had no clinically significant slit-lamp findings in 166 (99%) of 168 total observations (126).

DISINFECTION

Hydrogel contact lenses serve as an excellent culture medium for the growth of many different microorganisms (9, 111,118–134). When worn on the normal eye, lenses remain fairly free of microbial contamination, because antimicrobial agents found in tears, along with the mechanical flushing action of the lids, are known to help protect the lens from contaminants (135). Even so, it has been shown that bacteria colonizing normal skin and microbiota found in tap water appear to be transferred to the lens during wear (136). More significant risks of contamination can occur during lens care and maintenance procedures (28). Patient handling with improperly washed hands has been shown to be a major cause of lens microbial contamination (130,137). In addition, cosmetics and other applied or airborne products used near or about the eyes can be a potential source of microbial contamination (138,139). Consequently, lenses must be disinfected after each wearing to safeguard the eye from potential pathogens.

Terminology

Disinfection is defined as the process whereby vegetative or living microorganisms are completely killed or inactivated. This involves the destruction of microorganisms by attacking the cell wall or membrane, the inhibition of protein synthesis, or both (18). However, certain microorganisms are capable of producing spores that are not killed by a disinfection process (5,41,44,140–142). The implication is that the spores would be capable of germinating at some future point, which could lead to lens contamination and subsequent ocular infection. In contrast, *sterilization* refers to the process whereby all organisms, including spores, are completely inactivated, and there is no possibility for microbial growth.

Ideally, it would be beneficial to provide sterilization for all hydrogel contact lenses. This is especially true because 32% to 82% of patients are not totally compliant in how they care for their lenses (11,95,132,143–151). However, there are few commercially available contact lens sterilization units for practitioner or consumer use. Sterilization usually is achieved with an autoclave, which subjects the lens to a high temperature (115°–121°C) for 15 to 30 minutes under a pressure of 15 psi (141,142,152–154). This process is performed at the time a lens is manufactured; however, repeated autoclave cycles may hasten polymer degradation (7,44).

Hydrogel lenses must be disinfected after each wearing. Two primary methods have traditionally been used: thermal (heat) and chemical (nonheat). Both methods are safe and efficacious and have advantages and disadvantages. In the early 1980s, practitioners were equally divided in their preference. With the introduction of hydrogen peroxide systems and new preservatives, however, chemical disinfection has rapidly become the disinfection of choice.

Labeling

Current disinfecting products must pass specific FDA and International Organization for Standardization (ISO) microbiologic and cleaning efficacy tests in order to gain approval to use particular labeling (155). Upon passing the appropriate test, a solution may be designated a "multipurpose" solution (MPS), a "multipurpose disinfecting" solution (MPDS), or a "no rub required" disinfecting solution.

A test called the *Stand-Alone Test* has two standards, or criteria (156). The first, known as the primary criterion, is performed under laboratory conditions, using no lenses. Three specific bacteria *(Staphylococcus aureus, P. aeruginosa, Serratia marcescens)* and two fungi *(Candida albicans, Fusarium solani)* are soaked in the disinfection solution for the minimum recommended disinfection time. If a 3.0-log reduction in bacteria and a 1.0-log reduction in fungi occur, the solution is approved for use with the MPDS label.

The secondary criterion of the standalone test is similar in that it tests the same three bacteria and two fungi, but this criterion requires a total combined log reduction of at least 5.0 units, with at least a 1-log reduction for each individual bacterial strain tested and zero growth of the two fungi (156).

A solution meeting the second, but not the first, criterion of the Stand-Alone Test must also pass a *Regimen Test* to receive the MPS label. In the regimen test, lenses are used as inoculation vehicles. Four test lenses, representing each of the four categories of hydrogel lenses, are used to test the disinfectant. The lenses are inoculated with the test organisms and then cleaned, disinfected, and soaked according to the manufacturer's instructions. If the lenses are found to carry fewer than 10 microbiota of the original 100,000 to 1,000,000 inoculum, then the solution is approved for MPS labeling. This designation is given to describe solutions

that perform both the cleaning and disinfecting of lenses (135,153), but such solutions also may be used with separate cleaners for enhanced soil/deposit removal.

The most recent development in solution labeling is the so-called *no-rub* designation. Solutions that fall into this category have the most stringent test requirements (155–157); they need to pass both parts of the Stand-Alone Test as well as the Regimen Test to receive the no-rub label. Laboratory studies also must demonstrate the solution's cleaning ability. It is important to note that the no-rub designation does not necessarily streamline or simplify the steps required for proper lens care. Directions for the various no-rub formulations vary. Some require a prerinse as well as a postrinse, and the actual rinse times differ significantly among brands (57).

Types of Disinfection

Chemical Disinfection

Modern chemical disinfection systems offer the advantages of convenience and portability, with low incidences of sensitivity and toxicity responses (28,158–160). Solutions used for chemical disinfection contain either preservatives or hydrogen peroxide as antimicrobial agents. Earlier solutions in this category used preservatives such as thimerosal and chlorhexidine as antimicrobial agents. Whereas they were effective at disinfection, their small molecular size meant that they could penetrate the matrix of hydrogel lenses, thus increasing the risk of allergic or toxicity responses. Today's newer preservatives are of larger molecular size and are used in lower concentrations; thus, they provide effective disinfection activity with decreased adverse effects.

Factors described as having an impact on the effectiveness of a disinfection system include the concentration of disinfectant, the pH of the solution, the temperature at which the solution is stored, the ambient humidity, the length of storage time, and the composition and condition of the hydrogel material to be disinfected (161). To ensure the effectiveness of disinfecting systems in the presence of all of these variables, solutions are composed of complex combinations of preservatives, buffers, lubricants, ionic agents, and surfactants (135). Knowing the specific components of various care systems will help in prescribing the appropriate disinfecting system for a given patient.

Chemical systems usually require a 4-hour to overnight soak time to achieve antimicrobial effectiveness. Some studies have shown that even longer exposure times may be needed for certain disinfectants (162,163). At the end of the disinfection procedure, the disinfecting solution must be discarded. If the disinfectant is not changed with each disinfection cycle, it may lose its potency and even support microbial growth (3,11,42,70,164,165). Contact lenses can be stored in chemical disinfecting solutions as recommended in the manufacturer's package insert. Following the specific recommendations is important because microbial growth during storage can occur if directions are not followed (163).

The contact lens disinfection systems in use today are designed to maximize convenience and compliance. Some of these systems involve combinations of solutions that have specialized functions. Others are single-bottle systems, designed to clean, rinse, disinfect, and store lenses using only one solution. Systems falling into this second category are known as "multipurpose solutions" (MPS). They make the process of caring for lenses simpler than ever before. Despite their convenience, it should be noted that disadvantages of multipurpose systems have been identified (28). For example, it has been proposed that cleaners incorporated into MPSs may not be as effective as separate, specific-purpose surfactant cleaners (28), and because MPSs are more expensive than salines, it is possible that cost-conscious patients may use them more sparingly for prescribed rubbing or rinsing steps (28). Finally, patients who place lenses that have been soaked in MPSs directly into the eye may be vulnerable to subtle ocular responses that could lead to greater lens deposition (28). While acknowledging potential disadvantages of MPSs, practitioners appear to believe that their advantages of effectiveness and convenience greatly outweigh the drawbacks. This is reflected in the rapid growth of the MPS category, which comprised 80% of total chemical solutions sales in the United States by the late 1990s (166).

Two-Bottle Systems

Among solution systems, QuickCare 5 Minute System (CIBA Vision) is unique in that it cleans, disinfects, and conditions in less than 5 minutes (167). QuickCare consists of a starting solution, a finishing solution, and a disposable lens case. The solutions work together as a system and should not be substituted with other products. Key ingredients of the starting solution are isopropyl alcohol, which acts as a cleaner and antimicrobial agent; and 5% NaCl, which makes the solution hypertonic and thus causes osmotic desiccation of microbiota (57). The finishing solution contains perborate, a compound that releases low levels of peroxide. It functions as a preservative and serves to rinse and remove cleaning agents from the lens before insertion. These small quantities of peroxide are quickly neutralized by tear film enzymes upon lens insertion (168). One study revealed that the starting solution killed 80% of bacterial and fungal clinical isolates in 1 minute (162). During the initial phase of using QuickCare, patients may notice "fluted edges" because the starting solution is hypertonic. The lens will return to its normal shape after the soaking period in the finishing solution (169).

Multipurpose One-Bottle Systems

MPSs are single-bottle systems designed to clean, rinse, disinfect, and store lenses using only one solution. The simplic-

ity and convenience of one-bottle MPSs have made them a popular choice in today's contact lens marketplace. These solutions were first introduced in the late 1980s and are now the dominant players in the lens care market (156, 166). Current one-bottle disinfectants contain large molecular weight polymers with cationic (+) charges. They achieve a cidal effect by rapidly binding to the microbe cell surface, causing a loss of cell membrane integrity and resultant leakage of critical components (43). Some brands are approved with a digital rubbing step; others feature a no-rub option. Directions for the various no-rub formulations vary. Some require a prerinse as well as a postrinse, and rinse times vary significantly among brands (57).

Opti-Free Rinsing, Disinfecting, and Storage Solution (Alcon) contains polyquaternium-1 (Polyquad) as its preservative. Polyquad has a high molecular weight, which inhibits its ability to enter the matrix of hydrogel lenses (170). A study that examined the effect of preservative uptake by contact lenses on bactericidal activity concluded that very little Polyquad was absorbed into hydrogel lenses that were stored for a period of up to 14 days (165). The implication of this finding is that there is a reduced likelihood of solution-induced ocular irritation, because most of the preservative remains in the lens case. In addition, because the antimicrobial agent stays in the case, the solution maintains its ability to protect the case from contamination. Opti-Free Rinsing, Disinfecting, and Storage Solution originally was designed to be used with a separate cleaner. The solution also contains a citrate buffer system, which helps to make it compatible with all lens types (129,171). Clinical trials with Opti-Free conducted on nonpreservative- and preservative-sensitive patients demonstrated no irritation for all lens types (172–175). A 1-year study indicated that Opti-Free is compatible with CSI crofilcon A lenses (176).

Opti-One Multi-Purpose Solution (Alcon) is an MPS approved by the FDA for use with 2-week replacement contact lenses. Opti-One also contains Polyquad 0.001% as well as sodium citrate, NaCl, borates, mannitol, and edetate disodium. Citrate is a negatively charged sequestering agent (170) that contributes to the removal of dansyl-lysozyme deposits (177). It is postulated that citrate's mode of action involves ionic binding with, and displacement, of lens-adherent lysozyme (135,177). Addition of this chemical to a storage solution has been found to have a beneficial effect on lens cleaning in laboratory-based and clinical studies (28, 178). The citrate component allows Opti-One to have passive cleaning abilities (177). Opti-One also contains buffering agents, which are used to keep the solution at a pH near that of tears. Tear pH is noted to average 7.45, with a zone of ocular awareness outside the range of 6.6 to 7.8 (179). The pH for Opti-One averages 6.97 (179).

Opti-Free Express Multi-Purpose Disinfecting Solution (MPDS) (Alcon) contains Polyquad and sodium citrate, as well as additional agents for enhancing cleaning, disinfecting, buffering, and wetting properties. In the late 1990s, an antimicrobial agent called myristamidopropyl dimethylamine (Aldox) was added to the formulation of Opti-Free Express (180,181). With the addition of Aldox, Opti-Free Express was the first MPS in the United States to be designated as a "no-rub" solution for all lens types. This means that the traditional in-the-palm cleaning step has been replaced by a rinsing cycle (182). A study with Opti-Free Express has indicated that it is unlikely that stored hydrogel lenses take up the antimicrobial components of the solution (164). Thus, the solution in the case maintains its antimicrobial activity in the presence of lenses. Opti-Free Express contains a patented surfactant called Tetronic 1304, which aids in lipid removal (170) and helps to attract water molecules to the lens surface, thereby serving as a wetting agent as well. The buffering agents in Opti-Free Express MPDS help to maintain a stable pH of 7.3 (183). Lenses can be stored in Opti-Free Express for up to 30 days (184).

ReNu Multi-Purpose Disinfecting Solution (Bausch & Lomb) contains the chlorhexidine derivative polyaminopropyl biguanide (Dymed) 0.00005% as its preservative. Chlorhexidine derivatives are known by several names, including polyaminopropyl biguanide (PAPB), polyhexanide, polyhexamethylene biguanide (PHMB), and TrisChem (170). Differing antimicrobial effectiveness among such solutions is attributed to different concentrations of the preservative, as well as the presence of other formula ingredients—buffers, surfactants, salts, etc.—which are said to influence the antimicrobial activity of the disinfectant (43, 170,185). The unique structure of PAPB/PHMB enables it to attack cell walls of microorganisms without affecting cell walls of ocular structures (170). Dymed is stated to be noncytotoxic, nonirritating, and nonsensitizing, according to laboratory test results (186–188). Many studies involving ReNu have been performed (1,161,165,189–192). One study, sponsored by a competitor, suggested that PAPB is taken up by 55% water hydrogels in storage (165). Consequently, the bactericidal activity of PAPB in the case declined after 4 hours of hydrogel storage time and showed no activity after 3 days of storage (165). A retrospective study of 101 patients with 2 years' experience with ReNu Multi-Action (MPS) Solution revealed no clinically significant ocular changes among the patient population during the 2-year length of the study (189). A second study, using a sensitive grading scale designed to detect subtle tarsal changes, noted more significant tarsal changes in users of ReNu MPS compared with users of one other combination and two other hydrogen peroxide systems (190). A third study showed that ReNu Multi-Purpose Disinfecting Solution exhibited a greater effect on rabbit corneal epithelium and an increase in peeling cells when compared with AOSEPT and Opti-Free (191). However, this difference between solutions was significant by only one method of analysis; therefore, the relative lack of significance may indicate that the difference between these solutions is minimal

(191). ReNu MPS has an average pH of 7.18 (179). It continues to be a popular choice in care systems.

Bausch & Lomb also manufactures ReNu MultiPlus MPS-No Rub. Along with Dymed, the current formula includes the chelating agent hydroxyalkyl-phosphonate (Hydranate), which works similarly to citrate in that it ionically pulls protein molecules off the lens surface (135). *In vitro* tests suggest that this solution gave comparable cleaning performance to that achieved with a regular storage solution and an enzymatic cleaner (28,135). ReNu MultiPlus is a multipurpose disinfecting solution with the "no-rub" designation for lenses replaced in 30 days or less. It is an all-in-one solution designed to clean, disinfect, and rinse hydrogel contact lenses, and it requires no assistance from an enzymatic cleaner. Lenses can be stored for a maximum of 30 days in ReNu MultiPlus (193).

Complete Multi-Purpose Solution (Advanced Medical Optics) is another no-rub multipurpose care system for lenses replaced in 30 days or less. Complete contains the preservative TrisChem and the cleaning agent polaxomer 237 (194). This ingredient is a nonionic, lubricating surfactant. Also part of Complete's formula is an ingredient not previously used in MPSs. Hydroxypropyl methylcellulose (HPMC) is a lubricating agent that has been widely used in artificial tear preparations. HPMC is thought to bind to hydrogel lens surfaces during storage and is subsequently slowly released into the tear fluid during wear, reportedly promoting better wetting and prolonged comfort for the patient (155,170,195,196). Complete can be used for lens storage for up to 30 days (197).

SOLO-care Multi-Purpose Solution (CIBA Vision) is an all-in-one solution indicated for cleaning, rinsing, disinfecting, and storing of soft and gas permeable lenses. It contains poloxamer 407 as its surfactant and is preserved with polyhexanide (PHMB).

SOLO-care Plus Multi-Purpose Solution (CIBA Vision) is a new formulation specifically designed for both "no-rub" and "no-rinse" indications for all lenses replaced in 30 days or less (198). Key ingredients include a new biologic buffer system (Bis-Tris Propane), the preservative polyhexanide, a surfactant cleaner called Pluronic F127, and a lubricant called Aqualube (Cremophor RH40) (156). Cremophor RH40 is a derivative of castor oil produced from the palm plant family and is a tenacious wetting agent that works with EDTA to manage lens deposits (156). Its prolonged retention on the lens surface reduces protein adsorption and binding (156). The water-seeking part of Cremophor also promotes water retention and creates a moisture coating on the lens to keep it lubricated and maintain on-eye comfort (156). For added flexibility, the instructions for use offer the choice of two regimens: the no-rub, no-rinse option followed by a 4-hour soak; or the alternative 5-minute option. The latter caters to situations needing fast disinfection and calls for a 10-second rub on each side of the lens, then a thorough rinse followed by a 5-minute soak.

Lenses can be stored in SOLO-care Plus for a maximum of 30 days (198).

Although some practitioners and patients consider lens care solutions to be generally equivalent, products do vary significantly in their formulas (195). This is especially true in the MPS category, where slight differences in formulations can make big differences in patient performance (199). Given the wide variations in labeling and instructions among brands, practitioners and their staffs need to keep abreast of current products and be familiar with all product instructions for use. Special note should be made that instructions not only vary among MPS brands but also for a given brand from one country to another. This further adds to the complexity of the issue and mandates that the practitioner and staff personnel should frequently review proper lens care usage. Table 19.4 lists the major chemical disinfection systems currently available.

Chemical Hydrogen Peroxide Disinfection

Hydrogen peroxide offers many advantages over other chemical systems. It is safe, very effective, and does not contain sensitizing ingredients. Hydrogen peroxide penetrates into hydrogel lenses and is reported to provide deep-cleaning action by expanding the lens matrix and oxidizing foreign matter (200,201). There is no accumulation or binding of peroxide in a hydrogel lens as occurs with some of the other chemical systems. A retrospective study that surveyed records of patients using chemical (multipurpose) and peroxide systems in Hong Kong found that the incidence of corneal staining was greater and the severity of corneal staining was worse in patients using the combination systems versus those using peroxide (202).

A 3% concentration of peroxide has been determined to be the optimal concentration for disinfection of contact lenses (203). Hydrogen peroxide usually is hypotonic and has a pH of approximately 4.00 (4,204). These chemical properties result in lens expansion and contraction (accordion effect), which is believed to break protein and lipid bonds and may aid in the removal of trapped debris (5, 205). This may explain why some practitioners find less need for enzyme use when peroxide disinfection is used with hydrogel lenses.

Certain polymers change in base curve radius when exposed to long soak times in hydrogen peroxide (206). When

TABLE 19.4. CHEMICAL DISINFECTION SOLUTIONS

Product (Manufacturer)	Preservatives	Other Ingredients
Clear Conscience Multi-Purpose Solution (Clear Conscience)	Cosmocil CQ (polyhexamethylene biguanide) 0.0001%, edetate disodium	Polyoxyethylene-polyoxypropylene block copolymer, phosphate salt, sodium chloride
Complete Moisture PLUS Multi-Purpose Solution (Advanced Medical Optics)	Polyhexamethylene biguanide 0.0001%, edetate disodium	Hydroxypropyl methylcellulose, phosphate, taurine, propylene glycol, poloxamer 237, sodium chloride, potassium chloride
Complete Multi-Purpose Solution (Advanced Medical Optics)	Polyhexamethylene biguanide 0.0001%, edetate disodium	Hydroxypropyl methylcellulose, phosphate buffer, poloxamer 237, sodium chloride, potassium chloride
QuickCare 5 Minute System (CIBA Vision)		
QuickCare Starting Solution	—	Isopropanol, sodium chloride, polyoxypropylene-polyoxyethylene block copolymer, disodium lauro-ampho diacetate
QuickCare Finishing Solution	Antimicrobial buffer system generating up to 0.006% hydrogen peroxide	Sodium borate, boric acid, sodium perborate, phosphonic acid
Opti-Free (Alcon)	Polyquad (polyquaternium-1) 0.001%, edetate disodium 0.05%	Citrate buffer system, sodium chloride
Opti-Free Express (Alcon)	Polyquad (polyquaternium-1) 0.001%, Aldox (myristamidopropyl dimethylamine) 0.0005%, edetate disodium 0.05%	Sodium citrate, sodium chloride, boric acid, sorbitol, AMP-95, Tetronic 1304
Opti-One Multi-Purpose Solution (Alcon)	Polyquad (polyquaternium-1) 0.0011%, edetate disodium 0.05%	Pationic, Tetronic, sodium chloride, mannitol, borate and citrate buffers
ReNu MultiPlus (Bausch & Lomb)	Dymed (polyaminopropyl biguanide) 0.0001%, edetate disodium	Hydranate (hydroxyalkyl-phosphonate), poloxamine, boric acid, sodium borate, sodium chloride
ReNu Multi-Purpose Solution (Bausch & Lomb)	Dymed (polyaminopropyl biguanide) 0.00005%, edetate disodium	Boric acid, sodium borate, sodium chloride, poloxamine
Sauflon Lite Multi-Purpose Solution (Sauflon Pharmaceuticals)	Polyhexanide 0.0001%	Poloxamer, sodium phosphate, sodium chloride, disodium edetate,
SOLO-care PLUS (CIBA Vision)	Polyhexanide 0.0001%, edetate disodium 0.025%	Aqualube (Cremophor RH40), Bis Tris Propane, Pluronic F127, sodium chloride

this occurs, other physical characteristics of the lens change as well (207,208), thus potentially altering the fitting characteristics of the lens. All of these events are reversible, but recovery time is polymer-dependent (206). Neutral polymers (groups I and III) seem to be least affected by peroxide exposure, whereas high-water-content, ionic polymer lenses (group IV) containing methacrylic acid are the most affected (206,209). Another study concluded that high-water-content, nonionic polymer lenses (group II) also were compatible for use with peroxide systems, but use with group IV lenses may not be appropriate (210).

Hydrogen peroxide's antimicrobial effectiveness has been known for more than 100 years. It possesses broad-spectrum antibacterial activity (85,140,163,200,211–214), but exposure times of 45 to 60 minutes have been recommended to assure adequate antifungal activity (211,215). Hydrogen peroxide disinfection is much more effective against the mold *Beauvaria bassiana* than other chemical solutions (216).

There are some disadvantages associated with the use of hydrogen peroxide, such as the complexity of certain systems and the time considerations involved (217,218). A high concentration of hydrogen peroxide is irritating if it is instilled directly into the eye (204,205,219); therefore, it must be significantly reduced or eliminated before applying lenses safely to the eye. Concentrations of 50 or 60 parts per million (ppm) have historically been considered to be the threshold for ocular detection (203,204). Research has concluded that higher levels may be acceptable for certain patients (220,221).

Placing a lens directly on the eye immediately after using hydrogen peroxide solution will most likely cause ocular irritation. Clinical signs and symptoms include hyperemia, profuse tearing, epiphora, chemosis, burning, stinging, photophobia, and superficial punctate keratitis (203,222,223). Usually, only minimal corneal involvement occurs (200, 224). This most likely is because of the high corneal and conjunctival tissue levels of catalase, a naturally occurring enzyme that is capable of neutralizing peroxide extremely rapidly (225,226).

After the disinfection process is completed, three primary methods of neutralization are available to convert the peroxide into harmless byproducts (222,227–229). The neutralization methods consist of catalytic neutralizing agents, such as the enzyme catalase or a platinum disc (85,203,205,230, 231); reactive neutralizing agents, such as the chemicals sodium pyruvate (201) or sodium thiosulfate (200,232,233); and dilution/elution agents, such as saline (234,235). Residual hydrogen peroxide concentrations in solution and lenses after the neutralization process have been reported to be less than 1 ppm for systems that use a catalase neutralizer; 3 ppm or less for systems that use a sodium pyruvate neutralizer; and 12 ppm or less for systems that use a platinum disc (236).

Although hydrogen peroxide is known to be a very effec-

tive disinfectant, such solutions contain no preservatives [studies have shown that microbial regrowth can occur in the absence of preservatives (163), so storage in most neutralized hydrogen peroxide solutions is not recommended for more than 24 hours]. An exception to this is AOSEPT Clear Care (CIBA Vision), which contains a surfactant along with hydrogen peroxide in its formula. Lenses can be stored in neutralized Clear Care for up to 7 days following disinfection (237). Another hydrogen peroxide product, UltraCare (Advanced Medical Optics), also has been approved for 7-day storage, but UltraCare requires tablet neutralization and a separate mechanical cleaning step (238).

Peroxide systems are categorized as one- or two-step systems. In a two-step system, step 1 is the disinfection procedure (usually an overnight soak), and step 2 is the subsequent neutralization of the peroxide and reequilibration of the lens to its proper tonicity and pH. Depending on the system (brand), there are different disinfection times. These times reflect the amount of time required in a laboratory setting to completely eliminate all test microorganisms from a lens (239). Manufacturers of systems with longer disinfection times are specifically trying to address the issue of possible fungal contamination. With a two-step system, there usually are no major difficulties with fungal contamination because overnight disinfection most commonly is used. However, the clinical implication of a patient soaking the lenses on an overnight or long-term basis is that the patient may notice scalloped edges or lens curling because of the acidic pH of peroxide (240). To eliminate this situation, a longer soak time in the neutralizing agent should be recommended. This is not for the purpose of neutralizing the peroxide but to reequilibrate the lens to the proper parameters (209).

In one-step peroxide systems, the neutralizing agent is placed in the peroxide-filled case at the same time the lenses are placed in the solution. One-step systems use either a catalase tablet or a platinum disc as the neutralizing agent. Although one-step systems are simpler to use than their two-step counterparts, their antimicrobial efficacy may be lessened because neutralization of the hydrogen peroxide occurs more rapidly (170,241). Disinfection with a one-step system may be prolonged by delaying the addition of the neutralizing agent to the peroxide solution.

Advanced Medical Optics developed the UltraCare Disinfection/Neutralizer System, which uses a hydroxypropyl methylcellulose-coated catalase tablet for hydrogen peroxide neutralization (242). This delayed-release catalase has a vitamin B_{12} color reminder that turns the disinfectant solution pink if the neutralizing tablet has been added. The tablet is added to the 3% hydrogen peroxide solution at the beginning of the disinfection cycle. The coating on the catalase tablet delays neutralization, allowing the peroxide time to disinfect the lenses. As the coating dissolves, catalase comes in contact with the H_2O_2, neutralizing it into water and oxygen within 2 hours.

The AOSEPT Disinfection System (CIBA Vision) is a one-step hydrogen peroxide system that uses a platinum catalytic disc attached to a dome basket lens holder and a 3% hydrogen peroxide solution that is formulated in a buffered saline solution. As disinfection occurs, the catalytic disc simultaneously converts the hydrogen peroxide into preservative-free isotonic saline with a pH of 6.70. One study reported the residual peroxide level with AOSEPT at 1 month was 21 ± 9.4 ppm (243). At the end of 2 months, it was 36 ± 17.6 ppm, and at 3 months, when disc replacement was recommended, the residual peroxide level was 43 ± 4.7 ppm. The measured residual peroxide increased with time; however, these levels failed to induce any change in slit-lamp findings or symptoms (243). The major advantages of this system are its ease of use and absence of parameter changes (240,244) after overnight soaking because of the buffered nature of the solution.

CIBA Vision also manufactures a multipurpose peroxide system called Pure Eyes. This care system has two components: Pure Eyes Cleaner/Rinse, which contains an antimicrobial buffer system and the surfactant Pluronic 17R4; and Pure Eyes Disinfectant/Soaking Solution, which contains 3% hydrogen peroxide formulated in buffered 0.85% sodium chloride (245). Each package of Pure Eyes Disinfectant/Soaking solution includes a dome basket contact lens holder and case with built-in neutralizer (246). A study that tested the disinfecting efficacy of Pure Eyes Disinfectant, without the cleaning step, against *P. aeruginosa* found that the disinfectant was able to eradicate *P. aeruginosa* after 4- and 6-hour soaking periods (214). The authors suggest that use of the Pure Eyes system may add an extra margin of safety against microbial contamination for wearers who may be noncompliant with a cleaning step.

AOSEPT Clear Care Cleaning and Disinfecting Solution (CIBA Vision) is a one-bottle, peroxide-based system that cleans and disinfects. It carries the no-rub designation for all soft lenses. Ingredients include hydrogen peroxide 3% with a phosphate buffer system and a Pluronic surfactant cleaner. One study determined that MPS users who tried Clear Care for 1 month exhibited decreases in the frequency and intensity of dryness symptoms and increases in overall comfort as compared to the subjects' own MPSs (247). Of the 140 patients who completed the study, 113 (80.7%) preferred AOSEPT Clear Care over their previous multipurpose lens care systems. Table 19.5 lists the major hydrogen peroxide systems available, as well as their methods of neutralization.

Some reports of discomfort (stinging) with use of H_2O_2 disinfecting systems have appeared in the literature (248, 249). An *in vitro* double-masked placebo-controlled study with 361 patients was conducted using six commercially available systems (250). The results demonstrated that all of the hydrogen peroxide systems compared equally with each other and with a saline placebo with regard to comfort rating. A likely cause of ocular discomfort, if it does occur,

TABLE 19.5. HYDROGEN PEROXIDE SOLUTIONS

System (Manufacturer)	Disinfection Solution	Neutralization Method
AOSEPT Disinfectant (CIBA Vision)	AOSEPT (3% H_2O_2 + 0.85% sodium chloride)	Platinum catalyst
AOSEPT Clear Care Cleaning and Disinfecting Solution (CIBA Vision)	Clear Care (3% H_2O_2 + 0.85% sodium chloride)	Platinum catalyst
Pure Eyes (CIBA Vision)	Pure Eyes Disinfectant (3% H_2O_2 + 0.85% sodium chloride)	Platinum catalyst
UltraCare (Advanced Medical Optics)	UltraCare	Delayed-release catalase tablet

is a final solution pH after neutralization that is outside the ocular comfort range of 6.6 to 7.8 (248,249). This situation can be eliminated by rinsing the lens with a buffered saline solution before insertion.

Hydrogen Peroxide and the Eye The residual concentration of hydrogen peroxide in contact lenses after neutralization typically is less than 50 to 60 ppm, which is significantly below the apparent threshold for peroxide detection in eye drops or contact lenses (220,221,251). If low levels of peroxide are present at the time of lens insertion, they are rapidly neutralized. The rate of residual peroxide removal from hydrogel lenses *in vivo* has been shown to be less than 1 minute, presumably because of the presence of catalase and other antioxidants in the highly vascularized palpebral conjunctiva (225). More specifically, it has been shown that the majority of the hydrogen peroxide applied topically through contact lenses on rabbit eyes was neutralized by the conjunctival epithelium (252). The abundance of ocular catalase and other enzymes that naturally neutralize peroxide has been described and assayed (253–255). Nevertheless, it has been hypothesized that low levels of peroxide might cause damage to the corneal epithelium, stroma, endothelium, and tissues of the anterior chamber (222). This concern is raised by observations that increased concentrations of peroxide in the aqueous humor have been associated with cataract formation (256), and that exogenous H_2O_2 in experimental *in vitro* studies has been shown to affect the endothelium, crystalline lens, and iris.

Numerous studies have been conducted to further investigate the effect of peroxide on ocular tissue (257–259). To test the effect of H_2O_2 on the corneal epithelium, rabbit corneas were perfused with various concentrations of peroxide ranging from 0 to 235 ppm (260). Stromal swelling and anterior bright band swelling were compared for a single 10-minute pulse versus a 150-minute sustained dose. Results showed no significant swelling up to 235 ppm H_2O_2 in the

10-minute pulse dose. With the sustained dose, significant stromal swelling began between 72 and 153 ppm H_2O_2.

In another evaluation, contact lenses were soaked in hydrogen peroxide solutions with concentrations of 34 to 680 ppm and then placed on rabbit corneas to determine whether the peroxide could penetrate across the tissue (251). Corneas with intact epithelia allowed no hydrogen peroxide to cross, even with lenses containing the highest concentration. It was concluded that with normal contact lens use on an eye with an intact epithelium, there will be no corneal endothelial or other intraocular tissue damage by residual concentrations of hydrogen peroxide of up to 680 ppm, whether in single or daily events (251). These results suggest that peroxide disinfection systems do not expose the ocular tissue to peroxide doses at high enough concentration or long enough duration to affect the physiology of the cornea (251,260).

Heat Disinfection

Heat disinfection is a very effective but currently an infrequently used method of disinfecting contact lenses. It is safe, fast, and economical, but it is not compatible with all lens materials. It can destroy high-water-content polymer lenses if it is used on a repeated basis, and it bakes protein onto lenses, thereby decreasing lens life (4,10,11,44,56,261). Heat disinfection requires a temperature of 80°C for 10 minutes (44,45) and thus is not portable because it demands specific electric current requirements. It has been discovered that there is no guarantee that a heating unit actually is working. In some situations, an indicator light may come on, but the heating element itself can be burned out or not functioning properly. Traditional heat disinfection units that are older than 5 to 7 years should be checked to make sure that they are still functioning properly.

A newer heat disinfecting system called Earth Eyes Electronic Disinfecting Unit (Earth Eyes) may be more reliable because it is controlled by a computer chip (262). The chip is activated by plugging in the unit. Lenses are heat disinfected at 160°F (71°C) for 30 minutes, after which they are cooled for another 30 minutes. The EarthEyes system has been promoted as an economical, fast, and effective disinfection system for patients with low-water-content lenses (262).

From an efficacy standpoint, heat is very effective in killing microorganisms (44,45,216). Because of its disadvantages, however, practitioners now tend to dissuade patients from using heat disinfection.

Other Disinfection

Ultraviolet

Ultraviolet (UV) disinfection has been studied and is reported to be an effective method of soft and rigid gas-permeable contact lens disinfection. Sterilization occurs after 300 seconds or less of exposure to UV light (263). UV disinfection appears to be 10 times more effective than two-step hydrogen peroxide disinfection and 100 to 200 times more effective than other disinfection solutions (264). It is important, however, that sterile preservative-free saline solution be used because it transmits more than 90% of the UV radiation. Preservatives or other ingredients could interfere with the germicidal action of the UV light (264).

An automated system called the PuriLens Contact Lens Care System (PuriLens) is the first FDA-approved lens care regimen to use UV-C light for disinfection. PuriLens uses subsonic turbulence for cleaning and a patented lens holder that protects the lens from direct exposure to UV light, thereby preventing changes in lens parameters (265). It has been found to clean and disinfect after only 15 minutes (266). One study evaluated the system and reported cleaner lenses compared to ReNu Multi-Purpose (265). After 180 cycles, lenses were not adversely affected. The PuriLens system uses PuriLens solution, a nonpreserved sterile isotonic sodium chloride solution buffered with boric acid and sodium borate (265). This device disinfected challenged lenses inoculated with 2×10^6 *Aspergillus niger, Acanthamoeba castellani, P. aeruginosa,* and *Bacillus pumilus* in less than 10 minutes (266). Multiple studies have shown that using UV light is an effective alternative for lens cleaning and disinfecting (265–268). The PuriLens system has been recommended as a viable lens care option for patients requiring a simple, economical, and preservative-free mode of disinfection (269). Table 19.6 lists available UV radiation and ultrasonic disinfection devices.

Microwave

Use of microwave oven disinfection for contact lenses has been studied (270–276). Microwave irradiation is rapid and effective. Studies have shown that significant reductions in bacterial colony counts occur after 30 seconds of microwave exposure (270). Only a very small number of *S. aureus* survived after 60 seconds, and none of the bacteria tested survived 90 seconds of microwave exposure. In a study using low-power (10%) microwave disinfection, lenses challenged with *S. aureus, Staphylococcus epidermidis,* and *P. aeruginosa* were disinfected after 15 minutes of irradiation (272). Lens parameter changes may occur and are brand-specific (275) but for the most part usually are small and clinically insignificant (273,275), even after numerous cycles of disinfection.

TABLE 19.6. ULTRAVIOLET/SUBSONIC CLEANING AND ULTRASONIC DISINFECTING UNITS

System (Manufacturer)	Method of Disinfection
Lens Comfort (Best Health)	Ultrasonic
LensSoClean (Alpha Vista)	Ultrasonic
PuriLens Contact Lens Care System (PuriLens)	Ultraviolet radiation/subsonic turbulence

Salt crystal buildup has been reported to occur on some lenses and can lead to lens discomfort (274). A clinical trial of a patient-operated microwave care system found that after 1 and 3 months of using the microwave system, the overall incidence of clinical signs in the microwave group was not significantly greater than that in a control group (276). (The microwave-using group exhibited a significantly greater incidence of edema at 1 month, and the control group showed a significantly greater incidence of staining.) Further studies are needed to determine the long-term effects of microwave disinfection.

Mechanical Units

A device manufactured by LensCare, Ltd. that cleans by creating extreme amounts of turbulence within the lens case has been described in the literature as a simple and rapid method for disinfection (38). Saline can be used in the multidirectional vibration-generating device, but it is reported to be even more effective using an MPS (38). Little information regarding the clinical effectiveness of the device is available at this time. A couple of mechanical devices that utilize ultrasonic waves have been introduced in the market. Table 19.6 lists available ultrasonic cleaning and disinfecting units.

MICROBIOLOGIC CONSIDERATIONS

It is well known that a host of bacteria, viruses, and fungi are capable of causing ocular infection (277). Infections among contact lens wearers appear to be caused by different pathogens than those among non-contact lens wearers (278). *P. aeruginosa* accounts for approximately 60% of the contact lens-related cases of microbial keratitis (278). The human immunodeficiency virus (HTLV-III/AIDS) and *Acanthamoeba* have become particular concerns for the contact lens practitioner.

Isolation of HTLV-III retrovirus in the tears of a patient with AIDS raised concerns regarding the possible transmission of AIDS during contact lens fitting (279). There has been no documented case of a person transmitting AIDS by way of tears, but HTLV-III has been recovered from high-water content contact lenses or storage solution in four of six tested patients with AIDS or AIDS-related complex (41). Because of the implications of these findings, eye care practitioners are very concerned about safeguards that can be put into practice. The Centers for Disease Control (280) and others (281–283) have recommended disinfection by heat or 3% hydrogen peroxide as being effective in deactivating the AIDS virus.

The other microorganism of great concern is the protozoan *Acanthamoeba*. Fifteen different species have been reported (284). Five of these *Acanthamoeba* species have been found to cause corneal disease: *A. castellani, A. culbertsoni, A. hatchetti, A. polyphaga,* and *A. rhysodes* (285). A number of cases of *Acanthamoeba* keratitis in contact lens wearers

have been reported (94,96,97,99,100,102–104,106,150, 286). *Acanthamoeba* has been associated with improper use of salt tablet-prepared saline and patient noncompliance (287). This clinical entity is relatively rare when compared with the millions of people who wear contact lenses (288). Nevertheless, it is important for the contact lens patient to be prudent and prevent contamination because corneal infection by this microorganism is devastating.

Pathogenesis of *Acanthamoeba* keratitis may involve the contact lens acting as a mechanical vector for the protozoa to enter the eye. One study evaluated the differential adherence of *A. castellani* and *A. polyphaga* to different types of unworn hydrogel lenses (289). Results have shown that ionic and high-water content contact lenses were associated with an increased quantitative adherence of *Acanthamoeba* to the lens surface. Other researchers believe that binding of *Acanthamoeba* to the lens probably is affected mainly by surface tension, surface charge, and water content (290).

Acanthamoeba can exist in two forms: the free-living trophozoite and the cyst. The cyst is very resilient and resists extremes such as freezing, desiccation, and exposure to chlorine (96,291). Controversy exists regarding elimination of *Acanthamoeba* from the surface of contaminated lenses. In one of the first studies, results showed that heat disinfection was the only form of disinfection capable of killing both the trophozoite and cyst forms (291). It has been reported that longer soak times in hydrogen peroxide may be effective in killing *Acanthamoeba* (95,102,292–294). Other investigators, however, have found that soak times of up to 72 hours in hydrogen peroxide are not effective in eliminating the cyst form of *Acanthamoeba* (295). Studies on the effectiveness of the newer chemical (nonperoxide) disinfectants against *Acanthamoeba* have yielded mixed results. In one study, the efficacy of three widely used contact lens disinfection systems against an ocular isolate of *A. polyphaga* was compared (296). Another source reports favorable activity against *Acanthamoeba* cysts with 0.00005% polyhexanide (214). Comparing a one-step peroxide system against Opti-Free Express (Alcon) revealed minimal activity against *Acanthamoeba* cysts for the peroxide system compared with an average 2.4- to 3.2-log reduction after 6 hours of exposure to Opti-Free Express (286).

A study was conducted to determine the amoebicidal efficacy of different contact lens care products when using *A. castellani* (cysts and trophozoites) as the challenge organism (297). Only AOSEPT Clear Care (CIBA Vision) exhibited significant antimicrobial activity against the cyst form of *A. castellani.* Oxysept 1-Step (Advanced Medical Optics) showed mild activity against the cysts, and Opti-Free Express with Aldox (Alcon) showed virtually no anti-*Acanthamoeba* activity against the cyst form after 6 hours of exposure (297). Another investigation evaluated the effectiveness of three disinfection systems against *A. polyphaga* on the lens surface of worn lenses (298). Results indicated that all three systems, ReNu (Bausch & Lomb), Opti-Free (Alcon), and

AOSEPT (CIBA Vision), were highly effective against *Acanthamoeba* on the lens surface, although not 100%. In the absence of proper cleaning, AOSEPT was the most effective of the three. The results also showed the importance of thoroughly rubbing the lens surface to decrease the number of *Acanthamoeba*. In addition, different species of *Acanthamoeba* show varying susceptibilities to disinfection regimens (298). The amoebicidal activity of a contact lens MPS containing polyquaternium-1 and myristamidopropyl dimethylamine was compared to a disinfection/neutralization peroxide system against *A. castellanii* and *A. polyphaga* trophozoites and cysts (299). A quantitative microtiter technique was used for evaluation and revealed that the MPS showed similar amoebicidal activity to the peroxide system against trophozoites of both species and equal or more cidal activity against the cysts of both species.

Other studies compared the amoebicidal activity of the newer Opti-Free Express formula to a disinfection/neutralization peroxide system against species of *Acanthamoeba* (286,299). They found that Opti-Free Express showed similar activity to the peroxide system against trophozoites, and equal or more rapid activity against cysts of the *Acanthamoeba* species tested (286,299). Opti-Free Express also is noted for its activity against fungal contamination during soaking (170,183) and has been shown to retain its antimicrobial effectiveness under conditions of extreme heat (164, 181).

It has been shown that cleaning a lens by digital rubbing and mechanical action and subsequent rinsing dislodges *Acanthamoeba* if it is present on the surface of a lens (185, 195,298). Additional studies with *Acanthamoeba* tested several different cleaners (29). The results showed that Mira-Flow Extra-Strength Daily Cleaner (CIBA Vision), with isopropyl alcohol as an active ingredient, was capable of killing both the trophozoite and cyst forms of *Acanthamoeba*.

Because *Acanthamoeba* can have such devastating results, a number of authorities have made recommendations to minimize its occurrence (97,98,103–109,112). Patients must be educated on how they can avoid problems. They should adhere to the wearing schedule prescribed and wash their hands thoroughly before lens handling; not wear lenses while swimming; not wear lenses in hot tubs or spas; never use tap water, distilled water, mineral water, or saliva with contact lenses; use only sterile contact lens solutions; clean lenses each time they are removed; disinfect lenses each time they are removed; rinse lenses only with a sterile saline solution; use only sterile saline solution to dissolve enzyme tablets, not distilled water or tap water; never instill a nonsterile solution directly into the eye; and thoroughly clean the contact lens case daily by rinsing with fresh sterile saline or disinfecting solution and allow the case to air dry between uses. Soft lenses should never be rinsed with nonsterile solution, most specifically, salt-tablet saline. One study demonstrated the highly preventable nature of *Acanthamoeba* keratitis in that 91% of soft lens wearers could have avoided

this devastating disease by carrying out more effective disinfection and/or refraining from swimming while wearing lenses (150).

Microbial Efficacy

Rub and Rinse Systems

Lens care manufacturers must demonstrate that a disinfection system has an effective killing capability when challenged with microorganisms.

The effectiveness of a disinfection solution in killing the test microbes is described by a D-value, which represents the amount of time, in minutes, required to kill 90% (1 log) of the microorganisms that are inoculated initially on the lens (41,300). From these values, it can be approximated how well the disinfection agent itself actually is performing. The smaller the D-value, the quicker the disinfection solution is at killing microorganisms. Therefore, solutions with low D-values provide the greatest margin of error when patients are noncompliant (301). Conversely, solutions with high D-values require total patient compliance with directions, including the cleaning and rinsing steps.

Independent investigations have addressed the killing ability of certain disinfection agents. *S. marcescens* and *Aspergillus fumigatus* are among the most difficult of the challenge organisms to kill (185,302,303). An *in vitro* study evaluated the efficacy of a Polyquad-preserved disinfectant against four bacterial strains and showed that the solution prevented the proliferation of both *P. aeruginosa* and *Escherichia coli* (304). Only a few survivors of *S. epidermidis* were recovered. However, *S. marcescens* presented some resistance to the Polyquad solution (304). Published D-values have shown that the combination of chlorhexidine and thimerosal has very good effectiveness (212,302,305); however, chlorhexidine (0.005%) by itself appears to be ineffective against fungi (211,306) and *S. marcescens* (303). The effectiveness of different disinfectants also has been compared (301,307). Solutions tested included Dymed 0.00005% plus edetate disodium, Polyquad 0.001% plus edetate disodium 0.1%, and thimerosal 0.002% plus alkyltriethanol ammonium chloride and 3% hydrogen peroxide. Results showed that the thimerosal plus alkyltriethanol ammonium chloride disinfectant and 3% hydrogen peroxide were effective against all challenge organisms. The other disinfectants were not as effective because they did not kill *C. albicans* or *A. fumigatus*. The disinfecting efficacy of hydrogen peroxide and Polyquad against *P. aeruginosa* was compared at 4 and 6 hours (308). Results showed that both disinfectants were able to reduce the number of surviving organisms of *Pseudomonas* but to different degrees. Hydrogen peroxide was effective at eradicating the microorganisms, whereas with Polyquad the colony-forming units (CFUs) were too numerous to count (more than 200) for both soak times.

An extremely effective disinfectant system is the

QuickCare Cleaning and Disinfecting system (CIBA Vision). D-values are less than 5 seconds for bacterial and fungal microorganisms (309). One study revealed that the starting solution killed 80% of bacterial and fungal clinical isolates in 1 minute (162).

One case report documented a patient wearing a soft contact lens contaminated with fungal deposits of *Paecilomyces* species while using a Polyquad-preserved disinfection system (310). Another report presented a case of fungal contamination that occurred after disinfection with the Dymed disinfectant (311). The microbiologic effectiveness of hydrogen peroxide has been well documented (140,203, 211,212,239). D-value determination for hydrogen peroxide revealed bacterial organisms were killed rapidly, in less than 3 minutes, but 11 minutes was required for *Aspergillus* and 48 minutes for *Candida* (211). A direct antimicrobial evaluation over 6 hours compared three soft contact lens disinfection solutions: AOSEPT Disinfection Solution with AODISC Neutralizer (CIBA Vision), ReNu Multi-Purpose Solution (Bausch & Lomb), and Opti-Free (Alcon) (312). Inocula of 10^4 CFU per milliliter of *A. fumigatus, C. albicans, S. marcescens, P. aeruginosa,* and *S. epidermidis* were tested in 10-mL aliquots of each test solution. Samples of the test solution were taken at 2, 4, and 6 hours, and average counts of each microorganism were compared. AOSEPT Disinfection Solution with AODISC Neutralizer was more effective overall in killing the test organisms than either ReNu or Opti-Free. It was particularly efficacious against the fungal organisms at all time intervals (312); therefore, evidence suggests that, regardless of which disinfecting solution is used, most bacteria are killed in a fairly quick manner, but fungi require longer kill times to show even a minimal, if any, effect.

Once again, this emphasizes the importance of the concept of the contribution of elements. When the FDA grants marketing approval for a disinfection system, there is an implied assurance that it is safe and effective, provided the patient performs the care regimen precisely according to the instructions in the labeling. In other words, the patient must complete the cleaning, rinsing, and disinfecting steps thoroughly. Patients who start to break down in compliance obviously are at risk for problems. The contact lens practitioner needs to address those patients who do not properly care for their lenses and lens case because all types of microorganisms can be found. Also, patients with spare pairs of lenses can experience high contamination levels of microorganisms if lenses are stored for long periods of time without proper care.

Bacterial contamination of hydrogel lenses occurs more commonly than fungal contamination (44,212,215,239). It has been suggested, however, that the incidence of fungal lens spoilage will likely increase with the increased use of chemical disinfection systems with high D-values (310). The frequency of fungal contamination with soft lenses may be greatly underestimated because many cases are most likely mistaken for nonspecific or mucoprotein deposits (313). This is of concern because the growth of fungi on a lens may irritate the eye and even lead to a corneal ulcer (11,215,314,315). Investigations have indicated that the higher the water content of the lens, the greater the potential for fungal contamination and actual fungal invasion into the matrix (314). This most likely occurs because high-water-content lenses have larger pore sizes, which makes it easier for the hyphae of the fungi to invade into the matrix. Once fungal growth has penetrated the matrix of a hydrogel lens, it becomes difficult, if not impossible, to remove (9). In a situation where fungal contamination is involved, it is advisable to discard the lenses, solutions, and lens case and start anew.

No-Rub Systems

Patients using MPSs traditionally have been instructed that a "rub and rinse" step following lens removal is essential not only to remove debris and deposits but also to reduce bioburden as previously mentioned. All MPSs have some ability to remove a certain amount of deposits when used in a rub-and-rinse regimen (156). However, several MPSs recently have been approved for a "no-rub" indication and have undergone changes in their labeling and instructions. New solutions formulated specifically for use without rubbing also have been developed (156). As previously discussed, all contact lens disinfection systems must meet specific standards before they can be marketed. The current FDA Guidelines and ISO 14729 Standards specify five test organisms that must be used in assessing the disinfecting capabilities of individual products (156,164): *S. aureus, P. aeruginosa, S. marcescens, C. albicans,* and *F. solani*. Several different tests with detailed methodologies on how to conduct the testing are described in the guidelines (156,164). In the United States, the FDA permits contact lens products to be labeled as disinfecting solutions if they meet the primary criteria of the Stand-Alone Test for contact lens disinfectants against the five representative challenge microorganisms. This test does not use lenses, organic soil, or rub and rinse steps. Instead, products are tested after being inoculated with the challenge microorganisms. In contrast, the Regimen Test is performed with lenses in the presence of organic soil representing tear components. The lenses are inoculated with the test organisms and then are cleaned and disinfected according to the solution manufacturer's instructions. If the rub step is eliminated, then the product must be tested to determine the effect of the soil and to ensure product efficacy during consumer use (164).

It is important to note that the no-rub designation does not necessarily streamline or simplify the steps required for proper lens care, because the rubbing step is actually replaced by a rinsing step. Directions for the various no-rub formulations vary. Some require a prerinse as well as a post-rinse, and the actual rinse times differ significantly among brands (57). Because instructions for use may be subject to change, directions in the package insert should be reviewed periodically.

CLINICAL SELECTION CONSIDERATIONS

Selection of the appropriate disinfection system is best handled on an individual basis. Consideration must be given to the lens type, water content, ionic nature of the material, mode of wear, patient history, and patient needs, including costs (90,166,182,316,317). Numerous patient preference studies have been conducted (77,156,157,190,195,196, 247,318–323). These studies provide useful information but often are difficult to compare because of differences in test protocols. Maintaining current knowledge of the wide variety of solutions and the properties of their components will aid the practitioner in matching particular solution regimens to individual patients.

LENS LUBRICANTS, REWETTING DROPS, AND IN-EYE CLEANERS

Lens lubricants permit lubrication and rewetting of the lens while it is on the eye. Typically, they contain a low concentration of a nonionic surfactant to promote cleaning, a polymer to lubricate the lens, buffering agents, and preservatives (20). Lens lubricants are particularly helpful for wearers of extended wear lenses, but they also can be used by those with daily wear lenses. For the wearer of silicone hydrogel lenses, the use of lubricants upon awakening and at nighttime may decrease the formation of mucin balls beneath the lens (324). Drying out of the lens on the eye from exposure to wind, low humidity, and high temperatures also may be relieved by lens lubricants. Finally, patients who experience difficulty removing hydrogel lenses because of dehydration or who frequently damage their lenses on removal may benefit from the use of lens lubricants. Sales of lubricants have increased greatly in the past decade (166). Several reasons for the growth of this category of lens care products have been suggested (166). One is the belief that the trend is an indicator of increased lens discomfort among wearers. Other theories suggest that augmentation of the aging patient base or a greater awareness of lubricants among consumers may be responsible for their growing sales.

Lens Plus Rewetting Solution (Advanced Medical Optics) has the advantage of being packaged in a unit-dose format, allowing it to be preservative free. This is of tremendous value to those patients who have sensitivities to even some of the newer, nonirritating preservatives. One popular use for this particular product is in conjunction with disposable lenses because it assists in making the complete regimen disposable and preservative free.

CIBA Vision Lens Drops (CIBA Vision) incorporates the ingredient carbamide, which has the ability to temporarily expand the matrix of a hydrogel lens. This allows greater lens movement and thereby helps to flush debris out from under the lens (325).

Refresh Contacts (Advanced Medical Optics) has the same formula as the dry eye product Refresh Tears (Advanced Medical Optics). Refresh contains the mucomimetic agent hydroxypropyl methylcellulose (HPMC), which coats the lens and is slowly released into the tear fluid to promote long-lasting comfort (135,195,196). Another component, carboxymethylcellulose (CMC), is said to have cytoprotective properties (135,155). The lubricant's Purite preservative system is chemical free and buffered with lactate.

In-eye contact lens cleaners are a relatively recent development in contact lens care. These solutions rely on two components: chemical action of a surfactant and the physical action of the eyelid wiping across the lens (326). When the drop is applied to the lens surface, the surfactant ingredient reduces the surface tension in the overlying tear film. This allows the accumulated protein, lipid, and debris on the lens surface to mix more easily within the tears. The lids then help to wipe the lens clean (326).

Alcon's Clerz Plus is marketed as an "in-eye cleaner." Clerz Plus contains the surfactant cleaner PEG-11 lauryl ethyl carboxylic acid (Clens-100), which functions to clean debris and deposits from the lens surface during wear. A second surfactant, Tetronic, serves to reduce further binding of deposits (135,326).

Blink-and-Clean (Advanced Medical Optics) also is promoted as an in-eye cleaner. It contains the surfactant tyloxapol, which helps to remove lipid and debris, and the buffer tromethamine, which ionically displaces lysozyme deposits and then works to prevent further depositing by occupying protein binding sites. Blink-and-Clean also contains HPMC.

ReNu Preservative-Free Lubricating and Rewetting Drops (Bausch & Lomb) are packaged in single-dose containers. The formula contains HPMC and bendazal lysine. Benzadac lysine is reported to be a nonsteroidal antiinflammatory agent (NSAIA), which is described as having antioxidant as well as antiinflammatory properties (326). It functions mainly to prevent denaturation of proteins and previously has been proposed as a prophylactic treatment for cataract development or progression (326). It has been suggested that the compound might reduce deposit formation on contact lenses, presumably through prohibiting lysozyme denaturation on the lens surface (326).

AQuify Lens Drops (CIBA Vision) is a long-lasting comfort drop containing sodium hyaluronate, sodium chloride, sodium phosphate, and sodium perborate stabilized with phosphoric acid as a preservative (327). It is specially formulated to lubricate and moisten lenses to provide relief from dryness and irritation (327,328). Table 19.7 lists the lubricants and wetting solutions currently available.

Some other products occasionally used for lubricating

TABLE 19.7. LUBRICANTS AND WETTING SOLUTIONS

Product (Manufacturer)	Preservatives	Other Ingredients
AQuify Lens Drops (CIBA Vision)	Sodium perborate	Sodium hyaluronate, sodium chloride, sodium phosphate, phosphoric acid
CIBA Vision Lens Drops (CIBA Vision)	Sorbic acid 0.15%, edetate disodium 0.2%	Sodium chloride, borate buffer, CIBA E.A. (carbamide), poloxamer 407
Clear Eyes CLR (Ross)	Sorbic acid 0.25%, edetate disodium 0.1%	Borate, sodium chloride, hydroxypropyl methylcellulose, glycerin
Clerz Plus Lens Drops (Alcon)	Polyquad (polyquaternium-1) 0.001%, edetate disodium 0.05%	Citrate/borate buffer, sodium chloride, RLM-100 (PEG-11 lauryl ether carboxylic acid), Tetronic 1304
Complete Blink-N-Clean (Advanced Medical Optics)	Polyhexamethylene biguanide 0.0001%, edetate disodium	Sodium chloride, tromethamine, hydroxypropyl methylcellulose, tyloxapol
Complete Lubricating and Rewetting Drops (Advanced Medical Optics)	Polyhexamethylene biguanide 0.0001%, edetate disodium	Sodium chloride, tromethamine, hydroxypropyl methylcellulose, tyloxapol
Focus Lens Drops (CIBA Vision)	Sorbic acid 0.15%, edetate disodium 0.2%	Sodium chloride, borate buffer, OxyGentle (carbamide), LubriClens (polyoxyethylene/polyoxypropylene block copolymer)
Lens Plus Rewetting Drops (Advanced Medical Optics)	—	Sodium chloride, boric acid
Opti-Free Express Rewetting Drops (Alcon)	Polyquad (polyquaternium-1) 0.001%, edetate disodium 0.05%	Citrate buffer, sodium chloride
Opti-One Rewetting Drops (Alcon)	Edetate disodium 0.1%, Polyquad (polyquaternium) 0.01%	Citrate buffer, sodium chloride
Refresh Contacts (Allergan Optical)	Purite (stabilized oxychloro complex) 0.005%	Carboxymethylcellulose sodium, sodium chloride, boric acid, potassium chloride, calcium chloride
Refresh Contacts for Sensitive Eyes (Allergan Optical)	—	Carboxymethylcellulose sodium, sodium chloride, boric acid, potassium chloride, calcium chloride
ReNu MultiPlus Lubricating and Rewetting Drops (Bausch & Lomb)	Edetate disodium 0.1%, sorbic acid 0.1%	Povidone, boric acid, potassium chloride, sodium borate, sodium chloride
ReNu Preservative Free Lubricating and Rewetting Drops (Bausch & Lomb)		Borate buffer, bendazac lysine 0.25%, hydroxypropyl methylcellulose 0.25%, potassium chloride
ReNu Rewetting Drops (Bausch & Lomb)	Sorbic acid 0.15%, edetate disodium 0.1%	Boric acid, sodium borate, sodium chloride, poloxamine
Sensitive Eyes Drops (Bausch & Lomb)	Sorbic acid 0.1%, edetate disodium 0.025%	Boric acid, sodium borate, sodium chloride
Visine for Contacts (Pfizer)	Potassium sorbate, edetate disodium	Borate buffer, hydroxypropyl methylcellulose, glycerin

and rewetting hydrogel lenses have not been approved by the FDA for this indication. These include artificial tears or vitamin A preparations. Also, hypertonic saline has been used in an attempt to increase the duration of the improved comfort response (329). Because of the potential for ocular infection, only sterile solutions should be instilled directly into the eye.

CLINICAL PEARLS OF HYDROGEL LENS CARE

Diagnosis of Solution Sensitivities

Between 50% and 75% of patients who wear contact lenses have some symptoms or complaints of dryness (330,331). It has been reported that one of four patients must modify the wearing schedule because of dryness-related symptoms (332). Lens-wearing discomfort can occur for a number of reasons, one of which is sensitivity to a lens care solution.

The earliest chemical disinfection systems contained chlorhexidine and thimerosal as preservatives. These agents had excellent antimicrobial efficacy, but in some cases their use led to both acute and delayed hypersensitivity responses (332). Patients suffering from solution-related problems often presented with symptoms of dryness or irritation. Diagnosing the problem was relatively simple, because ocular manifestations of such reactions typically included obvious clinical signs, such as conjunctival injection, diffuse punctate keratitis, subepithelial infiltrates, and superior limbic keratitis (332). In the mid 1980s, newer solutions containing derivatives of chlorhexidine and other ingredients were released onto the market. Subsequently, surfactant cleaners were added to many disinfectant formulas, resulting in the so-called multipurpose disinfection systems of today (332). Use of the newer formulas has greatly decreased the number of clinical signs of solution sensitivity, but it also has created new diagnostic challenges for the practitioner.

When a contact lens wearer presents with dryness symptoms, solution sensitivity is one of the entities that must be considered in the differential diagnosis. Some of today's solutions have been shown to have cytotoxic potential (333, 334), but resulting inflammatory responses may be too subtle to detect in a biomicroscope examination. Certain MPSs have been shown to cause dry eye-type symptoms that result in a gradual decrease in wearing time (317). The name *multipurpose nonkeratitis* has been coined to describe the condition in which ocular symptoms of dryness develop during soft contact lens wear but no slit-lamp evidence of dryness is observed and a dry eye workup fails to detect abnormalities (265,332).

There are several options for addressing such symptoms. One is to switch the patient to a hydrogen peroxide system for a period of at least 10 days in order to determine whether symptoms improve (331). If symptoms abate, the diagnosis is confirmed. Comfort can be maintained by continuing with the hydrogen peroxide regimen or by trying other methods of chemical-free disinfection, such as heat and UV disinfection (269,331,333,335,336). Another suggested treatment is to remove the patient from solution exposure altogether by refitting to single-use disposable lenses (153, 331,336,337).

New lens wearers prone to dryness symptoms may be identified before being fit through the use of dry eye questionnaires (330,338). Those who are determined to be likely to suffer from symptoms can be started on a preservative-free care system at their initial dispensing or with single-use disposable lenses (153,331,336,337,339), thereby helping to increase the likelihood of successful lens wear.

Continuous Wear Care

The advent of silicone hydrogel contact lenses for up to 30 nights of continuous wear opens a new chapter in soft contact lenses. These new lens products are discussed in Chapter 37. However, not every patient will wear the lenses for the entire wearing period, thus necessitating lens care (340). If lens removal is due to ocular irritation, it is extremely important that the patient cleans and disinfects the lens prior to reinsertion, because physical irritation may cause a break in the corneal epithelium, thus increasing the risk of infection. It has been suggested that it may be preferable for the lenses not to be reinserted until the following morning (340). Because continuous wear patients are less likely to use large quantities of solution, they should be encouraged to purchase smaller bottle sizes and to replace the solution by its expiration date or at least annually (340). For those who take off their lenses only for cleaning, it is recom-

mended that the lenses also be disinfected before reinsertion, because contamination can occur during lens handling (28, 130,131,137). QuickCare (CIBA Vision) and SOLO-care (CIBA Vision) have been suggested as suitable options for this purpose, because they clean and disinfect in a matter of 5 minutes (340). The PuriLens Contact Lens Care System (PuriLens), which cleans and disinfects in 15 minutes, also has been suggested as an appropriate method of disinfection for this type of patient. The caveat with this system is that it must use nonpreserved solution, which should be discarded soon after opening. This may make it impractical for the intermittent use with continuous wear (340). Patients who wear silicone hydrogel lenses on a daily wear basis need to clean and disinfect their lenses after each removal according to the package inserts. Night & Day (CIBA Vision) lenses are compatible with all lens care systems. Pure Vision (Bausch & Lomb) lenses should not be used with Advanced Medical Optics's Ultracare hydrogen peroxide system or any of its components (341).

One author reported dense, coarse, diffuse superficial punctate staining in three patients who wore PureVision (Bausch & Lomb) silicone hydrogel lenses and used ReNu Multi-Purpose (Bausch & Lomb) (342). Another investigator reported a different staining pattern with daily wear of PureVision (Bausch & Lomb) lenses when they were disinfected with ReNu MultiPlus (Bausch & Lomb) (343). When staining was observed, it was invariably asymmetric: the center of the cornea was spared and the severity increased toward the periphery, resulting in circumferential staining (343). The staining was superficial, fairly dense, and cleared rapidly upon discontinuation of lens wear (343). Bausch & Lomb indicates that neither the clinical data nor the surveillance data available support the findings reported (344). One study used a double-masked, randomized, cross-over experimental design comparing subjective symptoms and signs in a group of 50 subjects wearing PureVision (Bausch & Lomb) silicone hydrogel lenses on a daily wear basis for two consecutive 1-month periods (345). During this time, the subjects used either Opti-Free Express (Alcon) or ReNu MultiPlus (Bausch & Lomb). Significant levels of relatively asymptomatic corneal staining were observed in subjects who used ReNu MultiPlus, with 37% of subjects demonstrating a level of staining consistent with a classic solution-based toxicity reaction. Only 2% of the subjects exhibited staining with Opti-Free Express. The researchers concluded that practitioners who fit silicone hydrogel contact lenses on a daily wear basis should be wary of the potential for certain polyaminopropyl biguanide (PHMB)-containing multipurpose care systems to invoke corneal staining. Even when used on a daily wear basis, silicone hydrogel lenses should be replaced every 30 days (341,346).

Lens Storage

If lenses are stored for prolonged periods, the storage solution should be replaced at regular intervals according to the recommendation of the solution manufacturer. In addition, it is essential that lenses be cleaned and disinfected immediately before reinitiating contact lens wear (18).

A direct antimicrobial evaluation over 28 days compared several soft lens solutions labeled for storage (137). The test solutions included three salines and a disinfectant solution: ReNu Saline (Bausch & Lomb), SoftWear Saline (CIBA Vision), Sensitive Eyes Saline (Bausch & Lomb), and Opti-Free Disinfecting Solution (Alcon). Results showed that the solutions varied greatly in their microbicidal activities against contaminants during storage. ReNu Saline, Soft-Wear Saline, and Opti-Free Disinfecting Solution showed short-term (1-week) storage properties superior to Sensitive Eyes Saline with respect to bacterial and yeast contaminants (137). SoftWear Saline provided markedly superior protection against fungal spores during long-term (2- to 4-week) storage (137). Another evaluation also revealed that chemical disinfectants retarded microbial growth, even after multiple recontamination (163). Storage in neutralized, nonpreserved hydrogen peroxide solution is not recommended for greater than 24 hours due to the risk of microbial regrowth (163). An exception to this is AOSEPT Clear Care (CIBA Vision), which has been approved to store contact lenses for up to 7 days following disinfection (237).

Multiple Pair Care

When advising patients how to care for their lenses, the contact lens practitioner usually follows the manufacturer's instructions for a given care regimen, but there is often no specific mention of care for multiple pairs of lenses. With the introduction of tinted lenses, it is not uncommon for patients to have two or three different pairs of colored lenses to complement their cosmetic wardrobe. Patients with spare pairs of lenses should follow certain procedures to safeguard against possible problems. Recommendations include cleaning and disinfecting the lenses immediately on removal, keeping lenses tightly sealed in the case, storing the case in the refrigerator, repeating the entire cleaning and disinfection procedure at least once a week, and repeating the cleaning and disinfection procedure within 24 hours of reapplication of lenses.

One additional caveat pertaining to spare pair care concerns the lens cases used. If a patient is using clear cases, it is easier to note which lenses (clear, green, or blue) are in a given case simply by looking through the clear plastic. However, if a patient is using identical opaque cases, it may be difficult to remember which lenses are in each case. In this situation, it is advantageous to use a permanent-ink marking pen to indicate on the top or bottom of the case which lenses (lens color) are stored within. This allows the case to remain tightly sealed at all times. Patients must be made aware of the fact that contamination can occur and that special procedures such as those described must be used when caring for multiple pairs of lenses.

Disposable Lens/Frequent Replacement Lens Care

Currently, the most popularly fit soft contact lenses fall into either the disposable or frequent replacement categories (151). These lenses are prescribed most often on a daily wear basis along with daily disinfection. Sometimes a simplified care regimen, without lens cleaning and rinsing, has been advocated for disposable and frequent replacement contact lenses in an attempt to improve patient compliance (312,347). This type of deviation from the product's package labeling is not advised if the solution is labeled with a rub or rinse step included. As previously discussed, the surfactant cleaning and rinsing steps are integral parts of the disinfection system. This is especially true when performing lens care with disinfectants that have low or questionable efficacy. There has been a report of three cases of *Pseudomonas* corneal ulceration occurring in patients who wore disposable lenses on a daily wear basis and practiced questionable lens care maintenance (347). A case-controlled study was performed in the United Kingdom to evaluate disposable lens use as a risk factor for microbial keratitis (348). Significant factors identified included "occasional" overnight use, use of a chloride-based disinfection system, poor storage case hygiene, and irregular disinfection (348). Other factors thought to be of significance in the development of ulcers include omission of cleaning, omission of the rub-and-rinse step, use of a disinfecting solution with marginal efficacy, use of a lens that attracts and rapidly deposits protein, and patient noncompliance (347).

MPSs approved with a "no-rub" indication still require a rinse step in order to adequately clean and disinfect the lenses. Directions for the various no-rub formulations differ. Some require a prerinse as well as a postrinse, and the actual rinse times vary significantly among brands (57).

For these reasons, it is important to educate patients on proper lens care and the use of a specific care system. Although the solutions in common use are designed for convenience, it is still essential to follow the cleaning, rinsing, and disinfecting guidelines for all care systems. Many systems are available for use with disposable/frequent replacement contact lenses. The key to success, however, is patient education and compliance.

In addition, lens case contamination can occur within short periods of time and serve to contaminate new, fresh lenses (349); therefore, even frequent replacement and disposable lenses need frequent replacement of lens storage cases.

In-Office Disinfection of Diagnostic Lenses

One of the most difficult clinical issues confronting the contact lens practitioner is the disinfection of trial or diagnostic lenses. Industry recommendations always have been to redisinfect open trial lenses on a periodic basis to prevent microbial growth of any contamination that may be present. One manufacturer has advised weekly redisinfection (350); however, little additional information is available in the literature.

Several years ago, different guidelines for in-office disinfection of hydrogel contact lenses were issued (351). These include the following:

1. The hands should be washed before lens handling occurs.

2. Mechanical cleaning with a surfactant cleaner should be conducted immediately after use.

3. Heat or cold (peroxide and nonperoxide) disinfection with an approved system should be completed immediately after the cleaning procedure.

4. All opened lenses should be redisinfected every 90 days.

5. Only new, factory-sealed lenses should be dispensed directly to patients.

A tracking system using three different colored dot stickers has been described (352). Once a month, all lenses with a certain color dot can be recleaned and redisinfected. In this way, each opened lens is cleaned and disinfected once every 3 months.

A combined prospective and retrospective study was conducted to evaluate the efficacy of in-office disinfection methods for hydrogel trial lenses (353). Two hundred twenty-one diagnostic lenses from seven test centers disinfected by four different disinfection regimens were collected and cultured for microbial contamination. After various storage times, a significant difference in the incidence of microbial contamination among the test centers for all storage times was found. Contamination of trial lenses in test centers using thermal disinfection with preserved SoftWear Saline (CIBA Vision) was negative, and thermal disinfection with nonpreserved Lens Plus Aerosol Saline (Advanced Medical Optics) was 8.7%. Lens contamination in test centers using chemical disinfection was significantly greater, with a rate of 13.6% with Dymed-preserved ReNu Multi-Purpose Solution (Bausch & Lomb) and 40.7% with Polyquad-preserved Opti-Free (Alcon). The degree of contamination encountered ranged from 10 to greater than 10 million CFU per milliliter of solution. As a result, it is suggested that all inventory trial lenses be disinfected at least once a month to minimize the risk of patient infection (353). In addition, for practitioners who choose to use chemical disinfection, it is recommended that trial lens vials be cultured periodically to monitor the system's efficacy (353).

Historically, the most common method used for in-office disinfection of trial lenses has been heat disinfection. Heat usually is acceptable for low-water-content materials. However, it is known that high-water-content lenses cannot routinely undergo repeated heat disinfection cycles (4,7,200); therefore, most practitioners use one of the chemical meth-ods for higher-water-content lenses (354). A number of practitioners use hydrogen peroxide for in-office disinfection of high-water content contact lenses because of the efficacy concerns previously mentioned. The procedure is conducted directly in the lens vial with any of the two-step peroxide systems that contain a preservative in the neutralizing solution. The reason is to make certain that lenses are stored in a preserved environment so that microbial growth would be minimized in the event of any contamination (163,355).

Additional methods may become available in the future. Microwave and UV radiation have been proposed as promising methods for in-office disinfection of lenses (263,264, 266–268,353).

Lens Case Care

A high degree of contamination of lens cases, which can lead to subsequent ocular infection, has been demonstrated (36,72,95,110,278,300,356–360). Contact lens wearers with eye infections are often found to have lens cases that are contaminated with the same organism as is involved in the eye infection. Regardless of the patient's reported level of compliance, the infecting agent usually is found as a contaminant in the patient's contact lens case and often is accompanied by other organisms (349). In one study, 43% (26/61) of lens cases were contaminated in asymptomatic patients who had worn hydrogel lenses for longer than 6 months (72). A breakdown by type of lens disinfection method revealed contamination in 32% (8/25) using heat disinfection, 44% (7/16) using chemical disinfection, and 44% (7/16) using hydrogen peroxide disinfection. All four cases in which no disinfection was used were contaminated. However, another study that evaluated lens cases from patients who had used the solution for at least 1 month found that lens cases from patients using peroxide-neutralizer systems tended toward heavier contamination (31.8%) than cases disinfected with a chemical system (20.3%) (163).

Other studies have shown a varying incidence of contaminated lens cases in the absence of any signs of ocular infection (43,72,130,349,361–365). The most frequently cited source of contamination of the lens case is the patient's own fingers (130). One evaluation found the degree of case contamination to be quite variable among patients, with a range of organisms from 0 to 10^4, even with carefully supervised hand washing as part of the lens removal protocol (349). Another source reports levels of microbial contamination of 10^8 CFU per milliliter and above (38). A prospective single-masked clinical study analyzed the microbial contamination of the overnight storage solution and biofilm in contact lens cases of patients who used either AOSEPT (CIBA Vision), ReNu (Bausch & Lomb), or Opti-Free (Alcon) lens care systems for 6 weeks (349). Results showed that after 6 weeks, the chemical systems had a significantly higher solution contamination level and a greater case wall biofilm formation than the peroxide system (349). The incidence of microbial contamination ranged from 0% to 85%, depending on the number of weeks of case usage and the disinfection system used (349). Further, there was a wide variance in the level of contamination among subjects. Another study showed that cases with contamination noted one week did not necessarily show it the next week or *vice versa* (304). In addition, the percentage of contaminated cases increased over a 6-week period from 30% at week 1 to 67% at week 6. Further, it has been suggested that case contamination can increase to an even higher level if patients become noncompliant by omitting lens cleaning or decreasing soak time in the storage solution (349).

The bacterial contamination rate of contact lens cases in different care systems was investigated and a comparison was made between hydrogen peroxide and chemical disinfection systems (364). Contact lens cases were collected from 39 hydrogen peroxide care system users and 14 chemical disinfection system users. The total contamination rate of all case samples was found to be 19% (10/53). Of the samples that were contaminated, 80% (8/10) were found to be positive for *P. aeruginosa.* There was no difference in contamination rate between the hydrogen peroxide and chemical disinfection systems. In another clinical evaluation, 42% of patients had bacteria growing in their contact lens cases even after having properly performed their disinfecting procedure (347). The bacteria most frequently isolated was the coagulase-negative staphylococcal organism. It is postulated that the bacteria present in contact lens cases are different from laboratory bacteria in that they protect themselves from the hostile environment of the case by living in a glycocalyx-protected biofilm, which is resistant to disinfecting procedures (363,366). A lens case contaminated with bacteria is an excellent growth medium for *Acanthamoeba* and favors the formation of trophozoites (298).

Lens cases should be cleaned regularly to prevent a buildup of mucoprotein material, which serves as a good culture medium for microbial growth. The best method for case cleaning was evaluated by inoculating lens storage cases with *P. aeruginosa* (367). Rinsing with hydrogen peroxide was the most effective (99.5%); however, significant residual hydrogen peroxide was detected in the case. Rinsing with hot water and air drying was the next most effective (94.7%). This suggests that regular case replacement and hot water rinsing with air drying is the most effective method for case cleaning. However, the risk of using water was not addressed in this study. In addition, the effectiveness of a chemical solution was not evaluated. In lieu of current knowledge regarding *Acanthamoeba,* manufacturers have changed product labeling, advising against rinsing with tap water. It is more appropriate to rinse the case thoroughly with sterile saline solution or with disinfecting solution on a daily basis and then allow the case to air dry. Other recommendations would be to boil the case once a week for a minimum of 10 minutes (131,364,368), shake the case or turn it upside down for a given amount of time (e.g., 60 seconds) (364), or heat the case with a hair dryer for at least 1 minute (364). In light of the evidence that a large number of lens cases are contaminated, patients must be educated regarding proper case hygiene. Lens cases should be examined at each visit. Certainly, all cases should be regarded as disposable items with a limited lifetime. Recommendations to replace the case on a minimum of a yearly basis would be prudent (369).

CIBA Vision supplies new lens cases with all SOLOcare Plus, QuickCare, AOSEPT Clear Care, and Pure Eyes products. By including a new lens case with every retail-sized bottle, it is a convenient and easy way for patients to remember to replace their lens cases often. This practice discourages overusing old, potentially contaminated lens cases. In the future, more frequent replacement and disposable lens cases may serve to decrease the potential for secondary ocular infection (18,242).

Solution Shelf Life

Lens care products are developed and tested in accordance with the standards set forth by the FDA and other regulatory bodies. Solution stability and sterility are among the many attributes that are evaluated. However, with any product, inappropriate use can result in contamination of the solution. In addition, a relationship between the etiologic agents isolated from ocular infections and those isolated from contaminated lens care solutions has been reported (370). Preventative measures include not touching the tip of the bottle to the hands, lens, or eye, and completely closing the bottle when it is not in use (340). Practitioners should routinely remind their patients to discard any solution that is beyond its expiration date (340).

Solution Misuse and Incompatibilities

With a number of solutions available to the contact lens wearer, the temptation is great to pick and choose or mix and match among all of the different products available. Although many contact lens solutions are reasonably compatible with different manufacturers' lenses and lens care products, some are not compatible.

It is important that practitioners, staff members, and patients read and follow manufacturers' directions for care products. All manufacturers adequately test for lens and eye compatibility with their recommended care regimens. However, with all of the solutions available, there is not adequate time or resources to allow for compatibility studies among all the different companies' products. Consequently, some incompatibilities do exist. Incompatibilities have been reported and usually are not severe enough to cause serious injury or damage to an eye, but often they may result in a nonusable lens. Examples of potential complications and incompatibilities reportedly associated with hydrogel contact lens care products are listed in Table 19.8.

Medication Interactions

Some systemic medications are excreted into the tears and may interact with soft contact lenses and the cornea (371, 372). Yellow to orange lens discoloration has been documented with certain drugs. Other medications used systemically also are suspected of causing undesired lens-related difficulties. Table 19.9 provides a listing of systemic drugs that have been reported as causing corneal and/or contact lens complications.

Cost of Lens Care

Practitioners and their staffs need to be aware of local solutions costs and the role that they may play in patient compliance. Annual costs of solutions can vary significantly. Prices differ from brand to brand, from retailer to retailer, and from one geographic region to another (316). Rapidly rising sales of private-label solutions suggest that certain patients may be price conscious in purchasing lens care products (166). Failure to adhere to a prescribed system, or to report problems that may arise as a result of changing solutions, can lead to adverse ocular consequences and, perhaps paradoxically, to greater expense for the patient. A patient in one reported case concluded that the annual cost of artificial tears used to ease her discomfort from a solution sensitivity was more than three times the annual cost of the solution itself (317).

Compliance

Ensuring compliance with a care regimen is one of the major challenges facing today's practitioner. The risk of corneal infection has been reported to be up to approximately 80 times greater for contact lens wearers versus non-contact lens wearers (219). Failure to adhere to prescribed lens care procedures can lead to a broad range of complications, ranging from mild symptoms of reduced vision and comfort to severe signs of infection and inflammation (219,348,373, 374). In the worst case scenario, improper lens care can result in sight-threatening consequences (150).

A number of surveys and studies indicate that 32% to 80% of patients do not care for their lenses in the manner prescribed by their practitioner or the solution manufacturer (11,95,104,110,132,143–147,150,151,375,376). Growing sales of private-label lens care products provide further evidence that patients are departing from practitioner recommendations and care kits (166). For the contact lens wearer, there are numerous avenues for deviating from a prescribed lens wear and care regimen (377–379). The most common practices associated with noncompliance are inadequate hand and lens case hygiene, overwearing of contact lenses, poor attendance at follow-up visits, omission or incorrect use of a daily cleaner, and other improper uses of solution systems (54,143,151).

Patients more likely to be noncompliant have been described as falling into particular groups (153). These include younger patients, long-time lens wearers, wearers who are refitted, extended wear patients, and patients who wear lenses for cosmetic rather than therapeutic purposes. Understanding why patients fail to follow proper lens care procedures is an important step in the prevention or remediation of behaviors that can have negative consequences for the lens wearer.

One reason for noncompliant behavior stems from inadequate or incomplete patient education regarding a selected solution system (166). Recommendations of practitioners are known to have a marked influence on patients' choices of solutions and their use (151,166), so it is essential that clinicians give patients clear instructions for wearing and caring for their lenses. First-time dispensings can be overwhelming experiences for patients. It is crucial to reinforce proper lens care procedures to the beginner so that improper usage of solutions does not develop into a habit (380). At all dispensing visits, previous and new wearers should receive a complete demonstration or explanation of their care system. It is important to note that patients who receive a complete demonstration of their recommended system have been shown to be among the least likely to change brands of solution (166).

Patient compliance also appears to improve when emphasis is placed on the interpersonal relationship between doctor and patient, namely, upon the tone of the interaction as well as the reciprocity of communication (381). Practitioners who invite their patients to participate in the decision-making process regarding their own therapy may be more likely to promote the patient's adherence to a care regimen (382). In the case of adolescent patients, practitioners should partner with the parents in the education process. One study evaluated the compliance of adolescent contact lens patients and found that, after 6 months, 85% could correctly identify the purpose of lens care solutions, 90% knew that daily cleaning was necessary, and 96% understood proper lens disinfection (383). These high compliance rates were attributed to the practitioner and the parents taking an active part in patient education, emphasizing the importance of understanding each aspect of lens care.

It has been shown that whereas 72% of practitioners instruct patients to clean contact lenses daily, fewer than 30% explain the potential outcomes of not doing so (384). The patient should be educated as to the importance of specific steps and the consequences of not following instructions. This approach will enhance the likelihood of the patient recognizing the significance of the care regimen and the regularity with which it should be performed (385). Patients are characterized as being much more likely to carry out procedures that will enhance comfort as opposed to

TABLE 19.8. POTENTIAL COMPLICATIONS AND INCOMPATIBILITIES REPORTEDLY ASSOCIATED WITH SOLUTIONS USED WITH SOFT CONTACT LENSES

Complication	Possible Causes
Lens Discoloration	
Mottled gray to black	Reuse of thimerosal-preserved solutions for heat disinfection (5,45)
	Use of thimerosal in lens case with rubber gaskets instead of silicone gaskets (5)
	Soaking of chemically disinfected lens in sorbate-containing solution without first purging (405,406)
Yellow to brown	Use of topical vasoconstrictors (93,407)
	Disinfection or storage of dirty lenses (protein coated) in sorbate-containing solutions (5,408–410)
	Heating of extended wear lenses in sorbate-containing solutions (4,408–410)
	Thermal disinfection of high water ionic lenses (411)
	Smoking (nicotine) (54,339)
Pink to brown	Use of generic hydrogen peroxide (drugstore brand) that contains colorants (203,412)
Yellow to green	Lens insertion too soon after fluorescein application (93)
	Use of products preserved with chlorhexidine (93)
Pink to rust	Reaction of hydrogen peroxide with sorbic acid-preserved saline solution (413,414)
Gray	Touching lenses with acne medication on hands (415)
Dark brown	Use of drops containing epinephrine (416)
Multiple colors (pink, yellow, brown, black, purple)	Switching from chemical disinfection system to hydrogen peroxide (411,417)
Clouding	Use of salt tablets (USP) that are not specifically formulated for soft contact lenses (411,418)
Opaque	Use of chemical disinfectants (e.g., chlorhexidine) in heat system (261,406)
	Switching from chemical disinfection to heat without first purging (405)
	Mixing of chlorhexidine and anionic detergents (5)
	Use of solutions past their expiration dates (406)
	Reaction to certain preservatives (5,54,83)
	Heating a soft lens in a soaking solution with a high-molecular-weight compound such as polyox (7)
	Heating lenses in solutions containing viscosity agents, such as polyvinyl alcohol or hydroxymethyl cellulose (419)
	Heating lenses in solutions containing PVP (261)
Gummy Residue on Lens	Mixing of polyvinyl alcohol and borate-buffered solutions (405,420)
	Heating of high-molecular-weight polymers, chemical disinfectants, surfactants (405,421)
	Using a daily cleaner as a soaking solution (421)
Fine Black Precipitate	Changing from a chemical disinfection system containing chlorhexidine to a hydrogen peroxide care system (417)
Water Insoluble Film/Precipitate	Mixing and matching cationic solutions (i.e., Opti-Soft, Opti-Free, Flexcare, ReNu) with anionic solutions (i.e., various Sensitive Eyes preparations) (411,418)
	Mixing of thimerosal and solutions with benzalkonium chloride (405)
Other Precipitates	pH incompatibilities from solution mixing (pH of eye solutions should typically be between 6.0 and 8.0) (422)
	Mixing of chlorhexidine with bicarbonates, borates, phosphates, or sulfates (5,306)
	Mixing a hydrogen peroxide neutralizer containing sodium thiosulfate with a neutralizer containing sorbate in the same lens case (418)
Fading of Tinted Lenses	Use of distilled water or tap water that contains chlorine (73,83), or chlorinated swimming pool water (339)
	Incomplete hand washing after use of acne preparations that contain benzoyl peroxide (83,339,423)
Incompatibility with Silicone Hydrogel Lenses	UltraCare (Advanced Medical Optics) system should not be used with Bausch & Lomb PureVision (balafilcon A) lenses (340)
Other Incompatibilities	Hydrogen peroxide incompatible with alkalis, ammonium carbonate, mercurous salts, organics (424)
	Generic hydrogen peroxide possibly contaminated by heavy metal: may have too low a pH and/or altered hydrogen peroxide concentration (5,83)
	Thimerosal degraded by hydrogen peroxide and heat (5)
	Borate buffer incompatible with alkali carbonates, acids, alkaloidal and metallic salts (424)
	Mixing and matching of solutions from different manufacturers could alter stability and chemical efficacy of the product (83)
	Mixing and matching of other chemical disinfecting solutions with chlorhexidine may cause the chlorhexidine to precipitate out of the solution and lose its effectiveness (417)
	Use of soaking solutions with alkyltriethanol ammonium chloride not recommended for lenses with >40% water content or for lenses made from silicone elastomers (7)

(continued)

TABLE 19.8. Continued

Complication	Possible Causes
Other Incompatibilities *(continued)*	Subtilisin enzyme tablets formulated for use in a heat disinfection case are not compatible with lenses made from glyceryl methacrylate (CSI) (79)
	Inability of certain contact lens case materials to withstand boiling (368)
	Papain-containing enzymatic cleaners not compatible with hydrogen peroxide used as the diluent (6,85)
	Polyquad-preserved borate-buffered solutions not recommended with ionic lenses of >50% water content (83,171)
	Polyquad-preserved solutions not compatible with solutions containing sorbic acid (83)
	Use of liquid hydrogen peroxide neutralizers in a case with a catalytic disc may gum up the disc (417)
Changes in Lens Parameters	Soaking of lenses that contain methacrylic acid (group IV) high water content for long periods of time in hydrogen peroxide causes transient effect, reversible with re-equilibration in neutralizer/saline solution (206,209)
	Heating lenses in chemical disinfectants causes permanent change (7,261)
	Substitution of traditional 3% hydrogen peroxide for AOSEPT Disinfection Solution (3% H_2O_2 + 0.85% NaCl) in a case with a platinum AODISC Neutralizer (417)
	Soaking lenses in cleaners with isopropyl alcohol (417)
Red Eye	Sensitivity to preservatives (3–5,83)
	Mixing of sorbate or chlorhexidine with quaternary ammonium compound (83)
	Mixing and matching of cold disinfection systems, particularly if one system contains chlorhexidine (83)
Corneal Staining	Mixing of thimerosal- and chlorhexidine-preserved solutions with those containing alkyltriethanol ammonium chloride (425)
	Use of thimerosal-preserved products in patients on tetracycline therapy (426)
	Use of alkyltriethanol ammonium chloride-preserved solution with glyceryl methacrylate lenses (CSI) (427)
	Use of OptiSoft solution with glyceryl methacrylate lenses (CSI) (176)
	Insufficient rinsing of lens cleaner (4,6,44,45)
	Insufficient removal of enzymatic cleaner (10,82,83)
	Storage of lenses in solution containing benzalkonium chloride (44,124,419)
	Failure to neutralize hydrogen peroxide before lens insertion (203,222,223)
	Use of ReNu Multi-Purpose Solution with silicone hydrogel lenses (342–345)
Perilimbal Conjunctival Injection and Corneal Edema	Mixing of Polyquad-preserved solutions and other disinfecting agents especially chlorhexidine (428)
Pseudodendrites	Toxic/hypersensitivity reaction to chemical disinfection compounds or corneal hypoxia (429–431)
Corneal "Pigmentation"	Swirl-shaped, reddish-brown pattern in central cornea; reported in patients using multipurpose chemical disinfection solutions (432–435)
Corneal Infiltrates	Use of certain chemical disinfection solutions (158,436,437)
Burning and Stinging	Insufficient rinsing of lens cleaner (4,6,44,45)
	Insufficient removal of enzymatic cleaner (10,80,83)
	Intolerance to buffering agents (114)
	Use of nonbuffered solutions (71,118,120)
	Use of solutions with pH <6.6 or >7.8 (420)
	Instillation into the eye of solutions with improper tonicity (124)
	Direct instillation into the eye of 3% hydrogen peroxide (189,226)
	Inadequate neutralization of hydrogen peroxide where ppm concentration is greater than the threshold level (220,221)
	Mixing H_2O_2 neutralizers of different peroxide systems in the same case (418)
Dry Spots	Use of chlorhexidine-preserved products (48,83)
Dry Eye Symptoms	Use of multipurpose solutions (MPS nonkeratitis) (265,269,331–333,335–337)

MPS, multipurpose solution.
Adapted from Lowther G, Shannon BJ, Weisbarth RE. *The pharmacist's guide to contact lenses and lens care.* CIBA Vision Corp., 1988.

safety (153). Thus, adverse outcomes described in terms such as "scratchiness" or "irritation" (symptoms a patient would wish to avoid) may be more effective than those referred to as an "infection" or "inflammation" (perceived as unlikely occurrences to them) (153).

It is the practitioner's responsibility to be well informed about the properties of solution system components and the steps required for the correct use of each. A small minority of patients may receive inadequate lens care instruction in the practitioner's office due to misinformation inadvertently communicated by the practitioner or staff. For example, it is believed that some clinicians may interpret the "no-rub" labeling of certain multipurpose disinfecting solutions to mean that a lens should be placed directly into solution after removal from the eye (182). In fact, a rinsing cycle replaces the traditional in-the-palm cleaning step of "no-

TABLE 19.9. POSSIBLE SYSTEMIC MEDICATION INTERACTION WITH SOFT CONTACT LENSES

Clinical Findings	Medication
Lens Discoloration	
Yellow to orange (339,371,372,438)	Nitrofurantoin
	Phenazopyridine
	Phenolphthalein
	Resorcinol
	Rifampin
	Rifadin
	Sulfasalazine
	Tetracycline
	Systemic β-blockers
Green (339)	Topical phenylephrine, epinephrine
Gray brown (339,438)	Dopamine
	Tetracycline
	Sulfasalazine
	Laxatives containing phenolphthalein or resorcinol
Brown (339)	
Pink (339)	Tetracycline when used with thimerosal-preserved products
Corneal Staining (426,438)	β-Blockers
	Acetylsalicylic acid (aspirin)
Contact Lens-Related	
Epithelial Irritation (371–372)	Antihypertensives
	Tricyclic antidepressants
Decreased Lens	Antihistamines
Wetting/Comfort (371,372,438)	Belladonnas
	Anticholinergics
	Oral contraceptives
	Conjugated estrogens
	β-Blockers
	Benzodiapines
	Phenothiazines
	Serotonin reuptake inhibitors
	Anticholesterol medications

rub" solutions. In a second example of practitioner misinformation, it was reported in one survey that approximately 15% of brands marketed for 2-week disposable use were recommended for replacement at intervals longer than 2 weeks (151). These cases illustrate the importance of the practitioner's staying current with new developments in the field so that complete and accurate information can be shared with the patient.

Patients who have received a thorough briefing on how to wear and care for their lenses may slip into noncompliant behaviors for a variety of reasons. One of these is cost. Studies have indicated that actual patient expenditures for lens care products are significantly less than theoretical predictions (316,382). Purchases of off-brand products have grown in the past decade, comprising a full one fourth of all soft lens solution sales by the late 1990s (166). These data suggest that patients are deviating from prescribed regimens in order to economize. Another important point to note, however, is that survey findings indicate that patients who are informed that the formula of an off-brand disinfec-

tant is different from that of their regular brand are much less inclined to switch solutions (166). It has been suggested that patients be educated about expected costs associated with proper lens care and maintenance in order to encourage consistent and compliant use (386). A candid discussion may help to accommodate patient needs for both convenience and cost (151).

Convenience is another factor in a patient's failure to comply with a prescribed care regimen. Patients who cannot readily find a recommended solution system in stores may opt on their own to purchase a more available system. Practitioners should be aware of the availability of solutions in their area and use this information as one factor in determining the appropriate solution system for their patients. One way of addressing this issue is for the practitioner to package solutions in bulk 3- to 4-month supplies for the convenience of the patient (387). An additional instance of noncompliance may occur when family members who have been assigned different solutions choose instead to purchase one brand for the entire household for the sake of convenience. It is useful for the clinician to inquire about solutions used by other family members when preparing to prescribe a regimen for a new contact lens-wearing patient. If the practitioner has a specific reason for choosing a different system, that reason should be communicated to the patient.

The patient's correct use of solutions should be monitored and reinforced at follow-up visits. A good approach to doing this is to request that the patient demonstrate the steps in the prescribed care regimen while explaining which solution is used for each (388,389). Open-ended inquiries should be used (for example, "Show me what you do with your lenses after taking them out.") rather than leading questions ("Do you rinse your lenses with solution before storing them in your case?"). Other strategies for encouraging compliance include written instructions (151); appointment reminders such as calendars, recall cards, telephone reminders, and stickers; and patient support programs that involve family members, support groups, reward systems, or frequent user awards (382). In addition, practitioners should routinely remind patients to discard old solutions or those beyond their expiration date, whenever the patients are in for a follow-up examination or lens purchase (340). Lastly, patients should always be encouraged to use the specific brand of solution recommended. Differences in performance of solutions labeled as having the same contents or with slight differences in formulation can occur from one patient to another (199,370).

Ensuring patient compliance is an ongoing challenge for practitioners, but it has been shown that practitioners who use vigorous efforts to improve patient compliance have greater levels of patient cooperation (385).

Patient Education

The importance of comprehensive patient education cannot be emphasized enough, especially because noncompliance can result in ocular complications. Patient education regarding the wear and care of contact lenses should follow four guidelines (381): (i) the patient should be able to understand the terminology the practitioner or staff member uses; (ii) information should be specific and to the point; (iii) the most important information should be presented at the beginning; and (iv) the practitioner should ask the patient to provide an overview of the information learned. The education should include a thorough review of the advantages and limitations of hydrogel lenses. All potential misconceptions regarding the nature of the lenses and their care need to be addressed. This discussion should be conducted in a relaxed fashion to provide reassurance before the actual education in the application and removal techniques and lens care procedures. Even with clear instructions, patients may alter their wear and care regimen (151); therefore, clear instructions should be given at the time patients are taught to insert and remove their lenses. These should clearly delineate the wearing, cleaning, and replacement schedule. On each subsequent visit, the wearing schedule, lens replacement frequency, and care regimen should be reviewed with the patient.

Hygiene

Good hygiene must be emphasized from the beginning. Cleanliness is one of the most important aspects of proper contact lens care. Hands always should be washed thoroughly with a mild soap, rinsed completely, and dried with a lint-free towel each time before handling the lenses. Antibacterial soaps have been shown to significantly reduce bacterial contamination (390). However, soaps containing cold creams, lotions, deodorant chemicals, antiseptics, or oily cosmetics should not be used because these substances may be absorbed by the lenses and interfere with successful lens wear (139,391–393). Also, liquid soaps are preferred over bar soaps, which can become contaminated more easily (154). Table 19.10 lists many of the commercial contact lens wearers' soaps currently available.

TABLE 19.10. CONTACT LENS WEARERS' SOAPS AND HYGIENE ACCESSORIES

Eyecare Special Hand Soap (Channel Laboratories, Ltd.)
Eyecare Lint-Free Towels (Channel Laboratories, Ltd.)
Contact Lens Wearers Glycerin Soap (Lobob Laboratories)
Optisoap (Optikem International)
Safe Scrub (Product Development Corporation)
OptiNaps (Professional Supplies)
Shield Optical Hand Soap (Shield Lens Care Products)
Pure & Natural Soap (The Dial Corporation)
Neutrogena (Neutrogena Corporation) (139,439)
Lobob clear glycerin bar soap (Lobob Laboratories) (139)
Ivory bar soap (The Proctor & Gamble Company) (139,439)
Dial bar, Dial pump (The Dial Corporation) (439)
Clear dishwashing detergent (Joy; The Proctor & Gamble Company) (439)

Handling of Lenses

Before handling lenses, the patient should be instructed to close the drain in the sink as a precaution against losing a lens. Inexpensive plastic drain guards can be purchased for this purpose. Patients should be instructed to develop the habit of consistently working with the right lens first to avoid mixing up lenses. Lenses should be handled with the fingertips, and care should be taken to avoid any contact with the fingernails. Fingernails should be short and smooth at all times. Lenses should be removed from the storage case and examined to make sure they are moist, clean, clear, and free of any nicks or tears.

Before its placement on the eye, the lens should be checked to make sure it is not inside-out. This is especially true for ultrathin and plus lenses. This determination can be made by placing the lens on the forefinger and observing its profile. If the lens assumes a natural, curved, bowlike shape, then it is right-side out. If the lens edges appear to point outward, then the lens is inside-out. Another method for determining lens orientation, sometimes referred to as the *taco test,* is performed by gently compressing the lens between the thumb and index finger or in a crease in the palm of the hand. If the edges of the lens are erect and point slightly inward when the lens is flexed, it is in the correct position (Fig. 19.3A). If the edges turn outward,

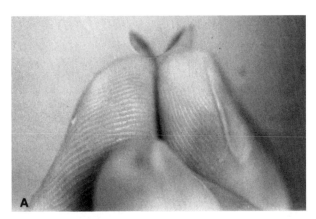

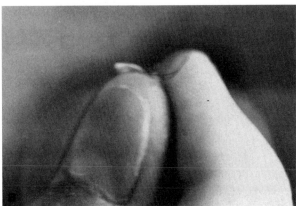

FIG. 19.3. A: Correct orientation of a hydrogel lens using the taco test. **B:** Inverted lens as demonstrated by the taco test.

folding back on the fingers, the lens is inside-out (Fig. 19.3B) and may be uncomfortable if placed on the eye.

Insertion of the Lens

Two different methods can be used for the application of a hydrogel lens. The method of choice varies depending on a number of factors, including patient apprehensiveness, palpebral aperture width, lid tonus, and lens diameter. With either technique, the lens should first be placed on the tip of the index finger. Care should be taken to make sure the index finger is dry, otherwise surface tension from any moisture present may prevent the lens from being transferred from the finger to the eye.

Method 1. After properly washing the hands, the lens should be placed on the tip of the index finger (the right index finger is used for the right lens and the left index finger is used for the left lens). The upper lid is retracted with the middle and index fingers of the opposite hand and the lower lid is depressed with the middle finger of the same hand used to insert the lens. With the patient looking up, the lens is placed on the inferior sclera (Fig. 19.4). The patient should slowly close the lids while changing fixation to a straight ahead gaze and the lens should position on the cornea. With the eye closed, the lids should be massaged to minimize bubble formation under the lens.

Method 2. This technique is identical to the one used for applying a rigid lens. Using the same hand control as in method 1, the lens is applied directly onto the cornea.

If there is an initial sensation of a foreign body, instruct the patient to look nasally and slide the lens off the cornea and onto the temporal bulbar conjunctiva. Next, the patient should look temporally until the lens repositions itself onto the cornea. If discomfort persists, the lens should be re-moved immediately. It should be inspected for debris or tears and reexamined to determine whether it is inside out.

If blurred vision is noted after the lens has been given time to settle, the lens should be removed and checked for the presence of oil or cosmetics. If the lens is clean, and if the patient's prescription is different between the two eyes, he or she may have inserted the lens into the incorrect eye. The patient should try inserting the lens onto the opposite eye to see if the vision becomes clearer.

Lens Removal

Lens removal is quite simple with hydrogel lenses. Once again, different methods can be used. Before lens removal, hands should be thoroughly washed and rinsed. If the lens feels dry, it should be rewetted with sterile saline or rewetting drops before lens removal. A dry lens is fragile and can easily be torn upon removal. The patient should always check to make sure the lens is centered on the cornea before attempting to remove it. A simple check is to monitor the vision in each eye separately before lens removal.

Method 1. With the patient looking up, the lower lid is retracted with the middle finger and the index fingertip is placed on the lower edge of the lens. Next, the lens is slid onto the inferior sclera where it is pinched off the eye with the thumb and index finger of the same hand (Fig. 19.5).

Method 2. With this method, the lens is pinched directly off the cornea with the thumb and forefinger (Fig. 19.6). However, care must be taken that the lens is positioned correctly on the cornea before starting, otherwise an abrasion can occur if removal is attempted.

Wearing Schedule

A wearing schedule can be developed in a fairly rapid fashion because a new wearer usually adapts to lens wear within a week. A representative wearing schedule would be as follows: day 1, 4 hours; day 2, 6 hours; day 3, 8 hours; day 4, 10 hours; day 5, 12 hours; and day 6, all waking hours. The patient should be instructed that the lenses can be removed sooner if they become uncomfortable before the end of a scheduled wearing time. Once lenses are dispensed, it is important for the patient to be evaluated on a regular basis. The contact lenses should be worn for several hours before scheduled follow-up visits. New wearers may need to be specifically reminded to wear their lenses into the office for scheduled appointments.

Lens Care

Instruction on proper use of each step in the lens care regimen is necessary. Clinical experience indicates that patients will follow a regimen more readily if they understand why they should perform specific steps in their lens care regimen

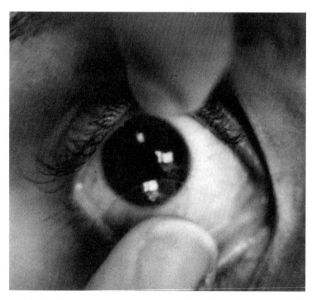

FIG. 19.4. Placement of a hydrogel lens directly onto the eye.

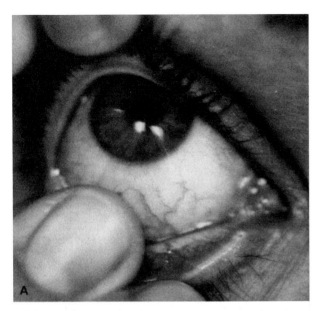

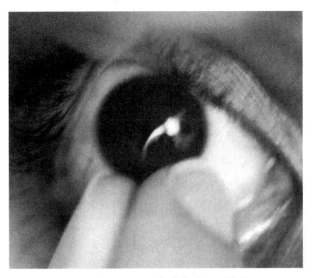

FIG. 19.6. Direct removal of the lens off the eye.

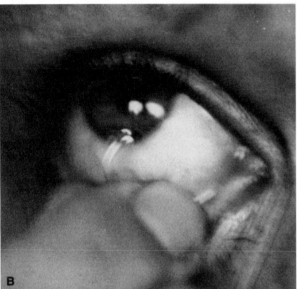

FIG. 19.5. A: Using the forefinger to push the lower lens edge inferiorly. **B:** Removing the lens off of the lower sclera by pinching the lens between the thumb and forefinger.

(318). Education should include advising patients of the following steps (394):

1. Wash hands before lens handling.
2. Clean and rinse lenses after each removal.
3. Use fresh solution in the lens cup/case each day.
4. Clean and/or replace the case periodically.
5. Avoid keeping open bottles of solution for too long.
6. Refrain from using tap water or saliva to moisten lenses
7. Seek immediate care if signs of inflammation or infection develop.

Cosmetics and Contact Lenses

Educating patients about the proper use of cosmetics is of the utmost importance (395). In general, cosmetics should be applied after hydrogel lenses have been applied. Complications can occur as a result of cosmetics coming into contact with the eye (396). Because many commonly used cosmetics contain ingredients such as preservatives, pigments, oils, and solvents, subjective discomfort and other problems can result (397). Cosmetics also can cause lens discoloration, damage, surface deposition, and contamination.

Mascara containing lash builders can cause severe problems (83,398). Such products have nylon or rayon fibers that may flake off into the tear film and cause a corneal abrasion. Waterproof mascara should be avoided as well, because it is difficult to remove with water and may stain contact lenses (399). Using sharp objects to separate lashes should be avoided; an eyelash brush is a safer option. Cosmetics can be a source of bacterial or fungal infection (400–403). A patient may transfer microorganisms from the lashes to the mascara wand and then to the mascara tube, where they colonize. Consequently, mascara and eyeliner should be replaced every 3 to 6 months. Eyeliner should not be applied to the inner lid margin because it could clog the meibomian glands, possibly resulting in a hordeolum, a chalazion, or blepharitis. Frosted, pearlized, iridescent, and other glittery types of eye shadow should be avoided because they contain ground oyster shells or tinsel, which could abrade the cornea (139). Pressed powders applied in small quantities are preferred over oily liquid or cream eye shadows (139). Cosmetic containers should be closed tightly and stored away from heat to help retard bacterial growth (139). Hairspray and other aerosol sprays can be absorbed by a hydrogel lens; these agents are difficult to remove. Using spray products before lens application will prevent this problem. If sprays must be used while lenses are in, the

TABLE 19.11. MANUFACTURERS OFFERING COSMETICS COMPATIBLE WITH CONTACT LENS WEAR

Almay Hypo-allergenic Cosmetics (Almay, Inc.)
Aziza Hypo-allergenic Contact Lens Cosmetics (Aziza)
Eye Society Cosmetics (Caesar Optical, Inc.)
Eye Care Cosmetics (ContraCare, Inc.)
Op-Tic Cosmetics (1 Tech)
For Your Eyes Only (Max Factor)
Eye Contact Cosmetics (Optical Cosmetic Labs)
Optique Cosmetics (Optique)
Physicians Formula Cosmetics (Physicians Formula)

wearer should close the eyes during spraying, then immediately step away from the mist. At the end of the day, lenses should be removed before removing makeup. An oil-free hypoallergenic remover should be used to remove cosmetics.

Numerous cosmetic products recommended for contact lens wearers are available. They contain no fragrances or fillers and are water-soluble. Cosmetics that are labeled "hypoallergenic," "for sensitive eyes," or "for contact lens wearers" are typically free of known irritants (139). Some practitioners dispense these products as part of the patient's care regimen. Table 19.11 lists some of the manufacturers of cosmetics who claim their products are compatible with contact lens wear. *Tyler's Quarterly* also carries a listing of contact lens-compatible makeup (404).

Patient Education Materials

Education can be enhanced by using a variety of approaches. Printed materials are likely the most common method and are available from many contact lens and lens care manufacturers. Supplemental comprehensive printed instructions can be useful but should be written in language that makes it easy for patients to read, understand, and comply with the information presented.

Other means of instructing patients include the use of audio tapes and video tapes. Audio tapes educating patients about proper lens care can be produced professionally in sufficient quantities at a reasonable cost; therefore, they can be provided as a supplement to the instruction materials for all new patients. Excellent video tapes are available from several sources. Instructional lens care video tapes can be obtained from many major corporations, including Advanced Medical Optics, Alcon, Bausch & Lomb, and CIBA Vision Corporation. Videos can be used for in-office or home viewing.

A compliance agreement signed in duplicate by the patient should be provided at dispensing visits. The agreement should indicate that the patient understands that successful contact lens wear is not guaranteed; that he or she knows what solutions must be used; that he or she is aware of the refund and replacement lens policies; and that he or she

agrees to adhere to the recommendations provided. One copy of the form should be kept in the patient's record.

SUMMARY

This chapter reviewed the various clinical and technical aspects of hydrogel lens care regimens and patient education. As hydrogel contact lens materials have advanced, the associated lens care products have grown in complexity. The multitude of products currently available often leads to patient confusion and bewilderment. Resultant improper lens care often interrupts normal lens wear and can lead to sight-threatening ocular infection. The knowledgeable contact lens practitioner can prevent these difficulties by thoroughly instructing patients on the use of lens care products and by regularly verifying continuing patient compliance.

ACKNOWLEDGMENT

The authors acknowledge the assistance of Audrey Manwell, Shannon Harper, and Cheryl Bergin in researching and formatting this chapter.

REFERENCES

1. Liu Y, Xie PY. Quantitative assay of protein deposits on hydrophilic contact lenses treated with ReNu and COMPLETE solutions. *Int Contact Lens Clin* 1999;26:15–20.
2. Bontempo AR, Rapp J. Protein and lipid deposition onto hydrophilic contact lenses in vivo. *CLAO J* 2001;27:75–80.
3. Lowther GE. Soft contact lens care: a review. *Rev Optom* 1982; 119:60–70.
4. Stein HA, Slatt BJ. Care systems for soft lenses. In: *Fitting guide for rigid and soft contact lenses: a practical approach.* St. Louis: CV Mosby, 1984:81–100.
5. Harris JK. Solutions for cleaning, disinfection and storage. In: Aquavella JV, Rao G, eds. *Contact lenses.* Philadelphia: JB Lippincott, 1987:226–262.
6. Mandell RB. Lens handling, care and storage. In: *Contact lens practice,* 4th ed. Springfield, IL: Charles C. Thomas, 1988: 568–597.
7. Morgan JF. Soft contact lens hygiene-clinical experience. In: Dabezies OH Jr, ed. *Contact lenses: the CLAO guide to basic science and clinical practice.* Orlando, FL: Grune & Stratton, 1988:40A.1–40A.19.
8. Rao G. Complications due to daily wear of soft contact lenses. In: Dabezies OH Jr, ed. *Contact lenses: the CLAO guide to basic science and clinical practice.* Orlando, FL: Grune & Stratton, 1984:42.1–42.7.
9. Tripathi RC, Tripathi BJ. Lens spoilage. In: Dabezies OH Jr, ed. *Contact lenses: the CLAO guide to basic science and clinical practice.* Orlando, FL: Grune & Stratton, 1984:45.1–45.35.
10. Wilson MS, Millis E. Contact lens care. In: Wilson MS, Millis E, eds. *Contact lenses in ophthalmology.* London: Butterworth & Co., 1988:20–22.
11. Roth HW. The etiology of ocular irritation in soft lens wearers: distribution in a large clinical sample. *Contact Intraoc Lens Med J* 1978;4:38–46.

12. Allansmith MR, Korb DR, Greiner JV, et al. Giant papillary conjunctivitis in contact lens wearers. *Am J Ophthalmol* 1977; 83:697–708.
13. Josephson JE, Caffery BE. Infiltrative keratitis in hydrogel lens wearers. *Int Contact Lens Clin* 1979;6:223–242.
14. Hill RM. Spoliation and its related implications. *Int Contact Lens Clin* 1981;8:44–46.
15. Hill RM. Nine lives of a gel-lens. *Int Contact Lens Clin* 1981; 8:42–43.
16. Lieblin JS. How important is enzymatic cleaning? An in-office evaluation. *Int Contact Lens Clin* 1979;6:151–153.
17. Fowler SA, Allansmith MR. The effect of cleaning soft contact lenses: a scanning electron microscopic study. *Arch Ophthalmol* 1981;99:1382–1386.
18. Efron N, Henriquez A, Merkx JTM, et al. Contact lens maintenance systems. *Int Contact Lens Clin* 1992;19:153.
19. Randeri KJ, Stark RL, Quintana RP, et al. Cleaning of contact lenses. In: Dabezies OH Jr, ed. *Contact lenses: the CLAO guide to basic science and clinical practice.* Orlando, FL: Grune & Stratton, 1984:30.1–30.9.
20. Lowther GE, Shannon BJ, Weisbarth RE. *The pharmacist's guide to contact lenses and lens care.* Atlanta, GA: CIBA Vision Corporation, 1988
21. Sibley MJ. Cleaning solutions for contact lenses. *Int Contact Lens Clin* 1982;9:291–294.
22. Boost M, Conway R, Shan ECT, et al. The antimicrobial effectiveness of a mechanical soft lens cleaning device. *Int Contact Lens Clin* 1994;21:137.
23. Phillips AJ, Czigler B. Polyclens (Opticlean): a further study. *Aust J Optom* 1985;68:36–39.
24. Fontana FD, Meier GD, Becherer PD. Opti-clean for hydrophilic lenses. *Contact Lens Forum* 1982;7:57–65.
25. Brazeau D, Gross M, Gellatly K, et al. Clinical evaluation of Opti-Free Daily Cleaner. *Contact Lens Spectrum* 1992;7:21.
26. Ghormley NR. MiraFlow: a new soft lens cleaner. *Int Eyecare* 1986;2:602.
27. Josephson JE, Caffery BE. Selecting an appropriate hydrogel lens care system. *J Am Optom Assoc* 1981;52:227–234.
28. Brennan NA, Coles C. Deposits and symptomatology with soft contact lens wear. *Int Contact Lens Clin* 2000;27:75–100.
29. Penley CA, Willis SW, Allen AW. Effects of cleaning and rinsing on the removal of Acanthamoeba from hydrogel lenses. Poster presented at the annual meeting of the American Academy of Optometry, Columbus, Ohio, December 1988.
30. Yamane SJ, Ghormley NR, Childress CW, et al. Miraflow: lens wearing time, visual acuity both increase. *Contact Lens Forum* 1987;65:56–64.
31. Jung J, Rapp J. The efficacy of hydrophilic contact lens cleaning systems in removing protein deposits. *CLAO J* 1993;19:47.
32. Simons PA, Sun CM, Yamamoto BA, et al. Comparison of surfactant cleaning times on protein deposit removal from hydrogel lenses. *Int Contact Lens Clin* 1995;22:16.
33. Shih KL, Hu J, Sibley MH. The microbiological benefit of cleaning and rinsing contact lenses. *Int Contact Lens Clin* 1985; 12:235–248.
34. Houslby RD, Ghajar M, Chavez G. Microbiological evaluation of soft contact lens disinfecting solutions. *J Am Optom Assoc* 1984;55:205–211.
35. Kreiner C. Microbiology and contact lenses. *Contact Lens J* 1978;7:6–18.
36. Hopkins GA. Drugs and solutions used in contact lens practice. *Contact Lens J* 1988;16:161–167.
37. Kaspar H. Binding characteristics and microbiological effectiveness of preservatives. *Aust J Optom* 1976;59:4–9.
38. Ifejika CP, McLaughlin-Borlace L, Lucas VJ, et al. Efficacy of a contact lens cleaning device and its enhancement of the

39. Landa AS, van der Mei HC, van Rij G, et al. Efficacy of ophthalmic solutions to detach adhering Pseudomonas aeruginosa from contact lenses. *Cornea* 1998;17:293–300.
40. FDA matrix guideline (contact lens). In: *Microbiological guidelines.* Silver Springs, MD: Center for Devices and Radiological Health, 1982.
41. Pepose JS. Contact lens disinfection to prevent transmission of viral disease. *CLAO J* 1988;14:165–167.
42. Shovlin JP. Resistant pathogens following disinfection: the significance of contribution of the elements. *Int Contact Lens Clin* 1989;16:126–128.
43. Hom MM, Simmons PA. Current multi-purpose solution concepts. *Contact Lens Spectrum* 2001;16:33–37.
44. Stewart-Jones JH, Hopkins GA, Phillips AT. Drugs and solutions in contact lens practice and related microbiology. In: Stone J. Phillips AJ, eds. *Contact lenses: a textbook for practitioner and student,* 2nd ed. London: Butterworth & Co., 1980:59–90.
45. Wechsler S, George NC. Disinfection of hydrophilic lenses. *J Am Optom Assoc* 1981;52:179–186.
46. Lowther GE. Effectiveness of an enzyme in removing deposits from hydrophilic lenses. *Am J Optom Physiol Opt* 1977;54: 76–84.
47. Hathaway RA, Lowther GE. Soft lens cleaners: their effectiveness in removing deposits. *J Am Optom Assoc* 1978;49:259–266.
48. Gold RM, Orenstein J. Surfactant cleaners vs. the enzyme cleaner. *Contact Lens Forum* 1980;5:39–41.
49. Ghormley NR. Contact lens enzyme cleaners. *Int Contact Lens Clin* 1987;14:384–385.
50. Huizinga L, Lowther GE. Comparison of care systems in cleaning hydrogel lenses. *Int Eyecare* 1986;2:620–624.
51. Karageozian HL, Walden PA, Boghosian MP. Cleaning soft contact lenses. *Int Contact Lens Clin* 1976;3:78–86.
52. Kleist FD, Thorson IC. How effective are soft lens cleaners? *Rev Optom* 1978;115:43–49.
53. Cumming JS, Karageozian H. "Protein" conjunctivitis in hydrophilic lens wearers. *Contact* 1975;19:8–9.
54. Franklin V, Tighe B, Tonge S. Contact lens deposition, discoloration and spoliation mechanisms. *Optician* 2001;222:16–20.
55. Ghormley NR. Soft contact lens cleaning and disinfection system evaluation. *Int Contact Lens Clin* 1987;14:48.
56. Maguen EM. Solutions and care regimens. In: Weinstock F, ed. *Contact lens fitting: a clinical text atlas.* Philadelphia: JB Lippincott, 1989:9.1–9.26.
57. Edrington TB, Barr JT. Keep up to date with changes in soft lens solutions. *Contact Lens Spectrum* 2002;17:46–47.
58. Jones L, Franklin V, Evans K, et al. Spoliation and clinical performance of monthly vs. three monthly group II disposable contact lenses. *Optom Vis Sci* 1996;73:16–21.
59. Maissa C, FranklinV, Guillon M, et al. Influence of contact lens material surface characteristics and replacement frequency on protein and lipid deposition. *Optom Vis Sci* 1998;75: 697–705.
60. Garrett Q, Laycock B, Garrett RW. Hydrogel lens monomer constituents modulate protein sorption. *Invest Ophthalmol Vis Sci* 2000;41:1687–1695.
61. Tsuda S, Tanaka K, Anan N, et al. Analysis of surface deposits and effective countermeasures. *Int Contact Lens Clin* 1981;8: 46–52.
62. Lasswell LA, Tarantino N, Kono D. Enzymatic cleaning of extended wear lenses: papain vs. pancreatin. *Int Contact Lens Clin* 1986;2:101–106.
63. Kotow M, Grant T, Holden BA. Evaluation of current care and maintenance systems for hydrogel extended wear. *Trans Br Contact Lens Assoc Conf* 1986;66–67.

64. Davis RL. Animal vs. plant enzyme. *Int Contact Lens Clin* 1983; 10:277–284.

65. Kjellsen T, Kiral R, Eriksen S. Single-enzyme vs. multi-enzyme contact lens cleaning system: speed and efficiency in removing deposits from hydrogel contact lenses. *Int Contact Lens Clin* 1984;11:660–671.

66. Kurashige LT, Kataoka JE, Edrington T, et al. Protein deposition on hydrogel contact lenses: a comparison study of enzymatic cleaners. *Int Contact Lens Clin* 1987;14:150–159.

67. Kjellsen T, Dziabo A, Kiral R. Enzyme vs. abrasive for removing protein deposits from hydrogel lenses. *Int Contact Lens Clin* 1986;2:579–581.

68. Schachet JL. Alcon's enzyme cleaner: a clinical study. *Contact Lens Forum* 1983;8:67–82.

69. Carmichael C. Safety and efficacy of a new enzyme cleaner. *Int Contact Lens Clin* 1983;10:286.

70. Houlsby RD, Ghajar M, Chavez G. Microbial quality of water used by pharmaceutical manufacturers and soft lens wearers. *Int Contact Lens Clin* 1981;8:9–14.

71. Jenkins C, Phillips Al. How sterile is unpreserved saline? *Clin Exp Optom* 1986;69:131–136.

72. Donzis PB, Mondino BJ, Weissman BA, et al. Microbial contamination of contact lens care systems. *Am J Ophthalmol* 1987; 104:325–333.

73. Liebetreu M, Hammack G, Lowther GE. Effect of chlorine on tinted lenses. *Int Eyecare* 1986;2:525–531.

74. Brazeau D. Preliminary study of the Opti-Tab system on soft colored lenses from Ciba. *Can J Optom* 1989;51:26–27.

75. Ghormley NR. Tinted soft contact lenses: lens care. *Int Contact Lens Clin* 1984;11:262.

76. Package insert for SupraClens Daily Protein Remover (340009-0798). Alcon Laboratories Inc., Fort Worth, Texas.

77. Lowe R, Coles MC, Brennan NA. Two different concentrations of Opti-Plus compared for daily protein cleaning of a disposable contact lens. *Int Contact Lens Clin* 1999;26:66–74.

78. Achieving compliance through new enzymes for contact lens cleaning (SL 7352). In: *Technically Speaking (Bulletin)*. Rochester, NY: Bausch & Lomb Personal Products Division, 1986.

79. Fontana F, Perry D. Coming trends in lens care. *Rev Optom* 1988;125:78–79.

80. Tarantino N, Courtney RL, Lasswell LA, et al. Simultaneous enzymatic cleaning and hydrogen peroxide disinfection of hydrogel lenses. *Int Contact Lens Clin* 1988;15:189–196.

81. Courtney RC, Tarantino N, Stubblefield D. Clinical evaluation of ultrazyme enzymatic cleaner used with AOSept. *Int Contact Lens Clin* 1989;16:40–47.

82. Binder PS, Rasmussen DM, Gordon M. Keratoconjunctivitis and soft contact lens solutions. *Arch Ophthalmol* 1981;99:87–90.

83. Rakow PL. *Contact lenses.* Thorofare, NJ: Charles Slack, 1988: 28–48.

84. Huth SW. Ultrazyme enzymatic cleaner dissolved in hydrogen peroxide: proposed mechanism of enhanced cleaning and disinfection. In: *Allergan Pharmaceutical Report Series 221.* Irvine, CA: Allergan Pharmaceuticals, 1988.

85. Janoff LE. The Septicon disinfection system-separating fact from fiction. *Rev Optom* 1984;12:79–82.

86. Campbell R, Caroline P. A strong case for enzymatic lens care compliance. *Contact Lens Spectrum* 1994;11:56.

87. Begley CG, Paragina S, Sporn A. An analysis of contact lens enzyme cleaners. *J Am Optom Assoc* 1990;61:190.

88. Larcabal JE, Hinrichs CA, Edrington TB, et al. A comparison study of enzymatic cleaners: papain versus subtilisin A. *Int Contact Lens Clin* 1989;16:318.

89. Bournakel G, Cushing G, Rigel L, et al. Normal use comfort comparison of two enzymatic cleaners. *Contact Lens Spectrum* 1990;5:51.

90. Fontana FD. Find the best solution for healthy lens wear. *Rev Optom* 1992;129:43.

91. Sibley MJ. The jungle of available lenses and care systems. *Ophthalmol Clin North Am* 1989;2:203–289.

92. Sibley MJ, Chu V. Nonenzymatic cleaning of protein and lipid from soft contact lenses. *Contact Lens Forum* 1982;7:35–39.

93. Kleist FD. Appearance and nature of hydrophilic contact lens deposits—part I: protein and other organic deposits. *Int Contact Lens Clin* 1979;6:49–59.

94. Shovlin JP, DePaolis MD, Edmonds SA, et al. Acanthamoeba keratitis: contact lenses as a risk factor-case reports and review of the literature. *Int Contact Lens Clin* 1987;14:349–358.

95. Key JE, Mobley CL. Preventing problems with the current care systems. *Ophthalmol Clin North Am* 1989;2:339–350.

96. Auran JD, Starr MB, Jakobiec FA. Acanthamoeba keratitis. *Cornea* 1987;6:2–26.

97. Moore MB, McCulley JP, Newton C, et al. Acanthamoeba keratitis: a growing problem in soft and hard contact lens wearers. *Ophthalmology* 1987;94:1654–1661.

98. Connor CG, Benjamin WJ. Reducing the risk of Acanthamoeba keratitis. *Contact Lens Spectrum* 1986;1:31–39.

99. Hirst LW, Green WR, Merz W, et al. Management of Acanthamoeba keratitis: a case report and review of the literature. *Ophthalmology* 1984;91:1105–1111.

100. Stinson EK. Acanthamoeba keratitis in soft contact lens wearers. *J Ophthalmic Nursing Tech* 1986;5:132–134.

101. Cohen EJ, Buchanan HW, Laughrea PA, et al. Diagnosis and management of Acanthamoeba keratitis. *Am J Ophthalmol* 1985;100:389–395.

102. Moore MB, McCulley JP, Luckenbach M, et al. Acanthamoeba keratitis associated with soft contact lenses. *Am J Ophthalmol* 1985;100:396–403.

103. Acanthamoeba keratitis in soft contact lens wearers. *MMWR CDC Surveill Summ* 1987;36:397–404.

104. Stehr-Green JK, Bailey TM, Brandt FH, et al. Acanthamoeba keratitis in soft contact lens wearers: a case control study. *JAMA* 1987;258:57–60.

105. Edmonds SA. Protecting your patients from Acanthamoeba. *Rev Optom* 1987;124:85–88.

106. Dornic DI, Wolf T, Dillon WH, et al. Acanthamoeba keratitis in soft contact lens wearers. *J Am Optom Assoc* 1987;58:482–486.

107. Acanthamoeba, the current situation (SL-7383). In: *Lens Care Research (Bulletin)*. Rochester, NY: Bausch & Lomb Personal Products Division, 1986.

108. *Acanthamoeba keratitis—CLAO policy statement.* New Orleans, LA: Contact Lens Association of Ophthalmology, 1988.

109. Benjamin WJ. Contact lens-associated Acanthamoeba keratitis. *Int Eyecare* 1986;2:490.

110. Bowden FW, Cohen EJ, Arensten JJ, et al. Patterns of lens care practices and lens product contamination in contact lens associated microbial keratitis. *CLAO J* 1989;15:49–54.

111. Silbert JA. Microbial disease and the contact lens patient. *Int Contact Lens Clin* 1988;15:221–224.

112. Moore MB. Early diagnosis: management of Acanthamoeba patients. *Contact Lens Forum* 1987;12:34–41.

113. Hill RM, Carney LG, Barr JT, et al. Soft lens solutions: a look at what's not on the label. *Contact Lens Spectrum* 1988;3:43–46.

114. Josephson JE, Caffery BE. Exploring the sting. *J Am Optom Assoc* 1987;58:288–289.

115. Hill RM, Carney LG, Barr JT, et al. The boric acid buffer questions. *Contact Lens Spectrum* 1988;3:44–46.

116. Mauger TF, Hill RM. The subtleties of saline. *Contact Lens Forum* 1983;8:104–105.

117. Carney LG, Brezinski SD, Hill RM. The pH question, and some answers. *Contact Lens Spectrum* 1986;1:63–65.
118. Edwards G. Saline pH value: a critical key to soft CL comfort. *Contact Lens Forum* 1986;14:40–42.
119. Hill RM. Salines and their pH problems. *Int Contact Lens Clin* 1991;18:203.
120. Carney LG, Hill RM. Other hydrophilic lens environments: pH. *Am J Optom Physiol Opt* 1976;53:456–458.
121. McCarey BE, Wilson LA. pH, Osmolarity and temperature effects on the water content of hydrogel contact lenses. *Contact Intraoc Lens Med* 1982;8:158–167.
122. Krezanoski JZ. Chemical buffering of contact lens solutions. *Contact Lens Forum* 1988;13:60.
123. Harris MG, Higa CK, Lacey LL, et al. The pH of aerosol saline solution. *Optom Vis Sci* 1990;67:84.
124. Bier N, Lowther GE. Solutions and containers. In: *Contact lens correction.* Boston: Butterworth & Co., 1977:92–102.
125. Shovlin JP, ed. Contact lens Q & A: a gas saving solution. *Rev Optom* 1989;126:93.
126. Zigler LG. Softwear saline and the sensitive patient. *Contact Lens Spectrum* 1990;5:50.
127. Christensen B, Janes JA. Clinical investigation of the new Softwear Saline. *Contact Lens Spectrum* 1990;5:37.
128. Fowler SA, Allansmith MR. Evolution of soft contact lens coatings. *Arch Ophthalmol* 1980;98:95–99.
129. Fowler SA, Greiner JV, Allansmith MR. Attachment of bacteria to soft contact lenses. *Arch Ophthalmol* 1979;97:659–660.
130. Hart DE, Shih KL. Surface interactions on hydrogel lenses: microflora and microfauna. *Am J Optom Physiol Opt* 1987;64:739–748.
131. Ward MA, Miller MJ. The microbiology of contact lens wear. *Contact Lens Forum* 1988;13:25–29.
132. Velasco J, Bermudez J. Comparative study of the microbial flora on contact lenses, in lens cases, and in maintenance liquids. *Int Contact Lens Clin* 1996;23:55–58.
133. Cabrera JV, Rodriguez JB. Ocular bacterial flora in contact lens wearers. *Int Contact Lens Clin* 1996;23:149–151.
134. Kumar R, Lloyd D. Recent advances in the treatment of Acanthamoeba keratitis. *Clin Infect Dis* 2002;35:434–441.
135. Watanabe R, Rah MJ. Preventative contact lens care: part III. *Contact Lens Spectrum* 2001;16:26–31.
136. Willcox MDP, Power KN, Stapleton F, et al. Potential sources of bacteria that are isolated from contact lenses during wear. *Optom Vis Sci* 1997;74:1030–1038.
137. Littlefield S, Bao N, Kreutzer P. Comparative antimicrobial capacity of soft contact lens storage solutions. *Int Contact Lens Clin* 1990;17:272.
138. Weissman BA, Schwartz C, Donzis PB, et al. The role of better care systems in assuring patient compliance. *Contact Lens Forum* 1989;14:44.
139. Contact lenses and cosmetics. Aarogya: *The Wellness Site,* July 4, 2002. Available at *http://www.aarogya.com/specialities/opthamalogy(sic)/contactlenses.asp.*
140. Sibley MJ. Soft contact lens hygiene: an overview. In: Dabezies OH Jr, ed. *Contact lenses: the CLAO guide to basic science and clinical practice.* Orlando, FL: Grune & Stratton, 1988:40.1–40.29.
141. Hill RM. To pasteurize. Sanitize. Asepticize, sterilize, or just disinfect? In: *Curiosities of the contact lens.* Chicago: The Professional Press, 1981:106–109.
142. Sherris JC. Microbial death: sterilization, pasteurization. disinfection, and sanitization. In: Sherris JC, ed. *Medical microbiology: an introduction to infectious disease.* New York: Elsevier, 1984:33–40.
143. Collins MJ, Carney LG. Patient compliance and its influence on contact lens wearing problems. *Am J Optom Physiol Opt* 1986;63:952–956.
144. Chun MW, Weissman BA. Compliance in contact lens care. *Am J Optom Physiol Opt* 1987;64:274–276.
145. Collins MJ, Carney LG. Compliance with care and maintenance procedures amongst contact lens wearers. *Clin Exp Optom* 1986;69:174–177.
146. Koetting RA, Castellano CF, Wartman R. Patient compliance with EW instructions. *Contact Lens Spectrum* 1986;1:23–30.
147. Phillips LJ, Prevade SL. Replacement and care compliance in a planned replacement contact lens program. *J Am Optom Assoc* 1993;64:201–205.
148. Turner FD, Gower L, Stein J, et al. Compliance and contact lens care: a new assessment method. *Optom Vis Sci* 1993;70:998.
149. Turner FD, Stein J, Sager DP, et al. A new method to assess contact lens care compliance. *CLAO J* 1993;19:108.
150. Radford CF, Lehmann OJ, Dart JKG (National Acanthamoeba Keratitis Study Group). Acanthamoeba keratitis: multicentre survey in England 1992–96. *Br J Ophthalmol* 1998;82:1387.
151. Coopersmith L, Weinstock FJ. Current recommendations and practice regarding soft lens replacement and disinfection. *CLAO J* 1997;23:172.
152. Charles AM. A comparison of some commercial methods for asepticizing and cleaning hydrogel lenses. *Contact* 1975;19:4–11.
153. Veys J, Meyler J, Davies I. Contact lens care systems. In: *Essential Contact Lens Practice.* Woburn, MA: Butterworth-Heinemann, 2002;72–79.
154. Veys J, Meyler J, Davies I. Basic contact lens practice: Part 10: contact lens care systems. *Optician* 2001;221:22–26.
155. Barr J. Contact lens solutions and lens care update. *Contact Lens Spectrum* 2001;16:26–33.
156. Amos C, Loveridge R. No rub, no rinse: a new line in multipurpose solutions. *Optician* 2002. Available at *http://www.optometryonline.net.*
157. Stiegmeier MJ. Solution drops digital cleaning step. *Contact Lens Spectrum* 2000;15:45–47.
158. Hood DA. Do soft lens solutions cause corneal infiltrates? *Contact Lens Spectrum* 1994;9:20.
159. Begley CG, Edrington TB, Chalmers RC. Effects of lens care systems on corneal fluorescein staining and subjective comfort in hydrogel lens wearers. *Int Contact Lens Clin* 1994;21:7.
160. Caffery BE. Diagnostic dilemmas: contact lens solution reactions vs. viral keratoconjunctivitis. *Rev Optom* 1996;133:87.
161. Lebow K, Christensen B. Cleaning efficacy and patient comfort: a clinical comparison of two contact lens care systems. *Int Contact Lens Clin* 1996;23:87–92.
162. Ajello L, Ajello M. A comparison of the anti-microbial spectra and kill rates of three contact lens care solutions: QuickCare Starting Solution, ReNu Multi-Purpose Solution, and Opti-Free Rinsing. Disinfecting & Storage Solution. *Int Contact Lens Clin* 1995;22:156.
163. Rosenthal R, Stein J, McAnally C, et al. A comparative study of the microbiologic effectiveness of chemical disinfectants and peroxide-neutralizer systems. *CLAO J* 1995;21:99.
164. Rosenthal RA, Henry CL, Buck SL, et al. Extreme testing of contact lens disinfecting products. *Contact Lens Spectrum* 2002;17:40–45.
165. Rosenthal RA, McDonald MM, Schlitzer RL, et al. Loss of bactericidal activity from contact lens storage solutions. *CLAO J* 1997;23:57–62.
166. Mummert R. Trends in lens care. *Contact Lens Spectrum* 1998;13[Suppl]:4s.
167. QuickCare roundtable. *Contact Lens Spectrum* 1994;9[Suppl]:1.

168. Simmons PA, Edrington TB, Pfondevida CJ, et al. Comparison between evening and morning surfactant cleaning of hydrogel lenses. *Int Contact Lens Clin* 1996;23:172–175.

169. Ghormley NR. QuickCare: a new soft lens disinfection system. *Int Contact Lens Clin* 1994;21:77.

170. Christie C. Contact lens care systems/part 8: a review of soft contact lens care systems. *Optician,* 2001;222:19–23.

171. McLaughlin R, Barr JT. Contact lens solution update. *Contact Lens Spectrum* 1989;4:21–26.

172. Davis R, Hansen D, Lowther GE, et al. Clinical evaluation of Opti-Free among preservative sensitive patients. *Contact Lens Spectrum* 1989;4:73–78.

173. Ghormley NR. Opti-Free: Alcon's new disinfection solution. *Int Contact Lens Clin* 1988;15:366.

174. Cedrone RM, Davis RL, Duryee J, et al. A clinical evaluation of the Opti-Free disinfecting system. *Contact Lens Forum* 1989; 14:62–68.

175. Schachet J, Lowther GE, Lavaux J, et al. Clinical evaluation of the Opti-Free disinfecting system. *Contact Lens Spectrum* 1990; 5:37.

176. Bournakel GS, Beale PV, Gibbs DE. The safety and patient acceptance of Opti-Free disinfecting system and CSI lenses: a one-year study. *Contact Lens Spectrum* 1989;4:56.

177. Hong B, Bilbault T, Chowhan M, et al. Cleaning capability of citrate-containing vs. non-citrate contact lens cleaning solutions: an in vitro comparative study. *Int Contact Lens Clin* 1994;21: 237.

178. Christensen B, Lebow K, White EM, et al. Effectiveness of citrate-containing lens care regimens: a controlled clinical comparison. *Int Contact Lens Clin* 1998;25:50–56.

179. Tang I, Wong DM, Yee DJ, et al. The pH of multi-purpose soft contact lens solutions. *Optom Vis Sci* 1996;73:746–749.

180. Lebow K. Moving from one care system to MPDS: a study. *Contact Lens Spectrum* 2000;15:45–48.

181. Schwartz CA. Industrial strength: contact lens update. *Optom Manage* 1999;34:31–37.

182. Johnson C, Kohler N, Bean B, et al. Rub vs. no rub: what are the costs? *Contact Lens Spectrum* 2002;17:24–30.

183. Christensen B. A new MPDS: effective and safe. *Contact Lens Spectrum* 1999;14[Suppl]:11s–12s.

184. Package insert for Opti-Free Express Multi-purpose Disinfecting Solution (340236–0502). Alcon Laboratories Inc., Fort Worth, Texas, 2002.

185. Connor CG, Presley L, Finchum SM, et al. The effectiveness of several current soft contact lens care systems against Aspergillus. *CLAO J* 1998;24:82–84.

186. Dymed: safe, gentle, and effective (SL 7497-1). In: *Lens Care Research (Bulletin).* Rochester, NY: Bausch & Lomb Personal Products Division, 1987.

187. Ghormley NR. ReNu multi-action disinfection solution-a new "cold" disinfection system. *Int Contact Lens Clin* 1987;14:428.

188. Bergmanson JPG, Ross R. A masked quantitative cytologic study of the safety of a multi-purpose contact lens solution applied to the in vitro rabbit eye. *J Am Optom Assoc* 1993;64: 308.

189. Leisring J, Gill L. The clinical safety of a new generation chemical disinfecting agent. *Contact Lens Spectrum* 1990;5:63.

190. Lofstrom T, Anderson JS, Kruse A. Tarsal abnormalities: a new grading system. *CLAO J* 1998;24:210–215.

191. Begley C, Waggoner P, Jani N, et al. The effects of soft contact lens disinfection solutions on rabbit corneal epithelium. *CLAO J* 1994;20:52.

192. Sakuma S, Reeh B, Dang D, et al. Comparative efficacies of four soft contact lens disinfection solutions. *Int Contact Lens Clin* 1996;23:234–239.

193. Package insert for ReNu MultiPlus Multi-purpose Solution (6486906). Bausch & Lomb Inc., Rochester, New York.

194. Fontana F. New solutions don't dilute the old rules. *Rev Opt* 1994;131:28.

195. Simmons PA, Donshik PC, Kelly WF, et al. Conditioning of hydrogel lenses by a multipurpose solution containing an ocular lubricant. *CLAO J* 2001;27:192–194.

196. Donshik P, Madden R, Simmons PA. Pursuing comfort in a multi-purpose solution. *Contact Lens Spectrum* 2000;15:33–36.

197. Package insert for COMPLETE brand Multi-Purpose Solution (71406US13K / 8941X). Advanced Medical Optics Inc., Irvine, California, April 2002.

198. Package insert for SOLO-care Plus with Aqualube Multi-Purpose Solution (S3411A). CIBA Vision—A Novartis Company, Atlanta, Georgia, September 2001.

199. Lebow KA. Are all multipurpose contact lens solutions created equal? *Optom Manage* 2002;10:45–48.

200. Gassett AR, Ramer RM, Katzin D. Hydrogen peroxide sterilization of hydrophilic contact lenses. *Arch Ophthalmol* 1975;93: 412–415.

201. Billig H, Bailey N, Fleischman W, et al. A new, rapid hydrogen peroxide system for contact lens disinfection. *CLAO J* 1984;10: 341–345.

202. Cho P, Lui T, Kee C. Soft contact lens care systems and corneal staining in Hong Kong-Chinese. *Contact Lens Anterior Eye* 1998;21:47–53.

203. Janoff LE. The Septicon system: a review of pertinent scientific data. *Int Contact Lens Clin* 1984;11:274–282.

204. Rogan M. Systems for hydrogen peroxide disinfection of soft contact lenses. *Transactions of the British Contact Lens Association Annual Clinical Conference,* Black-pool, England,1985:40–42.

205. Janoff LE. The effective disinfection of soft contact lenses using hydrogen peroxide. *Contact* 1979;12:37–40.

206. Janoff LE. The exposure of various polymers to a 24-hour soak in Lensept: the effect on base curve. *J Am Optom Assoc* 1985; 56:222–225.

207. Alvord LA, Walker V. The superposition of the effects of hydrogen peroxide tonicity and pH on contact lenses. Presented at the annual meeting of the American Academy of Optometry, Columbus, Ohio, December 1988.

208. Alvord LA, Walker V. The effect of hydrogen peroxide disinfection systems on properties of contact lenses. Presented at the annual meeting of the American Academy of Optometry, Denver, Colorado, December 1987.

209. Shovlin JP, ed. Contact lens Q & A: overnight in Oxysept? *Rev Optom* 1988;125:111.

210. Lowe R, Harris M, Lindsay R, et al. Hydration of high-water nonionic soft lenses during hydrogen peroxide disinfection. *Int Contact Lens Clin* 1993;20:145.

211. Penley CA, Llabres C, Wilson LA, et al. Efficacy of hydrogen peroxide disinfection systems for soft contact lenses contaminated with fungi. *CLAO J* 1985;11:65–68.

212. Penley CA, Ahearn DG, Wilson LA. Inhibition of fungi by soft contact lens solutions as determined by FDA-recommended tests. *Dev Ind Microbiol,* 1983;24:369–375.

213. Bilgin L, Manav G, Tutkun I, et al. Efficacy of a one-step hydrogen peroxide system for disinfection of soft contact lenses. *CLAO J* 1993;19:50.

214. Key JE, Monnat K. Comparative disinfectant efficacy of two disinfecting solutions against Pseudomonas aeruginosa. *CLAO J* 1996;22:118–121.

215. Wilson LA, Ahearn DG. Association of fungi with extended-wear soft contact lenses. *Am J Ophthalmol* 1986;101:434–436.

216. Richardson LE, Begley CG, Keck GK. Comparative efficacies of soft contact lens disinfection systems against fungal contaminant. *J Am Optom Assoc* 1993;64:210.

217. Perry DL, Turner FD, Stein JM, et al. Clinical comparison of Opti-Soft chemical to a hydrogen peroxide disinfection system. *Int Contact Lens Clin* 1989;16:12–19.

218. Ghormlev NR. Patient evaluation and the annual cost of soft contact lens care-revisited. *Int Contact Lens Clin* 1987;14:305–306.

219. Teenan DW, Beck L. Contact lens-associated chemical burn. *Contact Lens Anterior Eye* 2001;24:175–176.

220. Chalmers RL, McNally JJ. Ocular detection thresholds for hydrogen peroxide: lenses vs. drops. *Int Contact Lens Clin* 1988;15:351–357.

221. Paugh JR, Brennan NA, Efron N. Ocular response to hydrogen peroxide. *Am J Optom Physiol Opt* 1988;65:91–98.

222. Lowe R, Brennan NA. Hydrogen peroxide disinfection of hydrogel contact lenses: an overview. *Clin Exp Optom* 1987;70:190–197.

223. Knopf HLS. Reaction to hydrogen peroxide in a contact lens wearer. *Am J Ophthalmol* 1984;97:796.

224. Grant WM. *Toxicology of the eye,* 2nd ed. Springfield, IL: Charles C Thomas, 1974:559–560.

225. Chalmers RL, Tsao M, Scott G, et al. The rate of in vivo neutralization of residual H_2O_2 from hydrogel lenses. *Contact Lens Spectrum* 1989;4:21–26.

226. Chalmers RL. Hydrogen peroxide in anterior segment physiology: a literature review. *Optom Vis Sci* 1989;66:796–803.

227. Gyulai P, Dziabo A, Kelly W, et al. Relative neutralization ability of hydrogen peroxide disinfection systems. *Contact Lens Spectrum* 1987;2:61–68.

228. Sibley MJ. Hydrogen peroxide care systems. *Contact Lens Forum* 1987;12:57–63.

229. Krezanoski JZ, Houlsby RD. A comparison of new hydrogen peroxide disinfection systems. *J Am Optom Assoc* 1988;59:193–197.

230. Lutzi D, Callender M. Safety and efficacy of a new hydrogen peroxide disinfection system for soft lenses—in-a-wink. *Can J Optom* 1985;47:30–33.

231. Gyulai P, Dziabo A, Kelly W, et al. Efficacy of catalase as a neutralizer of hydrogen peroxide disinfecting solution for soft contact lenses. *Int Eyecare* 1986;2:418–422.

232. Ogunbiyi L. The use of sodium thiosulfate for inactivating residual hydrogen peroxide on contact lenses after disinfection. *Clin Exp Optom* 1986;69:16–21.

233. Callender MG. Clinical evaluation of Barnes-Hind hydrogen peroxide system. *Contact Lens Spectrum* 1988;3:58–61.

234. Sibley MJ, Shih KL, Hu J. Evaluation of a new thimerosal-free 5-minute hydrogen peroxide disinfection lens care regimen. *Can J Optom* 1983;44[Suppl]:3.

235. Sibley MJ. Hydrogen peroxide residues: a comparison between chemical and osmotic extraction. *Contact Lens Spectrum* 1988;3:39–43.

236. Kelly W, Ward G, Williams W, et al. Eliminating hydrogen peroxide residuals in solutions and contact lenses. *Contact Lens Spectrum* 1990;5:41.

237. Package insert for AOSEPT Clear Care Cleaning & Disinfecting Solution (S3345RID). CIBA Vision–A Novartis Company, Atlanta, Georgia, 2003

238. Package insert for UltraCare (7167X/9081X, 61963US14H). Advanced Medical Optics Inc, Irvine, California, August 2000.

239. "Quik-Step": why twenty minutes? (SL-7303). In: *Technically Speaking (Bulletin).* Rochester, NY: Bausch & Lomb Personal Products Division, 1986.

240. Weisbarth RE. Peroxide disinfection of contact lenses. Presented at British Contact Lens Association International Contact Lens Centenary Congress, London, United Kingdom, 1988.

241. Hiti K, Walochnik J, Haller-Schober EM, et al. Viability of Acanthamoeba after exposure to a multi-purpose disinfecting contact lens solution and two hydrogen peroxide systems. *Br J Ophthalmol* 2002;86:144–146.

242. Ghormley NR. Ultracare-disinfectant/Neutralizer. *Int Contact Lens Clin* 1992;19:6.

243. Kaplan EN, Gundel RE, Sosale A, et al. Residual peroxide as a function of platinum disc age. *CLAO J* 1992;18:149.

244. McKenney C, Payor R. Hydrogel diameter and base curve changes with hydrogen peroxide/catalase two step disinfection. Poster presented at the annual meeting of the American Academy of Optometry, Columbus, Ohio, December 1988.

245. Shovlin JP. Product report. Pure eyes from CIBA Vision. *Optom Today* 1995;3:115.

246. Iqbal Y. What's new in contact lenses. *Rev Ophthalmol* 1996;3:94.

247. Dillehay SM, McCarter H, The AOSEPT Clear Care Study Group, et al. A comparison of multi-purpose care systems. *Contact Lens Spectrum* 2002;17:30–36.

248. Harris MG, Torres J, Tracewell L. pH and H_2O_2 concentration of H_2O_2 disinfection systems. *Am J Optom Physiol Opt* 1988;15:527.

249. Harris MG, Hernandez GN, Nuno DM. The pH of hydrogen peroxide disinfection systems over time. *J Am Optom Assoc* 1990;61:171.

250. Melton JW, Phillips JH. Patient comfort comparison of hydrogen peroxide systems. *Contact Lens Spectrum* 1988;3:48.

251. Riley MV, Kast M. Penetration of hydrogen peroxide from contact lenses or tear-side solutions into the aqueous humor. *Optom Vis Sci* 1991;68:546.

252. Wilson G, Riley M. Does topical hydrogen peroxide penetrate the cornea? *Invest Ophthalmol Vis Sci* 1993;34:2752.

253. Atalla L, Fernandez MA, Rao NA. Immunohistochemical localization of catalase in ocular tissue. *Curr Eye Res* 1987;6:1181.

254. Bhuyan KC, Bhuyan DK. Regulation of hydrogen peroxide in eye humors. Effect of 3-amino-1 H-1, 2, 4-triazole on catalase and glutathione peroxidase of rabbit eye. *Biochem Biophys Acta* 1977;497:641.

255. Bhuyan KC, Bhuyan DK. Superoxide dismutase of the eye. Relative functions of superoxide dismutase and catalase in protecting the ocular lens from oxidative damage. *Biochem Biophys Acta* 1978;542:28.

256. Spector A, Garner WH. Hydrogen peroxide and human cataract. *Exp Eye Res* 1981;33:673.

257. Csukas S, Green K. Effects of intercameral hydrogen peroxide in the rabbit anterior chamber. *Invest Ophthalmol Vis Sci* 1988;29:335.

258. Riley MV, Giblin FJ. Toxic effects of hydrogen peroxide on corneal endothelium. *Curr Eye Res* 1982;2:451.

259. Giblin FJ, McCready JP, Reddy VN. The role of glutathione metabolism in the detoxification of H_2O_2 in rabbit lens. *Invest Ophthalmol Vis Sci* 1982;22:330.

260. Wilson GS, Chalmers RL. Effect of H_2O_2 concentration and exposure time on stromal swelling: an epithelial perfusion model. *Optom Vis Sci* 1990;67:252.

261. Morgan JF. Complications associated with contact lens solutions. *Ophthalmology* 1979;86:1107.

262. MacDonald WG, Martin WR. Electronic disinfection a possible remedy for red eye. *Contact Lens Spectrum* 2001;16:52.

263. Harris M, Fluss L, Lem A, et al. Ultraviolet disinfection of contact lenses. *Optom Vis Sci* 1993;70:839.

264. Lowe R, Vallas V, Brennan NA. Comparative efficacy of contact lens disinfection solutions. *CLAO J* 1992;18:34.

265. Choate W, Fontana F, Potter J, et al. Evaluation of the PuriLens contact lens care system: an automatic care system incorporating UV disinfection and hydrodynamic shear cleaning. *CLAO J* 2000;26:134–140.

266. Press L, Dagan J, Borovsky S. Purilens: a new integrated auto-

cleaning and disinfection method. *Contact Lens Spectrum* 1993; 8:33.

267. Admoni M, Bartolomei A, Qureshi MN, et al. Disinfection efficacy in an integrated ultraviolet light contact lens care system. *CLAO J* 1994;20:246.

268. Bartolomei A, Alcaraz L, Bottone E, et al. Clinical evaluation of Purilens, an ultraviolet light contact lens care system. *CLAO J* 1994;20:23.

269. Caroline PJ, Andre MP. The advantages of an ultraviolet disinfection system. *Contact Lens Spectrum* 2000;15:56.

270. Harris MG, Kirby JE, Tornatore CW, et al. Microwave disinfection of soft contact lenses. *Optom Vis Sci* 1989;66:82.

271. Harris MG, Gan CM, Grant T, et al. Microwave irradiation and soft contact lens parameters. *Optom Vis Sci* 1993;70:843.

272. Kastl PR, Maehara JR. Low-power microwave disinfection of soft contact lenses. *CLAO J* 2001;27:81–83.

273. Harris MG, Rechberger J, Grant T, et al. In-office microwave disinfection of soft contact lenses. *Optom Vis Sci* 1990;67:129.

274. Rohrer MD, Terry MA, Bulard RA, et al. Microwave sterilization of hydrophilic contact lenses. *Am J Ophthalmol* 1986;101: 49.

275. Crabbe A, Thompson P. Effects of microwave irradiation on the parameters of hydrogel contact lenses. *Optom Vis Sci* 2001; 78:610–615.

276. Crabbe A, Thompson P. Clinical trial of a patient-operated microwave care system for hydrogel contact lenses. *Optom Vis Sci* 2001;78:605–609.

277. Fedukowicz HB. *External infections of the eye: bacterial, viral and mycotic,* 2nd ed. New York: Appleton-Century-Crafts, 1978: 97–257.

278. Rosenthal RA, McAnally CL, Stone RP, et al. Disinfection efficacy of MPDS against Pseudomonas. *Contact Lens Spectrum* 2001;16:44–47.

279. Fujikawa LS, Palestine AG, Nussenblatt RB, et al. Isolation of human T-lymphotropic virus type III from the tears of a patient with the acquired immunodeficiency syndrome. *Lancet* 1985; 9:529–530.

280. Recommendations for preventing possible transmission of human T-lymphotrophic virus type III/lymphadenopathy-associated virus from tears. *MMWR CDC Surveill Summ* 1985;34: 533–534.

281. Martin LS, McDougal JS, Loskoski SL. Disinfection and inactivation of the human T-lymphotropic virus type III/lymphadenopathy-associated virus. *J Infect Dis* 1985;152:400–403.

282. Vogt MW, Ho DD, Bakar SR, et al. Safe disinfection of contact lenses after contamination with HTLV-III. *Ophthalmology* 1986;93:771–774.

283. Moore KB. Necessity and methods of HTLV-III inactivation in contact lens practice. *J Am Optom Assoc* 1987;58:180–186.

284. Benjamin WM. Acanthamoeba: not really a parasite. *Int Contact Lens Clin* 1988;15:70–71.

285. Wilhelmus KR. Microbial keratitis associated with contact lens wear. In: Dabezies OH Jr, ed. *Contact lenses: the CLAO guide to basic science and clinical practice.* Orlando, FL: Grune & Stratton, 1988:41.1–41.19.

286. Kilvington S. Reducing the risk of microbial keratitis in soft contact lens wearers. *Optician* 1998;5663:28–31.

287. Schnider CM. The quest for the ideal disinfection system. *Contact Lens Spectrum* 1989;4:20.

288. Trends in lens care. *Rev Optom* 1995;132[Suppl]:2.

289. Seal DV, Bennett ES, McFadyen AK, et al. Differential adherence of Acanthamoeba to contact lenses and effects of material characteristics. *Optom Vis Sci* 1995;72:23.

290. Raali E, Vaahtoranta-Lehtonen HH, Juhani Lehtonen O-P. Detachment of trophozoites of Acanthamoeba species from soft contact lenses with BEN22 detergent, BioSoak, and Renu Multi-Purpose solutions. *CLAO J* 2001;27:155–158.

291. Ludwig IH, Meisler DM, Rutherford I, et al. Susceptibility of Acanthamoeba to soft contact lens disinfection systems. *Invest Ophthalmol Vis Sci* 1986;27:626–628.

292. Meakin BJ. Contact lens care systems: an update. *BCLA J* 1989; 26–31.

293. Davies DJG, Anthony Y, Meakin BJ, et al. Anti-Acanthamoeba activity of chlorhexidine and hydrogen peroxide. *Transactions of the British Contact Lens Association, International Contact Lens Centenary Congress,* London, United Kingdom, May 1988: 60–62.

294. Moore MB. Early diagnosis and management of the Acanthamoeba patient. Paper presented at the 14th National Research Symposium on Contact Lenses, Washington, DC, August 1987.

295. Penley CA, Littlefield SA. Effects of hydrogen peroxide disinfection systems with hydrogel lenses contaminated with Acanthamoeba. Poster presented at annual meeting of American Academy of Optometry. Denver, Colorado, December 1987.

296. Liedel KK, Begley CG. The effectiveness of soft contact lens disinfection systems against Acanthamoeba. *J Am Optom Assoc* 1996;67:135.

297. Mowrey-McKee M.F. Contact lens solution efficacy against Acanthamoeba castellani. Poster presented at the annual meeting of The British Contact Lens Association. Birmingham, United Kingdom, May 2002.

298. Liedel KK, Begley CG. The effectiveness of soft contact lens disinfection systems against Acanthamoeba on the lens surface. *J Am Optom Assoc* 1996;67:135–142.

299. Buck SL, Rosenthal RA, Abshire RL. Amoebicidal activity of a preserved contact lens multi-purpose disinfecting solution compared to a disinfection/neutralization peroxide system. *Contact Lens Anterior Eye* 1998;21:81–84.

300. Penley CA, Schlitzer RL, Ahearn DG, et al. Laboratory evaluation of chemical disinfection of soft contact lenses. *Contact Intraoc Lens Med J* 1981;7:101.

301. Reinhardt DJ, Kaylor B, Prescott D, et al. Rapid and simplified comparative evaluations of contact lens disinfecting solutions. *Int Contact Lens Clin* 1990;17:9.

302. Penley CA, Ahearn DG, Schlitzer RL, et al. Laboratory evaluation of chemical disinfection of soft contact lenses. II. Fungi as challenge organisms. *Contact Intraoc Lens Med J* 1981;7: 196–204.

303. Ahearn DG, Penley CA, Wilson LA. Growth and survival of Serratia marcescens in hard contact lens wetting solutions. *CLAO J* 1984;10:172–174.

304. Merindano MD, Lluch S, Marques MS. The efficacy of the Opti-Free care system: a one-year study. *Contact Lens Spectrum* 1992;7:49.

305. Sibley MJ. Soft lens cold disinfection solutions: a comparative study. *Contact Lens Forum* 1981;6:41–49.

306. Erickson S, Dabezies OH. Preservatives. In: Dabezies OH Jr ed, *Contact lenses: the CLAO guide to basic science and clinical practice.* Orlando, FL: Grune & Stratton, 1984:28.1–28.9.

307. Reinhardt DJ, Kaylor B, Prescott D, et al. Rapid and standard evaluations of contact lens disinfecting solutions. Paper presented at the American Society for Microbiology Meeting, New Orleans, Louisiana, 1989.

308. Key JE, Monnat K. Comparative disinfectant efficacy of two disinfecting solutions against Pseudomonas aeruginosa. *CLAO J* 1996;22:118.

309. Schlesinger LM. Solutions update: reduced disinfection time improves patient convenience. *Optom Today* 1994;2:43.

310. Gnadt GR, Gordon A. Fungal contamination of soft contact lenses. *Int Contact Lens Clin* 1991;18:102.

311. Bergmanson JPG, Benjamin WJ. Fungal "deposition": a sign of the times? *Int Contact Lens Clin* 1990;17:42.

312. Sickler SG, Bao N, Littlefield SA. Comparative antimicrobial activity of three leading soft contact lens disinfection solutions. *Int Contact Lens Clin* 1992;19:19.

313. Churner R, Cunningham RD. Fungal-contaminated soft contact lenses. *Am Ophthalmol* 1983;55:724.

314. Yamaguchi T, Hubbard A, Fukushima A, et al. Fungus growth on soft contact lenses with different water contents. *CLAO J* 1984;10:166–170.

315. Wilhelmus KR, Robinson NM, Font RA. Fungal keratitis in contact lens wearers. *Am J Ophthalmol* 1988;106:708.

316. Schornack JA, Watanabe R, Dillehay SM, et al. Annual soft contact lens solution usage and costs. *Contact Lens Spectrum* 1998;13:43–48.

317. Caroline PJ, Andre MP. The cost of solution-induced dry eyes. *Contact Lens Spectrum* 2001;16:56.

318. Ghormley NR, Ardisson TJ. AOSEPT lens care system or Opti-Free system? *Contact Lens Spectrum* 1992;6:35.

319. Hammersla K, Coviello D. The consumer challenge: three care systems compared. *Contact Lens Spectrum* 1991;6:21.

320. Steel SA. Patient preference study compares top lens care systems. *Contact Lens Spectrum* 1990;5:56.

321. West W, Gallia M. Concept testing: what do patients want in a current lens care system? *Contact Lens Spectrum* 1993;8:49.

322. Hood D, Rigel L. A clinical comparison of multi-purpose solutions. *Contact Lens Spectrum* 1995;10:31.

323. Soni PS, Horner DG, Ross J. Ocular response to lens care systems in adolescent soft contact lens wearers. *Optom Vis Sci* 1996;73:70.

324. Dumbleton K, Jones L, Chalmers R, et al. Clinical characterization of spherical post-lens debris associated with lotrafilcon high-Dk silicone lenses. *CLAO J* 2000;26:186–192.

325. Package insert for CIBA Vision Lens Drops (S7127B). CIBA Vision–A Novartis Company. Atlanta, Georgia, 1993.

326. Hom M, Simmons P. In-eye contact lens cleaners. *Contact Lens Spectrum* 2002;17:33–38.

327. Package insert for AQuify (S7398A). CIBA Vision–A Novartis Company, Atlanta, Georgia, October 2002.

328. Amos C. In the blink of an eye: a multi-dose, preservative-free contact lens comfort drop. *Optician* 2003;5887:24–28.

329. Poster MG. Optical efficacy of rewetting and lubricating solutions. *Contact Lens Forum* 1981;6:25–31.

330. Doughty M, Fonn D, Richter D, et al. A patient questionnaire approach to estimating the prevalence of dry eye symptoms in patients presenting to optometric practices across Canada. *Optom Vis Sci* 1997;74:624–631.

331. Mathers WD, Caroline PJ. Broaden your working definition of dry eyes. *Refractive Eyecare Ophthalmol* 2001;7:26.

332. Caroline PJ, Andre MP. Profession still deciding between preservative-free and preserved-chemical disinfection. *Primary Care Optometry News* 1997;2:32.

333. Mowrey-McKee M, Sills A, Wright A. Comparative cytotoxicity potential of soft contact lens care regimens. *CLAO J* 2002;28:160–164.

334. Ruy T, McCanna DJ, Miller MJ. Comparison of contact lens multipurpose solutions by in vitro sodium fluorescein permeability assay. *CLAO J* 2002;28:151–156.

335. Campbell R, Caroline P. Multipurpose non-keratitis. *Contact Lens Spectrum* 1997;12:56.

336. Cosgrove J. Preventing contact lens dropouts. *Contact Lens Spectrum* 2001;16:32–36.

337. Robinson RS. When the solution is no solution. *Optom Manage* 2001;36:71–72.

338. McMonnies C, Ho A. Patient history in screening for dry eye conditions. *J Am Optom Assoc* 1987;58:296–301.

339. *Ocular Times,* July 4, 2002. Available at *http://www.geocities.com/oculartimes/cl.html.*

340. Bergenske P. Continuous wear lens care. *Rev CL's* 2002;7:10.

341. Package insert for PUREVISION (DP10016W0. Bausch & Lomb Inc., Rochester, New York, December 1999.

342. Epstein A. SPK with daily wear of silicone hydrogel lenses and MPS. *Contact Lens Spectrum* 2002;17:30.

343. Fonn D. Observations of corneal staining with MPS and silicone hydrogel lenses. *Contact Lens Spectrum* 2002;17:32.

344. Levy B. Contact lens and solution manufacturer responds with data. *Contact Lens Spectrum* 2002;17:34.

345. Jones L, MacDougall N, Sorbara G. Asymptomatic corneal staining associated with the use of balafilcon silicone-hydrogel contact lenses disinfected with a polyaminopropyl biguanide-preserved care regimen. *Optom Vis Sci* 2002;79:753–761.

346. Package insert for Focus Night & Day (lotrafilcon A) Soft Contact Lenses (D7348A/095617). CIBA Vision–A Novartis Company, Atlanta, Georgia, September 2001.

347. Efron N, Wohl A, Toma NG. Pseudomonas corneal ulcers associated with daily wear of disposable hydrogel contact lenses. *Int Contact Lens Clin* 1991;18:46.

348. Radford CF, Minassian DC, Dart JKG. Disposable contact lens use as a risk factor for microbial keratitis. *Br J Ophthalmol* 1998;82:1272–1275.

349. McKenney CD, Ajello M. Comparative case contamination: three disinfection systems. *Int Contact Lens Clin* 1991;18:14.

350. A reminder (instruction sheet) (SL-3599). Bausch & Lomb Inc., Rochester, New York, 1983.

351. Weiner B, Harris M, Josephson J, et al. Guidelines for in-office hydrogel lens disinfection. *Making Contact* 1992;11:20.

352. Shovlin J. How to keep trial lenses clean. *Optom Manage* 1991;26:67.

353. Callender MG, Charles AM, Chalmers RL. Effect of storage time with different lens care systems on in-office hydrogel trial lens disinfection efficacy: a multi-center study. *Optom Vis Sci* 1992;69:678.

354. Ghormley NR. Office contact lens inventory-storage & disinfection system? *Int Contact Lens Clin* 1984;11:650.

355. Jacob R. Principles of cleaning soft contact lenses. *Int Contact Lens Clin* 1988;15:317–325.

356. Pitts R, Krachmer J. Evaluation of soft contact lens disinfection in the home environment. *Arch Ophthalmol* 1979;97:470–472.

357. Barre ME, Cook ML. Microbial factors in contact lens fitting. *Am J Optom Physiol Opt* 1984;61:389–396.

358. Donzis R, Mondino B, Weissman BA. Bacillus keratitis associated with contaminated contact lens care systems. *Am J Ophthalmol* 1988;105:195–197.

359. Siwoff R, Haupt EJ. Bacterial growth on contact lens cases: do solutions make a difference? *Contact Lens Forum* 1986;11:47.

360. Pitts RE, Krachmer JH. Evaluation of soft lens disinfection in the home environment. *Arch Ophthalmol* 1979;97:470–472.

361. Callender MG, Tse LSY, Charles AM, et al. Bacterial flora of the eye and contact lens cases during hydrogel lens wear. *Am J Optom Physiol Opt* 1986;63:177.

362. Wilson LA, Sawant AD, Simmons RB, et al. Microbial contamination of contact lens storage cases and solutions. *Am J Ophthalmol* 1990;110:193.

363. Campbell RC, Caroline PJ. Inefficacy of soft contact lens disinfection techniques in the home environment. *Contact Lens Spectrum* 1990;5:17.

364. Simmons PA, Edrington TB, Hsieh L, et al. Bacterial contamination rate of soft contact lens cases. *Int Contact Lens Clin* 1991;18:188.

365. Midelfart J, Midelfart A, Bevanger L. Microbial contamination of contact lens cases among medical students. *CLAO J* 1996;22:21.

366. Caroline PJ, Campbell RC. Strategies of microbial cell survival in contact lens cases. *Contact Lens Spectrum* 1990;5:27.

367. Larragoiti N, Diamos M, Simmons P, et al. A comparative study of techniques for decreasing contact lens storage case contamination. *J Am Optom Assoc* 1994;65:161.

368. Amos C, Ward M. Thermal disinfection of contact lens cases. *Contact Lens Forum* 1988;13:59–63.

369. Ward M. Solutions and lens care. *Contact Lens Forum* 1989;14:11.

370. Durban JJ, Monteoliva-Sanchez M, Hita-Villaverde E, et al. Antimicrobial efficiency of hydrogel contact lens soaking solutions marketed in Spain. *Optom Vis Sci* 75:126–131.

371. Shovlin J. Systemic medications and their interaction with soft contact lenses. *Int Contact Lens Clin* 1990;17:250.

372. Lowther GE. Contact lens solutions in clinical practice. In: Bartlett JD, Janus SD, eds. *Clinical ocular pharmacology,* 2nd ed. Boston: Butterworth & Co., 1989:378–380.

373. Townsend WD. Managing those rare contact lens complications. *Contact Lens Spectrum* 1998;13:23–30.

374. Michaud L, Giasson CJ. Overwear of contact lenses: increased severity of clinical signs as a function of protein adsorption. *Optom Vis Sci* 2002;79:184–192.

375. Optimize your lens care options. *Contact Lens Spectrum* 1995;10:27.

376. Gower L. Stein J, Turner D. Compliance: a comparison of three lens care systems. *Optom Vis Sci* 1994;71:629.

377. Shannon BJ. Don't quit with the fit. *Contact Lens Forum* 1987;12:46–48.

378. Harris MG. Compliance in soft contact lens care. *Int Contact Lens Clin* 1988;15:143–145.

379. Weissman BA, Schwartz C, Donzis PB, et al. The role of better care systems in assuring patient compliance. *Contact Lens Forum* 1989;14:44–51.

380. Schwartz CA. What's on their minds when they don't comply. *Rev Optom* 1993;130:49.

381. Marren SE. Negotiating compliance with contact lens care. *Int Contact Lens Clin* 1990;57:63.

382. Trick LR. Patient compliance—don't count on it! *J Am Optom Assoc* 1993;64:264.

383. Soni PS, Horner DG, Jimenez L. Will young children comply with and follow instructions to successfully wear soft contact lenses? *CLAO J* 1995;21:86.

384. Schwartz CA. Convenience vs. compliance: you still have to teach 'em. *Rev Optom* 1996;133:32.

385. Bergmanson JPG, Snyder C, Lapple W, et al. Strategies for improving patient compliance with a case replacement regimen. *Contact Lens Spectrum* 1993;8:25.

386. Silbert JA, Gubman DT. Understanding cost differences among soft lens care systems. *Contact Lens Spectrum* 1993;10:46.

387. Barr JT, Bailey NJ. 1990 annual report. *Contact Lens Spectrum* 1991;6:32.

388. Schnider C. Part-time lens wear, full-time lens care. *Contact Lens Spectrum* 1994;9:17.

389. Schnider C. Old habits die hard. *Contact Lens Spectrum* 1994;9:17.

390. Barlow M, Plank D, Stroud S, et al. The effectiveness of typical hand-cleaning methods on hydrogel contact lenses. *Int Contact Lens Clin* 1994;21:232.

391. Hoffman WC, Cook SA. Reducing lens spoilage via contact lens wearers' hand soap. *Contact Lens Forum* 1986;11:44–45.

392. Ghormley NR. Contact lens care-hand soap? *Int Contact Lens Clin* 1984;11:318.

393. Bonsett-Veal JD. Cleaning hands with Opti-naps. *Contact Lens Forum* 1985;10:63.

394. Lowther GE. How safe are hydrogel disinfection systems? *Int Contact Lens Clin* 1991;18:124.

395. Ghormley NR. Cosmetics and contact lenses. *Int Eyecare* 1985;1:218.

396. Greco A. Cosmetics and contact lens wear. *Int Eyecare* 1985;1:41–45.

397. Baldwin JS. Cosmetics: too long concealed as culprit in eye problems. *Contact Lens Forum* 1986;11:38–41.

398. Bennett ES, Ghormley NR. Rigid extended wear: an overview. *Int Contact Lens Clin* 1987;14:319–331.

399. Contact lenses and cosmetics. American Optometric Association, July 3, 2002. Available at *http://www.aoa.org/conditions/contact lenses cosmetics.asp*.

400. Ng A, Mostardi B, Mandell RB. Adherence of mascara to soft contact lenses. *Int Contact Lens Clin* 1988;15:64–68.

401. Wilson LA, Ahearn DG. Pseudomonas-induced corneal ulcers associated with contaminated eye mascara. *Am J Ophthalmol* 1977;84:112–119.

402. Gassett AR, Mattingly TP, Hood I. Source of fungus contamination of hydrophilic soft contact lenses. *Am Ophthalmol* 1979;11:1295–1298.

403. Barr JT. How to protect patients from external hazards. *Contact Lens Spectrum* 1994;9:28.

404. Thompson TT. *Tyler's quarterly soft contact lens parameter guide.* Little Rock, AR: Tyler's Quarterly Inc., March 2003;20:61.

405. Boyd JR. Contact lens products. In: *Handbook of non-prescription drugs,* 8th ed, Washington DC: American Pharmaceutical Association, 1986:453–476.

406. Sibley MJ. Adverse effects of contact lenses-solution incompatibilities. *Audio-Digest Ophthalmol* 1986;24.

407. Gourley DR, Makoid MC. Ophthalmic products. In: *Handbook of non-prescription drugs,* 8th ed. Washington, DC: American Pharmaceutical Association, 1986:437–452.

408. Sibley MJ, Chu V. Understanding sorbic acid-preserved contact lens solutions. *Int Contact Lens Clin* 1984;11:531–542.

409. Wardlaw JC, Sarver MD. Discoloration of hydrogel contact lenses under standard care regimens. *Am J Optom Physiol Opt* 1987;63:403–408.

410. Stone RP, Mowery-McKee MF, Kreutzer P. Protein: a source of lens discoloration. *Contact Lens Forum* 1984;9:33–41.

411. Egan DJ, Myers RI. CL care systems: from regulations to elimination. *Contact Lens Forum* 1990;15:27.

412. Lowther GE. Disinfection of extended wear lenses. *Int Contact Lens Clin* 1984;11:14.

413. Dorman K, Scheid T. Unusual contact lens discoloration due to solution incompatibility. *Contact Lens Spectrum* 1992;7:19.

414. Shovlin JP, ed. Contact lens Q & A: the pink connection. *Rev Optom* 1986;123:115.

415. Dubow BW, ed. Contact lens Q & A: rose colored contacts. *Rev Optom* 1985;122:63.

416. Westerhout D. The use of soft lenses in ocular pathology. In: Stone J, Phillis AJ, eds. *Contact lenses: a textbook for practitioner and student,* 2nd ed. London: Butterworth & Co., 1981:613.

417. Rakow PL. Deciphering that solution confusion. *Vision Care Assistant* 1990;Sept/Oct:11.

418. Rakow PA. Solution confusion. *EyeQuest Magazine* 1991;1:28.

419. Jurkus JM, Cedarstaff TH, Nuccio RS. Solution confusion: photo documentation of what can happen. *Int Contact Lens Clin* 1981;8:47–56.

420. Lowther GE. Contact lens preparations. In: Barlett JD, Janus SD, eds: *Clinical ocular pharmacology.* Boston: Butterworth & Co., 1984:327–361.

421. Sibley MJ. Contact lens solution incompatibilities. *Contact Lens Forum* 1984;9:67–71.

422. Hill RM. pH and solution properties. *Int Contact Lens Clin* 1987;14:373–374.

423. Dubow BW, ed. Contact lens Q & A: fading away. *Rev Optom* 1985;122:89.
424. Windholtz M, Budavaris S, Blumetti R, et al. *The Merck index,* 10th ed. Rathway, NJ: Merck & Co., 1983.
425. Rakow PL. Solution incompatibilities. *Contact Lens Forum* 1988;13:41–46.
426. Crook TG, Freeman JJ. Reactions induced by the concurrent use of thimerosal and tetracycline. *Am J Optom Physiol Opt* 1983;60:759–761.
427. Gero G. Superficial punctate keratitis with CSI contact lenses dispensed with the Allergan Hydrocare cold kit. *Int Contact Lens Clin* 1984;11:674.
428. Roth HW. Polyquad-induced mixed solution syndrome in contact lens wear. *Contactologia* 1991;13:8.
429. Radoiu MC. Diagnostic dilemmas: CL-induced pseudodendrites vs. other dendriform mimickers. *Rev Optom* 1996;133:73.
430. Marguiles LJ, Mannus MJ. Dendritic corneal lesions associated with soft contact lens wear. *Arch Ophthalmol* 1983;101:1551.
431. Udel IJ, Mannus MJ, Meisler DM, et al. Pseudodendrites in soft contact lens wear. *CLAO J* 1985;11:51.
432. Professional newsletter: "vortex" patterns stirs up controversy. *Optom Manage* 1993;28:5.
433. Ditto K, Barr JT, Quinn T. Corneal update: Hudson-Stahli-like subepithelial observation. *Contact Lens Spectrum* 1993;8:20.
434. Shovlin JP, ed. Contact lens Q & A: it's a curious finding but not a serious one. *Rev Optom* 1993;10:89.
435. Reader's forum. Cause of pigmented verticillata keratopathy still unknown. *Contact Lens Spectrum* 1993;8:13.
436. Letter to the editor. *AOA News,* October 1, 1992:2.
437. Letter to the editor. Corneal infiltrate letter opens debate. *AOA News,* November 1, 1992:2.
438. Silbert JA. Medications and contact lens wear. *Contact Lens Spectrum* 2002;17:26–31.
439. Sindt C. Instructions for handling contact lenses. University of Iowa, July 4, 2002. Available at *www.vh.org/Patients/IHB/Ophth/handlingcontacts.html.*

HYDROGEL LENS SOLUTION CHEMISTRY

LEO G. CARNEY
JOSEPH T. BARR
AND RICHARD M. HILL

INTRODUCTION

Need for Lens Care Solutions

Successful contact lens wear depends on patient achievement of good vision, with comfort and safety. Choice of lens material, lens mechanical fit, and lens wearing modality are all clearly important. Attention to the care and maintenance of hydrogel lenses also is an integral element in the success of lens wear because it impacts on each of these three requirements of success (1,2). Therefore, the appropriate choice of lens care systems is an important step in achieving that success (3).

Care and maintenance of lenses is particularly relevant in avoiding the ocular complications of contact lens wear (4). Although the incidence of serious complications is low, the consequences can be serious; therefore, safe, clean, and comfortable lenses must remain the expectation. Careful attention to the choice of lens care and maintenance systems will reduce the potential for adverse ocular responses, patient error, and lens degradation (5).

The properties of contact lens solutions for hydrogel contact lens care, and the principles behind this development and application, are described in this chapter. The choice of care systems is considered elsewhere, because that depends not only on knowledge of solution properties but also of other lens (material and style) and patient (lifestyle, environment, and compliance) factors.

A complex array of solutions and procedures has evolved for lens care and maintenance over the years. Complexity has been compounded by the continual development of new products. The evolution of multipurpose solutions has counteracted this trend, although significant variations remain in the solution formulations that have been adopted (6,7).

Despite the plethora of formulations, solutions can be considered according to three underlying roles of solution use, namely, disinfecting, cleaning, and rehydrating or lubricating. Any solution may meet one specific role or some combination of roles (8).

The purpose of disinfection of lenses is the destruction of microorganisms and hence the reduction of the microbial load introduced by a contact lens into the eye. Contact lens wear of any type is known to increase the risk of ocular infection, although the likelihood of such an outcome remains low (4,9). The factors contributing to microbial keratitis are many, but contact lens wear can interfere with the known ocular defense mechanisms (10,11). Poor or no disinfection of lenses has been shown to contribute to the occurrence of microbial keratitis in contact lens wearers. Appropriate choice and use of a disinfection process is therefore an important element in the protection of the contact lens-wearing eye from infection.

Lens cleaning solutions and systems have the role of removing surface debris and preventing deposits (12). Maintenance of a clean lens surface is important for good vision, comfort, and prevention of infection; however, it also is an important element in the disinfection process (13). It acts to reduce the numbers of microorganisms adhering to the lens surface, thus enhancing the effectiveness of disinfection procedures.

Despite the development of new materials and the use of disposable lens wearing regimens, ocular discomfort, particularly symptoms of dryness, remains a common cause of patient failure with contact lens wear (14). Rewetting or lubricating solutions address this need by rehydrating lenses and modifying lens surface properties (15).

Rationale for Formulations

Solution components will be described in detail, and the solution formulation is designed to meet a number of characteristics. The most fundamental characteristic of any contact lens solution is that it is *efficacious* and meets its role(s) as described earlier. However, there are a number of other characteristics that the formulation of solutions must provide. In particular, solutions must be *safe* and nontoxic to ocular tissues (16–19). For example, it is well known that many solution components can disrupt epithelial cells and alter the epithelial barrier function. Solution *stability* is important so that solution efficacy is retained throughout its shelf life. Solutions must be *sterile* at the point of manufacture and be able to counteract microbial contamination throughout its use (20). Finally, the solution must be *compatible,* both with the contact lens material it was designed for and with other solutions with which it could reasonably be used in conjunction (21).

Developments in Solution Usage

Contact lens solutions, and their formulations, have continually changed and developed. The two most significant recent advances that have impacted on contact lens solution usage are the lens wearing modality itself and multipurpose solutions.

The use of disposable lenses, particularly daily disposable lenses, removes or at least modifies the need for and role of contact lens solutions (22). Extended wear similarly changes traditional dependence on lens care and maintenance (23).

The complex array of lens solutions of the past has to a large extent been replaced by the broad acceptance of multipurpose solutions. Formulations that are antimicrobial, clean lens surfaces, and provide rehydration and lubrication, all without compromising the safety of ocular tissues, are available (24–26). This assists patient compliance with solution use and reduces one source of patient error and adverse reactions. Significant differences remain in the approach to formulation of multipurpose solutions (7,27), and understanding the principles of lens care and solution components remains crucial.

DISINFECTION

Successful hydrogel lens wear requires control of microbial contamination of the lens. Thermal, ultraviolet, microwave, and ultrasonic techniques have been used for hydrogel lens disinfection (5), but by far the most common approach is chemical disinfection.

Chemical Disinfection

Although numerous antimicrobial agents are in common use, relatively few are suitable for use as disinfecting agents for hydrogel lenses (28). Some agents are toxic to ocular tissues at the concentrations required for effective disinfection of lenses, some can lead to lens degradation, and others are absorbed by or bound to the hydrogel lens matrix or surface deposits, leading to a build-up of concentrations and subsequent ocular reaction (29). Table 20.1 lists the classes of disinfecting agents, together with some examples of specific agents.

International Organization for Standardization (ISO)/United States Food and Drug Administration (FDA) procedure requires a lens care product to be labeled as a contact lens "disinfecting solution" if it can meet the primary crite-

TABLE 20.1. SOME COMMON ANTIMICROBIAL AGENTS

Quaternary ammonium compounds	Benzalkonium chloride (BAK)
	Akyltriethanol ammonium chloride
	Polyquaternium
Alcohols, acids, and related compounds	Chlorobutanol
	Sorbic acid
	Boric acid
	Chlorine
Mercurials	Thimerosal
Biguanides	Chlorhexidine
	Polyaminopropyl biguanide
	Polyhexamethylene biguanide
Oxidizers	Hydrogen peroxide
Chelating agents	Ethylenediaminetetraacetate (EDTA)

ria of the standalone test: the number of bacteria recovered per milliliter should be reduced by a mean value of not less than 3.0 logs within the recommended disinfection period. The number of yeast or mold recovered per milliliter should be reduced by a mean value of 1.0 log within the recommended disinfection time. Most solutions are very effective against bacteria but not as effective against yeast and mold. Manufacturers are required to test their solutions against standard organisms while the organisms in the real world may have adapted (30,31).

Quaternary ammonium compounds are cationic detergents that act by binding to bacterial cell membranes, causing disruption and lysis of the cellular contents (8,28). Benzalkonium chloride, a quaternary ammonium compound, is a commonly used preservative having both antifungal and antibacterial actions that also can be cytotoxic to corneal epithelium (32,33). Binding of this compound to the lens matrix, and subsequent release into the tears, can lead to toxic concentrations; therefore, it is not used in hydrogel lens solutions.

Alkyltriethanol ammonium chloride is chemically similar to benzalkonium chloride (34), but it is not as toxic to either epithelial or endothelial cells. Polyquaternium-1 (Polyquad) is a high-molecular-weight agent that has been found to be an effective disinfecting agent for hydrogel lenses when used at a concentration of 0.001%. It induces minimal tissue response and is less likely to cause lens discoloration (3,7).

Chlorobutanol (trichloroisobutyl alcohol) is a bacteriostatic agent present in some solutions used for rigid contact lenses, but it is not used in hydrogel lens solutions (34). Sorbic acid 0.1% is used in many solutions (especially saline) as a bacteriostatic (rather than bactericidal) agent, and its antimicrobial activity is enhanced when combined with the chelating agent ethylenediaminetetraacetate (EDTA). This is a well-known preservative, and the incidence of adverse ocular responses to EDTA is less than to other disinfecting agents. Adverse responses can still occur in some patients (34). Chlorine agents are other common preservatives in general use (35–37). Although they have been shown to induce low rates of adverse reactions in contact lens use, their effectiveness as lens disinfecting agents is questionable, and they have been linked to increased risk of microbial keratitis. Thimerosal, an organic mercury compound, is commonly used as a disinfecting agent and as a preservative. Unlike other organic mercurials (phenyl mercuric acetate or nitrate), it does not bind strongly to lens materials, although it can be bound to organic surface deposits. It is primarily bacteriostatic in action and has a wide spectrum of activity, although it is slow acting. Its action is enhanced by the chelating agent EDTA, and so both agents are usually present. It requires an alkaline pH for stability. Cytotoxic effects from thimerosal solutions are possible (38). More important in this context, however, the risk of hypersensitivity to thimerosal is high. The widespread use of organic mercurials in various proprietary solutions or long-term use of thimerosal-based contact lens solutions may sensitize patients, providing the basis for the familiar thimerosal hypersensitivity response (39).

Chlorhexidine is a biguanide antiseptic that acts by disrupting the plasma membrane of the bacterial cell. In the commonly used concentration of 0.005%, there is negligible cytotoxic effect (34). Toxic reactions to chlorhexidine compounds occasionally result in responses similar to those of thimerosal hypersensitivity. Chlorhexidine can bind to many polymers, and it may form complexes with tear proteins and mucin to produce lens surface deposits, further contributing to ocular irritation (2).

These drawbacks with the use of chlorhexidine for hydrogel contact lens disinfection have led to the development of high-molecular-weight derivatives under the alternative nomenclature of polyaminopropyl biguanide (PAPB, Dymed) and polyhexamethylene biguanide (PHMB, TrisChem) (7,8). These agents have markedly increased antibacterial effectiveness and can be used at concentrations that diminish the risk of adverse ocular responses. Typical concentrations of 0.00005% cause minimal ocular tissue responses.

Myristamidopropyl dimethylamine (Aldox) has been used in combination with polyquaternium-1 to provide a solution with low toxicity but continuous antimicrobial activity during lens storage (8).

EDTA is a chelating agent. It is relatively toxic and is used together with other disinfecting agents to enhance their antimicrobial activity.

Oxidizers, such as hydrogen peroxide, have been shown to be effective disinfection agents (40,41). Hydrogen peroxide, in the 3% concentration commonly incorporated in contact lens solutions, is usually considered to provide effective antimicrobial action. The major concern with the use of hydrogen peroxide solutions is the possibility of placing a contact lens containing residual hydrogen peroxide on the eye.

Hydrogen peroxide is toxic to the eye, and exposure of the ocular tissues to it will cause severe ocular reactions and discomfort, tearing, and tissue damage (42,43). Estimates of the threshold concentration for ocular responses vary and are dependent on additional factors, including pH of the solutions, but the concentration probably is approximately 100 parts per million or higher. Neutralization of residual hydrogen peroxide after disinfection has occurred can be achieved by any one of three processes: dilution (osmotic extraction), catalytic neutralization, or reactive neutralization (44,45).

Dilution neutralization was the first process used and the most prone to abuse. Multiple soaks and rinses with saline or rinsing solution are used to reduce the hydrogen peroxide levels. The number of required rinses makes the technique of dubious value in isolation, but it can be important as an adjunct procedure to other neutralization techniques.

In catalytic neutralization, various catalysts are incorporated into the process to bring about the decomposition of hydrogen peroxide to acceptable residual levels. Catalase, a naturally occurring biocatalyst, is one such agent used in hydrogel lens solutions. A second procedure using this principle is the platinum-coated catalytic disc. The catalytic action of this disc is slow to ensure adequate disinfection time before neutralization occurs.

Reactive neutralization uses chemical neutralizing agents, and several agents have been used. In each case, resultant byproducts, or remaining neutralizing agents, have the potential to cause ocular responses. The three chemical neutralizing agents that have been used in reactive neutralization are sodium thiosulfate, sodium sulfite, and sodium pyruvate.

Because attention to the procedure for neutralizing residual hydrogen peroxide is so important, the procedure to ensure patient compliance has been simplified. The original systems were "two-step," in which the neutralization process is initiated once disinfection is complete and prior to lens insertion into the eye. This system ensures high antimicrobial effectiveness, but it is complex and subject to wearer error. "One-step" systems allow the disinfection and neutralization processes to occur without the intervention of the wearer (46). Although more convenient for the wearer and less likely to lead to compliance problems, this system has decreased antimicrobial effectiveness because the lens is subject to high-concentration disinfection for a reduced time, and the lens is subsequently stored in neutralized solution that does not provide ongoing antimicrobial activity.

Physical Methods of Disinfection

Thermal disinfection is both effective and inexpensive. Thermal disinfection can be carried out using either preserved saline or preservative-free saline for patients who are sensitive to preservatives. Because use of thimerosal often leads to hypersensitivity responses, a range of nonthimerosal-preserved salines are available, using preservatives such as sorbic acid or polyquaternium-1. Of course, thermal disinfection procedures do not result in sterilization, and because ongoing disinfecting action is not provided, recontamination on storage is possible. Lens deposit formation during disinfection is another drawback.

A number of other physical alternatives to solution-based disinfection have been proposed. Ultraviolet radiation has general application for sterilization, but its efficacy in disinfecting surface-borne microorganisms on contact lenses is in doubt (47–49). The PuriLens ultraviolet disinfection system has been reported to improve efficacy (50). Ultrasound has been proposed as a cleaning and disinfection system for contact lenses (51,52), but studies have shown it has only limited effectiveness in disinfecting hydrogel lenses. Microwave radiation also has been suggested as providing an inexpensive alternative for lens disinfection, but there are few controlled studies on its effectiveness (53,54).

CLEANING

During both wear and handling, hydrogel lens surfaces become contaminated with ocular contaminants, such as proteins, mucus, lipids, and inorganic salts, and environmental contaminants, such as cosmetics, pollutants, and other debris. The composition and nature of the contamination and deposits are varied; consequently, a range of cleaning agents and processes has been developed to counteract them. These solutions primarily fall into the categories of surfactants, oxidizers, and enzymes (Table 20.2) for hydrogel lens use.

Daily use cleaning solutions may include surfactants, chelating agents, preservatives, buffers, and sometimes abrasives. The action of surfactants is to solubilize debris so that manual rubbing of the lens and rinsing will effectively remove the loosely bound surface debris. More tenacious forms of contamination, such as protein deposits, may require further action, including use of enzymatic cleaners.

Most cleaning solutions use nonionic surfactants that have limited interaction with polymers and few problems

with toxicity. Some amphoteric and anionic surfactants also are used.

Isopropyl alcohol is a lipid solvent that, in addition to its antimicrobial effect, is an effective lipid remover. The chelating agent EDTA sometimes is incorporated to complement this cleaning action. EDTA particularly contributes to control of protein deposit buildup through action on the calcium ion. Some cleaning solutions also incorporate abrasive agents or polymeric beads to give an added shearing component to the surface cleaning.

Preservatives, as described earlier, usually are incorporated in daily cleaning solutions to prevent microbial contamination of solutions once in use. Finally, buffering agents (such as borates and phosphates) can be included to ensure stability of the formulations or to assist with protein removal. Some solutions are formulated with increased tonicity as a further adjunct to the cleaning action of the surfactants.

Oxidizers such as hydrogen peroxide are primarily used for their disinfecting action, but they also provide cleaning action and assist in preventing surface deposit buildup (44, 46).

Tear film proteins, particularly lysozyme, accumulate on the surface of hydrogel lenses over time. These proteins become loosely attached to the lens surface on insertion and bind to the surface over time either as films or discrete deposits. Protein deposition can lead to decreased comfort and satisfaction with lens wear, loss of wearing time, vision decrements, and possibly atopic reactions (55). Bound protein is not removed from the lens surface by most surfactant cleaners. Proteolytic enzymes may be incorporated into cleaning regimens to remove proteinaceous deposits. Enzymatic cleaners lyse the bonds between protein molecules. This allows the deposited proteins to be removed by surfactant cleaners, together with the manual rubbing and rinsing included in most cleaning regimens. Three primary groups of proteolytic enzymes are used, namely papain, pancreatin, and subtilisin A. Pancreatin is a multiple enzyme that contains a protease, a lipase (for action on lipids), and an amylase (for actions on polysaccharides). It is available as a liquid.

Disposable lenses and planned replacement programs have lessened dependence on protein removal treatments, which should be used regularly for lenses that will be worn for longer than 1 month. Inclusion of hydroxyalkyl phosphonate, a sequestering agent that binds calcium and so indirectly minimizes protein absorption and adsorption, in multipurpose solutions also has diminished the need for separate enzymatic cleaning (56).

LUBRICANTS

It is not unusual for hydrogel lenses to require lubrication and rehydration while they are being worn. In fact, symptoms of dryness and discomfort are common and are the

TABLE 20.2. SOME CLEANING AGENTS AND ADJUNCT CHEMICALS

Surfactants	Nonionic
	Amphoteric
	Anionic
Lipid solvents	Isopropyl alcohol
Chelating agents	Ethylenediaminetetraacetate (EDTA)
Preservatives	Polyquaternium-1
	Sorbic acid
Buffers	Borate
	Phosphate
Oxidizers	Hydrogen peroxide
Enzymatic cleaners	Papain
	Pancreatin
	Subtilisin A

most cited cause of discontinuing lens wear (57). These symptoms often are managed by the use of rewetting solutions or lubricants (15).

Sterile physiologic saline can be used for this purpose. Preserved or unpreserved saline should be used only in unit-dose form (20).

Solutions offering longer contact times, together with the potential additional action of hindering debris accumulation on the lens surface, are sometimes indicated. Although use of such lubricating solutions is common, there is evidence that their effect on dryness symptoms is little different from that of saline (58).

In addition to sodium chloride, lubricants contain wetting agents, viscosity builders, preservatives, and buffers (Table 20.3). Wetting agents reduce surface tension, making the surface more wettable. Wetting agents contained in lubricants include polyvinyl alcohol, polyvinyl pyrrolidone, poloxamer 407, PEG-11 lauryl ester carboxylic acid, and Tetronic 1304.

To extend the contact time of the instilled solutions with contact lenses, viscosity-building agents are incorporated in the formulation. The most common viscosity builders are cellulose derivatives, such as methyl cellulose, hydroxyethyl cellulose, hydroxypropylmethyl cellulose, and carboxymethyl cellulose. Preservatives also are included to minimize microbial contamination while the lenses are in use. Preservatives must be present only in concentrations that will not cause epithelial cell damage, even with extended contact time, because the solution is instilled directly into the eye. Sorbic acid and polyquaternium-1 are two examples of preservatives often included in lubricating solutions (15). Finally, buffers are included to maintain solution pH at an appropriate level. Sometimes, a nonphysiologic pH is needed for optimum preservative action. The buffering system must be adequate to maintain the required pH in this case, but it also must be capable of moving toward tear pH levels when instilled into the eye. Conversely, solutions at physiologic pH may be more strongly buffered to retain

that pH. Commonly used buffering agents are the borates, phosphates, and nitrates.

MULTIPURPOSE SOLUTIONS

Solution formulations designed to clean, rinse, and disinfect hydrogel lenses were described earlier. Multipurpose solutions combine these three actions (24,26,59). Although separate cleaners have been required in some systems, many multipurpose solutions are complete in their actions and provide an answer to the issue of noncompliance with lens care. Multipurpose solutions are the most common care systems in current usage (60,61). They may contain preservatives, surfactants, lubricants, sequestering agents, and buffers.

The two most common preservatives in multipurpose solutions are PHMB (or polyhexamide) and polyquaternium-1 (7). Both are high-molecular-weight preservatives that provide high antimicrobial effectiveness together with little risk of adverse ocular responses at the concentrations in use. More recently, myristamidopropyl dimethylamine has been incorporated as an additional preservative to enhance the disinfecting action of these multipurpose solutions (25,62).

Multipurpose solutions include cleaning agents in their formulations, usually surfactants, in order to assist with removal of debris from the lens surface (63). As well as surfactants, citrate has been included to provide an additional cleaning effect and reduce protein deposition (64). Enzymatic cleaning usually is provided as an additional step, although the availability of liquid pancreatin is another option for simpler enzymatic cleaning.

Multipurpose solutions may include EDTA as a chelating agent to increase the antimicrobial effectiveness of the preservatives. Hydroxyalkyl phosphonate is a sequestering agent that binds calcium and so indirectly minimizes protein absorption and adsorption. Buffers ensure that solution pH is maintained at levels that will ensure preservative effectiveness.

Although most multipurpose solutions retain manual rubbing as part of the cleaning process, some solutions may have adequate effectiveness without the need for mechanical dislodgment of materials (65,66). This is a further improvement in multipurpose solution development and, together with the use of disposable lenses, offers practitioners ways to effectively manage noncompliance. Nevertheless, although modern multipurpose solutions may be approved without a rubbing step, optimal lens care still includes this step in the lens care regimen.

OTHER PHYSIOCHEMICAL CHARACTERISTICS

Nonlabel Features

The labeled formula of each solution informs the practitioner of its active and inactive ingredients. Most contact

TABLE 20.3. COMMON COMPONENTS OF LUBRICANTS

Wetting agents	Polyvinyl alcohol
	Polyvinyl pyrrolidone
	Poloxamer 407
	PEG-11 lauryl ester carboxylic acid
	Tetronic 1304
Viscosity builders	Methyl cellulose
	Hydroxyethyl cellulose
	Hydroxypropylmethyl cellulose
	Carboxymethyl cellulose
Preservatives	Sorbic acid
	Polyquaternium-1
Buffers	Borate
	Phosphate
	Nitrate

lens fitters make the tacit assumption that each class of hydrogel lens care product (cleaning, disinfecting, lubricating) also has a set of fundamental physical and chemical attributes that make it suitable to meet its mission ideally. A corollary to this notion is that there then would be an *ultimate* formulation from which the ideal solution would result (67). These fundamental characteristics, which rarely are listed on the labels of the solutions, include osmolality, pH, buffering capacity (the ability to resist pH change), and viscosity.

A reasonable question to ask, therefore, is just what range of characteristics of hydrogel lens care solutions exists in the marketplace. We have studied the four characteristics mentioned earlier for representative solutions with varying uses and have grouped the results for solutions designed for direct in-eye use and those designed for use with hydrogel lenses but off-eye (34). The resulting values are shown in Fig. 20.1 as average and range values for in-eye and off-eye use.

Of the four characteristics, osmolality of any solution

will have an immediate effect on the hydration level of a hydrogel lens, so it might be expected to be tightly controlled. However, a surprising range of values exists for these solutions, namely, from 0.83% to 1.23% NaCl. Even more surprisingly, these extremes are encountered not only in solutions used just before a reequilibrating step but also in solutions designed for direct in-eye use. Whereas other advantages of these solutions are inherent in the formulation, these findings suggest that there are no long-term disadvantages to the osmolality extremes. If ocular or visual consequences result from the use of any given solution, conversely, reequilibration of the contact lens with a solution of a different osmolality may be required. Unfortunately, the absence of information available to fitters concerning this characteristic of one lens solution forces decision making about alternatives into a *trial-and-error* process.

The pH or relative acidity of these solutions can affect hydrogel lens values (34,68,69), yet deviations from the normal tear pH of 7.4 are surprisingly characteristic of these solutions. The material characteristics of some lenses are

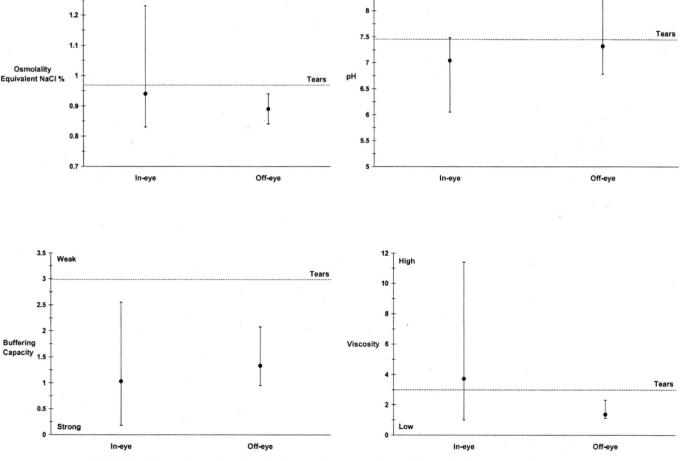

FIG. 20.1. Comparison of nonlabel features of representative solutions for in-eye and off-eye use. Values are shown as average and range for each solution group. *Top left* is osmolality (as equivalent % NaCl), *top right* is pH, *bottom left* is buffering capacity (as pH shift to a standard alkali challenge), and *bottom right* is viscosity (relative to water).

susceptible to pH shifts; fitting and oxygen delivery characteristics both can be compromised. Again, if relative acidity is implicated as a mechanism for lack of hydrogel lens wearing performance, equilibration with solutions of different pH can be attempted.

The buffering capacity, or ability to resist pH change, of these solutions will influence the equilibration of the contact lens with a tear environment on insertion into the eye. When a nonphysiologic solution pH value is a characteristic of the solution (e.g., to protect preservative efficacy), poorly buffered formulas typically are used to allow rapid adjustment to the ocular conditions. Intolerance to particular buffering chemicals occasionally occurs; a care system using alternative buffering chemicals then can be recommended.

Viscosity normally would not be considered a particularly critical characteristic for hydrogel lens care solutions (unlike the case for rigid lens solutions), and the low values typically measured support this theory. Occasionally, high viscosities are encountered, however, so the possibility of adverse effects on lens wear or, conversely, an enhanced lubrication effect by such solutions should be considered.

Other Clinical Implications

Over the years, each of the solutions represented here has achieved a place in current practice. In that sense, each is a successful solution that must meet the needs of at least some patients. Despite this, the findings for these representative solutions are notable for their wide range of values. Therefore, the concept of a "right" solution is not a viable one. Given the individuality of the eye's needs and responses, the range of attributes among these solutions is both explicable and necessary. Subtleties of combinations and features, as well, are likely to be the most critical determinants of the efficacy of any given solution.

These variabilities do not lessen the need for vigilance by the practitioner in interpreting incompatibilities that may surface, even with the general acceptance of multipurpose solutions. The knowledgeable practitioner will recognize solution, eye, or lens incompatibilities. Appropriate action often requires more information than usually is given on a solution's label, however, and this chapter is aimed at filling in some of the information gaps.

Matching solution systems to specific eye and lens combinations could be useful in the same way. If achieved, improved compliance should result. Unfortunately, recognition of mismatching still relies on rapid and early detection of adverse responses through symptomatology and biomicroscopy evaluation.

COMPLIANCE

Impressive advances have been made in the development of solutions with improved efficacy and ease of use. Avoiding failures is, however, still dependent on lens wearers using their prescribed care and maintenance systems in the intended manner. Unfortunately, compliance with instructions is poor among wearers of contact lenses, in common with many health care situations (70,71).

To contact lens wearers, loss of comfort is more of a stimulus to compliance than the potential for complications. Compliance among contact lens wearers is known to diminish with duration of lens use, indicating a need for increased vigilance among practitioners in the case of long-term lens wearers (72). In general, compliance also decreases with the complexity of any intervention, so the use of multipurpose solutions is to be encouraged when noncompliance is suspected (70,71,73).

CONCLUSION

Availability of disposable and extended wear contact lenses has altered the dependence of some lens wearers on care and maintenance of their contact lenses. Development of new, highly efficacious, and yet tissue-compatible disinfecting and other agents has likewise reduced the prospect of adverse ocular responses. The acceptance of the simplified care systems offered by multipurpose solutions has improved the prospect of compliance and reduced the likelihood of complications. Despite these undoubted gains, the contact lens practitioner must remain knowledgeable on solution components and their relative merits.

The patient's individual tolerances and the contact lens material tolerances remain the overriding factors that require a variety of active and inactive ingredients and their combinations, as well as ranges of physical and chemical attributes in hydrogel lens care solutions. The *right* solution may not exist, but knowledgeable use of the solutions available allows optimization of any eye–contact lens–solution combinations.

REFERENCES

1. International Committee on Contact Lenses. Contact lens maintenance systems. *Int Contact Lens Clin* 1992;19:153–156.
2. Morgan PB. Soft lens care systems. In: Efron N, ed. *Contact lens practice.* Boston: Butterworth Heinemann, 2002.
3. Veys J, Meyler J, Davies I. *Essential contact lens practice.* Boston: Butterworth Heinemann, 2002;133–149.
4. Brennan NA. Is there a question of safety with continuous wear? *Clin Exp Optom* 2002;85:127–140.
5. Stapleton F, Stechler J. Contact lens care systems and solutions used by the practitioner. In: Ruben M, Guillon M, eds. *Contact lens practice.* London: Chapman and Hall, 1994;529–558.
6. Jones L, Jones D, Houlford M. Clinical comparison of three polyhexanide preserved multi-purpose contact lens solutions. *Contact Lens Anterior Eye* 1997;20:23–30.
7. Franklin V, Tighe B, Tonge S. Disclosure—the true story of multi-purpose solutions. *Optician* 1995;200:25–28.

8. Watanabe RK, Rah MJ. Preventative contact lens care: part III. *Contact Lens Spectrum* 2001;16:26–31.

9. Giese MJ, Weissman BA. Contact lens associated corneal infections. Where do we go from here? *Clin Exp Optom* 2002;85:141–148.

10. Ward MA. The microbiology of contact lens wear. *Contact Lens Spectrum* 1997;12:23–29.

11. Lowe R, Vallas V, Brennan NA. Comparative efficacy of contact lens disinfection solutions. *CLAO J* 1992;18:34–40.

12. Keith D, Stein J, Christensen M, et al. Which products keep deposits under control? *Contact Lens Spectrum* 1999;14:38–40.

13. Shih KL, Hu J, Sibley M. The microbiological benefit of cleaning and rinsing contact lenses. *Int Contact Lens Clin* 1985;12:235–142.

14. Begley CG, Caffery B, Nichols KK, et al. Responses of contact lens wearers to a dry eye survey. *Optom Vis Sci* 2000;77:40–46.

15. Doughty MJ. Re-wetting, comfort, lubricant and moisturizing solutions for the contact lens wearer. *Contact Lens Anterior Eye* 1999;22:116–126.

16. Sivak JG, Herbert KL, Fonn D. In vitro ocular irritancy measure of four contact lens solutions: damage and recovery. *CLAO J* 1995;21:169–174.

17. Begley CG, Waggoner PJ, Jani NB, et al. The effects of soft contact lens disinfection solutions on rabbit corneal epithelium. *CLAO J* 1994;20:52–58.

18. Geerling G, Daniels JT, Dart JKG, et al. Toxicity of natural tear substitutes in a fully defined culture model of human corneal epithelial cells. *Invest Ophthalmol Vis Sci* 2001;42:948–956.

19. Bergmanson JPG, Ross RN. A masked quantitative cytologic study of the safety of a multipurpose contact lens solution applied to the in vivo rabbit eye. *J Am Optom Assoc* 1993;64:308–314.

20. Sweeney DF, Wilcox MDP, Sansey N, et al. Incidence of contamination of preserved saline solutions during normal use. *CLAO J* 1999;25:167–175.

21. Barr JT. What you need to know about solution interactions. *Contact Lens Spectrum* 1994;9:15–21.

22. Edwards K. Lens care with frequent replacement lenses. *Optician* 1998;215:32–34.

23. Sweeney DF, Keay L, Carnt N, et al. Practitioner guidelines for continuous wear with high Dk silicone hydrogel contact lenses. *Clin Exp Optom* 2002;85:161–167.

24. Lever AM, Miller MJ. Comparative antimicrobial efficacy of multi-purpose lens care solutions using the FDA's revised guidance document for industry: stand-alone primary criteria. *CLAO J* 1999;25:52–56.

25. Rosenthal RA, McAnally CL, McNamee LS, et al. Broad spectrum antimicrobial activity of a new multi-purpose disinfecting solution. *CLAO J* 2000;26:120–126.

26. Guillon M, Maissa C. Clinical acceptance of two multipurpose solutions: MPS containing HPMC versus citrate-based MPS without rubbing. *CLAO J* 2002;28:186–191.

27. Rosenthal RA, McAnally CL, Stone RP, et al. Disinfection efficacy of MPDS against pseudomonas. *Contact Lens Spectrum* 2001;16:44–47.

28. Ward MA, Barr JT. Contact lens care systems and solutions. *Contact Lens Spectrum* 1998;13:9s–18s.

29. Rosenthal RA, McDonald MM, Schlitzer RL, et al. Loss of bactericidal activity from contact lens storage solutions. *CLAO J* 1997;23:57–62.

30. International Organization for Standardization. Ophthalmic optics—contact lens care products—microbiological requirements and test methods for products and regimens for hygienic management of contact lenses. ISO/FDIS 14729. 2000.

31. Food and Drug Administration. Guidance for industry: premarket notification (510[k] guidance document for contact lens care products. US Department of Health and Human Services, Food and Drug Administration, Center for Devices and Radiological Health, May 1997.

32. Simmons PA, Clough SR, Teagle RH, et al. Toxic effects of ophthalmic preservatives on cultured rabbit epithelium. *Am J Optom Physiol Opt* 1988;65:867–873.

33. Collin HB, Grabsch BE, Carroll N, et al. The effects of benzalkonium chloride on in vitro corneal endothelium and keratocytes. *Int Contact Lens Clin* 1982;9:237–243.

34. Carney LG, Barr JT, Hill RM. Lens solution chemistry. In: Bennett ES, Weissman BA, eds. *Clinical contact lens practice.* Philadelphia: JB Lippincott Company, 1991; chapter 35, 1–7.

35. Rosenthal RA, Schlitzer RL, McNamee LS, et al. Antimicrobial activity of organic chlorine releasing compounds. *J Br Cont Lens Assoc* 1992;15:81–84.

36. Christie C. Solutions: same or different? *Optician* 1999;218:20–24.

37. Copley CA. Chlorine disinfection of soft contact lenses. *Clin Exp Optom* 1989;72:3–7.

38. Burton GD, Hill RM. Aerobic responses of the cornea to ophthalmic preservatives, measured in vivo. *Invest Ophthalmol Vis Sci* 1981;21:842–845.

39. Wilson LA, McNatt J, Reitschel R. Delayed hypersensitivity to thimerosal in soft contact lens wearers. *Ophthalmology* 1981;88:804–809.

40. Miller MJ, Callahan DE, McGrath D, et al. Disinfection efficacy of contact lens care solutions against ocular pathogens. *CLAO J* 2001;27:16–22.

41. Janoff LE. Origin and development of hydrogen peroxide disinfection systems. *CLAO J* 1990;16:S36–S42.

42. Paugh JR, Brennan NA, Efron N. Ocular response to hydrogen peroxide. *Am J Optom Physiol Opt* 1988;65:91–98.

43. Tripathi BJ, Tripathi RC. Hydrogen peroxide damage to human corneal epithelial cells in vitro. *Arch Ophthalmol* 1989;107:1516–1519.

44. Senchyna M. Contact lens care: biochemistry of antimicrobial agents used in contact lens care solutions. *Optician* 2001;221:36–41.

45. Lowe R, Brennan NA. Hydrogen peroxide disinfection of hydrogel contact lenses. *Clin Exp Optom* 1987;70:190–197.

46. Christie CL, Meyler JG. Contemporary contact lens care products. *Contact Lens Anterior Eye* 1997;20:S11–S17.

47. Palmer W, Scanlon P, McNulty C. Efficacy of an ultraviolet light contact lens disinfection unit against microbial pathogenic organisms. *J Br Cont Lens Assoc* 1991;14:13–16.

48. Admoni MM, Bartolomei A, Qureshi MN, et al. Disinfection efficacy in an integrated ultraviolet light contact lens care system. *CLAO J* 1994;20:246–248.

49. Harris MG, Fluss L, Lem A, et al. Ultraviolet disinfection of contact lenses. *Optom Vis Sci* 1993;70:839–842.

50. Choate W, Fontana F, Potter J, et al. Evaluation of the Purilens contact lens care system: an automatic care system incorporating UV disinfection and hydrodynamic shear cleaning. *CLAO J* 2000;26:134–140.

51. Fatt I. Physical limitation to cleaning soft contact lenses by ultrasonic methods. *J Br Cont Lens Assoc* 1991;14:135–136.

52. Scanlon P. Microbiological aspects of combined ultrasonic contact lens disinfection units. *J Br Cont Lens Assoc* 1991;14:55–59.

53. Kastl PR, Maehara JR. Low-power microwave disinfection of soft contact lenses. *CLAO J* 2001;27:81–83.

54. Harris MG, Gan CM, Grant T, et al. Microwave irradiation and soft contact lens parameters. *Optom Vis Sci* 1993;70:843–848.

55. Meisler DM, Keller WB. Contact lens type, material, and deposits and giant papillary conjunctivitis. *CLAO J* 1995;21:77–80.

56. Simmons PA, Ridder WH, Edrington TB, et al. Passive protein removal by two multipurpose lens solutions: comparison of ef-

fects on in vitro deposited and patient-worn hydrogel contact lenses. *Int Contact Lens Clin* 1999;26:33–37.

57. Vajdic C, Holden BA, Sweeney DF, et al. The frequency of ocular symptoms during spectacle and daily soft and rigid contact lens wear. *Optom Vis Sci* 1999;76:705–711.

58. Golding TR, Efron N, Brennan NA. Soft lens lubricants and prelens tear film stability. *Optom Vis Sci* 1990;67:461–465.

59. Donshik P, Madden R, Simmons PA. Pursuing comfort in a multi-purpose solution. *Contact Lens Spectrum* 2000;15:33–36.

60. Morgan PB, Efron N, Helland M, et al. How does the UK market compare with other countries? *Optician* 2001;221:26–32.

61. Woods C, Morgan PB. Contact lens prescribing in the Australian states and territories 2001. *Clin Exp Optom* 2002;85:279–283.

62. Rosenthal RA, Buck S, McAnally C, et al. Antimicrobial comparison of a new multi-purpose disinfecting solution to a 3% hydrogen peroxide system. *CLAO J* 1999;25:213–217.

63. Franklin VJ. Cleaning efficacy of single-purpose surfactant cleaners and multi-purpose solutions. *Contact Lens Anterior Eye* 1997; 20:63–68.

64. Christensen B, Lebow K, White EM, et al. Effectiveness of citrate-containing lens care regimens: a controlled clinical comparison. *Int Contact Lens Clin* 1998;25:50–57.

65. Barr JT. Contact lens solutions and lens care update. *Contact Lens Spectrum* 2001;16:26–33.

66. Stiegmeier MJ. Solution drops digital cleaning step. *Contact Lens Spectrum* 2000;15:45–47.

67. Hill RM, Carney LG, Barr JT, et al. Soft lens solutions: a look at what's not on the label. *Contact Lens Spectrum* 1988;3:43–46.

68. Montes I Mico R, Lopez-Alemany A. Comparative study of the pH over time of use of contact lens saline solutions. *Int Contact Lens Clin* 1998;25:9–15.

69. Harris MG, Hale B, Lee D, et al. Discovering the effect of temperature on a solution's pH. *Contact Lens Spectrum* 1999;14: 41–44.

70. Collins MJ, Carney LG. Patient compliance and its influence on contact lens wearing problems. *Am J Optom Physiol Opt* 1986; 63:952–956.

71. Collins MJ, Carney LG. Compliance with care and maintenance procedures among contact lens wearers. *Clin Exp Optom* 1986; 69:174–177.

72. Radford CF, Woodward EG, Stapleton F. Contact lens hygiene compliance in a university population. *J Br Contact Lens Assoc* 1993;16:105–111.

73. Claydon BE, Efron N, Woods C. Non-compliance in optometric practice. *Ophthalmic Physiol Opt* 1998;18:187–190.

DISPOSABLE AND FREQUENT REPLACEMENT HYDROGEL CONTACT LENSES

MELISSA W. CHUN
LISA BARNHART FOX
AND ALANA J. ZHOU

"All contact lenses are disposable, it is just a matter of the frequency of replacement" (1). Conventional, or "reusable," hydrogel lenses have normally been replaced on an approximately annual basis. With the introduction of "disposable" hydrogels by Vistakon (Johnson & Johnson Vision Care, Inc., Jacksonville, FL, USA) in 1987, however, the practice of planned or frequent replacement became not only economically feasible but created a new classification of contact lens wear. A variety of frequent replacement and disposable contact lenses have entered the contact lens field since 1987. Of note, the introduction of daily wear disposable lenses in 1994 and the recent United States Food and Drug Administration (FDA) approval in 2001 of silicone hydrogel lenses for up to 30 nights of continuous wear necessitates precise use of contact lens nomenclature in describing these different contact lens modalities. The FDA originally defined a disposable lens as a "single use lens, which, when removed, is discarded and never used again." Hence, the term *disposable lens* refers to lenses worn once and then disposed of upon removal from the eye, regardless of whether the lens is worn on a daily wear basis or a 1-week or 30-day extended wear schedule. A frequent replacement contact lens refers to all contact lenses that are cleaned, disinfected, and reused whether they are replaced every 2 weeks, monthly, quarterly, and so forth (2).

Approximately 32 million ametropic patients in the United States wore contact lenses in 2001 (3). Clinical experience has shown that satisfied contact lens wearers can provide considerable revenue to the eye care practitioner, if their loyalty can be maintained (4).

As early as 1991, frequent replacement lenses were recognized to have a positive impact on the contact lens industry. One industry publication even nominated disposable and frequent replacement lenses as "the contact lens event of the year" (5,6). With almost five million additional patients interested in wearing disposable contact lenses (market research in 1990) (7), some then predicted that a frequent replacement modality would constitute 50% to 75% of the contact-lens-wearing market, whereas disposable lens use might show a decline without another breakthrough due to cost. These predictions were made even though the contact lens market showed a decline in growth by the early 1990s. According to the Contact Lens Manufacturers Association (CLMA), contact lens sales in 1991 were down 5% from previously consistent growth (8). It was not until the first half of 1996 that the expanding disposable and frequent replacement lens brought the industry out of the "flat market" and showed strong growth. In the same year, the concept of disposable lenses was saluted by the White House, and Vistakon was awarded a National Medal of Technology for several novel products including 1-Day Acuvue (9). By 1996, nearly half, or 45%, of soft contact lens wearers were in a disposable or frequent replacement modality. In 2001, more than a decade later, at least 65% of soft contact lens wearers were using a disposable or frequent replacement modality, thus meeting earlier market predictions. For new contact lens patients, the use of a frequent replacement toric lens modality showed a 15% increase in the first half of 2001 (3). (A "new" patient is defined as either someone new to contact lenses or a previous lens wearer refit into a different lens.) For over a decade, frequent replacement lenses have changed the traditional distribution pattern for contact lenses; they should continue to have a substantial positive impact on the contact lens industry.

A PANACEA?

Are disposable and frequent replacement lenses a panacea? This concept has been promoted in the media as healthier, more comfortable, and more convenient to the "consumer." Practitioners have been informed that these lenses are a more profitable alternative, increasing both patient compliance and retention. The primary advantages of frequent replacement are reduced lens soilage and any associated adverse ocular complications. A psychological advantage lies in increased convenience. Research indicates that daily wear disposable lenses clearly cause the lowest incidence of contact lens complications (10,11) and are the safest option of all available contact lens modalities (12). One study conducted in Italy compared the bacterial and protein load on contact lenses worn on a daily wear disposable schedule versus a daily wear 15-day replacement schedule. Even on a short 15-day regimen, the natural flora of the ocular surface environment was altered compared to eyes using a daily wear disposable lens. They found through impression cytology a decline in the ocular surface quality in eyes that wore the 15-day lenses. They attributed this decline to the disinfection solutions and the preservatives in those solutions. In addition, the quantity of protein deposits on the lenses was directly proportional to the aging of the lens. Their findings suggest that daily wear disposable lenses are safer and more likely to maintain the normal physiologic environment of the ocular surface (13). That said, no modality of contact lens wear eliminates all risks. Incidents of daily wear disposable contact lens-related complications have been reported. Hingorani et al. (14) reported in 1995 a case of ulcerative keratitis in a 27-year-old woman on a 5-day trial of 1-Day Acuvue. The lens was worn on a daily wear basis and discarded (14). Choi et al. (15) reported in 2001 a case of fungal keratitis in a young female wearing daily wear disposable contact lenses. This patient also had no history of overnight wear of the lens or of ocular trauma. These are unusual occurrences, but they serve as a reminder of potential risks, and patients need to be properly advised in the informed consent process.

Extended wear disposable hydrogel lenses, on the other hand, have not proven to reduce the risk of infection and corneal ulceration (16–18). In fact, some studies cite equal if not greater rates of corneal ulcers in patients wearing extended wear disposable hydrogel lenses (17). Studies from the Cornea and Contact Lens Research Unit (CCLRU) at the University of New South Wales, Australia, indicated that the corneal infection rate with disposable lenses remains similar to that found in extended wear conventional lenses (19). Case reports by Dunn et al. (16) and Buehler et al. (17) also showed that sight-threatening central bacterial corneal ulcers still occurred with extended wear disposable hydrogel lenses. The relationship between contact lens wear and ulcerative keratitis has been studied since a correlation between the two was noted in the 1970s. In the 1980s, it was suggested that the cause of microbial keratitis and corneal ulceration among contact lens wearers could be linked to the wearing of contact lenses exposed to contaminated exogenous sources, such as cleaning, rinsing, and/or disinfecting solutions, contact lens cases, cosmetics, and eye drops. There is a high frequency of storage case and care solution microbial contamination even among asymptomatic contact lens wearers. The frequency of contamination was found to be higher in extended wear patients, presumably because the solutions last longer than those used by daily wear patients (20). It was erroneously thought that a dispos-

TABLE 21.1. FACTORS CONTRIBUTING TO CONTACT LENS CONTAMINATION

Soiled hands and fingers
Cosmetic debris
Foreign particles
Environmental pollutants (dust, smoke)
Toxic fumes
Ultraviolet radiation

From Marshall EC. Disposable vs. non-disposable contact lenses—the relative risk of ocular infection. *J Am Optom Assoc* 1992;63:28.

able lens would reduce the problems of contamination from solutions and handling, resulting in safer extended wear (Tables 21.1 and 21.2). The primary culprit for the heightened risk of infection appears to be a cascade of events produced by hypoxia (21). Until recently, most extended wear hydrogel lenses, including disposables, have similar oxygen transmissibility (Dk/t) values. As discussed in other chapters, the optimal daily wear Dk/t value to meet the oxygen requirements of the cornea was suggested by Holden and Mertz (22) to be 25×10^{-9} cm mL O_2/s mL mm Hg. Disposable hydrogel lenses meet this requirement. However, the minimal "compromise" extended wear Holden/Mertz criterion of Dk/t of 34×10^{-9} cm mL O_2/s mL mm Hg is not met. These authors believed that to achieve no excess nighttime swelling under the closed eyelid, a Dk/t of 87×10^{-9} cm mL O_2/s mL mm Hg would be required (22). Furthermore, Harvitt and Bonanno (23) established that to prevent anoxia throughout the entire corneal thickness, the Dk/t requirements are 35 for the open eye and 125 for the closed eye. These limitations, however, very likely will be overcome with the use of extended wear disposable silicone hydrogel lenses. The silicone hydrogel lenses recently approved for up to 30 nights of continuous wear have a nominal Dk/t value of 110×10^{-9} cm mL O_2/s mL mm Hg for balafilcon A (PureVision, Bausch & Lomb, Rochester, NY, USA) and 175×10^{-9} cm mL O_2/s mL mm Hg for lotrafilcon A (Focus Night and Day, CIBA Vision Care, Duluth, GA, USA). As discussed elsewhere in this volume, it is possible that extended wear disposable lenses of silicone hydrogel polymers may reduce the incidence of corneal infection and ulceration associated with

TABLE 21.2. COMPLICATIONS SECONDARY TO LENS CONTAMINATION

Decreased wettability
Surface irregularities
Distortion and decreased visual acuity
Ocular irritations and hyperemia
Infectious and allergic conjunctivitis
Epithelial hypertrophy
Keratitis/corneal ulceration

From Marshall EC. Disposable vs. non-disposable contact lenses—the relative risk of ocular infection. *J Am Optom Assoc* 1992;63:28.

extended wear. They certainly have demonstrated negligible corneal neovascularization and hypoxic effects in subjects on a 30-night extended wear schedule for an average duration of 9 months (24,25). A 1-year prospective study found that signs of hypoxia-induced changes in the cornea were virtually nonexistent in patients wearing silicone hydrogel lenses for 30 nights of continuous wear compared with patients wearing hydrogel lenses for 1-week extended wear (26). Last year, the FDA approved silicone hydrogel contact lenses for up to 30 nights of continuous wear. These lenses should be replaced every month. Once the lenses are removed, the eyes should have a rest without lens wear for at least one night. Due to known complications with extended wear, the FDA is requiring that the manufacturers of silicone hydrogel lenses perform postmarketing surveillance to monitor the long-term safety of these devices (3).

EVOLUTION OF FREQUENT REPLACEMENT

The development of frequent replacement and disposable contact lenses was a direct result of the trend toward preventative medicine in the 1990s. This era was evidenced by the vast array of disposable products available to the consumer, ranging from razors to cameras. In the medical environment, disposability (i.e., syringes, thermometers) is associated with improved health protection. This proactive philosophy has led to more preventative lens maintenance (Table 21.3).

The disposable and frequent replacement modalities were not so much revolutionary in material chemistry as they were innovative marketing and packaging concepts. When this was supplemented with an improvement in manufacturing ability that provides inexpensive yet highly reproducible lenses of excellent optical quality and design, disposable and frequent replacement programs become a practical reality for most hydrogel lenses. In 1987, Vistakon (formerly Frontier Contact Lenses) test marketed the first extended wear disposable contact lens (Acuvue) in Florida.

TABLE 21.3. ADVANTAGES OF FREQUENT REPLACEMENT/DISPOSABLE LENSES

Insertion of a sterile lens
Decreased lens surface deposits, biofilm, and microorganisms
Decreased opportunity for lens damage and discoloration
Decreased incidence of toxicity and hypersensitivity reactions to solutions
Decreased cost associated with reduced need for chemical solutions
Increased comfort
Increased convenience for daily activities
Decreased in-office lens disinfection procedures
Decreased chair time associated with fewer complaints-related office visits
Increased patient compliance

The lens was released nationwide in June 1988. The Acuvue lens was based on the work of Danish ophthalmologist and entrepreneur Michael Bay. Bay's system created a reproducible product, although it lacked quality control. Vistakon refined the product after analyzing the growth potential of this expanding market.

The Acuvue lens was introduced as a single-use product, requiring no disinfecting or cleaning. The lens was intended to be used for extended wear for a maximum of 1 week, then discarded and replaced with a new lens. Demand and acceptance as an extended wear lens, however, were relatively low. As discussed in this volume, the unprecedented growth in the use of hydrogel lenses for both daily wear and extended wear resulted in an increase in ocular complications by the mid 1980s. The most feared of these complications was and still is corneal infection. Practitioners preferred to recommend daily wear use of lenses for their patients because patients and practitioners alike were conscious of media information regarding contact lens problems. A poll by the Gallup organization found that most contact lens wearers are well-educated young adults ranging in age from 25 to 40 years. This poll indicated 82% of those questioned could cite some disadvantages of wearing contact lenses, and 7% specifically mentioned infection. In another separate Gallup poll, 69% of Americans wearing a vision correction device expressed awareness about disposable contact lenses (27). In response to these concerns, Vistakon obtained FDA approval for daily wear use of the Acuvue lens in 1990.

Once considered a novelty, the idea of contact lenses that can be discarded on a daily basis became a reality in 1994. The daily wear disposable lens was first introduced in five blister-pack strips packaged as a box of 30 lenses to provide the patient fresh, sterile lenses for daily wear use. The lenses would be discarded at the end of the wearing day and new sterile lenses used for the next wearing period, whether this was the following day or the following week. This modality eliminates the need for any daily cleaning, disinfecting, and enzymatic solutions. From the patient's point of view, the convenience of daily wear disposable contact lenses is the primary advantage. From the clinician's point of view, the decreased risk of compromised ocular health secondary to contact lens wear is the leading reason to prescribe daily wear disposable contact lenses. With this method, the doctor is assured that a fresh and sterile lens is always on patients' eyes, thus minimizing the effects of contact lens deposits and improper cleaning techniques. Irritations, allergies, and giant papillary conjunctivitis (GPC) associated with lens wear are reduced when there is a clean, sterile lens surface each day. Furthermore, the side effects of contaminated solution bottles, soiled storage cases, and sensitivities to solutions and preservatives are eliminated. In terms of lifestyle, disposable lenses are ideal for those who travel frequently or tend to lose lenses. For example, it is important to ensure that all patients involved in athletics, whether on a collegiate, professional, or recreational level, have replacement lenses with them, or on the sidelines, at all times. If the lens is disturbed by the athletic environment, it will be disposed of at the end of the day, if not immediately. It is easy and inexpensive to provide these patients with disposable lenses. This practice also eliminates the long-term consequences of contact lens exposure to dirt, dust, chalk, sweat, or ocean or pool water. For the patient interested in the occasional use of contact lenses for social or athletic use, the single-use packaging eliminates the problem of storing the lens safely between prolonged wearing periods.

Daily wear disposable contact lenses are a viable option for many contact lens wearers. The ability to better maintain ocular health, vision, comfort, and convenience at an optimal level offsets the cost and parameter limitations for most contact lens patients. In a multisite comparison between disposable and conventional daily wear contact lens regimens, previously successful contact lens wearers were fit with one or the other contact lens modalities (28). Follow-up visits were conducted at weeks 1, 4, 12, 26, and 52. At all examinations, daily wear disposable lens patients surpassed daily wear conventional lens patients with regard to Snellen acuity, subjective vision, contact lens comfort, ocular symptomatology, lens deposits, and overall satisfaction. When the results of follow-up examinations from weeks 1 and 52 were compared, improvement was noted for the daily wear disposable lens patients but regression was noted for the daily wear conventional lens patients. This demonstrates that patients are more likely to develop ocular and visual complications as their conventional lens ages. This study also reported that the daily wear disposable lens patients were much less likely to return for an unscheduled examination and presented with fewer serious ocular health problems compared with the daily wear conventional patients. The results of this study support the intuitive notion that a new contact lens worn each day is more likely to provide better vision, comfort, and ocular health than is a daily wear "reusable" or "conventional" lens, when both are worn for 1 year.

Noncompliance in lens care is reduced with daily wear disposable lens wear. When comparing compliance between daily wear disposable and daily wear conventional contact lens wear, the compliance rate is strikingly higher: 96% compliance with daily wear disposable versus 50% with daily wear conventional contact lenses (29). The only way a patient can be noncompliant with daily wear disposable contact lenses is by not disposing of the lenses on a daily basis, which, in effect, eliminates the concept of daily wear disposable contact lenses altogether.

There are significant numbers of contact lens dropouts who can be reintroduced to a safer, more convenient system of hydrogel contact lens wear (1). Additionally, in one study, 9 of 10 eye care professionals reported a lower dropout rate and an increased number of patient referrals from patients using disposable lenses (30). In 1990, a manufacturer's an-

nual consumer survey suggested that 37% of contact lens dropouts discontinued contact lens wear secondary to lens deposits. This may have been the first quantitative evidence that disposable lens patients will be less likely to drop out of contact lens wear (31).

Studies have shown that clinicians can decrease the number of complications associated with the use of extended wear hydrophilic bandage lenses for therapeutic purposes by recommending that a daily wear disposable lens be worn on an extended wear basis as the bandage lens of choice. Each practitioner must decide whether to use any contact lens modality that is not FDA approved (32). Bandage contact lenses are generally prescribed on an extended wear basis, subjecting the patient to the same risks associated with cosmetic extended wear. Preexisting corneal and anterior segment pathology, however, can increase these risks. Disposable bandage contact lenses have demonstrated a high level of subjective and objective therapeutic efficacy and a low complication rate. In the mid 1990s, CIBA Vision introduced the 55% water content, ProTek therapeutic lens of vifilcon A material specifically for use as a bandage contact lens after refractive surgery. The plano power only lens is available in two base curves of 8.9 and 9.2 mm (14.5-mm diameter). Focus Night & Day (CIBA Vision) received the CE Mark for therapeutic use this year. European eye care practitioners now can use the silicone hydrogel lens as a bandage lens. The role of disposable bandage lenses may increase with the introduction of new lens materials and adjunct pharmaceutical agents (33).

Initially, the technologic constraints of disposable/frequent replacement manufacture limited the range of parameters available. This limitation is decreasing as products are introduced in expanded parameters and designs, including toric and multifocal lenses. Frequent replacement toric lens new fits increased nearly 15% in the first half of 2001, and bifocal lens patients increased almost 20% in that time (3). The practitioner now has the option to replace lenses daily, weekly, monthly, or at 3-, 4-, or 6-month intervals. In fact, disposable and frequent replacement soft contact lenses are the predominant lens type in the United States and Europe (21).

LENS PARAMETERS
Daily Wear Disposable Lenses

Currently, three brands of daily wear disposable contact lenses are on the market. These lenses are to be worn for 1 day and then disposed. Vistakon's 1-Day Acuvue lens was introduced in 1994. The 1-Day Acuvue is a mid-water content (58%) etafilcon A, HEMA-based ionic lens material. It comes in two base curves: 8.5 and 9.0 mm (14.2-mm diameter). Power availability ranges from +6.00 D to −12.0 D (in 0.50-D steps above −6.00 D). 1-Day Acuvue comes in a light blue visibility tint and with an inversion indicator "123" on the front surface. As with all the Acuvue lenses, the 1-Day Acuvue also contains ultraviolet (UV) blocker. The 1-Day Acuvue lens was redesigned in 2001 with a monocurve back-surface design presumably to improve handling. The 1-Day Acuvue lenses are available in 30-packs. Focus Dailies lenses are manufactured by CIBA Vision Care. It is a high-water (69%), nonionic polyvinyl alcohol (PVA)-based lens made of nelfilcon A. Available base curve is 8.6 mm (13.8-mm diameter); power ranges from $+6.00$ D to -10.00 D (in 0.50-D steps above -6.00 D). Bausch and Lomb's daily wear disposable lens, SofLens 1-day disposable contact lens, is made of a 70% water content, hilafilcon A nonionic material. It comes in a 8.6-mm base curve (14.2-mm diameter), and power ranges from $+6.50$ D to -9.00 D (in 0.50-D steps above -7.00 D). The lenses are visibility tinted and are available in 15-packs and 90-packs.

Two studies have been published comparing 1-Day Acuvue and Focus Dailies in terms of fitting characteristics, comfort, user preference, and complication rates with diametrically opposing results. A multinational study, conducted in Canada, Norway, and the United Kingdom, found a strong subjective wearer preference for the Dailies lens (34). Their subjects cited lens comfort and insertion handling as the primary reasons for lens preference. The second study performed in Japan reported a statistically significant preference for the 1-Day Acuvue lens (35). The major reasons cited were comfort and the greater ease of removal of the 1-Day Acuvue lens. However, both studies found that the Focus Dailies lenses are easier to handle on insertion, and the 1-Day Acuvue lens is easier to remove at the end of the day. The recently redesigned 1-Day Acuvue lens should have improved handling, and with this modification, differences in handling on insertion may be reduced.

In fitting patients, we practice a right versus left eye comparison of the daily wear disposable lenses under consideration if all other factors are even. This approach takes up minimal chair time to assess the best fitting lens. Schwallie and Bauman (36) have suggested that the optimal time for evaluating lens centration and movement of Focus Dailies, a PVA-based contact lens, is during the first 5 minutes of wear as opposed to the traditional 10 to 30 minutes of equilibration time recommended by most fitting guides, and that evaluating lens movement at approximately 5 minutes is generally more representative of typical lens movement found after 8 hours of contact lens wear. Furthermore, they conclude that their results agree with previous studies indicating a strong similarity in the time course of equilibration between PVA lenses and other low- and high-water HEMA-based hydrogel contact lenses (37).

Frequent Replacement Spherical Lenses

The original "disposable lens," Acuvue, is a mid-water content (58%) etafilcon A, stabilized, soft-molding processed

lens. It has a light blue tint and UV filter, is approved for daily and extended wear use, and is designed for 1- to 2-week replacement. The lenses are supplied in six-packs. The Acuvue lens is a thin, usually comfortable lens, but it may present handling difficulty to first time lens wearers, hyperopes, presbyopes, and patients with dexterity problems. The Surevue lens, approved for daily wear and designed for 2-week replacement, was introduced by Vistakon to address these issues. The Acuvue lenses are generally successful with patients needing a thin (0.07 mm at -3.00 D), mid-water-content lens, especially in plus power. The Acuvue lens is available in base curves of 8.4 and 8.8 mm (14.0-mm diameter), in powers ranging from -0.50 D to -6.00 D in 0.25-D steps and from -6.50 D to -9.00 D in 0.50-D steps. The 8.8-mm base curve lens also is available up to -11.00 D in 0.50-D steps. In plus power, the lens has a 9.1-mm base curve (14.4-mm diameter) and is available in powers ranging from $+0.50$ D to $+6.00$ D in 0.25-D steps and from $+6.50$ D to $+8.00$ D in 0.50-D steps. The Acuvue lens contains an "AV" inside-out marker. The thicker (0.105 mm centrally at -3.00 D) daily wear Surevue is generally successful with first-time lens wearers and is available in 8.4-mm and 8.8-mm base curves, in powers ranging from -0.50 D to -6.00 D in 0.25-D steps and from -6.50 D to -9.00 D in 0.50-D steps. The Surevue 9.1-mm base curve (14.4-mm diameter) lenses are available from $+0.50$ D to $+6.00$ D power in 0.25-D steps. However, we have found that if the patient does not have difficulty in handling the thinner Acuvue lenses, the Acuvue lenses are more comfortable than the Surevue lenses. The lenses are approved for cleaning and disinfection with chemical or hydrogen peroxide systems. The Acuvue 2 lens, introduced in 1999, is available in two base curves of 8.3 and 8.7 mm (14.0-mm diameter), with power ranges from $+8.00$ D to -12.00 D in 0.50-D steps above ±6.00 D. The lens contains a "123" inversion mark on the front surface. All Acuvue, Acuvue 2, and Surevue lenses are available in six-packs. They are all available with a light blue visibility tint and with UV blocker. The Acuvue 2 Colours opaque and enhancer tinted lenses are available in an 8.3-mm base curve (14.0-mm diameter) from plano to -6.00 D. The enhancer tints of blue, green, and aqua also are available in a 8.7-mm base curve.

The Optima FW (Bausch & Lomb), previously the See-Quence 2/Medalist lens, is based on a low-water-content (38%) polymacon material approved for both daily and extended wear. The lenses are packaged for 2-week replacement in six-packs or 3-month replacement in four-packs; it also is available in 30-lens value packs. The lens has a light blue visibility tint and a "B & L" inversion indicator. The system is available in three base curves: 8.4, 8.7, and 9.0 mm (14.0-mm diameter). The powers range from -9.00 D to $+4.00$ D in 0.25-D steps. This lens can be disinfected with chemical, heat, or hydrogen peroxide systems and is approved for enzymatic cleaning. The original SeeQuence lens, a 38% water content lens of polymacon material, is a spin-cast lens with a blue-green visibility tint and an inversion mark. It is available from −0.50 D to −9.00 D in 0.25-D steps. The Bausch & Lomb Soflens 66 is a 66% water content, alphafilcon A material lens approved for both daily wear and extended wear. It is a cast-molded lens available in two base curves (14.2-mm diameter). The steep/medium (S/M) curvature has an equivalent base curve (EBC) of 8.1 (actual central base curve of 8.5) and F/M (flat/medium) curvature has an EBC of 8.4 (actual central base curve is 8.7). It is available from +6.00 D to −6.00 D in 0.25-D steps and from −6.50 D to −9.00 D in 0.50-D steps. It has been approved for heat, chemical, or hydrogen peroxide disinfection and has a light blue handling tint. The lenses are available in six-packs and 30-packs. The Bausch & Lomb Two Week lens is a cast-molded lens made of hilafilcon B (59%) nonionic material. This lens is available only in a 8.6-mm base curve (14.2-mm diameter). It is approved for daily wear and can be disinfected with chemical or oxidation systems. The six-pack is the least expensive frequent replacement option.

The Focus 1–2 Week (formerly NewVue; CIBA Vision) is a 55% water content, vifilcon A lens with a blue visibility tint. It is approved for extended and daily wear use and is designed for 1- to 2-week replacement, respectively. It is available in base curves of 8.4 and 8.8 mm (14.0-mm diameter), in powers ranging from +4.00 D to −6.00 D steps and from −6.50 D to −10.00 D in 0.50-D steps. The Focus 1–2 Week SoftColors have the same base curves and diameter and are available in translucent royal blue, aqua, and evergreen with powers of +4.00 D to −6.00 D. The Focus Monthly lens is the same material and comes in base curves of 8.6 and 8.9 mm, with power ranges from +6.00 D to −8.00 D in 0.25-D steps and from −8.50 D to −15.00 D in 0.50-D steps. The lens is packaged in six-packs and recommended for monthly replacement. The Focus Monthly SoftColors lens also is the same material and is available in aqua, royal blue, and evergreen enhancing tints. These tinted lenses are helpful for hyperopes, presbyopes, and patients with visual acuity or dexterity limitations. Power availability ranges from +6.00 D to −8.00 D in 0.25-D steps. Any CIBA disinfection systems can be used for Focus lenses. The FreshLook series of lenses (acquired from Wesley Jessen) is made of a 55% phemfilcon A ionic material and approved for flexible wear. They are available in transparent colors, FreshLook Color Enhancers, and opaque colors, FreshLook Color Blends and FreshLook Colors. Lens diameter is 14.5 mm with a 5.0-mm pupil and 12.5-mm iris diameter; base curve is 8.6 mm. Power ranges from +6.00 D to −8.00 D in 0.25-D steps. The lenses include an "FL" inversion mark and are available in six-packs. Recommended disinfection method is chemical or oxidation. The FreshLook Color Enhancers come in blue, green, and aqua. The FreshLook Color Blends are available in blue, turquoise, gray, brown, honey, green, and amethyst.

Available colors for the FreshLook Colors include blue, green, hazel, and violet. The Precision UV lens, acquired by CIBA Vision, is a 74% water content vasurfilcon A material recommended for a 2-week replacement schedule for daily wear users and a 1-week replacement schedule for extended wear users. The 8.7-mm base curve (14.4-mm diameter) is available in powers ranging from +10.00 D to −16.00 D (0.50-D steps above +5.00 D and −6.00 D); the 8.4-mm base curves comes in powers ranging from +8.00 D to −10.00 D (0.50-D steps above +5.00 D and −6.00 D). Plano powers are not available in either base curve. The lenses are packaged as six-packs.

The ProClear Compatibles lens from CooperVision (previously from Biocompatibles, Norfolk, VA, USA) is a 62% water content lens made from omafilcon A with phosphorylcholine. It is a cast-molded lens with a light blue handling tint and is available in two base curves of 8.2 and 8.6 mm (14.2-mm diameter) in a power range of plano to −10.00 D. The 8.6-mm base curve is also available from plano to +10.00 D. ProClear Compatibles has been approved for chemical and hydrogen peroxide disinfection; they do not need enzymatic cleaning. The lenses are available in six-packs. The lens can be considered for patients experiencing dry eyes with lens wear and may provide improved comfort for mild dry eye symptoms (38). The Preference DW/FW lens, from CooperVision (Fairport, NY, USA), is a 43% water content, tetrafilcon A, low-water nonionic polymer lens. It is approved for daily and extended wear use and designed for quarterly replacement. The lens has a light blue handling tint and is available in two base curves: 8.4 and 8.7 mm (14.4-mm diameter). Power ranges from −0.25 D to −6.25 D in 0.25-D steps and from −6.50 D to −10.00 D in 0.50-D steps. The Preference Standard daily wear lens is made of the same material, has the same design, and is available in 8.3-mm and 8.6-mm base curves (14.0-mm diameter) and a 8.7-mm base curve (14.4-mm diameter). Power ranges from +6.00 D to −6.25 D in 0.25-D steps and from −6.50 D to −10.00 D in 0.50-D steps. The center thickness for Preference and Preference Standard is 0.04 and 0.07 mm, respectively, for −3.00 D. The lenses can be heat disinfected or disinfected with the standard chemical and hydrogen peroxide systems. Both the Frequency 55 EW and the Frequency 55 Aspheric FW are a 55% water content, methafilcon A lens with recommended monthly replacement. The Frequency 55 EW parameters are 8.7-mm base curve (14.2-mm diameter), with power ranges from +8.00 D to −10.00 D (0.50-D steps above −8.00 D). Both the 8.4-mm and 9.0-mm base curves come in minus powers only from 0.25 D to −8.00 D in 0.25-D steps. The parameters for the Frequency 55 Aspheric FW are the same, except that the 9.0-mm base curve is not available. The Frequency 55 Aspheric FW lens is designed to reduce or eliminate spherical aberration. The Ascend Aspheric FW lens also is designed to reduce or eliminate spherical aberration. Made of the same methafilcon A material, the base curve is 8.6 mm (14.5-mm diameter). Power ranges from $+8.00$ D to -10.00 D (0.50-D steps above -8.00 D). A second base curve of 8.3 mm is available for minus powers up to -8.00 D. The Ascend Aspheric FW lens is also a monthly replacement lens. The Hydrasoft Standard lens (acquired from formerly Coast Vision) is available as a multipack. After determining the fit and power of the first lens, a multipack can be ordered at a reduced price to provide patients with a frequent replacement plan.

The Edge III Proactive lens, from Ocular Sciences (San Francisco, CA, USA), is a 38% water content, polymacon lens approved for daily wear use and designed for 1-, 2-, or 3-month replacement. It is available in three base curves: 8.4, 8.7, and 9.0 mm (14.0-mm diameter). Powers range from -0.25 D to -6.00 D in 0.25-D steps and from -6.50 D to -8.00 D in 0.50-D steps. Plus powers range from $+0.25$ D to $+5.00$ D in the 8.7-mm base curve only. The lenses are available in three-packs or two-packs (under the packaging of Edge III Proactive XT). The Hydrogenics 60 UV (Ocular Sciences) is made of a 60% water content, ocufilcon F material. It is available in a single base curve with a 3.75-mm sagittal depth in the minus powers and a 3.74-mm sagittal depth for the plus powers. All lenses are 14.1-mm diameter. The minus powers range from -0.25 D to -6.00 D; the plus powers range from $+0.25$ D to $+5.00$ D. The Hydron Biomedics 55 UV is a 55% water content, ocufilcon D lens available in a 8.6-mm base curve (14.2-mm diameter). Power ranges from $+5.00$ D to -10.00 D in 0.50-D steps above -6.00 D. The minus powers also come in a 8.9-mm base curve; the plus powers are available in an additional base curve of 8.8 mm. Both the Hydrogenics 60 UV and the Hydron Biomedics 55 UV are approved for chemical and hydrogen peroxide disinfection. Packaged in six-packs, the lenses can be disposed of every 2 weeks.

Extreme H_2O (Hydrogel Vision Corp., a division of Benz Research & Development, Sarasota FL, USA) is a 59% water content, hioxifilcon A nonionic lens. It is available in a 14.2-mm diameter with an 8.6-mm base curve for minus lenses and an 8.8-mm base curve for plus lenses. Power ranges from $+6.00$ D to -8.00 D (in 0.50-D steps above -6.00 D). The lens can be disinfected using all three systems: heat, chemical, and oxidation. It is packaged in six-packs.

A number of companies are offering their conventional lenses in multipacks. Typically, a second lens or a multipack can be ordered at a reduced pricing following the completion of the fitting process and determination of the necessary parameters for the patient. Companies offering these lens replacement programs include Alden Optical (Alden, NY, USA), Flexlens Products (Duluth, GA), and Opti-Centre Laboratories, Inc. (Sherbrooke, Quebec, Canada). If a frequent replacement schedule is desired for patients currently wearing a conventional lens, consider contacting the manufacturer to determine if such a program is available.

All contact lenses begin to accumulate debris from the moment they are placed on the eye. The visible deposits and coatings are minimized with frequent replacement, increasing the potential for long-term success with daily wear. Noncompliance with lens replacement and/or cleaning and disinfection negates the advantage of cleaner and more frequently replaced lenses and may lead to an increase in possible adverse side effects. One study of 50 daily wear patients found that 40% were noncompliant; 13 of the 50 patients believed they were following the prescribed regimen (39). Many patients may wear their lenses longer than the prescribed regimen in an attempt to save money on lens replacement costs. A recent study showed that the overwear of both a daily wear disposable and a frequent replacement lens significantly increased the amount of protein bound on the lens and the degree of upper conjunctival papillae, upper lid conjunctival hyperemia, and limbal congestion (40). We believe it is of utmost importance for both practitioner and patient to determine and adhere to the optimal wearing and replacement schedule.

Protein and lipid interaction with contact lenses are material dependent. The key factors are the material ionicity for protein deposition and the material chemical composition for lipid deposition. Three high-water-content contact lens materials were tested: netrafilcon A (FDA group 2, Gentle Touch, now discontinued), etafilcon A (group 4, Acuvue), and vifilcon A (group 4, Focus). Significantly more proteins were deposited on the ionic materials than on the nonionic materials. Among the ionic materials, the higher the ionicity, the higher the level of protein deposition. There were significantly more surface proteins on the ionic material after 3 months than after 1 month of wear, but no difference over time was demonstrated for the nonionic materials. Significantly more lipids were deposited onto the surface of vifilcon A than the other two materials, due primarily to the presence of vinyl pyrrolidone in the vifilcon A formulation. The protein and lipid interactions with contact lenses were also found to be time dependent. Group 4 (ionic) lenses need to be replaced more often than group 2 (nonionic) lenses, which showed greater deposit resistance. The optimum performance was achieved for the large majority of patients with a 3-month replacement regimen for group 2 contact lenses and with a monthly replacement regimen for group 4 contact lenses (41).

Many materials are now available with UV radiation blocker. A number of frequent replacement lenses were tested for their UV transmittance, including the Acuvue lens, Precision UV (CooperVision), Specialty Sport (Specialty UltraVision, no longer available), and Surevue. All of the UV-absorbing lenses provided better protection from sunlight UV exposure than lenses without UV absorber. In addition, there was good agreement with published spectral transmittance curves and the actual UV transmittance of the lenses studied. Finally, of the four hydrogel lenses studied, the Surevue lens performed the best with transmittance of less than 1% in the 280- to 348-nm waveband and had the longest safe exposure duration for the crystalline lens and cornea (42).

Visibility tinted disposable lenses have little effect on the visible spectrum, except for a slight decrease in overall light transmittance. Enhancement tinted lenses (NewVues Soft-Colors were specially studied in this case) decreased the transmittance of wavelengths in the spectral range of the complementary color of the lens tint. For example, the royal blue showed approximately a 10% drop in the orange and yellow range (43). More recently, Diego et al. (44) compared visual performance in subjects wearing tinted soft contact lenses (specifically Optima Colors, Bausch & Lomb). They found no statistical difference in visual performance assessed, including contrast sensitivity, color vision, and subjective vision, between wearing the tinted lenses and not wearing lenses. The only statistically significance measured in subjects wearing tinted lenses was in static perimetry at eccentricities greater than 30 degrees (44).

Toric Contact Lenses

The improvement in technology, the low cost production methods, and the growth of the frequent replacement hydrogel market translate into greater options of frequent replacement toric hydrogel lenses for astigmatic patients. A daily wear conventional toric lens wearer can now enjoy improved ease of care and comfort along with enhanced ocular health with a frequent replacement lens. Practitioners now have the option to replace toric hydrogel lenses weekly, monthly, or quarterly. The range of cylinder power correction extends from −0.50 D to −9.75 D of power at any axis. The expansion of parameters makes fitting a high cylinder correction a viable option. Colored toric hydrogel lenses are offered for astigmatic patients in limited parameters. These advancements make frequent replacement toric hydrogel lenses a reality for astigmatic patients (Tables 21.4–21.6).

The surge of frequent replacement toric hydrogel lenses brought on a wave of studies on the quality, reproducibility, and clinical performances of these lenses. Lens reproducibility is regarded as a key in the success of these toric lenses (45). Some studies have shown that variations exist in manufacturing quality and clinical performance of toric lens designs (46–49). Other studies have shown that these variations can affect visual performance. For example, one masked randomized study evaluated the effect of manufacturing variability on the clinical performance of three frequent replacement toric soft contact lenses: Acuvue Toric (Vistakon), Focus Toric (CIBA Vision), and FreshLook Toric (Wesley Jessen, now CIBA Vision) (50). The results concluded that the variability in clinical performance appears to be linked to the variability of manufacturing output, and better reproducibility is needed for toric lenses used on a frequent replacement basis. An inventory sample study calculated that 83.5% of a sample of Focus Toric lenses was accurate enough to give visual acuity within one line of best corrected visual acuity (51). It estimated the clinical problem rate associated with inaccurate lens power was 3.3%, which equated to one problem pair every 30

TABLE 21.4. TWO-WEEK REPLACEMENT TORIC LENSES

Manufacturer	Lens	BC	Sphere Power	Cylinder Power	Axis	Stabilization Method	Toric Marking
Bausch & Lomb	Soflens 66 Toric	8.5	+6.00 to −9.00 (0.5 D steps above −6.00)	−0.75, −1.25, −1.75, −2.25	Full circle in 10-degree steps	Lo-Torque cast mold	3 marks: 5, 6, 7 o'clock
Ciba Vision	Fresh Look Toric	Median	+4.00 to −6.00	−0.75, −1.25, −1.75	Full circle in 10-degree steps	Back surface thin zones	FTL: T at 6 o'clock
	Fresh Look Colorblend Toric	Median	PL to −4.00	Same as above	180 ± 20, 90 ± 20 in 10-degree steps	Back surface thin zones	FTL: T at 6 o'clock
Cooper Vision	Encore Toric	8.6	+4.00 to −8.00	−0.75, −1.25, −1.75, −2.25	Full circle in 10-degree steps	Back surface prism ballast	1 mark at 6 o'clock
Ocular Science	Biomedic Toric	8.7	PL to −6.00	−0.75, −1.25, −1.75	Full circle in 10-degree steps	Cast molded	1 mark at 6 o'clock
Vistakon	Acuvue Toric	8.7	PL to −6.00	−0.75, −1.25, −1.75	Full circle in 10-degree steps	Double slab off prism	6 marks: 3 and 9 o'clock
			−6.50 to −9.00 (0.50 D step)	−1.25, −1.75	180 ± 20, 90 ± 20 in 10-degree steps	Double slab off prism	6 marks: 3 and 9 o'clock
			+0.25 to +6.00	−1.25, −1.75	180 ± 20, 90 ± 20 in 10-degree steps	Double slab off prism	6 marks: 3 and 9 o'clock

From Tyler Thompson TT, ed. *Tyler's quarterly soft contact lens parameter guide.* Little Rock, AK: Tyler's Quarterly Inc., June 2002.

TABLE 21.5. MONTHLY REPLACEMENT TORIC LENSES

Manufacturer	Lens	BC	Sphere Power	Cylinder Power	Axis	Stabilization Method	Toric Marking
Ciba Vision	Focus Toric	8.9, 9.2	+4.00 to −6.00	−1.00, −2.00	Full circle in 10-degree steps	Cast molded	3 marks: 3, 6, 9 o'clock
			PL to −6.00	−2.50	Full circle in 10-degree steps		
Cooper Vision	Freq 55 Toric	8.4, 8.7	+6.00 to −8.00 (0.50 D steps above −6.50)	−0.75, −1.25, −1.75, −2.25	Full circle in 10-degree steps	Back surface prism ballast	1 mark at 6 o'clock
	Freq 55 Toric XR	8.4, 8.7	+6.00 to −8.00 (0.50 D steps above −6.50)	−2.75, −3.25, −3.75, −4.25, −4.75, −5.25, −5.75	Full circle in 10-degree steps	Back surface prism ballast	1 mark at 6 o'clock
	Proclear Toric	8.8	+4.00 to −6.00	−0.75, −1.25, −1.75	Full circle in 10-degree steps	Prism ballast	3 marks at 6 o'clock

From Tyler Thompson TT, ed. *Tyler's quarterly soft contact lens parameter guide.* Little Rock, AK: Tyler's Quarterly Inc., June 2002.

months for a lens replaced monthly. It seems that the variability in manufacturing and lack of reproducibility can potentially increase the chance of patients experiencing problems.

In summary, despite the variable visual problems arising from the manufacturing process and the lack of reproducibility, frequent replacement toric hydrogel lenses are a viable option for practitioners and astigmatic patients because they offer ease of care, good comfort, and maintenance of optimal ocular health when the lenses are replaced as recommended. If the patient is noncompliant, the potential benefits of frequent replacement lenses are negated. Practitioners must better educate their patients on the importance of compliance with replacement schedule, proper lens care, and timely follow-up examination.

Multifocal Lenses

The presbyopic population is the largest untapped portion of the contact lens market; only 7% of the "over 40" population wears contact lenses. A survey by the CCLRU, however, showed that over 25% of these presbyopes are interested in contact lenses (52). According to The Gallup Quarterly Study of the Consumer Contact Lens Market, the multifocal and monovision market could increase up to 34% as the baby boomer generation matures. The projected 40% increase in the number of people ages 50 to 64 by the year 2005 would result in an increase from 1.4 million multifocal/monovision contact lens wearers in 1996 to 1.9 million in the year 2005. Many of these baby boomers have worn contact lenses as their primary visual correction most of their adult life and do not desire to discontinue contact

TABLE 21.6. MONTHLY REPLACEMENT TORIC LENSES

Manufacturer	Lens	BC	Sphere Power	Cylinder Power	Axis	Stabilization Method	Toric Marking
Bausch & Lomb	Gold Medalist Toric	8.3, 8.6	+4.00 to −6.00	−0.75, −1.25, −1.75	180 and 90 ± 20 in 10-degree steps	Lathe cut prism ballast	3 marks: 5, 6, 7 o'clock
	Optima Toric	8.3, 8.6, 8.9	+6.00 to −9.00	−0.75 to 4.25 in 0.50 D steps	Full circle in 5-degree steps	Lathe cut prism ballast	3 marks: 5, 6, 7 o'clock
CooperVision	Hydrasoft Toric	8.3, 8.6, 8.9, 9.2	+20.00 to −20.00	Custom	Custom	Lathe cut prism ballast	1 mark at 6 o'clock
	Preference Toric	8.4, 8.7	+6.00 to −8.00 (0.50 D steps above −6.50)	−0.75, −1.25, −1.75	Full circle in 5-degree steps	Lathe cut prism ballast	1 mark at 6 o'clock
	Preference Toric XR	8.4, 8.7	+6.00 to −9.50 (0.50 D steps above −6.50)	−2.75 to −9.75	Full circle in 5-degree steps	Lathe cut prism ballast	1 mark at 6 o'clock

From Tyler Thompson TT, ed. *Tyler's quarterly soft contact lens parameter guide.* Little Rock, AK: Tyler's Quarterly Inc., June 2002.

lens wear because of presbyopia (7). Monovision, one of the more successful contact lens options for presbyopes, is simple to offer the patient on a trial basis because of the low cost of diagnostic frequent replacement lenses to the practitioner. New technology is producing improved multifocal lenses as an alternative to monovision. Early presbyopes may adapt well as long as the patient's specific visual demands, expectations, and motivation are determined (53).

The multifocal hydrogel lenses have become more available in different designs and replacement modules in recent years (Table 21.7). Practitioners can choose between the aspheric and concentric designs in several frequent replacement options (54). The aspheric design can have a center-near or center-distance design. The center-near aspheric lenses include Focus Dailies Progressive (CIBA Vision), Focus Progressive Visitint (CIBA Vision), Sunsoft Additions (Ocular Sciences, Inc.), Quattro (Blanchard Contact Lens, Inc, Manchester, NH, USA), and EMA (Unilens Corp., Largo, FL, USA) (54). Occasions Multifocal (Bausch & Lomb) is a center-distance aspheric design lens. The new type of multizone multifocal lens improves on the conventional bizone concentric design (55). It has a center-distance surrounded by multiple peripheral zones. The leading example is the Acuvue Bifocal lens (Vistakon), which has a center-distance with five alternating distant and near zones. Life Style MV2 (Life Style Co., Morganville, NJ, USA) is another multizone lens but has a center-intermediate design. The distance lens has a center-intermediate zone (the intermediate power is +0.50 D over the distance prescription) and a distance surround. The near lens has a center-intermediate zone (intermediate power is −1.25 D over the near prescription) and a near surround (54). The new Frequency 55 Multifocal (CooperVision) is a progressive design, with a D lens for the dominant eye and an N lens for the nondominant eye. The D lens has a spherical center-distance; the N lens is designed with a spherical center-near. An aspheric intermediate zone and a spherical outer ring surround the central zone (54). The Ultra Vue 2000 4-cycle (Opti-Centre Laboratories) similarly has a center-distance design for the dominant eye and a center-near design for the nondominant eye (54). Another category of multifocal lenses worth mentioning is the toric multifocal lenses. The majority of the lenses offered are replaced annually, except for the Lifestyle Toric Multifocal (Life Style Co.), which can be replaced quarterly or annually. The design is similar to the Lifestyle MV2 Multifocal (38). Manufacturers may offer toric multifocal lenses in a frequent replacement modality as they attempt to capture more of the presbyopic population.

The new generation of multifocals has a better success rate than the first-generation alternating, aspheric, or concentric designs (56–59). The clinical performance and patient satisfaction of these lenses are comparable to the traditional monovision fitting method as reported by some studies. No statistical significant difference was found between the Sunsoft Multifocal and monovision in clarity of distance and near vision, comfort, lens handling, and overall

TABLE 21.7. MULTIFOCAL LENSES

Manufacturer	Lens	BC	Power	Adds	Designs	Replacement
Bausch & Lomb	Occasions Multifocal	8.6	+6.00 to −9.00	+1.50 D	Aspheric center-distance	Quarterly
Blanchard	Quattro	8.4, 8.8	+6.00 to −7.00	Progressive up to +2.25	Aspheric center-near	Quarterly
CIBA	Focus Dailies Progressive	8.6	+5.00 to −6.00	Progressive up to +3.00	Aspheric center-distance	Daily
	Focus Progressive	8.6, 8.9	+6.00 to −7.00	Progressive up to +3.00	Aspheric center-distance	Monthly
Coopervision	Frequency 55 Multifocal	8.7	+4.00 to −6.00	+1.50 +2.00 +2.50	Progressive	Monthly
Lifestyle	MV2	8.5, 8.8	+5.00 to −8.00	Add up to +2.50	Concentric central area in both distance and near	Monthly
Ocular Science	Sunsoft Addition	8.4, 8.7	+6.00 to −6.00	Add A: +0.75 to +1.25 Add B: +1.50 to +2.00 Add C: +2.25 to +2.50	Aspheric center-near	Quarterly
Unilen	EMA	8.5, 8.8	+6.00 to −10.0	Low add up to +1.50 High add +1.75 to 2.00	Aspheric center-near	6 months
Vistakon	Acuvue Bifocal	8.5	+6.00 to −9.00	+1.00, +1.50, +2.00, +2.50	Concentric center-distance 5 alternating zones	1 week extended wear 2 week daily wear

From Tyler Thompson TT, ed. *Tyler's quarterly soft contact lens parameter guide.* Little Rock, AK: Tyler's Quarterly Inc., June 2002.

satisfaction (60). A group of previous monovision patients, when switched to Acuvue Bifocal, experienced a statistically significant decrease in the interocular difference between distant and near visual acuity. This increased binocularity, including stereoacuity (61). Another study found a 53% success rate with the same lens (55). Reports on their performance and patient satisfaction are encouraging. With the continued growing demands of the presbyopic population and with the newly improved multifocals, it is foreseeable that more practitioners will attempt to fit multifocal lenses. These lenses can be an alternative to monovision and can be successful if the patient's specific visual demands, motivation, and expectations are determined (53).

FITTING

As discussed in other chapters, a preliminary evaluation should be performed to determine the patient's refractive error, corneal curvature, and ocular health. The practitioner should rule out any contraindications to contact lens wear. Careful evaluation of the patient's ocular health, lifestyle, and motivation lead to proper placement of the patient in the most suitable lens replacement program and should facilitate long-term compliance.

Many patients are attracted to disposable lenses because of the perceived "hassle" in caring for traditional lenses. Convenience may attract a patient to daily wear disposable contact lenses, but cost is the primary reason that dissuades some of them (31). The annual cost of frequent replacement lenses is slightly less than or equal to the cost of conventional lenses when one considers the cost of care systems. The cost of disposable lenses is relatively higher. Consider, however, a report in 2001 comparing the cost of lens care products and frequent replacement lenses versus the cost of daily wear disposables. Mai-Le and Caroline (62) calculated the average annual cost of multipurpose disinfection products to be $138 and of hydrogen peroxide disinfection products to be $315. They calculated that the cost of replacement contact lenses (2-week) and multipurpose solutions is only approximately 10% less than the cost of a year's supply of daily wear disposables. The cost of lenses and hydrogen peroxide disinfection actually is more than a year's worth of supplies for daily wear disposable lenses even if the lenses are replaced on a monthly basis (62). Regional differences in products pricing, however, need to be taken into consideration. We have found it best to discuss the cost of the disposable lenses on a per day basis rather than describing an annual total. Many practitioners set fees for professional services at a reasonable level and position lens replacement cost in close proximity to material cost. The patient often is aware of the actual cost of lenses because wholesale prices are found in many health and consumer publications and online.

After review of the patient's ophthalmic findings and history, a diagnostic lens with the appropriate parameters is placed on the eye and allowed to equilibrate for approximately 5 minutes (37). Space-efficient diagnostic lens sets are available from most manufacturers. These sets allow the practitioner to make adjustments in base curve, power, diameter, material and water content, and even tint, during the trial fitting. With the significantly expanded parameters now available in disposable and frequent replacement lenses, the vast majority of spherical lens patients are prescribed such a system. In our practice, practically all new hydrogel lens patients, including refittings, are evaluated with some sort of frequent replacement lens. New hydrogel lens wearers are given an extra pair of trial lenses to use in the event of damage or loss. At the progress evaluation visit, the replacement schedule is determined. If indicated, the lens type or material is changed to optimize the fitting.

Most manufacturers will supply fitting sets that provide for most, if not all, of the available parameter range, allowing precise fitting and dispensing at the same visit. This saves valuable chair time for both the practitioner and the patient. If the lens fits too loosely, exhibiting decentration or excessive edge lift, one proceeds to a steeper base curve or a lens with a larger diameter. If the lens is too tight, exhibiting movement that is less than acceptable, one can proceed to a flatter base curve or a lens with a smaller diameter. If a substantial spherocylindrical overrefraction is present, one proceeds to toric lenses. If the patient is interested in enhancing or changing his or her eye color, this can be performed in the office the same day. A clinical comparison of the fitting characteristics of 1-Day Acuvue in the original 9.0-mm base curve and 14-day Acuvue lenses indicated that there should be no clinically significant difference in the movement or centration of the two lenses. It is still recommended that a diagnostic fitting be performed; however, the refitting time should be minimal (63).

Our lens of choice tends to be a 2-week frequent replacement lens worn on a daily wear basis (Table 21.8). In a masked study comparing daily wear disposable lenses with biweekly replacement lenses, the differences were not as conclusive (64). SeeQuence 2, now known as Optima FW (Bausch & Lomb), lenses worn for 1 day only on one eye were compared with SeeQuence 2 lenses worn 2 weeks on the fellow eye. The age of the lens on a particular eye was masked; there were no appreciable biomicroscopic differences in lens centration, movement, or condition, or in

TABLE 21.8. RELATIVE INDICATIONS FOR FREQUENT REPLACEMENT/DISPOSABLE LENSES

Heavy lens surface deposition
Patient noncompliance
Frequent lens loss or damage
Use of ocular medication
Ocular systemic disease considerations
Avocational or vocational needs for decreased lens care or less
   frequent replacement

corneal or bulbar conjunctival fluorescein staining. Measurements of corrected visual acuity and subjective ratings of comfort and clarity of vision also showed no statistically significant differences. Although SeeQuence 2 lenses are not daily wear disposable contact lenses, the results of this study underscore the fact that there may not be as much of a difference between biweekly lens replacement and daily wear disposable lens wear. Patients on a 2-week replacement schedule seem to show little change in their ocular surface (65), although there is another study favoring a daily wear disposable regimen in maintaining the normal physiologic environment of the ocular surface (13). A 2-week replacement schedule also results in a lower incidence of GPC. Porazinski and Donshik (66) found that patients who replaced their contact lenses every 4 weeks or longer had a 36% incidence of GPC. Patients who replaced their contact lenses more frequently (at least every 2 weeks) had only a 4.5% incidence of GPC. Of note, a history of allergy was more prevalent, and was statistically significant, in patients who developed GPC. No significant difference in average daily wearing time, FDA classification of contact lens material, or parameters and fitting characteristics of the contact lenses were found. For patients who are at high risk for GPC, these authors recommend replacing lenses at least every 2 weeks. This appears to offer a better strategy for avoiding GPC than incorporating enzymatic cleaning into the care system (66). Once a patient develops GPC, a 2-week replacement lens can be used to manage the GPC. A study at Johns Hopkins University also showed that patients who develop GPC can switch to frequent replacement lenses rather than discontinue contact lens wear. This study involved 25 patients who were refit and showed decreased clinical signs of GPC after 3 to 6 months. It was advised that once the GPC resolved, patients should not return to traditional daily or extended wear lenses (67).

As other risks enter the equation, daily wear disposable lens wear should be favored. Studies demonstrate a significant clinical benefit, by symptom analysis, associated with frequent lens replacement in patients with environmental allergies. This trend persists even when comparing daily replacement to weekly replacement (68). For the patient who wears contact lenses on an occasional basis with prolonged periods of no lens wear, daily wear disposable lenses are prescribed. Those patients whom we consider to be at higher risk for contact lens-related complications (such as microbial infection) because of the concerns about the wearing environment, compliance, or ocular and systemic health considerations also are fit with disposable lenses. This includes children, athletes, and patients with a history of noncompliance, GPC, allergies, or infection. Patients with ocular surface irregularities due to dry eye, corneal dystrophy, thyroid eye disease, scarring, or refractive surgery also are included. Persons who are immunocompromised, such as those with diabetes or AIDS, are carefully educated as to the risks of contact lens wear, are fit only with daily wear

disposable lenses, and are carefully monitored. If the patient has dry eyes and cannot comfortably wear disposable lenses, a lens with lower water content, with hydrogen peroxide disinfection, and enzymatic cleaning is generally quite successful. For all patients expressing an interest in refractive surgery, particularly due to previous failure or dissatisfaction with contact lenses, we recommend a trial with daily wear disposable lenses or extended wear disposable silicone hydrogel lenses as a noninvasive alternative to refractive surgery.

CARE

A care system must provide safety, convenience, and simplicity. The introduction of hydrogel lenses in the early 1970s sparked regulatory concern for potential infection and thus a recommendation for heat disinfection. Heat disinfection is thought by some practitioners to be the most effective lens care regimen; unfortunately, however, the manufacturing of heat disinfection units has been discontinued. Many practitioners have switched their patients to chemical or hydrogen peroxide disinfection to increase patient compliance and prolong lens life.

Many chemical care systems have evolved over the past 2 decades. There is an optimal balance between antimicrobial effectiveness and minimal potential for ocular irritation. Early chlorhexidine- and thimerosal-based disinfection and irrigation solutions could result in ocular irritation, sensitivity, and allergic response. This led to the development of new chemical systems showing better acceptance by ocular tissues and alternative hydrogen peroxide-based disinfection (69).

Hydrogen peroxide (H_2O_2) care systems have been evolving for 20 years. They now have a high level of effectiveness and can be used on most hydrogel lenses. Some criticisms of the early care systems involved their complexity and their effect on compliance. Significant improvements, such as neutralizing tablets with slowly dissolving color-coded coatings that indicate complete neutralization and self-contained neutralizing discs, have been made in these systems.

Multipurpose solutions have regained popularity with the introduction of frequent replacement systems. They were developed to provide convenience and simplicity in disinfection. This is consistent with the philosophy of frequent replacement lenses. However, because they are chemical care systems, the same inherent problems in such systems are not resolved. Many researchers have pointed out the reduced efficacy of multipurpose solutions for disinfection, removal of deposits, and adverse reactions such as stinging and allergic reaction (70). Products such as SupraCLENS (Alcon, Fort Worth, TX, USA) help enhance certain aspects of such systems, acting as a liquid daily protein remover (70). Several manufacturers, including Alcon, Allergan, and

CIBA Vision, have bottled their multipurpose solutions under private label for retail sale (71). Also available are disinfection systems using ultrasound and microwave. Current research involves the use of UV and electrochemical devices for disinfection (72). Differences in patient attention to proper solution handling, in addition to differences in patient/lens tolerance and shifts in solution characteristics such as pH, buffering ability, osmolality (tonicity), and refractive index, can be sources of unsuspected patient difficulty (Table 21.9). Education on proper lens handling, cleaning, disinfection, and storage is crucial. All hydrogel lenses that are removed nightly or reused require mechanical cleaning and disinfection. Proper disinfection is not achieved without daily cleaning due to the high number of microorganisms bound to the lens. Ninety percent of these microorganisms are removed with daily cleaning and rinsing (73,74). The increased replacement of lenses in many cases (i.e., 2-week replacement) may minimize or eliminate the need for enzymatic cleaning. Many practitioners prescribe one-step "no-rub" chemical disinfection, but we believe rubbing and rinsing is still important. For 2-week replacement with the mid-water-content lenses, we recommend a multipurpose solution such as No Rub Opti-Free Express (Alcon Laboratories, Ft. Worth, TX, USA) or Renu Multiplus (Bausch & Lomb). If the patient requires a fast-acting system due to an infrequent wearing schedule, we recommend Quick-Care (CIBA Vision), a 5-minute cleaning and disinfecting system.

As discussed in another chapter, small variations in the tonicity of the lens solutions and individual tear composition may cause slight changes in the fitting characteristics, such as diameter, base curve, thickness, and oxygen transmissibility. All hydrogel lenses dehydrate on the eye, and the amount of dehydration depends upon the lens material type. The practitioner should be aware that the group 4 materials in particular tend to undergo greater dehydration compared with group 1 lens materials. Several of the hydrogen peroxide systems have been approved for use with disposable lenses; however, one study has indicated parameter changes, especially among group 4 materials, with two-step H_2O_2 disinfection (75).

As more disposable/frequent replacement lenses are prescribed, the environmental impact of the discarded plastic and foil containers must be considered. Most of these lenses are packaged in buffered saline in a sealed polypropylene

TABLE 21.9. INITIAL DISADVANTAGES OF FREQUENT REPLACEMENT/DISPOSABLE LENSES

Lens handling difficulties
Patient noncompliance with lens care and replacement schedule
Possible lens distribution by nonlicensed facilities
Increased practitioner paperwork and inventory
Perceived high cost to patient
Medical-legal liability

blister pack. This packaging consists of five layers, which provide a sterile environment and a 4-year shelf life. The packaging must be leakproof, clearly labeled, easily opened, and preferably environmental friendly. Vistakon changed the original six-pack plastic Acuvue container to cardboard, and Bausch & Lomb became the first contact lens manufacturer to introduce an environmentally friendly biodegradable lens shipping package made of 100% recyclable molded paper fiber. Bausch & Lomb also added universally accepted recycling codes to its solution product bottles. Most blister packs now are coded for proper recycling. CIBA Vision redesigned the packaging of the Focus multipacks to a more compact design that is approximately half the size and weight of the original New Vue packaging. The blister pack also has been reconfigured for easier opening and handling.

CLINICAL CONCERNS AND MANAGEMENT

The volume of information required for each patient can present practice management difficulties. Many practitioners have developed simple forms that include the fees, wearing schedule, replacement schedule, number of lenses dispensed, recall and follow-up visits, and informed consent. Manufacturers of daily wear disposable contact lenses send their lenses directly to the patient. This has the advantage of eliminating the large storage space necessary to inventory lenses. The method of delivery directly to the patient has its drawbacks: it decreases the doctor's control over contact lens distribution, it provides companies with customer addresses and thus an avenue to solicit their future business, and it raises the issue of doctor/patient confidentiality because names, addresses, and prescriptions are given to a third party. The growing practice of patients obtaining frequent replacement lenses via mail order or the Internet has reduced practitioner profit. In 1996 it was estimated that 1% to 15% of patients obtain their contact lenses by mail order (4,71). This practice likely will increase as practitioners must provide patients with their contact lens prescription after the completion of the fitting process starting January 2004. We reinforce the importance of regular checkups and warnings about brand substitution specifically on our contact lens prescription forms. An FDA Internet posting provides consumer advice and guidelines for purchasing lenses, including the importance of regular checkups, the need for a current prescription, and warnings about brand substitution. The site also provides an opportunity for consumers to report problems with Internet vendors (3). To learn more, visit *www.fda.gov/cdrh/consumer/buycontactqa.html.* The promotion of eye health and education must supplement the promotion of disposable and frequent replacement lenses for the practitioner to continue to provide optimal care and consultation to patients. One manufacturer revised its distribution agreement to limit distribution of lenses to locations with facilities to fit the lenses. It was thought that this action (if other manufacturers followed suit) would reduce the mail-order distribution of lenses. However, there have been several class action lawsuits claiming restraint of trade in contact lenses, including a federal lawsuit filed in 1994 in 32 states against three contact lens manufacturers, seven contact lens organizations, eight optometrists, and their state associations and the American Optometric Association (AOA) (76,77). The lawsuits claim that defendants have conspired to limit consumer access to contact lens prescriptions and availability of lenses to mass merchandise outlets, buying groups, and mail-order companies, keeping contact lens prices artificially high. The manufacturers denied these allegations and defended their right to limit distribution of contact lenses in the best interest of the patient. According to the AOA, "the earlier suits and the multistate suit are not well-founded and are based on a serious misinterpretation of the facts" (77). However, *Business Week* published a commentary stating that the lawsuits are consumer friendly: "The pressure is having a positive effect on a system that needs changing" (78). The lawsuits eventually were settled, with each manufacturer agreeing to sell lenses to alternative providers who followed state laws on filling contact lens prescriptions. Cash rebates and discounts on lenses and eye examinations were made available to consumers who had purchased lenses since 1998. One manufacturer settled a second lawsuit that claimed its daily wear disposable and 2-week replacement lenses were the same lenses. The manufacturer substantiated the difference between the two products; however, it agreed to remove the words "disposable" and "for single use" from the packaging. Subsequently, cash rebates and discounts were provided to consumers who had purchased the lenses (3).

According to product liability law, the seller of the contact lens, namely the practitioner, is potentially liable for defects in the lenses that cause injury (79). With conventional lenses, the practitioner is expected to inspect or verify the lenses both initially and at periodic (i.e., 6-months) intervals. We believe that patients should be advised to inspect each lens before placing it on the eye, and that they should remove and inspect it again if a problem arises. Current manufacturing techniques ensure good reproducibility, but the number and the clinical significance of minor lens defects, when present, have yet to be determined. A study by Efron and Veys (80) focused on defects found in one type of disposable hydrogel lens, the Acuvue lens, and suggested that these defects could lead to ocular irritation. At the time, the article received considerable attention and resulted in a debate pertaining to the clinical significance of small but "statistically significant" ocular complications caused by defects. It should be noted that other brands probably also will be found to have occasional defects. Practitioners on both sides of the debate agreed that the clinical performance of the Acuvue lenses, based on visual acuity, comfort, and patient satisfaction, is quite good, but the clinical impact of lens defects should become more apparent

with further investigation. The defect debate highlights the importance of having the practitioner advise his or her patients to inspect each and every lens before insertion.

FUTURE OUTLOOK

Ocular Science has announced plans for a daily wear disposable lens.

CIBA Vision has launched the first daily wear disposable contact lens for astigmatism, Focus Dailies Toric, in Switzerland. The company says the lenses will be available in other countries in the near future. The back-surface toric lens is available with -0.75 D cylinder. Base curve is 8.6 mm, diameter is 14.2 mm, and spherical powers range from -0.50 D to -6.00 D in 0.25-D steps, in axis 180 and 90 degrees. The lenses will be available in packs of 30.

SUMMARY

Practitioners and patients alike have enthusiastically embraced the disposable/frequent replacement concept as an advance in eye care and a welcome addition to our contact lens armamentarium. The frequent replacement of lenses is an effective modality that enhances public health by decreasing the incidence of adverse ocular reactions to hydrogel lenses, especially when lenses are worn on a daily wear basis.

However, even these lenses are not a substitute for good patient care or for monitoring physiologic response during fit and follow-up care. The potential benefits from disposable/frequent replacement contact lens wear may be negated if patients are noncompliant, and poor personal hygiene and overwear can still occur. A noncompliant patient creates problems in any type of contact lens system. It is important for manufacturers and clinicians to keep necessary restraints on marketing contact lenses to the public and to set and maintain high ethical standards. Practitioners must instill in their patients the importance of patient compliance with replacement schedule, proper lens care, lens inspection, and follow-up examination.

REFERENCES

1. Harrison KW, Stein HA. Daily wear disposable lenses. *Contact Lens Spectrum* 1991;5:37.
2. Doughman DJ, Massare JS. Defining contact lens terminology. *CLAO J* 1996;22:228–229.
3. Barr JT. Contact lenses 2001. *Contact Lens Spectrum* 2002. Available at *http://www.clspectrum.com/archiveresults.asp?article = 12083&iss = 1/1/02.* Accessed July 19, 2002.
4. *The contact lens marketplace. Trends in lens care 1996.* Bausch & Lomb North American Vision Care, Volume 3, 1996.
5. Barr JT, Bailey NJ. 1991 annual report. *Contact Lens Spectrum* 1992;7:23.

6. Barr JT. The Contact Lens Spectrum contact lens event of the year. *Contact Lens Spectrum* 1992;7:8.
7. Vistakon literature, data on file, 1997.
8. Coopersmith LW, Arons I. The trends of the 1990's. *Optom Econ* 1992;2:23.
9. Acuvue cited by White House in award to J&J. *AOA News* 1996; 35:14.
10. Solomon OD, Freeman MI, Boschnick EL, et al. A 3-year prospective study of the clinical performance of daily disposable contact lenses compared with frequent replacement and conventional daily wear contact lenses. *CLAO J* 1996;22:250.
11. Suchecki JK, Ehlers WH, Donshik PC. A comparison of contact lens-related complications in various daily wear modalities. *CLAO J* 2000;26:204–213.
12. Hamano H, Watanabe K, Hamano T, et al. A study of the complications induced by conventional and disposable contact lenses. *CLAO J* 1994;20:103–108.
13. Alongi S, Rolando M, Macri A, et al. Bacterial load and protein deposits on 15-day versus 1-day disposable hydrophilic contact lenses. *Cornea* 1998;17:146–151.
14. Hingorani M, Christie C, Buckley RJ. Ulcerative keratitis in a person wearing daily disposable contact lenses. *Br J Ophthalmol* 1995;79:1138.
15. Choi DM, Goldstein MH, Salierno A, et al. Fungal keratitis in a daily disposable soft contact lens wearer. *CLAO J* 2001;27: 111–112.
16. Dunn JP, Mondino BJ, Weissman BA, et al. Corneal ulcers associated with disposable hydrogel contact lenses. *Am J Ophthalmol* 1989;108:113.
17. Buehler PO, Schein OD, Stamler JF, et al. The increased risk of ulcerative keratitis among disposable soft contact lens users. *Arch Ophthalmol* 1992;110:1555.
18. Matthews TD, Frazer DG, Minassian DC, et al. Risks of keratitis and patterns of use with disposable contact lenses. *Arch Ophthalmol* 1992;110:1559.
19. Schnider C. How safe are EW disposables? *Contact Lens Spectrum* 1991;5:16.
20. Donzis PB, Mondino BJ, Weissman BA, et al. Microbial contamination of contact lens care systems. *Am J Ophthalmol* 1987;104: 325.
21. McMahon TT, Zadnik K. Twenty-five years of contact lenses. *Cornea* 2000;19:730–740.
22. Holden BA, Mertz GW. Critical oxygen levels to avoid corneal edema for daily and extended wear contact lenses. *Invest Ophthalmol Vis Sci* 1984;25:1161–1167.
23. Harvitt DM, Bonanno JA. Re-evaluation of the oxygen diffusion model for predicting minimum contact lens Dk/t values needs to avoid corneal anoxia. *Optom Vis Sci* 1999;76:712–719.
24. Covey M, Sweeney DF, Terry R, et al. Hypoxic effects on the anterior eye of high-Dk soft contact lens wearer are negligible. *Optom Vis Sci* 2001;78:95–99.
25. Dumbleton KA, Chalmers RL, Richter DB, et al. Vascular response to extended wear of hydrogel lenses with high and low oxygen permeability. *Optom Vis Sci* 2001;78:147–151.
26. Brennan NA, Coles CC, Comstock TL, et al. A 1-year prospective clinical trial of balafilcon A (PureVision) silicone-hydrogel contact lenses used on a 30-day continuous wear schedule. *Ophthalmology* 2002;109:1172–1177.
27. Asbell PA. Understanding the risk of corneal ulcerations. *Contact Lens Spectrum* 1992;7:25.
28. Nason RJ, Boschnick EL, Cannon WM, et al. Multisite comparison of contact lens modalities. Daily disposable wear vs. conventional daily wear in successful contact lens wearers. *J Am Optom Assoc* 1994;65:774.
29. Kame RT. Are your patients ready for daily disposables? *Contact Lens Spectrum* 1994;9:26.
30. New survey shows disposable wearers dropout far less. *Making Contact* 1992;10:17.
31. You and your practice. *Making Contact* 1992;10:18.
32. Weiner BM. How and when to prescribe bandage contact lenses. *Rev Optom* 1996;133:38.
33. Lindahl KJ, DePaolis MD, Aquavella JV, et al. Applications of hydrophilic disposable contact lenses as therapeutic bandages. *CLAO J* 1991;17:241.
34. Land JK, Bauman RE, Reichner M, et al. Multi-national clinical comparison of two daily disposable lenses. *Int Contact Lens Clin* 1977;24:20–27.
35. Inaba M. 1-day Acuvue vs. Focus Dailies: a comparison of comfort, user preference, and incidence of corneal complications. *CLAO J* 2000;26:141–145.
36. Schwallie JD, Bauman RE. Fitting characteristics of Dailies daily disposable hydrogel contact lenses. *CLAO J* 1998;24:102–106.
37. Brennan NA, Lindsay RG, McGraw K, et al. Soft lens movement temporal characteristics. *Optom Vis Sci* 1994;71:359–363.
38. Tyler Thompson TT, ed. *Tyler's quarterly soft contact lens parameter guide.* Little Rock, ARK: Tyler's Quarterly Inc., March 2002.
39. Chun MW, Weissman BA. Compliance in contact lens care. *Am J Optom Physiol Opt* 1986;64:274.
40. Michaud L, Giasson CJ. Overwear of contact lenses: increased severity of clinical signs as a function of protein adsorption. *Optom Vis Sci* 2002;79:184–192.
41. Maissa C, Franklin V, Guillon M, et al. Influence of contact lens material surface characteristics and replacement frequency on protein and lipid deposition. *Optom Vis Sci* 1998;75:697–705.
42. Quesnel NM, Fares F, Verret E, et al. Evaluation of the spectral transmittance of UV-absorbing disposable contact lenses. *CLAO J* 2001;27:23–29.
43. Harris MG, Haririfar M, Hirano KY. Transmittance of tinted and uv-blocking disposable contact lenses. *Optom Vis Sci* 1999; 76:177–180.
44. Diego CA, Montes-Mico R, Pons AM, et al. Influence of the luminance level on visual performance with a disposable soft cosmetic tinted contact lens. *Ophthalmic Physiol Opt* 2001;21: 411–419.
45. Hodd NF, Josephson JE. Toric hydrogel lenses. In: Ruben M, Guillon M, eds. *Contact lens practice.* London: Chapman and Hall, 1994:649–683.
46. Hanks AJ, Weisbarth RE, McNally JJ. Clinical performance comparisons of toric soft contact lens designs. *Int Contact Lens Clin* 1987;14:16–21.
47. Weisbarth RE, Clutterbuck TA, Shannon BJ. Comparison of toric hydrogel contact lens designs. *Int Contact Lens Clin* 1987; 14:225–231.
48. Davies IP. A comparison of the reproducibility of soft toric lenses. *Contact Lens Spectrum* 1990;5:79–82.
49. Young G, Hickson-Curran S, Lewis Y, et al. Process capability measurement of toric soft contact lenses. *Contact Lens Anterior Eye* 2001;24:25–33.
50. Young G, Coleman S, Hickson-Curran S. Clinical evaluation of toric soft lens reproducibility. *Optom Vis Sci* 2002;79:321–328.
51. Payor RE, Robird SR, Zhange X, et al. Soft toric lens power accuracy and reproducibility. *CLAO J* 1995;21:163–168.
52. Kuhl SA, Henry VA, Bennett ES. Clinical evaluation of fitting presbyopic patients with contact lenses. *J Am Optom Assoc* 1992; 63:182.
53. Bailey ES. Soft multifocal lens fitting. *Optom Today* 1997;5:37.
54. Benoit, DP. Multifocal contact lens update. *Contact Lens Spectrum* November 2001. Available at *http://www.clspectrum.com/pfarticle.asp?article=12050.* Accessed on May 30, 2002.
55. Key, JE, Yee, JL. Prospective clinical evaluation of the Acuvue bifocal contact lens. *CLAO J* 1999;25:218–221.

56. Bierly JR, Ferguson TG, Litteral G, et al. Clinical experience with Simulvue soft bifocal contact lens. *CLAO J* 1995;21:96–98.

57. Gussler CH, Solomon KD, Gussler JR, et al. A clinical evaluation of two multifocal soft contact lenses. *CLAO J* 1992;18:237–239.

58. Key JE, Morris K, Mobley CL. Prospective clinical evaluation of Sunsoft multifocal contact lens. *CLAO J* 1996;22:179–184.

59. Shapiro MB, Bredeson DC. A prospective evaluation of Unilens soft multifocal contact lenses in 100 patients. *CLAO J* 1994;20:189–191.

60. Gromacki, SJ, Nilsen E. Comparison of multifocal lens performance to monovision. *Contact Lens Spectrum* May 2001. Available at *http://clspectrum.com/pfarticle.asp?article=11968*. Accessed May 30, 2002.

61. Kirschen DG, Hung CC, Nakano TR. Comparison of suppression, stereoacuity, and interocular differences in visual acuity in monovision and Acuvue Bifocal contact lenses. *Optom Vis Sci* 1999;76:832–837.

62. Mai-Le K, Caroline P. The cost of lens care vs. daily disposable contact lenses. *Contact Lens Spectrum* 2001. Available at *http://www.clspectrum.com/archiveresults.asp?article=archive\2001\July\0701031.htm*. Accessed October 17, 2001.

63. Le AH, Liem SE, Su JL, et al. Fitting characteristics of 1-Day and 14-Day Acuvue disposable contact lenses. *Optom Vis Sci* 1996;73:750.

64. Snyder C, Hammack GG. Daily disposed hydrogel lenses-a comparison with biweekly replacement. *J Am Optom Assoc* 1994;65:164.

65. Connor CG, Campbell JB, Steel SA. The effects of disposable daily wear contact lenses on goblet cell count. *CLAO J* 1997;23:37–39.

66. Porazinski AD, Donshik PC. Giant papillary conjunctivitis in frequent replacement contact lens wearers: a retrospective study. *CLAO J* 1999;25:142–147.

67. Study proves disposables help GPC. *Optom Manage* 1992;27:3.

68. Bucci FA, Myers PJ, Evans RE, et al. Clinical and overnight corneal swell comparison of the 1-day Acuvue lens versus the Medalist, Surevue, Biomedics, and Acuvue lenses. *CLAO J* 1997;23:103–112.

69. Aquavella JV. Controlling contact lens-related infection. *Contact Lens Spectrum* 1992;7:13.

70. Thomas E, Stein H, Cox D, et al. A new standard in lens hygiene. *Contact Lens Spectrum* 1996;11:32.

71. Barr JT. Contact lenses and vision—the annual report. *Contact Lens Spectrum* 1997;12:21.

72. Harris MG, Kirby JE, Tomatore CW, et al. Microwave disinfection of soft contact lenses. *Optom Vis Sci* 1989;66:82.

73. Houlsby RD, Ghajar M, Chavez G. Microbiological evaluation of soft contact lenses disinfection solutions. *J Am Optom Assoc* 1984;55:205.

74. Woods CA. A disposable contact lens in independent practice: three years on. *J Br Contact Lens Assoc* 1991;14:207.

75. Harris MG, Brennan NA, Lowe R, et al. Hydration changes of Acuvue disposable contact lenses during disinfection. *Clin Exp Optom* 1989;72:159.

76. Appeals deadline passes in Tennessee CL court case. *AOA News* 1996;35:4.

77. Antitrust suits proliferate. *Contact Lens Spectrum* 1997;12:3.

78. Blair A. Keeping in contact. *Optom Today* 1997;5:10.

79. Snyder RP. Stop disposable lens patients from walking. *Optom Manage* 1992;27:31.

80. Efron N, Veys J. Defects in disposable contact lenses can compromise ocular integrity. *Int Contact Lens Clin* 1992;8:8.

HYDROGEL CONTACT LENS FOLLOW-UP CARE AND PROBLEM SOLVING

JENNIFER SMYTHE
PETER D. BERGENSKE
AND PATRICK J. CAROLINE

Follow-up care is considered an integral component of contact lens patient management. Daily wear of modern hydrogel lenses most often is relatively problem free. Routine monitoring of lens tolerance and patient compliance, however, as well as other aspects of general ocular health, are considered standard of care (1). Although daily wear is generally very safe and well tolerated by most patients, as many as two million patients discontinue lens wear each year due to dissatisfaction with dryness, comfort, wearing time, convenience, or vision.

Patients may present for routine evaluation and monitoring visits, in which case all that is needed is to verify that the patients are as successful in their contact lens wear as they feel they are. Patients who are symptomatic pose an additional challenge in that the clinician must determine the cause of the symptoms in order to alleviate them.

Contact lenses disturb the ocular environment. This is evident from the increased frequency of complaints of dryness, redness, and gritty sensation compared with spectacle wearers (2). Although soft contact lenses have a reputation for initial comfort, in fact, adapted rigid lens wearers are not significantly more symptomatic than are soft lens wearers.

After the initial fitting, or refitting, of the hydrogel lens patient, planned evaluation of the outcome typically is scheduled within the next 1 to 2 weeks to ensure the patient is able to successfully and safely wear the lenses. Problems related to dehydration, tightening (or excessive looseness), or sensitivity to solution systems often can be elicited only after the patient has worn lenses for, at minimum, several days, and has had the lenses on the eyes for several hours.

For routine planned evaluation of daily wear of hydrogel lenses, a first visit may be scheduled between 7 and 10 days after the dispensing visit. For lenses designed for 2-week replacement and daily wear, this allows evaluation of the initial pair within the time frame they are expected to be used and allows adequate time to supply the patient with a supply of lenses. A shorter period between dispensing and evaluation may be indicated in some situations. Patients fit

with single-use lenses realistically need only a few days in which to determine effectiveness, and reducing the length of time until follow-up decreases the need for use of large numbers of trial lenses. Patients fit with toric or multifocal hydrogel lenses who, although they may need more time to completely adapt visually, typically know if they can be expected to adapt to a given correction in just a few days. If the dispensed lenses are not successful, it is likely the patient will tolerate wearing them for no more than a few days, and if follow-up is scheduled too far into the future, it is likely they will return without the lenses on the eyes. In this situation, the clinician loses time and information that could have been gained by observing the lenses on the eyes. For these reasons, it is suggested that a follow-up visit of patients for whom vision is likely going to present a challenge should occur within 4 or 5 days of dispensing.

PLANNED FOLLOW-UP EXAMINATION

The patient who returns for planned routine evaluation should be evaluated after lenses have been on the eyes for, at minimum, 1 hour to allow equilibration. Fit characteristics of hydrogel lenses may change with wearing time due to effects of dehydration (3). This can be particularly important with toric hydrogels, as this may affect orientation of cylinder axis. The routine evaluation consists of the following components to be discussed.

Contact Lens History

The patient is interviewed with regard to subjective symptoms and impressions of the success of the contact lens fitting. It often is preferable that this be approached in an open-ended fashion so that the patient is asked to report any symptoms but is not given a list of possible symptoms to which to respond. More specific questions may be necessary if the patient has symptoms or complaints. In general, the patient is asked if vision and comfort are satisfactory. The number of hours the lenses have been worn at the time of the visit and the maximum hours of comfortable wear on previous days should be noted. It is expected that patients will be satisfied with vision and comfort, and that they are able to wear lenses, at minimum, 12 hours without significant difficulty.

Lens handling can be a challenge for new wearers of hydrogel lenses; thus, patients are asked if they are having any difficulty with insertion or removal of lenses. Lens care procedures are reviewed to reinforce instructions given at the dispensing. It is a particularly effective and revealing technique to ask the patient to explain their lens care procedures, rather than repeating them to the patient.

Vision Evaluation

Visual acuity is measured binocularly and then under monocular conditions. In the event that the vision is at expected levels, an overrefraction may not be necessary. Simple overrefraction with hand-held +0.50 D spherical trial lenses (which should cause slight distance vision blur) allows rapid confirmation that the lens power is proper.

When vision is less than expected, a spherical overrefraction is attempted first. If this does not result in adequate improvement, a spherocylinder overrefraction is indicated. Although hydrogel lenses are thought to "drape" the cornea evenly, irregularity can be induced by lenses that are excessively tight or loose. Retinoscopy and keratometry performed with the lens in place are beneficial in evaluating the lens/eye system for optical quality and stability (Fig. 22.1).

Lens-to-Cornea Fitting Evaluation

The follow-up visit is a particularly good time for evaluation of the lens-to-cornea fitting relationship, as the lens has been on the eye for a sufficient period of time that some dehydration has occurred and the post-lens relationship of lens and eye has had time to equilibrate. Although the exact reason is unclear, it is established that hydrogel lenses tighten after being on the eye for, at minimum, 5 minutes (3–6).

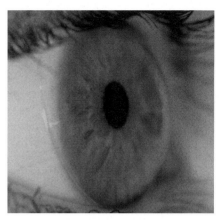

FIG. 22.2. Loose-fitting soft lens.

Evaluation of hydrogel lens fit involves assessment for centration, limbal coverage, and movement. Although centration is noted, typically decentration is acceptable as long as there is complete limbus-to-limbus coverage despite asymmetric overlap. Exceptions to this pertain to both multifocal lenses, which may be very dependent on position relative to the pupil, and opaque tinted lenses, which may induce unacceptable cosmesis when decentered. Centration may be improved by steepening the base curve radius or increasing lens diameter (Figs. 22.2 and 22.3).

Terminology borrowed from gas-permeable (GP) lens fitting may be applied to hydrogel lenses, such that the fitting relationship can be characterized as flat or steep; however, it is perhaps more appropriate to consider hydrogel lenses as simply loose or tight. Movement is assessed by observing lens behavior as the patient blinks. Typically very little (0.25 mm) movement is expected in primary gaze. On upgaze, movement with the blink increases slightly. As the patient views superiorly, a slight inferior decentration is often noted. Excessive movement of 1 mm or greater may be associated with discomfort and vision disturbance. In the event of little or no observed movement upon blinking,

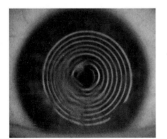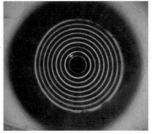

FIG. 22.1. Soft lens-induced corneal distortion.

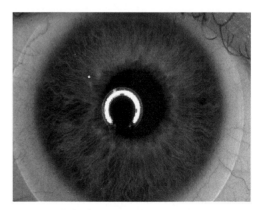

FIG. 22.3. Well-fitted soft lens.

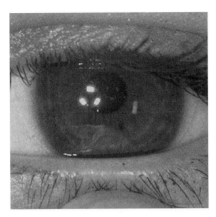

FIG. 22.4. Push-up test for lens tightness.

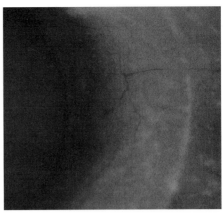

FIG. 22.5. Conjunctival impingement caused by tight-fitting soft lens.

lens tightness is best evaluated by the "push-up" test. The clinician observes the lens on the eye in primary gaze and attempts to move the lens by applying finger pressure to the lower lid (Fig. 22.4).

Evaluation of Ocular Response

Once vision and fit have been addressed, ocular response is evaluated. Although much can be observed at the biomicroscope with lenses in place, removal allows optimal examination of the anterior segment, both with and without fluorescein.

After lens removal, a systematic examination is used to search for evidence of lens-induced complications. Use of a standardized grading scale such as the Efron and Cornea and Contact Lens Research Unit (CCLRU) scale is recommended for consistent and accurate record keeping (7). Complications can be mechanical, inflammatory, or physiologic.

Mechanical complications can result from fit or condition of the lens. A lens that is too loose or too tight may cause chafing or binding that leads to localized disruption of corneal or conjunctival epithelium. Such areas will stain with fluorescein and may result in patient discomfort. Likewise, a cracked or torn lens can abrade the cornea or conjunctiva. Such complications are remedied by improving the lens-to-cornea fitting relationship or by replacing the damaged lens (Fig. 22.5).

The superior epithelial arcuate lesion (SEAL) is believed to be caused by a lens fitting relationship that is too tight, although the phenomenon is also reported to occur with loose fits (8). Hence, resolution of SEAL may involve either flattening or steepening the fit to alleviate the chafing that apparently causes it. When mechanical factors cause a break(s) in the corneal epithelium, prophylaxis with an appropriate antibiotic often is indicated until the break is resolved (Fig. 22.6).

Contact lens-associated papillary conjunctivitis (CLPC) may be caused by mechanical irritation by the edge or anterior lens surface. The cause of CLPC is multifactorial, including both mechanical irritation and inflammatory response, most likely due to denatured tear proteins on the lens surface. This has been less common since the introduction of disposable hydrogel lenses, and pure mechanical causes warrant careful scrutiny. Mechanical complications are discussed more comprehensively in Chapter 41 (Fig. 22.7).

Inflammatory responses may be characterized by conjunctival redness and swelling, as well as corneal staining and infiltration. For the hydrogel contact lens wearer presenting for routine evaluation with limbal or conjunctival redness, the first concern should be directed at solution toxicity. Solution reactions may present as conjunctival redness (particularly superior tarsal) with or without accompanying corneal staining. Occasionally such reaction will manifest only trace signs; however, patient symptoms of dryness

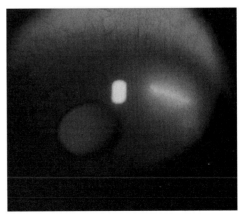

FIG. 22.6. Superior epithelial arcuate lesion (SEAL).

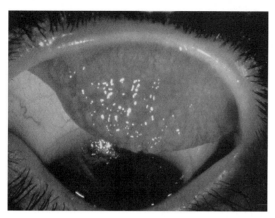

FIG. 22.7. Contact lens-induced papillary conjunctivitis.

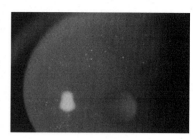

FIG. 22.9. Epithelial microcysts induced by overnight wear of low-Dk soft lens.

should raise suspicion of solution sensitivity. Management should primarily concentrate on elimination of preservative-based solutions from lens care. A comprehensive discussion of inflammatory complications is given in Chapter 39 (Fig. 22.8).

Physiologic complications are largely associated with oxygen deprivation, manifested by signs of corneal edema, including microcyst formation and corneal striae. Long-standing oxygen deprivation can result in corneal vascularization and possible myopic refractive shift. Management is aimed at increasing oxygen supply to the cornea by changing to a lens of higher oxygen transmissivity or by reducing the wearing schedule (Figs. 22.9 and 22.10; see Color Plate 22.10).

In addition to biomicroscope evaluation, a number of examination tools are used in the follow-up care of the hydrogel contact lens patient. Keratometry and topography are beneficial in evaluation for suspected corneal distortion, which can be associated with long-term use of low-oxygen transmissivity lenses (9). Pachymetry is a relatively simple

and sensitive means of assessing swelling resulting from hydrogel lens wear (10).

Refraction following lens removal is expected to be essentially the same as it was prior to lens wear. Unexpected changes are a sensitive indicator of corneal swelling or distortion. Changes in refraction that are not expected due to normal changes with age could be representative of physiologic compromise, indicating the need for greater oxygen supply to the corneal surface.

Routine follow-up examination of the hydrogel contact lens wearer who does not wear lenses overnight can prudently be scheduled on an annual basis. Patients with specific risk factors, a history of problems, or who engaged in overnight wear may justify more frequent monitoring. At such visits, the patient's vision, lens fit, ocular response, and compliance should all be reevaluated.

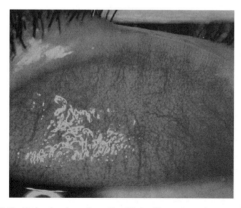

FIG. 22.8. Palpebral conjunctival injection secondary to solution sensitivity.

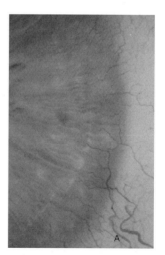
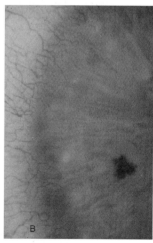

FIG. 22.10. Peripheral neovascularization **(A)** subsequent to long-term wear of low-Dk soft lens and **(B)** 30 days after refitting with high-Dk lens. (See Color Plate 22.10.)

PROBLEM SOLVING

Dryness

Reports documenting reasons for discontinuing contact lens wear conclude that symptoms of dryness are the number one contact lens-related complaint (2,11). Both by subjective complaint and physical findings, the "dry eye" contact lens patient differs significantly from the true dry-eye patient. Most often the contact lens patient has neither complaint of ocular dryness nor clinical signs of dry eye when not wearing lenses, but the patient finds that *symptoms* of dryness limit the ability to comfortably wear lenses. The cause of this traditionally has been attributed to lens dehydration; however, no such correlation has been demonstrated (12). Other possible causes of dryness symptoms include elevated tear osmolarity, hypoxia (13), tear evaporation (14), and solution sensitivity. In one report, the most frequent complaint of contact lens dry eye patients was "dryness," followed by blurry and changeable vision (11). In contrast, the true dry-eye patient does not need contact lenses to stimulate symptoms, and the complaints most frequently are of dryness, but also of soreness (15).

For many contact lens dry-eye patients, the problem becomes worse later in the day, although patients wearing lenses on an overnight basis also may complain of dryness upon awakening. Clinicians and patients alike quickly learn that the simple use of lens rewetting drops at the onset of symptoms is a disappointingly short-lived solution to the problem. Use of rewetting agents at regular intervals (every 3 hours throughout the day) does provide relief to many patients, but this regimen is expensive, particularly when preservative-free preparations are used.

It is known that all soft lens materials dehydrate *in vivo* (16), most likely through evaporation. Unfortunately, rewetting agents only minimally relieve symptoms. Significantly more effective is removal of the lens for brief immersion in saline or multipurpose solution, allowing the lens to fully rehydrate. For many patients, this allows a noticeably longer relief of symptoms than does the use of rewetting drops. The "5 o'clock, 5-minute soak" is a simple and effective strategy for the contact lens patient who has a long evening ahead. (Patients who wear lenses on an overnight basis should be advised to properly clean and disinfect lenses after any removal prior to sleeping with lenses.)

When simple rehydration by drops or soaking is ineffective, the clinician must consider that dryness symptoms may not be due to the effects of evaporation and must consider other factors, such as oxygen transmission and solution hypersensitivity reactions. A solution hypersensitivity reaction also causes symptoms of dryness and, in some cases, may result in a punctate keratitis (17). Conversely, absence of significant staining does not rule out solution sensitivity. A trial with a preservative-free disinfection system (such as peroxide or ultraviolet [UV]-C) is indicated. Another alter-

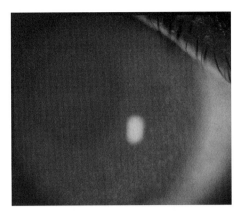

FIG. 22.11. Solution-induced superficial punctate keratitis.

native is elimination of preservatives by trial with single-use lenses (Fig. 22.11.

Another approach to the rehydration challenge is to use lenses that are less prone to dehydration. The silicone hydrogels are low-water-content, high-oxygen permeability materials for which evaporation and dehydration appear to be significantly less of a problem than with conventional hydrogel lenses. Both PureVision (36% water) and Focus Night & Day (24% water) lenses are reported to provide relief for many patients suffering from dryness symptoms with conventional soft lenses. In addition to the reduction of dehydration as a contributor to the syndrome, these lenses have surface properties that reduce binding of protein, likely resulting in less preservative uptake. Finally, the high-oxygen transmission is associated with less ocular redness and may be a contributing factor (Fig. 22.12) (18,19).

If low-water content is an answer, GP lenses are a viable option. GP materials offer the benefits of essentially no evaporation, no preservative uptake, and high-oxygen transmission. For the contact lens dry-eye patient, GP lenses can be a very successful alternative and should be considered, particularly when other attempts fail.

Punctal occlusion, a mainstay of dry eye treatment, is notably ineffective for many soft lens dry-eye patients. Because these patients are not actually tear-deficient, this should come as no surprise. Rigid lens patients with dryness may benefit from punctal occlusion because they are more

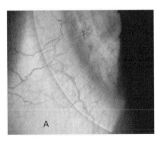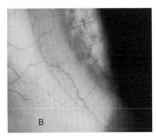

FIG. 22.12. Limbal injection **(A)** with low-Dk soft lens and **(B)** with high-Dk silicone hydrogel.

likely to have true dryness. For soft lens wearers, rehydration, preservative elimination, and changing to a silicone hydrogel material all should be attempted prior to consideration of punctal occlusion. Success with punctal occlusion in soft lens wearers occurs, but the reason for success remains unclear. In many cases the benefits appear to decrease over a few months' time, leading to greater skepticism over the true benefit of this procedure (20,21).

Guidelines for managing contact lens patients with symptoms of dryness include the following:

1. If lubricants are used, they should be preservative-free and used frequently throughout the day, prior to onset of symptoms.
2. Removal for lens rehydration is suitable for daily wear patients.
3. Eliminate preservative-based solutions from the care regimen.
4. Use low-water lenses, such as silicone hydrogels and GP lenses.

Discomfort

Hydrogel contact lenses, if nothing else, are expected to be comfortable. Discomfort of the eye must be differentiated from lens awareness, a determination that is readily made most often by simple removal of the lens. Diagnosis of the problem is necessary in order to arrive at a solution.

Lens discomfort that occurs only when the lens is worn is indicative of a damaged or poorly fitting lens. A loose-fitting lens will move excessively and, in some cases, may result in lid sensation due to edge lift. If the lens previously exhibited a good lens-to-cornea fitting relationship, the problem most likely is an inverted lens. Another possible explanation for the onset of such lens movement and awareness is development of CLPC.

A cracked or torn lens can create lid or ocular surface irritation. Lens replacement is the only and obvious solution. A common presentation is that of a distressed patient who claims he or she was able to remove only part of a torn lens from the eye. Instillation of fluorescein often will aid greatly in locating the remaining fragment(s), which most likely will have migrated to the superior fornix.

Foreign matter beneath a hydrogel lens typically is a problem only at the time of lens insertion. Removal and reinsertion of the lens usually are adequate to resolve this. Alternatively, it often is possible to displace small amounts of foreign matter by sliding the lens off of the cornea to the inferior or temporal conjunctival surface, then sliding the lens back over the cornea. When successful, this results in an immediate improvement in comfort.

Stinging or burning upon insertion typically indicates a chemical irritation that may be due to solution sensitivity or transfer by the patient of some other irritating substance, such as soap, to the lens. Persistent stinging or burning

warrants review of the patient's lens care practices. In the event of a suspected solution sensitivity, trial with a preservative-free care system or single-use lenses is advisable.

Discomfort that increases with lens removal most often indicates either epithelial break or presence of a foreign body. Instillation of fluorescein and careful biomicroscope examination, including eversion of the lids, are indicated.

Poor Compliance

Patient compliance with lens care and lens replacement schedules, in general, leave much to be desired. Self-reporting of compliance indicates that patients often fail to wash hands prior to handling lenses, and they fail to fully comply with approved lens care procedures. Industry data as well as patient survey data indicate that a significant number of patients fail to replace lenses according to an approved and prescribed schedule (22).

Patient confusion over proper lens care practice and products poses a challenge to the practitioner. Poor compliance with care systems can lead to contamination of lenses and cases, thus increasing the likelihood of ocular infection and irritation. Estimates of patient noncompliance with lens care systems range from 40% to 70% (23–25). Studies evaluating patients with contact lens-related microbial keratitis have concluded that as many as 90% of these patients are noncompliant (26,27).

Factors that have been shown to positively affect patient compliance include the quality of the patient–practitioner relationship and the degree of patient education. Reinforcement of instructions at follow-up visits has been shown to be particularly effective in increasing compliance (28).

In order to optimize compliance, patient education must not only be provided but also reinforced with printed materials and repetition. The assumption that patients are routinely caring for contact lenses in the manner they have been instructed will mislead the practitioner and places the patient at increased risk. The patient history performed at each contact lens follow-up examination should include a review of lens care practices. A particularly revealing interrogation technique is to ask the patients to explain in their own words how they take care of their lenses.

Blurred Vision

Determining the cause of blurred vision in symptomatic patients begins with ascertaining when the problem began and differentiating between constant and intermittent blur.

Constant Blur

Lens Reversal/Defects

When a patient presents with reduced vision that occurs suddenly and is constant throughout the contact lens wear time, it is prudent to first verify that the lenses have not been inadvertently switched between eyes. Other causes of sudden constant blur that should be ruled out include lens inversion or lens defects. Generally, both of these scenarios would also induce a foreign body sensation or some form of discomfort and are easily confirmed during a slit-lamp examination. For some very thin lenses, an inverted lens may be surprisingly comfortable, yet the vision can be adversely affected, particularly with multifocal designs.

Refractive Error Changes and Residual Astigmatism

Refractive error change should be suspected if the visual symptoms occurred gradually over a period of time and can be confirmed through a careful overrefraction as described previously. A simple change in spherical refractive error can be accommodated by a trial with a new lens power. Residual astigmatism typically manifests as a symptom of blur at both distance and near; and a significant amount of cylinder in the overrefraction indicates the need for another form of contact lens correction, such as GP or soft toric lenses. For low-astigmatic patients, some practitioners have reported success with single-vision aspheric hydrogel lenses. These lenses incorporate aberration-reducing optics, and although measured visual acuity or residual astigmatism may not change, subjectively, patients have reported improved vision while wearing these designs (29,30).

Physiologic Changes

If visual acuity is not improved through a spherical or spherocylindrical overrefraction, a physiologic change, such as corneal edema, should be suspected. Significant corneal edema, which may be due to a tight-fitting or low-Dk lens, can cause decreased visual acuity (31). A careful slit-lamp examination is necessary to ascertain corneal transparency and integrity. Epithelial edema may result from solution sensitivity and has been shown to adversely affect vision (32). Topographical changes as a result of edema also can be revealed with corneal mapping, although the effect can be subtle (33). Management of physiologically induced symptoms of blur require eliminating the cause by refitting the patient with a higher–oxygen-permeable lens material, ensuring an appropriate lens fit and/or reducing lens wear time.

Surface Deposits/Soiled Lenses

Although less common with the trend toward more frequent lens replacement schedules, lens surface deposition can cause symptoms of blur. The most common deposits are organic in nature; however, inorganic films from cosmetics or even air pollution can adhere to a soft contact lens (34, 35). Differentiation of the type of deposit on the lens is best accomplished by inspection of the lens on the eye with the slit lamp. This allows observation of surface wetting patterns after each blink. Inspection also can be performed with a magnifying loupe after first drying the lens with a

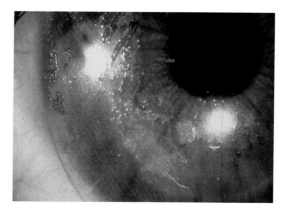

FIG. 22.13. Lipid deposition on soft contact lens.

lint-free tissue. Often these deposits are either protein-based or lipid-based (Fig. 22.13).

Protein Deposits Lysozyme-based protein deposits from the normal tear film is the most common type of lens deposition. Protein should be suspected if the deposit appears as a sticky film or in a small "beaded" pattern. The film is typically hazy gray or white, and the tear film breaks up immediately over the surface. Prolonged or frequent exposure to denatured protein on the surface of a contact lens is associated with the development of CLPC (36). High-water-content, ionic lens materials are more frequently associated with lysozyme adherence; therefore, when frequent lens replacement is not a viable option for specific patients, refitting with a low-water, nonionic lens material may result in a lower incidence of deposits (Fig. 22.14) (34).

Enzymatic cleaners have been historically considered the most effective way to accomplish protein hydrolysis and the ultimate removal of the deposit. Modern care products are designed to help prevent binding of protein to the lens surface. Patients who are prone to this type of deposition are best managed by increasing the frequency of lens replacement, including daily replacement, when feasible.

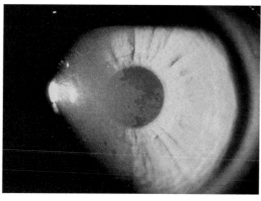

FIG. 22.14. Protein deposits.

Lipid Deposits and Calcium/Lipid Complexes Lipid deposition is possible, both into the lens matrix as well as on the surface. Greasy-appearing, discrete nodular deposits are commonly referred to as *jelly bumps.* The deposits are primarily lipid in nature. They also can form complexes with calcium. Deposition in the center of the lens can cause visual disturbance. Unfortunately, jelly bumps cannot be removed by standard cleaning techniques without leaving a defect in the lens. It is not uncommon for patients to have a foreign body sensation or report that they have a "spot" on the lens that they are unable to remove. Lens replacement is indicated when their presence is detected.

The primary source of the lipid is meibomian gland secretions. Patients who are prone to these complex deposits should use a frequent lens replacement schedule. Alcohol-based cleaners are effective in solubilizing lipid and are indicated when a more frequent lens replacement schedule is not an option.

Intermittent Blur

Fluctuating visual acuity can be attributed to several causes. Patients may report vision that "blurs and clears" after blinking when a lens fit is excessively flat and decenters. This is especially true for toric and multifocal soft contact lenses. With multifocal lenses, centration is critical to achieve the simultaneous vision effect. With a soft toric lens, excessive lens movement can result in unstable orientation of the cylinder axis. Spherical lenses that display excessive lag in alternating positions of gaze can affect the consistency and clarity of vision as the optic zone of the contact lens is not centered adequately.

Lenses that are fitted excessively tight can induce intermittent blur. As wear time increases during the day, a soft contact lens may dehydrate and further tighten in the periphery. This can result in lens vaulting and irregular draping effects that distort the optics, causing intermittent late-day blur.

Finally, if intermittent blur is instantaneous after lens insertion, especially if accompanied by a physical lens awareness, an inverted lens should be suspected as described previously (Fig. 22.15).

Ocular Redness

Ocular redness is a common finding and complaint with soft contact lens wearers (37). However, it is critical to delineate more serious causes of ocular redness, such as infectious or inflammatory adverse responses. A comprehensive case history and observation of additional signs aids in differentiating a potentially serious adverse response from more routine causes of redness. Conditions such as contact lens acute red eye; microbial keratitis; contact lens peripheral ulcer; bacterial, viral, and allergic conjunctivitis; and symptomatic

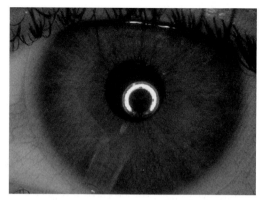

FIG. 22.15. Inverted soft lens may give rise to lens movement, increased awareness, and possible blurred acuity.

infiltrative keratitis all can cause redness and are discussed thoroughly in other chapters.

It now is accepted that limbal hyperemia (the filling and engorgement of limbal blood vessels) often is related to the oxygen permeability of the lens material. The high-Dk fluoro-silixone and silicone hydrogel contact lenses reduce limbal hyperemia (18,19). Limbal hyperemia is thought to be a precursor to neovascularization. Identifying patients with this common finding and refitting them into a high-Dk lens material will lower the risk of corneal vascularization, and patients will enjoy cosmetically "whiter" eyes.

Finally, conjunctival redness can occur in response to a mechanical insult from a defective or poorly fitting lens or toxic reaction to lens care products. Typically, with each of these scenarios, the patient also will experience lens discomfort and/or dryness symptoms. Once again, a case history combined with careful slit-lamp evaluation will aid in the diagnosis. It is important to include an evaluation of the cornea and conjunctiva with sodium fluorescein, cobalt blue light, and a Wratten no. 12 filter to assess staining patterns that often are an indication of mechanical insult or solution toxicity. Diffuse corneal staining across several regions of the cornea combined with ocular redness and dryness or discomfort may indicate a hypersensitivity or toxic reaction to lens care products. In contrast, a localized area of corneal or conjunctival staining combined with a symptom of discomfort with the lens on the eye most likely would occur with a defective lens or grossly inappropriately fitted lens.

REFERENCES

1. Classe J. Clinicolegal problems in contact lens practice. In: *Legal aspects of optometry.* Stoneham, MA: Butterworths, 1989: 373–388
2. Vajdic C, et al. The frequency of ocular symptoms during spectacle and daily soft and rigid contact lens wear. *Optom Vis Sci* 1999; 76:705–711.
3. Pritchard N, Fonn D. Dehydration, lens movement and dryness ratings of hydrogel contact lenses. *Ophthalmic Physiol Opt* 1995; 15:281–286.

4. Golding TR, et al. Soft lens movement: effect of blink rate on lens settling. *Acta Ophthalmol Scand* 1995;73:506–511.

5. Golding TR, et al. Soft lens movement: effects of humidity and hypertonic saline on lens settling. *Acta Ophthalmol Scand* 1995;73:139–144.

6. Brennan NA, et al. Soft lens movement: temporal characteristics. *Optom Vis Sci* 1994;71:359–363.

7. Efron N. *Contact lens complications.* Stoneham, MA: Butterworth-Heinemann,1999.

8. Holden BA, et al. Superior epithelial arcuate lesions with soft contact lens wear. *Optom Vis Sci* 2001;78:9–12.

9. Holden BA. The Glenn A. Fry Award lecture 1988: the ocular response to contact lens wear. *Optom Vis Sci* 1989;66:717–733.

10. Herse P, Akakura N, Ooi C. Topographical corneal edema. An update. *Acta Ophthalmol (Copenh)* 1993;71:539–543.

11. Begley CG, et al. Responses of contact lens wearers to a dry eye survey. *Optom Vis Sci* 2000;77:40–46.

12. Fonn D, Situ P, Simpson T. Hydrogel lens dehydration and subjective comfort and dryness ratings in symptomatic and asymptomatic contact lens wearers. *Optom Vis Sci* 1999;76:700–704.

13. Gilbard J, Rossi S, Gray K. Mechanisms for increased tear film osmolarity. In: Cavanagh HD, ed. *The cornea: transactions of the World Congress on the Cornea III.* New York: Raven Press, 1988:5–7.

14. Cedarstaff TH, Tomlinson A. A comparative study of tear evaporation rates and water content of soft contact lenses. *Am J Optom Physiol Opt* 1983;60:167–174.

15. Nichols KK, Begley CG, Caffery B, et al. Symptoms of ocular irritation in patients diagnosed with dry eye. *Optom Vis Sci* 1999;76:838–844.

16. Efron N, Young G. Dehydration of hydrogel contact lenses in vitro and in vivo. *Ophthalmic Physiol Opt* 1988;8:253–256.

17. Begley CG, Edrington TB, Chalmers R. Effect of lens care systems on corneal fluorescein staining and subjective comfort in hydrogel lens wearers. *Int Contact Lens Clin* 1994;21:7–13.

18. Papas EB, et al. High-oxygen-transmissibility soft contact lenses do not induce limbal hyperaemia. *Curr Eye Res* 1997;16:942–948.

19. Papas E. On the relationship between soft contact lens oxygen transmissibility and induced limbal hyperaemia. *Exp Eye Res* 1998;67:125–131.

20. Slusser TG, Lowther GE. Effects of lacrimal drainage occlusion with nondissolvable intracanalicular plugs on hydrogel contact lens wear. *Optom Vis Sci* 1998;75:330–338.

21. Virtanen T, et al. Lacrimal plugs as a therapy for contact lens intolerance. *Eye* 1996;10:727–731.

22. Coopersmith L, Weinstock FJ. Current recommendations and practice regarding soft lens replacement and disinfection. *CLAO J* 1997;23:172–176.

23. Collins MJ, Carney LG. Patient compliance and its influence on contact lens wearing problems. *Am J Optom Physiol Opt* 1986;63:952–956.

24. Chun MW, Weissman BA. Compliance in contact lens care. *Am J Optom Physiol Opt* 1987;64:274–276.

25. Sokol JL, et al. A study of patient compliance in a contact lens-wearing population. *CLAO J* 1990;16:209–213.

26. Bowden FW 3rd, et al. Patterns of lens care practices and lens product contamination in contact lens associated microbial keratitis. *CLAO J* 1989;15:49–54.

27. Radford CF, et al. Risk factors for acanthamoeba keratitis in contact lens users: a case-control study. *BMJ* 1995;310:1567–1570.

28. Wilson LA, et al. Microbial contamination of contact lens storage cases and solutions. *Am J Ophthalmol* 1990;110:193–198.

29. Edrington TB, Barr JT. Creating a better locus of focus. *Contact Lens Spectrum* 2002:44.

30. Snyder C. Aspheric hydrogels "correct" minimal astigmatism? *Contact Lens Spectrum* 2000:15.

31. Binder PS. The physiologic effects of extended wear soft contact lenses. *Ophthalmology* 1980;87:745–749.

32. Pinckers A, et al. Contact lens induced severe epithelial disruption. A case report. *Int Ophthalmol* 1989;13:229–232.

33. Lowther GE, Tomlinson A. Clinical study of corneal response to the wear of low water content soft lenses. *Am J Optom Physiol Opt* 1979;56:674–680.

34. Tomlinson A, Caroline P. Comparative evaluation of surface deposits on high water content hydrogel contact lens polymers. *CLAO J* 1990;16:121–127.

35. Fowler SA, Allansmith MR. Evolution of soft contact lens coatings. *Arch Ophthalmol* 1980;98:95–99.

36. Allansmith MR, et al. Giant papillary conjunctivitis in contact lens wearers. *Am J Ophthalmol* 1977;83:697–708.

37. Sweeney DF, Gauthier C, Terry R. The effects of long-term contact lens wear on the anterior eye. *Invest Ophthalmol Vis Sci* 1992;33[S]:1293.

ADVANCED CONTACT LENS APPLICATION

TEARS, DRY EYE, AND MANAGEMENT

**BARBARA CAFFERY AND
JERRY R. PAUGH**

Practitioners are familiar with increased symptoms of ocular "dryness" with which many contact lens wearers present (1–3). In one large survey, patients chose dryness as the most common reason for discontinuation of contact lens wear (4). Some practitioners believe that disturbances in the intimate and active relationship between the preocular tear film and contact lenses, causing dry eye symptoms, often determines the success or failure of contact lens wear. In order to avoid or treat dry eyes during contact lens wear and to screen contact lens candidates, practitioners should have a solid understanding of the preocular tear film and its interactions with the ocular surface, contact lenses, and their solutions (Figs. 23.1 and 23.2).

This chapter begins with a review of preocular tear film composition, production, function, and biochemical characteristics. Tear film changes that occur with contact lens wear are discussed, and an approach to clinical care is presented.

PREOCULAR TEAR COMPOSITION AND STRUCTURE

The ocular surface is bathed in constantly replenishing tears. This thin liquid layer is essential for clear vision, epithelial cell health, and protection of the ocular surface. The healthy tear film creates a smooth refracting surface, washes debris from the surface, provides antimicrobial protection, and supplies nutrients to the surface cells. Homeostasis of the tear film involves a complex neuronal and hormonal regulatory balance. Sex hormones, particularly androgens, modulate the immune system, trophic functions of the lacrimal gland, and functioning of the meibomian glands. The cornea, lacrimal glands, goblet cells, and meibomian glands are all richly innervated, and parasympathetic, sympathetic, and sensory nerves play key roles in tear film regulation. As if this were not enough complexity, practitioners place contact lenses with various thicknesses, materials, and edge designs (Fig. 23.3) on patients' eyes to challenge all of these systems.

At one time, the tear film was believed to have three distinct layers: mucin, aqueous, and lipid. The thickness was estimated as 7 μm or greater (5,6). Recent research suggests a more complicated thin film system of six layers but only 3 μm for average tear film thickness (7). Although we will continue to discuss the tear film as a three-layered structure, the reader is encouraged to keep in mind the more complex six-layer theory (8–12) and that a significant percentage of the volume of the tear film is found in the menisci or tear lakes at the upper and lower lid margins (Fig. 23.4; see Color Plate 23.4).

Epithelium and Mucous Layer

The tear film resides on an ocular surface composed of conjunctival and cornea epithelial cells. Although clinicians tend to think of the corneal surface as smooth, microscopi-

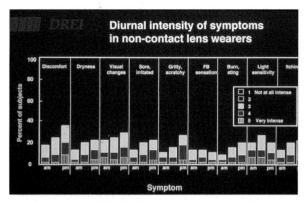

FIG. 23.1. Diurnal intensity of symptoms in non-contact lens wearers. (Reprinted with permission from Begley C, Chalmers R, Mitchell L, et al. Characterization of ocular surface symptoms from optometric practices in North America. *Cornea* 2001;20: 610–618.)

cally the surface is extremely convoluted. The apical (or outward facing) sides of the epithelial cells have specialized surface ridges called *microplicae* (see Chapter 2). Healthy epithelial cells secrete the correct amount and type of mucin to allow the tear film to run a smooth course over their surfaces. Unhealthy cells, not covered with mucus, are observed clinically as red stained spots when rose bengal is instilled (13).

Mucous layer components are created by, and lie in, intimate contact with the surface epithelial cells. Mucins are secreted by the goblet cells of the conjunctiva, the epithelial cells of the conjunctiva and cornea, and the lacrimal gland. Goblet cells are former epithelial cells that create gel-forming mucins such as MUC 5AC (13,14). Corneal and conjunctival epithelial cells contribute to the mucous layer by expressing transmembrane mucins, such as MUC 1, 2, and 4, which maintain the wettability of the apical side of the cell walls (15). These transmembrane mucins, together with the mucinlike proteins found in the vicinity of cell membranes, make up the glycocalyx.

The mucin layer interacts with the microplicae of the ocular surface cells, facilitating the spread of the remaining

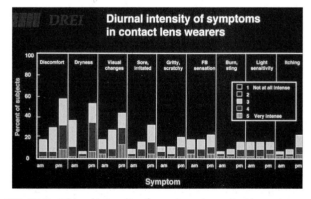

FIG. 23.2. Diurnal intensity of symptoms in contact lens wearers. (Reprinted with permission from Begley C, Chalmers R, Mitchell L, et al. Characterization of ocular surface symptoms from optometric practices in North America. *Cornea* 2001;20:610–618.)

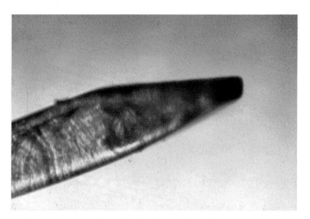

FIG. 23.3. Blunt edge of a hydrogel lens. (Courtesy of J.E. Josephson.)

aqueous and lipid components of the tear film over the ocular surface and lubricating lid movement. The mucous layer also acts as a mechanism to eliminate debris by bundling dead cells and foreign objects into mucous threads for removal.

The mucin layer also plays a major role in contact lens wear. Mucous coats lenses to enhance lens wettability. However, these coatings also might contribute to the development of giant papillary conjunctivitis (16).

Aqueous Layer

The aqueous layer is the thickest layer of the tear film. It is primarily secreted by the lacrimal gland, with some participation from the glands of Krause and Wolfring. This layer contains inorganic salts, glucose, biopolymers, proteins, and glycoproteins.

Control of the rate and composition of lacrimal gland secretion is the result of an interplay between direct neural influences, via autonomic and peptidergic nerve fiber endings on the lacrimal gland secretory cells, and hormones reaching the lacrimal gland cells via the circulation (17).

Hormones, especially androgens, modify lacrimal gland secretions (18,19). Lower secretory function is observed in

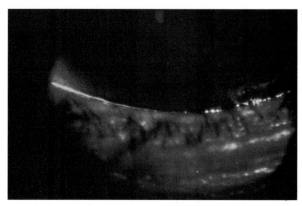

FIG. 23.4. Unsaturated tear meniscus. (Courtesy of J.E. Josephson.) (See color Plate 23.4.)

postmenopausal women, especially those using estrogen-only hormone replacement therapy (20) and those suffering from Sjögren syndrome. Sjögren syndrome is a disease mainly of females (21) that is diagnosed by a clinical triad of dry eye, dry mouth, and autoimmune markers in the serum. These patients also have depressed circulating androgen levels (22,23).

The lacrimal gland responds to the sensory nerves of the ocular surface. At one time, basic secretions were thought to be produced by the noninnervated accessory lacrimal glands, whereas reflex tearing was believed to result from sensory stimulation of the ocular surface. A newer paradigm, however, suggests that all tearing is reflex tearing. Basal secretion is considered the result of minimal sensory stimulation, whereas active tearing is the result of maximal stimulation (24). In this model, the initial stimulus of secretion is found on the ocular surface, e.g., a rigid lens is placed on the eye of a novice wearer and copious tears stream down the patient's cheeks in response. Corneal and conjunctival sensory nerves regulate tear flow during normal daily activities in a more subtle fashion, such as when a cold wind hits the eye.

A contact lens has several potential effects on the aqueous layer. First, changes in volume and perhaps composition are likely to occur due solely to the presence of a foreign body. Also, the aqueous layer becomes divided between the lens' front and back surfaces, and there is little exchange of the post-lens tear volume, at least with hydrogel lenses (25). Stimuli to the corneal sensory nerves change. Hydrogel lens wearers do not usually respond with reflex tearing when exposed to irritating fumes, such as raw onions, and adapted rigid contact lens wearers eventually cease foreign body-related copious tearing (26,27).

Lipid Layer

The lipid layer is the outermost layer of the tear film. It is primarily secreted by the meibomian glands of the upper and lower lids, but also in part by the accessory glands of Zeis. Observed using interferometry or a biomicroscope, this colorful layer intrigues the observer with beautiful patterns. It is a complex layer of two phases dependent upon each other for stability.

More polar lipids (phospholipids, fatty acids, and free cholesterol) lie deeper in the tear film, adjacent to the aqueous-mucin phase upon which the nonpolar lipids reside. The relatively less polar lipids (cholesterol esters) form a thicker outer phase to interface with the atmosphere (28, 29). Any alteration in the makeup of the lipid secretions alters the tear film. The interrelation of the lipid classes present, length of fatty acids and alcohols, and their relative saturation and hydroxylation are important for maintaining good barrier properties, thus protecting the tear layer from skin lipids. Contamination leads to a rapid tear breakup. A

healthy lipid layer retards evaporation of the underlying aqueous phase (30,31).

The lipids of the tear film are secreted and distributed with the blink. In an ideal situation, the complete blink will cause a droplet of clear baby oil-like secretion from the meibomian glands onto the surface of the eye to replenish the lipid layer (32). Meibomian glands are affected by hormones, particularly androgens, and by systemic diseases such as rosacea (33–36), and can become colonized with surface bacteria such as *Staphylococcus epidermis* leading to abnormal secretions contaminated with bacterial exotoxins. The glands also can deteriorate and become nonsecreting (Fig. 23.5).

Lipid layer patterns and colors have been studied extensively by McDonald (36,37) Guillon (38), Hamano et al. (39,40), Josephson (41), and Doane (42). Hamano first described the typical surface patterns of tears using interferometry. He observed marmoreal, flow, and amorphous patterns (39,40). Guillon (38) added a fourth pattern called *colored fringe* (Figs. 23.6 and 23.7; see Color Plate 23.7).

The marmoreal pattern appears to be the most common, a gray marblelike structure observed with or without contamination. It represents a lipid layer 13 to 70 nm thick. The amorphous pattern is the next most common, appears blue gray in white light, and is 70 to 90 nm thick. The flow pattern is less common, distinguished by its wavy pattern caused by spreading of various lipids of different thicknesses from 10 to 90 nm. The colored fringe pattern is most rare. This indicates a layer thickened to 86 to 170 nm. Often there are dark spots in the pattern indicating mucous strands or lumps.

The lipid pattern may predict contact lens success. Patients with amorphous patterns, for example, show good tolerance to lens wear, as do those with flow patterns (38). Patients with contaminated marmoreal patterns, however, often show excess surface drying and deposits on lenses (38). Those with colored fringe patterns are unlikely to be suc-

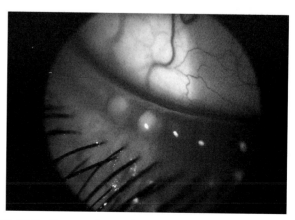

FIG. 23.5. Nonsecreting meibomian glands. (Courtesy of J.E. Josephson.)

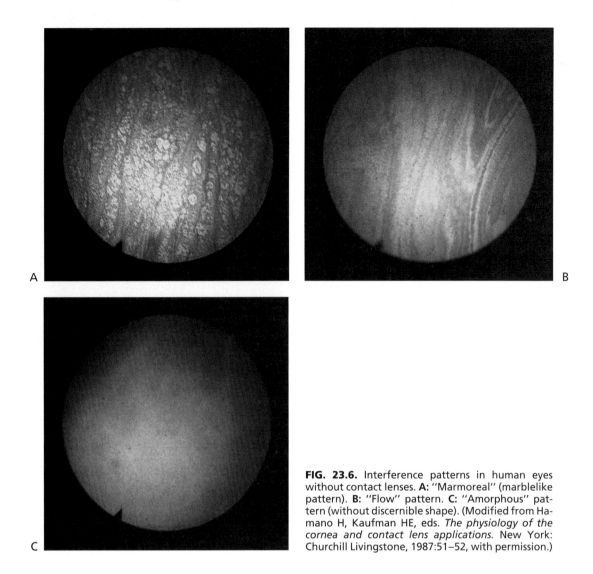

FIG. 23.6. Interference patterns in human eyes without contact lenses. **A:** "Marmoreal" (marblelike pattern). **B:** "Flow" pattern. **C:** "Amorphous" pattern (without discernible shape). (Modified from Hamano H, Kaufman HE, eds. *The physiology of the cornea and contact lens applications.* New York: Churchill Livingstone, 1987:51–52, with permission.)

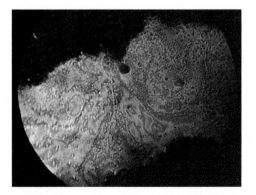

FIG. 23.7. "Colored fringe" interference pattern. (From Josephson JE. Appearance of the preocular tear film lipid layer. *Am J Optom Physiol Opt* 1983:60:885, with permission.) (See Color Plate 23.7.)

cessful because the pattern usually indicates blepharitis and meibomian gland dysfunction.

TEAR FILM CHARACTERISTICS

Evaluation of the tear film is difficult. It is dynamic, changing with each blink and affected by general health, environment, and hormone status. Although only a few characteristics of the tear film have established norms, some have been correlated with contact lens success.

The tear film is compressed and disrupted by the lid movement each blink. As the lids lift, a new tear film must develop. It takes from 3 to 10 seconds for the tear layer to establish itself (43–45). Mucus is balled up and removed, debris is pushed to the meniscus, the goblet and epithelial cells secrete more mucins, the aqueous is replenished, and the lipid layer spreads over the surface. At this point the tear film begins to decay and the process begins again.

Tear Film Breakup Time

Clinicians routinely observe breakup of the tear film, either when attempting to determine the suitability of a patient for contact lens wear or to establish a dry eye diagnosis. The test is easy to perform when using sodium fluorescein instilled into the eye to highlight the tear film. The physical phenomenon of film breakup has a subjective corollary. If we hold our eyes open for a long time, we eventually feel burning and stinging associated with rupture of the tear film. Clinical wisdom suggests that our ocular surfaces will remain moist, and we will not feel symptoms if tears are stable between blinks. Similarly, we believe that a precontact lens tear film that remains intact between blinks will keep the surface of the lens wetted and thereby reduce symptoms of dryness induced by a lid rubbing over a dry lens. Rolando and Refojo (46) found a higher tear evaporation rate in eyes with keratoconjunctivitis sicca. Although this finding has been contested by Hamano et al. (47), it seems clinically intuitive that thinner and less well-made tear films would evaporate more quickly and produce symptoms and signs of dry eye.

Cessation of blinking eventually leads to the breakup of the tear film. Mishima (48) proposed that disruption was a result of a discontinuity of the lipid layer. Holly (49) and Lemp et al. (50) suggested that the surface lipids naturally and rapidly migrate to the aqueous–mucus interface. This changes the hydrophilic nature of the mucus layer–epithelial cell interface and creates hydrophobic spots on the corneal epithelium. More recently, Sharma and Ruckenstein (51) proposed, like Lin and Brenner (52), that van der Waals dispersion forces explain tear breakup and that the lipid layer is an unimportant element in the process. Blink action exerts a shear force across the tear film to redistribute and smooth the mucus layer onto the corneal surface. The aqueous layer then begins its normal thinning process, as does the underlying mucus layer. The mucus layer is particularly vulnerable to thinning in areas where the aqueous layer is somewhat thinner. If another blink does not occur, interface perturbations cause the mucus layer to rupture, the aqueous phase comes into contact with the exposed epithelium, and tear breakup occurs.

Alternatively, Liotet et al (53) proposed that the key structure in breakup of the tear film is the glycocalyx rather than the mucus or lipid layers. Development of a dry spot on the cornea results from interference with the ability of epithelial cells to form a proper glycocalyx. There are no sites to which mucous proteins adhere and the cell becomes hydrophobic.

Whatever its cause, tear film breakup is most easily observed by adding fluorescein dye to the ocular surface. The patient is asked to cease blinking. The clinician watches the ocular surface through the biomicroscope, counting seconds or timing with a stopwatch until the first rupture of the tear film (seen as a black spot) appears. This technique is fraught with error, however, as the very addition of fluid and dye to the eye automatically disrupts its normal state (54).

The normal tear film breakup time (BUT), using fluorescein, ranges from 10 to 40 seconds. Norn (55) observed BUTs of 25 to 30 seconds. Lemp et al. (50) found a low BUT of 10 seconds or less in dry eye patients. Evidence in Hong Kong Chinese (56) suggests that mean BUT in normals, at least in this ethnic group, may be less than 10 seconds. A generally accepted value of 5 seconds or less is often used by clinicians to classify a tear film as unstable.

Mengher et al. (57) found that instillation of fluorescein itself reduces corneal tear film stability. This group introduced the use of a grid pattern projected onto the eye, observed through a biomicroscope, to quantify a noninvasive BUT. This instrument has become known as the *xeroscope*. BUTs increased to 40 to 150 seconds with this technique (58).

Patel et al. (59) developed another noninvasive technique of measuring BUT using a grid attached to a keratometer. They observed average breakups of 18 seconds and found reduced BUTs when fluorescein was instilled. Guillon (38) developed a technique using a hand-held interferometer to measure noninvasive BUT. The lipid layer is visible with this technique, and normal breakup of the tears is 45 seconds or more.

Given the variability of the BUT, should clinicians continue to perform this test? It definitely is one of many observations that we should make. Tear BUT is quite simple and provides an estimate of the stability of the tear film, at least at the particular time that we are assessing it.

Tear Flow

Clinicians also estimate tear flow. This is a difficult measurement because every test may induce excess tearing that probably exaggerates true tear flow. The Schirmer test is most commonly used (60): a filter paper strip is placed into the inferior lacrimal prism for five minutes. Schirmer 1 uses no anesthetic and is subject to higher readings because of reflex tearing. Schirmer 2 is performed after instillation of anesthetic. This test cannot measure normal tear flow because corneal sensory stimulation is one of the triggers for lacrimal gland flow. Irritative reflex tearing, however, is eliminated (Fig. 23.8).

Schirmer measurements of less than 10 mm in 5 minutes are considered suspect for dry eye. Certainly measures of less than 5 mm in 5 minutes are very suggestive.

The phenol red thread test is an alternative tear flow evaluation that uses a much less irritating thread for a reduced period of time (15 seconds) (61). It is unclear, however, what the phenol red test is really measuring. Tomlin-

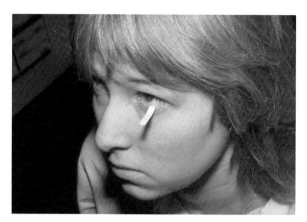

FIG. 23.8. Schirmer tear test *in vivo*.

son et al. (62) found no correlation to either tear turnover rate or tear volume (as measured with fluorophotometry), or to tear meniscus height (measured using a reticule eyepiece) in normal eyes (Fig. 23.9).

Tear clearance rates recently have been suggested as a measure of tear flow. This measurement is greatly affected by the outflow system. For example, patients with punctal occlusion (or naturally small puncta) have reduced tear outflow that may increase the time of tear clearance, but not because of increased or normal tear flow. Fluorometric techniques have been used to measure tear clearance by evaluation of fluorescein decay with sophisticated instruments. The clinician can simulate the results using a series of Schirmer strips and observing the color change of the strips over time (63–65). Macri et al. (66) suggested a six-level visual scale to judge tear clearance. This approach involves instillation of 5 μL of 2% sodium fluorescein and observation of the lateral lower tear meniscus after 15 minutes. Normal tear flow measured using fluorophotometry is 0.5 to 2.2 μL/min, and normal tear volume is 4 to 13 μL (12, 67).

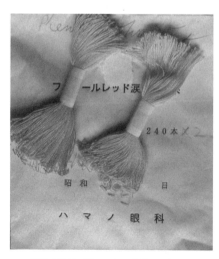

FIG. 23.9. Phenol red thread test.

Should clinicians continue to assess the rate of tear flow despite the vagaries of the results? The answer is "yes" because a measured observation of tear flow is part of the information stream describing the dynamics of any individual's tear film. Schirmer tests are quick and easy to perform. A low finding is very useful in explaining symptoms of dryness and may deter us from providing contact lenses to affected patients. Moreover, Pflugfelder et al. (68) suggest using tear flow, measured clinically, as a key test to differentiate the aqueous tear-deficient dry eye from those involving meibomian gland disease.

Tear Protein Composition

There may come a day when a clinician can take a tear sample from a prospective contact lens wearer and determine, in office, whether the tear film composition is suitable and, if so, which lens type would be most appropriate. Until that time, protein analysis of the tear film is an academic pursuit. Understanding the composition of the tear film is valuable, however, as background to our paradigm of the normal tear film.

Accuracy and reproducibility of tear protein measurements currently are poor because both collection methods and natural compositional changes make describing a normal state difficult. Confounding variables (such as collecting from more than one layer of the tear film or from the lid itself, incomplete mixing of the tears, and various rates of drainage) interfere with establishing normative values. Any minor irritation or infectious process will alter secretions.

The aqueous portion of the tear film is approximately 98% water and 2% solids. Solids include proteins, such as lysozyme, albumin, and globulin (69), and inorganic electrolytes such as sodium, potassium, and calcium chloride and bicarbonate. The lacrimal gland produces many of the tear film proteins, including tear albumin, β_2-globulin, lysozyme, and secretory IgA and IgG. Serum proteins make up about 1% of the total proteins in the tear film in a noninflamed eye. These proteins include albumin, haptoglobin, IgG, IgA, IgM, and IgE, α_2-macroglobulins, complement-derived proteins, transferrin, α_1-antitrypsin, and β_2-microglobulin. The mix of proteins continually changes as some stimuli increase lacrimal gland production while others increase dilation of conjunctival vessels to increase serum proteins.

The amount and ratio of these components alter tear structure and effect. Serum proteins such as IgG and IgM increase dramatically in inflammatory states and participate in the cascade of events that leads to sore, red, and swollen eyes. Inflammatory products are also in the tear film of dry eye patients with Sjögren syndrome. These defense chemicals stimulate the nerve endings of the ocular surface to produce symptoms of discomfort. Conceivably, contact lenses, especially if soiled or damaged, could induce such compositional changes leading to dryness symptoms.

Tear Osmolarity

Tear film osmolarity helps to maintain the health of the ocular surface cells and is also altered in dry eye states. Tear osmolarity measurement is difficult and requires elaborate instruments and trained technicians. Both Gilbard (70) and Farris (71) found that normal tear osmolarity averages 302 mOsm/L, whereas osmolarity of dry eyes ranges from 330 to 340 mOsm/L.

Several factors contribute to hyperosmolarity. Tear film turnover declines in aqueous-deficient conditions, allowing more time for evaporation to concentrate the preocular tear film. As the total tear volume declines, evaporation has an increased effect on the tear film. Rolando and Refojo (46) found increased evaporation in keratoconjunctivitis sicca patients. Increased osmolarity increases cell desquamation (72), loss of microplicae (73), cell membrane disruption, and decreases intracellular cytoplasmic density (74).

A contact lens divides the tear film, thereby thinning at least the pre-lens tear film and increasing osmolarity. The cells under the contact lens will be bathed in a post-lens tear film that is likely to be more stagnant and, therefore, *probably* hyperosmolar (75). The lens edge tear meniscus will be thin during rigid lens wear. Will this lead to increased evaporation and increased local osmolarity? Surely some of these changes will affect the comfort and wearability of contact lenses.

TEAR FILM CHANGES WITH CONTACT LENS WEAR

Much work has been done in an attempt to study contact lens caused changes in the precorneal tear film. Unfortunately, results of this research are contradictory and, often, patient specific.

Changes During Adaptation

Increased tear volume occurs with insertion of a foreign body (such as a contact lens), leading to lowered concentrations of many tear components followed by a return to homeostasis, or even an up-regulation of the secretion of a particular component.

Mucous Layer in Contact Lens Wear

Foreign objects inserted to the body are actively coated in biofilm so that our bodies find them like "self." This coating is made up of many components, especially mucus. A contact lens is such a foreign body. Because the surface upon which the upper lid rubs is biofilm, this is what will influence the patient's perception of dryness and discomfort when wearing contact lenses.

Greiner and Allansmith (76) noted that nongoblet epi-thelial cells of the conjunctiva start to create mucous vesicles in lens wearers. An up-regulation of mucous production will affect tear film characteristics and coatings on lenses. Practitioners have discovered that contact lenses left for months and years under the upper lid are thickly coated with mucus.

The type and design of a contact lens affect the amount of mucus produced by the ocular surface and the characteristics of the contact lens biofilm coating. Normal mucus is thin and uniform over a non–lens-wearing cornea. Guillon (38) observed tear mucous layers over *in situ* contact lenses using a modified specular microscope. Mucus appeared in patchy nonuniform patterns on surfaces of hydrogel lenses, but no mucus was observed on rigid contact lens surfaces.

Aqueous Layer in Contact Lens Wear

Tearing with insertion of a contact lens is a normal response for a novice wearer, especially during rigid gas permeable (GP) lens fitting. Tearing decreases with GP lens adaptation, and normal tear production rates have been found in both adapted soft (61,77) and rigid lens wearers (78).

These findings may be surprising given that corneal sensitivity decreases during contact lens wear, suggesting decreased stimulus to lacrimal secretion. Perhaps the presence of the foreign body and its interaction with the upper lid counteracts reduced corneal sensitivity, thereby maintaining normal tear flow.

Lipid Layer in Contact Lens Wear

Guillon (38) described the appearance of the tear film in the presence of various types of contact lenses. The lipid pattern differs with lens type, material, and thickness. The amorphous pattern is present in stable pre-lens tear films. Guillon commonly observed a thin lipid layer in a marmoreal or flow pattern during hydrogel lens wear. Higher-water-content materials caused less stable and thinner patterns. Young and Efron (79) did not confirm this report, however. These authors found absent or very thin lipid layers on all hydrogel lens types except those of very high water content. PHEMA lenses had the most stable and thickest pattern, most similar to the non–lens-wearing preocular tear film.

Polymethyl methacrylate (PMMA) lenses had thin surface aqueous layers but no visible lipid layers, even though the tear film away from the lens was normal (38). GP rigid lenses provided more wettable surfaces over which aqueous and lipid layers remain fairly stable. Most often the pre-lens pattern was marmoreal, with islands of thicker lipid.

Lens design has been found to affect lipid patterns. Standard-thickness hydrogel lenses cause more stable tear patterns than do ultrathin lenses (38). Lens movement affects the pattern. Excessive lens movement induces disruption of the tear film. Lens size and fit also affect the pre-lens tear film pattern. Larger lenses that sit under the upper lid allow more normal pre-lens tear films. Lid-lens apposition prevents the major disruption of the tear film that occurs at the remaining edges of the lens. Our choice of lens type and design, therefore, influences tear film stability and no doubt our patients' sense of comfort and lens wettability when wearing contact lenses as well.

Tear Composition During Contact Lens Wear

Tear film composition has been measured during adaptation to lens wear. A rigid lens placed on a novice eye will increase tear production and decrease certain tear components, but a "normal' state is reestablished after adaptation. Tear chloride (80), sodium (81), potassium (82), cholesterol (83), and total protein (84) have all been studied and found to follow this adaptive course to homeostasis.

The protein content of the tear film is complex and has two major sources. The lacrimal gland produces tear-specific pre-albumin, lysozyme, and lactoferrin. The most frequent serum derived proteins are albumin, IgG, and transferring IgA. Lacrimal gland proteins tend to stay at the same concentration with reflex tearing, whereas serum-derived proteins are naturally found in lesser concentrations.

Clinicians are more concerned with changes in the tear film after adaptation, which are less well described in the literature. Farris (85) found no differences in tear lactoferrin, lysozyme, and albumin in long-term hard and soft lens wearers.

Several researchers hint at increased inflammatory tear proteins during contact lens wear, particularly with use of soft lenses and for extended wear. Serum albumin and IgG increase (86), as does the ratio of IgG to IgA (87). Vinding et al. (88), however, found decreased secretory IgA during primarily hydrogel contact lens wear, a finding that may be related to infectious complications. Greiner and Allansmith (76) and Allansmith et al. (89) reported up-regulated mucous production relative to contact lens wear.

The dry eye literature suggests that dry eye disease may be an inflammatory process, and inflammatory mediators are believed to alter epithelial cell health (90). Can contact lens wear cause sufficient inflammation to induce a dry eye-like state? This seems particularly possible with soiled lenses or giant papillary conjunctivitis. Perhaps this also can occur to a lesser degree in apparently "successful" patients who later present with symptoms of dryness.

pH of Tears in Contact Lens Wear

The normal human tear pH varies from 6.93 to 7.83 (91–94), fluctuating diurnally and with pH measurement technique. Contact lens wear influences tear pH in some studies but not in others. Carney and Hill (95) found no difference between PMMA lens wearers prefit and postfit

tear pH. They found a decrease in pH, however, in the closed-eye state, whether or not soft lenses were worn (96). Browning and Foulks (97) alternately found no trend in pH changes in lens wear. Hamano (98) and Chen and Maurice (99) found a reduction in pH (thus a shift toward more acidic tears) in lens wearers. They suggested that lactic acid increase under the contact lens (because of hypoxia-induced anaerobic metabolism of the cornea) produces the acidic shift in tear pH. Lattimore (100) measured a pH change from 6.99 to 7.43 on contact lens surfaces during 7 days of wear. This suggests that lactic acid buildup under a contact lens can induce a pH gradient across the contact lens. Generally, it is believed that pH is not greatly altered by contact lens wear because of tear buffering capacity.

Osmolarity and Contact Lens Wear

Tear osmolarity is critical to the health of the ocular surface cells and increases in both dry eye states and contact lens wear (85,101,102). Normal tear osmolarity is 308 mOsm/L, whereas the tears of rigid daily and soft lens extended wearers were measured at 316 and 318 mOsm/L, respectively (85). Gilbard et al. (101) proposed that reduced corneal sensation of lens wearers produces a reduction in tear flow (not confirmed by tear flow testing). Combined with increased tear film evaporation (103) that appears to be common during contact lens wear, a concentrated and, therefore, highly osmolar tear film occurs.

Tear Evaporation in Contact Lens Wear

Tear evaporation is believed to be responsible for 10% to 40% of total tear loss from the ocular surface (104). Tears also normally drain through the canaliculus. The lipid layer normally protects the tears from evaporation (30,105), but contact lenses change the lipid layer to increase tear evaporation and thereby induce dry eye symptoms and signs (103). All types of contact lenses produce the same results (106).

CLINICAL ASPECTS OF FITTING CONTACT LENSES WHEN TEARS ARE NOT NORMAL

Prefitting Evaluation

Contact lens practitioners should understand the condition of the tear film and the ocular surface prior to fitting a patient. Careful observation will allow the practitioner to choose whether or not to fit, determine which type of lenses might be most appropriate, and predict with some accuracy the likelihood of success. Choice of care system and wearing schedule for the individual may be enhanced as well.

Minimal testing for a prefit evaluation should include the following:

1. History
2. Observation of the blink

3. White light observation of the tear film
4. Schirmer test
5. Fluorescein staining and BUT
6. Observation of the lid margins and meibomian gland function

At the conclusion of this evaluation, the practitioner should consider the following questions:

1. Does this patient have dry eye disease?
2. Is the condition mild, moderate, or severe?
3. What is the likely cause of the condition?
4. Should this patient wear contact lenses?

History

Taking a careful history is one of the most important steps in evaluating a potential contact lens wearer. Several systemic factors are known risk factors for dry eye disease that will complicate contact lens wear. Autoimmune disease, hypertension, and diabetes are three of the most common systemic conditions. Lifestyle factors such as smoking may be problematic. The hormone status of females is of major concern because both low and high estrogen states can cause symptoms of dry eye disease.

It is important to conduct a history specific to dry eye disease. The McMonnies dry eye questionnaire has been a standard screening tool for some time and can help to identify patients with dry eye and/or risk factors for dry eye (107). As with all questionnaires in this field, however, it often fails to predict objective ocular signs. Begley et al. (4) discussed a new dry eye questionnaire (in development) that may enhance screening for dry eye.

A recent study identified histories positive for smoking tobacco or caffeine use, arthritis, thyroid disease, gout, and diabetes as strong risk factors for dry eye. Use of medications such as antihistamines, parasympathetics, antidepressants, diuretics, and antiemetics, alcohol consumption, and (surprisingly) the intake of multivitamins also were included (108).

Many clinicians have their patients complete such questionnaires prior to clinical evaluation. As this information is reviewed with patients, the clinician should observe the frequency and completeness of blinking. Blinking is an important part of contact lens success. The clinician also should observe the patient's facial skin during this interview. It is important to look for flushing and redness across the nose, which may be signs of rosacea. Because rosacea often affects the meibomian glands, the index of suspicion of dry eye disease should increase when any of these signs are noted.

Observations of the Ocular Surface with White Light

It is prudent to observe the ocular surface before instilling drops or manipulating the lids. Observe the tear meniscus with very low-level light. Is it thick and continuous, or broken and thin? The height of the tear meniscus suggests adequacy of resident tear volume (Fig. 23.4) (109).

It is important to note particles in the tear meniscus and to observe their movement to the puncta. This observation can provide an estimate of tear film viscosity. Highly viscous tears will cause particles to move slowly, whereas particles move swiftly to the puncta in low-viscosity tears. The appearance of foam in the tear margin indicates a malfunction of the meibomian glands and blepharitis.

The tearscope is a valuable instrument to assess the lipid layer pattern (38). Categorizing the lipid layer before fitting will assist estimation of potential lens success. The tearscope uses a cold cathode source of light that does not dry the ocular surface. The pattern and color of the lipid layer can be categorized as: marmoreal open or closed, flow, amorphous, color fringe, or other (see earlier). This categorization is listed from thinnest to thickest lipid layer (Fig. 23.10).

Tear Flow

The Schirmer tear (Fig. 23.8) test should be performed, usually without anesthetic (e.g., Schirmer 1) (60). This test, although not accurate when results are above 20 mm, will capture many patients with reduced lacrimal gland function. Any finding of less than 10 mm after 5 minutes of testing suggests poor lacrimal function. Some practitioners prefer to use anesthetic for this test (Schirmer 2), and there is continuing controversy as to which may be the best approach.

Tear Volume

The phenol red thread test (Fig. 23.9) is not a substitute for the Schirmer test, but it is less irritating (110). Testing time is 15 seconds and eyes remain closed. The normal wetting is 16.7 mm. Values less than 9 mm increase suspicion of dry eye. This test probably measures the amount of tear film in the meniscus rather than tear flow (62).

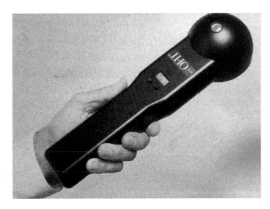

FIG. 23.10. Tearscope.

Fluorescein and the Ocular Surface

Installation of fluorescein to the ocular surface creates a very visible new world. Use of a cobalt blue filter combined with a yellow Wratten filter allows the practitioner to assess many aspects of the ocular surface.

Breakup Time

Following fluorescein instillation, invasive BUT should be assessed. The patient is first asked to blink normally, then stop blinking while the observer measures the time to the first corneal surface black spot (55). Note that tears are disrupted by instillation of the drop (57). Some researchers, therefore, suggest using a standardized drop of liquid fluorescein to improve repeatability. Korb invented a strip that ensures less liquid is instilled with the fluorescein to increase the chances of repeatable findings (54).

Most practitioners continue to use a standard fluorescein strip and find some value in the gross observation of BUT. BUTs less than 10 seconds are considered suspect of an unstable tear film, with times less than 5 seconds (average of three measurements) very likely indicative of a true tear film instability situation.

Fluorescein Vital Staining

Fluorescein highlights areas of epithelial defects as it pools in areas of missing cells or divots. It penetrates to the stroma if the Bowman layer is broken (111). Fluorescein also enters cells that are devitalized (112). It creates black spots seen as nonwetting areas of the cornea in dystrophies. Normal eyes often show small areas of punctate staining but never localized clusters or larger stained areas (113). Central cornea staining may indicate dry eye disease, whereas inferior staining is most often seen in blepharitis and lagophthalmos (Fig. 23.11).

Fluorescein also stains conjunctiva, but this tissue is better observed with the use of rose bengal or lissamine green. Use of a diagram as suggested by Josephson and Caffery

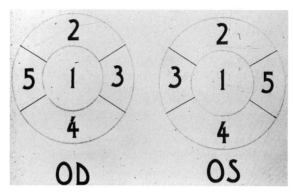

FIG. 23.12. Corneal staining diagram.

(114) and a grading scale of 1 to 3 facilitates baseline documentation (Fig. 23.12).

Rose Bengal Vital Stain

Rose bengal staining is not an essential test for prefit screening. It is useful when the diagnosis of dry eye is entertained, however, and when the practitioner is unsure of the cause of dryness symptoms. Rose bengal is an iodine derivative of fluorescein that stains epithelial cells that are devitalized, as well as those cells that do not have a normal mucous coating (Fig. 23.13) (13,115,116).

Normal eyes show little to no staining with rose bengal. Staining of the interpalpebral conjunctiva and central cornea, however, are characteristic of dry eye disease.

Instillation of this dye is problematic. Liquid rose bengal (which produces the best stain) is very irritating to dry eye patients. Insufficient stain often results with use of strips, however, and many false-negative results are found (117).

This dye is observed with white light or, preferably, using the green (red free) filter on the biomicroscope light tower. Having a prepared diagram for documenting staining grades is helpful. For example, the National Eye Institute/Industry Workshop report recommended a six-zone system for conjunctival rose bengal staining characterization (118). The van Bijsterveld diagram and three-point scoring system is also commonly reported in the literature.

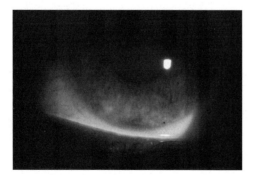

FIG. 23.11. Inferior corneal staining with fluorescein.

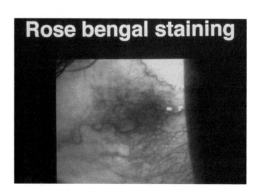

FIG. 23.13. Rose bengal staining of the conjunctiva.

Lissamine Green Vital Stain

Lissamine green dye stains degenerated epithelial cells and mucus in the same pattern as rose bengal but does not cause stinging (119). White light is used to observe this staining pattern, or a red free filter can be used. Use of the van Bijsterveld diagram and grading system facilitates documentation (Fig. 23.14).

Observations of the Lid Margin

It is important to carefully observe the lid margins. The eyelid margin should be considered as anterior (lashes) and posterior (meibomian gland orifices) zones to facilitate differentiation of anterior and/or posterior blepharitis (120).

It is important to look for erythema and foam at the lid margin. Vascular injection often occurs in meibomian gland dysfunction and anterior blepharitis. Foaming occurs when the meibomian glands secrete abnormal lipids that undergo saponification when in touch with the calcium of the tear film. The lash line should be observed and any cuffing or flaking noted. This is indicative of active anterior blepharitis, usually of *Staphylococcus* sp origin.

The lid margins should be felt to obtain a sense of their thickness. As meibomian glands deteriorate, lids may thicken. The meibomian glands should be pressed upon to determine how much force is required to express their oils, and the quantity and quality of these secretions should be noted (Fig. 23.15) (120,121).

The percentage of glands that secrete, how difficult it was to make them secrete, and the quality of the secretions should all be noted and recorded. The presence or absence of anterior lid thickening, erythema, or flaking likewise should be observed and recorded.

CLINICAL ASSESSMENT

Now the practitioner can consider the important questions listed at the beginning of this section. Any combination of

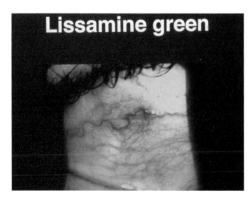

FIG. 23.14. Lissamine green staining of the conjunctiva.

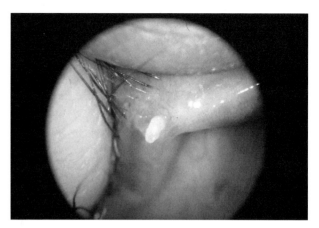

FIG. 23.15. Inspissated material expressed from the meibomian gland.

symptoms, tear film abnormalities of quality or quantity, ocular surface staining, and lid disease will lead to the diagnosis of dry eye syndrome. The severity of the condition can be estimated by the extent of ocular surface staining, symptoms, reduced tear flow, and extent of lid disease. The patient's clinical history may provide clues for dry eye cause, be it simple age or autoimmune disease.

Patients with severe dry eye, i.e., Schirmer less than 5 mm in 5 minutes, significant rose bengal staining of the interpalpebral conjunctiva, and a poorly wetting cornea, should be advised that contact lenses are not a good option for them. This statement does not consider unusual dry eye cases in which contact lenses are the only way comfort can be achieved. This group is described in the section on Contact Lenses for the Severe Dry Eye Patient.

Many patients have marginal dry eyes. It is important to treat them before fitting the patients with contact lenses. Treat initially with simple but intensive lid care. One of the most rewarding efforts of the contact lens practitioner is to diagnosis common blepharitis and meibomian gland dysfunction, treat with simple techniques of lid scrubs and hot soaks, and observe a very positive subjective response. It has been demonstrated that an intensive 2-week treatment of lid massage and warm compresses can increase BUT by clinically and statistically significant amounts (~4 seconds) (122). Sometimes the situation is severe enough to warrant adjunctive use of topical or oral medications for a period of time (usually 4–6 weeks) (120).

If mild corneal staining is observed (Fig. 23.11), you can attempt to determine the cause. Is the problem blink frequency or completeness? Computer-related reduced blinking induces corneal staining that worsens at the end of a long day of work. Such patients occasionally can be trained to think about their blinks and to perform this activity regularly. Use of a tear substitute to increase flushing of the ocular surface by rewetting the eye regularly usually is helpful.

Applicable general health issues can be discussed. Patients

should be advised to intake sufficient water during the day. Consumption of a large bottle of water each day is helpful. Smokers should be counseled to quit to enhance general health as well as to address contact lens problems. Patients should be advised to consume a healthy diet, with fresh vegetables and fruits. This may make a difference in the health of their mucous membranes, including the ocular surface and the secretion of tears, as well as decrease the risks of macular degeneration and cataracts.

FITTING OF THE LESS THAN PERFECT EYE

Contact Lenses for the Severe Dry Eye Patient

A small number of patients with severe keratoconjunctivitis sicca or Sjögren syndrome inexplicably wear contact lenses well. The usual route to fitting these patients begins when every other effort to relieve symptoms has proven inadequate.

Severe dry eye patients have constant discomfort and often function poorly at their jobs and within their social world because of ocular symptoms. They often have filamentary keratitis. It is the author's (B.C.) opinion that the presence of filaments in dry eye patients should be an indication that contact lenses may enhance function. Contact lens wear, however, is an exercise of last resort in these patients because of the increased risk of complications, especially corneal infection.

The patient must be educated as to the increased risk of infection during contact lens wear due to poor tear flow and compromised epithelia. Formal informed consent is essential. Diagnostic contact lens application determines the comfort level anticipated. Some patients respond with immediate relief. Those who note improved ocular comfort can be considered candidates. Others find the foreign object unbearable, and fitting such patients should be abandoned.

The choice of contact lenses is important. One of the authors (B.C.) has found through clinical experience that thin hydrogel lenses are not effective. Standard-thickness lenses with low to medium water content appear to be most effective. Some success also is possible with the new silicone hydrogel materials.

Whatever the final choice, these patients must be followed closely. Lenses should be removed in the evening and a nonpreserved solution system used. Some elderly patients, especially those with severe rheumatoid arthritis, will have a difficult time handling lenses. In these circumstances, a family member can be trained to help them.

These patients may benefit from additional lenses. Insertion of a fresh lens mid-day will help them to remain comfortable longer. They should use unpreserved artificial tear supplements hourly. They should replace lenses frequently.

Risks and failures are high in this patient group. However, the rewards for both patient and practitioner are very high when success is achieved.

Contact Lenses for the Marginal Dry Eye Patient

Patients with marginal dry eye are at increased risk for many complications of lens wear. Their ocular surfaces are compromised, and wearing a lens can further increase corneal staining (123). Patients with poor tear composition, reduced tear proteins, and poor tear volume and turnover are intuitively at greater risk for infection. Poor tear quality will increase lens deposits, leading to ocular irritation and inflammation. In each case, the risk-to-benefit ratio should be assessed.

Clinicians are often amazed at the surprising number of marginal dry eye patients who wear lenses well. This phenomenon suggests the amazing adaptability of the ocular surface and the power of the immune system (124).

If the decision is made to fit a patient, how does one go about this risky business?

Patient Education

The most important undertaking for a clinician prior to fitting a marginal dry eye patient is to discuss the issues with the patient. It is important to make the patient well aware of his or her chances of failure, risks for infection, prescribed reduced wear time, and increased need for lens replacements and more frequent care visits. If the patient understands these risks and costs and is a willing participant in the journey, the fit can begin.

Choosing the Contact Lens

The next decision is whether to prescribe rigid or soft contact lenses. Rigid lenses enhance tear exchange, are less likely to soil with deposits, and are associated with less risk for infection (125). They also do not absorb tears and therefore leave whatever is available on the surface of the eye. Many marginal dry eye patients, however, have sensitive eyes and are unwilling or unable to adapt to rigid lens wear. If the situation warrants rigid lens fitting, the fit and selection of materials are important. Lower-Dk fluorinated materials are the material of choice because they deposit less readily. The authors have found that "Korb design" lenses, in which the lens positions under the upper lid and moves as if attached with each blink, can be a beneficial beginning (126). This design minimizes edge lift, reducing corneal desiccation symptoms and discomfort (127).

Because marginal dry eye patients often are sensitive to lens coatings and solution preservatives, daily disposables are a good initial choice if soft lenses are to be worn. Daily disposable soft lenses eliminate problems of deposits and solution reactions. Because many of these patients do not wear lenses full time, daily disposable lenses are advantageous in that they are never left in a potentially contaminated contact lens case for long periods of time between wear.

Daily disposables do not necessarily provide all of the parameters we may need to care for marginal dry eye patients. Lower water content and lenses with greater center thicknesses appear to provide the greatest comfort to dry eye patients (128,129). Finnemore (124) advocates the use of thicker lenses and even suggests that prism ballast in spherical lenses, with increased inferior thickness. suppress symptoms. Very thin, high-water-content lenses should be avoided because they can produce significant corneal desiccation in dry eye patients (129).

At least one contact lens material, Proclear by Biocompatibles, has achieved United States Food and Drug Administration (FDA) approval as beneficial for dry eye symptoms (130); omafilcon A material contains phosphorylcholine to promote retention of water. Another brand, "Xtreme H2O," has been promoted to decrease symptoms of dryness. Silicone hydrogel lenses (CIBA Focus Night & Day and Bausch and Lomb's PureVision) also dehydrate minimally during wear and may be beneficial.

Care Systems for Marginal Dry Eye Patients

Patients with marginal dry eyes are less able to flush solutions from the surface of their eyes; therefore, preservatives found in contact lens solutions remain in higher concentrations and for longer times on the ocular surface. Because chemical preservatives are associated with surface desiccation (131), many practitioners prescribe nonpreserved lens care systems. These are more cumbersome than simple multipurpose systems but often relieve dryness symptoms.

Patients wearing rigid lenses must use preserved solutions. The chemicals in these products are not absorbed but can be adsorbed to the lens surface and certainly are splashed onto the ocular surface with lens insertion. Patients with very reactive eyes may benefit from rinsing lenses well with nonpreserved saline prior to insertion. Although this reduces the wetting effect on the surface of the lens, it also reduces the concentration of the preservatives and other ingredients presented to the ocular surface and, therefore, secondary reactions. Sometimes, a simple change of care systems decreases stinging on lens insertion, dryness symptoms, and corneal staining.

Hydrogel lens-wearing patients who use preserved systems and present with irritation and corneal staining may be experiencing solution reactions. Substitution of nonpreserved systems and follow-up care will determine if the solutions were the cause. If a multipurpose system is to be used, the practitioner might consider products that contain methylcellulose, also used in tear substitutes recognized for treatment of dry eye disease.

Importance of the Blink

The tear film cannot maintain itself on the ocular surface without regular replenishment and turnover. The most important element in this system is the blink. The upper eyelid moves downward, compressing the lipid layer between the two lid edges. Blinking is essential for the secretion of the meibomian glands and the replenishment of the lipid layer, the washing away of debris from the ocular surface, and the spreading of the complete tear film over the ocular surface (132–134).

Improper blinking is known to cause changes in tear structure and stability of the tear film (135). A normal blink rate, in the absence of contact lens wear, is about 12 blinks per minute (136).

Patients may decrease their blink rate after contact lens fitting so as to avoid the feeling of the lens or because of the reduced corneal sensitivity caused by the lack of exposure of the corneal epithelium or edema induced by lens wear (137). Other studies suggest an increase in blinking in adapted hard and soft lens wearers from 12 to 20 blinks per minute (138), but these blinks may be incomplete (139).

Drops and Contact Lenses

When a patient has been well fitted with contact lenses and has the proper wearing schedule and care system but still presents with symptoms of dryness, clinicians often prescribe artificial tear drops or lubricants. Tear evaporation rates, however, may increase after instillation of eye drops (140) because of interruptions in the lipid layer. Neither saline nor lubricant drops improve the pre-lens tear film for longer than 5 minutes (141). Patients report relief for a maximum of 10 minutes after instillation (142).

Success of drops during contact lens wear is difficult to assess. What happens to the drop? Does it disrupt the already disrupted pre-lens tear film? Does it wipe away deposits on the lens surface and change the nature of the surface coating on the contact lens? Does it do this for the better or for worse? Does any of it get under the contact lens? If so, does it remove some of the stagnant tear film from under the lens? Does it penetrate the lens matrix and change the water content of the lens? Some patients do very well and obtain good relief with their use. They also often have a much better effect with one drop compared to another. Some patients find only a momentary relief and then a rebound effect that makes their eyes feel even more dry (143).

Clinically, offering the patient two types of contact lens-approved drops is a good way to begin the process of determining whether drops will help this particular patient. First teach the patient how to use the drops. The patient should make a "pocket" of the lower lid, add the drop, and gently squeeze their nasal puncta closed for a count of 10 seconds. Patients should use the drops on a routine basis of 3 to 4 times per day. Use one type of drop for 1 week and the other for the next week and determine which drop provides the most subjective relief. If irritation continues, a nonpreserved tear supplement should be considered. One must consider the possibility that ocular tear lubricant preservatives may cause irritation, but the amount and type of preservatives used today are less problematic than previously encountered (144).

Punctal Occlusion

Dry eye disease often is treated by punctual occlusion. Sjögren syndrome patients who have their puncta cauterized often report a significant decrease in dryness symptoms (145). Practitioners must be cautious, however, about the use of punctual occlusion in patients with better tear films. Patients who have almost normal tear flow may develop epiphora after insertion of the plugs and, therefore, should be fitted with the easily removed silicone plugs. Those who have epiphora immediately after insertion of the plugs and then adapt to the point where they no longer experience overflow tearing are an interesting group. Some form of feedback must have occurred to reduce tear flow. Is this desirable, and will tearing return to normal if the plugs are removed? If contact lens wear is not essential, should we be interfering with the normal tear flow feedback mechanism by this procedure? (Fig. 23.16).

Both the inflammatory aspects of dry eye and the additive effect of contact lens wear suggest that inflammatory mediators may increase in the tears of symptomatic lens wearers. We might, therefore, desire tear layers that actively flush the eye and do not stagnate on the ocular surface. Will insertion of punctal plugs be advantageous under these circumstances? Practically, lens wearers with symptoms of dryness often achieve reduced symptoms after silicone intracanalicular occlusion, especially if supplementary drops are continued. Unfortunately, the clinical effect diminishes over time in a large number of subjects (146).

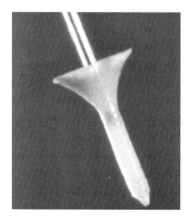

FIG. 23.16. Punctal plug.

EVALUATION OF THE CURRENT LENS WEARER WHO PRESENTS WITH DRYNESS

Contact lens practice is filled with consultations for current lens wearers who are not satisfied with their comfort levels. These patients may be our own failures, patients with changing symptoms related to aging, or new consultations from other practices. As with all presenting clinical problems, we must approach each case with an open mind and a broad differential diagnosis.

It is best to have patients wear their contact lenses into the office on the day of the consult. If possible, it is important to evaluate them later in the day when irritation is likely to be greater and clinical signs more obvious. You can begin with a comprehensive history that concentrates on any new health conditions or medications, recent changes in job description, the design of lenses used, how often the lenses are replaced, and which solutions are used. While interviewing a patient, note his or her blink pattern.

History: The Essential Questions

1. When did the symptoms begin, and when are they the worst?
2. Did this occur at a time when your health changed?
3. Do you have a change in medications?
4. Do you have new visual tasks?
5. For how many years have you been wearing contact lenses?
6. How old are your lenses?
7. Have you changed your solution system?
8. How often do you replace you lenses?
9. Show me exactly how you remove and care for your lenses.

Always perform a careful visual acuity and overrefraction. Patients with poor or inconsistent vision will become much more aware of their eyes and, therefore, feel more discomfort or even a sense of dryness while wearing contact lenses. Solving a vision problem such as presbyopia often will enhance contact lens comfort and tolerance. Intermittent blurring can be a result of either poor lens condition or a dry eye problem.

At this point it is important to look at the lens condition, the mechanical "fit," and the ocular surfaces. Both ocular surface debris and lens damage should be carefully evaluated. Is there sufficient contact lens movement? Is the limbal area covered? It also is important to look carefully at the limbal vessels for dilation. Is there evidence of corneal edema?

If a rigid lens is being worn, fluorescein can be instilled at this point to evaluate lens surface wettability, tear exchange under the lens, and whether there is 3- to 9-o'clock staining. If a hydrogel lens is being worn, the lens should be removed and fluorescein added. Lens-associated staining patterns, such as a perilimbal rings, superior arcuate stain, inferior smile stain, or foreign body staining, are the main concerns. The upper lids should be everted to evaluate the patient's tarsal conjunctivae for papillae (giant or otherwise), follicles, and scars, whether rigid or hydrogel lenses are being used.

If dry eye disease is suspected, lissamine green stain can be used to assess the conjunctiva. The lid margins should be inspected for evidence of meibomian gland dysfunction and blepharitis.

Schirmer testing should be considered. One of the authors (B.C.) generally notes suppressed Schirmer results following lens removal and therefore usually defers Schirmer testing to a follow-up visit. Because patient time is always an issue, however, if the test is performed at this point, results should be considered with additional caution. Perhaps a low finding would prompt a return to the office for a second test.

The practitioner should now have a good idea of the issues surrounding the discomfort and dryness symptoms with which the patient has presented. In most cases there is more than one cause for the symptoms, and many steps may have to be taken before the situation is resolved.

Differential Diagnosis When Dryness Is the Presenting Symptom

1. Poorly fit lenses
2. Damaged or soiled lenses
3. Solution reaction
4. Wrong choice of lens materials
5. Poor choice of lens modality
6. Contact lens overwear
7. Systemic diseases leading to dry eye
8. Medications leading to dry eye
9. Dry eye disease of unknown etiology

Management Plans

The best initial management decision is often to discontinue lens wear and allow the eye to recover. This is not often popular with patients but may solve the acute problem. After 1 month of spectacle wear, the tear tests and observations of the ocular surfaces should be repeated to establish a new baseline. At this point, the patient may be refitted with a more appropriate lens design and/or material, utilizing a more frequent replacement plan, with use of nonpreserved solutions, reduced daily wear time, and new instructions on the care and handling of the lenses. Any confounding visual problems should be eliminated by use of GP, toric design, and/or bifocal lenses, or reading glasses as appropriate. Adjunctively the patient should be educated about drinking enough fluids, eating healthy foods, reducing the intake of drying chemicals, blinking regularly, reducing computer use, and humidifying home and work environments.

SUMMARY

Contact lens practice currently is filled with the complications of lens wear associated with dry eye symptoms. Successful clinicians will have the knowledge, time, and patience to assess potential lens wearers for their suitability for such wear and the ability to diagnose and treat causes of symptoms of dryness when patients who wear lenses present with decreased tolerance.

REFERENCES

1. Brennan NA, Efron N. Symptomatology of HEMA contact lens wearers. *Optom Vis Sci* 1989;66:834–836.
2. du Toit R, Situ P, Simpson T, et al. The effects of six months of contact lens wear on the tear film, ocular surfaces, and symptoms of presbyopes. *Optom Vis Sci* 2001;78:455–462.
3. Begley C, Caffery B, Nichols KK, et al. Responses of contact lens wearers to a dry eye survey. *Optom Vis Sci* 2000;77:40–46.
4. Begley C, Chalmers R, Mitchell L, et al. Characterization of ocular surface symptoms from optometric practices in North America. *Cornea* 2001;20:610–618.
5. Wolff E. The mucocutaneous junction of the lid margin and the distribution of tear fluid. *Trans Ophthalmol Soc UK* 1946; 66:291–308.
6. Holly FJ, Lemp MA. Tear physiology and dry eyes. *Surv Ophthalmol* 1977;22:69–87.
7. King-Smith PE, et al. The thickness of the human precorneal tear film: evidence from reflection spectra. *Invest Ophthalmol Vis Sci* 2000;41:3348–3359.
8. Tiffany JM. Tear stability and contact lens wear. *J Br Contact Lens Assoc* 1988;11[Suppl.]:35–38.
9. Holly FJ. Tear film physiology. *Am J Optom Phys Opt* 1980; 57:252–257.
10. Maurice D. The dynamics and drainage of tears. *Int Ophthalmol Clin* 1973;13:103–116.
11. Holly FJ. Tear film physiology and contact lens wear, I. Pertinent aspects of tear film physiology. *Am J Optom Physiol Opt* 1981;58:324–330.
12. Mishima S, et al. Determination of tear volume and tear flow. *Invest Ophthalmol* 1966;5:264–276.
13. Feenstra R, Tseng SC. What is actually stained by rose bengal? *Arch Ophthalmol* 1992;110:984–993.
14. Inatomi T, Spurr-Michaud S, Tisdale AS, et al. Expression of secretory mucin genes by human conjunctival epithelia. *Invest Ophthalmol Vis Sci* 1996;37:1684–1692.
15. Watanabe H. Significance of mucin on the ocular surface. *Cornea* 2002;21[2 Suppl. 1]:S17–S22.
16. Allansmith MR, Korb DR, Greiner JV. Giant papillary conjunctivitis induced by hard and soft contact lens wear: quantitative histology. *Trans Am Acad Ophthalmol Otolaryngol* 1978;85: 766–778.
17. Dartt D. Cellular control of protein, electrolyte and water secretion by the lacrimal gland. In: Holly FJ, ed. *The preocular tear film in health, disease and contact lens wear*. Lubbock, TX: Dry Eye Institute, 1986:358–370.
18. Warren D. Hormonal influences on the lacrimal gland. *Int Ophthalmol Clin* 1994;34:19–25.
19. Sullivan DA, Bloch KJ, Allansmith MR. Hormonal influence on the secretory immune system of the eye: androgen regulation of secretory component levels in rat tears. *J Immunol* 1984;132: 1130–1135.
20. Schaumberg D, Buring JE, Sullivan DA, et al. Hormone re-

placement therapy and dry eye syndrome. *J Am Med Assoc* 2001; 286:2114–2119.

21. Molina R, Provost TT, Arnett FC, et al. Clinical serologic and immunogenic features. *Am J Med* 1986;80:23–31.

22. Sullivan D, Krenzer KL, Sullivan BD, et al. Does androgen deficiency cause lacrimal gland inflammation and aqueous tear deficiency? *Invest Ophthalmol Vis Sci* 1999;40:1261–1265.

23. Sullivan DA, Wickham LA, Rocha EM, et al. Androgens and dry eye in Sjogren's syndrome. *Ann NY Acad Sci* 1999;876: 312–324.

24. Jordan A, Baum JL. Basic tear flow: does it exist? *Ophthalmology* 1980;87:920–930.

25. McNamara NA, Polse KA, Brand RJ, et al. Tear mixing under a soft lens: effects of lens diameter. *Am J Ophthalmol* 1999;127: 659–665.

26. Millodot M. Effect of soft lenses on corneal sensitivity. *Acta Ophthalmol* 1974;52:603–608.

27. Millodot M. Does the long term wear of contact lenses produce a loss of corneal sensitivity? *Experientia* 1977;33:1475–1476.

28. McCulley JP, Shine W. A compositional model for the tear film lipid layer. *Trans Am Ophthalmol Soc* 1997;95:79–88, discussion 88–93.

29. Records R. Tear film. In: Records R, ed. *Physiology of the eye and visual system.* Hagerstown, MD: Harper and Rowe, 1979: 47–67.

30. Mishima S, Maurice DM. The oily layer of the tear film and evaporation from the corneal surface. *Exp Eye Res* 1961;1: 39–45.

31. Korb DR, Baron DF, Herman JP, et al. Tear film lipid layer thickness as a function of blinking. *Cornea* 1994;13:354–359.

32. Sullivan DA, Sullivan BD, Evans JE, et al. Androgen deficiency, meibomian gland dysfunction, and evaporative dry eye. *Ann NY Acad Sci* 2002;966:211–222.

33. Sullivan DA, Sullivan BD, Ullman MD, et al. Androgen influence on the meibomian gland. *Invest Ophthalmol Vis Sci* 2000; 41:3732–3742.

34. Krenzer K, Dana MR, Ullman MD, et al. Effect of androgen deficiency on the human meibomian gland and ocular surface. *J Clin Endocrinol Metab* 2000;85:4874–4882.

35. Esmaeli B, Harvey JY, Hewlett B. Immunohistochemical evidence for estrogen receptors in meibomian glands. *Ophthalmology* 2000;107:180–184.

36. McDonald JE. Surface phenomena of tear films. *Trans Am Ophthalmol Soc* 1968;66:905–939.

37. McDonald JE. Surface phenomena of the tear film. *Am J Ophthalmol* 1969;67:56–64.

38. Guillon JP. Tear film structure and contact lenses. In: Holly FJ, ed. *The preocular tear film in health, disease and contact lens wear.* Lubbock, TX: Dry Eye Institute, 1986:914–939.

39. Hamano H. The change of precorneal tear film by the application of contact lenses. *Contact Intraoc Lens Med J* 1981;7: 205–209.

40. Hamano H, Kaufman HE, eds. *The physiology of the cornea and contact lens applications.* New York: Churchill Livingstone, 1987:100.

41. Josephson J. Appearance of the preocular tear film lipid layer. *Am J Optom Physiol Opt* 1983;60:883–887.

42. Doane MG. An instrument for tear film interferometry. *Optom Vis Sci* 1989;66:383–388.

43. Benedetto D, Clinch TE, Laibson PR. In vivo observation of tear film dynamics using fluorophotometry. *Arch Ophthalmol* 1984;102:410–412.

44. Brown S, Dervichian DG. In vitro study of the interaction of the superficial oily layer and tears. *Arch Ophthalmol* 1969;82: 541–547.

45. Nemeth J, Erdelyi B, Csakany B, et al. High speed videotopo-

graphic measurement of tear film build-up time. *Invest Ophthalmol Vis Sci* 2002;43:1783–1790.

46. Rolando M, Refojo, MF. Increased tear evaporation in eyes with keratoconjunctivitis sicca. *Arch Ophthalmol* 1983;101: 557–558.

47. Hamano H, Hori M, Mitsunaga S. Measurement of evaporation rate of water from the precorneal tear film and contact lenses. *Contacto* 1981;25:7–14.

48. Mishima S. Some physiological aspects of the tear film. *Arch Ophthalmol* 1965;73:233–241.

49. Holly FJ. Formation and rupture of the tear film. *Exp Eye Res* 1973;15:515–525.

50. Lemp M, Dohlman CH, Holly FJ. Corneal desiccation despite normal tear volume. *Ann Ophthalmol* 1970;2:258–261.

51. Sharma A, Ruckenstein E. Mechanism of tear film rupture and its implications for contact lens intolerance. *Am J Optom Physiol Opt* 1985;62:246–253.

52. Lin S, Brenner H. Tear film rupture. *J Colloid Interface Sci* 1982;89:226–231.

53. Liotet S, van Bijsterveld OP, Kogbe O, et al. A new hypothesis on tear film stability. *Ophthalmologica* 1987;195:119–124.

54. Korb D, Greiner JV, Herman J. Comparison of fluorescein break-up time measurement reproducibility using standard fluorescein strips versus the Dry Eye Test (DET) method. *Cornea* 2001;20:811–815.

55. Norn MS. Desiccation of the pre-corneal tear film: I. Corneal wetting time. *Acta Ophthalmol* 1969;47:856–880.

56. Cho P, Brown B. Review of the tear break-up time and a closer look at the tear break-up time of Hong Kong Chinese. *Optom Vis Sci* 1993;70:30–38.

57. Mengher LS, et al. Effect of fluorescein instillation on the precorneal tear film stability. *Curr Eye Res* 1985;4:9–12.

58. Mengher LS, et al. A non-invasive instrument for clinical assessment of the pre-corneal tear film stability. *Curr Eye Res* 1985; 4:1–7.

59. Patel S, et al. Effects of fluorescein on tear breakup time and on tear thinning time. *Am J Optom Physiol Opt* 1985;62:188–190.

60. Halberg GP, Berens C. Standardized Schirmer tear test kit. *Am J Ophthalmol* 1961;51:840–842.

61. Hamano H, et al. A new method of measuring tears. *CLAO J* 1983;9:281–289.

62. Tomlinson A, Blades KJ, Pearce EI. What does the phenol red thread test actually measure? *Optom Vis Sci* 2001;78:142–146.

63. Xu K, Yagi Y, Toda I, et al. Tear function index: a new measurement of dry eye. *Arch Ophthalmol* 1995;113:84–88.

64. Xu K-P, Tsubota K. Correlation of tear clearance rate and fluorophotometric assessment of tear turnover. *Br J Ophthalmol* 1995;79:1042–1045.

65. Prabhasawat P, Tseng SCG. Frequent association of delayed tear clearance in ocular irritation. *Br J Ophthalmol* 1988;182: 666–675.

66. Macri A, Rolando M, Pflugfelder S. A standardized visual scale for evaluation of tear fluorescein clearance. *Ophthalmology* 2000; 107:1338–1343.

67. Occhipinti JR, et al. Fluorophotometric measurement of human tear turnover rate. *Curr Eye Res* 1988;7:995–1000.

68. Pflugfelder SC, Tseng SCG, Sanabria O, et al. Evaluation of subjective assessments and objective diagnostic tests for diagnosing tear-film disorders known to cause ocular irritation. *Cornea* 1998;17:38–56.

69. Fullard R, Snyder C. Protein levels in non-stimulated tears of normal subjects. *Invest Ophthalmol Vis Sci* 1990;31:1119–1126.

70. Gilbard JP. Tear film osmolarity and keratoconjunctivitis sicca. In: Holly FJ, ed. *The preocular tear film in health, disease and contact lens wear.* Lubbock, TX: Dry Eye Institute, 1986: 127–139.

71. Farris R. Tear osmolarity variation in the dry eye. *Trans Am Ophthalmol Soc* 1986;84:250–268.

72. Abdel-Khalek L, Williams J, Lee WR. Morphological changes in the human conjunctival epithelium. II. In keratoconjunctivitis sicca. *Br J Ophthalmol* 1978;62:800–806.

73. Beitch I. The induction of keratinization in the corneal epithelium: a comparison of the "dry" and vitamin A-deficient eyes. *Invest Ophthalmol* 1970;9:827–843.

74. Maudgal P. The epithelial response in keratitis sicca and keratitis herpetica (an experimental and clinical study). *Doc Ophthalmol* 1978;45:223.

75. Little SA, Bruce AS. Osmotic determinants of postlens tear film morphology and hydrogel lens movement. *Ophthalmic Phys Opt* 1995;15:117–124.

76. Greiner JV, Allansmith MR. Effect of contact lens wear on the conjunctival mucous system. *Ophthalmology* 1981;88:821–832.

77. Sorenson T, Taagehoj F, Christensen U. Tear flow in soft lenses. *Acta Ophthalmol* 1980;58:182–187.

78. Puffer M, Neault RW, Brubaker RF. Basal precorneal turnover in the human eye. *Am J Ophthalmol* 1980;89:369–376.

79. Young G, Efron N. Characteristics of the pre-lens tear film during hydrogel contact lens wear. *Ophthalmic Phys Opt* 1991;11:53–58.

80. Schmidt P, Hill RM. Tear chloride as an adaptive index. *Am J Optom Physiol Opt* 1980;57:25–28.

81. Lowther GE, Miller RB, Hill RM. Tear concentrations of sodium and potassium during adaptation to contact lenses; 1. Sodium observations. *Am J Optom Arch Am Acad Optom* 1970;47:266–275.

82. Miller RB. Tear concentrations of sodium and potassium during adaptation to contact lenses. II. Potassium observations. *Am J Optom Arch Am Acad Optom* 1970;47:773–779.

83. Young WH, Hill RM. Tear cholesterol levels and contact lens adaptation. *Am J Optom Arch Am Acad Optom* 1973;50:12–6.

84. Callender M, Morrison PE. A quantitative study of human tear proteins before and after adaptation to non-flexible contact lenses. *Am J Optom Physiol Opt* 1974;51:939–945.

85. Farris RL. Tear analysis in contact lens wearers. *CLAO J* 1986;12:106–111.

86. Lundh RL, Liotet S, Pouliquen Y. Study of the human blood-tear barrier and the biochemical changes in the tears of 30 contact lens wearers (50 eyes). *Ophthalmologica* 1984;188:100–105.

87. Jones B, Sack R. Immunoglobulin deposition on soft contact lenses: relationship to hydrogel structure and mode of use and giant papillary conjunctivitis. *CLAO J* 1990;16:43–48.

88. Vinding T, Eriksen JS, Nielsen NV. The concentration of lysozyme and secretory IgA in tears from healthy persons with and without contact lens use. *Acta Ophthalmol (Copenh)* 1987;65:23–26.

89. Allansmith MR, et al. Giant papillary conjunctivitis in contact lens wearers. *Am J Ophthalmol* 1977;83:697–708.

90. Creuzot-Garcher C. Ocular surface in dry eye syndrome. In: Hoang-Xuan T, Baudouin C, Creuzot-Garcher C, eds: *Inflammatory diseases of the conjunctiva*. Stuttgart: Thieme, 1998:149.

91. Andres S, et al. Tear pH, air pollution, and contact lenses. *Am J Optom Physiol Opt* 1988;65:627–631.

92. Carney LG, Hill RM. Human tear pH. Diurnal variations. *Arch Ophthalmol* 1976;94:821–824.

93. Coles WH, Jaros PA. Dynamics of ocular surface pH. *Br J Ophthalmol* 1982;94:549–552.

94. Fischer FH, Wiederholt M. Human precorneal tear film pH measured by microelectrodes. *Graefes Arch Clin Exp Ophthalmol* 1982;218:168–170.

95. Carney LG, Hill RM. Tear pH and the hard (PMMA) contact lens patient. *Int Contact Lens Clin* 1976;3:27–30.

96. Carney LG, Hill RM. Tear pH: hydrophilic lenses and the closed eye. *Int Contact Lens Clin* 1976;3:30–31.

97. Browning DJ, Foulks GN. Tear pH in health, disease and contact lens wear. In: Holly FJ, ed. *The preocular tear film in health, disease and contact lens wear.* Lubbock, TX: The Dry Eye Institute, 1986:954.

98. Hamano H. Fundamental researches on the effects of contact lenses on the eye. In: Ruben M, eds. *Soft contact lens clinical and applied technology.* New York: John Wiley and Sons, 1978:35.

99. Chen FS, Maurice DM. The pH in the precorneal tear film and under a contact lens measured with a fluorescent probe. *Exp Eye Res* 1990;50:251–259.

100. Lattimore MRJ. Contact lens anterior surface pH. *Int Contact Lens Clin* 1990;17:228–231.

101. Gilbard JP, Gray KL, Rossi SR. A proposed mechanism for increased tear-film osmolarity in contact lens wearers. *Am J Ophthalmol* 1986;102:505–507.

102. Martin DK. Osmolality of the tear fluid in the contralateral eye during monocular contact lens wear. *Acta Ophthalmol (Copenh)* 1987;65:551–555.

103. Tomlinson A, Cedarstaff TH. Tear evaporation from the human eye: the effects of contact lens wear. *J Br Contact Lens Assoc* 1982;5:141–150.

104. Milder B. The lacrimal apparatus. In: Moses RA, Hart WM, eds: *Adler's physiology of the eye,* 8th ed. St. Louis: CV Mosby, 1987:15–35.

105. Iwata S, et al. Evaporation rate of water from the precorneal tear film and cornea in the rabbit. *Invest Ophthalmol Vis Sci* 1969;8:613–619.

106. Cedarstaff TH, Tomlinson A. A comparative study of tear evaporation rates and water content of soft contact lenses. *Am J Optom Physiol Opt* 1983;60:167–174.

107. McMonnies CW. Key questions in a dry eye history. *J Am Optom Assoc* 1986;57:512–517.

108. Moss SE, Klein R, Klein BE. Prevalence of and risk factors for dry eye syndrome. *Arch Ophthalmol* 2000;118:1264–1268.

109. Port MJA, Asaria TS. The assessment of human tear volume. *J Br Contact Lens Assoc* 1990;13:76.

110. Hamano H. Tear secretion test (preliminary report). *J Contact Lens Soc* 1982;24:103–107.

111. Maurice D. The movement of fluorescein and water in the cornea. *Am J Ophthalmol* 1960;49:1011–1016.

112. Wilson G, Ren H, Laurent J. Corneal epithelial fluorescein staining. *J Am Optom Assoc* 1995;66:435–441.

113. Norn MS. Vital staining of cornea and conjunctiva. Fluorescein-rose bengal mixture and tetrazolium-Alcian blue mixture. *Acta Ophthalmol Suppl* 1972;113:3–66.

114. Josephson JE, Caffery BE. Corneal staining after instillation of topical anesthetic (SSII). *Invest Ophthalmol Vis Sci* 1988;29:1096–1099.

115. van Bijsterveld OP. Diagnostic tests in the sicca syndrome. *Arch Ophthalmol* 1969;82:10–14.

116. Norn MS. Rose bengal vital staining. Staining of cornea and conjunctiva by 10 percent rose bengal, compared with 1 percent. *Acta Ophthalmol* 1970;48:546–559.

117. Snyder C, Paugh JR. Rose bengal dye concentration and volume delivered via dye-impregnated paper strips. *Optom Vis Sci* 1998;75:339–341.

118. Lemp M. Report of the National Eye Institute/Industry workshop on clinical trials in dry eyes. *CLAO J* 1995;21:221–232.

119. Norn MS. Lissamine green. Vital staining of cornea and conjunctiva. *Acta Ophthalmol* 1973;51:483–491.

120. Korb DR, Henriquez AS. Meibomian gland dysfunction and contact lens intolerance. *J Am Optom Assoc* 1980;51:243–251.

121. Hom MM, Silverman MW. Displacement technique and meibomian gland expression. *J Am Optom Assoc* 1987;58:223–226.

122. Paugh JR, et al. Meibomian therapy in problematic contact lens wear. *Optom Vis Sci* 1990;67:803–806.

123. Lemp MA. Is the dry eye contact lens wearer at risk? Yes. *Cornea* 1990;9[Suppl. 1]:S48–S50, discussion S54.

124. Finnemore VM. Is the dry eye contact lens wearer at risk? Not usually. *Cornea* 1990;9[Suppl. 1]:S51–S53, discussion S54.

125. Stapleton F, Dart JK, Minassian D. Risk factors with contact lens related suppurative keratitis. *CLAO J* 1993;19:204–210.

126. Korb DR, Korb JE. A new concept in contact lens design. Parts 1 and 2. *J Am Optom Assoc* 1970;41:1023–1026.

127. Bennett ES, Gordon JM. The borderline dry eye patient and contact lens wear. *Contact Lens Forum* 1988;14:52–73.

128. Sorbara LG, Talsky C. Contact lens wear in the dry eye patient: predicting success and achieving it. *Can J Optom* 1988;50:234–241.

129. Orsborn GN, Zantos SG. Corneal desiccation staining with thin high water content contact lenses. *CLAO J* 1988;14:81–85.

130. Lemp MA, et al. Omafilcon A (Proclear) soft contact lenses in a dry eye population. *CLAO J* 1999;25:40–47.

131. Burstein NL. The effects of topical drugs and preservatives on the tears and corneal epithelium in dry eye. *Trans Ophthalmol Soc UK* 1985;104[Pt. 4]:402–409.

132. Holly FJ. Tear film formation and rupture: an update. In: Holly FJ, ed. *The preocular tear film in health, disease and contact lens wear.* Lubbock, TX: Dry Eye Institute, 1986:634–645.

133. Berger RE, Corrsin S. A surface tension gradient mechanism for driving the pre-corneal tear film after a blink. *J Biomech* 1974;7:225–238.

134. Doane MG. Interactions of eyelids and tears in corneal wetting and the dynamics of the normal human eyeblink. *Am J Ophthalmol* 1980;89:507–516.

135. Abelson MB, Holly FJ. A tentative mechanism for inferior punctate keratopathy. *Am J Ophthalmol* 1977;83:866–869.

136. Carney LG, Hill RM. The nature of normal blinking patterns. *Acta Ophthalmol (Copenh)* 1982;60:427–433.

137. Holly FJ. Tear film physiology and contact lens wear. II. Contact lens-tear film interaction. *Am J Optom Physiol Opt* 1981;58:331–341.

138. Carney LG, Hill RM. Variation in blinking behavior during soft lens wear. *Int Contact Lens Clin* 1984;11:250–253.

139. Hill RM. The quantitative blink. *Int Contact Lens Clin* 1984;11:366–368.

140. Trees GR, Tomlinson A. Effect of artificial tear solutions and saline on tear film evaporation. *Optom Vis Sci* 1990;67:886–890.

141. Golding TR, Efron N, Brennan NA. Soft lens lubricants and tear film stability. *Optom Vis Sci* 1990;67:461–465.

142. Efron N, Golding TR, Brennan NA. The effect of soft lens lubricants on symptoms and lens dehydration. *CLAO J* 1991;17:114–119.

143. Tomlinson A. Tear film changes with contact lens wear. In: Tomlinson A, ed. *Complications of contact lens wear.* St. Louis: Mosby, 1992:159.

144. Tomlinson A, Trees GR. Effect of preservatives in artificial tear solutions on tear film evaporation. *Ophthalmic Physiol Opt* 1991;11:48–52.

145. Lemp MA. General measures in management of the dry eye. *Int Ophthalmol Clin* 1987;27:36–43.

146. Slusser TG, Lowther GE. Effects of lacrimal drainage occlusion with nondissolvable intracanalicular plugs on hydrogel contact lens wear. *Optom Vis Sci* 1998;75:330–338.

24

HYBRID MATERIALS AND DESIGNS

MICHAEL D. DEPAOLIS
JOSEPH P. SHOVLIN
DWIGHT H. AKERMAN AND
GAROLD L. EDWARDS

Since the introduction of polymethylmethacrylate (PMMA), manufacturers have pursued many alternatives in polymer development in an attempt to enhance contact lens performance. The result actually has been a plethora of hybrid materials. The mixed composition of gas-permeable and hydroxyethylmethacrylate (HEMA) copolymers are, by definition, hybrids. However, the clinical interpretation of a hybrid contact lens is more limited. In this chapter we will discuss hybrid materials and designs, present and future.

MATERIAL TECHNOLOGY

Through many years of research and development, contact lens manufacturers have recognized tremendous physiologic improvements with the introduction of new materials. As impressive as these strides have been, we are still in search of the ideal contact lens material. Improved corneal physiology, because of increased oxygen transmission and improved biocompatibility, in conjunction with excellent comfort and visual performance remain primary priorities. As hydrogel lenses continue to maintain the majority of the domestic marketplace (1), research continues. Historically, hydrophilic lenses have achieved higher oxygen transmission because of greater water content and thinner designs (2). It may be impossible to develop a pure hydrogel lens, using HEMA as a primary base, with no hypoxic impact (3). Furthermore, there is a limitation to this strategy, as critical performance variables, such as refractive capabilities and durability, often are compromised. Because of the inherent limitations of existing hydrogel materials, many manufacturers have looked to new hybrids. One such example is the incorporation of biodegradable components, such as collagen. A nontraditional matrix of collagen and a synthetic hydrogel material offers certain benefits, including increased oxygen transmission (4); however, the limitations of a protein-based polymer also must be considered. Biodegradation, potential allergenicity, and the potential for microbial growth are present-day concerns. These concerns have been the basis for investigation of other potential hybrids including silicone hydrogels. The concept of combining traditional rigid monomers with traditional hydrogel monomers is one such avenue. Blending silicone and HEMA, for example, proved to be beneficial in providing the excellent oxygen permeability of the former, while maintaining the durability, ease of manufacture, and hydrophilicity of the latter. A complete discussion of recently approved silicone hydrogels including indications and clinical implications can be found in Chapter 18. This same rationale applies to the concept of combining certain fluorinated materials with existing hydrogel materials.

FLEXIBLE FLUOROPOLYMERS

A category of materials encouraged by hybrid technology has been the development of flexible fluoropolymer lenses. This technology deviates from traditional hydrogel and rigid gas permeable in that there is no carbon-carbon backbone structure (5). This class is based primarily on a polyperfluoroether component, having a carbon-oxygen-carbon backbone. In addition, methylmethacrylate imparts flexural resistance while N-vinyl-pyrrolidone enhances wettability. The net effect is a fluorine-containing material with a nonacrylic backbone and without silicone. Clinically, this results in a lens with excellent oxygen permeability and wettability and a modulus of elasticity between that of rigid and hydrogel lenses. Limitations, to date, have been the difficulties in lens manufacturing.

The first flexible fluoropolymer lens made available in the United States was the Allergan Advent lens. Manufactured by 3M, the lens was a molded pentacurve design. The reported oxygen permeability (Dk) value was in the range of 100, assuring a reasonable physiologic response in the event of overnight wear (6). Of all the materials previously introduced, only the silicone elastomer lens offers higher oxygen permeability. An additional attribute of this lens involves surface reactivity. Much information has been reported in the literature pertaining to the poor wettability and propensity toward deposits in silicone-containing polymers (7), thus resulting in their early demise.

Although the aforementioned material is a true example of a hybrid, traditional clinical interpretation has been somewhat different. The remainder of this chapter will be devoted to traditional hybrid contact lens practice, namely implementation of two-phase technology, as well as utilization of piggyback technology.

TWO-PHASE TECHNOLOGY

Two-phase contact lens technology first appeared in the United States marketplace as the Saturn II lens. Consisting of a rigid gas-permeable center surrounded by a soft hydrophilic skirt, this material, synergicon A, offers the advantages of rigid lens optics and soft lens comfort (9–12; Boucher J, Powell J. Personal communication, 1989). The lens technology was developed at Precision-Cosmet Company in Minnesota, and joined the Sola/Barnes-Hind family of lenses in 1986. SoftPerm was introduced to the marketplace in the fall of 1989 and is now marketed by Ciba Vision.

HISTORY

In 1977, Precision-Cosmet acquired the rights to a hard/soft bonding concept developed by Erikson and Neogi (13). The Erikson patent described a process for the cross-linking of a soft hydrophilic plastic to a rigid plastic. The early research performed in Minnesota was undertaken using a HEMA-based hydrogel and PMMA materials (13). However, the appearance of rigid gas-permeable lens materials on the horizon forced the investigators first to develop a rigid gas-permeable lens material to be used in the center of this as yet unnamed lens. This research was initiated in 1978 and, in 1980, a final formulation for the center material, pentasilcon P, was developed.

Much of 1981 was dedicated to developing the bonding technology outlined in the Erikson patent and developing a manufacturing system for the production of a two-phase contact lens material. An additional 14 months were devoted to developing possible design parameters for the lens and in March of 1982, the US Food and Drug Administration (FDA) clinical evaluations were initiated. The FDA guidelines required the study of 400 eyes wearing the Saturn lenses for a period of 6 months. In April 1984, the Ophthalmic Advisory Panel of the FDA recommended premarket approval of the Saturn II lens, and in January 1985, the FDA granted premarket approval status for the lens.

CHEMISTRY

The Saturn contact lens is one lens in two phases: a rigid gas-permeable phase and a soft hydrophilic phase (9,10,14,15). It is not a hard lens material with a soft lens glued to it. It is made from a single button and the finished lens has two distinct phases with a transitional zone. The lens is lathe-cut on both front and back surfaces.

The center material, pentasilcon P, was marketed for a period of time as Opus III, a rigid gas-permeable lens. The specifications of pentasilcon P are provided in Table 24.1. The low specific gravity and high index of refraction allow for lens designs with minimal average thickness, thus maximizing oxygen transmission in a relatively low-Dk material.

Pentasilcon P has a very interesting surface chemistry (5,15). In order to overcome the problems of wettability experienced with silicone/acrylate lens materials, some features are incorporated into pentasilcon P to enhance its wettability. Figure 24.1 is a schematic representation of pentasilcon P. Three features to note are the anhydride group, tertiarybutyl styrene, and siloxane.

Tertiarybutyl styrene is part of the material because of its lightweight strength and its oxygen-transmission qualities. The anhydride group, on exposure to an aqueous solution, will open up as shown in Fig. 24.2 to expose polar hydrophilic sites. It also can be observed that the siloxane group has disappeared from the picture.

When exposed to an aqueous environment, the siloxane group will, with time, hydrolyze from the surface of pentasilcon P leaving a polar hydrophilic site. By eliminating silicone from the surface of the lens, the problems of hydrophobicity and lipophilicity are overcome, resulting in a hydrophilic, lipophobic surface. The hydrolysis of siloxane and the anhydride is a characteristic of the surface chemistry of pentasilcon P, while the matrix of the lens is tightly cross-linked to prevent the lens from dissolving while in an aqueous solution. When the lens is scratched, however, exposing the unhydrolyzed siloxane, those groups will hydrolyze off after a period of time in an aqueous solution (14,16). A lens with a large number of scratches still can be worn comfortably and with little effect on visual acuity because of the hydrolysis of the siloxane and anhydride groups (Boucher J. Personal communication, 1989). It is important to note that the hydrophilicity of the surface of pentasilcon P is a quality of the surface chemistry of the lens and is not a surface treatment provided to the lens during the manufacturing process.

TABLE 24.1. PHYSICAL CHARACTERISTICS OF SOFTPERM RIGID CENTER

Dk	Specific Gravity	Index of Refraction
14×10^{-11} @ 35c	1.05	1.53

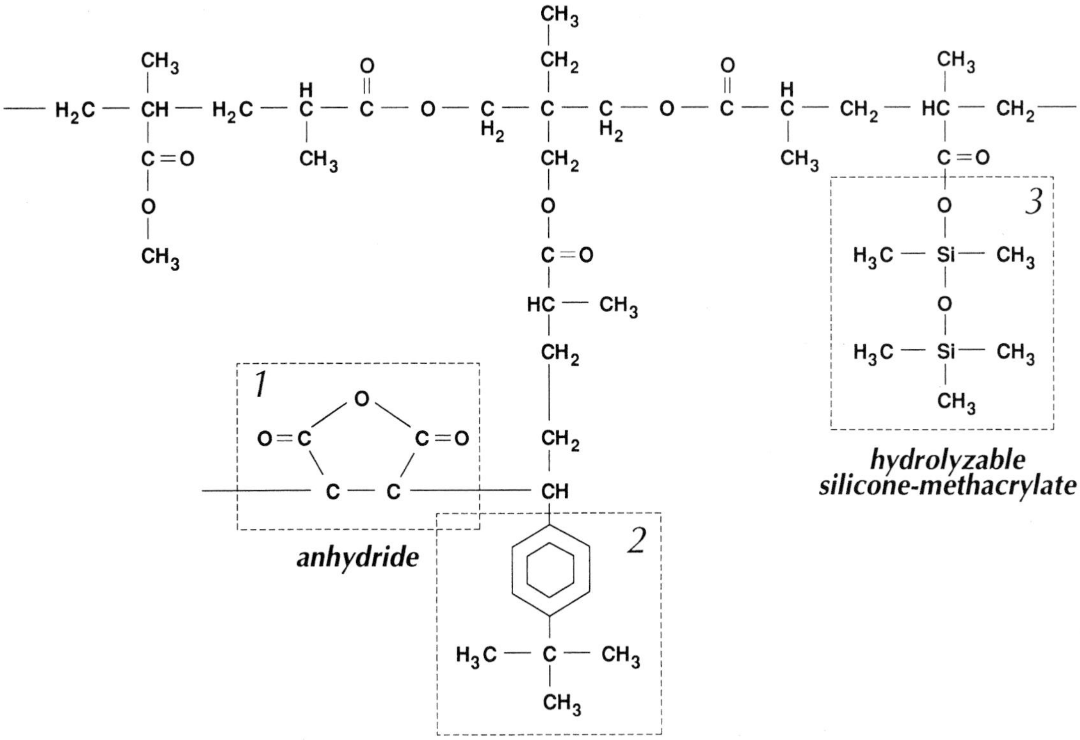

FIG. 24.1. SoftPerm rigid gas-permeable center prior to hydrolysis.

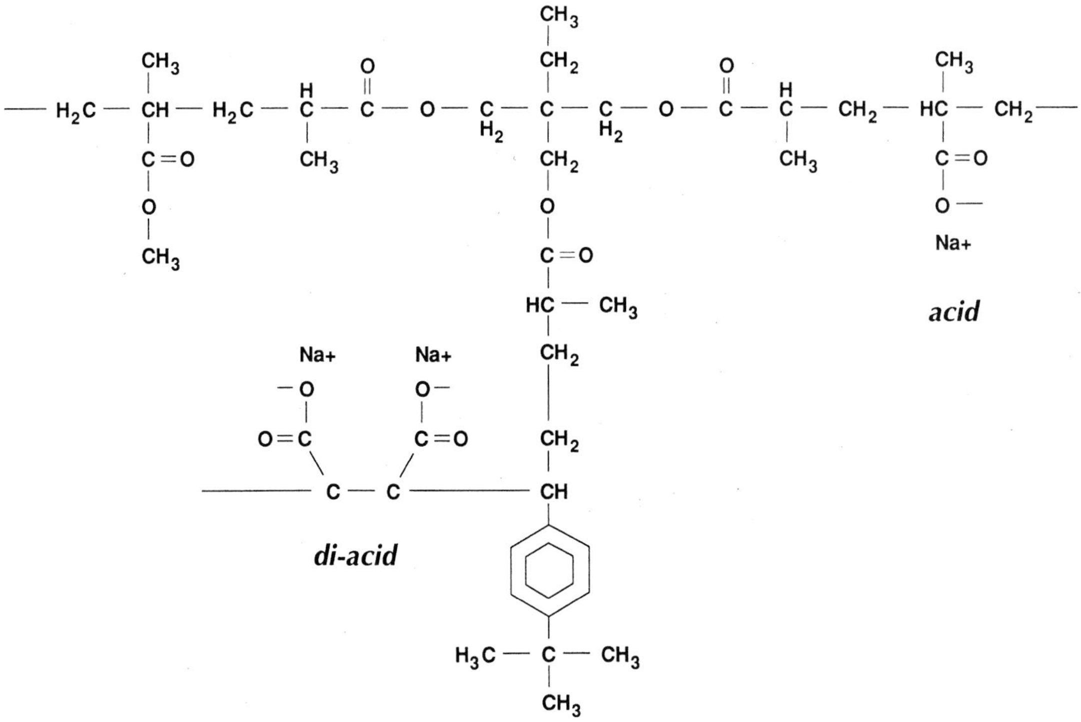

FIG. 24.2. SoftPerm rigid gas-permeable center post hydrolysis.

The skirt, or flange, of the lens is a HEMA-based hydrogel material with a water content of approximately 25%. The relatively low water content of the skirt provides a very durable material, which gives support to the rigid phase of the lens The flange provides more than comfort to the wearer; its interaction with the cornea contributes greatly to the fitting characteristics of the lens (10).

The transition zone is a very narrow band lying between the rigid center and the soft hydrophilic skirt that can be observed with the biomicroscope. It consists of a combination of pentasilcon P and the skirt materials. The transition zone is not glue; it is a cross-linking or a molecular interweaving of the center and skirt materials (9,10,14,15).

SATURN II LENS

In 1981, when the original design work was being undertaken with Saturn II, the investigators chose a balance between rigid and hydrogel lens fitting and selected 13.0 mm as the optimum overall diameter for the lens. After many trials, a rigid center size of 6.5 mm was chosen. Because the only purpose of the rigid center was to provide good optics to the system, the size of the center was kept at a minimum. The rigid center of the Saturn II is single cut, having no peripheral curves. As a well-fitting Saturn II lens generally centers very well and provides minimal movement, few complaints of glare or haloes have been reported. However, we have observed that some patients with very large pupils have reported a rainbow effect, especially with night driving, when the pupil dilates beyond the hard/soft transition zone. This appears to be the result of a prismatic effect at the transition zone between the center and skirt materials.

Because Saturn II was made up of a comparatively rigid material, it was possible to cut the center thickness of it quite thin. Center thicknesses ranged from 0.16 to 0.08 mm in powers of plano to -4.50 D, and the center thickness remained constant at 0.08 mm from -4.50 D to the highest minus-power lenses.

While the fit of Saturn II is controlled both by the center and the skirt of the lens, it was found that a large number of base curve radii would be necessary to fit the greatest number of patients. Saturn II entered the market with an 11-lens diagnostic set with base curve radii ranging from 7.20 to 8.20 mm in 0.1-mm increments.

Since the introduction of soft hydrophilic lenses, there has been a desire to produce a lens with the comfort of hydrogel contact lens and with the visual acuity of a rigid lens material. Besides providing the comfort of a hydrogel contact lens, the Saturn II has other advantages to offer. A well-fit Saturn II typically provides excellent centration in all lens powers on any corneal topography. Patients with moderate-to-high degrees of corneal astigmatism or an irregular corneal topography benefit from the centration characteristics of Saturn II. The lenticular edge design allows for good comfort and good corneal physiologic response, even in highly ametropic patients. As the rigid center of the lens corrects astigmatism with a tear lens, Saturn II often shows an advantage over toric hydrogel contact lenses, providing good stability of vision even with lens movement and rotation.

Despite the numerous theoretic advantages of this two-phase technology, the Saturn II lens experienced certain clinical limitations. Lens tearing, at the transition zone, has been problematic with lens handling. Lens adherence with attending edema often occurs during wear. These limitations ultimately resulted in a redesigning of the Saturn II lens and the introduction of the SoftPerm lens.

SOFTPERM LENS

Research work with the original Saturn lens revealed that stresses developed in the lens material during the button manufacturing process. These stresses could be observed in finished lenses by examining the lens profile. Figure 24.3 shows a profile of the Saturn II lens. Modifications to refine the button manufacturing process were initiated in order to prevent those stresses from occurring. A profile of SoftPerm with design changes incorporated is shown in Fig. 24.3.

Many design challenges were presented in developing measurements for the SoftPerm lens. While the same center and skirt materials as those in Saturn II are used, the *unstressed* material provided the investigators with greater freedom in redesigning the lens. Unlike a hydrogel lens, however, the rigid center of this material contributes its own unique qualities to the fit. It is necessary to balance optimum center and skirt diameters with the proper intermediate and peripheral curve configurations in both materials.

The overall diameter of a SoftPerm lens is 14.3 mm with an 8.0-mm rigid center. In order to promote better lens movement with the SoftPerm lens, some edge lift has been provided in both the rigid center and the soft portion of the lens. By providing a pool of tears at the rigid-soft interface, the lens shows less tendency toward diminished movement with wear due to dehydration of the hydrophilic skirt. Future variations of this design will likely include the use of more oxygen permeable materials using a silicone hydrogel skirt.

SoftPerm Fitting

A ten-lens diagnostic set is recommended for the fitting of the SoftPerm lens; a Saturn II fitting set (13.0-mm diameter) cannot be substituted for the 14.3-mm-diameter SoftPerm lens.

Fluoresoft (Holles Laboratories), a macromolecular fluorescein, is a useful tool in a SoftPerm-lens diagnostic fitting. Before placement on a patient's eye, the diagnostic lens should have a drop of Fluoresoft placed into the concave

IMPROVED HARD\SOFT JUNCTION

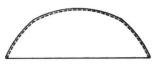

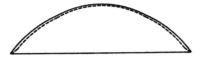

SATURN II
ENHANCED SATURN II

FIG. 24.3. Cross-sectional profile comparison of Saturn II and SoftPerm.

surface of the lens. It may be helpful to balance the lens between the index and the middle fingers before placing it on the patient's eye, because the solution inside the lens may make it difficult to balance on one fingertip.

The first lens of choice for use on the patient with low-to-moderate astigmatism will have a base curve radius on the flat K to 0.1 mm steeper than K (16). In cases of increased corneal astigmatism, a steeper diagnostic lens is indicated. Because of the dynamics of the rigid-soft material interaction on the cornea, a lens fit too flat may show decreased movement. It is desirable to provide a near-alignment fit with both the rigid center and the soft skirt materials in order to distribute the lens bearing area evenly on the cornea. The recommended base curve radius is based on the selection chart seen in Table 24.2 (15).

A lens that is fit too flat loses support of the hydrophilic skirt in the periphery and may show bearing in the transition zone (Fig. 24.4). This bearing at the transition zone can create a negative pressure behind the rigid center and decrease movement. Refitting with a steeper base curve radius may enhance lens mobility. With more support from the skirt, a more uniform layer of tears lies behind the entire lens (Fig. 24.5). Comfort often is compromised in a flat-fitting lens. A very flat lens may move excessively and exhibit edge standoff, especially on upward gaze.

The fluorescein pattern in a flat-fitting lens may show apical touch in the gas-permeable center. There also can be the initial presence of significant inferior tear pooling, which can give the false impression of a steep-fitting skirt. How-

ever, unlike tear entrapment in a steep-fitting lens, tear exchange is free and rapid with the blink in a flat-fitting lens.

If a diagnostic lens is too steep, a relatively thick tear pool behind the lens will provide a large amount of movement on insertion. After equilibration, however, the lens will tighten on the cornea, as will any soft contact lens that is fit too steeply. An excessively steep lens may show only minimal movement, or movement with conjunctival drag. The fluorescein pattern will show significant apical clearance in the gas-permeable center, as well as a pool of trapped tears under the skirt (Fig. 24.6). The trapped tears will dissipate only slowly with blinking. In this case, a flatter base curve should be selected.

After a 15- to 20-minute equilibration period, the lens should be assessed for movement and centration. In most cases, the SoftPerm lens will demonstrate excellent centration, even on highly ametropic eyes. A decentered lens with minimal movement often is fit too flat. Movement of about 0.50 mm or more should be seen after equilibration, but movement of 0.25 mm or less often is acceptable.

When the best-fitting SoftPerm diagnostic lens has been selected and allowed to equilibrate, an overrefraction and visual acuities should be performed. If the fitter is concerned about flexure in the rigid center of the lens, this can be verified by overkeratometry and by spherocylindrical over-refraction. Flexure generally is not predictable without a

TABLE 24.2. SELECTION CHART FOR BASE CURVE RADII

Corneal Toricity (D)	Base Curve (mm)
1.37 or less	On K to 0.1 steeper than K
1.50–2.75	0.1–0.2 steeper than K
Over 2.75	0.2–0.3 steeper than K

If deviations from the above base curve selection table are considered, it is best to err slightly on the steep side. Thus, the final base curve should be within the recommended range or perhaps 0.1 mm steeper. (From *SoftPerm fitting guide.* Sola/Barnes Hind, Inc., 1989, with permission).

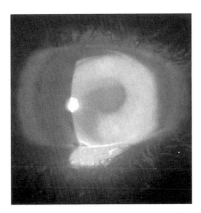

FIG. 24.4. Flat-fitting SoftPerm lens. (Courtesy of James Boucher. OD, Laramie, Wyoming.)

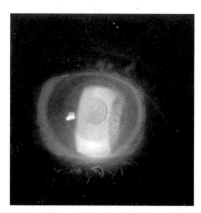

FIG. 24.5. Optimum-fitting SoftPerm lens. (Courtesy of James Boucher, OD, Laramie, Wyoming.)

diagnostic fitting because it is related not only to central corneal astigmatism, but also to peripheral corneal topography and individual lid interactions. In most cases, SoftPerm lenses will mask as much corneal cylinder as other rigid gas-permeable lenses. If significant residual astigmatism is found, the fitter should try flattening the base curve by 0.1 mm. This can be a viable solution only if lens movement and patient comfort are preserved.

SoftPerm lenses generally behave in a predictable fashion on the eye. Movement of 0.50 mm, characteristic of a well-fit soft lens, can be expected with SoftPerm lenses. Macromolecular fluorescein will reveal an alignment-type pattern across the back surface of the lens. The design provides a good physiologic fit on the eye initially and with prolonged wear, making the practitioner's job easier in a diagnostic fitting.

SoftPerm Dispensing

At the dispensing evaluation, care must be taken to instruct each patient properly in insertion and removal. For example, excessive pressure at 3- and 9-o'clock on lens removal may

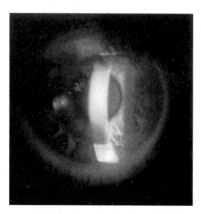

FIG. 24.6. Steep-fitting SoftPerm lens. (Courtesy of James Boucher, OD, Laramie, Wyoming.)

contribute to premature lens breakage. This can be avoided by removing the lens at the 5- and 7-o'clock positions.

If a tear develops in a lens, the patient usually will observe a foreign-body sensation on insertion. At the dispensing evaluation, the wearer must be instructed to remove the lens, clean, rinse, and reinsert it if this occurs. If the irritation persists, the patient must be cautioned to remove the lens immediately and not reinsert it until an evaluation has been performed in the fitter's office.

Because of the relatively low water content of the skirt and oxygen permeability of the center, a conservative wearing schedule should be used initially, even with experienced contact lens wearers. It has been recommended to start with 4 hours the first day and add 1 hour to a maximum of 12 hours. After the first progress evaluation, the wearing schedule can be adjusted to meet individual patient needs.

Lens Care

Because of the nature of the lens material, heat disinfection is not recommended with the SoftPerm lens. Surfactant cleaning and cold chemical or hydrogen peroxide disinfection are indicated on a daily basis. Weekly intensive cleaning also is recommended.

An interesting effect of the combination rigid and soft materials is the fact that the two materials may not exhibit an equal attraction for deposits from the patient's tears (10; Boucher J, Powell J. Personal communication, 1989). The rigid center, with most patients, has been shown to be quite resistant to deposits. The soft skirt, conversely, may accumulate debris from the tears and the fingers at a greater rate. Whereas, in a standard hydrogel contact lens, deposits will result in an adverse effect on vision, this may not be the case with the SoftPerm lens. It is possible for the patient to show an accumulation of debris on the skirt of the lens without any visual disturbance. This buildup of debris can, of course, create or exacerbate physiologic problems, such as giant papillary conjunctivitis. Therefore, patient compliance in lens care and cleaning, both on a daily and a weekly intensive basis, is extremely important.

SoftPerm Follow-up

As with most contact lens patients, it is best to perform a follow-up evaluation after, at minimum, 4 hours of wear. With the lens in place, it can be inspected with a biomicroscope for nicks, tears, and scratches. The transition zone should be inspected carefully for a break or tangential tear in the soft skirt (Fig. 24.7). If a tear in this area is not full thickness, the patient may be unaware of any discomfort. Nevertheless, this lens should be discarded and a new one dispensed.

Lens movement should now be evaluated. A well-fitting SoftPerm lens should show about 0.50 mm of movement with a normal blink. Movement to a greater or lesser degree

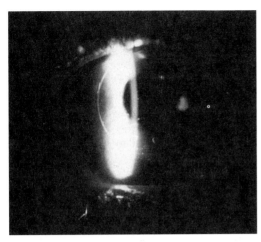

FIG. 24.7. Tangential tear at rigid-soft interface of original Saturn II design.

is not a contraindication provided corneal health and integrity are maintained. Movement is assessed most easily in the up-gaze position. Next, the lens should be removed and the tears stained with fluorescein. The cornea should be inspected for signs of staining. If staining is observed, the type and pattern should be noted. Three types of staining are observed most often.

1. *Stipple staining* is a characteristic of mechanical irritation or low oxygen flux reaching the cornea. This pattern generally appears behind the rigid center of the lens and may be related to poor tear exchange behind the rigid center of the lens.
2. *Abrasion* is caused by a tear in the soft material at the transition zone. This appears as an arcuate defect in the midperiphery of the cornea.
3. *Ring staining* is not a true stain, but a pooling of fluorescein on the cornea. In appearance, this is not unlike the lens adhesion staining pattern observed with patients wearing rigid gas-permeable extended wear lenses. Generally short-lived, this pattern typically disappears in 5 to 15 minutes.

While a tear at the transition zone may still precipitate a corneal abrasion, the incidence of stippling and ring staining is significantly less with the SoftPerm lens than with the Saturn II lens.

PIGGYBACK DESIGN

The concept of integrating multiple contact lens systems simultaneously originated over two decades ago. The initial piggyback application was one of employing two PMMA lenses simultaneously for the correction of presbyopia. In the early 1970s, Baldone (17) pioneered the idea of piggybacking a rigid lens over an underlying hydrogel lens. The potential benefits of simultaneously using hydrogel and rigid technology are obvious. The improved comfort and stability provided by hydrogel lenses in conjunction with the crisp optics of rigid lenses have made piggyback combinations the logical choice for many complex cases. However, until recently the limited corneal physiologic response and difficulty in achieving an acceptable fit in certain patients have been documented as well (18,19).

Applications

Traditional applications for hydrogel/rigid piggyback designs have included irregular corneal topography with an associated complex refractive error. Often the patient who has this profile has a history of corneal disease, trauma, or surgical misadventures. A partial list of these conditions is provided in Table 24.3. For those individuals with anisometropia or irregular astigmatism, traditional spectacle correction is not beneficial. Application of a hydrogel lens may improve topographic irregularity and lessen anisometropia, but often fails to maximize restoration of visual acuity. Spectacle overcorrection of residual refractive error may be helpful (20). However, this also often results in inadequate visual performance. A rigid contact lens may provide an excellent correction of refractive error. However, *in vivo* flexure and decentration can be limiting factors in visual performance. The potential for flexure and lens instability in this group is much greater because of corneal irregularity. Lens instability becomes the primary concern; the end result is poor patient comfort and contact lens intolerance. The potential is for poor visual result or limited tolerance. The potential for poor visual result or limited tolerance is exacerbated by the attendant compromised patient profile.

For the patient with irregular corneal topography and attendant refractive error, a piggyback system offers a logical solution. As this system is not without limitations, an initial trial with hydrogel (with or without spectacles) and rigid lens options is warranted. The primary benefit of this system compared to hydrogel and rigid lenses used alone is the ability to provide the potentiality of improved stability, comfort, and vision. A well-fit hydrogel lens will provide good corneal surface symmetry, thus preventing areas of harsh bearing between the rigid lens and cornea. In addition, rigid lens tolerance often is greatly improved because

TABLE 24.3. APPLICATIONS OF THE PIGGYBACK LENS SYSTEM

Trauma	Corneal Disease	Post
Perforation	Keratoconus	Aphakia
Laceration	Furrow dystrophy	Penetrating keratoplasty
Burns	Pterygia	
Contact lenses	Ulceration	Lamellar keratoplasty
	Bullous keratopathy	

of the bandage effect of a hydrogel lens. The overlying rigid lens will complete the system by correcting for the irregular astigmatism originating from the anterior corneal surface.

Appropriate utilization of a piggyback system involves proper patient selection and skillful clinical application. Only when the use of hydrogel (with or without spectacles) and rigid lenses has failed should one consider simultaneous lens systems.

Fitting Considerations

Successful application of a piggyback system necessitates a basic understanding of soft and rigid lens fitting, as well as how the two interact. As the candidate for a piggyback system often has a complex history, special consideration must be given to preexisting ocular pathology. The elderly patient with aphakia who has undergone a penetrating keratoplasty and necessitates a piggyback combination must be evaluated differently than the young patient with advanced keratoconus who desires this alternative in lieu of a penetrating keratoplasty. In addition to reviewing the uniqueness of clinical presentation, each candidate for a piggyback system needs to be evaluated in three phases: first, selection and evaluation of the appropriate soft lens; second, selection and evaluation of the appropriate rigid lens; and third, long-term monitoring of the combination.

Initial selection of a soft lens is the result of many factors, including preexisting pathology, corneal topography, and refractive status. As a general rule, materials must be fairly durable and highly oxygen permeable. Low water (<45%) ultrathin and midwater (45% to 55%) thin lens materials perform successfully for many myopic refractive errors. Silicone hydrogels are tried first since they have excellent physiologic characteristics and are generally well tolerated by the cornea. Unfortunately, they may not always fit properly due to limited parameters available. In addition, the unique topography that is being fitted often presents a challenge. The patient with advanced keratoconus who has a steep corneal profile and a highly myopic refractive error generally will only have success with a high-minus ultrathin design lens (21). These lenses have an extremely thin center thickness for maximum oxygen transmission and also are easier to handle in comparison to their low-minus counterparts. In addition to providing improved comfort and stability for the overlying rigid lens, these lenses allow edge thickness to be maintained at a minimum value. However, the elderly aphakic patient with penetrating keratoplasty requires a different approach. This patient may have a relatively flat plateau topography that requires a high-plus correction. For this patient, a high water (<60%) aphakic carrier lens or a moderately plus power silicone hydrogel is recommended. This will provide a steeper optic cap on which to fit the overlying rigid lens. The result is a much more stable fit than is achievable by fitting a rigid lens alone. An additional benefit to this approach pertains to the patient's ability to

function without the overlying rigid lens. If the patient is monocular, the rigid lens can be removed at bedtime permitting overnight wear of the hydrogel lens. Therefore, the patient is able to function in the case of emergencies during the night. This approach must be viewed cautiously, however, as the use of extended wear lenses in patients with penetrating keratoplasty has certain risks, which is discussed later.

The primary objectives in soft lens fitting are good centration and adequate movement. Centration improves the potential of a successful rigid lens fit, and adequate movement minimizes retrolens debris stagnation of tears. Whenever possible, retrolens bubble formation should be avoided as a secondary consideration. Relative to traditional soft lens fitting, slightly more movement is desired in the diagnostic assessment of the piggyback hydrogel lens alone. The presence of a rigid lens usually will immobilize the underlying soft lens to varying degrees. By achieving slightly greater movement when evaluating the soft lens alone, the potential for tight lens sequelae in the piggyback phase can be minimized.

Once the appropriate soft lens has been selected and a diagnostic evaluation has been completed, overkeratometry should be performed. The presence of irregular astigmatism and the attending limitations of this procedure can adversely affect accuracy. As a rule, the accuracy of overkeratometry can be increased when assessing a clean lens, with an even tear film, and without infringement from the upper or lower tear meniscus. This can be best accomplished immediately after the blink in the patient with a wide aperture. In many situations, such as a scarred cornea or advanced keratoconus, the clarity and quality of mires will be improved greatly when compared to baseline keratometry. The results then can be used in selection of an initial diagnostic rigid lens.

As is true when selecting a soft lens, the material and design of the rigid piggyback lens must be considered. With the introduction of rigid gas-permeable materials in the late 1970s, the physiologic viability of piggyback options increased dramatically. The selection of a high-Dk material is indicated, as edema-related complications are almost certain when using a low-Dk rigid lens in a piggyback combination. Selection of a highly oxygen permeable silicone/acrylate or fluoro-silicone/acrylate lens will optimize corneal physiology. Care must be taken, however, that flexure and visual performance are not compromised by this strategy. Overkeratometry and static retinoscopy with the rigid lens in place are indicated. Initial design selection can be performed in a traditional fashion. Evaluating palpebral aperture, horizontal visible iris diameter, and overkeratometry assist in overall diameter, optical zone diameter, and base curve radius selection. In addition to a good visual response, primary objectives include optimum centration and movement. High molecular weight fluorescein will assist in evaluation of the soft-rigid lens interface. This interface is critical to the possibility of this system adversely affecting both physiology and vision. Excess apical clearance with attending interlens tear stagnation can result in variable vision, debris entrapment, and possible reduced oxygen transmission. Excessive apical touch with attending inferior decentration and pseudoadherence can be equally detrimental. Whenever achievable, an aligned fluorescein pattern with optimum centration should be present. This often can be obtained by overall diameter, optic zone diameter, and base curve radius manipulation during diagnostic fitting. If this cannot be resolved through use of varying rigid lens measurements, reevaluation of the soft lens may be necessary. By altering the design and prescription of the soft lens, the optic cap dimension on which the rigid lens will be fit can be changed effectively. This is demonstrated most dramatically when working with patients who have had penetrating keratoplasty and flat, plateaulike corneal topographies. By altering the prescription in the soft lens from a low-minus to midrange plus, the optic cap topography often can be improved and better rigid lens centration obtained.

With the piggyback combination in place, a spherocylindrical overrefraction will determine the final power requirements of the system. Please note that a soft lens power change will not have the same effect as a rigid lens change. A necessary additional spherical prescription can be incorporated in either component of the system. Residual cylindrical prescription and bifocal additions can be incorporated in spectacles worn over the contact lens combination.

Another alternative for an improved lens fit pertains to the FlexlensR (22) piggyback carrier lens. This lathe-cut, hefilcon A lens features a recessed bed for application of the rigid lens. The diameter of the recess can vary from 7.5 to 9.5 mm to accommodate a wide variety of rigid lens diameters. The recess depth varies from 0.19 to 0.24 mm to assure rigid lens stability. Although this is a good alternative for assuring lens stability, one must be aware of the possible compromises in corneal physiologic response resulting from using a thick carrier lens.

Lens Care and Ancillary Considerations

Certainly, a limitation of piggyback lens systems pertains to lens care. As a general rule, each component should be maintained with its own system. The soft lens care system should consist of a daily surfactant, sterile saline care with heat, chemical, or oxidative disinfection on a nightly basis. The use of a weekly surfactant or enzyme, as well as rewetting drops, on an as-needed basis is also recommended. The rigid-care system should include cleaning daily with a surfactant and a disinfecting solution. Where complexity of compliance may become a problem, a hydrogel surfactant and disinfectant can be used, with heat being an obvious exception. Of course, should this not prove efficacious for optimum cleaning, a rigid lens system is necessary. The use of a weekly surfactant or enzymatic cleaner can be employed on an as-needed basis; an adjunct lubricant similarly can be used. Care must be exercised in the indiscriminate use of benzalkonium chloride because of the toxicity associated with this preservative and hydrogel lens materials.

Piggyback lens system insertion involves the traditional technique with each lens being applied separately. Lens removal often is best accomplished by removing the soft lens in the usual fashion, with the overlying rigid lens simultaneously removed. The instillation of a rewetting drop prior to removal facilitates the process. Also, using a tinted hydrogel lens may facilitate handling.

The wearing schedule can vary depending on patient demands and the corneal physiologic response. Patients are encouraged to remove the overlying rigid lens later in the day if an ability to function with the hydrogel lens alone is demonstrated. A pair of spectacles over the hydrogel lens alone may enhance visual performance if the corneal physiologic response is compromised by all-day piggyback wear.

Complications

As is true of any contact lens application, the potential for complications exists. This is especially evident when using a piggyback lens system. The combination of lenses in the presence of a compromised ocular environment greatly increases the risk for complications. To manage these patients effectively, one must be aware of various complications that may occur during the wearing of multiple lenses.

Hypoxia

Certainly one of the most common concerns when using a piggyback system pertains to induced corneal hypoxia and attendant sequelae. The effects of lens-induced hypoxia on the corneal epithelium, stroma, and endothelium have been well documented (23). In recent years, many researchers have developed oxygen-transmission guidelines commensurate with hypoxia-free daily lens wear (24). Manufacturers have responded with materials and designs that meet these requirements for the average patient. Unfortunately, employing multiple lenses simultaneously can create certain problems. In addition to the reduced oxygen transmission associated with wearing two types of contact lenses, there is the concern of a significantly thick tear film at the soft-rigid lens interface. This tear film may further impede oxygen transmission. Management of the patient using a piggyback system and manifesting corneal edema can be difficult. Indeed, the patient with penetrating keratoplasty and marginal graft viability may be reluctant to comply with all therapy. Other individuals can be managed more successfully by selecting alternate materials, improving design, and limiting wearing time. For some patients, such as those with endstage keratoconus for whom penetrating keratoplasty is imminent, management of piggyback lens-induced corneal edema may be temporary. For the post–penetrating keratoplasty patient, however, edema management and graft maintenance can be a lifelong commitment.

Corneal Neovascularization

Perhaps the most potentially significant sequela of long-term hypoxia is the potential for corneal neovascularization. Although this entity is not thought to be purely hypoxia mediated, the role of hypoxia in its pathogenesis is evident (25). Neovascularization is a major concern for many candidates for the piggyback system. Eyes that have been traumatized, diseased, or surgically altered often manifest a history of edema, inflammation, and other stimuli necessary for neovascularization. This is frequently observed in the patient with penetrating keratoplasty and neovascularization to the graft or host junction, or in the patient with a corneal laceration and neovascularization along the wound edge. Since these changes are evident in the prefit phase, it becomes very important for the clinician to photodocument this activity and proceed cautiously. Management of contact lens-induced vascular ingrowth must be directed at minimizing hypoxia, inflammation, and perhaps a yet-undetermined variable (26). The selection of lens material, design, and wearing time becomes very important. By altering lens material and design selection, the oxygen transmission can be increased. Equally important is achieving sufficient movement to assure adequate tear exchange, thus preventing retrolens debris entrapment.

Retrolens Debris

Another possible adverse response pertains to inadequate lens system movement and the attending retrolens debris entrapment. An acute red-eye response, commonly observed in hydrogel lens extended wear, may occur in the patient using a piggyback system as well. Although the pathogenesis of this condition is not fully understood, the role of inadequate lens movement and retrolens debris entrapment is a possible contributing factor (27). Patient symptomatology and the overall clinical picture can be quite variable, often easily confused with other non–lens-related entities. The differential diagnosis is important, particularly in the patient with penetrating keratoplasty who may be manifesting incipient graft rejection. Management of the piggyback lens-induced acute red eye is twofold. First, all efforts should be made to assure sufficient movement of both lenses in the system. Second, long-term maintenance, especially good lens hygiene, frequent instillation of lens rewetting drops, and frequent replacement of the hydrogel carrier lens can minimize this condition.

Papillary Conjunctivitis

Another complication, secondary to inflammation, that is associated with soiled lens wear is contact lens papillary conjunctivitis. The exact variables in the pathogenesis of this disease remain somewhat obscure, although the presence of patient predisposition, lid trauma, and lens deposits is evident (28). The patient using a piggyback system may be particularly at risk as a result of an existing patient profile. Patient status of post-penetrating keratoplasty or repair of corneal laceration may already manifest suture-induced superior tarsal papillary changes. The patient with keratoconus, with a history of atopy and of having worn thick-edged high-minus contact lens correction for a number of years, may also manifest tarsal papillary conjunctivitis. Management must be directed toward lessening lid trauma and minimizing deposits. A certain amount of lid trauma is imminent during blinking, but careful attention to edge profile in both the hydrogel lens and the rigid lens can be beneficial. Lens deposits can be managed effectively through maximum lens hygiene and frequent lens replacement. Whenever possible, disposable lenses should be employed to minimize solution related problems. The use of enzymatic cleaner, at minimum once per week, is recommended. Frequent hydrogel lens replacement and routine rigid lens polishing, although less critical, should be considered in the management.

Adherence

A *pseudoadherence* can occur, in which the rigid lens decenters and becomes immobilized on the hydrogel lens, although this is not the same as the true adherence syndrome associated with rigid lens wear (29). Retained interlens debris can reduce vision and the immobile rigid lens can manifest tight-lens symptoms. Management of this phenomenon is difficult at best. Strategies such as reducing overall diameter, flattening the base curve, and increasing axial edge lift have met with some success (30). If positive signs and symptoms persist, discontinuation may be the only option.

Reduction in Vision

The visual response of a piggyback system is often quite satisfactory. Variable vision may be associated with surface contamination or interlens debris entrapment and can be managed as discussed earlier. *In vivo* flexure occasionally can interfere with visual performance as well. Management of this problem lies primarily in lens design. If the astigmatism is with-the-rule, a lid attachment design, increased center thickness, flatter base curve radius, or smaller optical zone diameter may be beneficial (31). As the astigmatism is often irregular and oblique, the only viable strategy may be increased center thickness or movement to a more flexural-resistant material. However, the selection of this material may result in reduced oxygen transmission and possible long-term physiologic complications.

As is true of any contact lens application, complications are minimized by appropriate diagnostic evaluation, careful follow-up, and full patient participation. A complete understanding of lens handling, lens hygiene, wearing schedule, and warning symptoms is mandatory. The piggyback lens patient generally is sensitive to these issues, as this modality may be their only option.

SUMMARY

The development of hybrid materials and designs has made a significant impact on contact lens practice. Commensurate with more sophisticated options has been the ability to provide contact lens correction for a larger segment of the population. However, the development of new technology also has mandated a more advanced approach to contact lens fitting. This trend will continue as more hybrid options are developed in the years to come.

REFERENCES

1. Barr JB, Bailey NJ. 1989 annual report: part 1. *Contact Lens Spectr* 1989;1:39.
2. Hill RM. Hydrophilic "horse trades." *Int Contact Lens Clin* 1984; 1:190.
3. Fatt I. Gas transmission properties of soft contact lenses. In: Ruben M, ed. *Clinical and applied technology.* New York: John Wiley & Sons, 1978:106.
4. Hill RM, Brezinski SD. The great water race. *Contact Lens Spectr* 1986;9:21.
5. Isaacson W, Rodrigues O. Flexible fluoropolymer. *Contact Lens Spectr* 1989;1:60.
6. Brennan N, Efron N, Holden B. Oxygen permeabilities of hard gas permeable contact lens materials. *Clin Exp Optom* 1986;69: 82.
7. Grohe R, Caroline P. Rigid gas permeable non-wetting lens syndrome. *Contact Lens Spectr* 1989;3:32.
8. McMonnies C. How well do high Dk lenses correct astigmatism? Paper presented at: Bausch & Lomb National Research Symposium; August 1987; Washington, DC.
9. *Saturn II professional fitting guide.* Precision-Cosmet Company, Inc., 1985.
10. Zilliox J. Fitting the Saturn II. *Contact Lens Forum* 1985;12:54.
11. Hartstein J. Contact lens update. *Ocul Surg News* 1985:2.
12. Soper J. Fitting keratoconus with piggy-back and Saturn II. *Contact Lens Forum* 1986;8:25.
13. Saturn II [package insert]. Precision-Cosmet Company, Inc., 1985.
14. Powell J. Saturn II technology. Paper presented at: Saturn II Educational Seminar; April 1985; Phoenix, AZ.
15. *SoftPerm fitting guide.* Sola/Barnes Hind, Inc., 1989.
16. Winegar W. A management overview of the keratoconus patient. *Contact Lens Forum* 1989;2:28.
17. Baldone J. Piggyback fitting in keratoconus. In: Gassett AR, Kaufman HE, eds. *Soft contact lenses.* St. Louis: CV Mosby, 1972: 167.
18. Romanchuk K, Braun D. Piggyback fitting in a case of corneal scarring. *CLAO J* 1987;13:177.
19. Soper J, Paton D. A piggyback contact lens system for corneal transplants and other cases with high astigmatism. *Contact Lens Intraocul Lens Med J* 1980;6:132.
20. Mannis M. Indications for contact lens fitting after keratoplasty. *CLAO J* 1986;12:225.
21. Weissman BA. An old-new piggyback fit. *Contact Lens Forum* 1982;6:71.
22. Caroline P, Doughman D. A new piggyback lens design for correction of irregular astigmatism: a preliminary report. *Contact Lens J* 1979;5:40.
23. Holden BA et al. Effects of long term extended contact lens wear in the human cornea. *Invest Ophthalmol Vis Sci* 1985;26:1489.
24. Holden BA, Sweeney DF, Sanderson G. The minimum precorneal oxygen tension to avoid corneal edema. *Invest Ophthalmol Vis Sci* 1984;25:476.
25. Baum JL, Martola EL. Corneal edema and corneal neovascularization. *Am J Ophthalmol* 1968;65:881.
26. Robin JB et al. The histopathology of corneal neovascularization inhibitory effects. *Arch Ophthalmol* 1985;103:284.
27. Weissman BA, Mondino BJ. Complications of extended wear contact lenses. *Int Eyecare* 1985;1:230.
28. Allansmith MR. Palpebral conjunctivitis: Factors associated with papillary response and contact lens wear. *J Am Optom Assoc* 1984; 55:199.
29. Kenyon E, Polse KA, Mandell RM. Rigid contact lens adherence: incidence, severity, and recovery. *J Am Optom Assoc* 1988;59: 168.
30. Swarbrick HA. A possible etiology for RGP lens binding (adherence). *Int Contact Lens Clin* 1988;15:13.
31. Herman JP. Flexure of rigid contact lenses on toric corneas as a function of base curve fitting relationships. *J Am Optom Assoc* 1983;54:209.

RIGID CONTACT LENSES AND ASTIGMATISM

JOEL A. SILBERT

The critical goals of contact lens design are to appropriately meet the physical and physiologic requirements of the cornea while concomitantly addressing the visual requirements of the eye. Eyes that exhibit large amounts of residual astigmatism or high corneal toricity present practitioners with formidable challenges. Most of these challenges are surmountable, however, with an orderly and logical approach to lens design.

Corneal toricity is often the major component contributing to a patient's total refractive astigmatism. Total refractive astigmatism, however, is influenced by numerous other factors. This may explain why refractive astigmatism (that astigmatism manifested in the best subjective refraction) may be more or less than that exhibited by the cornea, and may assume a different axis as well (1). The practitioner must therefore distinguish between the physical challenges of corneal toricity and the optical challenges presented by the type of contact lens employed.

RESIDUAL ASTIGMATISM

The contact lens practitioner must consider the possibility of each patient potentially having a *residual* astigmatic refractive error remaining when a contact lens is applied to the cornea to correct an existing ametropia. It has become commonplace to use the term *residual astigmatism* to pertain to the residual refractive error present with a spherical contact lens (1). It should be noted, however, that residual astigmatism is a generic term, and may encompass residual astigmatic errors differing in magnitude depending on the nature of the lens used (i.e., spherical rigid lens, spherical soft lens, rigid toric lens). Thus, one should more accurately speak of a residual astigmatism present *with* a particular lens type.

For example, the residual astigmatism present with a spherical rigid lens on the eye is approximately the difference between the corneal astigmatism and the refractive astigmatism of the eye. Yet, the residual astigmatism of a spherical hydrogel lens is simply the same as the refractive astigmatism itself.

There are two general sources of residual astigmatism,

the first being the components of the eye's refractive system. As such, this is termed *physiologic residual astigmatism,* which may arise from any or all of the following (2,3):

1. Contributed power from the posterior cornea–aqueous interface
2. Contributed power from the different meridians of the crystalline lens interfaces
3. Tilt of the crystalline lens
4. Variations in refractive index of the cornea, lens, and other media
5. The fluid lens not fully neutralizing the anterior corneal surface astigmatism
6. Obliquity of light incident to the cornea
7. Irregularities in shape or eccentricity of the fovea

As the physiologic astigmatism may result from cornea, lens, vitreous, or retinal sources, it should be clear that clinically the astigmatism cannot be distinguished among these sources, nor is that necessary. Together they constitute the *total physiologic residual astigmatism,* over which there is no control.

Physiologic astigmatism may be exacerbated by or diminished by the *induced residual astigmatism,* the second source of residual cylinder. The induced residual astigmatism is that astigmatic error contributed by the presence of the lens itself on the eye, and may result from lens warpage (4), lens flexure on the eye (5–8), lens decentration (as illustrated by a high-riding lens inducing with-the-rule cylinder), contact lens tilt (inducing radial astigmatism, especially in highly powered lenses) (9), and toric anterior and/or posterior curvatures on a rigid contact lens (10,11).

Residual astigmatism, therefore, made up of both physiologic and induced components, may decrease the visual performance of a contact lens. This may have the effect of reducing visual acuity and possibly initiating asthenopic symptoms. If either of these problems occurs, then residual astigmatism must be corrected or a different type of lens chosen that produces less physiologic astigmatism.

Calculated Residual Astigmatism

The approximate amount of residual astigmatism that may be observed in a patient wearing a rigid spherical lens can be predicted by calculation, if the keratometric reading and spectacle refraction are known. In its simplest terms, the *calculated residual astigmatism* (CRA) is the difference between the keratometric cylinder (ΔK) and the spectacle cylinder or *total refractive astigmatism* (TRA), as shown in the following examples:

CRA = TRA − ΔK

Example:
Spectacle Rx −1.00 −2.00 × 90
Keratometer 44.00 @ 90 / 45.00 @ 180

CRA = TRA − ΔK
     = −2.00 × 90 − (−1.00 × 90)
     = −1.00 × 90

Note that for a *spherical* hydrogel, the CRA is simply equal to the refractive astigmatism (in other words, CRA = TRA) or − 2.00 × 90, whereas the CRA for a rigid spherical lens is − 1.00 × 90.

Example:
Spectacle Rx −3.00 −0.50 × 90
Keratometer 43.50 @ 180 / 43.50 @ 90 (spherical)
(On inspection, note that there is no cylinder in the tear lens. Thus, CRA = − 0.50 × 90)
   or

CRA = TRA − ΔK
     − 0.50 × 90 − [0]
     = − 0.50 × 90

Example:
Spectacle Rx +1.75 − 2.75 × 180
Keratometer 42.00 @ 180 / 44.00 @ 90

CRA = TRA - ΔK
     = − 2.75 × 180 − [−2.00 × 180]
     = − 0.75 × 180

Example:
Spectacle Rx − 1.50 −1.50 × 015
Keratometer 41.00 @ 015 / 44.00 @ 105

CRA = TRA − ΔK
     = − 1.50 × 015 − [−3.00 × 015]
     = + 1.50 × 015
Transpose: + 1.50 −1.50 × 105
CRA = − 1.50 × 105

Note that if the patient's spectacle prescription is high (over ± 4.00 D.), then vertex distance adjustments must be made in *each major meridian* before calculating the residual astigmatism, as illustrated in the following example:

Example:
Spectacle Rx + 12.00 −3.00 × 180
Spectacle vertex: 12 mm
Keratometer 42.00 @ 180 / 45.00 @ 90
 At the corneal plane:
the adjusted power effective at 180° = + 14.00 D

the adjusted power effective at 90° = + 10.00 D
Thus, the corneal plane Rx is

+ 14.00 = − 4.00 × 180
CRA = TRA - ΔK
     = − 4.00 × 180 − [−3.00 × 180]
     = − 1.00 × 180

Note that in this example, if the vertex distance calculations had been ignored, the CRA would be predicted to equal *zero*. Vertex power adjustments must be made whenever the power of either principal meridian in the spectacle prescription is equal or greater than ± 4.00 D.

Measured Residual Astigmatism

Studies have shown that while there is a low positive correlation between the CRA and the actual or *measured residual astigmatism* (MRA), there can be a significant variance between them, with the MRA often being less than the CRA (12).

For example, Sarver (13) determined the mean CRA for 408 eyes wearing spherical polymethylmethacrylate (PMMA) lenses to be approximately 0.50 D against-the-rule, with the mean MRA equaling approximately 0.25 D against-the-rule. Such studies have led to the possibility of predicting the MRA from the CRA using regression equations (10,13). However, the range of predicted values for any given patient, using such a technique, can be quite large. Thus, from a clinical standpoint, a refraction performed over spherical diagnostic lenses is preferred to determine whether a significant residual astigmatism exists, and whether it will adversely affect a patient wearing spherical rigid lenses.

There are a number of causes for the differences found between CRA and MRA. The first is based on an assumption, namely that the keratometric values for corneal curvature are accurate measures of radius of curvature of the major meridians for that part of the cornea used to form a foveal image. This assumption is further based on an assumption that the corneal *cap* is spherical along each meridian (14). In reality, most of the cornea is aspheric in shape (15) and there is no anatomical corneal cap. In addition, the keratometer reading is based on only two points in each principal meridian, approximately 3 mm apart, which is averaged to produce the spherical reading observed on the instrument drum. Unlike corneal topography, the keratometer inherently assumes sphericity between these points, which is not the case. Thus, keratometric values that are intended to give an accurate measure of "*K*" have a number of intrinsic inaccuracies.

Secondly, astigmatic errors are introduced whenever incidence of light on the anterior cornea is oblique to this surface. This error, which may occur with angles of oblique incidence as little as 3 to 5 degrees, is a common one with ophthalmic measuring instruments and may add 0.50 D or more of against-the-rule astigmatism with horizontal plane errors (16).

Furthermore, the sources of contact lens–induced residual astigmatism discussed earlier may all add inaccuracies to the CRA value. For example, it is assumed that a rigid lens is not itself bending on the cornea, and thus does not introduce a cylindrical error. However, thin lenses do flex on toric corneas. When this occurs, a 0.25-D cylindrical error is introduced for each 0.25 D of flexure (6).

Incidence

The incidence of residual astigmatism is rather high among patients wearing spherical contact lenses. Bailey (17) found that 66% of 105 subjects fitted in this manner showed at least 0.50 D of residual astigmatism in one or both eyes, and 37% of the 208 eyes in the study demonstrated 0.75 D or more.

Sarver (14), in a study involving 250 patients with 408 eyes wearing spherical lenses, found a mean value of -0.23 D axis 90 $\pm$ 30 degrees, with a standard deviation of $\pm$ 0.30 D. In this study, 34% of the eyes showed residual astigmatism of 0.50 D or more.

Although residual astigmatism is common, the practitioner fitting a patient who has a CRA of -1.00×90 should not assume that this patient's use of spherical rigid lenses will fail. As we have seen, actual astigmatism or MRA is often less than the CRA for patients with against-the-rule astigmatism. Indeed, this patient may exhibit an MRA of 0.50 D or less at axis 90, and may see satisfactorily. Thus, it is wise to evaluate such a patient with a diagnostic spherical lens for optical considerations, and not only for physical fit.

When the MRA is 0.75 D or higher, the clinician should become more concerned, as reduced visual acuity and/or asthenopia may result. A decision must be made by the clinician on whether to proceed with a spherical lens design or a more complex lens. Some patients may not require critical vision as, for example, when wearing lenses for social activities. Under these circumstances, uncorrected residual astigmatism may be tolerated as long as it does not cause eyestrain. On the other hand, should the uncorrected MRA reduce the acuity to unsatisfactory levels, then the practitioner must seek to correct it. Most patients with an MRA of 0.50 D or less function extremely well with spherical rigid lenses, experiencing neither asthenopia nor reduced visual acuity. For patients with an MRA of 0.75 D or higher, even if acuity levels appear to be satisfactory at first, as the lenses are worn regularly asthenopia usually develops. As lenses are worn more regularly, the accommodative system is probably overactivated in an unconscious and futile attempt to stabilize the *interval of Sturm,* which is created by the residual astigmatic error. For these patients, and any others who do a lot of extended near work, the residual astigmatism may be corrected by:

1. Spectacles worn over spherical contact lenses to correct the residual error.
2. Special lens design, such as a front-surface toric rigid lens, or a toric soft lens.
3. The use of spherical rigid lenses with nonstandard lens thickness, when appropriate, either to increase or decrease lens flexure, thus modifying the amount of measured residual astigmatism.

LENS DESIGN

Flexure

Rigid spherical lenses demonstrate a property known as *flexure* in which the plastic may flex or conform somewhat to the underlying corneal toricity. Rigid spherical lenses are only *rigid* in the true sense of the word in the upper thickness ranges used by the manufacturers. For any lens material, there is a *critical thickness* below which flexure begins to become clinically significant. These amounts are generally small, but may become meaningful as the lens is made thinner. Indeed, for some patients, using too thin a lens, especially if gas permeable (GP), may increase flexure to a degree that negates the optical value of using a rigid lens, as when corneal and refractive astigmatism are present in the same amount and axis, which is the ideal circumstance for use of a nonflexing lens. This is why GP lenses usually are made with greater center thickness than PMMA lenses of similar design.

Flexure thus can be harmful to visual acuity if it increases the amount of unwanted residual astigmatism. On the other hand, flexure can be quite advantageous in those instances where a lens can be made thinner and still maintain optical stability, and when used on corneas of certain toricity. This is particularly useful, as flexure is a function not only of lens thickness, but also of a given material and lens-cornea fitting relationship. *Planned flexure* can be a valuable tool for the practitioner when used appropriately to correct all or part of a patient's residual astigmatism.

The clinician can observe contact lens flexure on the eye by taking a keratometric reading of the lens while worn by the patient. Such an "over-K" measurement may demonstrate lens flexure in a rigid lens if there is a significant difference found in the radii of the principal meridians of the cornea and if the lens is manufactured thinner than its critical thickness.

Harris and co-workers (18,19) showed that PMMA has the highest resistance to flexure of several lens materials investigated, with a critical thickness of 0.12 mm. Flexure of PMMA lenses begins when center thickness is less than this value, with an inverse relationship that more flexure occurs as the lens is made thinner. Flexure also increases proportionally to corneal toricity (Figs. 25.1 and 25.2).

Many of today's GP lens materials (silicone acrylates and fluoro-silicone acrylates) have higher critical thicknesses

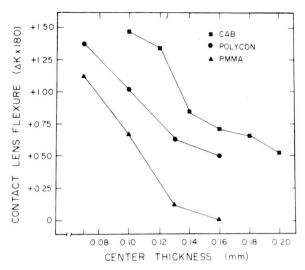

FIG. 25.1. Mean contact lens flexure found with cellulose acetate butyrate, Polycon, and PMMA lenses as a function of lens center thickness. (Reproduced with permission from Harris MG, Sweeney KE, Rocchi S. et al. Flexure and residual astigmatism with cellulose acetate butyrate (CAB) contact lenses on toric corneas. *Am J Optom Physiol Opt* 1982;59:859–862.)

than PMMA. In other words, GP lenses will typically begin to show flexure at lens thicknesses where PMMA would not, which accounts for some of the optical drawbacks of these materials when lenses are made too thin. Thus, many first- and second-generation GP lens materials must be made somewhat thicker (on the order of 0.02 to 0.04 mm) to reduce this increased flexure characteristic. However, making lenses thicker may in turn make the lens design less than desirable owing to increased weight and edge thickness, and perhaps reduced oxygen transmissivity. Newer third-

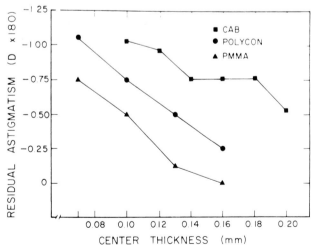

FIG. 25.2. Mean induced residual astigmatism with cellulose acetate butyrate, Polycon, and PMMA lenses. (From Harris MG, Sweeney KE, Rocchi S, et al. Flexure and residual astigmatism with cellulose acetate butyrate (CAB) contact lenses on toric corneas. *Am J Optom Physiol Opt* 1982;59:859–862, with permission.)

generation lens materials have recently been introduced that once again have allowed the practitioner to prescribe a thin GP lens that does not exhibit the optical problems of flexure. The clinician who prescribes GP lenses must not only be familiar with the optics of these lenses, but must also become familiar with these material properties, when selecting the right material for his or her patient.

The work of Harris and co-workers (18,19) described above can be summarized as follows:

1. Spherical lenses that are fit on spherical corneas should produce no lens flexure if the lens is centered.
2. Thinner lenses will flex in the direction of the corneal toricity, in the amounts seen in Figs. 25.1 and 25.2.

Pole (9) measured flexure and residual astigmatism in 12 eyes with with-the-rule corneal toricities wearing Polycon I lenses, ranging from 1.00 D *steeper than K* to 1.00 D *flatter than K* fits. Those lenses fit steeply flexed more than lenses fit *on K* or flatter than K (Fig. 25.3).

Herman (20) showed that flexure may be controlled further by the lens-cornea fitting relationship, such that flexure may be increased or decreased if a lens does not center. This may be seen in Fig. 25.4, in which a flat fit using a 9.5-mm Polycon lens, which leads to a high riding, lid-attachment fit on a with-the-rule cornea, will actually reduce lens flexure. Flexure is probably reduced because the lens rides higher, thereby moving closer to the flatter peri-limbal region, and thus reduces the difference between the two principal flexure meridians. Thin lens design thus can be used *without* the accompanying problems of lens flexure, if designed by the fitter in this fashion. If the clinician were to disregard this and fit this lens too steeply, it would work against lid attachment and higher lens positioning, thus *increasing* lens flexure on with-the-rule astigmatic corneas and likely reducing visual acuity. By the same token, if the clinician wishes lens flexure to occur, a modified fitting strategy of fitting the patient with a small and very thin lens steeper than K should produce the desired result. The opposite effects are illustrated in Fig. 25.4 for against-the-rule corneas.

Prior to the introduction of GP lenses, many clinicians recognized the improvement in physical fit and physiology that was possible with the use of ultrathin PMMA lenses (lenses made below 0.12 mm in thickness). These typically small diameter (8.0 to 8.5mm) lenses were thin and lightweight, centered well, and often were fitted steeper than K. Of interest was the observation that many patients had less than desirable visual acuity, obviously caused by lens flexure in the direction of the patient's corneal toricity. This flexure-induced reduction in acuity was resolved only when the practitioner remade the lens somewhat thicker and larger (above the critical thickness for PMMA). Indeed, a review of these cases would demonstrate that these patients had about the same amount of corneal and refractive astigmatism, thus requiring a rigid or nonflexing lens to correct the refractive astigmatism.

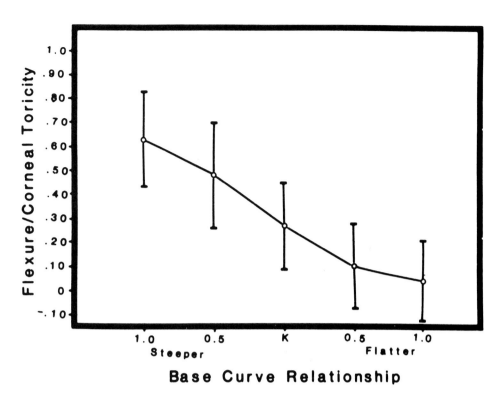

FIG. 25.3. Amount of lens flexure as a function of base curve relationship. (From Pole JJ. The effect of the base curve on the flexure of Polycon Lenses. *Int Cont Lens Clin* 1983;10: 49–52, with permission.)

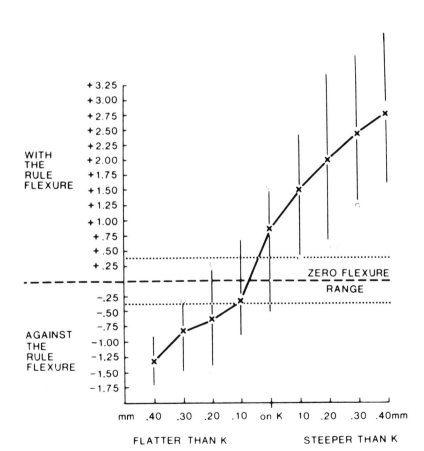

FIG. 25.4. Flexure results of 9.5-mm Polycon I and II inventory design lenses on corneas ranging in toricity from 0.75 D to 5.00 D with-the-rule as a function of base curve fitting relationship. (From Herman JP. Flexure of rigid contact lenses on toric corneas as a function of base curve fitting relationship. *J Am Optom Assoc* 1983;54:209–213, with permission.)

However, some patients who previously experienced reduced visual acuity with rigid, nonflexing spherical lenses as a result of internal, physiologic astigmatism were found to achieve excellent visual acuity when ultrathin flexing lenses were used. This paradox can easily be explained by recognizing that flexible lenses can represent either a "boon or bane" depending on whether flexure is desired or not. The use of spherical, ultrathin lenses can indeed be very helpful as a clinical tool for dealing with residual astigmatism, *if and when* certain conditions are met:

1. The corneal toricity demonstrates significant with-the-rule astigmatism
2. The refractive astigmatism demonstrates substantially less with-the-rule. (In other words, the patient demonstrates against-the-rule residual astigmatism when wearing a spherical rigid, nonflexing lens.)

The following example shows how "planned flexure" using an ultrathin spherical lens can be used to correct for the above problem:

Example:
Spectacle Rx $-2.00 - 1.00 \times 180$
Keratometer 43.00 @ 180 / 45.00 @ 90

$$\text{CRA} = \text{TRA} - \Delta K \text{ (for rigid spherical lenses)}$$
$$= -1.00 \times 180 - (-2.00 \times 180)$$
$$= +1.00 \times 180$$

Transpose: $+1.00 - 1.00 \times 90$
CRA = -1.00×90 (for a rigid spherical lens)

However, if a Polycon II interpalpebral design (8.5 to 9.0 diameter) is chosen with a center thickness of 0.09 mm, the lens will flex approximately 30% of the corneal toricity (19) in the direction of the with-the-rule cornea and even more so if we fit *steeper than K*. As the lens flexes about 30% of the corneal toricity (0.3×2.00 D), then 0.60 D of the previously calculated residual cylinder will be eliminated, leaving the patient with less than 0.50 D of residual astigmatism at axis 90. Thus, the use of an ultrathin lens in this scenario provides *planned flexure* of a desirable type to reduce residual astigmatism to a clinically acceptable level, and thus greatly enhances visual acuity. It can also be seen from this example that planned flexure, using an ultrathin design, can negate the need for more complex methods of correcting residual astigmatism. The material chosen must of course be compatible with the use of very thin center thicknesses, thus making this impractical for the hyperopic patient. Polycon II material, however, is an example of a low-Dk GP material that is stable when cut to thicknesses such as those illustrated above for myopia, and lends itself well to this approach.

Residual Astigmatism with Spherical Soft Lenses

One also must look at predicted residual astigmatism for each patient by a considering the value of soft lenses over rigid lenses. As noted earlier, residual astigmatism for a soft spherical contact lens is equal to the patient's refractive astigmatism. Thus, as the refractive astigmatism approaches zero, the patient becomes an excellent candidate for spherical soft lenses, as optimal visual acuity would be achieved.

For a spherical soft lens, CRA = TRA

Example:
Spectacle Rx $-2.00 - 0.25 \times 180$
Keratometer 43.00 @ 180 / 44.50 @ 90

$$\text{CRA} = \text{TRA} - \Delta K \text{ for a rigid lens}$$
$$= -0.25 \times 180 - (-1.50 \times 180)$$
$$= +1.25 \times 180$$

Transpose: $+1.25 - 1.25 \times 90$)
Thus, TRA = -1.25×90 for a rigid spherical lens
But,

CRA = TRA for a soft spherical lens:
CRA = -0.25×180

Thus, the use of a spherical soft lens will provide much better visual acuity than the use of a rigid spherical lens, and will avoid the problems associated with complex front toric rigid lenses.

Soft Toric Lenses

While this chapter is devoted to rigid lens alternatives for correcting toric corneas and astigmatic refractive errors, it should be noted that perhaps the best method available today for correcting *refractive astigmatism* is the soft toric lens. With superior manufacturing techniques, including toric generated curves, slaboff thin zones, edge chamfers, eccentric lenticulation, and isometric ballasting, today's soft toric lenses provide good comfort, crisp optics, and a high degree of reproducibility. The use of diagnostic fitting sets makes the fitting of such lenses (discussed in detail in Chapter 26) relatively simple, and many newer designs are so stable in lens orientation that they may be designed empirically. In addition, the large range of *stock* parameters available, including correction of as low as 0.75-D cylinder errors, is ideal for the correction of residual astigmatism present with spherical lenses.

Furthermore, the ability of the practitioner to obtain customized soft toric lenses in round-the-clock axes and in almost unlimited refractive powers allows the use of such lenses for the correction of high-corneal and refractive astigmatism, as well as for use in postsurgical applications. However, as lens powers become higher, it becomes more difficult to control variations in meridional edge thickness. This increases the probability that custom soft toric lenses may mislocate from the desired axis, leading to blurred vision, instability of vision, or both. For this reason, rigid toric lenses are often a more useful option for the correction of high corneal astigmatism.

FRONT TORIC LENSES

When toric soft lenses cannot be used, or when other spherical lens options have been considered and found to be non-applicable, the practitioner may wish to design a front surface rigid toric lens for the correction of residual astigmatism. It should be emphasized from the outset that the use of such lenses is only for optical reasons, as they employ spherical base curve radii and, from the standpoint of physical fit, are no better (and perhaps may be worse) than conventional spherical lenses.

Front toric lenses are indicated for low-to-moderate degrees of corneal toricity (usually 2 D or less) and when there is a significant degree of residual astigmatism with spherical lenses. In addition to a spherical back curvature, this lens design incorporates base down prism and a toric front surface that generates the required degree of astigmatic correction. The prism is incorporated in order to reduce lens rotation triggered by the action of the lids (Fig. 25.5). As the blink normally causes the lower portion of the lens to rotate toward the nose, the incorporation of an adequate degree of prism ballast works to control and retard the degree of lens torque, thus keeping the front surface cylinder in a reasonably stabilized position.

Prism produces a continuous variation in thickness across the lens surface. The superior portion of the lens, or apex, is the thinnest part while the inferior base is the thickest. GP lens materials are necessary for good physiologic tolerance with front toric lenses, as corneal edema often is found with low-riding, ballasted lenses that may not exchange tears as readily.

Front toric lenses may be either *circular* or *truncated* (Fig. 25.6), and only rarely are double truncated. Truncation is added to front toric lens designs as another method of increasing lens stability. If not properly designed and fabricated, however, truncation may produce just the opposite effect and defeat the best intentions of the fitter.

Truncated Prism-ballasted Lenses

These lenses are indicated for patients with normal-to-high positioning lower lids, and upper lids at or near the limbus (Fig. 25.7). The basic lens design including overall diameter, base curve optic radius (BCR), and peripheral curve radii, is similar to that selected for conventional spherical lens design, but the overall diameter chosen is not large or lid controlled. The lens should lift with the blink and then settle inferocentrally. Except during blinking, the lens should not be in contact with the upper lid. Typically, vertical diameters are 8.7 to 9.2 mm, with horizontal diameters usually 0.4 to 0.5 mm greater. The vertical size of the lens must be large enough to extend beyond the superior edge of the pupil in dim illumination; usually 1 mm is adequate.

As the upper edge of the lens is thin, it must be well rounded and polished, so that it does not irritate the limbus. The truncation, designed to match the contour of the lower lid, must have a base edge that is properly shaped. This means that if the lens is designed to ride on the lower lid margin and not slip under it, then the edge should be broadly flat to increase the distribution of lens pressure across the maximum surface area of the lid (Fig. 25.8). Anterior tapering of the truncated edges should be avoided, as this will allow the lens to slip under the lower lid. Posterior tapering of the edge from back to front should also be avoided, as this places all the pressure of the lens on a small area of the lid, greatly increasing discomfort.

Because of the presence of truncation, the fitter should remember that significant ballast effect is lost in higher-minus prescriptions (and much less so in higher-plus prescriptions). The reduction in weight might allow the truncated base to lift off the lower lid instead of remaining in the desired position. Thus, more prism needs to be used in truncated lenses of higher-minus prescription to compensate for this loss. (Fig. 25.9) Typically, truncated prism-ballasted lenses require at least 1.50 to 1.75 prism diopters (21).

In order to maximize success with truncated design lenses, two additional features are essential. First, the optic zone (OZ) of the lens should be decentered upward about 0.5 mm to offset the relative geometric lowering of the OZ created by the truncation. This helps reduce flare and maintains better overall centration of the lens (Fig. 25.10). When flare persists, a larger vertical lens diameter must be used. Second, the fitter must remember to order the lens with the truncation *temporal to the base apex line* (22). This is necessary because prism-ballasted lenses typically ride with their base-apex line rotated nasally, approximately 15 to 20 degrees. If the lenses were truncated perpendicularly to the base-apex line, then the resulting lens would still rotate nasally (as this is determined by the prism base) and the truncation thus would not rest along the lower lid (Fig. 25.11). By truncating the lens temporally to the base-apex line by the amount of degrees of kick towards the nose (this

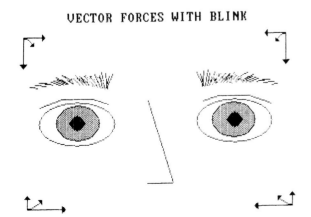

VECTOR FORCES WITH BLINK

FIG. 25.5. Tendency for nasalward lens rotation by lid forces during the blink.

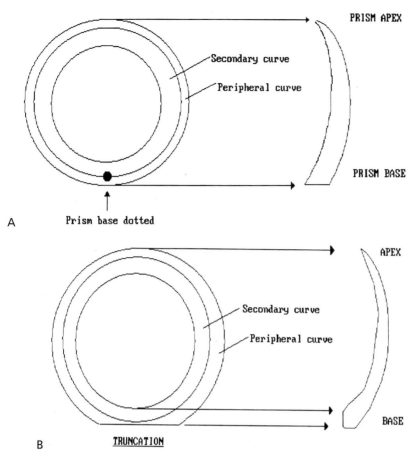

A

Prism base dotted

B   TRUNCATION

FIG. 25.6. (A) Circular, prism-ballasted front toric lens. (B) Truncated, prism-ballasted front toric lens.

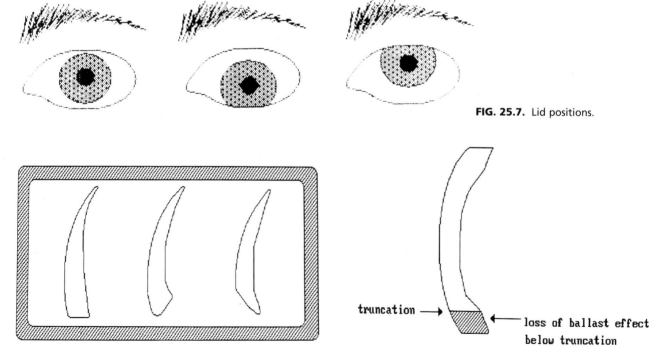

FIG. 25.7. Lid positions.

FIG. 25.8. Shape and contour of truncation in a front toric lens. Edge should be square, with little anterior or posterior tapering.

FIG. 25.9. Loss of ballast effect in truncation of higher-minus prescriptions.

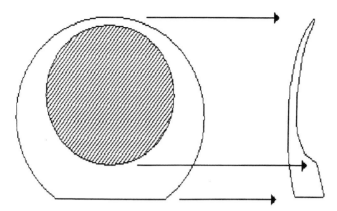

FIG. 25.10. Upward decentration of optic zone, in a truncated, prism-ballasted front toric lens.

can either be estimated at 15 to 20 degrees, or be measured more accurately using diagnostic prism lenses with their base apexes dotted), the finished lens will rest evenly along the lower lid. (Note that while the truncation rests more evenly along the lower lid, the prism base still will be rotated nasally.)

The practitioner who requires a truncated, prism-ballasted lens for a patient would benefit by contacting the laboratory for use of a spherical power prism-ballast diagnostic set, or the use of loaner lenses when designing the lens. This not only allows for more accurate observations of lens movement, torsion, and overall lens–cornea relationship through the use of fluorescein patterns, but also allows the practitioner to make a more accurate spherocylindrical overrefraction (23).

A spherical ballasted diagnostic lens is chosen with the BCR and other lens parameters as close as possible to the final design. The lens should be marked with the base-apex line dotted, and then carefully measured for drift angle of the prism base, in the same manner as is performed with soft toric lenses. This is conveniently done with a thin vertical parallelopiped beam of the biomicroscope placed in the cen-

ter of the lens, with the illumination system in click-stop position, normal to the cornea. The illuminating beam is rotated until it is perpendicular to the prism base of the lens, and the degrees of rotation read off the protractor scale of the illumination housing, or from an eyepiece reticule. If neither of these is available, a trial frame with a plano lens marked across its surface with a line, matches the position of the prism base of the contact lens, and the orientation is read off the trial frame axis scale (24) (Fig. 25.12). The fabricating laboratory is given a complete set of lens specifications, including the final spherocylindrical Rx and a description or diagram of the base-apex orientation.

The Circular Prism-ballasted Lens

A much simpler front-toric lens design for the correction of residual astigmatism is the circular prism-ballasted lens. It is indicated when patients have lower lids at or below the lower limbus, when there are large palpebral apertures, with loose lids, and, in general, when there are comfort problems associated with the truncated variety of lens.

In this design, there are fewer variables with which to be concerned. The lens has a centered optic zone, and less prism is required than with truncated lenses. Bailey (4) suggests the use of 0.75 to 1 prism diopter of ballast for moderate- to high-powered minus lenses. For plus as well as low-minus lenses, both of which have relatively thinner edges, Bailey (4) suggests the use of 1.25 to 1.5 prism diopters. The use of lower amounts of prism makes these lenses more comfortable and better tolerated physiologically. A conventional spherical diagnostic lens may be used to design the basic lens parameters, but again, the use of a prism-ballasted spherical diagnostic lens is preferable, as it allows the fitter to assess more accurately the lens dynamics, including actual lens rotation and the vertical position of the lens.

The techniques for measuring rotation have been de-

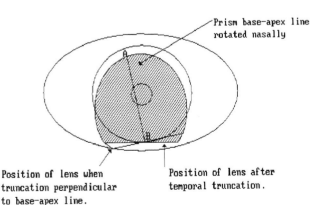

Prism base-apex line
rotated nasally

Position of lens when
truncation perpendicular
to base-apex line.

Position of lens after
temporal truncation.

FIG. 25.11. Truncation should be temporal to the base-apex line to allow the truncation to rest evenly along the lower lid.

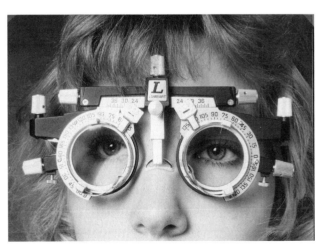

FIG. 25.12. Trial frame worn to measure angular rotation of a prism-ballasted lens.

scribed previously. In the absence of a prism lens, the fitter may use an average of 15 degrees as a reasonable estimate of lens rotation and proceed on this basis with the understanding that, for each patient, numerous variables exist that may make this estimate unreliable.

A careful spherocylindrical overrefraction is performed and added to the power of the spherical diagnostic lens. As with soft toric lenses, the practitioner must *compensate* for the number of degrees of angular rotation or drift angle of the prism base when determining the final contact lens prescription. The traditional LARS method (left add, right subtract) works well here, as it does with soft toric lenses:

For example, if the right lens were found to rotate 15 degrees toward the nose (or counterclockwise rotation) and the right subjective refraction axis was at 80 degrees, the right lens axis would be decreased by 15 degrees, resulting in a lens to be ordered at 65 degrees. Similarly, if the left lens were found to rotate 10 degrees toward the nose (or clockwise rotation) and the left subjective axis was at 90 degrees, the left axis would be increased by 10 degrees, resulting in a lens to be ordered at 100 degrees (Fig. 25.13).

Diagnostic lenses range in overall diameter from 8.8 mm (for steeper base curve radii) to 9.2 mm (for flatter curves), with standard spherical Rx power (e.g., −2.00 D or −3.00 D). Optic zones are 1.2 mm smaller than the overall diameter, peripheral curve radii of standard tricurve design, and each lens should have 1 prism diopter of ballast with the prism base dotted.

Bailey (4) uses similar lenses to design a spherical prism-ballasted lens that is fit to the patient's eye using the higher-minus meridian sphere power. Only after patient adaptation, when the lens is fully stabilized, is the process of deter-

mining the cylinder power and axis completed. Using special equipment, the same lens is modified with the necessary cylinder, or a final lens is reordered (25,26).

Circular prism-ballasted lenses will position inferocentrally, but should lift with the blink to assure adequate tear exchange. Vision will be comfortable if the pupil is covered adequately by the optic zone, if the correct refraction is used, and if lens torsion remains stable within ± 5 degrees. Excessive lens torque dictates that increased prism or other parameter modifications be considered (i.e., increase sagittal depth), as blurred vision will result after each blink. This is caused by obliquely crossed cylinders (the MRA and the front toric cylinder) altering the spherocylindrical equation.

Verification of Front Toric Lenses

To verify the power of a front toric lens, the clinician needs to follow certain steps:

1. Place the lens convex side up (as with spectacles or any back vertex measurement) against the lensometer stop.
2. Rotate the lens until the target mires show maximum base-down prism (i.e., axis 90 degrees).
3. Read sphere, cylinder, and axis in the usual manner.
4. Read the amount of prism, with the lens centered over the stop.

Note that as the thickness of the lens changes from its apex to its base, there is a gradual change in power, resulting from more vergence coming from the thicker portion. Prism lenses increase in plus power approximately 0.25 D per 0.1-mm increase in lens thickness (27). Thus, it may be difficult to obtain the target pattern in sharp focus because of this problem, as well as from other optical aberrations and manufacturing inaccuracies. Sarver (28) suggested a technique to reduce the aperture stop. He drilled a 3- or 4-mm hole through a thin layer of opaque plastic, which was then placed over the lensometer stop to reduce peripheral aberrations.

Prism Ballast and Binocularity

A front toric lens with prism for weighting purposes also produces vertical prism power before the eye. As most cases of residual astigmatism are bilateral (29), the corresponding bilateral vertical prism produces no significant effect on the underlying binocular system. However, if a prism-ballasted front toric lens were to be used on one eye only, there likely would be a need to incorporate prism in the fellow lens to avoid inducing or exacerbating a vertical phoria.

Sarver and Mandell (28) have shown that the prismatic effect of a plano-power contact lens varies across its surface, unlike plano-power flat prisms. Thus, a given prism contact lens does not have a specific prism power, as the prism power varies with regard to lens position on the eye. Furthermore, when spherical prescription power exists in a

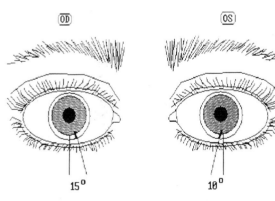

FIG. 25.13. LARS method of axis compensation. *(Left, right-eye diagram)* If subjective refraction axis is 80 degrees and 15 degrees rotation to the right is observed, *subtract* and order axis 65 degrees. *(Right, left-eye diagram)* If subjective refraction axis is 90 degrees and 10 degrees rotation to the left is observed, *add* and order axis 100 degrees.

prism-ballast lens, both base-up and base-down prism effect on either side of the optical center are generated. Lens position on the eye will determine both the type and magnitude of the actual prism effect (Fig. 25.14). Thus, in a unilateral prism lens fitting, lens position, although typically inferior, needs to be known in order to evaluate whether the lens prism effect will be beneficial or harmful to the patient's binocular status.

Nonprismatic Ballasted Lens Designs

There are two additional methods of lens stabilization worthy of note for the correction of residual astigmatism that do not require the incorporation of prism ballast.

Periballasted Lens

The periballast lens is made from a lenticulated lens with a high-minus carrier (30), the superior portion of which has been largely removed (Fig. 25.15).

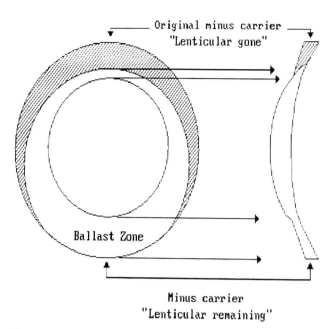

FIG. 25.15. The periballast lens. (From Wechsler S. The periballast lens for correcting residual astigmatism. *Rev Optom* 1979; 116:45–46, with permission.

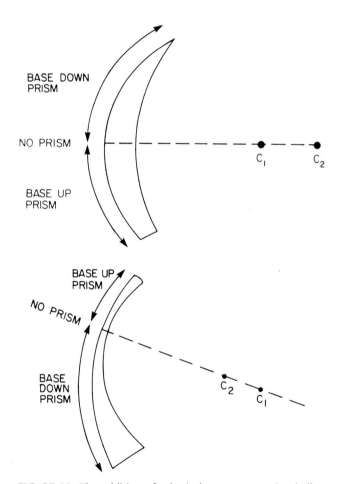

FIG. 25.14. The addition of spherical power to a prism-ballast contact lens changes the position of the optic center (*top*). A plus-power lens has base down prism above the optical center, and (*bottom*) a minus-power lens has base up prism. The prism is reversed below the optical center. (From Mandell RB. *Contact lens practice,* 4th ed. Springfield: Charles C Thomas, 1988:290, with permission.)

This leaves a finished lens with an inferior zone that is, in effect, ballasted, but which has no prism throughout the optical portion of the lens. This design has particular advantages in managing monocular residual astigmatism, as it avoids the inducement of vertical imbalance, which is potentially inherent with the use of a single prism-ballasted front toric lens. The optical quality of the lens is also superior to a prism-ballasted lens, as the dioptric powers are unchanging throughout the optical zone. In addition, as there is no prism, there are reduced optical aberrations (31). The periballast lens, since it is a lenticular design, can be made considerably thinner than the often thickly fabricated prism-ballast lens. This can be a major benefit in improved physiologic tolerance, especially when combining this design with rigid GP materials. Drawbacks to this design include inadequate stabilization in some patients with resulting visual blurring from the obliquely crossed cylinder effect, and lower lid discomfort.

It should be remembered that if the periballast lens rides on the lower lid, it will behave in the fashion of a prism-ballast lens and rotate nasally. Thus, measurement and compensation for this rotation must be made when ordering the final cylinder axis, in the manner previously described. However, if the lens is supported by the upper lid, as is likely with reduced-mass lenses, then it is probable that no axis compensation will be necessary.

Double Truncation

Although not commonly attempted, there are reports of using a spherical BCR with double truncation as a means

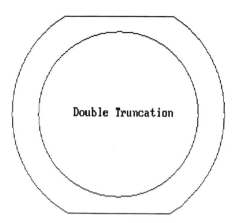

FIG. 25.16. Rendition of a spherical lens with double truncation.

of cylinder stabilization (Fig. 25.16). Fairmaid (32) reported a high degree of success with 82% of a patient study sample of 53 patients who had achieved spectacle-quality visual acuity. In this study, no compensating allowance was used for rotation, as the lenses consistently oriented within a few degrees of the horizontal axis. Base curve radii were chosen for a minimal apical clearance design. The use of a 9.0- to 9.6-mm horizontal diameter range was recommended, with a vertical diameter range of 7.7 to 8.2 mm, varying with the pupil and palpebral aperture dimensions. Small optical zones of 6.8 to 7.0 mm were advised, as the double truncations removed a sizable portion of the lens.

Pole (33) described an in-office procedure for modifying a Polycon 9.5-mm diameter lens to a double truncated lens with an 8.0-mm vertical diameter. This technique was recommended as being helpful in stabilizing lenses on against-the-rule corneas.

CORRECTION OF HIGH ASTIGMATISM

Toric back-surface corneal lenses have been underutilized since their initial introduction nearly 50 years ago (34,35). This is all the more perplexing given the knowledge that has developed throughout years of clinical and laboratory research (11,36–38). The routine use of GP materials today has minimized any concerns regarding physiologic intolerance to toric lenses, unlike previous experiences with PMMA lenses. Perhaps the greatest impediment to their use has been the optics, which can be made to appear both mystifying and complex, but which are in reality rather straightforward and easily mastered (39–41).

Indications

When a spherical base lens used on a toroidal cornea is unable to provide either an acceptable lens-cornea bearing relationship, or an acceptable physiologic result, then a toric back-surface lens is indicated. It should be emphasized that

the *primary* use of such a lens is to improve the physical fit on a toric corneal surface and not for optical correction of residual astigmatism. However, when residual astigmatism is present in a patient requiring a toric back-surface lens, the correction can be factored into the design of the lens.

Spherical Lenses

Although low degrees of corneal toricity are desirable when fitting spherical rigid lenses, larger degrees present a problem. The goal of alignment fitting becomes progressively more difficult to achieve as corneal toricity increases. Instead of paralleling the corneal contour, the spherical lens aligns with the flat meridian, leaving excessive clearance in the steeper meridian. Despite claims by some manufacturers that spherical GP lenses can fit up to 3.00 or 4.00 D of corneal toricity, the majority of patients fitted in such a manner will have difficulties. Although good visual acuity may be possible with the use of a spherical lens on a highly toric cornea, many patients will develop limbal and conjunctival injection, unnatural blink patterns and head postures, 3- and 9-o'clock staining, and visual disturbances related to flare and decentered lenses (Fig. 25.17).

The decision whether or not to use a spherical lens should not be based strictly on keratometric readings as the peripheral corneal toricity may differ significantly from the central values. The analysis of fluorescein patterns using diagnostic spherical lenses should be undertaken to observe the topographic features of the cornea. When the corneal toricity is significant, the spherical lens will result in a fluorescein pattern exhibiting base curve alignment with the flat corneal meridian and excessive clearance in the steep corneal meridian.

A with-the-rule toric cornea will show a horizontal bearing area across the flat axis (Fig. 25.18). Deep pooling can be seen at the 6- and 12-o'clock positions in the meridian of steep corneal curvature, with excessive lens standoff.

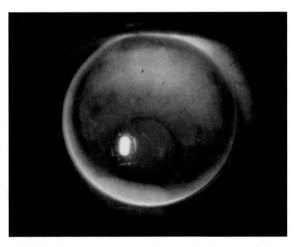

FIG. 25.17. Spherical base curve radius lens on a with-the-rule toric cornea. Note the low lens position.

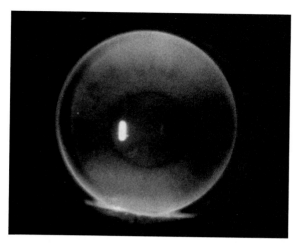

FIG. 25.18. Spherical base curve radius rigid lens on a 3-D with-the-rule toric cornea. Note horizontal bearing across the flat axis, and standoff in the steep meridian.

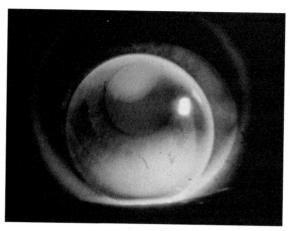

FIG. 25.20. Same lens as seen in Fig. 25.19, shortly after the blink. Note excess fluorescein pooling, low position, and potential problems of flare and lens loss.

Blinking causes the spherical lens to rock across the horizontal axis, with the lid often grabbing the lens into a high-riding position (Fig. 25.19). As the lower edge is lifted away, small bubbles may be seen frothing at the lens edge where the surface tension of the precorneal tear film may be broken. The patient often visualizes flare with the high optical zone bisecting the pupil. If the lens is not large enough, or if the lid action is not strong enough, the lens will pull away from the upper lid and fall onto the lower lid, bearing on the central cornea and exacerbating an inferior pooling (Fig. 25.20). The rapid drop of the lens can lead to excessive blinking, tearing, discomfort, and even lens decentration and loss.

Attempts to compensate for the corneal astigmatism by fitting the spherical BCR lens *steeper than K* to improve centration may lead to other problems, such as limbal hyperemia, inadequate tear exchange, and corneal staining. These complications are often caused by lens compression of the cornea at the periphery of the flat meridian (Fig. 25.21).

Spherical lenses fit on against-the-rule corneas will show a band of corneal touch in the vertical meridian. Here, the lens will rock on a vertical axis, leading to excessive lens translation and lateral lag. These problems are encountered more frequently when spherical lenses used in corneal astigmatism are in excess of 2.00 D.

While the use of a spherical lens should not be ruled out in patients with corneal astigmatism above 2.00 D, careful assessment, using fluorescein analysis and lens observation, should be made. This evaluation may include having the patient wear spherical lenses for a reasonable time to allow the practitioner to assess adequately the optical, physical, and physiologic performance.

Kame and Hayashida (42) have pointed out that fluorescein analysis of a spherical rigid lens may demonstrate that a moderately toric cornea (as measured by the keratometer) may have considerably less toricity in the periphery. As a

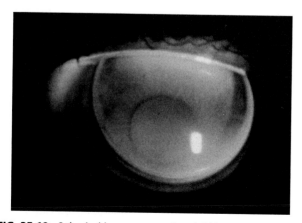

FIG. 25.19. Spherical base curve radius rigid lens on a 3-D with-the-rule toric cornea. Note excess edge standoff, which may lead to superior malpositioning, excessive movement, discomfort, and flare.

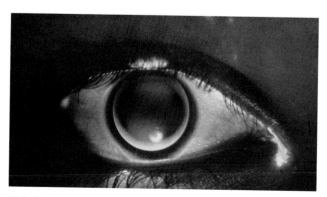

FIG. 25.21. Same patient as seen in Figs. 25.19 and 25.20 fit with a spherical base curve radius lens 0.50 D steeper than K. Note dumbbell or H pattern of bearing zones, as well as compression at 3 and 9 o'clock.

result, the use of a spherical-base lens may be the best option.

As an alternative to spherical lenses, which manifest harsher bearing zones on toric corneas, the practitioner may also consider the use of a lens with an *aspheric* BCR. Aspheric lenses, which typically have ellipsoidal eccentricity values that more effectively parallel the natural flattening of the cornea, are often better choices for fitting the moderately astigmatic cornea than using spherical lenses. They may be considered with corneal astigmatism up to 2.5 or even 3.0 D.

Although GP lens materials are routinely used, one should remember that a good lens fit is more than the absence of corneal edema. Fitting GP spherical lenses regardless of corneal toricity ignores the lens-cornea relationship, and will produce clinical success on a haphazard basis. On the other hand, fitting a more expensive lens, with greater complexity and taking more chair time than is necessary is neither a service to the patient nor a benefit to the practitioner. Whenever there are doubts about the efficacy or safety of a spherical lens for a cornea with significant corneal toricity, then a toric back-surface lens is warranted.

Back-surface Toric Lenses

Back-surface toric lenses are used when it is desirable to align the corneal contour more closely in moderate-to-high corneal astigmatism. Traditional fitting philosophies for back-surface toric lenses were developed using PMMA lenses, the only material available during the many years when toric lenses were being studied and evaluated. These designs included full corneal alignment (43), *flatter-than-K* techniques (41,44), as well as undercorrection methods (45–47).

Prior to the availability of toric diagnostic lens sets, clinicians often fit toric lens empirically, by providing keratometer and refraction measurements to the laboratory, which would make up a tentative lens design. In other cases, keratometer and refractive findings were placed on optical crosses, in order to generate a tentative lens prescription.

Fittings based primarily on keratometric readings can result in significant inaccuracies in toric lens design, as the keratometer measures only a small central area of the cornea over an approximate 3-mm diameter (11,41,44). In addition, the effects of lid tension, lid position, contact lens edge thickness and clearance, and other variables can greatly affect lens centration and movement. Whenever possible, diagnostic lens evaluation is preferable in rigid lens design, whether fitting spherical-base or toric-base lenses. As discussed later, the use of a well-designed toric fitting set can provide the practitioner with a powerful tool for very accurate design of back-surface toric lenses of any type.

Examples of keratometer methods for back-surface toric design are illustrated in Table 25.1, which compares toric base curve selection for PMMA, using the techniques of Remba (40,44) and Goldberg (12). A description of Goldberg's method of lens diameter and optical zone selection is given in Table 25.2, based on varying degrees of toricity as measured by the keratometer (12).

When designing a back-surface toric curvature, the clinician should be aware that there should be an appropriate balance between physical fit and physiology. A lens that too closely aligns the toric surface of the cornea will interfere with tear and metabolic exchange in the same manner that a spherical lens can be too closely aligned to a spherical cornea. Back-surface toric lenses inherently will fit more tightly than spherical lenses on toric corneas, and with less rotation and lag. The lens must be designed carefully to ensure a proper degree of tear venting, while at the same time correcting enough of the corneal toricity to improve the overall bearing relationships as well as lens centration.

The Rear Surface Curvature

Whether prescribing toric-base lenses with spherical front surfaces, or bitoric lenses (i.e., a toric-base with a toric-front surface), the design principles of the posterior or fitting curvature are the same. Silbert (48) described two options for designing the rear surface curvature: the *saddle fit* and the *low toric simulation*.

TABLE 25.1. TORIC BASE CURVE INITIAL DESIGN, BASED ON KERATOMETER VALUES

	Corneal Toricity (ΔK)	Flat Meridian Compared to K	Steep Meridian Compared to K
Remba (40,44)			
	2.00 D	0.25 D flatter	0.25 D flatter
	3.00 D	0.25 D flatter	0.50 D flatter
	4.00 D	0.25 D flatter	0.75 D flatter
	5.00 D	0.50 D flatter	0.75 D flatter
Goldberg (12)			
	2.00–4.00 D	0.50 D steeper	(Steeper curve is flattened by one half the difference of the meridians)
	4.25–6.00 D	0.75 D steeper	
	>6.00 D	1.00 D steeper	

K, keratometer value.

TABLE 25.2. SELECTION OF OPTICAL ZONE DIAMETER AND OVERALL DIAMETER BASED ON LENS TORICITY, USING GOLDBERG'S TECHNIQUE (12)

Lens Toricity	Lens Base Curve (in D)		
	40.00–41.75 D	42.00–43.75 D	44.00–45.75 D
2.00 D	9.4/8.0 mm	9.2/8.0 mm	9.0/7.6 mm
3.00 D	9.2/7.8 mm	9.0/7.8 mm	8.8/7.4 mm
4.00–6.00 D	9.0/7.6 mm	8.8/7.6 mm	8.6/7.2 mm

The Saddle Fit Design

The *saddle fit* technique acquires its name from the description of full alignment of the principal corneal meridians, that is, an on-K fit of each meridian. As this design tends to create more tightly fitting lenses, smaller lenses are recommended. Typically, diameters range from 8.5 to 9.0 mm, with optic zones of 7.2 to 7.6 mm. The saddle fit design is best used with corneal toricities of 2.50 D or less, in which a toric lens is preferred over a spherical lens. Because a minimum of 2.00 D of corneal toricity usually is necessary for a toric-base lens to maintain rotational stability (13), full meridional alignment generally is required when working with these lower degrees of corneal toricity. The saddle fit design offers good torsional stability along with simple lens optics and closely aligned fluorescein patterns (Fig. 25.22).

A disadvantage of the saddle fit design when used in corneal toricity above 2.5 D is that it may ultimately prove to be too closely aligned with the cornea, preventing adequate tear exchange. Another potential disadvantage is related to its maximal correction of the corneal toricity, as this produces higher-powered lenses, which, in turn, become thicker, heavier, and less oxygen transmissive.

Low Toric Simulation

This design, based on undercorrection of the corneal cylinder, should produce a fluorescein pattern aligning the flat corneal meridian, but allowing for mild clearance in the steeper meridian (Fig. 25.23).

As its name suggests, this technique, in effect, converts the patient's high corneal toricity to the *fitting equivalent* of a patient with low corneal toricity, a highly desirable fitting condition for rigid spherical lenses. The net result is to create a *simulation of low toricity*, regardless of the degree of corneal cylinder. This design creates a small degree of lens *rock* about the flatter meridian, which assists in venting tears and debris. In addition, lenses constructed in this fashion will be thinner, lighter, and more oxygen transmissive than their counterparts in the saddle fit design.

The flat meridian of the lens typically should be fit on-K, or within ±0.25 D. of the flat K. The steeper meridian is then *undercorrected* (i.e., fit *flatter* than the steep corneal meridian) by approximately one third of the difference between the major corneal meridians. An alternate approach would be to undercorrect the steep corneal meridian by about 1.00 D regardless of the amount of corneal astigmatism. This alternate method of undercorrection works satisfactorily for lower to moderate amounts of corneal cylinder, but is more likely to create a tighter fitting relationship if used on higher degrees of corneal toricity.

For example, one would select an initial lens to undercorrect a 3.00 D corneal astigmatism with 2 D of rear surface toricity (fitting the flat meridian nearly on-K and the steep corneal meridian 1.00 D flatter than its respective K mea-

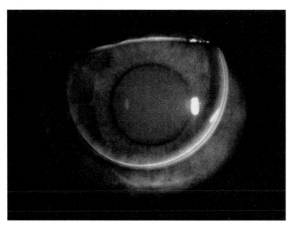

FIG. 25.22. A toric-base lens fit by the saddle fit method, on a cornea with 3.50 D of with-the-rule toricity. Note the close alignment of the principal corneal meridians.

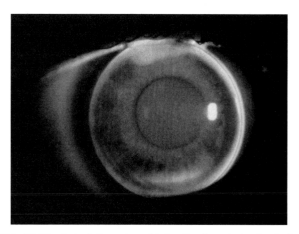

FIG. 25.23. A toric-base lens fit by the low toric simulation method, on the same patient with 3.50 D of with-the-rule toricity. Note the increased clearance in the steeper (vertical) meridian.

BCR	SCR(W)		PCR(W)		OAD	OZD	Rx	CT
8.00/7.50	9.00/8.50	(0.5)	11.0/10.5	(0.3)	9.2	7.6	-1.00/-4.00	0.17

FIG. 25.24. Example of prescription order for a lens with a toric base curve and with toric peripheral curves. Note that the same toric difference is kept in the peripheral radii as in the base curve. The finished lens will have a circular-shaped optical zone.

surement). However, to design a low toric simulation lens for a 5.00-D corneal astigmatism, a 3.5-D rear surface toricity is recommended (fitting the flat meridian nearly on-K but undercorrecting the steep meridian by approximately one third, or 1.50 D flatter than the steep K meridian). These guidelines are helpful when designing a lens empirically, or when deciding what diagnostic lens to select initially from for evaluation on the eye.

The low toric simulation can be ordered in larger OAD, because it does not create as tight a fit as the saddle fit design. As a result, overall diameters ranging from 9.0 to 9.4 mm and optical zones ranging from 7.6 to 8.0 mm are recommended. A typical lens has a 9.2-mm OAD with a 7.8-mm optical zone diameter.

Peripheral Curve Radii

There appears to be little agreement among clinicians on the choice of spherical versus toric peripheral curve radii for back-surface toric lenses. Advocates of spherical peripheral radii feel that they are acceptable, despite producing oval-shaped optical zones. Also, they are easier to modify in the office should an adjustment become necessary (44, 49,50). Advocates of toric peripheries feel that they provide improved rotational stability (51). In addition, toric peripheral radii used on a toric base lens produce *circular-shaped* optical zones.

Silbert (48) prefers the use of spherical peripheral radii when designing *saddle fit* lenses and when corneal toricity is less than 3.00 D. The spherical peripheral radius is satisfactory, especially when lens diameters are smaller, as there will not be excessive peripheral clearance in the steep corneal meridian. When larger diameters are employed, and when corneal toricity is 3.00 D or higher, as is usually the case when the *low toric simulation* design is used, then the use of toric peripheral curves is preferred. This is necessary to

prevent significant *ovalization* of the optical zone, and to reduce edge clearance in the steeper corneal meridian. Typically, a tricurve design is used [BCR, secondary curve radius (SCR), peripheral curve radius (PCR)] and axial edge lift preferably should be controlled such that it does not exceed 0.12 mm (52). When ordering toric peripheral curves, the same toric difference should be maintained between the secondary and peripheral curve principal meridians as is used in the base curve radii (Figs. 25.24 and 25.25).

The Optics of Toric-base Lenses

A back-surface toric lens may demonstrate excellent alignment properties on the cornea, but will rarely provide adequate visual acuity. This results from certain inherent optical characteristics of toric lenses that must be understood in order to provide good vision for the patient.

The Induced Cylinder

When a back-surface toric lens with a spherical front surface is placed on the eye, it induces a cylindrical-power optical error. This unwanted *induced cylinder* results from the difference in index of refraction of the lens plastic (typically $n = 1.49$ for PMMA, and $n = 1.47$ to 1.48 for many GP lens materials) compared with the index of refraction of tears in the precorneal fluid lens ($n = 1.336$). The induced cylinder typically acts as an additional error in the refractive system, comparable to the optical effect of additional residual astigmatism (53). However, the induced cylinder is *not* the patient's physiologic residual astigmatism, which may or may not be present. The induced cylinder acts to compound whatever physiologic astigmatism may already exist, thus rarely allowing adequate visual acuity to prevail.

The induced cylinder is always a *minus cylinder,* of the same axis as the flatter principal meridian of the toric-base

BCR	SCR(W)		PCR(W)		OAD	OZD	Rx	CT
8.00/7.50	9.00	(0.4)	11.0	(0.3)	9.0	7.6	-1.00/-4.00	0.17

FIG. 25.25. Example of prescription order for a lens with a toric base curve and a spherical peripheral curve. The finished lens will have an oval-shaped optical zone.

TABLE 25.3. SUMMARY OF CYLINDER RELATIONSHIPS IN TORIC BASE, SPHERICAL FRONT SURFACE LENSES (N = 1.49)

Rule of $\frac{1}{2}$	
Induced cylinder (*in situ*)	= 0.456 × ΔK cl (radiuscope value)
	= ~ $\frac{1}{2}$ contact lens toricity
Rule of $\frac{1}{3}$	
Induced cylinder (*in situ*)	= 0.314 × air cylinder (lensometer value)
	= ~ $\frac{1}{3}$ air toricity
Rule of $1\frac{1}{2}$	
Air cylinder (lensometer)	= 1.456 × ΔK cl (radiuscope value)
	= ~ $1\frac{1}{2}$ × contact lens toricity

Note: The above relationships of induced cylinder-to-contact-lens toricity and to the air cylinder can be visualized more easily by the following:

1	–	2	–	3
(induced cylinder)		(rear surface cylinder radiuscope)		(air cylinder lensometer)

contact lens. On the eye, the power of the induced cylinder is equal to 0.456 times the toricity of the rear surface curvature (i.e., ΔK cl), and equals 0.314 times the power of the *air cylinder* (the toricity of the lens when measured *in air*, as in a lensometer).

For quick in-office clinical estimates, clinicians may approximate the above values by the *rule of $\frac{1}{2}$* or the *rule of $\frac{1}{3}$*, in which the induced cylinder can be estimated at slightly less than one half or 50% of the contact lens toricity (ΔK cl), or slightly less than one third of the air cylinder (Tables 25.3 and 25.4). It should be noted that these values are for PMMA lens material, in which the index of refraction is 1.49. When GP plastics are used, the somewhat lower index typically found with these materials will create a slightly lower percentage of induced cylinder. However, the approx-

imation formulae are clinically useful with either category of lens materials.

The Air Cylinder

The *air cylinder* (lensometer reading) for toric-base spherical front curve lenses equals 1.456 times the contact lens toricity (ΔK cl). This is often approximated clinically as the *rule of $1\frac{1}{2}$*, in which the lensometer reading (air cylinder) equals about one and one half times the radiuscope reading (ΔK cl). These relationships can be summarized and more easily visualized in Table 25.3. For example, consider a back-toric lens fitted on K in a saddle fit design, with the following radii:

7.50 mm (45.00 D) axis 180
6.89 mm (49.00 D) axis 090

This 4.00 D back-toric lens will *induce* an error cylinder of −1.80 D axis 180, on the eye. (By the *rule of $\frac{1}{2}$*, this error would be estimated to be approximately 2.00 D). It is this cylinder that will degrade the patient's visual acuity (in addition to any physiologic residual astigmatism that might also be present). Off the eye, this same lens will have an air cylinder power of −5.80 D axis 180. By the rule of $1\frac{1}{2}$, the air cylinder or lensometer cylinder would be estimated to be approximately 6.00 D of toricity).

In summary, the optics of back-surface toric lenses have essentially a simple relationship that can be reduced to the ratio of 1:2:3 in which the induced cylinder may be considered equal to 1 unit, the rear surface toricity (or radiuscope value) equal to 2 units, and the air cylinder (or lensometer value) equal to 3 units (Table 25.3).

Because an induced cylinder in most cases has a harmful effect on visual acuity, back-toric lenses must be compensated to counter these adverse effects. This is done by applying a *front surface cylinder,* in essence leading to a *bitoric* lens. Bitoric lenses, therefore, should thus be used by clinicians in most instances.

TABLE 25.4. DERIVATION OF CONVERSION FACTORS

Index (*n*)
  Air = 1.0
  Plastic = 1.490
  Tears = 1.336
  Keratometer = 1.3375

A. Induced Cylinder = 0.456 × ΔK cl

$$\frac{n_{tears} - n_{plastic}}{n_{air} - n_{Keratometer}} = \frac{1.336 - 1.490}{1.0 - 1.3375} = 0.456$$

B. Induced Cylinder = 0.314 × *air cylinder*

$$\frac{n_{tears} - n_{plastic}}{n_{air} - n_{plastic}} = \frac{1.336 - 1.490}{1.0 - 1.490} = 0.314$$

C. Air Cylinder = 1.456 × ΔK cl

$$\frac{n_{air} - n_{plastic}}{n_{air} - n_{keratometer}} = \frac{1.0 - 1.490}{1.0 - 1.3375} = 1.456$$

Back-Toric Lens Applications

From the previous discussion, it might seem that there is no use for a back-toric lens construction. When might a back-toric lens alone be used? Only when the error created by the induced cylinder can be used as a *correcting lens* for the patient's physiologic residual astigmatism. This occurs infrequently, but there are two examples that illustrate how back-toric lenses may be used for this purpose.

Case 1

A patient whose refractive (spectacle) with-the-rule cylinder is significantly greater than the corneal with-the-rule cylinder (an unusual case in which the patient manifests with-the-rule residual astigmatism).

> Spectacle Rx $-1.00 = -4.50 \times 180$
> Vertex adjusted Rx $-1.00 = -4.00 \times 180$
> Keratometer 41.00 @ 180 / 44.00 @ 90
>
> CRA = TRA $- \Delta$ K
>   = $-4.00 \times 180 - (-3.00 \times 180)$
>   = -1.00×180

If a back-toric lens is designed with 2.00 to 2.50 D of toricity, it will create an induced cylinder of about -0.75 to -1.00×180. Thus, the induced cylinder power, created when the back toric is on the eye, will serve well as a correcting lens for the patient's with-the-rule physiologic astigmatism, and will produce good visual acuity as long as the lens remains rotationally stable.

Case 2

In this example (54), a patient's refractive against-the-rule astigmatism is significantly greater than the corneal against-the-rule cylinder. (This follows the more typical clinical pattern of against-the-rule physiologic astigmatism.)

> Spectacle Rx $-1.00 = -3.00 \times 90$
> Keratometer 44.00 @ 180 / 42.00 @ 90
>
> CRA = TRA $- \Delta$ K
>   = $-3.00 \times 90 - (-2.00 \times 90)$
>   = -1.00×90

Here, the predicted physiologic residual astigmatism is -1.00×90. If a toric-base lens is designed with 2.00 D toricity, it will induce a cylindrical error of just under -1.00×90. This *error cylinder* can serve nicely as a correcting lens for the patient's residual astigmatism.

Note that in both of the previous examples, the total refractive astigmatism (TRA) was about one third greater than the patient's corneal astigmatism, and both shared the same axis. If these conditions are present, then back-toric lenses can produce good visual acuity. However, the author's experience suggests that these conditions are met in-

frequently, and that in the vast majority of cases back-toric lenses will not suffice. It is also interesting to note that the clinician can *influence* the amount of induced cylinder created by the selection of the degree of rear surface toricity in the contact lens ordered, since the induced cylinder is a function of the back surface toricity (ΔK cl) and *not* the corneal toricity. This can be beneficial by allowing the clinician to adjust the fitting curves (within reason) in these special cases to correct for a patient's physiologic residual astigmatism (55).

Even in these few cases in which back-toric lenses are used to correct for patients' physiologic astigmatism, the lens must maintain excellent meridional stability in order for visual acuity to be stable. If the lens were to rotate because of lid forces, or from an inadequate amount of toricity on the rear surface, then visual acuity would be reduced or would become unstable during the blink. This is because a new cylinder error would form as a result of obliquely crossed cylinders (induced cylinder versus physiologic residual astigmatism).

Bitoric Lenses

As noted, back-toric lenses typically fail to correct astigmatism adequately. As a result, a front surface cylinder needs to be applied to correct for the induced cylinder, as well as for any significant physiologic residual astigmatism.

There are essentially two methods for determining the power specifications of a bitoric lens:

1. Design by empirical calculation

In this method, data are collected regarding the patient's spectacle prescription and adjusted for vertex distance to the corneal plane as necessary, keratometer reading, and whether the final bitoric lens is fitted *on K* in each meridian or some variation thereof in which case a lacrimal lens would then apply. These data are then determined for each meridian, either by optical cross diagrams or by alternative template technique to produce the final bitoric prescription. In essence, this method treats each meridian as if it were a separate spherical contact lens.

Example 1

A patient with a K reading of 42.00 @ 180 /46.00 @ 90, and a spectacle prescription of $-2.00 = -5.00 \times 180$ is being fitted with a toric lens. It is determined that a lens with a toric base curve dioptric equivalent of 42.00 / 46.00 is required (a *saddle fit*). Determine the final lens powers.

Step 1: The spectacle prescription of $-2.00 = -5.00 \times 180$ first must be vertexed to the corneal plane, as the power of one of the principal meridians is greater than 4 D. The adjusted prescription power is thus noted as $-2.00 = -4.50 \times 180$, or as seen on an optical cross as:

$$(180) \quad \overset{-7.00}{+} \quad -2.00 \quad \Rightarrow \quad \overset{-6.50}{+} \quad -2.00$$
$$(90)$$

Spectacle Rx   Vertex-adjusted Rx

Step 2: Calculate the lacrimal lens by relating the base curve radii (in dioptric equivalents) to the keratometer dioptric readings:

$$(180) \quad \overset{46.00}{+} \quad 42.00 \quad \overset{46.00}{+} \quad 42.00 \quad \Rightarrow$$
$$(90)$$
K   Ordered B.C.

$$\overset{PL}{+} \quad PL$$
Lacrimal Lens

Step 3: Determine the final bitoric lens prescription by adding the powers of the vertexed spectacle prescription to the compensatory powers for the lacrimal lens (in Example 1 there is no need to add a compensatory power adjustment for the lacrimal lens as the lens was fit on K in both meridians):

$$(180) \quad \overset{-6.50}{+} \quad -2.00 \quad + \quad \overset{PL}{+} \quad PL \quad =$$
$$(90)$$
Spectacle Rx   Lacrimal Lens
(vertex adjusted)   Compensation

$$\overset{-6.50}{+} \quad -2.00$$
Final CL Rx

The final lens powers to be given to the laboratory will be either the actual powers in each respective meridian, as −2.00 D flat meridian (180) and −6.50 D steep meridian (90), or the optical prescription may be given as one would write a spectacle prescription, as follows: −2.00 = −4.50 × 180. This may also be written as −2.00 = −4.50 × flat meridian. It is important that a confirmation be made with the fabrication laboratory, and a mutually agreeable method of giving the prescription developed, so that there is no confusion. As all of these prescriptions are correct and provide the same information, it is simply a matter of form and standardization.

Example 2

The same patient, with K readings of 42.00 @ 180 / 46.00 @ 90 and a spectacle prescription of −2.00 −5.00 × 180 is now fitted with a *low toric simulation* design. The toric base curve dioptric equivalents are fit 0.25 flatter than K in the flat meridian, and undercorrected by 1 D in the steep meridian, producing a final rear-surface toric curvature of

41.75 @ 180 and 45.00 @ 90. Determine the final toric lens prescription powers.

Step 1: As in the previous example, the spectacle prescription (− 2.00 − 5.00 × 180) is once again vertexed to the corneal plane:

$$(180) \quad \overset{-7.00}{+} \quad -2.00 \quad \Rightarrow \quad \overset{-6.50}{+} \quad -2.00$$
$$90$$
Spectacle Rx   Vertex-adjusted Rx

Step 2: Calculate the lacrimal lens by relating the base curve radii (in dioptric equivalents) to the keratometer dioptric readings:

$$(180) \quad \overset{46.00}{+} \quad 42.00 \quad \overset{45.00}{+} \quad 41.75 \quad \Rightarrow$$
$$(90)$$
K   Ordered B.C.

$$\overset{-1.00}{+} \quad -0.25$$
Lacrimal Lens

Step 3: Determine the final bitoric lens prescription by adding the powers of the vertexed spectacle prescription to the compensatory powers for the lacrimal lens:

$$(180) \quad \overset{-6.50}{+} \quad -2.00 + \quad \overset{+1.00}{+} \quad +0.25 \quad =$$
$$(90)$$
Spectacle Rx   Lacrimal Lens
(vertex adjusted)   Compensation

$$\overset{-5.50}{+} \quad -1.75$$
Final CL Rx

Here, in the low toric simulation, the final toric lens prescription may be written as − 1.75 flat meridian (180) and −5.50 steep meridian (90). Or, it may be given in spectacle Rx form:

−1.75 −3.75 × 180

Or, it may also be given as:

−1.75 −3.75 × flat meridian

The use of optical crosses has often been perceived by clinicians as being time-consuming and confusing, despite their rather straightforward application. This has led some clinicians to abandon bitoric lenses, despite the fact that they are essential to proper contact lens design. To address this issue, Mandell and Moore (56) developed a template or *bitoric lens guide* which assists the practitioner in inserting the respective values of the K readings, spectacle powers for each principal meridian, and the *fit factors,* resulting in the final bitoric contact lens prescription (Figs. 25.26 and

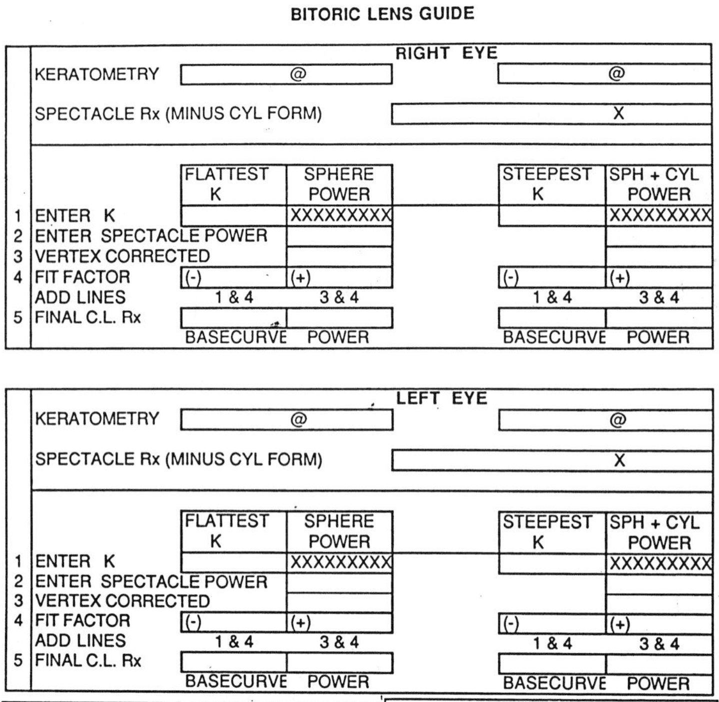

BITORIC LENS GUIDE

RIGHT EYE

| KERATOMETRY | @ | | @ | |
| SPECTACLE Rx (MINUS CYL FORM) | | | X | |

		FLATTEST K	SPHERE POWER	STEEPEST K	SPH + CYL POWER
1	ENTER K		XXXXXXXX		XXXXXXXX
2	ENTER SPECTACLE POWER				
3	VERTEX CORRECTED				
4	FIT FACTOR	(-)	(+)	(-)	(+)
	ADD LINES	1 & 4	3 & 4	1 & 4	3 & 4
5	FINAL C.L. Rx				
		BASECURVE	POWER	BASECURVE	POWER

LEFT EYE

| KERATOMETRY | @ | | @ | |
| SPECTACLE Rx (MINUS CYL FORM) | | | X | |

		FLATTEST K	SPHERE POWER	STEEPEST K	SPH + CYL POWER
1	ENTER K		XXXXXXXX		XXXXXXXX
2	ENTER SPECTACLE POWER				
3	VERTEX CORRECTED				
4	FIT FACTOR	(-)	(+)	(-)	(+)
	ADD LINES	1 & 4	3 & 4	1 & 4	3 & 4
5	FINAL C.L. Rx				
		BASECURVE	POWER	BASECURVE	POWER

VERTEX DISTANCE CORRECTION

4.00	3.75	8.00	7.25	12.00	10.50	16.00	13.25
4.25	4.00	8.25	7.50	12.25	10.75	16.25	13.50
4.50	4.25	8.50	7.75	12.50	10.75	16.50	13.75
4.75	4.50	8.75	8.00	12.75	11.00	16.75	13.75
5.00	4.75	9.00	8.00	13.00	11.25	17.00	14.00
5.25	5.00	9.25	8.25	13.25	11.25	17.25	14.00
5.50	5.25	9.50	8.50	13.50	11.50	17.50	14.25
5.75	5.50	9.75	8.75	13.75	11.75	17.75	14.50
6.00	5.50	10.00	9.00	14.00	12.00	18.00	14.50
6.25	5.75	10.25	9.00	14.25	12.00	18.25	14.75
6.50	6.00	10.50	9.25	14.50	12.25	18.50	15.00
6.75	6.25	10.75	9.50	14.75	12.50	18.75	15.00
7.00	6.50	11.00	9.75	15.00	12.50	19.00	15.25
7.25	6.75	11.25	10.00	15.25	12.75	19.25	15.50
7.50	7.00	11.50	10.00	15.50	13.00	19.75	15.75
7.75	7.00	11.75	10.25	15.75	13.00	20.00	16.00

FIT FACTOR

CORNEAL CYL	FLAT MERIDIAN	STEEP MERIDIAN
2.0 DIOP	ON K	.50 FLATTER
2.5 "	.25 FLATTER	.50 "
3.0 "	.25 "	.75 "
3.5 "	.25 "	.75 "
4.0 "	.25 "	1.00 "
5.0 "	.25 "	1.25 "

If the spectacle lens power is less than 4.00 diopters then line 5 = line 4. Otherwise: For **minus** power spectacle lenses find the power in the left side of the column and convert to the power in the right side, but retain the minus sign. For **plus** power spectacle lenses find the power in the right side of the column and convert to the power in the left side, but retain the plus sign.

FIG. 25.26. Mandell-Moore bitoric lens guide (From Mandell RB, Moore CF. A bitoric lens guide that really is simple. *Contact Lens Spectr* 1988;3:83–85, with permission.)

25.27). The fit factor provides the clinician with values to fit each meridian relative to the keratometric measurements, so that an appropriate lens-cornea relationship is maintained for each meridian. In its most recent version, the fit factor for the steep meridian (where most undercorrection occurs) is 0.50 D flatter than K for up to 2.5 D of corneal cylinder, and 0.75 D flatter than K for all higher degrees of corneal astigmatism (Fig. 25.28). The guide is easy to use, saves time for the busy clinician, and practically precludes the practitioner from making an error as long as each step is followed in sequence according to the instructions. Vertex tables are included as well. The template is, in essence, the optical cross method demonstrated earlier, but is made much easier in this new format.

Pitts et al. (57) did a retrospective analysis of 33 successful bitoric GP lens wearers fit at a university optometric contact lens clinic, and compared the final base curve radii for each patient's flat and steep contact lens meridians with values predicted by the Mandell-Moore bitoric lens guide. Success was defined as having both a clinically acceptable fluorescein pattern and visual acuity within one line of the best-corrected spectacle visual acuity. Although small statistical differences were found in comparisons of the flat meridian radii, and in the steep meridian powers, these values were clinically insignificant. The study concluded that the guide was an efficient tool with which to accurately and quickly design an initial bitoric lens and had a high likelihood of clinical success.

2. Design by diagnostic lenses

The second method for determining the power and curvature specifications of a bitoric lens employs the use of diagnostic contact lenses. In prior years, some clinicians advocated the use of back toric lenses (spherical front surface) for determining the best physical fitting relationship, and then performed a spherocylindrical overrefraction while the back toric lens was in place. The contact lens specifications, lens orientation measurements, and overrefraction data were then supplied to laboratories for what the clinicians hoped would be good results (50,58,59). Unfortunately, such a technique requires laborious measurements, particularly for

BITORIC LENS GUIDE

RIGHT EYE

		FLATTEST K	SPHERE POWER		STEEPEST K	SPH + CYL POWER
(1)	KERATOMETRY	*42.50 @ 180*			*46.50 @ 90*	
(2)	SPECTACLE Rx (MINUS CYL FORM)				−*3.00* −*3.25* X *180*	
(3)	ENTER K	*42.50*	▓▓▓		*46.50*	▓▓▓
(4)	ENTER SPECTACLE POWER	−*3.00*				−*6.25*
(5)	VERTEX CORRECTION	−*3.00*				−*5.75*
(6)	ADD FIT FACTOR	(−) *0.25*	(+) *0.25*		(−) *1.00*	(+) *1.00*
	ADD LINES	3 & 6	5 & 6		3 & 6	5 & 6
(7)	FINAL C.L. Rx	K *42.25*	Rx −*2.75*		K *45.50*	Rx −*4.75*

LEFT EYE

		FLATTEST K	SPHERE POWER		STEEPEST K	SPH + CYL POWER
(1)	KERATOMETRY	*43.50 @ 180*			*41.50 @ 90*	
(2)	SPECTACLE Rx (MINUS CYL FORM)				−*1.00* −*2.00* X *90*	
(3)	ENTER K	*41.50*	▓▓▓		*43.50*	▓▓▓
(4)	ENTER SPECTACLE POWER	−*1.00*				−*3.00*
(5)	VERTEX CORRECTION	−*1.00*				−*3.00*
(6)	ADD FIT FACTOR	(−) *0*	(+) *0*		(−) *0.50*	(+) *0.50*
	ADD LINES	3 & 6	5 & 6		3 & 6	5 & 6
(7)	FINAL C.L. Rx	K *41.50*	Rx −*1.00*		K *43.00*	Rx −*2.50*

VERTEX DISTANCE CORRECTION

−4.00 +3.75	−8.00 +7.25	−12.00 +10.50	−16.00 +13.25
−4.25 +4.00	−8.25 +7.50	−12.25 +10.75	−16.25 +13.50
−4.50 +4.25	−8.50 +7.75	−12.50 +10.75	−16.50 +13.75
−4.75 +4.50	−8.75 +8.00	−12.75 +11.00	−16.75 +13.75
−5.00 +4.75	−9.00 +8.00	−13.00 +11.25	−17.00 +14.00
−5.25 +5.00	−9.25 +8.25	−13.25 +11.25	−17.25 +14.00
−5.50 +5.25	−9.50 +8.50	−13.50 +11.50	−17.50 +14.25
−5.75 +5.50	−9.75 +8.75	−13.75 +11.75	−17.75 +14.50
−6.00 +5.50	−10.00 +9.00	−14.00 +12.00	−18.00 +14.50
−6.25 +5.75	−10.25 +9.00	−14.25 +12.00	−18.25 +14.75
−6.50 +6.00	−10.50 +9.25	−14.50 +12.25	−18.50 +15.00
−6.75 +6.25	−10.75 +9.50	−14.75 +12.50	−18.75 +15.00
−7.00 +6.50	−11.00 +9.75	−15.00 +12.50	−19.00 +15.25
−7.25 +6.75	−11.25 +10.00	−15.25 +12.75	−19.25 +15.50
−7.50 +7.00	−11.50 +10.00	−15.50 +13.00	−19.75 +15.75
−7.75 +7.00	−11.75 +10.25	−15.75 +13.00	−20.00 +16.00

FIT FACTOR

CORNEAL CYL	FLAT MERIDIAN	STEEP MERIDIAN
2.0 DIOP	ON K	.50 FLATTER
2.5 "	.25 FLATTER	.50 "
3.0 "	.25 "	.75 "
3.5 "	.25 "	.75 "
4.0 "	.25 "	1.00 "
5.0 "	.25 "	1.25 "

If the spectacle lens power is less than 4.00 diopters then line 5 = line 4. Otherwise: For **minus** power spectacle lenses find the power in the left side of the column and convert to the power in the right side, but retain the minus sign. For **plus** power spectacle lenses find the power in the right side of the column and convert to the power in the left side, but retain the plus sign.

FIG. 25.27. Calculations of toric lens specifications using the Mandell-Moore bitoric lens guide for a with-the-rule toricity (right eye) and for an against-the-rule toricity (left eye). (From Mandell RB. *Contact lens practice*, 4th ed. Springfield: Charles C Thomas, 1988:303, with permission.)

torsional characteristics, and overly relies on the abilities of a laboratory to put all these variables together.

The Spherical Power Effect Bitoric

Many patients require toric-base lenses for proper fit, but do not have problems associated with physiologic astigmatism. That is, these patients would see well with a spherical lens correcting their refractive error, if only the lens could be made to fit the shape of the toroidal cornea. It was Sarver (60) who, in 1963, realized that just such a lens could be easily manufactured. He proposed a lens that could combine the excellent fitting qualities of a toric-base lens with the optics of a spherical lens. It took over 20 years for his elegant

idea to take hold among contact lens practitioners, who have now recognized that this design will easily handle the optical needs of patients without significant physiologic residual astigmatism. In addition, the use of such lenses in a diagnostic set can provide accurate lens design and optical correction, not only for patients benefiting from spherical lens optics, but also for patients requiring the most complex bitoric lens constructions.

The *spherical power effect* (SPE) bitoric lens has a toric base curve, but with one important distinction: The induced cylinder that normally would be produced on the eye is instead countered by an equal but opposite *plus cylinder* generated on the front surface, the axis of which is made coincident with the axis of the flatter toric meridian (42). As the back surface toricity is always known, then the labora-

RGP Lens Institute

Mandell-Moore Bitoric Lens Guide - Per eye

	Flattest K	Sphere Power	Steepest K	Sph + Cyl Power
1 Keratometry	@		@	
2 Spectacle Rx (Minus Cyl Form)			x	
3 Enter K		✕		✕
4 Enter Spectacle Power				
5 Vertex Adjust Line 4				
6 Insert Fit Factor	(-)	(+)	(-)	(+)
Add Line	3&6	5&6	3&6	5&6
7 Final CL Rx	Base Curve	Power	Base Curve	Power

Bitoric Lens Fit Factor		
Corneal Cyl	Fit Flat Meridian	Fit Steep Meridian
2.0 Diopters	On K (0 D)	0.50D Flatter
2.5 Diopters	0.25D Flatter	0.50D Flatter
3.0 Diopters	0.25D Flatter	0.75D Flatter
3.5 Diopters	0.25D Flatter	0.75D Flatter
4.0 Diopters	0.25D Flatter	0.75D Flatter
5.0 Diopters	0.25D Flatter	0.75D Flatter

Instructions

1. On line 1 and 2 enter the patient Keratometry readings and Spectacle Rx respectively.
2. On line 3 enter the flattest K in the box on the left side and the steepest K in the box on the right.
3. On line 4 enter the sphere power in the box on the left and the sphere power plus the cylinder power in the box on the right.
4. If the powers noted in line 4 are greater than or equal to +/- 4.00 D an adjustment for vertex distance is entered in line 5. Vertex adjusted powers are used to complete the remaining calculations.
5. Use the Fit Factor Chart above for the values needed to be entered into line 6. The amount of corneal cyl will determine the Fit Factor for the flat and steep meridians. "On K" has a 0 Fit Factor.
6. Add/subtract the lines as noted and enter the results in line 7. These are the actual numbers that you will give the lab to manufacture your bitoric lens. They are referred to as drum value.
7. Go to **www.rgpli.org** and see detailed examples.

For more RGP fitting information visit our
Practitioner website – www.rgpli.org

FIG. 25.28. Newest version of the Mandell-Moore bitoric lens guide (reprinted with permission from the RGP Lens Institute). Note the revised values for the steep meridian in the fit factor.

tory knows the magnitude of the induced cylinder and will produce a compensating front surface cylinder to cancel it, thus producing an *optically spherical* system.

For example, a patient with 4.00 D of corneal astigmatism and 4.00 D of refractive astigmatism of similar axis would see well with spherical lenses (if the side effects of poor lens centration, lens rock, and flare from a spherical base lens are ignored). A conventional back toric lens would produce poor acuity from the induced cylinder. Thus, an SPE bitoric is ideal, for it allows the patient to be fitted with a toric posterior curvature while producing the excellent visual acuity expected with a spherical optical system.

Another advantage of this lens is that its power can be determined *without regard for its meridional orientation.* Rotation of an SPE bitoric lens on the cornea produces no change in the patient's vision, similar to the effects of rotation of spherical base lenses, and unlike other toric base lenses (61). This is because the plus cylinder, which exactly neutralizes the effect of the induced cylinder, continues to do so in whatever rotational position the lens is in while on the cornea.

The air cylinder of an SPE bitoric lens is equal to one times the back surface toricity (unlike a toric-base, spherical front surface lens, in which the air cylinder equals 1.456 times the back surface toricity). The reason for this difference now becomes clear: *with an SPE bitoric, there is now effectively no induced cylinder.* As a result, to determine the powers of an SPE bitoric lens, the air power of the flat principal meridian must first be determined. This is performed either by spherical refraction through a spherical trial lens (whose BCR is the same as that of the flatter meridian of the ordered toric curvature), or through spherical refraction through a diagnostic SPE bitoric lens.

If performed through a spherical base trial lens, the power of the steeper meridian is then determined simply by adding the power of the contact lens toricity (i.e., the air cylinder or ΔK cl) to the flat meridian power previously determined. The steep meridian is always more minus power (or less plus) than the flat meridian power.

Example:
Spectacle Rx: $-2.00 -4.25 \times 180$
K reading: 43.00 @180 / 47.00 @ 90
(Note that there is close agreement between the amount of corneal and refractive astigmatism).

A spherical base curve trial lens of 7.85 mm radius (43.00 D) is selected and placed on the cornea. Spherical overrefraction confirms a total power of -2.00D, although the spherical lens is rocking and does not fit well on this toric cornea.

The total amount of corneal cylinder will be undercorrected by approximately one third; thus, a lens with only 3 D of rear surface cylinder (ΔK cl $= -3.00$ D) will be empirically ordered for this patient.

Spherical trial lens BCR is 7.85 or 43.00 D (on K in

flat meridian). Thus, air power of the flat meridian $=$ -2.00 D.

To determine the air power of the steep meridian, simply add the air cylinder to the flat meridian:

$-2.00 + (-3.00) = -5.00$ D. Thus, the air power of the steep meridian $= -5.00$ D.

The final SPE bitoric Rx can be written as:

$$
\begin{array}{c}
-5.00 \\
(7.85) \ \text{FM} \ \vphantom{|} {\underset{(7.34)}{\overset{}{\mid}}} \ -2.00 \quad \text{or} \quad -2.00 -3.00 \times \text{FM} \\
\text{SM}
\end{array}
$$

SPHERICAL POWER EFFECT DIAGNOSTIC SETS

Because of their simple and elegant design, SPE bitoric lenses lend themselves easily to diagnostic fitting. In fact, the use of a diagnostic set in which each lens has spherical power effect but varies only in BCR or toricity, allows for a rapid clinical method of bitoric design. These lenses provide the clinician with a straightforward, reliable device through which an overrefraction can be performed, thus eliminating the need for optical crosses and computations.

The use of SPE diagnostic sets of 10 to 12 lenses each, and having 2.00 D and 3.00 D of back-surface toricity, respectively, will allow up to 90% of all patients with high astigmatism to be fit effectively (62). For most clinicians, having even one diagnostic set of 2.00-D toricity lenses would be very beneficial, as it could be used to design lenses for corneas ranging in toricity from 2.00 D to as high as 3.50 D. Table 25.5 shows a typical format for the design of such sets, each with a flat meridian power of plano.

It should be remembered that because SPE bitoric lenses are optically spherical, they will be no better at correcting a patient's residual physiologic astigmatism than would a conventional spherical base lens. However, the SPE lens can be used to determine whether residual astigmatism is present, and if so, to incorporate a correction for it in the final lens design (63).

Assuming that diagnostic SPE bitoric lenses are available, the following steps should be followed to design the lens specifications:

1. Obtain K readings and refraction.
2. Decide on *saddle fit* or *low toric simulation* design for the patient, and select the closest diagnostic set available.
3. Within the chosen set, select a lens with flat meridian closest to the patient's flat K.
4. Evaluate the fluorescein pattern. There should be general alignment with adequate peripheral clearance. Closer alignment with saddle fit is to be expected. Some undercorrection with low toric designs would be desirable (see Figs. 22 and 23).

TABLE 25.5. TEMPLATE DESIGN FOR SPE BITORIC DIAGNOSTIC SETS

Diameter/OZD: 9.0/7.6 mm or 9.2/7.8 mm
Flat meridian air power: Plano
Steep meridian air power: If 2.00 D bitoric set: −2.00 D
                                  If 3.00 D bitoric set: −3.00 D

Toric Base Curves	
2.00 D Bitoric	3.00 D Bitoric
39.50 × 41.50	39.50 × 42.50
40.00 × 42.00	40.00 × 43.00
40.50 × 42.50	40.50 × 43.50
41.00 × 43.00	41.00 × 44.00
41.50 × 43.50	41.50 × 44.50
42.00 × 44.00	42.00 × 45.00
42.50 × 44.50	42.50 × 45.50
43.00 × 45.00	43.00 × 46.00
43.50 × 45.50	43.50 × 46.50
44.00 × 46.00	44.00 × 47.00
44.50 × 46.50	44.50 × 47.50
45.00 × 47.00	45.00 × 48.00

OZD, optical zone diameter.

5. If the initial diagnostic lens is not correcting enough cylinder (excessive clearance in steep meridian), the next highest SPE set should be used and evaluated. If only one set is available, then a lens with greater toricity than that used in the diagnostic lens should be ordered.
6. If instead, the fluorescein shows optimal correction of toricity as expected, but is simply showing apical clearance or conversely apical bearing, then the next-flatter or next-steeper lens, respectively, within the same diagnostic set should be used, until the optimal pattern is seen (Figs. 25.29 and 25.30). These lens changes can be made rapidly between assessments.
7. The fluorescein pattern should be evaluated to determine if the degree of toricity in the diagnostic lens is excessive.

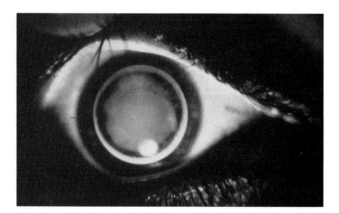

FIG. 25.29. Example of diagnostic spherical power effect lens, which has adequate rear surface toricity for the corneal astigmatism, but is too steep, causing apical clearance. The next-flattest lens in the set should be tried, and the lens reevaluated.

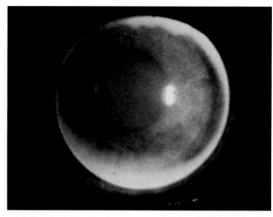

FIG. 25.30. Example of diagnostic spherical power effect lens, which has an adequate degree of toricity for the corneal astigmatism, but is too flat, causing apical bearing and decentration. The next-steeper lens in the set should be tried and reevaluated.

If so, a lens set should be used with less toricity, or if only one set is available, a lens with less toricity than that used in the diagnostic lens should be ordered (Fig. 25.31).

8. A spherical overrefraction should be performed. If visual acuity is good, the overrefraction is simply added to *each meridian's* air power, which is listed on the diagnostic lens package.

Example:
Diagnostic SPE 42.00 × 45.00 toric base
Diagnostic SPE Plano/ − 3.00 air powers
Overrefraction: − 3.00 D
(add to each meridian)
  Final ordered air powers: − 3.00(flat)/ − 6.00 (steep)
or
 − 3.00 − 3.00 × flat meridian

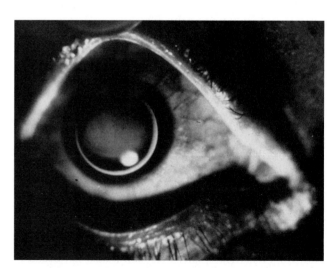

FIG. 25.31. Example of diagnostic spherical power effect lens with an excessive degree of rear surface toricity for the corneal astigmatism. Excessive compression of the steeper corneal meridian can be seen, necessitating a change to a set with lower toricity. (Courtesy of Gerald E. Lowther, OD, PhD.)

9. Vertex adjustment must be made if the overrefraction exceeds 4.00 D.
10. If, however, visual acuity is poor with a spherical overrefraction, this indicates that the patient has residual astigmatism. A *spherocylindrical* overrefraction is then performed. If the axes are at or near the principal corneal meridians, the appropriate power in the refraction is added to the air power of the corresponding meridian in the diagnostic lens, and the lens is ordered. This will produce a *CPE bitoric* (or cylindrical power effect) lens.

Example:
Diagnostic SPE 42.00 × 45.00 toric base
Diagnostic SPE Plano/ − 3.00 air powers
Overrefraction − 1.00 − 1.25 × 180
Observing the rules of prescription power meridians, − 1.00 D is added to the 180th meridian, and − 2.25 D is added to the 90th meridian.

Final ordered air powers:

$$- 1.00(\text{flat}) \: / \: - 5.25(\text{steep})$$

or

$$- 1.00 \: - 4.25 \times \text{flat meridian}$$

Note that in this example the resultant CPE air powers are actually the same as would have been created using a true back toric only.

$$
\begin{aligned}
\text{Air power of back toric} &= 1.456 \times \Delta K \text{ cl} \\
&= 1.456 \times 3.00 \text{ D} \\
&= 4.25\text{-D cylinder}
\end{aligned}
$$

A back toric is actually what would be manufactured based on the powers ordered coincidentally in this particular case. Thus, it can be seen that diagnostic SPE lenses can be used to design any type of toric-base lenses (SPE, CPE, or back toric). The clinician, however, once satisfied with the corneal fit, should only be concerned with designing a lens that properly corrects the patient's vision, and not what form the final toric lens ultimately takes.

Diagnostic SPE bitoric fitting sets should be made in GP materials of lower-to-moderate Dk for optical stability, and should be carefully fabricated by a skilled laboratory. Verification of these lenses, as well as of any ordered lens, is essential for good lens performance. Contact lens practitioners who like to use the Burton lamp for fluorescein pattern analysis will prefer to have their bitoric fitting sets made in GP materials without UV absorptive additives. Such additives are commonly incorporated today in many GP materials, but will prevent the fluorescein pattern from being seen when using a Burton lamp (all lenses regardless of how they are fit will appear black). Use of a Wratten 12 yellow filter held over the objective lens in the biomicroscope will greatly facilitate fluorescein pattern analysis with any GP lens, including those with ultraviolet absorptive additives.

When bitoric GP lenses are used for the correction of high astigmatism, these lenses may have rather high prescription powers, and correspondingly the lens thickness will be substantial. In *with-the-rule* corneas the steep or vertical meridian will have the highest refractive power and the greatest edge thickness for myopic patients. This may result in more upper lid discomfort, excessive movement and inferior positioning in interpalpebral fits (64), or even in high-riding lens positioning in larger diameter lenses. Although heavier edge tapering and the use of CN bevels is frequently used, plus-edge lenticulation (myolenticulation) becomes especially important in these cases, and should be employed when powers approach or exceed − 7 or − 8 D in either meridian. Plus-edge lenticulation will provide greater overall lens comfort and assist in keeping lenses centered. For highly hyperopic patients, bitoric lenses may position inferiorly because of increased center thickness and a low center of gravity in the lens. The use of minus-carrier lenticulation is helpful in these cases, in facilitating good lens centration, in preventing stagnation of the post–lens tear film and debris, and in preventing lens adherence. Additionally, lens mass reduction from plus-edge or minus-carrier lenticulation will increase oxygen transmission (Dk/t). When ordering lenses for a patient with a high prescription, the use of high-Dk lens materials becomes more important in order to provide satisfactory levels of oxygen to the cornea and to prevent hypoxic consequences (65).

Although a very successful lens design for moderate to high corneal astigmatism, bitoric lenses may fail despite the most diligent attempts by the practitioner. This usually occurs when there is misalignment between the axis of the spectacle correction and the keratometer axis, misalignment between the axis of the residual astigmatism and the spectacle cylinder axis, or when lens rotation occurs in the presence of front surface cylindrical correction of residual astigmatism in CPE bitoric lenses.

According to Korb (10), 10% of patients requiring bitoric lenses fall into this general failure category, because of the inability to resolve resultant astigmatism from obliquely crossed cylinders. Newer technology today in the generation of toric curvatures may allow a number of these patients to be fit satisfactorily by the use of crossed cylinders in the final lens. That is, the generation of a toric base curve with a toric front curve that is not at the same axis (66).

Verification of Toric-base Lens Designs

For verification of the BCR of any toric-base lens, rotate the lens in its radiuscope holder until the principal meridians are aligned, to allow for a contiguous mire reading. When the vertical image of the star mire pattern becomes sharp, focused, and contiguous, it has measured the horizontal radius, and vice versa (Fig. 25.32). To verify the air powers of a toric-base, spherical front surface lens, remember that

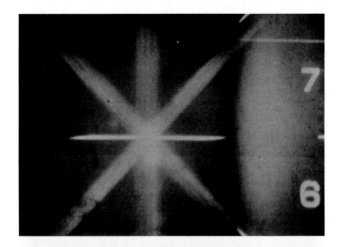

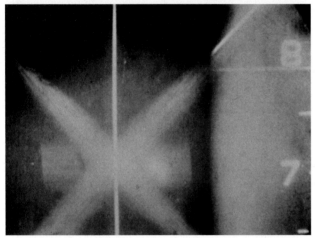

FIG. 25.32. Radiuscope mire patterns of a toric base lens.

the cylinder power in air (lensometer cylinder) should be 1.456 times the radiuscope toricity.

For SPE bitoric lenses, the cylinder power in air must precisely equal the toricity measured in the radiuscope. For CPE bitoric lenses, compare the measured air powers of the major meridians to the ordered powers in those respective meridians.

Toric Peripheral Curves with Spherical Base Curve

There are times when a spherical-base lens can be made to fit a toric cornea in a manner that reduces lens instability and improves the lens-cornea bearing relationship (67). This is accomplished by using a spherical-base lens, with toric peripheral curves. Such a lens can be used on corneas with over 2.00 D of toricity for improved centration, as the lens more closely aligns with the peripheral cornea, reducing peripheral clearance and bubble formation commonly observed with spherical-base lenses. This lens is also indicated for corneas that are relatively spherical, but which become more toric in the periphery. This situation is sometimes

observed in routine fluorescein pattern analysis using conventional spherical diagnostic lenses.

Base curve radii are often designed with moderate apical clearance, steeper than the flat corneal meridian. Combining this with a toric periphery reduces edge lift in the steep corneal meridian, and will produce an ellipsoidal or oval-shaped optical zone (Fig. 25.33) (68). The smaller optic zone diameter corresponds to the flatter secondary curve, and these orient along the flatter principal meridian of the cornea. The lens can achieve good stability with little torsion if the peripheral curve radii are made wide enough and have sufficient toricity.

An example of a lens ordered in the above fashion is illustrated below:

Spectacle prescription: $-1.50 -2.00 \times 180$
Keratometer: 42.00 @ 180 / 43.75 @ 90
Spherical diagnostic lens with spherical peripheral curves is evaluated: BCR 7.94 mm (42.50); -2.00 D
Overrefraction: PL -0.25×180

The diagnostic lens decenters inferiorly, rocking on the horizontal meridian of the cornea. The fluorescein pattern shows horizontal meridian alignment and excess peripheral clearance at the 12-o'clock and 6-o'clock vertical meridian.

Instead of ordering a conventional spherical-base lens, or even a bitoric lens, a spherical-base with a toric periphery may be ordered, with the following design (Fig. 25.33):

BCR 7.94 mm
SCR 9.0/8.6 mm
PCR 11.0/10.6 mm
Overall diameter 9.2 mm
Optical zone diameter 8.0/6.8 mm
Back vertex power -2.00 D

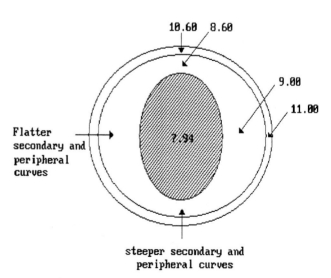

FIG. 25.33. Oval-shaped optical zone with a spherical-base lens with toric peripheral curves.

REFERENCES

1. Bier N, Lowther GE. *Contact lens correction.* Boston: Butterworth & Co., 1977:299.
2. Michaels DD. *Visual optics and refraction*, 2nd ed. St. Louis: CV Mosby Co., 1980:524.
3. Borish IM. *Clinical refraction*, 3rd ed. Chicago: Professional Press, 1970:982.
4. Bailey NJ. Residual astigmatism with contact lenses. Part 3: possible sites. *Rev Optom* 1961;98: 31–32.
5. Harris MG. Contact lens flexure and residual astigmatism on toric corneas. *J Am Optom Assoc* 1970;41:247–248.
6. Harris MG, Chu CS. The effect of contact lens thickness and corneal toricity on flexure and residual astigmatism. *Am J Optom Physiol Opt* 1972;49:304–307.
7. Herman JP. Flexure of rigid Lenses on toric corneas as a function of base curve fitting relationship. *J Am Optom Assoc.* 1983;54: 209–213.
8. Pole JJ. The effect of the base curve on the flexure of Polycon lenses. *Int Cont Lens Clin* 1983;10:49–52.
9. Sarver MD. The effect of contact lens tilt upon residual astigmatism. *Am J Optom Physiol Opt* 1963;40:730–744.
10. Korb DR. A preliminary report on toric contact lenses. *Optom Wkly* 1960;51:2501–2505.
11. Goldberg JB. Clinical application of toric base contact lenses. *Optom Wkly* 1962;53:1911–1915.
12. Dellande WD. A comparison of predicted and measured residual astigmatism in corneal contact lens wearers. *Am J Optom Physiol Opt* 1970;47:459–463.
13. Sarver MD. A study of residual astigmatism. *Am J Optom Physiol Opt* 1969;46:578–582.
14. Mandell RB. Reflection point ophthalmometry. *Am J Optom Physiol Opt* 1962;39:513–537.
15. Mandell RB, St Helen R. Mathematical model of the corneal contour. *Br J Physiol Opt* 1971;26:183–197.
16. Mote HG, Fry GA. The relation of the keratometric findings to the total astigmatism of the eye. *Am J Optom Physiol Opt* 1939; 16:402–409.
17. Bailey NJ. Residual astigmatism with contact lenses. Part I: incidence. *Opt J Rev Optom* 1961;98:30–31.
18. Harris MG, Sweeney KE, Rocchi S, et al. Flexure and residual astigmatism with cellulose acetate butyrate (CAB) contact lenses on toric corneas. *Am J Optom Physiol Opt* 1982;59:858–862.
19. Harris MG, Sweeney KE, Rocchi S, et al. Flexure and residual astigmatism with Polycon and polymethyl methacrylate lenses on toric corneas. *Am J Optom Physiol Opt* 1982;59:263–266.
20. Herman JP. Flexure of rigid contact lenses on toric corneas as a function of base curve fitting relationship. *J Am Optom Assoc* 1983;54:209–213.
21. Ewell DG, Gates H, Remba MJ. The prism ballast contact lens principle. In: Haynes P, ed. *Encyclopedia of contact lens practice*, Vol 2. South Bend, IN: International Optics, 1959–1963: 31–38.
22. Bier N, Lowther GE. *Contact lens correction.* Boston: Butterworth & Co, 1977:305.
23. Sarver MD, Mandell RB. Toric lenses. In: Mandell RB, ed. *Contact lens practice*, 4th ed. Springfield: Charles C. Thomas, 1988: 286–287.
24. Goldberg JB. A clinical procedure to determine the effective cylinder axis for prism ballast lenses. In: Haynes P, ed. *Encyclopedia of contact lens practice*, Vol 3. South Bend, IN: International Optics, 1959–1963: 31–38.
25. Borish IM. Cylinder lenses. Marian, IN: Indiana Contact Lens Co., 1960: Bulletin No. 4.
26. Borish IM. The Max Schapero Memorial Lecture, American Academy of Optometry Annual Meeting; December 1987; Denver, CO.
27. Sarver MD, Mandell RB. Toric lenses. In: Mandell RB, ed. *Contact lens practice*, 4th ed. Springfield: Charles C Thomas, 1988: 291.
28. Sarver MD. Astigmatism. In Mandell RB, ed. *Contact lens practice*, 3rd ed. Springfield: Charles C. Thomas, 1981:259.
29. Hofstetter HW, Baldwin W. Bilateral correlation of residual astigmatism. *Am J Optom Physiol Opt* 1957;34:388–391.
30. Wechsler S. The Periballast lens for correcting residual astigmatism. *Rev Optom* 1979;116:45–46.
31. Braff S.M. A new corneal contact lens design for the correction of residual astigmatism. *Optom Wkly* 1970;61:24–25.
32. Fairmaid JA. The correction of residual astigmatism with double truncated front surface toric micro-lenses: A report of 50 cases. *Aust J Optom* 1967;50:33–38.
33. Pole JJ. Double truncated front surface toric gas permeable (Polycon) lens used in the correction of astigmatism. *Optom Mon* 1983;74:34–37.
34. Schapero M. A review of a new corneal contact lens. *Optom Wkly* 1952;43:713–716.
35. Schapero M. The fitting of highly toric corneas with toric corneal contact lenses. *Am J Optom Physiol Opt* 1953;30:157–160.
36. Wesley NK. A new contact lens for toroidal eyes. *Opt J Rev Optom* 1960;97:39–43.
37. Korb DR. A preliminary report of continuing performance of toric inner surface contact lenses. *Contacto* 1961;5:317–323.
38. Goldberg JB. Clinical application of toric base curve contact lenses. *Optom Wkly* 1962;53:1911–1915.
39. Sarver MD. Calculation of the optical specifications of contact lenses. *Am J Optom Physiol Opt* 1963;40:20–28.
40. Remba MJ. The ABCs of toric contact lens fitting. *Opt J Rev Optom* 1962;99:25–30.
41. Neefe CW. Prescribing torics: easy as 1:2:3. *Contact Lens Forum* 1981;6:59–65.
42. Kame RT, Hayashida JK. A simplified approach to bitoric gas permeable lens fitting. *Int Cont Lens Clin* 1988;15:53–58.
43. Platt WD. The saddle fit for toric corneas. *Contact Lens Forum* 1981;6:47–51.
44. Remba MJ. Contact lenses and the astigmatic cornea. *Contacto* 1967;11:38–43.
45. Goldberg JB. Toroidal cornea lens designing. *J Am Optom Assoc* 1967;38:213–216.
46. Goldberg JB. Toric and bitoric corneal lenses-Part I. *Optom Wkly* 1976;67:39–41.
47. Goldberg JB. Toric and bitoric corneal lenses-Part II. *Optom Wkly* 1976;67:53–55.
48. Silbert JA. Prescribing gas permeable bitoric lenses. In: Haynes P, ed. *Clinical issues in cornea and contact lens*, Vol 2. Newtown, PA: Associates in Medical Marketing, Cooper Vision Monograph, 1988:1–8.
49. Blackstone MR. Toroidal micro-corneal lenses. *Optician* 1968; 155:235–238.
50. Sellers FJE. Fitting of toric corneal contact lenses. *Am J Optom Physiol Opt* 1969;46:127–130.
51. Bayshore CA. Toric contact lens fitting. *Contacto* 1967;11: 35–36.
52. Bennett ES, Sorbara L. Lens design, fitting, and evaluation. In: Bennett ES, Henry VA, eds. *Clinical manual of contact lenses*, 2nd ed. Philadelphia: Lippincott Williams & Wilkins, 2000:101.
53. Bier N, Lowther G. *Contact lens correction.* Boston: Butterworth & Co, 1977:35–36.
54. Sarver MD. Astigmatism. In: Mandell RB, ed. *Contact lens practice*, 3rd ed. Springfield, Charles C. Thomas, 1981:268.
55. Gordon S. The correction of residual astigmatism through toric inside contact lenses. *Optom Wkly* 1961;3:11–12.
56. Mandell RB, Moore CF. A bitoric lens guide that really is simple. *Contact Lens Spectr* 1988;3:83–85.

57. Pitts K, Pack L, Edmondson W, Pack CE. Putting a bitoric RGP lens fitting guide to the test. *Contact Lens Spectr* 2001;16:34–40.

58. Capelli QA. Determining the final power of bitoric lenses. *Br J Physiol Opt* 1964;21:356–363.

59. Morrison RJ, Kaufman KJ, Seruly E. Oblique bitorics: a method to calculate and/or check prescriptions as indicated on the lensometer. *J Am Optom Assoc* 1965;36:1068–1069.

60. Sarver MD. A toric base corneal contact lens with spherical power effect. *J Am Optom Assoc* 1963;34:1136–1137.

61. Silbert JA. Take the bother out of bitorics. *Rev Optom* 1986;123:75–82.

62. Sarver MD, Kame RT, Williams CE. A bitoric gas permeable hard contact lens with spherical power effect. *J Am Optom Assoc* 1985;56:184–189.

63. Silbert JA. RGP Correction of High Astigmatism. *Contact Lens Spectr* 1990;5:25–31.

64. Benjamin WJ. Bitoric rigid gas permeable lenses. In: Schwartz CA, ed. *Specialty contact lenses: a fitter's guide.* Philadelphia: WB Saunders, 1996:35.

65. Benjamin WJ. EOP and Dk/L: the quest for hyper transmissibility. *J Am Optom Assoc* 1993;643:196.

66. Harmon MG, Dill GL, Carter WD. Residual astigmatism: the lab can make the difference. *Contact Lens Spectr* 1988;3:68–70.

67. Greenman N. Toric periphery lens fitting. *Contacto* 1967;11:9–15.

68. Haynes PR. Corneal contact lenses with toric peripheral curves. In: *Encyclopedia of contact lens practice*, Vol 1(B). South Bend, IN: International Optics, 1959–1963:26–32.

HYDROGEL TORIC CONTACT LENS CORRECTION

**ARTHUR B. EPSTEIN AND
MELVIN J. REMBA**

As we enter the 21st century, the hydrogel toric contact lens (HTCL) is well established as an essential part of contemporary contact lens practice. The success of the HTCL is a direct result of steady improvement since its initial introduction in the 1980s. Improved clinical performance combined with greater practitioner fitting skills and comfort have played an important role in the growth of this design. Modern HTCLs are available in a wide range of lens designs and modalities, including conventional daily and extended wear, frequent replacement and disposable modalities, specialty combination designs like multifocal torics, and more recently, single-use disposable HTCLs.

Manufacturing and fitting of early HTCLs was a hit or miss proposition, both costly and complex. Lenses were often inaccurate or unstable and reproducibility was elusive. Despite significant flaws in first generation HTCLs, the need for hydrogel astigmatic correction drove their continued development. Several studies report that as much as 45% of the contact lens-seeking population has an astigmatic correction of 0.75 D or greater (1,2), supporting earlier estimates (3–5). Despite the potential demand, toric lens fabrication is complex and lenses evolved slowly. It took well over a decade until HTCLs became consistently reproducible and fitting "practitioner-friendly."

HTCLs emerged slowly during the 1970s, principally in Europe and Australia. Development progressed more rapidly during the 1980s, as both large and small contact lens manufacturers in the United States showed increased interest in both standard and specialty lens production reflecting overall industry expansion. Improvements in lens designs and trends toward more frequent replacement modalities fueled significant growth in the HTCL segment, over 15% of all hydrogel lens sales in 2002 (6). Much of this growth has been in monthly and 2-week replacement lenses that increasingly replaced quarterly and traditional replacement HTCL modalities. More stable and predicable HTCL designs inspired practitioners to fit more low-cylinder patients, further expanding the market.

HTCLs currently represent more than 20% of all new hydrogel lens fits in the United States. While this seems impressive, it still represents less than half of the projected 45% of potential patients who could benefit from HTCLs. Opportunity for growth in the HTCL market therefore still exists. Reflecting changing prescribing trends, in 1995 frequent replacement lenses represented only 23% of all toric lenses dispensed. By 1997 this percentage was up to 40% and in 2002 it had risen to over 80% of HTCLs dispensed (7). Despite the availability of improved lenses, and greater market acceptance, surprisingly, consumers still lack knowledge about the benefit and availability of toric lenses. Approximately 40% of vision corrected consumers know they have astigmatism, but just over 20% are aware that contact lenses can correct this condition (8).

HTCLs are a fascinating part of contact lens art and science. Despite two decades of existence, HTCL designs and our ability to successfully fit them continue to improve. In this chapter we present an in-depth overview and an update of current HTCL technology with a special focus on clinical application.

ASTIGMATISM DEFINITIONS

Various types of astigmatism can be defined in both physiologic and optical terms. The following are definitions of astigmatism that specifically pertain to clinical contact lens applications.

- *Astigmatism:* a condition of refraction that causes light rays to be focused as two line images instead of a single point.
- *Toricity:* the geometric (physical) description of a surface with two primary curvatures (major and minor meridians), usually at right angles to each other.
- *Corneal astigmatism:* the astigmatic component produced by the toricity of the corneal surface. Corneal astigmatism is the primary contributor to refractive astigmatism.
- *Internal astigmatism:* the astigmatic component produced by optical elements behind the anterior corneal surface. Primarily lenticular in origin, this is also termed "calculated residual astigmatism."

- *Refractive astigmatism:* the astigmatism found on refraction that represents the combination of internal and corneal astigmatism. This is also termed "total" astigmatism.
- *Residual astigmatism:* manifest (by calculation or overrefraction) astigmatism remaining after correction with a contact lens.
- *Induced astigmatism:* astigmatism caused by soft contact lens flexure or by the tear-lens when a toric rigid lens is on the eye.
- *Irregular astigmatism:* astigmatism where the major and minor axes are not perpendicular and thus not likely correctable using a simple toric refractive surface.

PRINCIPLES OF CORRECTING ASTIGMATISM WITH SOFT LENSES

Traditionally, HTCL fitting relies on four basic assumptions:

1. The lenses provide the proper *in situ* meridional back vertex powers needed to correct the eye's refractive error including astigmatism.
2. The lenses conform to the shape of the central cornea without irregular draping or tear film effects that induce additional refractive power.
3. The lenses orient as anticipated.
4. The lenses remain stable and nonrotating.

In clinical practice these basic elements are rarely achieved without the application of considerable professional expertise, especially when higher amounts of astigmatism are present. Despite steady improvements in technology and manufacturing techniques, HTCLs remain relatively complicated medical and optical devices. Hydrogel-lens flexure, and incomplete draping and axis mislocation caused by unanticipated lens rotation, can combine to significantly complicate the fitting process. In essence, the art and science of HTCL management requires a fine balance between simple optics and the dynamics of a complex lens in an inherently unstable environment. Proper patient and contact lens selection can minimize many of the potential problems that face the HTCL fitter.

PATIENT SELECTION AND SPECIFIC INDICATIONS FOR HTCLS

As is true of all contact lens fitting, patient needs are central to this process. HTCL fitting begins with a thorough understanding of all patient-related factors as well as the specific performance characteristics of each type of HTCL. Clinical success with HTCLs demands the same physical and physiologic performance that other lenses require, combined with specialized visual requirements unique to toric lenses. Visual requirements include the following:

1. Good vision maintained in all directions of gaze.
2. Stable vision, minimally affected by lid actions, lens fit factors, or eye movement.
3. Sustained vision minimally affected by environmental or physiologic factors that may affect meridional orientation or the optical characteristics of the lens.

Careful patient selection and proper choice of lens type or brand can maximize the probability of success. The following patient characteristics should be considered.

PATIENT HISTORY

Patients being considered for HTCLs should be good candidates for hydrogel lenses in general. Relative contraindications for hydrogel soft lens wear include ocular surface disease, dry eye, severe allergy, chronic infection, or prior history of multiple serious complications associated with hydrogel lenses. The physiologic limitations inherent in current hydrogel materials may preclude some patients from safely wearing presently available HTCLs. Newer materials such as silicone hydrogels will expand safety and physiologic tolerance profiles significantly when they become available in toric designs. Motivated patients who were unable to adapt to rigid gas-permeable (GP) lenses because of general discomfort or edge awareness are usually excellent candidates for HTCLs. These patients are typically more willing to accept the minor visual compromise that may occur with HTCLs. GP wearers with astigmatism who have chronic 3- and 9-o'clock staining, corneal warpage, excessive lens movement or decentration, lens-induced visual disturbance, persistent lens coating, or poor lens wetting may also be good candidates for HTCLs.

Astigmatic first-time contact lens wearers now benefit from a large number of possible choices encompassing both GP and HTCL designs. HTCLs include conventional and a growing number and variety of frequent replacement-disposable lenses. The relative advantages and disadvantages of each type of lens must be considered with regard to the patient's needs and expectations. The most effective way of selecting the best lens for a specific patient is through diagnostic evaluation and a thorough discussion with the patient about the relative merits of each lens type. For example, rigid GP lenses may provide better and more consistent acuity but may not be appropriate when initial comfort is an important issue for the patient (9,10). Patients who participate in active sports may prefer HTCLs because of their greater corneal coverage and reduced potential for displacement during physical activity. Despite significant advances in lens construction and much improved ease of fit, diagnostic evaluation of lenses on patients' eyes remains the best method of selecting the appropriate lens type, and also assists in rapidly determining lens specifications.

SOFT LENS CORRECTION OF ASTIGMATISM

Amount of Astigmatism

Tolerance for uncorrected astigmatism generally increases with greater total refractive error. Uncorrected refractive astigmatism greater than 0.75 D is unacceptable to many patients with low spherical refractive errors (5). Such patients typically have acceptable uncorrected acuity and tend to be less tolerant of visual compromise and inconsistency that may result from the use of HTCLs. In contrast, patients who present with greater overall spherical refractive errors usually tolerate uncorrected cylinder with less difficulty. Despite significant improvements in HTCL optical power range, stability, and ease of fit, when the astigmatic correction is less than 25% of the spherical correction, several authorities believe it is advisable to first assess the performance of a spherical hydrogel lens (particularly with high minus, where magnification also benefits the clinician) (11, 12). Spherical lenses in higher power ranges, of thicker construction, and those made from less pliant materials incompletely drape over a toric cornea and may neutralize some corneal toricity. This cylinder-masking effect can provide acceptable visual performance for patients with mild and, in some cases, even moderate astigmatism. Patients with small degrees of against-the-rule astigmatism have also been successfully corrected with spherical prism hydrogel lenses with 2.0 Δ of base-down prism (13). The refractive effect of a tilted prismatic surface combined with the lens thickness differential produces a cylindrical power effect on the eye that can correct up to 0.75 D of against-the-rule cylinder.

Single use disposable toric lenses have recently been introduced for patients with low degrees of astigmatism. Focus DAILIES, manufactured by Ciba Vision, is a back-surface toric employing double thin zones and a tricurve design. It is currently available in an 8.6 base curve (BC), 14.2-mm overall diameter (OAD) with only a −0.75-D cylinder power in two axes: 180 and 90 degrees. Currently, spherical powers range from −0.50 to −6.00 D in 0.25-D steps. Parameter expansion in the near future is likely.

Moderate astigmatism (1.25 to 2.50 D), which is most common, is easily managed with many of the available frequent replacement or disposable HTCLs. Highly astigmatic corrections will generally require custom HTCLs; however, several frequent replacement lenses are now available in higher cylinder powers. Special custom toric designs are available in cylinder powers of up to −16.00 D. Despite their greater sensitivity to rotation or axis mislocation, they provide a viable option for high astigmatism regardless of axis (14,15).

Axis of Astigmatism

The cylindrical axis plays a dual role in HTCL correction. For patients with myopic astigmatism, uncorrected oblique and against-the-rule astigmatism can cause more visual distress and asthenopia than will uncorrected with-the-rule astigmatism. This occurs because the predominant (perceptual) requirement is that vertical lines be in focus; the least minus focal line falling on the retina provides the preferred visual result in cases of myopic astigmatism (16). Thus, HTCL correction of with-the-rule astigmatism is easier to achieve. The correcting cylinder axis itself can affect HTCL orientation and stability. Torquing effects of the blink tend to cause more rotation and instability in oblique cylinder lenses because of lid-lens interaction occurring at the meridian with the thickest edge profile (most minus power). Modern HTCL designs, however, minimize lid interaction by equalizing edge thickness around the full circumference of the lens (12,14,17). Rigid GP lenses tend to be more difficult to fit on against-the-rule corneas, often positioning laterally, and HTCLs may be more stable and less problematic in these cases (7,8).

TORIC SOFT LENS FITTING GUIDELINES

Some general rules may be helpful in initial lens selection. A quantitative comparison of the relative amount of corneal toricity to refractive astigmatism is helpful whenever the use of a toric lens is contemplated. This simple calculation will predict any residual astigmatism and assist in the selection of the least complex and most appropriate GP or hydrogel lens design. If calculated residual astigmatism is significant, a HTCL is usually preferred. It automatically corrects the internal cylinder that would be manifest if a spherical rigid GP lens were used, and eliminates the need for a more complex prism-ballast front toric, or bitoric rigid lens design. Internal astigmatism is most commonly found with spherical corneas or moderately against-the-rule corneas, typically in the range of −0.75 to −1.50 D at axes of 90 ± 15 degrees. Corneal toricity can negate or add to internal astigmatism. When refractive astigmatism is *significantly less* or *significantly greater* than the corneal toricity, a HTCL design usually provides the least complex contact lens option. A spherical GP lens would create significant residual astigmatism in either situation.

When the axes of the principal corneal meridians do not coincide with the refractive axes, HTCL correction may be unpredictable. The contact lens tends to align with the primary corneal meridians instead of the refractive axis. This can induce a cross cylinder effect and significant oblique residual astigmatism, especially when a back-surface HTCL has been fitted (18). In such situations a GP lens may be preferable (15), although a HTCL design may still be effective if the lens remains stable. GP lenses may also be preferable for patients who are overly sensitive to axis mislocation caused by HTCL instability. The *Becherer twist test* evaluates a patient's visual sensitivity to axis rotation (8). This test is performed by rocking the patient's refractive cylinder axis in a trial frame or phoropter until the patient first reports blur. A report of blur with less than 5 degrees of axis rotation is not likely to result in successful soft toric lens wear. Despite reduced clarity compared to rigid lenses, many patients report an overall preference for HTCLs (19).

When calculating the cylinder power of an HTCL, only the total refractive cylinder needs to be considered. The relationship of the cornea and the posterior contact lens surface does not create a significant tear lens as occurs with GP lenses. Rotational and flexure effects of toric soft lenses may affect the final prescription, however, and require lens power or axis compensation.

Lid Configuration and Anatomy

Since the dynamics of lid action is one of the principal causes of lens axis mislocation and undesired rotation, eyelid anatomy and function are critical when fitting toric lenses (20). The ideal eye has a relatively wide aperture, normal lid tension, complete closure, a lower lid that positions at the inferior limbus, and no elevated or redundant conjunctival tissue or scars that might interfere with lens positioning or movement. Lids that are unusually tight or eyes that have small palpebral apertures can exert excessive force on the lens, resulting in unpredictable orientation. A lower lid positioned higher than 2 mm above the limbus or sharply angled from the horizontal plane may cause undesired axis mislocation. Lid anatomical angles and aperture size were recently found to play a significant role in lens fit and stability. Specifically, greater upward incline of the temporal lids was associated with increasing inferior-temporal lens orientation, and smaller palpebral aperture size was associated with more stable lens orientation (21). Racial variation may also play a role in HTCL fitting and success (22).

An incomplete blinking pattern can adversely affect HTCL performance because of localized dehydration and deposit buildup on the inferior lens surface (Fig. 26.1). Re-

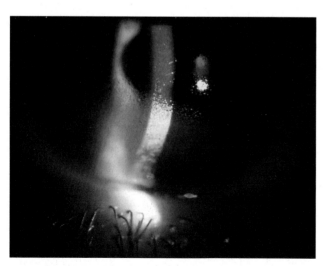

FIG. 26.1. Dense mixed protein and mineral coating characteristic of a conventional prism ballasted (nonrotating) toric hydrogel worn for an extended period.

duced tear volume or an unstable tear film may also induce unwanted lens rotation as a result of lens dehydration during wear, with subsequent changes in lens-cornea adherence.

Special Considerations

The use of HTCLs may be unacceptable for patients with intolerance to slight prescription changes or for people who have critical visual requirements. Patients with early presbyopia require special consideration. Lens axis shifts in the down gaze position can affect visual acuity, which can further strain an already stressed accommodative system. Prescribing HTCLs for presbyopic patients using a monovision approach can be successful but may require several refinements to optimize the correction. Several manufacturers now produce toric hydrogel multifocal lenses, which offer presbyopic patients with astigmatism a possible contact lens option. When early presbyopic patients need only minor astigmatic correction and comfort is an important factor, a nontoric HTCL may be the best choice. When vision is the overriding concern, however, GP lenses are usually preferred (8).

Irregular astigmatism, distorted corneal topography, and keratoconus also typically require GP lenses for best correction (23), although HTCLs may be successfully fitted when GP lenses are not tolerated. HTCLs may not provide visual acuity equal to that of GP lenses in these cases, yet some patients will find HTCL visual performance adequate in light of enhanced comfort. For more advanced keratoconus patients, HTCLs have generally been advocated as a last resort or as alternate "relief" lenses. Despite the unusually steep central corneal topography of most keratoconus patients, a median base curve often fits acceptably. Soft lenses are semiscleral designs with relatively large sagittal heights and, therefore conform well to the usually normal peripheral corneal topography. Pellucid marginal degeneration (PMD) is another indication for HTCL correction. Inferior thinning can result in GP inferior decentration and visual compromise. Prism-ballasted HTCLs are often surprisingly stable, and because the central topography is usually regular, provide adequate visual correction. Recently, keratoconus- and PMD-specific HTCLs have become available (e.g., SUPER NOVA HydroKone Toric; Innovations in Sight, Front Royal, VA). These lenses work surprisingly well for many patients.

HTCLs can also be extremely helpful in managing post–penetrating keratoplasty (24) and post–refractive surgery contact lens fitting (25). Physiologic limitations of current hydrogel lens materials and the risk of potentially serious complications, however, make caution prudent. Trial fitting is crucial in these complex patients and an accurate overrefraction is essential. Aberrant topography may produce a refractive resultant that is unexpected, but overall visual results are often remarkably functional. Because of their complexity, use of custom HTCLs for patients with keratoconus or other topographic irregularities is often complicated by refinements leading to the need for reordered lenses in effort to achieve a satisfactory visual result.

LENS DESIGN AND STABILIZING TECHNIQUES

Rotational stability is critical requirement for a successful HTCL design. The methods used to stabilize HTCLs include prism ballasting, truncation, dynamic stabilization with double-thin zones, periballasting, eccentric lenticulation, back-surface toricity, and combinations of all of the above. No matter which method of stabilization is used, orientation is achieved as a result of a thickness differential between the superior, central, and inferior portions of the lens. Currently, in the United States, there are at least 27 manufacturers fabricating 73 different toric soft lenses, many of which are very similar to each other in basic construction and design (26). The various methods used to achieve rotational stability are discussed below.

Prism Ballasting

Incorporating 0.75 to 2.0 D of base-down prism can stabilize a hydrogel lens and allow it to resist rotational forces. One theory is that prism stabilizes a lens by its lower center of gravity (27). Prism stability is more accurately explained, however, by the *watermelon seed principle* (28). This concept, elaborated by Hanks (29), is analogous to the engineering principle describing pressure effects on wedges. If a moist wedge is squeezed, the resultant action is for the wedge to be expelled by the pressure in a direction away from the wedge apex. Lid pressure squeezes the lens into the base-down direction, thus stabilizing it. The principle works in a similar way for both prism and nonprism toric lenses. Nonprism, double-thin zone designs are thinned superiorly and inferiorly and have greater thickness in the center. This creates a *biprism* effect with bases joined along the horizontal plane at the center of the lens. Lid pressure keeps the lens stabilized within the open aperture. Because the insignificant role gravity plays in stabilizing the lens compared to lens-cornea adherence and lid forces, HTCLs usually do not rotate while patients lie on their sides. This is occasionally observed with prism-ballasted GP lenses (where gravity effects are more significant).

Research in Australia recently evaluated several HTCL characteristics and on-eye performance. The result of this research was the design of a new 2-week disposable HTCL with a variety of enhanced characteristics (30). Specifically, the new design optimized prism ballast thickness and position for improved comfort and orientation stability. Uniform horizontal ballast thickness and a wide ballast band evenly distribute lens mass and minimize thickness differen-

tials. Additionally, constant ballast between powers eases fitting and enhances lens consistency.

Truncation

Although truncated lenses were common some years ago, they have fallen out of favor and are now of greater historical than practical interest. Advances in HTCL design provide much of the stability of truncated designs without the common comfort problems. Truncated lenses are made by removing 0.5 to 1.5 mm of plastic from the lower lens edge. Larger truncations are used with larger overall lens diameters. Truncation stabilizes the lens by alignment with the lower lid margin. This technique is still currently used in the fabrication of rigid translating segmented-bifocal lens designs. While truncation effectively raises the lens' center of gravity, rotational stability is minimally affected because of the minor role gravity plays. Although double truncation had been attempted, it was found to be uncomfortable and of no clinical advantage (60).

Truncation adds stability to a prism-ballasted lens, provides an easily observable reference for axis position at 90° to the prism base-apex line, and has an anchoring effect between the lobes or ends of the truncation and the bulbar conjunctiva (9). A slight loosening of the fit can enhance the inherent stabilizing effects of this design, and the formation of a tear meniscus along the truncation promotes better tear exchange and aids in the flushing of metabolic byproducts and debris (31). Since the truncated edge remains aligned with the lower lid margin, nasal torquing is minimized when the eye is lowered and converged to a reading position. Truncation should ideally parallel the lid margin and in contact with the lid, except for a brief, post-blink vertical movement. Compensation of the correcting cylinder must be made if the lower lid slope is other than 180 degrees since the lens usually will orient along the angle of the lid margin. Patients with lower lids positioned below the inferior limbus are generally poor candidates for truncated lens designs.

Dynamic Stabilization: Thin-zone Design

Thinning both upper and lower sections of a lens causes the thickest portion of the lens to be its center. Thin zones at the top and bottom are covered by the lids and, because of the *watermelon seed principle* described previously, the thicker center can be expected to position horizontally between the lids. This "dynamic stabilization" was first developed in Europe and a viable design was marketed called the "Titmus Eurocon thin zone lens." Thin-zone stabilization is currently used alone and in combination with other stabilization methods by several manufacturers in the United States and abroad. These stabilization zones are beveled equally or are double slaboff in form resulting in a nonprismatic lens. *Thin-zone* designs are more successful when the horizontal and vertical lens profiles have their greatest thickness differential, such as in higher myopic corrections or with against-the-rule cylinder patients that maximize the previously described wedge effect. Plus lenses in this design are inherently less stable, but incorporating a minus carrier before the thin zones are added, artificially creates a thickness differential that works in much the same way as it does for minus toric lenses. The *thin-zone* construction usually provides good comfort, good optics, but occasionally unpredictable axis location despite reasonably good stability (32).

When a toric lens on one eye produces a clinically significant vertical imbalance (induced by the lens' prism ballast), using a double thin-zone design, which contains no prism, may be beneficial. Symptomatic induced vertical imbalance while very rare has been reported (33). The effective prismatic power of a contact lens on the eye is related to the position of the visual axis relative to its geometric center, and its refractive power (34). Thus, the effective prism power of a prism contact lens varies along its vertical meridian and also depends upon the refractive index of the surrounding media.

Periballasting

The periballasted design differs from prism-ballasted designs by limiting the prism ballast to the lens periphery only, excluding it from the optical zone. A true periballasted lens is fabricated by removing the superior portion of a high-minus lenticular carrier, which reduces lid-lens edge interaction and produces a peripheral-ballast in the inferior area of the lens. By eliminating prism in the optical zone, center thickness is reduced and optical quality improved (35). Several current HTCL designs mimic periballasting by eliminating prism from optical zone.

Eccentric Lenticulation

This is a front-surface, off-center (eccentric) lenticular cut in the direction of the prism apex, similar to a periballast. Removal of this "excess" material from the lens' anterior surface provides several benefits. Among them are reduced differential edge thickness (which increases both stability and comfort), reduced lens mass (which better replicates the behavior of a spherical soft lens), and better limbal-scleral draping (to minimize compression of the conjunctiva).

Eccentric lenticulation is especially beneficial with front toric lens construction, where edge thickness can vary significantly. Increased stability is particularly evident with oblique astigmatic corrections where, upon eye closure, the descending lid margin will first meet an offset thickened portion of a lens at an oblique angle to cause torsional mislocation (1). Eccentric lenticulation creates superior and inferior thin portions on the lens, and thereby equalizes the thickness of the lens periphery (with the prism remaining only in the central two thirds of the lens). Many laboratories and manufacturers making modern HTCLs incorporate eccentric lenticulation into their designs, a concept that was initially pioneered by Ewell (13).

Back Toricity

Some clinicians report that back cylinder construction enhances HTCL stability, especially on eyes with corneal toricity greater than 3.00 D (9,36,37). Studies have not been performed to isolate back toricity as a major stabilizing feature; however, it seems logical to expect that the same "saddle fitting the horse" or wrapping effect observed with toric GP lenses is present and leads to this conclusion. Many modern toric lenses and most custom HTCLs are now made with back toricity, with toric zones limited to central optic areas. Toric curves that are confined to the central optic zone reduce differential edge thickness, which again minimizes lid-blink–related torsional effects. Whether by design or manufacturing skill, back surface toric designs function very well in terms of predictable axis location and nonrotation, but only when combined with prism ballasting. As a rule of thumb, many clinicians believe that corneas with low toricities are best fit with front toric designs and moderate and high corneal toricities (1.50 D and up) are best fit with back toric designs (32). Unlike toric GP lenses (where the difference can be significant), there is little functional difference or advantage to either front or back toric construction in terms of toric soft lens optical performance.

TORIC LENS FABRICATION

Presently available HTCLs use the design features described earlier in various combinations (except for obsolete truncation). Production methods can be categorized into three basic groups: wet and dry cast molding, lathe-cut/crimped, or lathe-cut/toric-generated. Several HTCL designs combine molding and lathing (discussed in Chapter 18).

Traditional toric-specific lathe-cutting/crimping techniques produce either a front or back toric surface. The lens' optical zone is cut and polished while the button is kept under controlled pressure in a crimped state; the lens is then removed and allowed to "relax," generating toric surface(s). Used most frequently with back toric constructions, a toroidal oval shape is generated in the central optical zone only, which helps minimize asymmetric edge thickness. The other surface curvature (usually the front of the lens) is calculated for the spherical power required and is lathed spherically, by "offset cutting," to produce the prism. Crimping is still widely used by several manufacturers, especially for custom toric lens designs in higher cylinder powers.

A direct toric-generating process was first introduced by Bausch & Lomb with its "Optima" HTCL. Without the need for crimping, and secondary plastic fatigue and stress, optical quality and power predictability (yield) all improve. Computer lathing also produces a desirable relatively thin lens profile. Modern computer controlled lathes produce complex nonrotationally symmetrical surfaces by synchronized controlled movement of both the cutting tool and the lens holding spindle. More traditional "fly cutting," which is commonly used in the spectacle lens industry, produces complex curves by moving the rotating cutting tool through a controlled arc. Computer-controlled lathing produces excellent optical surfaces and a thin, uniform edge profile without the need for additional finishing. However, the amount of toricity that can be practically generated is limited by the size of the optical zone of the lens.

Polishing a toric surface (or any nonspherical surface) is difficult and can compromise optical surface quality and resultant clarity; modern technology has now minimized this problem. Although traditional techniques like crimping are still commonly in use, recent advances in computer controlled toric lathing, improved molding techniques and combinations of both, have revolutionized HTCL manufacture to provide reliable and reproducible lenses with excellent optical and physical qualities.

FITTING PRINCIPLES AND PROBLEM SOLVING

Axis Location and Orientation

Under ideal circumstances, HTCLs position predictably and without rotation. In practice, this is not always the case (38). Lens rotation results from the combined effects of several factors. Of these, the primary influence on lens orientation is from the torsional forces of the lids applied to the lens during a blink. Lid closure is a complex motion (39) that creates a tendency for nasal up-rotation (encyclorotation) of a contact lens, a movement that is commonly observed with GP lenses. Blinking, therefore, can destabilize an HTCL (40). Lid shape, anatomy, as well as movement, lid tightness against the globe, size of the aperture, the dynamics of lid closure, lens lifting effects upon lid opening, and the lid-lens edge interaction also play important but variable roles (21).

Lens design, prescription, and fitting parameters influence lens stability (41). Specific factors include overall lens thickness and mass, the construction of the lens such as front versus back toricity or lenticulation, the amount and position of any prism, adherence between the lens and eye (determined by the lens-eye fitting relationship), lens material characteristics (flexure and elasticity), and tear film dynamics such as capillary attraction and lubricity. Other factors, including peripheral corneal topography (42), a variety of topographic descriptors including asymmetry (43), and the effects of gravity on the lens, play important roles in lens orientation. Ocular cyclorotation may influence lens

orientation and stability (44). All of these factors combine to produce a complex ballet of forces and motion.

With this litany of potential destabilizing factors, it is surprising how little most modern HTCLs rotate (45–49), yet rotation leading to axis mislocation remains the major cause of inadequate HTCL visual acuity (1,50). The term mislocation describes a consistent lens rotation to some resting position other than that desired or anticipated. This occurs more frequently with tightly fitting lenses, tight lids or inadequately ballasted lenses (21). The less common problem of blink-induced rotation or rocking usually occurs because of a loose fit or insufficient lens stabilization features or forces. The amount of visual disruption produced by an unstable lens depends on the power of the cylinder, the degree of rocking, and speed of recovery as the lens regains its resting position following a blink or change of gaze. Selecting a different base curve, increasing lens overall diameter, or selecting a lens design of greater prism ballast often resolves dynamic stability problems.

Axis misorientation invariably produces an optical spherocylindrical miscorrection. Since this effect can be substantial, especially with higher cylinder powers, most clinicians believe it necessary to evaluate and compensate for axis misorientation. This requires trial fitting of a similar contact lens so that lens alignment and stability can be observed. Although time consuming, trial fitting also provides important information about lens fit, position, stability, and patient comfort.

Determining the Appropriate Toric Soft Lens Parameters

Despite improvements in design and more consistent manufacturing, HTCLs remain complex optical devices that must be specified precisely. Empirical fitting is technically the easiest way to order lenses since it initially requires no chair time beyond a conventional ocular examination without trial lens fitting. This method has become increasingly attractive with the emergence of frequent replacement and more predictable disposable HTCLs. While numerous studies suggest that direct empirical ordering based only on a spectacle refraction and keratometry provides an acceptable result (51–56), other studies indicate that trial lens fitting with subsequent calculation of the appropriate lens powers is more effective (33,57–59). Recent advances in lens design and manufacturing enhance fitting success using an empirical approach for direct ordering or fitting from an in-office lens bank (30).

Direct Ordering

Proponents of direct ordering cite simplicity and convenience. Lenses are ordered directly from the patient's spectacle prescription (compensated for vertex distance effects) or selected from a bank of stocked "trial" lenses. Keratometer readings uncommonly help select lens fitting characteristics. Alternatively, examination results can be provided to the HTCL manufacturer where consultants determine the appropriate powers and fit. Computer lens design programs may be used to assist in selecting lens specifications. Some clinicians automatically compensate for anticipated nasal lens rotation, although the value of this is uncertain.

The direct order method appears to be successful. One study found that 75% of eyes achieved acuity equal to that of the patient's best corrected spectacle acuity, and 95% of eyes achieved acuity equal to or within one line of the optimal spectacle acuity with empirically ordered HTCLs (61). A more recent study looked at empirical fit success with a newer HTCL design and reported a resultant difference (between the actual and predicted OR) of only +0.35D sphere and −0.18 cylinder (30). Another study found that a lens manufacturer using empirical data designed a lens yielding better clinical results than that achieved by two experienced contact lens practitioners (53). An Internet-based survey of optometrists' toric lens ordering preferences generated responses from 106 optometrists in five countries (62); 55% direct-ordered HTCLs. Most clinicians automatically consider the initial empirically ordered lens as a diagnostic lens if it performs poorly, using it to help determine the appropriate reorder.

Diagnostic Lens Fitting

Diagnostic lens fitting serves several purposes. It is the only way to evaluate lens alignment and stability, and provides important information about lens position and comfort. Lens rotation causes axis misorientation that in turn produces spherocylindrical miscorrection. Although some patients will tolerate small degrees of misorientation (63), others, especially those who have higher amounts of cylinder, will find uncompensated lens axis mislocation unacceptable. To ensure that the diagnostic lens will function in a similar fashion to the final lens, diagnostic lenses should be of the same brand, overall diameter, and base curve. Diagnostic fitting using a similar lens design in a different material may be useful if the exact lens or design is unavailable. Parameters should be relatively close to the desired sphere and cylinder powers and especially astigmatic axis (about 20 degrees). Ideally, the clinician should allow 15 to 20 minutes for lens equilibration before evaluating the fit and overrefraction. The final lens can be determined from the trial lens in one of three ways:

Rotational Compensation

A popular method of compensating for axis misorientation is to apply a trial lens to determine rotation and to then adjust for the order, commonly referred to as the "LARS" method (left add, right subtract). A recent survey suggests that more than 70% of optometrists who trial fit HTCLs

use LARS (54). The method requires that any misrotation be *stable* and referenced to the examiner's right or left. If the lens marking rotates to the examiner's left, the amount of rotation is *added* to the correction. If to the right, the amount of rotation is *subtracted*. Another approach uses the patient's nose as the reference point: if the bottom of the lens rotates inward (toward the patient's nose), the new axis is specified "out" by an equal amount and vice versa. Both methods share the same objective: compensation for lens rotation by specifying a new astigmatic axis, equal in amount but opposite in direction to the observed rotation. For example, using LARS, if a −1.00 −1.00 × 180 HTCL in the left eye rotates 10 degrees to the right, the amount of rotation would be subtracted and an axis 170 would be ordered. Using the nose as a reference, a right lens axis 180 that rotates "in" 10 degrees should be reordered at axis 170 (10 degrees out). To understand why these simple approaches work, consider that a cylinder of axis 180 rotating 10 degrees counterclockwise would actually be orienting at axis 10. To compensate, the lens should be ordered at axis 170 so that after the 10 degrees counterclockwise rotation the cylinder would position at the desired axis of 180. Important but "hidden" sources of potential error with positional approaches like LARS include any inaccuracies in marked or measured cylinder power/axis, prism base markings, or in estimating the amount of rotation.

Several methods can measure lens rotation. A trial frame with a low-powered cylindrical trial lens marked along its axis, or a biomicroscope/slit-lamp narrow beam, can be aligned with the markings on the diagnostic HTCL and measured. Alternatively, the biomicroscope/slit lamp can be modified by use of a protractor reticule mounted in one of the microscope oculars. Most oculars are designed so that such a measuring reticule can be inserted within the optical system (64). Some biomicroscopes allow an optional eyepiece marked with radial reticules that allow accurate measurements while viewing the eye and the lens under magnification.

The aximeter is a simple but very useful device that can aid in measuring with accuracy of 20 degree rotation. A focusing rod is inserted in the biomicroscope calibration rod mount which has a protractor etched onto its head (65). After aligning a narrow slit lamp beam with the lens axis marking, the beam is superimposed onto the aximeter head for accurate axis measurement.

A simpler approach, used by many practitioners, is to grossly estimate the amount of rotation. Although this would appear to be inaccurate, one study found that estimates were generally within 20 degrees of the actual rotation (66). No difference was noted in accuracy when different lens marking methods were compared in this study.

Computational Compensation

Under ideal circumstances, a HTCL with an on-the-eye back vertex power equal to the patient's refraction at the ocular plane should produce a Plano overrefraction. Any deviation caused by lens misorientation, incorrect power, or other unanticipated factors will generate a spherocylindrical resultant that can be measured by overrefraction. Thus, overrefraction serves as an excellent way to assess the clinical performance of a lens and define any required correction. HTCL axis misorientation produces a spherocylinder with the amount of the cylinder double the power of the spherical component but of opposite sign (1). Other potential sources of HTCL miscorrection include initial refraction or overrefraction errors, lens parameter miscalculation, marking or fabrication errors and unexpected power induced by lens flexure, draping and tear film effects (67–69). Power effects directly caused by lens flexure are generally insignificant. However, a small minus-power tear film lens may be created beneath the thicker meridian due to reduced meridional conformity (70). This effect increases with greater cylinder power and would be further exaggerated by prism ballast in a lens that corrects with-the-rule astigmatism. Although subject to some debate, (71) the presence of a meridional minus tear lens has been cited as a rationale for reducing the amount of cylinder power when prescribing HTCLs (50). Several contact lens manufacturers provide a chart to suggest compensation for these effects (Table 26.1). On highly astigmatic corneas, especially when the refractive and corneal cylinders do not align, draping of a toric soft lens can induce a bitoric-like effect. In such cases, the lens may appear to be in alignment, but the induced off-axis cylinder may produce a new and significantly different resultant axis (50). Toric lens computation based on overrefraction intrinsically compensates for these factors. By comparison, rotational compensation alone does not.

Experienced clinicians often treat the overrefraction and the power of the correcting lens *in situ* as crossed cylinders and apply the sum of the crossed cylinders formula to calculate a resultant spherocylindrical power. The spherocylindrical resultant of the trial lens power and the overrefraction represents a combination of the effects of axis mislocation, trial lens power, and any meridional power differences between the trial lens and actual patient refraction. It also yields an approximation of the power of the new lens to be ordered. Axis mislocation by itself in a properly powered lens produces an overrefraction with a spherical equivalent

of zero. However, errors in contact lens power will produce a spherical equivalent unequal to zero (72). An alternative approach to mathematically calculating the spherocylindrical resultant is to combine the original lens power (*oriented at the specified axis*) with the overrefraction in a trial frame using trial lenses. The resultant power is read directly from a lensometer.

Despite any inherent inaccuracy in this method of calculation, a study that compared the LARS method with computer calculation using trial lens overrefraction showed that overrefraction produced close to a one line increase in Snellen acuity performance (73). Other studies validate use of spherocylindrical overrefraction as an accurate predictor of HTCL performance (33,74). Toric lens calculation using a handheld computer combined with autorefraction over known diagnostic lenses is generally an effective and efficient means of determining HTCL parameters (75). Several contact lens manufacturers advocate this computational approach to lens ordering and offered inexpensive preprogrammed handheld computers or, more recently, personal digital assistant-based or desktop-based programs that can be utilized to make the necessary calculations (Fig. 26.2). Under most circumstances, calculated compensation is reasonably accurate. Perfecting a HTCL prescription, however, may still involve a series of refinements in lens power and orientation.

Until recently, the majority of clinicians assumed that use of the crossed cylinders' formula applied to sum the trial

TABLE 26.1. RECOMMENDED CYLINDER POWER COMPENSATION FOR MYOPIC CORRECTIONS

Cylinder Power	Add to Spectacle Cylinder Rx
−1.00 to −2.00	+0.25
−2.25 to −3.50	+0.50
−3.75 to −5.75	+0.75
−6.00 to −7.00	+1.00

Compensation is not necessary for hyperopic corrections. Reprinted with permission of Sunsoft.

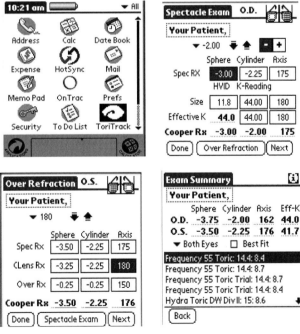

FIG. 26.2. Four sample screen shots of Palm-based "ToriTrack" program for calculating hydrogel toric contact lens overrefraction-based resultant optical powers and appropriate CooperVision products. (Compliments of and with permission from CooperVision.)

contact lens prescription and the resultant spherocylindrical overrefraction automatically compensated for lens rotation. Koers and Quinn demonstrated, however, the need to account for lens rotation while making this calculation (76). Comparing HTCL parameters calculated by using a preprogrammed toric lens computer to values obtained by applying the LARS method, they mathematically established that failure to account for rotation could result in significant error (Table 26.2), and these authors recommend first compensating for any trial lens rotation by using RALS (right add, left subtract) and then applying the sum of the crossed cylinders formula using the compensated axis The result of this series of calculations invariably concurs with results obtained by using the LARS method.

Although somewhat complicated, this rotationally compensated approach of calculation may also be accomplished using trial lenses in a lensometer. The technique is the same as described previously, only trial lens rotation needs to be factored in when aligning the lenses in the lensometer and LARS applied to the resultant. Several computer programs are now available that compensate for lens rotation when calculating the appropriate HTCL to be ordered (Fig. 26.2).

Matrix optics have been proposed as a more accurate way to determine axis misalignment and power errors of HTCLs (64,77). This method calculates the appropriate effective back vertex power of the trial lens by subtracting any overrefraction from the patient's refraction. By comparing the calculated back vertex power to the specified back vertex power of the lens, the amount of axis mislocation

and the appropriate HTCL powers can be determined. Toric lens calculation using matrix optics can be made using a Java applet located (at the time of publication of this text) at: http://www.optometry.unimelb.edu.au/misc/OphthalmiCalc/OphthalmiCalc.html.

Evaluating Toric Lens Performance

The accuracy of any calculation or compensation for HTCL rotation is only as accurate as its individual elements. When using the LARS approach, accurate lens marking and accuracy in measuring lens rotation are both critical. Calculated solutions, regardless of method used, will be accurate only if flexure, tear film effects, lens rotation, and other relevant factors remain consistent between the trial and the ordered lens. Other sources of error include trial lens mislabeling or mismarking; so-called target labeling used by some manufacturers, (73) errors in overrefraction and in the accuracy of the initial refraction; and even the 0.25-D steps that are most commonly used to overrefract can result in miscalculation (69). When meridional powers have been correctly calculated and these other factors remain constant, any residual overrefraction is likely caused by rotation inconsistent with the anticipated position. In combined approaches, both observational and computation factors can adversely affect accuracy. The majority of patients seem unaffected, however, by this inherent inaccuracy (39). With the limited amount of mislocation commonly observed with modern lenses, many clinicians and contact lens manufacturers believe that

TABLE 26.2. COMPARISON OF TORIC LENS ROTATION, RESULTANT OVERREFRACTION, THE LENS ORDER SUGGESTED BY THE SUM OF CROSS-CYLINDER FORMULA (TRIAL LENS + OVERREFRACTION) AND THE LENS ORDER SUGGESTED BY LARS COMPENSATION IN A PATIENT WITH A PL −2.00 × 180 REFRACTION

Lens Rotation	Pl−2.00 × 180 Aligns at Axis	Patient's Overrefraction	Sum of Crossed Cylinder Result	After LARS Compensation
0°	180	Plano	Pl −2.00 × 180	Pl −2.00 × 180
+10°	10	+0.35 −0.69 × 50	Pl −2.00 × 10	Pl −2.00 × 10
+20°	20	+0.68 −1.37 × 55	Pl −2.00 × 20	Pl −2.00 × 20
+30°	30	+1.00 −2.00 × 60	Pl −2.00 × 30	Pl −2.00 × 30
+40°	40	+1.29 −2.57 × 65	Pl −2.00 × 40	Pl −2.00 × 40
+50°	50	+1.53 −3.06 × 70	Pl −2.00 × 50	Pl −2.00 × 50
+60°	60	+1.73 −3.46 × 75	Pl −2.00 × 60	Pl −2.00 × 60
+70°	70	+1.88 −3.76 × 80	Pl −2.00 × 70	Pl −2.00 × 70
+80°	80	+1.97 −3.94 × 85	Pl −2.00 × 80	Pl −2.00 × 80
+90°	90	+2.00 −4.00 × 90	Pl −2.00 × 90	Pl −2.00 × 90
−80°	100	+1.97 −3.94 × 95	Pl −2.00 × 100	Pl −2.00 × 100
−70°	110	+1.88 −3.76 × 100	Pl −2.00 × 110	Pl −2.00 × 110
−60°	120	+1.73 −3.46 × 105	Pl −2.00 × 120	Pl −2.00 × 120
−50°	130	+1.53 −3.06 × 110	Pl −2.00 × 130	Pl −2.00 × 130
−40°	140	+1.29 −2.57 × 115	Pl −2.00 × 140	Pl −2.00 × 140
−30°	150	+1.00 −2.00 × 120	Pl −2.00 × 150	Pl −2.00 × 150
−20°	160	+0.68 −1.37 × 125	Pl −2.00 × 160	Pl −2.00 × 160
−10°	170	+0.35 −0.69 × 130	Pl −2.00 × 170	Pl −2.00 × 170
0°	180	Plano	Pl −2.00 × 180	Pl −2.00 × 180

(Adapted from Holden [1].)

using the obliquely crossed cylinders formula and trial lens overrefraction provides sufficient accuracy for clinical use.

Lens fitting characteristics can impact lens orientation and stability. Steeply fitting lenses tend to lock at unpredictable and incorrect orientations or will slowly rotate in one direction (78). Lenses that move freely will respond properly to the orientation forces that stabilize them. In contrast, loose fitting lenses often result in poor vision from blink-induced variable rotation (79). Rotational velocity should be checked at the lens edge. This is the speed with which a poorly oriented toric lens will rotate in its effort to recover and to reorient (31). Following deliberate mislocation (by dialing about 45 degrees using a finger-tip or a cotton-tipped applicator) and release, the lens should to return to its initial stable orientation within 15 seconds (with normal blinking). A rapid return is desirable and is particularly important for patients with demanding sports or occupational vision requirements. Tight lids can impede proper lens orientation. Patients with tight lids should be instructed to insert their lenses with careful attention to the prism markings (80).

Equilibration (a "settling" time) of about 20 minutes should be adequate for a reliable assessment of the fit of most HTCL designs; note that lenses made of lower water content plastics are generally believed to require less time. If a lens shows unpredictable rotation or mislocation of greater than 30 degrees after equilibration, a base curve change, a larger diameter, or a different type of toric lens should be considered. Small degrees of mislocation or rocking (0 to 5 degrees) are visually acceptable to most patients, especially in cylinder powers of -2.00 D or less (55). Greater amounts of mislocation must be corrected using axis compensation. Some clinicians have suggested undercorrecting the cylinder, since this would decrease sensitivity to shifts of axis and variable vision from cross-cylinder effects (62). Undercorrecting the cylinder by 20% with a corresponding increase in the sphere power is a sometimes-helpful strategy, especially with high cylinder powers and oblique axes.

Increasing the amount of prism can often solve mislocation problems. Lenses having against-the-rule cylinders usually require less prism because the horizontal meridian is the thickest, allowing the thin-zone effect to aid stability. Several manufacturers make toric soft lenses with customized parameters including variable amounts of prism. Prism amounts greater than 2Δ are rarely needed.

MANAGING TORIC SOFT LENS PERFORMANCE PROBLEMS AND COMPLICATIONS

Poor Visual Response

HTCLs, even when optimally fitted, sometimes result in inferior visual quality and acuity compared to an equivalent spectacle correction. This possibility should be explained to patients in advance to preclude unrealistic expectations.

Modern HTCLs should correct a patient's vision to a consistent 20/20 acuity, and most unexpected visual responses can be managed. Common reasons for poor visual performance during the early fitting phase include axis mislocation, incorrect sphere or cylinder power, poor centration (which creates noncoincidence of visual axis and lens optical center), flexure related power and lens surface effects (caused by incomplete or irregular draping), irregular astigmatism or topographic abnormality, corneal curvature change, corneal edema, lens dehydration, and optically poor or mismarked (defective) lenses (81). Abnormal or unusual ocular anatomy or corneal topography may also create unstable on suboptimal visual results.

Several simple diagnostic tests may be used to isolate the factors causing the reduced vision. First, the correct axis location should be verified by relocating or dialing the base to either side of its stabilized position. This test should be routinely performed with underperforming lenses that have small amounts of prism ballasting because of possible decreased stability and a reduced impetus to reorient. The effect on vision should be noted as the lens is moved off axis and then allowed to return to its original position. If a slight off-axis movement reduces visual acuity significantly and equally on either side of the shift, then the axis is correctly positioned. If axis location is correct and consistent, a spherical overrefraction should be performed to verify the spherical power. Finally, the cylinder power should be verified using a handheld flip cylinder. When poor optics or insufficient cylinder are suspected as the cause of reduced visual acuity and verified by relative insensitivity to large axis shifts (produced by "dialing"), lens optical powers and clarity should be checked using a lensometer.

Verification of suspect or poorly performing HTCLs by standard lensometry is advisable in order to identify the offending element in a HTCL failure. To do this, the lens is prepared by lightly "blot" drying it with a lint-free cloth. The lens then should be geometrically centered over the lensometer stop, convex side up, with the prism base or lens marking positioned in the base-down position. The use of a smaller aperture (3 to 4 mm) stop attachment to the vertically mounted lensometer is beneficial and decreases peripheral aberration effects to allow more accurate power and axis measurements. Inexpensive plastic mounts are available for most lensometers. Measuring with the lens ocular surface down (back vertex) will yield the true axis, cylinder, and sphere. If the lens is placed convex down on the aperture stop, the measured axis will be complementary or mirror reversed from the true axis (i.e., axis 80 degrees will be read as axis 100 degrees).

The retinoscopic reflex can be used by the clinician to help assess the effective optical quality of a HTCL on the eye. A distorted reflex may be caused by an incorrect base curve relationship (usually too steep) or irregular wrapping of the back surface around the central cornea. Improperly draping lenses also distort vision, which varies during the blink (82). This phenomenon also may be observed using overkeratometry, noting the change in the shape and clarity of the mires immediately following the blink (73) or by using handheld or photokeratoscopy. Computerized topography can also be used to observe such distortion. Although the view is static, the increased sensitivity of the instrument can still reveal underlying distortion quite adequately. HTCLs will typically show some residual surface astigmatism (83). The best fit is the flattest lens that allows good alignment and centration with regular lens wrapping over the central cornea and no edge buckling.

In general, eyes with refractive astigmatism equal to corneal toricity may be best fitted with a back-toric design while eyes that have refractive astigmatism with minimal or no corneal toricity may be best fitted with a front-toric construction lens. However, the improved stability of modern toric soft lens designs blur these distinctions. HTCL flexure should transfer toricity to either surface, from the back surface to the front surface, thus creating a bitoric form on the eye. Theoretically, a properly draped toric lens will induce no significant unexpected optical power effects *in situ*. Power changes caused by flexure sometimes occur although they cannot always be quantified in clinical practice. The general rules for power compensation (i.e., adding plus sphere and reducing cylinder power) have been gleaned from clinical experience. Many manufacturers' fitting guides contain power compensation suggestions for their specific lens material, type and thickness.

Fitting corneas with irregular astigmatism, however, may yield unpredictable refractive results. This may be especially true of patients who have undergone refractive surgery (25). Ideally, overall diameters of such lenses should be large to assist stability. Thicker HTCLs usually have some additional masking effect of underlying topographic irregularity; (19) however, this should be verified in each such case by diagnostic fitting. In some eyes, a steeper base curve may mask additional surface irregularity by vaulting over areas of distortion (which are then filled in by tears). While such masking effects can be clinically significant, they are still substantially less than that observed with rigid lenses.

Induced Power Changes

The wrapping characteristics (or flexure) of a hydrogel lens, when placed on an eye, can change its effective refractive power. This is of significant clinical importance when attempting to achieve first lens-final fit success. There are several theories that attempt to explain and predict how hydrogel front and back radii change when placed on the eye (84). A modification of the "beam-bending" hypothesis may apply to HTCLs, which are generally thicker than spherical lenses (59), wherein lens thickness prevents the front surface from stretching enough to allow complete flexure. This would occur most dramatically with thicker, and

especially with plus optically powered lenses. Since the front surface does not flex completely, the net effect is to increase the effective minus power of the contact lens on the eye. Lens flexure for HTCLs is further complicated by other factors, including two primary power meridians, the differential bending of the prism containing (vertical) meridian, regional lens thickness differences, the elasticity of the material, and anatomic (topographic) variations of the corneal and limbal contours.

There has been speculation regarding the existence of a minus powered tear-lens under hydrogel lenses. Holden and Zantos (85) and Chaston and Fatt (86) suggested that the posterior surfaces of thin spherical hydrogel lenses closely align with anterior corneal surfaces, resulting in thin-tear lenses of no effective power. Weissman and Gardner (87) presented evidence that thicker (and low-plus powered) lenses may not align quite as well thereby generating low-minus–powered tear layers. These phenomena may explain clinical observations that thicker plus, aphakic, or prism-ballasted HTCLs often provide less effective plus power than predicted by empirical fitting or calculation, even after proper vertex power adjustment. The combined effects of flexure and a minus-tear lens, therefore, suggest that a slight increase in plus sphere power should be incorporated when prescribing these types of contact lenses, and this rationale is apparently equally applicable with HTCLs.

Although no precise data are available on how to adjust or compensate for flexure changes with HTCLs, clinical observations suggest some general guidelines for empirical prescribing. Thinner HTCLs that are constructed with no prism, and all HTCLs in low-power corrections ($+2.00$ to -3.00 standard thickness), require little, if any, power compensation. Thicker prism-ballasted designs should be adjusted by $+0.25$ D to $+0.50$ D in spherical power. In higher corrections (about 5.00 D), this power and adjustment should increase to $+0.50$ D to $+1.00$ D. The spherical power compensation component should be considered relative to the amount of cylinder. It appears that higher cylinders (3.00 D) result in more flexure effects, requiring less cylinder power, and manufacturers recommend compensating for the spherical power with an additional $+0.25$ D for these higher cylinders (Table 26.1). The cylinder power correction of the ordered lens should be reduced whenever possible by 15% to 20% to allow for flexure effects and to minimize the effect of variable vision caused by rotation or rocking. In general, the lower the amount of cylinder possessed by an HTCL, the less its meridional sensitivity. If the patient's astigmatism falls between the stock cylinder measurements of a given brand, the lower cylinder power should be used. Compensating for vertex distance in both primary meridians is important in higher powers. Since HTCLs are expressed in minus cylinder form, there is an increase of cylinder at the corneal plane in patients with hyperopia and a decrease of cylinder at the cornea in patients with myopia. For example, for a spectacle prescription of $-6.00 -2.50 \times 180$ (13 mm) at the cornea $-5.50 -2.12 \times 180$, the ordered lens powers would be $-5.00 -1.75 \times 180$ if no axis compensation is needed.

The enhanced accuracy and reproducibility of modern manufacturing methods have improved the reliability of labeled lens parameters, especially compared to the "snowflake" lenses that early HTCL fitters initially encountered. This provides greater confidence when the initial lens specifications or lens reordering is based on a toric-diagnostic or first ordered lens and overrefraction data. A recent analysis of Focus Toric (Ciba Vision) HTCLs, using acuity as a criterion, found that 83.5% ± 1.7% of the lenses were accurate enough to deliver one line or less loss of visual acuity compared to spectacle correction (88). Reproducibility is critically important with frequent replacement and disposable HTCLs since lens performance is not routinely evaluated with every lens replacement (81). Most manufacturers provide liberal exchange policies and allow for often-needed fitting refinements without increased cost. Fitting sets of frequent replacement and disposable HTCLs are commonplace and many patients leave the office wearing lenses immediately after the initial consultation and fitting. Fitting sets have increased accuracy, decreased chair time and dramatically increased patient satisfaction (60,89). Despite improvements in lens construction, refinement of axis and lens power is still often necessary. Several studies report use of 1.4 to 1.6 toric lenses per eye to achieve clinical success (90,91). Recent clinical experience suggests that for all but the most complex patients, the number of lenses required has diminished substantially along with the amount of chair time necessary to achieve an accurate and acceptable fit.

Using Keratometry and Corneal Topography for Troubleshooting

Several reports suggest overkeratometry aids determining the lens cornea relationship, although this keratometric technique for confirming HTCL fit has not been widely applied (82,92). There may be value, however, in assessing overkeratometry measurements and mire quality for some hydrogel lenses. The clarity, shape and consistency of the mires, reflecting from the anterior lens surface, can be informative and useful in certain problem situations. Patients complaining of visual fluctuation with lenses that are otherwise stable may have a steep fit or irregular lens wrapping. In steep-fitting situations, overkeratometry or keratoscopy will reveal distorted mires that become more regular as the eye remains open (and the lens regains its shape) between blinks. Flat-fitting lenses will reflect clear mires immediately after a blink, but will show increased distortion as the eye remains open. With irregular lens wrapping, overkeratometry, or computerized topography over the lens *in situ* will show more consistent distortion and toricity of the mires that are inconsistent with underlying corneal curvatures and

axes. Theoretically, an eye with refractive astigmatism equal to the corneal toricity, wearing a properly fitting HTCL, should produce an overkeratometry reading (or corneal topography) that is spherical and clear. Only when internal astigmatism is present *should* the readings show definite and appropriate residual cylinder over the lens. However surface toricity is clinically observed using topography over all toric soft lenses (74). When patients complain of asthenopia and inconsistent vision and any unusual over the lens toricity or mire fluctuation related to the blink is observed, a change in physical fit of the lens or the lens material is indicated. Overlens keratometry or topography, therefore, can be an extremely helpful clinical tool in troubleshooting difficult cases.

Front Versus Back Toricity Effects

When using modern relatively thin HTCLs, in the common cylinder powers of 0.75 to 2.50 D, there appears to be no significant advantages to either front or back surface toric construction. HTCLs assume a bitoric configuration when draping over the toric cornea and, if properly prescribed, result in a spherical power effect on the eye (10). Hydrogel lens toricity *in situ* is transferred from one surface to the other. Using conventional manufacturing techniques, a front-toric design is less complex. Back-toric fabrication requires more steps, but lenses can be made with higher cylinders more easily and probably more accurately. This has become less of an issue with modern toric-generator lathes and molding techniques.

There are special considerations, however, when toric lens designs are used on nearly spherical corneas and in cases of high or oblique corneal toricity. It has been suggested that a back-toric lens may provide better wrap and stability in highly toric corneas, and conversely, front-toric construction may perform better on near spherical corneas with significant internal astigmatism (93). Although not a common problem, the unusual flexure that may occur with a back-toric design on a nearly spherical cornea, could adversely affect the quality of vision. Gundel et al. (94) found a measurable decrease in contrast sensitivity as a result of fitting patients who had slight astigmatism with spherical hydrogel lenses. This decrease, however, could not be attributed solely to hydrogel lens wear or to the presence of an uncorrected cylinder. It was suggested that the flexure of a soft lens on the cornea could degrade optical image quality. Investigation, using computerized corneal topography over HTCLs, revealed that front and back-toric lenses possess different draping characteristics (Shovlin JP. Personal communication, 1990). The results suggested that variation in draping can cause subjective and clinically significant visual problems, and in these cases an appropriate (front or back) toric design performed better in patients where irregular draping lowered vision significantly. It seems reasonable then to assume that spherical corneas may be best corrected by front-toric designs and corneas with significant toricity (2.00 D) may be best fit with back-toric designs. If neither front nor back-design toric soft lenses yield acceptable quality of vision when all other criteria are met, then it is advisable to consider rigid GP lenses. Thinner HTCL designs are less affected by unusual draping problems and there are brand differences in visual performance. However, further research regarding HTCL flexure is needed before optical behavior can be predicted in every situation.

Physiologic Problems

An HTCL should meet the same physiologic requirements as a spherical hydrogel lens. In addition to the complications and adverse reactions that occur with spherical lenses, there are problems unique to HTCL. The addition of cylinder and prism ballasting increases toric lens thickness both centrally and regionally throughout most of the lens profile. Oxygen transmission and hypoxia varies with regional lens thickness despite the averaging that occurs beneath the entire lens (95,96). Studies have shown an increase in corneal swelling response induced by prism, compared to nonprism lenses (97). The added thickness and increased mass of HTCLs suggest that they may impair normal corneal metabolism more often than spherical hydrogel lenses (98).

Superficial punctate keratitis (SPK), when it occurs with HTCLs is usually observed in the inferior cornea (99). Edema, if present, is also more frequently observed within the lower hemisphere (100). A probable cause of this SPK, in addition to localized hypoxic edema, is localized dehydration of toric lenses (57). With toric (nonrotating) lenses, dehydration is more common in the inferior region as evidenced by a tendency to form surface deposits in this area (Fig. 26.1) (91). This problem is more common in patients with incomplete blinking patterns or meibomian gland dysfunction leading to evaporative dry eye and concentration of tear proteins. In addition, the flushing of tear debris may be impaired by nonrotating lenses and this increases the likelihood of epithelial staining.

Conjunctival or scleral indentation from the pressure of lens edges is observed with larger lenses, thicker edge designs, tight fits, and base-curve steepening caused by lens aging. If not resolved, mechanical compression can lead to perilimbal congestion, limbal swelling, or an acute red eye response.

Corneal epithelial edema is a concern because of the increased thickness of toric lenses. This is especially true of lenses with a lower water content or increased thickness. Pachymetric studies have shown that corneal swelling of 2.6% to 4.9% occurs after 3 hours of lens wear with some currently available HTCLs (29). Although most patients using HTCLs tolerate their lenses well when using a reasonable (daily wear) schedule, for the more sensitive or more oxygen demanding cornea, a thinner (e.g., "extended-wear design"), HTCL or GP lens should be considered.

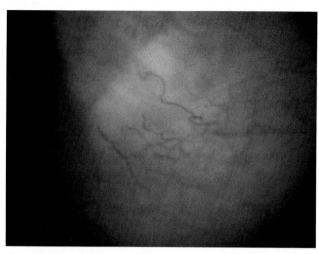

FIG. 26.3. Localized peripheral corneal neovascularization due to low oxygen tension beneath the thick prism ballast of a toric hydrogel lens.

Neovascularization can be a response to a variety of factors, such as hypoxia (and local edema), mechanical irritation, infection, allergy or toxin exposure. The decreased oxygen transmission that occurs with thicker HTCL designs increases the risk of neovascularization of the inferior cornea (93). Inferior neovascularization occurs more commonly in patients wearing prism-ballasted lenses (Fig. 26.3) (101). The amount of ingrowth can be substantial, especially with myopic and thick toric lenses. Patients must be carefully monitored to prevent vessel encroachment into the visual axis or hemorrhage especially from deeper stromal vessels (102). Again, the use of lenses with smaller diameters, thinner profiles and highest transmission of oxygen may help prevent vascular-invasion of the cornea.

Extended-wear HTCLs are available and have similar risks and benefits to spherical extended-wear lenses. When contemplating extended wear of HTCLs the relative risks and benefits should be discussed with the patient. HTCLs made using silicone hydrogel materials are on the immediate horizon and should increase oxygen availability to the cornea and hopefully improve overall HTCL safety substantially.

CONCLUSION

Not long ago, early HTCL fitters jokingly referred to these lenses as "snowflakes" because no two were alike. Fitting HTCLs was complicated, unpredictable, and often so unprofitable that it was essentially the exclusive domain of a small number of determined specialists. Today, modern HTCLs are firmly entrenched in modern contact lens practice. This would not be the case had significant advances in design and manufacture paved the way. Modern lenses are far more practitioner and patient friendly than their early predecessors. Except for the most esoteric custom designs, current HTCLs are also so reproducible that they can be dispensed with care similar to that required of a spherical lens.

The past quarter century has been one of exciting development of HTCLs. The near future should be even more interesting for the HTCL fitter. New materials will revolutionize HTCL fitting, making it yet safer and more convenient; ultimately providing an attractive yet reversible continuous wear alternative to refractive surgery. Single-use daily disposable toric lenses have just become available and will likely become popular. As has been true in the past, technology and science will drive the future of HTCLs. New insight and appreciation of optical aberration will increase interest in wavefront correcting contact lenses. At the next revision of this chapter, it is conceivable that HTCLs will have become a subset of universal aberration-correcting lenses that correct astigmatism in addition to other optical aberrations. Despite major technological advances, the most critical element in successfully prescribing complex lenses remains practitioner skill and problem solving ability. It is our sincere hope that this chapter expands the reader's ability to master HTCL application.

REFERENCES

1. Holden BA. The principles and practice of correcting astigmatism with soft contact lenses. *Aust J Optom* 1975;58:279.
2. Secor, GB. Contact lenses for astigmatism: better than ever. *Contact Lens Spectr* 1998;13:14.
3. Duke-Elder SW. *Systems of ophthalmology*, Vol 5. London: H Kimpton, 1970.
4. Gerber PC. Prescribing soft toric lenses for the low astigmat. *Contact Lens Forum* 1990;11:50–53.
5. Dabkowski JA, Roach MP, Begley CG. Soft toric versus spherical contact lenses in myopes with low astigmatism. *Int Contact Lens Clin* 1992;19:252.
6. HPR data provided courtesy of Dr. Nikki Iravani, Cooper Vision, Inc.
7. CLI data provided courtesy of Dr. Nikki Iravani, Cooper Vision, Inc.
8. Data from Bausch & Lomb. *Trends in contact lenses and lens care,* December 2001.
9. Quinn TG. Choosing between soft torics and RGPs. *Contact Lens Spectr* 1995;10:15.
10. Andrasko, G. Are you going soft on astigmats? *Contact Lens Spectr* 1995;10:19.
11. Remba M. Part II: Clinical evaluation of toric hydrophilic contact lenses. *J Am Optom Assoc* 1981;52:220.
12. Hanks AJ, Weisbarth RE. Troubleshooting soft toric contact lenses. *Int Contact Lens Clin* 1983:10:305.
13. Ewell D. Clinical application of toric soft lenses. *Contact Lens Forum* 1980;5:23.
14. Blaze P, Downs S. Fitting toric soft lenses in high astigmats. *J Am Optom Assoc* 1984;55:12.
15. Snyder C. Evaluation of high-cylinder toric soft contact lenses. *Int Contact Lens Clin* 1997;24:160.
16. Gasson A. Correction of astigmatism and hydroflex toric soft lenses. *Contact Lens J* 1979;8:3.
17. Dain SJ. Over refraction and axis mislocation of toric lenses. *Int Contact Lens Clin* 1979;6:57.
18. Bergenske PD. A guide to prescribing toric lenses (Part 2). *Contact Lens Spectr* 1996;11:30.
19. Snyder C, Wiggins NP, Daum KM. Visual performance in the correction of astigmatism with contact lenses: spherical RGPs versus toric hydrogels. *Int Contact Lens Clin* 1994;21:127.
20. Tomlinson A, Bibby MM. Lid interaction and toric soft lens axis location. *Am J Optom Physiol Opt* 1982;59:60.
21. Young G, Hunt C, Covey M. Clinical evaluation of factors influencing toric soft contact lens fit. *Optom Vis Sci* 2002;79: 11–9.
22. Wong MK, Lee TT, Poon MT, Cho P. Clinical performance and factors affecting the physical fit of a soft toric frequent replacement contact lens. *Clin Exp Optom* 2002;85:350–7.
23. Griffiths M, Zahner K, Collins M, Carney L. Masking of irregular corneal topography with contact lenses. *CLAO J* 1998;24: 76.
24. Epstein AB. Post-penetrating keratoplasty lens fitting. In: Schwartz CA, ed. *Specialty contact lenses: the fitters guide.* Philadelphia, PA: WB Saunders 1996;210.
25. Alio JL, Belda JI, Artola A, Garcia-Lledo M, Osman A. Contact lens fitting to correct irregular astigmatism after corneal refractive surgery. *J Cat Refract Surg* 2002;28:1750–1757.
26. Thompson TT. *Tylers Q* 1998: March.
27. Ott W. Soft toric contact lenses. *Optician* 1978;4534:29.
28. Knoll HA. The stability of the shape of the human cornea. *Am J Optom Physiol Opt* 1976;53:360.
29. Hanks A. The watermelon seed principle. *Contact Lens Forum* 1983;8:31.
30. Epstein AB, Freedman JM. Putting the biomedics toric to the test. *Rev Contact Lens* 2001;November:32–33.
31. Tomlinson H, Bibby M. Movement and rotation of soft contact lenses: effect of fit and lens design. *Am J Optom Physiol Opt* 1980;57:275.
32. Hanks AJ, Weisbarth RE, McNally JJ. Clinical performance comparisons of toric soft contact lens designs. *Int Contact Lens Clin* 1987;14:16.
33. Staarmann H, Andrasko G. Vertical imbalance induced by a unilateral prism-ballasted contact lens. *Int Eyecare* 1985;1:310.
34. Mandell RB. *Contact lens practice.* Springfield, IL: Charles C Thomas, 1988:961–996.
35. Bralf SM. A new corneal contact lens design for the correction of residual astigmatism. *Optom Wkly* 1970;61:24.
36. Strachan JPF. Further comments on the fitting of spherical hydrophilic lenses and the correction of astigmatism with toric lenses. *Contacto* 1971;20:22.
37. Maltzman BA, Rengel A. Soft toric lenses: correcting cylinder greater than sphere. *CLAO J.* 1989;15:196.
38. Myers RI, Castellano C, Becerer PD, Walter DE. Lens rotation and spherocylindrical over-refraction as predictors for soft toric lens evaluation. *Optom Vis Sci* 1989;66:573.
39. Remba M. Clinical evaluation of contemporary soft toric lenses. *Optician* 1986;192:17–24.
40. Tomlinson A, Ridder WH III, Watanabe R. Blink-induced variations in visual performance with toric soft contact lenses. *Optom Vis Sci* 1994;71:545.
41. Castellano CF, Myers RI, Becerer PD, Walter DE. Rotational characteristics and stability of soft toric lenses. *J Am Optom Assoc* 1990;61:167.
42. Reddy T, Szczotka LB, Roberts C. Peripheral corneal contour measured by topography influences soft toric contact lens fitting success. *CLAO J* 2000;26:180–5.
43. Szczotka LB, Roberts C, Herderick EE, Mahmoud A. Quantitative descriptors of corneal topography that influence soft toric contact lens fitting. *Cornea* 2002;21:249–55.
44. Baron WS. Cyclorotation impacts on toric contact lens fitting and performance. *Optom Vis Sci* 1994;71:350.

45. Jurkus JM, Furman DW, Colip MK. Stability characteristics of toric soft lenses. *Int Contact Lens Clin* 1993;20:65.

46. Myers RI. Off-axis fitting of soft toric contact lenses. *Int Eyecare* 1985;1:486.

47. Goldsmith WA, Steel S. Rotational characteristics of toric contact lenses. *Int Contact Lens Clin* 1991;18:227.

48. Ames KS, Erickson P, Medici L. Factors influencing hydrogel toric lens rotation. *Int Contact Lens Clin* 1989;16:221. 49. Bucci FA, Tanner JB, Moody KJ, Myers PJ. Clinical performance of the OptimaJ toric contact lens versus the CSI-T toric contact lens. *CLAO J* 1997;23:43.

50. McMonnies C, Parker D. Predicting the rotational performance of toric soft lenses. *Aust J Optom* 1977;135.

51. Remba MJ. Evaluating the Hydrasoft Toric. *Contact Lens Forum* 1987;12:45.

52. Silbert J, Ghormley NR, Hankin B, et al. An evaluation of empirically fitting a posterior toric hydrogel contact lens. *J Am Optom Assoc* 1992;63:170.

53. Leiblein JS, Wells MM. To trial fit torics or not. *Contact Lens Spectr* 1991;6:35.

54. Studebaker JR. A planned replacement toric soft lens in trial and practice. *Contact Lens Spectr* 1997;12:47.

55. Kleinstein RN. Simplified fitting procedures for toric soft contact lenses. *J Am Optom Assoc* 1984;55:777.

56. Englehart K, Finley T, Geller J, et al. Empirical fitting with a toric soft lens. *Contact Lens Spectr* 1996;11:42.

57. Blaze P. Refining toric soft lens correction. *Contact Lens Forum* 1988;13:53.

58. Edrington TB, Ackely KD. Evaluation of the Toric Tamer. *Contact Lens Spectr* 1989;4:77.

59. Hallak J. Standard soft toric lenses: a problem of orientation. *Int Contact Lens Clin* 1982;9:250.

60. Bayshore CA. Astigmatic soft contact lenses: a report on 88 patients. *Int Contact Lens Clin* 1975;2:68.

61. Silbert J, Ghormley NR, Hankin B, et al. An evaluation of empirically fitting a posterior toric hydrogel contact lens. *J Am Optom Assoc* 1992;63:170.

62. Epstein AB. Optcomlist internet based survey, Winter 1997.

63. Myers RI. Off-axis fitting of soft toric contact lenses. *Int Eyecare* 1985;1:486.

64. Malin AH, Kohler J. Measuring soft toric rotation. *Contact Lens Forum* 1981;6:17.

65. Clompus R. Custom correction for astigmats and soft torics. *Rev Optom* 1986;23:51.

66. Snyder C, Daum KM. Rotational position of toric soft contact lenses on the eye: clinical judgments. *Int Contact Lens Clin* 1989;16:146.

67. Holden BA, Siddle JA, Robson G, et al. Soft lens performance models: the clinical significance of the flexure effect. *Aust J Optom* 1975;58:279.

68. Weissman BA, Gardner KM. Flexure effects of double-thin zone toric soft contact lenses. *Am J Opt Physiol Opt* 1984;61:465.

69. Weissman BA, Gardner KM. Power and radius changes induced in soft contact lens systems by flexure. *Am J Opt Physiol Opt* 1984;61:239.

70. Weissman BA. Theoretical optics of toric hydrogel contact lenses. *Am J Optom Physiol Opt* 1986;63:536.

71. Gundel RE. Determining appropriate cylinder correction with soft toric lenses. *J Am Optom Assoc* 1988;59:206.

72. Long WF. Lens power matrices and the sum of equivalent spheres. *Optom Vis Sci* 1991;68:821.

73. Edrington TB, Ackely KD. Evaluation of the toric tamer. *Contact Lens Spectr* 1989;4:77.

74. Myers RL, Jones DH, Meinell P. Using overrefraction for problem solving in soft toric fit-tact lens designs. *Int Contact Lens Clin* 1987;14:16.

75. Purcell H, Teig D, Eiden B, et al. How to fit true specification labeled torics. *Contact Lens Spectr* 1993;8:21.

76. Koers DM, Quinn TG. How to ensure accuracy with toric soft lens prescriptions. *Contact Lens Spectr* 1997;12:36.

77. Lindsay RG, Bruce AS, Brennan NA, Pianta MJ. Determining axis misalignment and power errors of toric soft lenses. *Int Contact Lens Clin* 1997;24:101.

78. Jurkus J, Tomlinson A, Gilbault D, et al. The effect of fit and parameter changes on soft lens rotation. *Am J Optom Phys Opt* 1979;56:734.

79. Quinn TG. Troubleshooting with soft toric contact lenses. *Contact Lens Spectr* 1995;10:17.

80. Rakow PL. Problem solving with toric hydrogels. *Contact Lens Forum* 1990;11:29-36

81. Young G, Coleman S, Hickson-Curran S. Clinical evaluation of toric soft lens reproducibility. *Optom Vis Sci* 2002;79:321–8.

82. Eiden SB. Precision management of high astigmats with toric hydrogel contact lenses. *Contact Lens Spectr* 1992;7:43.

83. McCarey BE, Amos CF. Topographic evaluation of toric soft contact lens correction. *CLAO J* 1994;20:261.

84. Janoff L, Dabezies O. Power change induced by soft contact lens flexure. *CLAO J* 1983;9:32.

85. Holden BA, Zantos S. On the conformity of soft lenses to the shape of the cornea. *Am J Optom* 1981;58:139.

86. Chaston J, Fatt I. The change in power of soft lenses. *Optician* 1980;180:12.

87. Weissman BA, Gardner KM. Power and radius changes induced in soft contact lens systems by flexure. *Am J Optom Physiol Opt* 1984;61:239.

88. Payor RE, Robirds SR, Zhang X. Soft toric lens power accuracy and reproducibility. *CLAO J* 1995;21:163.

89. Epstein AB. Don't be forced into torics. *Optom Manage* 1997; 32:S2.

90. Remba MJ. Clinical evaluation of contemporary soft toric lenses. *Int Contact Lens Clin* 1985;12:294.

91. Kennedy JR. Clinical consideration of sub 'K' findings. *Contacto* 1972;21:25.

92. Janoff LE, Skolnick S. Predicted and measured over-keratometer readings on soft lenses. *Int Contact Lens Clin* 1975;2:74.

93. Maltzman B, Rengel A. Soft toric lenses: an update. *CLAO J* 1985;11:335.

94. Gundel R, Kirschen S, Dillergillio D. Changes in contrast sensitivity induced by spherical soft lenses on low astigmats. *J Am Optom Assoc* 1988;59:336.

95. White P, Miller D. Corneal edema. In: *Complications of contact lenses*. Boston: Little Brown & Co, 1981;3–12.

96. Eghbali F, Hsui EH, Eghbali K, Weissman BA. Oxygen transmissibility at various locations in hydrogel toric prism-ballasted contact lenses. *Optom Vis Sci* 1996;73:164.

97. Soni P, Borish I, Keech P. Ballasted contact lenses: topographical comparative changes in corneal thickness. Paper presented at: 5th National Research Symposium on Contact Lenses; August 1978; Boston, MA.

98. Hallak J, Cohen H. Localized edema with soft toric contact lenses. *J Am Optom Assoc* 1985;56:12.

99. Nichols KK, Mitchell GL, Simon KM, Chivers DA, Edrington TB. Corneal staining in hydrogel lens wearers. *Optom Vis Sci* 2002;79:20–30.

100. Maltzman BA. Lipid protein precipitates in toric soft lenses. *Contact Lens Forum* 1988;13:74.

101. Westin EJ, McDaid K, Benjamin WJ. Inferior corneal vascularization associated with extended wear of prism-ballasted toric hydrogel lenses (a case report). *Int Contact Lens Clin* 1989;16: 20.

102. Epstein AB. Contact lens complications. In: Schwartz CA, ed. *Specialty contact lenses: the fitters guide.* Philadelphia, PA: WB Saunders, 1996;281.

PRESBYOPIC CORRECTION

EDWARD S. BENNETT AND
JANICE M. JURKUS

Presbyopia as a result of a gradual decrement in visual function at near is one of the most prevalent conditions causing patient concern and complaints in the 40 and older age group. The presbyopic patient also represents the largest growing segment of the population in the United States, as well as the largest untapped segment of the contact lens market. With approximately 78 million "baby boomers" (i.e., individuals born in the United States between 1946 and 1964), there is a large group of potential bifocal contact lens wearers (1). However, of these individuals, only approximately 3% wear some form of presbyopic contact lens correction (2,3). It is evident that practitioners are reluctant to provide this option even though this cohort potentially can benefit greatly from the visual freedom and cosmesis provided by contact lenses. It also is evident that, although changes in tear volume can result in greater symptoms of dryness with contact lens wear, presbyopic patients still are viable candidates for contact lens wear (4).

It is becoming evident that contact lens practitioners can successfully build their practice by offering presbyopic contact lens designs—both gas-permeable (GP) and soft—as well as myopia reduction designs (i.e., corneal reshaping). With this potential demand in mind, manufacturers are introducing many new GP and soft bifocal designs, and many others are being patented and are under clinical investigation. As a result of factors such as cost, perceived design and fitting complexity, limited success, and the wealth of spectacle lens advertising, the numbers of bifocal or multifocal contact lenses fitted traditionally have been low. However, this is beginning to change as manufacturing technology improves, new and better designs replace older ones, and consumer confidence in the improved lenses and fitting skills of practitioners is established.

DEFINITIONS

Bifocal contact lenses typically are defined as lenses that provide two corrections: distance and near. *Multifocal lenses* provide a correction for more than two distances, often in a progressive manner. These designs use either the simul-taneous vision or the alternating vision technique, and they are available in soft and GP lens materials. *Monovision* pertains to prescribing a power for the contact lens in one eye that optimally corrects distance vision and prescribing a power for the contact lens in the other eye that optimally corrects near vision.

PATIENT SELECTION

Fitting a patient into bifocal/multifocal contact lenses or monovision depends upon a comprehensive preliminary evaluation that includes a thorough consultation with the patient.

PRELIMINARY EVALUATION
Normal Aging Changes

Most notable of the changes associated with age is decrease in tear volume, possibly resulting in dryness symptoms with contact lens wear. Goblet cells of the conjunctiva and the mass of the lacrimal glands decrease with age, resulting in a progressive reduction of tear production (5). Therefore, these patients, especially if an extended wear schedule is prescribed, should be advised against sleeping under a ceiling fan and should avoid any forms of air drafts during the day, which typically act to evaporate tear fluid (6). With the thicknesses often required in these lenses, a daily wear schedule is often indicated. Careful evaluation of tear film quality and quantity is essential and assists in selecting the appropriate lens type and material. Because reduced tear flow results in an increase in the amount of lens surface deposition, which leads to blurred vision, discomfort, and possible papillary hypertrophy, the selection of a wettable lens material and a wearing schedule compatible with tear film function is important. Frequent use of ocular lubricants is often necessary. If a soft multifocal lens design is prescribed, a planned replacement or disposable lens program is indicated.

Other changes that occur with age include an increased likelihood for pingueculae and pterygia formation, which can decrease comfortable contact lens wear. Loss of eyelid tonicity also occurs, which can make it challenging for translating bifocal designs to be successful in some cases. In addition, the quality of vision tends to be compromised over time as a result of changes in the crystalline lens.

Tests

Good candidates for presbyopic contact lens correction are essentially similar to those individuals who are good candidates for contact lens wear in general. It is important to determine the patients' goals: what distance(s) is most important to them, what are the activities they spend much of their time involved in, and how they desire the contact lenses to help them.

The patient should be asked about his or her medication history. Specifically, is the patient taking any medications that would reduce tear volume (i.e., antihistamines)? Any previous surgeries should be discussed as well. Cosmetic lid surgery, in particular, can affect GP bifocal and multifocal lens positioning by causing excessive lifting and superior decentration with the blink.

Anatomical measurements should be carefully performed. In particular, it is important to note pupil size, both in room illumination and with the lights dimmed (Fig. 27.1). The presence of a large pupil in normal room illumination (i.e., >5 mm)—although not highly common in the presbyopic population—would contraindicate an aspheric GP multifocal lens design because of the glare and ghost images the patient would experience under low-illumination conditions. The lid-to-limbus relationship should be noted, particularly the position of the lower lid. Individuals with a low-positioned lower lid (i.e., >1 mm below the inferior limbus) will not be good candidates for a translating GP lens design.

As with any patient, tear quality and volume should be assessed. As tear volume decreases with age, this is especially important to evaluate in determining if the patient is a good candidate for contact lens wear in general. A tear breakup time of 5 seconds or less typically contraindicates contact lens wear. Likewise, a value of less than 9 mm with the Zone-Quick (Menicon/Allergan) phenol red thread test for tear volume assessment should contraindicate lens wear (7). Corneal integrity should be evaluated, and the lids should be assessed for signs of papillary and follicular hypertrophy.

The visual status should be determined. The best candidates for bifocal/multifocal contact lenses should have >1 D of hyperopia or >1.25 D of myopia (8). If the patient is amblyopic, fitting of multifocal and monovision lenses should be discouraged because of the potential for further compromise in distance vision.

Corneal topography evaluation is beneficial as well. Although a videokeratography (VKG) instrument is not required when fitting a presbyopic patient with contact lenses, it does have several benefits. Patients with irregular corneas and/or keratoconus can be diagnosed; typically, these patients are not good candidates for bifocal, multifocal, or monovision contact lens correction. The location of the apex can be determined. A centrally located apex lends itself well to multifocal designs, whereas an inferior positioned apex lends itself to lenses in which an inferior position is desired (i.e., translating designs). Important preliminary tests and procedures for the potential presbyopic contact lens patient are listed in Table 27.1.

Consultation

If the patient is determined to be a viable contact lens candidate, it is important to review all of the options available to him or her. These options include single-vision lenses in combination with over-near spectacles, monovision correction, and GP and GP bifocal/multifocal contact lenses. The latter category should be especially emphasized.

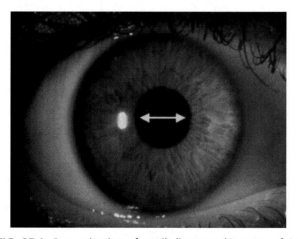

FIG. 27.1. Determination of pupil diameter. (Courtesy of Dr. Peter Kollbaum.)

TABLE 27.1. TESTS AND EVALUATION PROCEDURES FOR THE POTENTIAL PRESBYOPIC CONTACT LENS PATIENT

Case history
- Surgical history
- Medications
- Primary visual requirements and goals
- Occupational requirements

Anatomical/external measurements
- Pupil size (room illumination/dim illumination)
- Lid position and tonicity
- Vertical fissure size
- Blink rate/quality

Tear quality and volume
Corneal integrity
Manifest refraction
Keratometry/corneal topography

The patient's goals and expectations should be discussed. As mentioned earlier, it is important to determine the patient's occupational and recreational visual needs and whether bifocal contact lenses will meet those needs. What is the patient's goal from wearing contact lenses? Patients must understand that these lenses differ from spectacles. The dynamics of lens movement on the eye must be explained such that they understand that the stability of visual correction obtained with spectacles is not the same with GP bifocal and multifocal designs. They may experience transient blur in certain directions of gaze. It is important to mention that some visual compromise may be present compared with spectacles such that the patient who desires good vision at all distances during all activities should be told he or she is not a good candidate for this modality. The goal of presbyopic contact lens wear should be to satisfy "most of the visual needs, most of the time, or essentially to reduce, rather than eliminate, the need for supplemental near correction" (9,10). Intermediate distance correction during prolonged computer use may be necessary for a GP bifocal (not multifocal) wearer with presbyopia, or a + 1.00 D spectacle correction for prolonged reading of small print may be needed for the patient with absolute presbyopia who is an aspheric multifocal GP wearer. Fortunately, these scenarios typically are the exception to the rule. However, the practitioner is more likely to be successful and patient confidence in the practitioner maintained if practitioners "underpromise and overdeliver" (11).

A realistic approach to GP bifocal adaptation should include a discussion of the time frame for adaptation, including the possible need for lens exchanges. It is preferable to indicate to a patient that it could take up to 6 weeks to achieve success than to have a patient return after 1 week dissatisfied because his or her expectations included a perception that success would be easily and quickly obtained. However, the patient can be reassured that if he or she is patient and motivated, the lenses likely will be successful (12).

Several contact lens options for the presbyope will be discussed, including: (i) single-vision contact lens wear and reading glasses, (ii) monovision, and (iii) bifocal/multifocal contact lenses.

SINGLE-VISION CONTACT LENS WEAR AND READING GLASSES

The use of single-vision lenses (GP or hydrogel) in combination with reading glasses provides the following benefits (13): (i) good bilateral vision at both distance and near, (ii) simplicity of fit, and (iii) low costs. The over-spectacles typically are single-power plus lenses but may be a progressive addition, especially to assist with intermediate correction. In some cases, minimal add powers are used to enhance the reading ability of emerging presbyopes. However, patients with varied near and distance tasks will complain of the inconvenience of frequent application and/or removal of spectacles. In addition, many patients desire contact lenses with the intent of cosmetically eliminating the need for spectacles. Nevertheless, it is important that the single-vision/over-spectacles option be presented to all potential presbyopic contact lens wearers. Some patients will prefer to begin with this most basic option; however, ultimately— for the aforementioned reasons—they will change to one of the other presbyopic contact lens systems discussed with them at the original fitting/consultation visit.

MONOVISION

The anisometropic contact lens correction, monovision, is one of the most successful methods used to provide presbyopic patients with clear vision at both near and distance. Success rates between 60% and 80% have been reported (14). By prescribing the contact lens power for one eye to correct the distance refractive error while using the near power for the other eye, patients are able to see both distances as long as they keep both eyes open.

The origin of monovision is unclear. The use of the monocle in the 1800s certainly was an early method of monovision correction. Using contact lens in this fashion was first attributed to Westsmith about 40 years ago (15). The advantages of the monovision system are many and include the following: (i) use of conventional lenses so that special lens designs rarely are necessary; (ii) decreased professional time; (iii) less expense for the patient; (iv) thinner lenses that are more physiologically acceptable to the cornea typically are utilized; (v) only one contact lens need be changed for continuing distance vision lens wearers; and (vi) avoidance of many of the symptoms/compromises associated with bifocal contact lenses, including ghost images, reduced illumination, reduced contrast sensitivity, and fluctuating vision related to pupil size changes.

Concerns about the lack of balanced binocular vision cannot be ignored. A literature review of monovision by Johannsdottir and Stelmach (16) indicates that monovision may stress the visual system, impair stereoscopic depth perception, and affect performance on complex spatial-motor tasks such as driving. Before the challenges of the monovision system are discussed in detail, it is important to review patient selection and prescription techniques.

Patient Selection

In monovision, as with all contact lenses, the patient's ocular health must be sufficient to support a contact lens. Care should be taken to investigate the presbyope's tear layer, because dry eyes are a common part of aging. Lid tonicity also should be considered because aging may produce a looser lid but cosmetic blepharoplasty may create a very taunt lid.

The lifestyle of the patient, as well as his or her visual needs, must be considered when prescribing monovision. A motivated person with visual needs equally distributed between far and near distances is preferred (1). Various studies looked at personality and psychological factors of successful monovision wearers. Cattell's 16 Personality Factor (16PF) test showed that patients with realistic expectations and the willingness to persevere, the "Factor G superego strength score," could predict monovision success (17). Adaptable, holistic people with an optimistic attitude toward treatment had high potential for success. A person's self-efficacy expectation to succeed with monovision is a predictor of success (14).

The age and add powers of the patient also are predictive of success (10,14). Younger presbyopes are more successful than older presbyopes; add powers of +1.25 to +2.00 are more readily accepted than higher adds. Schwartz (18) recommends monovision screening criteria that evaluate age, add, distance prescription, prior use of contact lenses, motivation, pupil size, occupational and avocational needs, and apprehension of handling lenses. Once the initial screening has been completed, the best predictor of success with monovision is a trial period using the appropriately selected lens powers. Good and poor candidates for monovision are listed in Table 27.2.

Lens Selection

Because monovision can be prescribed with either GP or soft lenses, the fitter's usual criteria for lens type remain the same for monovision. It is the power selection that is different in monovision and must be carefully determined. Cerebral cortex binocular cells have identical receptive fields for detection of size, orientation, motion sensitivity, and directionality. The inputs from the two eyes do not produce identical influences on the cortical cells. One eye produces a dominant response. This creates ocular dominance (19,

TABLE 27.2. GOOD AND POOR CANDIDATES FOR MONOVISION

Who are Good Monovision Candidates?
- Early presbyopes who have a significant refractive error are generally better candidates than emmetropes or previously uncorrected hyperopes, low myopes
- People who read in positions other than the standard downward gaze, such as office workers, executives, auto mechanics, and pharmacists
- Current contact lens patients
- Highly motivated patients

Who are Poor Monovision Candidates?
- Someone with concentrated, specific visual needs
- A "dry" eye complainer
- Someone who wants "perfect" vision

20). As noted by Jain et al. (14), the dominant eye was corrected for distance vision in 95% of the monovision papers reviewed. Ocular dominance can be determined via the hole in the hand test or asking the patient which eye he or she uses to sight a camera. The alternate introduction of a plus lens over the best corrected distance correction while viewing at near also can be used to determine the eye that most readily accepts plus add with minimal disruption of vision (21). The plus lens power can be determined by performing a plus buildup, using age-determined add charts. An easy way to determine the add power is described by Jurkus and Nichols (22). Using the patient's age as a base, subtract 35 and multiply by 0.1 (Add power = [age − 35] × 0.1]). A +1.50 D lens is commonly used to evaluate the subjective response. The eye looking through the plus lens that notices little or no distance vision disruption when binocularly viewing the distance chart should be corrected for near. The full distance and near powers are generally prescribed. The concept of "cutting the power" to minimize the dioptric span may alter the suppression pattern. It is advantageous if constant interocular suppression of blur is present, as in patients with no sighting preferences. Patients with strong sighting preferences have reduced interocular blur suppression and decreased binocular depth of focus. This strong dominancy may make it difficult for the patient to learn to ignore the out-of-focus monovision image (23).

Lens Type

The monovision technique is applicable to both rigid and soft contact lenses. Lens parameters such as size, base curve, and material are dependent on the ocular findings. Care should be taken when deciding on the type of lens to prescribe, as well as the power differential. One must remember that significant anterior segment changes occur as the eye ages. Dry eyes, reduced lid tonicity, and decreased corneal sensitivity often are evident in the presbyopic population (22). In addition to the anatomical challenges presented by the presbyopic patient, handling of lenses must be considered because near tasks, such as checking if the lens is inside-out, can be difficult for the presbyope. The use of handling tints as well as lenses that are less "floppy" help the monovision wearer get the lenses in the eyes. Use of daily disposable or continuous wear lenses allows the monovision wearer greater ease of care.

Fitting Procedure

Once the lens design and powers are determined, trial lens fitting can proceed. Trying to explain the concept of monovision to a patient can be challenging. It often is more efficient to actually demonstrate the system. After placing the appropriate lens powers on each eye, ask the patient to read the distance chart with both eyes open. If using a Snellen projection chart, having 20/25 as the "bottom line" can give the patient comfort that his or her vision is good at far. Offering the patient a magazine or type of reading material that he or she is accustomed to reading offers the patient a real-world view of his or her near vision. The patient should be queried as to the comfort of the vision, not only the quantitative value. If the patient reports he or she feels off balance or that a headache is starting, monovision should be reconsidered. Before discarding the monovision concept, it may be beneficial to switch the eye powers, but if the initial acceptance of monovision is lacking, it may not be successful. Full adaptation to the monovision system can take 2 to 3 weeks (14).

A benefit of monovision is the ability to modify the system. The initial full-distance and near powers can be altered to provide more comfortable vision. For example, if a patient reports that distance vision is not comfortable and becomes better when the near eye is covered, consider reducing the plus power on the near eye to minimize the add power difference. After determining the lenses for the patient, always show the new monovision wearer what monocular and binocular acuity is like. Fitting and prescribing guidelines for presbyopia are given in Table 27.3 (6).

Monovision Challenges

Monovision may present some visual challenges. Identifiable visual changes with monovision include a small reduction in high-contrast visual acuity, such as that required for reading or viewing the Snellen chart. There also is a loss of contrast sensitivity function that is proportional to amount of add.

One of the biggest questions with monovision is if there is a change in depth perception due to the anisometropic correction. Monocular clues and binocular clues are used to judge depth and distance. The monocular clues are unchanged with monovision. These include object interposition hiding parts of an object, judging the customary object size, color and clarity of objects, lines convergence to a vanishing point, and shadows.

Although monocular clues for depth perception are present, monovision can reduce stereoacuity. The normal aging process reduces the mean angle of stereopsis from 20 to 58 arc seconds. Monovision further reduces stereoacuity. Stereopsis in monovision ranged from 23 to 73 arc seconds for distance and 50 to 113 arc seconds for near (14,16). Although there is generally no significant effect on peripheral visual acuity, low-contrast binocular distance acuity may be reduced with monovision. This visual change may interfere with the patient's ability to judge distances while driving at night. Woods et al. (21) compared monovision contact lens correction to binocular spectacle correction while patients performed various aspects of daytime driving, such as sign recognition, mirror checks, lane keeping, driving time, speed estimation, and ability to park. They

TABLE 27.3. FITTING AND PRESCRIBING CONSIDERATIONS IN MONOVISION

1. Fit patients who do not require long periods of critical distance vision.
2. Perform binocular function testing to determine the effect of monovision on stereopsis.
3. Demonstrate the add power effect to the patient; subjective reaction to plussing one eye may help determine the preferred distance corrected eye.
4. Select the proper eye for near; as it is most important for distance vision to be less impaired, the near eye typically represents the nondominant and/or the eye in which vision is reduced relative to the other eye. If the patient is anisometropic, the higher myopic eye should be considered for near, all other factors being equal.
5. Prescribe the full amount of correction; it is tempting to underplus the near eye and overplus the distance eye to lessen the anisometropia. However, for optimum near and distance vision, it is preferable to prescribe the full add amount.
6. Strongly encourage—if not require—monovision patients to purchase either a pair of "driving" spectacles (that is, minus power over near eye) or a second distance contact lens for use while driving. The patient also should be encouraged to first be a passenger in the car to experience the monovision effect prior to driving.
7. An informed consent that discusses the benefits and limitations of monovision in addition to discussing alternative forms of presbyopic correction (contact lens and spectacle) should be reviewed and signed by the patient.
8. Although most patients adapt to monovision within 2 weeks, they nevertheless should be told it could take up to several weeks for complete adaptation. If they experience difficulty in adapting, consider changing lenses (i.e., "distance" lens on previous "near" eye and vice versa).

From Bennett et al. (20).

concluded that an adapted monovision wearer showed no differences in driving performance. They suggest that stereoacuity is not critical for distances greater than 20 feet. They also recognize that night driving conditions may offer different challenges to the monovision wearer. As a precaution, it is wise to caution new monovision wearers regarding possible distance perception changes and suggest that they may want to be a passenger while in the car to allow them to become accustomed to perception changes. If they are unable to adapt, prescription of distance glasses to correct the near eye may be desirable. To make these spectacles useful in situations other than night driving, a photochromatic tint can be prescribed, and the glasses can also be used on sunny days while the patients are at the beach.

Some monocular suppression of blur occurs in monovision, which is desired; however, the blurred eye will still contribute to binocular summation (24). The degree of suppression usually increases as the add increases (25). It also has been observed that residual astigmatism caused a significantly greater reduction of binocular visual acuity in the monovision condition than in normal binocular conditions. This effect appears to be related to a process of meridional interocular suppression (25). Development of anisometropia occurred significantly more often among monovision wearers than in controls wearing spectacles or contact lenses. Changes in anisometropia of 0.50 D or greater, with amounts up to 1.25 D, occurred in 29% of monovision wearers (26). Contrast sensitivity function is reduced in monovision, and, in high adds, binocular summation is difficult to achieve (27–29). Although visual performance of monovision patients is comparable to that of nonabsolute presbyopic patients with balanced binocular corrections, in photopic conditions, blurring one eye for distance, especially in advanced presbyopia, can result in significant compromise in critical distance vision-related tasks, including night driving and some occupations (16, 29).

It certainly is possible that a practitioner could be liable for any injury for which a monovision prescription is a contributing factor (30). The report of an aviation accident in which the pilot was wearing a monovision correction—which is prohibited by the Federal Aviation Administration—heightened consumer awareness of possible compromise with this form of correction (31). All contact lens patients should be made aware of potential problems that may occur with wearing of contact lenses. The monovision wearer must be particularly aware of the induced vision change and how it may affect perception. Each patient should be presented with other vision correction options and participate in the modality selection. In their review of legal liabilities regarding monovision, Harris and Classe (30) suggest that the patient be carefully selected, have a demonstration of vision with monovision, and be aware of the adaptation period. Risk and benefits of correcting the pres-

byope with all types of lenses must be considered. Monovision is one of the most effective options currently available. It also has become a popular option for the refractive surgery candidate who is presbyopic.

Specific monovision complaints generally are related to either the quality or the quantity of the wearer's vision. Changing the power or prescribing a modified monovision using a single-vision lens on one eye and a multifocal on the other can minimize the visual problems. Table 27.4 lists common monovision problems and recommended solutions (32).

BIFOCAL CONTACT LENS DESIGNS

Use

Of the one million presbyopes wearing a presbyopic contact lens correction, only 30% wear bifocal contact lenses; the other 70% wear monovision (2,3). There are numerous reasons why this figure is so low. First, there is a certain level of practitioner apprehension about the complexity and expense of the designs and the potential length of time for the fitting/refitting and adaptation. Patients are often told that "bifocal lenses do not work" or "they are not perfected yet." One of the comments most frequently submitted by consumers to a popular contact lens website *(www.contactlenses.org)* is their inability to find a practitioner to fit these lenses or that they were informed that bifocal contact lenses either do not work or are not very successful (33). It certainly can be argued by bifocal contact lens fitters that the visual performance of these designs, in addition to the visual freedom enjoyed by lens wearers, is a powerful benefit if the patient is aware of this option and the practitioner is willing to provide it.

Definitions

Bifocal contact lenses typically are defined as those having multiple powers that are positioned within the pupil, thus the term *simultaneous vision designs,* which are available in soft and GP lens materials, and those that shift upward or translate, which often result in only one corrective power in front of the pupil at any one time. The latter translating or alternating designs are limited to GP lens designs.

Simultaneous Vision

Simultaneous vision (also termed *bivision)* pertains to the vision achieved when the distance and near-power elements are positioned within the pupillary opening at the same time; therefore, light rays from both distance and near targets are imaged on the retina. The patient will selectively suppress the most blurred images that are not desired for a given visual task. This concept functions on the basis of blur interpretation and/or blur tolerance of superimposed

---

TABLE 27.4. MONOVISION PROBLEM SOLVING

Far Vision Problem
- Fuzzy OU, clear when near eye is covered
  - Change eyes near to far
  - Reduce plus power on near eye
  - Fit simultaneous vision bifocal, "pushing plus" on the near eye
- Fuzzy all the time
  - Check for residual cylinder
  - Evaluate lens wetting and cleanliness
  - Reassess distance power

Near Vision Problem
- Fuzzy OU, clear with distance eye covered
  - Switch lenses in eyes
  - Increase plus on distance eye
  - Multifocal lens on distance eye
  - Prescribe half eyes with plus power over far eye

Headaches or Dizziness
- Adaptation may take up to 2 weeks
- Reduce power span
- Consider alternate type of correction

OU, each eye.

multiple images on the retina, which are formed by the various powers of the lens (34). For true simultaneous vision, the two primary segments must remain within the pupillary boundary in all positions of gaze and, in order to give equally bright images, the distance and near areas of the lens should cover nearly equal areas of the pupil. Three designs using the simultaneous vision concept are (i) aspheric, (ii) concentric/annular (or target), and (iii) diffractive. Aspheric lens designs have a gradual change of curvature along one of their surfaces based on the geometry of conic sections. This rate of flattening (or eccentricity) is much greater than with aspheric single vision lenses and creates a plus add power effect. In some aspheric multifocals, eccentricity is located on the posterior surface and increases in plus power from the center to the periphery. Conversely, center-near aspherics have their maximum plus power at the center, which then gradually decreases away from the geometrical center. Concentric or annular lens designs are structured with a small (typically two thirds to three fourths the size of the pupil in normal room illumination) annular central zone that, in most designs, provides the distance vision correction; the near correction is ground on the annulus that surrounds the distance zone. Both aspheric and concentric near zone lenses do gain some additional near power via slight shifting or translating of the lens upward with downward gaze for reading. The only designs with true equality of near and distance powers are those with diffractive properties. Diffractive lenses function through a central diffractive zone plate that focuses images at distance by refraction of light and near through diffraction principles created by the zone eschelettes. This design is pupil-independent, as equal amounts of light pass though both the distance and near-power elements of the lens for all normal pupil opening diameters. Currently this is available only in a soft lens design in the United States. All three of these "simultaneous vision" lens designs must center.

Alternating/Translating Vision

Alternating vision pertains to lens designs and function in which vertical movement or translation results in only one power zone to position in front of the pupil (or visual axis) at any one time (that is, ideally the distance zone is in front of the pupil when viewing at a distance and the near zone when viewing is at near). Essentially there is an intentional shifting of lens position in which separate, discrete images formed by the two power segments in the lens focus on the retina with a change of gaze from distance (up) to near (down) or vice versa. Typically these designs are nonrotating by prism ballast construction, sometimes in combination with inferior truncation, which stabilizes the lens and allows a smooth translation from the superior distance zone to the inferior near zone when the gaze is lowered in order to read. These nonrotating segmented designs typically are similar to spectacle bifocals. Several types of GP prism ballast lenses have been developed through the years, including decentered concentric, one-piece segmented, and fused crescent and segmented. They are most commonly crescent or executive style and are used with GP lens materials, although several attempts have been made to create translating ballasted hydrogel bifocals with only very limited success. It is imperative for alternating bifocal lenses to translate sufficiently when the patient shifts gaze from one distance to another, and this translation is attained much more easily with rigid lenses than with hydrogels. For these reasons, simultaneous image designs have been more successful when incorporated into soft ,lenses and translating designs are rarely used today and will not be discussed in this chapter.

GAS-PERMEABLE BIFOCAL AND MULTIFOCAL DESIGNS

As a result of advancements in manufacturing technology, a number of new and improved lens designs have been introduced in recent years. These have included higher add aspheric multifocal designs, monocentric optics alternating designs, and alternating designs with an intermediate aspheric correction. As a result, a trend toward GP multifocal and bifocal lens fitting and away from monovision was demonstrated in the results of a recent survey of Diplomates in the Cornea and Contact Lens Section of the American Academy of Optometry (35) and in a recent *Review of Optometry* online survey (36).

Simultaneous Vision

Although a few GP concentric designs are still available, the most common form of simultaneous vision correction pertains to aspheric multifocals. It would be a misnomer, however, to indicate that these designs are strictly simultaneous vision in nature. To be successful, it is important that these lens designs exhibit some upward shift or translation on downward gaze.

Aspheric Lens Designs

Numerous presbyopic designs have an entirely (that is, not peripheral only) aspheric back-surface geometry. The peripheral flattening of the back surface provides a continuously variable near addition. To provide the maximum near addition, a high degree of peripheral curvature flattening or asphericity must be used. This departure from spherical shape is known as *eccentricity* or *e factor*. The first designs introduced were fit as much as 3 D steeper than "K." These lenses had a very high e value, and some designs are still in common use today. Because of the back-surface geometry, only slight apical clearance would be present with fluores-

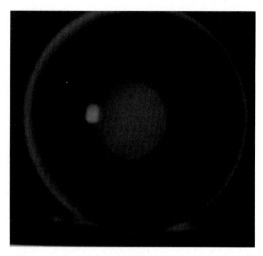

FIG. 27.2. High-eccentricity aspheric lens showing mild apical clearance. (Courtesy of Dr. Peter Kollbaum.)

cein application (Fig. 27.2). In recent years, many designs with a lower eccentricity have been introduced. These lenses are commonly fit approximately 1 to 1.5 D steeper than K. However, as a result of the aspheric geometry and rate of flattening, an alignment or slight central clearance fluorescein pattern will be present (Fig. 27.3).

The best candidates for these lenses are individuals who are not good candidates for translating design bifocals. With aspheric GPs, it is difficult to generate the necessary add power within the pupillary zone without inducing disturbing aberration effects on distance vision; therefore, early or emerging presbyopes are the best candidates. Several lens designs now incorporate higher add powers, often via a smaller effective distance optical zone and/or a modification of the front surface resulting in increased plus power. However, it still is difficult to achieve greater than a +1.75 to +2.00 D effective add power. Other candidates include patients with any one of the following anatomical characteristics:

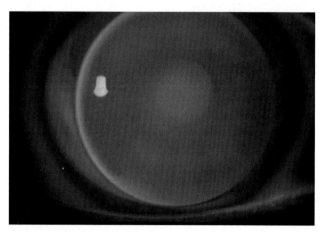

FIG. 27.3. Optimum fitting aspheric gas permeable multifocal lens.

1. Lower lid margin well above or below limbus
2. Small-to-average pupil size; a larger than normal pupil size is a contraindication because of the aberrations induced, particularly at night
3. Loose lids that will not support prism ballast lenses
4. Steep corneal curvatures

The benefits of aspheric designs include the absence of prism and truncation in their construction. Therefore, the thickness profile is similar or better than conventional single-vision lenses, which makes this a good option for the single-vision GP wearer who has entered presbyopia. In fact, when the decision has been made to fit GP multifocals, it is recommended to fit single-vision–wearing presbyopes initially before progressing onto translating or other, more challenging, presbyopic GP fits. Because these lenses, if fit properly, exhibit little movement, the presbyopic athlete also can benefit from them. Good intermediate vision often is obtainable because of the progressive add feature that benefits the computer user. This design is not recommended for patients who have very critical distance vision demands, a large pupil size, or are not motivated for a GP lens design.

When fitting these lenses, a well-centered fitting relationship with minimal movement with the blink is desired. Once experience has been gained via diagnostic fitting (with the ease of fitting these lenses), an empirical method is recommended (37). This has the benefit of allowing the new multifocal wearer to experience the potential visual benefits immediately, which, in turn, may lessen his or her perception of initial awareness. The use of a topical anesthetic at the initial application will be beneficial in enhancing the patient's initial experience (38). The use of either loose trial lenses or ±0.25/0.50 D flip lenses is preferred to a phoropter for overrefracting. Likewise, it is important to have the patient walk around the office and perform common tasks (i.e., look at a magazine, at a computer, off at a distance) to determine his or her initial level of satisfaction and perhaps what improvements may be necessary. These are fitting pearls that would benefit any new bifocal contact lens wearer. A list of fitting pearls is given in Table 27.5.

Excessive decentration and/or excessive movement will result in variable and generally unsatisfactory vision at all distances. When this occurs, steepening the base curve by, at minimum, 0.50 D may solve the problem. Increasing the overall diameter may likewise be beneficial. Another problem pertains to the presbyopic patient who requires a higher effective add power than the lens is able to provide. Many designs now provide multiple add powers. For example, Conforma Laboratories manufactures a popular high-eccentricity design (VFL 3) that also is available in a "Super Add." A representative low-eccentricity lens design is the Essentials Multifocal (Blanchard), which has Series I (low add), Series II (medium add), and Series III (high add) lens designs. Nevertheless, particularly for advanced presbyopes and those exhibiting a smaller than average pupil size, it

TABLE 27.5. BIFOCAL/MULTIFOCAL CONTACT LENS FITTING GUIDELINES

- Explain all of the options to a potential presbyopic contact lens patient; emphasize the bifocal option.
- When fitting bifocal/multifocal lenses, begin with patients who have great potential for success (i.e., highly motivated individuals; patients who presently are contact lens wearers and who are entering presbyopia) before fitting more challenging patients.
- Be sure to indicate to the patient the differences between the selected contact lens bifocal and spectacles. Some vision compromise may exist, and it may take a few lenses to achieve the best fit and quality of vision.
- Whenever possible, provide lenses in their prescription so that they can comment on what they feel are strengths and weaknesses. Likewise, it is important to have patients walk around the office and simulate tasks that they commonly perform on a daily basis and determine their level of satisfaction with their vision and possible areas of improvement.
- Use trial lenses or ± 0.25/0.50 D flip lenses as opposed to a phoropter to overrefract.
- Check vision binocularly to simulate a real-world environment.
- Determine what the patient's primary visual goals are and attempt to meet them; although not commonly necessary, the patient should be told that spectacles may be necessary for occasional tasks. Your goal is to meet, at minimum, 80% of the patient's visual needs and goals.
- Allow sufficient time (15–20 minutes) for the lenses to settle prior to assessing the lens-to-cornea fitting relationship.
- Be willing to try different types (gas permeable and soft) of lenses to achieve success.
- Do not hesitate to prescribe unequal adds.

often is difficult to achieve a sufficient effective add for near work; therefore, a "modified bifocal" approach is recommended. This could include any one of the following approaches:

1. Use a lower add bifocal on one eye (i.e., Series II) and a higher add on the other eye (i.e., Series III)
2. If step 1 is not sufficient, slightly over-plus one eye for optimum near vision while only slightly compromising distance vision
3. Prescribe low plus power reading spectacles for occasional use (i.e., small print, low illumination)

Alternating Vision

There are two types of alternation (translating) bifocal GP designs. They are used more commonly than the simultaneous type bifocals just discussed and include concentric and segmented lens designs.

Annular/Concentric

Front- or back-surface concentric designs, also know as *target* bifocals, typically have a 3- to 5-mm central distance

zone that is decentered to the superior part of the lens. Prism and truncation are often present to prevent lens rotation and to facilitate translation when shifting gaze (Fig. 27.4). For example, a common design incorporates 1 to 1.5 prism diopters with a small amount of truncation. The distance zone is decentered 1 to 2 mm superiorly.

When the patient shifts gaze inferiorly to read, the near zone of the lens should translate into the proper position in front of the pupil as the lens is held by the lower lid margin and the eye rotates downward. This is the mechanism by which all translating lenses function.

Good candidates for this design, as well as for all other prism ballast segmented bifocals, include patients having a lower lid margin tangent to, or slightly above, the lower limbus (or no more than 1 mm below the limbus), an 8.5-mm or larger vertical fissure size, normal (not loose) lid tension, and myopic/low hyperopic refractive powers. The benefits of these lenses include the ability to achieve precise correction and good vision at distance and near unaccompanied by secondary images, assuming proper fit, minimal lens rotation, and consistent translation. In addition, any amount of presbyopic adds can be corrected successfully. The disadvantages include the increased center thickness required with a prism ballast, although the translating concentrics are the thinnest of the prism ballast bifocals. With annular segments, it is important to specify a distance zone large enough to minimize distance flare. Finally, image jump, due to prismatic effects resulting from the bicentric construction of these lenses, can result in patient problems during gaze shift with concentric, translating bifocals. Some representative fitting problems and methods of managing them, applicable to all types of prism ballast lenses, including segment type bifocal GPs, are given in Table 27.6.

These lenses often are fitted slightly flatter than "K" because heavy GP lenses tend to decenter inferiorly when a flat base curve is selected. This is a desirable characteristic

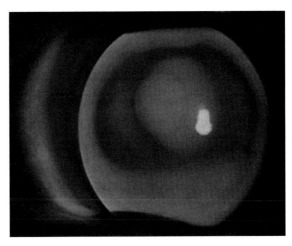

FIG. 27.4. DeCarle-style concentric bifocal with a decentered distance zone. (Courtesy of Dr. Peter Kollbaum.)

TABLE 27.6. TROUBLESHOOTING GAS-PERMEABLE TRANSLATING BIFOCAL LENS DESIGNS

Problem	Management Strategies
Poor translation	1. Flatten BCR 0.50 D or flatten peripheral curve to increase edge clearance 2. Increase prism or truncation 3. Change to another lens design (i.e., flaccid lids)
Excessive rotation	1. Flatten BCR 0.50 D if WTR cyl; steepen 0.50 D if ATR cyl 2. Offset prism if upswept lower lid; order prism at 105 degrees OD and 75 degrees OS
Superior decentration (lens picked up high with the blink)	1. Increase prism by 0.50Δ 2. Flatten BCR by 0.50 D
Poor distance vision	1. Superior decentration: increase prism by 0.50 Δ 2. Inadequate pupil coverage: increase OAD ≥0.5 mm 3. If seg height into pupil: reduce seg height
Poor near vision	1. Poor lens translation: manage as indicated above 2. Too low seg height: increase seg height 3. Excessive rotation: manage as indicated above 4. Patient is dropping head, not eyes, to read: educate patient appropriately
Poor intermediate vision	1. Over-spectacles for intermediate distance (i.e., for computer use) 2. Select a gas permeable translating bifocal lens with an intermediate correction

with a translating lens design because it is important for the inferior edge to position adjacent or very close to the lower lid. A new concentric annular design, the Mandell Seamless Bifocal (Con-Cise), provides an aspheric transition zone between the distance and near annular zones. It is a front-surface concentric design with central distance zone diameters ranging from 3.0 to 3.8 mm and an average overall diameter of 9.8 mm (39–42).

Segmented

Although more complex in design, perhaps the most successful bifocal contact lenses from a visual standpoint are the GP segmented translating designs. These lenses have had a long history of development and refinement during the polymethyl methacrylate (PMMA) years from 1960 to 1980. Segmented one-piece GP bifocals utilizing monocentric optics are now available.

Monocentric means that the optical centers of the lens power zones are coincident and "image jump" when viewing from one section of the lens to another is eliminated. At one time, this benefit was limited to fused bifocal designs. However, as a result of the difficulty in fusing the softer GP lens materials, due to the pioneering work of George Tsuetaki of Fused Kontacts, the near and distance optical centers were manufactured to be coincident at a tangent at the segment line. Thus, introduction of the Tangent Streak (Firestone Optics) lens in the 1980s repopularized segmented translating bifocals. The Tangent Streak, like all prism ballasted designs, typically is provided in a high Dk material (often Fluorex 500 or 700) to provide sufficient oxygen transmission. A full range of powers and geometries are available because the lenses are custom designed by the clinician. It is heavily prism ballasted (often between 1.75 and 3.00Δ) and truncated. The segment shape is similar to an "executive" bifocal; the seg can be ordered at any height, and a trifocal version of this lens is available.

The following diagnostic lens specifications are recommended (20 lenses) by the manufacturer:

BCR: 41.00–45.50 D
Seg height: 4.2 mm
Power: ±2.00 D
Add: +2.00 D
OAD: 9.4/9.0 mm

Many of the same fitting principles (i.e., anesthetic use (for a new wearer), loose trial lenses, or flipper bars) used with aspheric patients also apply to the alternating design patient. However, these lenses, like all alternating designs, are fit slightly flatter than "K." The lens rests on the lower lid during distance gaze, and the seg line should be positioned at or slightly below the lower pupil margin (Fig. 27.5). The lens must decenter (translate) 2 mm or more on downward gaze to position a sufficient amount of the near point region in front of the pupil while near point tasks are being performed.

The lens should ride with its lower edge supported by the lower lid margin. With the patient fixating straight

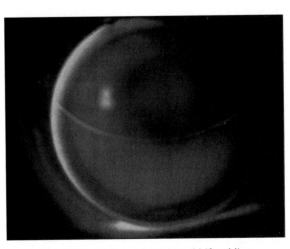

FIG. 27.5. Optimum positioned bifocal line.

ahead, the lens usually is picked up 1 to 2 mm on the blink and then drops back to the lower position quickly.

Several popular segmented lens designs include the Metro-Seg (Metro Optics), Solitaire II (Tru-Form Optics), and Solutions (X-Cel). The latter design is a representative example of current efforts to make these designs easy to fit. It is a crescent design that is fit similarly to the Tangent Streak in terms of base curve radius and seg position. However, it is available in only three prism amounts (low, medium, and high) and five seg heights. The standard design is not truncated, and the diagnostic set has medium prism, an intermediate seg height, a 9.6-mm overall diameter, and similar distance and near powers as the Tangent Streak diagnostic set.

Good candidates for this design are similar to those for other translating bifocals and include: (i) early and advanced presbyopes, (ii) lower lid above, tangent to, or no more than 0.5 mm below the limbus (Fig. 27.6), (iii) myopia and low hyperopic powers, (iv) normal-to-large palpebral fissure sizes, and (v) normal-to-tight lid tension.

Patients with high hyperopia may have more difficulty because of the increased thickness of the prism ballasted plus lenses. Individuals with loose lids may not be able to maintain proper alignment of the thicker inferior edge on the lower lid margin with downward gaze. The advantages of this design are the same as the translating concentric designs; however, the segmented designs have the advantages of having a larger distance zone and absence of image jump. The disadvantages primarily pertain to the thickness inherent in their construction and the importance of achieving translation with downward gaze.

Troubleshooting translating lens designs primarily pertains to the following three potential problems (11):

1. Excessive rotation with the blink. This is often the result of a base curve radius that is too steep. Flattening the base curve radius by 0.50 D will often allow the lens to fall quicker to the lower lid and not be prone to the rotational effects of the upper lid.

2. Insufficient or lack of translation. This may be resolved by increasing the amount of edge clearance to allow the lens edge to exhibit more contact with the lower lid. This can be accomplished by selecting a flatter base curve lens or, alternatively, flattening the peripheral curve radius. If this change is not beneficial and the lens is still not translating, it most likely is the result of a flaccid lower lid that becomes more problematic with age.

3. The lens exhibits excessive movement with the blink. If the lens is picked up too superiorly with the blink, increasing the prism should result in less upward displacement (Fig. 27.7).

Another problem with segmented translating designs is the absence of an intermediate correction for the advanced presbyope. A few of the segmented bifocal lens designs also are available in a trifocal (i.e., Tangent Streak Trifocal from Firestone Optics and both Llevations and Solitaire I from Tru-Form Optics). Several recently introduced lens designs also have eliminated this problem. The Presbylite lens (Lens Dynamics) is a nontruncated lens design with 1.5Δ. This lens design incorporates a spherical distance zone, spherical near zone, and unique triangle-shaped aspheric intermediate zone (Fig. 27.8) (39). The Solitaire II (Tru-Form Optics) is a nontruncated executive design that incorporates a small aspheric zone on the front of the lens in between the near and distance zones for intermediate vision. The X-Cel ES-Sential-Solution segmented aspheric multifocal is the result of a combined effort of two of the leading GP bifocal manufacturers (X-Cel and Blanchard) (12). The posterior geometry of this design generates about 1.00 D of add power. The front surface is similar to the X-Cel Solutions Bifocal with a crescent-shaped segment configuration.

Translating GP lenses yield the highest success rate of any contact lens bifocals available today, but their fitting requires precise measurement of anterior eye anatomy, familiarity with the translating concept, use of a reliable diag-

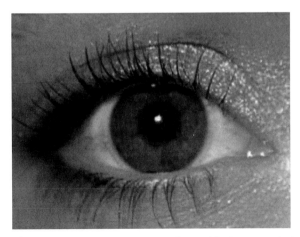

FIG. 27.6. Optimum lid-to-cornea relationship for a translating bifocal design. (Courtesy of Dr. Peter Kollbaum.)

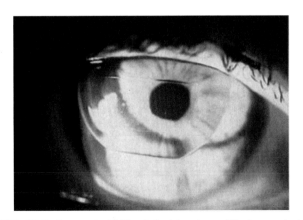

FIG. 27.7. Segmented bifocal that has been lifted excessively with the blink.

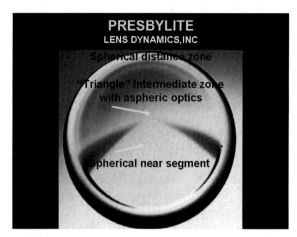

FIG. 27.8. Presbylite segmented multifocal lens design.

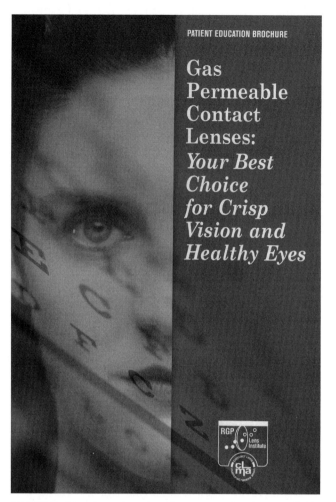

FIG. 27.9. Myopia and presbyopia consumer brochure available from the Gas Permeable Lens Institute.

nostic lens, and a willingness to consult with the experts at the fabricating laboratory. Many resources (e.g., Clinical Management Guide, laminated pocket card, fitting and problem-solving video tape, and C/D-ROM) as well as a listing of all of the CLMA member laboratories and the bifocal and multifocal lens designs they manufacture are available from the GP Lens Institute *(www.rgpli.org)* (Table 27.7). A consumer brochure on myopia and presbyopia and the contact lens applications also is available (Fig. 27.9).

SOFT BIFOCAL/MULTIFOCAL DESIGNS

Soft bifocal and multifocal lens designs have certain limitations compared to their GP counterparts. The quality of vision is somewhat compromised as a result of both the water content and the dependence upon the simultaneous vision concept. In fact, the term "20/happy" has been ascribed to these lenses because the best corrected vision may be reduced compared to the best spectacle corrected acuity but the patient is satisfied. It is important to note that some presbyopes are so motivated not to wear spectacles that they would be satisfied with a multiple line Snellen acuity reduction; however, this becomes an ethical issue for the practitioner. Likewise, the inability of these designs to translate (with one exception to be discussed) negates an important benefit for optimizing near vision with GP designs.

TABLE 27.7. BIFOCAL/MULTIFOCAL RESOURCES AVAILABLE FROM THE GP LENS INSTITUTE (WWW.RGPLI.ORG)

1. GP Correction of Presbyopia CD-ROM
2. GP Bifocal Fitting and Problem-Solving Video
3. "Correcting Presbyopia" Laminated Pocket Card
4. GP Clinical Management Guide
5. GPL:I On-Line Symposia (available at *www.rgpli.org*)
6. GP Product Directory

However, numerous improvements in both lens design and replacement have resulted in greater use and success with soft lenses than in the past. Perhaps the most important change has been the availability of these designs in disposable and frequent replacement modalities. Because tear volume decreases with age, it is important to minimize the impact of deposits on both ocular health and quality of vision. In addition, although these designs utilize the simultaneous vision principle, the ability to vary the design—between eyes—to optimize vision at various distances is present. In addition, patients can trial these lenses for limited time periods while the practitioner adjusts the design to optimize both the fitting relationship and vision at all distances. This is important due to the large number of single vision soft lens wearers who would prefer to continue soft lens wear as they enter presbyopia.

Good candidates for soft bifocal lenses include current single-vision soft lens wearers who have entered presbyopia, dissatisfied monovision wearers, those with low (or no) refractive astigmatism, and individuals who do not have a critical distance vision demand.

Several lens designs currently are available. The easiest method of differentiating commonly used soft bifocal and multifocal designs is whether the design is center-distance or center-near.

Center-Distance

Center-distance lens designs can be either aspheric or concentric, although most are concentric in design. Common designs in this category include the Acuvue Bifocal (Vistakon), Frequency 55 Multifocal (CooperVision), and Ultra Vue (Acuity One).

A popular center-distance concentric design is the Acuvue Bifocal. In lieu of a more conventional two-zone design, this lens is multizone with five alternating distance and near zones (Fig. 27.10) (43,44). The multizone design enhances distance and near power coverage of the pupil as it dilates or constricts with contact lens movement. It is available in 0.25 D increments from +4.00 to −6.00 D with +1.00 D to +2.50 D adds in 0.50 D increments. It is disposed of every 2 weeks.

As with other frequent replacement lenses, the benefits to this lens design include the ability to fit directly from inventory and allow the patient to trial the lenses for a designated time period (often 1 week). The lens can be fine tuned at that time if a change is indicated. According to Rigel (45), approximately half (51%) will be successful with the "full binocular" approach; 32% were successful with a "modified bifocal" approach (adding plus power to the distance prescription of the nondominant eye to enhance near vision; and 17% were fitted with the "enhanced monovision" approach (fitting the nondominant eye with a single vision lens for near and reducing the add power of the Acuvue Bifocal in the dominant eye). Lee (46) recommends

TABLE 27.8. ACUVUE BIFOCAL PROBLEM SOLVING

1. Distance single vision Acuvue on dominant eye and Acuvue Bifocal on nondominant eye for patients with critical distance vision demands
2. Acuvue Bifocal on the dominant eye and Acuvue single vision lens in dominant eye for patients with extremely fine near work
3. Both eyes wearing Acuvue Bifocals with less add on the dominant eye to provide greater intermediate correction if needed
4. Fit Acuvue Bifocals on both eyes but increase the distance plus power on the nondominant eye (i.e., "modified monovision") to increase the effective add
5. Use a single Acuvue Bifocal contact lens on the dominant eye of low myopes or on the nondominant eye of low hyperopes

(From [46].)

the guidelines given in Table 27.8 for problem-solving reduced vision with the Acuvue Bifocal. The important factor is altering the design to be consistent with the patient's goals and needs (i.e., distance single-vision Acuvue on dominant eye and Acuvue Bifocal on nondominant eye for patients with critical distance vision demands; Acuvue Bifocal on the dominant eye and a single-vision lens on the nondominant eye for patients with extremely fine near work). It is important to emphasize that 75% of successfully fitted patients have a distance prescription within ±0.25 D of the best corrected sphere (47).

Modified Monovision

The Frequency 55 Multifocal is derived from the UltraVue lens design from Acuity One. This design combines multifocal optics with monovision. The intention is to have the

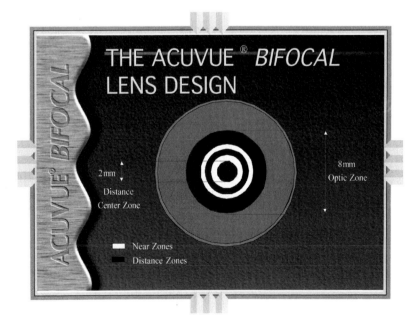

FIG. 27.10. Acuvue Bifocal lens design.

LENS DESIGN – D LENS

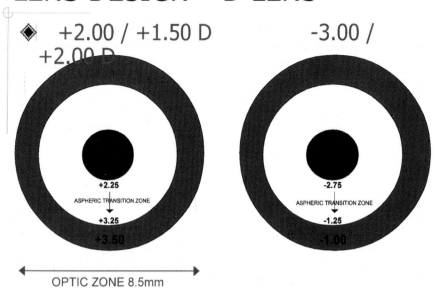

FIG. 27.11. Frequency 55 Multifocal "D" lens design.

ease of fitting (i.e., monovision) with the little-compromised visual acuity of all distances with binocular vision corrections (36,48). A center distance (D) lens, which transitions through an aspheric intermediate to an outer near zone, is placed on the dominant eye (Fig. 27.11). A center near (N) lens, which transitions through an aspheric intermediate to a spherical peripheral distance zone, is placed on the nondominant eye (Fig. 27.12) (48–50). It is hoped that binocular summation will occur, providing acceptable vision at all distances under binocular conditions. The central zone sizes are different between the D lens (2.3 mm) and the N lens (1.7 mm) to emphasize the visual performance at the emphasized vision demand zone.

Like the Acuvue Bifocal, it is available in one overall diameter and base curve. It is available in +1.50, +2.00, and +2.50 D adds and is recommended for monthly replacement. In a multicenter study, on average, patients had 0.12 D greater add with the Frequency 55 Multifocal nondominant lens compared to their vision with spectacles in the same eye (48). It has been recommended that the patient be advised about possible shadowing and ghost images, which may be adaptational, and return in 4 to 7 days (50). Changes in lens design can be expected with 20% to 40% of the patients at the first follow-up visit.

The UltraVue lens design is similar to the Frequency 55 lens. The Ultravue P lens (add in the periphery) is designed for the dominant eye and has a spherical central zone for distance vision (51). The central zone is surrounded by an

LENS DESIGN – N LENS

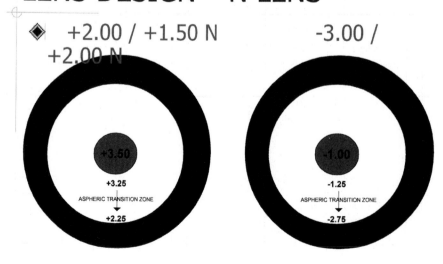

FIG. 27.12. Frequency 55 Multifocal "N" lens design.

aspheric annular zone that creates a gradual refractive shift toward plus power and offers intermediate and near visual function. The UltraVue C lens (add in the center) is designed with a spherical central near vision zone surrounded by an aspheric annular zone that creates a gradual refractive shift toward minus power and offers intermediate and distance visual function. The goal is to achieve 20/20 distance vision and 20/40 near vision out of the UltraVue P lens and vice versa out of the UltraVue C lens.

Center-Near

There are several aspheric or progressive near-center lens designs. A representative example of this design is the Focus Progressive (Ciba Vision). This is a center-near aspheric lens design with a 2-week to 1-month replacement schedule (Fig. 27.13) (42,43). It is approved for up to 6 nights of extended wear and has two base curve radii. The add is reported to be a nominal add that could provide up to 3 D, although it is not often that advanced presbyopes need to add + 0.50 to 0.75 D over the nondominant eye (52). In a comparison study, the Focus Progressives resulted in significantly better distance vision and was rated higher in comfort and handling by patients compared to the Acuvue Bifocal (53). These results were not consistent, however, with the results of a study by Guillon et al. (54). Ciba Vision recently unveiled Focus Dailies Progressive, which is available in one base curve and discarded daily.

Diffractive Bifocals

The only diffractive bifocal lens design available today is the Echelon (Ocular Sciences). This design utilizes uses a diffraction zone plate to equally separate light rays to both the distance and the near focal images. The distance power is refracted, and the near power is achieved by the diffractive principles. The major advantage of this design is pupil size

independence. The near diffractive power is achieved through the circular annular grooves (echelettes) on the back surface of the lens and the refractive index of the tear layer that pools behind the grooves. The radii and spacing of the annular grooves determine the add power of the lens. This posterior diffractive zone is approximately 4.00 to 4.5 mm in diameter, located at the center of the line, and the entire lens contains the distance power. The central zone plate can easily be observed against the dark background of the pupil with biomicroscopy. When fitting this lens, the use of trial lenses to assess fit, centration, and power determination by overrefraction is essential (55). If only slight decentration is present, the patient can still be successful with the Echelon lens; however, more add power may be required in this case. In addition, because at minimum one half of the illumination is lost to higher orders of diffraction, the illumination should be high when the patient is performing near tasks. However, whereas the Echelon and other simultaneous vision soft bifocal/multifocal lenses compromise distance binocular contrast sensitivity, two experimental diffractive/refractive soft multifocal lens designs from Austria were recently found to result in no compromise in this function (56).

Translating

The one exception to the absence of translating soft lenses is the Triton Translating Soft Bifocal Lens from Gelflex. It is a back-surface design that allows for translation with truncation and a biprism design to allow for lens stability and location (57,58). The lens has an overall size in the horizontal meridian of either 14.5 or 15.0 mm, with 14.5 mm being the most common. The larger lens is recommended for low positioned lower lids (i.e., 2 mm below the lower limbus). The Triton fitting set includes six lenses of two base curve radii and vertical sizes that vary from 11.4 to 13.9 mm in 0.5-mm steps. It has two location dots engraved at the 3- and 9-o'clock positions at the periphery of the lens, which are on line with the geometrical center of the lens. The near power segment is positioned 1 mm below the geometrical center.

Toric Bifocal Designs

A limitation to the aforementioned lens designs is the correction of astigmatism. Several lens designs are available, although they are custom and not available in planned replacement or disposable forms. The Horizon 55 BiCon Toric (Westcon Contact Lens) is a concentric center-near lens that can correct as much as %.00 D of astigmatism and + 3.00 D of add (41,43). The UCL Multifocal Toric (United Contact Lens) has an aspheric back surface that results in a center-distance design. The Essential Soft Toric Multifocal (Blanchard Contact Lens) has a front aspheric, center-near design with posterior astigmatic correction and anterior double slaboff for stability. The UltraVue 2000

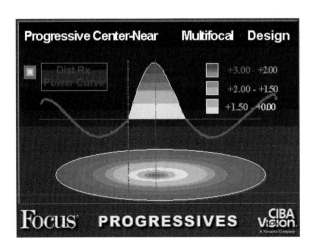

FIG. 27.13. Focus Progressive multifocal design.

Multifocal Progressive Toric (Opti-Centre Laboratories) is available with a center-distance design and a center-near design for dominant and nondominant eyes with up to +3.50 D add power.

LENS SELECTION

Success Rates

The low lens cost, east of fitting, and relatively high success rates (often 70%–90%) achieved with monovision have made it a popular technique for presbyopic contact lens correction among practitioners (8,59,60). A comparable, if not higher, success rate (75%–86%) appears to be present with GP multifocal and bifocal lens designs (61–65). Most traditional soft bifocal studies resulted in a success rate of only 40% to 50% (66–69). However, with the introduction of innovative new designs and frequent replacement modalities, this success rate currently is higher (70). Nevertheless, the need to screen patients and use an adequate and reliable diagnostic set of the desired bifocal lens design is imperative.

It is evident in comparison studies, however, that when patients are given a choice, bifocal contact lenses are often preferred to monovision and exhibit improved objective performance. Kirschen et al. (71) found that Acuvue Bifocal lenses provided a lower interocular difference in visual acuity than monovision, which resulted in improved stereoacuity and a lower prevalence of suppression at distance and near. Johnson et al. (72) fit subjects with GP monovision for 6 weeks followed by 6 weeks of the Boston Multivision GP aspheric design (or vice versa). At the conclusion of the study, 75% of the subjects preferred the multifocal design. Therefore, if given the choice, patients likely will prefer a multifocal/bifocal lens design. It also is evident that experts in the field are recommending that bifocal contact lenses be positioned ahead of monovision when presenting presbyopic contact lens options to interested patients (35,58).

Rajagopalan et al. (73) assessed the contrast sensitivity function of subjects wearing GP multifocals, soft bifocals, and GP monovision. The results showed that GP multifocal wearers exhibited the highest contrast sensitivity function at all spatial frequencies. Soft bifocal wearers exhibited a significantly lower contrast sensitivity function; however, their performance was significantly improved compared to monovision. Several recent studies have found subjective preference to be similar between soft bifocals and monovision, with the latter requiring fewer lenses to achieve an optimum fit (74,75).

Factors Important to Patient Success

The most important considerations for patient success are the visual demands and expectations of the patient (8). The first lens of choice for individuals who lower their gaze to perform their work is a translating GP segment design. Patients who need intermediate and/or near vision while viewing in the primary position of gaze would benefit from a simultaneous bifocal such as an aspheric or annular design. Aspheric GP multifocals or soft lens designs, often used in some form of "modified bifocal" technique, are popular for most patients who do not have a critical distance vision demand and perform tasks (e.g., computer use) that require intermediate correction. Anatomical considerations, such as pupil size and lower lid position, are critical when fitting a GP lens design. It is preferable to attempt to simulate the patients' working environment during the screening visit when determining the type and powers of a presbyopic contact lens correction with the aid of trial lenses. At minimum, one translating GP trial set, one aspheric GP trial set, and two or three different soft simultaneous design trial sets/inventories should be sufficient for good patient screening and success assessment. Initially, it is desirable to order lenses on a warranty basis; once experience has been gained with a particular GP bifocal lens, the additional fee for a warranty may not be necessary. For the many patients who are entering presbyopia and are long-term successful single-vision contact lens wearers, it is best to stay with the same lens material, GP or soft, when refitting with a multifocal lens.

What about the role of monovision? Certainly, the controversy continues as to how monovision should be positioned in the practice, whether as a first or last choice. Although monovision is a viable option, unless definite contraindications are found, it is a good idea to assess patient response to a bifocal diagnostic lens fitting prior to choosing monovision empirically as the first presbyopic contact lens option.

PATIENT EDUCATION AND FOLLOW-UP CARE

Presbyopic patients, especially new contact lens wearers, need to be thoroughly educated about proper lens care and handling. Contact lens wear can be intimidating for the patient who not only has experienced 45 or more years without lens wear but who also may have been exposed to negative experiences/complications from friends and relatives. In addition, these individuals need to be monitored closely because of possible complications that may arise from the aforementioned physiologic changes of the aging eye, as well as to reinforce compliance to lens care procedures.

Care and Handling

The keys for successful handling of contact lenses by the presbyopic patient are patience and reassurance. Older individuals, especially novice wearers, will be apprehensive and lack confidence. No matter how frustrating it is to the individual performing the instruction, that feeling of frustration must not be conveyed to the patient. The instructions must be provided slowly and on a one-to-one basis. The patient should never have the perception that the optometrist has lost confidence in his or her ability to handle the lenses properly; otherwise, feeling of failure and surrender may result. Conversely, if the patient feels confident about handling the lenses, the feeling of accomplishment improves the motivation to succeed. It is important that the patient leaves the office feeling confident in the handling of his or her lenses.

In addition to instructions on handling, the patient needs to be instructed on the functions of the various solutions and how to properly use them. The most important information contained in the manual or patient brochure should be discussed with the patient, and the patient can be encouraged to ask questions. In fact, the patient should be asked to review how to use the solutions to ensure compliance with cleaning, rinsing, and disinfection steps. Finally, lens care instructions and care compliance should be reinforced at every follow-up visit. For example, patients should be asked to repeat the name and use of the solutions they are currently using, if they have any questions about handling, the condition of their case if available (the practitioner may want to replace the case at regular intervals), how they are caring for the lenses, and the wearing schedule.

Presbyopic contact lens patients should be monitored regularly, preferably every 6 months. As a result of their predisposition for dryness-related problems, a careful silt-lamp evaluation with contact lens wear is important. The surface condition and wettability of the worn lens should be evaluated carefully, and aging deposited lenses must be replaced. If feasible (that is, monovision), a 1- to 3-month planned replacement program should be used with soft lens wearing patients. With lenses off, the cornea should be evaluated with fluorescein dye and the upper eyelids everted to rule out papillary changes. In addition, because the bifocal lens designs often are thicker that their single-vision counterparts, the cornea should be evaluated for the presence of corneal edema resulting from possible hypoxia. If striae, central corneal clouding, or another form of edema is present, a thinner design and higher oxygen transmissible material are indicated. Keratometry/corneal topography and refraction also should be performed during follow-up visits, notably with patients wearing the thicker bifocal designs, in which undesirable curvature and refractive changes may occur.

PRESBYOPIA SUMMARY

The presbyopic contact lens market is growing every year. It appears that numerous companies are developing new multifocal lenses in hopes of capturing the "baby boomers" who have reached, or are reaching, presbyopic age. The cosmetic and sometime functional benefits of contact lenses should make them a recommended option for every contact lens-using presbyopic patient and for the many who are becoming aware of multifocal contact lenses. Every presbyopic patient should not automatically be considered for monovision; in fact, a bifocal diagnostic fitting should be considered as the first option for most presbyopes. Finally,

comprehensive education and follow-up care should be performed to ensure patient confidence with care and handling, verify compliance with the care regimen, and minimize the risks associated with contact lens wear.

ACKNOWLEDGMENTS

The authors thank Courtney Westrich and Cheryl Bergin for their contributions to this chapter.

REFERENCES

1. Schwartz CA. Portrait of a presbyope in 1999. *Optom Today* 1999;(Suppl):5–7.
2. Wooley S. "Doctor, do I have to give up my contact lenses just because I need bifocals?" *Optom Today* 1998;6:40–42.
3. Rigel LE, Castellano CF. How to fit today's soft bifocal contact lenses. *Optom Today* 1999;7(Suppl):45–51.
4. Du Toit R, Situ P, Simpson T, et al. The effects of six months of contact lens wear on the tear film, ocular surfaces, and symptoms of presbyopes. *Optom Vis Sci* 2001;78:455–462.
5. Weale RA. *A biography of the eye: development, age, and growth.* London: HK Lewis, 1982.
6. Bennett ES, Jurkus JM, Schwartz CA. Bifocal contact lenses. In: Bennett ES, Henry VA, eds. *Clinical manual of contact lenses,* 2nd ed. Philadelphia: Lippincott Williams & Wilkins, 2000: 410–449.
7. Sakamoto R, Bennett ES, Henry VA, et al. The phenol red thread test: a cross-cultural study. *Inv Ophthalmol Vis Sci* 1993;34: 3510–3514.
8. Josephson JE, Caffery BE. Hydrogel bifocal lenses. In: Bennett ES, Weissman BA, eds. *Clinical contact lens practice.* Philadelphia: JB Lippincott, 1990:43-1–43-20.
9. Erickson DB. Self-efficacy may determine monovision success. *Contact Lens Spectrum* 1995;10:51.
10. Erickson P, McGill EC. Role of visual acuity, stereoacuity, and ocular dominance in monovision patient success. *Optom Vis Sci* 1992;69:761–764.
11. Bennett ES, Hansen DW. Presbyopia: gas permeable bifocal fitting and problem-solving. In: Bennett ES, Hom MM, eds. *Manual of gas permeable contact lenses,* 2nd ed. St. Louis: Elsevier Science, 2004:324–356.
12. Norman CW. Combining simultaneous and alternating vision GP concepts. *Contact Lens Spectrum* 2003;18:21.
13. Bennett ES, Weissman BA, Remba MJ. Contact lenses and the elderly patient. In: Rosenbloom A, eds. ???? *(In press).*
14. Jain S, Arora I, Azar DT. Success of monovision in presbyopes: review of the literature and potential applications to refractive surgery. *Surv Ophthalmol* 1996;40:491–499.
15. Fonda G. Trans Ophthalmologic Society of Australia XXV. 1966;46–50.
16. Johannsdottir KR, Stelmach LB. Monovision: a review of the scientific literature. *Optom Vis Sci* 2001;78:646–651.
17. Du Toit R, Ferreira JT, Nel ZJ. Visual and nonvisual variables implicated in monovision wear. *Optom Vis Sci* 1998;75:119–125.
18. Schwartz CA. Presbyopia: monovision. In: Schwartz CA, ed. *Specialty contact lenses: a fitter's guide,* 1st ed. Philadelphia: WB Saunders, 1996:85–93.
19. Michaels DD. Ocular dominance. *Surv Ophthalmol* 1974;17: 151–163.
20. Pearlman A. The central visual pathways. In: Moses RA, Hart WM, eds. *Adler's physiology of the eye: clinical application.* St. Louis: CV Mosby, 1987:583–618.

21. Woods JM, Wick K, et al. The effect of monovision contact lens wear on driving performance. *Clin Exp Optom* 1998;81:100–103

22. Jurkus JM, Nichols SL. Contact lenses and the aging eye. *Optom Today* 1999;4(Suppl):53–60.

23. Schor C, Landsman L. Ocular dominance and the interocular suppression of blur in monovision. *Am J Optom Physiol Opt* 1987;64:723–730.

24. Westendorf DH, Blake R, Sloane M, et al. Binocular summation occurs during interocular suppressions. *J Exp Psychol* 1982;8:81–90.

25. Collins MJ. Goode A. Brown B. Distance visual acuity and monovision. *Optom Vis Sci* 1993;70:723–728.

26. Wick B. Westin E. Change in refractive anisometropia in presbyopic adults wearing monovision contact lens correction. *Optom Vis Sci* 1999;76:33–39.

27. Loshin DS, Loshin MS, Comer G. Binocular summation with monovision contact lens correction for presbyopia. *Int Contact Lens Clin* 1982;9:161–165.

28. Collins MJ, Brown B, Bowman KJ. Contrast sensitivity with contact lens correction for presbyopia. *Ophthalmic Physiol Opt* 1989;9:133–138.

29. Rajagopalan AS, Bennett ES, Lakshminarayanan V, et al. Performance of presbyopic contact lenses under mesopic conditions. Presented at ARVO, Fort Lauderdale, Florida, April 2003.

30. Harris MG, Classe JG. Clinicolegal considerations of monovision. *J Am Optom Assoc* 1988;59:491–495.

31. Nakagawara VB, Veronneau SJH. Monovision contact lens use in the aviation environment: a report of a contact lens-related aircraft accident. *Optometry* 2000;71:390–395.

32. Schwartz CA, Jurkus JM. Trouble-shooting the monovision fit. *Contact Lens Forum* 1991;16:24–26.

33. Bennett ES, Hansen DW, Baker R. GPs and presbyopes: why today's designs are easier to fit. *Rev Optom* 2003;140.

34. Benjamin WJ, Borish IM. Physiology of aging and its influence on the contact lens prescription. *J Am Optom Assoc* 1991;62:743–752.

35. Bergenske PD. The presbyopic fitting process. *Contact Lens Spectrum* 2001;16:34–41.

36. Shovlin JP, Eisenberg JS. Monovision vs. multifocal. Which would you choose? *Rev Optom* 2003;140:36–38.

37. Ames K. Fitting the presbyope with gas permeable contact lenses. *Contact Lens Spectrum* 2001;1642–45.

38. Bennett ES, Smythe J, Henry VA, et al. The effect of topical anesthetic use on the initial patient satisfaction and overall success with rigid gas permeable contact lenses. *Optom Vis Sci* 1998;75:800–805.

39. Davis R. Pinpoint success with GP multifocal lenses. *Contact Lens Spectrum* 2003;18.

40. Mandell RB. A new concept in GP bifocal contact lenses. *Contact Lens Spectrum* 2002;17.

41. Hansen DW. Multifocal contact lenses: the next generation. *Contact Lens Spectrum* 2002;17:42–47.

42. Shovlin JP. Extended wear for presbyopes? *Rev Optom* 2002139:55.

43. Benoit DP. Multifocal contact lens update. *Contact Lens Spectrum* 2001;16.

44. Ghormley NR. The new Acuvue Bifocal contact lens. *Int Contact Lens Clin* 1998;25:71,72.

45. Rigel LE. What to expect from the Acuvue Bifocal. *Optom Today* 1998;6:26–27.

46. Lee WC. Factors for fitting success. *Contact Lens Spectrum* 1999;14:7a.

47. Lloyd M. Fitting a soft disposable bifocal lens. *Optician* 1999;217:18–22.

48. Iravani N. New multifocal offers best of both worlds. *Contact Lens Spectrum* 2002;17.

49. Quinn TG. Making sense of frequent replacement soft multifocals. *Contact Lens Spectrum* 2002;17.

50. Wan L. Take some frustration out of multifocal fitting. *Contact Lens Spectrum* 2003;18.

51. Bridgewater BA, Farkas B, Toscano F. A hydrogel system for the correction of presbyopia. *Contact Lens Spectrum* 1999;14:41–44.

52. Quinn TG. The monovision vs. multifocal debate. *Contact Lens Spectrum* 2002;17.

53. Fisher K, Bauman E, Schwallie J. Evaluation of two new soft contact lenses for correction of presbyopia: the Focus Progressives Multifocal and the Acuvue Bifocal. *Int Contact Lens Clin* 1999;26:92–103

54. Guillon M, Maissa C, Cooper P, et al. Visual performance of a Multi-zone Bifocal and a Progressive Multifocal Contact lens. *CLAO J* 2002;28;88–93.

55. Vehige JG. Hydron Echelon lens fitting guide, part III: fitting factors for success. *Contact Lens Spectrum* 1992;7:39–46.

56. Soni PS, Patel R, Carlson RS. Is binocular contrast sensitivity at distance compromised with multifocal soft contact lenses used to correct presbyopia? *Optom Vis Sci* 2003;80:505–514.

57. Ezekiel DF, Ezekiel DJ. A soft bifocal lens that does not compromise vision. *Contact Lens Spectrum* 2002;17.

58. Barr JA. Bifocals, multifocals, monovision: what works today. *Contact Lens Spectrum* 2003;18:41–45.

59. Collins M, Bruce A, Thompson B. Adaptation to monovision. *Int Contact Lens Clin* 1994;21:218–224.

60. Weinstock FJ. Presbyopic correction with contact lenses. *Ophthalmol Clin North Am* 1996;111–116.

61. Remba MJ. The Tangent Streak rigid gas permeable bifocal contact lens. *J Am Optom Assoc* 1988;59:212–216.

62. Kirman ST, Kirman GS. Tangent Streak Bifocal contact lenses. *Contact Lens Update* 1990;9:65–69.

63. Woods C, Ruston D, Hough T, et al. Clinical performance of an innovative back surface multifocal contact lens in correcting presbyopia. *CLAO J* 1999;25:176–181.

64. Byrnes SP, Cannella A. An in-office evaluation of a multifocal RGP lens design. *Contact Lens Spectrum* 1999;14:29–33.

65. Lieblein JS. Finding success with multifocal contact lenses. *Contact Lens Spectrum* 2000;14:50–51.

66. Donshik PC, Luistro A. Soft bifocal contact lens fitting with the Alges lens. *CLAO J* 1987;13:174–176.

67. Hanks A. Contact lenses for presbyopia. *Eye Contact* 1984;9–14.

68. Edwards K, Haig-Brown G. An evaluation of bifocal contact lens performance and the design of a new fitting protocol. *Trans BCLA* 1987;30–34.

69. Herrin S. How to fit the new bifocal soft lenses. *Rev Optom* 1989;126:57.

70. Odineal C. Fitting a soft disposable bifocal contact lens. *Contact Lens Spectrum* 2001;16.

71. Kirschen DG, Hung CC, Nakano TR. Comparison of suppression, stereoacuity, and interocular differences in visual acuity in monovision, and Acuvue bifocal contact lenses. *Optom Vis Sci* 1999;76:832–837.

72. Johnson J, Bennett ES, Henry VA, et al. MultiVision™ vs. monovision: a comparative study. Presented at the Annual Meeting of the Contact Lens Association of Ophthalmologists, Las Vegas, Nevada, February 2000.

73. Rajagopalan AS, Bennett ES, Lakshminarayanan V, et al. Contrast sensitivity with presbyopic contact lenses. Presented at the American Academy of Optometry, Dallas, Texas, December 2003.

74. Gromacki SJ, Nilsen E. Comparison of multifocal lens performance to monovision. *Contact Lens Spectrum* 2001;16.

75. Fonn D, Dutoit R, Situ P, et al. Determination of lens prescription for monovision and Acuvue Bifocal contact lenses. Presented at the Annual Meeting of the American Academy of Optometry, December 2000.

CONTACT LENS APPLICATIONS FOR OCULAR TRAUMA, DISEASE, AND SURGERY

TIMOTHY T. MCMAHON AND LORETTA B. SZCZOTKA-FLYNN

The irregular cornea (postoperative and otherwise) poses interesting challenges to the contact lens clinician. This chapter chronicles these challenges and offers clinical techniques to address them. The strategies described herein share substantial similarities across ocular conditions, dependent on the shape characteristics of the cornea involved. An oblate cornea produced by an excimer laser, for example, is likely to be addressed in a common manner to other oblate corneas. The contact lens fitter's challenge is to identify the major corneal shape factors and pair them with the most appropriate lens fitting strategies, taking into account the vagaries associated with each particular ocular condition. Our effort presented here will hopefully lessen the burden of these challenges.

THE OPTICAL REASONS FOR USING CONTACT LENSES

Contact lenses are prescribed for a variety of reasons in corneal disease, and following trauma, infection, and surgery. Indications include high refractive error, regular and irregular astigmatism, anisometropia with or without secondary asthenopia, post–refractive surgery residual refractive error with the patient's preference for contact lens use, and poor surface healing requiring bandage lens therapy. Spectacles are often of limited value and usefulness will vary with the underlying corneal condition. Optical shortfalls of spectacles include: (a) inability to correct significant irregular astigmatism; (b) aniseikonia induced from spectacle corrected anisometropia; (c) barrel and pin cushion distortions in highly myopic and hyperopic prescriptions, respectively; (d) visual distortion in highly astigmatic corrections; (e) induced prism in peripheral gaze; and (f) image magnification or minification secondary to high prescriptions.

Following corneal shape alterations, whether induced by corneal scarring, surgery, or ectasia, anisometropia can far exceed that found in the normal patient population resulting in exaggerated spectacle-corrected image size difference (aniseikonia) between the eyes. Most patients can only tolerate up to a 3% magnification difference between the eyes; estimate 1% magnification per diopter of refractive difference. Aniseikonia can present with symptoms of headache, photophobia, reading difficulties, nervousness, nausea, diplopia, distortion, decreased sensory fusion, and/or a decreased perception of space. Anisometropia, in general, can be either refractive or axial but corneal shape change always induces refractive anisometropia. A patient's symptoms are usually proportional to the image size differential. It is not uncommon for diseased, traumatized, or postsurgical cases to experience greater than a 5% image difference. Contact lenses are the treatment of choice as relative spectacle magnification is minimized with correction in the corneal plane.

Irregular astigmatism (also known as higher-order optical aberrations) is an indication for gas-permeable (GP) contact lenses in visual management of corneal diseases, trauma, and following surgery. GP contact lenses should neutralize the image degradation effects of these aberrations.

GENERAL FITTING ISSUES

Corneal Shape Assessment

Keratometry is of limited value in the analysis of corneal cylinder and shape in diseased or injured eyes. The keratometer measures only two points in a given meridian approximately 3 to 3.5 mm apart in the paracentral cornea (1) and assumes that the cornea is spherocylindrical, orthogonal, and symmetrical, a set of conditions which is uncommon in irregular corneas. As overall corneal shape data is critical in determining the best lens design for a given contour, corneal topography is superior to keratometry. Peripheral and midperipheral corneal shape abnormalities are also best imaged with this technology.

Five major post–penetrating keratoplasty (PKP) corneal shapes were described by Waring et al. (2): prolate, oblate, mixed prolate and oblate, asymmetric, and steep to flat (Fig. 28.1; see Color Plate 28.1). Although this organization was

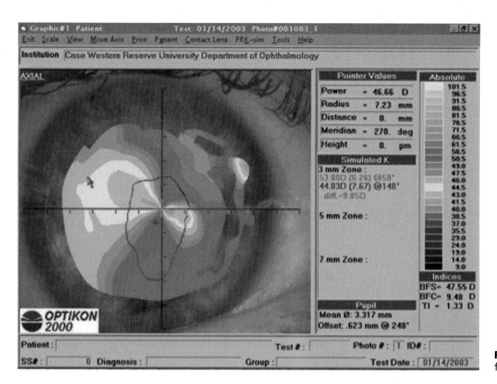

FIG. 28.1. Example of a steep-to-flat graft tilt. (See Color Plate 28.1.)

intended to describe post-PKP eyes, these shape categories apply to many other corneal conditions. The prolate shape is described as that portion of an ellipse steeper in the center and flatter in the periphery (Fig. 28.2; see Color Plate 28.2) (positive shape factor) and is most similar to the asphericity of the normal human cornea. On a standard topographic color map, this corneal shape commonly shows a symmetric red bow tie pattern. Warm colors (red tones) denoting steeper curvatures are seen centrally with cooler colors (blue tones) in the periphery. An oblate shape (negative shape factor) refers to that portion of an ellipse flatter in the center and steeper in the periphery (Fig. 28.3; see Color Plate

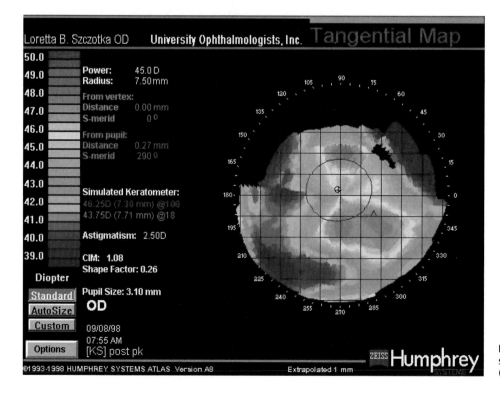

FIG. 28.2. Example of a prolate shape after corneal transplantation. (See Color Plate 28.2.)

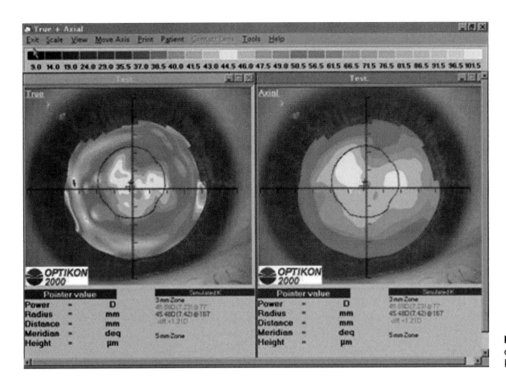

FIG. 28.3. Example of an oblate corneal shape after penetrating keratoplasty. (See Color Plate 28.3.)

28.3). This cornea features regular central astigmatism described as a symmetric blue bow tie pattern, with cooler colors centrally and warmer colors (steeper curvatures) toward the periphery. The mixed prolate and oblate shape is a regular astigmatic pattern with a red bow tie intercepted by a blue bow tie at 90 degrees to each another. In the asymmetric pattern, the principle semi-meridians are not described by any previous shape factor, and the distinguishing feature is two steep hemi-meridians that are not 180 degrees apart. In the steep-to-flat pattern, the steepest hemi-meridian is located 180 degrees from the flattest hemi-meridian of the cornea. Table 28.1 displays the prevalence of each pattern in PKP eyes.

General Contact Lens Considerations

Soft lenses, either spherical or toric, are suitable for patients whose refractive errors are spherical ametropias and/or regular astigmatism. Post–corneal trauma cases, patients suffering from epithelial surface problems, and disorders causing minimal corneal irregularity only occasionally fall into this group. Bandage and piggyback bottom roles of soft lenses,

TABLE 28.1. POST–PENETRATING KERATOPLASTY CORNEAL SHAPES

Prolate shape factor	31.0%
Oblate shape factor	31.0%
Mixed (prolate and oblate)	17.8%
Asymmetric	8.7%
Steep to flat	13.5%

however, are more common and are discussed both below and in Chapter 33.

GP contact lenses should be considered as the initial lens of choice for all patients with irregular corneas. GP lenses offer high oxygen transmissibility, decreased bacterial and protein adherence, optical rigidity, dynamic tear exchange, and ease of care and handling. The thought process supporting GP design selection based on topography follows physical, mechanical, and centration considerations. Modern corneal topography systems have been shown to evaluate a large enough area of the cornea to describe corneal shape and identify steep/flat hemi-meridians in most patients (2). A critical analysis of topography results may limit the number of necessary diagnostic GP lenses (3,4) as preliminary classification of shape allows rational selection of GP lens design. For example, an *in situ* GP contact lens usually assumes the position of least mechanical resistance to center over any steep hemi-meridian (5,6). Topographic analysis identifies such steep meridians and highlights other obstacles to contact lens fitting such as areas of irregularity, and thereby aids qualitative preliminary contact lens design. Table 28.2 lists lens design recommendations for each of the five topographic irregular cornea patterns.

Most eyes benefit visually with spherical rigid lenses. Rarely will residual astigmatism be present over a standard GP, as most astigmatism is refractive. Front surface toric or cylindrical power effect bitoric GPs are, therefore, only occasionally beneficial.

Prolate cornea shapes can be fit with standard lens designs including spherical, aspheric, or bi-aspheric, since this shape resembles normal corneal asphericity. If the degree

TABLE 28.2. LENS TYPES SEGREGATED BY CORNEAL SHAPE

Shape	Suggested GP Designs
Prolate	Aspheric
	Bispheric
	Bitoric
	Keratoconus design
	Standard spherical posterior curves
Oblate	Reverse-geometry lens
	Bitoric
Mixed asymmetric	Bitoric
	Aspheric
	Biaspheric
	Keratoconus design
	Standard spherical posterior curves
Steep to flat	Large-diameter and optic zone
	Standard spherical posterior curves
	Aspheric periphery

GP, rigid gas permeable.

TABLE 28.3. LENS DESIGN BY LOCATION OF STEEP HEMIMERIDIAN

Location of Steep Hemimeridian	Design Options
Inferior	Minus carrier lenticular
	Flatter base curve
	Large diameter/optic zone
Nasal/temporal	Large diameter/optic zone
	Aspheric possible
Superior	Prism ballast
	Nonlenticular or plus carrier lenticular
	High specific gravity

of central corneal steepening is excessive, however, a keratoconic design may be indicated to limit apical bearing and perhaps even vault the steep central apex.

Oblate corneal shapes are best fit with one of the reverse geometry (RG) GP designs. Initially used in orthokeratology, RG lenses have "plateau" shapes, with secondary curves 2 to 5 D steeper than the central posterior curve of the optic zone to better align with the oblate corneal contour. Standard posterior curve designs could result in excessive and stagnant tear layer formation centrally that trap debris, bubbles, and ultimately may decrease corneal integrity if fit steep enough to align with the peripheral cornea. They may also develop excessive edge lift if fit flat enough to align with the central curves. Fitting techniques for oblate corneas are further discussed in the following section on fitting GPs after refractive corneal surgery, and concepts can be applied to the post-PKP oblate eye as well.

If astigmatism, whether corneal shape is prolate or oblate, is minimal, and localized to the central 5 mm of the graft, it may be possible to vault the entire astigmatic area with a standard spherical lens design. If astigmatism is regular and expands into the midperiphery, however, the cornea is classified as "mixed prolate and oblate," and a bitoric lens design is indicated. A bitoric lens design improves lens centration, tolerance, and minimizes excessive impingement in the flat meridian.

GP lenses may not center well with the asymmetry of the steep-to-flat and asymmetric patterns that account for an estimated 22% of post-PKP topographies. As noted earlier, GP lenses tend to center on steep corneal locations. Consideration of design options that limit decentration is, therefore, an important part of the prefitting process. Such contact lens design options are listed in Table 28.3 (which refer to the steep portion of the graft as denoted by topography).

One hybrid design on the US market at the present time is the SoftPerm from Ciba Vision (Duluth, GA). This lens uses a low-Dk rigid GP center (n-butyl-styrene) and a low-Dk hydrogel skirt. This lens should be ideal for many irregular corneas as it offers the comfort and stability of a soft lens with the optics of a rigid lens. Unfortunately, its oxygen transmissibility is so low that secondary corneal edema and occasional neovascularization limit use to very specific circumstances where benefits outweigh risks.

Scleral lenses, and their smaller counterparts, the semiscleral lens designs, can be excellent choices to treat both markedly distorted corneas and ocular surface disease. The learning curve for using these designs is steep, however, and limits popular use.

The list of ocular conditions where contact lenses are potentially beneficial is lengthy. Further, in this chapter we will discuss several major entities and address most of the issues one would consider in the care of patients who have specific disorders. The conditions discussed are ocular trauma, post–refractive surgery, post-PKP, keratoconus, and anterior corneal dystrophies.

OCULAR TRAUMA

Ocular injuries occur everyday throughout the world, ranging from assault, to accident, to intentional self-induced injury. Missiles, electromagnetic energy, chemicals, sharp instruments, and blunt objects all have been implicated in ocular trauma. Contact lenses can be both causal agents of trauma and participate in rehabilitation.

Incidence and Prevalence

Estimates vary from approximately 1 to 2.4 million eye injuries per year in the United States (7–14). Categorization differences and the tendency for regional reporting leads to this wide variance. Many minor injuries are treated in private doctor's offices or go untreated and thus not identified but Klopfer et al. (7) estimated 29.1 cases per 100,000 hospital admissions have ocular trauma as either a primary or secondary diagnosis. This suggests 20,000 to 68,000 cases per year are hospitalized with serious vision-threatening eye injuries. Males were admitted for eye trauma three times more frequently than females, and young adults were involved much more frequently than older adults. Dannenberg et al. (15) (National Eye Trauma System data) found 635 (22%) eye injuries in the work place from a total of 2,939 cases collected from 48 regional eye trauma centers in the United States. They noted that 75% of individuals injured were younger than 40 years of age and 97% were male.

The National Society to Prevent Blindness reported that eye injuries were second only to cataract in producing a visual impairment in the US population (16). Almost 1 million people were estimated to have visual impairments caused at some time by eye injuries as of 1977, with a projected annual incidence of visual impairment estimated to be 40,000 per year. Seven percent had a severe visual impairment; 79% were blind in one eye; 75% of cases reported were under age 65; and 78% were male.

Etiology

The causes of eye injuries span the range from assault to bizarre circumstance. Projectile injuries are prevalent (457 of 635 cases, 71.9%) in the workplace (17). In assault, however, the fist is the most common weapon (15). Sporting injuries are commonly associated with baseball. Home products are the source for most injuries in the United States (16), and eye injuries (80%) are the most common of product-related injuries. Home workshop materials and equipment, home and family maintenance, and personal use items are the three most common product groups associated with eye injuries. Contact lenses (as a personnel use product) are specifically cited as of one of three types of products most frequently linked with eye injuries; metallic injuries and motor vehicle accidents are the other two.

Corneal Topography

Alterations of the ocular surface from penetrating trauma and subsequent repair will have the greatest effect at the site of the injury and immediately adjacent to it. The greater the insult, the greater the effect on the immediate area and the further from the site one can find effects on the ocular surface contour. Tissue loss, long corneal lacerations (greater than two thirds the corneal diameter), and corneoscleral lacerations have the greatest impact on corneal contour. Generally, full thickness punctures and lacerations will have a greater influence on topography than partial thickness injuries (Figs. 28.4 and 28.5). Suturing a wound has a profound effect on topography and, therefore, the importance of good technique in wound repair cannot be overstated (18,19).

Corneal lacerations affect vision more by irregular sur-

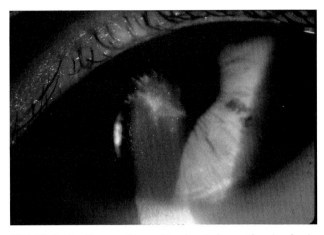

FIG. 28.4. Small corneal laceration located near the visual axis.

faces than scarring (20). Scars from healed peripheral lacerations affect vision via corneal topography alterations that extend into the visual axis. The density of the scar may be important to vision, however, if it is located in the visual axis and if it occludes the vast majority of that space.

The Role of Contact Lenses in Ocular Trauma

Estimates suggest that more than 35 million Americans (and perhaps 80 people million worldwide) wear contact lenses. The clinician must recognize the high prevalence of contact lens wear among the general population when confronted with a head trauma patient and, more specifically, the eye injury patient. Both injuries in general and eye injuries in particular, and contact lens wear, are all quite prevalent in the same young adult age group. Contact lenses may therefore be an unimportant bystander in the injury process or may add to or be the cause of injury.

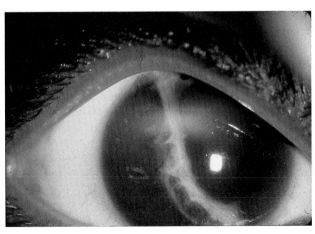

FIG. 28.5. Large, limbus-to-limbus corneal laceration.

Ocular Trauma: Contact Lens Induced

Trauma induced by contact lens wear is common (16). These devices represent the most prevalent source of product subgroup injuries among 15- to 24-year-olds and the second most common subgroup for the 25- to 64-year-old age group. Mishandling of lenses is one common source of injury, leading to abrasion of either cornea or conjunctiva. Corneal abrasions directly or indirectly from material under worn lenses, and chemical burns from certain contact lens disinfection solutions such as hydrogen peroxide and some surfactants used for cleaning, are also common. Most surface abrasions and solution-related injuries, though often painful, are not vision threatening. Soft lens–related superior limbic keratoconjunctivitis linked to thimerosal in lens care solutions, is the only contact lens solution associated toxic trauma demonstrated to cause a permanent loss in vision (requiring a corneal transplant to rehabilitate vision) in the contact lens domain (21). Interestingly, rigid lens–induced corneal lacerations rarely are reported, even though contact lenses have been worn during profound trauma.

Circumstances where a rigid lens appears to offer some protection are documented (22,23). We have observed two such cases. A middle-aged female laboratory assistant splashed a chemical (weak acid) in one of her eyes while at work. She was wearing GP contact lenses at the time and they were still in place when she arrived at the office. After lens removal and irrigation, slit-lamp examination demonstrated peripheral corneal and conjunctival staining but the central corneas (previously under lenses) were without injury or defect. Another case involved a young child shot in the eye with a small disk-shaped projectile. His GP contact lens fractured into five pieces. The cornea demonstrated only mild superficial punctate staining with fluorescein dye despite the impact and lens fragments removed from his conjunctiva and cul-de-sac. One should not construe an inherent protective benefit of wearing contact lenses in all cases. To inform individuals of a protective value from contact lens wear against traumatic injury would overstate what is clinically observed and may give patients a false sense of protection.

Minor conjunctival lacerations have been rarely reported in the literature (22,24). A 19-year-old woman, for one example, suffered a partial thickness corneal laceration from her contact lens as a consequence of a motor vehicle accident (25). This patient eventually recovered 20/30 visual acuity. Either the relative lack of reports of corneal lacerations secondary to contact lens wear represents the rare nature of such complications or many events have gone undetected or unreported. Corneal abrasions associated with contact lens wear are common (22,24,26). Long-term retention of contact lenses, both rigid and soft, rarely have led to more serious scleral erosion (27), migration of the lens into the eyelid substance (28–31), formation of cysts (32), and even migration into the orbit (33,34).

Contact Lenses in Posttrauma Care and Rehabilitation

Although prominent authorities occasionally expound on the dangers and complications of contact lens use, it can be stated paradoxically that these same "dangerous" devices are extremely useful tools to heal corneal and conjunctival wounds and aid in the visual rehabilitation of the patient who has experienced ocular trauma. The role for contact lenses following trauma extends to the management of aphakia, irregular astigmatism, iris/pupil abnormalities, ocular disfigurement, amblyopia management, and wound healing.

Aphakia

Aphakia is a common end-stage result of both penetrating and severe blunt trauma. The crystalline lens can be lost or subluxed, be necessarily removed during the repair process, or become cataractous at some later stage to require removal. The more severe the injury, in general, the more likely aphakia will result in the long run. If ocular anatomy is sufficiently disturbed by injury, an intraocular lens implant will be contraindicated. Aphakia also generates special concern for children in the amblyogenic age range. Combined with a corneal laceration, management of optical correction and treatment of amblyopia in a child can be a major clinical challenge.

Contact lens correction for aphakia following trauma is almost always monocular in nature. The most common rationale for using a contact lens is to manage anisometropia due to unilateral aphakia. The clinician has the option of utilizing either hydrophilic lenses or GP lenses even with concomitant low-to-moderate corneal and refractive astigmatism. Soft lenses are quite effective in these cases for two reasons. The first is initial comfort. Unilateral contact lens wear is more difficult to tolerate physically; therefore, soft lenses offer a comfort advantage. The second reason is ocular protection. All posttrauma patients should be encouraged to wear protective eyewear, but those who have been rendered aphakic or who have lost some or all of their vision in the injured eye should be instructed to wear protective eyewear full-time. If a part of the visual correction is placed in the protective spectacles (low-to-moderate astigmatic correction, residual spherical power that would be cosmetically desirable or necessary to balance anisometropia, and any necessary add), compliance is encouraged.

A GP corneal lens is lens of choice in circumstances where the primary goal of both clinician and patient is to maximize visual rehabilitation. The optical performance advantage of rigid lenses becomes even more evident in the presence of irregular astigmatism. Aphakic soft lenses will only mask small amounts of irregular and regular astigmatism, but GP lenses will accomplish this task in a far superior manner.

The clinical decision to select the class of lens design used should therefore be a joint decision between the patient and the clinician. For example, if the best acuity attained with an aphakic soft lens in an injured eye is 20/200, including any cylinder overcorrection in glasses and is 20/100 with a GP lens, and the uninjured eye was 20/20, then the optical advantages of the GP lens would not likely prove to be a sufficient advantage over the comfort of a soft lens. If acuity improves to 20/40 with a GP lens, then it would have a clear visual advantage over a soft lens, suggesting that adaptation may be worth the patient's effort. Management of comfort issues is as important as vision issues to long-term success.

Irregular Astigmatism

Immediately following injuries of virtually every type, the corneal surface becomes irregular. The permanence, location, and degree of the irregularity are ultimately the important issues. Transient corneal irregular astigmatism occurs with minor chemical burns, abrasions to the cornea, nonpenetrating blunt trauma, and in some lid lacerations. These typically resolve without sequelae. Some corneal abrasions, more severe chemical burns and all penetrating and perforating corneal trauma as well as some perforating scleral injuries result in permanent alteration to corneal shape and irregular astigmatism.

Contact lenses play a very important role in the visual rehabilitative process in the presence of irregular corneal astigmatism post ocular trauma. Thick soft lenses only provide a fair degree of masking of mild degrees of astigmatism. GP lenses, however, both corneal and scleral, remain the gold standard in optical masking of corneal curvature irregularities.

Iris/Pupil Abnormalities and Gross Disfigurement

Blunt nonpenetrating trauma and penetrating trauma of all varieties commonly disturbs large portions of the anterior segment of the eye including the iris. Damage can be divided into two groups: cosmetic disfigurement and optical problems.

Ocular disfigurement has five origins: corneal opacities, mature cataract, and physical damage to the iris, scleral/conjunctiva, and/or eyelid. Iris damage causes disfigurement through nerve damage to the sphincter muscles, dilating the pupil; or through tears of the sphincter muscle and in the body of the iris leaving unintentional iridectomies. Whole sections of iris may be lost or atrophy due to injury or subsequent repair. Many of these can be cosmetically unsightly, particularly to the patient with light-colored irides (such as blue, green, or hazel). The physical appearance can be the major concern of the patient, far outweighing concerns about vision. Contact lenses, principally prosthetic soft lenses, frequently manage many of the cosmetic prob-

lems, especially corneal opacities, iris damage, and mature but inoperable cataract.

Dyscoric pupils and polycoria produce optical problems. Multiple images, glare, and photophobia are likely complaints associated with these defects. A contact lens can serve as a new optical diaphragm creating an artificial pupil. By limiting the light or image to a portion of the visual space or by covering extraneous optical openings, extra images can be muted or removed entirely. Lid and scleral/conjunctival damage is not approachable with prosthetic soft lenses but can, at times, be aided with scleral prostheses.

Amblyopia Management

The role for contact lenses in amblyopia management following trauma is straightforward: a contact lens will provide optimum optics for the eye of an individual in the amblyogenic age range. Children with irregular astigmatism in the amblyopic eye should, therefore, be provided contact lenses that adequately mask surface irregularities (e.g., GP lenses) unless there are extenuating reasons to contraindicate these devices.

Another, somewhat controversial, indication for a contact lens in amblyopia management is to serve as a patch on the normal eye. This approach enhances cosmetic acceptance and is difficult for a young child to learn to remove. Risk is increased, however, in that the better of the two eyes is now being exposed to infection or other lens-related complications. These risks are relatively small, but they are real. An additional concern is that, to date, no study has been published demonstrating the comparative efficacy of opaque or inappropriately high-optical–powered contact lenses in amblyopia management to patching.

Lens Selection and Fitting Procedures

Selection of contact lens types for patients with irregular corneas spans the entire range of available materials and designs. Each has its benefits and shortcomings and will be discussed in turn for each ocular condition, beginning with ocular trauma.

Bandage Lenses

Bandage lenses first assist in the healing process after trauma to provide tectonic support for perforations, punctures, and partial-thickness lacerations, or serve as a protective barrier when corneal gluing is performed. Bandage soft lenses secondarily are the bottoms of piggyback systems, providing additional stability and comfort when rigid corneal lenses are not suitable by themselves.

Bandage soft contact lens fitting after trauma is similar to treatment of recurrent erosions. Many practitioners utilize commonly available disposable hydrogel lenses that are inexpensively replaced after short-term use. Choice of bandage lens involves the selection of water content, thickness, and dehydration characteristics. Thin (<0.07-mm center thickness), high-water-content (usually >50%) hydrogel lenses often are the best option, in attempt to limit movement and leave the underlying epithelium undisturbed (34). Lower-water-content or thicker lenses may move too much to achieve the planned effect. Collagen shields have also been used with some success, to simultaneously protect and lubricate the eye. Bandage lens use is more completely discussed in Chapter 33.

Optical Soft Lenses

Soft lenses should not be overlooked as a refractive option in the posttrauma vision rehabilitation plan. The key positive features of hydrogel lenses are comfort and stability. The almost instantaneous comfort of a soft lens is particularly advantageous in the care of children. The principle disadvantages of soft lenses are their failure to mask much visual astigmatism, regular or irregular, and a tendency to promote vascularization of corneal scars.

Soft lens application to the posttrauma patient has been enhanced with readily available disposable spherical and toric lenses (if the prescription falls within available parameters). This first analysis of the soft lens on an injured eye is important because unexpected mechanical and optical results are often observed. The authors' preference is to use moderately thick, medium-water-content lenses (disposable or conventional) that afford moderate gas transmissibility, dimensional stability, slightly better optics than thin lenses, and good handling characteristics. Complete corneal coverage and some blink dependent movement are required as in other soft lens fitting paradigms.

Soft toric lens designs often are particularly frustrating after trauma. The unique nature of eye trauma leads to unpredictable soft toric lens behavior, and unpredictable behavior usually leads to an unsatisfactory mechanical and, most importantly, visual outcome.

Patients should be monitored on a regular basis if corneal scarring is present. This is particularly important for patients with corneoscleral lacerations and those with iris material entrapped in wound sites as these patients can develop new blood vessels racing up their corneal scars. At times these vessels may branch out and/or leak lipids into clear cornea to cause further opacity.

Spherical Rigid Lenses

Spherical GP contact lenses are the mainstay of contact lens use for patients with corneal lacerations and represent the visual benchmark to which all other approaches will typically be compared. GP corneal lenses offer the greatest benefit ratio for eyes with irregular astigmatism, aphakia, mild-to-moderate corneal astigmatism, and reasonably intact irides/pupils. The challenge is to design a lens that is comfort-

able, mechanically behaves in predictable manner, is physiologically well-tolerated by the damaged tissues, and also remains in place.

The art of our science is surely tested with this group of patients. There are no firmly established rules and therefore decisions are, to a great extent, empirical. The following guidelines are used by the authors in making fitting decisions.

Overall diameters between 9.0 and 11 mm are the most commonly used, with 9.5 mm having the greatest frequency, as large overall diameters enhance lens stability and allow optics to cover irregular and large pupils.

Lenses should be fit with base curves steeper than usual to account for the elevation of the corneal scar. Fluorescein patterns will typically look irregular and often are difficult to interpret, but the goal is to avoid harsh bearing on the scar. Fluorescein pooling adjacent to the scar is the rule, but one should attempt to minimize chronic bubbles (leading to dimple veil stain) within the pool. Both excessive edge bearing and gaping should be minimized while maintaining both good edge lift and tear exchange.

Lens position ideally should be central to superior central, although perfect centration is uncommon. The lens will generally center about the highest landmark unless that landmark is in the far corneal periphery (Fig. 28.6). If a GP lens cannot center, it slides "downhill" from the high point in the opposite direction. Approach the concept of centration from the perspective of function, not beauty. Good centration delivers the optics of the lens to the visual space and avoids harsh limbal impact. If a lens decenters, the question of whether the optical zone covers the pupillary space should arise. If the optical zone bisects the pupil, optical zone and overall diameter should be increased. If the lens behaves erratically, lens overall diameter should be

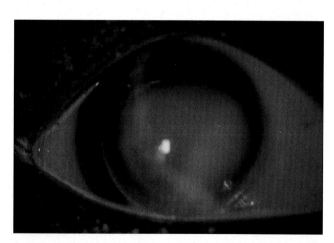

FIG. 28.6. Fluorescein pattern of a rigid corneal lens on the same eye shown in Fig. 28.5. Note the relatively gentle bearing of the lens over the scarred region. This feature tends to result in a steep-looking fit. Attention should be placed also on the peripheral clearance of the lens edge and tear exchange.

increased initially. Adjustments of the base curve, optic zone and peripheral curves may also prove helpful.

Toric Rigid and Soft Toric Lenses

Toric lenses, both rigid and soft, are used in managing significant astigmatism. GP toric lenses are best suited for patients with large amounts of "global" corneal astigmatism, principally regular. The term "global" refers to the predominance of the astigmatism over the corneal surface (Fig. 28.7; see Color Plate 28.7). Astigmatism can also cover a relatively small area of the corneal surface, termed "local" astigmatism (Fig. 28.8; see Color Plate 28.8). Corneal topography displays these corneal features well. A spherical or aspheric base curve GP will often better treat area(s) of local astigmatism than a toric base curve design.

Combination (Hybrid) Designs

Hybrid lenses combine the comfort and centering capabilities associated with silicone and hydrogel lenses with the visual acuity offered by a rigid lens (36). The SoftPerm Lens (Ciba Vision) is made of a low-Dk styrene core surrounded by a hydrophilic skirt. This design is an extremely attractive concept that, unfortunately, has problems leading to limited usefulness. The design is attractive because it offers the overall diameter and supple edges, and hence tolerance, of a soft lens with the optics of a rigid lens. Problems result from limited parameter selection, unpredictable fitting characteristics (often leaving a lens fitting very tightly), poor oxygen transmission, limited masking of astigmatism, and frequent

ripping or splitting of the soft lens skirt near the rigid lens center. At present, therefore, this design should be considered one of last resort.

Piggyback Fitting

Piggyback lens systems have value from four perspectives: (a) providing comfort, (b) improving rigid lens stability and predictability, (c) bandage lens characteristics, and (d) in circumstances where both improved cosmesis and rigid lens optics are needed.

Except in cases where a prosthetic soft lens is needed, a piggyback system should be considered after a trial of a rigid corneal lens alone. Experience with GP lenses will help define the soft lens role and the choice of soft lens will be guided by its purpose.

When the soft lens cushions lens-cornea contact to improve tolerance, a thin "membrane" lens is often most useful. Possible "membranes" include most disposables soft lenses. In cases where the soft lens is being used to affect lens behavior on the eye, thicker, conventional lenses are often superior. Patients should be counseled on both the fairly high damage rate of soft lenses and to use soft lens solutions with both lenses. Silicone hydrogel lenses may be ideal piggyback bottom lenses because of their high Dk values and good handling characteristics.

Prosthetics

Corneal opacities and/or iris irregularities are both common sequelae of ocular injury. When these are unsightly or affect

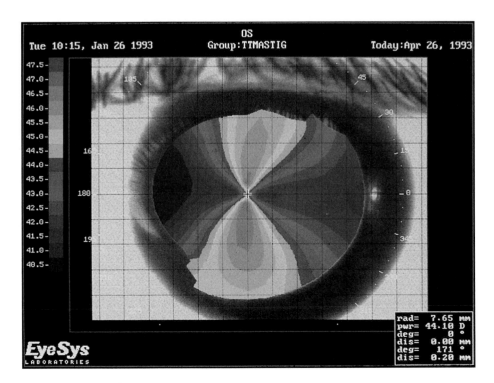

FIG. 28.7. Global astigmatism. With-the-rule astigmatism topographic pattern involving virtually the entire mappable surface. (See Color Plate 28.7.)

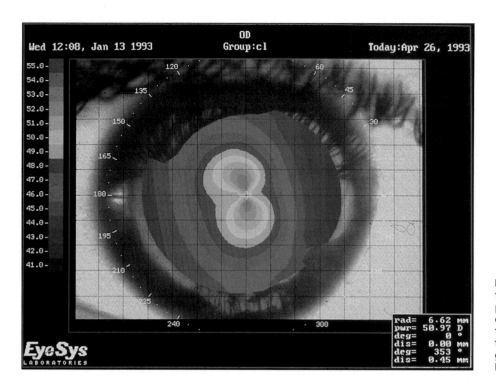

FIG. 28.8. Focal astigmatism. With-the-rule astigmatism topographic pattern primarily involving a 4-mm central zone. Note the lower amplitude oval-shaped global astigmatism pattern by observing just the green and blue colors. (See Color Plate 28.8.)

function, a prosthetic soft lens can be used, either with optics or in combination with a rigid lens. The two most common reasons to use a prosthetic soft lens are management of iris-related optical problems (such as photophobia or multiple images through multiple iris apertures) and cosmetic enhancement of a disfigured eye. Prosthetic hydrogel lenses can be obtained with spherical or astigmatic powers when indicated, or a plano prosthetic lens may be used as the soft lens base of a piggyback system.

POST–PENETRATING KERATOPLASTY

Penetrating keratoplasty (PKP) is performed for optical, tectonic, therapeutic, and cosmetic indications. By far the most common indication for keratoplasty is for optical purposes. Some of the more common conditions that benefit from full thickness corneal transplantation include: (a) aphakic or pseudophakic bullous keratopathy (the most common indication for corneal grafting in the United States); (b) Fuchs' endothelial dystrophy; (c) keratoconus; (d) previous graft failure; (e) interstitial keratitis or herpes keratitis; and (f) corneal stromal dystrophies.

Tectonic procedures refer to grafting for reparative or structural purposes such as in marginal thinning at the corneal limbus. Therapeutic procedures are a form of therapy to remove actively diseased tissues. Cosmetic procedures remove an unsightly corneal opacity for cosmetic purposes only.

Modern PKP has a very high rate of graft survival owing to advances in corneal preservation techniques, surgical

techniques, and postoperative medications, with over 90% of avascular grafts remaining clear (37), but graft rejection and failure were previously common complications. Common current complications include both regular and irregular postoperative astigmatism and anisometropia limiting successful spectacle wear. Contact lenses remain the best possible optical correction in many cases.

Surgical Management of Refractive Error

Regardless of differences in suturing and grafting techniques among corneal surgeons, postoperative astigmatism remains a major PKP complication today, averaging 4 to 5 D per eye (37,38). Management of refractive error begins with donor-recipient trephination techniques, optimal suture placement, and suture removal. Refractive surgical techniques can limit corneal cylinder as well decreasing postoperative spherical ametropia. Contact lens fitting is recommended once other techniques have been exhausted or are contraindicated.

A variety of suturing techniques are described in the literature. The most common techniques are single or double running sutures, combination interrupted and running sutures, and interrupted sutures alone. The combination of interrupted and one running suture technique is probably the best technique to allow for control of postoperative astigmatism. Suture removal is best determined with both corneal topography and manifest refraction (Fig. 28.9; see Color Plate 28.9) (39). Interrupted sutures can be removed as soon as 3 months postsurgically if only interrupted sutures are used, or as early as 1 month postoperatively if

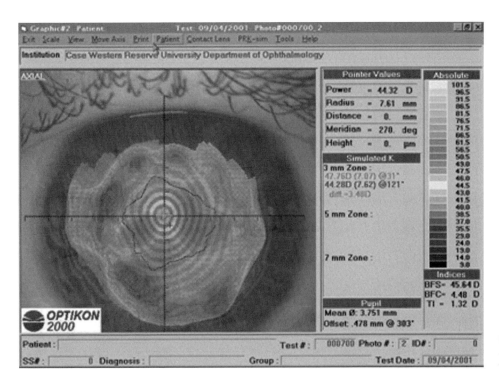

FIG. 28.9. Example of tight sutures at 8 o'clock causing localized steepening. (See Color Plate 28.9.)

a continuous running suture has also been placed. Most topographic changes occur within 3 to 5 weeks after suture removal, a recommended time interval after individual suture removal to determine the resultant corneal topography (39).

Once suture removal has been exhausted, refractive surgical techniques may be attempted in cases of high astigmatism or ametropia. Common surgical techniques for reduction of astigmatism include relaxing incisions, compression sutures, or laser photoablation procedures. Relaxing nearly full corneal thickness arcuate incisions placed along the steep meridian, usually central to the graft-host interface, or less commonly within the graft-host interface, flatten the steep meridian. This procedure also steepens the flatter meridians in an equal amount, to result in a negligible spherical dioptric change. Paired relaxing incisions usually correct 4 to 5 D of postkeratoplasty astigmatism but may correct up to 10 D (40). Although a relatively popular and simple technique for an experienced corneal surgeon, its major disadvantage remains significant undercorrection or overcorrection as results do not faithfully follow any known nomogram. Compression sutures compliment relaxing incisions. Such sutures are placed on either side of the graft-host interface 90 degrees away from the relaxing incision and augment by further steepening the flat meridian.

Laser-assisted *in situ* keratomileusis (LASIK) is becoming a more accepted option for the correction of both regular astigmatism and anisometropia after PKP, and is often considered for contact lens–intolerant patients. Considerable reduction of spherical equivalent and cylindrical refractive errors is achieved with very few, if any, complications.

Spherical equivalents reduced from a range of almost −8.00 to −0.75 D, and astigmatism decreased from approximately 6.5 D to under 2 D, in several series (41–43). Best-corrected visual acuity most often remains unchanged, but has been reported to improve in 37% of eyes in one study (42). Correction of irregular astigmatism by LASIK remains challenging and treated under investigational procedures at the current time (44). One study, using topographically guided ablation, was able to increase regularity in 66% of PKP eyes, allowing average uncorrected vision to improve from 20/200 to 20/50 (45).

The wedge resection technique is reserved for correction of high post-PKP cylinder. A full-thickness crescentric incision around 25% of the graft circumference is made, an angled wedge of tissue is removed, and then the wound is sutured. This technique steepens the flatter meridian approximately twice as much as it flattens the steep meridian; therefore, the net effect is a slight increase in myopia. Although wedge resections are capable of correcting up to 20 D of astigmatism, it is rarely used because multiple sutures are required (which can induce significant corneal irregularity with longer postoperative rehabilitation).

Contact Lens Management of Refractive Error

Contact lenses are an accepted treatment of residual ametropia after PKP (46), with success rates as high as 84% in the literature (47,48). Between 31% and 56% of patients who undergo PKP to treat keratoconus, for example, return to contact lens wear after surgery (49,50). The greatest percentages of contact lens failures occur secondary to allograft rejection, contact lens intolerance, or excessively difficult contact lens fittings leading to abandonment of the fit by the practitioner. Allograft rejections are usually not attributed to the use of the contact lenses, but such episodes may prevent future contact lens wear (50,51).

Contact lens wear after PKP has not been shown to induce significant long-term graft complications. No difference was found in graft endothelial cell density three years after fitting when post-PKP patients who became contact lens wearers were compared to those who did not (52). Both polymegethism and pleomorphism are still expected in the contact lens–wearing group, an effect likely attributable to corneal hypoxia. Long-term graft stability after contact lens wear has been documented; corneal curvatures derived from topography as well as corneal symmetry remained stable after GP fitting (53–55). Well-centered GP lenses may increase regularity and decrease asymmetry in grafts (38,56), suggesting a beneficial "splint" or mold effect. This corneal molding effect has been attributed to post-PKP stromal wound healing. Long-term prospective studies of fitting GP lenses after surgery to intentionally induce regularity have been postulated but have not been performed.

Examination of the Patient (Specific to Post-PKP Patients)

Anatomical and Neurologic Findings

Reduced corneal sensitivity secondary to surgically induced denervation after PKP is a major factor in contact lens fitting and may be a mixed blessing, allowing the patient to adjust rapidly to lenses; but also encouraging overwear and diminishing early awareness of complications. Since lid margins remain sensitive, some aspects of lens awareness and adaptation remain typical of the normal contact lens patient.

Post-PKP patients often have concurrent preexisting external ocular conditions such as keratitis sicca or tear insufficiency, blepharitis, insufficient lid apposition and, in rare cases, cicatricial disease. These prefitting complications require careful management and monitoring during the prefitting and postfitting phases.

Since initial contact lens management can begin as early as 3 months postoperatively, with sutures present, all sutures should be examined and documented prior to initiating contact lens fitting. Most surgeons believe that remaining sutures are not a contraindication to contact lens fitting unless suture removal is soon planned. Contact lenses can be safely fit over sutures as long as they are completely covered by epithelium, and all knots are buried.

Lens Selection and Fitting Procedures

Bandage Lenses

Bandage soft lenses are often indicated in the immediate postoperative period to treat persistent epithelial defects

(>7 days) and delayed wound healing, epithelial filaments, or extreme height discrepancies at the host-graft junction inducing poor healing (35,57). Extended-wear complications such as microbial ulcers, and "tight lens syndromes" are the most serious complications. Silicone hydrogel lenses have been suggested as alternative bandage lenses to minimize hypoxia (58).

Soft Lenses

The use of soft contact lenses for vision should be limited after PKP (63). Hydrophilic contact lenses do not effectively correct astigmatism, and especially if used for extended wear, have been thought to cause corneal neovascularization and possible subsequent rejection (35,59,60). The transplanted central cornea is normally an avascular, immunologically privileged area. Host immune mechanisms fail to "see" this tissue. Graft vascularization can compromise immune privilege.

Soft lenses also have increased infection rates compared to GPs, more so in extended wear (61). Since the donor cornea of the post-PKP patient is desensitized, the patient may not detect early symptoms of this and other corneal complications. The soft lens–wearing post-PKP patient should, therefore, be monitored closely and extended wear for refractive purposes is contraindicated.

High-Dk silicone hydrogel lenses may be beneficial if the spherical contact lens power is a satisfactory visual alternative; toric lenses are not available in these polymers at the current time.

Gas-permeable Lenses

If the steepest area of the graft is inferior, several design options can be incorporated in GP lenses proactively to attempt lid attachment and alignment along the flatter superior cornea. These include minus carrier lenticular, or flatter posterior lens curvature. If the lens continues to decenter inferiorly, then design options to decrease the mass of the GP lens may promote centration.

If the steep area of the graft is nasal or temporal, then a decentered lens position is often unavoidable. As in the posttraumatic eye, the fitting philosophy should be guided at stabilizing lens movement and providing sufficient pupil coverage to minimize glare. Large overall and optic zone diameters may aide in centration and pupillary coverage. Aspheric lenses have been suggested to improve centration; if an aspheric lens remains decentered, however, visual acuity will diminish secondary to eccentric viewing through the aspheric periphery. The Boston Envision lens is a bi-aspheric lens that has been reported successful in a series of post-PKP eyes (62). The lens design incorporates an elliptical optic zone followed by a hyperbolic peripheral curve.

If the steepest area of the graft is superior, it may be difficult to clear the superior steep zone without causing inferior lens impingement. Lens design options may be incorporated to promote improved centration, however, including: prism ballast, a high specific gravity lens, and/or nonlenticular design which all can increase the mass of a lens.

Posterior lens curvature selection follows standard GP fitting philosophies once the corneal shape has been determined. Overall lens diameters are typically large (9.2 to 11.0 mm), usually to incorporate optic zones wider than the graft itself (which typically measures 7.0 to 8.5 mm in diameter) (46,63). Peripheral curve systems depend on the chosen design, but they should remain flat enough in the periphery to promote good tear exchange, yet snug enough to promote centration and align along the host corneal periphery (63). Exact parameters are best determined during diagnostic fitting using detailed peripheral curve data. Optical power must be determined by spherocylindrical overrefraction with the best-fit diagnostic lens on the eye.

Contact lens software modules are available with most modern corneal topography systems. Although the contact lens modules have been tested on normal eyes with good results, the tear layer and resultant lens power calculations have not been designed for use with irregular corneal surfaces (64). The contact lens modules are, therefore, most useful as a qualitative analysis of corneal topography rather than to provide lens selection. Although some manufacturers promote their topography software to fit irregular corneas, no peer-reviewed literature exists that supports the success of such programs for this purpose. Topography maps, however, may be used quantitatively for: (a) analysis of overall corneal astigmatism, (b) selection the optical zone size required to vault the greatest portion of irregularity, and (c) curvature data in the mid-to-far periphery to help choose peripheral curve systems.

Combination (Hybrid) Designs

The SoftPerm lens should be used with special caution after PKP due to the potential for inflammation from entrapped tear film debris, neovascularization from its low oxygen permeability and poor tear exchange, or to the possibility of a "steep lens syndrome" characterized by a bound lens leading to subsequent keratoconjunctivitis. The fitting technique involves selecting a base curve slightly steeper than the mean keratometric curvature and analyzing the resultant high molecular weight fluorescein pattern (65). Steepening a SoftPerm base curve is said to contraintuitively increase movement, as it reduces lens flexure (36).

Piggyback Fitting

Piggyback systems should also be used with caution in post-PKP patients because of anticipated decreased oxygen supply leading to neovascularization, which can induce rejection. Piggyback systems are indicated in cases of persistent epithelial staining secondary to mechanical trauma during GP wear or for the rigid lens intolerance patient. Because of anticipated increased oxygen supply, new silicone hydrogels may prove very beneficial in the bottom lens role when long-term management with this system is anticipated.

Scleral Lenses

Scleral contact lenses, originally manufactured from non–oxygen-permeable polymethylmethacrylate (PMMA), have essentially disappeared from use. Their predominant complications were corneal hypoxia leading to conjunctival injection, corneal edema and neovascularization. Recently, scleral lenses have been redesigned in high-Dk GP materials with a series of successful therapeutic refits reported (66). Indications for GP scleral lenses for visual rehabilitation include significant corneal irregularity necessitating GP vision correction concomitant with corneal surfaces that cannot tolerate the friction of a corneal lens, or whose anterior segment topography does not allow adequate corneal lens centration or stability (see Chapter 34).

Semiscleral and limbus-to-limbus GP lens designs are also now available form a variety of manufacturers. The Macrolens (C&H Labs, Dallas, TX) and the Dyna Intralimbal Lens (Lens Dynamics, Golden, CO) are two such designs that have been successful in the authors' experiences. They can be manufactured in almost any GP material, including high-Dk polymers, and at times are the only lens option that may be successful for some irregular corneas.

Postfitting Management

The contact lens clinician must not take any eye complaints lightly, and this is especially true with the post-PKP patient. All episodes of decreased vision, photophobia, pain, and conjunctival redness, which are symptoms of many contact lens problems like refractive change and relatively benign abrasion as well as graft rejection or corneal infection, should be evaluated promptly.

Four types of corneal graft rejection have been recognized: epithelial rejection, subepithelial infiltrates, stromal rejection, and endothelial rejection (57). Epithelial rejection is characterized by the appearance of an elevated epithelial rejection line that stains with fluorescein which represents destruction of donor epithelial cells. Stromal rejections usually present as a sudden onset of peripheral full thickness haze and circumcorneal injection in a previously clear graft. Subepithelial infiltrates randomly distributed immediately below Bowman's layer in the donor tissue can occur in either or both epithelial or stromal rejection. Endothelial rejection presents as a "Khoudadoust" line advancing across the posterior cornea over a period of a few days; full-thickness corneal stromal edema is left in its wake (57). Pigmented keratic precipitates are also often present in endothelial rejection. Diffuse endothelial rejection may occur as well. Graft failure occurs as well, without accompanying inflammation, due to simple compromise to the graft endothelium through aging and other etiologies (e.g., herpetic keratitis).

Patients may first present to the contact lens practitioner because of recent onset of contact lens intolerance, decreased visual acuity, or ocular pain and redness, which the patient attributes to contact lens wear. The underlying condition may be contact lens related, or a surgical complication including a broken suture, a secondary effect of the ophthalmic medications, or an early graft rejection. It is surprising how many patients are unaware of remaining sutures. Informing the patient that sutures are still present is critical so that possible suture breakage may be detected early. Loose sutures should be promptly removed to avoid a source of infection and a stimulus to neovascularization and/or infection and secondary rejection.

Patients should be professionally monitored every 4 to 6 months (for the first year) after contact lens fitting because many early complications of both lens wear and corneal surgery may be asymptomatic due to reduced corneal sensitivity. Among the possible contact lens–induced complications, the most often encountered include chronic epithelial staining, epithelial defects, lens adherence, epithelial or stromal edema, deposits, and solution sensitivity. However, if appropriately managed, the patient should enjoy many years of successful contact lens wear.

POSTREFRACTIVE SURGERY

Fitting contact lenses to the refractive surgery patient who presents with complications or a poor visual result postoperatively can be challenging due to the physical attributes of the cornea as well as the psychological attributes of the patient. Although the primary purpose of cosmetic refractive surgery is to eliminate the requirement of spectacle or contact lens wear, a patient may be encouraged to seek contact lens correction to manage unanticipated postoperative overcorrections or under corrections or irregular astigmatism.

Contact lens considerations following myopic (and astigmatic) refractive procedures vary depending on the major corneal surface tissue alterations desired and achieved. Tissue removal (keratectomy) procedures such as photorefractive keratectomy (PRK), automated lamellar keratoplasty (ALK), LASIK, and laser subepithelial keratomileusis (LASEK) should be differentiated from surface incisional procedures such as radial keratotomy (RK) and astigmatic keratotomy (AK). Comprehension of respective corneal contour changes are critical to understanding the corneal topography and secondary optical complications which may necessitate the use of spectacle or contact lens correction. Lastly, tissue addition procedures exist such as epikeratoplasty and intrastromal corneal rings. Epikeratoplasty is rarely performed today due to optical problems (67). Intrastromal corneal rings (Intacs) are a newer procedure origi-

nally approved but now rarely used for myopia, yet gaining favor as an experimental procedure in the correction of keratoconus (68). Contact lens fittings after tissue addition procedures are more rare than the procedures themselves, and will not be covered here.

Incisional Procedures

A diamond knife is used to make partial corneal thickness incisions in RK and AK that flatten the corneal curvature in all meridians or in a selected meridian, respectively. Although these procedures are now rarely performed as standalone procedures for myopia and astigmatism, they are still used in conjunction with other refractive and surgical techniques. A large percentage of patients presenting for contact lens correction after refractive surgery in our practices are those that had RK when it was popularized in the early 1980s. Many patients, most of whom are now presbyopic or in the early stages of cataract, are now symptomatic from overcorrections and hyperopic drifts since their original procedure. The Prospective Evaluation of Radial Keratotomy (PERK) study reported that 58% of patients felt some type of optical correction was required 10 years postoperatively with 23% of patients being overcorrected (induced hyperopia greater than 1 D) and 17% undercorrected (residual myopia greater than 1 D) (69). Conditions and complications that may benefit from contact lens use postincisional refractive surgery are listed in Table 28.4.

Persistent visual fluctuation may occur (due to diurnal changes in stromal hydration) throughout the day (70). Glare can be induced by incisions extending into the visual axis, poor wound healing, or irregular astigmatism. Irregular astigmatism can result from an eccentric optical zone, uneven healing, unintentional incisions across the visual axis, microperforations or macroperforations, or intersecting radial and tangential incisions (71). Crossing corneal incisions produce excessive corneal flattening resulting in focal irregularity. Although a patient with intersecting incisions benefits with significantly improved visual acuity after GP fitting, the fitting is commonly challenging because of lens centration difficulties caused by elevated pivot points created at the intersecting sites (72).

TABLE 28.4. COMPLICATIONS OF INCISIONAL PROCEDURES TREATED WITH CONTACT LENSES

Overcorrection
Undercorrection
Anisometropia with possible secondary aniseikonia
Residual and induced astigmatism
Irregular astigmatism
Visual fluctuation
Glare
Monocular diplopia

Tissue-Removal Procedures

The excimer laser ablates Bowman's layer and the anterior corneal stroma in PRK. Alternatively, an initial lamellar keratotomy is performed with a mechanically driven microkeratome creating a hinged corneal flap 160 or 200 μm deep, and folded on itself either nasally or superiorly, in both ALK and LASIK. A secondary stromal lenticula is mechanically removed in ALK while the excimer laser produces the refractive cut in the stromal bed in LASIK, and then the corneal cap is replaced. LASEK purportedly combines the advantages of LASIK and PRK. Like LASIK, it employs a "flap" and consequently has the advantages of faster visual recovery, less postoperative pain, reduced stromal haze, and faster epithelial healing than PRK. Conversely, like PRK, because the procedure is performed on the anterior cornea, there are virtually no flap- or interface-related complications per se (73). After PRK, LASIK, LASEK, or ALK, conditions that may benefit from contact lens use are far fewer than after RK/AK (see Table 28.5).

Irregular astigmatism after PRK is either a result of a decentered ablation, persistent central islands, or rarely corneal stromal haze. Stromal haze is less frequent after LASIK and LASEK than after PRK. Irregular astigmatism is most often secondary to cap misalignment or loss, epithelial ingrowth, or corneal perforation improper assembly of the microkeratome after LASIK.

Physiologic Factors Affecting Contact Lens Fitting

Post-RK corneas suffer from epithelial, stromal, and endothelial changes. Physiologic changes include uneven tear film due to an irregular corneal surface, transient basement membrane changes (74), spontaneous epithelial erosions (75), misdirected epithelial regeneration, loss of sensory innervation from severed corneal nerves, impaired wound healing after epithelial insult, and stromal hypercellularity. Scanning electron microscopy suggests alteration and ridges in the portions of Descemet's membrane underlying the stromal incisions and, therefore, possible mild endothelial cell damage (76). No known corneal cellular changes have been yet found secondary to the laser energy with photoablative procedures. Improvements in the shape and size of the cells of the endothelium were observed, however, perhaps an effect of contact lens discontinuation.

The additional effect of contact lens wear may add stress

TABLE 28.5. COMPLICATIONS OF TISSUE REMOVAL PROCEDURES TREATED WITH CONTACT LENSES

Undercorrection
Overcorrection
Residual and induced regular astigmatism
Irregular astigmatism

to an already compromised cornea, so the authors suggest prescription of GP lenses with moderate-to-high oxygen transmissibility (Dk >40 barrers) to enhance oxygen transmissibility (Dk/t) (77).

Lens Selection and Fitting Procedures

Bandage Lenses

Bandage contact lenses are widely prescribed immediately postoperative in PRK to protect loosely adhered healing epithelium. The epithelium should be completely intact (about 3 days postoperative) before the bandage lens is removed (78,79). Thin, mid to high-water-content lenses are successful in this role because of their limited movement on the eye (which helps prevent mechanical trauma to protect immature epithelium). Patients require supervision; postoperative topical acidic medications can dehydrate a lens causing a "steep lens syndrome." Ciba Vision Ophthalmics intentionally designed their ProTek Lens (ionic hydrogel vifilcon A of 55% water content) as a post-PRK bandage. This lens has an ultrathin center and base curves of 8.9 or 9.2 mm to conform to the PRK contour. Standard extended wear disposable lenses have also been used with good results, although they have not been specifically approved by the US Food and Drug Administration (FDA) for therapeutic purposes (80,81).

Soft Lenses

Since most patients proceeding to elective refractive surgery have been prescreened for concurrent external ocular diseases, they should have no specific contraindications to contact lens wear. Hydrophilic contact lenses are often requested by patients to correct any residual postoperative refractive error, especially in cases of presurgical GP lens intolerance. The desire to fit soft lenses as the initial lens of choice should be discouraged after RK, however, as hypoxia from their chronic use has been reported to lead to neovascularization along the incision lines in up 50% of patients (75,82–84). Lens-induced hypoxia concerns extend to both hybrid designs (SoftPerm) and low-Dk piggyback lenses. Cosmetic use of soft lenses to correct residual ametropias after LASIK is more accepted than after RK since there are only superficial incisions paracentrally and corneal neovascularization has not been reported.

Soft lens use can be considered after refractive surgery for occasional wear, and for problem solving such as managing epithelial erosions or masking glare with opaque iris tints (85). For the patient with residual, regular astigmatism, soft toric lenses are often considered but can be difficult to fit because of poor lens back–surface-to-cornea fitting relationships and subsequent rotational instability and unpredictable lens rotation.

Since the entire central cornea has flattened postoperatively with RK, a good rule of thumb is to flatten the base curve radius from the preoperative value if using standard hydrogel lenses. Larger-overall-diameter lenses (>15 mm) should be considered in an attempt to vault the corneal-scleral junction and decrease limbal compression, which can be a stimulus to neovascularization. As the central cornea flattens more than the periphery, relative peripheral corneal steepening occurs, significantly altering expected lens-to-cornea fitting relationships (72,86). The relative steepening of the corneal contour averages 2.8 ± 2.2 D of increasing dioptric power from the center to the periphery. At least 79% of corneas have oblate corneal shapes after RK.

Knowledge of the early healing response is important in fitting contact lenses after PRK because it gives the contact lens fitter a good indication of the integrity of the patient's epithelium and stroma. Classification into one of the three post-PRK identified healing responses is beneficial because it may encourage or contraindicate future contact lens wear, or it may dictate the selection of postoperative lens alternatives. For example, the Type I healing response (observed in 95% of patients), is characterized by a slight hyperopic refraction at approximately 30 days postoperatively, with the development of progressive corneal haze and regression towards emmetropia in the next few months (78). Normal-thickness epithelial regeneration occurs after approximately 6 months, and soft or rigid contact lens wear can be initiated by 9 months.

Early therapeutic use of hydrogel lenses may be beneficial for a Type II healer, which presents in only 2% to 3% of cases. The Type II response, characterized by inadequate healing, presents with suppressed inflammation (no stromal haze), excessive corneal flattening, and secondary hyperopia at 1 to 3 months. Contact lens wear may be encouraged early in the healing phase to purposefully stimulate a mild inflammatory reaction through mild corneal irritation. Some advocate the use of an extended-wear soft contact lens worn for up to 3 months in an attempt to initiate healing and accelerate the desired correction (78).

Early use of contact lenses is contraindicated in the Type III "aggressive" healing response, detected in 1% to 3% of patients (78). The Type III healing response usually presents at 1 to 3 months with significant undercorrection and marked corneal haze. Among other causes, excessive corneal irritation (including contact lens wear) has been suggested as a potentiator of this effect. A patient with a Type III healing response may seek early contact lens correction for residual myopia; however, the additional irritation may stimulate a further regression of the refractive effect. All contact lens wear should, therefore, be postponed until, at minimum, 2 years after surgery in a Type III healer.

The healing response is not as important in LASIK as in PRK. No specific post-LASIK stromal healing types have been identified, although there may be a slight tendency of a myopic drift (<1 D) in some highly myopic patients without haze formation ("regression without haze"). Refractions

are relatively stable within 2 weeks of LASIK and a contact lens can be fit as soon as 3 weeks postoperative for patients who decline surgical enhancement to treat residual ametropia.

The only FDA-approved soft lens in the United States for the correction of ametropia following refractive surgery is the Flexlens Harrison Post Refractive Lens (Excel). This lens is indicated for patients whose corneal topography has been altered following RK, PRK, LASIK, and other refractive procedures that produce oblate corneal shapes. The lens functions like a reverse-geometry GP in that its central optical portion is flatter than its midperiphery.

Gas-permeable Lenses

The lens of choice for irregular astigmatism remains an GP because of material rigidity, potential high oxygen transmissibility, removal of corneal by-products and tear debris through efficient tear exchange, and absorption of diurnal visual fluctuations (for post-RK patients) through the formation of a posterior lens tear pool. The most comfortable GP fit occurs when the lens rests in a slightly superior position and receives support from the upper lid. After procedures that create oblate corneal shapes, the contact lens vaults the flatter central cornea resulting in fluorescein pooling and an optically plus-powered lacrimal lens (Fig. 28.10; see Color Plate 28.10). Additional minus power must therefore be provided in the GP lens, ironically resulting in a lens power similar to the patient's preoperative power. Some patients wear the same GP contact lens postoperatively as they did preoperatively.

Traditional GP concepts for base curve, overall diameter, and peripheral curve selection are only rarely appropriate for postoperative oblate corneal shapes (after RK, or myopic PRK, ALK, LASIK, or LASEK). Initial GP base curve selection in these cases varies depending on the method of corneal curvature assessment: preoperative keratometry, postoperative keratometry, or postoperative topography. Some fitters advocate preoperative keratometry readings (82).

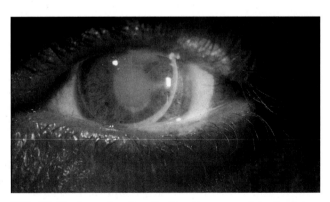

FIG. 28.10. Example of optically plus-powered lacrimal lens (formed beneath an rigid gas-permeable lens after radial keratotomy). (See Color Plate 28.10.)

Keratometry of the unoperated fellow eye is, therefore, an option if preoperative measurements are not available. Initial trial base curve is selected 0.5 to 1.0 D flatter than the flat preoperative keratometry "K" and the fit is then titrated according to clinical observation. Others report that empirical lens fitting based upon the flat postoperative keratometry is successful, although the base curves of the final GP lenses are usually steeper than the postoperative flat "K." (87). Due to the disproportionate amount of central corneal flattening and relative peripheral steepening (compared to an unoperated eye), a contact lens fit near the average or flat central postoperative "K" will usually be unacceptably flat and unstable in our experience, due to little or no midperipheral bearing. The base curve radius should therefore be, at minimum, 1.0 to 1.5 D steeper than the postoperative flat "K." This lens is then titrated to achieve the goal of midperipheral corneal alignment and central pooling. Ward also suggested an initial base curve selection steeper than the mean postoperative keratometric power (approximately 2.1 D) (88).

Peripheral keratometry readings (87,88) can be used to estimate the midperipheral topography (approximately 3 mm from corneal apex). Four targets placed 4 mm from the edge of the keratometer viewing port to serve as fixation points. As the patient changes fixation from one to the other, the clinician can respectively measure nasal, temporal, superior, and inferior corneal mid-peripheral keratometry. Campbell and Caroline (88) suggest the selection of an initial base curve should be equal to the temporal reading, although others have averaged four lateral readings with successful results.

Corneal topography is the most sophisticated method of assessing corneal curvature after refractive surgery and is arguably the most appropriate method for contact lens fitting. Important data retrievable from topography includes the qualitative shape, quantitative values of optical zone size, simulated central keratometry, axial midperipheral curvature, and the dioptric curvature change across the "knee" or "bend" or the transition zone.

Roberts documented abrupt curvature changes and oblate patterns following RK, apparent on corneal topography maps, and differences between midperipheral corneal curvatures when comparing axial and instantaneous reconstruction algorithms (89). A very defined steep transitional ring surrounds the central flat zone on instantaneous radius of curvature maps. On axial maps, however, only a central flat zone is often noted due to the averaging nature of the axial algorithm (Fig. 28.11; see Color Plate 28.11). Although instantaneous curvatures are proportional to the true local curvatures of a given peripheral corneal location, these values are not applicable to GP contact lens fitting. Global or "averaged" curvatures provided by axial displays are most appropriate for selecting a GP lens base curve, which is fit globally and not locally to a given cornea. Figure 28.12 (see Color Plate 28.12) shows a post ALK eye imaged by both the instantaneous and axial reconstruction algorithms. Note the cursor positioned over the same location on each map reads significantly different values in the midperiphery between the two displays.

Corneal topography after myopic PRK, ALK, or LASIK helps determine the quality and stability of the treatment zone, the diameter and centration of the surgical zone, the

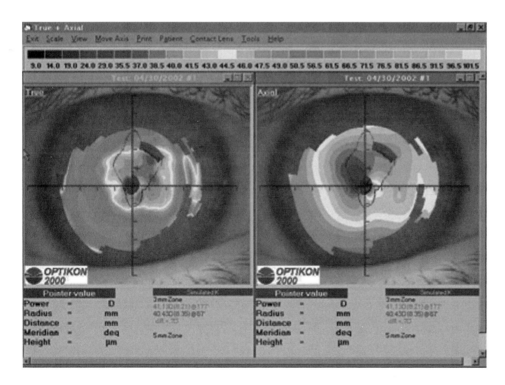

FIG. 28.11. Topographical differences noted on axial versus tangential maps after radial keratotomy. (See Color Plate 28.11.)

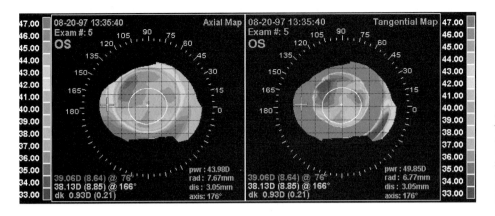

FIG. 28.12. Topographical differences noted on axial versus tangential maps on the same eye after automated lamellar keratoplasty. Note the cursor positioned over the same point on the two different maps results in very different corneal curvature readings. (See Color Plate 28.12.)

mean central curvature, and the peripheral corneal curvatures. Laser ablation of the central cornea produces a flattened optical zone with a smooth power transition to the peripheral cornea (90). The predominant postoperative contour is the oblate configuration observed in more than 98% post-PRK corneas (91). The corneal periphery is essentially unaltered outside of the ablation zone, in contrast to RK, which shows both large central and peripheral topographic variations from preoperative topography and more abrupt and irregular curvature changes at the transition zone.

For any oblate corneal shape, select a standard GP design base curve equal to the corneal curvature value 3.5 to 4.0 mm superior to the visual axis on axial computerized videokeratograph (82). The so-selected GP lens should exhibit midperipheral corneal alignment and adequate but not excessive central pooling. The GP base curve is, therefore, chosen similar in curvature to that of the midperipheral cornea at the inflection point on the axial map.

Larger overall diameter lenses than typically used for normal eyes encourages lens centration. Common overall diameters range from 9.2 to 10.2 mm, with optical zones typically 1 to 3 mm smaller than the overall diameter. Optical zone size varies much more among RK patients than post PRK or LASIK patients. Studies show that there is often a sharp inflection point on axial topography maps after RK, denoting the edge of the surgical optical zone, approximately 2.7 mm (range, 1.75 to 3.3 mm) from the center of the cornea (84). The posterior contact lens optical zone should vault the RK optical zone; therefore, determining this topographic landmark may be beneficial in GP lens design.

As these refractive procedures produce a relative steepening of peripheral versus central corneal topography, a reverse geometry (RG) lens, which better conforms to the relatively steeper corneal periphery is often beneficial. RG lenses incorporate secondary curvatures 3 to 5 D steeper than their central curvatures, and are most used in our practices to assist in lens centration after RK or PKP. Isolated steep areas surrounding the RK optical zone are common due to

uneven incisions, and GP lens decentration often occurs over the steepest hemi-meridian of the cornea. Decentration can be managed by better alignment along the midperipheral cornea with an RG design. Several designs have been developed, many of which are currently advocated for corneal refractive therapy (orthokeratology).

The selection of secondary curves in RG fitting depends on the axial dioptric change across the knee of the transition zone. This measurement is facilitated by moving the interactive cursor on topography instruments across the "bend" of the surgical optical zone to measure the dioptric change across the transition. If the change noted is 3 D, a secondary curve 2 to 3 D steeper than the base curve is suggested. Since the intermediate curves have been specifically designed for midperipheral alignment, the base curve can be selected 1 D steeper than the post operative simulated flat "K," or the average keratometry reading (if greater than 2 D of corneal astigmatism persists) (92).

Some clinicians believe RG lenses are unnecessary after myopic photoablation procedures, and advocate the use of standard GP designs (93). Improved centration than occurred with the preoperative lenses might be observed because of increased negative pressure created by the central apical clearance, and no asymmetric steepening surrounding the treatment zone (as may occur after RK) is observed (93). We have fit more reverse geometry lenses after ALK and LASIK than after PRK, however, because we note that use of the microkeratome causes an immediate and more abrupt curvature change surrounding the corneal cap versus PRK (Fig. 28.13; see Color Plate 28.13) (94). All 13 eyes studied in one series were successfully fit postoperative with standard aspheric designs; the base curve was an average of 0.065 mm flatter (range 0.05 mm steeper to 0.2 mm flatter) then the pre-PRK GP base curve (93). Several lenses were even fit with the same base curve as the preoperative GP! Preoperative keratometry readings can, therefore, reasonably predict initial diagnostic lens base curve after LASIK, PRK, ALK, or LASEK.

Temporary or permanent corneal molding may occur after GP lens fitting. GP lenses have even been applied in

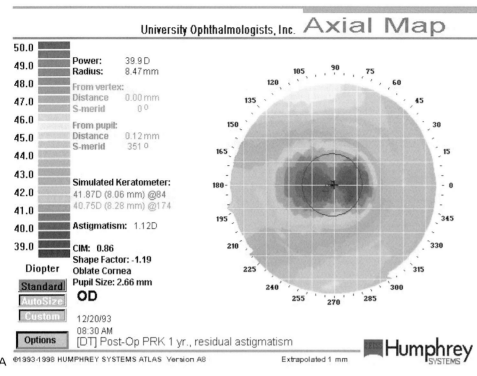

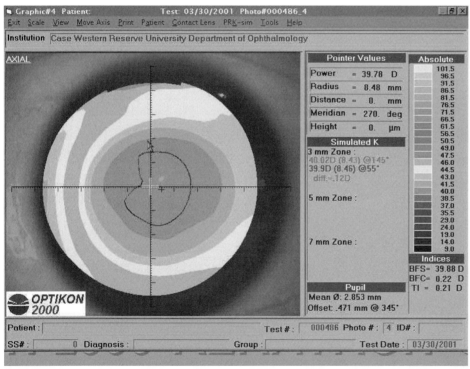

FIG. 28.13. Example of topography after photorefractive keratectomy and LASIK. **(A)** This eye underwent photorefractive keratectomy and has a symmetrical peripheral cornea surrounding the ablation. **(B)** This eye underwent laser-assisted *in situ* keratomileusis and has more asymmetry surrounding the ablation zone. (See Color Plate 28.13.)

the early postoperative phase to intentionally reshape an overcorrected eye. Because the cornea may be unstable and in its preliminary stages of healing, an over corrected patient may benefit from intentional corneal steepening from the retained shape of a steep fit GP lens (97). Other than a small series of cases, this procedure has not been reported

in a controlled study to date. With three months of healing, the cornea is far more firm and stable, and such corneal molding effects are minimal and temporary.

Corneas altered by either incisional or lamellar refractive surgery techniques are indeed more challenging to fit with contact lenses than "normal" eyes, requiring more lenses and chair time, while resulting in slightly poorer contact lens corrected visions and more failures (96).

KERATOCONUS

Overview

Keratoconus is typically classified as an asymmetric, noninflammatory, and progressive ectasia of the cornea characterized by thinning, steepening, and scarring of the central cornea (97). Because of distortion and secondary irregular astigmatism as the disease progresses, affected patients experience a decrease in best-corrected spectacle acuity. Clinical data and diagnostic examinations reveal several characteristic signs and symptoms that become more prevalent as the disease progresses. These include worsening of best corrected spectacle acuity (97), fluctuating visual acuity (98), increased regular and irregular corneal astigmatism, an inferiorly thinned and displaced ectasia of the cornea, deposition of iron in a ring or ring segment in the corneal epithelium surrounding the base of the cone (Fleisher's ring), Vogt's striae in the posterior corneal stroma, and central corneal scarring.

The cause of keratoconus remains unknown, although metabolic/chemical changes that occur in the corneal tissue have been documented (99). The disease has been associated with atopy (100), connective tissue disorders (101), eye rubbing (102), inheritance (103), and contact lens wear (104).

Lens Design and Fitting

Keratoconus Contact Lens Fitting

The global shape of the cornea with keratoconus is that of an irregular prolate ellipse. The corneal apex is frequently displaced inferiorly, although central steepening and steepening in the upper half of the cornea may present. The role for contact lenses in keratoconus has been a topic of some controversy over the past 30 to 40 years. Many ways to fit rigid contact lenses have been advocated. The goals fitters wish to achieve are varied and have substantially contributed to the above-mentioned controversies. Generally, there are three "philosophies" into which virtually all fitting strategies can be grouped: (a) reshape or splint methods, (b) the three-point-touch method, and (c) the apical clearance method. Each has its ardent supporters and none has solid clinical or experimental evidence to support superiority.

Those that support the reshape or splint philosophy seek to either restore a more normal corneal shape to the keratoconic cornea or attempt to use the lens to reshape the ectatic cornea by using the rigid lens as a splint. They believe that the thinned and weakened cornea will behave more normally in an optical sense (and possibly be less likely to change) if it is "supported" by a rigid lens. This thinking has significant intuitive and emotional value: one is treating

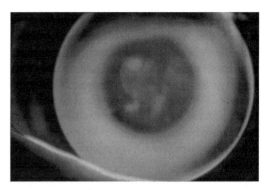

FIG. 28.14. Large, flat-fitted lens on an eye with keratoconus. (See Color Plate 28.14.)

the disease, not just merely correcting refractive error. Unfortunately, results of such fittings have not been studied or presented in refereed journals but have been disseminated by word of mouth and during continuing education lectures. At present there is no evidence, beyond unsupported anecdotal comments, that this philosophy has any merit, despite a significant number of ardent believers. The rigid lenses employed are typically large in diameter and fitted quite flat in order to achieve their goals (Fig. 28.14; see Color Plate 28.14). Korb (105), however, suggested that this flat fitting method may actually be harmful rather than beneficial.

The three-point-touch method is also a flat-fitting method, originally described by Arias (106). The goal is to achieve mild apical touch and then midperipheral touch on the slopes of the cone. This approach achieves a distribution of load bearing across a relatively large area, reducing the likelihood of excessive pressure in a single area (Fig. 28.15; see Color Plate 28.15). Subtleties of how much bearing and how large or small the midperipheral bearing areas should be, are as varied as the practitioners who employ this method. We believe that this is the most common means of fitting lenses to the keratoconus patient. Two large stud-

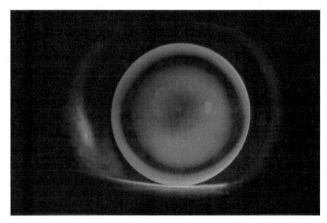

FIG. 28.15. "Three-point-touch" fluorescein pattern in keratoconus. (See Color Plate 28.15.)

ies (107,115) suggest that the vast majority of patients are fitted flat in the US (88%).

The third method is the apical clearance method. Adherents of this philosophy believe the thinned corneal apex should not be assaulted with the mechanical rubbing of a lens. Rather, the lens should vault over this area and the bearing or contact areas should be either on the slope of the cone or further distal to the apex (Fig. 28.16; see Color Plate 28.16 (109,110). In our experience, fitters who follow this philosophy are passionate about preserving the apex from harm, believing that apical contact by a lens will increase the likelihood for corneal scarring. Korb's series (105) is commonly used as a foundation for their belief.

Despite the myriad of lens fitting strategies that have been used since the advent of the rigid corneal lens, and the passion with which respective supporters defend their philosophies, there is a glaring paucity of evidence that any one method is any better than the next. We believe that fitters should select the approach with which they are most comfortable. We also believe that the proven role for lenses in the keratoconic eye is to improve visual function. Until such time as lens wear is proven to be of therapeutic assistance to these patients, claiming such seems to be nothing more than wishful thinking.

Soft Lenses

Soft lenses can be used in keratoconus for piggybacking and in those cases where spherical spectacle lenses produce reasonably good vision. Soft lenses have little benefit over spectacles and, therefore, are an alternative to glasses, just as in normal corneas. Toric soft lenses may be more beneficial than spheres but cylinder axes tend to be oblique, suggesting that a lens that is rotationally very stable should be the lens of choice.

Rigid Corneal Lenses

Rigid corneal lenses are the principal means for managing visual impairment produced by keratoconus. As with other conditions mentioned, the anterior surface of the lens optically behaves like a new smooth cornea, improving visual function substantially. These lenses may be fit steep or flat, large or small in overall diameter, all achieving the same effect. Several technical details are common to all of the fitting strategies described over the ages. The first issue is centration. Because keratoconus quite often results in a decentered apex, there is a profound tendency for a corneal lens to decenter in the direction of the apex. This can be unsettling to an inexperienced clinician who was previously admonished by his or her instructors to strive for a well-centered lens. Except in the very mildest of cases, decentration is part of the picture and the fitter should not spend undue time and effort attempting to defeat this tendency. Rather the goal should be to provide good optics over the entrance pupil so that the visual function goals can be met. In cases where decentration is a significant issue, a larger overall diameter will be required in order that the entrance pupil is adequately covered.

The second important issue is optic zone size. Manipulation of the size of the posterior optic zone (POZ) is an extremely powerful tool in the fitting process. Most fitters tend to standardize the size of the optic zone for normal corneas or link it to the overall diameter of the lens. For example, a 9.5-mm lens would have a 8.1-mm optic zone and a 9.0-mm lens would have a 7.6-mm optic zone. In these cases 1.4 mm is available for peripheral curves. In keratoconus, the POZ can make or break the fit. In Fig. 28.17 (see Color Plate 28.17), a medium-size lens (8.6 mm) with a 7.6-mm POZ is shown on a keratoconic cornea. Apical touch, midperipheral clearance, and peripheral impingement is illustrated. This fitting pattern is rare in normal corneas but is a common presentation for keratoconic eyes. Figure 28.18 demonstrates the limited effect of flattening the peripheral curves. There is an increase in apical bearing and only a minimum increase in edge lift. If the POZ is decreased, as viewed in Fig. 28.19, however, the

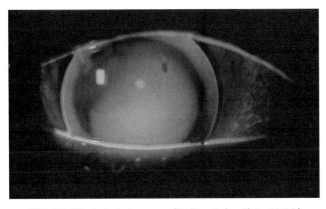

FIG. 28.16. Apical clearance fit. (See Color Plate 28.16.)

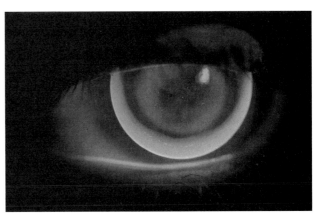

FIG. 28.17. Overall diameter/posterior optic zone: 8.6/7.6-mm gas-permeable lens shown on a keratoconus cornea. (See Color Plate 28.17.)

peripheral bearing areas can be moved up the slope of the cone, giving the peripheral curves an opportunity to provide edge clearance.

The third issue is edge clearance. We feel this is one of the most important features in a well-fitted lens in keratoconus. Patients who are comfortable in their lenses have one distinguishing feature, there is adequate edge clearance all around the lens. Experienced keratoconus fitters recognize this and spend considerable attention in efforts to provide appropriate edge clearance for their patients' corneas.

The last issue is optical design. Toric designs are rarely needed in keratoconus, even if there is substantial cylinder in the refraction and keratometry. Back-toric and bitoric lens designs are beneficial in the presence of global regular astigmatism, not in irregular or atypical corneal shapes such as those found with keratoconus. We also rarely will consider aspheric optics. We prefer spherical optical designs as experience has shown that visual acuity is better with spherical optics than with aspheres with this disorder. Lenticular designs are frequently used to control anterior edge shape and edge thickness. Ectasia of the cornea and steepened curvature commonly results in highly myopic refractive errors in these eyes.

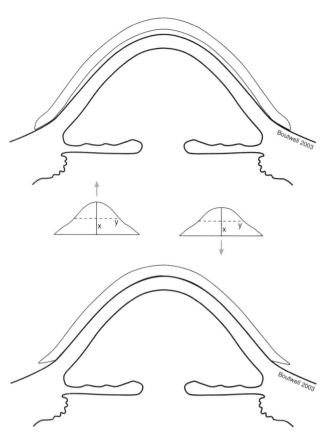

FIG. 28.19. Effect of decreasing the optical zone size in keratoconus.

Piggyback Lens Fitting

Piggyback fitting can be extremely beneficial in keratoconus, primarily to enhance rigid lens tolerance. A soft lens is placed on the eye first with a rigid lens then placed over it. The soft lens acts as a cushion and barrier reducing corneal nerve stimulation. The soft lens does not help if the lens intolerance is eyelid related, and thereby diagnostically identifies the discomfort. The rigid lens is fitted using customary methods. A low-minus soft lens, normally a disposable of relatively steep base curve, is then added. Piggybacking is rarely an initial approach to fitting, rather it is a means of rescuing a patient from lens intolerance. We make every effort to improve the rigid lens fit before resorting to a piggyback. Although piggybacking is a wonderful adjunct for the fitter, it is quite inconvenient for the patient. Keep in mind that the patient is now manipulating two lenses per eye each and every day. When we use a piggyback, we tend to use it in an "on demand" basis; namely, patients can use this option when they feel like it. Most use it regularly initially, but over time rely on it less and less.

Scleral and Semiscleral Lenses

Scleral lenses predate all the other lens types described in this section and chapter. Similar to scleral lenses is a rela-

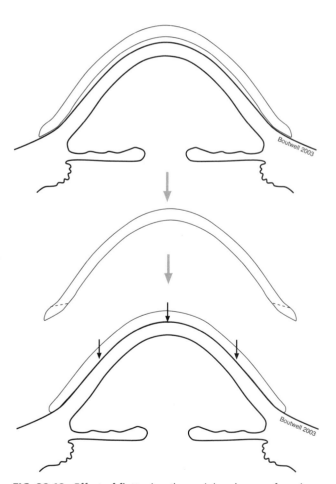

FIG. 28.18. Effect of flattening the peripheral curves for a lens with a tight periphery on a keratoconic cornea.

tively new class referred to as semisclerals. Scleral lenses are rarely used in the United States. A minor resurgence of preformed GP scleral lenses has recently occurred in both the United States and particularly in the United Kingdom (111–113), but these lenses are very costly and arduous to fit and are normally reserved for very advanced keratoconus cases where the other designs no longer are tolerated or remain on the eye and the patient declines PKP. In cases where PKP is less likely to succeed, such as in pellucid marginal degeneration, Terrien's degeneration, cornea disease with limbal stem cell failure, cicatricial diseases, corneal burns, or inflammatory corneal melts; however, scleral lenses for vision rehabilitation may be a reasonable option (see Chapter 34).

The Collaborative Longitudinal Evaluation of Keratoconus Study

The CLEK study is an 8-year observational study of the characteristics and progression of keratoconus and provides the best current information on this disease. A total of 1,209 eligible patients were enrolled between May 31, 1995 and June 29, 1996 at 16 CLEK-participating clinics (114).

Most CLEK subjects utilized contact lenses for visual correction. Sixty-five percent of the patients wore GP contact lenses in both eyes while 94 (8%) wore a GP lens in one eye only, and most of these patients (73%) reported that their lenses were comfortable. Twelve percent of GP-wearing eyes were using lenses fitted with apical clearance based upon the clinician's fluorescein pattern interpretation. The remainder (88%) was wearing lenses fitted with apical touch. For mild (steep keratometric reading <45 D) keratoconus, the mean estimate of the base curve to cornea-fitting relationship was 1.18 D flat (SD ± 1.84 D). In moderate disease (steep keratometric reading: 45 to 52 D), corneas were fitted on average 2.38 D flat (SD ± 2.56 D) while severe (steep keratometric reading > 52 D) disease had lenses fitted an average of 4.01 D flat (SD ± 4.11 D) (116).

Other visual options included both spectacles and hydrogel contact lenses either separately or in combination with GP lenses, or PKP in advanced disease. Prevalence of various visual or surgical options has been described in the literature, usually in retrospective evaluations or as reported in trends of clinical management. We are prospectively monitoring trends in clinical management in CLEK, and measuring variability of important clinical measures that influence prescribing habits and decision making.

Disease severity or progression in keratoconus is typically measured by keratometry or videokeratography. Repeatability of both these techniques has been reported in normals, but the CLEK Study Group is the first to report on the repeatability in keratoconus patients (116–118). There was a high correlation with both steep ($r = 0.89$; $p = 0.0001$) and flat keratometric readings ($r = 0.83$; $p = 0.0001$) and a CLEK-designed custom diagnostic rigid lens evaluation

of corneal sagittal depth (these lenses were termed "FDACL" for "first definite apical clearance lens"). The FDACL technique was developed for the CLEK Study for assessment of disease severity and progression as well as a benchmark for ascertaining how flat or steep a patient's current lenses are fitted. The FDACL was found to be a repeatable, reliable new procedure for determining disease severity, and a quantifiable, indirect estimation of apical curvature in keratoconus. In fact, the FDACL technique was found to be more repeatable than keratometry in the advanced stages of the disease. This was evidenced by consistent FDACL readings across the spectrum of curvatures found in keratoconus, whereas keratometry becomes less repeatable in the advanced stages, which limits the usefulness of the keratometer to document disease progression.

The FDACL technique also allows an analysis of the current community standard of care with regard to the apical fitting relationship of GP lens fitting. By comparing the FDACL base curve to the patient's habitual GP lens parameters, an estimate of how steep or flat patient's eyes were fitted could be determined. Although the influence of flat-fitting contact lenses on corneal scarring in keratoconus is frequently debated (specifically the potential risk for corneal scarring imposed by flat-fitting rigid contact lenses (107), the large majority of CLEK study patients wear flat-fitting lenses. Overall, rigid lenses were fitted an average of 2.86 D (SD ± 3.31 D) flatter than the FDACL, but patients were fit relatively flatter in advanced disease. In fact, some eyes with severe keratoconus were fit more than 10 D flatter than FDACL (116).

CORNEAL DYSTROPHIES

Corneal dystrophies frequently result in irregular corneal surfaces affecting vision. The corneal dystrophies are generally grouped into epithelial, stromal and endothelial categories. Of the epithelial dystrophies, epithelial basement membrane dystrophy (map-dot-fingerprint) and Reis-Bucklers dystrophy at times may benefit from contact lenses.

Epithelial Basement Membrane (Map-Dot-Fingerprint) Dystrophy

Contact lenses are beneficial in two roles for this dominantly inherited disorder. The first role is as a bandage when recurrent erosions occur. Due to the weakened attachment of the epithelium as a result of the aberrant basement membrane some individuals experience erosive episodes. Hydrogel lenses have been used as bandages in these cases with mixed results. In our experience, about 50% of patients obtain relief from pain and a decreased frequency of events with bandage lenses but the other patients are more irritated with lens wear than without. Bandage use can either be designed for short-term (days) management of acute erosions or longer-term prevention. For short-term use, thin membrane lenses are preferred. The lens should be fit so that there is little movement, but flat enough to avoid tight lens signs and symptoms. The bandage lens should be observed on-eye in office for a half hour to an hour. Significant symptomatic relief should be observed and lens movement maintained without tight lens signs prior to discharge. The patient should be evaluated in 24 hours and then every 3 or 4 days until the epithelium is healed. We recommend observing the patient without removing the lens and without fluorescein. This requires a very careful slit-lamp examination. The lens should be left in place for 3 to 7 days after symptoms and signs are absent.

For long-term preventive management, silicone hydrogels are preferred. Lenses are often left in place as long as they remain clean or for 30 days, whichever is shorter. The goal is 6 to 12 months of continuous wear. After this period of time, most patients with recurrent erosions from this dystrophy can go symptom-free for many months.

Bandage lenses secondly can address mild visual impairment due to irregular corneal surfaces. This occurs when abnormal basement membrane builds up in some regions more than others. Buildup reflects to the surface resulting in irregular astigmatism and reduced visual acuity. A thick hydrogel or a rigid lens may be used to mask the astigmatism and provide an improvement in vision. If there is no history of erosions a corneal lens may be fitted. If a patient has a history of both erosions and irregular astigmatism, a semiscleral lens is preferred. These lenses move very little and can provide a bandage effect as well as improved optics. The semiscleral lens should be fit with minimal apical clearance in the central and midperipheral cornea.

Reis-Bucklers Dystrophy

Reis-Bucklers dystrophy is an uncommon bilateral corneal disorder resulting in frequent episodes of photophobia and erosions. Anterior stromal and subepithelial scarring develops over time to result in visual impairment. Contact lens issues and approaches are equivalent to epithelial basement membrane dystrophy except that long-term bandage lens use is generally not advisable.

The Stromal Dystrophies

The stromal dystrophies, of which granular, macular and lattice are the best known, result in corneal opacity and surface irregularities. Although patients with these dystrophies have a varied frequency of spontaneous erosions, contact lenses can assist with the irregular astigmatism common to these disorders. Rigid lenses can be used in the native cornea, and in eyes that have undergone lamellar keratectomy, phototherapeutic keratectomy and PKP for stromal dystrophic disease.

Corneal GP lenses should be fitted large in overall diameter (9.5 to 11.0 mm) and minimally steep in base curve to limit harsh bearing over the central cornea. For very distorted corneas centration and lens stability can be problems requiring a semi-scleral lens design.

Fuchs Dystrophy

Patients with Fuchs endothelial dystrophy suffer from loss of vision initially due to an accumulation of pigmented or nonpigmented guttata, followed by diminished corneal clarity from corneal edema and finally pain associated with bullous keratopathy. Contact lenses are most beneficial in pain management in cases where PKP is inadvisable. A high-water-content hydrogel or a silicone hydrogel can be placed for a week to a month at a time. The lens reduces the pain remarkably. Management of these patients involves long-term care. Fortunately, after 1 or 2 years, most of these patients can cease lens wear without further discomfort. Over time, chronic low-grade inflammation that accompanies the bullae leads to subepithelial fibrosis and reduced or stable bullae.

SUMMARY

Specialty contact lens fitters who provide care for patients suffering from forms of irregular cornea face complicated corneal contours that fall outside of the "normal" contact lens population. Fitting these patients requires skill and a solid understanding of both corneal shape and contact lens mechanical principles. The application of basic fitting techniques, combined with recent developments in the contact lens industry, should allow successful fitting of these patients.

REFERENCES

1. Mandell RB. A guide to videokeratography. *Int Contact Lens Clin* 1996;23:205–228.
2. Waring GO III, Hannush S, Bogan S, Maloney R. Classification of corneal topography. In: Schanzlin DJ, Robin JB, eds. *Corneal topography: measuring and modifying the cornea.* New York: Springer-Verlag. 1992:70–71.
3. Millin JA, Maguire LJ. Developing entry criteria for studies of severe postkeratoplasty astigmatism. *Am J Ophthalmol* 1991; 112:666–670.
4. Stevenson RW CM, O'Brart DP, Rosen ES. Corneal topography in contact lens practice. *Eur J Implant Ref Surg* 1995;7: 305–317.
5. Szczotka LB, Reinhart W. Computerized videokeratoscopy contact lens software for RGP fitting in a bilateral postkeratoplasty patient: a clinical case report. *CLAO J* 1995;21:52–56.
6. Caroline P, Andre MP, Norman CW. Corneal Topography and Computerized Contact Lens Fitting Modules. *Int Contact Lens Clin* 1997;21:185–195.
7. Klopfer J, Tielsch JM, Vitale S, et al. Ocular trauma in the United States. Eye injuries resulting in hospitalization, 1984 through 1987. *Arch Ophthalmol* 1992;110:838–842.

8. Parver LM. Eye trauma. The neglected disorder. *Arch Ophthalmol* 1986;104:1452–1453.

9. Parver LM, Dannenberg AL, Blacklow B, et al. Characteristics and causes of penetrating eye injuries reported to the National Eye Trauma System Registry, 1985–91. *Public Health Rep* 1993;108:625–632.

10. White MF Jr, Morris R, Feist RM, et al. Eye injury: prevalence and prognosis by setting. *South Med J* 1989;82:151–158.

11. Tielsch JM, Parver L, Shankar B. Time trends in the incidence of hospitalized ocular trauma. *Arch Ophthalmol* 1989;107:519–523.

12. Morris RE, Witherspoon CD, Helms HA, Jr., et al. Eye Injury Registry of Alabama (preliminary report): demographics and prognosis of severe eye injury. *South Med J* 1987;80:810–816.

13. Glynn RJ, Seddon JM, Berlin BM. The incidence of eye injuries in New England adults. *Arch Ophthalmol* 1988;106:785–789.

14. Liggett PE, Pince KJ, Barlow W, et al. Ocular trauma in an urban population. Review of 1132 cases. *Ophthalmology* 1990;97:581–584.

15. Dannenberg AL, Parver LM, Brechner RJ, et al. Penetration eye injuries in the workplace. The National Eye Trauma System Registry. *Arch Ophthalmol* 1992;110:843–848.

16. *Vision problems in the US: data analysis.* New York: National Society to Prevent Blindness, 1980.

17. Dannenberg AL, Parver LM, Fowler CJ. Penetrating eye injuries related to assault. The National Eye Trauma System Registry. *Arch Ophthalmol* 1992;110:849–852.

18. McMahon TT. Corneal topography following traumatic corneal lacerations. In: Shanzlin D, Robin J, eds. *Corneal topography.* New York: Springer-Verlag, 1991:95–104.

19. Rowsey JJ. Ten caveats in refractive surgery. *Ophthalmol* 1983;90:95–104.

20. McMahon TT, Devulapally J, Rosheim KM, et al. Contact lens use after corneal trauma. *J Am Optom Assoc* 1997;68:215–224.

21. Stenson S. Superior limbic keratoconjunctivitis associated with soft contact lens wear. *Arch Ophthalmol* 1983;101:402–404.

22. Brown DVL. Traumatic fracture of plastic contact lens. *Arch Ophthalmol* 1964;72:319–322.

23. Gyorffy ST. Das verhalten der kontaktschale bei augenverletzungen. *Ophthalmologica* 1951;122:344–347.

24. Lubeck D, Greene JS. Corneal injuries. *Emerg Med Clin North Am* 1988;6:73–94.

25. O'Rourke PJ. Traumatic fracture of contact lens with corneal injury. *Br J Ophthalmol* 1971;55:125–127.

26. Reiss GR, Dyer JA. Corneal abrasion secondary to a malpositioned contact lens. *Am J Ophthalmol* 1985;99:598.

27. Brown SI, Rosen J. Scleral perforation. A complication of the soft contact lens. *Arch Ophthalmol* 1975;93:1047–1048.

28. Michaels DD, Zugsmith GS. An unusual contact lens complication. *Am J Ophthalmol* 1963;55:1057–1058.

29. Oshima T. A case of foreign body granuloma due to a contact lens retained long in the upper fornix. *Bull Jpn Ophthalmol* 1966;17:103–106.

30. Bellan L, Buffam F. The "O" sign—clue to a lost lens. *Can J Ophthalmol* 1990;25:348–350.

31. Kao CS, Shih YF, Ko LS. Embedded hard contact lens: reports of a case. *J Formos Med Assoc* 1990;89:234–236.

32. Glatt HJ. Periocular pseudocyst caused by a displaced contact lens: CT appearance. *AJR Am J Roentgenol* 1992;159:435–436.

33. Roberts-Harry TJ, Davey CC, Jagger JD. Periocular migration of hard contact lenses. *Br J Ophthalmol* 1992;76:95–97.

34. Nicolitz E, Flanagan JC. Orbital mass as a complication of contact lens wear. *Arch Ophthalmol* 1978;96:2238–2239.

35. Beekhuis WH, van Rij G, Eggink FA, et al. Contact lenses following keratoplasty. *CLAO J* 1991;17:27–29.

36. Binder PS, Kopecky L. Fitting the SoftPerm contact lens after keratoplasty. *CLAO J* 1992;18:170–172.

37. Perlman EM. An analysis and interpretation of refractive errors after penetrating keratoplasty. *Ophthalmology* 1981;88:39–45.

38. Manabe R, Matsuda M, Suda T. Photokeratoscopy in fitting contact lens after penetrating keratoplasty. *Br J Ophthalmol* 1986;70:55–59.

39. Strelow S, Cohen EJ, Leavitt KG, et al. Corneal topography for selective suture removal after penetrating keratoplasty. *Am J Ophthalmol* 1991;112:657–665.

40. Maguire LJ, Bourne WM. Corneal topography of transverse keratotomies for astigmatism after penetrating keratoplasty. *Am J Ophthalmol* 1989;107:323–330.

41. Donnenfeld ED, Kornstein HS, Amin A, et al. Laser in situ keratomileusis for correction of myopia and astigmatism after penetrating keratoplasty. *Ophthalmol* 1999;106:1966–1975.

42. Nassaralla BR, Nassaralla JJ. Laser in situ keratomileusis after penetrating keratoplasty. *J Refract Surg* 2000;16:431–7.

43. Koay PY, McGhee CN, Weed KH, Craig JP. Laser in situ keratomileusis for ametropia after penetrating keratoplasty. *J Refract Surg* 2000;16:140–147.

44. Kremer F, Aronsky M, Bowyer B, et al. Treatment of corneal surface irregularities using biomask as an adjunct to excimer laser phototherapeutic keratectomy. *Cornea* 2002;21:28–32.

45. Knorz MC, Jendritza B. Topographically-guided laser in situ keratomileusis to treat corneal irregularities. *Ophthalmology* 2000;107:1138–1143.

46. Maeyens E, Houttequiet I, Missotten L. Corneal grafts and contact lens fitting. *Contacologia* 1994;16E:96–100.

47. Genvert GI, Cohen EJ, Arentsen JJ, et al. Fitting gas-permeable contact lenses after penetrating keratoplasty. *Am J Ophthalmol* 1985;99:511–514.

48. Mannis MJ, Zadnik K, Deutch D. Rigid contact lens wear in the corneal transplant patient. *CLAO J* 1986;12:39–42.

49. Lass JH, Lembach RG, Park SB, et al. Clinical management of keratoconus. A multicenter analysis. *Ophthalmology* 1990;97:433–445.

50. Silbiger JS, Cohen EJ, Laibson PR. The rate of visual recovery after penetrating keratoplasty for keratoconus. *CLAO J* 1996;22:266–269.

51. Vail A, Gore SM, Bradley BA, et al. Clinical and surgical factors influencing corneal graft survival, visual acuity, and astigmatism. Corneal Transplant Follow-up Study Collaborators. *Ophthalmology* 1996;103:41–49.

52. Bourne WM, Shearer DR. Effects of long-term rigid contact lens wear on the endothelium of corneal transplants for keratoconus 10 years after penetrating keratoplasty. *CLAO J* 1995;21:265–267.

53. Gomes JA, Rapuano CJ, Cohen EJ. Topographic stability and safety of contact lens use after penetrating keratoplasty. *CLAO J* 1996;22:64–69.

54. Lopatynsky M, Cohen EJ, Leavitt KG, et al. Corneal topography for rigid gas permeable lens fitting after penetrating keratoplasty. *CLAO J* 1993;19:41–44.

55. Sperber LT, Lopatynsky MO, Cohen EJ. Corneal topography in contact lens wearers following penetrating keratoplasty. *CLAO J* 1995;21:183–190.

56. Wilson SE, Friedman RS, Klyce SD. Contact lens manipulation of corneal topography after penetrating keratoplasty: a preliminary study. *CLAO J* 1992;18:177–182.

57. Wilson SE, Kaufman HE. Graft failure after penetrating keratoplasty. *Surv Ophthalmol* 1990;34:325–356.

58. Lim L, Tan DT, Chan WK. Therapeutic use of Bausch & Lomb PureVision contact lenses. *CLAO J* 2001;27:179–185.

59. Lemp MA. The effect of extended-wear aphakic hydrophilic

contact lenses after penetrating keratoplasty. *Am J Ophthalmol* 1980;90:331–335.

60. Mannis MJ, Matsumoto ER. Extended-wear aphakic soft contact lenses after penetrating keratoplasty. *Arch Ophthalmol* 1983; 101:1225–1228.

61. Poggio EC, Glynn RJ, Schein OD, et al. The incidence of ulcerative keratitis among users of daily-wear and extended-wear soft contact lenses. *N Engl J Med* 1989;321:779–783.

62. Weiner BM, Nirankari VS. A new biaspheric contact lens for severe astigmatism following penetrating keratoplasty. *CLAO J* 1992;18:29–33.

63. Koffler BH, Clements LD, Litteral GL, et al. A new contact lens design for postkeratoplasty patients. *CLAO J* 1994;20:170–175.

64. Szczotka LB. Clinical evaluation of a topographically based contact lens fitting software. *Optom Vis Sci* 1997;74:14–19.

65. Maguen E, Caroline P, Rosner IR, et al. The use of the SoftPerm lens for the correction of irregular astigmatism. *CLAO J* 1992; 18:173–176.

66. Schein OD, Rosenthal P, Ducharme C. A gas-permeable scleral contact lens for visual rehabilitation. *Am J Ophthalmol* 1990; 109:318–322.

67. Spitznas M, Eckert J, Frising M, et al. Long-term functional and topographic results seven years after epikeratophakia for keratoconus. *Graefes Arch Clin Exp Ophthalmol* 2002;240: 639–643.

68. Holmes-Higgin DK, Burris TE, Lapidus JA, et al. Risk factors for self-reported visual symptoms with Intacs inserts for myopia. *Ophthalmology* 2002;109:46–56.

69. Waring GO III, Lynn MJ, McDonnell PJ. Results of the prospective evaluation of radial keratotomy (PERK) study 10 years after surgery. *Arch Ophthalmol* 1994;112:1298–1308.

70. MacRae SM, Rich LF. Long-term effects of radial keratotomy on the corneal endothelium. *J Refract Surg* 1998;14:49–52.

71. McDonnell PJ, Caroline PJ, Salz J. Irregular astigmatism after radial and astigmatic keratotomy. *Am J Ophthalmol* 1989;107: 42–46.

72. McDonnell PJ, McClusky DJ, Garbus JJ. Corneal topography and fluctuating visual acuity after radial keratotomy. *Ophthalmology* 1989;96:665–670.

73. Dastjerdi MH, Soong HK. LASEK (laser subepithelial keratomileusis). *Curr Opin Ophthalmology* 2002;13:261–263.

74. Nelson JD, Williams P, Lindstrom RL, et al. Map-fingerprint-dot changes in the corneal epithelial basement membrane following radial keratotomy. *Ophthalmology* 1985;92:199–205.

75. Waring GO III, Lynn MJ, Gelender H, et al. Results of the prospective evaluation of radial keratotomy (PERK) study one year after surgery. *Ophthalmology* 1985;92:177–198, 307.

76. Eiferman RA, Schultz GS, Norquist RE, et al. Corneal wound healing and its pharmacologic modification after refractive keratotomy. In: Waring GO III, ed. *Refractive keratotomy for myopia and astigmatism*. St. Louis: Mosby Yearbook, Inc., 1992: 749–780.

77. Mizutani Y, Matsutaka H, Takemoto N, et al. The effect of anoxia on the human cornea. *Acta Soc Ophthalmol Jpn* 1987; 9:644–649.

78. Karpecki PM, Smith JM, Durrie DS. What can you do to improve PRK outcomes. *Rev Optom* 1996;133:127–133.

79. Komarnicky GS. Day three post PRK: what can you expect? *Rev Optom* 1996;133:68–72.

80. Srur M, Dattas D. The use of disposable contact lenses as therapeutic lenses. *CLAO J* 1997;23:40–42.

81. Weiner B. How and when to prescribe bandage contact lenses. *Rev Optom* 1996;133:38–42.

82. McDonnell PJ, Garbus JJ, Caroline P, et al. Computerized analysis of corneal topography as an aid in fitting contact lenses after radial keratotomy. *Ophthalmic Surg* 1992;23:55–59.

83. Shivitz IA, Arrowsmith PN, Russell BM. Contact lenses in the treatment of patients with overcorrected radial keratotomy. *Ophthalmology* 1987;94:899–903.

84. Waring GO III, Lynn MJ, Culbertson W, et al. Three-year results of the Prospective Evaluation of Radial Keratotomy (PERK) study. *Ophthalmology* 1987;94:1339–1354.

85. Walline J, Zadnik K. Opaque soft contact lens to mask glare secondary to radial keratotomy: A case Report. *Optom Vis Sci* 1996;12s:236.

86. Bogan SJ, Maloney RK, Drews CD, et al. Computer-assisted videokeratography of corneal topography after radial keratotomy. *Arch Ophthalmol* 1991;109:834–841.

87. Lee AM, Kastl PR. Rigid gas permeable contact lens fitting after radial keratotomy. *CLAO J* 1998;24:33–35.

88. Campbell MD, Caroline P. A unique technique for fitting post RK patients. *CLAO J* 1998;12:56.

89. Roberts C, Cuff S, Kelley CG. Comparison of characteristic corneal topography patterns following radial keratotomy. *Invest Ophthalmol Vis Sci* 1997;38:s921.

90. Wilson SE, Klyce SD, McDonald MB, et al. Changes in corneal topography after excimer laser photorefractive keratectomy for myopia. *Ophthalmology* 1991;98:1338–1347.

91. Hersch PS, Schwartz BH. Corneal topography of stage III excimer laser photorefractive keratectomy. *Ophthalmology* 1995; 102:963–978.

92. *Menicon Plateau fitting guide.* Clovis, CA: Menicon USA.

93. Schipper I, Businger U, Pfarrer R. Fitting contact lenses after excimer laser photorefractive keratectomy for myopia. *CLAO J* 1995;21:281–284.

94. Edwards KH, Hough DA, Kersley HJ. Designing rigid lenses for the post PRK eye. *Optom Vis Sci* 1995;72(12 suppl):13. 95. Hannigan J. RGP lens to the rescue of a post-op RK patient. *Rev Optom* 1996;133:114–116.

95. Hannigan J. RGP lens to the rescue of a post-op RK patient. *Rev Optom* 1996;133:114–116.

96. Yeung KK, Olson MD, Weissman BA. Complexity of contact lens fitting after refractive surgery. *Am J Ophthalmol* 2002;133: 607–612.

97. Krachmer JH, Feder RS, Belin MW. Keratoconus and Related Non-inflammatory corneal thinning disorders. *Surv Ophthalmol* 1984;28:293–322.

98. Zadnik K. Contact lens fitting relation and visual acuity in keratoconus. *Am J Optom Physiol* Opt 1987;64:698–702.

99. Kenney CM, Brown DJ, Rajeev B. The Elusive Causes of Keratoconus. *CLAO J* 2000;26:10–13.

100. Harrison RJ, Easty DL, Manku M, et al. Association between keratoconus and atopy. *Br J Ophthalmol* 1989;73:816–822.

101. Ihalainen A. Clinical and epidemiological features of keratoconus: genetic and external factors in the pathogenesis of the disease. *Acta Ophthalmol* 1986;suppl 178:1–64.

102. Ridley F. Eye rubbing and contact lenses. *Br J Ophthalmol* 1961; 45:631.

103. Rabinowitz Y. Keratoconus. *Surv Ophthalmol* 1998;42: 297–319.

104. Macsai MS VG, Krachmer JH. Development of keratoconus after contact lens wear. *Arch Ophthalmol* 1990;108:435–538.

105. Korb DR, Finnemore VM, Herman JP. Apical changes and scarring in keratoconus as related to contact lens fitting techniques. *J Am Optom Assoc* 1982;53:199–205.

106. Arias C. A new technique of fitting contact lenses on keratoconus. *Contacto* 1959;3:393–415.

107. Zadnik K, Barr J, Edrington T, et al. Baseline findings in the collaborative longitudinal evaluation of keratoconus (CLEK) study. *Invest Ophthalmol Vis Sci* 1998;39:2537–2546.

108. Zadnik K, Barr JT, Gordon MO, et al. Biomicroscopic signs and disease severity in keratoconus. Collaborative Longitudinal

Evaluation of Keratoconus (CLEK) Study Group. *Cornea* 1996; 15:139–146.

109. Raber IM. Use of CAB Soper Cone contact lenses in keratoconus. *CLAO J* 1983;9:237–240.

110. Spring TF. The Soper keratoconus lens. *Trans Aust Coll Ophthalmol* 1970;2:48–49.

111. Tan DT, Pullum KW, Buckley RJ. Medical applications of scleral contact lenses: 1. A retrospective analysis of 343 cases. *Cornea* 1995;14:121–129.

112. Tan DT, Pullum KW, Buckley RJ. Medical applications of scleral contact lenses: 2. Gas-permeable scleral contact lenses. *Cornea* 1995;14:130–137.

113. Pullum KW, Buckley RJ. A study of 530 patients referred for rigid gas permeable scleral contact lens assessment. *Cornea* 1997; 16:612–622.

114. Edrington T, Zadnik K, et al. Standardized rigid contact lens fitting protocol for keratoconus. *Optom Vis Sci* 1996;73: 369–375.

115. Edrington T, Barr J, et al. Rigid contact lens fitting relationships in keratoconus. *Optom Vis Sci* 1999;76:692–699.

116. Edrington T, Begley C, et al. Repeatability and agreement of two corneal-curvature assessments in keratoconus: keratometry and the first definite apical clearance lens (FDACL). *Cornea* 1998;17:267–277.

117. Raasch TW, McMahon TT, Friedman NE, et al, and the CLEK Study Group. Repeatability of topography measurement in keratoconus. *Optom Vis Sci* 1998;12s:22.

118. McMahon TT, Anderson RJ, Joslin CE, et al. Precision of three topography instruments in keratoconus subjects. *Optom Vis Sci* 2001;78:599–604.

CONTACT LENS CORNEAL RESHAPING

MARJORIE J. RAH AND
JOHN MARK JACKSON

Contact lens corneal reshaping (orthokeratology) is defined as the planned application of specially designed gas-permeable (GP) contact lenses to reshape the cornea, temporarily reducing myopic refractive error and improving unaided visual acuity. The goal of this procedure is to allow patients to see well enough to perform daily tasks without the need for spectacle or contact lens correction for at least part of the day. Although this procedure has been practiced in one form or another for nearly 40 years, the efficacy and safety of the procedure remains somewhat controversial.

Overnight wear of contact lenses for corneal reshaping is a relatively recent development in the use of the procedure. Traditionally, the lenses were worn for several hours during the day to produce and maintain the treatment effects. With the advent of modern highly oxygen-permeable rigid lens materials, overnight wear of the lenses has become a viable option for patients. Overnight wear may represent a more attractive modality for most patients, as the lenses are only worn during sleep to produce and maintain the treatment effect. Patients remove the lenses shortly after awakening and theoretically have acceptable uncorrected visual acuity for most waking hours. Patients are thus able to avoid the inconvenience of spectacles and the potential inconvenience and discomfort of daytime wear of contact lenses. Alternatively, overnight wear of corneal-reshaping lenses may put the patient at undue risk for adverse events such as infection or corneal hypoxia.

Corneal-reshaping fitting techniques are vastly different today than when the procedure was first introduced. While there were a variety of fitting methods employed when the procedure was young, the majority of practitioners used a series of standard rigid lenses to progressively flatten the cornea. Initially the lenses were only moderately flatter than the patient's cornea, and as refractive error changes occurred and stabilized, new lenses were used that were slightly flatter than the previous pair. This process continued until the desired refractive error changes were induced. However, using standard lens designs that were significantly flatter than the normal corneal curvature often resulted in poorly centered lenses and induced irregular astigmatism. As a re-

sult, the treatment was generally limited to low amounts of myopic correction. Also, using a series of lenses in this manner made the procedure very time-consuming, often taking months to achieve the desired results.

Modern corneal reshaping employs reverse-geometry lenses to produce the desired corneal shape changes. These lenses have secondary peripheral radii of curvature that are steeper than the back optic zone radius of curvature. This alteration in lens design allows the lens to re-approach the cornea beyond the base curve, resulting in greatly improved lens centration. It is also thought that this steeper secondary curve causes the corneal tissue to redistribute radially from the center of the cornea, causing the central corneal epithelium to thin and the peripheral epithelium to thicken, leading to the refractive changes observed [1]. The use of reverse-geometry designs allows for more rapid changes in refractive error and fewer lens changes. In theory, a single lens is needed to produce the desired changes instead of a series of lenses as used previously; however, it is not unusual to make minor changes in the lens parameters to improve the treatment outcome.

This chapter describes the history of contact lens corneal reshaping, current fitting procedures, and patient management strategies.

HISTORY OF CONTACT LENS CORNEAL RESHAPING (ORTHOKERATOLOGY)

Early Use of Orthokeratology

The early use of corneal contact lenses generally utilized a flatter lens-to-cornea fitting relationship than the original scleral contact lenses. While scleral lenses were typically fitted with apical corneal clearance, the smaller corneal lens design was typically fit 1 to 2 D flatter than the flat keratometry reading [2]. This was performed to facilitate tear flow under the lens to provide oxygen to the cornea and to flush away debris trapped behind the lens. When patients removed their lenses after several hours of wear, many were left with blurry vision while wearing their eyeglasses. This phenomenon, likely due to a combination of corneal edema from the polymethylmethacrylate (PMMA) lens material and central corneal flattening from the flat lens, became known as "spectacle blur." Upon observing these accidental changes, a number of practitioners attempted to purposefully alter corneal shape to change refractive error. Jessen (3) in 1962 appears to be the first to describe this intentional change in the cornea, calling the technique "orthofocus." Other similar reports soon followed (4–6). Many terms have been used to describe the procedure throughout the past 30 years. In 1986, El Hage and Baker (7) coined the term "controlled kerato-reformation" for a corneal-reshaping technique using corneal topography and shape factor instead of traditional keratometry. "Precision corneal molding" is also used by some practitioners. Most recently, the term "corneal refractive therapy" has been used by Paragon Vision Sciences (Mesa, AZ).

Early Clinical Trials in Orthokeratology

Previous studies of orthokeratology vary widely in their methods and conclusions about this procedure. The earliest controlled studies were performed in the mid-1970s and early 1980s (8–20). All of these studies used traditional rigid lenses worn during the day and showed a mean refractive error change of approximately 1 D. They generally concluded that the procedure was capable of producing impressive changes, but that these changes were mostly temporary, minimal, unpredictable, and unstable. They did, however, all agree that the procedure appeared to be no more harmful than wearing standard, daily-wear, rigid contact lenses.

Newer studies of corneal reshaping using the reverse-geometry lens designs show an overall increase in the amount of myopia that is correctable. Many of these studies were compromised by small sample sizes or lack of standardized procedures. The corneal-reshaping literature within the last 10 years has focused on looking for mechanisms and predictive factors for patient outcomes as well as reporting efficacy and safety (1,21–25). However, there is still no clear picture of what factors may be used to predict success with the procedure. Long-term safety, particularly in overnight wear, is still an unanswered question.

The first large-scale, controlled clinical trial was performed by Kerns (1976, 1977) at the University of Houston College of Optometry (13–20). The goal of this study was to investigate the efficacy, predictability, safety, and permanency of the procedure. The subject groups included a control group of non–contact lens wearers, a group of conventional, alignment-fitted rigid contact lens wearers, and an orthokeratology group. The orthokeratology group underwent a modified May-Grant fitting technique (described later in the chapter). Subjects were followed for 1,000 days of lens wear and for 60 days after lens wear was discontinued. Kerns found that many orthokeratology patients were able to achieve desirable and impressive results, but that many showed little to no change at all. The mean reduction

in spherical equivalent for the orthokeratology group was 0.98 D, with results taking between 200 to 300 days to achieve. It was noted that the corneal shape factor played a greater role than the base curve-to-cornea relationship. This study also noted that as fits became flatter to achieve the desired results, the corneal responses became more variable and with-the-rule astigmatism increased. Kerns noted that the amount of corneal flattening measured by keratometry was usually less than the refractive error change. After discontinuation of lens wear, visual acuity and refractive error regressed toward baseline levels but did not return completely in some individuals.

Another early study, performed by Binder et al. (11), compared an orthokeratology group to a group of cosmetic rigid lens wearers for 40 months. The mean refractive change in the orthokeratology group was 1.60 D. They reported three levels of response to orthokeratology: no response, variable response, and good response. No response was defined as an improvement in unaided visual acuity of less than or equal to three lines, while good response was defined as an endpoint of 20/20 Snellen visual acuity. Those in the no-response category tended to have high amounts of initial myopia (mean of -3.95 D), while those in the variable-response and good-response categories had lower amounts of initial myopia (means of -1.98 D and -2.03 D, respectively). They also reported that, similar to Kerns' findings, predictability was poor, with-the-rule astigmatism increased, and vision and corneal measurements generally returned to baseline amounts when lens wear was discontinued. Interestingly, some orthokeratology patients complained of a decrease in the quality of their uncorrected vision while undergoing treatment, claiming it was similar to "a dirty windshield." No lasting detrimental corneal effects were reported, however.

The Berkeley Orthokeratology study was conducted by Polse et al. (8–10,26) in the early 1980s. The study compared a group of orthokeratology patients to a group of cosmetic rigid lens wearers. The patients were followed for 1.5 years. The lens material for this study was primarily PMMA, but some patients were refitted into Polycon GP material if hypoxic effects were noted. A mean refractive change of approximately 1.00 D was observed, with 40% of patients achieving more than this amount. It took approximately 130 days of therapy to achieve the results. It was also noted that vision without contact lenses was variable between subjects and that those subjects reporting good results stated that their vision fluctuated daily. After discontinuation of lens wear, it took approximately 90 days for the maximum amount of regression toward baseline measurements. In the orthokeratology group, the mean sphere after discontinuation was within 0.2 D of the original mean sphere, a clinically insignificant finding.

Coon (12) conducted an investigation evaluating the Tabb fitting philosophy (described later in the chapter) at Pacific University in 1984. Patients were followed for a total of 728 days. Maximum change occurred at approximately three months. A mean change in myopia of 0.73 D was observed. No significant increases in astigmatism were noted in this sample. The study also found central corneal thinning and peripheral corneal thickening.

Early Orthokeratology Fitting Philosophies

Jessen's orthofocus technique appears to be the earliest orthokeratology method described in the literature (3,27). This method utilized a plano-powered contact lens fitted flatter than the flat keratometry reading by the amount of the refractive error. In this manner, the tear layer under the contact lens provided the appropriate amount of refractive power to correct the patient's myopia. As the patient's cornea flattened and the refractive error was reduced, the tear lens was also reduced in power until the patient reached the maximum amount of correction possible. This technique suffers from the difficulty in obtaining and maintaining centration with very flat traditional lenses. The lenses were reported to be uncomfortable as well. For these reasons, success was usually limited to low amounts of refractive error. This technique for base curve selection is still used with some of the modern, reverse-geometry lenses to be described later.

Grant and May (28) in 1971 developed a somewhat different method of fitting rigid lenses for corneal reshaping. Instead of using very flat fitting lenses, they used a series of gradually flatter-fitting lenses until they achieved their results. Initially lenses were fit in alignment with the flattest K reading and the power determined from the vertex-adjusted spectacle refraction. Lens thickness was a key factor in their success. Thicker lenses were thought to be necessary to avoid lens flexure and to induce the desired flattening. Plano lenses had center thicknesses of 0.18 mm, and for each diopter of minus required the lens was thinned by 0.01 mm to avoid an uncomfortably thick lens edge. When a 0.50 D flattening of the cornea was noted, or when the patient accepted a plus power overrefraction, the lenses were exchanged for a pair fitted 0.50 to 1.50 D flatter than the new flat K reading. Once a desired endpoint was reached, a retainer lens had to be worn to maintain the effect, as the cornea would regress towards the original shape when lens wear was discontinued. Other fitting philosophies popular in the early years of orthokeratology utilized a similar technique (4–6, 29).

Tabb (12) utilized a somewhat unique method for performing orthokeratology. It had been noted that very flat-fitting lenses tended to increase with-the-rule astigmatism, due to the tendency for very flat lenses to decenter on the cornea. Tabb's method instead used steeper-than-K lenses (12). Patients with less than 1.00 D of astigmatism were initially fit 0.25 D steeper than flat K, and those with more than 1.00 D were fit 0.50 to 0.75 D steeper than flat K.

Tabb believed that the manipulation of fluid forces beneath the lens was the important factor in success, not simply having a very flat-fitting lens. This was manipulated in his lenses by careful design of the peripheral curve system of the lenses. Intermediate and peripheral curves were designed to occupy 32.5% of the posterior lens surface. As lens changes were needed, the base curve and diameter of the lens were kept constant, but the peripheral curves were widened until they occupied 45% of the lens. This method was reported to decrease the inducement of with-the-rule astigmatism, possibly due to the improved centration of the lenses (12).

Reverse-geometry Lens Designs

Reverse-geometry lens designs have a curvature profile that is "reversed" from traditional rigid lens designs. Traditional lens designs have secondary and peripheral curves that are progressively flatter than the central (base) curve of the lens. This design allows for tear exchange under the lens and prevents the periphery of the lens from rubbing and irritating the cornea. Reverse-geometry lenses have secondary curves that are steeper than the base curve instead of flatter. The peripheral curve design varies but usually is flatter than the secondary curve, and is designed to contour the peripheral cornea. The unique design of the reverse-geometry lens allows for improved centration on the eye and allows the corneal tissue to redistribute into the corneal periphery as the central cornea flattens (1,30).

The first mention of the use of a reverse-geometry design was by Fontana (31), although he did not use the term. He described his use of a "one piece bifocal" that had a back optic zone diameter of 6.0 mm and a secondary curve radius 1.00 mm steeper than the base curve. The lens was initially fitted 1.00 D flatter than the flat keratometry reading and was fit progressively flatter until the desired changes were achieved. The lens was reported to achieve good centration even when fit quite flat and allegedly prevented unwanted astigmatism.

Dr. Richard Wlodyga (32), a Detroit optometrist, first began working with reverse-geometry designs in 1989. He teamed with Nick Stoyan of Contex Laboratories (Sherman Oaks, CA) to develop what became known as the "OK" series of lenses for orthokeratology (2). They noted that the amount of change achievable with this type of design was greater than with traditional designs and was also more rapid. The term accelerated orthokeratology was coined to describe the procedure using reverse-geometry lenses for corneal reshaping. Orthokeratology with traditional designs could take many months to achieve the desired effect, whereas with accelerated orthokeratology it was claimed that results could be achieved in days to weeks. It was believed that the steeper secondary zone created a "tear reservoir" under the lens that served several purposes. This reservoir of tears was thought to enhance the delivery of oxygen to the cornea and to provide room for the peripheral cornea to steepen as the central cornea flattened while still allowing the lens to maintain good centration on the cornea (32). Many other laboratories have since created their own reverse-geometry lens designs for corneal reshaping. Although these designs all have unique, proprietary characteristics, they are all based on the original reverse-geometry concepts.

Overnight Contact Lens Corneal Reshaping (Orthokeratology)

Advances in contact lens materials have led to the introduction of highly oxygen-permeable materials. In the early days of orthokeratology, PMMA was the only material available. As GP materials were introduced in the 1980s, daytime lens wear became safer, with less resulting corneal edema from nonpermeable PMMA. As the permeability of materials increased, extended-wear of rigid lenses became a viable option. Night therapy was born out of these advancements. According to Grant (33), overnight wear of reverse-geometry lenses has numerous advantages over daytime wear, including:

- convenience for the patient, as (theoretically) no optical devices are required during the course of the day;
- better ocular health, as the wearing time of the lenses is decreased;
- little lens adaptation is required, as lens irritation is reduced during the closed-eye sleeping situation;
- increased effectiveness, as there is increased eyelid pressure from closed eyes and rapid eye movement during sleep; and
- may retard or stop the progression of myopia if used in children.

These claims for overnight corneal reshaping have not been substantiated by large-scale university-based clinical trials. However, in June 2002, Paragon Vision Sciences (Mesa, AZ) became the first manufacturer to receive approval from the US Food and Drug Administration for a lens designed for overnight corneal reshaping.

Mechanism

Early studies of orthokeratology attributed the changes to several factors, including axial length changes (4), although this was later refuted (34), and reduction of ciliary spasm (35). Recent efforts have produced more compelling explanations, though more research is needed. Swarbrick et al. (1) used optical pachymetry to measure corneal thickness at various points in the central and peripheral cornea before and after daily wear of corneal-reshaping lenses. Statistically significant central corneal epithelial thinning on the order of 7 μm and midperipheral stromal thickening were observed. Munnerlyn's formula, used in laser refractive surgery to calculate the depth of the ablation, was used to calculate the expected change in refraction based on the change in corneal sagittal height observed. It was concluded that the change in sagittal height can account for the refractive change, and concluded that the changes to the cornea are an anterior corneal phenomenon rather than an overall bending of the cornea. The changes in thickness noted were likely due to a redistribution of tissue from the central to midperipheral cornea. Nichols et al. (23) performed a similar study of thickness changes associated with overnight orthokeratology. The Orbscan Slit Scan Corneal Topography/Pachometry System Analyzer (Bausch & Lomb, Rochester, NY) was used to measure corneal thickness. A statistically significant central corneal thinning was observed. Swarbrick and Alharbi (30) repeated the previous study using overnight lens wearers and found similar results.

Predictive Factors

Contact lens corneal reshaping can produce impressive results with reverse-geometry lens designs, but individual patient responses are somewhat variable. If corneal reshaping is to be accepted by the ophthalmic community, clinicians will need to be able to better predict how patients will respond to treatment in order to properly counsel them on their likely success.

The most commonly cited factor thought to be predictive of change in corneal reshaping is the baseline corneal eccentricity value. It has been noted that with corneal reshaping, the cornea changes from an oblate ellipselike shape (central corneal curvature is steeper than the peripheral corneal curvature) to a more spherical shape (13,36). Several models have been developed, the most notable being that of Mountford (37), which states that a reduction in eccentricity by 0.2 leads to a change of 1.00 D in refractive error. However, Joe et al. (25) did not find a significant correlation between eccentricity and refractive error change. In a more recent study, Liu et al. (21) did find baseline eccentricity to be a useful prediction factor, but only in a multiple-factor model.

Other predictive factors suggested have been ocular rigidity (25), baseline refractive error (36), and baseline corneal thickness (21). Liu found no predictive value in ocular rigidity, but did find that baseline corneal thickness was somewhat predictive of the amount of change possible. Using a multiple-factor model, a combination of eccentricity and corneal thickness was most predictive of the refractive change, but it was not a strong indicator.

Efficacy

Studies of reverse-geometry lenses in corneal reshaping have shown various levels of change in refractive error. Soni and Horner (38) showed a maximum reduction in spherical equivalent (SE) of about 2.50 D, and a 40% reduction of astigmatism. Joe et al. (25) reported an SE mean change of 2.23 D, Mountford (37) showed an SE reduction of 2.19 D, and Nichols et al. (24) found an SE change of 1.83 D, but none of these studies described changes in astigmatism. Most recently, Liu et al. (21,22) showed a mean reduction of 1.50 D in the spherical component, an increase of less than 0.25 D of astigmatism, and a reduction in the SE of 1.45 D. All of these studies had a wide range of responses, partly depending on the initial refractive errors of the subjects, but generally ranged from 1.00 to 5.00 D of improvement of myopia.

Rah et al. (39) has conducted a multicenter pilot study to evaluate the safety and efficacy of overnight contact lens corneal reshaping in a sample of 60 adult patients. The patients were examined upon awakening and at least 6 hours following completion of the morning examination. Unaided and best-spectacle corrected logMAR visual acuities were recorded at each visit along with keratometry, corneal topography, refraction, and biomicroscopy. Of the 60 patients who began the study, 27 completed a 6-month evaluation. Some reasons for discontinuation from treatment were as follows:

- Residual astigmatism
- Poor comfort
- Treatment failure
- Unable to achieve adequate lens fit
- Poor motivation

A mean reduction in spherical equivalent manifest refraction of 2.15 ± 1.01 D was noted in the right eyes and 2.30 ± 1.06 D in the left eyes. A mean resultant spherical equivalent refractive error of 0.07 ± 0.59 D was attained in the right eyes and 0.05 ± 0.68 D in the left eyes of the 27 patients. High contrast visual acuity of at least 20/20 was achieved in 74.1% of patients. Fluorescein staining of the cornea was present in 76% of the right and left eyes of the patients; however, only one patient had staining above a grade 2 in the right eye and two patients had staining above a grade 2 in the left eye.

SAFETY

Overnight Gas-permeable Lens Wear Complications

Overnight GP lens wear is associated with numerous ocular health complications. Although these complications may be somewhat rarer than those encountered with overnight soft lens wear (40), a review of the major adverse responses to GP wear is needed to understand the potential impact of overnight corneal reshaping on eye health.

The majority of ocular complications from extended wear are the result of hypoxia. Hypoxia occurs when the oxygen demands of corneal metabolism are not adequately met as a result of decreased oxygen supply. As the cornea is avascular, the normal supply of oxygen to the cornea comes from the atmosphere via the tear film (41). When the eye is closed, however, the oxygen supply comes from diffusion from the capillary plexus of the tarsal conjunctiva, greatly diminishing the amount of available oxygen (42). A contact lens acts as a physical barrier to oxygen for the cornea, and has the potential to limit the oxygen supply enough to result in hypoxia. Short-term hypoxia to the cornea manifests itself in many ways. Clinically, the most commonly observed complications of short-term hypoxia include epithelial and stromal edema, infection/ulceration, contact lens-induced acute red eye (CLARE), neovascularization, infiltrative keratitis, epithelial microcysts and vacuoles, and the endothelial bleb response (43). Long-term hypoxia has been shown to produce stromal thinning (44), reduced sensitivity (45), poor adherence of epithelial cells to the basement membrane (46), delayed wound healing (47), and endothelial polymegethism and pleomorphism (48).

Many of the hypoxic effects of extended wear can be reduced with lenses that provide adequate oxygen supply to the cornea. Holden and Mertz (49) in 1984 conducted the landmark study on the lens material requirements for oxygen delivery to the cornea. They determined that, for overnight wear, a lens with a Dk/t value of 87.0×10^9 (cm $\times$ mL O_2)/(sec $\times$ mL $\times$ mm Hg), an equivalent oxygen percentage (EOP) of 18%, was needed to limit overnight swelling to 4% (the amount of normal overnight swelling without lens wear). However, as no hydrogel lenses were available at the time with this transmissibility, a compromise Dk/t of 35×10^{-9} (cm $\times$ mL O_2)/(s $\times$ mL $\times$ mm Hg), an EOP of 12%, was suggested. This EOP limited overnight swelling to approximately 8%, which allowed the cornea to revert back to normal thickness within a short time after eye opening.

Overnight GP wear has several complications not normally seen in hydrogel wear. These include corneal molding and distortion (50), lens adherence (51), and 3- and 9-o'clock staining (52). For orthokeratology, corneal molding is a desired outcome of lens wear, but in standard lens wear it should be avoided. Lens adherence presents a potentially significant complication, as removal of the lens can cause an epithelial abrasion and can lead to infection (52). Many GP wearers have mild 3- and 9-o'clock staining, but the incidence appears to be higher with overnight wear (52). As the staining persists and worsens, it can lead to erosion, dellen formation, and vascularized limbal keratitis (53). For all of these complications, design and/or material changes have been suggested to alleviate the problems, but the mechanisms for occurrence are still not completely understood.

In summary, overnight wear of contact lenses can increase the risk of ocular health complications. The risks can be minimized with careful lens design and monitoring by the clinician, but the potential benefits of overnight wear, including orthokeratology, must be carefully weighed against the risks. It is important to note that overnight lens wear with orthokeratology is not the same as extended wear of traditional rigid lens designs. Unlike extended wear, in overnight corneal reshaping the lenses are removed upon awakening and the eye is able to recover from the hypoxic state on a daily basis.

Overnight Contact Lens Corneal-reshaping Complications

Only a few adverse responses to overnight corneal reshaping have been reported in the literature. Gupta and Weinreb (54) reported a patient with an infection of a filtering bleb for glaucoma treatment in a patient undergoing orthokeratology. The authors acknowledged that any contact lens wear should be contraindicated in these patients and that corneal reshaping was not necessarily the sole reason for the infection. Levy (55) described a patient with permanent corneal warpage from orthokeratology treatment.

Chen et al. (56) described a case of a 9-year-old boy in Taiwan who experienced a corneal ulcer after approximately 8 months of orthokeratology lens wear. Less serious conditions such as clinically significant fluorescein staining of the cornea (24), imprinting, contact lens adherence, and epithelial microcysts may also result from overnight orthokeratology lens wear (39).

Recently, deposition, presumably of iron, in the corneal epithelium has been noted in patients undergoing overnight corneal-reshaping treatment. The deposition is arcuate or circular in appearance and occurs in the midperipheral cornea in the area corresponding to the reverse curve of the lens (Fig. 29.1). It is similar in appearance to findings seen in patients who have undergone surgical corneal-refractive procedures (57–64). The deposition is not sight-threatening and does not require treatment. In fact, one hypothesis is that it is a variation of the Hudson-Stahli line, a normal physiologic change seen in many normal patients (65).

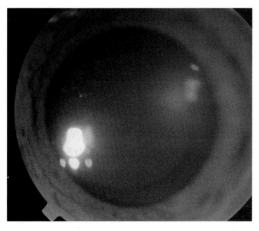

FIG. 29.1. Iron deposition in the midperipheral cornea of a patient undergoing overnight corneal-reshaping treatment.

None of the studies mentioned here reported any significant safety risks to using orthokeratology. Comparisons of corneal staining, edema, and other corneal health measures showed no difference between orthokeratology and standard contact lens wear. However, as Swarbrick (1) has concluded, any procedure that induces dramatic changes in corneal thickness like orthokeratology must be viewed with caution (1). As night wear of orthokeratology lenses increases, the potential for complications may increase.

Patient Selection

Selecting the best candidate for treatment is a critical factor in the success of contact lens corneal reshaping. It is important to perform a comprehensive case history and determine the expectations of the patient. It can take anywhere from 1 week to 1 month for treatment with orthokeratology to be effective, depending on the initial refractive error and the corneal response to treatment. Multiple visits may be necessary to achieve the best possible treatment outcome. These aspects of the procedure should be communicated to the patient prior to lens fitting. If the patient is aware of these considerations, it is more likely that the treatment will be successful.

When selecting patients for orthokeratology, the following should be considered. The patient must be motivated to wear the lenses and must be willing to agree to the necessary follow-up schedule. Orthokeratology is most successful for low-to-moderate amounts of myopia (up to -6.00 D) and with-the-rule astigmatism (up to -1.75 D). It is not as successful for high myopia, high astigmatism, or moderate-to-high amounts of against-the-rule astigmatism. To maximize success, especially in patients with against-the-rule astigmatism, any predicted residual astigmatism should be demonstrated to the patient prior to initiation of treatment.

It has not been determined to what extent orthokeratology is effective in the treatment of astigmatic refractive errors. Against-the-rule astigmatism is often internal rather than corneal and cannot be treated by flattening the cornea. For this reason, when selecting patients for the procedure, it is best to limit the amount of against-the-rule astigmatism to that which a patient can tolerate uncorrected. Limiting treatment to patients with 1 D or less of against-the-rule astigmatism is a good guideline for success.

Good lens centration is also critical for success with orthokeratology treatment. The optic zone (which creates the treatment zone on the cornea) must be centered over the pupil to achieve the best visual outcome. Patients with greater than 2 D of corneal astigmatism often require toric base curves in traditional rigid lens designs to maintain acceptable lens to cornea apical fitting relationships and adequate lens centration (66). Although some orthokeratology lens designs can be manufactured with toric peripheral radii of curvatures, it is best to limit the amount of corneal astigmatism to 2 D of with-the-rule astigmatism.

Pupil size is also an important consideration for corneal-reshaping treatment. Patients with large pupils are more likely to experience glare or halos in dim lighting conditions and may have difficulty with night driving.

FITTING PROCEDURES

Basic Lens Terminology

Modern contact lens corneal reshaping involves the use of reverse-geometry lenses to achieve the desired shape change and vision improvement. The concept was first introduced by Fontana (31) when he described the use of his "one-piece" bifocal lens. The design was later improved upon by Contex Labs (Sherman Oaks, CA) and other laboratories. Since the introduction of this basic concept in the 1980s, advances in corneal topography, manufacturing technology, and the basic science behind this procedure have resulted in greatly improved lens designs and reproducibility of lenses.

Today's reverse-geometry lenses are comprised of essentially three distinct zones. A commonly used way to illustrate these zones is with a "top-hat" or "bottle-cap" type of drawing, as shown in Fig. 29.2 (67–69). From center to periphery, the zones are often called the Base Curve or Treatment Zone, the Reverse Zone, and the Alignment Zone. The exact terminology is somewhat inconsistent, as various manufacturers have their own names for these areas of the lens. There is much variation in the actual number of curves and techniques used to generate them (spherical, aspheric, or other configurations). However, the basic concepts the clinician needs to know are essentially the same for all lenses.

Base Curve/Treatment Zone

The base curve or treatment zone of the lens corresponds to the optic zone of a standard rigid lens. This central portion of the lens is usually fit flatter than the corneal curvature to provide a "mold" for the desired corneal shape change. The exact amount of flatness will vary with the fitting technique or system, but it is usually chosen to be flatter than the patient's flat keratometry value by the amount of myopia to be treated (and usually an additional 0.50 to 0.75 flatter to allow for regression of refractive error throughout the day) if the desired endpoint of treatment is emmetropia to low hyperopia. The treatment zone is usually about 6 mm in diameter.

For many designs, the base curve is calculated based on the Jessen technique using the spherical portion of the refractive error, the flat keratometry reading, and an allowance for regression throughout the day (3,27). For example, if a patient is a −3.00 D myope with keratometry readings of 43.00/44.00 @ 090, and you predict the patient's treatment will regress approximately 0.5 D throughout the day, the following base curve should be selected if the desired endpoint is emmetropia to low hyperopia:

43.00 (flat keratometry reading)
−3.00 (sphere of spectacle refractive error)
−0.50 (allowance for regression)
────────────────────────────────
39.50 = initial base curve selection

Once the base curve has been calculated, it should not be modified to improve the lens fit. Changes should only be made in the base curve radius in instances of under-treatment or poor retention throughout the day.

Reverse Zone

The secondary or reverse zone is designed to bring the lens back towards the cornea just beyond the end of the treatment zone. The reverse zone is often 1 to 2mm in diameter. In a standard tricurve rigid lens design, if the central lens curvature were much flatter than the corneal curvature, the lens would teeter and rock on the corneal apex, causing it to decenter. By having the second zone of the lens contour back towards the cornea, this problem is minimized. This configuration is responsible for the ring of fluorescein pooling seen in the paracentral zone of well-fitted reverse-geometry lenses (Fig. 29.3; see Color Plate 29.3).

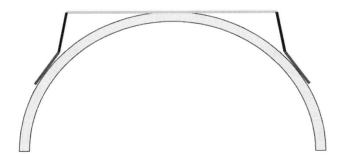

FIG. 29.2. "Bottle-cap" illustration of an ideal fit of a reverse-geometry lens on a cornea.

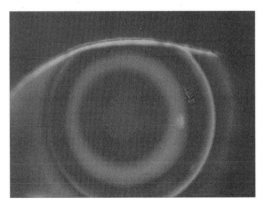

FIG. 29.3. Fluorescein pattern of an ideal fit of a reverse-geometry lens design. (See Color Plate 29.3.)

After the base curve has been calculated, trial fitting is conducted to determine the proper reverse zone for the lenses. Each lens design follows a slightly different procedure for lens fitting; however, in most instances the resulting fluorescein patterns are similar to that shown in Fig. 29.3.

Alignment Zone

The peripheral or alignment zone of the lens is designed to flatten the periphery of the lens after the steep reverse zone and contour the peripheral cornea. This configuration adds to the stability of the lens on the cornea and aids in lens centration. This zone is observed as the broad area of touch in the periphery of a well-fitting lens (Fig. 29.3). The addition of the alignment zone usually results in an overall diameter of reverse-geometry lenses equal to 10 to 11mm in diameter. The lens diameter is based on the horizontal visible iris diameter and is approximately 90% of this measurement.

In summary, Figs. 29.2 and 29.3 show an "ideal" fit of a reverse-geometry lens for corneal reshaping. The diagram shows the lens just returning to the cornea at the outer edge of the reverse zone, and the alignment zone of the lens is parallel to the cornea.

Basic Fitting Concepts

Lens Design Method Options

As with any rigid lens fit, a reverse-geometry lens can be designed in one of two ways: empirically, using the patient's refraction, keratometry values, and corneal topography; or diagnostically, using trial sets of known lenses and fluorescein pattern analysis to determine the appropriate lens parameters for a given patient. Both techniques have merits and flaws, but in either case, the practitioner must be able to understand the basic characteristics of how these lenses perform on the patient's eye.

Empirical fitting has a number of advantages, including reduced chair time for the clinician, fewer lenses to try on the eye, and a reasonable rate of first-time fit success. Each lens laboratory has a unique method of designing lenses based on the patient's data, but most use sophisticated computer technology to determine the correct lens parameters. By examining the contours of the cornea from corneal topography, these programs are able to make lenses that closely evaluate the sagittal depth of the cornea and theoretically predict a precise fit.

There are several problems with empirical fitting. As precise as modern topographers are, there is still potential for measurement error with these instruments. Each topographer and lens software package is only as good as the computational algorithms with which it is programmed. All such programs are subject to the programmers' assumptions and bias to some degree. They also do not allow the clinician

to assess movement of the lens on the eye and any interaction with the lid that may occur.

Diagnostic fitting is useful for many practitioners. Diagnostic fitting allows the clinician to assess lens movement, positioning, and bearing pattern with each lens. By interpretation of fluorescein patterns, the lens fit can be altered until an adequate fit is obtained.

Diagnostic fitting has limitations as well. Multiple lenses may be required to obtain the correct fit, increasing chair time for the clinician. This method has also been criticized as being less accurate, as the differences in fluorescein patterns among trial lenses are subtle and may be difficult for the clinician to assess (70).

Regardless of the method used to select an initial lens, requesting a summary of the lens parameters from the laboratory is important with empirical fitting. If problems arise, knowing the original parameters of the lenses is beneficial for troubleshooting problems during follow-up.

Characteristics of a Good Reverse-geometry Lens Fit

Centration

Lenses for corneal reshaping must center well over the pupil immediately after a blink. Lenses with poor centration do not applanate the cornea over the appropriate area. This results in a decentered treatment zone, which is likely to cause induced astigmatism and halos or ghosting in dim illumination. This effect is similar to a decentered ablation in refractive surgery. Good centration is essential for success in contact lens corneal reshaping.

Central Bearing

In a well-fitted reverse-geometry lens, there is usually about 4 to 5 mm of central bearing in the treatment zone of the lens. Inadequate central bearing will likely result in undertreatment.

Paracentral Ring of Fluorescein Pooling

As the reverse zone of the lens reapproaches the cornea, there is a space created in the paracentral area of the lens that fills with tears. This produces the ring of fluorescein pooling just beyond the treatment zone of the lens. Depending on the lens design, this area of pooling should be between 1 and 2 mm in width.

Peripheral Touch and Edge Clearance

A properly designed alignment zone will show bearing in the periphery of the lens upon fluorescein evaluation. In addition, the lens should also show an adequate amount of fluorescein pooling under the edge of the lens (edge lift) to allow for tear exchange. Evaluation of edge lift can also be used as an indicator of appropriate alignment zone fit. An appropriate amount of edge pooling is approximately 0.25 mm.

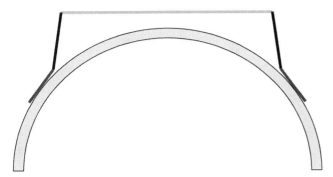

FIG. 29.4. Illustration of excessive sagittal depth from a steep reverse zone.

Overall Diameter

Most reverse-geometry lenses are large compared to traditional rigid lens designs. The large diameter aids in centration of the lens. A rule-of-thumb is to design a lens with a total diameter that is approximately 90% of the horizontal visible iris diameter. This usually results in an overall diameter of 10.5 to 11.5 mm.

Troubleshooting

Excess Sagittal Depth: Steep Reverse Curve

The reverse curve serves to bring the lens back towards the cornea beyond the flat base curve. If the reverse curve is too steep, the result is a lens with excessive sagittal depth that does not provide adequate central touch, shown in Figs. 29.4 and 29.5 (see Color Plate 29.5) (67–69). The lens shown in Fig. 29.5 shows good centration but only approximately 3 mm of central touch, indicating the overall sagittal depth is excessive. The small bubble in the reverse zone in Fig. 29.5 is also an indicator of excessive sagittal depth.

A lens that has excessive sagittal depth will result in a treatment zone with an inadequate diameter, little to no change in refraction and topography, or can result in a "central island" topography pattern (Fig. 29.6; see Color Plate 29.6). Excessive sagittal depth can also result in an increase in myopia.

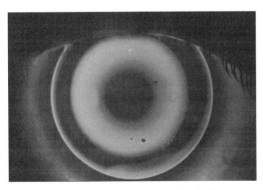

FIG. 29.5. Photo of a lens with sagittal depth that is too deep. (See Color Plate 29.5.)

Inadequate Sagittal Depth: Flat Reverse Curve

If the reverse curve is too flat, the lens fails to approach the cornea in the reverse zone, as shown in Fig. 29.7. This results in an insufficient sagittal depth and a lens that will teeter on the apex of the cornea and decenter, as shown in Fig. 29.8 (see Color Plate 29.8) (67–69). A decentered lens will result in a decentered area of applanation on the cornea, and subsequently a decentered treatment zone (Fig. 29.9; see Color Plate 29.9). This results in symptoms of halos and ghosting in dim illumination, and can produce induced astigmatism.

Flat Alignment Curve

An inappropriate alignment zone curvature will result in a poor lens fit. Note that in Figs. 29.5 and 29.7, there is good touch in the alignment zone and each lens has about 0.25 mm of pooling under the edge, indicating an appropriate alignment curve configuration. Figures 29.10 and 29.11 (see Color Plate 29.11) show a lens with a flat alignment zone, resulting in inadequate touch in the periphery of the lens and excessive edge lift (67–69). This causes excessive lid interaction and results in a decentered lens.

Steep Alignment Curve

If the alignment curve is too steep, the lens will have excessive bearing in the far periphery of the lens and cause the lens to bridge centrally, resulting in an excessive sagittal depth, and minimal edge lift as seen in Figs. 29.12 and 29.13 (see Color Plate 29.13) (67–69). Although there appears to be fluorescein under the edge of this lens, it is actually pooling around the perimeter of the lens, rather than under the edge; this indicates the alignment curve is too steep. Also note the bubble seen in the reverse zone of the lens. This is also indicative of the subtle "bridging" seen with this type of fit.

When fitting traditional rigid lenses, a common way to alter the centration of a lens is to adjust the base curve. Changes to the base curve should generally not be made with reverse-geometry lenses to improve lens centration for corneal reshaping. The base curve is calculated to achieve the desired refractive results. The other zones of the lens are used to control the overall sagittal depth of the lens to achieve the proper centration. Changes in the secondary curve, alignment zone and overall diameter are necessary to provide better lens centration.

Epithelial Disruption with Fluorescein Staining of the Cornea

Epithelial disruption with fluorescein staining of the cornea is common in patients undergoing overnight orthokeratology treatment. If corneal staining occurs, look for mechanical trauma or lack of tear exchange under the lens. A review of proper lens care is also important to make sure the patient is compliant with lens cleaning and disinfecting. Addition of an enzymatic cleaner may also aid in protein removal. If

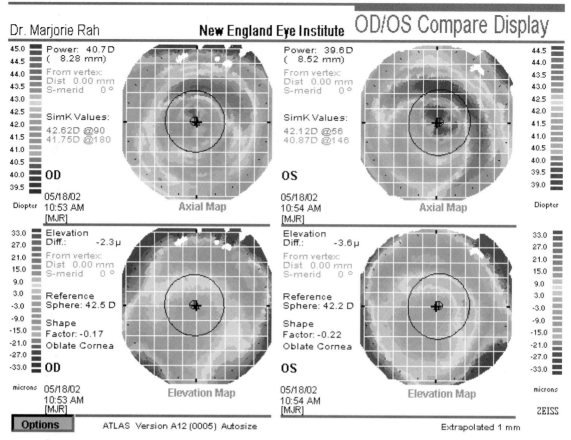

FIG. 29.6. Central island corneal topography caused by a lens with excess sagittal depth. (See Color Plate 29.6.)

the problem persists, it may be necessary to refit the contact lens. Use of a lens material with a higher Dk may be necessary. In addition, modifying the peripheral curve of the lens may help to increase tear flow.

Lens Adherence

Lens binding is not uncommon in orthokeratology and is usually detected early in the treatment. The patient should be instructed on how to remove the lens if lens binding

occurs. Rewetting drops should be applied, and the patient should gently manipulate the edge of the lens with the eyelid until the lens loosens. If lens binding becomes a chronic problem, the lens should be refitted. Some suggestions include using a contact lens material with a higher Dk value, decreasing the diameter of the lens, flattening the alignment

FIG. 29.7. Illustration of a lens with insufficient sagittal depth from a flat reverse zone.

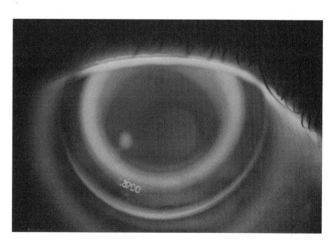

FIG. 29.8. Photo of a lens with sagittal depth that is too shallow. (See Color Plate 29.8.)

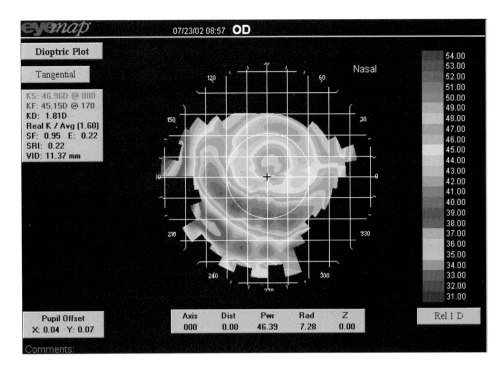

FIG. 29.9. Topography map from a lens with shallow sagittal depth. (See Color Plate 29.9.)

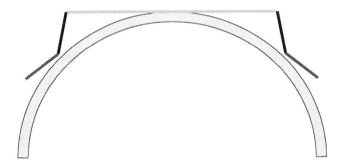

FIG. 29.10. Illustration of a lens with a flat alignment zone.

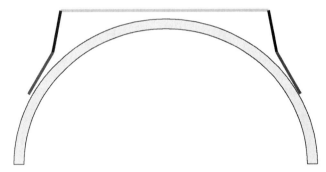

FIG. 29.12. Illustration of a deep lens from a steep alignment curve.

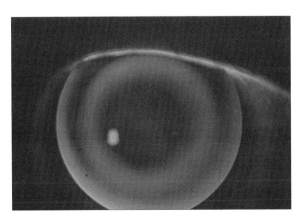

FIG. 29.11. Decentered lens due to a flat alignment zone. (See Color Plate 29.11.)

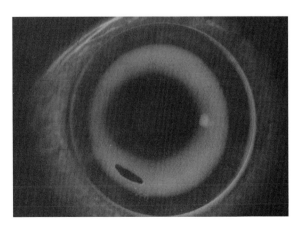

FIG. 29.13. Photograph of a lens with a steep alignment zone. (See Color Plate 29.13.)

and/or peripheral curve radius, and using artificial tears (71).

FOLLOW-UP CARE

It is best to examine the patient the first morning following overnight wear to assess lens fit, comfort, and corneal physiology, especially if the patient is new to overnight lens wear. The purpose of the 1-day visit is to assess the contact lens fit, evaluate the ocular health, and answer any questions or concerns the patient may have. Early signs of adherence or poor lens centration may be evident and can be corrected at this visit. Although it is not expected that the uncorrected visual acuity will be greatly improved at this time, some change in corneal shape and refraction will be noticeable even after one night of lens wear with a proper lens fit. The patient should be educated that the unaided vision will most likely regress significantly throughout the first day.

Depending on initial refractive error and whether some type of transitional correction is necessary, the patient is next examined 3 days to 1 week following dispensing of the treatment lenses. Testing at each follow-up visit should include entrance visual acuity, unaided visual acuity, refraction, biomicroscopy, corneal topography and an assessment of the contact lens-to- cornea fitting relationship. Symptoms of glare and/or halos are often reported at early visits. The patient should be reassured that most, but not all, of the glare will improve over the course of the treatment.

After 2 weeks of treatment, significant changes in corneal shape, unaided visual acuity and refraction should be evident and the patient should again be examined. In some patients, the treatment effect will occur rapidly, while in others corneal changes may occur gradually over the first 2 or 3 weeks. During this transitional period, disposable hydrogel lenses may be worn to improve vision. If significant change is not observed after two weeks of treatment, changes in one or more parameters of the lens should be considered. Changes in lens design should not be made prior to this point unless the fit is compromising corneal physiology or no treatment effect has been observed. Once successful treatment has been achieved, follow-up at 6-month intervals is recommended.

Patients undergoing contact lens corneal reshaping can benefit from purchasing a spare pair of treatment lenses. Unlike patients fitted with traditional contact lens designs, orthokeratology patients are greatly inconvenienced by a lost or broken treatment lens. Traditional lens wearers have the option of wearing spectacles while waiting for a new lens. A corneal-reshaping patient, however, has a limited period of time without treatment lenses before visual acuity regresses. To avoid this inconvenience to the patient, offer the option of ordering a spare pair of lenses once the final lens parameters are established and a good endpoint of treatment has been attained.

CASE REPORTS

Case 1

A 31-year-old Asian man, MSR, presented to the New England Eye Institute for treatment with overnight contact lens corneal reshaping. A pretreatment manifest refraction of $-3.25 -0.75 \times 090$ in the right eye and $-4.25 -0.75 \times 110$ in the left eye was obtained. Corrected Snellen visual acuity was 20/20 in each eye. Baseline keratometry readings were 43.50/42.62 @ 120 with clear and regular mires in the right eye and 43.12/43.37 @ 030 with clear and regular mires in the left eye. The patient was fitted with Paragon CRT lenses (Paragon Vision Sciences, Mesa, AZ). After 3 weeks of treatment, unaided visual acuity was 20/25 in both eyes. The patient's refractive error had improved to $+0.50 -0.50 \times 060$ in the right eye and $+0.50 -1.00 \times 120$ in the left eye. The patient complained of significant glare and halos, especially at night. Corneal topography showed treatment zones that were centered, but smaller than the pupil diameter (Fig. 29.14; see Color Plate 29.14). Upon examination of the fluorescein pattern of the treatment lenses, it was determined that the sagittal depth of the lenses was too deep. The secondary curve was changed to decrease the sagittal depth by 0.025 mm (25 μm) in both eyes. Unaided visual acuity with the new lenses was 20/25 in each eye. A spectacle refraction of $+0.75 -1.00 \times 090$ in the right eye and $+0.75 -1.00 \times 105$ in the left eye was achieved with the new lenses. Larger treatment zones were evident upon corneal topography with the new treatment lenses (Fig. 29.15; see Color Plate 29.15).

Case 2

A 24-year-old Asian man, NAB, presented to the Southern College of Optometry contact lens service desiring overnight contact lens corneal reshaping. A pretreatment manifest refraction of -3.00 sphere in the right eye and -3.25 sphere in the left eye was obtained. Corrected Snellen visual acuity was 20/20 in each eye. Baseline keratometry readings were 40.50/41.00 @ 090 with clear and regular mires in the right eye and 40.50/41.25 @ 090 with clear and regular mires in the left eye. Baseline topography is seen in the top two maps of Fig. 29.16 (see Color Plate 29.16). The patient was fitted with Paragon CRT lenses (Paragon Vision Sciences). He returned for examination the first morning after beginning overnight lens wear. At that visit, the refraction was -2.00 sphere in the right eye and the -2.25 sphere in the left eye, both corrected to 20/20. Corneal topography (bottom maps in Fig. 29.16) showed the beginnings of central flattening and midperipheral steepening with a well-centered treatment in both eyes. The patient was instructed to continue overnight lens wear.

At the 1-week follow-up appointment, the refraction was $-0.50 -0.25 \times 180$ in the right eye and $-0.75 -0.25 \times 180$ in the left eye, both corrected to 20/20. The topogra-

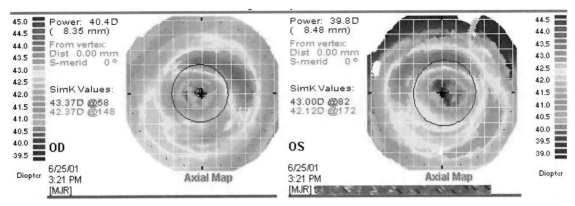

FIG. 29.14. Topography pattern for Case 1 depicting a small treatment zone from a lens with excessive sagittal depth. (See Color Plate 29.14.)

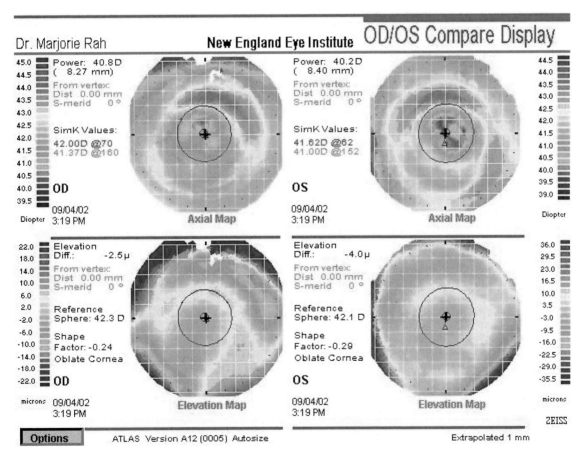

FIG. 29.15. Corneal topography for Case 1 following a change in contact lens parameters to increase the treatment zone diameter. (See Color Plate 29.15.)

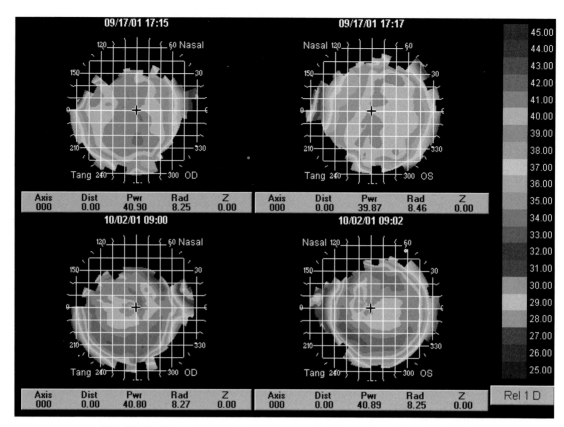

FIG. 29.16. Baseline corneal topography for Case 2. (See Color Plate 29.16.)

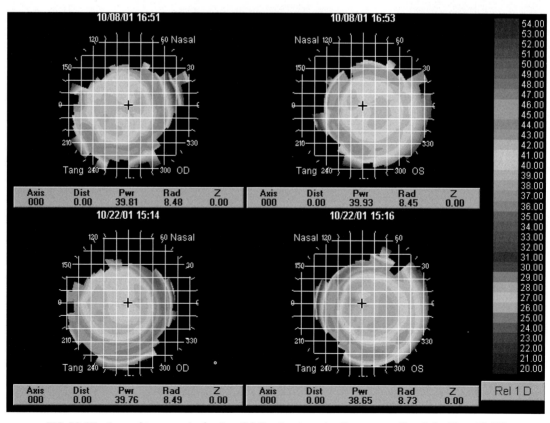

FIG. 29.17. Corneal topography for Case 2 following 1 week of treatment. (See Color Plate 29.17.)

phy maps (top of Fig. 29.17; see Color Plate 29.17) continued to show an adequate central flattening pattern. The patient reported acceptable comfort with the lenses and was pleased with the results.

At the 2-week follow up appointment, the refraction was +0.75 sphere in the right eye and +0.50 −0.25 × 180 in the left eye, both corrected to 20/20. Unaided acuities in each eye were 20/20. The patient reported good acuity all waking hours with treatment. The patient was instructed to continue lens wear every night and to report any problems.

Case 3

A 24-year-old white woman, CMA, presented to the Southern College of Optometry contact lens service desiring overnight contact lens corneal reshaping. A pretreatment manifest refraction of −4.50 −1.00 × 075 in the right eye and −4.50 sphere in the left eye was obtained. Corrected Snellen visual acuity was 20/20 in each eye. Baseline keratometry readings were 45.50/45.00 @ 090 with clear and regular mires in the right eye and 45.00/45.50 @ 090 with clear and regular mires in the left eye. Baseline topography is seen in the top two maps of Fig. 29.18 (see Color Plate 29.18). The patient was fitted with Paragon CRT lenses

(Paragon Vision Sciences). She returned the first morning after beginning lens wear. At that visit, the refraction in the right eye was −7.75 −1.00 × 075 and the refraction in the left eye was −3.00 sphere, both corrected to 20/20. Corneal topography (bottom maps of Fig. 29.18) revealed a central island pattern in the right eye, corresponding to the increase in myopia, and a normal central flattening pattern in the left eye, corresponding to the decrease in myopia in that eye. Lens wear was discontinued in the right eye until it returned to baseline; treatment continued in the left eye.

On the third day of treatment, the right eye had returned to baseline and the left eye continued to improve, as can be seen in the top maps in Fig. 29.19 (see Color Plate 29.19). At this visit, the refraction had returned to −4.75 −1.00 × 060 in the right eye and the left eye had improved to −0.50 sphere, both corrected to 20/20. The right lens was refitted with the same parameters as the left lens and provided an adequate fit.

Both eyes made steady progress after the right eye was refitted. At the two-week visit, the refraction was +0.50 −0.50 × 060 in the right eye and +0.50 sphere in the left eye at 4:00 p.m. Both eyes had an uncorrected visual acuity of 20/20. Topography maps (bottom of Fig. 29.19) showed a centered treatment zone with peripheral steeping.

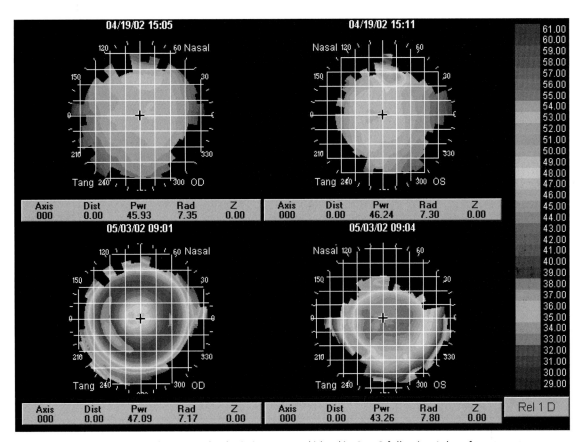

FIG. 29.18. Corneal topography depicting a central island in Case 3 following 1 day of treatment. (See Color Plate 29.18.)

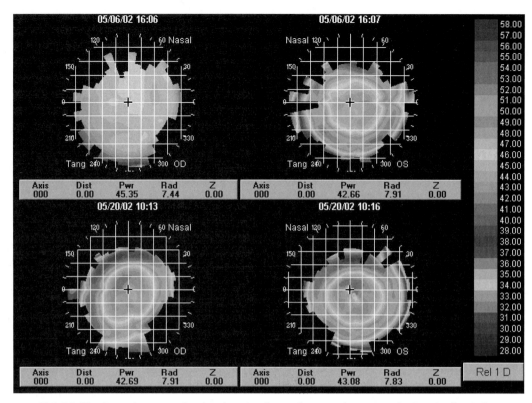

FIG. 29.19. Corneal topography showing the change in corneal curvature in Case 3 after 3 days of treatment. The central island has resolved, the right eye had returned to baseline values, and the left eye showed improved progress of the treatment. (See Color Plate 29.19.)

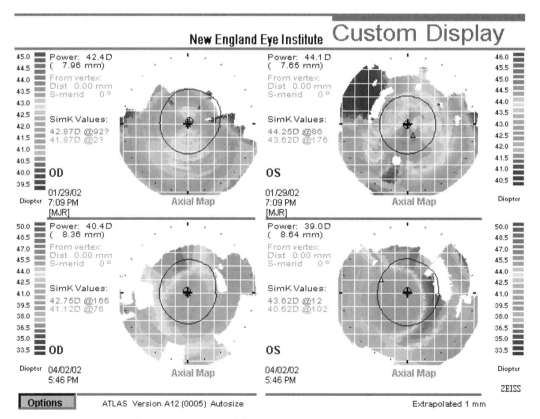

FIG. 29.20. Corneal topography maps following treatment with overnight corneal-reshaping contact lenses in Case 4. (See Color Plate 29.20.)

The patient continued to wear the lenses each night and maintained good visual acuity for all waking hours.

This case illustrates a central island topography. The lens parameters in the right lens were changed to decrease the overall sagittal depth of the lens. The sagittal depth of the secondary zone was decreased by 0.025 mm (25 μm) and the alignment/landing zone of the lens was flattened. This allowed the lens to applanate the central cornea more efficiently and improved the performance of the lens.

Case 4

A 12-year-old Asian boy, BL, presented to the New England Eye Institute interested in overnight contact lens corneal reshaping. A pretreatment manifest refraction of − 4.25 sphere in the right eye and − 4.25 − 0.50 × 150 in the left eye was obtained. Corrected Snellen visual acuity was 20/20 in each eye. Baseline keratometry readings were 44.00/44.75 @ 090 with clear and regular mires in the right eye and 43.50/44.75 @ 090 with clear and regular mires in the left eye. Baseline topography is seen in the top two maps of Fig. 29.20 (see Color Plate 29.20). The patient was fitted with DreimLens design lenses.

At the 1-week follow-up appointment, the refraction was + 0.25 sphere in the right eye and − 0.25 sphere in the left eye, both corrected to 20/20. Unaided visual acuities were 20/20 in each eye. At the two week follow up appointment, the refraction was plano in the right eye and + 0.50 sphere in the left eye, both corrected to 20/20. Unaided acuities in each eye were 20/20. The patient reported good acuity all waking hours with treatment. The patient was instructed to continue lens wear every night and to report any problems. The final topography maps are provided in the bottom two maps of Fig. 29.20.

CONCLUSION

Children can be excellent candidates for contact lens corneal reshaping. Many children are active in sports or other activities in which wearing glasses or contact lenses can be bothersome. Overnight contact lens corneal reshaping may be a good alternative for this population. Care should be taken to instruct the child and parents concerning proper handling and care of the treatment lenses.

REFERENCES

1. Swarbrick HA, Wong G, O'Leary DJ. Corneal response to orthokeratology. *Optom Vis Sci* 1998;75:791–799.
2. Winkler TD, Kame RT. *Orthokeratology handbook,* 1st ed. Boston: Butterworth-Heinemann, 1995.
3. Jessen GN. Orthofocus techniques. *Contacto* 1962;6:200–204.
4. Nolan JA. Orthokeratology. *J Am Optom Assoc* 1971;42: 355–360.
5. Ziff SL. Orthokeratology. II. *J Am Optom Assoc* 1968;39: 243–254.
6. Ziff SL. Orthokeratology. 1. *J Am Optom Assoc* 1968;39: 143–147.
7. El Hage SG, Baker RN. Controlled kerato-reformation for postoperative radial keratotomy patients. *Int Eyecare* 1986;2:49–53.
8. Polse KA, Brand RJ, Schwalbe JS, Vastine DW, Keener RJ. The Berkeley Orthokeratology Study, Part II: Efficacy and duration. *Am J Optom Physiol Opt* 1983;60:187–198.
9. Polse KA, Brand RJ, Keener RJ, Schwalbe JS, Vastine DW. The Berkeley Orthokeratology Study, part III: safety. *Am J Optom Physiol Opt* 1983;60:321–328.
10. Polse KA, Brand RJ, Vastine DW, Schwalbe JS. Corneal change accompanying orthokeratology. Plastic or elastic? Results of a randomized controlled clinical trial. *Arch Ophthalmol* 1983;101: 1873–1878.
11. Binder PS, May CH, Grant SC. An evaluation of orthokeratology. *Ophthalmology* 1980;87:729–744.
12. Coon LJ. Orthokeratology. Part II: evaluating the Tabb method. *J Am Optom Assoc* 1984;55:409–418.
13. Kerns RL. Research in orthokeratology. Part III: results and observations. *J Am Optom Assoc* 1976;47:1505–1515.
14. Kerns RL. Research in orthokeratology. Part II: experimental design, protocol and method. *J Am Optom Assoc* 1976;47: 1275–1285.
15. Kerns RL. Research in orthokeratology. Part I: introduction and background. *J Am Optom Assoc* 1976;47:1047–1051.
16. Kerns RL. Research in orthokeratology. Part VII: examination of techniques, procedures and control. *J Am Optom Assoc* 1977; 48:1541–1553.
17. Kerns RL. Research in orthokeratology. Part VI: statistical and clinical analyses. *J Am Optom Assoc* 1977;48:1134–1147.
18. Kerns RL. Research in orthokeratology. Part V: results and observations—recovery aspects. *J Am Optom Assoc* 1977;48:345–359.
19. Kerns RL. Research in orthokeratology. Part IV: results and observations. *J Am Optom Assoc* 1977;48:227–238.
20. Kerns RL. Research in orthokeratology. Part VIII: results, conclusions and discussion of techniques. *J Am Optom Assoc* 1978;49: 308–314.
21. Lui WO, Edwards MH. Orthokeratology in low myopia. Part 1: efficacy and predictability. *Contact Lens Anterior Eye* 2000;23: 77–89.
22. Lui WO, Edwards MH. Orthokeratology in low myopia. Part 2: corneal topographic changes in safety over 100 days. *Contact Lens Anterior Eye* 2000;23:90–99.
23. Lui WO, Edwards MH, Cho P. Contact lenses in myopia reduction: from orthofocus to accelerated orthokeratology. *Contact Lens Anterior Eye* 2000;23:68–76.
24. Nichols JJ, Marsich MM, Nguyen M, Barr JT, Bullimore MA. Overnight orthokeratology. *Optom Vis Sci* 2000;77:252–259.
25. Joe JJ, Marsden HJ, Edrington TB. The relationship between corneal eccentricity and improvement in visual acuity with orthokeratology. *J Am Optom Assoc* 1996;67:87–97.
26. Brand RJ, Polse KA, Schwalbe JS. The Berkeley Orthokeratology Study, Part I: General conduct of the study. *Am J Optom Physiol Opt* 1983;60:175–186.
27. Jessen GN. Contact lenses as a therapeutic device. *Arch Am Acad Optom* 1964;41:429–435.
28. Grant SC, May CH. Orthokeratology control of refractive errors through contact lenses. *J Am Optom Assoc* 1971;42:345–359.
29. Neilson RH, Grant SC, May CH. Emmetropization through contact lenses. *Contacto* 1964;8:20–21.
30. Swarbrick HA, Alharbi A. Overnight orthokeratology induces central corneal epithelial thinning. *Invest Ophthalmol Vis Sci* 2001;42:S597.

31. Fontana AA. Orthokeratology using the one piece bifocal. *Contacto* 1974;18:45–47.
32. Wlodyga RJ, Bryla C. Corneal molding: the easy way. Contact Lens Spectrum 1989;4:58–62.
33. Grant SC. Orthokeratology night therapy and retention. *Contacto* 1995;35:30–33.
34. Erickson PM. Accounting for refractive change in orthokeratology. *Contacto* 1978;22:9–12.
35. Grant SC, May CH. Orthokeratology: a therapeutic approach to contact lens procedures. *Contacto* 1970;14:3–16.
36. Carkeet NL, Mountford JA, Carney LG. Predicting success with orthokeratology lens wear: a retrospective analysis of ocular characteristics. *Optom Vis Sci* 1995;72:892–898.
37. Mountford J. An analysis of the changes in corneal shape and refractive error induced by accelerated orthokeratology. *Int Contact Lens Clin* 1997;24:128–143.
38. Soni P, Horner D. Orthokeratology. In: Bennett ES, Weissman B, eds. *Clinical contact lens practice.* Philadelphia: Lippincott-Raven, 1997:49-1–49-7.
39. Rah MJ, Jackson JM, Jones LA, Marsden HJ, Bailey MD, Barr JT. Overnight orthokeratology: preliminary results of the lenses and overnight orthokeratology (LOOK) Study. *Optom Vis Sci* 2002;79:598–605.
40. Schnider CM. Rigid gas permeable extended-wear lenses. In: Silbert JA, ed. *Anterior segment complications of contact lens wear,* 2nd ed. Boston: Butterworth-Heinemann, 2000:309–328.
41. Lemp MA, Wolfley DE. The lacrimal apparatus. In: Hart WMJ, ed. *Adler's physiology of the eye.* 9th ed. St. Louis: Mosby-Year Book, 1992.
42. Pepose JS, Ubels JL. The cornea. In: Hart WMJ, ed. *Adler's physiology of the eye.* 9th ed. St. Louis: Mosby-Year Book, 1992.
43. Bruce AS, Brennan NA. Corneal pathophysiology with contact lens wear. *Surv Ophthalmol* 1990;35:25–58.
44. Holden BA, Sweeney DF, Vannas A, Nilsson KT, Efron N. Effects of long-term extended contact lens wear on the human cornea. *Invest Ophthalmol Vis Sci* 1985;26:1489–1501.
45. Millodot M. Effect of long-term wear of hard contact lenses on corneal sensitivity. *Arch Ophthalmol* 1978;96:1225–1227.
46. Madigan MC, Holden BA, Kwok LS. Extended wear of contact lenses can compromise corneal epithelial adhesion. *Curr Eye Res* 1987;6:1257–1260.
47. Mauger TF, Hill RM. Corneal epithelial healing under contact lenses. Quantitative analysis in the rabbit. *Acta Ophthalmol (Copenh)* 1992;70:361–365.
48. Schoessler JA. Corneal endothelial polymegathism associated with extended wear. *Int Contact Lens Clin* 1983;10:148–155.
49. Holden BA, Mertz GW. Critical oxygen levels to avoid corneal edema for daily and extended wear contact lenses. *Invest Ophthalmol Vis Sci* 1984;25:1161–7.
50. Key JE, Mobley CL. Paraperm EW lens for extended wear. *CLAO J* 1989;15:134–137.
51. Kenyon E, Polse KA, Mandell RB. Rigid contact lens adherence: incidence, severity and recovery. *J Am Optom Assoc* 1988;59:168–174.
52. Schnider CM, Zabkiewicz K, Holden BA. Unusual complications associated with RGP extended wear. *Int Contact Lens Clin* 1988;15:124–128.
53. Levy B. Rigid gas-permeable lenses for extended wear: a 1-year clinical evaluation. *Am J Optom Physiol Opt* 1985;62:889–894.
54. Gupta N, Weinreb RN. Filtering bleb infection as a complication of orthokeratology. *Arch Ophthalmol* 1997;115:1076.
55. Levy B. Permanent corneal damage in a patient undergoing orthokeratology. *Am J Optom Physiol Opt* 1982;59:697–699.
56. Chen KH, Kuang TM, Hsu WM. Serratia Marcescens corneal ulcer as a complication of orthokeratology. *Am J Ophthalmol* 2001;132:257–258.
57. Ozdamar A, Aras C, Sener B, Karacorlu M. Corneal iron ring after hyperopic laser-assisted in situ keratomileusis. *Cornea* 1999;18:243–245.
58. Ozdamar A, Aras C, Ustundag C, Bahcecioglu H, Ozkan S. Corneal iron ring associated with iatrogenic keratectasia after myopic laser in situ keratomileusis. *J Cataract Refract Surg* 2000;26:1684–1686.
59. Probst LE, Almassway MA, Bell B. Pseudo-Fleischer ring after hyperopic laser in situ keratomileusis. *J Cataract Refract Surg* 1999;25:868–870.
60. Molina CA, Agudelo LM. Corneal iron pigmentation after LASIK for hyperopia. *J Cataract Refract Surg* 2000;16:755–756.
61. Nagy ZZ, Krueger RR, Hamberg-Systrom H, Fust A, Kovacs A, Kelemen E, et al. Photorefractive keratectomy for hyperopia in 800 eyes with the Meditec MEL 60 laser. *J Cataract Refract Surg* 2001;17:525–533.
62. Koenig SB, McDonald MB, Yamaguchi T, Friedlander M, Ishii Y. Corneal iron lines after refractive keratoplasty. *Arch Ophthalmol* 1983;101:1862–1865.
63. Assil KK, Quantock AJ, Barrett AM, Schanzlin DJ. Corneal iron lines associated with the intrastromal corneal ring. *Am J Ophthalmol* 1993;116:350–356.
64. Fink AM, Gore C, Rosen ES. Corneal changes associated with intrastromal corneal ring segments. *Arch Ophthalmol* 1999;117:282.
65. Rah MJ, Barr JT, Bailey MD. Corneal pigmentation in overnight orthokeratology: a case series. *Opt JAOA* 2002;73:425–434.
66. Edrington TB. Rigid gas permeable lenses for astigmatism. In: Hom MM, ed. *Manual of contact lens prescribing and fitting with CD-ROM,* 2nd ed. Boston: Butterworth-Heinemann, 2000:143–166.
67. Jackson JM. Ortho-k fits: the good, the bad, and the ugly, part III. *Contact Lens Spectr* 2002;17:21.
68. Jackson JM. Ortho-k fits: the good, the bad, and the ugly, part I. *Contact Lens Spectr* 2002;17:21.
69. Jackson JM. Ortho-k fits: the good, the bad, and the ugly, part II. *Contact Lens Spectr* 2002;17:21.
70. Mountford J, Caroline P, Noack D. Corneal topography and orthokeratology: pre-fitting evaluation. *Contact Lens Spectr* 2002;17:38–44.
71. Hom MM, Watanabe R. Rigid Gas-Permeable Cases. In: Hom MM, ed. *Manual of contact lens prescribing and fitting with CD-ROM,* 2nd ed. Boston: Butterworth-Heinemann, 2000:419–422.

APHAKIA

LARRY J. DAVIS
CHERYL BERGIN
AND EDWARD S. BENNETT

Removal of a cataractous crystalline lens continues to be one of the most frequently performed surgical procedures throughout the United States. The number of surgeries, including implantation of an intraocular lens (IOL), have been increasing rapidly during the past two decades. However, the number of patients who remain aphakic following surgery has been declining during this time period for the same reason. This is the result of a combination of factors such as the quality of IOLs, improved surgical techniques, and low incidence of complications associated with this modality (1).

It is apparent that as the number of individuals requiring optical correction of surgical aphakia is dwindling. The pool of patients with aphakia comes primarily from the existing population, from those patients where an IOL is contraindicated, or from "secondary aphakia" in patients who have demonstrated the need for removal of a primary implant and are considered poor candidates for a secondary implant. Contact lens manufacturers have responded to this trend of fewer patients with aphakia by not including aphakic powers in their application for US Food and Drug Administration approval for new materials (2).

The most frequent, yet controversial, contraindication for implantation of an IOL is a young age. Recent advances in surgical technique, technology of IOL design, and practitioner philosophy have altered the accepted age standard in the decision whether or not to place an IOL. In addition, concern has been expressed pertaining to the refractive power changes that are expected with axial length changes. However, this concern has been alleviated by considering the expected rate of myopic shift that occurs in the growing eye when deriving the power in the IOL (1,3,4).

However, in addition to the relative youth of a patient, an unplanned occurrence during a primary cataract extraction can complicate implantation and the long-term success of an IOL. Also, many patients who have developed crystalline lens opacification, secondary to blunt or penetrating injury, are frequently considered poor candidates for implantation of an IOL. Other factors to consider include diabetic retinopathy, uncontrolled glaucoma, aniridia, a chronically infected eye, and one-eyed patients (5,6).

Prior to the introduction of the corneal contact lens, the primary mode of correction for the large hyperopic refractive error resulting from cataract surgery was spectacles. Aphakic spectacle correction results in specific physical and optical problems, which make them a less desirable mode of correction compared to contact lenses. Spectacle lenses for aphakia demonstrate all the various imperfections of any thick spectacle lens (7).

These high-powered lenses (usually between + 10 D and + 14 D) demonstrate significant chromatic and spherical aberration, distortion, prismatic affect, restriction of visual field, and, when used for the correction of monocular aphakia, diplopia. These properties usually make spectacle correction of aphakia undesirable with few exceptions (Fig. 30.1) (7–9). In addition to optical problems, these thick lenses have physical disadvantages as well. The heavy weight of the spectacles makes them very difficult for patients to tolerate for long periods of wear. Proper lens position in most frames is very difficult. Even under the best conditions of frame choice, lens manufacturer, and lens positioning, patients frequently have difficulty maintaining the critical vertex distance throughout the wearing day resulting in periods of reduced visual acuity.

These optical and physical problems make spectacle correction of unilateral aphakia in patients whose paired eye has good visual function virtually contraindicated. Spectacle correction of bilateral aphakia can be successful and tolerated quite well. However, these spectacles are cosmetically unattractive, making the wearer's eyes unusually magnified.

The current method of choice for correction of aphakia is the use of contact lenses. This chapter will describe various considerations when prescribing contact lenses for the correction of aphakia. When fitting contact lenses for aphakia, practitioners are faced with two initial questions: daily wear versus extended wear, and gas permeable (GP) versus hydrogel. These decisions must include an evaluation of various patient, optical, and physiologic considerations. Following a discussion of these topics, lens design and fitting are reviewed.

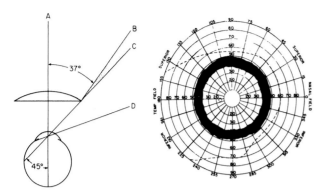

FIG. 30.1. Ring scotoma secondary to wearing aphakic spectacle lenses. (From Borish IM. Aphakia: perceptual and refractive problems of spectacle correction. *J Am Optom Assoc* 1983;54:701–711, with permission.)

PATIENT CONSIDERATIONS

Lens opacification, sufficient enough to result in decreased vision, can occur in all ages. However, the great majority of cataract surgeries are performed for elderly patients (10). Patients in this age group can demonstrate various eyelid, cornea, conjunctiva, and tear-film abnormalities, which should be considered prior to fitting a contact lens (11). Some patients may acquire a postsurgical ptosis, which can affect the dynamics of the contact lens on the eye. Eyelid elasticity may be lowered in these patients and result in specific fitting problems related to lens movement and adequate lens position (12). Alterations in tear film including a decrease in lacrimation and meibomian gland abnormalities are not uncommon with aging and may influence long-term success with contact lenses (13–15). These problems can be worse in cases of relatively poor hygiene. Evaluation for various corneal complications including guttata, scars, degenerations, dystrophies, and persistent epithelial defects should be considered prior to fitting contact lenses. Conjunctival changes, including superior limbic keratoconjunctivitis and pinguecula, can affect the success of contact lens wear (16).

Perhaps the most important consideration resulting from age is the patient's manual dexterity. This is an important observation during the initial fitting to determine whether a daily wear lens or an extended wear lens is indicated. In addition to problems with physical dexterity, many patients demonstrate a psychological reluctance to allow contact lens wear, or take control of lens care (11,16). When patients do not take an active role with lens care, their social situation and availability of assistance can further complicate successful lens wear. It is very tempting for the doctor to provided the patient with "an easy way out" and prescribe an extended-wear form of contact lens in these cases. However, the success of this form of correction is frequently short-lived, resulting in various lens-related complications, particularly if a non–silicone-based lens material is used (17–19).

Insertion, removal, and lens maintenance provided by a friend or family member should be considered for these patients.

While patients having bilateral aphakia may tolerate spectacle correction quite well, patients demonstrating unilateral aphakia tend to have more success with contact lens wear. For bilateral aphakia, the significant optical blur resulting when both contact lenses are removed can make it difficult for patients to perform lens insertion and removal. This also can occur when the paired eye is nonseeing. Highly motivated patients, however, may be successful. One technique is to provide a magnifying mirror and bright illumination to assist in visualizing the contact lens (20). Some bilateral aphakic patients benefit from using "limited" extended wear by removing one lens, on an alternate eye basis, each night. This prevents the disturbing optical blur that occurs when both lenses are removed. It also is helpful in patients are already familiar with contact lens care and insertion/removal prior to surgery. We prefer to reserve extended wear lenses with monthly in office cleanings for those limited number of patients who demonstrate the inability or lack of motivation to perform lens care and do not have a friend or family member to assist them in doing so.

Patients with glaucoma who are receiving topical medications may be poor candidates for hydrogel lenses. These lenses not only discolor with the use of some medications (21), but the lens may interfere with penetration of the drug and reduce its therapeutic effect (22–24). For example, with regard to drug delivery via hydrogel contact lenses, it has been found that the maximal effect occurs if lenses are soaked in the medication rather than having the medication dropped on top of the contact lens (23,24). One recommendation for glaucoma patients using daily wear soft contact lenses for aphakia and administering a drop of medication twice a day is to be told to wait 15 minutes after the A.M. drop to insert the lens, and to remove the lens prior to the P.M. drop. Lens removal prior to applying medication would be impractical for patients receiving a four-times-daily dose. A GP lens would be expected to have less influence on the efficacy of medications.

Some preservatives, such as benzalkonium chloride, chlorhexidine, and chlorbutanol, may become bound in the hydrogel lens material and result in keratitis (25–27). Some authors, therefore, have recommended that nonpreserved medications should be used with bandage soft contact lenses (28,29). Other authors have presented conflicting opinions regarding the risk of preservative keratitis with the use of topical medications while wearing hydrogel lenses (30,31).

Patients with dry eye who require frequent tear supplements should use a preservative-free solution while wearing a hydrogel lens. Frequent use of any preserved solution has the potential for resulting in toxicity, allergic reactions, and keratitis. The use of vasoconstrictors with hydrogel lens wear should be discouraged. Contact lens–related complications will be masked, preventing early intervention. Rebound hyperemia may occur on discontinuation of some sympatho-mimetic agents.

OPTICAL FACTORS

The primary goal of any form of optical correction following cataract surgery is to provide the wearer with the best potential visual acuity. Various optical considerations can influence the decision regarding the type of contact lens correction. These include refractive astigmatism, clarity of the media, pupil configuration, refractive error of the paired eye, and the potential visual acuity.

Perhaps the most important consideration when selecting the type of contact lens correction for aphakia is the degree and type of postoperative astigmatism. During the immediate postoperative period, it is not uncommon for the cornea to manifest 3 to 4 D of with-the-rule astigmatism. At 6 to 8 weeks after surgery, wound healing has reduced the astigmatism and the cornea is usually sufficiently stable to consider the fitting of a contact lens (32). Newer surgical techniques have reduced the large changes in postoperative astigmatism, as well as the time required for would healing and stabilization.

After deciding to proceed with contact lens fitting, the amount of final corneal astigmatism, and the patient's best potential visual acuity, can influence the amount of effort one gives to providing a full correction of the refractive error. A good estimate of the expected refractive astigmatic error is obtained from keratometry readings. Without the contribution of the crystalline lens, the cornea is likely to be the sole element contributing to the refractive astigmatism. The amount of acceptable residual astigmatism varies inversely with the potential visual acuity. In cases of significantly reduced, best-corrected visual acuity, the manifest refraction should include evaluating the results of undercorrecting the refractive astigmatism. Many of these patients do not benefit from the full astigmatic correction provided by a GP contact lens. This poor visual potential also can complicate attempts to achieve a daily lens wear schedule.

Many patients acquire alterations in iris anatomy during surgery. If they become sensitive to the conditions of high illumination, a darkly tinted hydrogel lens can be applied. These tinted lenses typically are not available using GP lens materials. Hydrogel lenses are tinted relatively easily with many companies making custom lenses (2,33). Contact lens tints sufficient to reduce glare in bright illumination will reduce vision at night during reduced lighting. Tints in the form of sunglasses may be more desirable. Many patients with rather dramatic alterations in iris structure, however, are virtually asymptomatic.

A GP contact lens can be applied in those patients who have more than 1 D of astigmatism and good potential visual acuity. This can be very beneficial if the paired eye requires no visual correction. This is the lens of choice if the patient shows any irregular astigmatism; however, this is rare following uncomplicated planned cataract extraction.

An alternate method of correction for astigmatism can include the use of spectacles over a soft lens. This can be very beneficial in patients who are unable to adapt to GP lens wear, who have corneal curvatures that complicate fitting of a rigid lens, or who are apprehensive regarding rigid contact lenses. In patients who require optical correction of the paired eye, one should attempt to balance an overcorrection in the aphakic eye. This can help provide better-quality binocular vision by creating approximately equal magnification between the eyes (34).

The contact lens-corrected aphakic eye demonstrates approximately 5% to 9% magnification compared to the phakic eye (Appendix 1). While this is greatly reduced from the 20% to 30% of that experienced with aphakic spectacle correction, some patients will be symptomatic (35,36). An iseikonic lens has been demonstrated to be beneficial for some patients with unilateral aphakia, with some obtaining subjective improvement by overcorrection of the aphakia, resulting in a minus-power spectacle correction at distance (37).

PHYSIOLOGIC CONSIDERATIONS

All contact lens wear can affect the integrity and physiology of the cornea, conjunctiva, and ocular tear surface (38). A complete discussion of these effects is found in other chapters. A discussion of a few frequently observed complications follows.

Perhaps the most significant effect resulting from contact lens wear for aphakia is a result of the relative barrier to oxygen transmission secondary to the thick lens. Corneal hypoxia can result from all contact lens wear. Some investigators have demonstrated decreased corneal edema in aphakic eyes compared to normal eyes under equal hypoxic stress (39–41). This reduced corneal edema in aphakic eyes has occurred without an accompanying decrease in the oxygen uptake rate at the corneal epithelium (40,41).

As a result of the limited oxygen permeability and great thickness of these lenses, all patients wearing hydrogel aphakic designs demonstrate significant corneal edema, which is particularly excessive in extended wear. Patients who have experienced prolapsed vitreous fluid into the anterior chamber, which makes contact with the endothelium, may develop dramatically increased corneal edema with extended wear lenses and a daily wear lens should be considered (42, 43). Holden and Mertz (44) have estimated the required oxygen transmissibility (Dk/L) for zero swelling with cosmetic daily wear as 24×10^{-9} (cm $\times$ m^{102}) / (s $\times$ mL $\times$ mm Hg). To achieve no residual corneal swelling (i.e., no swelling several hours upon awakening), a Dk/L of 34×10^{-9} (cm $\times$ m^{102}) / (s $\times$ mL $\times$ mm Hg) is needed. Finally, to achieve 4% overnight (zero extra) swelling during cosmetic extended wear, a requirement of 87.0×10^{-9} (cm $\times$ m^{102}) / (s $\times$ mL $\times$ mm Hg) is estimated. Figure 30.2 demonstrates relative comparisons of an average Dk/L for aphakic contact lenses manufactured from various GP and hydrogel contact lens materials. It is evident that hydrogel lenses fall far short of the 34 value for no residual swelling with overnight wear while hyper-Dk GP materials either fall slightly short (i.e., Boston XO) or slightly above (i.e., Menicon Z) this criterion. However, these materials benefit from the significant contributions of the tear pump in reducing edema in the open eye environment. The only lens material that approximates the criterion for zero induced overnight swelling is the Silsoft silicone lens from Bausch & Lomb.

Giant papillary conjunctivitis, comprehensively described elsewhere, is found relatively more often with extended-wear lenses for aphakia than with daily wear contact lens correction for aphakia. It has been reported to be less common in extended lens wear for aphakia than extended contact lens wear for myopia (46). This may be a result of the relatively reduced activity of the elderly immune system or the thin edge design of a plus lens, reducing the mechanical irritation for the lens edge. The incidence of giant papillary conjunctivitis in GP lens daily wear is relatively low.

The risk of microbial keratitis has been demonstrated to be greater for patients who sleep wearing their lenses. Weissman and associates (47) found a risk of approximately 0.5% for patients without aphakia using daily wear, and 3% for those using extended wear. Noncompliance and longer periods of wear before removal are associated with a greater incidence of infection. Elderly patients may have lowered rates of healing, and those with diabetes are believed to be especially at risk (17). The incidence of ulcers with use of extended-wear lenses for aphakia was recently reported to be 0.5%, while the rate of serious adverse reactions was 2% (48).

The adverse effects of acute exposure to ultraviolet light have been will documented (49), but some data on the ocular effects of chronic exposure are equivocal (50–52). While ultraviolet (UV)-induced crystalline lens changes can

be managed with surgery, the effect on the macula photoreceptors and pigment epithelium can be devastating (53). With regard to retinal damage, Young (50) has recommended that all wavelengths below 510 nm should be attenuated maximally. Currently, several GP lens materials available in aphakic powers for contain a UV-absorbing chromophore. These materials include FluoroPerm 30, 60, 90, and 151 and Paragon HDS (all manufactured by Paragon Vision Sciences), Boston XO UV (Polymer Technology Corporation), Fluorex 300, 500, and 700 (all manufactured by Lifestyle Co., Inc.) (2,3,54). This protection is beneficial but should be considered inadequate, because it does not cover the entire cornea and only attenuates wavelengths from 400 nm and below. At this time, none of the UV-absorbing hydrogel materials has been used for the manufacture of aphakic lens powers. It is, therefore, prudent to recommend good quality sunglasses that have, at minimum, 97% absorbance at 400 nm for all patients with aphakia.

PREFIT ASSESSMENT

It is important to perform a comprehensive prefit assessment prior to making the decision to fit contact lenses and also to determine which lens material to fit. This assessment would include a careful history, evaluation of the lids, lashes, tear film, conjunctiva and sclera, limbus, cornea, pupil, retina, corneal curvature and manifest refraction (3). Although determining if a patient is a good contact lens candidate is, for the most part, the same as that indicated in Chapter 9, there are some characteristics fairly unique to the aphakic and/or elderly patient that need to be evaluated.

As the lids tend to become more flaccid with age, lid tension should be evaluated. Loose lids can make GP lens lift and centration difficult. Limbal neovascularization, surgical incisions, residual suturing, and any bleb formation along the limbus should also be noted. Tear-film volume and quality should be evaluated to ensure they will be able to tolerate contact lens wear. The cornea should be evaluated for any existing scars, dystrophies, and surgically rendered of contact lens–induced endothelial changes. The location, shape, and size of the pupil should be recorded, with special attention to noting any presence of a keyhole pupil or encroaching iridectomy that is not covered by the lids.

A very careful manifest refraction should be performed to achieve the best-possible spectacle-corrected visual acuity. The vertex distance should be accurately determined as well. Baseline keratometry or corneal topography measurements should be made; likewise, these measurements should be made at regular intervals to monitor the healing process and ultimately arrive at stabilization. The use of a corneal topography instrument is valuable to evaluate postoperative changes in corneal shape, possibly resulting from tight sutures, and to identify any areas of corneal irregularity (55).

Once the prefitting evaluation has been completed, the examination findings can be reviewed with the patient and

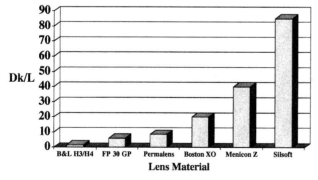

FIG. 30.2. Oxygen transmission of common soft and GP lens materials in aphakia.

a decision made about the viability of contact lenses and which material would be preferable. It is important for the practitioner to determine the patient's goals, expectations and motivation for wearing contact lenses prior to continuing with this process.

LENS MATERIALS, DESIGNS, AND FITTING

Gas Permeable

The introduction of hyperpermeable GP lens materials (i.e., Dk ≥ 100) has great applications in aphakic contact lens correction and, in fact, these should be the only GP lens materials used with aphakic patients (1,56). These include materials such as Boston XO (Polymer Technology Corporation), Paragon HDS 100 and FluoroPerm 151 (both from Paragon Vision Sciences) and Menicon Z (Menicon) (2). At the thicknesses required for high plus powers, these lenses should exhibit good stability. However, with the decreased tear volume—in combination with the high Dk associated with these materials, regular replacement of these materials (typically annually)—is recommended.

The use of a topical anesthetic is always recommended prior to the initial application of a GP lens although the effect of the anesthetic should be allowed to wear off while the lens is still on the eye such that the patient can gradually experience some awareness. However, it must also be considered that corneal sensitivity decreases with age. In addition, cataract surgery can result in a reduction of as much as 50% in corneal sensitivity because of severed afferent sensory nerve fibers (57). Adaptation to a rigid lens, therefore, is easier for the aphakic patient.

A well-fit GP contact lens demonstrates good centration of the optics, 2 to 3 mm of excursion with a blink, and an alignment lens-to-cornea fitting relationship without areas of significant pooling (standoff) or touch. The ability to achieve such a fit is influenced by the corneal radius of curvature, corneal astigmatism, position and tonicity of the upper lid, lens base curve radius and overall diameter, and lens design.

Perhaps the best candidates for optimum fitting GP contact lenses are those patients who have a relatively flat corneal curvature with very little astigmatism. In addition, an upper lid at or below the limbus, which demonstrates good elasticity, is desirable. For patients with corneal curvatures of 43.00 D or less and 1.50 D or less with-the-rule corneal astigmatism, a lens that is "on K" to slightly steeper than "K" with an overall diameter of approximately 9.5 mm with an optical zone of 7.8 to 8.0 mm is recommended. All these lenses tend to demonstrate better centration with a minus carrier design. This results in reduced center thickness, reduced overall mass, and a movement of the center of gravity from the anterior lens surface toward the posterior lens surface (58,59). The design of the carrier portion varies depending on laboratory procedures. It has been demonstrated previously that the radius of the anterior surface carrier has a significant influence on lens position and comfort. Flatter anterior radii, while providing a more central to superior fit, result in more lens awareness, discomfort, and possibly intolerance (60). In addition to the better lens centration, other advantages of a large diameter lens are enhanced comfort and reduction of 3- and 9-o'clock corneal staining. Diagnostic fitting is important to provide an accurate estimate of the best fit and lens power. If a high-plus-power fitting set is needed, a CLMA member laboratory can be contacted for the possibility of providing a diagnostic set for purchase or loan. Recommended lenticular and single-cut diagnostic sets are given in Tables 30.1 and 30.2.

TABLE 30.1. RECOMMENDED LENTICULAR APHAKIA DIAGNOSTIC LENS SET

Base Curve (D) Radius	Overall Diameter (mm)	Optical Zone Diameter (mm)	Back Vertex Power (D)	Secondary Curve Radius/Width (mm)	Peripheral Curve Radius/Width (mm)	CT (mm)	Flange (mm)
39.00	9.50	8.0	+13.00	BCR +1.0/0.4	SCR +1.5/0.35	0.44	+1.5
40.00	9.50	8.0	+13.00	BCR +1.0/0.4	SCR +1.5/0.35	0.44	+1.5
40.50	9.50	8.0	+13.00	BCR +1.0/0.4	SCR +1.5/0.35	0.44	+1.5
41.00	9.50	8.0	+13.00	BCR +1.0/0.4	SCR +1.5/0.35	0.44	+1.5
41.50	9.50	8.0	+13.00	BCR +1.0/0.4	SCR +1.5/0.35	0.44	+1.5
42.00	9.50	8.0	+13.00	BCR +1.0/0.4	SCR +1.5/0.35	0.44	+1.5
42.50	9.50	8.0	+13.00	BCR +1.0/0.4	SCR +1.5/0.35	0.44	+1.5
43.00	9.30	7.8	+13.00	BCR +1.0/0.4	SCR +1.5/0.35	0.42	+1.5
43.50	9.30	7.8	+13.00	BCR +1.0/0.4	SCR +1.5/0.35	0.42	+1.5
44.00	9.30	7.8	+13.00	BCR +1.0/0.4	SCR +1.5/0.35	0.42	+1.5
44.50	9.30	7.8	+13.00	BCR +1.0/0.4	SCR +1.5/0.35	0.42	+1.5
45.00	9.50	7.6	+13.00	BCR +1.0/0.4	SCR +1.5/0.3	0.40	+1.5
45.50	9.50	7.6	+13.00	BCR +1.0/0.4	SCR +1.5/0.3	0.40	+1.5
46.00	9.50	7.6	+13.00	BCR +1.0/0.4	SCR +1.5/0.3	0.40	+1.5
47.00	9.50	7.6	+13.00	BCR +1.0/0.4	SCR +1.5/0.3	0.40	+1.5
48.00	9.30	7.6	+13.00	BCR +1.0/0.4	SCR +1.5/0.3	0.40	+1.5

TABLE 30.2. RECOMMENDED SINGLE-CUT APHAKIA DIAGNOSTIC LENS SET

Base Curve (D)	Overall Diameter (mm)	Optical Zone Diameter (mm)	Back Vertex Power (D)	Secondary Curve Radius/Width (mm)	Peripheral Curve Radius/Width (mm)	CT (mm)
45.00	9.00	7.6	+13.00	BCR +1.0/0.4	SCR +1.5/0.3	0.40
45.50	9.00	7.6	+13.00	BCR +1.0/0.4	SCR +1.5/0.3	0.40
46.00	9.00	7.6	+13.00	BCR +1.0/0.4	SCR +1.5/0.3	0.40
46.50	9.00	7.6	+13.00	BCR +1.0/0.4	SCR +1.5/0.3	0.40
47.00	9.00	7.6	+13.00	BCR +1.0/0.4	SCR +1.5/0.3	0.40
48.00	9.00	7.6	+13.00	BCR +1.0/0.4	SCR +1.5/0.3	0.40

An acceptable lens fit can be made more difficult when the corneal curvatures are above 43.00 D, demonstrate greater than 1.5 D of with-the-rule corneal astigmatism, or manifest any amount of against-the-rule corneal astigmatism. A good starting point of these relatively steep corneas include selecting a base curve radius slightly "steeper than K" with an overall diameter of 9.0 mm and an optical zone of 7.8 mm or less. Changing to a steeper base curve radius will provide better centration with more stability. A lens that is excessively steep may promote 3- and 9-o'clock staining and corneal edema with central superficial punctate keratitis resulting from poor tear exchange. Again, a minus lenticular design usually is indicated.

In some cases of very steep corneal curvature (greater than 45.00 D) and extremely tight lid structure, single cut lens designs can be successful. In general, these lenses need to be fit "steeper than K" with a relatively smaller diameter than the lenticular lens designs. Edge thicknesses smaller than .12 mm may result in frequent lens breakage, especially with the hyper Dk materials.

It is important to always consider the impact of effective power in aphakia. The power at the corneal plane is, at minimum, two diopters greater than at the spectacle plane (Appendix 2). In addition, both sphere and cylinders powers increase as you approach the corneal plane. It is also important to specify whether the power to be ordered for an aphakic lens is the front surface or back surface power. The back surface power is typically 0.50 to 0.75D greater than the front surface power. It has become customary to order these lenses specifying the back vertex power (Appendix 3).

Proper lens care for GP lenses is vital to their success and for long-term patient comfort. Cleaning in the palm of the hand immediately following lens removal with an abrasive surfactant is indicated. Deposits may develop at the anterior junction zone on a lenticular design requiring extended cleaning or special attention with a cotton swab applicator (61) (Fig. 30.3).The use of a liquid enzymatic cleaner is indicated for these patients.

Hydrogel

A well-fitting hydrogel lens, whether aphakic or nonaphakic, includes a diameter sufficient to provided limbal-to-limbal coverage, good optical centration, and movement after the blink equal to 1 to 2 mm. Lenses having low, medium, and high water content are available. Lens dehydration may result in significant base curve and power changes (62,63). A slightly increased movement is indicated

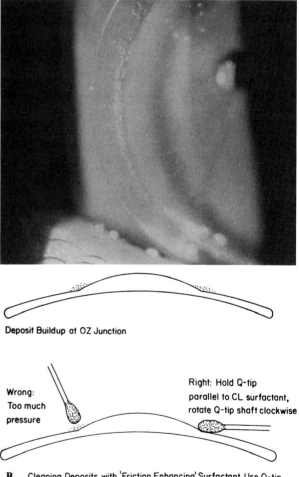

FIG. 30.3. A. deposits on lenticular junction of aphakic contact lens. B. Method of removal for lens deposits at lenticular junction. (From Grohe RM. Aphakia. In Bennett ES, Grohe RM, eds. *Rigid gas permeable contact lenses.* New York: Professional Press, 1986: 423, with permission.).

in medium- and high-water-contact lenses due to lens dehydration resulting in a relatively tighter-fitting lens. When fitting patients with hydrogel lenses having a water content greater than 40%, allow approximately 1 hour of in-office lens wear prior to evaluating the fit of the lens. Also, patients who are prone to develop significant corneal edema while wearing hydrogel lenses may demonstrate a relatively tighter lens-to-cornea fitting relationship after a few hours of lens wear. This edema is consistent with the poor oxygen transmissibility in the thick lens designs and as a result of minimal tear exchange.

The Silsoft lens (Bausch & Lomb), from an oxygen standpoint, is preferable to the non—silicone-containing hydrogel lenses. It also has the benefits of low water content and the ability for use of ocular medications (6). For the pediatric aphake it is available in one diameter, 11.3 mm, and three base curve radii, 7.5, 7.7, and 7.9 mm. The adult version of this lens is available in both 11.3-mm and 12.5-mm diameters (2). At minimum, 1 mm of movement with the blink is desirable. The primary limitations to this design are the hydrophobicity of the lens surface, necessitating frequent replacement, especially for the adult aphake, and the high expense associated with this custom lens.

Gas Permeable versus Hydrogel Lenses

When making the initial decision on fitting a hydrogel or GP lens, practitioners must evaluate the significance of various considerations (Table 30.3). I prefer, with few exceptions, to begin with a GP lens design (Fig. 30.4). The advantages of better corneal physiology, ease of care, and better optical correction with GP lens correction cannot be ig-

TABLE 30.3. FACTORS TO CONSIDER FOR LENS MATERIAL SELECTION

Lens Material	Advantages	Disadvantages
Hydrogel	More forgiving fit	Deposits/contamination
	Decreased fitting time	Hypoxia (exception: silicone)
	Initial comfort	Acute red eye, infiltrates
	Extended wear (silicone)	Neovascularization
GP	Quality of vision	Initial comfort
	Increased tear exchange	Lens mass, decentration
	Low risk of hypoxia with hyperpermeable materials	Increased fitting time
	Less limbal complications	
	Decreased contamination	
	Ease of care	

GP, gas-permeable.

nored. Changing from a GP to a soft lens in the event of a poor fit or intolerance can be achieved relatively easily. When indicated, changing from a soft lens to a GP lens can be difficult due to the increased lens awareness with rigid lenses.

Perhaps the most significant adverse reaction to aphakic contact lens correction is corneal hypoxia. This is reduced as a result of wearing a GP lens for the better tear exchange and oxygen transmissibility of these lens materials or via the application of a silicone-based lens material. However, some

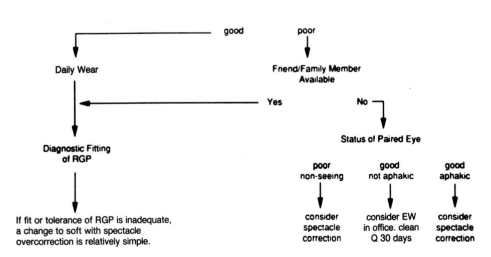

FIG. 30.4. Factors influencing initial lens of choice for contact lens correction of aphakia.

patients with aphakia will be unable to obtain satisfactory comfort secondary to a poor-fitting lens. In these cases, a hydrogel lens may be desirable. Complications with hydrogel lenses worn on a daily wear basis are significantly fewer than with the use of extended wear lenses.

An indication for use of extended-wear lenses on patients with aphakia is poor dexterity, with the patient demonstrating an inability to maintain lens care and perform insertion and removal. Many of these patients will have a friend or family member who can provide lens care for them. A select few patients will demonstrate the inability to maintain lens care and require in-office removal and cleaning. Monthly examinations with lens removal, cleaning, and disinfection are indicated for these patients. Comprehensive evaluation of any lens-related complications is also recommended.

SUMMARY

It has been suggested that the patients with aphakia can be the most challenging and least grateful of the practitioner encounters (8). In order to promote successful lens wear for them, practitioners should be prepared to perform a comprehensive evaluation and provide an initial lens fit that is likely to result in good visual acuity and lens comfort, with the least patient inconvenience. In addition to this, informing the patient of the type of lens care needed and the possible ways to enhance wearability and reduce the inconvenience of lens wear, can improve success with this unique patient group.

APPENDIX 1: SPECTACLE VERSUS CONTACT LENS MAGNIFICATION

The magnification can be determined for spectacles and contact lenses via the following formula:

$$SM = \frac{1}{1 - t/nF1} \times \frac{1}{1 - dFv'}$$

Where:

F1 = power of front surface
Fv' = back vertex power of lens
t = lens thickness (meters)
n = lens index of refraction
d = distance from back of lens to eye's entrance pupil (meters)

If for example, a spectacle lens power is +13.00 D and the power at the corneal plane is +15.50 D with a front surface power of +16.50 D, the following magnifications will result:

Magnification: spectacle lens

$$\frac{1}{1 - 0.007/1.49\,(+16.50D)} \times \frac{1}{1 - 0.015 \times (13)}$$

Where:

t = 7.0 mm
n = 1.49
d = 12 + 3 mm
= 1.085 × 1.242 = 1.34 or 34% magnification

Magnification: contact lens

$$\frac{1}{1 - 0.0005/1.47\,(+77.00D)} \times \frac{1}{1 - 0.003 \times (15.50)}$$

Where:

F1 = +77.00 D
Fv' = +15.50 D
t = 0.50 mm
n = 1.47
d = 3 mm
= 1.027 × 1.05 = 1.08 or 8% magnification

This example shows that contact lenses result in less than one fourth the magnification of spectacle lenses in aphakic powers.

APPENDIX 2: EFFECTIVE POWER

The aphakic eye will need a much greater plus power incorporated into a contact lens as compared to a spectacle lens due to the fact that when a lens is moved from the spectacle plane toward the cornea, the effective vergence of the light is altered such that greater plus correction is necessary. The following equation is used to determine the effective power:

$$Fe = \frac{F}{1 - dF}$$

Where:

F1 = +77.00 D
Fe = effective power (diopters)
F = back vertex power of lens (diopters)
d = vertex distance, or distance lens is moved in meters' (+) if lens is moved toward cornea; (−) if lens is moved away from the cornea.

For example, if a spectacle lens power of +13.00 D would be equal to approximately +15.50 D at the corneal plane if the vertex distance is 12 mm.

$$Fe = \frac{+13}{1 - 0.012(13)} = +15.40\ D$$

or approximately +15.50 D

Therefore, a contact lens with a power of +15.50 D would

be necessary to provide a correction for a patient with an effective spectacle lens power of + 13.00 D.

APPENDIX 3: VERTEX POWER

Although contact lenses are much thinner than spectacle lenses, as the lens shape is a meniscus [front surface has a positive (+) power, the back surface has a negative (−) power], the vertex power is different when measuring from a reference point on the front of the lens as opposed to the back of the lens (1). The values of front vertex power and back surface will be significantly different in an aphakic lens and depend upon the center thickness, according to the following equations:

$$\text{Front Vertex Power (Fv)} = \frac{F2}{1 - t/n \, F2} + F1$$

$$\text{Back Vertex Power (Fv')} = \frac{F1}{1 - t/n \, F1} + F2$$

Where:

$$
\begin{aligned}
F1 &= +77.00 \text{ D} \\
F1(\text{air}) &= +77.00 \text{ D} \\
F2(\text{air}) &= -64.00 \text{ D} \\
N(\text{air}) &= 1.47 \\
Ct &= 0.5 \text{ mm } (0.0005 \text{ m})
\end{aligned}
$$

$$(Fv') = \frac{+77.00}{1 - 0.0005/1.47 \, (77.00)} + -64.00 = +15.07 \text{ D}$$

$$(Fv) = \frac{-64.00}{1 - 0.0005/1.47 \, (64)} + 77.00 = +14.38 \text{ D}$$

In this example, there is a difference of 0.69 D between back and front vertex power, making it important to both order the lenses and verify the lenses using the same power measurement, which is typically back vertex power.

REFERENCES

1. Davis LJ. Aphakia. In: Bennett ES, Henry VA, eds. *Clinical manual of contact lenses,* 2nd ed. Philadelphia: Lippincott Williams & Wilkins, 2000:477–492.
2. Thompson TT. Tyler's Quarterly soft contact lens parameter guide. *Tylers Q* 2003;20(2).
3. Luk BMW, Grohe RM. Aphakia. In: Bennett ES, Hom MM, eds. *Manual of gas permeable contact lenses,* 2nd ed. St. Louis: Elsevier Science, 2004:357–379.
4. Cassidy L. Pediatric cataract. *OT* 2001;9:27–31.
5. Jaffe NS. The way things were and are: changing indications for intraocular lens implantation. *Ophthalmology* 1983;90:318–320.
6. Zikoski E. Aphakia. In: Schwartz CA, ed. *Specialty contact lenses: a fitter's guide.* Philadelphia; WB Saunders, 1996:165–174.
7. Davis JK, Torgersen DC. The properties of lenses used for the correction of aphakia. *J Am Optom Assoc* 1983;54:685–693.
8. Borish I. Aphakia: Perceptual and Refractive Problems of Spectacle Correction. *J Am Optom Assoc* 1983; 54:701.
9. Kumar D. Management of aphakia. *Contact Lens J* 1985;13:4–7.
10. McCarthy EM, Pokras R, Moien M. National trends in lens extraction 1965–1985. *J Am Optom Assoc* 1988;59:31–35.
11. Mannis MJ, Zadnik K. Contact lenses in the elderly patient. *Geriatr Ophthalmol* 1986;2:23–27.
12. Newell FW. Ophthalmology principles and concepts. In: Newell FW. *Eyelids,* 6th ed. St. Louis: C.V. Mosby, 1986:201.
13. Holly FJ, Lemp MA. Tear physiology and dry eyes. *Surv Ophthalmol* 1977;22:69–87.
14. Kohlhaas M. Corneal sensation after cataract and refractive surgery. *J Cataract Refract Surg* 1998;24:1399–1209.
15. Sakamoto R, Bennett ES, Henry VA, et al. The phenol red thread test: a cross-cultural study. *Invest Ophthalmol Vis Sci* 1993;34:3510–3514.
16. Blaydes JE, Minor RH, Mozzocco TR. Prefitting evaluation. In: Dabezies OH, ed. *Contact lenses: CLAO guide to basic science and clinical practice.* New York: Grune & Stratton, 1984:21.1–21.7.
17. Eichenbaum JW, Feldstein M, Podos SM. Extended wear aphakic soft contact lenses and corneal ulcers. *Br J Ophthalmol* 1982;66:663–666.
18. Salz JJ, Schlanger JL. Complications of aphakic extended wear contact lenses encountered during a seven-year period in 100 eyes. *CLAO J* 1983;9:241–244.
19. Graham CM, Dart JK, Buckley RJ. Extended wear hydrogel and daily wear hard contact lenses for aphakia. *Ophthalmology* 1986;93:1489–1494.
20. Scott CA. A practical mirror for aphakic contact lens wearers. *Rev Optom* 1978;115:84.
21. Sugar J. Adenochrome pigmentation of hydrophilic lenses. *Arch Ophthalmol* 1974;91:11–12.
22. McCarey BE, et al. Gentamicin diffusion across hydrogel bandage lenses and its kinetic distribution on the eye. *Curr Eye Res* 1984;3:977–989.
23. Podos SM, Becker B, Asseff C, Hartstein J. Pilocarpine therapy with soft contact lenses. *Am J Ophthalmol* 1972;73:336–341.
24. Hull DS, Edelhauser HF, Hndiuk RA. Ocular penetration of prednisolone and the hydrophilic contact lens. *Arch Ophthalmol* 1974;92:413–416.
25. Gasset A. Benzalkonium chloride toxicity to the human cornea. *Am J Ophthalmol* 1977;84:169–171.
26. Mondino BJ, Groden LR. Conjunctival hyperemia and corneal infiltrates with chemically disinfected soft contact lenses. *Arch Ophthalmol* 1980;98:1767–1770.
27. Burstein NL. Cornea cytotoxicity of topically applied drugs, vehicles, and preservatives. *Surv Ophthalmol* 1980;25:15–30.
28. Gasset AR, Kaufman HE. Therapeutic uses of hydrophilic contact lenses. *Am J Ophthalmol* 1970;69:252–259.
29. Lerman S, Sapp G. The hydrophilic corneoscleral lens in the treatment of bullous keratopathy. *Ann Ophthalmol* 1970;2:142–144.
30. Aquavella JV. Chronic corneal edema. *Am J Ophthalmol* 1973;76:201–207.
31. Lemp MA. Bandage lenses and the use of topical solution containing preservatives. *Ann Ophthalmol* 1978;10:1319–1321
32. Jaffe NS. *Cataract surgery and its complications,* 4th ed. St. Louis: CV Mosby, 1984:320–323.
33. Meshel L. Prosthetic contact lenses. In: Dabezies OH, ed. *Contact lenses: CLAO guide to basic science and clinical practice.* New York: Grune & Stratton, 1984:59.1–59–8.
34. Katsumi O et al. Binocular function in unilateral aphakia. *Ophthalmology* 1988;95:1088–1093.
35. Ogle KN et al. On the correction of unilateral aphakia with contact lenses. *Arch Ophthalmol* 1958;59:639–652.
36. Dyer JA, Ogle KN. Correction of unilateral aphakia with contact lenses. *Am J Ophthalmol* 1960;50:11–17.
37. Enoch JM. A spectacle-contact lens combination used as a reverse

Galilean telescope in unilateral aphakia. *Am J Optom Arch Am Acad Optom* 1968;45:231–240.

38. Holden BA, Brennan NA, Efron W, Swarbrick HA. The contact lens: Physiological considerations. In: Aquavella JV, Rao GN, eds. *Contact lenses.* Philadelphia: JB Lippincott, 1987:1–38.

39. Korb DR, Richmond PP, Herman JP. Physiological response of the cornea to hydrogel lenses before and after cataract extraction. *J Am Optom Assoc* 1980;51:267–270.

40. Guillon M, Morris JA. Corneal response to a provocative test in aphakic patients. *J Br Contact Lens Assoc* 1981;4:162–167.

41. Polse KA, Holden BA, Sweeney D. Corneal edema accompanying aphakic extended lens wear. *Arch Ophthalmol* 1983;101: 1038–1041.

42. Irvine SR. A newly defined vitreous syndrome following cataract surgery. *Am J Ophthalmol* 1953;36:599–619.

43. Vail D. After results of vitreous loss. *Am J Ophthalmol* 1965;59: 573–586.

44. Holden BA, Mertz GW. Critical oxygen levels to avoid corneal edema for daily and extended wear contact lenses. *Invest Ophtalmol Vis Sci* 1984;25:1161–1167.

45. Chaston J, Fatt I. Design criteria for a high plus contact lens that fulfills the oxygen needs of the cornea in the aphakic eye. *J Am Optom Assoc* 1981;52:237–241.

46. Lembach RG, Wilson CA. Extended wear contact lenses. In: Dabazies OH, ed. *Contact lenses: CLAO guide to basic science and clinical practice.* New York: Grune and Stratton, 1984:61-1–61-17.

47. Weissman BA, Remba MJ, Fugerly E. Results of the extended wear contact lens survey of the Contact Lens Section of the AOA. *J Am Optom Assoc* 1987;58:166–171.

48. MaCrae S. Contact lens as a corneal time bomb, abstracted. Presented at: Research to Prevent Blindness Seminar, Arlington, VA, September 25–28, 1988:12–13.

49. Young RW. Solar radiation and age related macular degeneration. *Surv Ophthalmol* 1988;32:253–269.

50. West SK et al. Exposure to sunlight and other risk factors for age-related macular degeneration. *Arch Ophthalmol* 1989;107: 875–879.

51. Taylor HR, West SK et al. Effect of ultraviolet radiation on cataract formation. *N Engl J Med* 1988;319:1429–1433.

52. Bochow TW, West SK et al. Ultraviolet light exposure and risk of posterior subcapsular cataract. *Arch Ophthalmol* 1989;107: 369–372.

53. Weissman BA. Contact Lens Application in Aphakia. In: London R, Harris MG eds. *Mosby's optometric problem-solving series: contact lenses for pre- and post-surgery.* St. Louis: Mosby, 1997:67–96.

54. *GP materials and products guide.* Available at: www.rgpli.org. Accessed January, 2004.

55. Corbett MC, Rosen ES. Lens replacement: corneal topography in cataract surgery. In: Yanoff M, Duker JS, eds. *Ophthalmology.* London: Mosby, 1999:4.15.1–4.15.6

56. Bennett ES, Levy B. Material selection. In: Bennett ES, Henry VA, eds. *Clinical manual of contact lenses,* 2nd ed. Philadelphia: Lippincott Williams & Wilkins, 2000:59–74

57. Phillips LJ, Soltis GG. Intraocular lenses: an update. *J Am Optom Assoc* 1983;54:697–700.

58. Polse KA. Hard lens aphakic fitting procedures. *Int Contact Lens Clin* 1975;2:44–50.

59. Pullum K. Handling high power prescription contact lenses. *Optician* 1987;193(5083):21–25.

60. Polse KA. Aphakia. In: Mandell RB, ed. *Contact lens practice,* 4th ed. Springfield, IL: Charles C. Thomas, 1988: 732–769.

61. Grohe RM. Aphakia. In: Bennett ES, Grohe RM, eds. *Rigid gas permeable contact lenses.* New York: Professional Press Books/ Fairchild Publications, 1986:411–429.

62. Fatt C, Chaston J. Response of vertex power to change in dimensions of hydrogel lenses. *Int Contact Lens Clin* 1981;8: 22–28.

63. McCaney BE, Wilson LA. PH osmolarity, and temperature effects in the water content of hydrogel contact lenses. *Contact Intraocul Lens Med J* 1982;8:158–167.

31

PEDIATRIC CONTACT LENSES

JEFFREY JAY WALLINE

The developing visual system of young children requires appropriate, nearly constant correction in order to maximize children's visual potential and binocularity. Contact lens correction may play a vital role in correcting children's vision because spectacles may be cosmetically unappealing, uncomfortable to wear, visually disturbing, and too easy for a young child to remove.

Even infants and toddlers can benefit from contact lens wear. Contact lenses are less easy to remove than spectacles, so children who consistently remove their glasses and require constant visual correction can be fitted with contact lenses. Parents must care for the contact lenses when children are this age, but children quickly learn to tolerate people inserting and removing contact lenses on a daily basis.

Children older than 7 years of age may be capable of handling the responsibility of contact lens wear (1,2), and they can be fitted using techniques similar to what would be performed on adult patients. Although these children are capable of caring for their contact lenses independently, adult supervision may improve hygiene and lower contact lens replacement rates due to loss or breakage.

INDICATIONS

Children may benefit from contact lens wear for a variety of reasons (3), ranging from correction of refractive error to vision therapy. Children may be fitted with contact lenses available for the general population or they may require custom made contact lenses, depending on the reason for contact lens wear and the anatomy of the child's eyes and adnexa. Occasionally contact lens wear is medically necessary, but typically contact lens wear in children is elective. The purpose of the contact lens may be to improve vision or it may be to improve the child's appearance. Disfigured eyes or unappealing spectacles may be very traumatic for a young child; therefore, contact lenses should be considered by the parents and the practitioner. Many parents do not realize that children are able to wear contact lenses or that contact lenses may mask a disfigured eye. The practitioner should make parents aware of the contact lens treatment options that are available in order to provide the optimal care for the child.

REFRACTIVE ERROR

The distribution of refractive error at birth is relatively normally distributed and centered at about +2.00 D. During the early elementary years, the refractive error distribution narrows considerably and centers closer to emmetropia (Fig. 31.1). Although the majority of children have a refractive error that does not require vision correction, children with refractive errors in the tails of the distribution require vision correction to develop maximal vision and to optimize formal education.

Each type of refractive error uniquely affects vision and visual development. Prescribing of vision correction depends on the type of refractive error, the age of the child, the needs of the child, and the motivation of the parent.

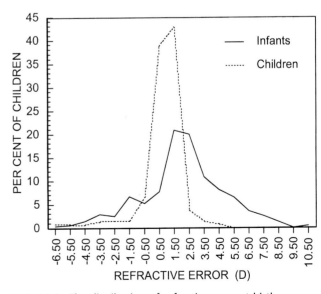

FIG. 31.1. The distribution of refractive error at birth narrows and shifts toward emmetropia during the first few years of life. (Reprinted from Zadnik K. *The ocular examination: measurements and findings,* 1st ed. Philadelphia: WB Saunders, 1997:55, with permission).

Myopia

During infancy, myopia is very rare and may be associated with premature birth or systemic disease (4,5). By the time children enter elementary school, approximately 2% are myopic (6). Myopia typically progresses through age 15 years for girls and 16 years for boys (7), until approximately 15% of the children are myopic (8).

Low-to-moderate myopia does not typically result in amblyopia, and the vision loss associated with high myopia is typically due to retinal detachment, macular problems, chorioretinal degeneration, or increased spacing between photoreceptors. Although amblyopia does not typically occur, myopia should be corrected in young children to maximize their vision. Spectacle correction of high myopia results in image minification, peripheral distortion, and reduced field of view. Contact lenses can minimize all of these effects (Fig. 31.2).

Rigid contact lenses may also slow the progression of myopia in children (9–13), but soft contact lenses have been shown to have no effect on long-term myopia progression in children (14). Annual myopia progression rates of children enrolled in controlled studies are shown in Table 31.1.

Rigid contact lenses have been thought to slow the progression of myopia in children, but a current study of myopia control with rigid gas-permeable contact lenses in children does not provide confirmation. Although previous studies did not measure all of the ocular parameters, evidence suggested that rigid gas-permeable contact lens wear could slow axial growth (11). Although many of the studies showed evidence that rigid contact lenses slow myopia progression on average, none of them was able to predict individuals who will benefit most from decreased myopia progression. When discussing treatment options with parents, the practitioner should state that rigid contact lenses are a standard treatment option for myopia, and they may have an additional benefit of possibly slowing myopia progression in children.

Hyperopia

Many infants and children are hyperopic, but vision correction is not necessary for all hyperopic refractive errors. In fact, practitioners' opinions vary greatly about the level of hyperopic refractive error that requires correction (15,16). The majority of eye care practitioners would prescribe vision correction for a 6-month-old child with no other ocular problems beginning at 5 to 6 D, and between 3 and 4 D for 4-year-old children free of other eye problems (15).

Approximately 2% to 3% of children have esotropia (17–19), and approximately one third of these children have accommodative esotropia (20). Prescribing for hyperopia greater than +3.50 D may (21) or may not (22) prevent the onset of accommodative esotropia. Some practitioners do not prescribe for hyperopia because they believe that children are likely to naturally emmetropize, but evidence shows that children with +2.00 D or more hyperopia are unlikely to emmetropize (Fig. 31.3) (23), and refractive error correction does not alter emmetropization (24).

Spectacle lenses with high hyperopia correction are heavy, they magnify the eyes of the patient and the object being viewed, and they distort the peripheral vision. Contact lenses can provide optimal vision as well as improved cosmesis and comfort for children. High-plus contact lenses are thick, and they allow less oxygen to reach the eye. Contact lenses with high oxygen permeability should be fitted, and parents should be advised to remove the contact lenses nightly so that children are not harmed by long-term contact lens wear.

Astigmatism

Large amounts of astigmatism are more common in infants, but the magnitude of the astigmatism decreases over the first 2 to 5 years of life (18,25,26). Approximately 30% of infants between birth and 4 weeks have greater than 1.00 D of astigmatism, and the prevalence increases up to approximately 60% at 17 to 32 weeks. The prevalence then decreases to approximately 40% from 2.5 to 5 years of age (27). After age 5 years, the prevalence of astigmatism further decreases to adult levels of approximately 10% (28).

Astigmatism is primarily against-the-rule in children under 1 year of age (29,30), but the magnitude of against-the-rule astigmatism decreases rapidly over the first 3 years of life (31). With-the-rule astigmatism is more common by the time children enter elementary school (30). The astigmatism that is present at birth and decreases over time appears to be primarily due to corneal toricity (29).

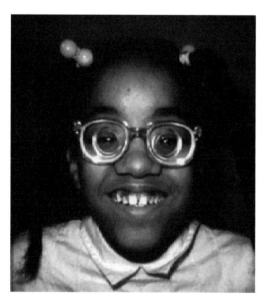

FIG. 31.2. Spectacle correction for high myopia can be uncomfortable and can distort the visual field considerably. Contact lenses may decrease the visual distortion.

TABLE 31.1. ANNUAL MYOPIA PROGRESSION RATE FOR CHILDREN ENROLLED IN CONTACT LENS MYOPIA CONTROL STUDIES WITH CONTROL GROUPS

Author (year)	Contact Lens Type	Contact lenses	Spectacles	% Difference
Baldwin (1969)	PMMA	−0.59	−0.43	37.2
Stone (1976)	PMMA	−0.10	−0.35	71.4
Perrigin (1990)	RGP	−0.16	−0.51	68.6
Khoo (1999)	RGP	−0.42	−0.78	46.2
Horner (1999)	Soft	−0.36	−0.31	13.8
Levy (2001)	RGP	−0.67	−0.64	4.7

PMMA polymethyl methacrylate; RGP rigid gas permeable.

The astigmatism that is present in infants typically resolves spontaneously, and it usually does not significantly affect vision, so refractive error correction may not be necessary. Children with greater than 3.00 D of astigmatism are less likely to experience spontaneous regression (32), so one may consider prescribing a correction. Against-the-rule astigmatism detected in infancy is more likely to diminish than oblique astigmatism and with-the-rule astigmatism. Children below the age of 3 years do not need correction for against-the-rule astigmatism less than 3.00 D. Because the magnitude of oblique and with-the-rule astigmatism is less likely to decline, one may consider prescribing for lower amounts if the visual acuity is affected and the refractive error is stable. After 3 years of age, all astigmatism that affects visual acuity should be corrected.

Children who have against-the-rule astigmatism should be examined every 3 to 4 months because it is more likely to change with age. Oblique and with-the-rule astigmatism is more stable and needs to be examined every 6 months.

When astigmatism influences visual acuity, the eye care practitioner should prescribe the full correction. Many eye care practitioners prescribe less than the full amount of astigmatism because they believe children are less likely to adapt to full astigmatism correction and therefore less likely to wear their visual correction. Children are very capable of adapting to a new refractive error prescription, so one should not be wary of prescribing the full amount of astigmatism correction necessary to optimize visual acuity.

Because astigmatism rarely affects visual acuity significantly and because spectacles are not overly uncomfortable, even for higher amounts of astigmatism, spectacles are typically the first line of visual correction. However, children who have significant myopia or hyperopia associated with the astigmatism or children who refuse to wear spectacles

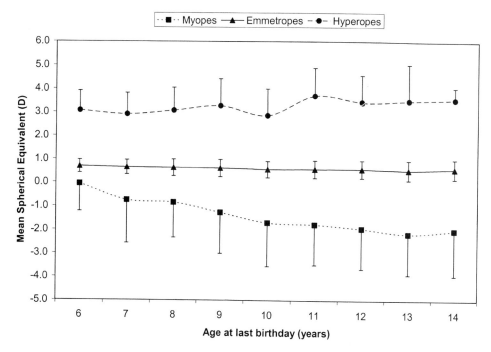

FIG. 31.3. The refractive error of children who are hyperopic at age 6 years is relatively stable through age 14 years. (From Karla Zadnik, OD, PhD, with permission.)

may benefit from contact lens wear. Astigmatism is rarely of visual consequence for infants, so by the time children need astigmatism correction, they can typically wear contact lenses designed for adults. Either rigid gas-permeable or soft toric contact lenses are appropriate for children.

Anisometropia

Visual correction for anisometropia should be considered when the refractive error difference between the two eyes is 1 D or more. Approximately 3% of preschool children have anisometropia (33). Careful evaluation of an anisometropic child's vision and binocular status should be made every 6 months. Although a child may not present with symptoms, anisometropia can result in amblyopia if not corrected.

When both eyes have low-to-moderate myopia, amblyopia typically does not develop because the less myopic eye will view distance objects and the more myopic eye will view near objects. Refractive error correction may not be necessary for lower amounts of myopia. When both eyes are hyperopic, the more hyperopic eye is rarely used due to increased accommodative demand. The more hyperopic eye will therefore often become amblyopic, so refractive error correction should be provided as soon as hyperopic anisometropia is detected. Amblyopia usually does not develop in children with antimetropia because the myopic eye is usually used for near vision and the hyperopic eye is used for distance viewing. In order to equalize the accommodative demand between the two eyes, visual correction should be provided when the refractive error becomes stable. Spectacle lenses that correct hyperopia increase the retinal image size, and myopic spectacle lenses decrease retinal image size. Therefore, spectacle lenses that vary in prescription may create retinal images that differ in size. When the size difference is 5% or greater, it is difficult to fuse the two images. If the refractive error is due to a longer or shorter eye (axial myope or axial hyperope), the retinal image size of a spectacle-corrected patient is the same as an emmetropic patient, but the retinal image size of a contact lens-corrected patient is larger for a myope and smaller for a hyperope than an emmetrope. If the refractive error is due to a difference in something other than the axial length (a difference in corneal curvatures, for example) the patient is a refractive myope or a refractive hyperope. The retinal image size of a refractive myope corrected with spectacles is smaller, and the retinal image size of a refractive hyperope corrected with spectacles is larger than the retinal image size of an emmetropic patient (Table 31.2).

Anisometropic patients with refractive myopia or hyperopia should, therefore, be corrected with contact lenses to reduce retinal image size differences.

When viewing an off-axis object, a spectacle lens creates a prismatic effect. An off-axis object viewed through a plus lens results in a prismatic effect that is opposite of an off-axis object viewed through a minus lens (Fig. 31.4). If the prismatic effects of the lenses differ substantially, visual symptoms such as headaches, distorted vision, and "swimming" images may occur. Because contact lenses move freely with the rotation of the eye, one always views through the optical center of the lens so the prismatic effectivity of the lens is reduced. When patients with anisometropia complain of visual symptoms while wearing spectacles, contact lens correction should be considered to improve visual comfort.

TABLE 31.2. RETINAL IMAGE SIZES RELATIVE TO AN EMMETROPIC PATIENT

	Contact Lens Correction	Spectacle Correction
Refractive myope	Similar	Smaller
Refractive hyperope	Similar	Larger
Axial myope	Larger	Similar
Axial hyperope	Smaller	Similar

Adapted from Keating MP, ed. *Geometric, physical, and visual optics*, 1st ed. Boston: Butterworth Publishers, 1988.

APHAKIA

Congenital cataracts occur in approximately 1.6 per 10,000 live births in the United States (34). They are usually quite dense, and they may substantially affect vision. Although congenital cataracts are relatively rare, they are a leading cause of visual impairment among children.

Infants and children develop cataracts due to a large variety of etiologies, and the cataracts may be unilateral or bilateral. Bilateral cataracts are typically hereditary. They are not usually associated with other ocular or systemic diseases, but they have been noted in children with a variety of problems (Table 31.3). Congenital cataracts associated with galactosemia may be reversible if diagnosed and treated early.

Unilateral cataracts are typically secondary to persistent hyperplastic primary vitreous or trauma. The incidence of trauma increases dramatically after children become ambulatory, and trauma is the most common cause of cataracts in children.

Cataracts can have devastating effects on a very young, developing visual system. The only way to avoid amblyopia if the cataract is deemed "visually significant" is to surgically remove the cataract as soon as possible.

Intraocular lenses may be implanted at the time of cataract removal, but controversy still exists as to whether this is the most appropriate treatment alternative (35–40). Intraocular lenses do not allow the optics of the eye to compensate for the rapid axial elongation (41), so frequent replacement of the intraocular lens may be necessary.

Spectacles may be an acceptable form of vision correction

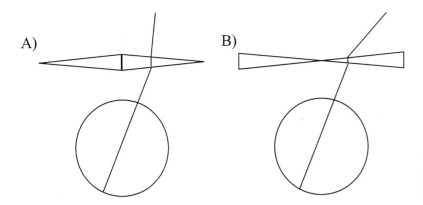

FIG. 31.4. Plus lenses **(A)** act as prisms with the base at the center of the lens, and minus lenses **(B)** act as prisms with the base at the periphery of the lens, when objects are viewed off-axis through the lens.

if aphakia is bilateral, but peripheral distortion and image magnification complicate visual input, even in bilateral spectacle wear. Unilateral aphakia results in extreme aniso-metropia and aniseikonia, so spectacle correction may result in visual symptoms and poor development of visual acuity and binocular vision. Children's frames may also be uncomfortable for the child because they are difficult to keep adjusted appropriately. The visual distortion and relatively poor comfort may cause young children to repeatedly remove the spectacles. If children do not receive nearly constant visual correction, amblyopia may result.

In the early 1980s, epikeratophakia was a treatment for aphakia (42), but it is rarely performed now due to relatively poor long-term visual acuity results (43) and improvements in intraocular lens implantation procedures.

Contact lenses are commonly prescribed for aphakia (38, 39,44,45), because the power of the contact lenses can be easily changed to adjust to the rapidly changing refractive error. They also provide constant visual correction because a child cannot remove them as easily as glasses. Conversely, contact lenses may require more effort for the parent and the child and more out-of-pocket expenses than intraocular

TABLE 31.3. MOST COMMON CAUSES OF CONGENITAL CATARACTS

Unilateral	Bilateral
Persistent hyperplastic primary vitreous	Genetics
Trauma	Maternal infection
	Rubella
	Herpes simplex
	Cytomegalovirus
	Syphilis
	Down syndrome
	Stickler's Syndrome
	Lowe's Syndrome
	Metabolic disease
	Hypoglycemia
	Galactosemia
	Fabry's disease
	Refsum's disease
	Prematurity

lenses due to the routine care and potential for loss or breakage of the contact lenses.

Rigid gas-permeable contact lenses and soft contact lenses are available for aphakia. Rigid gas-permeable contact lenses are less expensive, they provide clearer vision, and they afford greater ocular health benefits than soft contact lenses. Soft contact lenses are more likely to stay in the eye, and parents are typically more comfortable handling soft contact lenses because of the perceived comfort and greater likelihood of experiencing soft contact lens care. Each of these benefits should be discussed with the parents prior to the contact lens fitting in order to determine the most appropriate correction and to maximize the potential for success once the contact lenses are dispensed.

Contact lenses should be dispensed as soon after the cataract surgery as both the contact lens practitioner and the surgeon (when these are not the same individual) feel comfortable. Fitting the contact lenses on the day of the cataract surgery decreases the time that the child's vision is not corrected and eliminates an unnecessary administration of general anesthesia. When fitting the contact lenses in the operating room, the main priority is to determine the appropriate power of the contact lens. The best method to determine the power is to place a contact lens on the eye that approximates the resulting refractive error of the child (approximately +35 D). Retinoscopy should be performed over this contact lens using refractive trial lenses to determine the most appropriate power. Placing a high plus contact lens on the eye reduces the error potentially induced by the variable working distance of a high plus refractive trial lens. It may be necessary to stand on a stool or a short ladder in order to achieve the appropriate working distance on a child lying on an operating room table.

An infant's visual world is very close, so prescribing approximately +3.00 D greater than the child's refractive error may enhance the visual experience that the child receives. The power of the contact lens should be reduced to correct the child to emmetropia as the child begins to walk and requires greater viewing distances.

Over the first 1 or 2 years, the hyperopic refractive error reduces rapidly as the eye grows. The child should be examined every week for the first month or two of contact lens wear, then every 1 to 3 months until the child reaches school age. The power of the contact lenses should be checked at each visit and a new power should be provided as needed. The fit of the contact lens may also change as the eye continues to grow, so the diameter and base curve may need to be adjusted accordingly. A smaller diameter contact lens may be necessary for infants, but the size of the contact lens should increase to approximately adult size by the time the child is two years old. Larger contact lenses are less likely to become displaced when the child rubs the eyes.

Most children, especially children with unilateral aphakia, will require vision therapy to treat amblyopia. Vision therapy should begin at as early an age as possible and continue until about age 8 years. Consistent patching is very important to the development of functional binocular vision. If the child does not tolerate adhesive eye patches, an opaque contact lens may be fitted on the sound eye to provide visual rehabilitation (46).

Although continuous wear contact lenses are available in soft and rigid gas-permeable contact lenses, daily wear should be recommended except in rare cases. Daily wear contact lenses decrease the potential for serious complications of contact lens wear, such as neovascularization or infection. Daily wear is also the preferred mode of contact lens wear because parents and children are better able to adapt to the routine care of contact lenses if they perform it daily, and there will be fewer hassles with contact lens wear when the infant becomes a toddler. Silicone contact lenses are available for extended wear, but they are available in a limited range of powers, they are more expensive than many contact lenses, and they may deposit heavily.

Rigid contact lenses for aphakia should be ordered with a lenticular design. Without the lenticular design, the contact lenses are very thick, and the center of gravity is more anterior so the lens tends to fall to the inferior lid. Lenticular lenses are thinner and they center better on the eye. To improve lid attachment, minus carrier lenses should be ordered to increase the edge thickness of the lens (Fig. 31.5).

Glaucoma may occur in about 10% of children following cataract removal (47). Glaucoma is difficult to diagnose in young children because they cannot perform visual fields, intraocular pressures are difficult to measure, and reliable views of the optic nerve are difficult to obtain. Examinations on aphakic children should include routine intraocular pressure checks and dilated optic nerve assessments.

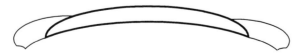

FIG. 31.5. A minus-carrier lenticular lens designs increases edge thickness of a plus lens to promote lid attachment.

TRAUMA

Trauma is a very common cause of contact lens wear in young children (3), and it can be a very challenging contact lens problem. Contact lenses are often necessary if the cornea is affected or if the crystalline lens develops a cataract or becomes dislodged. Irregular corneas in children can present an even more challenging situation, and they often require rigid gas-permeable contact lens correction to maximize vision.

Children who are aphakic following trauma should be fitted with contact lenses as soon as possible after the insult to reduce the potential for permanent vision loss. The practitioner should fit the child as discussed in the previous section on aphakia, keeping in mind that the cornea is likely to have irregular astigmatism. Thick, soft contact lenses may correct some of the irregular astigmatism, but rigid gas-permeable contact lenses are typically the most appropriate correction in terms of maximizing vision and health of the eye.

Fitting contact lenses on an eye after trauma is often done by trial and error. While keratometry performed on the fellow eye may provide some helpful information for the initial fitting, only evaluation of a trial contact lens on the eye will provide sufficient information to order a contact lens. Careful consideration of the centration of the lens on the eye must be made, because the contact lens may center over the scarred part of the cornea and not provide adequate coverage over other parts of the eye. Quite often, large-diameter (9.5 mm or larger) rigid gas-permeable contact lenses provide the best fit on an irregular cornea.

Trauma may also result in disfigured eyes that are cosmetically unappealing. Contact lenses may be prescribed to mask scarring that a causes a child to feel self-conscious. Because they provide greater corneal coverage and because they move less, soft contact lenses are typically fitted to mask disfigured eyes. They can be ordered with or without refractive correction, and they may custom made to match the fellow eye.

VISION THERAPY

Contact lenses can be a very useful adjunct in a vision therapy practice. Children who are noncompliant with an adhesive patching regimen may benefit from an opaque occluder contact lens (46). Study of a case series of 13 patients who were previously unsuccessful with adhesive patching suggested that one third of the children were successful with occluder contact lenses, one third of the children were successful with occluder contact lenses until the children determined how to dislodge the lenses themselves, and one third were never successful with occluder contact lenses. The authors found that dispensing high-plus contact lenses decreased the number of lost or torn lenses, and contact lenses were replaced on average every 3 months due to lost or torn contact lenses. Because the contact lenses are only worn for short periods during waking hours, the potential side effects of corneal hypoxia with high plus contact lenses are dramatically reduced. While opaque occluder contact lenses may not be a primary regimen for patching therapy, they provide an additional option to treat noncompliant patients.

Visual penalization with atropine has been shown to be successful for the visual rehabilitation of low to moderate amblyopia (48). Children may also be corrected with contact lenses that have high plus powers to achieve visual penalization. Contact lenses allow the patching regimen to be tailored to individual children, and the potential for photophobia complaints is lower than for children using atropine. Children with severe amblyopia may still prefer to fixate with the nonamblyopic eye, even when the power of the contact lens is +30.00 D greater than their refractive error (49).

Patching with contact lenses should be prescribed for a minimum of 4 hours of wear every day, and the child should be given specific visual tasks to perform while wearing the patch. Potential complications with occluder contact lenses are the same as all contact lenses, so the child should be monitored regularly for contact lens complications as well as progress with visual therapy.

COSMETIC AND PROSTHETIC CONTACT LENSES

Contact lenses may be used to improve the outward appearance of a patient with disfigured eyes, and they may improve the vision of people suffering from severe photophobia due to albinism (50), iris deformities (51,52), or achromatopsia (53).

Cosmetic contact lenses that translate well on the eye may reduce the appearance of nystagmus, which can have profound effects on a child's self-esteem. Contact lenses

TABLE 31.5. COMPANIES THAT WILL PAINT CONTACT LENSES TO MATCH THE FELLOW EYE (57)

Company	Location	Telephone
Adventures in Colors Technology	Golden, CO	(800) 537-2845
Crystal Reflections International, Inc.	Green Valley, AZ	(800) 807-8722
Custom Color Contacts	New York, NY	(800) 598-2020
Innovations in Sight, Inc.	Front Royal, VA	(877) 853-1509
Prosthetic Soft Lens Corporation	Englewood, CO	(800) 574-2581
Specialty Tint	Escondido, CA	(800) 748-5500

have also been shown to reduce the magnitude of nystagmus, which results in visual improvement (54,55).

Commercially available trial lens sets may be used to match the fellow eye (Table 31.4), or pictures may be provided to custom paint a contact lens eye to match the fellow eye (Table 31.5). Prosthetic contact lenses worn to mask a disfigured eye are typically expensive, and they require greater commitment by the patient and the practitioner to fit properly, but they are usually worth the added time and expense for the patient.

Prosthetic contact lenses should be fitted slightly tighter than other soft contact lenses in order to maintain the proper centration on the eye. The fit of the contact lens may also need to be altered once the proper color match is made, so the patients should be monitored regularly.

FITTING PROCEDURE

Contact lens fitting can be very traumatic for a young child because it is a new experience. When communicating with a young patient, a direct approach is often best but is not universally appropriate. While preparing to insert a contact

TABLE 31.4. COSMETIC AND PROSTHETIC CONTACT LENSES (57)

Company	Lenses	Telephone
Alden Optical	Alden HP, Alden Classic Tinted Toric, Alden Classic Prosthetic, Alden HP Prosthetic	(800) 253-3669
Bausch & Lomb	Optima 38 Natural, Natural Tint-B3, Natural Tint-U3, Natural Tint-U4, Natural Tint-03, Natural Tint-04	(800) 828-9030
CIBA Vision Corporation	Focus Softcolors, Fresh Look Color Blends, Fresh Look Colors, Fresh Look Color Enhancers, Focus Monthly Softcolors, Fresh Look Color Blends Toric, Fresh Look Toric, CIBASoft Softcolors, Durasoft 2 Colors, Illusions, Durasoft 3 Colorblends, Durasoft 3 Complements (D3•CO), Durasoft 3 Colors (D3•OP), Durasoft 2 Colors (D2•OP), Wild Eyes, Durasoft 3 Optifit Toric Colors MTO, Durasoft 2 Optifit, Durasoft 2 Optifit	(800) 241-5999
CooperVision	Vantage Accents DW, Vantage Thin Accents FW, Natural Touch Opaque, Crazy Lenses, Standard Prosthetic DW, Clear Periphery Lens DW, Custom/Prosthetic Lens DW	(800) 341-2020
Innovations in Sight	Super Nova Lenses	(877) 533-1509
Metro Optics	Metrotint	(800) 223-1858
Ocular Sciences, Inc.	Hydron Versa-Scribe Softints (FW)	(800) 628-5387

lens, the child may be told, "I am going to put a contact lens in your eye. It will feel like getting an eyelash or a piece of dust in your eye. After you wear the lens for one or two weeks, you probably won't feel it in your eye any more." The questions should be limited before putting the contact lens in the eye and it is important to not wait too long before inserting the contact lens because anxiety is a major factor in the child's ability to initially tolerate a contact lens. As soon as the contact lens is inserted, the child can be told that it is already in the eye. Generally the child is surprised at how easy it is to put the contact lens in the eye.

Infant

Initial fitting of contact lenses on infants (and possibly toddlers) is typically performed in the operating room while the child is under general anesthesia. The equipment necessary for fitting an infant under general anesthesia is listed in Table 31.6. Refractive error correction is the most important aspect of the infant's contact lens fitting. Retinoscopy should be performed under cycloplegia while a trial contact lens with a prescription close to the child's refractive error is on the eye. The overrefraction helps to reduce the error that can be induced by changing the vertex distance of a high power refractive trial lens. The complete procedure of fitting an infant with contact lenses while under anesthesia is described in the previous section on aphakia.

Toddler

Fitting a toddler with contact lenses can be one of the most challenging procedures for a contact lens practitioner. Infants are easier to control than toddlers, and it is easier to allay an older child's anxiety than a toddler's. There are no universal procedures to fit toddlers with contact lenses, so the practitioner must be very adept at several methods. When fitting in the examination room is unsuccessful, a fitting under general anesthesia should be considered.

The most important part of fitting a toddler with contact

TABLE 31.6. EQUIPMENT NECESSARY FOR FITTING A CHILD UNDER GENERAL ANESTHESIA WITH CONTACT LENSES

Retinoscope
Refractive lenses
Trial contact lenses
Portable slit lamp, Burton lamp, or a direct ophthalmoscope and condensing lens
Cobalt filter (GP contact lens fitting)
Fluorescein strips (GP contact lens fitting)
Lid speculum
Multipurpose contact lens solution
Handheld keratometer (if available)

GP, rigid gas permeable.

lenses is parent education. The parents must be told prior to the fitting that the child will kick and scream, but the contact lenses are necessary to prevent permanent vision loss. The parents must be taught how to insert and remove contact lenses, how to care for the contact lenses, and to be aware of any signs or symptoms of potential problems. The parents should also be educated about the cost of the contact lenses and the likelihood of frequent replacements.

Occasionally, a toddler must be restrained to be fitted with contact lenses (Fig. 31.6). This can be accomplished by having the parent hold the child, by wrapping a sheet around the child, or by straddling the child while he or she is lying on the floor. At least one extra pair of hands is necessary to provide assistance with the equipment necessary to conduct the fitting.

An eye care practitioner may consider having an office assistant insert the contact lens in the child's eye. Children may not trust the person who inserts the first contact lens for some time, so evaluation of the contact lens prescription may become very difficult. Once the child calms down, the eye care practitioner should evaluate the prescription and fit of the contact lens using retinoscopy over the contact lens and a slit-lamp examination. A slit-lamp examination

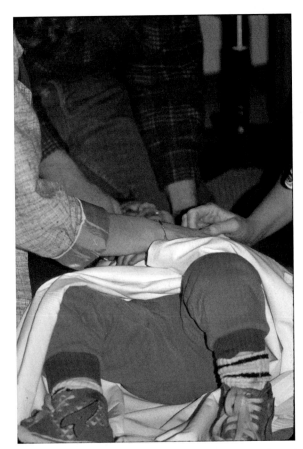

FIG. 31.6. Toddlers may need to be restrained with a sheet during a contact lens fitting, and extra hands can be very helpful (photo courtesy of Karla Zadnik, OD, PhD).

may be made easier by having the child pretend that the slit lamp is a motorcycle and by having the parent help hold the child steady in the chin rest.

Children

Once children enter first grade, they are capable of performing most of the test procedures similar to adults. The primary difference is that young children have shorter attention spans, they may be more nervous about visiting the doctor, and they may be less disciplined than an adult. As long as the examination is efficient, a child's contact lens fitting does not differ greatly from an adult's fitting.

Soft Contact Lenses

Soft contact lenses are initially more comfortable than rigid gas-permeable contact lenses, they require less time and effort to fit properly, and they can be dispensed at the fitting visit. Thus, they are fitted much more often than rigid gas-permeable contact lenses. When fitting young children with contact lenses, parents may have to be involved in the daily contact lens care, including insertion and removal. Because most parents who wear contact lenses have soft contact lenses, children may be fitted with soft contact lenses in order to alleviate some of the concerns about contact lens care for the parent. The parent will be more comfortable using a contact lens that is similar to the one she is wearing.

Although keratometry should be performed before all contact lens fittings, keratometry readings are not particularly useful for soft contact lens fittings. In order to reduce chair time and stress for the child, the practitioner should try a different base curve on each eye to determine the most appropriate fit of the contact lens. A soft contact lens should cover the entire cornea, and it should move 0.50 to 1.25 mm with each blink. If the base curve is too steep, the contact lens will not move sufficiently to provide adequate tear exchange. If the base curve is too loose, the edge of the contact lens may fold and be uncomfortable, or the contact lens will move too much and result in variable vision.

An overrefraction is easier to conduct on a new soft contact lens fit than on a new rigid gas-permeable contact lens fit because the soft contact lenses are initially more comfortable. Generally, the spherical equivalent of the manifest refraction will provide optimal vision and can be ordered without performing an overrefraction.

The diameter choice of soft contact lenses is limited, but they are nearly always sufficient to provide complete coverage of the cornea if the contact lens centers well. Each soft contact lens typically only comes in one diameter, so if the overall diameter is not adequate, a different brand of contact lens may be necessary.

Soft contact lenses are available in standard daily wear, frequent replacement, 2-week disposable, daily disposable, and 30-day continuous wear modalities. Children are likely to benefit from frequent replacement or disposable contact lenses because spare lenses are readily available should the lenses be lost or torn. Daily disposable contact lenses eliminate the need to clean contact lenses and are therefore easier to care for, but they are rarely fitted due to higher cost. While 30-day continuous wear contact lenses also reduce the hassle of daily contact lens care, caution should be used in fitting novice wearers with them. When complications do arise, the wearer must be adept at removing the contact lenses. Children may not become adept at removing the contact lenses if continuous wear contact lenses are dispensed before confirming that the child is capable of daily contact lens insertion and removal over a 3- to 6-month-period.

A number of children were switched from rigid gas-permeable contact lens wear to soft contact lens wear during the Contact Lens and Myopia Progression (CLAMP) study (2). Anecdotally, most of the children complained vehemently about the difficulty inserting and removing the soft contact lenses after adapting to rigid gas-permeable contact lens wear. When the children returned to the office 1 week after wearing soft contact lenses, few complained about insertion or removal, and most were satisfied with their soft contact lenses.

Rigid Contact Lenses

Rigid gas-permeable contact lenses may provide clearer vision than soft contact lenses, especially when worn to correct astigmatism caused by corneal toricity. Rigid gas-permeable contact lenses also allow improved tear flow and oxygen under the contact lens, thereby providing ocular health benefits to the long-term contact lens wearer. Anecdotally, rigid gas-permeable contact lenses are easier to handle because they cannot invert or fold as soft contact lenses do, and less contact time with the eye is necessary to allow the lens to settle. Myopic children may also benefit from a reduction in the progression of myopia due to the influence of rigid contact lens wear (10–12).

When fitting children with rigid gas-permeable contact lenses, there are many tips to make the process easier for the child and for the practitioner. Bennett et al. (56) reported the use of topical anesthetic at the fitting and dispensing visits improves adaptation to rigid contact lens wear. To prevent putting an additional drop in a child's eyes, the drop of anesthetic can be placed in the contact lens prior to insertion. After instilling the drop on the contact lens, a finger can be placed in the contact lens to displace most of the liquid, but the anesthetic effect still occurs. The anesthetic improves the child's disposition as well as the practitioner's ability to evaluate vision and lens fitting with fluorescein due to reduced tearing.

Children often squirm to avoid having the contact lens inserted in the eye. Avoid chasing the child by having the child fixate on a target, firmly holding the eyelids open, and

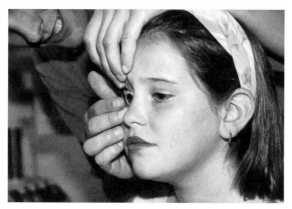

FIG. 31.7. A firm grasp of the child's head will make the contact lens insertion quicker and less stressful for the child.

stabilizing the head (Fig. 31.7). A quick insertion of the contact lens will make the entire fitting process much easier for the child and the doctor.

There are few differences between an adult and a child when deciding the lens parameters to order. Most children can be fitted with a 9.2-mm-diameter contact lens and a 7.8-mm optic zone diameter. Some practitioners like to fit children with smaller contact lenses because the palpebral aperture is smaller, and some practitioners like to fit children with larger-diameter contact lenses because they may fall out of the eye less often. The philosophy to be selected is an individual decision, but a 9.2-mm diameter may be a good compromise.

The base curve for the initial trial lens is based on keratometry readings and the standard fitting guide found in contact lens text books (Table 31.7). It may be difficult to get accurate keratometry readings on a child fidgeting in the chair, but verification that the readings are correct if the two eyes have similar readings, if the keratometry readings are similar to simulated keratometry readings from a corneal topographer, or if two measurements of the same eye are similar.

A slit-lamp assessment of the anterior segment and the fit of the contact lens must be performed at the initial fitting. An alignment-fitted contact lens should result in a refraction that is equal to the spherical component of the manifest refraction, so an empirical power determination is appropriate given a good lens-to-cornea fitting relationship. A spherical overrefraction is not necessary.

TABLE 31.7. GUIDE TO DETERMINE THE BASE CURVE FROM KERATOMETRY READINGS

Corneal Toricity	Base Curve
Spherical	0.50 D flatter than flat K
≤0.75 D toricity	0.25 D flatter than flat K
0.87–1.37 D	Fit on flat K
≥1.50 D toricity	0.33 times the toricity steeper than flat K

Depending on the child's motivation, the dispensing visit may be exciting or scary. One way to alleviate some of the anxiety is to instill a drop of topical anesthetic at the dispensing visit. The drop will help alleviate some of the child's fears and allow for a more proper assessment of the fit and prescription of the contact lens. Insertion and removal training takes more than 15 minutes, so corneal sensation will return to normal levels by the time the child leaves the office.

Children often find it fun to remove contact lenses by pulling temporally on the lateral canthus and blinking the lens out of the eye. Occasionally, children are not able to open their eyes wide enough or their lids will not "pop" the contact lens out of the eye with blinking. When this happens, the children should be taught to remove their contact lenses using one hand to hold the contact lens in place with the top eyelid and pushing under the contact lens with the other hand on the lower eyelid. A third alternative involves using a plunger to pull the contact lens out of the eye. Small plungers used for this purpose are available from DMV Corporation (Zanesville, OH).

Children have a steep learning curve when it comes to handling rigid gas-permeable contact lenses. They regularly lose or break at least one lens in the first week, but the number of lost or damaged lenses decreases dramatically after 2 weeks. Consider ordering a spare pair of contact lenses with the initial order. Most lenses will fit appropriately and provide good vision, and a contact lens lost in the early stages dramatically extends the adaptation period.

When checking the refraction over the contact lenses, the child may accept +0.50 to +1.00 D of additional sphere power without a reduction in acuity. When this happens, ask the child to blink hard, then recheck the power immediately. You will probably find that the child will no longer accept the plus power. Even if the child accepts up to +1.00 D over the contact lens power at the initial dispensing visit, wait to recheck the power in 1 week. The acceptance of additional plus power may be due to excess tearing, so after 1 week of adaptation, children typically experience poorer vision with a +0.25 D over refraction.

SUCCESSFUL RIGID GAS-PERMEABLE CONTACT LENS WEARERS

Some four out of every five children adapt to rigid gas-permeable lens wear (2). Knowing how to predict which children can successfully wear contact lenses will save both you and the child many problems.

Young girls are typically more mature than boys of a similar age. While maturity plays a role in the success rate of rigid gas-permeable contact lens wearers, 8- to 11-year-old boys and girls are equally successful at adapting to rigid contact lens wear. However, more girls attempt to wear

TABLE 31.8. CONSTRAINTS TO DISCUSS WITH PARENTS WHEN DISPENSING TOPICAL ANESTHETIC

The bottle of anesthetic should be in the parent's possession only

Limit the administration of anesthetic to one drop per eye per day

The child must attempt insertion for 5 minutes per eye prior to anesthetic installation

Weekly examinations are necessary until the child is able to insert contact lenses without anesthetic

If the child is not able to insert contact lenses without anesthetic after 2 weeks, then the child will not be able to wear rigid contact lenses

The bottle of anesthetic must be returned to the practitioner at the end of the trial

contact lenses, and they may account for three fifths of the patients who adapt to rigid contact lens wear.

Maturity is primarily an issue at the fitting visit rather than the dispensing visit. Some 8-year-old subjects are not able to distinguish the initial discomfort from pain. They are not able to comprehend that the sensation of the eyelids rubbing on the edge of the contact lenses is temporary, so they cry or refuse to wear contact lenses. A child's ability to handle or care for rigid gas-permeable contact lenses is not dependent on the child's age. Nearly all of the 8- to 11-year-old children can insert, remove, and care for contact lenses without assistance from their parents.

It is often believed that the motivation to wear lenses must belong solely to the contact lens wearer. When young lens wearers are involved, parents must also be motivated. Once outside of the office, parents must encourage the child to insert the contact lenses every day and help with problems that may be encountered during the adaptation period. Parents must also be willing to allow the child to learn alone

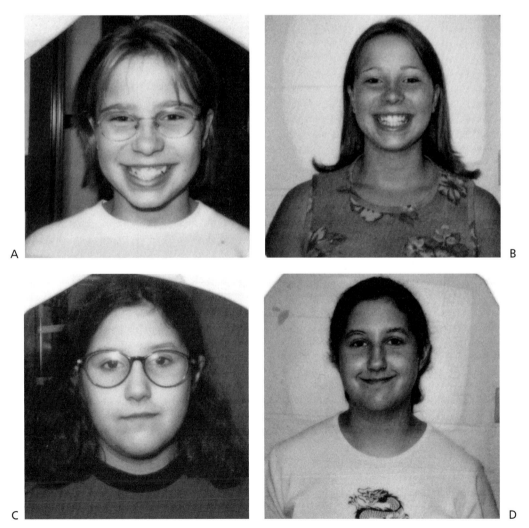

FIG. 31.8. The most rewarding aspect of fitting children is watching them grow up to be happy contact lens wearers.

and must tolerate the additional time necessary to insert or remove lenses.

In-office indicators of success include the child's ability to tolerate eye drops and holding of the eyelids by the practitioner. Children who run to "mommy" for a hug between each eye drop or are not able to answer your questions on their own are less likely to become successful rigid gas-permeable contact lens wearers.

Occasionally a successful contact lens wearer may experience a traumatic situation such as inserting the lens without rinsing off all of the soaking solution. This single event may cause a mental block that is very difficult for the child to overcome. The child may want to insert the contact lenses but be unable to because he or she subconsciously fears it will hurt again. When a parent reports that the child does great once the contact lenses are worn, but the child does not like to put them in, the problem is typically due to a mental block. The mental block may be due to one traumatic event or irritation upon insertion due to solution allergies. The eye care practitioner's reassuring affirmation and individual coaching or changing solutions often helps the child overcome the mental block.

If the child is not able to overcome a mental block after changing solutions and coaching from an experienced individual, dispensing topical anesthetic may be considered. A child who cannot insert a contact lens alone will often insert the contact lens on the first attempt after instillation of a drop of topical anesthetic. Due to the potential abuse of topical anesthetic, several constraints on dispensing should be discussed with the parents (Table 31.8).

Unfortunately, no universal predictors of success exist. Children may become successful rigid lens wearers despite initial signs that indicate the child may not be a good candidate. Fortunately, two thirds of the children who cannot adapt to rigid contact lens wear do not report to the 1-week check. Most children who are not able to wear rigid lenses realize it in a relatively short period of time, which is beneficial to the practitioner because it reduces time and resources necessary for the child to learn to care for contact lenses.

SUMMARY

Fitting children with contact lenses can be a challenging yet extremely rewarding experience. By fitting children with contact lenses, the clinician can expand his or her practice by tapping into a new population of contact lens wearers. The experience can be enjoyable for both patient and doctor when the examination is efficiently conducted, with little time for the child to worry about what might happen next. The clinician must always be completely straightforward with both parents and the child/patient about what to expect regarding the examination and future contact lens care. By following these two previous critical pieces of advice, the clinician will often enjoy watching young children grow up as very happy contact lens wearers (Fig. 31.8).

REFERENCES

1. Soni PS, Horner DG, Jimenez L, Ross J, Rounds J. Will young children comply and follow instructions to successfully wear soft contact lenses? *CLAO J* 1995;21:86–92.
2. Walline JJ, Mutti DO, Jones LA, et al. The Contact Lens and Myopia Progression (CLAMP) Study: design and baseline data. *Optom Vis Sci* 2001;78:223–233.
3. Shaughnessy MP, Ellis F, Jeffery AR, Szczotka L. Rigid gas-permeable contact lenses are a safe and effective means of treating refractive abnormalities in the pediatric population. *CLAO J* 2001;27:195–201.
4. Thomann KH, Marks ES, Adamczyk DT. *Primary eyecare in systemic disease,* 2nd ed. New York, NY: McGraw-Hill Medical Publishing Division, 2001.
5. Curtin B. *The myopias: basic science and clinical management.* Philadelphia: Harper & Row Publishers, Inc., 1985.
6. Blum H, B P, Bettman J. *Vision screening for elementary schools: the Orinda Study.* Berkeley: University of California Press, 1959.
7. Goss DA. Cessation age of childhood myopia progression. *Ophthalmic Physiol Opt* 1987;7:195–197.
8. Sperduto RD, Seigel D, Roberts J, Rowland M. Prevalence of myopia in the United States. *Arch Ophthalmol* 1983;101:405–407.
9. Morrison RJ. Contact lenses and the progression of myopia. *Optom Wkly* 1956;47:1487-1488.
10. Perrigin J, Perrigin D, Quintero S, Grosvenor T. Silicone-acrylate contact lenses for myopia control: 3-year results. *Optom Vis Sci* 1990;67:764–769.
11. Khoo CY, Chong J, Rajan U. A 3-year study on the effect of RGP contact lenses on myopic children. *Singapore Med J* 1999;40:230–237.
12. Stone J. The possible influence of contact lenses on myopia. *Br J Physiol Opt* 1976;31:89–114.
13. Baldwin WR, West D, Jolley J, Reid W. Effects of contact lenses on refractive corneal and axial length changes in young myopes. *Am J Optom Arch Am Acad Optom* 1969;46:903–911.
14. Horner DG, Soni PS, Salmon TO, Swartz TS. Myopia progression in adolescent wearers of soft contact lenses and spectacles. *Optom Vis Sci* 1999;76:474–479.
15. Lyons SA, Carlson NB, Moore BD, et al. The Hyperopic Infants Study: a survey of clinical prescribing philosophies. *Optom Vis Sci* 1999;76(suppl):140.
16. Miller JM, Harvey EM. Spectacle prescribing recommendations of AAPOS members. *J Pediatr Ophthalmol Strabismus* 1998;35:51–52.
17. Kornder LD, Nursey JN, Pratt-Johnson JA, Beattie A. Detection of manifest strabismus in young children. 2. A retrospective study. *Am J Ophthalmol* 1974;77:211–214.
18. Ingram RM, Barr A. Changes in refraction between the ages of 1 and 3 1/2 years. *Br J Ophthalmol* 1979;63:339–342.
19. Nixon R, Helveston E, Miller K, Archer S, Ellis F. Incidence of strabismus in neonates. *Am J Ophthalmol* 1985;100:798–801.
20. Fletcher MC, Silverman SJ. Strabismus. I. A summary of 1,110 consecutive cases. *Am J Ophthalmol* 1966;61:86–94.
21. Atkinson J, Braddick O, Robier B, et al. Two infant vision screening programmes: prediction and prevention of strabismus and amblyopia from photo- and videorefractive screening. *Eye* 1996;10:189–198.
22. Ingram RM, Arnold PE, Dally S, Lucas J. Results of a randomised trial of treating abnormal hypermetropia from the age of 6 months. *Br J Ophthalmol* 1990;74:158–159.

23. Zadnik K, Mitchell GL, Jones LA, Mutti DO. Ocular component development as a function of refractive error. *Optom Vis Sci* 2001; 78(Suppl):237.
24. Atkinson J, Anker S, Bobier W, et al. Normal emmetropization in infants with spectacle correction for hyperopia. *Invest Ophthalmol Vis Sci* 2000;41:3726–3731.
25. Mohindra I, Held R, Gwiazda J, Brill J. Astigmatism in infants. *Science* 1978;202:329–331.
26. Atkinson J, Braddick OJ, Durden K, Watson PG, Atkinson S. Screening for refractive errors in 6–9 month old infants by photorefraction. *Br J Ophthalmol* 1984;68:105–112.
27. Mohindra I, Held R. Refraction in humans from birth to five years. *Doc Ophthalmol Proc* 1981;28:19–27.
28. Attebo K, Ivers RQ, Mitchell P. Refractive errors in an older population: the Blue Mountains Eye Study. *Ophthalmology* 1999; 106:1066–1072.
29. Howland HC, Sayles N. Photorefractive measurements of astigmatism in infants and young children. *Invest Ophthalmol Vis Sci* 1984;25:93–102.
30. Dobson V, Fulton AB, Sebris SL. Cycloplegic refractions of infants and young children: the axis of astigmatism. *Invest Ophthalmol Vis Sci* 1984;25:83–87.
31. Gwiazda J, Scheiman M, Mohindra I, Held R. Astigmatism in children: changes in axis and amount from birth to six years. *Invest Ophthalmol Vis Sci* 1984;25:88–92.
32. Atkinson J, Braddick O, French J. Infant astigmatism: its disappearance with age. *Vision Res* 1980;20:891–893.
33. Fern KD, Manny RE, Garza R. Screening for anisometropia in preschool children. *Optom Vis Sci* 1998;75:407–423.
34. Cotlier E, Lambert S, Taylor D. *Congenital cataracts.* Austin, TX: R.G. Landes Company, 1994.
35. Ainsworth JR, Cohen S, Levin AV, Rootman DS. Pediatric cataract management with variations in surgical technique and aphakic optical correction. *Ophthalmology* 1997;104:1096–1101.
36. Basti S, Ravishankar U, Gupta S. Results of a prospective evaluation of three methods of management of pediatric cataracts. *Ophthalmology* 1996;103:713–720.
37. Braverman DE. Pediatric contact lenses. *J Am Optom Assoc* 1998; 69:452.
38. Ozbek Z, Durak I, Berk TA. Contact lenses in the correction of childhood aphakia. *CLAO J* 2002;28:28–30.
39. Chia A, Johnson K, Martin F. Use of contact lenses to correct aphakia in children. *Clin Exp Ophthalmol* 2002;30:252–255.
40. Buckley EG. Scleral fixated (sutured) posterior chamber intraocular lens implantation in children. *J AAPOS* 1999;3:289–294.
41. McClatchey SK, Parks MM. Myopic shift after cataract removal in childhood. *J Pediatr Ophthalmol Strabismus* 1997;34:88–95.
42. Morgan KS, McDonald MB, Hiles DA, et al. The nationwide study of epikeratophakia for aphakia in children. *Am J Ophthalmol* 1987;103:366–374.
43. Hiatt RL. Rehabilitation of children with cataracts. *Trans Am Ophthalmol Soc* 1998;96:475–515.
44. Ellis P. Extended wear contact lenses in pediatric ophthalmology. *CLAO J* 1983;9:317–321.
45. Cutler SI, Nelson LB, Calhoun JH. Extended wear contact lenses in pediatric aphakia. *J Pediatr Ophthalmol Strabismus* 1985;22: 86–91.
46. Joslin CE, McMahon TT, Kaufman LM. The effectiveness of occluder contact lenses in improving occlusion compliance in patients that have failed traditional occlusion therapy. *Optom Vis Sci* 2002;79:376–380.
47. Magnusson G, Abrahamsson M, Sjostrand J. Glaucoma following congenital cataract surgery: an 18-year longitudinal follow-up. *Acta Ophthalmol Scand* 2000;78:65–70.
48. Pediatric Eye Disease Investigator Group. A randomized trial of atropine vs. patching for treatment of moderate amblyopia in children. *Arch Ophthalmol* 2002;120:268–278.
49. Moore BD. *Eye care for infants & young children,* 1st ed. Boston: Butterworth-Heinemann, 1997.
50. Rakow PL. Making miracles with prosthetic soft lenses. *J Ophthalmic Nurs Technol* 1999;18:120–122.
51. Jurkus JM. Contact lenses for children. *Optom Clin* 1996;5: 91–104.
52. Burger DS, London R. Soft opaque contact lenses in binocular vision problems. *J Am Optom Assoc* 1993;64:176–180.
53. Schiefer U, Kurtenbach A, Braun E, Kraus W, Zrenner E. Centrally tinted contact lenses. A useful visual aid for patients with achromatopsia. *Ger J Ophthalmol* 1995;4:52–56.
54. Allen ED, Davies PD. Role of contact lenses in the management of congenital nystagmus. *Br J Ophthalmol* 1983;67:834–836.
55. Enoch JM, Windsor CE. Remission of nystagmus following fitting contact lenses to an infant with aniridia. *Am J Ophthalmol* 1968;66:333–335.
56. Bennett E, Smythe J, Henry V, et al. Effect of topical anesthetic use on initial patient satisfaction and overall success with rigid gas permeable contact lenses. *Optom Vis Sci* 1998;75:800–805.
57. Thompson TTT. Soft contact lens parameter guide. *Tylers Q* 2001;18:2–68.

THERAPEUTIC CONTACT LENSES

**WING-KWONG CHAN AND
BARRY A. WEISSMAN**

A therapeutic or "bandage" contact lens may be defined as any transparent material placed between the eye and the lids for the purpose of treating a pathological ocular condition. A bandage contact lens exerts a protective and therapeutic effect on the eye, either by itself or with additional medication (1).

Celsus has been credited with the first use of such an eye bandage: a honey-soaked linen placed in the inferior fornix of a patient to prevent the formation of symblepharon (2). Contact lenses were first used in the treatment of ocular diseases at their inception, about a century ago. Fick in Paris, Kalt in Zurich, and Muller in Weisbaden all independently produced glass contact lenses and used them to improve vision in traumatized and irregularly surfaced corneas (e.g., keratoconus) and to prevent corneal desiccation (3, 4). Virtually any and all contact lens designs have been used to treat ocular disease: rigid [both conventional (5) and glued onto the stroma (1,6)], scleral (1,3), and recently gas-permeable scleral lenses (7) (for additional information, see Chapter 33), hydrogel (8,9), silicone (10,11), and collagen contact lenses (12).

Hydrogel contact lenses have been the principle devices used in the bandage lens role since they first became available (8). Several hydrogel contact lens designs received specific US Food and Drug Administration (FDA) approval for such use. These lenses include those made from low-water (e.g., Bausch & Lomb Piano T, B4, U3, 04, and the CSI T), medium-water (Sofcon and Protek), and high-water-content materials (Permalens); oxygen transmissibility varies from very low ($\sim 5 \times 10^{-11}$ cm^2 mL O$_2$/s mL mm Hg) through modest ($\sim 25 \times 10^{-11}$ cm^2 mL O$_2$/s mL mm Hg) to high (Ciba Night and Day silicone hydrogels with Dk of 140×10^{-11} cm^2 mL O$_2$/s mL mm Hg) depending upon polymer and lens thickness values (see below). These lenses are usually prescribed in an afocal design so as to provide a parallel-sided uniform thickness shell of gel plastic (13). Patients continue to wear their normal spectacle correction, if any, for vision correction.

There is no physiologic reason, however, to restrict bandage lenses solely to special designs. Many of the various "cosmetic" contact lenses can be used in a "custom device" role to meet specific therapeutic requirements of patients. To this end, optical correction can be provided at the same time as "bandaging" the eye: the clinician must remember, however, that the addition of optics imparts increased lens thickness, centrally for plus-powered and peripherally for minus-powered lenses, and thereby may decrease oxygen flux to the cornea (14,15). The distribution of new silicone-hydrogel contact lenses for cosmetic wear (16) allows clinicians access to contact lenses of very enhanced oxygenation (Dk of 100 to 170×10^{-11} cm^2 mL O$_2$/s mL mm Hg) indeed, whether used for cosmetic devices or bandages.

The introduction of much less costly, but physiologically comparable, "disposable" hydrogel lenses in 1988 almost immediately inspired their utilization as therapeutic lenses. Although most of these have not been specifically approved by the FDA for the bandage lens role, it is clear that these inexpensive lenses are being widely used currently as bandage lenses (9,17,18) (Ciba Vision's "Protek" design, however, has such FDA approval).

Silicone rubber lenses have had a particular role to play when hydrogel lenses prove difficult to use: severely dry eyes, decompensated and vascularized corneas, and corneal surfaces so flat or irregular that other modalities are unusable (10,11,19). Scleral lenses have also been useful with these patients (7,20).

GOALS OF THERAPEUTIC (BANDAGE) CONTACT LENSES

The major goals, or clinical benefits, sought from the use of therapeutic (bandage) contact lenses are

- Reduction of pain associated with corneal epithelial defects and abnormalities.
- Healing of corneal epithelial defects.
- Protection of the cornea from drying and mechanical trauma (e.g., entropion or trichiasis).
- Sealing of small corneal wounds and perforations by splinting the wound, thereby restoring the anterior chamber.

- Optical enhancement by providing a new smooth anterior air/cornea interface over corneal surfaces made irregular by trauma, surgery, or disease (e.g., keratoconus). (This aspect has been well described elsewhere in this text; see Chapter 28.)

FITTING PRINCIPLES

Base Curve and Total Diameter

Bandage hydrogel lenses should be applied, by the appropriate selection of base curve and diameter during a diagnostic fitting, to achieve lens centration and modest movement. Achieving such a fit is more an act of matching sagittal depths than base curve/diameters to corneal surfaces. Additionally, the movement of a bandage lens on the ocular surface should probably be somewhat less than that optimally desirable for a cosmetic fitting. Minimization of lens movement is believed to facilitate patient acceptance by decreasing lid sensations and is also helpful in decreasing mechanical trauma to fragile, healing epithelial cells (21).

Many clinicians use a single design for most of their bandage hydrogel lens dispensing, but adding 1.0 mm to the mean keratometry measurement can assist in the selection of initial base curve (the curvature of the contralateral "normal" eye may prove more helpful than the often distorted values of the eye being treated). Corneal protection demands full corneal coverage; therefore, most clinicians select initial hydrogel lens diameters about 1.0 mm larger than the visible horizontal corneal diameter. Bandage lenses should be slightly steeper in base curve than cosmetic design lenses, and have larger (14.5 to 16.0 mm) rather than smaller (13 mm) overall diameters. (Occasionally, however, small diameters may be necessitated by specific ocular conditions; e.g., when the perilimbal bulbar conjunctiva is distorted, redundant, and irregular following surgery or trauma.) Hydrogel bandage lenses should not be fit so tight, however, that they indent the sclera, blanch conjunctival blood vessels, cause central air bubbles, or ripple the conjunctiva (22). Such observations are not in themselves serious problems, but hydrogel lenses, especially if used for extended wear, may tighten further with dehydration, changes in pH, or aging, and may subsequently induce a "tight lens syndrome," wherein the eye becomes painful and inflamed (23,24).

Lens Thickness

Lens thickness should be minimized to optimize oxygenation, promote epithelial healing (25) and maintain other aspects of corneal physiology especially if extended wear is necessary or desirable during the treatment of a specific condition. If hydrogel lenses are to be worn for daily wear, handling may be improved by use of a thicker lens at the sacrifice of some oxygen flux. Some clinicians have advocated ultrathin "membrane" bandage hydrogel contact lenses in instances of minimal inflammation, while thicker high water content bandage hydrogels are suggested for use in eyes with substantial inflammation (26). Use of silicone rubber, silicone hydrogel, rigid gas-permeable, and scleral lenses will require consideration of the individual material characteristics and ocular situations to determine appropriate lens thicknesses.

Water Content

The optimum water content of a hydrogel bandage lens remains an area of some controversy. Thoft (27) suggested that high-water-content hydrogels were helpful in the treatment of dry-eye conditions by providing a fluid reservoir. Others alternatively proposed that evaporation from the anterior surface of hydrogel lenses will draw water from the precorneal tear film and underlying epithelial surface, perhaps further dehydrating the cornea; such effects will be enhanced with increasing lens water content and decreasing lens thickness (28,29). This effect, if it exists, might be beneficial in the management of bullous keratopathy but problematic in cases of dry eye (1).

Oxygen Transmissibility

Oxygen has been shown to be essential for the maintenance of normal corneal physiology (30,31). The oxygen transmissibility (Dk/t) (see Chapters 4 and 35 for more complete discussions of this topic) of a hydrogel contact lens may be optimized either by increasing the water content of the hydrogel plastic or by decreasing the lens thickness (32). Dk is the oxygen permeability of the contact lens plastic, which is determined by the water content of a hydrogel or the silicone content of a silicone material. It is an intrinsic property of the material and is independent of lens thickness. The t is lens thickness. Research suggests minimal Dk/t values to maintain corneal physiology for normal eyes under both daily and extended wear at about 25 and 90 × 10^{-9} cm mL O_2/s mL mm Hg respectively (33), but no such values have been established for treatment of any of the various diseased corneal states.

Wearing Schedule

If it is at all possible for a patient to manage a contact lens on a daily wear basis, and if the disease being managed is such that extended wear is not necessarily desirable or essential, daily wear is preferable. Daily wear should reduce risks of severe complications (especially microbial infection and neovascularization) (34–37). Thin, but not ultrathin, low-water-content lenses facilitate daily patient care and handling of the lenses. High-water-content and/or thinner hydrogel lenses, or silicone hydrogel lenses (thereby enhancing

Dk/t), should be used when extended wear is elected or necessitated by the specific ocular disease being managed.

Lens-cleaning routines as appropriate should be employed as frequently as the disease process and the patient's particular situation allow. Certainly every time the lens is removed from the eye it should be cleaned and disinfected prior to reinsertion. To optimize antimicrobial efficiency while minimizing reactions, lens care should primarily utilize peroxide systems as appropriate for the specific contact lens material and patient situation as heat disinfection has been discontinued and chemical lens care systems have been more associated with hypersensitivity reactions. Disposable (single use) hydrogel lenses may therefore prove particularly helpful, eliminating the need for any disinfection process.

Evaluation Schedule

Frequent professional evaluations are essential in the continuing management of all therapeutic contact lens–wearing patients, particularly if patients are managed with extended wear. Also, concomitant medical, and perhaps surgical, treatment is often required.

Following application of the contact lens, the patient should be examined at the biomicroscope after a few minutes, then again after about an hour of wear to confirm the continued appropriate mechanical fit, patient comfort, and to observe and address any acute physiologic distress. Lens changes are not uncommon at this point to refine the mechanical fit. The appropriate progress visit schedule varies with the situation being managed, but in general, patients should be seen the day following initial application, 3 or 4 days later, and then at intervals ranging from weekly to monthly until the patient's particular situation has stabilized. Some situations require therapeutic lens management for only short intervals, for days or weeks, while healing occurs, while other situations require that a bandage lens remain on an eye for months to years, or even indefinitely. Patients who are unable to care for their lenses, and who have no family or friends to fulfill this role, may need to visit the clinician's office to obtain contact lens care on a periodic basis.

INDICATIONS FOR THE THERAPEUTIC USE OF HYDROGEL LENSES

Corneal Erosions

Recurrent corneal erosions are known to follow trauma to the epithelial basement membrane (e.g., from fingernail or paper-cut abrasions), or are secondary to the anterior corneal dystrophies (the fairly common Cogan's map-dot-fingerprint, Reis-Buckler's, or the rare Meesman's dystrophies); corneal degenerations (e.g., Salzmann's degeneration); stromal dystrophies (such as lattice, granular, or macular); and metaherpetic ulcers or other scars. Initial therapy includes patching the eye and use of hypertonic saline drops and/or ointment. If this treatment is unsuccessful, bandage hydrogel lenses have been found to reduce acute foreign body sensation, pain, photophobia and tearing, and promote long-term healing (8,38,39). There may be some visual benefit as well, as a hydrogel lens may smooth the irregular anterior corneal surface. Achieving optimal vision, however, demands a rigid contact lens. This form of therapy is usually on an extended wear basis and continued for several months to permit healing and subsequent epithelial stabilization (27), but the success rate of this therapy appears to only be about 50% (38,40–44).

Bandage contact lenses have been similarly used to patch epithelial defects following excimer laser photorefractive keratectomy (PRK) (45,46) for myopia and phototherapeutic keratectomy (PTK) for superficial corneal scars. Hydrogel lenses, of slightly steep base curves, are applied immediately after these laser procedures and are usually removed 3 to 5 days postoperatively, once the corneal epithelium has healed. Following the success of this application, some clinicians have used bandage hydrogel lenses with adjunctive non-steroidal antiinflammatory drops as an alternative to pressure patching in the treatment of other corneal abrasions to good result (47).

Chronic Epithelial Defects

Large chronic epithelial defects following herpetic and other infectious diseases, chemical (particularly alkali) bums, topical anesthetic abuse, Stevens-Johnson syndrome, neurotrophic or postradiation keratitis, or surgery [e.g., diabetic vitrectomy (48) and corneal grafts], are dangerous because both stromal melting and infection may occur. Such lesions have been treated with bandage contact lenses used on an extended-wear basis (49–51). In this role, the contact lens is again an alternative to a pressure patch intended to heal the epithelium. It must be recognized that healing alone does not address the underlying epithelial abnormality. Ali and Insler (52) questioned the efficacy of this approach. Recent research also suggests that some epithelial defects may be associated with destruction of the limbus based epithelial "stem" cells and that limbal stem cell grafting may be a more appropriate and effective treatment (53,54). Bandage hydrogel contact lenses are similarly known to improve patient comfort and promote epithelial healing in cases of Thygeson's superficial punctate keratitis (55,56).

Bullous Keratopathy

Bandage hydrogel contact lenses provide symptomatic relief for patients suffering from painful corneal decompensation secondary to corneal endothelial failure (e.g., Fuchs' dystrophy, aphakic or pseudophakic bullous keratopathy, Chandler's iridocorneal-endothelial syndrome, and corneal hydrops secondary to severe keratoconus) (8,21,34,43,50,

57–66). Severe corneal edema results in epithelial blistering which induces foreign-body sensation, pain, and photophobia upon rupture (Fig. 32.1). A bandage hydrogel lens reduces these effects by providing a tamponade to the corneal surface, reinforcing the damaged tissues and protecting any exposed nerve endings from the abrasive actions of the lids (9). Healing may also be assisted, but corneal infection (67) and vascularization often complicate long-term care. Vascularization of the cornea, should it occur, may secondarily compromise the success of future keratoplasty. Hovding's data suggested a modest improvement in attainable vision, and he indicated that a decrease in corneal thickness could be achieved with the concomitant use of topical hypertonic saline (65), but review of the literature suggests such results are inconsistent (40). Some feel this role is best served by thicker, high-water-content lens designs, fitted relatively flat, which then mechanically press down upon and flatten the bullae. As mentioned previously, dehydration of the epithelium through a high-water-content lens may serve as an additional therapeutic factor (1). For most cases of chronic bullous keratopathy, however, therapeutic hydrogel lenses are a temporizing measure while awaiting more definitive surgical intervention such as a conjunctival flap for eyes with poor visual potential or a corneal transplant for those eyes which have potentially useful vision.

Mechanical Trauma

Both hydrogel and scleral bandage contact lenses are often used to protect the cornea from mechanical damage due to inwardly misdirected eyelashes (entropion or trichiasis) (34), rubbing of sutures (e.g., following lid surgery), keratinization of the posterior lid margins in atopic keratoconjunctivitis (68), giant papillae [e.g., in vernal keratoconjunctivitis (57)], and similar changes in the palpebral

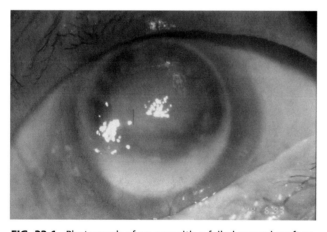

FIG. 32.1. Photograph of an eye with a failed corneal graft resulting in bullous keratopathy. A bandage contact lens helps alleviate the ocular pain and irritation that frequently accompany bullous keratopathy.

conjunctiva, or from inflammation [e.g., superior limbic keratoconjunctivitis (58)].

Dry Eyes and Filamentary Keratitis

Mild dry eye is often treated by lid hygiene, artificial tear supplements during the day and ointments at bedtime. The corneal surface may be protected from more severe dry eye conditions by the presence of a hydrogel contact lens, usually with the continued use of artificial tears and ocular lubricants (8,27,63,69). A similar indication is described after damage to cranial nerves V or VII (50). This role is somewhat controversial as the hydrogel lenses tend to dry out (1,69,70). These patients are then at greater risk for corneal infection (34,35). Bandage hydrogel contact lenses should be considered in cases of severe dry eye; therefore, only if other methods, such as supplementary lubrication, punctal occlusion, or moisture chambers have failed. Adjunctive care includes close professional supervision and often concomitant topical antibiotics.

Filamentary keratitis can occur following any process that damages the integrity of the corneal epithelium (e.g., superior limbic keratoconjunctivitis or recurrent corneal erosion) but is particularly common with severe dry eyes (keratitis sicca). Filaments have been successfully treated with bandage hydrogel contact lenses (60,71,72).

Bullous Diseases of the Conjunctiva

The management of bullous diseases of the conjunctiva, such as ocular cicatricial pemphigoid and Stevens-Johnson syndrome, may be assisted either by bandage hydrogel (73) or by scleral lenses (20). Contact lenses serve in multiple roles in these diseases, protecting the corneal epithelium from both drying and mechanical damage due to eyelid abnormalities (e.g., entropion or trichiasis). The lenses themselves may also work as a mechanical barrier to the formation of symblepharon and progressive forniceal shallowing.

Structural Reinforcement of the Cornea

Bandage hydrogel contact lenses have been used as structural reinforcement to promote sealing, healing and vascularization of small (<3 mm), suitably positioned corneal perforations or wound dehiscence (e.g., in a corneal graft), in the absence of incarceration or prolapse of the uvea or crystalline lens (74–76). The clinician should note a rapid reformation of the anterior chamber under such conditions. Laibson (77) advises that such contact lens application should preferably begin within the first 72 hours after perforation.

Larger wounds that have been sealed with sutures or tissue adhesives (78) are often co-treated with bandage hydrogel lenses to provide support, smooth the anterior surface of the eye, and thereby improve patient comfort and toler-

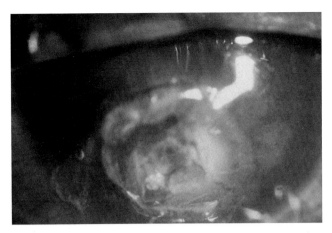

FIG. 32.2. Photograph of an eye with a corneal perforation after trauma. Tissue glue has been applied to seal the perforation, and a bandage contact lens has been applied. The contact lens improves patient comfort and prevents the lids from rubbing the glue off.

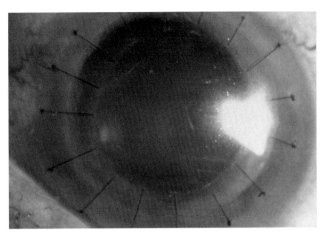

FIG. 32.4. Photograph of an eye after penetrating keratoplasty. A bandage contact lens is used here to promote healing of the corneal epithelium and to protect the eye from the irritative effects of the exposed suture knots.

ance (Fig. 32.2). Similarly, such lenses can occasionally serve to support threatening descemetoceles (74,79,80) and other corneal thinning disorders [e.g., Mooren's ulcer (81)], often to temporize while waiting for more definitive surgical repair (Fig. 32.3).

Following Ocular Surgery

Oversized hydrogel contact lenses (diameters ranging from 16 to 24 mm) have been used following glaucoma filtration surgery to tamponade bleb leaks and allow conjunctival closure of the wound (82,83). These lenses also prevent overfiltration either by decreasing the hydraulic conductivity or by mechanically pressing on the scleral flap to close the sclerostomy, but do not necessarily raise intraocular pressure or reverse maculopathy (84). The earliest use of a contact lens in this role was with an oversized rigid contact lens

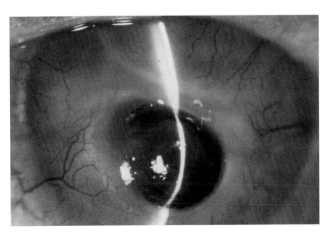

FIG. 32.3. Photograph of an eye with a descemetocele. A bandage contact lens can provide structural support and protect the cornea until definitive surgical repair.

(Simmon's shell) with an elevated platform on its concave surface to be positioned over the site to be tamponaded (85). Topical pharmaceuticals are used with these devices: steroids and cycloplegics to reduce inflammation and pain, and antibiotics, which are employed in the hopes of precluding infection (86).

During and immediately after surgery, contact lenses have been used:

1. to protect the eye [e.g., during lid procedures (87)],
2. to aid in visualization during vitreoretinal surgery,
3. to promote healing of the epithelium and pain relief after PRK as well as to protect the eye from the irritative effects of exposed suture knots (Fig. 32.4) after penetrating keratoplasty (88), and
4. following laser *in situ* keratomileusis, where they are used to stabilize the corneal flap in the early postoperative period, and also serve to decrease the occurrence of inadvertent flap dislodgement, striae formation, and epithelial ingrowth.

CONTRAINDICATIONS

Contraindications to therapeutic (bandage) contact lens wear are considered relative and not absolute, in that treatment of disease should be guided by what appears to the clinician to be in each individual patient's best interest given the specific circumstances. The reader must also recall that contact lens wear is contraindicated, according to the package inserts which accompany most of the contact lenses distributed in the United States, in the presence of dry eyes and any active disease (e.g., infection/inflammation) of the anterior ocular surface—precisely those situations in which bandage lenses are most often used.

Therapeutic hydrogel contact lenses should probably not

be used, or only used cautiously, in the presence of active microbial infection of the eye. Also, during an active infection of one eye, contact lens wear should probably be discontinued for both eyes (if possible) to preclude the spread of infection to the second eye. Patients with hypoesthetic or anesthetic corneas, dry eyes, or exposure keratitis present a particularly increased risk for concomitant corneal infection.

A therapeutic lens probably should not be used when a patient is unwilling or unable to return for appropriate and timely professional care, or unable to comply with reasonable care guidelines. Not only should patients be willing and able to present for scheduled visits, but patients should also be advised to present immediately should they experience any symptoms of pain, discharge, injection of the conjunctival vasculature, or subjective reduction in vision between scheduled examinations. The participation of family members and other caregivers in contact lens maintenance and compliance is helpful and should be encouraged.

Additional relative contraindications include other aspects of concern that apply to contact lens wear: dusty, polluted environments; poor personal hygiene; concomitant lid diseases like blepharitis; and obstruction or infection of the lacrimal drainage system. Filtering blebs have long been considered a contraindication as they have been thought to serve as a potential pathway for infection to spread from the surface of the eye to the inner structures leading to endophthalmitis (89); a recent article, however, has questioned this concern (90).

DRUG DELIVERY

The standard approach for drug delivery to the anterior segment of the eye is with the use of topically applied solutions, suspensions, and ointments. It is known that this method of pharmaceutical application results in a repetitive series of biphasic pulses: initial overdosage, then underdosage. This is repeated after every drop or set of drops. Several attempts have therefore been made to arrive at improved ophthalmic drug delivery systems, including suspensions of liposomes, ocular inserts, iontophoresis, and more recently intracameral vehicles such as the Surodex steroid-delivery system (91).

Sedlacek (92) was perhaps the first to propose that hydrogel contact lenses could be used to provide topical drug therapy. Wattman and Kaufman (93) thought that hydrogel contact lenses enhanced drug contact time and thereby promoted drug penetration into the cornea and anterior segment of the eye. The total amount of drug delivered was found to be dependent upon the concentration of the drug in the preapplication soaking solution (93–96), although one would expect that water solubility, molecular weight (97,98), and ionic state of the lens' molecules would play some role as well.

Hydrogel contact lenses have a dimensional structure where effective pore size is dependent upon water content (99). Drug absorption and release were therefore also found to be dependent to a certain extent on this parameter. Higher-water-content hydrogel lenses absorb more water-soluble drug and release it more quickly than do lower-water-content hydrogel lenses (93). Thicker, higher-water-content hydrogel lenses were also found to deliver more drug than thinner, lower-water-content lenses (97).

Many drugs have been used in hydrogel contact lens–delivery systems over the succeeding years (95–101), including pilocarpine (95,102–104), acetazolamide and methazolamide (105), cysteine hydrochloride (106) and acetylcysteine (107), corticosteroids (98), and antibiotics such as chloramphenicol (108), tetracycline (108), bacitracin (109), polymyxin B (109), gentamicin (110), and idoxuridine (111). EDTA (ethylenediaminetetraacetic acid) has also been incorporated in hydrogel lenses for the treatment of alkali burns (106).

It was difficult to substantiate that hydrogel contact lenses offered clinical advantages as drug-delivery systems compared to the logistically simpler use of topical pharmaceuticals. Nearly all the drug absorbed by presoaked hydrogel lenses was found to be released within the first few hours of elution (94,98,111), and the enhanced effect originally observed was eventually attributable to bolus administration rather than a sustained release (100,101).

Collagen shields were developed and used to promote corneal wound healing (12). Collagen shields have also largely supplanted hydrogel lenses in the drug-delivery role. When a collagen shield becomes hydrated in a solution containing a water-soluble drug, the drug becomes trapped within and evenly bound to the collagen (112). The drug is then released as the shield dissolves on the eye. A great variety of ophthalmic drugs have been delivered by collagen shield (112–125) with only rare reports of toxicity [from the co-use of antibiotics and steroids (126)]. Drug delivery by collagen shields has been found to be comparable or even superior to eyedrop therapy or subconjunctival injection across a wide range of studies (112–125). A disadvantage is that vision is usually reduced, to perhaps 20/80 to 20/200 (127), and not improved as might be possible with an appropriately optically powered hydrogel contact lens.

COMPLICATIONS

All the known complications of contact lens wear can be encountered during therapeutic applications, but severity and prevalence may increase when the cornea and/or anterior segment of the eye have already been compromised by disease. Infective keratitis is of greatest concern. In this setting, cultures are more commonly positive for either fungi or gram-positive bacteria (37,128) rather than for the gram-negative bacteria (more commonly found in association with cosmetic contact lens wearers). Corneal neovascularization is another major concern.

Neovascularization of the normally avascular cornea may be desirable in certain circumstances (to promote healing) but may eventually result in visual loss from stromal opacification (129) and can compromise the survival of a future corneal transplant.

The clinician should also be alert to the potential for other complications of contact lens wear. Giant papillary conjunctivitis is particularly common during the wear of bandage lenses of all varieties, where longer wearing periods are the rule and less attention is paid by the patient or practitioner to minor symptoms like itch and mucous. Sterile infiltrates (34) and corneal wrinkling (22) are additional concerns. Postkeratoplasty patients must be followed for corneal vascularization, loose sutures, or graft rejection. Such patients may also be more prone to corneal abrasions.

CONCLUSION

Therapeutic (bandage) contact lenses are widely used to provide pain relief from corneal epithelial defects and bullous keratopathy; promote healing of corneal epithelial defects; sealing and tamponade of small corneal perforations; after corneal surgery such as corneal transplantation and PRK; and to protect the cornea from mechanical trauma. Bandage lenses are usually hydrogel soft lenses and can be custom made for the role or are "cosmetic" contact lenses (especially the disposable lenses), which are the main type of hydrogel lenses used in this role today. The newer silicone and hydrogel hybrid lenses with very high oxygen transmissibility, such as Bausch & Lomb's PureVision (130) and Ciba's Night and Day contact lenses have also found application as bandage lenses.

Careful and stringent assessment of the patient and the eye is of utmost importance in determining if a bandage contact lens will benefit the ocular condition being treated. All the complications associated with the use of contact lenses can occur with increased prevalence and severity due to the pre-existing pathological status of the eye. More frequent than usual evaluation of the patient using a bandage lens is therefore necessary to detect and treat complications such as giant papillary conjunctivitis, corneal neovascularization and infective keratitis. When they are used appropriately, fitted correctly and managed well, bandage contact lenses are a useful, effective, and safe modality in the management of a wide variety of ocular surface and corneal conditions.

REFERENCES

1. Kaufman HE. Therapeutic use of soft contact lenses. In Dabezies OH, ed. *Contact lenses: the CLAO guide to basic science and clinical practice.* Orlando: Gruen and Stratton, 1984: 46.1–46.11.
2. Arrington GE. *A history of ophthalmology.* New York: MD Publishers, 1959.
3. Obrig TE. *Contact lenses.* Philadelphia: Chilton, 1942.
4. Bailey NJ. The genesis. *Contact Lens Spectr* 1987;2:23–26.
5. Genvert Gl, Cohen EJ, Arentsen JJ, et al. Fitting gas permeable contact lenses after penetrating keratoplasty. *Am J Ophthalmol* 1985;99:511–514.
6. Dohiman CH, Carroll J, Ahmad B, et al. M. Replacement of the corneal epithelium with a contact lens. *Trans Am Acad Ophthalmol Otolaryngol* 1969;73:482–493.
7. Ezekiel D. Gas permeable haptic lenses. *J Br Contact Lens Assoc* 1983;6:158–161.
8. Gasset AR, Kaufman HE. Therapeutic uses of hydrophilic contact lenses. *Am J Ophthalmol* 1970;69:252–259.
9. Lindahl KJ, DePaolis MD, Aquavella JV, et al. Applications of hydrophilic disposable contact lenses as bandages. *CLAO J* 1991;17:241–243.
10. Woodward EG. Therapeutic silicone rubber lenses. *J Br Contact Lens Assoc* 1984;7:39–40.
11. Bacon AS, Astin C, Dart JKG. Silicone rubber contact lenses for the compromised cornea. *Cornea* 1994;13:422–428.
12. Aquavella JV, del Cerro M, Musco PS, et al.. The effect of collagen bandage lens on corneal wound healing; a preliminary report. *Ophthalmic Surg* 1987;18:570–573.
13. Weissman BA. Designing uniform thickness contact lens shells. *Am J Optom Physiol Opt* 1982;59:902–903.
14. Weissman BA, Pham C. The L in Dk/L. *Optom Vis Sci* 1992; 69:639–644.
15. Fatt I, Weissman BA, Ruben CM. Areal differences in oxygen supply to a cornea wearing an optically powered hydrogel contact lens. *CLAO J* 1993;19:226–234.
16. Montero Iruzubieta J, Nebot Ripoll JR, Chiva J, et al. Practical experience with a high Dk lotrafilcon A fluorosilicone hydrogel extended wear contact lens in Spain. *CLAO J* 2001;27:41–46.
17. Tanner JB, DePaolis MD. Disposable contact lenses as alternative bandage lenses. *Clin Eye Vis Care* 1992;4:159–161.
18. Bouchard CS, Trimble SN. Indications and complications of therapeutic disposable Acuvue contact lenses. *CLAO J* 1996; 22:106–108.
19. Jackson AJ, Sinton JE, Frazer DG, et al. Therapeutic contact lenses and their use in the management of anterior segment pathology. J Br Cont Assoc 1996;19:11–19.
20. Schein OD, Rosenthal P, Ducharme C. A gas-permeable scleral contact lens for visual rehabilitation. *Am J Ophthalmol* 1990; 109:318–322.
21. Aquavella JV. Chronic corneal edema. *Am J Ophthalmol* 1973; 76:201–207.
22. Mobilia EF, Yamamoto GK, Dohiman CH. Corneal wrinkling induced by ultrathin soft contact lenses. *Ann Ophthalmol* 1980; 12:371–375.
23. Murphy GE. A case of sterile endophthalmitis associated with the extended wear of an aphakic soft contact lens. *Cont Intraocul Lens Med J* 1981;7:5–7.
24. Snyder DA, Litinsky SM, Calender H. Hypopyon iridocyclitis associated with extended wear soft contact lenses. *Am J Ophthalmol* 1982;93:519–520.
25. Mauger TF, Hill RM. Corneal epithelial healing in hypoxic environments. *Invest Ophthalmol Vis Sci* 1987;28(Suppl):2.
26. Bodner BI. Selection of therapeutic lenses. In: Dabezies OH, ed. *Contact lenses: the CLAO guide to basic science and clinical practice.* Orlando: Grune and Stratton, 1984:47.1–47.9.
27. Thoft RA. Therapeutic soft contact tenses. In Smolen G, Thoft RA, eds. *Cornea.* Boston: Little-Brown, 1983.

28. Baldone JA, Kaufman HE. Soft contact lenses in clinical disease. *Am J Ophthalmol* 1983;95:851–852.

29. Zantos S, Orsborn GN, Walter HC, et al.. Studies on corneal staining with thin hydrogel contact lenses. *J Br Contact Lens Assoc* 1986;9:61–64.

30. Smelser G, Ozanics V. Importance of atmospheric oxygen for maintenance of the optical properties of the human cornea. *Science* 1952;115:140.

31. Poise KA, Mandell RB. Critical oxygen tension at the corneal surface. *Arch Ophthalmol* 1970;84:505–508.

32. Fatt I. Gas transmission properties of soft contact lenses. In: Ruben M, ed. *Soft contact lenses.* New York: J Wiley & Sons, 1978:83–110.

33. Holden BA, Mertz GW. Critical oxygen levels to avoid corneal edema for daily and extended wear contact lenses. *Invest Ophthalmol Vis Sci* 1984;25:1161–1167.

34. Dohiman CH, Boruchoff SA, Mobilia EF. Complications in use of soft contact lenses in corneal disease. *Arch Ophthalmol* 1973;90:367–371.

35. Brown SJ, Bloomfield S, Pearce DB, Tragakis M. Infections with the therapeutic soft lens. *Arch Ophthalmol* 1974;91: 275–277.

36. Lemp MA. The effect of extended wear aphakic hydrophilic contact lenses after penetrating keratoplasty. *Am J Ophthalmol* 1980;90:331–335.

37. Kent HD, Cohen EJ, Laibson PR, et al.. Microbial keratitis associated with therapeutic soft contact lenses. *CLAO J* 1990; 16:49–52.

38. Mobilia EF, Foster CS. The management of recurrent corneal erosions with ultra-thin lenses. *Contact Intraocul Lens Med J* 1985.;4:25–29.

39. Gans LA. Eye lesions in epidermolysis bullosa. Arch Dermatology 1988;124:762–764.

40. Zadnik K. Therapeutic soft contact lenses. In: Harris MG, ed.: *Problems in Optometry: contact lenses and ocular disease.* Philadelphia: JB Lippincott, 1990:632–641.

41. Langston RHS, Machmer CJ, Norman CW. Soft lens therapy for recurrent corneal erosion syndrome. *Ann Ophthalmol* 1978; 10:875–878.

42. Williams R, Buckley RJ. Pathogenesis and treatment of recurrent erosion. *Br J Ophthalmol* 1985;69:435–437.

43. Hull DS, Hyndiuk RA, Chin GN, et al. Clinical experience with therapeutic hydrophilic contact lens. *Ann Ophthalmol* 1975;7: 555–562.

44. Liu C, Buckley R. The role of therapeutic contact lenses in the management of recurrent corneal erosions: a review of treatment strategies. *CLAO J* 1996;22:79–82.

45. Cherry PM, Tutton AK, Adhikary H, et al. The treatment of pain following photorefractive keratectomy. *Refract Corneal Surg* 1994;10(2 Suppl):S222–S225.

46. Arshinoff S, D'Addario D, Sadler C, et al. Use of topical nonsteroidal anti-inflammatory drugs in excimer laser photorefractive keratectomy. *Refract Corneal Surg* 1994;10(2 Suppl): S216–S222.

47. Donnenfeld ED, Selkin BA, Perry HD, et al. Controlled evaluation of a bandage contact lens and a topical non-steroidal anti-inflammatory drug in treating traumatic corneal abrasions. *Ophthalmology* 1996;102:979–984.

48. Mandelcorn MS, Blankenship G, Machemer R. Pars plana vitrectomy for the management of severe diabetic retinopathy. *Am J Ophthalmol* 1976;81:561–570.

49. Liebowitz HM, Rosenthal P. Hydrophilic contact lenses in corneal disease. I. Superficial, sterile indolent ulcers. *Arch Ophthalmol* 1971;85:163–166.

50. Espy JW. Management of corneal problems with hydrophilic contact lenses. *Am J Ophthalmol* 1972;72:521–526.

51. Brown SI, Tragakis MP, Pearce DB. Treatment of the alkali-burned cornea. *Am J Ophthalmol* 1972;74:316–320.

52. Ali Z, Insler MS. A comparison of therapeutic bandage lenses, tarsorrhaphy, and antibiotic and hypertonic saline on corneal epithelial wound healing. *Ann Ophthalmol* 1986;18:22–24.

53. Schermer A, Galvin S, Sun TT. Differentiation related expression of a major 64K corneal keratin in vivo and in culture suggests limbal location of corneal epithelial stem cells. *J Cell Biol* 1986;103:49–62.

54. Kenyon KR, Tseng SCG. Limbal autograft transplantation for ocular surface disorders. *Ophthalmology* 1989;96:709–723.

55. Forstot SL, Binder PS. Treatment of Thygeson's superficial punctate keratitis with soft contact lenses. *Am J Ophthalmol* 1979;88:186–189.

56. Goldberg DB, Schanzlin DK, Brown SI. Management of Thygeson's superficial punctate keratitis. *Am J Ophthalmol* 1980;89:22–24.

57. Levinson A, Weissman BA, Sachs U. Use of a Bausch & Lomb PlanoT contact lens as a bandage. *Am J Optom Physiol Opt* 1977;54:97–103.

58. Mondino BJ, Zaidman GW, Salamon SW. Use of pressure patching and soft contact lenses in superior limbic keratoconjunctivitis. *Arch Ophthalmol* 1982;100:1932–1934.

59. Lerman S, Sapp G. The hydrophilic (Hydron) corneoscleral lens in the treatment of bullous keratopathy. *Ann Ophthalmol* 1970;2:142–144.

60. Aquavella JV, Jackson GK, Guy LF. Therapeutic effects of Bionite lenses: mechanisms of action. *Ann Ophthalmol* 1971;3: 1341–1350.

61. Takahashi GH, Leibowitz HM. Hydrophilic contact lenses in corneal disease III. Topical hypertonic saline therapy in bullous keratopathy. *Arch Ophthalmol* 1971;86:133–137.

62. Leibowitz HM, Rosenthal P. Hydrophilic contact lenses in corneal disease. II. Bullous keratopathy. *Arch Ophthalmol* 1971; 85:283–285.

63. Leibowitz HM. The soft contact lens II. Therapeutic experience with the Soflens. *Int Ophthalmol Clin* 1973;13:179–191.

64. Ruben M. Soft contact lens treatment of bullous keratopathy. *Trans Ophthalmol Soc U K* 1975;95:75–78.

65. Hovding G. Hydrophilic contact lenses in corneal disorders. *Acta Ophthalmol* 1984;62:566–576.

66. Buxton JN, Locke CR. A therapeutic evaluation of hydrophilic contact lenses. *Am J Ophthalmol* 1972;72:532–535.

67. Luchs JI, Cohen EJ, Rapuano CJ, et al. Ulcerative keratitis in bullous keratopathy. *Ophthalmology* 1997;104:816–822.

68. Kieselbach GF, Gensluckner W. Die behandlung der atopischen keratokonjunktivitis im kindesalter. *Klin Monatsb Augenheilkd* 1987;191:380–381.

69. Mackie IA. Contact lenses in dry eyes. *Trans Ophthalmol Soc UK* 1985;104:477–483.

70. Cederstaff TH, Tomlinson A. A comparative study of tear evaporation rates and water content of soft contact lenses. *Am J Optom Physiol Opt* 1983;60:167–174.

71. Lemp M. Therapeutic lens use with dry eye syndromes. In: *Therapeutic use of soft lenses in anterior segment diseases.* Phoenix: Syntex Ophthalmics, 1982:10–12.

72. Bloomfield SE, Gasset AR, Forstot SL, et al. Treatment of filamentary keratitis with soft contact lenses. *Am J Ophthalmol* 1973;76:978–980.

73. Mondino BJ, Weissman BA, Manthey R. Therapeutic soft contact lenses. In: Stenson S, ed. *Contact lenses: a guide to selection, fitting and management of complications.* Norwalk: Appleton and Lange, 1987:155–183.

74. Leibowitz HM. Hydrophilic contact lenses in corneal disease IV. Penetrating corneal wounds. *Ann Ophthalmol* 1972;88: 602–606.

75. Hirst LW, Smiddy WE, Stark WJ. Corneal perforations: changing methods of treatment 1960–1980. *Ophthalmology* 1982;89: 630–634.

76. Mannis MJ, Zadnik K. Hydrophilic contact lenses for wound stabilization in keratoplasty. *CLAO J* 1988;14:199–202.

77. Laibson PR. Surgical approaches to the treatment of active keratitis. *Int Ophthalmol Clin* 1973;13:65–74.

78. Weiss JL, Williams P, Lindstrom RL, et al. The use of tissue adhesives in corneal perforations. *Ophthalmology* 1983;90: 610–616.

79. Arentsen JJ, Laibson PR, Cohen EJ. Management of corneal descemetoceles and perforations. *Trans Am Ophthalmol Soc* 1984;82:92–105.

80. Leibowitz HM, Berrospi AR. Initial treatment of descemetocele with hydrophilic contact lenses. *Ann Ophthalmol* 1975;7: 1161–1166.

81. Joondeph HC, McCarthy WL, Rabb M, et al. Mooren's ulcer: two cases occurring after cataract extraction and treated with hydrophilic lens. *Ann Ophthalmol* 1976;8:187–194.

82. Blok MDW, Kok JHC, Nan Mil C, et al. Use of Megasoft bandage lens for treatment of complications after trabeculectomy. *Am J Ophthalmol* 1990;110:264–268.

83. Smith MF, Doyle JW. Use of oversized bandage soft contact lenses in management of early hypotony following filtration surgery. *Ophthalmic Surgery and Lasers* 1996;27:417–421.

84. Nuyts RM, Greve EL, Geijssen HC, et al. Treatment of hypotenous maculopathy after trabeculectomy with mitomycin C. *Am J Ophthalmol* 1994;118:322–331.

85. Simmons RJ, Kimbrough RL. Shell tamponade in filtering surgery for glaucoma. *Ophthalmic Surg* 1979;10:17–34.

86. Melamed S, Hersh P, Kersten D, et al. The use of glaucoma shell tamponade in leaking filtration blebs. *Ophthalmology* 1986; 93:839–842.

87. Guibor P, Gould H, Smith B. Contact lenses and oculoplastic surgery. *Contact Lens Med Bull* 1973;6:15–19.

88. Aquavella JV, Shaw EL. Hydrophilic bandages in penetrating keratoplasty. *Ann Ophthalmol* 1976;8:1207–1219.

89. Bellows AR, McCulley JP. Endophthalmitis in aphakic patients with unplanned filtering blebs wearing contact lenses. *Ophthalmology* 1981;88:839–843.

90. Lois N, Dias JL, Cohen EJ. Use of contact lenses in patients with filtering blebs. *CLAO J* 1997;23:100–102.

91. Tan DTH, Chee SP, Lim L, et al. Randomized clinical trial of a new dexamethasone delivery system (Surodex) for treatment of post-cataract surgery inflammation. *Ophthalmology* 1999;106: 223–231.

92. Sedlacek J. Possibility of the application of ophthalmic drugs with use of gel contact lenses. *Cesk Oftal* 1965;21:509–512.

93. Waltman SR, Kaufman HE. Use of hydrophilic contact lenses to increase ocular penetration of topical drugs. *Invest Ophthalmol Vis Sci* 1970;9:250–255.

94. Leaders FE, Hecht G, VanHoose M, et al. New polymers in drug delivery. *Ann Ophthalmol* 1973;5:513–522.

95. Kaufman HE, Utoila MH, Gassett AR, et al. The medical uses of soft contact lenses. *Trans Am Acad Ophthalmol Otolaryngol* 1971;75:361–373.

96. Podos SM, Becker B Asseft C, et al. Pilocarpine therapy with soft contact lenses. *Am J Ophthalmol* 1972;73:336–341.

97. Aquavella JV. New aspects of contact lenses in ophthalmology. *Adv Ophthalmol* 1976;32:2–34.

98. Hull DS, Edelhauser HF, Hyndiuk RA. Ocular penetration of prednisolone and the hydrophilic contact lens. *Arch Ophthalmol* 1974;92:413–416.

99. Fatt I. Water flow conductivity and pore diameter in extended wear gel lens materials. *Am J Optom Physiol Opt* 1978;55:43–47.

100. McDermott ML, Chandler JW. Therapeutic uses of contact lenses. *Surv Ophthalmol* 1989;33:381–394.

101. Bartlett JD, Cullen AP. Clinical administration of ocular drugs. In: Bartlett JD, Jaanus SD. *Clinical ocular pharmacology,* 2nd ed. Boston: Butterworths, 1989:29–66.

102. Maddox YT, Bernstein HN. An evaluation of the Bionite hydrogel contact lens for use in a drug delivery system. *Ann Ophthalmol* 1972;4:789–802.

103. Ruben M, Watkins R. Pilocarpine dispensation for the soft hydrophilic contact lens. *Br J Ophthalmol* 1975;59:455–458.

104. Hillman JS. Management of acute glaucoma with pilocarpine soaked hydrophilic lens. *Br J Ophthalmol* 1974;7:674–679.

105. Friedman Z, Alien RC, Ralph SM. Topical acetazolamide and methazolamide delivered by contact lenses. *Arch Ophthalmol* 1985;103:963–966.

106. Krejci L, Brettschneider L, Praus R. Hydrophilic gel contact lenses as a new drug delivery system in Ophthalmology and as a therapeutic bandage lenses. *Acta Univ Carol Med Monogr* 1975;21:387–396.

107. Shaw EL, Gasset AR. Management of an unusual case of keratitis mucosa with hydrophilic contact lenses and N-Acetylcystein. *Ann Ophthalmol* 1974;6:1054–1056.

108. Praus R, Brettscheider L, Krejci L, et al.. Hydrophilic contact lenses as a new therapeutic approach for topical use of chloramphenicol and tetracycline. *Ophthalmologica* 1972;165:62–70.

109. Brettschneider L, Praus R, Krejci L, et al. Intraocular penetration of bacitracin and polymyxin B after administration by means of hydrophilic gel contact lenses. *Ophthalmol Res* 1975; 7:296–302.

110. Busin M, Spitznas M. Sustained gentamicin release by presoaked medicated bandage contact lenses. *Ophthalmology* 1988; 95:796–798.

111. Wilson LE. Therapeutic use of soft contact lenses. *Royal Soc Med Proc* 1975;68:55–56.

112. Phinney RB, Schwartz SD, Lee DA, et al. Collagen shield delivery of gentamicin and vancomycin. *Arch Ophthalmol* 1988;106: 1599–1604.

113. Sawusch MR, O'Brien TP, Dick JD, et al. Use of collagen shields in the treatment of bacterial keratitis. *Am J Ophthalmol* 1988;106:279–281.

114. Unterman SR, Rootman DS, Hill JM, et al. Collagen shield drug delivery. Therapeutic concentrations of tobramycin in the rabbit cornea and aqueous humor. *J Cataract Refract Surg* 1988; 14:500–504.

115. O'Brien TP, Sawusch MR, Dick JD, et al. Use of collagen corneal shields vs soft contact lenses to enhance penetration of topical tobramycin. *J Cataract Refract Surg* 1988;14:505–507.

116. Hobden JA, Reidy JJ, O'Callaghan RJ, et al.. Treatment of experimental Pseudomonas keratitis using collagen shields containing tobramycin. *Arch Ophthalmol* 1988;106:1605–1607.

117. Hobden JA, Reidy JJ, O'Callaghan RJ, et al. Quinolones in collagen shields to treat aminoglycoside-resistant pseudomonal keratitis. *Invest Ophthalmol Vis Sci* 1990;31:2241–2243.

118. Schwartz SD, Harrison SA, Engstrom RE, et al.. Collagen shield delivery of amphotericin B. *Am J Ophthalmol* 1990;109: 701–704.

119. Gussler JR, Ashton P, VanMeter WS, et al. Collagen shield delivery of trifluorothymidine. *J Cataract Refract Surg* 1990;16: 719–722.

120. Hwang DG, Stem WH, Hwang PH, et al. Collagen shield enhancement of topical dexamethasone penetration. *Arch Ophthalmol* 1989;107:1375–1380.

121. Sawusch MR, O'Brien TP, Updegraff SA. Collagen corneal shields enhance penetration of topical prednisolone acetate. *J Cataract Refract Surg* 1989;15:625–628.

122. Murray TG, Stern WH, Chin DH, et al. Collagen shield hepa-

rin delivery for prevention of postoperative fibrin. *Arch Ophthalmol* 1990108:104–106.

123. Hagenah M, Lopez JG, Insler MS. Effects of EGF, FGF and collagen shields on corneal epithelial wound healing. *Invest Ophthalmol Vis Sci* 1990;31(Suppl):225.

124. Reidy JJ, Gebhardt BM, Kaufman HE. The collagen shield. A new vehicle for delivery of cyclosporin A to the eye. *Cornea* 1990;9:196–199.

125. Chen YF, Gebhardt BM, Reidy JJ, et al.Cyclosporine-containing collagen shields suppress corneal allograft rejection. *Am J Ophthalmol* 1990;109:132–137.

126. Pflugfelder SC, Murchison JF. Corneal toxicity with an antibi-

otic-steroid soaked collagen shield. *Arch Ophthalmol* 1992;110:2.

127. Hill JM, O'Callaghan RJ, Hobden JA, et al. Corneal collagen shields for ocular delivery. In: Mitra AK, ed. *Ophthalmic drug delivery systems.* New York: Marcel Dekker, 1993.

128. Schein OD, Ormerod LD, Barraquer E et al. Microbiology of contact lens related keratitis. *Cornea* 1989;8:281–285.

129. Rozenmann Y, Donnenfeld ED, Cohen EJ, et al.. Contact lens related deep stromal neovascularization. *Am J Ophthalmol* 1989;107:27–32.

130. Lim L, Tan DTH, Chan WK. Therapeutic use of Bausch & Lomb PureVision contact lenses. *CLAO J* 2001;27:179–185.

3 3

SCLERAL LENSES

KENNETH W. PULLUM

Scleral contact lenses retain a small but uniquely valuable place in contact lens practice; there are instances when visual rehabilitation is only possible by their application. Professional instruction on scleral lens practice has become a low priority in recent years, most likely due to the perception of a cumbersome fitting processes and anticipation of complications. Clinicians therefore do not appreciate the unique advantages of scleral lenses and they are rarely recommended. The author acknowledges corneal neovascularization (CNV) is a particular problem but can personally report cases where no corneal vascularization has occurred with up to 50 years of polymethylmethacrylate (PMMA) scleral lens wear. It is also worth noting that CNV also occurs secondary to the use of other contact lens types, and in many cases when the indication for contact lens wear is a cosmetic one only. This chapter provides both an introduction to the clinical application of scleral contact lenses and a description of recent developments.

Historical Background

The original blown-glass scleral contact lenses of the 1880s (1–3) were commendable early efforts, but both lack of knowledge of mechanical fitting principles and oxygen deprivation were limiting factors. Rudimentary preformed fitting sets were first produced in the 1920s. Impression techniques were described and developed by a number of workers, in particular Dallos and Obrig, in the 1930s. PMMA was introduced in the 1940s: its machinability and thermoplastic properties allowed both more precise manufacturing of preformed lenses and more versatility for fitting from impressions. Fenestration (4), which was not feasible in glass, resolved some oxygen problems but also complicated fitting. PMMA also made corneal lens manufacture possible, and hydrogels followed a few years later. Once both alternatives were established, the primary role of sclerals became as a "last resort" for very advanced ocular pathology—when all other options had totally failed—preceding corneal transplantation. The introduction of gaspermeable (GP) materials in the mid-1980s (5) to improve tolerance and simplify fitting, however, has increased interest in scleral lens practice.

Advantages of Scleral Lenses

- Scleral lenses are almost never dislodged because they are large enough to fit under both eyelids.
- They are dimensionally stable and robust.
- Because of their size, insertion and removal may be easier for less dexterous patients.
- Maintenance is simple. The cleaning and surface conditioning procedures applicable to corneal lenses are also appropriate for sclerals, and dry storage is satisfactory even for GP sclerals.
- Lid sensation is minimal.
- Foreign bodies do not lodge behind the lens during wear.
- An extensive power range is possible without lid traction and center-of-gravity effects.

Disadvantages of Scleral Lenses

- PMMA scleral lenses are occlusive to gaseous exchange even if skillfully fitted.
- They are labor intensive to produce compared to other lens types.
- Their physical size intimidates some patients.
- While lid sensation may be reduced, some patients are conscious of the sensation and appearance of bulk.
- Fenestrations in scleral lenses admit air bubbles to the precorneal reservoir causing visual disturbances and localized dehydration.
- Fenestrations in scleral lenses also cause settling back on the globe.
- The visual result may not be as good as with corneal lenses in some cases.

Indications

Scleral lenses are indicated as an alternative to surgery in many anterior segment ocular disease states if there is sufficiently good contact lens visual potential. If their unique attributes can be harnessed, however, they can also serve as an alternative to corneal lenses at much lower levels of pathology. There is also a significant role in post transplant management and for high refractive errors. Retention of a

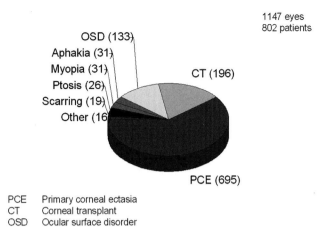

1147 eyes
802 patients

OSD (133)
Aphakia (31)
Myopia (31)
Ptosis (26)
Scarring (19)
Other (16)
CT (196)
PCE (695)

PCE   Primary corneal ectasia
CT   Corneal transplant
OSD   Ocular surface disorder

FIG. 33.1. Referrals for initial scleral lens assessment or continued management 1999 to 2002.

precorneal reservoir to maintain corneal hydration in some ocular surface disorders and mechanical protection from irregular lids and misdirected lashes are two particular therapeutic applications. Occasionally scleral lenses are also used to provide a ptosis prop. Figure 33.1 shows the major underlying indications from a series of 800 cases referred in the last 3 years to a dedicated scleral lens clinic at Moorfields Eye Hospital, United Kingdom, for initial assessment or continued management. Some clinical examples are illustrated later in this text.

SCLERAL LENS FITTING PRINCIPLES

The general objective is to achieve scleral zone alignment without corneal contact, but such perfection is rarely achieved as the sclera and cornea are not symmetrical about the geometric axis of the eye. Figure 33.2 illustrates the optimum mechanical fit, but in practice, acceptable departures from this ideal still yield successful outcomes.

Preformed and Impression Scleral Lenses

Scleral lens fitting can be approached either by using diagnostic preformed lenses of known specifications or by taking an impression of the eye. Preformed fitting has limitations

if the eye is too irregular, but impression lenses enable a near glove fit over the sclera and more uniform optic zone clearance with any ocular topography. As topographically abnormal eyes have constituted the major scleral lens requirement in recent years, fitting by impression has been the preferred method, at least in countries where contact lens practitioners use topical anesthetics.

Ventilation

A means of ventilation to provide fresh oxygenated tears to the underlying cornea is a prerequisite for a PMMA scleral lens, but how it is achieved has a profound effect on the fit of the lens. The discussion relating to ventilation is, therefore, central to the fitting processes.

Fenestrations
Fenestrating, usually at the temporal limbus, is a simple process and can be used for impression or preformed lenses. The precorneal fluid reservoir is disrupted, and there is usually an air bubble trapped behind the lens, which is acceptable if it is not too large and does not cross the visual axis. The positive pressure of the reservoir is also relieved by fenestrating, and the lens may settle onto the globe. Figure 33.3 illustrates a fenestration and the theoretically ideal associated crescent shaped bubble, and Fig. 33.4 (see Color Plate 33.4) is an example of such a lens *in situ*. If the bubble is too large, vision is affected and there may be some corneal dehydration.

Channels
Channels (Figs. 33.5 and 33.6) can be worked into the scleral zone to provide tear flow from the edge of the lens into the optic zone. The lens must be inserted filled with

FIG. 33.2. Optimum scleral zone alignment and full optic zone clearance.

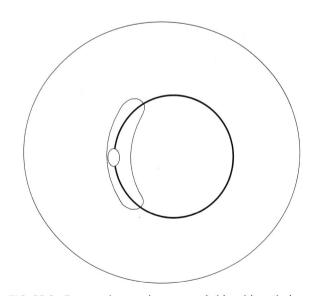

FIG. 33.3. Fenestration on the temporal side with typical crescent-shaped bubble.

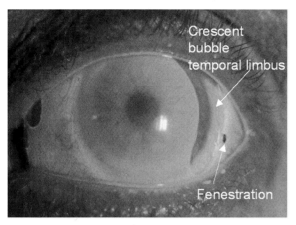

FIG. 33.4. Fenestrated scleral lens *in situ*. Note the crescent shaped bubble on the temporal side and reduced clearance on the nasal side. (See Color Plate 33.4)

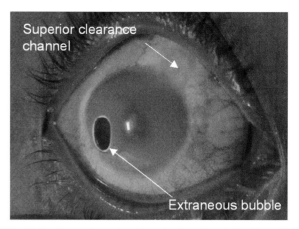

FIG. 33.7. Channeled scleral lens *in situ*. (See Color Plate 33.7)

saline to avoid trapping an air bubble under the lens. The rate of tear exchange is slower than would be expected via a fenestration, but there is less disruption of the precorneal fluid reservoir, reducing both problems of air bubbles and settling back. Figure 33.7 (see Color Plate 33.7) is an example of a channeled lens *in situ*. Effective channeling depends on a closely aligned scleral zone, and upon a critical depth of the channel. If too shallow, they are not patent; if too deep, air bubbles are admitted behind the lens. If the depth is just right, it is possible to give excellent fluid coverage with very irregular corneal topographies. As the sclera is not symmetrical, any rotation affects the precise positioning of a channel, so it is only an option for impression lenses.

Slotted Scleral Lenses

Slotted sclerals (6) (Figs. 33.8 and 33.9) enhance tear circulation, and provide both an escape route and an entry point for air bubbles. Slots are usually sited just at the superior

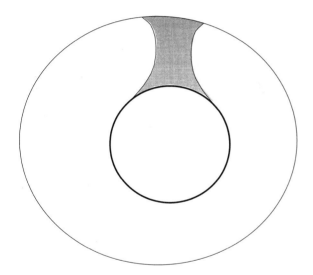

FIG. 33.5. Superior channel between optic zone and lens edge.

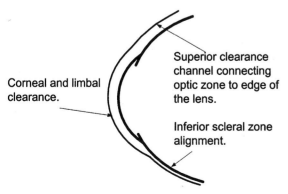

FIG. 33.6. Superior channel in cross section.

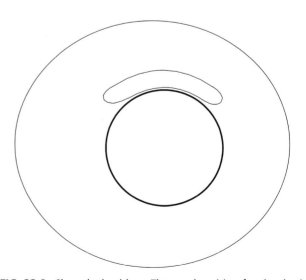

FIG. 33.8. Slotted scleral lens. The usual position for the slot is just outside the upper limbus.

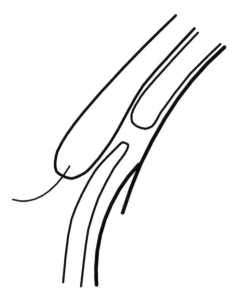

FIG. 33.9. Slotted scleral lens. Cross section to show the slot profile shaped to reduce lid sensation.

limbus, as illustrated in Fig. 33.10 (see Color Plate 33.10). As preformed lenses are subject to rotation and decentration, slotted sclerals must be fitted by impression.

Corneal Clearance

Fenestrated PMMA Preformed Sclerals
The corneal portion of a fenestrated PMMA scleral should clear the corneal apex by 0.1 mm and the limbus by between 0.15 and 0.2 mm. Greater clearance can result in air bubbles trapped between the lens and the ocular surface. Too little clearance leads to corneal touch when the lens settles. Preformed scleral lenses tend to decenter temporally and downwards; hence the axes of symmetry of the eye and the lens are rarely coincident. Consequently, there can be quite large

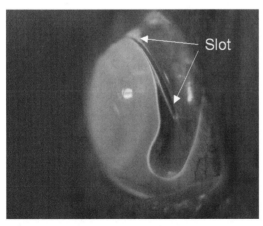

FIG. 33.10. Slotted scleral lens *in situ* fitted to a highly protrusive keratoglobus. Even a thinly cut slot, as shown here, enables excellent tear coverage. (See Color Plate 33.10)

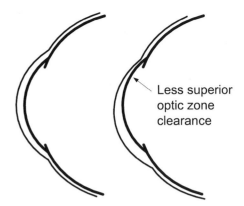

FIG. 33.11. Uneven precorneal reservoir depth as the lens decenters downwardly to favored position.

variations in the depth of the precorneal reservoir, as shown in Fig. 33.11, which further increases the chances of trapping air bubbles in the deeper areas.

Impression Sclerals
A more uniformly deep precorneal fluid reservoir is possible with impression compared to preformed scleral lenses as the lens is fabricated from a cast of the eye as a starting point. Centration is also improved, further reducing variations in depth. The greater tear catchment possible with slotted lenses may enable increased apical and limbal clearance compared to fenestrated scleral lenses. As there is minimal disruption of the precorneal fluid reservoir with a channeled scleral, even more clearance is usually possible.

Gas-permeable Scleral Lenses

The introduction of rigid GP materials has now shifted the emphasis away from impression and back to preformed lens designs for two reasons:

- GP materials are not sufficiently thermoplastic to heat mold; therefore, although GP sclerals from impressions are possible to manufacture (7,8), the process is more cumbersome than for preformed scleral lenses.
- Research suggests that sealed (i.e., nonfenestrated), high-Dk GP scleral lenses cause corneal edema at a level comparable with normal overnight swelling (9–13). Figure 33.12 shows corneal swelling following three hours wear of sealed PMMA scleral lenses and sealed GP sclerals of different oxygen transmissibilities (Dk/t). Sealed lenses circumvent the drawbacks of fenestrations. Settling back is minimized and air bubbles are eliminated from the precorneal reservoir in most instances even with a variable precorneal fluid reservoir of depth over 1 mm, with the result that there is a vast increase in latitude at the initial fitting stage.

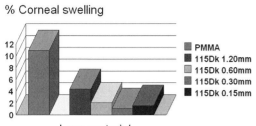

% Corneal swelling

Lens material
PMMA and RGP compared, 3 normal subjects.
Data published, BCLA journal, 1990 and 1991

FIG. 33.12. Corneal swelling following polymethylmethacrylate (PMMA) and rigid gas permeable (RGP) sealed scleral lens wear. From left to right: first PMMA, and then RGPs (115 Dk) 1.20-mm, 0.6-mm, 0.30-mm, and 0.15-mm thick, respectively. A mean swelling of 11% is seen to occur with PMMA, but less than 4% occurs with even the 1.20-mm-thick RGP lens, which is similar to normal overnight swelling without a lens in place. There is no significant difference between the swelling induced by the lenses of 0.6, 0.3, and 0.15 mm in thickness, all producing approximately 2% cornea swelling. The diminishing return is probably an indication of the boundary layer effect on oxygen transmission. As it is not feasible to produce GP lenses less than 0.6 mm in thickness, this is an encouraging result.

Sealed or Fenestrated?

There remains some debate on this subject. Sealed GP scleral lenses are increasingly being fitted (14–23) with encouraging results, although some [including Ezekiel (24)] suggest that fenestrations remain helpful even for GP scleral lenses. Mountford et al. (25) found fenestrated GP scleral lenses induced less corneal swelling than fenestrated PMMA sclerals. In the author's opinion, increased tear flow and secondary oxygenation allowed by fenestrations does not compensate for their disadvantages. However, there are good reasons at times, irrespective of the corneal oxygenation issue, for at least investigating the option of fenestrating.

To Regulate a Persistent Air Bubble

The precorneal fluid reservoir under a sealed lens remains air-free in most cases, but if a bubble is admitted behind the lens because the sclera is insufficiently regular, it may be more troublesome than with an optimally fitted fenestrated lens. If the corneal topography is reasonably regular, and the lens is centered well enough so that the precorneal fluid reservoir is sufficiently uniform in depth, a fenestration allows some escape facility as well as the entry point for the bubble.

For Easier Handling

Sealed lenses have to be inserted filled with saline, so the patient must lean forward with his or her head horizontal so that the saline stays in the lens. Some patients do not master the technique, or it may be impossible in some cases if, for example, the patient has a back or neck disorder.

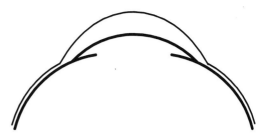

FIG. 33.13. Scleral zone fitting shell. The optic zone is well clear of the cornea to allow independent assessment of the scleral zone.

Fenestrated lenses can be inserted with a normal head posture.

Traditional PMMA Preformed Fitting Methods

The future of scleral lens practice undoubtedly lies primarily with GP sclerals, but traditional PMMA fitting principles assists the understanding of modern methods. Three variables must be considered: the back scleral radius (BSR), the back optic zone radius (BOZR), and the back optic zone diameter (BOZD). The diameter has some impact on the apical clearance but is a much less predictable variable. Fenestrated preformed scleral lens fitting is achieved either with a system that evaluates the optic and scleral zones independently or one that varies scleral and optic zone dimensions simultaneously.

Independent Optic and Scleral Zone Fitting

Scleral Zone Fitting

There is no method currently available to measure the scleral contour: the only way is to select a lens with a known BSR and inspect it *in situ*. It is necessary to ensure that the optic zone is well clear of the cornea (Fig. 33.13) to eliminate the possibility of the whole lens standing off the sclera because of optic zone contact (Fig. 33.14). If the BSR is too steep, the lens may vault the whole anterior eye, extending the precorneal reservoir towards the periphery of the lens, as shown in Fig. 33.15. This is easily observed with fluores-

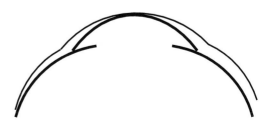

FIG. 33.14. The possible consequence of optic zone contact when the scleral zone is being evaluated is that there may be stand-off, giving a confused appearance of a flat-fitting lens.

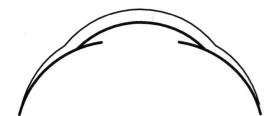

FIG. 33.15. Steep fitting scleral zone. The whole lens vaults from the periphery, giving rise to increased apical clearance.

FIG. 33.17. The reduced bearing surface may lead to increased settling back with reduction of apical and limbal optic zone clearance at a later stage.

cein dye. If the BSR is too flat, the periphery of the scleral zone stands off the globe, allowing fluorescein to encroach under the periphery. A BSR that is too flat does not affect apical clearance, but the lens may settle back more because of a narrower bearing surface (Figs. 33.16 and 33.17).

Conjunctival vessels blanch with compression. Peripheral blanching (Fig. 33.18) indicates the BSR is too steep. If in the midperiphery (Fig. 33.19), the BSR is too flat. A normal sclera is not symmetrical about the geometric axis (26), so some localized conjunctival blanching may be acceptable. If blanching is unavoidable, it is preferable to be more peripheral.

The BSR ranges from 12.50 to 14.50 mm in 0.25-mm steps, but as the scleral zone fit is at best an approximate match, the author's view is that 0.50-mm steps are more appropriate. BSRs of 13.50 or 14.00 mm are successful for the majority of eyes. A radius of 13.50 mm errs on the steep side, increasing limbal clearance, so is as good a first choice as any. A radius of 14.00 mm and sometimes 14.50 mm are frequent second choices if 13.50 mm seems to be too steep, but radii steeper than 13.50 mm are less common.

Use of Fenestrated Lenses for Optic Measurement (FLOMs) to Vary the Apical and Limbal Clearance

Corneal clearance is determined by the use of FLOMs (4), which vary the BOZR and the BOZD. FLOMs have a narrow and flat scleral zone with an unblended transition (Fig. 33.20) to ensure scleral stand off and to allow optimum assessment of the optic zone parameters. This may cause some discomfort, so a topical anesthetic may be required to reduce excessive reflex lacrimation.

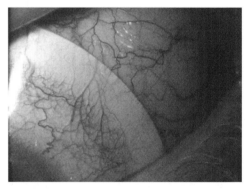

FIG. 33.18. Conjunctival blanching at the periphery with a steep fitting scleral zone.

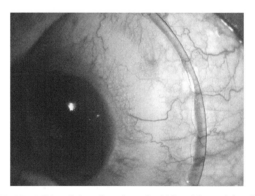

FIG. 33.19. Midperipheral conjunctival blanching with a flat fitting scleral zone.

FIG. 33.16. A lens with a flat-fitting scleral zone stands off the globe, but the optic zone clearance is unaffected in the first stages of the fitting process.

FIG. 33.20. Fenestrated lens for optic measurement *in situ*. The narrow and flat scleral zone eliminates any chance of scleral zone vaulting.

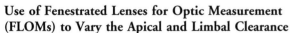

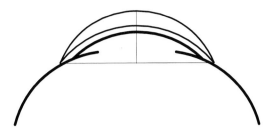

FIG. 33.21. Variation of optic zone clearance by steepening or flattening the back optic zone radius. The limbal clearance is virtually unchanged.

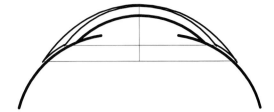

FIG. 33.23. Clinical equivalent designs. The apical clearance is unchanged but the limbal clearance is increased with a flatter back optic zone radius and a wider back optic zone diameter.

The usual range of parameters for the BOZR is 7.50 to 9.50 mm, and for the BOZD 12.50 to 14.50 mm, both in 0.25-mm steps. Steepening the BOZR with an unchanged BOZD or widening the BOZD with an unchanged BOZR increases the apical clearance, as in Figs. 33.21 and 33.22. Steepening the BOZR by 0.25 mm is comparable to widening the BOZD by 0.50 mm. Widening the BOZD also increases limbal clearance while steepening the BOZR has little effect on limbal clearance. A lens with the BOZR flattened by 0.25 mm and the BOZD widened by 0.50 mm are clinical equivalents; i.e., a design retaining the same apical clearance, as shown in Fig. 33.23. The optimum appearance is a uniform fluid coverage of the optic zone with a crescent shaped bubble at the limbus.

A Four-step Method for Using FLOMs

- A FLOM from the middle of the range is selected. Keratometry has limited value, but if corneal topography is "normal," the first FLOM can be appropriately to the steep or the flat side of the mean by 0.25 mm.
- If apical corneal contact occurs, a steeper BOZR with the same BOZD increases apical clearance. If there is a central bubble, a flatter BOZR reduces clearance.
- If steepening the BOZR by 0.25 mm converts apical contact to excessive clearance, the original (flatter) BOZR but with a BOZD widened by 0.25 mm should provide a smaller apical clearance increment.
- When apical clearance is optimal, limbal clearance is refined by using clinical equivalents. Of two clinical equivalent FLOMs, the one with the larger diameter has greater limbal clearance.

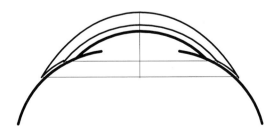

FIG. 33.22. Variation of optic zone clearance by widening the back optic zone diameter. Note the increased depth and breadth of the limbal clearance.

Limitations of Separate Optic and Scleral Zone Fitting
Changing the BOZR alone gives a precisely calculable increase in corneal clearance as it is unaffected by the scleral curvature (Fig. 33.21), but the relationship between apical clearance increments and the BOZD (Fig. 33.22) is an estimation based on a schematic scleral curve. The bearing surface of the FLOM is just a narrow annulus and its mechanical effect is quite different than that of a finished lens: the final fitted lens is never seen until it is ready to be dispensed. Linking up the estimated parameters for the two zones does not always give the anticipated result because there may have been some scleral zone vaulting which the practitioner did not observe, or for which an accurate allowance could not be made. In the author's opinion, FLOM fitting is too complex and unpredictable for use as a first choice method of fitting preformed scleral lenses.

Simultaneous Scleral and Optic Zone Fitting

If the two zones are assessed together, the final trial lens is the same as the finished lens. There are many permutations of the three variables, but it is reasonable to use a large BOZD with a flat BOZR and a smaller BOZD with a steeper BOZR, so some combinations can be omitted from a fitting set.

Wide-angle Lenses
Wide-angle lenses have been successfully used as a simultaneous fitting system (27). The BOZR and BSR are both spherical with a conical transition. The cone angle is calculated for each BOZR to give a tangential junction. As there is only one possible calculated BOZD for each combination of BOZR and BSR, the term is not used in the defining parameters of the lenses, but is replaced by the corneal and limbal chords, which are 11.50 mm and 16.00 mm, respectively, for all lenses in the system. The design of a wide-angle lens is illustrated in Fig. 33.24.

The scleral zone is assessed as described previously, but lenses from the fitting set are used rather than fitting shells that are dedicated to fitting the scleral zone only. The BOZR of the first lens should be steep enough to ensure optic zone clearance. Having established the optimum BSR, the optic zone can be assessed. A central spherical bubble

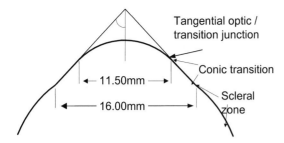

FIG. 33.24. Wide-angle scleral lens design. The back optic zone diameter is replaced by the optic and limbal chords. The cone angle gives a tangential junction for each back optic zone radius.

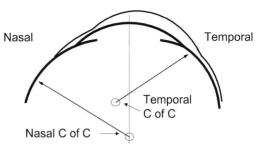

FIG. 33.26. The center of curvature (C of C) for the temporal sclera is offset contralaterally, giving a less pronounced limbus compared to the nasal side. A lens dislodges towards the temporal side due to the flatter nasal sclera contour, leading to increased depth of the precorneal fluid reservoir on the temporal side.

is trapped beneath the lens if clearance is excessive, in which case a flatter BOZR is evaluated. To alleviate central contact, a steeper BOZR is needed. Fluorescein covers the cornea, extending about 2 mm beyond the limbus, when clearance is optimum. A crescent-shaped peripheral bubble 4 to 8 mm is a usual appearance, but it is not possible to refine limbal clearance as the BOZD cannot be varied.

Other Parameters

Diameter

Medial and lateral recti muscle insertions are about 24 mm apart, so 23 mm is a good standard initial diameter, but it can be varied when indicated. A patient with small, recessed eyes may find removal difficult; hence, a smaller diameter may be required while larger may be necessary if the eye is exophthalmic. However, care is necessary when specifying larger diameters as small changes give rise to a relatively large increase in the bearing surface (Fig. 33.25). Peripheral scleral topography is usually more irregular, so the lens may bear on nodules that cause the lens to vault the whole anterior eye.

If smaller, the lens edge may snag on the lid, but otherwise, moderate diameter reductions, for example, from 23 mm to 21 mm or even 20 mm, would not usually have much impact on the scleral zone bearing, hence apical clearance, other than to possibly increase settling back. Further reductions, say to approximately 18 mm, may eliminate the bearing surface almost completely causing an immediate reduction in optic zone clearance. Such a lens would have

to be specifically designed to account for the bearing surface situated in closer proximity to the limbus compared to a full-diameter scleral.

Thereafter, still further diameter reductions, perhaps in the order of just 1 mm, that would not have affected the fit of a full-diameter (23 mm) lens, may cause problems. When diameter is reduced to as small as 15 mm, with scleral zones only 1.5 to 2 mm wide, limbal clearance may be virtually nonexistent. So although the lens is just encroaching onto the sclera, it would be more appropriately described as a corneoscleral lens, for which the fitting rationale is not the same as for a scleral.

Decentration of the Optic Zone

Scleral contour is flatter nasally than in the other three quadrants (26), and the typical temporal scleral contour has a center of curvature offset to the contralateral side, further accentuating differences between the temporal and nasal scleral surfaces. The flat nasal sector causes the lens to decenter to the temporal side (Fig. 33.26). Horizontal eye movements often cause the conjunctiva to bunch up at the caruncle. It is, therefore, usually beneficial to decenter the optic 1 to 1.5 mm towards the nasal side (Fig. 33.27) to reduce the width of the nasal scleral zone and to minimize rotation of the lens.

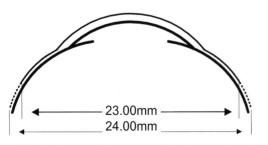

FIG. 33.25. An increased diameter of just 1 mm gives rise to a large increase in the bearing surface of a scleral lens.

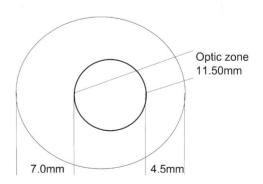

FIG. 33.27. Optic zone displacement 1.0 to 1.5 mm nasally is usual to improve lens centration *in situ*.

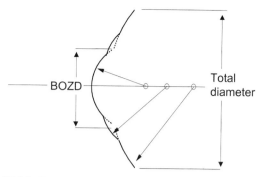

FIG. 33.28. Transcurve cross section showing the optic zone, transition, and scleral zone centers of curvature.

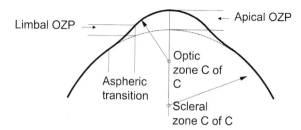

FIG. 33.29. Rigid gas-permeable scleral lens design with limbal and optic zone projection.

Transition Curves

Specifications for a finished lens specified other than from the wide-angle system would normally include a transition curve approximately midway between the BOZR and the BSR, as shown in Fig. 33.28, to "soften" the optic / scleral junction. The name "transcurve" has been given to a scleral incorporating such a transition curve of specific radius.

Specifying the Power

The back vertex power (BVP) is derived from a simple spherical overrefraction making appropriate allowances for the back vertex distance (BVD). If the overrefraction is too great, the practitioner may prefer to use a lens having a BVP nearer to that estimated for the final lens.

Sealed Gas-permeable Fitting Methods

As previously discussed, sealed GP sclerals eliminate air bubbles from the precorneal reservoir in most instances. Settling back is also minimized, so there is more latitude in final corneal clearance both apically and at the limbus compared to fenestrated PMMA scleral lenses. Matching the corneal curvature is therefore less important than establishing the optimum apical clearance.

Optic Zone Sagitta

Visser (14) and Schien et al. (15) described use of trial transcurve GP sealed lenses as an integrated scleral and optic zone fitting system including combinations of BOZRs and BOZDs to vary the sagittal depth. More recent designs have smoother and less demarcated transitions between the optic and scleral curves. Differences between the sagittal depths for each lens can be calculated, or a table included providing this information may be included in the fitting set.

Optic Zone Projection

An alternative method is to vary corneal clearance by changing the forward projection of the optic zone from the plane

of the scleral curve extended to its apex (28), as in Fig. 33.29. Each lens is defined by three parameters:

- BSR
- Optic zone projection (OZP) from the extrapolation of the scleral curve at the apex
- OZP measured at the limbus

The fitting system is dedicated to the whole range of normal and topographically abnormal eyes. To indicate the value of OZPs typically required, between 1.00 mm and 2.00 mm clear topographically normal corneas, but in excess of 4.00 mm is required for some advanced keratoconic or globic corneas. OZP increments of approximately 0.25 mm are just clinically significant, thereby keeping the fitting system within manageable proportions. The lens parameters are interdependent, enabling assessment of the scleral radius and the apical clearance simultaneously. As the scleral contour is normally asymmetric, and because the precorneal fluid reservoir has a certain cushioning effect, two standard variables for the BSR, 13.50 mm and 14.50 mm give a clinically significant difference for the scleral zone.

Initial Lens Selection

A steeper BSR is the preferred first choice as a certain amount of midperipheral vaulting improves limbal clearance, and blanching is peripheral. If the lens is not sufficiently sealed on the sclera to exclude air bubbles, a lens with a flatter scleral curve may be better because a bearing surface closer to the limbus tends to avoid peripheral scleral irregularities. As discussed above, some conjunctival blanching is expected, but the cushioning effect of the precorneal fluid reservoir reduces scleral compression. Keratometry and corneal topography are of little to no value in selection of the optic zone parameters because neither gives any information about the corneal profile at the limbus. A better indicator is a simple assessment of the corneal profile (Fig. 33.30).

Choice of Subsequent Lenses

A diagnostic lens filled with fluoresceinated saline is used to establish the optic zone parameters. Contact zones are

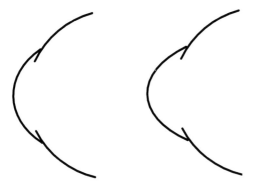

FIG. 33.30. Shallow and deep corneal projection from the scleral plane.

observed using cobalt blue light, and a white light slit lamp optical section gives an estimate of corneal clearance by comparing the depth of the precorneal fluid reservoir with the corneal thickness (Fig. 33.31). Approximately 0.25 mm (i.e., about half the thickness of a normal cornea) is optimal. Figure 33.32 illustrates the alleviation of corneal contact with a corneal clearance increment. Some clinical examples appear later in the text.

Interaction of Scleral Radius and OZP

Partial scleral zone vaulting increases limbal clearance, so this may be a beneficial fitting feature. Apical clearance can be reduced with a reduced apical OZP while retaining an unchanged BSR to maintain a greater limbal clearance (Fig. 33.33) or with a flatter BSR, giving a closer fit at the limbal area (Fig. 33.34).

Impression Fitting

The need for impression fitting has dramatically reduced, in the author's estimation, to approximately 5% of scleral lens fittings, with the introduction of GP materials. The primary indications are poor scleral zone sealing, when air bubbles are admitted into the precorneal fluid reservoir, or excessive localized scleral compression.

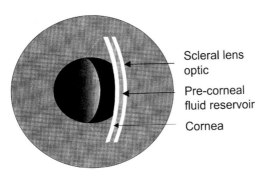

Scleral lens optic

Pre-corneal fluid reservoir

Cornea

FIG. 33.31. Optical section showing depth of the precorneal fluid reservoir compared to the corneal thickness.

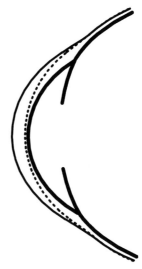

FIG. 33.32. Central contact zone (dotted line) alleviated by a single optic zone projection increment (solid line).

Impressions give the closest possible match to the underlying scleral topography and establish the optimum starting point for removal of substance from the optic zone to provide a precorneal fluid reservoir when the lens is placed onto the eye. A PMMA scleral ventilated in the appropriate method, a duplicate of a final fitted PMMA lens in a GP material, or a thermally molded PMMA scleral zone with an GP optic zone button cemented in place are feasible options. A GP duplicate can be sealed or fenestrated, but the drawbacks of fenestrating, as previously described, still apply. A channel in the PMMA model would be reproduced in the GP duplicate, but cutting a slot into a GP scleral is a precarious exercise due to the fragility of the materials. There is a better likelihood of a successful outcome fenes-

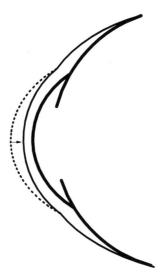

FIG. 33.33. Corneal clearance reduced by reducing the optic zone projection (dotted line to solid line) but retaining an unchanged back scleral radius.

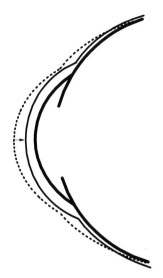

FIG. 33.34. Corneal clearance reduced by switching to a flatter back scleral radius (dotted line to solid line). Note the limbal clearance is reduced in depth and breadth compared to when the optic zone projection is reduced with an unchanged back scleral radius.

trating an impression lens compared to preformed because the back surface of the lens is a better match to the ocular topography, so the depth of the precorneal fluid reservoir is more uniform.

Impression Materials and Trays

Impression Trays

A selection of impression trays with diameters ranging from 21 to 25 mm in diameter is adequate for most eyes, although special sizes can be made. The nasal and inferior sectors are about 2 mm smaller than the temporal and superior sectors. The tray is about 0.8 mm thick to prevent flexure. A tubular handle about 25 mm long and 5 mm in diameter is attached (Fig. 33.35).

Impression Materials

Suitable dental alginate and polyvinylsiloxane (PVS) have been used for many years. Both separate easily from the cornea and conjunctiva without causing serious corneal abrasions.

Alginate Kromopan has been used extensively for ophthalmic work, but the formulation of the current version has recently been changed causing some adverse corneal reactions. Orthoprint has been used as an alternative without problems for five years at the time of writing. The optimum consistency is achieved by mixing 2 g powder with 7 mL of fresh distilled water or sterile nonpreserved saline.

Polyvinylsiloxane Most scleral lens practitioners in the United Kingdom currently use PVS for eye impressions. Water is not needed for mixing PVS, so it is not subject to dehydration and has a longer shelf life compared to alginate. Storey (29) described the use of Panasil C, but this has been superseded by Panasil light-body grade (Fig. 33.36).

Polyvinylsiloxane or Alginate? Alginate impressions dehydrate after a few minutes, and therefore must be cast immediately. PVS impressions retain their shape indefinitely, so casting can be delayed if desired, or a second cast can be made if necessary. Alginate is hygroscopic, so it deteriorates after the container is opened, affecting the quality of the impression. Humid conditions speed up the gelling process so that it may be necessary to use refrigerated water or saline. By contrast, PVS is unaffected by ambient atmospheric conditions. Flexible rubber or plastic bowls, measuring flasks or spoons and spatulas are necessary for mixing alginates. Mixing equipment provided with PVS kits (Fig. 33.37) provides the right consistency every time. PVS is more expensive but so much more convenient that it is, without doubt, the more suitable choice unless the individual practitioner is comfortable with alginate.

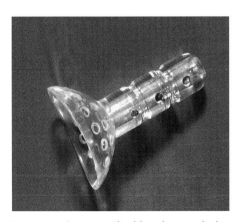

FIG. 33.35. Impression tray. The blue dots mark the top for a left eye. Three dots indicate it is the largest size.

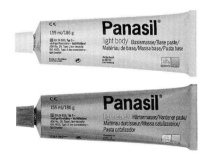

FIG. 33.36. Panasil light body (Panadent Ltd, Kent, UK). Equal volumes of the paste base and hardener give an optimum consistency for taking impressions.

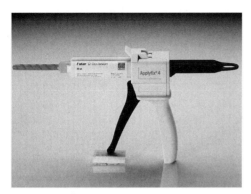

FIG. 33.37. Use of a mixing gun (Applyfix) is the simplest and most accurate way to mix equal volumes of Panasil.

Taking Impressions

The patient should be relaxed, sitting upright, but with his or her head supported comfortably. Topical anesthetic is instilled: up to four drops, as incomplete anesthesia is unpleasant and may result in upwards rotation of the globe. The eye should be in the primary position, but as the impression material obscures the eye, correct positioning is achieved by positioning the fellow eye. The patient fixates on the index finger, or on an alternative suitable fixation point, while the impression is taken. Gelling takes only a few seconds so the items of equipment must be neatly laid out in advance.

The impression material is transferred to a 10-mL syringe and injected through the tubular handle of the tray. Moving the tray in all directions during injection helps to fill the space between the tray and the eye. The tray rests on the globe at its extremities only, clearing the cornea and sclera elsewhere (Fig. 33.38). The paste extrudes through the holes in the tray, locking the impression to the tray.

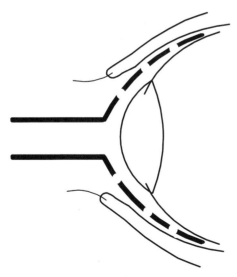

FIG. 33.38. Impression tray on the eye. Bearing at the edge only ensures that the back surface does not otherwise touch the eye while the impression is taken.

After gelling, the lower lid is pulled down and pressed gently underneath the tray to relieve suction and allow the impression to slide out. The top is recorded with a fiber marking pen and any excess impression material removed. The anterior segment should be inspected to reveal any abrasion or retained bits of impression material. The eye is irrigated with saline and a prophylactic antibiotic instilled if necessary.

Important Cautionary Note with Impression Taking

Dental materials manufacturers decline to sanction use of their products outside dentistry. Some packaging states the product is for dental use only and some specifically indicate: "Keep away from eyes." Thousands of impressions for either scleral lens or prosthetic fitting, however, have been safely performed in the United Kingdom alone over the last four decades. Taking an impression may lead to an irritable eye for a while, but the risk of significant injury is minimal. Impressions have become less often necessary with the introduction of GP materials, but the alternative is usually contact lens failure in cases when success is most needed. Further options may be surgical, and therefore with attendant risks clearly greater than those attached to taking an impression.

Casting the Impression

Dental stone powder and cold water are mixed to form a creamy homogeneous paste that is lowered into the impression, taking care to avoid trapping bubbles, and left to set, usually after about an hour. The back of the cast is marked at the top with "R" or "L" appropriately, dated, and identified with the patient's name, then separated from the impression. Surplus material, such as that generated by the conjunctival folds, is scraped away with a plaster knife. Plaster of Paris is useful for making a solid base and to repair minor flaws. Plaster of Paris is softer than dental stone and can be cut or shaped as it sets. Figure 33.39 shows a cast

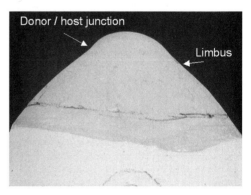

FIG. 33.39. Dental stone cast of a eye having undergone corneal transplantation. The donor–host junction is clearly visible, but the limbus is barely detectable by comparison.

of an eye having undergone a corneal transplant mounted on a plaster base.

Essential Manufacturing Procedures

Either a cast of the eye or a PVS impression can be sent to a competent scleral lens manufacturer. For successful results, a sound working relationship between practitioner and laboratory is essential.

Selection of Primary BOZR

Keratometry and corneal topography are of little value for the reasons discussed earlier. Deriving optic zone parameters from preformed lenses is not feasible because scleral zone fitting characteristics of preformed and impression lenses are completely different. A skilled technician producing the primary shell is better placed than the practitioner to decide on the optic zone curvature. The primary back optic curvature is selected by lightly grinding the optic zone of the flush shell with spherical diamond stones on a vertical bench spindle. The optimal curve touches the midperiphery first, and then cuts into the surface simultaneously towards the center and the periphery. Sometimes a multi-curve design may be necessary to create the optimum apical and limbal clearance. Spherical cloth covered brass or specially cut wax tools are used to polish the BOZR.

Removal of Optic Zone Substance

Apical optic zone clearance for a fenestrated PMMA scleral is approximately 0.1 mm for normal corneal topography. Greater clearance allows space for an air bubble to form across the visual axis. Limbal clearance approaching 0.2 mm is necessary to avoid tightness after the lens has fully settled. If the corneal profile is abnormally protrusive or irregular, there is greater variation in the depth of the precorneal fluid reservoir. Just enough substance is removed so that the optimum back surface radius skims the most prominent point of the shell, with a view to carrying out further optic zone grind outs after the shell has been evaluated *in situ*.

Ventilation

The position of any fenestrations, slots or channels should be specified, unless inspection of the lens before ventilating is considered necessary.

Power Specification for Impression Lenses

As lenses have not been seen *in situ* during the course of impression fitting, the laboratory needs refractive data (i.e., the BOZR and BVP of a lens used for a vision trial, and the over-refraction required for optimum correction). An appropriate power allowance can be calculated if the BOZR of the test lens is different from the finished lens, which is usually the case. The test lens should preferably be a scleral or a large diameter corneoscleral lens. Recent corneal lens specifications can be used, but there is more potential for

error as the optic zones of corneal lenses are much smaller than those of sclerals. A scleral should always be used for power prescribing in the case of GP impression sclerals, as the less they are modified, the better.

The negative liquid lens entrapped behind a scleral can be up to −4.00 D with normal corneal topography and even higher in cases of corneal ectasia, so the BVP for a scleral is usually more positive than that for a corresponding acceptable fit of a corneal lens. Adding minus power to a positive powered lens is a technically simple process compared to adding further positive power, so erring towards extra positive with a view to adding minus is advisable. If a lens does not quite meet the prescribed power, it is as well to check the over-refraction *in situ* before returning to the laboratory to effect any change.

Modifications to Finished Lenses

Impression PMMA Lenses

An impression PMMA lens that is currently being worn should never be modified, even if it is clear that there is room for improvement. Scleral lens wearers tend to have a distinct preference for an old favorite lens and its preservation is essential. Modifying is unpredictable, so it should be implemented on a new shell pressed over a cast of the original lens. Every modification reduces substance; hence, all entail a risk of increasing settling back on the globe, not least an optic zone grind-out because apical contact may limit settling back. Reducing the diameter may cause the edge to catch on the lower lid, but diameter reductions may be necessary if the shell impinges against the inferior fornix or the inner canthus, or if there are persistent difficulties with insertion or removal. Sometimes just the superior scleral zone may be reduced to improve lens removal.

Preformed PMMA Scleral Lenses

Modification to preformed scleral lenses should not be necessary because the specifications are selected following observations after a reasonable settling back period. Refitting or starting again with an impression is preferable with a poorly fitting scleral zone. The only feasible modifications to a preformed lens are optic zone or transition grind-outs if there is sufficient substance, or diameter reductions. An optic grind out of 0.10 mm is the minimum worth considering.

Gas-permeable Sclerals

Practitioners should not attempt to modify GP sclerals. There is a risk of distortion and it is difficult to re-establish an acceptable surface. Diameter reductions can be made, but it is advisable only if the practitioner has first evaluated the effect of such a change with a trial lens made to the smaller diameter. Before requesting any modification, it is worthwhile having a second inspection of the lens *in situ*: it is surprising how often its value may be questioned on further reflection. Fortunately, the need for modification is less with sealed GP scleral lenses because the settling back is considerably reduced compared to fenestrated lenses.

Power Changes with BOZR Alterations

It is worth noting that the power formula may change as a consequence of optic zone modifications. The approximate rule of thumb for power allowances is to add -0.50 D for every 0.10-mm radius steepening, but this is not a linear relationship across the range of radii required for scleral lenses. Steepening the BOZR from 6.10 mm to 6.00 mm requires nearly -1.00 D to compensate, while 9.60 mm to 9.50 mm needs only -0.25 D.

Solutions and Maintenance of Sclerals

PMMA Scleral Lenses

Maintenance procedures for PMMA scleral lenses are the easiest and most economical of all lens types. Dry storage is perfectly adequate, and any contact lens cleaner can be used. Wetting solutions used just prior to insertion help cushion the lenses, but some scleral lens wearers do not like the increased viscosity, preferring to use just sterile nonpreserved saline.

Rigid Gas-permeable Scleral Lenses

The choice of cleaning and wetting solutions can make a difference to successful wear with GP scleral lens wear. These surfaces attract more lipid and protein compared to PMMA, and a tear film is not retained as well. Due to the greater substance and rigidity of scleral lenses, dry storage does not cause a loss of dimensional stability. Application of a cleaning solution and rinsing with saline just prior to inserting may be all that is necessary. Soaking solutions can be added to the regime if the surface does not wet adequately, but in the author's experience it does not make much difference.

Gas-permeable sealed scleral lenses have to be inserted filled with saline, so preservatives are retained by the precorneal reservoir for long periods. Therefore, wearers may encounter certain brands of solutions that cause problems. Saline from aerosol cans is unsuitable because it is too gassy. If time is given for the bubbles to disappear, the front surface of the lens begins to dry out. Ultrafiltered unit dose saline is the best preparation for filling lenses. Some patients also report "favorite" solutions, or preferred ways to modify the regular recommended modality of use. For example, if they may find normally available wetting agents too viscous, multifunctional soft lens solutions may be preferable for wetting

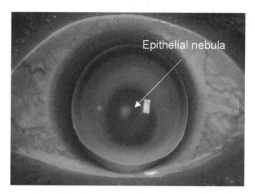

FIG. 33.40. A proud central nebula with corneal lens wear in keratoconus. Apical contact with the lens abrades the delicate surface. (See Color Plate 33.40)

prior to insertion. The practitioner may have to spend some time working through the options to establish the best combination for each patient.

MANAGEMENT OF REFRACTIVE CONDITIONS WITH SCLERALS

Primary Corneal Ectasia

Since the introduction of GP materials, in addition to being an alternative to a corneal transplant, scleral lenses have become an option available to all grades of keratoconus and other forms of primary corneal ectasia (PCE). Many moderate PCE patients complain of excessive corneal lens mobility, lid sensation, foreign bodies behind lenses, or dislodging. GP scleral lenses offer a potential remedy for all these frequently encountered complaints. Epithelial erosions (Fig. 33.40; see Color Plate 33.40) cause persistent discomfort with long-term corneal lens wear, but may resolve while maintaining functional contact lens wear with use of GP sealed scleral lenses that minimize corneal contact. Some patients alternate variously between corneals and scleral lenses to good effect.

The fitting principles are similar for GP sealed scleral lenses irrespective of corneal topography. Figure 33.41 is

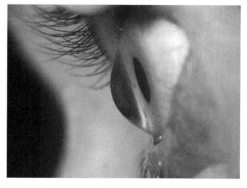

FIG. 33.41. Primary corneal ectasia, conic-type profile with nearly central apex.

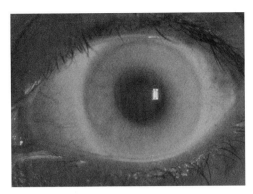

FIG. 33.42. The same eye as shown in Fig. 33.41 fitted with a scleral lens with central contact zone. There is good limbal clearance, but note that the contact zone extends more to the nasal side than to the temporal side. (See Color Plate 33.42)

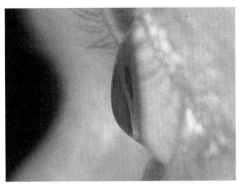

FIG. 33.44. Moderately advanced primary corneal ectasia profile with a downwardly displaced apex.

an example of what could be described as a moderate PCE with minimal eccentricity of the apex. Figure 33.42 (see Color Plate 33.42) illustrates a GP sealed scleral *in situ* with a central contact zone corresponding to the cone apex. Minimum apical clearance is achieved with an apical OZP increment of 0.24 mm (Fig. 33.43; see Color Plate 33.43). Corneal clearance is usually better tolerated, although visual acuity is sometimes considerably better with a visual axis contact zone.

When the corneal apex is eccentric, there is more corneal clearance at the visual axis than at the apex. If the apical contact is alleviated excessively, any bubbles or mucus strands which have otherwise been restricted to the limbal region cross the visual axis. Figure 33.44 illustrates a PCE with its apex nearer the limbus than the geometric center of the cornea, and Fig. 33.45 (see Color Plate 33.45) an off-axis contact zone with a GP scleral lens.

Corneal Transplant

Corneal profile ectasia following transplantation is quite variable, but topographies are usually more symmetrical

about the visual axis compared to PCE. High astigmatism is common after surgery. While usually reasonably regular, high astigmatism—even after repeated posttransplant refractive surgery—may remain in some cases. Figure 33.46 shows a protrusive transplant profile with astigmatism greater than 20.00 D, and Fig. 33.47 (see Color Plate 33.47) a sealed GP scleral lens with a spherical BOZR. There is a contact zone at the superior limbus, but otherwise nothing indicates such high astigmatism in the fluorescein pattern. Most posttransplant scleral lens fitting tends to have a similar appearance whether astigmatism is 2.00 D or 20.00 D.

Aphakia and Myopia

Scleral lenses have a role in the management of high myopia and aphakia when corneal or hydrogel lenses are unsuccessful. Elderly patients in both groups may find large scleral lenses easy to handle and tolerate. Fenestrated PMMA may be preferable to GP lenses for these patients. They do not have to be inserted filled with saline, and maintenance is simple. The cornea is more likely to be regular in both groups, so these patients are good candidates for an integrated optic/scleral zone preformed fitting system. Long-term contact lens–induced changes are less of a problem in

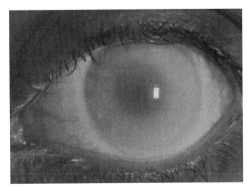

FIG. 33.43. One significant OZP increment of 0.24 mm gives minimum apical clearance. The upper nasal quadrant clearance is still noticeably less than the inferior temporal quadrant. (See Color Plate 33.43)

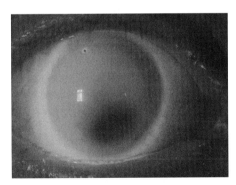

FIG. 33.45. Same eye as shown in Fig. 33.44 fitted with a rigid gas-permeable sealed scleral giving apical contact but clearance at the visual axis. (See Color Plate 33.45)

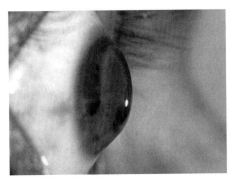

FIG. 33.46. Protrusive and highly astigmatic (over 20.00 DC) posttransplant corneal profile.

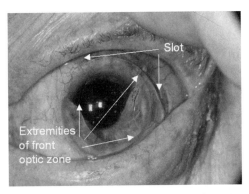

FIG. 33.48. Elderly aphakic patient fitted with an impression PMMA scleral lens. The slot enabled insertion without the need to fill the lens with saline. Fitting by impression allowed more accurate positioning of the optic, as the pupil was displaced upwards.

older patients as their life expectancy is shorter. GP scleral lenses are indicated if signs of hypoxia became apparent, or for younger myopes undergoing scleral lens fitting. Impression fitting is indicated in the event of poor centration or an inadequate scleral zone fit with preformed. Figure 33.48 shows an elderly aphake fitted with an impression slotted PMMA scleral.

Traumatic cataract may also have other incidental problems such as corneal irregularity subsequent to scarring, pupil displacement, or iris loss. A cosmetic iris can be encapsulated into PMMA or the optic can be surface tinted. A full-diameter front optic zone that completely covers the pupil may reduce photophobia and glare from incidental iris injuries. An impression lens provides the best opportunity of achieving this objective because of the improved centration.

Therapeutic applications and management of ocular surface disorders with scleral lenses

Hydrogel or silicone rubber lenses are used extensively for corneal protection or hydration, but are subject to surface

degradation. There is, therefore, a role for scleral lenses that has been enhanced with the advent of GP materials.

Tear Fluid Retention in Dry-eye Pathology and Exposure Keratitis

Scleral lenses should be considered for corneal protection and hydration in some serious dry-eye conditions such as exposure keratitis, Stevens-Johnson syndrome (SJS), and ocular cicatrizing pemphigoid. As well as corneal hydration they provide full protection from lashes which are misdirected or metastatic, i.e., emergent from the meibomian glands or the tarsal plate, and commonly encountered in SJS. Normal fitting procedures can be adopted in many cases, but small diameter sclerals of 18 to 20 mm may be useful if the fornix is shrunken. Fenestrated lenses may be necessary sometimes if inserting a sealed lens is difficult due to the shrunken fornix. Symblepharon in close proximity to the limbus more or less precludes GP scleral fitting unless it is feasible to surgically remove them, but it may be possible to make a functional lens by impression. Figure 33.49 (see Color Plate 33.49) illustrates a scleral *in situ* in a case of SJS, showing corneal decompensation and disease process CNV.

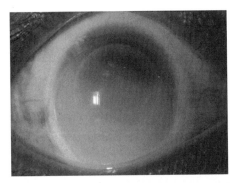

FIG. 33.47. Same eye as shown in Fig. 33.46 fitted with a sealed rigid gas-permeable scleral lens giving full clearance except at the upper limbus and just inside. Typically, nearly all the astigmatism is corrected by the precorneal fluid reservoir without a visual axis contact zone, as is often necessary with some forms of primary corneal ectasia fitted with scleral lenses prior to a transplant. Achieving visual axis clearance is not usually a problem because of the symmetry about the geometric axis. Superior contact may be difficult to avoid with such a protrusive profile because the tendency for the lens to displace downwards and temporally. (See Color Plate 33.47)

Epithelial Defects and Dysplasia

Poor healing epithelial defects may also benefit from continual bathing in the precorneal fluid reservoir retained by a GP sealed scleral, with simultaneous protection from the sloughing action of the lids (19,21–23,30). A fluid reservoir entrapped by a scleral may be indicated both for visual improvement and for alleviation of discomfort. Figure 33.50 (see Color Plate 33.50) shows a serious corneal lesion consequent to neurotrophic keratopathy in a young diabetic patient, and Fig. 33.51 (see Color Plate 33.51) its reduction in size following 2 weeks of GP sealed scleral lens wear.

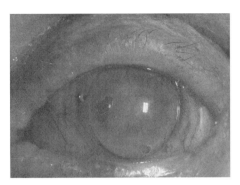

FIG. 33.49. A patient with Stevens-Johnson syndrome fitted with a fenestrated rigid gas-permeable scleral lens. In this example there is a fenestration at the nasal limbus, one just above the lid on the temporal side and a third (unseen) just under the upper lid in the upper temporal quadrant. The corneal surface is not distended, as is often the case with primary corneal ectasia or postoperative transplant, but the surface is still irregular. An area of clearance can be seen over the inferior half of the cornea, and a contact zone over the superior half. The small bubbles trapped under the optic are not a problem, but their presence suggests there could not be much more clearance if the lens is to retain a functional precorneal fluid reservoir. The corneal neovascularization is also clearly visible: this is part of Stevens-Johnson syndrome disease process and was present before scleral lens fitting was undertaken. (See Color Plate 33.49)

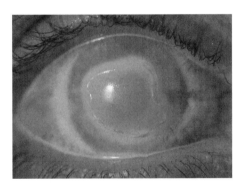

FIG. 33.50. A massive neurotrophic epithelial defect that was refractory to treatment. (See Color Plate 33.50)

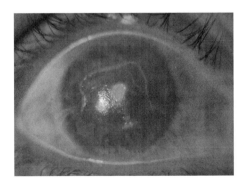

FIG. 33.51. The same lesion following 3 weeks day wear of a rigid gas-permeable scleral lens. The defect has almost resolved, although its original margin is still clearly visible. (See Color Plate 33.51)

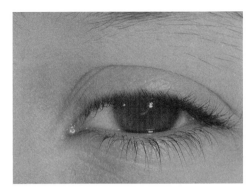

FIG. 33.52. Ptosis following cataract surgery in a young teenager.

Ptosis

A shelf to prop up the upper lid can be cemented onto the front of a scleral or fabricated by cutting through a thick shell. Sometimes just a thicker lens gives sufficient bulk to open the palpebral aperture. Figures 33.52 and 33.53 show a young patient with a ptosis, and a functional increase in the vertical palpebral aperture with a GP scleral of thickened scleral zone.

Overnight Use of Sclerals for Therapeutic Applications

The introduction of gas-permeable materials has also enabled the application of scleral lenses for overnight use to manage painful or progressive ocular surface disorders if necessary (18,21,23,30). Corneal exposure consequent to injury, the aftermath of lid surgery, or following surgical removal of cerebral tumors such as acoustic neuroma remains round the clock if there is poor night-time lid closure. Occasionally it may be a night-time requirement only, with no need to use the lens during the waking hours if there are no symptoms. However, removal of the lens by the patient or an assistant for regular cleaning to remove surface deposits or mucus behind the lens usually is required in the morning and just before bedtime. Thus, there is a clear distinction between continuous and overnight wear.

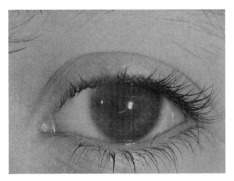

FIG. 33.53. A thick (approximately 1.5 mm) sealed rigid gas-permeable scleral lens has a significant upper lid–propping effect.

There is a potential hypoxia problem associated with overnight wear of any contact lens, but the observation that GP sclerals appear to provide an environment for epithelial healing indicates a sufficiently high level of corneal metabolism when the lids are closed during sleep. Overnight lens wear can be recommended when it is considered that the benefits of continuous corneal hydration and protection provided by a scleral lens outweighed the anticipated effects of overnight hypoxia. There have been few corneal metabolism studies during wear of sclerals with a closed eye to confirm this, but one study suggests that, albeit proceeding with caution, overnight wear can be justified if there is a strong clinical indication (31).

Cosmetic Shells

Hydrogel lenses can incorporate iris patterns, but a superior cosmetic result is sometimes possible with a cosmetic scleral shell (e.g., conjunctival blood vessels can be simulated). Such prosthetic scleral lenses also may last many years with minimum maintenance costs. They make the treated eye look larger than the fellow eye, which may be desirable (to give the illusion of normality for phthisical eyes) or undesirable. They are also more time consuming to fit and cannot be made from GP materials at present.

COMPLICATIONS OF SCLERAL LENS WEAR

PMMA is very inert, wets well *in situ*, and is subject to very little deterioration, as is proven by the fact that some patients have worn the same lens for many years. GP scleral lenses can be effectively cleaned, so there are few problems with contaminated solutions and little risk of infections. However, they do not wet as well *in situ* as PMMA, hence lens surface–eye interaction is more of a problem.

Contact Zones

PMMA scleral lenses are commonly fenestrated, leading to settling back on the globe and almost invariably contact between the cornea and lens back surface. Contact with GP materials appear to be more problematic than with PMMA. Figure 33.54 (see Color Plate 33.54) shows a contact zone and a corresponding confluent epithelial stain. Fortunately, controlled clearance fitting avoids such contact in most cases. Abrasions may also occur with clumsy insertion or if contact occurs against an especially delicate cornea.

Upper Tarsal Plate Changes

Giant papillary conjunctivitis (GPC) is not common, but may increase with GP scleral lens wearers in the author's experience, consistent with reports of more GPC with GP

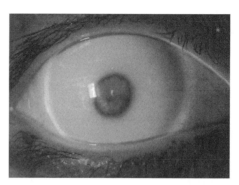

FIG. 33.54. A rigid gas-permeable scleral lens fitted for primary corneal ectasia with a central apex. Corneal stain is visible within the contact area. (See Color Plate 33.54)

corneal lens wearers. This is a minor issue when set against the benefits of increase oxygen permeability.

Mucus

Overproduction of mucus is a common problem with sealed GP scleral lenses. While not a sight-threatening complication, it is a major nuisance and some patients give up wear because the problem becomes intractable. Accumulation occurs in the precorneal reservoir and is visually disruptive (Fig. 33.55). A different material may assist, but there is no satisfactory way to predict the outcome of such a change. It is worth refitting in "old style" PMMA if there is a strong indication for scleral lens management.

Bunching of the Limbal Conjunctiva

The conjunctiva is relatively flaccid and tends to be pushed over the limbus during scleral lens wear (Fig. 33.56). This is more noticeable with GP sealed scleral lenses as compared to PMMA. As soon as the lens is removed, the conjunctiva returns to its normal position and there does not seem to

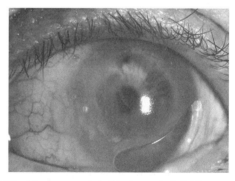

FIG. 33.55. Mucus strands behind a sealed rigid gas-permeable scleral lens fitted after a corneal transplant. The lens had to be repeatedly removed and cleaned to enable clear vision. There is also a bubble at the lower temporal limbus, but this did not cause a problem.

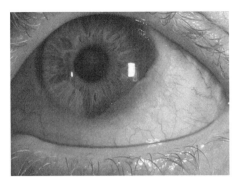

FIG. 33.56. Conjunctival fold displaced over the inferior temporal limbus during sealed rigid gas-permeable scleral lens wear. It is a common phenomena, but does not seem to be uncomfortable, and reverts to normal when the lens is removed.

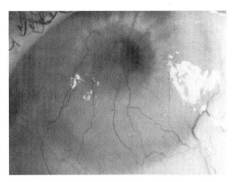

FIG. 33.58. Sight-threatening visual axis corneal neovascularization and lipid leakage in an only eye following 30 years of fenestrated polymethylmethacrylate lens wear. The underlying condition was acne rosacea keratitis. A scleral lens had been the only option to maintain functional vision for the patient's adult life, therefore the vascularization should be judged to be acceptable sequelae as there was no feasible alternative.

be any adverse effects, but patients sometimes remark on the appearance.

Corneal Hypoxia in Corneal Transplant

A major problem during PMMA scleral lens management of postoperative corneal transplant was that the endothelial cell loss as a consequence of surgery lowered the threshold at which contact lens wear lead to corneal edema from hypoxia. This has been reduced with the introduction of GP materials, but if there are insufficient endothelial cells to allow normal metabolic processes after the surgical procedure there are still some instances when hypoxia causes misty vision.

Corneal Neovascularization

Corneal neovascularization is recognized as a serious complication with PMMA scleral lens management. Some patients are only diagnosed late, after noting visual deterioration. Others develop incipient CNV that is not necessarily sight-threatening in its own right, but enough to jeopardize

the survival of a future transplant (a particular concern in PCE patients).

It is important to not overstate the threat. CNV is detectable in its early stages if patients present appropriately for after-care consultations. It is also a complication of other lens types, when the onset can be quite rapid. Long-term scleral lens induced CNV is not necessarily sight-threatening, considering the patient's expected lifespan, or may be self-limiting. Figure 33.57 shows peripheral, non–sight-threatening CNV following 40 years of PMMA sealed scleral lens wear.

Tan et al. (17) illustrated that long-term PMMA scleral lens induced CNV and that subsequent lipid leakage can be reversed by refitting with GP scleral lenses, leaving just ghost vessels. Figures 33.58 and 33.59 show an example. This does not prove CNV is no longer a complication of scleral lens wear, but does indicate that the threat is reduced.

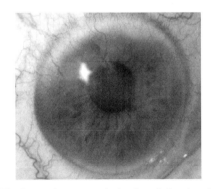

FIG. 33.57. Corneal neovascularization following 50 years of sealed PMMA scleral lens wear. The longest fronds have just reached the visual axis, but as the patient was older than 80 years, it was not considered to be sight-threatening.

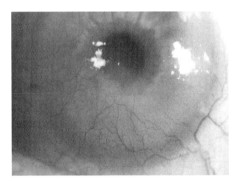

FIG. 33.59. The eye was refitted as a matter of urgency with a duplicated rigid gas-permeable scleral, as soon as they had become available since it was entirely necessary to maintain scleral lens wear. It was hoped that further progress of the vessels would be retarded, but the outcome was better than expected as the vessels actually regressed and some of the lipid absorbed after about 4 months, giving a significant improvement in visual acuity.

CONCLUSION

Scleral lenses are often indicated when a result is needed more than at any other time, so it is clearly advisable that the professions preserve clinical and manufacturing skills. Since the introduction of GP materials these lenses can be applied at all grades of pathology, wherever benefits are anticipated. Although only a small number of active practitioners are needed to maintain a functional service, those who are not directly involved should also be aware of the significant developments in recent years in this subspecialty of contact lens practice.

ACKNOWLEDGMENT

The author is indebted to the cornea consultants at Moorfields and Oxford Eye Hospitals, United Kingdom, in particular to Professor Roger Buckley, for many years of support for the development of a modern scleral lens unit.

REFERENCES

1. Kalt E. Reported by Panas P. *Bull Aced Med* 1888;19:400. [English translation by Pearson RM, Kalt E. Keratoconus and the contact lens. *Am J Optom Vis Sci* 1989;66:643.]
2. Muller A. Brillenglaser und hornhautlinsen [inaugural dissertation]. University of Kiel. 1889:20.
3. Fick AE. A contact lens [translation by May CH]. *Arch Ophthalmol* 1888;19:215–226.
4. Bier N. The practice of ventilated contact lenses. *Optician* 1948; 116:497–501.
5. Ezekiel D. Gas permeable haptic lenses. *J Br Contact Lens Assoc* 1983;6:158–161.
6. Pullum KW, Trodd TC. Development of slotted scleral lenses. *J Br Contact Lens Assoc* 1984;7:28–38, 92–97.
7. Pullum KW. Feasibility study for the production of gas permeable scleral lenses using ocular impression techniques. Trans Br Contact Lens Association Annual Conference 1987.
8. Lyons CJ, Buckley RJ, Pullum KW, et al. Development of the gas-permeable impression-moulded scleral contact lens. A preliminary report. *Acta Ophthalmol* 1989;67(Suppl 192):162–164.
9. Ruben M, Benjamin WJ. Scleral contact lenses: preliminary report on oxygen-permeable materials. *Contact Lens* 1985;13: 5–10.
10. Bleshoy H, Pullum KW. Corneal response to gas permeable impression scleral lenses. *J Br Contact Lens Assoc* 1988;11:31–34.
11. Pullum KW, Hobley AJ, Parker JH. Dallos award lecture part two. Hypoxic corneal changes following sealed gas permeable impression scleral lens wear. *J Br Contact Lens Assoc* 1990;13: 83–87.
12. Pullum KW, Hobley AJ, Davison C. 100 + Dk: does thickness make much difference? *J Br Contact Lens Assoc* 1991;6: 158–161.
13. Pullum KW, Stapleton FJ. Scleral lens induced corneal swelling: what is the effect of varying Dk and lens thickness? *CLAO J* 1997;23:259–263.
14. Schein OD, Rosenthal P, Ducharme C. A gas-permeable scleral contact lens for visual rehabilitation. *Am J Ophthalmol* 1990;109: 318–322.
15. Visser R. Een nieuwe toekomst hoogzuurtofdoorlatende scleralenzen bij verschillende pathologie. *Nederl Tijdsch Optom Contactol* 1990;3:10–14.
16. Kok JHC, Visser R. Treatment of ocular surface disorders and dry eyes with high gas-permeable scleral lenses. *Cornea* 1992;11: 518–522.
17. Tan DTH, Pullum KW, Buckley RJ. Medical applications of scleral contact lenses: 2. Gas-permeable scleral contact lenses. *Cornea* 1995;14:130–137.
18. Pullum KW, Buckley RJ. A study of 530 patients referred for rigid gas permeable scleral contact lens assessment. *Cornea* 1997; 16:612–622.
19. Cotter M, Rosenthal P. Scleral contact lenses. *J Am Optom Assoc* 1998;69:33–40.
20. Romero-Rangel T, Stavrou P, Cotter JM, et al. Gas-permeable scleral contact lens therapy in ocular surface disease. *Am J Ophthalmol* 2000;130:25–32.
21. Rosenthal P, Cotter JM, Baum J. Treatment of persistent corneal epithelial defect with extended wear of a fluid-ventilated gas-permeable scleral contact lens. *Am J Ophthalmol* 2000;130: 33–41.
22. Segal O, Barkana Y, Hourovitz D, et al. Scleral contact lenses may help where other modalities fail. *Cornea* 2003;22:308–310.
23. Rosenthal P, Cotter J. The Boston Scleral Lens in the management of severe ocular surface disease. *Ophthalmol Clin N Am* 2003;16:89–93.
24. Ezekiel DF. Gas permeable scleral lenses. *Spectrum* 1991;July: 19–24.
25. Mountford J, Carkeet N, Carney L. Corneal thickness changes during scleral lens wear: Effect of gas permeability. *ICLC* 1994; 21:19–21.
26. Marriott PJ. An analysis or the global contours and haptic lens fitting. *Br J Physiol Optics* 1966;23:3–40.
27. Cowan JM. The wide angle contact lens. *Optician* 1948;115: 359.
28. Pullum KW. In: Phillips A, Speedwell L, eds. *Contact lenses. A text book for practitioner and student.* 4th ed. Butterworth-Heinemann, 1997:566–608.
29. Storey JK. The use of Panasil C silicone rubber impression material in contact lens work. *Optom Today* 1987;27:711–714.
30. Tappin MJ, Pullum KW, Buckley RJ. Scleral contact lenses for overnight wear in the management of ocular surface disorders. *Eye* 2001;15:168–172.
31. Smith GTH, Mireskandari K, Pullum KW. Corneal swelling with overnight wear of scleral contact lenses. *Cornea* 2004;23: 1,29–34.

EXTENDED WEAR: PHYSIOLOGIC CONSIDERATIONS

HELEN A. SWARBRICK

INTRODUCTION

The cornea and its associated tissues are remarkably resilient to environmental stresses, such as those imposed by eye closure and contact lens wear. This resilience to induced stress is primarily directed at maintaining corneal transparency, without which the more complex task of visual perception of the surrounding world is severely compromised.

In many respects the physiologic challenge associated with contact lens wear resembles that imposed by eye closure. During sleep, oxygen availability from the atmosphere is reduced, carbon dioxide accumulates in the tissue, and the flushing of debris and resurfacing of the cornea are impeded. The corneal response to these environmental changes during eye closure is well documented; epithelial metabolic activity slows, corneal sensitivity is reduced, the cornea swells slightly, and stromal pH falls. Corneal recovery is rapid on eye opening with a resurgence in metabolic activity and initiation of blinking, which removes accumulated debris and reforms the tear film.

In the short term, contact lens wear induces similar environmental changes and the cornea shows a similar short-term response. The challenge imposed by contact lens wear, however, can be both more chronic and more intense than during eye closure. As a result, long-term contact lens wear can eventually induce more extensive and profound changes in corneal structure and function. During daily wear, these changes result from the presence of a contact lens during a period when the cornea usually would be exposed to a normal environment. Extended wear imposes an even greater stress, because the changes in environment are more extreme during eye closure than those normally experienced, and also more prolonged, because the continual presence of the lens inhibits recovery on eye opening.

As well as exacerbating normal environmental changes, contact lens wear presents some unique challenges. The presence of the contact lens can exert localized pressure on the cornea and act as a stimulus to the defense mechanisms of the cornea and adnexa. Contact lens wear also increases the risk of corneal infection. Thus, contact lens wear can induce corneal responses that are otherwise rarely observed in the absence of active disease or damage. This is particularly so during extended wear, when the stresses are more prolonged and intense.

The purpose of contact lens research and development is to identify the factors that precipitate acute and chronic changes in corneal structure and function during contact lens wear, and to develop materials and strategies that will reduce or avoid these changes. As a result of increasing knowledge of corneal physiology and the effects of contact lenses, requirements for successful extended contact lens wear can be defined. These include providing adequate oxygen during open and closed eye lens wear to maintain normal levels of epithelial metabolic activity; minimizing corneal pH changes by reducing lactate and carbon dioxide accumulation in the tissue; facilitating the removal of debris and contaminants from the corneal surface, and allowing regular resurfacing of the cornea; minimizing physical stresses by ensuring even pressure distribution; and reducing inflammatory and infective stimuli associated with the lens.

The recent introduction of highly oxygen-transmissible silicone hydrogel lenses represents a major breakthrough in satisfying corneal requirements for successful extended wear. Clinical reports to date indicate that these lenses provide adequate oxygen to avoid acute and chronic hypoxic stress (1–5) and minimize corneal acidosis (6), confirming earlier clinical results with high-Dk/t gas-permeable (GP) extended wear (7,8). The challenges of enhancing post–lens tear exchange, avoiding pressure effects and minimizing corneal inflammation and infection remain, however, and will continue to drive contact lens research and development in the quest for truly safe lenses for extended wear.

In this chapter, the nature of environmental changes and stresses associated with eye closure and contact lens wear will be discussed, and the short- and long-term physiologic changes that occur in response to this challenge will be described.

OXYGEN

Corneal Oxygen Supply and Utilization

In common with other body tissues, the cornea requires energy to support normal cellular functions such as replication, growth, and maintenance. This energy is obtained by metabolism of glucose, which is supplied principally from the aqueous (9) and glycogen that is stored in the epithelium (10). Carbohydrate metabolism in the corneal tissues functions most efficiently in the presence of oxygen, which is supplied to the anterior cornea principally from the atmosphere when the eyes are open (11,12) and from the capillary plexus of the upper palpebral conjunctiva during eye closure (13). Little oxygen is available from other sources such as the limbal blood vessels (14).

The relative oxygen consumption rates of the epithelium: stroma:endothelium are in the ratio of 40:39:21 (15). On the basis of tissue volume, however, the epithelium consumes oxygen 10 times faster than the stroma (15). While this indicates that the epithelium is more metabolically active than the stroma, stromal keratocytes may consume glucose at a faster rate per cell than the epithelial cells (16). Despite this, the direct effect of hypoxia on stromal keratocytes has received little attention, and it is generally considered that the epithelium is the tissue layer most directly affected by changes in ambient oxygen levels at the anterior corneal surface. Although the endothelium appears to consume even more oxygen than the epithelium on a tissue-volume basis, the importance of atmospheric oxygen in maintaining endothelial metabolic activity is uncertain. In the open eye, atmospheric oxygen reaches the endothelium and aqueous humor (17–19) and when access of atmospheric oxygen is impeded, such as during eyelid closure or contact lens wear, oxygen levels in the aqueous fall (19–21). Under these conditions, however, the aqueous can still sup-

ply the endothelium with some oxygen diffusing from iris blood vessels and other surrounding tissues (19,21).

Contact lenses act as a barrier impeding the supply of oxygen to the anterior corneal surface. During open-eye lens wear, oxygen may reach the cornea by dissolving and mixing in the tear fluid layer between lens and cornea. Lens movement, activated by blinking, is a necessary factor in maximizing oxygen availability by this route. Thus, hydrogel lenses, which generally exhibit less lens movement than rigid lenses, provide considerably less oxygen via the tear pump (22). During closed-eye lens wear, oxygen provision via the blink-activated tear pump is believed to be minimal (23).

Oxygen also reaches the cornea during contact lens wear by diffusion through the lens material itself. The amount of oxygen provided by this route is dependent on the oxygen transmissibility (Dk/t) of the lens. Oxygen diffusion through a contact lens is also limited by the oxygen availability at the front surface of the lens (24). In the closed eye, therefore, the level of oxygen reaching the anterior corneal surface will be limited further in the presence of a contact lens because of the reduced oxygen availability from the palpebral conjunctival vascular plexus.

Under normal (non–lens-wearing) circumstances, the cornea is exposed to atmospheric levels of oxygen immediately on eye opening. Although the indirect effects of reduced oxygen levels during eye closure may persist for some time, normal epithelial aerobic activity is rapidly reestablished and increased energy is available to support normal cellular functions.

When a contact lens has been worn overnight, oxygen availability also increases significantly immediately on eye opening. More oxygen is available from the atmosphere to diffuse through the lens material, and the circulation of oxygenated tears behind the lens resumes as soon as lens movement is triggered by blinking. However, the presence of the contact lens impedes oxygen supply compared to the no-lens situation and, consequently, normal aerobic metabolic activity is slower to resume. If lens movement is inadequate or the Dk/t of the lens is low, insufficient oxygen may be supplied to allow the resumption of normal levels of aerobic metabolic activity. In this situation, epithelial energy supplies are chronically reduced while the lens is worn and epithelial integrity may be compromised in the long term.

Effects of Reduced Oxygen Availability

Epithelium

The reduction in epithelial metabolic activity associated with contact lens–induced hypoxia has a number of immediate physiologic effects. In general, the extent of these effects is directly related to the relative degree of oxygen deprivation. Thus, polymethylmethacrylate (PMMA) lenses, which do not transmit oxygen through the lens material but rely on tear pumping to supply the cornea with oxygen, produce the most rapid and dramatic effects. In contrast, lenses with high oxygen transmissibility, such as silicone hydrogels and high-Dk/t GP lenses, produce minimal changes.

The decreased rate of aerobic metabolism under hypoxic conditions is reflected directly in reduced levels of adenosine triphosphate (ATP) (25,26) and alterations in the epithelial mitochondrial redox state (27,28). The levels of enzymes associated with metabolic activity are also affected. Lactate dehydrogenase, an enzyme that potentiates the conversion of pyruvate to lactate, accumulates in the basal layer (29), while the concentration of succinic dehydrogenase, a Krebs cycle enzyme, also varies but in a more complex manner (30). In addition, glycogen stores in the epithelium are mobilized to fuel anaerobic glycolysis (10,25,31).

Maintenance of epithelial structural and functional integrity is compromised as a result of the reduction in energy available for normal cellular processes. With short-term contact lens wear the rate of cellular mitosis is dramatically reduced (32,33), and other cellular regulatory functions, such as synthesis of cell components and waste removal, are similarly affected. This is evidenced by distortion of epithelial cells, degenerative intracellular changes, the formation of lipidlike bodies within cells, and the loosening of tight junctions between epithelial cells (34,35). Intercellular and intracellular fluid accumulation has also been observed (34); however, this epithelial edema may be attributable not only to hypoxic stress (36) but also to influx of water because of excessive or hypotonic tearing stimulated by lens wear (37). There is also a significant fall in transcorneal potential (35,38), which may represent an increase in passive ion flux due to the compromised epithelial barrier in association with a decrease in active cation pumping because of the reduced energy availability (39). Interestingly, short-term hypoxia (using gas-goggles) does not appear to increase epithelial permeability to fluorescein (40), suggesting that increases in permeability found after short-term hydrogel lens wear (41) may reflect physical interactions between the lens and the epithelium.

Recovery from these acute changes is rapid once normal oxygen supplies become available and aerobic metabolism resumes. However, chronic reduction in oxygen availability, as may occur during extended contact lens wear, results in more long-term epithelial changes, which can severely compromise the epithelial barrier function and ultimately threaten corneal integrity.

The epithelium reacts to a chronically reduced oxygen supply in the long term by decreasing its oxygen utilization. This is demonstrated by a gradual decrease in oxygen consumption rate over the first few months of lens wear (42) and a significantly lower consumption rate after several years of hydrogel extended lens wear (Fig. 34.1) (43). Although the mechanism for this response is unclear, it may reflect either a chronic reduction in the level of metabolic activity

within individual epithelial cells, or an overall reduction in cell numbers because of the decrease in mitotic rate. Certainly, the number of epithelial cell layers can decrease with short-term contact lens wear, although this may be attributable partially to pressure effects (44,45). However, epithelial thinning has also been reported after several years of hydrogel extended lens wear (Fig. 34.1) (43). This is thought to be a result of the reduced mitotic rate and tissue synthesis under chronic hypoxic conditions.

Chronic hypoxia leads to the development of epithelial microcysts (Fig. 34.2). These small inclusions, 15 to 50 μm in diameter, are usually distributed in an annulus in the corneal midperiphery and appear after approximately 3 months of hydrogel extended lens wear (46,47). The level of microcystic development has proven a useful clinical index of the degree of chronic hypoxic stress experienced by the cornea during extended lens wear (48). Although their exact nature is unclear, epithelial microcysts are thought to comprise pockets of disorganized cellular material (49) or apoptotic cells (50) and, as such, reflect the reduced efficiency of epithelial functioning under hypoxic conditions (43). The fact that microcysts take several months to develop, and to disappear after cessation of lens wear, indicates that they represent relatively fundamental changes in tissue synthesis processes in the epithelium.

Other long-term changes in epithelial structure and function under chronic hypoxic conditions may affect epithelial barrier function and thus render the epithelium more susceptible to damage and infection. Superficial epithelial cells tend to survive longer before sloughing into the tear film. Reduced rates of epithelial cell desquamation have been reported in association with hypoxia induced under gas-goggles (51) and by contact lens wear (45,52,53). In addition, the average cell size on the epithelial surface is increased with contact lens wear (45,51–55), suggesting that surface cells are older than in the non–lens-wearing eye. This may represent a compensatory mechanism for the reduced cell production and turnover rate but, as a result, the vitality of the surface epithelial cells may be compromised. In particular, epithelial fragility is increased (56), potentiating the risk of epithelial injury. At the same time, epithelial sensitivity is reduced (57,58). This effect appears to be directly attributable to hypoxia (58) and is thought to reflect a reduction in the concentration of the neurotransmitter acetylcholine in the epithelium (59).

The integrity of the physical barrier is also compromised in the long term by a reduction in the density of hemidesmosomes, which anchor the basal cell layer to the basement membrane (60). This results in a significant reduction in epithelial adhesion (60,61), further increasing the risk of significant epithelial damage. A syndrome characterized by spontaneous loss of large areas of epithelium has been described in association with chronic lens-induced hypoxia (62,63). Once corneal damage has been sustained, epithelial wound healing is inhibited under contact lenses (64,65).

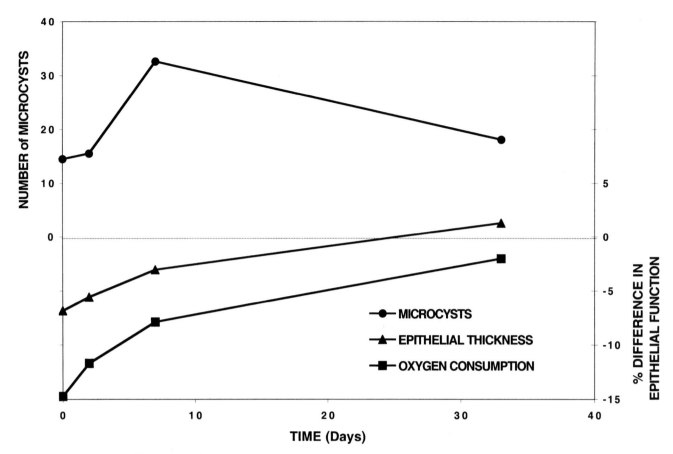

FIG. 34.1. Mean changes in epithelial oxygen uptake, epithelial thickness, and epithelial microcysts after cessation of long-term extended wear of high water content hydrogel contact lenses. Data on day 0 were obtained within 2 hours of lens removal. (Redrawn from Holden BA, Sweeney DF, Vannas A, et al. Effects of long-term extended contact lens wear on the human cornea. *Invest Ophthalmol Vis Sci* 1985;26:1489, with permission. © Association for Research in Vision and Ophthalmology.)

There is increasing evidence that chronic hypoxia may also affect the ability of bacteria, in particular *Pseudomonas aeruginosa,* to bind to the epithelial surface (66,67). Cavanagh and colleagues (45,52,53) have established a clear relationship between lens Dk/t and the level of bacterial binding to exfoliated epithelial cells. Bacterial binding is significantly reduced after wear of silicone hydrogel lenses in extended wear compared to hydrogel lenses (Fig. 34.3). (53,68). Interestingly, less bacterial binding was found with GP compared to soft lens wear independent of Dk/t (45,53), suggesting that lens movement and post–lens-tear flow also play an important role in maintaining epithelial defenses against bacterial invasion, possibly by maintaining the integrity of the protective mucus layer of the tear film (see later discussion).

Stroma

Altered epithelial metabolism under hypoxic conditions has an important indirect effect on the corneal stroma. Anaerobic glycolysis produces lactate as a by-product; under aerobic conditions lactate is converted to pyruvate in the tricarboxylic acid cycle, but in a hypoxic environment excess lactate accumulates in the tissue as it is gradually eliminated into the aqueous (13,69). The increased concentration of lactate in the epithelium and stroma has two important consequences; corneal pH is reduced (70), and the osmotic pressure in the stroma increases. According to the theory of Klyce (71), this increased osmotic pressure causes an influx of water into the tissue, resulting in stromal swelling or edema.

Stromal edema is frequently used as an index of the level of acute hypoxia experienced by the tissue during eye closure and contact lens wear. Of particular clinical relevance is the level of edema induced during overnight wear of contact lenses (72). The cornea is able to eliminate only 8% edema during the day after overnight wear of hydrogel lenses (73) and approximately 10% after overnight GP lens wear (74, 75). Lenses that induce levels of overnight edema greater than this will consequently cause persistent residual daytime edema while the lens is worn (73). This implies that the cornea is experiencing chronic hypoxic stress, which in turn will precipitate associated long-term corneal changes.

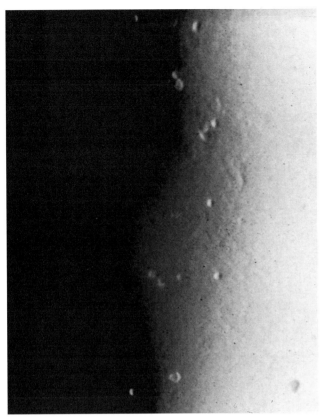

FIG. 34.2. Slit-lamp photograph of epithelial microcysts in the corneal epithelium of a lens-wearing eye. Note that the microcysts display reversed illumination (i.e, the distribution of light within the microcysts is opposite to that of the background). This suggests that the microcysts represent pockets of cellular debris. Original magnification 100×. (Modified from Holden BA, Sweeney DF, Vannas A, et al. Effects of long-term extended contact lens wear on the human cornea. *Invest Ophthalmol Vis Sci* 198526:1489, with permission. © Association for Research in Vision and Ophthalmology.)

Apart from its usefulness as an index of hypoxic stress, the direct effects of chronic stromal edema on the corneal tissue are unclear. It has been suggested that in the short term, acute high levels of stromal edema may be associated with the induction of epithelial edema because of a rapid osmotically driven influx of water into the tissue from the tears (76). High levels of stromal edema may also cause leaching of stromal glycosaminoglycans (77); this may represent the mechanism for the gradual thinning of the stroma reported with long-term hydrogel lens extended wear (43, 78). Corneal molding associated with GP extended wear may also be exacerbated by softening of the cornea due to persistent edema (79).

Endothelium

The direct effects of reduced oxygen at the anterior corneal surface on endothelial structure and function are unclear. Although all layers of the cornea receive oxygen from the atmosphere while the eyes are open (17–19), oxygen levels

at the endothelium–aqueous interface are reduced under hypoxic conditions (19–21). Whether this reduction in available oxygen has a significant direct effect on endothelial structure and function has yet to be resolved.

The observation of the appearance of small nonreflective areas scattered over the endothelial mosaic shortly after insertion of a contact lens (80) was initially thought to represent an endothelial response to reduced oxygen availability (81). These so-called endothelial blebs (Fig. 34.4B) have also been reported in association with eye closure (82), providing support for this hypothesis. However, Holden and associates (83) have established that the endothelial bleb response is more probably induced by changes in stromal pH, because blebs are also produced by exposure of the cornea to nonhypoxic stimuli such as carbon dioxide/oxygen gas mixtures.

Similarly, it has been thought that more chronic changes in endothelial morphology that develop with long-term contact lens wear are induced by chronic hypoxia. However, there is increasing evidence that these changes may also be attributable to chronic corneal acidosis. Consequently, these endothelial changes will be discussed in more detail later.

Recovery from Chronic Hypoxic Stress

Once normal levels of oxygen become available from the atmosphere, aerobic metabolism can be reestablished. However, if the hypoxic stress has been persistent, corneal recovery is not immediate. Holden and co-workers (43) found that after 5 years of extended hydrogel lens wear, epithelial oxygen consumption and thickness took approximately 1 month to return to pre–lens-wearing levels (Fig. 34.1). The gradual recovery of the epithelium from chronic hypoxic stress is also reflected in a dramatic increase in the number of epithelial microcysts in the first week after cessation of hydrogel extended lens wear (Fig. 34.1) and a subsequent reduction in numbers over the following months (48,84). A similar effect has been reported in patients refitted with silicone hydrogel lenses after hydrogel extended wear (1, 85). The sudden increase in microcyst numbers over the first week is thought to represent a resurgence in epithelial metabolic activity and a consequent increased rate of cellular waste removal from the compromised epithelial layer.

The recovery of other epithelial alterations, such as increased superficial epithelial cell size, increased fragility and reduced epithelial adhesion, after relief from chronic hypoxic stress has yet to be documented. However, it is reasonable to assume that once normal epithelial metabolic activity resumes, the synthesis of intracellular and extracellular components would return to normal levels, and the epithelium would recover gradually to its previous non–lens-wearing status. Recovery of corneal sensitivity, however, is slow, and normal touch thresholds may not be regained for some months (86). The reasons for this relatively slow rate of recovery are uncertain.

During extended lens wear, the stroma typically exhibits

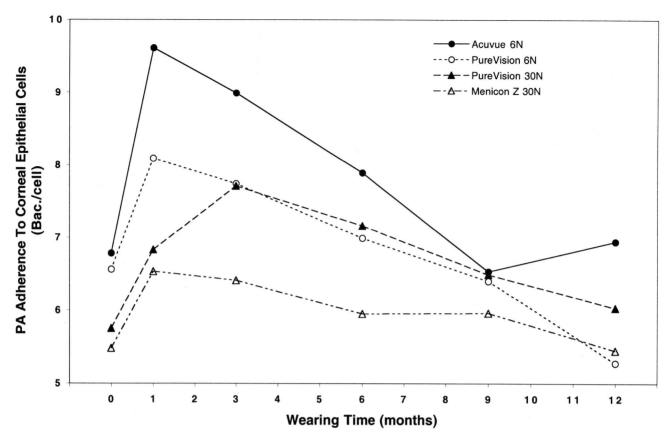

FIG. 34.3. *Pseudomonas aeruginosa* (PA) adherence to exfoliated corneal epithelial cells after extended wear of hydrogel (Acuvue), silicone hydrogel (PureVision), and gas-permeable (Menicon Z) contact lenses. (Redrawn from Ren DH, Yamamoto K, Ladage PM, et al. Adaptive effects of 30-night wear of hyper-O_2 transmissible contact lenses on bacterial binding and corneal epithelium. *Ophthalmology* 2002;109:27, with permission.)

overnight swelling, and unless high-Dk/t silicone hydrogel or GP lenses are worn, some edema generally persists during the day (73). On cessation of lens wear, the edema resolves rapidly as excess lactate produced during anaerobic metabolism is metabolized in aerobic pathways and progressively eliminated from the tissue. Once the edema has resolved, however, the stroma is thinned relative to the pre–lens-wearing condition (Fig. 34.5) (43,78). This thinning is thought to represent leaching of substance from the stroma. Because of the low metabolic rate of the stroma, replacement of this lost bulk is slow, and measurable stromal thinning persists for up to 6 months after cessation of extended lens wear (84).

Oxygen Levels Required to Avoid Hypoxic Effects

Because the measurement of stromal edema provides a useful index of the degree of acute hypoxic stress experienced by the cornea, the level of oxygen required at the anterior corneal surface to avoid measurable edema can give an indication of the minimum oxygen levels required by the epithe-lium to sustain normal aerobic metabolic activity. It is now well established that, on average, at least 10% oxygen must be delivered to the anterior cornea to avoid measurable stromal edema (87,88). There is considerable individual variation in this critical oxygen level (87,89), with some individuals exhibiting edema with very slight reductions in ambient oxygen, confirming earlier results demonstrating significant individual variation in corneal oxygen consumption rates (90,91).

Because corneal edema is a secondary effect of epithelial hypoxia, it is not surprising that more sensitive measures of epithelial metabolic disturbance give higher estimates of the minimum corneal oxygen requirement. Hamano and colleagues (35) have measured accumulation of lactate in the anterior chamber and suppression of epithelial mitosis when anterior oxygen levels fall below 13% oxygen. Williams (92) reports that an endothelial bleb response is generally observable at oxygen levels below 15% oxygen. It is likely that, at least for some patients, any reduction in anterior corneal oxygen levels below 21% oxygen can adversely affect epithelial metabolic activity (87).

During closed-eye contact lens wear, when oxygen avail-

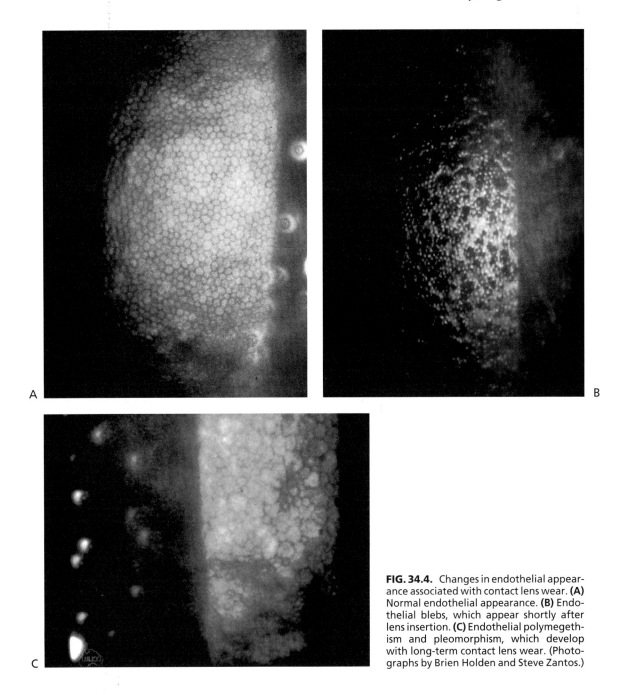

A

B

C

FIG. 34.4. Changes in endothelial appearance associated with contact lens wear. **(A)** Normal endothelial appearance. **(B)** Endothelial blebs, which appear shortly after lens insertion. **(C)** Endothelial polymegethism and pleomorphism, which develop with long-term contact lens wear. (Photographs by Brien Holden and Steve Zantos.)

ability is reduced, lenses must be able to transmit considerably more oxygen in order to avoid hypoxic stress. In 1984, Holden and Mertz (93) derived the critical lens oxygen transmissibility required to limit overnight corneal edema to 4%, the level experienced when lenses are not worn during sleep (94). They found that a lens that provides 18% oxygen during open-eye lens wear would satisfy this criterion. In practice this can be achieved when lens Dk/t exceeds 87×10^{-9} (cm.mL O$_2$)./(s.mL.mm Hg).

The Holden-Mertz criterion has recently undergone refinement. Sweeney and colleagues (1) have suggested that a critical Dk/t of 125×10^{-9} (cm.mL O$_2$)./(s.mL.mm Hg) would be required to avoid lens-induced overnight edema if

an average of 3.2% overnight edema in non–lens-wearing eyes, as reported by La Hood et al (72), is assumed. Mean overnight edema levels substantially lower than this have since been reported in non–lens-wearing eyes (95). Clearly the definition of "normal" overnight edema levels will strongly influence the derived critical Dk/t to avoid lens-induced edema during overnight lens wear.

At the same time, Harvitt and Bonanno (96) have determined that corneal acidosis increases corneal oxygen consumption. They incorporated this novel finding into a recalculation of the distribution of oxygen through the corneal tissues during hypoxia (97) (Fig. 34.6) using a refinement of Fatt's early model (98). Interestingly, they derived a criti-

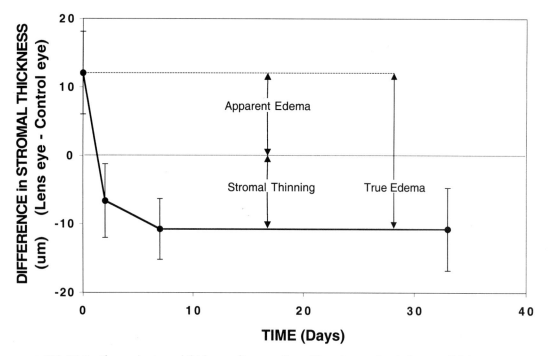

FIG. 34.5. Change in stromal thickness after cessation of long-term extended wear of high-water content hydrogel contact lenses. Data on day 0 were obtained immediately following lens removal. The apparent edema, stromal thinning, and true edema are indicated. (Adapted from Holden BA, Sweeney DF, Vannas A, et al. Effects of lens-term extended contact lens wear on the human cornea. *Invest Ophthalmol Vis Sci* 1985;26:1489, with permission. © Association for Research in Vision and Ophthalmology.)

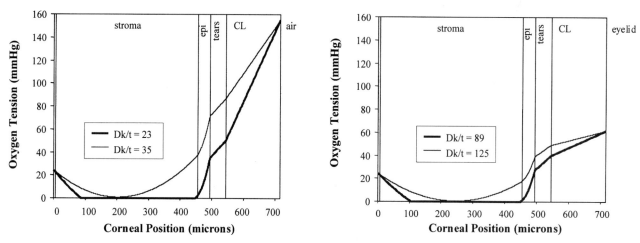

FIG. 34.6. Model predictions of the distribution of oxygen across the cornea and contact lens for the human eye, accounting for the effect of pH on oxygen consumption. **(A)** For the open eye, Dk/t values of 23 and 35 allow the oxygen tension to remain above zero at the stroma–epithelial boundary and throughout the cornea, respectively. **(B)** For the closed eye, Dk/t values of 89 and 125 are necessary. (From Harvitt DM, Bonanno JA. Re-evaluation of the oxygen diffusion model for predicting minimum contact lens Dk/t values needed to avoid corneal anoxia. *Optom Vis Sci* 1999;76:712, with permission. © American Academy of Optometry.)

cal lens Dk/t to avoid anoxia at the basal epithelium of 89 $\times 10^{-9}$ (cm.mL O_2)/(s.mL.mm Hg), reflecting the earlier Holden-Mertz criterion. To avoid anoxia in the mid-stroma, however, the critical Dk/t was 125×10^{-9} (cm.mL O_2)/(s.mL.mm Hg). The physiological impact of midstromal hypoxia is poorly understood, and its clinical effects are likely to be subtle relative to the effects of epithelial hypoxia. The significance of the coincidental agreement with Sweeney's recalculated critical Dk/t is also unclear.

From a clinical viewpoint, it is important to remember that theoretical critical Dk/t determinations represent average values and do not reflect the large individual variation in corneal oxygen requirements. Furthermore, because a standard lens thickness profile (typically −3.00 D) is assumed in calculations of critical lens material Dk, higher-Dk materials than predicted may be required to provide adequate oxygen beneath lenses of greater overall or regional thickness, such as hyperopic, toric, and bifocal lenses (99).

Although refinement of theory is important in furthering our understanding, clinical evidence is also relevant in defining minimum corneal oxygen requirements. Clinical reports to date indicate that signs of corneal hypoxia, such as edema, striae, and microcysts, are significantly reduced or absent with current silicone hydrogel extended wear, using lenses with nominal Dk/t (at −3.00 D) of 110 (PureVision, Bausch & Lomb) and 175 (Focus Night & Day, Ciba Vision) (1–5). This reflects earlier clinical results with high Dk/t GP extended wear (7,8). Although overnight edema levels, measured immediately on eye opening, may be marginally higher than non–lens-wearing levels (1,95), recovery from this slight edema is swift and clinical signs of edema are rarely observed.

In summary, it is apparent that the corneal epithelium is extremely sensitive to reduced oxygen availability. Recovery from short-term hypoxia, as occurs during normal sleep, is rapid. However, chronic hypoxic stress, as occurs during daily wear with low-Dk/t lenses and hydrogel lens extended wear, induces long-term changes that exhibit slow recovery once normal oxygen levels are restored. Clinical reports indicate that currently available high-Dk/t silicone hydrogel and GP lenses minimize acute and chronic hypoxic effects and thus can be considered to meet the corneal oxygen requirements of the majority of patients during extended wear.

CORNEAL ACIDOSIS

Carbon Dioxide Efflux and Accumulation

In the normal open-eye situation, a carbon dioxide gradient exists through the corneal tissue from the aqueous fluid, where carbon dioxide tension is approximately 40 mm Hg (100) to the atmosphere where carbon dioxide partial pressure is close to zero (98). In addition to this passive outward flux from the interior of the eye, carbon dioxide produced as a by-product of corneal metabolism also leaves the cornea

across the epithelium. When the eye is closed, carbon dioxide efflux is impeded, although efflux into the palpebral conjunctival vessels and the aqueous may occur (98). The resultant increase in carbon dioxide concentration in the cornea during normal sleep has received little attention, and it was assumed until recently that the associated decrease in corneal stromal pH was of little significance.

For many years it was also assumed that carbon dioxide efflux from the cornea is not significantly attenuated during contact lens wear. This belief was based on the supposedly high carbon dioxide transmission properties of hydrogel lenses (101). However, in 1987 Holden and co-workers (102) reported a significant increase in carbon dioxide partial pressure at the anterior corneal surface after only 10 minutes wear of hydrogel lenses with a center thickness as thin as 0.035 mm. A similar buildup of carbon dioxide at the anterior corneal surface was demonstrated after short periods of eye closure. Accumulation of carbon dioxide at the anterior corneal surface has since been confirmed for both hydrogel and GP lens wear, and has been shown to be related to the lens Dk/t (103).

Increased concentration of carbon dioxide within the corneal tissue would be expected to be associated with a decrease in corneal pH, because of the formation of carbonic acid. Bonanno and Polse (70,104) have demonstrated such a pH shift in the stroma soon after the insertion of contact lenses (Fig. 34.7), and with eye closure. Their studies implicate both carbon dioxide and lactate accumulation as contributing causative factors. Giasson and Bonanno (105,106) have since measured epithelial and endothelial acidosis with contact lens wear in rabbits. Thus, it is now apparent that contact lens wear can induce acidosis of all corneal layers for the period that the lens is worn. Extended contact lens wear, in particular, provides no opportunity for the cornea to recover from this acidic shift within the tissue, leading to chronic corneal acidosis.

Effects of Corneal Acidosis

In vitro studies have demonstrated that the corneal epithelium and endothelium are both sensitive to acute changes in ambient pH. With decreasing pH, epithelial chloride transport is inhibited (107) and endothelial sodium flux, fluid transport, and transendothelial potential are also reduced (108,109). Gonnering and associates (110) have demonstrated gross morphologic changes in endothelium on exposure to relatively large shifts in pH. Acidosis also increases corneal oxygen consumption (96). This effect may represent activation of cellular pH regulatory mechanisms such as Na^+/H^+ exchange, which in turn increases ATP utilization (96).

Although corneal acidosis does not affect the resting thickness of the cornea (92), the corneal edema response to hypoxia is reduced (111). Interestingly, recovery from induced edema is also slower in an acidic environment

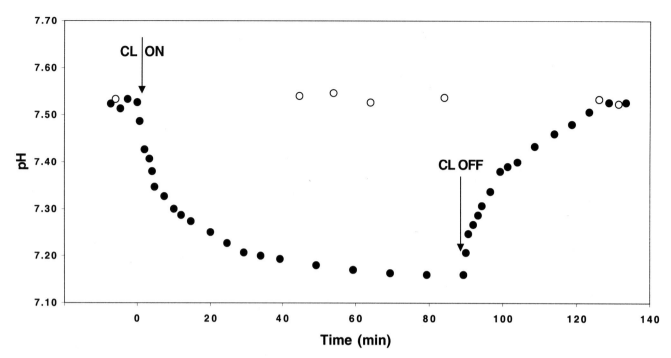

FIG. 34.7. Effect of contact lens wear on human in vivo stromal pH. A thick (0.4 mm) low-water-content (38%) hydrogel lens was placed on the cornea and the stromal pH determined by measuring the fluorescence intensity ratio from excitation of stromal fluorescein at 490 and 450 nm. Arrows indicate lens on and lens off. Filled circles, lens-wearing eye; open circles: non–lens-wearing eye. (Redrawn from Bonanno JA, Polse KA. Corneal acidosis during contact lens wear: effects of hypoxia and CO_2. *Invest Ophthalmol Vis Sci* 28: 1514, 1987, with permission. © Association for Research in Vision and Ophthalmology.)

(112), implicating endothelial acidosis as a possible factor. The endothelial bleb response, observed soon after insertion of a contact lens, is also thought to be caused by endothelial acidosis. Holden and co-workers (83) found that a bleb response could be induced not only by reducing available oxygen, but also by exposing the cornea to a gaseous mixture containing increased levels of carbon dioxide mixed with normal atmospheric levels of oxygen. They concluded that pH shifts in the vicinity of the endothelium caused by increased stromal lactate or carbonate concentration were responsible for this characteristic transient endothelial response.

The demonstrated sensitivity of the endothelium to changes in pH has promoted speculation that more long-term endothelial changes associated with extended lens wear may represent a response to chronic corneal acidosis rather than hypoxia, as had been generally believed. Schoessler and Woloschak (113) first reported increased endothelial polymegethism (variation in cell size) and pleomorphism (variation in cell shape) (Fig. 34.4C) after long-term PMMA lens wear; this finding has since been confirmed by many investigators in association with both daily (114,115) and extended hydrogel lens wear (43,116). Silicone elastomer (117) and silicone hydrogel lenses (5), with their high oxygen transmissibility, do not appear to induce these long-term changes; however, these lenses also readily transmit carbon dioxide, and would thus be unlikely to cause significant pH shifts in the tissue. Endothelial polymegethous changes may be measurable 2 or 3 months after commencing daily wear of low-Dk/t lenses (118), but as soon as 2 to 4 weeks after initiating extended hydrogel lens wear (84).

It is interesting to note that endothelial polymegethism has also been demonstrated to increase gradually with age (119). Schoessler and Orsborn (120) have reported significantly increased endothelial polymegethism in one eye of a patient with long-standing unilateral ptosis. It is tempting to speculate, therefore, that endothelial changes with aging are induced by corneal acidosis associated with repeated eye closure during sleep.

The relationship between the transient bleb response and more long-term changes in endothelial cell size and shape is not clear. The endothelial bleb response is thought to represent localized cell edema, which disrupts the specular reflex from the endothelium (121). The nature of endothelial polymegethous changes is less clear. Bergmanson (122) suggests that polymegethism may represent a change in the alignment of cell walls without a change in cellular volume. However, it is difficult to reconcile this with the clusters of small cells observed in high levels of polymegethism (123). An overall reduction in endothelial cell density with increased polymegethism has not been demonstrated (43,113, 124), suggesting that cell loss is an unlikely explanation for the observed changes in cell morphology. However, some long-term contact lens wearers show a tendency toward reduced endothelial cell density (115,125), suggesting that severe polymegethism and pleomorphism may precede cell loss in susceptible individuals. Further work to clarify our understanding of this phenomenon is clearly needed.

Recovery from Chronic Corneal Acidosis

On cessation of extended lens wear, carbon dioxide gradients across the cornea rapidly return to normal. Bonanno and Polse (70) have demonstrated a return to normal pH in the corneal tissue within approximately 40 minutes after short-term contact lens wear. It is reasonable to assume that even after long-term lens wear, normal corneal pH would be restored quite rapidly following lens removal, and acute changes in cellular function would recover.

The presumed effects of chronic contact lens–induced corneal acidosis do not show such rapid recovery. Indeed, the weight of evidence suggests that endothelial changes associated with long-term contact lens wear are irreversible, even after many years of no lens wear (115,124). Although the apparent permanent nature of these lens-induced changes is cause for concern, there are conflicting views whether endothelial polymegethism is associated with clinically significant compromise of endothelial function.

Evidence has been presented suggesting that patients with high degrees of contact lens–induced polymegethism may show slower recovery from corneal edema, suggesting reduced endothelial pump function (125,126). Increased endothelial permeability has also been reported in long-term contact lens wearers (127,128). However, a clear causal link between changes in endothelial morphology and these functional deficits has yet to be established. Perhaps the best direct evidence comes from Sweeney (129), who has described a corneal exhaustion syndrome in long-term contact lens wearers demonstrating intolerance to continued lens wear; these patients typically exhibit high degrees of endothelial polymegethism.

Rao and associates (130) have reported that patients who show high levels of preoperative polymegethism are more likely to experience complications after intraocular lens implantation. This suggests that endothelial morphologic changes may compromise the functional reserve of the endothelium, making it more susceptible to the added stress of surgery. However, others have not been able to confirm this observation (131). The functional significance of lens-induced endothelial polymegethism may thus not be clear for many years, until the responses of long-term contact lens wearers to stresses such as ocular surgery can be assessed.

EYELID ACTION

Role of Normal Eyelid Action

The anterior surface of the cornea is covered with a complex tear fluid layer that maintains the integrity of the epithelium and provides a smooth primary optical surface for the ocular refractive system. The integrity of this fluid layer is maintained primarily by eyelid action. Blinking serves to remove debris and contaminants from the corneal surface, and acts to resurface the epithelium with mucin and respread the aqueous and lipid layers smoothly over this hydrophilic base.

The presence of the tear film is vital for maintenance of epithelial integrity. Localized disruption of the tear film rapidly leads to damage and/or death of superficial epithelial cells and associated fluorescein staining. If sustained, disruption of the tear film can result in dellen formation caused by thinning of the epithelial layer (132), increasing the risk of opportunistic corneal infection. In addition, the tear layer supplies some of the essential corneal metabolites necessary for cell growth and repair (133,134). Also of considerable importance is the presence of antibacterial agents in the tears, such as lysozyme, lactoferrin, lipocalin, and beta lysin, which provide a significant primary defense against invading pathogens (135).

The normal eyelid action plays an important role in spreading aqueous and lipid in a smooth film over the cornea, as well as removing foreign material and cellular wastes from the anterior corneal surface. Blinking spreads mucin produced in the conjunctival goblet cells over the corneal surface. The corneal and conjunctival epithelial cells also secrete mucin from intracellular vesicles (136,137), forming the glycoprotein-rich glycocalyx that covers the anterior surface of the epithelium (138,139). The glycocalyx acts as a hydrophilic base that potentiates the even spread of the aqueous and mucous tear layers over the essentially hydrophobic epithelial cells (140). The glycocalyx and associated mucin are rich in receptors that bind bacteria, preventing their passage to the epithelial cells (67,141). In addition, because of its intensely hydrophilic nature, mucin traps lipids, phospholipid-rich cell debris, and other foreign material in the tear layer, in the process of which it rapidly becomes more viscid and hydrophobic in nature (142). This contaminated mucus conglomerates and rolls into strands under the influence of the shear imparted by eyelid action, and is gradually pushed to the lower fornix to form a mucous thread, which is expelled, together with the contaminating material, at the inner canthus (143,144).

The shear force exerted on the corneal epithelium by blink action is also thought to play a role in epithelial cell shedding or exfoliation. Increasing shear forces increase the rate of cell shedding (145,146), while damping of shear forces, such as occurs during contact lens wear, reduces the exfoliation rate (45,52). It has been suggested that epithelial surface cell shedding represents a form of apoptosis or programmed cell death, which is dependent on shear forces for its activation and maintenance (146).

The nature of the tear film is dramatically altered when the eye is closed during sleep. There is evidence to suggest that the closed eye is a relatively dry eye (147), primarily because of reduced aqueous tear production. The reasons for this are unclear; it has been suggested that open-eye tear production is essentially reflex in nature (148), stimulated by subtle environmental stimuli that are absent to a large extent during eye closure (149).

When the eyes are closed, the lipid layer is compressed between the lid margins (142); thus the closed eye tear film consists primarily of aqueous and mucous components. Evaporation from the tear film, which in the open eye is inhibited by the presence of the oily lipid layer (150), is absent during eye closure, resulting in a decrease in tear tonicity (151). Tear pH also decreases slightly (152) because of the inhibition of carbon dioxide efflux from the anterior corneal surface (104). In addition, there is a slight increase in temperature under the closed lid, from approximately 34°C to 36°C (153). The effects of these environmental changes on corneal physiology are minor compared to the effects of reduced oxygen availability, but they may contribute to the slight (3% to 4%) overnight corneal swelling response (72,94).

The absence of eyelid action during sleep results in an accumulation of cell debris and contaminated mucus in the closed eye tear film, and a dramatic increase in the number of inflammatory cells (154,155). There is also an increase in the levels of normal ocular microbiota, which can readily proliferate in the warm undisturbed closed-eye environment (156). Immediately on eye opening a surge in aqueous tear production, together with renewed eyelid action, rapidly flushes these accumulated contaminants from the eye. The initiation of blinking also resurfaces the cornea with fresh mucin, allowing the re-formation of a stable tear film.

Role of Lens Movement

The presence of a contact lens on the eye disrupts the complex structure of the tear film, and inhibits normal tear spreading and circulation. Furthermore, the action of the eyelid is dampened, reducing the spreading of mucin over the ocular surface, and the rate of removal of debris and contaminants. These effects are compensated for, to some extent, by lens movement, which pumps tears under the lens and thus allows tear circulation to areas of the cornea covered by the lens. The efficiency of the lid-activated tear pump is dependent on lens type. Rigid lenses generally allow tear exchange of 10% to 20% with each blink, dependent to a large extent on lens design and fitting characteristics (157). However, the hydrogel lens tear pump is considerably less efficient, with a tear exchange per blink of as low as 1% (158,159). This is because of the flexible nature of these lenses and their large diameter, which result in much reduced lens movement compared to rigid lenses.

Maintenance of lens movement during open-eye lens wear is important for several reasons. First, circulation of oxygenated tears behind the lens helps to maintain normal epithelial metabolism, particularly if insufficient oxygen is transmitted through the lens material to adequately meet epithelial oxygen needs. The role of tear circulation in the provision of tear-borne metabolites is also probably significant, although smaller ions can probably diffuse through a soft contact lens to reach the epithelial surface (160). Lens movement also physically aids the removal of exfoliated epithelial cells, contaminated mucus and debris from behind the lenses, partially compensating for the loss of normal shear action of the eyelid during blinking.

During rigid lens wear in particular, even tear spreading across the corneal surface may be disrupted at the lens edge by meniscus formation, which can draw tears from areas adjacent to the lens edge, resulting in localized tear thinning and break-up (138,161). Furthermore, a bridging effect at the lens edge may inhibit the ability of the lid to spread mucin over the corneal surface at this point (162,163). Adequate lens movement partially compensates for this localized drying, by allowing continual rewetting of these areas.

Lens movement during closed-eye lens wear is believed to be minimal, although some movement of the lenses across the corneal surface may occur during the rapid eye movement phase of sleep (164). Because tear circulation is minimal during eye closure when lenses are not worn, the lack of lens movement during closed-eye lens wear is probably of little significance in terms of further inhibition of tear circulation. However, because the lens is relatively immobile, significant localized lens pressure against the cornea may develop.

Tear circulation resumes and debris and contaminants are removed from behind the lens once lens movement is initiated by eye opening and subsequent eyelid action. However, on eye opening, both hydrogel and GP lenses may be adherent to the cornea (165–168), with consequent stasis of the tear film between lens and cornea. The mechanism for this adherence is believed to be thinning of the post–lens tear film as a result of eyelid pressure during sleep, potentiated by the reduced tear production and consequent dry closed eye (166,169). The consequences of persistent lens adherence will be discussed below.

Effects of Inadequate Lens Movement

Inadequate lens movement reduces the circulation of oxygenated tears behind the lens. If oxygen transmission through the lens is insufficient to supply corneal oxygen needs, epithelial metabolism is affected, with consequences such as those discussed in detail earlier. This is of particular significance immediately on eye opening after overnight wear of lenses. Rigid lenses rapidly resupply the epithelium with oxygen because of their efficient tear pumping mechanism, allowing rapid and more complete recovery from overnight corneal edema (Fig. 34.8). Thus, with rigid lenses, up to 10% overnight edema can be eliminated during daytime lens wear (74,75), as compared to an average of 8% edema with hydrogel lenses (73). Furthermore, corneal cov-

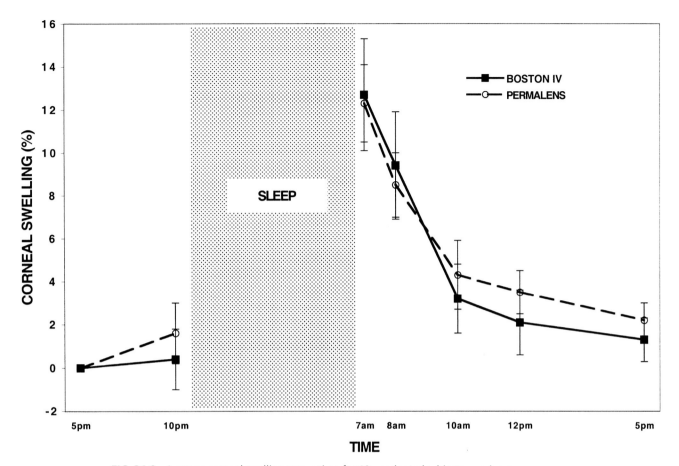

FIG. 34.8. Average corneal swelling versus time for 10 unadapted subjects wearing a gas-permeable lens (Boston IV) in one eye and a soft lens (Permalens) in the other eye over a 24-hour wake/sleep cycle. (Redrawn from Holden BA, Sweeney DF, La Hood D, Kenyon E. Corneal deswelling following overnight wear of rigid and hydrogel contact lenses. *Curr Eye Res* 1988;7:49, with permission.)

erage is less with GP lenses. Consequently, extended wear of rigid lenses induces less overall hypoxic stress than extended wear of soft lenses with equivalent oxygen transmission characteristics.

While the contribution of lens movement in providing oxygen to the cornea immediately on eye opening is certainly significant with low-Dk/t lenses, the role of tear circulation in supplementing oxygen supply has become less critical with the development of high-Dk GP and silicone hydrogel lens materials, which transmit considerably more oxygen by diffusion through the lens material. However, inadequate lens movement still can have marked effects on the cornea, particularly if lens movement is not initiated soon after eye opening.

Lens adherence or binding after overnight lens wear is a relatively common occurrence during GP extended wear, with an overall incidence of 40% to 50% (168). Although most adherent lenses show spontaneous lens movement within a few minutes after eye opening, lenses may remain adherent for many hours (166). While the lens is adherent, tear circulation behind the lens is absent, and debris and

contaminated mucus remain trapped in the stagnant post–lens tear pool (Fig. 34.9) (166). Transient lens adherence is also frequently noted immediately on eye opening following overnight hydrogel lens wear (167,169). Because hydrogel lenses may tighten during overnight wear, lens movement may remain inadequate for some time after eye opening, resulting in prolonged entrapment of contaminants between lens and cornea.

Debris retained in the post–lens tear film may give rise to corneal epithelial compromise and staining with fluorescein (170). Silicone hydrogel lens wear, in particular, precipitates a particular type of post–lens tear film debris, termed "mucin balls," (1,3,171), previously known as lipid plugs in association with rigid and hydrogel lens wear (172). It is thought that the relatively high incidence of mucin balls with silicone hydrogel lenses relates to the greater stiffness of these materials (173), or to factors associated with the lens surface treatment (1) that induce the ocular mucins, in combination with tear proteins and lipid, to roll up into spherical bodies under the shear force of lens movement (1, 3,174). These remain trapped behind the lens, indenting

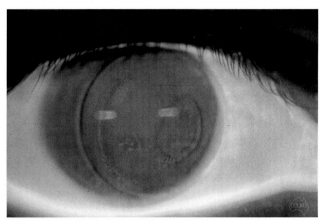

FIG. 34.10. Disruption of the mucus layer immediately following removal of an adherent gas-permeable lens. (From Swarbrick HA. A possible etiology for RGP lens binding (adherence). *Int Contact Lens Clin* 1988;15:13, with permission.)

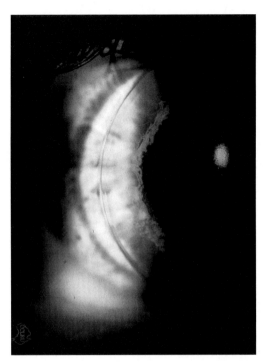

FIG. 34.9. Tear film debris and mucus trapped behind the midperiphery of an adherent gas-permeable lens. (Photograph by Robert Terry.)

the epithelium (175). After lens removal, the transient indentations pool fluorescein, giving rise to an appearance similar to fine dimple veiling. Mucin balls cause few symptoms and appear to be of little clinical consequence (1,3, 174).

Zantos and Holden (176) have suggested that toxins released by the breakdown of contaminants trapped between the lens and cornea provide the stimulus for the contact lens–induced acute red eye (CLARE) reaction, also known as the tight lens syndrome and nonulcerative keratitis. The recovery of large numbers of inflammatory cells, together with mucus and epithelial cell debris, from the post–lens tear pool of a CLARE patient supports this view (177). If the patient has not removed the lens, lens movement is often minimal or absent, with flakes of debris trapped between lens and cornea. On lens removal, epithelial staining corresponding to the pattern of trapped debris may be noted. The inflammatory nature of the response is further reinforced by the typical presence of infiltrates, which represent the invasion of polymorphonuclear (PMN) leukocytes into the cornea from the limbal blood vasculature (178).

The incidence of CLARE reactions is significantly higher with soft, compared to GP, extended wear (179). Several factors may account for this, in addition to the lower average rate of tear exchange and debris removal with hydrogel lenses. The greater propensity for these lenses to attract and bind deposits and to absorb and retain chemicals from lens care solutions probably contributes to the higher incidence of inflammatory reactions. It is interesting to speculate on

reasons for the surprisingly low incidence of CLARE reactions with adherent GP lenses (180), given the relatively high incidence of this phenomenon. Presumably, the lower propensity for lens spoliation provides a partial explanation. However, GP lens adherence rarely persists throughout the day, allowing the release of entrapped contaminants in most cases before eye closure the following night.

During lens wear, the sweeping action of the eyelid over the corneal surface is inhibited because of the presence of the lens, and consequently the epithelium under the lens is not resurfaced with fresh mucin from the conjunctival goblet cells. During extended wear, this resurfacing is absent for a considerable period; in particular, hydrogel lenses prevent resurfacing of any portion of the cornea because of their large diameter. Following lens removal, poor corneal wetting and transient disruption of the mucus layer are often observed, particularly if the lens has been immobile or adherent (166,181) as shown in Fig. 34.10. It is possible that the nonrenewal of this important protective layer of the tear film, together with the dampened sweeping action of the eyelid, may compromise the barrier preventing adherence and invasion of the cornea by pathogenic microorganisms. Chemical removal of the mucus layer dramatically increases adherence of microorganisms, in particular *P aeruginosa*, to the cornea (182), and contact lens wear appears to thin the mucin-rich glycocalyx, resulting in closer association between bacterial receptors and the superficial epithelial cell membrane (141). Further work is clearly needed to determine the relative significance of hypoxia, disruption of epithelial defenses such as mucin, and other factors in the pathogenesis of contact lens–related corneal infections.

PRESSURE

During normal blinking, the eyelid moves over the cornea with the eyelid margin held against the corneal surface because of tension in the orbicularis oculi muscle. The pressure applied against the cornea during blinking varies depending on the force and completeness of the blink, and reaches between 1 g_f and 5 g_f for a normal complete blink (183). Doane (184) and Lydon and Tait (183) have demonstrated that this force is dampened to some extent by movement of the globe into the orbit.

Similar eyelid pressures are exerted with eye closure during sleep. When a lens is present on the eye during sleep, pressure exerted on the cornea may be increased slightly compared to the non–lens-wearing situation, but this is unlikely to have significant consequences as long as the pressure is evenly distributed. However, if there are localized areas of pressure, particularly if the lens is immobile and the pressure persistent, the epithelium can show marked localized thinning and cell movement away from the pressure point (185,186). This is observed most dramatically in the corneal indentation accompanying GP lens adherence, where the edge of the immobile lens applies considerable localized pressure against the cornea (Fig. 34.11) (166). The rapid recovery of the corneal epithelium, once lens mobility resumes, provides an insight into the remarkable recuperative powers of the epithelium (167,168).

More subtle changes in corneal shape associated with uneven pressure distribution have been found following long-term GP lens extended wear. Sphericalization of mild-to-moderate toric corneas fitted with spherical lenses, and slight overall flattening of corneal curvature suggest corneal molding towards the back surface shape of the contact lens (187,188). The oxygen transmissibility of the lens also appears to influence the extent of corneal distortion, with lenses of higher Dk/t tending to induce less marked corneal molding (79).

The effects of rigid lenses on corneal shape are deliberately exploited in the technique of orthokeratology. Reverse-geometry lenses, designed purposefully to apply pressure to the central cornea, induce rapid central corneal flattening (189) and thus reduce the manifest myopic refractive error (190–192). This is achieved by epithelial thinning rather than overall corneal bending (193,194), although the exact mechanisms are yet to be elucidated. Interestingly, these reverse-geometry lenses, which create a midperipheral annulus of post–lens tear pooling due to their steeper secondary curve, induce midperipheral corneal steepening and stromal thickening (193,194). It is thought that this may arise due to negative pressures generated in the midperipheral tear film reservoir. Although orthokeratology lenses are increasingly worn in an overnight modality, the potential role of corneal edema in modulating the corneal shape change is not yet understood (195). Overnight orthokeratology lenses are removed on awakening, with no lens wear during the day, thus minimizing many of the other effects and risks of extended wear.

Because of the flexible nature of hydrogel lenses, there is less opportunity for significant localized areas of pressure to develop. Consequently, regular and irregular corneal distortion and molding are less marked with these lenses, although both corneal steepening (196–198) and flattening (198) have been reported with hydrogel lens wear. Most typically there is a slight myopic shift in refraction accompanying mild corneal steepening, implicating hypoxia-induced central corneal edema rather than pressure as the primary factor. Although the absence of such changes with silicone hydrogel lenses (1,3,199) and the slight myopic regression and corneal flattening noted when patients move from hydrogel to silicone hydrogel lens wear (1) support this hypothesis, the stiffer nature of the silicone hydrogel material may also play a role (199).

Superior epithelial arcuate lesions (SEALs) have been reported with hydrogel lenses (200–202), but are more frequent with silicone hydrogel extended wear (202). This condition is thought to be induced by abrasive shear force applied by the back surface of the lens against the peripheral corneal epithelium, and can be attributed to a combination of factors including lens design, rigidity and surface characteristics, and individual variables including peripheral corneal topography and tear film properties (202). Lens-related factors, including material stiffness and surface treatment (173), may thus explain the higher incidence of SEALs with silicone hydrogel lenses.

Conjunctival staining and indentation, as shown in Fig. 34.12, may occur if a tightly fit soft lens edge applies significant pressure against the conjunctival surface (203), particularly during eye closure when lens movement is minimal and the pressure persistent. This type of conjunctival staining has also been reported with prototype designs of the

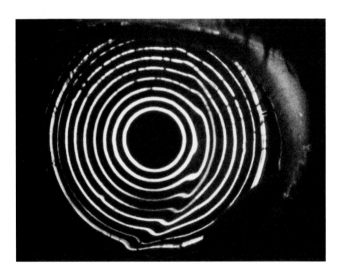

FIG. 34.11. Photokeratoscopic image showing corneal distortion associated with corneal indentation induced by the edge of an adherent gas-permeable lens. Complete recovery is usually noted within 4 hours after lens removal. (From Swarbrick HA, Holden BA. Rigid gas permeable lens binding: significance and contributing factors. *Am J Optom Physiol Opt* 1987;64:815, with permission. © American Academy of Optometry.)

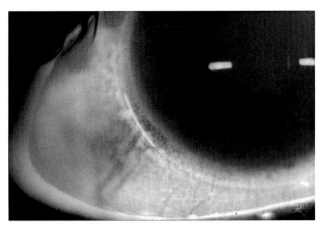

FIG. 34.12. Conjunctival indentation induced by a tight hydrogel lens worn overnight. (Photograph by Timothy Grant.)

stiffer silicone hydrogel lenses (5). Changes in soft lens parameters in response to the modified environment under the closed lid may exacerbate this problem.

In summary, contact lens wear can cause corneal changes due to localized or generalized pressure exerted against the epithelium. Localized pressures induce local effects (e.g., lens edge indentation, SEALs), whereas more generalized or regional pressures (e.g., in orthokeratology) can induce overall corneal shape changes. Lens rigidity plays a major role in determining the severity of such changes. GP lenses are more likely to induce changes in corneal shape than soft lenses, and the stiffer silicone hydrogel lenses appear to induce more frequent pressure-related effects than hydrogel lenses. In extended lens wear the lenses are immobile in a dry environment during sleep, allowing more persistent pressures to develop and inducing more rapid and severe changes in corneal shape.

INFLAMMATION

Inflammation represents a tissue's response to challenge by a stimulus that is recognized as threatening to the integrity of the tissue. The response of the tissue is aimed at interrupting, neutralizing and eliminating the inflammatory stimulus and effecting repair to damaged tissue. Typically, the inflammatory response follows a pattern of vasodilation, increased permeability of the vasculature, and the release of immunogenic mediators, antibodies, and inflammatory cells into the extravascular spaces, and is characterized by hyperemia, edema, heat and pain.

In the non–lens-wearing eye, anterior segment inflammation may be triggered by a number of stimuli of exogenous or endogenous origin, including physical and toxic trauma, invasion by pathogens, and allergenic stimuli that may precipitate a hypersensitivity reaction. The presence of a contact lens on the eye provides many subtle and unique stimuli that increase the potential for triggering an inflammatory response. Such responses during extended wear tend to be more frequent and severe than during daily wear because of the chronic presence of the stimulus, and also because the tissue may be compromised by the physiologic stresses imposed by extended wear. An inflammatory response may be triggered directly during contact lens wear by a complex diversity of stimuli, including mechanical trauma, chemicals leaching from the lens, deposits on the lens surface, debris trapped behind the lens, and the presence of bacteria contaminating the lens. Repeated or continual contact with chemicals or lens deposits, for example, may induce an immediate or delayed hypersensitivity reaction, whereas debris trapped behind a lens may induce an acute inflammatory episode particularly when the lens is worn during sleep. The level of response may vary from mild conjunctival and limbal hyperemia to marked corneal infiltration, neovascularization, and stromal scarring. Individual susceptibility, particularly in terms of the general state of health, is also an important factor influencing both the occurrence and severity of the inflammatory response.

Several inflammatory mediators have been found in the tear fluid in the quiet eye and during inflammatory episodes, including immunoglobulins sIgA and IgG (135), plasmin (204), complement proteins (205), vitronectin (206), histamine (207), cytokines such as interleukins IL-6 and IL-8 (208), and arachidonic acid metabolites such as leukotriene LTB_4 (208). The roles and interplay of these substances in regulating and modulating the inflammatory response are complex. While some of these mediators are present normally in tear fluid, others are recruited only after the occurrence of injury or immunogenic challenge (135,209). Some (e.g., sIgA, IL-8) are produced locally by lacrimal gland, corneal, or other tissues, whereas others (e.g., vitronectin, complement proteins) are derived from serum and reach the cornea and tear film from engorged and leaky limbal and conjunctival blood vessels. Many of these mediators act to recruit PMN leukocytes into the tear film to aid in ocular defense (135).

The concentration of many of these inflammatory substances in the tear film varies on a diurnal cycle (155). During eye closure, the tear film becomes stagnant due to the absence of normal reflex tear production from the lacrimal gland (210). The concentrations of sIgA and albumin increase dramatically (210) (Fig. 34.13), complement (210) and plasminogen (204) are activated, and PMN cells invade the tear film in large numbers (154,155). Other inflammatory mediators such as histamine, vitronectin, IL-8, and LTB_4 are also found in increased concentrations in the closed eye (206,208). Together, these changes in tear film composition during eye closure suggest that the closed eye is in a state of subclinical inflammation (210). This may represent a protective mechanism to combat the threat posed by bacterial proliferation in the closed-eye environment, but may also render the closed eye susceptible to acute

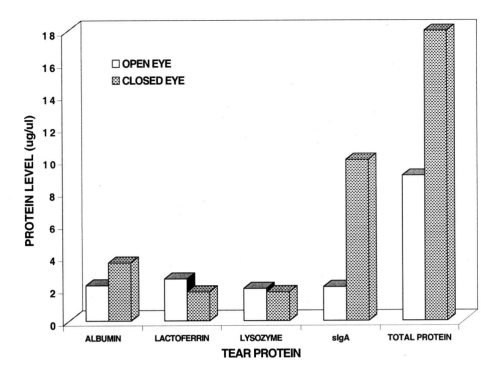

FIG. 34.13. Differences in protein composition of the open-eye and closed-eye tear fluid. Together with increased plasmin activity, conversion of complement C3 to C3c, and the presence of large numbers of polymorphonuclear cells in the closed-eye tear film, these changes suggest that the closed eye may be in a state of subclinical inflammation. Albumin includes prealbumin; the levels of albumin are negligible in the open eye but comprise the dominant portion in the closed eye. (Data from Sack RA, Tan KO, Tan A. Diurnal tear cycle: evidence for a nocturnal inflammatory constitutive tear fluid. *Invest Ophthalmol Vis Sci* 1992;33:626.)

inflammatory responses in the presence of inflammatory stimuli.

The effects of contact lens wear on this normal pattern of diurnal variation are subtle. Although the concentrations of the major tear proteins such as lysozyme and lactoferrin appear to be unaffected by lens wear (211), there is a slight decrease in the concentration of sIgA with both hydrogel and silicone hydrogel lens wear (135,212,213). The concentration of IL-8, which normally acts to recruit PMN cells, also increases in contact lens wearers (208) and increased numbers of PMN cells are found in the tear film of novice lens wearers, although there appears to be a downregulation of PMN cell recruitment in long-term wearers (214). Interestingly, Langerhans cells, which normally reside in the limbal region, may be recruited into the cornea during lens wear (215), suggesting that the lens-wearing cornea may become more susceptible to inflammatory responses as a result.

During eye closure, there is a slight increase in limbal and bulbar hyperemia that resolves rapidly on eye opening. Contact lens wear may also stimulate increased ocular hyperemia, particularly during adaptation, in response to the "foreign body" effect of the lens. During long-term hydrogel extended wear, the chronic presence of the lens can also stimulate chronic conjunctival and limbal hyperemia, and increased limbal vessel penetration into the cornea (216). This chronic hyperemia has been thought to represent a low-grade inflammatory response to the presence of the foreign body, exacerbated by pressure exerted on the limbal vessels by the lens edge. Recent work by Papas (217, 218), however, has provided strong evidence that contact

lens–induced limbal hyperemia may represent a response to hypoxia rather than an inflammatory response. Significantly reduced levels of limbal hyperemia have been reported with silicone hydrogel compared to hydrogel lenses (1,217–219).

There is little doubt that the presence of infiltrates in the cornea represents an inflammatory response (178,220). Corneal infiltrates comprise PMN cells invading the cornea from the limbal blood vessels, and possibly the tears, in response to inflammatory stimulation (178,221). The severity of this response varies considerably, from subtle, asymptomatic idiopathic infiltrates, which are relatively common even in non–lens-wearers, to rare but severe infiltrative events characterized by marked limbal and conjunctival hyperemia, pain, and widespread infiltration of the epithelium and anterior stroma (201). Such episodes are much more common in contact lens wearers than in the general population, and are more frequent in extended than daily lens wear (222–224).

The CLARE response is an acute inflammatory reaction that appears to be specific to extended lens wear (201), and thus probably represents an overstimulation of the normal subclinical inflammatory status of the closed eye environment, triggered by the introduction of inflammatory stimuli associated with the lens. As discussed earlier, it has been suggested that toxins released by entrapped post–lens tear debris may act as a trigger for this acute response (176,177). There is increasing evidence, however, that lens-associated bacteria are more likely to act as the inflammatory stimulus, through the release of toxins such as lipopolysaccharide, enzymes and other bacterial byproducts (135). Patients exhibiting CLARE responses have been shown to be more

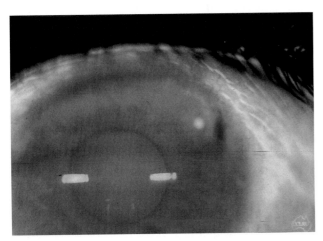

FIG. 34.14. Contact lens-induced peripheral ulcer (CLPU) in a patient using hydrogel extended-wear lenses, showing intense uptake of fluorescein at the site of the lesion. (Photograph by Mee Sing Chong.)

likely to harbor large numbers of gram-negative bacteria on their lenses (225,226), and Holden et al. have reported an unusually high occurrence of CLARE responses after inadvertent lens contamination with gram-negative bacteria (227). Gram-positive bacteria are also implicated in some of these acute inflammatory episodes (135,228). The particular bacterial strain contaminating the lens may also be significant. Distinct strains of *P aeruginosa* have been demonstrated, some of which induce frank infection whereas others are unable to infect the cornea but induce an acute inflammatory response in the mouse model (229). Thus, less virulent inflammatory strains of bacteria may be responsible for the relatively limited nature of the CLARE response in extended lens wearers, compared to the potentially devastating response that can occur in the presence of invasive or cytotoxic bacterial strains.

Contact lens–induced peripheral ulcers (CLPU) are another acute inflammatory response seen predominantly in extended lens wear (201,224) (Fig. 34.14). These small midperipheral ulcers are relatively asymptomatic, and can be distinguished from early microbial keratitis by their characteristic circumscribed appearance, size and location, and the absence of pain, mucopurulent discharge, and anterior chamber reaction (230,231). As with CLARE, bacterial lens contamination has been implicated in this response (135, 232,233). The bacteria do not appear to infect the ulcer; scrapes taken from the ulcer bed have proved to be culture-negative, and histologic examination of the ulcers has shown a classic acute PMN infiltrative response, but with no evidence of the presence of microorganisms (234).

Acute inflammatory responses such as infiltrative keratitis, CLARE and CLPU have been reported to occur in both hydrogel and silicone hydrogel extended lens wear (224). This suggests that these responses are independent of the hypoxic challenge faced by the cornea during closed-eye lens wear, and thus are not exacerbated by hypoxic corneal compromise. Similar levels of bacterial lens contamination have been reported for silicone hydrogel as for hydrogel lenses (235,236), also suggesting that these inflammatory responses are likely to occur with both lens types. Further developments in contact lens technology will clearly be needed to combat these relatively uncommon but clinically significant challenges to ocular health.

During contact lens wear, the palpebral conjunctiva may display a characteristic inflammatory response involving hyperemia, edema, and subsequent papillary hypertrophy if the inflammatory stimulus is chronic. This reaction gives rise to the classic symptoms and signs associated with contact lens–induced papillary conjunctivitis (CLPC) (Fig. 34.15A). Left untreated, the condition can progress to the more florid presentation of giant papillary conjunctivitis

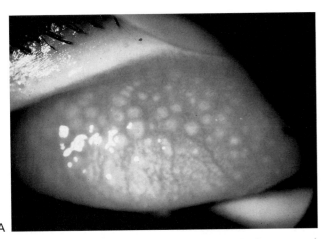
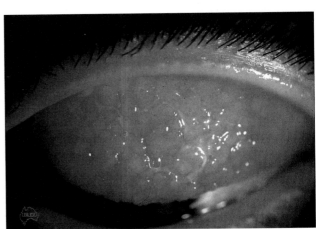

A

B

FIG. 34.15. Papillary changes in the upper palpebral conjunctiva induced by long-term hydrogel lens wear. **(A)** In the early stages, this reaction can be classified as contact lens-induced papillary conjunctivitis (CLPC). **(B)** Continuation of lens wear may lead to the development of giant papillary conjunctivitis (GPC), characterized by more extreme papillary hypertrophy and eventual scarring. (Photographs by Timothy Grant.)

or GPC (Fig. 34.15B); if this occurs, the patient becomes intolerant to continuing lens wear. CLPC has been reported with both rigid and soft lenses worn for daily and extended wear (180,201,237–240), although the incidence appears to be higher, and the time to onset shorter, with soft lenses and with extended lens wear (224).

Allansmith and associates (238), who first described this condition in detail, considered that papillary conjunctivitis represents a cutaneous basophilic hypersensitivity reaction potentiated by antigens produced in response to lens deposits. Others have suggested that an IgE-mediated immediate hypersensitivity response may be involved (240). Histopathologic analysis reveals the presence of mast cells, eosinophils, and basophils in the conjunctival epithelium and substantia propria (241). Because the condition may also be stimulated by chronic low-grade trauma [e.g., from exposed suture ends after anterior segment surgery (242)] or the use of ocular prostheses (243), a mechanical component also has been established (244). It is hypothesized, therefore, that irritation of the palpebral conjunctiva, by contact with the lens edge or surface deposits, allows access of the antigen to the mucous membrane, initiating the hypersensitivity reaction (245). Skotnitsky and colleagues (246) have described a localized form of the condition which may be induced primarily by mechanical factors, as compared to the more widespread presentation which may represent a more classic immunologic response in susceptible individuals. The tendency for silicone hydrogel lenses to attract fewer protein deposits than hydrogel lenses (247) and their greater rigidity (173) might be expected to lead to a higher incidence of the local mechanically induced form of CLPC with these lenses, although further studies are needed.

INFECTION

Corneal infection, or microbial keratitis, is the most serious adverse response associated with contact lens wear. Before 1980, microbial keratitis was rarely seen in otherwise healthy eyes and was typically associated with trauma or corneal surface disease. With the increasing popularity of contact lens wear, the incidence of this complication has increased dramatically in the contact lens–wearing population, and it is now recognized that contact lens wear, and in particular hydrogel lens extended wear, is a significant risk factor in the development of corneal infection. Up to two thirds of cases of microbial keratitis seen in major eye hospitals in the United States and United Kingdom are now contact lens–related (248,249). It has been demonstrated convincingly that, compared with daily wear of rigid or hydrogel lenses, hydrogel extended wear carries a two- to fifteen-fold increase in risk of corneal infection (250–257), and that this risk is exacerbated as the number of consecutive nights of lens wear increases (251,252). Despite these alarming figures, it must be borne in mind that contact lens–rel-

ated microbial keratitis is rare; annualized incidences for hydrogel extended wear of approximately 0.05% to 0.5% have been reported from large-scale studies (224,252,256, 257).

The inflammatory process accompanying corneal infection follows a typical course: hyperemia, tearing, and pain may progress rapidly to corneal infiltration, epithelial edema, and erosion, associated with mucopurulent discharge. In many cases, a uveal response characterized by aqueous flare may be observed, while severe infection may initiate a hypopyon. Corneal vascularization may also be stimulated. Tissue lysis as a result of bacterial activity, and also because of the release of lysosomal enzymes from inflammatory cells, may result in rapid stromal excavation and perforation in extreme cases. When corneal infection involves the stroma, scarring remains after resolution of the infection; if the scarring is located centrally, vision will be reduced and surgical intervention may be required to restore useful vision.

Corneal infection can be initiated by a number of pathogens, many of which are present in the normal conjunctival flora. The pathogens most frequently associated with infections during extended lens wear are gram-negative bacteria, in particular *P aeruginosa* (249,258–260). *P aeruginosa* is an opportunistic organism commonly found in water, sewage, and soil, and is known to contaminate bathroom areas such as basins and toilets. Cytotoxic and invasive strains of this bacterium have been implicated in microbial keratitis (261), whereas less virulent strains are more likely to provoke inflammatory reactions rather than frank corneal infection (229). Although in most cases a break in the epithelium is necessary before bacterial infection (262,263), invasive bacterial strains have been demonstrated to invade intact epithelial cells both *in vitro* and *in vivo* (264,265). Cytotoxic strains, although unable to penetrate the intact epithelial barrier, can nevertheless induce significant epithelial cell damage, thus potentiating the disease process (266). Unfortunately, this virulent pathogen shows a rapid course of infectious process after inoculation, and can have extremely devastating consequences, in the worst case resulting in perforation of the globe and loss of the eye within as little as 24 hours (267).

Extended hydrogel lens wear carries an enhanced risk of serious corneal infection compared to daily hydrogel or rigid lens wear. The reasons for this have been under active investigation over the last decade, and many of the recognized contributing factors have already been discussed in this chapter. Under the chronic hypoxic conditions induced by hydrogel extended wear, the epithelium becomes thinner (43) and more prone to damage (56,60,61), there is a reduction in corneal sensitivity (57), and corneal wound healing slows (64,65). The normal rates of mitosis of basal epithelium (32,33) and exfoliation of surface epithelial cells (52, 53) are reduced and cells retained on the ocular surface are larger, and possibly older, than in non–lens-wearing eyes

(54,55). The chronic presence of the lens on the eye also disrupts the normal eyelid-mediated cleansing processes of the eye. In particular, the integrity of the protective mucus layer is compromised (181) and bacterial receptors normally present to entrap bacteria in the ocular mucus become more closely associated with the epithelial surface (141). Bacteria are able to attach more avidly to epithelial cells following extended wear (66,67), and this effect has been demonstrated to be related to lens Dk/t (52,53,68). With the enhanced oxygen performance of silicone hydrogel lenses, it is hoped that many of these hypoxia-related factors might be eliminated, thus reducing the risks of microbial keratitis in extended wear. The outcomes of large-scale studies and longer real-world experience are awaited to determine if this is so. Some cases of microbial keratitis have already been reported with silicone hydrogel lens extended wear (268, 269), however, emphasizing the complex nature of predisposing factors in the pathogenesis of microbial keratitis.

Although contamination of lens care solutions may provide a source for the infecting organism, the significance of this route is unclear during extended wear when lenses only intermittently undergo lens care, or may be disposed of at the end of the extended wearing period. Patient reports and case studies have implicated patient noncompliance as a contributing factor in individual cases (270,271), but case–control studies have not identified noncompliance with normal lens care as an obligatory risk factor (248,251, 253). Contamination during lens handling is also less likely during extended compared with daily wear, and it has been suggested that, in any case, the normal antimicrobial action of tear components such as lysozyme and lactoferrin may be sufficient to reduce the microbial load introduced by this route (272). Willcox and colleagues (273) have suggested that the water supply may provide a significant source for lens contamination by gram-negative organisms, whereas gram-positive organisms are more likely to gain access to the eye from the surrounding skin and eyelid margins. It is known that the closed-eye environment encourages the proliferation of the normal conjunctival microbiota (156), suggesting that entrapped pathogens may also be able to replicate rapidly in this warm, stagnant, and nutrient-rich environment.

Because extended wear lenses are not removed for cleaning and disinfection as often as during daily wear, pathogens introduced to the eye have an increased opportunity for adhesion and replication on the lens surface. In common with other slime-producing bacteria, *P aeruginosa* is known to elaborate a glycocalyx, which aids in adhesion of the bacteria to the lens surface and protects the proliferating organisms from the host defenses (274,275). In the stagnant post–lens tear film environment that prevails during extended wear, bacteria have a greater chance to develop colonies in this fashion, thus creating a reservoir of pathogens available to invade the compromised cornea.

It has been suggested that lens wear may alter the normal spectrum of commensal bacteria present in the eye, thus allowing growth of pathogenic organisms. Research findings in this area have been conflicting, with some studies showing little effect (276,277), and others reporting significant changes in the spectrum and levels of microbial contamination of external ocular sites, contact lens cases or the contact lens itself with various modalities of lens wear (278,279), and even after cessation of lens wear (280). Large-scale clinical studies indicate an increase in lid and conjunctival microbial colonization with long-term daily wear and an increase in the incidence of pathogenic organisms with extended wear (281), but little change in the incidence of lens contamination over time with either modality (282), a finding recently confirmed with silicone hydrogel lenses (235,236).

Alternatively, it has been suggested that lens wear may alter the subtle balance of antimicrobial tear film constituents, compromising the host defense system and thus potentiating infection. However, despite considerable deposition of tear film components such as lysozyme on contact lens surfaces, the eye seems to be able to maintain the concentrations of these defensive proteins during lens wear, resulting in no significant changes in tear film protein profile, even with extended wear (211,214). Conversely, subtle changes in the concentrations of certain inflammatory mediators, such as IL-6, IL-8, and LTB_4, have been demonstrated after overnight lens wear (283). Differential effects with novice as opposed to adapted lens wearers suggest some alteration in the inflammatory mediator profile in tears over time, but further research is needed to elucidate the time course and clinical significance of such changes.

Several other factors appear to increase the risk of a severe progression of corneal infection during extended wear, including aphakia (284) and diabetes (285,286) (where the cornea is compromised by surgical intervention or an underlying abnormal condition), delay in removing lenses and seeking treatment when symptoms arise (287,288) lens wear in warm climates (289), and the initiation of inappropriate antibiotic (259) or corticosteroid (250) therapy.

CONCLUSION

In this chapter, the physiologic challenges and stresses imposed by contact lens wear, particularly during closed-eye or extended wear, have been discussed and the ocular responses to these challenges have been described. Our increasing knowledge of the physiologic response to lens wear allows us to define the requirements for successful extended wear. These include:

- Providing sufficient oxygen to maintain normal epithelial metabolic activity
- Allowing carbon dioxide efflux from the cornea to avoid corneal acidosis

- Maintaining adequate tear circulation behind the lens to allow flushing of debris and contaminants
- Minimizing localized pressures applied by the contact lens against the ocular surface
- Reducing or avoiding inflammatory and infective stimuli associated with the lens

The availability of silicone hydrogel and GP lenses with high oxygen (and carbon dioxide) transmissibility has revolutionized extended wear. Although we await the outcomes of long-term, real-world clinical experience with silicone hydrogel lenses in extended wear, it is becoming clear that these lenses avoid many of the chronic hypoxic effects found previously with hydrogel extended wear. Because of the critical role that chronic hypoxia plays in compromise of epithelial integrity, it is hoped that these lenses will also reduce the incidence of microbial keratitis with extended wear. Although further evidence from large-scale studies is still required, early signs are promising.

It is clear, however, that many challenges remain in our quest for safe extended wear. Current research efforts to better understand the importance of post–lens tear circulation, the protective role of the mucus layer of the tear film, and the subtle effects of lens pressures will provide guidance in this quest. Greater understanding of the complexities of inflammatory responses seen in extended wear and the pathogenesis of contact lens-induced corneal infections is also clearly needed. These challenges will continue to drive research and development towards the ultimate goal of truly safe extended wear.

REFERENCES

1. Sweeney DF, Keay L, Jalbert I, et al. Clinical performance of silicone hydrogel lenses. In: Sweeney DF, ed. *Silicone hydrogels: the rebirth of continuous wear contact lenses.* Oxford: Butterworth-Heinemann, 2000:90.
2. Fonn D, MacDonald KE, Richter D, Pritchard N. The ocular response to extended wear of a high Dk silicone hydrogel contact lens. *Clin Exp Optom* 2002;85:176.
3. Morgan PB, Efron N. Comparative clinical performance of two silicone hydrogel contact lenses for continuous wear. *Clin Exp Optom* 2002;85:183.
4. Brennan NA, Coles MLC, Comstock TL, Levy B. A 1-year prospective clinical trial of balafilcon A (PureVision). silicone hydrogel contact lenses used on a 30-day continuous wear schedule. *Ophthalmology* 2002;109:1172.
5. Covey M, Sweeney DF, Terry R, et al. Hypoxic effects on the anterior eye of high-Dk soft contact lens wearers are negligible. *Optom Vis Sci* 2001;78:95.
6. Lin MC, Graham AD, Polse KA, et al. The effects of one-hour wear of high-Dk soft contact lenses on corneal pH and epithelial permeability. *CLAO J* 2000;26:130.
7. MacKeen DL, Sachdev M, Ballou V, Cavanagh HD. A prospective multicenter clinical trial to assess safety and efficacy of Menicon SF-P RGP lenses for extended wear. *CLAO J* 1992;18:183.
8. Holden BA, Grant T, Kotow M, et al. Epithelial microcysts with daily and extended wear of hydrogel and rigid gas permea-
ble contact lenses. *Invest Ophthalmol Vis Sci* 1987;28(Suppl):372.
9. Riley MV. Glucose and oxygen utilization of the cornea. *Exp Eye Res* 1969;8:193.
10. Smelser GK, Ozanics V. Structural changes in corneas of guinea pigs after wearing contact lenses. *Arch Ophthalmol* 1953;49:335.
11. Smelser GK, Ozanics V. Importance of atmospheric oxygen for maintenance of the optical properties of the human cornea. *Science* 1952;115:140.
12. Hill RM, Fatt I. How dependent is the cornea on the atmosphere? *J Am Optom Assoc* 1964;35:873.
13. Langham M. Utilization of oxygen by the component layers of the living cornea. *J Physiol* 1952;117:461.
14. Maurice DM. The cornea and sclera. In: Davson H, ed. *The eye,* Vol 1. London: Academic Press, 1969:489.
15. Freeman RD. Oxygen consumption by the component layers of the cornea. *J Physiol* 1972;225:15.
16. Zurawski CA, McCarey BE, Schmidt F. Glucose consumption in cultured corneal cells. *Curr Eye Res* 1989;8:349.
17. Kwan M, Niinikoski J, Hunt TK. In vivo measurements of oxygen tension in the cornea, aqueous humor, and anterior lens of the open eye. *Invest Ophthalmol* 1972;11:108.
18. Barr RE, Hennessey M, Murphy VG. Diffusion of oxygen at the endothelial surface of the rabbit cornea. *J Physiol* 1977;270:1.
19. McLaren JW, Dinslage S, Dillon JP, et al. Measuring oxygen tension in the anterior chamber of rabbits. *Invest Ophthalmol Vis Sci* 1998;39:1899.
20. Barr RE, Silver IA. Effects of corneal environment on oxygen tension in the anterior chamber of rabbits. *Invest Ophthalmol* 1973;12:140.
21. Stefansson E, Foulks GN, Hamilton RC. The effect of corneal contact lenses on the oxygen tension in the anterior chamber of the rabbit eye. *Invest Ophthalmol Vis Sci* 1987;28:1716.
22. Efron N, Carney LG. Effect of blinking on the level of oxygen beneath hard and soft gas-permeable contact lenses. *J Am Optom Assoc* 1983;54:229.
23. Benjamin WJ, Rasmussen MA. The closed-lid tear pump: oxygenation? *Int Eyecare* 1985;1:251.
24. Fatt I, St. Helen R. Oxygen tension under an oxygen-permeable contact lens. *Am J Optom Arch Am Acad Optom* 1971;48:545.
25. Thoft RA, Friend J. Biochemical aspects of contact lens wear. *Am J Ophthalmol* 1975;80:139.
26. Ichijima H, Imayasu M, Tanaka H, et al. Effects of RGP lens extended wear on glucose-lactate metabolism and stromal swelling in the rabbit cornea. *CLAO J* 2000;26:30.
27. Masters BA. Effects of contact lenses on the oxygen concentration and epithelial mitochondrial redox state of rabbit cornea measured noninvasively with an optically sectioning redox fluorometer microscope. In: Cavanagh HD, ed. *The cornea: transactions of the World Congress on the Cornea III.* New York: Raven Press, 1988:281.
28. Tsubota K, Laing RA. Metabolic changes in the corneal epithelium resulting from hard contact lens wear. *Cornea* 1992;11:121.
29. King JE, Augsburger A, Hill RM. Quantifying the distribution of lactic dehydrogenase in the corneal epithelium with oxygen deprivation. *Am J Optom Arch Am Acad Optom* 1971;48:1016.
30. Hill RM, Rengstorff RH, Petrali JP, Sim VH. Critical oxygen requirement of the corneal epithelium as indicated by succinic dehydrogenase activity. *Am J Optom Physiol Opt* 1974;51:331.
31. Burns RP. Meesman's corneal dystrophy. *Trans Am Ophthalmol Soc* 1968;66:530.
32. Hamano H, Hori M, Hamano T, et al. Effects of contact lens wear on mitosis of corneal epithelium and lactate content of aqueous humor of rabbit. *Jpn J Ophthalmol* 1983;27:451.
33. Ladage PM, Yamamoto K, Ren DH, et al. Proliferation rate of

rabbit corneal epithelium during overnight rigid contact lens wear. *Invest Ophthalmol Vis Sci* 2001;42:2804.

34. Bergmanson JPG, Chu LW-F. Corneal response to rigid contact lens wear. *Br J Ophthalmol* 1982;66:667.

35. Hamano H, Hori M, Hirayama K, et al. Influence of soft and hard contact lenses on the cornea. *Aust J Optom* 1975;58:326.

36. O'Leary DJ, Wilson G, Henson DB. The effect of anoxia on the human corneal epithelium. *Am J Optom Physiol Opt* 1981;58:472.

37. Krutsinger BD, Bergmanson JPG. Corneal epithelial response to hypotonic exposure. *Int Eyecare* 1985;1:440.

38. Hamano H, Komatsu S, Hirayama K. Influence of oxygen deficiency on corneal potential. *Contacto* 1969;13:14.

39. Kwok S. The effects of contact lens wear on the electrophysiology of the corneal epithelium [Review]. *Aust J Optom* 1983;66:138.

40. McNamara NA, Chan JS, Han SC, et al. Effects of hypoxia on corneal epithelial permeability. *Am J Ophthalmol* 1999;127:153.

41. McNamara NA, Fusaro RE, Brand RJ, Polse KA. Epithelial permeability reflects subclinical effects of contact lens wear. *Br J Ophthalmol* 1998;82:376.

42. Carney LG, Brennan NA. Time course of corneal oxygen uptake during contact lens wear. *CLAO J* 1988;14:151.

43. Holden BA, Sweeney DF, Vannas A, et al. Effects of long-term extended contact lens wear on the human cornea. *Invest Ophthalmol Vis Sci* 1985;26:1489.

44. Bergmanson JPG, Ruben CM, Chu LW-F. Epithelial morphological response to soft hydrogel contact lenses. *Br J Ophthalmol* 1985;69:373.

45. Ladage PM, Yamamoto K, Ren DH, et al. Effects of rigid and soft contact lens daily wear on corneal epithelium, tear lactate dehydrogenase, and bacterial binding to exfoliated epithelial cells. *Ophthalmology* 2001;108:1279.

46. Humphreys JA, Larke JR, Parrish ST. Microepithelial cysts observed in extended contact-lens wearing subjects. *Br J Ophthalmol* 1980;64:888.

47. Zantos SG. Cystic formations in the corneal epithelium during extended wear of contact lenses. *Int Contact Lens Clin* 1983;10:128.

48. Holden BA, Sweeney DF. The significance of the microcyst response: a review. *Optom Vis Sci* 1991;68:703.

49. Bergmanson JPG. Histopathological analysis of the corneal epithelium after contact lens wear. *J Am Optom Assoc* 1987;58:812.

50. Madigan MC. Cat and monkey as models for extended hydrogel contact lens wear in humans [PhD thesis]. Sydney: University of New South Wales, 1989

51. Ren DH, Petroll WM, Jester JV, et al. Short-term hypoxia downregulates epithelial cell desquamation in vivo, but does not increase *Pseudomonas aeruginosa* adherence to exfoliated human corneal epithelial cells. *CLAO J* 1999;25:73.

52. Ren DH, Petroll WM, Jester JV, et al. The relationship between contact lens oxygen permeability and binding of *Pseudomonas aeruginosa* to human corneal epithelial cells after overnight and extended wear. *CLAO J* 1999;25:80.

53. Ren DH, Yamamoto K, Ladage PM, et al. Adaptive effects of 30-night wear of hyper-O_2 transmissible contact lenses on bacterial binding and corneal epithelium. *Ophthalmology* 2002;109:27.

54. Lemp MA, Gold JB. The effects of extended-wear hydrophilic contact lenses on the human corneal epithelium. *Am J Ophthalmol* 1986;101:274.

55. Tsubota K, Hata S, Toda I, et al. Increase in corneal epithelial cell size with extended wear soft contact lenses depends on continuous wearing time. *Br J Ophthalmol* 1996;80:144.

56. O'Leary DJ, Millodot M. Abnormal epithelial fragility in diabetes and in contact lens wear. *Acta Ophthalmol* 1981;59:827.

57. Millodot M. Effect of soft lenses on corneal sensitivity. *Acta Ophthalmol* 1974;52:603.

58. Millodot M, O'Leary DJ. Effect of oxygen deprivation on corneal sensitivity. *Acta Ophthalmol* 1980;58:434.

59. Mindel JS, Szilagyi PIA, Zadunaisky JA, et al. The effects of blepharorrhaphy induced depression of corneal cholinergic activity. *Exp Eye Res* 1979;29:463.

60. Madigan MC, Holden BA. Reduced epithelial adhesion after extended contact lens wear correlates with reduced hemidesmosome density in cat cornea. *Invest Ophthalmol Vis Sci* 1992;33:314.

61. Madigan MC, Holden BA, Kwok LS. Extended wear of contact lenses can compromise corneal epithelial adhesion. *Curr Eye Res* 1987;6:1257.

62. Wallace W. The SLACH syndrome. *Int Eyecare* 1986;1:220.

63. Lindsay R, Lakkis C, Brennan NA. Focal loss of epithelium associated with hydrogel contact lens wear and trigeminal nerve defect. *Int Contact Lens Clin* 1993;20:234.

64. Zimny ML, Salisbury C. Effects of soft contacts on corneal wound healing in rabbits. *Cornea* 1982;1:301.

65. Mauger TF, Hill RM. Corneal epithelial healing under contact lenses: quantitative analysis in the rabbit. *Acta Ophthalmol* 1992;70:361.

66. Klotz SA, Misra RP, Butrus SI. Contact lens wear enhances adherence of *Pseudomonas aeruginosa* and binding of lectins to the cornea. *Cornea* 1990;9:266.

67. Fleiszig SMJ, Efron N, Pier GB. Extended contact lens wear enhances *Pseudomonas aeruginosa* adherence to human corneal epithelium. *Invest Ophthalmol Vis Sci* 1992;33:2908.

68. Cavanagh HD, Ladage PM, Li SL, et al. Effects of daily and overnight wear of a novel hyper oxygen-transmissible soft contact lens on bacterial binding and corneal epithelium. *Ophthalmology* 2002;109:1957.

69. Smelser GK, Chen DK. Physiological changes in cornea induced by contact lenses. *Arch Ophthalmol* 1955;53:676.

70. Bonanno JA, Polse KA. Corneal acidosis during contact lens wear: effects of hypoxia and C02. *Invest Ophthalmol Vis Sci* 1987;28:1514.

71. Klyce SD. Stromal lactate accumulation can account for corneal oedema osmotically following epithelial hypoxia in the rabbit. *J Physiol* 1981;321:49.

72. La Hood D, Sweeney D, Holden BA. Overnight corneal edema with hydrogel, rigid gas-permeable and silicone elastomer contact lenses. *Int Contact Lens Clin* 1988;15:149.

73. Holden BA, Mertz GW, McNally JJ. Corneal swelling response to contact lenses worn under extended wear conditions. *Invest Ophthalmol Vis Sci* 1983;24:218.

74. Andrasko GJ. Corneal deswelling response to hard and hydrogel extended wear lenses. *Invest Ophthalmol Vis Sci* 1986;27:20.

75. Holden BA, Sweeney DF, La Hood D, Kenyon E. Corneal deswelling following overnight wear of rigid and hydrogel contact lenses. *Curr Eye Res* 1988;7:49.

76. Cox IG. Vision with soft contact lenses [PhD thesis]. Sydney: University of New South Wales, 1988.

77. Kangas TA, Edelhauser HF, Twining SS, O'Brien WJ. Loss of stromal glycosaminoglycans during corneal edema. *Invest Ophthalmol Vis Sci* 1990;31:1994.

78. Holden BA, Sweeney DF, Efron N, et al. Contact lenses can induce stromal thinning. *Clin Exp Optom* 1988;71:109.

79. Polse KA, Rivera RK, Bonanno J. Ocular effects of hard gas-permeable-lens extended wear. *Am J Optom Physiol Opt* 1988;65:358.

80. Zantos SG, Holden BA. Transient endothelial changes soon

after wearing soft contact lenses. *Am J Optom Physiol Opt* 1977; 54:856.

81. Holden BA, Zantos SG. Corneal endothelium: transient changes with atmospheric anoxia. In: *The cornea in health and disease (VIth Congress of the European Society of Ophthalmology), Royal Society of Medicine International Congress and Symposium Series No. 40.* London: Academic Press and Royal Society of Medicine, 1981:79.

82. Khodadoust AA, Hirst LW. Diurnal variation in corneal endothelial morphology. *Ophthalmology* 1984;91:1125.

83. Holden BA, Williams L, Zantos SG. The etiology of transient endothelial changes in the human cornea. *Invest Ophthalmol Vis Sci* 1985;26:1354.

84. Holden BA, Vannas A, Nilsson K, et al. Epithelial and endothelial effects from the extended wear of contact lenses. *Curr Eye Res* 1985;4:739.

85. Keay L, Sweeney DF, Jalbert I, et al. Microcyst response to high Dk/t silicone hydrogel contact lenses. *Optom Vis Sci* 2000;77:582.

86. Millodot M. Effect of long-term wear of hard contact lenses on corneal sensitivity. *Arch Ophthalmol* 1978;96:1225.

87. Holden BA, Sweeney DF, Sanderson G. The minimum precorneal oxygen tension to avoid corneal edema. *Invest Ophthalmol Vis Sci* 1984;25:476.

88. Mizutani Y, Matsunaka H, Takemoto N, Mizutani Y. The effect of anoxia on the human cornea. *Jpn Soc Acta* 1983;87:644.

89. Sarver M, Polse K, Baggett D. Intersubject difference in corneal edema response to hypoxia. *Am J Optom Physiol Opt* 1983;60:128.

90. Larke JR, Parrish ST, Wigham CG. Apparent human corneal oxygen uptake rate. *Am J Optom Physiol Opt* 1981;58:803.

91. Brennan NA, Efron E, Carney LG. Corneal oxygen availability during contact lens wear: a comparison of methodologies. *Am J Optom Physiol Opt* 1988;65:19.

92. Williams LJ. Transient endothelial changes in the in vivo human cornea [PhD thesis]. Sydney: University of New South Wales, 1986.

93. Holden BA, Mertz GW. Critical oxygen levels to avoid corneal edema for daily and extended wear contact lenses. *Invest Ophthalmol Vis Sci* 1984;25:1161.

94. Mertz GW. Overnight swelling of the living human cornea. *J Am Optom Assoc* 1980;51:211.

95. Fonn D, du Toit R, Simpson TL, et al. Sympathetic swelling response of the control eye to soft lenses in the other eye. *Invest Ophthalmol Vis Sci* 1999;40:3116.

96. Harvitt DM, Bonanno JA. pH dependence of corneal oxygen consumption. *Invest Ophthalmol Vis Sci* 1998;39:2778.

97. Harvitt DM, Bonanno JA. Re-evaluation of the oxygen diffusion model for predicting minimum contact lens Dk/t values needed to avoid corneal anoxia. *Optom Vis Sci* 1999;76:712.

98. Fatt I, Bieber MT, Pye SD. Steady state distribution of oxygen and carbon dioxide in the in vivo cornea of an eye covered by a gas-permeable contact lens. *Am J Optom Physiol Opt* 1969; 46:3.

99. Smith BJ, Fink BA, Hill RM. Dk/L: into the ultra-high zone. *CL Spectrum* 1999;14:31.

100. Gamm E. The dependence of acid-base balance in the aqueous humor on carbon dioxide and oxygen diffusion through the cornea. *Albrecht Von Graefes Arch Klin Ophthalmol* 1980;214:101.

101. Fatt I. Gas transmission properties of soft contact lenses. In: Ruben M, ed. *Soft contact lenses.* London: Balliere Tindall, 1978:108.

102. Holden BA, Ross R, Jenkins J. Hydrogel contact lenses impede carbon dioxide efflux from the human cornea. *Curr Eye Res* 1987;6:1283.

103. Efron N, Ang JHB. Corneal hypoxia and hypercapnia during contact lens wear. *Optom Vis Sci* 1990;67:512.

104. Bonanno JA, Polse KA. Measurement of in vivo human corneal stromal pH: open and closed eye. *Invest Ophthalmol Vis Sci* 1987;28:522.

105. Giasson C, Bonanno JA. Corneal epithelial and aqueous humor acidification during in vivo contact lens wear in rabbits. *Invest Ophthalmol Vis Sci* 1994;35:851.

106. Giasson C, Bonanno JA. Acidification of rabbit corneal endothelium during contact lens wear in vitro. *Curr Eye Res* 1995; 14:311.

107. Fischer F, Wiederholt M. The pH dependency of sodium and chloride transport in the isolated human cornea. *Invest Ophthalmol Vis Sci* 1978;17:810.

108. Green K, Cheeks L, Hull DS. Effect of ambient pH on corneal endothelial sodium fluxes. *Invest Ophthalmol Vis Sci* 1986;27:1274.

109. Fischbarg J, Lim JJ. Role of cations, anions and carbonic anhydrase in fluid transport across rabbit corneal endothelium. *J Physiol* 1974;241:647.

110. Gonnering R, Edelhauser HF, Van Horn DL, Durant W. The pH tolerance of rabbit and human corneal endothelium. *Invest Ophthalmol Vis Sci* 1979;18:373.

111. McNamara NA, Polse KA, Bonanno JA. Stromal acidosis modulates corneal swelling. *Invest Ophthalmol Vis Sci* 1994;35:846.

112. Cohen SR, Polse KA, Brand RJ, Bonanno JA. Stromal acidosis affects corneal hydration control. *Invest Ophthalmol Vis Sci* 1992;33:134.

113. Schoessler JP, Woloschak MJ. Corneal endothelium in veteran PMMA contact lens wearers. *Int Contact Lens Clin* 1981;8:19.

114. Hirst LW, Auer C, Cohn J, et al. Specular microscopy of hard contact lens wearers. *Ophthalmology* 1984;91:1147.

115. MacRae SM, Matsuda M, Shellans S, Rich LF. The effects of hard and soft contact lenses on the corneal endothelium. *Am J Ophthalmol* 1986;102:50.

116. Schoessler JP. Corneal endothelial polymegethism associated with extended wear. *Int Contact Lens Clin* 1983;10:148.

117. Schoessler JP, Barr JT, Freson DR. Corneal endothelial observations of silicone elastomer contact lens wearers. *Int Contact Lens Clin* 1984;11:337.

118. Yamaguchi H, Ogihara K, Kajita M, et al. Corneal endothelial cell change in the early stage of contact lens wear. *J Jpn CL Soc* 1993;35:146.

119. Laing RA, Sandstrom M, Berrospi A, Liebowitz H. Changes in corneal endothelium as a function of age. *Exp Eye Res* 1976;22:587.

120. Schoessler JP, Orsborn GN. A theory of corneal endothelial polymegethism and age. *Curr Eye Res* 1987;6:301.

121. Vannas A, Holden BA, Makitie J. The ultrastructure of contact lens induced changes. *Acta Ophthalmol* 1984;62:320.

122. Bergmanson JPG. Histopathological analysis of corneal endothelial polymegethism. *Cornea* 1992;11:133.

123. Stevenson RWW, Kirkness CM. Corneal endothelial irregularity with long-term contact lens wear. *Cornea* 1992;11:600.

124. Yamauchi K, Hirst LW, Enger C, et al. Specular microscopy of hard contact lens wearers II. *Ophthalmology* 1989;96:1176.

125. McMahon TT, Polse KA, McNamara N, Viana MAG. Recovery from induced corneal edema and endothelial morphology after long-term PMMA contact lens wear. *Optom Vis Sci* 1996;73:184.

126. Polse KA, Brand RJ, Cohen SR, Guillon M. Hypoxic effects on corneal morphology and function. *Invest Ophthalmol Vis Sci* 1990;31:1542.

127. Lass JH, Dutt RM, Spurney RV, et al. Morphologic and fluorophotometric analysis of the corneal endothelium in long-term hard and soft contact lens wearers. *CLAO J* 1988;14:105.

128. Dutt RM, Stocker EG, Wolff CH, et al. A morphological and fluorophotometric analysis of the corneal endothelium in long-term extended wear soft contact lens wearers. *CLAO J* 1989; 15:121.

129. Sweeney DF. Corneal exhaustion syndrome with long-term wear of contact lenses. *Optom Vis Sci* 1992;69:601.

130. Rao GN, Aquavella JV, Goldberg SH, Berk ML. Pseudophakic bullous keratopathy: relationship to preoperative corneal endothelial status. *Ophthalmology* 1984;91:1135.

131. Bates AK, Cheng H. Bullous keratopathy: a study of endothelial cell morphology in patients undergoing cataract surgery. *Br J Ophthalmol* 1988;72:409.

132. Mackie IA. Localised corneal drying in association with dellen, pterygia and related lesions. *Trans Ophthalmol Soc U K* 1971; 41:129.

133. O'Leary DJ, Wilson G, Bergmanson J. The influence of calcium in the tear-side perfusate on desquamation from the rabbit corneal epithelium. *Curr Eye Res* 1985;4:729.

134. Bachman WG, Wilson G. Essential ions for maintenance of the corneal epithelial surface. *Invest Ophthalmol Vis Sci* 1985; 26:1484.

135. Willcox M, Sankaridurg PR, Lan J, et al. Inflammation and infection and the effects of the closed eye. In: Sweeney DF, ed. *Silicone hydrogels: the rebirth of continuous wear contact lenses.* Oxford: Butterworth-Heinemann, 2000:45.

136. Dilly PN. Contribution of the epithelium to the stability of the tear film. *Trans Ophthalmol Soc U K* 1985;104:381.

137. Watanabe H, Fabricant M, Tisdale AS, et al. Human corneal and conjunctival epithelia produce a mucin-like glycoprotein for the apical surface. *Invest Ophthalmol Vis Sci* 1995;36:337.

138. Holly FJ, Lemp MA. Tear physiology and dry eyes. *Surv Ophthalmol* 1977;22:69.

139. Nichols B, Dawson CR, Togni B. Surface features of the conjunctiva and cornea. *Invest Ophthalmol Vis Sci* 1983;24:570.

140. Holly FJ, Lemp MA. Wettability and wetting of corneal epithelium. *Exp Eye Res* 1971;11:239.

141. Latkovic S, Nilsson SEG. The effect of high and low Dk/L soft contact lenses on the glycocalyx layer of the corneal epithelium and on the membrane associated receptors for lectins. *CLAO J* 1997;23:185.

142. Holly FJ. Tear film physiology. *Am J Optom Physiol Opt* 1980; 57:252.

143. Norn MS. Mucus flow in the conjunctiva: rate of migration of the mucous thread in the inferior conjunctival fornix towards the inner canthus. *Acta Ophthalmol* 1969;47:129.

144. Adams AD. The morphology of human conjunctival mucus. *Arch Ophthalmol* 1979;97:730.

145. Ren H, Wilson G. Apoptosis in the corneal epithelium. *Invest Ophthalmol Vis Sci* 1996;37:1017.

146. Ren H, Wilson G. The effect of a shear force on the cell shedding rate of the corneal epithelium. *Acta Ophthalmol* 1997;75: 383.

147. Kurihashi K. Diagnostic tests of lacrimal function using cotton thread. In: Holly FJ, ed. *The preocular tear film in health, disease and contact lens wear.* Lubbock, TX: Dry Eye Institute, 1986: 89.

148. Jordan A, Baum J. Basic tear flow: does it exist? *Ophthalmology* 1980;87:920.

149. Baum JL. Clinical implications of basal tear flow. In: Holly FJ, ed. *The preocular tear film in health, disease and contact lens wear.* Lubbock, TX: Dry Eye Institute, 1986:646.

150. Mishima S, Maurice DM. The oily layer of the tear film and evaporation from the corneal surface. *Exp Eye Res* 1961;1:39.

151. Terry JE, Hill RM. Human tear osmotic pressure: diurnal variation and the closed lid. *Arch Ophthalmol* 1978;96:120.

152. Carney LG, Hill RM. Human tear pH. *Arch Ophthalmol* 1976; 94:821.

153. Fatt I, Chaston J. Temperature of a contact lens on the eye. *Int Contact Lens Clin* 1980;7:195.

154. Wilson G, O'Leary DJ, Holden BA. Cell content of tears following overnight wear of a contact lens. *Curr Eye Res* 1989;8:329.

155. Tan KO, Sack RA, Swarbrick HA, Holden BA. Temporal sequence of changes in tear film composition during sleep. *Curr Eye Res* 1993;2:1001.

156. Ramachandran L, Sharma S, Sankaridurg PR. Examination of the conjunctival microbiota after 8 hours of eye closure. *CLAO J* 1995;1:195.

157. Fatt I. Oxygen tension under a contact lens during blinking. *Am J Optom Physiol Opt* 1969;6:654.

158. Polse KA. Tear flow under hydrogel contact lenses. *Invest Ophthalmol Vis Sci* 1979;8:409.

159. McNamara NA, Polse KA, Brand RJ, et al. Tear mixing under a soft contact lens: effects of lens diameter. *Am J Ophthalmol* 1999;27:659.

160. Wilson G. The epithelium in extended wear. In: Sweeney DF, ed. *Silicone hydrogels: the rebirth of continuous wear contact lenses.* Oxford: Butterworth-Heinemann, 2000:22.

161. McDonald JE, Brubaker S. Meniscus-induced thinning of tear films. *Am J Ophthalmol* 1971;72:139.

162. Graham R. Persistent nasal and temporal stippling. *Contacto* 1968;12:20.

163. Lemp MA, Holly FJ. Recent advances in ocular surface chemistry. *Am J Optom Arch Am Acad Optom* 1970;47:669.

164. Benjamin WJ. The closed-lid tear pump during rigid extended wear. *Int Eyecare* 1986;2:224.

165. Zantos SG, Zantos PO. Extended wear feasibility of gas-permeable hard lenses for myopia. *Int Eyecare* 1985;1:66.

166. Swarbrick HA. A possible etiology for RGP lens binding (adherence). *Int Contact Lens Clin* 1988;15:13.

167. Kenyon E, Polse KA, Mandell RB. Rigid contact lens adherence: incidence, severity and recovery. *J Am Optom Assoc* 1988;59: 168.

168. Swarbrick HA, Holden BA. Rigid gas-permeable lens adherence: a patient-dependent phenomenon. *Optom Vis Sci* 1989;66:269.

169. Bruce AS, Brennan NA. Hydrogel lens binding and the post-lens tear film. *Clin Eye Vis Care* 1992;4:111.

170. Lin ST, Mandell RB. Corneal trauma from overnight wear of rigid or soft contact lenses. *J Am Optom Assoc* 1991;62:224.

171. Pritchard N, Jones L, Dumbleton K, Fonn D. Epithelial inclusions in association with mucin ball development in high-oxygen permeability hydrogel lenses. *Optom Vis Sci* 2000;77:68.

172. Fleming C, Austen R, Davies S, et al. Pre-corneal deposits during soft contact lens wear. *Optom Vis Sci* 1994;71(Suppl):152.

173. Tighe B. Silicone hydrogel materials: how do they work? In: Sweeney DF, ed. *Silicone hydrogels: the rebirth of continuous wear contact lenses.* Oxford: Butterworth-Heinemann, 2000:1.

174. Dumbleton K, Jones L, Chalmers R, et al. Clinical characterization of spherical post-lens debris associated with lotrafilcon high-Dk silicone lenses. *CLAO J* 2000;26:186.

175. Ladage PM, Petroll WM, Jester JV, et al. Spherical indentations of human and rabbit corneal epithelium following extended contact lens wear. *CLAO J* 2002;28:177.

176. Zantos SG, Holden BA. Ocular changes associated with continuous wear of contact lenses. *Aust J Optom* 1978;61:418.

177. Mertz GW, Holden BA. Clinical implications of extended wear research. *Can J Optom* 1981;43:203.

178. Josephson JE, Caffery BE. Infiltrative keratitis in hydrogel lens wearers. *Int Contact Lens Clin* 1979;6:223.

179. Holden BA, Sweeney DF. Ocular requirements for extended wear. *Contax* 1987;May:10.

180. Schnider CM, Zabkiewicz K, Holden BA. Unusual complica-

tions associated with RGP extended wear. *Int Contact Lens Clin* 1988;15:124.

181. Faber E, Golding TR, Lowe R, Brennan NA. Effect of hydrogel lens wear on tear film stability. *Optom Vis Sci* 1991;68:380.

182. Fleiszig SMJ, Zaidi TS, Ramphal R, Pier GB. Modulation of *Pseudomonas aeruginosa* adherence to the corneal surface by mucus. *Infect Immunol* 1994;62:1799.

183. Lydon D, Tait A. Lid-pressure: its measurement and probable effects on the shape and form of the cornea-rigid contact lens system. *J Br CL Assoc* 1988;11:11.

184. Doane MG. Interaction of the eyelids and tears in corneal wetting and the dynamics of the normal human eyeblink. *Am J Ophthalmol* 1980;89:507.

185. Holden BA, Collin HB, Sweeney DF. The effects of silicone elastomer lens binding on corneal structure. *Am J Optom Physiol Opt* 1988;65(Suppl):133P.

186. Holden BA, Sweeney DF, Collin HB. The effects of RGP and silicone elastomer lens binding on corneal structure. *Invest Ophthalmol Vis Sci* 1989;30(Suppl):481.

187. Polse KA, Sarver MD, Kenyon E, Bonanno J. Gas permeable hard contact lens extended wear: ocular and visual responses to a 6-month period of wear. *CLAO J* 1987;13:31.

188. Henry VA, Bennett ES, Forrest JF. Clinical investigation of the Paraperm EW rigid gas-permeable contact lens. *Am J Optom Physiol Opt* 1987;64:313.

189. Sridharan R, Swarbrick HA. Corneal response to short-term orthokeratology lens wear. *Optom Vis Sci* 2003;80:200.

190. Mountford J. An analysis of the changes in corneal shape and refractive error induced by accelerated orthokeratology. *Int Contact Lens Clin* 1997;24:128.

191. Nichols JJ, Marsich MM, Nguyen M, et al. Overnight orthokeratology. *Optom Vis Sci* 2000;77:252.

192. Rah MJ, Jackson JM, Jones LA, et al. Overnight orthokeratology: preliminary results of the Lenses and Overnight Orthokeratology (LOOK) study. *Optom Vis Sci* 2002;79:598.

193. Wong G, Swarbrick HA, O'Leary DJ. The corneal response to orthokeratology. *Optom Vis Sci* 1998;75:791.

194. Alharbi A, Swarbrick HA. The effects of overnight orthokeratology lens wear on corneal thickness. *Invest Ophthalmol Vis Sci* 2003;44:2518.

195. Alharbi A, Swarbrick HA, La Hood D. Overnight orthokeratology suppresses the overnight central corneal edema response. *Invest Ophthalmol Vis Sci* 2003;44(Suppl):3704.

196. Hill JF. A comparison of refractive and keratometric changes during adaptation to flexible and non-flexible contact lenses. *J Am Optom Assoc* 1975;46:290.

197. Harris MG, Sarver MD, Polse KA. Corneal curvature and refractive error changes associated with wearing hydrogel contact lenses. *Am J Optom Physiol Opt* 1975;52:313.

198. Grosvenor T. Changes in corneal curvature and subjective refraction in soft contact lens wearers. *Am J Optom Physiol Opt* 1975;52:405.

199. Dumbleton KA, Chalmers RL, Richter DB, Fonn D. Changes in myopic refractive error with nine months' extended wear of hydrogel lenses with high and low oxygen permeability. *Optom Vis Sci* 1999;76:845.

200. Hine NA, Back A, Holden BA. Aetiology of arcuate epithelial lesions induced by hydrogels. *Trans BCLA Conference* 1987:48.

201. Sankaridurg PR, Sweeney DF, Sharma S, et al. Adverse events with extended wear of disposable hydrogels: results for the first 13 months of lens wear. *Ophthalmology* 1999;106:1671.

202. Holden BA, Stephenson A, Stretton S, et al. Superior epithelial arcuate lesions with soft contact lens wear. *Optom Vis Sci* 2001;78:9.

203. Robboy M, Cox I. Assessment of conjunctival staining in soft contact lens wearers. *Am J Optom Physiol Opt* 1988;65:119P.

204. Vannas A, Sweeney DF, Holden BA, et al. Tear plasmin activity with contact lens wear. *Curr Eye Res* 1992;11:243.

205. Willcox MDP, Morris CA, Thakur A, et al. Complement and complement regulatory proteins in human tears. *Invest Ophthalmol Vis Sci* 1997;38:1.

206. Sack RA, Underwood PA, Tan KO, et al. Vitronectin: possible contribution to the closed-eye external host defense mechanism. *Ocular Immunol Inflamm* 1993;1:327.

207. Abelson MB, Soter NA, Simon MA, et al. Histamine in human tears. *Am J Ophthalmol* 1977;83:417.

208. Thakur A, Willcox MDP, Stapleton F. The proinflammatory cytokines and arachidonic acid metabolites in human overnight tears: homeostatic mechanisms. *J Clin Immunol* 1998;18:61.

209. Thakur A, Willcox MD. Cytokine and lipid inflammatory mediator profile of human tears during contact lens associated inflammatory diseases. *Exp Eye Res* 1998;67:9.

210. Sack RA, Tan KO, Tan M. Diurnal tear cycle: evidence for a nocturnal inflammatory constitutive tear fluid. *Invest Ophthalmol Vis Sci* 1992;33:626.

211. Carney FP, Morris CA, Willcox MDP. The effect of hydrogel lens wear on the major tear proteins during extended wear. *Aust N Z J Ophthalmol* 1997;25(Suppl):s36.

212. Pearce DJ, Demirci G, Willcox MD. Secretory IgA epitopes in basal tears of extended-wear soft contact lens wearers and in non-lens wearers. *Aust N Z J Ophthalmol* 1999;27:221.

213. Willcox MD, Lan J. Secretory immunoglobulin A in tears: functions and changes during contact lens wear. *Clin Exp Optom* 1999;82:1.

214. Stapleton F, Willcox MDP, Morris CA, Sweeney DF. Tear changes in contact lens wearers following overnight eye closure. *Curr Eye Res* 1998;17:183.

215. Hazlett LD, McClellan SM, Hume EBH, et al. Extended wear contact lens usage induces Langerhans cell migration into cornea. *Exp Eye Res* 1999;69:575.

216. Holden BA, Sweeney DF, Swarbrick HA, et al. The vascular response to long-term extended contact lens wear. *Clin Exp Optom* 1986;69:112.

217. Papas EB, Vajdic CM, Austen R, Holden BA. High-oxygen-transmissibility soft contact lenses do not induce limbal hyperemia. *Curr Eye Res* 1997;16:942.

218. Papas E. On the relationship between soft contact lens oxygen transmissibility and induced limbal hyperemia. *Exp Eye Res* 1998;67:125.

219. Dumbleton K, Chalmers RL, Richter DB, Fonn D. Vascular response to extended wear of hydrogel lenses with high and low oxygen permeability. *Optom Vis Sci* 2001;78:147.

220. Gordon A, Kracher GP. Corneal infiltrates and extended wear contact lenses. *J Am Optom Assoc* 1985;56:198.

221. Thakur A, Willcox MD. Chemotactic activity of tears and bacteria isolated during adverse responses. *Exp Eye Res* 1998;66:129.

222. Bates AK, Morris RJ, Stapleton F, et al. Sterile corneal infiltrates in contact lens wearers. *Eye* 1989;3:803.

223. Stapleton F, Dart J, Minassian D. Nonulcerative complications of contact lens wear: relative risks for different lens types. *Arch Ophthalmol* 1992;110:1601.

224. Holden BA, Sankaridurg PR, Jalbert I. Adverse effects and infections: which ones and how many? In: Sweeney DF, ed. *Silicone hydrogels: the rebirth of continuous wear contact lenses*. Oxford: Butterworth-Heinemann, 2000:150.

225. Baleriola-Lucas C, Grant T, Newton-Howes J, et al. Enumeration and identification of bacteria on hydrogel lenses from asymptomatic patients and those experiencing adverse responses with extended wear. *Invest Ophthalmol Vis Sci* 1991;32(Suppl):739.

226. Sankaridurg PR, Willcox MDP, Sharma S, et al. *Haemophilus*

influenzae adherent to contact lenses is associated with the production of acute ocular inflammation. *J Clin Microbiol* 1996; 34:2426.

227. Holden BA, La Hood D, Grant T, et al. Gram-negative bacteria can induce contact lens related acute red eye (CLARE). responses. *CLAO J* 1996;22:47.

228. Sankaridurg PR, Sharma S, Willcox M, et al. Colonization of hydrogel lenses with *Streptococcus pneumoniae:* risk of development of corneal infiltrates. *Cornea* 1999;18:289.

229. Cole N, Willcox MDP, Fleiszig SMJ, et al. Different strains of *Pseudomonas aeruginosa* isolated from ocular infections or inflammation display distinct corneal pathologies in an animal model. *Curr Eye Res* 1998;17:730.

230. Grant T, Chong MS, Vajdic C, et al. Contact lens induced peripheral ulcers (CLPUs) during hydrogel contact lens wear. *CLAO J* 1998;24:145.

231. Stein RM, Clinch TE, Cohen EJ, et al. Infected vs sterile corneal infiltrates in contact lens wear. *Am J Ophthalmol* 1988;105:632.

232. Willcox MDP, Sweeney DF, Sharma S, et al. Culture negative peripheral ulcers are associated with bacterial contamination of contact lenses. *Invest Ophthalmol Vis Sci* 1995;36(Suppl):152.

233. Jalbert I, Willcox MDP, Sweeney DF. Isolation of *Staphylococcus aureus* from a contact lens at the time of a contact lens-induced peripheral ulcer: case report. *Cornea* 2000;19:116.

234. Holden BA, Reddy MK, Sankaridurg PR, et al. Contact lens-induced peripheral ulcers with extended wear of disposable hydrogel lenses: histopathologic observations on the nature and type of corneal infiltrate. *Cornea* 1999;18:538.

235. Keay L, Willcox MD, Sweeney DF, et al. Bacterial populations on 30-night extended wear silicone hydrogel lenses. *CLAO J* 2001;27:30.

236. Willcox MD, Harmis NY, Holden BA. Bacterial populations on high-Dk silicone hydrogel contact lenses: effect of length of wear in asymptomatic patients. *Clin Exp Optom* 2002;85:172.

237. Spring TF. Reaction to hydrophilic lenses. *Med J Aust* 1974;1: 449.

238. Allansmith MR, Korb DR, Greiner JV, et al. Giant papillary conjunctivitis in contact lens wearers. *Am J Ophthalmol* 1977; 83:697.

239. Alemany AL, Redal P. Giant papillary conjunctivitis in soft and rigid lens wear. *Contactologia* 1991;13:14.

240. Barishak Y, Zavaro A, Samra Z, Sompolinsky D. An immunological study of papillary conjunctivitis due to contact lenses. *Curr Eye Res* 1984;3:1161.

241. Allansmith MR, Korb DR, Greiner JV. Giant papillary conjunctivitis induced by hard or soft contact lens wear: quantitative histology. *Ophthalmology* 1978;85:766.

242. Sugar A, Meyer RF. Giant papillary conjunctivitis after keratoplasty. *Am J Ophthalmol* 1981;91:239.

243. Srinivasan BD, Jakobiec FA, Iwamoto T, et al. Giant papillary conjunctivitis with ocular prosthesis. *Arch Ophthalmol* 1979;97: 892.

244. Reynolds RMP. Giant papillary conjunctivitis: a mechanical aetiology. *Aust J Optom* 1978;61:320.

245. Molinari JF. Giant papillary conjunctivitis [Review]. *Aust J Optom* 1983;66:59.

246. Skotnitsky C, Sankaridurg PR, Sweeney DF, Holden BA. General and local contact lens induced papillary conjunctivitis (CLPC). *Clin Exp Optom* 2002;85:193.

247. McKenney C, Becker N, Thomas S, et al. Lens deposits with a high Dk hydrophilic soft lens. *Optom Vis Sci* 1998;75:276.

248. Dart JKG, Stapleton F, Minassian D. Contact lenses and other risk factors in microbial keratitis. *Lancet* 1991;338:651.

249. Schein OD, Ormerod LD, Barraquer E, et al. Microbiology of contact lens-related keratitis. *Cornea* 1989;8:281.

250. Chalupa E, Swarbrick HA, Holden BA, Sjostrand J. Severe cor-

251. Schein OD, Glynn RJ, Poggio EC, et al. The relative risk of ulcerative keratitis among users of daily-wear and extended-wear soft contact lenses. *N Engl J Med* 1989;321:773.

252. Poggio EC, Glynn RJ, Schein OD, et al. The incidence of ulcerative keratitis among users of daily-wear and extended-wear soft contact lenses. *N Engl J Med* 1989;321:779.

253. Buehler PO, Schein OD, Stamler JF, et al. The increased risk of ulcerative keratitis among disposable soft contact lens users. *Arch Ophthalmol* 1992;110:1555.

254. Matthews TD, Frazer DG, Minassian DC, et al. Risks of keratitis and patterns of use with disposable contact lenses. *Arch Ophthalmol* 1992;110:1559.

255. Stapleton F, Dart JKG, Minassian D. Risk factors with contact lens related suppurative keratitis. *CLAO J* 1993;19:204.

256. Poggio EC, Abelson M. Complications and symptoms in disposable EW lenses compared with conventional soft DW and soft EW lenses. *CLAO J* 1993;19:31.

257. Nilsson SEG, Montan PG. The hospitalised cases of contact lens induced keratitis in Sweden and their relation to lens type and wear schedule: results of a three year retrospective study. *CLAO J* 1994;20:97.

258. Adams CP, Cohen EJ, Laibson PR, et al. Corneal ulcers in patients with cosmetic extended-wear lenses. *Am J Ophthalmol* 1983;96:705.

259. Galentine PG, Cohen EJ, Laibson PR, et al. Corneal ulcers associated with contact lens wear. *Arch Ophthalmol* 1984;102: 891.

260. Weissman BA, Mondino WC, Pettit TH, Hofbauer JD. Corneal ulcers associated with extended-wear soft contact lenses. *Am J Ophthalmol* 1984;97:476.

261. Fleiszig SMJ, Zaidi TS, Preston MJ, et al. Relationship between cytotoxicity and corneal epithelial cell invasion by clinical isolates of *Pseudomonas aeruginosa. Infect Immunol* 1996;64:228.

262. Stern GA, Weitzenkorn D, Valenti J. Adherence of *Pseudomonas aeruginosa* to the mouse cornea. *Arch Ophthalmol* 1982;100: 1956.

263. Stern CA, Lubniewski A, Allen C. The interaction between *Pseudomonas aeruginosa* and the corneal epithelium. *Arch Ophthalmol* 1985;103:1221.

264. Fleiszig SMJ, Zaidi TS, Fletcher EL, et al. *Pseudomonas aeruginosa* invades corneal epithelial cells during experimental infection. *Infect Immunol* 1994;62:3485.

265. Fleiszig SMJ, Zaidi TS, Pier GB. *Pseudomonas aeruginosa* invasion of and multiplication within corneal epithelial cells in vitro. *Infect Immunol* 1995;63:4072.

266. Fleiszig SMJ, Lee EJ, Wu C, et al. Cytotoxic strains of *Pseudomonas aeruginosa* can damage the intact corneal surface in vitro. *CLAO J* 1998;24:41.

267. Raber IM, Laibson PR, Kurz GH, Bernardino VB. *Pseudomonas* corneoscleral ulcers. *Am J Ophthalmol* 1981;92:353.

268. Lim L, Loughnan MS, Sullivan LJ. Microbial keratitis associated with extended wear of silicone hydrogel contact lenses. *Br J Ophthalmol* 2002;86:355.

269. Holden BA, Sweeney DF, Sankaridurg PR, et al. Microbial keratitis and vision loss with contact lenses. *Eye & Contact Lens* 2003;29(Suppl):S131.

270. Dunn JP, Mondino BJ, Weissman BA, et al. Corneal ulcers associated with disposable hydrogel contact lenses. *Am J Ophthalmol* 1989;108:113.

271. Mondino BJ, Weissman BA, Farb MD, Pettit TH. Corneal ulcers associated with daily-wear and extended-wear contact lenses. *Am J Ophthalmol* 1986;102:58.

272. Mowrey-McKee MF, Sampson HJ, Proskin HM. Microbial contamination of hydrophilic contact lenses. Part II: Quantifi-

cation of microbes after patient handling and after aseptic removal from the eye. *CLAO J* 1992;18:240.

273. Willcox MDP, Power KN, Stapleton F, et al. Potential sources of bacteria that are isolated from contact lenses during wear. *Optom Vis Sci* 1997;74:1030.

274. Stapleton F, Dart JK, Matheson M, Woodward EG. Bacterial adherence and glycocalyx formation on unworn hydrogel lenses. *J Br CL Assoc* 1993;16:113.

275. Stapleton F, Dart J. *Pseudomonas* keratitis associated with biofilm formation on a disposable soft contact lens. *Br J Ophthalmol* 1995;79:864.

276. Rauschl RT, Rogers JJ. The effect of hydrophilic contact lens wear on the bacterial flora of the human conjunctiva. *Int Contact Lens Clin* 1978;5:56.

277. Tragakis MP, Brown SI, Pearce DB. Bacteriologic studies of contamination associated with soft contact lenses. *Am J Ophthalmol* 1973;75:496.

278. Callender MG, Tse LSY, Charles AM, Lutzi D. Bacterial flora of the eye and contact lens cases during hydrogel lens wear. *Am J Optom Physiol Opt* 1986;63:177.

279. Larkin DFP, Leeming JP. Quantitative alterations of the commensal eye bacteria in contact lens wear. *Eye* 1991;5:70.

280. Fleiszig SMJ, Efron N. Conjunctival flora in extended wear of rigid gas permeable contact lenses. *Optom Vis Sci* 1992;69:354.

281. Stapleton F, Willcox MDP, Fleming CM, et al. Changes to the ocular biota with time in extended- and daily-wear disposable contact lens use. *Infect Immunol* 1995;63:4501.

282. Gopinathan U, Stapleton F, Sharma S, et al. Microbial contamination of hydrogel contact lenses. *J Appl Microbiol* 1997;82: 653.

283. Thakur A, Willcox MD. Contact lens wear alters the production of certain inflammatory mediators in tears. *Exp Eye Res* 2000; 70:255.

284. Graham CM, Dart JKG, Wilson-Holt NW, Buckley RJ. Prospects for contact lens wear in aphakia. *Eye* 1988;2:48.

285. Eichenbaum JW, Feldstein M, Podos SM. Extended-wear aphakic soft contact lenses and corneal ulcers. *Br J Ophthalmol* 1982; 66:663.

286. Spoor TC, Hartel WC, Wynn P, Spoor DK. Complications of continuous-wear soft contact lenses in a nonreferral population. *Arch Ophthalmol* 1984;102:1312.

287. Cooper RL, Constable IJ. Infective keratitis in soft contact lens wearers. *Br J Ophthalmol* 1977;61:250.

288. Lemp MA, Blackman HJ, Wilson LA, Leveille AS. Gram-negative corneal ulcers in elderly aphakic eyes with extended-wear lenses. *Ophthalmology* 1984;91:60.

289. Sjostrand J, Linner E, Nygren B, et al. Severe corneal infection in a contact lens wearer. *Lancet* 1981;17:149.

GAS-PERMEABLE EXTENDED WEAR

EDWARD S. BENNETT
CAROL TAM
CRISTINA M. SCHNIDER
ROBERT M. GROHE
AND RAJNI SINGH

The introduction of gas-permeable (GP) extended-wear contact lens materials has provided practitioners with a potentially safer, healthier alternative than presently available (nonsilicone) hydrogel lens materials. Many GP extended-wear lens materials recently have been introduced to practitioners, with one being approved by the US Food and Drug Administration (FDA) for 30-day continuous wear. This chapter will describe the clinical applications, fitting, care, and complications associated with this modality.

CLINICAL APPLICATIONS AND BENEFITS

Patient and practitioner interest in extended wear, which was quite high in the 1980s, decreased in the following decade, primarily as a result of reports hydrogel lens–induced complications (1–3). However, the recent introduction of silicone hydrogel and GP lenses for continuous wear appears to have resulted in worldwide growth in this modality although GP extended wear represents only 2% of GP lenses prescribed in the United States (4).

The primary reason given for the low rate of use of GP lenses for extended wear is the relative ease of fitting hydrogel lenses compared to GP lenses. Other factors may include a practitioner unwillingness to ask the patient to undergo even a brief period of adaptation with new GP lenses and because of patient apprehension to wear GP lenses overnight.

Gas-permeable lenses offer a number of advantages over hydrogel lenses, particularly for extended wear (5). These include superior optics and visual performance; verifiable and reproducible parameters that can be modified, if needed, to improve fit, vision, and comfort; easier (and potentially safer) care regime, improved physiologic performance; and durability (5,6). Table 35.1 compares the various features of hydrogel and GP extended-wear materials.

The most important advantage of GP extended-wear lens materials over their hydrogel counterparts is safety. Hydrogel lens-induced complications are primarily the result of four limitations of the materials and designs used: (7)

■ Insufficient oxygen transmission
■ Lens surface deposition/contamination
■ Limbal compression/seal-off
■ Porous polymer composition

Insufficient oxygen transmission results in corneal hypoxia, which can be manifested in several forms (microcystic edema, edematous corneal formations) (8,9). However, whereas non–silicone-containing hydrogel lenses are limited by having to depend on the specific water content for oxygen permeability, GP lens materials can incorporate several "dry" monomers that can provide much higher oxygen permeability.

Hydrogel lens surface contaminations, particularly mucoprotein complexes, have been associated with giant papillary conjunctivitis (GPC) (10). They also have been shown to act as a substrate for bacterial adherence (11). GPC leads to decreased wearing time or discontinuation from lens wear for an indefinite period of time and is the leading cause of discontinuing hydrogel contact lens extended wear (12). Deposits are not as adherent to GP lens materials nor do they invade the matrix of the lens and, therefore, they are more easily removed. This characteristic of GP lens materials probably lessens the probability of GPC as well as of serious eye infections.

Limbal compression by a hydrogel extended-wear lens also has ocular health implications. Acute red eye, a nonulcerative keratoconjunctivitis, characterized by marked conjunctival hyperemia, corneal infiltrates, pain, photophobia, and lacrimation, generally noted in the early morning (12), is postulated to be the result of debris accumulated beneath an immobile lens. Because of the better exchange of tears and debris during open-eye periods with GP lenses, a red eye is not usually a problem, despite the fact that GP lenses do adhere to the cornea to some degree during sleep. Fur-

TABLE 35.1. COMPARISON OF BENEFITS HYDROGEL VERSUS GP EXTENDED WEAR

	Hydrogel	Rigid
Parameter availability	Limited	Unlimited
Manufacturing reliability, verifiability	Poor–good	Good–excellent
Fitting expertise required	Minimal	Moderate Good–excellent
Visual performance	Fair–good	Good–excellent
Oxygen transmission	Poor–fair (hydrogel) to excellent (S-H)	
Initial comfort	Good–excellent	Poor–good
Long-term comfort	Fair–good	Good
Replacement frequency	1 week to 3 months	6 months to 2 years
Modification possible	None	In most cases
Dehydration	Significant	Minimal
Soilage	Progressive	Manageable

GP, gas permeable.

thermore, the smaller-diameter GP lens does not usually impinge on the limbus.

Finally, dehydration of a hydrogel lens material can both provide a steeper fitting relationship and reduce oxygen transmission through the lens (13). As GP lens materials absorb very little water, dimensional stability (base curve) changes are very uncommon, except in cases of inappropriate handling.

PATIENT SELECTION

Patient Requirements

Perhaps the most important factor in achieving a successful GP extended-wear lens experience is to prescreen the potential patients properly. Studies have shown a very strong link between patient factors (compliance with lens regimen, personal hygiene, and habits such as smoking) and serious corneal complications resulting from extended wear (2,14,15). Some of the more important factors are discussed below.

Vision Correction

Extended wear may be deemed a visual luxury item. Patient attitudes can be somewhat causal when determining need based on visual correction factors alone. However, the increased rate of complications with this modality should more than justify a careful assessment of the appropriateness of extended wear for visual need (16).

Extended wear should be limited to the use of materials that meet the corneal oxygen demand (to be discussed) as many lens materials today—predominantly hydrogel—do not provide adequate oxygen to the cornea throughout the wearing cycle, and evidence suggests that oxygen deprivation damage is irreversible to a large degree. Daily wear should, therefore, be the primary recommendation and extended wear should be prescribed—in a highly oxygen-transmissible material—to patients who demonstrate, not only desire, but some vocational, avocational, or medical need.

Binocular status can create a dilemma for teenagers and young adults. The desire for hassle-free lens wear for this very active age group is high, yet this is also the prime time of myopia onset and progression. A careful binocular assessment should be made on patients with low or suspected myopia progression before contact lenses are prescribed. Many low myopes who habitually read without spectacles can be pushed over the edge binocularly when contact lenses are prescribed for full-time wear. Extended wear may add even more opportunities for stress in a fragile visual system. The increase in accommodative demand for moderate and high degrees of myopia, especially for patients nearing the age of 40 years or with poor binocular skills, may be another contraindication to lens wear generally, and extended wear in particular.

The visual needs of some patients with high myopia, hyperopia, and aphakia often are particularly suited to extended wear, in view of the optical distortion inherent in spectacle prescriptions (17). However, these prescriptions result in thicker lenses and are often accompanied by poorer physiologic performance. GP lenses are particularly advantageous for the hyperopic patient as a result of high oxygen transmission (18). These patients should be informed by the practitioner of the physical limitations of their lenses, as well as their relative advantages.

Vocational Needs

Contact lenses are often viewed in terms of social advantages, without consideration for their function in a work environment. Extended wear requires assessment of the needs and potential hazards in the work place. While a number of studies and case reports have documented the protective ability of GP contact lenses in industrial accidents (19), they are not substitutes for safety goggles or spectacles. In some places of business, contact lenses are actually forbidden in the work place, while in others their use is only restricted to persons with minimal level of uncorrected visual acuity. Generally, dusty environments or those with noxious fumes and vapors are not conducive to GP lens wear.

Less threatening, but probably more troublesome in the work place, are air conditioning systems, computer terminals, and forced-air heating or ventilation systems. All are instrumental in decreasing the ambient humidity or altering the blink rate of contact lens wearers, leading to signs and symptoms of dryness and lens intolerance. Adequate instructions in maintaining normal blink habits, in-eye lubricants, or a humidifier often are effective in reducing or eliminating these problems.

Motivation

A suitably motivated patient makes every practitioner's work easier. Whatever the reason for the motivation, such patients are more likely to take an active part in the lens care process and often will gladly endure minor difficulties in the fitting and adaptation process. However, this motivation sometimes can be misdirected and result in some abuse of wearing schedules and follow-up care. All patients must be made aware of the responsibilities that accompany wearing an extended-wear lens, and should be encouraged to report any unusual occurrence.

Patient Expectations and Experience

A clear understanding of the patient's perception of extended wear is necessary to provide an optimal extended-wear experience. Non–lens-wearers may be anxious about the insertion and removal process, while experienced wearers are more likely seeking a minimal maintenance care regimen. Both types of patients must be informed of the need for good lens handling and care, regardless of frequency of removal. Previous lens wearers should be questioned carefully about the reason for desiring a change in wearing schedule. Problems relating to hydrogel lenses, such as edema, lid problems, and poor vision often are eliminated when switching to GP lenses. However, previous rigid lens problems, such as dryness, may be magnified with extended wear. In the case of previous GP failure, a trial period of daily wear using the extended-wear material is essential. If material-related problems (deposit, drying) can be overcome, extended wear may be successful. Discomfort and poor adaptation with GP lenses sometimes can be overcome with extended wear by having the patient remove, rinse, soak, then reinsert the lenses just prior to retiring, since movement is minimal during sleep, making the lenses quite comfortable. While daily-wear adaptation prior to beginning extended wear is preferable, this technique can help a sensitive wearer accelerate the adaptation period.

Practitioner Assessment

Selection of patients for extended wear requires careful inspection and consideration of all factors involved in the normal daily wear assessment. A discussion of several factors follows.

Ocular and General Health Questions

The same questions required for daily-wear assessment apply to GP extended wear, but may be even more significant in this modality. While allergies alone do not preclude extended wear, the use of antihistamines may cause unacceptable alterations in the tear film, leading to problems such as staining and binding. Diabetes or any other conditions associated with poor wound healing, depression sensitivity, or immunosuppression should rule out extended wear. Patients with ocular abnormalities, such as keratoconus, or postsurgical, such as penetrating keratoplasty or LASIK, also are not suited to extended wear. Other poor candidates for GP extended-wear lenses may be those who have experienced multiple corneal abrasions or scarring.

Ocular Topography

This should include the entire anterior bulbar surface, including the sclera and limbus in addition to the cornea. While unusual corneal topography typically can be managed with the appropriate lens design, limbal and scleral abnormalities, such as pingueculae and pterygia can pose more difficult problems (20). The presence of a pterygium generally contraindicates a GP extended-wear schedule, because of the proximity of vascular elements and the increased inflammatory potential. Patients with pingueculae may be successful in extended wear, but should be followed closely on a daily-wear schedule prior to commencement of extended wear. Significant peripheral corneal or conjunctival staining, ocular redness, or engorgement of limbal vessels that cannot be managed with a change in diameter or edge configuration indicate a poor prognosis for extended wear.

Tear Layer Characteristics

Because of the less frequent cleaning inherent in an extended-wear schedule, a good tear layer is essential. Observation of the oily layer using specular reflection, or the Guillon apparatus, can be particularly useful (21). An excess of lipid or debris, evidenced by deeply colored fringes and dark globules in the marbled appearance of the oil layer of the tears, can be a sign of a potentially heavy lipid depositor. When generally evident with daily wear, the dry ocular environment during sleep and with decreased frequency of cleaning with extended wear can exacerbate the problem. Patients with mucous- or aqueous-deficient tear films typically represent poor extended-wear candidates.

Lid Appearance

Careful documentation of lid redness and smoothness must be made prior to initiation of an extended-wear schedule. Lid problems can flare up quite suddenly with extended wear, particularly in patients with a prior history of lid inflammation with GP or hydrogel lenses.

Signs of chronic blepharitis, such as scaliness of the lids and lashes and hordeola may indicate the potential for a secondary staphylococcal keratitis. These patients should be successful with an intensive lid hygiene regimen prior to considering extended wear.

Corneal Physiological Status

This assessment must include limbus-to-limbus, epithelium-to-endothelium examination of the cornea with both white light and fluorescein. The presence of significant ghost vessels, neovascularization, or limbal engorgement with GP daily wear may signal the potential for more rapid vascular response following future insult. Signs of possible high oxygen demand include epithelial microcysts, increased visibility of epithelial and stromal nerve fibers, decreased transparency of the stroma, and polymegethism of the endothelium. All these findings are frequently observed in cases of long-term chronic hypoxia as well as corneal dystrophies. Hypoxic changes indicate the need for very high oxygen-transmissibility levels in the lens material, while extended wear should be avoided completely with dystrophies.

Corneal staining should be minimal prior to commencing extended wear. The presence of any significant staining, whether large in extent or coalescent over a smaller area, should be viewed as a contraindication of extended wear. Heavy or localized conjunctival staining may indicate a marginal dry eye and, therefore, also a guarded prognosis for extended wear. The use of a yellow Wratten #12 gelatin filter over the objective or eyepieces of the slit lamp greatly enhances the appearance of fluorescein with cobalt blue light and is invaluable in accurately assessing corneal and conjunctival staining and fluorescein patterns.

MATERIAL SELECTION, LENS DESIGN, AND FITTING

Selection of suitable lens for each patient involves not only consideration of lens design and fit, but also of lens material, which will influence several other characteristics. The increase in oxygen permeability available with the newer GP materials is a result of either the introduction of new fluorinated polymer components or a change in the formulation ratio of components used in lower permeability materials.

Material Characteristics and Selection

The primary criterion for GP material selection should pertain to meeting the Holden-Mertz criteria for no residual corneal swelling (i.e., no corneal swelling within a few hours of awakening) (22). Therefore, the lens material should have an oxygen transmission (Dk/t) of, at minimum, 34. This can typically be achieved with a high-Dk [51 to 99] material for myopic extended wear and a hyper Dk [≥ 100] for a hyperopic patient (23). It is important to understand that a +3.00 D lens is about two times the center thickness of

a −3.00 D lens. If center thickness (not average thickness) is used and Dk/t equals the material oxygen permeability divided by the thickness (in mm) times 10, the following example demonstrates the importance of hyper Dk materials in hyperopia. If the center thickness of a −3.00 D high [60] Dk lens is 0.15 mm and of a +3.00 D hyper [120] Dk lens material is 0.30 mm, the oxygen transmission of both lenses is 40 as shown below:

* High-Dk −3.00 D Myope: $60/0.15 \times 10 = 40$
* Hyper-Dk +3.00 D Hyperope: $120/0.30 \times 10 = 40$

Therefore, in both cases, these lenses meet the Holden-Mertz criterion. Extended-wear lens materials are listed in Table 35.2 (24).

The Berkeley Contact Lens Extended Wear Study (CLEWS) found equivalence, when comparing the success rate of medium-Dk versus high-Dk GP lens materials over a 12 month period (25,26). However, it was important to note that the lens discontinuation from contact lens–associated keratopathies was over three times higher in the medium-Dk group.

Several hyper-Dk lens materials are FDA approved for extended wear. Representative examples include Boston XO (Polymer Technology Corporation, Rochester, NY), Paragon HDS 100 (Paragon Vision Sciences, Mesa, AZ) and Menicon Z (Menicon Co., Ltd., Nagoya, Japan, manufactured in the United States by Con-Cise Contact Lens Co., San Leandro, CA). The Boston XO is one of the lens materials introduced in recent years by Polymer Technology (other materials include Boston EO and Boston ES) utilizing their AEROCOR process, which results in a lower silicone content while providing an oxygen-permeable backbone and an oxygen-permeable cross-linker relative to their previous materials (27). The Paragon HDS 100 is one of a series of lens materials recently introduced by Paragon Vision Sciences (also including Paragon Thin and Paragon HDS) using their hyperpurification process, which, in effect, sorts silicone molecules to select more oxygen-efficient silicone (28).

The Menicon Z lens material is a derivative of fluoromethacrylate in combination with siloxanylstyrene and benzotriazol (an ultraviolet light absorber) (29). The Menicon Z has the additional benefit of being FDA approved for up to 30 days of continuous wear (30,31). In a comparison of the success rate between the Menicon Z, worn for 30 days of continuous wear, and the Acuvue, worn for 7 days of extended wear, an equal percent of patients completed the 12-month investigation (32). However, the Acuvue lens resulted in a greater incidence of adverse events, notably, bacterial infections. In addition, the Acuvue lens resulted in greater corneal swelling (by an average of 3%), increased striae and microcysts, and polymegethism (33,34). The Menicon Z lens did not result in significant endothelial morphology changes. It was also important to note that two thirds of the Menicon Z wearers were able to wear their

TABLE 35.2. GAS-PERMEABLE EXTENDED-WEAR LENS MATERIALS

Lens	Manufacturer	Composition	Dk
Menicon Z*	Menicon/Concise Contact Lens Lab	FS/A	163–250
Fluoroperm 151†	Paragon Vision Science	FS/A	151
Equalens II†	Polymer Technology Corp.	FS/A	85
Paragon HDS 100†‡	Paragon Vision Science	FS/A	100
Boston XO	Polymer Technology Corp.	FS/A	100
Fluoroperm 92†	Paragon Vision Science	FS/A	92
Fluoroperm 60†	Paragon Vision Science	FS/A	60
Fluorocon	Ciba Vision	FS/A	60
Paragon HDSc	Paragon Vision Science	Paflufocon B	58
Paraperm EW†	Paragon Vision Science	S/A	56
Equalens†	Polymer Technology Corp.	FS/A	47

FS/A, fluorosilicone/acrylate; S/A, silicone/acrylate.
* FDA approved for 30-day extended wear.
† FDA approved for 7-day extended wear.
‡ FDA approved for overnight CRT use.
From Thompson TT. *Tyler's Quarterly* soft contact tens, parameter guide. *Tylers Q* 2003; 20: 52, 53, 56, with permission.

lenses, at minimum, for 22 days continuously. In fact, it was found that, in addition to silicone hydrogel lens materials, 30 nights of continuous wear of these lens materials did not result in a significant increase in *Pseudomonas aeruginosa* binding to the lens surface after 12 months (35). It was concluded that these lens materials may decrease the risk for microbial infections by 10 to 40 times.

It is important to select a highly oxygen-transmissible lens material that will result in stable, comfortable vision for the patient (36). For that reason it is advantageous to diagnostically fit the same material as the one to be ordered for the extended-wear GP patient. As these lenses are softer and more flexible than their lower-Dk counterparts, the possibility of flexure is present. It has been found that fitting a lens with apical alignment to slight apical bearing will minimize flexure (37–39). For patients with with-the-rule (WTR) astigmatism, the lid tends to exert an against-the-rule force on a lens, versus the WTR pull of corneal forces. This is in contrast to increasing lens thickness, which has an adverse effect on oxygen transmission and is, therefore, not a desirable option for extended-wear lenses. Flexure can be assessed by performing keratometry over the lens; if the values are toric, flexure is present.

Lens Design and Fitting

Gas-permeable lenses for extended wear must be designed and fitted to control a number of factors, including comfort, vision, physiology, and corneal topography. By using the same material and design for both diagnostic fitting and ordering, lens flexure, wetting, and centration characteristics of the patient's lenses should be similar to the diagnostic fit. To confirm the presence of flexure during the fitting, it is recommended that keratometry and retinoscopy be performed over the diagnostic lenses, especially if a spherical

overrefraction provides reduced acuity when compared to the best-corrected spectacle visual acuity (40,41). A base curve radius that is too steep can result in flexure-related visual acuity reduction and midperipheral bearing with resultant peripheral corneal staining. In addition, it has also been suggested that poorly wetting lenses may be associated with increase in 3- and 9-o'clock staining (42).

The choice of lens design is largely individual but not too dissimilar than that recommended for a daily-wear design (see Chapter 13). Certainly, there have been numerous recommendations for the fitting philosophy of these designs (43–46). A patient having an upper lid overlapping the superior limbus can benefit from a large diameter (≥ 9.4 mm), tucked underneath the upper lid or lid attachment alignment fitting relationship, to optimize initial comfort and minimize flare (47,48) (Fig. 35.1). This typically requires a base curve radius equal to, or slightly flatter than,

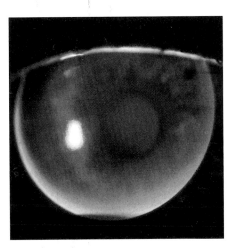

FIG. 35.1. Optimum rigid extended-wear fit and fluorescein pattern.

the flattest corneal meridian. For highly positioned upper lids, a smaller-diameter (i.e., typically 8.8 to 9.0 mm) lens, fit steeper than "K" to achieve an interpalpebral fitting relationship, is recommended. A bitoric lens may be necessary with patients exhibiting two or more diopters of astigmatism. This design can provide better centration and comfort than a spherical design and theoretically, better oxygen transmission as well (49). A steeper base curve radius may be necessary to obtain good centration with patients who are hyperopic. The edges should be thin and not interfere with the normal blinking process. Flexure should not be a consideration with the center thickness necessary for plus power lenses.

A well-centered lens is also important. This can be optimized by ordering the lens at a minimal thickness (but thick enough to offset the effects of flexure). The use of a minus lenticular edge is recommended for all plus and low-minus powers and a plus lenticular for all high-minus lenses for the same purpose.

An important factor for a successful fitting relationship is good tear exchange. This minimizes adherence as well as disruption of the corneal epithelial cell layer (50). To minimize focal bearing areas and promote free exchange of tears and flushing of debris, lenses should be well-blended at all peripheral curve junctions. The amount of edge lift desirable for extended wear is a hotly debated topic among panels of experts. Literature on daily wear suggests maintaining a thin edge and minimum edge lift to minimize lid gap and, therefore, peripheral staining (51). However, studies that target known stainers support a different conclusion for extended wear. These studies have reported that incidence of severe staining was higher for designs with a lower edge lift (42, 52). It has also been shown that as edge clearance decreases, the incidence of lens adherence increases (46). The effect of edge width on peripheral staining also is very significant, and a wide (0.4 mm), well-blended edge with moderate clearance is advocated. This can be achieved with a well-blended tricurve or tetracurve design as described in Chapter 13.

It should be noted, however, that specifying a design in the absence of information about corneal shape is not ideal. A cornea that tends to be more spherical than average may show excessive amounts of edge clearance with these designs when fitted to give apical alignment. Similarly, a cornea with a high degree of asphericity may display insufficient edge clearance and/or midperipheral bearing, as edge lift calculations (axial or radial) assume a spherical cornea, while actual clearances include variations in corneal shape factor. The use of a corneal topography system provides more valuable information for fitting purposes than the standard keratometer.

As noted before, the center thickness ordered for rigid extended-wear lenses should be great enough to minimize flexure, but not so thick that it compromises oxygen transmission. Verification of center thickness is an important part of the lens evaluation process. As mass increases with increasing center thickness, this can adversely affect fitting and performance characteristics. Fortunately, advances in polymer chemistry and lens manufacturing have resulted in the introduction of hyper-Dk lens materials that can be manufactured in center thicknesses not much greater than low-Dk materials.

Finally, the edge configuration and finish are extremely important in assuring good comfort with GP lenses. An ideal thickness has been reported to be approximately 0.09 mm, but a large variation of tolerance has been observed (53). A centrally or posteriorly placed apex was found to be more comfortable than one that was placed anteriorly, and it was found that a gradual taper from the edge (thus voiding a sharp angle on the anterior lens surface) is a key factor for improving lens comfort. However, since oxygen permeable lens materials require careful machining because of their softer composition, the possibility of edge defects must be ruled out. Careful inspection of every lens edge in both the frontal plane and in profile is recommended. Once again, however, in recent years manufacturing advancements have resulted in more consistent and reproducible high- and hyper-Dk lenses.

PATIENT EDUCATION AND FOLLOW-UP CARE

Frequent and thorough patient education and follow-up care is essential to the success of any contact lens patient, but particularly so in the case of extended wear. This permits early detection of potential problems to allow for modification in lens fit, material or wearing schedule to avoid more serious consequences.

Patient Education

Proper patient education must begin at the first moment of contact with the patient. A thorough exploration of the patient's expectations should occur, followed by a complete discussion of the concept of extended wear, its risk, and its responsibilities. Extended wear requires even more attention to detail than daily wear, and noncompliant daily-wear lens patients are, therefore, not good candidates.

Instructional slides, photographs, CD-ROMs, or videotapes can be employed to enhance patient education as described elsewhere. The written instructions should include application and removal techniques, cleaning and disinfection solutions and procedures, cosmetics, wearing schedule, and, ideally, should contain a consent agreement. The latter is particularly important for both patient compliance and legal purposes. Patients should read and sign a consent form that details the problems and complications that can occur with extended-wear lenses, as well as the number of follow-up visits to be scheduled (54). This form could be in duplicate at the back of the instruction booklet with one copy for placement in the patient record.

Follow-up Schedule

A necessary prerequisite for GP lens extended wear should be successful GP lens daily wear. Therefore, first-time wearers should be allowed to adapt to their lenses on a daily-wear basis before beginning an extended-wear schedule. Previous polymethylmethacrylate (PMMA) or hydrogel lens patients also generally benefit from daily-wear adaptation, although the process may be more rapid in these persons. Daily wear adaptation allows a period of time for patients to gain confidence and proficiency in lens care and handling and an opportunity to identify any contraindication to extended wear.

Many practitioners recommend a gradual increase in wearing time, from 4 hours the first day, increasing 1 hour each day. However, it is unlikely that oxygen deprivation will be a problem with GP extended-wear materials, as is the case with very-low-Dk GP and PMMA lenses. Therefore, the patient can be advised to build up wearing time on an as-tolerant basis to a maximum period of 8 to 12 hours, with certain restrictions. Alterations in blink habits and tear film stability are not unusual with new wearers, and most often result in signs and symptoms of dry eyes. If the eyes become red, itchy, dry, or scratchy, lens-rewetting drops should be instilled. If relief occurs, lens wear may be continued. If signs and symptoms are not alleviated by the use of drops, the lenses should be removed, and lens wear resumed later in the day or on the following day. If symptoms persist, despite removal of the lenses, or if wearing time cannot be increased each day, the patient should contact their practitioner. Under no circumstances should the patient exceed the recommended maximum wearing time, even if the lenses are comfortable.

At every progress examination, the following procedures should be performed:

1. Pertinent case history
2. Visual acuity
3. Overrefraction
4. Overkeratometry
5. Biomicroscopy with lenses on (white light and fluorescein)
6. Biomicroscopy with lenses off (white light and fluorescein)
7. Visual acuities through baseline (pre–extended-wear) refraction
8. Refraction and visual acuity
9. Keratometry
10. Lens inspection/verification

The case history should include information pertaining to vision, including extent and duration of any morning blur (a symptom of excessive overnight swelling), comfort,

care regimen and wearing schedule, patient detection of lens adherence (obvious immobility of lens on awakening, redness, marked decreased lens sensation in the morning), and overall satisfaction.

Visual acuity, overrefraction, and over-Ks should be compared to baseline (lens issue) findings to identify possible lens flexure or warpage problems. Biomicroscopy with white light should be performed with lenses on to assess wettability and front- and back-surface deposits and debris. An increase in front-surface deposits can lead to undesirable lid changes (12,55). Heavy back-surface deposits and debris can be signs of poor cleaning techniques (20) or lens adherence (46). Fluorescein should then be instilled to allow observation of fitting patterns, tear flow characteristics, and the relationship of any staining to lens position and movement.

Examination of the lids and lash margins, palpebral and bulbar conjunctiva, limbal vasculature, and cornea should be performed, both with white light and fluorescein with the Wratten #12 and cobalt light. Red-free filters may enhance the appearance of the vascular tissues. The presence of any conjunctival chemosis, loss of clarity of the cornea, epithelial wrinkling, epithelial microcysts, striae, folds or endothelial blebs or polymegethism should be noted, along with a grading of lid hyperemia and papillae. Any staining of the cornea or conjunctiva should be graded and described or drawn. Careful observation of the pattern of tear film breakup may show evidence of lens binding. (Observation of an arcuate area of tear film breakup in a consistent location may be a subtle sign of lens adherence.) Fluorescein assessment of the lids is often helpful in highlighting lumps and bumps of the palpebral conjunctiva.

Prior to performing a postrefraction, visual acuity performed through the baseline (pre–extended-wear fit) refraction should be recorded to assess possible spectacle blur. A reduction of greater than one line from the original value may signal undesirable corneal changes caused by poor fit or physiology (56). A full refraction and visual acuities should follow. A decrease in WTR astigmatism or sphericalization of the cornea is expected with any rigid lens. However, other significant refractive changes should not occur in most persons.

Keratometry should be performed on lens removal, with a notation made on mire clarity (related to regularity of the tear film) and distortion (related to corneal regularity). Corneal topography images are especially valuable in detecting signs of lens adherence. Keratometric changes should be limited to primarily to the aforementioned sphericalization of the cornea.

Inspection of the lens for cleanliness, base curve stability, and surface and edge integrity should be performed routinely, and in any case of unexplained poor vision or comfort. Base curve radius change, typically flattening or warpage, can occur with high-Dk GP lenses.

A follow-up visit after approximately 1 week of daily wear should be scheduled, preferably at a time near the end of the recommended wearing time. If there are no contraindications to extended wear at this visit, the patient should be scheduled for an early morning visit following the first night of lens wear. Patients who are experiencing adaptation problems on daily wear, or lens deposits, should not begin extended wear until or unless these problems are rectified.

The first morning visit should be scheduled within 2 hours of eye opening, as signs of excessive overnight swelling and lens binding are more difficult to detect after this time. If any signs or symptoms of these conditions are elicited, a second visit should be scheduled for mid-to-late morning and if signs are still present, a change in material or wearing schedule (for edema) or return to daily wear (for binding) is indicated. Additional extended wear visits should be scheduled at 1 week, 2 weeks, 1 month, and 3 months after initiating extended wear, and every 3 months thereafter. Patients should remove the lenses overnight for cleaning and disinfection at least once a week, although some patients may require additional cleaning or overnight removals. It is advisable to have the patient select a specific night(s) for removal to facilitate setting a routine.

Frequent lens replacement should help minimize deposit- and warpage-related problems (36,57). With hyper-Dk lens materials, at minimum, replacement every 12 months is recommended.

Care Regimen

As lens materials become more complex, so does the accompanying care system. While it can be said generally that solution systems that are suitable for daily wear should be acceptable for extended wear, there are some notable exceptions. Because of the high-Dk FS/A polymers are chemically distinct from S/A and PMMA materials (and often even from each other), each will react slightly differently to exposure of different solutions. Therefore, the use of the manufacturer's recommended care system is the safest option, and deviation from the prescribed regimen may invalidate any warranty claims.

Perhaps the most important part of the care regimen is proper cleaning. The lens should be cleaned with surfactant cleaner immediately after removal to remove loosely bound deposits before they dry and become more adherent. Cleaning in the palm, as with hydrogel lenses, is preferred to "between the fingers" because of the possibility of lens warpage or breakage. Patients wearing a hyper-Dk lens material who have been previous PMMA or early-generation GP lens wearers may be especially prone to problems with care systems, because of long-standing poor care habits. Studies have shown a significantly higher percentage of warpage with previous PMMA lens wearers refitted into GP extended-wear materials than former GP lens, hydrogel lens, or new lens wearers (55,58). Problems with warpage may necessitate use of a cotton swab for cleaning or the mechanical cleaning machines. Other recommended cleaning proce-

dure should be considered as well. These are discussed in Chapter 14.

Because of the lowered affinity of F-S/A materials for protein, enzymatic cleaning may not be required for all patients. Observation of a matte texture or chalky white film on the lens surface is an indication of a protein buildup and shows the need for more frequent or vigorous cleaning or the addition of an enzyme cleaner to the regimen. Surfactant cleaners with friction enhancing agents (i.e., the Boston Cleaner, Polymer Technology Corp.) or sponge (Menicon) may help alleviate the buildup, although care should be taken not to exert excessive pressure with these methods as a change in power or surface characteristics may result.

The application of rewetting drops or saline is important both to rinse away trapped debris at bedtime and to enhance lens movement and comfort on awakening. In addition, the use of drops during the day for deposit-prone patients will both rinse away debris and rewet the lenses (59). Nonpreserved drops are recommended for frequent use.

Cosmetics can be a particular problem with GP extended-wear lenses, as lanolin, oils, perfumes, and any gel-like substance can easily coat the surface and result in hydrophobic wetting surfaces. Likewise, mascara can become trapped under the lens, possibly resulting in a foreign body–induced corneal abrasion. Cosmetics should be applied after lens insertion with one of the hand soaps formulated for contact lens wearers.

Modification

Whether or not GP extended-wear lens materials should be modified in the office is a matter of debate (60,61). However, if special precautions are taken, it is likely that the particular modification will be successful. During each modification procedure, a slow spindle speed ($\leq$ 1,000 rpm), application of light pressure, and the liberal use of polish are recommended in an effort to reduce the effects of heat, which can affect the surface wettability of the lens and result in surface cracking or crazing (61,62).

COMPLICATIONS

Studies of patients wearing GP extended-wear lenses have shown a very low complication rate, especially when compared to those studying hydrogel extended-wear lens materials (32,63,64). Frequently reported hydrogel extended-wear complications, such as GPC, corneal infiltrates, acute red eye, and corneal neovascularization, are rare with GP materials, and are generally more easily predicted and managed when they do occur.

Discomfort

Two clinical studies in which patients were fitted with one GP and one hydrogel extended-wear lens resulted in patients preferring the comfort and performance of the GP lens after adaptation was achieved, although it is important to note that these studies were performed prior to the introduction of disposable lenses (5,65). In one study, seven patients preferred the comfort of the hydrogel lens, one the GP lens, and two had no preference at the 1-week visit. However, at the exit examination at 6 months, five patients preferred the comfort of the GP lens, three the hydrogel lens, and two had no preference. Rating for overall preference at the final examination were nine in favor of the GP lens, with only one in favor of the hydrogel lens. Better visual acuity, easier handling, and long-term comfort were cited as advantages of the GP material.

Nevertheless, minor awareness during the first week or two of lens wear for nonadapted wearers is expected. Studies have demonstrated that the use of a positive attitude when presenting GPs, avoiding terms such as discomfort and pain, complemented by the application of a topical anesthetic immediately prior to the initial application, have a significant impact in optimizing the initial GP experience as well as the patient's attitude about adaptation (66–68).

Irritation that persists or worsens with lens wear implies causes other than normal adaptive processes. The first step in such cases is to define the problem adequately with a good history relating to the time of onset, accompanying environmental influences (i.e., air conditioning, dust), nature of discomfort, and what, if anything, provides relief.

Irritation from lens dryness with a particular polymer can often be rectified by improved cleaning, blinking habits, or selecting an alternate material. A persistent lid sensation, or inhibition of the blink, may be caused by poorly shaped or beveled edge. Intermittent sharp pains or burning may result from a sharp edge. Careful inspection of the entire edge profile with a handheld loupe, or preferably, a projection magnifier, should identify any edge imperfection.

Acute onset discomfort in an adapted wearer also can signal a lens defect, such as edge chips, surface scratches or a more serious problem, such as an epithelial abrasion. Inspection of the lens on and off the eye, as well as of the cornea, lids, and conjunctiva usually will provide the differential diagnosis. Foreign body sensation can be much more bothersome to high-Dk GP lens patients, particularly in the case of previous lens wearers, as the increased oxygen availability allows the return of some corneal sensitivity. Significant foreign body staining necessitates lens removal, particularly if the object is or was embedded, causing a full thickness epithelial defect. Lens wear generally can be assumed the day following epithelial healing when the cornea demonstrates uniform surface wetting.

The observation of epithelial erosion, not accompanied by other staining or obvious irritation, raises the suspicion of a basement membrane dystrophy or defect. A patient who shows recurrent erosions or a persistent area of cloudiness or microcysts should be considered a dystrophy suspect and should not continue in extended wear. Daily wear also may be impossible if the erosions continue.

Late-onset, gradual, or chronic discomfort may indicate lid problems, solution intolerance, lens deposits, or dry eye. The first step should be to clean the lenses thoroughly, and change solution systems if possible, to rule out solution sensitivity. Lens replacement as a second step should be considered if symptoms do not abate. The diagnosis of dry eyes often is made by default in these cases. Increasing the number of overnight removals, returning to a daily wear schedule, or lens removal for 15 minutes during the day may be necessary.

Vision Complaints

Even when an adequate visual result is achieved at the fitting visit, vision problems can surface at later visits. Fogginess or blur on insertion often indicates poor lens wetting or surface contamination. Adequate soaking prior to lens issue can help this problem. If contamination is noted, use of an approved in-office cleaner is indicated.

Onset of the above symptoms after a period of wear generally is related to poor surface wettability caused by a dry environment, poor blinking, or lens deposits. Rewetting or cleaning should solve the problem. If problems with visual acuity or poor contrast have resulted from a change in residual astigmatism, lens flexure usually is the cause, and performing keratometry over the lens will confirm the result. The preferred solution is to alter lens fitting characteristics, center thickness or material to optimize lens flexural characteristics.

Poor visual acuity that cannot be correlated with overrefraction often is associated with lens warpage. A warped lens will give a spherical reading on the lensometer, but a toric base curve reading on the radiuscope. The lens should be replaced and the patient reinstructed on lens care and handling if warpage is observed.

Hypoxia

There are many signs of corneal hypoxia that occur with lens wear, some of which are very subtle. Central corneal clouding is seldom observed with modern-day GP lenses, even on extended wear. Also, La Hood and associates (69) noted that fewer GP lens patients, when studied on awakening, exhibited vertical striae than soft lens patients with similar levels of overnight swelling. Therefore, the presence or absence of striae may not be a reliable indicator of unacceptable corneal swelling. Pachometric measurement of corneal thickness is the only reliable method of ascertaining the true level of corneal swelling, but is not practical in most clinical situations. Therefore, aside from the patient's report of persistent morning blur or observation of striae and folds, we may not be able to monitor adequately hypoxia in its acute stages.

Chronic changes, however, are much better indicators of insufficient oxygen levels in the cornea. The first, and most obvious sign of hypoxia occurs after approximately 3 months of extended wear. Epithelial microcysts are tiny pockets of cellular debris that are formed in the basal layer of the epithelium during periods of corneal stress (70). They appear as refractile bodies and characteristically exhibit reversed illumination in retro-illumination caused by greater refractive index of the microcyst versus a lower surrounding corneal refractive index. These small cystic formations then migrate through to the anterior layers of the epithelium, erupt through the anterior layers, and can be observed as small epithelial disruptions that stain with fluorescein. Microcysts appear and disappear in cycles; therefore, the number may vary considerably from visit to visit, but the presence of more than 10 at any given time is a sign of some level of corneal distress. Numbers exceeding 50 indicate a need for a change of wearing schedule or material. It should be noted that microcysts often increase in number for 2 or 3 months following cessation of extended wear, or a change in material, as they work their way through the epithelial tissue layers.

A less obvious, but detectable, change caused by hypoxia is endothelial polymegethism, or changes in the regularity of the size of endothelial cells, which is accompanied by pleomorphism, a change in cell shape (71). A simple analogy can be made to chicken wire: the normal young cornea appears as a uniform hexagonal array of roughly equal size and shape, much like chicken-wire mesh. As polymegethism increases, some cells increase in size while others decrease, until daisylike clusters appear, reminiscent of flower pop art from the 1960s and early 1970s. Observation of the endothelium requires specular reflection and high magnification ($\times 30$ to $\times 45$), or a specular microscope.

Although the consequences of long-term chronic hypoxia and polymegethism are still being investigated, the possibility of intraocular cataract surgery increases as a large segment of the population becomes older and medical science is better able to prolong life. Therefore, it seems prudent to protect patients from premature aging of the corneal tissue whenever possible. Fortunately, it is evident that the more recently introduced hyper-Dk and silicone hydrogel lens materials appear to result in very mild—and possibly insignificant—long-term change in corneal swelling and endothelial cell alteration (35).

Staining

The most common type of corneal staining seen with GP lens extended wear is peripheral corneal desiccation, or 3- and 9-o'clock staining. Occasional foreign body, indentation, or exposure staining is observed in some patients as well, but these generally do not represent major problems. Peripheral corneal desiccation staining can account for up to

one third of all lens–related discontinuations from extended wear, and while initially superficial, the staining can coalesce with accompanying engorgement of adjacent conjunctival blood vessels. In the most severe cases, peripheral corneal thinning occurs with ulceration, vascularization, and scarring (13,41). Patients who exhibit repeated occurrences of 3- and 9-o'clock staining of greater than grade 2 on the scale listed below should be returned to daily wear.

The following is a corneal desiccation grading system: (58)

0 = no staining
1 = widely scattered, discrete punctate spots
2 = scattered punctate spots with mild coalescence
3 = moderate coalescence
4 = severe coalescence, dellen, opacification, or neovascularization

Mild desiccation staining often can be managed with the frequent addition of rewetting drops and improved blinking habits. Moderate staining requires modification of lens design, while severe staining should contraindicate extended wear, and in some cases, daily wear as well.

Schnider (42,72) and Andrasko (52) recommended a slight increase in edge width or depth in chronic heavy stainers. In fact, it has been recommended that patients displaying significant levels of corneal staining not proceed to extended wear (72). Businger and associates (73) have developed an entire schema for managing 3- and 9-o'clock staining. Because of the difficulties in defining average edge lift, no one rule will always apply. However, the following considerations apply in most cases:

1. The anterior tear film must remain intact. Tapering the anterior edge, decreasing edge lift or changing diameter to minimize lid gap and facilitate proper blinking, or changing lens polymer to enhance lens wetting may provide some improvement.
2. The posterior tear film must be allowed to flow unrestricted. Maintenance of an uninterrupted tear film behind the lens by fitting to achieve apical alignment, blending to provide a smooth transition between peripheral curves, and widening or flattening the edge curve to provide a good tear meniscus may achieve these desired results.
3. Disruption to the mucus layer of the cornea must be avoided. Minimizing lens bearing on the corneal surface by avoiding excessively flat or steep fits, and designing the lens to traverse both horizontally and vertically across the entire corneal surface during normal blinks and eye movements should minimize staining.

Another more unusual observation on fluorescein evaluation is the corneal mosaic pattern, also referred to as the Fischer-Schweitzer pattern. This polygonal pattern does not

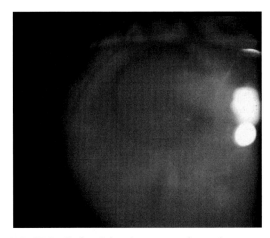

FIG. 35.2. Fischer-Schweitzer corneal mosaic pattern.

represent epithelial cell loss as with true staining, but instead a result of lens compression against the cornea (Fig. 35.2). It is often present on awakening, but usually disappears within a few hours. It may be related to corneal rigidity or the amount of corneal swelling.

Lens Adherence

Adherence of the lens to the cornea during sleep, or lens binding, has been reported in up to 50% of patients in GP lens extended-wear studies, (46,74,75) and probably occurs on a transient basis in nearly 100% of patients at some time (76). Lens-to-cornea adherence in the absence of lens movement with blinking was first described in 1979 with silicon rubber lenses (77). It was described as a contact adhesion of the lens to the cornea resulting in a suction effect. It was suggested that the primary factors responsible for lens adherence were negative pressure of the lens against the eye and surface hydrophobicity or poor quality of the precorneal tear film, and it was proposed that a large tear volume between the back surface of the lens (i.e., a steep central fit) and the front of the eye produced adherence via the negative centration forced exerted by the high pressure (78). Tears then were believed to be forcefully expelled from underneath the lens by the lid action, with the initial contact site being the midperipheral portion of the lens, eventually progressing to corneal seal off. A steep-fitting relationship could easily create the physical space capable of allowing a suction effect to occur. However, the most likely explanation for GP lens adherence pertains to changes in the tear film (79). Thinning of the post–lens-tear film during sleep leaves a very thin, highly viscous layer of mucus rich tears between the lens and cornea. On eye opening, the force imparted by the eyelid may be insufficient to initiate lens movement and the lens still remain bound until the mucus film is diluted and thinned by the gradual penetration of

aqueous tears. In clinical situations, both negative suction pressure and post–lens-tear film thinning may occur.

The patient with a bound lens is often asymptomatic, but may experience dryness or be aware of lens *sticking*. In fact, some patients report improved comfort when the lenses are bound. The adherent lens usually is located in a decentered position, often with the edge crossing the limbus (80). However, as most lenses begin moving spontaneously within 15 minutes of eye opening, observation of an immobile lens in the office is rare. Other slit-lamp signs of lens binding (in order of frequency or occurrence) include full or partial indentation ring (Fig. 35.3), central punctate keratitis, and peripheral arcuate staining.

When indentation rings form within the epithelium patients may become very uncomfortable. The use of a corneal topography system can be particularly helpful in identifying even mild corneal distortion caused by lens binding.

Most of the above signs disappear within 2 hours of the time that the lens begins to move, so morning aftercare visits should be scheduled as early as possible to maximize detection of lens adherence. Holden and associates (81) have documented severe disruption to the epithelium and stroma following long-term lens binding in cats. It also has been noted that lens binding is largely a patient dependent phenomenon and that lens design and material have little or no effect on the severity or frequency of binding in persons prone to binding (82). Lens binding has been associated with acute red eye reactions (13) and corneal ulceration (13,83). Therefore, patients who show persistent or severe binding should not continue in extended wear.

Adherence can be minimized by proper patient education. Patients should instill rewetting drops soon after awakening and use gentle pressure through the lower lid to nudge the lens and break any adherence that may be present. Cleaning the lenses and replacing as instructed by the practitioner will minimize posterior surface deposit-induced adherence. Maintaining the center thickness to a minimum and utilizing lenticulated designs will optimize centration, thereby reducing the potential for adherence.

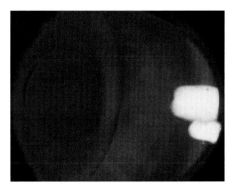

FIG. 35.3. An indentation ring present upon removal of a gas-permeable extended-wear lens.

Lid Changes

Giant Papillary Conjunctivitis

While a frequent complication with hydrogel lens extended wear, GPC is rarely reported with use of GP lenses, except in cases of heavy anterior lens surface deposits (13,55). However, as GP lenses become more commonly used and are worn for longer periods of time, GPC may become more prevalent in the GP population. Giant papillary conjunctivitis in rigid-lens wearers follows a different course than with hydrogel lenses (84). An increase in hyperemia and papillae is first seen near the lid margin (Allansmith's area 3) and changes progress toward the fold (area 1). These changes are reversed rapidly when lens wear is discontinued or a new, nondeposited lens is issued, but they also can appear and progress very rapidly. A thorough examination of the upper palpebral conjunctiva at each visit is required to minimize lid complications. Any increase in hyperemia or papillae should be managed by a more frequent and vigorous cleaning routine (addition of enzymes or adjunct cleaning materials) or lens replacement. Patients with previous hydrogel lens-induced lid complications may experience a recurrence of symptoms on GP extended wear, but return to daily wear often solves the problem.

Ptosis

Although the long-term significance of this problem is unknown, ptosis, induced by GP extended-wear lenses worn for a 2-month period in 5 to 11 patients, has been reported (85). In all cases, the ptosis resolved quickly after cessation of lens wear.

Vascularization

While extended-wear hydrogel lens patients have experienced various degrees of contact lens–related vascularization (86,87), GP extended wear patients have enjoyed a relative absence of vascular response. Previous reports in the literature of rigid lens vascularization have pertained primarily to PMMA lenses (88,89). However, a condition that appears to be predominantly extended wear in etiology is termed vascularized limbal keratitis (VLK) (90). Patients experiencing VLK manifest extensive staining of the corneal epithelium, limbus, and conjunctiva. There also are significant amounts of superficial and deep vascularization of the cornea. If the condition progresses, there will be a heaping of hyperplastic corneal epithelium, as noted in Fig. 35.4, which can form an infiltrate and eventually degenerate into peripheral corneal erosion. Any GP lens patient with active VLK will be very symptomatic with increased lens awareness, localized ocular pain, and reduced wearing time. Also, the patient will visualize a very red eye with an elevated corneal mass when looking into a mirror during self-inspection.

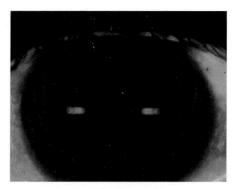

FIG. 35.4. Heaping mass of hyperplastic corneal epithelium in a patient with vascularized limbal keratitis.

Since the condition of VLK can progress through four stages (hyperplasia, inflammation, vascularization, erosion) it is important for the clinician to observe and monitor GP extended-wear patients routinely for any early signs or symptoms of VLK. It is important to note that in VLK patients, an inflammatory response in the form of an infiltrate and conjunctival hyperemia precedes the appearance of corneal vascularization. The inflammatory response appears to be mediated by a chronic mechanical insult to the limbus with resulting limbal and corneal desiccation.

Vascularized limbal keratitis appears to be independent of GP lens materials since all patients were successfully refit with the same material. There is one report by Elie (91) of a material-related vascular formation with a corneal nebula in a GP extended-wear patient. Regression of the lesion occurred only when there was a change in GP materials from low Dk to high Dk. There does, however, appear to be a strong association between VLK and GP lens designs that consist of a large diameter, a steep fitting relationship, and a very low edge clearance.

Treatment for VLK consists of discontinuation of lens wear from 2 days to 2 weeks, depending on the severity of the condition. A combination steroid–antibiotic should be prescribed during this time and the patient should be evaluated at 24 hours and frequently thereafter. A thorough evaluation of the lens-to-cornea fitting relationship should be performed, with particular emphasis given to the central and peripheral curve bearing relationships. If an existing lens has insufficient edge clearance, a peripheral curve modification may be all that is needed. If the base curve or diameter is viewed as the cause, it is best to redesign a new lens(es). Additional treatment for VLK can include the liberal use of lubricating drops, such as decongestants or antioxidants. Usually the best results are achieved when a lens is redesigned to a smaller diameter as shown in Fig. 35.5. This effectively reduces the mechanical irritation to the limbus and peripheral cornea.

The key goal in treatment is to remove the mechanical irritation (lens) and regress both the infiltrate and vasculari-

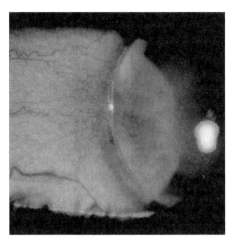

FIG. 35.5. A small-diameter gas-permeable lens designed to minimize and eliminate the clinical signs of vascularized limbal keratitis.

zation. This usually can be achieved within a 7- to 10-day period of no lens wear.

Corneal Topographical Changes

Early GP extended-wear clinical studies have shown a trend toward significant corneal flattening during the first month of wear, followed by steepening toward the baseline, with a vertical meridian flattening of 1.00 D reported (58,74, 92,93). As the horizontal meridian does not flatten as much, a sphericalization effect often results. Typically, there is also an accompanying reduction in myopia. However, studies with higher-oxygen-permeable materials have demonstrated fewer keratometric and refractive changes (75,94). As mentioned earlier, changes that result in sphericalization of the cornea with less than one line of change in visual acuity through the baseline spectacle prescription are probably acceptable. Any significant increase in myopia, astigmatism, or reduction in best-corrected spectacle acuity should warrant a change in design or material. The use of a corneal topography system can assist in determining any lens-induced changes in corneal shape as well as—via design software—recommend a lens design that may alleviate the problem.

SUMMARY

Gas-permeable extended-wear lenses have many advantages over their hydrogel lens counterparts, including ocular health, quality of vision, durability, ease of lens care, availability of custom designs, and ability to modify. However, any extended-wear material is only as successful as the ability of the practitioner to fit the lenses properly, educate the patient, and monitor ocular health. Many of the lens-in-duced problems are easily controlled if patients are carefully monitored on a regular basis.

REFERENCES

1. Review of Optometry brief article, " Patient sues Sterling," B& L 1985;122:3.
2. Schein OD, Glynn RJ, Poggio EC, et al. The relative risk of ulcerative keratitis among users of daily wear and extended wear soft contact lenses: a case control study. *New Engl J Med* 1989; 321:773–778.
3. Poggio EC, Glynn RJ, Schein OD, et al. The incidence of ulcerative keratitis among users of daily wear and extended wear soft contact lenses. *New Engl J Med* 1989;321:779–783.
4. Morgan PB, Efron N, Woods CA, et al. International contact lens prescribing in 2003. *Contact Lens Spectr* 2004;19:34–37.
5. Fonn D, Holden BA. RGP vs. hydrogel lenses for extended wear. *Am J Optom Physiol Opt* 1988;65:545–551.
6. Maehara J, Kastl P. Rigid gas permeable extended wear. *CLAO J* 1994;20:139–143.
7. Bennett ES, Ghormley NR. Rigid extended wear: an overview. *Int Contact Lens Clin* 1987;14:319–332.
8. Brennan NA, Coles MLC. Extended wear in perspective. *Optom Vis Sci* 1997;74:609–623.
9. Chahine T, Weissman B. Peripheral corneal furrow staining: a sign to discontinue hydrogel contact lens use. *Int Contact Lens Clin* 1996;23:229–233.
10. Fowler SA, Greiner JV, Allansmith MR. Soft contact lenses from patients with giant papillary conjunctivitis. *Am J Ophthalmol* 1987;8:1956.
11. Aswad M, Barza M, Kenyon K, et al. Bacterial adherence to extended wear soft contact lenses. *Invest Ophthalmol Vis Sci* 1989; 27(Suppl):166.
12. Grant T, Holden BA, Recgberger J, Chong MS. Contact lens related papillary conjunctivitis (CLPC): influence of protein accumulation and replacement frequency. *Invest Ophthalmol Vis Sci* 1989;30(Suppl):166.
13. Schnider CM, Zabkiewicz K, Holden BA. Unusual complications associated with RGP extended wear. *Int Contact Lens Clinic* 1988;15:124–129.
14. Cutter GR, Chalmers RL, Roseman M. The clinical presentation, prevalence, and risk factors of focal corneal infiltrates in soft contact lens wearers. *CLAO J* 1996;22:30–37.
15. Andrasko GJ. The amount and time course for soft contact lens dehydration. *J Am Optom Assoc* 1982;53:207.
16. Chalupa E, Swarbrick HA, Holden BA, Sjostrand S. Severe corneal infection associated with contact lens wear. *Ophthalmology* 1987;94:17–22.
17. Gurwood AS. Prescribing contact lenses for aphakes. *Contact Lens Spectr* 1995;10:17–23.
18. Gordon JM, Bennett ES. Dk revisited: the hypoxic corneal environment. Paper presented at: Annual Meeting of the American Academy of Ophthalmology, Chicago, IL, November 1993.
19. Rengstorff RH. Eye protection from contact lenses. *J Am Optom Assoc* 1974;45:274–275.
20. Terry R, Schnider C, Holden B. Maximizing success with rigid gas permeable extended wear lenses. *Int Contact Lens Clin* 1989; 16:169–175.
21. Guillon JP, Guillon M. Tear film examination of the contact lens patient. *Contax* 1988:14–18.
22. Holden BA, Mertz GW. Criteria oxygen levels to avoid corneal edema for daily and extended wear contact lenses. *Invest Ophthalmol Vis Sci* 1984;25:1161–1167.
23. Bennett ES. Gas permeable materials. In: Bennett ES, Hom MM,

eds. *Manual of gas permeable contact lenses,* 2nd ed. St. Louis: Elsevier, 2004:48–56.

24. Thompson TT. *Tyler's Quarterly* soft contact lens parameter guide. *Tylers Q* 2003;20:52,53,56.

25. Polse KA, Graham AD, Fusero RE, et al. The Berkeley contact lens extended wear study: part I. *Ophthalmology* 2001;108: 1381–1388.

26. Polse KA, Graham AD, Fusero RE, et al. The Berkeley contact lens extended wear study: part II. *Ophthalmology* 2001;108: 1389–1399.

27. Bennett ES, Levy B. Material selection. In: Bennett ES, Henry VA, eds. *Clinical manual of contact lenses,* 2nd ed. Philadelphia: Lippincott Williams & Wilkins, 2000:59–74.

28. Schachet JL, Rigel LE, Reeder KM et al. Rethinking the link between RGP lens performance. *Contact Lens Spectr* 1998;13: 43–47.

29. Menicon Z Web site [www.menicon.com]. Accessed July 2003.

30. Gleason W, Tanaka H, Albright R, et al. A 1-year prospective clinical trial of Menicon Z 30-day rigid gas permeable contact lenses worn on a continuous wear schedule. *Eye Contact Lens* 2003;29(1 Suppl):S2–S9.

31. Kogan BA. The benefits of oxygen permeable contact lenses. *Optom Management* 2002;37:57–58.

32. Gleason W, Albright R. Menicon Z 30-day continuous wear lenses: a clinical comparison to Acuvue 7-day extended wear lenses. *Eye Contact Lens* 2003;29(1 Suppl):S149–S152.

33. Pall B, Barr J, Szczotka L, et al. Corneal thickness results in the Menicon Z 30-day continuous wear and Acuvue 7-day extended wear contact lens clinical trial. *Eye Contact Lens* 2003;29(1 Suppl):S10–S13.

34. Barr JT, Pall B, Szczotka LB, et al. Corneal endothelial morphology results in the Menicon Z 30-day continuous wear contact lens clinical trial. *Eye Contact Lens* 2003;29(1 Suppl):S14–S16.

35. Ren DH, Yamamoto K, Ladage PM, et al. Adaptive effects of 30-night wear of hyper-02 transmissible contact lenses on bacterial binding and corneal epithelium. *Ophthalmology* 2002;109: 27–40.

36. Siedlecki I, Bennett ES. Gas permeable extended wear. In: Bennett ES, Hom MM, eds. *Manual of gas permeable contact lenses,* 2nd ed. St. Louis: Elsevier, 2004:380–395.

37. Harris MG, Chu CS. The effects of contact lens thickness and corneal toricity on flexure and residual astigmatism. *Am J Optom Arch Am Acad Optom* 1972;49:304–307.

38. Herman JP. Flexure of rigid contact lenses on toric corneas as a function of base curve fitting relationship. *J Am Optom Assoc* 1983;54:209–213.

39. Pole JJ. The effect of base curve on the flexure of Polycon lenses. *Int Contact Lens Clin* 1983;10:49–52.

40. Egan DJ, Bennett ES. Trouble-shooting rigid contact lens flexure: a case report. *Int Contact Lens Clin* 1985;12:147–149.

41. Bennett ES, Egan DJ. Rigid gas permeable lens problem-solving. *J Am Optom Assoc* 1986;57:504–511.

42. Schnider CM, Terry RL, Holden BA. Clinical correlates of peripheral corneal desiccation. *Invest Ophthalmol Vis Sci* 1988; 29(Suppl):336.

43. Jones L, Woods CA. Contact lens fitting and design. *Optician* 1992;203:16–22.

44. Morgan P. Advanced contact lens fitting: Part one: extended wear RGP lenses. *Optician* 1997;5595:20–26.

45. Sorbara L, Fonn D, Holden BA et al. Centrally fitted versus lid-attached rigid gas permeable lenses Part II: A comparison of the clinical performance. *Int Contact Lens Clin* 1996;23:121–126.

46. Swarbrick HA, Holden BA. Rigid gas permeable lens binding: significance and contributing factors. *Am J Optom Physiol Opt* 1987;64:815–823.

47. Bennett ES, Sorbara L. Lens design, fitting and evaluation. In:

48. Bennett ES, Henry VA, eds. *Clinical manual of contact lenses,* 2nd ed. Philadelphia: Lippincott Williams & Wilkins, 2000:75–124.

48. Bennett ES. Silicone/acrylate lens design: *Int Contact Lens Clin* 1985;12:45–53.

49. Weissman BA, Fatt I. In situ oxygen transmissibility of rigid gas-permeable contact lenses. *Am J Optom Physiol Opt* 1988;65:402.

50. Lin MC, Graham AD, Fusaro RE, Polse KA. Impact of rigid gas-permeable contact lens extended wear on corneal epithelial barrier function. *Invest Ophthalmol Vis Sci* 2002;43:1019–1024.

51. Holden T, Bahr K, Koers D, et al. The effects of secondary curve liftoff on peripheral corneal desiccation. *Am J Optom Physiol Opt* 1987;64:113.

52. Andrasko GJ. Clinical implications of 3 & 9 o'clock staining. Paper presented at: First Annual RGP Lens Institute Symposium, St. Louis, MO, July 1989.

53. Andrasko GJ. What makes RGP lenses comfortable? Paper presented at: First Annual RGP Lens Institute Symposium, St. Louis, MO, July 1989.

54. Classe JG, Harris MG. Liability and extended wear contact lenses. *J Am Optom Assoc* 1987;58:848–854.

55. Ghormley NR. Rigid EW lenses: complications. *Int Contact Lens Clin* 1987;14:219.

56. Schnider CM, Terry RL. Evaluation of success rate for RGP EW contact lenses: survival versus clinical criteria. *Invest Ophthalmol Vis Sci* 1989;30(3 Suppl):258.

57. Woods CA. Efron N. Regular replacement of extended wear rigid gas permeable contact lenses. *CLAO J* 1996;22:172–178.

58. Henry VA, Bennett ES, Forrest JF. Clinical investigation of the Paraperm EW rigid gas-permeable contact lens. *Am J Optom Physiol Opt* 1987;64:313–320.

59. Shovlin J, Christensen B, De Paolis MD, et al. How to fit rigid gas permeable extended wear lenses. *Rev Optom* 1987;24:69–80.

60. Grohe RM, Caroline PJ, Norman CW. The role of in-office modification for RGP surface defects. *Contact Lens Spectr* 1988; 3:52–60.

61. Morgan BW, Henry VA, Bennett ES, Caroline PJ. The effect of modification procedures on rigid gas permeable lenses: the UM-St. Louis study. *J Am Optom Assoc* 1992;63:201–214.

62. Bennett ES, Clompus RJ, Hansen DW. A hands-on approach to RGP modification. *Rev Optom* 135(1):88–96, 1998.

63. Schnider CM. An overview of RGP extended wear. *Contax* 1987; May:10–12.

64. Weissman BA, Remba MJ, Fugedy E. Results of the extended wear contact lens survey of the contact lens section of the American Optometric Association. *J Am Optom Assoc* 1987;58: 166–171.

65. Weiss L. Clinical study of extended wear lenses: hydrogel versus gas permeable. *Contact Lens Forum* 1987;12:41–46.

66. Bennett ES, Stulc S, Bassi CJ, et al. Effect of patient personality profile and verbal presentation on successful rigid contact lens adaptation, satisfaction and compliance. *Optom Vis Sci* 1998;75: 500–505.

67. Schnider CM. Anesthetics and RGPs: crossing the controversial line. *Rev Optom* 1996;133:41–43.

68. Bennett ES, Smythe J, Henry VA et al. The effect of topical anesthetic use on initial patient satisfaction and overall success with rigid gas permeable contact lenses. *Optom Vis Sci* 1998;75: 800–805.

69. LaHood D, Grant T, Holden BA. Characteristics of the overnight corneal edema responses caused by RGP and soft contact lenses. *Am J Optom Physiol Opt* 1987;64:99.

70. Zantos SG. Cystic formations in the corneal epithelium during extended wear of contact lenses. *Int Contact Lens Clin* 1983;10: 128.

71. Holden BA, Sweeney DF, Vannas A, et al. Effects of long term

extended contact lens wear on the human cornea. *Invest Ophthalmol Vis Sci* 1985;26:1489–1501.

72. Schnider CM, Terry RL, Holden BA. Effect of patient and lens performance characteristics on peripheral corneal desiccation. *J Am Optom Assoc* 1996;67:144–150.

73. Businger U, Treiber A, Flury C. The etiology and management of three and nine o'clock staining. *Int Contact Lens Clin* 1989; 16:132–140.

74. Polse KA, Sarver MD, Kenyon E, et al. Gas-permeable hard contact lens extended wear: ocular and visual responses to a 6-month period of wear. *CLAO J* 1987;13:31–38.

75. Polse KA, Rivera RK, Bonanno J. Ocular effects of hard gas permeable-lens extended wear. *Am J Optom Physiol Opt* 1988; 65:358–364.

76. Swarbrick HA, Holden BA. The incidence of RGP lens adherence: experimental vs. clinical findings. *Invest Ophthalmol Vis Sci* 1989;30(3 Suppl):166.

77. Fatt I. Negative pressure under silicone rubber contact lenses. Contacto 1979;23:6–8.

78. Bennett ES, Grohe RM. How to solve stuck lens syndrome. *Rev Optom* 1987;124:51–52.

79. Swarbrick HA. A possible etiology for RGP lens binding (adherence). *Int Contact Lens Clin* 1988;15:13–19.

80. Kenyon E, Polse KA, Mandell RB. Rigid contact lens adherence: incidence, severity and recovery. *J Am Optom Assoc* 1988;59: 168–174.

81. Holden BA, Sweeney DF, Collin HB. The effects of RGP and silicone elastomer lens binding on corneal structure. *Invest Ophthalmol Vis Sci* 1989;30(3 Suppl):481.

82. Swarbrick HA, Holden BA. Rigid gas-permeable lens adherence: a patient-dependent phenomenon. *Optom Vis Sci* 1989;66: 269–275.

83. Levy B. Rigid gas-permeable contact lenses for extended-wear: a 1-year clinical evaluation. *Am J Optom Physiol Opt* 1985;62: 889–894.

84. Korb DR, Allansmith MR, Greiner JV, et al. Prevalence of conjunctival changes in wearers of hard contact lenses. *Am J Ophthalmol* 1980;90:336–341.

85. Fonn D, Holden BA. Extended wear of hard gas-permeable contact lenses can induce ptosis. *CLAO J* 1986;12:93–94.

86. Holden BA, Sweeney DF, Swarbrick HA, et al. The vascular response to long term extended contact lens wear. *Clin Exp Optom* 1986;69:112–119.

87. McMonnies CW, Chapman-Davies A, Holden BA. The vascular response to contact lens wear. *Am J Optom Physiol Opt* 1982;59: 795–799.

88. Korb DR, Korb JME. Corneal staining prior to contact lens wearing. *J Am Optom Assoc* 1970;41:2–6.

89. Finnemore V. Factors in contact lens failure. *Am J Optom Physiol Opt* 1973;50:50–55.

90. Grohe RM, Lebow KA. Vascularized limbal keratitis. *ICLC* 1989; 16:197–209.

91. Elie G. Gas Permeable extended wear lenses: an excellent solution for aphakic patients. *CLAO J* 1986;12:51–53.

92. Sevigny J. Clinical comparison of the Boston IV contact lens under extended wear vs the Boston II lens under daily wear. *Int Eyecare* 1986;2:260–264.

93. Iskeleli G, Oral AY, Celikkol L. Changes in corneal radius and thickness in response to extended wear of rigid gas permeable contact lenses. *CLAO J* 1996;22:133–135.

94. Bennett ES, Tomlinson A, Mirowitz MC, et al. Comparison of overnight swelling and lens performance in RGP extended wear. *CLAO J* 1988;14:94–100.

36

SILICONE HYDROGEL LENSES FOR CONTINUOUS WEAR

DEBORAH F. SWEENEY
NICOLE A. CARNT
RÈNÈE DU TOIT
SERINA STRETTON
CHERYL SKOTNITSKY
JUDITH STERN
LISA KEAY
AND BRIEN A. HOLDEN

INTRODUCTION

Lenses made from high-oxygen-permeability (Dk) silicone hydrogel materials provide patients with the convenience of continuous wear and have the potential to change the contact lens industry worldwide. The ongoing increase in the number of patients wearing silicone hydrogels, and the increase in the number of eyecare practitioners that are willing to prescribe these lenses, suggest that continuous wear is having a resurgence despite its previous problems. The use of silicone hydrogel lenses however is not restricted to continuous wear. These lenses also offer the potential for a flexible wear schedule. These lenses are being used as an "alternative" lens for daily wear and the flexibility in the number of nights that these lenses can be worn is an advantage for those who prefer the benefits of silicone hydrogels and for those who use silicone hydrogels for therapeutic indications. (In Europe, silicone hydrogels are approved for a range of therapeutic indications.) Estimates from current lens sales data indicate that there are nearly three quarters of a million patients wearing silicone hydrogels worldwide.

Why Continuous Wear?

Consumers are enormously interested in a convenient form of vision correction. A Bausch & Lomb survey (Bases International) indicates that up to 66% of spectacle wearers and more than 81% of contact lens wearers across Europe would probably or definitely buy a continuous-wear lens, providing it was recommended by their eye care practitioner (1). Since the late 1980s, surveys of prospective patients from the Cornea and Contact Lens Research Unit (CCLRU) have found that patients consistently want the convenience of extended or continuous wear (2). Up to 77% of our patients indicated that they would use continuous wear if it were available, 21% desired occasional extended wear and the remainder preferred daily wear. Many patients have considered laser surgery to give them the 'continuous vision' that they seek because they are dissatisfied with their current forms of vision correction. Principally they complain that they cannot see in the morning, or that their contact lens routines interfere with their lifestyles (3). Our patients are aware, however, of the risks of permanent forms of vision correction such as laser surgery.

HYDROGEL EXTENDED WEAR

Soft contact lenses were promoted for use on both extended and continuous-wear regimens in the 1970s and 1980s. The lenses were primarily composed of hydroxyethylmethylacrylate (HEMA) materials (Chapter 17) and the convenience of extended/continuous wear initially made these "hydrogel" lenses very popular. De Carle (4) launched continuous-wear contact lenses in the early 1970s and reported on hundreds of patients using continuous wear without any side effects. It was not long after, however, that the reports of adverse responses and the sight-threatening problems with infections began to pervade both the scientific and public literature.

Ruben (5), and Cooper and Constable (6) were the first to report that extended wear could cause serious ocular problems. Soon after, Holden and Zantos (7) reported a high adverse reaction rate in 35 patients wearing 71%-water contact lenses on a continuous-wear basis. The numerous adverse reactions associated with continuous and extended wear of these early-generation materials are listed in Table

36.1 and include not only the serious sight-threatening infections (8–11), but also other inflammatory adverse responses such as acute red eyes (7), giant papillary conjunctivitis (12), chronic edema (7), corneal neovascularization, and infiltrates (13).

The long-term effects of chronic edema associated with hydrogel extended wear on all the layers of the cornea were detailed in the Gothenburg study conducted in Sweden. Holden and colleagues (14,15) reported that chronic hypoxia produced a 15% decrease in oxygen uptake of the epithelium and 85% of patients exhibited significant levels of microcysts (mean of 17 ± 21). The epithelium thinned by 6% and the stroma thinned by 2.3% (measured at 7 days, after the immediate edema of 2.5% had subsided). The majority (95%) of patients had increased endothelial polymegethism with a mean increase over the group of 22%. Holden et al. (15) also found that long-term extended wear with hydrogel lenses caused increased conjunctival injection and neovascularization (15).

Although infections associated with continuous wear were exacerbated by poor compliance (6,8,9,16), it was the increasing number of reports making headlines in the media (17,18) coupled with the previously described morphologic changes to the cornea that halted the widespread use of contact lenses on an extended or continuous-wear basis. By the late 1980s, the number of extended wearers had decreased dramatically. Only 20% to 30% of contact lens wearers in the United States and Sweden were using extended wear, and in other countries extended-wear lenses were responsible for only 2% to 15% of new fits (2). The average number of nights of wear for patients in extended wear was also on the decrease in the United States and other countries and occasional extended wear was becoming a much more common modality. It was at this time that the concept of "flexible" extended wear was popularized (19).

The introduction of regular replacement of lenses every 1 to 3 months was followed closely by the concept of the disposable extended-wear lens (replacement every 7 to 14 days). It was hoped that frequent replacement would reduce the effect of handling, deposits, and other contaminants, and that elimination of the need for cleaning and disinfection of lenses would improve patient compliance (20,21). It was soon evident, however, that these strategies were not as effective as envisioned. Work by Kotow, Grant and colleagues (22,23) indicated that, while the risk and possibly the severity of adverse responses such as contact lens–induced acute red eye (CLARE) or contact lens–induced papillary conjunctivitis (CLPC) could be reduced significantly with regular replacement, they were not eliminated. The overall long-term effects on the cornea described by Holden et al. (14) also remained. Grant et al. (23,24) showed that the rates of contact lens–induced peripheral ulcers (CLPUs) were equivalent between conventional and regularly replaced lenses. Sankaridurg et al. (25) also found that frequent replacement of hydrogel lenses during extended wear did not eliminate many of the adverse events, particularly infiltrative events, and that CLPC resulted in a significant number of discontinuations. Finally, Schein (26) reported that the threat of serious corneal infections was not reduced with the use of disposable hydrogel lenses and suggested that overnight wear was the overriding risk factor.

Why Hydrogel Extended Wear Was Not a Success

Although the early work of Polse, Mandell, and Farrell (27, 28) suggested that an atmospheric level of oxygen of 2% to 5% was adequate to avoid cornea edema, it became clear from the experience with hydrogel extended wear, that lenses made from low-Dk materials did not provide sufficient oxygen to the eye when worn on an extended-wear basis. Consequently, the work of Holden (29), Mizutani (30), Hamano and colleagues (31), and Bonanno and Polse (32) established that the eye's need for oxygen was much higher than initially thought.

Holden and Mertz (33) set the criterion for the critical level of oxygen required to avoid overnight corneal edema. The criterion was based on Mertz's estimate of overnight swelling of the human cornea from 10 non–lens-wearing subjects (4.1%) (34), and established that a lens should have oxygen transmissibility (Dk/t) of 87×10^{-9} (cm $\times$ mL O_2)(s $\times$ mL $\times$ mm Hg)$^{-1}$ if overnight edema is to be avoided. La Hood et al. (35) later revised the average overnight corneal edema for non–lens wearers to 3.2% using data from a greater number of subjects ($n = 41$). This revised value means that the minimum Dk/t to prevent overnight corneal edema with lens wear can be shifted to approximately 125×10^{-9} (cm $\times$ mL O_2)(s $\times$ mL $\times$ mm Hg)$^{-1}$.

Harvitt and Bonnano's mathematical model (36) estimates that a minimum lens Dk/t of 125×10^{-9} (cm $\times$ mL O_2)(s $\times$ mL $\times$ mm Hg)$^{-1}$ is required to allow normal

TABLE 36.1. ADVERSE REACTIONS OBSERVED WITH EARLY HYDROGEL EXTENDED WEAR

Limbal hyperemia	Corneal distortion
Neovascularization	Endothelial polymegethism
Bulbar hyperemia	Endothelial blebs
Conjunctival staining	Corneal infiltrative events
Corneal edema, striae, and folds	Contact lens–induced acute red eye (CLARE)
Epithelial and stromal thinning	Contact lens–induced peripheral ulcer (CLPU)
Altered epithelial adhesion	Superior epithelial arcuate lesions (SEALs)
Reduced epithelial mitosis	Infiltrative keratitis
	Erosions
Epithelial microcysts and vacuoles	Contact lens papillary conjunctivitis (CLPC)
Epithelial staining	Microbial keratitis

oxygen delivery to the entire stroma. It estimates the oxygen distribution across all the layers of the cornea, tear layer, and contact lens, and also incorporates the effects of acidosis on oxygen consumption with lens wear. In attempting to understand the relationship between oxygen supply and limbal redness normally associated with hydrogel contact lens wear, Papas (37) also established that 125×10^{-9} (cm $\times$ mL O_2)(s $\times$ mL $\times$ mm Hg)$^{-1}$ is required to eliminate limbal hyperemia during extended wear.

Conventional hydrogel materials used in the late 1970s and 1980s, and even current polymers used for frequent replacement or disposable extended wear, have poor Dk values because the plastic, primarily HEMA, has little affinity for oxygen. In theory, a 100%-water-content material can only have a maximum Dk of 80×10^{-11} (cm^2 $\times$ mL O_2)(s $\times$ mL $\times$ mm Hg)$^{-1}$ (Fig. 36.1). Although attempts were made to increase the Dk/t of lenses manufactured from these materials by reducing lens thickness or increasing the water content of the polymers, the actual oxygen delivered was much less than the established criterion.

Can We Avoid Hypoxia and Other Problems?

By the mid-1980s, some lens materials and lenses were available that could satisfy the oxygen needs of the cornea during overnight wear. La Hood and colleagues (35) reported that some gas-permeable (GP) lenses produced overnight corneal swelling close to the levels seen without a lens, and Sweeney and Holden (38) reported that the overnight corneal swelling with silicone elastomer lenses was even less than the levels observed without a lens.

Although the vast majority of patients could wear GP and silicone elastomer lenses, there were some major disadvantages that prevented them from becoming a convenient

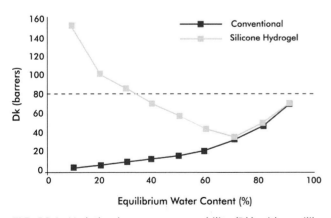

FIG. 36.1. Variation in oxygen permeability (Dk) with equilibrium water content for conventional hydrogel and silicone hydrogel materials. (From Tighe B. Silicone hydrogel materials: how do they work? In: Sweeney DF, ed. *Silicone hydrogels: the rebirth of continuous wear contact lenses.* Oxford: Butterworth-Heineman, 2000:1–21, with permission.)

lens for continuous wear. Silicone elastomer lenses have exceptional Dk/t and durability but tend to bind to the cornea. In addition, the higher modulus of elasticity of silicone elastomer lenses in comparison to conventional hydrogels contributed to the discomfort that wearers experienced. GP lenses have high Dk/t and provide superior optics, visual performance, and durability. However, the market for GP lenses for extended wear has remained low primarily because patients do not find GP lenses to be comfortable immediately after insertion and because practitioners have the perception that these lenses are difficult to fit.

The lens needed by patients and practitioners for continuous wear is one that provides the necessary oxygen requirements for the closed eye [Dk/t of at least 87×10^{-9} (cm $\times$ mL O_2)(s $\times$ mL $\times$ mm Hg)$^{-1}$] while maintaining the comfort, fitting, and surface characteristics of conventional hydrogels. The ideal lens should have good movement and simple fitting procedures, good wettability, and be resistant to deposits.

CLINICAL PRACTICE WITH SILICONE HYDROGEL LENSES

Silicone Hydrogel Materials

Such importance is placed on corneal oxygen supply that material Dk was rated as the most important lens characteristic ahead of surface biocompatibility, lens movement, dehydration resistance, wettability, and elastic modulus in a survey of contact lens practitioners (3). The inability to design polymers to meet corneal oxygen criteria has impeded development of hydrogel lens materials for extended wear for nearly 30 years.

Silicone hydrogels combine the high Dk of silicone with other material characteristics of conventional hydrogel materials that facilitate fluid transport and lens movement. This combination has not been easy to achieve, because such monomers typically have little affinity for one another and the components have had to be combined in two-phase structures to allow their coexistence.

Pure silicone rubber has a Dk in excess of 400×10^{-11} (cm^2 $\times$ mL O_2)(s $\times$ mL $\times$ mm Hg)$^{-1}$, which ensures that silicone hydrogel lenses have Dk/t of at least 110 to 175×10^{-9} (cm $\times$ mL O_2)(s $\times$ mL $\times$ mm Hg)$^{-1}$. The incorporation of silicone, however, results in a lens with poor wettability, greater lipid interaction and stiffer mechanical properties. The surfaces of silicone hydrogel lenses are treated to make them more hydrophilic and therefore more biocompatible (39). Surface treatments do not significantly impact the Dk/t of the lens, and during continuous wear this results in lenses with extremely low protein deposition (40) and wettability characteristics similar to conventional hydrogels.

Silicone hydrogel lenses have excellent handling characteristics because they are "stiffer" than conventional hy-

TABLE 36.2. PROPERTIES OF SILICONE-HYDROGEL LENSES IN COMPARISON TO CONVENTIONAL HYDROGEL LENSES

	Pure Vision	Focus Night & Day	Acuvue
Material name	Balafilcon A	Lotrafilcon A	Etafilcon
Manufacturer	Bausch & Lomb	CIBA Vision	Vistakon
Water content	36%	24%	58%
Oxygen permeability (DK)*	99	140	22
Oxygen transmissibility (Dk/t)†	110	175	31
Center thickness @ −3.00 D (mm)	0.09	0.08	0.07
Modulus (g/mm²)	110	120	35
Surface charge	Surface slightly ionic	Surface slightly ionic	Surface highly ionic
Surface treatment	Plasma oxidation producing glassy islands	25-nm plasma coating with high refractive index	No treatment

$* \times 10^{-11} (cm^2 \times ml\ O_2)(s \times ml \times mm\ Hg)^{-1}$
$\dagger \times 10^{-9} (cm \times ml\ O_2)(s \times ml \times mm\ Hg)^{-1}$ measured at 35°C.

drogels; however, the disadvantages of a stiffer lens are the potential difficulties with lens fit and mechanical effects of the lens on the cornea and conjunctival tissue during wear.

Currently, the two silicone hydrogels for continuous wear that are commercially available on the worldwide market are Ciba Vision's Focus Night & Day lens (lotrafilcon A) and Bausch & Lomb's PureVision lens (balafilcon A). Details of the various material properties of the currently available silicone hydrogels are compared to a conventional hydrogel in Table 36.2.

Patient Selection

Correct patient selection is important to achieving successful contact lens wear with silicone hydrogels. The criteria are very to similar to those used for conventional hydrogel lenses and rely on attention to general health and ocular status, patient history, ands motivational, personality, lifestyle, and demographic factors.

Silicone hydrogels are currently only available in the spherical form, and therefore are not suitable for patients with astigmatism greater than 1 D (Table 36.3). The high Dk/t of silicone hydrogels means high myopes and hyperopes now have the option of choosing continuous wear. Motivational factors also assist in the selection of a suitable patient. The magnitude of refractive error is the most apparent factor linked to motivation (41); however, vocational, lifestyle, recreational, and self-image factors also play a role.

A detailed patient history should be conducted before contact lens fitting commences to determine any contraindications or issues that need to be considered when contemplating wear schedules for silicone hydrogel wear. For example, patients who have compromised immunity, severe allergies, or who use systemic medication should probably avoid extended wear altogether. Patients that have had a history of inflammatory events or contact lens intolerance such as CLPC may be at greater risk of developing further events (42); therefore, patients should be informed about the risk of repeat events. Given both the modulus and surface characteristics of high-Dk silicone lenses, patients with any signs and symptoms of CLPC should not be considered as candidates for either extended or continuous wear.

It is also important to be cautious of existing patients that experience problems with daily wear of contact lenses or that cannot maintain a 6-night extended-wear schedule with conventional hydrogel lenses (42). Some of these patients may find that the higher Dk/t and generally lower water content of silicone hydrogels may be advantageous, but there are no guarantees of success. Discomfort is strongly correlated with symptoms of dryness (43), and discomfort and dryness are the major reasons that patients discontinue from wearing soft contact lenses (44–46). Our studies indicate that symptoms of dryness may be reduced with silicone hydrogels compared to conventional hydrogel lenses, possibly because of the lower water content of the silicone hydrogel material. Chalmers and colleagues (47)

TABLE 36.3. SILICONE-HYDROGEL LENS PARAMETERS

	Pure Vision	Focus Night & Day
Base curve (mm)	8.6	8.4, 8.6
Diameter (mm)	14.00	13.8
Power availability	+0.50 to +6.00; −0.50 to −6.00; −6.50 to −12.00	+0.25 to +6.00; −0.25 to −8.00; −8.50 to −10.00

have shown symptoms of dryness significantly improve in patients who are refitted with silicone hydrogels after wearing conventional hydrogel lenses.

Even a normally compliant daily wear patient will occasionally sleep in their lenses, and the percentage of patients who report sleeping in their lenses is always higher when asked by a third party in contrast to their practitioner (48). Therefore the flexibility in wear schedule that silicone hydrogel lenses provide may be beneficial to those patients who need the convenience and benefit of higher Dk/t. Silicone hydrogels should also be considered as problem solvers for patients that have high oxygen demands (possibly as suggested by corneal neovascularization or high levels of microcysts) or those who need to wear their lenses for more than 12 to 14 hours per day. Parents and practitioners may also appreciate the added benefits of high oxygen supply when considering silicone hydrogel lenses for children and teenagers.

Hygiene and compliance issues must always be addressed. While the convenience of continuous wear is an important motivational factor, the desire for convenience per se is not sufficient for fitting continuous wear. This is because the desire for convenience may be linked to a trend toward noncompliant behavior. Noncompliance can be a major issue in the development of contact lens complications (26,49,50). It is therefore essential that clinicians educate patients on the importance of lens hygiene and correct maintenance procedures.

Brennan and Coles (51) have devised a checklist of prefit ocular health conditions, which can be used as a guideline before prescribing silicone hydrogels. Table 36.4 presents a modified version of this checklist, which uses many of the CCLRU grading scales shown in Fig. 36.2. It has been suggested that an edema stress test may be useful for predicting a patient's success in extended wear (52); however, as silicone hydrogels eliminate hypoxic stress, such tests may now be unnecessary.

Biomicroscopic assessment of the anterior eye and tear layer should be performed to detect any contraindications to contact lens wear. There should be no irregular corneal distortion. The quality of the tear layer is an important factor in the success of any contact lens wearer, and the practitioner should avoid continuous wear for patients with poor tear quality, excessive contamination or insufficient tears. Any significant degree of corneal staining or infiltration should be resolved before contact lens wear commences and certainly before a patient progresses to continuous wear. Some level of corneal staining is expected in many patients. As the work of Norn and others (53,54) have shown, over 20% of patients without any other signs or symptoms will exhibit minor corneal staining. Any confluent areas of macropunctate staining, epithelial loss, or abrasions, although unlikely, should be allowed to resolve before initiating lens wear. Our clinical experience has indicated that if any significant event involving corneal infiltration does not resolve completely before the patient recommences lens wear, a flare up of the condition often occurs.

TABLE 36.4. PREFIT OCULAR HEALTH CHECKLIST FOR REFITTING WITH SILICONE HYDROGELS

Characteristic	Requirement
*Hypoxic effects**	
Microcysts*	Any level
Vacuoles*	Any level
Striae or edema	No visible signs at time of commencing wear
Endothelial polymegethism	Any level
Bulbar/limbal conjunctiva	≤Grade 2 (no adverse response at time of refitting)
Limbal vascularization	Any level
Other physiologic effects	
Corneal staining	≤Grade 1
Conjunctival staining	≤Grade 1
Corneal curvature*	Any irregularity or warpage
Palpebral conjunctival papillae	No significant papillae
Palpebral redness	≤Grade 2
Infiltrates	None
Vision and subjective responses	
Visual acuity	Within 1 line of BCVA
Overall vision	≥80 (1 to 100)
Overall comfort	≥80 (1 to 100)

*Existing wearers, particularly those using low-Dk hydrogels, may show some signs of microcysts, vacuoles, bulbar and limbal redness, limbal vascularization, corneal warpage, and/or endothelial polymegethism. Clinical judgement should be used and these signs should regress with silicone-hydrogel wear.
BCVA, best-corrected visual acuity.

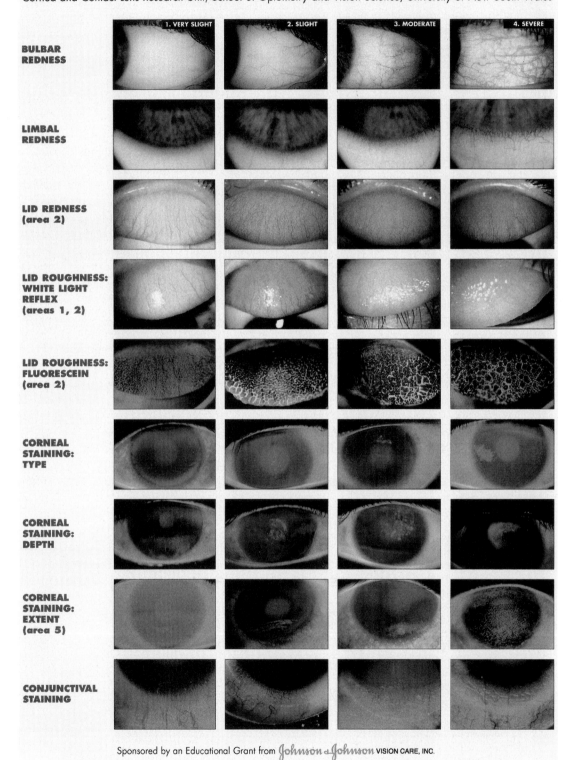

FIG. 36.2. Cornea and contact lens research unit grading scales. From Sweeney DF, Keay L, Jalbert I, et al. Clinical performance of silicone hydrogel lenses. (In: Sweeney DF, ed. *Silicone hydrogels: the rebirth of continuous wear contact lenses.* Oxford: Butterworth Heinemann, 2000:90–149, with permission.)

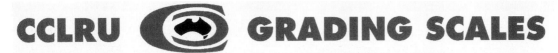

CCLRU GRADING SCALES

APPLICATION OF GRADING SCALES

- Patient management is based on how much the normal ocular appearance has changed.
- In general, a rating of slight (grade 2) or less is considered within normal limits (except staining).
- A change of one grade or more at follow up visits is considered clinically significant.

PALPREBRAL CONJUNCTIVAL GRADES

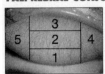

- The palprebal conjunctiva is divided into five areas to grade redness and roughness.
- Areas 1, 2 and 3 are most relevant in contact lens wear.

ADVERSE EFFECTS WITH CONTACT LENSES

CLPC CONTACT LENS PAPILLARY CONJUNCTIVITIS

Inflammation of the upper palprebal conjunctiva

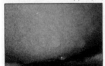

Signs
- Redness
- Enlarged papillae
- Excess mucus

Symptoms
- Itchiness
- Mucus strands
- Lens mislocation
- Intolerance to lenses

INFILTRATES

Accumulation of inflammatory cells in corneal sub-epithelial stroma. Inset: high magnification view

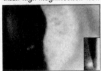

Signs
- Whitish opacity (focal) or grey haze (diffuse)
- Usually confined to 2-3mm from limbus
- Localized redness

Symptoms
- Asymptomatic or scratchy, foreign body sensation
- Redness, tearing and photophobia possible

CLARE CONTACT LENS REDUCED RED EYE

An acute corneal inflammatory episode associated with sleeping in soft contact lenses

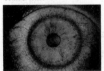

Signs
- Unilateral
- Intense redness
- Infiltrates
- No epithelial break

Symptoms
- Wakes with irritation or pain
- Photophobia
- Lacrimation

CORNEAL STAINING GRADES

- Staining assessed immediately after single instillation of fluorescein using cobalt blue light and wratten 12 (yellow) filter over the slit lamp objective.
- The cornea is divided into five areas. The type, extent and depth of staining are graded in each area.

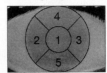

Type
1 Micropunctate
2 Macropunctate
3 Coalescent macropunctate
4 Patch

Extent: Surface area
1 1 – 15%
2 16 – 30%
3 31 – 45%
4 > 45%

Depth*
1 Superficial epithelium
2 Deep epithelium, delayed stromal glow
3 Immediate localized stromal glow
4 Immediate diffuse stromal glow

*Based on penetration of fluoroscein and slit lamp optic section

EROSION

Full thickness epithelial loss over a discrete area

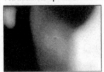

Signs
- No stromal inflammation
- Immediate spread of fluoroscein into stroma

Symptoms
- Can be painful
- Photophobia
- Lacrimation

CLPU CONTACT LENS PERIPHERAL ULCER

Round, full thickness epithelial loss with inflamed base, typically in the corneal periphery which results in a scar. Insets: with fluorescein, scar

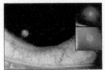

Signs
- Unilateral, "white spot"
- Localized redness
- Infiltrates
- Post healing scar

Symptoms
- Varies from foreign body sensation to pain
- Lacrimation and photophobia may occur

INFECTED ULCER

Full thickness epithelial loss with stromal necrosis and inflammation, typically central or paracentral

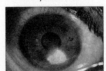

Signs
- Intense redness
- "White patch" (raised edges)
- Infiltrates
- Epithelial and stromal loss
- Anterior chamber flare
- Conjunctival and lid edema

Symptoms
- Pain, photophobia
- Redness, mucoid discharge
- VA (if over pupil)

POLYMEGETHISM

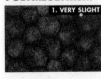
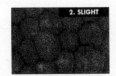
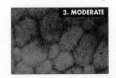
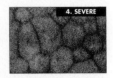

VASCULARIZATION

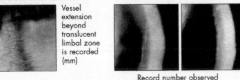

Vessel extension beyond translucent limbal zone is recorded (mm)

STROMAL STRIAE and FOLDS

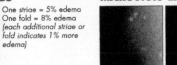

One striae = 5% edema
One fold = 8% edema
(each additional striae or fold indicates 1% more edema)

Record number observed

MICROCYSTS and VACUOLES

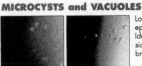

Located in epithelium. Identified by side showing brightness.

Microcyst
Vacuoles
reversed
unreversed

Record number observed

Sponsored by an Educational Grant from *Johnson & Johnson* VISION CARE, INC.

FIG. 36.2. Continued.

Lens Selection and Fitting

When prescribing silicone hydrogels, it is important to ensure that patients have well-fitted lenses to ensure optimum comfort and to minimize the risk of mechanically induced adverse responses. Trial lens fitting should always be performed and, if there is any problem with fit, then an alternative design or product should be assessed. We recommend that trial fitting should begin with the flatter base curve if more than one base curve is available for a particular lens type.

After a minimum of 5 minutes of equilibration (to allow the lens to "settle")—as long as there is no reflex tearing—the lens mechanical fit can be assessed. Assessment involves evaluation of lens centration, corneal coverage and lens movement. Ideally, silicone hydrogel lenses should be slightly loose (45% to 50% tightness) when assessed with the push-up test (55), and have 0.2 to 0.3 mm movement and good limbal coverage in all gaze positions. As mentioned previously, silicone hydrogels move more than most other spherical soft lenses and may result in a temporary increase in lens awareness in patients that are refitted from conventional hydrogel lenses.

The goal of mechanical lens fit is to maximize lens movement to allow for tear exchange. This is not for the purpose of oxygenation, but to encourage the removal of debris (and bacteria) from under the lens. It is generally considered good practice to fit extended-wear and/or continuous-wear lenses as mobile as possible, while maintaining good initial comfort.

The primary sign of poorly fitting silicone hydrogels is lens "fluting," whereas insufficient limbal coverage and decentration are the primary sign of poorly fitting conventional hydrogels. Lens fluting is a buckling of the lens edge, which occurs when the lens is too flat relative to the curvature of the cornea. It can be detected by observing the lens edge as it moves over the limbal area near the lower lid. In some patients, the fluting maybe minimal or intermittent and the diagnostic dye fluorexon, a high-molecular-weight fluorescein, may be needed to improve visualization (Fig. 36.3). Lens fluting causes a foreign body–like discomfort and will not decrease significantly with wear. Patients do not adapt to this interaction of the lens edge with the lower lid margin. If fluting or edge lift does occur, even intermittently, the trial lens fitting should be considered unacceptable.

Dumbleton and colleagues (42) have recommended that eyes with steeper corneal curvature (over 45.50 D) may achieve a more comfortable fit with the 8.4 mm base curve option for lotrafilcon A lenses. They also report that approximately 75% of patients in their trial could be fitted optimally with the 8.6 mm base curve and that 98% could be satisfactorily fitted with either the 8.4 or 8.6 mm base curve.

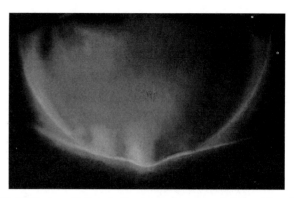

FIG. 36.3. Lens fluting indicating an unsuccessful fit with a silicone hydrogel-lens. Visualization is improved with fluorexon, a high-molecular-weight fluorescein.

Wear Schedule

Silicone hydrogels are suitable for wear for up to 30 nights continuously but can be worn for either flexible extended wear or daily wear, depending on a patient's suitability and requirements. Lenses should be replaced monthly according to manufacturer's guidelines, regardless of the wear schedule used. Patients should be encouraged to remove their lenses as often as necessary, particularly if they are unwell or simply feel the need for a break from lens wear. Lenses that are removed temporarily should be rinsed or cleaned before reinsertion, and if they are removed overnight or for any significant period of time must be disinfected properly before they are reinserted. We strongly recommend that patients rinse their lenses with unpreserved unit doses of saline or lubricants morning and night. We find that 50% of our patients comply with these instructions and are able to relieve symptoms of dryness and improve comfort upon waking and in the evenings.

Aftercare

Patients who have not worn contact lenses previously should undergo a brief period (minimum of 1 week) of adaptation to silicone hydrogels on a daily-wear schedule prior to initiating either extended or continuous wear. This is to circumvent any difficulties that patients may have with regard to lens handling and/or care procedures before progressing to continuous wear. This also gives the practitioner the opportunity to confirm the mechanical lens fit and assess both corneal integrity and response to lens wear.

In the first month of continuous wear, practitioners should have frequent contact with the patient. We recommend an assessment after the first night of sleeping in lenses, if at all possible, regardless of whether patients have had previous extended-wear experience. This allows the practitioner to assess the response of the eye to overnight wear with silicone hydrogels and gives the patient the opportunity to discuss any concerns they may have about sleeping in their lenses.

The next visit should be scheduled after the first week of wear, then the first month, 3 months, and every 3 to 6 months thereafter. As much as possible, the appointments should be made early in the morning, to allow the practitioner to assess the eye when it is most illustrative of the potential stress that continuous wear can induce. If possible, the supply of lenses should coincide with the scheduled aftercare visits to further encourage patient compliance. The visit after the first week of extended wear enables the practitioner to determine whether there are any responses that may prevent the patient from progressing with continuous wear (for instance, significant levels of lens deposition).

Overall aftercare visits should entail a thorough patient history that discusses wear time and symptoms (including comfort and vision ratings), as well as an assessment of the patient's ocular appearance and visual acuity. It is important to include subjective refraction, particularly for those patients who have been refitted after long-term wear of conventional hydrogels on a daily- or extended-wear basis, as regression of myopic creep has been reported in patients within the first 6 months of initiating continuous wear with silicone hydrogel lenses (56,57). Hypoxic effects, degree of vascularization, and endothelial polymegethism should be measured and corneal and conjunctival staining and bulbar redness should be assessed. There should be a less than 1 grade increase in papillae or redness of the eyelid (CCLRU grading scales from 0 to 4) and no significant increase in ocular redness or neovascularization (58,59).

Some of the adverse responses associated with silicone hydrogel wear, such as CLPC and superior epithelial arcuate lesions (SEALs), are potentially driven by mechanical interaction of the lens with the ocular surface and can be asymptomatic in the early stages. Assessment of the upper tarsal conjunctiva and the superior cornea for early signs of interaction can minimize development of these events.

It is also important to assess the wettability of the lens surface and to detect any signs of deposits on either the front or back surface. There have been no reports of problems with durability or surface deterioration of silicone hydrogel lenses. Patients should bring their cleaner, disinfectant, unit dose saline, and lens case to each aftercare visit so that their care and maintenance procedures can be appraised and so that the practitioner can ensure that care solutions are being replaced regularly.

Patient Education and Support

To minimize potential problems, practitioners should communicate well with their patients and continuously educate them on the use and handling of contact lenses. Patients should also be actively involved in monitoring their own ocular health. To do this, patients should be encouraged to check every morning and night to ensure that their eyes "Look Good, Feel Good, and See Well" (60). If any problems such as redness, watering, discomfort, or pain occur, then patients should remove their lenses and contact their practitioner as soon as possible. Importantly, patients should not sleep in lenses if they feel unwell, as they may be at higher risk of adverse events such as CLARE (61).

The importance of patient compliance should be reiterated at every visit. Patients should be reminded of the potential risks of continuous wear and the steps needed to avoid problems. They should also be reminded that their wear schedule is flexible, and that they should remove their lenses whenever necessary. It should be emphasized that lens care solutions are still needed and that an up-to-date pair of spectacles should always be available if lenses need to be removed. We also recommend to our patients to always swim with goggles when wearing contact lenses.

To minimize the effects of complications, it is vital that patients have access to care 24 hours a day. Contact procedures should be established by the practitioner to ensure a rapid response, or it may be advisable to organize a local practitioner network. We recommend that practitioners provide a credit card–sized card that lists the following:

- Practitioner contact numbers
- An emergency clinic number (this must be a pager service)
- Address details for your clinic
- Address and contact details for an ophthalmic registrar (cornea specialist/ophthalmologist) from the local hospital, preferably who is aware of contact lens complications
- Details of the patient's lenses, wear and removal schedule, and care and maintenance systems

In addition, the card can include a reminder for patients to check their eyes every day. At CCLRU, we also provide refrigerator magnets to our patients with this information.

Clear documentation should be provided for patients that includes an information brochure on care of contact lenses and continuous wear in layman's terms, and evidence of discussion confirming that they have understood the risks and procedures described to them. Many clinics involved in extended or continuous wear provide the following information to all patients:

- Information brochure
- Practitioner/patient agreement
- Instruction sheet: "Do's and Don'ts" with contact lenses
- Question and answer sheet
- Informed consent
- Emergency documentation

Finally, patient education must occur at every aftercare visit. To ensure that this occurs, we use in-office posters and take-home material to remind our patients of the potential risks of contact lens wear if they do not remain vigilant.

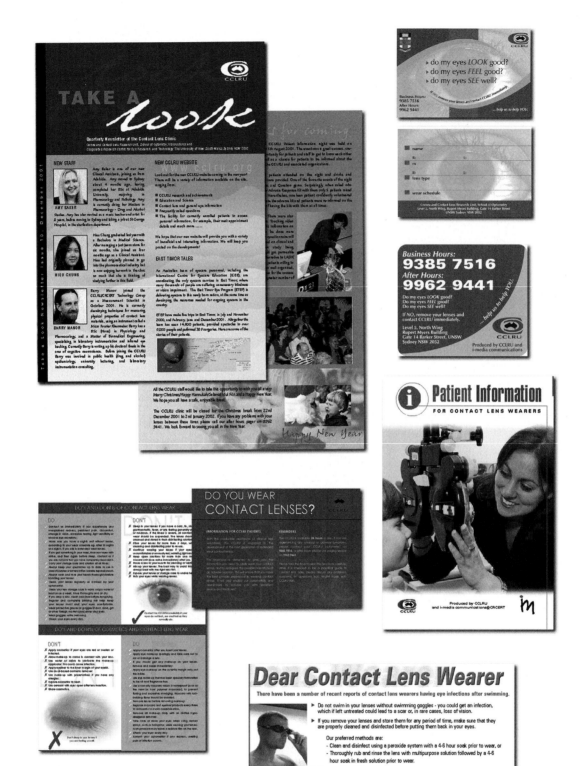

FIG. 36.4. Patient educational and support materials used by the Cornea and Contact Lens Research Unit (CCLRU).

Figure 36.4 illustrates a range of patient education and support materials used by the CCLRU.

The office should also be equipped for continuous wear. An in-office system for recall of patients is essential. Where possible, appointments for the following 12 months should be scheduled with the patient in advance. If possible, patients should be contacted either by phone or e-mail the day before their appointment to remind them and reschedule if necessary. If a patient fails to make an appointment they must be contacted by phone or, if necessary, in writing to make a further appointment. This letter should emphasize the need for regular monitoring even if the patient is not experiencing any problems.

It is important to maintain good clinic records. Clear guidelines should be used for establishing suitability of patients for daily versus flexible versus extended versus continuous wear. Standard procedures for aftercare and for appraising a patient's ability to continue with extended or continuous wear should be used. An important part of accurate record keeping is the use of a grading scale system. Two grading scales with illustrated representations are available for use, the CCLRU grading scale system (Fig. 36.2) and the Efron grading scales for contact lens practice (62).

The liability of fitting continuous wear ultimately rests with the practitioner. As such, practitioners must try to minimize the extent of legal liability by adopting the appropriate standard of care. Many of the steps and suggestions outlined previously for patient documentation and staff education are part of such standard of care. It is important that all staff from the office, including technical and administrative support, be well informed about the advantages of continuous wear and how to manage any potential problems. In addition, all members of a network of practitioners for out-of-hours service or designated ophthalmic registrars/ophthalmologists, need to be well informed regarding the handling and fit of lenses, wear schedules, issues of care and maintenance, and potential problems that can occur.

CLINICAL PERFORMANCE

Edema

A number of researchers (63–66) have investigated overnight corneal edema with the two commercially available silicone hydrogels, and have contrasted the results to those found with no lens wear and conventional low-Dk hydrogels (Table 36.5). These studies all clearly demonstrate that central corneal swelling is significantly reduced with silicone hydrogel lenses in comparison to conventional hydrogels used for extended wear and is similar to the levels of overnight edema observed with no lens wear.

Although these results are very encouraging, it is important to remember that the overnight edema response varies for individuals within the population. Comstock et al. (65) reported that over 10% of wearers can experience greater than 7.7% overnight corneal edema after wearing lenses made from balafilcon A. Further, Mueller et al. (67) compared overnight edema with lenses made from lotrafilcon A, balafilcon A, and no lens wear and found significant differences between balafilcon A lenses and no lens wear. Mueller concluded that the differences in response to the two lenses can be linked to the differences in Dk/t, and in part may be associated with the variation in edema within the normal population. This variation in overnight edema should also be considered as we initiate prescribing these lenses not only for our low myopic patients, but also for high myopes and hyperopes.

Generally, we find a relatively low number of striae in our patients, even when they are observed immediately after opening the eye. However, if striae are observed at early morning aftercare visits, an afternoon appointment should be scheduled to confirm that the edema has resolved. If any signs of edema persist, then patients should be advised to change to daily wear and only wear lenses overnight occasionally.

TABLE 36.5. OVERNIGHT CORNEAL EDEMA WITH SILICONE-HYDROGEL AND CONVENTIONAL-HYDROGEL LENSES

Lens Type	Overnight Edema (mean ± SD)	Subjects	Reference
Silicone hydrogels			
Prototype A	3.8 ± 1.8	10 non–lens wearers	CCLRU Studies
Prototype B	3.9 ± 1.3	9 non–lens wearers	CCLRU Studies
Prototype C	3.6 ± 2.3	7 non–lens wearers	CCLRU Studies
Balafilcon A	2.8 ± np	20 adapted soft-lens wearers	MacDonald et al. (63)
Balafilcon A	3.1 ± 4.8	10 not specified	Bullimore et al. (64)
Balafilcon A	2.9 ± 2.7	10 adapted soft-lens daily wearers	Comstock et al. (65)
Lotrafilcon A	2.7 ± 1.9	20 non–lens wearers	Fonn et al. (122)
Conventional low-Dk hydrogels			
Etafilcon A	9.0 ± 4.1	10 not specified	Bullimore et al. (64)
Etafilcon A	10.0 ± 1.6	7 non–lens wearers	La Hood et al. (35)
Etafilcon A	8.7 ± 2.8	20 non–lens wearers	Fonn et al. (122)
No lens	**3.2 ± 1.6**	**41 non–lens wearers**	**La Hood et al. (35)**

CCLRU, Cornea and Contact Lens Research Unit; np, not provided.

Microcysts

Microcysts are small (typically 10 to 15 μm), irregularly shaped, and highly refractive inclusions that form in the basal layers of the epithelium and with time move toward the anterior surface of the cornea. They are probably the most clinically useful marker of chronic hypoxic stress.

Microcysts are observed using marginal retroillumination with, at minimum, ×16 magnification. Once observed, magnification is increased to ×20 to ×40 while keeping the inclusion centered in the beam and are confirmed if the inclusion shows reversed illumination.

The number of microcysts that are observed during lens wear is inversely proportional to the Dk/t of lenses worn (68,69). Relatively low numbers of microcysts (fewer than 10) are observed in patients wearing silicone hydrogels if they are new to contact lens wear or have been wearing these lenses for several months or longer (70). Generally, the number of microcysts observed with silicone hydrogel lenses is similar to the number seen with no lens wear or with daily wear of lenses.

Large numbers of microcysts will be observed within the first month of wear in approximately 50% of patients that are refitted from conventional hydrogel lenses to silicone hydrogels, particularly if the hydrogel lenses were worn on an extended-wear basis (Fig. 36.5). Keay and colleagues (70) have shown that this spike or rebound effect is temporary, and that the number of microcysts will decrease to low levels between 1 and 3 months of continuous wear. Such a trend has also been observed when patients are discontinued from conventional hydrogel extended wear. It has been suggested that this rebound phenomenon is related to reoxygenation of the corneal surface, which results in recovery of epithelial metabolism and subsequent clearance of extracellular debris trapped in the deeper basal layers of the epithelium. The large numbers of microcysts can occur across the cornea or may aggregate in a ring in the corneal midperiphery. As microcysts move to the anterior surface of the cornea, areas of negative staining, or black spots, may be observed. These are best observed after instillation of fluorescein using a cobalt blue illumination with a Wratten yellow filter.

When observing the corneal epithelium, it is important to ensure that microcysts are differentially diagnosed from the many other presentations with which they may be confused. Table 36.6, adapted from Keay et al. (71), details a number of conditions that can have a similar appearance to microcysts and the primary features that distinguish them from microcysts.

Limbal and Bulbar Redness and Ghost Vessels

A masked, prospective study conducted at the CCLRU/CRCERT (72) demonstrated that the eyes of patients wearing silicone hydrogel lenses on a continuous-wear basis show

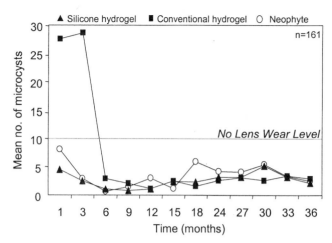

FIG. 36.5. Comparison of the mean number of microcysts between groups of subjects wearing silicone hydrogel lenses. Subjects had a history of wearing silicone hydrogel lenses, a history of wearing conventional hydrogel lenses, or had no previous lens-wear experience.

no differences in bulbar or limbal redness when compared with age- and gender-matched non–lens wearing eyes. There were no differences in the number of microcysts or level of endothelial polymegethism, and it was not possible to distinguish the clinical appearance of lens wearers from non–lens wearers in this study. These studies confirmed the findings of Papas (37) and later studies by Dumbleton et al. (73) that the level of limbal redness is associated with the Dk/t of the lens edge.

Papas et al. (74) showed that limbal hyperemia occurs to a lesser degree in eyes wearing silicone hydrogel lenses than in eyes wearing conventional hydrogel lenses. Differences were most marked following periods of eye closure and lens wear (for further discussion, see Chapter 38).

Limbal hyperemia has also been shown to recover to baseline levels more rapidly after overnight eye closure with silicone hydrogels compared with lenses of lower Dk/t (75). Within 3 hours of eye opening, the limbal hyperemia in eyes wearing silicone hydrogels returns to baseline levels. Eyes wearing lenses made from lower-Dk materials still show significantly more limbal hyperemia 3 hours after eye opening than is recorded at baseline.

Long-term data from CCLRU/CRCERT studies with conventional hydrogel lenses confirm that low levels of redness continue to be observed across time (3). As with microcysts, the level of redness induced by previous low-Dk lens wear decreases after patients are refit with silicone hydrogel lenses. Similar reductions have been found in overall bulbar redness, but this response is not as consistent as that seen for the limbal vasculature.

As well as a reduction in the overall level of limbal redness, it has been proposed that the unfilling (or "ghosting") of limbal vessels observed during silicone hydrogel lens wear is associated with high Dk/t in the peripheral area of the

TABLE 36.6. DIFFERENTIAL DIAGNOSIS OF MICROCYSTS AND MUCIN BALLS

	Size (μm)	Appearance	Cause
Recurrent corneal erosion	15–100	Clear cysts	Trauma, often unknown
Microcystic edema	20–50	Clear cyst surrounding epithelial haze, >200	Inflammatory origin
Epithelial infiltrates	100–500	Granular, dense center	Chemotactic stimulus
Vacuoles	20–50	Round, bubblelike, unreversed illumination	Hypoxia
Mucin balls	<100	Spherical balls	Surface interaction between lens and cornea
Punctate corneal staining	10–50	Fine opaque dots, positive stain	Epithelial trauma (e.g., toxin or dehydration)
Microcysts	10–50	Small, irregularly shaped dots; reversed illumination (negative stain)	Hypoxia

From Keay L, Jalbert I, Sweeney DF, et al. Microcysts: clinical significance and differential diagnosis. *Optometry: J Am Optom Assoc* 2001;72:452–560, with permission.

lens. Dumbleton and coworkers (73) have shown that there is no increase in corneal neovascularization after 9 months of continuous wear with silicone hydrogel lenses, whereas moderate levels of neovascularization develop after only 3 months of extended wear with conventional hydrogels. A brief case history is provided that illustrates the "unfilling" of limbal vessels in a silicone hydrogel lens wearer following a long history of daily wear with conventional hydrogel lenses (Figs. 36.6 and 36.7).

Refractive Error

Myopic creep, the need for additional minus power, has been reported to accompany both daily and extended wear of conventional hydrogels (76,77). Several studies have now

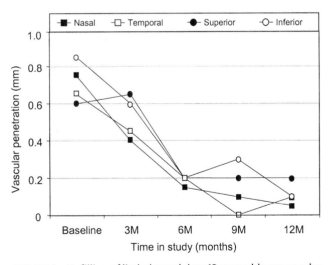

FIG. 36.6. Unfilling of limbal vessels in a 42-year-old woman who completed 12 months of extended wear with silicone hydrogel lenses. The patient had worn conventional hydrogel lenses with daily wear for 15 years (baseline) before being refitted with silicone hydrogel lenses. After 6 months there was a significant reduction filling of the limbal vessels.

reported that this induction of myopia does not occur with silicone hydrogel lens wear and can be reversed in wearers with a history of conventional extended wear. As a result, it has been postulated that hypoxia plays a major role in the topographic changes induced by contact lens wear. When McNally and Mc Kenney (48) reviewed data from the 59 practices that were involved in Food and Drug Administration (FDA) approval of lotrafilcon A in the United States, they found that 1.5% of subjects wearing etafilcon A had an increase in myopia greater than 1.00 D over 12 months, whereas no silicone hydrogel wearer showed such an increase (Fig. 36.8).

Jalbert et al. (57) found that extended wear with conventional hydrogel lenses was associated with an increase in myopia and corneal steepening, whereas continuous wear with silicone hydrogel lenses did not cause any changes in refractive error or corneal curvature in subjects with no previous lens-wear experience. In fact, continuous wear with silicone hydrogels was associated with a decrease in myopia and corneal flattening in subjects with a previous conventional hydrogel experience. Dumbleton and co-workers (56) found similar results with myopic creep after, at minimum, 9 months of lens wear.

Lens Surface Performance

Lens wettability is assessed using a combination of factors including the pattern, size, and speed of tear breakup, stability of the tear film, and the lipid layer appearance. The grading system used at the CCLRU is based on a comparison of the wettability seen with HEMA lens surfaces and a normal healthy cornea. The grade ranges from 0 to 5, where 0 corresponds to a totally nonwetting surface, 1 corresponds to patches of nonwetting after blinking, 2 corresponds to the appearance equivalent to a HEMA lens surface, 3 corresponds to more wettable than a HEMA lens surface, 4 corresponds to an appearance approaching a healthy cornea, and

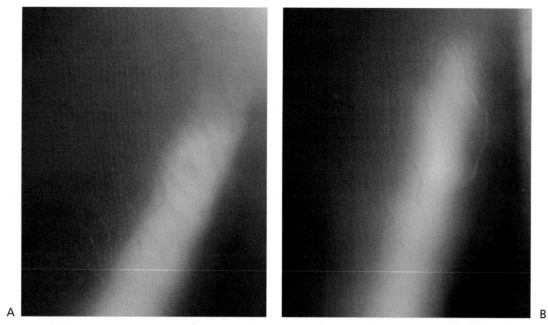

FIG. 36.7. Limbal vascularization in a 42-year-old woman after 15 years of daily wear with conventional hydrogel lenses (**A**), and reduction in filling of the limbal vessels after 12 months of silicone hydrogel lens wear (**B**).

5 corresponds to an appearance that is equivalent to a healthy cornea (3).

Lens surface deposits are best observed immediately following a blink. A medium parallelepiped at a magnification of ×16 to ×25, and with both direct and retroillumination is used while scanning across the lens surface. An optic section can be used to determine if deposits are on the front or back surface of the lens. Back-surface deposits should be differentiated from debris and mucin balls. Debris is loose

under the lens and moves with a blink or when the lens is pushed. Our clinical studies, and those of other researchers, demonstrated that the level of deposition with currently available silicone hydrogels is minimal and similar to conventional hydrogels and wettability is similar to that of HEMA lenses (3,78–82).

The deposits that form on silicone hydrogels usually have a film or hazy appearance. Film or haze appears as a streaky or meshwork layer of fine white or grayish material on the

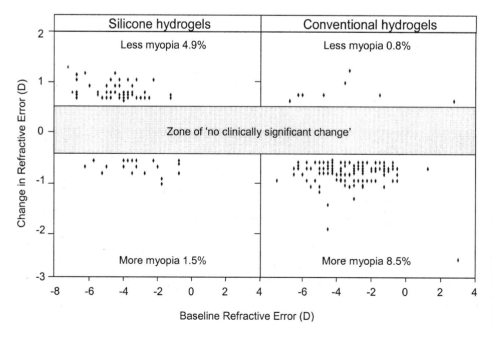

FIG. 36.8. Comparison of the change in refractive error after 12 months of continuous wear with silicone hydrogel lenses ($n = 966$) and conventional hydrogel lenses ($n = 1158$). From McNally J, Chalmers R, McKenney C. Factors associated with change in refractive error during a year of 6 night or 30 night extended wear. (Paper presented at: Annual Meeting of the Association for Research in Vision and Ophthalmology, 2002, with permission.)

lens surface. These deposits are observed on all types of lenses, but may be more prevalent on silicone hydrogels. A buildup of material resembling, small-to-medium–sized grayish globules may also adhere to silicone hydrogel lenses. Haze and globule-type deposition (Fig. 36.9) generally occurs at higher levels on the front compared to the back surface of lenses.

Some patients may be predisposed to develop higher levels of deposition more rapidly. This may be due to the interaction of factors such as tear film composition, ocular surface, environment, the lens material, the relative stiffness of the lenses, and contaminant characteristics.

When these deposits are severe, patients may report symptoms such as blurry or misty vision, discomfort, and irritation. Deposits can be removed easily, however, by rubbing and rinsing the lens with a cleaning surfactant. If the deposit cannot be removed after cleaning, the lens should be replaced. Some patients tend to develop lens deposits rapidly, regardless of whether they are wearing the lenses on a 6- or 30-night schedule, and may need to clean their lenses by as much as every 2 or 3 days. In our experience, development of deposits does not preclude the patient from continuous wear with silicone hydrogel lenses. Biochemical analyses suggest that the deposits on silicone hydrogels are primarily comprised of lipid, and that only very small amounts of protein are deposited in comparison to conventional lenses (80,83).

Mucin Balls

Although mucin balls have been described as a new phenomenon accompanying silicone hydrogel lens wear, they have also been observed in varying number with both conventional hydrogels and GP lenses. Mucin balls are spherical structures that range in size and clarity (Fig. 36.10). Typically, smaller mucin balls are sized from 10 to 20 μm in diameter and are translucent whereas larger mucin balls

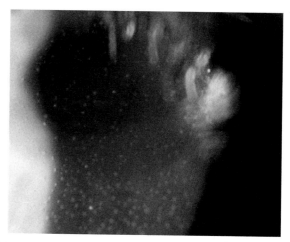

FIG. 36.10. High numbers of mucin balls in a patient wearing silicone hydrogel lenses.

range from 40 to 120 μm and are more opalescent. Although the composition of mucin balls is unknown, they are thought to be composed primarily of mucin, tear proteins, and small amounts of lipid.

Mucin balls can be observed very rapidly following lens insertion and tend to increase in size and number with lens wear. They can be seen scattered beneath the lens or clumped and are frequently observed near the resting position of the upper lid.

Tan and colleagues (84) found that a subpopulation of lens wearers is predisposed to develop mucin balls and that this predisposition appears to exist irrespective of lens type. Higher numbers of mucin balls occur in predisposed subjects when wearing silicone hydrogel lenses in comparison to conventional hydrogel lenses (Fig. 36.11).

The predominant hypothesis for the formation of mucin balls is that mechanical interaction of the lens with the ocular surface results in shear and tension forces that cause post tear film debris to form into spherical bodies as the lens moves. The role of the interaction between the lens and ocular surfaces in mucin ball formation has been confirmed by Tan et al. (84), who found a relationship between increasing lens wettability and higher numbers of mucin balls in both high- and low-Dk soft lens wearers. In addition, both Dumbleton et al. (85) and Tan et al. (84) found higher numbers of mucin balls in wearers with relatively steeper corneas, which further supports role of mechanical interaction of the lens and ocular surfaces in the formation of mucin balls.

It is important to differentiate mucin balls from punctate staining, post–lens-tear debris, microcysts, and vacuoles (Table 36.6). Typically, mucin balls do not move with the lens during a blink but remain attached or embedded in the underlying epithelium (86). When the lens is removed, the mucin balls may stay attached to the cornea for a few blinks. Indentations of mucin balls can be observed in the

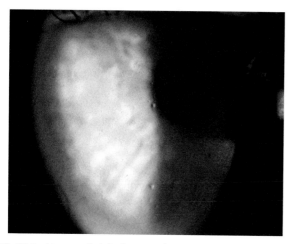

FIG. 36.9. Haze and globules-type deposits seen during continuous wear with silicone hydrogel lenses.

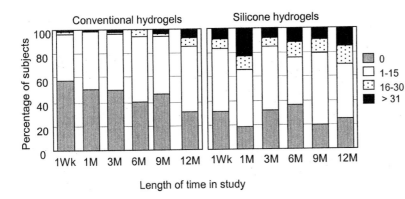

FIG. 36.11. Frequency of subjects with mucin balls while wearing conventional hydrogel for extended wear (*n* = 69) or silicone hydrogels for continuous wear (*n* = 70). (From Tan J, Keay L, Jalbert I, et al. Mucin balls with wear of conventional and silicone hydrogel contact lenses. *Optom Vis Sci* 2003;80: 291–297, with permission.)

corneal epithelium immediately after instillation of fluorescein; however, these indentations rapidly resolve.

No study to date has found a link between the formation of mucin balls and any adverse effect. Vision and comfort are not compromised, even in those individuals that have very high numbers of mucin balls [>200]. Pritchard et al. (87) have reported one case where a mucin ball appears to have become embedded within the corneal epithelium; however, the patient showed no deleterious effects.

Corneal and Conjunctival Staining

Generally levels of both corneal and conjunctival staining are low and comparable to those levels observed with conventional hydrogels. Morgan and Efron (40) have reported that staining can increase with wear of silicone hydrogels and indicated that staining might be higher than that observed with conventional hydrogel daily wear lenses. Our studies indicate that staining with silicone hydrogels is not characteristic of the dehydration type of staining seen with conventional extended-wear lenses, possibly because of the lower water content of silicone hydrogel lenses.

A recent study has examined the compatibility of silicone hydrogels with daily cleaning agents and has found that 37% of wearers develop corneal staining when using polyaminopropyl biguanide (PHMB)-containing multipurpose care systems whereas only 2% develop staining when using a non-PHMB system (88). The staining is characteristic of solution-based toxicity and can be accompanied by a stinging sensation after lens insertion.

Patient Responses: Comfort, Vision, and Compliance to Wear Schedule

Over 80% of patients on a continuous-wear schedule in studies at CCLRU rate their overall satisfaction with silicone hydrogel lenses at 85 or above out of 100. Overwhelmingly, 88% of these patients describe convenience as the primary reason for their satisfaction followed by the ability to see in the morning (7%) and comfort (5%).

Studies that assess the response of both existing and new

lens wearers to silicone hydrogels have found that both groups report that these lenses offer excellent levels of initial and ongoing comfort (89). Our 3-year data suggest that initial comfort might be slightly lower than ongoing comfort as there appears to be greater lens awareness in the early stages of lens wear, particularly for previous lens wearers. We find that comfort on waking and at the end of the day are also slightly lower than overall comfort for wearers on 6- and 30-night wear schedules (Fig. 36.12). However, this is to be expected with all contact lens wear and can be alleviated with saline rinses on waking and before sleep.

Results from the FDA trial in the United States also indicate that symptoms of dryness occur less frequently with wear of silicone hydrogels compared with conventional hydrogel lenses (48). This includes significantly fewer overall complaints of dryness, less dryness upon awakening, and fewer unscheduled removals because of dryness. Short-term nondispensing studies by Fonn and Dumbleton (90), however, have not found any differences in reporting of symptoms of dryness among silicone hydrogel and conventional hydrogel lens wearers. The difficulties in assessing patients' subjective responses to lens wear and differences in sample sizes and study length may account for the differences between these studies. Overall, it is clear that comfort and dryness are still the major causes of dissatisfaction in silicone hydrogel lens wearers and improved methods of measuring these responses are needed if we are to improve comfort during wear.

CCLRU research consistently finds that subjects are satisfied with vision when wearing silicone hydrogels. In the FDA trial, 83% of wearers had 20/20 or better visual acuity at all visits, whereas data from FDA trials for laser *in situ* keratomileusis (LASIK) show that only 65.2% of patients have acuity of 20/25 or better (48). Further, there was no loss of two or more lines of best-corrected visual acuity (BCVA) with silicone hydrogel extended wear, whereas 1.2% of patients lost two or more lines of BCVA in the LASIK trial. Our surveys indicate that while 66% of patients will consider refractive surgery as a permanent means of correcting their vision, only 32% are still interested in laser surgery after using silicone hydrogels on a continuous-wear basis (91).

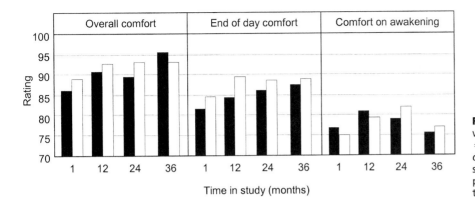

FIG. 36.12. Ratings of comfort in subjects wearing silicone hydrogels for 6 nights (*n* = 36, *filled columns*) or 30 nights (n = 93, *open columns*). Comfort was rated on a scale of 0 to 100, where 0 corresponded to pain and 100 corresponded to cannot feel the lens.

There is very little difference in the performance of silicone hydrogel lenses when they are worn on 6- or 30-night wear schedules. Parameters such as lens deposition, indicators of hypoxia, rates of discontinuation, subjective responses, and inflammatory adverse responses are all equivalent. The 6-night wear schedule does not appear to offer any advantages over the 30-night schedule, in terms of reducing lens spoilage or improving corneal physiology.

A useful indicator of the relative success of different wear schedules is a measure of the percentage of patients that are able to complete their assigned wear schedule. The percentage of patients who only removed their lenses at scheduled times was high for both groups. Over an average of 27 months, we found that 90% of our patients (*n* = 815) can wear their lenses for 21 to 30 consecutive nights and 67% of patients did not remove their lenses overnight during their wear schedule (92). We infer that the majority of patients are able to maintain a 30-night wear schedule with minimal interruption.

Adverse Responses

Silicone Hydrogels and Bacteria

A range of different bacteria can cause corneal infiltrative adverse events. Microbial keratitis for example, is most commonly caused by colonization of contact lenses with *Pseudomonas aeruginosa* (93), a gram-negative bacterium found in many environments, including water. Historically, *Pseudomonas* infections that develop during daily wear have been associated with poor hygiene practices. CLARE is associated with colonization of contact lenses by a range of both gram-negative (in particular *Haemophilus influenzae*) and gram-positive (*Streptococcus pneumoniae*) bacteria and there appears to be an association between the bacteria associated with these events and the general health status of patients in whom these events develop (61,94). *H influenzae* and *S pneumoniae* are commonly isolated from the throat, especially after acute flu-like symptoms. Thus it is important to be careful with recommendations for patients who have upper respiratory tract conditions, or who are at risk of such

infections. In contrast, CLPU is produced by gram-positive colonization of contact lenses, with *Staphylococcus aureus* being the most commonly associated bacterium (95,96). This highlights the importance of vigilance when treating patients with blepharitis, a condition caused by such gram-positive bacteria. Causes of infiltrative keratitis (IK) and asymptomatic infiltrates (AI) appear to be multifactorial, but include colonization of the lens by large numbers of gram-negative bacteria for IK and large numbers of gram-positive bacteria for AI.

Studies by Keay and other researchers (97,98) have shown that there are very few differences in the numbers and type of bacteria found on the lens or ocular surfaces with wear of silicone hydrogels in comparison to conventional hydrogels. This result holds true for asymptomatic or symptomatic wear.

Microbial Keratitis

With all contact lens wear, the adverse response with the most significant outcome is microbial keratitis. It is a rare but potentially devastating complication that threatens the sight of our patients. Estimates of the annualized incidence of microbial keratitis with conventional hydrogel lenses in the United States (99,100), United Kingdom (101), Europe (102,103), and Hong Kong (49) are surprisingly consistent and range from 9.3 to 20.9 per 10,000 extended wearers per year and from 2.2 to 5.2 per 10,000 daily wearers per year. In addition, the rate of loss of BCVA is estimated at 1 in 300 extended wearers and 1 in 25,000 daily wearers per decade (104). For comparison, the rate of loss of BCVA following excimer laser surgery is estimated at 1 in 100 to 500 per decade.

The presentation of microbial keratitis can vary depending on the type of microorganism involved, its pathogenicity and the stage at which the patient presents. In general, excavation of the corneal epithelium, Bowman's layer and stroma is observed, with serious necrosis and infiltration of the underlying tissue (105). The shape of the lesion is usually irregular and "satellite" lesions (smaller lesions adjacent to the primary site of infection) may be present. The bulbar conjunctiva is generally very red. Anterior chamber reaction is often observed in the active stage. Prompt attention and treatment are mandatory as infection associated with more pathogenic microorganisms can progress and cause severe destruction of the cornea within 24 hours. Conjunctival swabs and a corneal scrape will help to determine the type of microorganism involved. Aggressive antibiotic therapy delivered topically at frequent intervals is then the usual approach, however treatment can vary according to the stage and severity of the condition. Once the type of microorganism has been identified, the treatment may then be modified to better target antibiotic sensitivities. Early differential diagnosis of microbial keratitis from CLPU is important for effective treatment (Table 36.7).

TABLE 36.7. DIFFERENTIAL DIAGNOSIS OF MICROBIAL KERATITIS–AND CONTACT LENS–INDUCED PERIPHERAL ULCERS

	Microbial keratitis (MK)	Contact lens–induced peripheral ulcer (CLPU)
Definition	Infection of the cornea by microbes, characterized by excavation of the corneal epithelium, Bowman's layer, and stroma, with infiltration and necrosis of the tissue	Inflammatory reaction of the cornea, characterized in its active stage by focal excavation of the epithelium, infiltration and necrosis of the anterior stroma; Bowman's layer is intact
Occurrence	Incidence of MK in lens and nonlens wearers is limited to few individuals per 10,000 wearers (4 or 5 events with daily wear; 20 or 21 with low-Dk extended wear)	Rare in non–lens wearers; 25 times more frequent with daily wear in comparison to MK; 50 times more frequent with extended wear in comparison to MK (CCLRU/LVPEI data)
Symptoms	Moderate to severe pain of rapid onset, severe redness ("meaty" appearance), decreased visual acuity if the lesion is on the visual axis, discharge (mucopurulent), tearing, photophobia, puffiness of lids	Ranges from moderate to severe pain, foreign body sensation, irritation to asymptomatic, moderate to severe redness, tearing to asymptomatic
Signs		
Infiltrate		
Size	Commonly >1 mm, can be multiple focal infiltrates	Usually small, single, circular, focal infiltrate (up to 2 mm)
Shape	Any shape; commonly irregular	Circular, well-circumscribed
Location	Mainly central or paracentral, sometimes peripheral	Peripheral or midperipheral
Depth	Anterior to midstroma, may involve entire depth	Anterior stroma (subepithelial)
Surrounding cornea	Involved, ranges from edema with diffuse infiltrates to satellite lesions or ring infiltrate	Diffuse infiltrates limited to anterior stroma
Overlying epithelium	Full thickness loss (when active)	Full thickness loss (when active)
Endothelial involvement	Ranges from none to endothelial dusting with cells, keratic precipitates/plaques	None
Anterior chamber reaction	Common, ranging from flare to hypopyon	Only if severe; flare and cells
Lid edema	Usual	Rare
Bulbar and limbal redness	Severe	Moderate, localized
Unilateral/bilateral	Usually unilateral	Usually unilateral
Aetiology	Microbial invasion and infection (bacteria, fungus, parasites)	Toxins released by *Staphylococcus aureus* colonizing the contact lens surface; bacteria not found on scraping or biopsy
Risk factors	Trauma, poor contact lens hygiene, overnight contact lens wear, immunocompromised states, swimming	Overnight contact lens wear, lens material interaction with corneal surface
Course and management	Immediately discontinue lens wear	Discontinue lens wear until resolution
	Progressively worsens without treatment	Normally heals rapidly without intervention
	Corneal scrapings and antimicrobial therapy (e.g., fluoroquinolones) mandatory	Close monitoring required (e.g., within 24 h on day 1)
	Monitor daily	Antibiotics (if monitoring not possible)
	Resolves with scar, may be vascularized, vision loss may occur	Resolves with scar ("bullseye" appearance)

From Aasuri M, Venkata N, Kumar V. Differential diagnosis of microbial keratitis and contact lens-induced peripheral ulcer. *Eye Contact Lens* 2002;29 (IS):S60–S62, with permission.
CCLRU, Cornea and Contact Lens Research Unit.

The hypothesis for the association of silicone hydrogels with an improved risk of microbial keratitis is based on the virtual elimination of the clinical signs of hypoxic effects of continuous wear. Improved corneal epithelial physiology and subsequent improved barrier function is hoped to be associated with a protective effect against microbial keratitis. The work of Ren et al. (106) offers support for this hypothesis. These investigators found that there is less binding of *P. aeruginosa* to human epithelial corneal cells during wear of high-Dk silicone hydrogel and GP lenses in comparison to wear of conventional hydrogel lenses. Interestingly, the bacteria isolated from silicone hydrogel cases of microbial keratitis are similar to the bacteria responsible for culture-proven cases of microbial keratitis with conventional hydrogel lenses (Table 36.8). Therefore, it will be of interest to determine whether the incidence of microbial keratitis with silicone hydrogel lenses is lower than the incidence with conventional hydrogels.

Although elimination of the signs of hypoxia is a very significant step forward, it is unlikely to totally eliminate the occurrence of microbial keratitis. Other risk factors that also play a significant role include the interaction of bacteria with lenses and the cornea during closed-eye conditions, the other effects of lens wear on the cornea and host defense mechanisms as well as the role of the patients and possible issues related to noncompliance. To date, the CCLRU has collated summaries of 26 cases of presumed microbial keratitis associated with silicone hydrogel lens wear around the world including six cases from Australia. By reviewing these case histories, Holden and colleagues (107) suggested risk factors that maybe associated with the development of microbial keratitis with silicone hydrogels (Table 36.9).

Noninfectious Corneal Infiltrative Events

The signs and symptoms of CLARE, CLPU, and IK are similar between silicone hydrogel and conventional hydrogel lens wearers (108) (Fig. 36.13). Although the majority of these events are not severe, it is essential that practitioners do not become complacent as severe cases can still occur (109). The 3-year comparative studies of 6- versus 30-night wear schedules with silicone hydrogels at CCLRU have shown that the rate of inflammatory adverse events (CLPU, CLARE, and IK) is identical with both wear schedules. The rate of inflammatory events is low and is no different from the rate observed with conventional hydrogel extended wear.

Accurate diagnosis of corneal infiltrative events enables us to identify possible causes and risks, to decide whether treatment is necessary, and to gauge the time to resolution. By understanding the differences between corneal infiltrative events we can better inform patients of the likely amount of time they are to be out of lens wear, the chances of recurrence, and strategies to reduce risk. Recurrence of inflammatory complications in individual patients found in this and other studies suggests that a predisposition to inflammation or sensitization can exist among certain individuals (110). Bates (111) reported that sterile epithelial

TABLE 36.8. MICROORGANISMS ISOLATED FROM CULTURE-PROVEN MICROBIAL KERATITIS IN CONTINUOUS WEAR OF SILICONE HYDROGELS AND EXTENDED WEAR OF CONVENTIONAL HYDROGELS

	Percentage of Culture-positive Events	
Microorganism	Silicone Hydrogel (*n* = 14)	Conventional Hydrogel (*n* = 100)
Total gram-negative bacteria	**79% (11)**	**73%**
Pseudomonas sp (including *P. aeruginosa*)	50% (7)	66%
Serratia marcescens	7% (1)	4%
Alcaligenes xylosoxidans	7% (1)	—
Acinetobacter sp	7% (1)	—
Haemophilus influenzae	—	1%
Morganella morgagni	—	1%
Escherichia coli	—	1%
Unidentified gram-negative sp	7% (1)	—
Total gram-positive bacteria	**21% (3)**	**25%**
α-hemolytic streptococci	14% (2)	—
Coagulase-negative staphylococci	—	13%
Staphylococcus aureus	—	6%
Corynebacterium sp	7% (1)	3% (mixed)
Propionibacterium sp	—	3%
Bacillus cereus	—	1%
Other organisms		
Aspergillus fumigatus	7% (1)	—

From Fiona Stapleton, Cornea and Contact Lens Research Unit (CCLRU), with permission.

TABLE 36.9. POSSIBLE RISK FACTORS FOR MICROBIAL KERATITIS WITH SILICONE-HYDROGEL LENSES*

Risk Factors	Number of Patients
Smoker	3
Swam in lenses before event (<2 weeks)	7
Poor health	
Flu/cold symptoms	2
Other	2
Noncompliance	
Wore same lenses for >30 nights	2
Slept in lenses despite discomfort	2
Not disinfecting lens before reinserting	1
Other	
Dry-eye patient—inappropriate wear schedule	1

* Of the 26 cases to date, 17 patients were identified as having at least one risk factor and of these, 3 had two risk factors.

infiltrates are four times more likely to recur in contact lens patients than in non–contact lens wearers. Therefore patients must be counseled about the possibility of an inflammatory event recurring to ensure they follow the appropriate steps toward treatment.

Mechanically Driven Adverse Events

The mechanically driven adverse events that are associated with silicone hydrogel lenses include CLPC, SEALs, and erosions, and some cases of CLPU and IK may also be triggered by mechanical events. The 3-year comparative studies of 6-night versus 30-night wear schedules with sili-

cone hydrogels at CCLRU have shown that there are no differences in the rate of mechanically driven adverse events with either wear schedule.

SEALs

SEALs present as a thin white arcuate lesion in the superior cornea, with significant overlying staining and possible underlying diffuse infiltrates. Approximately 40% of cases have underlying infiltrates and a third exhibit stromal glow with fluorescein. The edges of the lesion are often irregular and may be slightly roughened or thickened. Approximately one third are asymptomatic in silicone hydrogel extended wear,

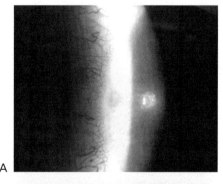

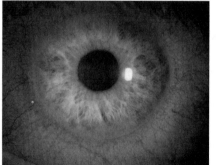

FIG. 36.13. Typical appearance of a contact lens–induced peripheral ulcer (**A**), hyperemia seen with contact lens induced acute red eye (**B**), and diffuse and focal infiltration seen infiltrative keratitis (**C**).

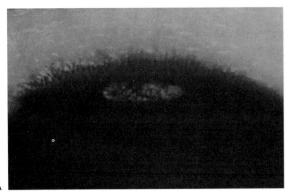 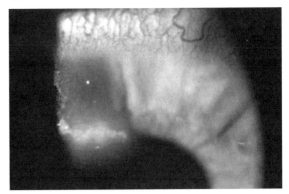

FIG. 36.14. Superior epithelial arcuate lesions seen with silicone hydrogel lens wear in the limbal (**A**) and paralimbal (**B**) regions.

and if symptoms are present, the most common are foreign body sensation or irritation.

In silicone hydrogel wear, SEALs tend to occur in two locations: limbal (immediately adjacent to the limbus) and paralimbal (approximately 1 mm from the limbus) (Fig. 36.14). The paralimbal lesions are more likely to be associated with infiltrates and cause symptoms (112). Time of occurrence of the first event varies widely, and in studies at the CCLRU, the time of onset has ranged from 1 to 20 months.

SEALs are hypothesized to have a multifactorial etiology. Identified risk factors include steep corneas, tight eyelids, Asian eye shape, presbyopia, and male gender (113). In case–control studies of silicone hydrogel wearers, poor wettability and tight fitting lenses lend support to the hypothesis that mechanical chaffing due to a thinning tear film in the superior cornea are major factors in the development of SEALs (114).

The recommended management of SEALs involves discontinuation of lens wear until the epithelial lesion, including any infiltrates has resolved. Resolution usually occurs within 24 to 48 hours, but may take 1 or 2 days longer if infiltrates are present. SEALs tend to recur in approximately 50% of cases, but the time to recur varies widely among patients. There is generally no scarring associated with the events on resolution or after repeated events.

CLPC

CLPC is commonly referred to in the literature as giant papillary conjunctivitis (GPC). Studies at CCLRU indicate that there may be two distinct categories of CLPC: general and local (Fig. 36.15).

General CLPC is the form with which most practitioners are familiar. It involves large, raised papillae of a cobblestone appearance with moderate to severe hyperemia across the entire tarsal plate. General CLPC is characterized by moderate-to-severe patient symptoms, including itching or irritation, a stringy or ropy discharge, excessive movement of the lens, and blurred vision due to this movement or coatings/discharge on lenses. General CLPC occurs at a similar rate during continuous wear with silicone hydrogels and during extended wear with conventional hydrogels. In our experience, CLPC develops after an average of 11 months of silicone hydrogel lens wear and ranges from 6 to 17 months.

The etiology of CLPC remains uncertain, but it has been

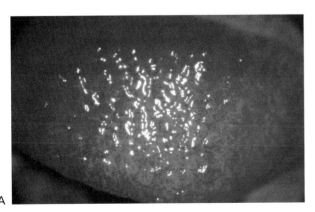 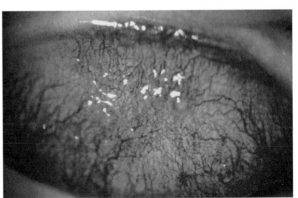

FIG. 36.15. General (**A**) and local (**B**) contact lens papillary conjunctivitis seen with silicone hydrogel lens wear.

hypothesized that it is a delayed or immediate type of hypersensitivity reaction, possibly in response to proteinaceous lens deposits (115). Younger patient age, increased periods of lens wear, infrequent replacement of lenses, and the wear of larger lenses have also been suggested as risk factors (116, 117). Mechanical irritation due to front-surface deposition may also play a role.

Management options for general CLPC include frequent cleaning and replacement of lenses to reduce deposits, a decrease in wear time, or a change in mode of wear (extended wear to daily wear), lens type, or material. Mast cell inhibitors in conjunction with steroids are used in some cases to manage recurrent events. Tarsal redness decreases significantly, but does not tend to return to baseline levels, despite successful management. Papillae also may remain dispersed over the entire tarsus, but are significantly smaller.

Local CLPC involves papillae and hyperemia confined to one or two areas of the upper tarsus only, usually in the central region nearest the lid margin (118). The symptoms of local CLPC can be much milder than general CLPC, with slight irritation or foreign body sensation often the only symptoms. Preliminary evidence indicates that patients wearing silicone hydrogel lenses are more disposed to local CLPC than conventional hydrogel lens wearers (119). Local enlarged papillae are also found in patients with sutures and ocular prostheses, etc., suggesting that mechanical trauma has a role in the etiology of local CLPC (115). However it is possible that hypersensitivity reactions to deposits also play a role in local CLPC. Local CLPC can occur very quickly after a patient initiates silicone hydrogel lens wear, but in others, there may be no significant papillae for at least 2 years of lens wear.

Following discontinuation of lens wear, tarsal redness usually resolves in 2 to 4 weeks; however, the papillae, while smaller, tend to remain. In our experience, local CLPC has a tendency to recur in approximately 50% of cases and if a second episode occurs in the same eye, then the current management strategy is to change the patient to frequent replacement conventional daily wear or daily disposable lens wear, which is usually successful. Refitting with a steeper base curve may be beneficial for some patients (119).

Erosions

A small number of corneal erosions can be observed with silicone hydrogel wear (Fig. 36.16). Corneal erosions or abrasions can occur due to mechanical trauma (fit, lens defect, trapped foreign body, or on insertion and removal) and the damage is usually limited to anterior to the Bowman's layer. The signs and symptoms can vary widely depending upon the cause. If the depth of the abrasion is limited to the superficial one to three layers of the epithelium, the event is often asymptomatic. However, if the erosion is deeper, then moderate to severe pain, watering and blepharospasm may be present (120). If infiltrates are pres-

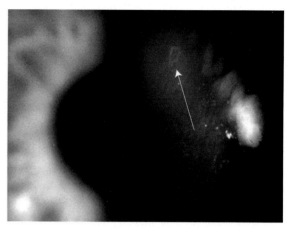

FIG. 36.16. Corneal erosion in the superior cornea seen with silicone hydrogel lens wear.

ent, the event becomes infiltrative keratitis, and is categorized as such with the appropriate management strategy followed.

If the erosion or abrasion is small (<0.5 mm), lens wear should be discontinued for 12 to 24 hours and the patient should be monitored. For large (>0.5 mm) abrasions or erosions, lens wear should be discontinued for, at minimum, 24 hours and not resumed until complete resolution. It is important not to patch the eye as this significantly increases the risk of secondary infection (121). Prophylactic antibiotics may be used in severe cases; however, preservatives in these solutions can delay healing. Artificial tears or lubricants can be used if discomfort is present.

THE FUTURE

Silicone hydrogel contact lenses perform well for up to 30 nights of continuous wear because they have overcome the difficulties associated with hypoxia. A major advantage of these lenses is the flexibility that they offer in terms of wear schedule. Although many patients prefer the convenience of 30 nights of continuous wear, practitioners should use their discretion to determine a wear schedule that best suits the patient and should ensure that patients have appropriate instructions for their care regimen and follow proper procedures if they have any trouble with the lenses.

Practitioners need to consider how to integrate these products into their practices and how to offer this exciting development in vision correction to patients. Silicone hydrogels play an excellent role in therapeutic uses and are being considered more for use with children, even on a daily-wear regimen.

We await the outcomes of the FDA surveillance studies and other studies that are being conducted worldwide to determine if indeed a healthier cornea results in a reduction in the incidence of microbial keratitis with silicone hydrogel lenses. Although the lower water content of silicone hydrogels compared with hydrogels leads us to believe that dryness is less problematic in these lenses, in our experience dryness is still the most common symptom of silicone hydrogel lens wear that leads to patient discomfort. Therefore, the next generation of products to be developed will aim at improving biocompatibility and comfort. In addition a reduction in bacterially driven adverse responses should be possible through improved biocompatibility and possibly incorporation of antibacterial substances. Further increased biocompatibility in association with improved designs will also help reduce the mechanically driven adverse responses that accompany silicone hydrogel wear.

Acknowledgment: The authors thank the Australian Federal Government for their support through the Cooperative Research Centres Program, and acknowledge the assistance of the following people from the CCLRU/CRCERT: Jerome Ozkan (particularly for assistance with figures), Padmaja Sankaridurg, Katie Edwards, Angela Kalliris, Nina Tahhan, Isabelle Jalbert, Robert Terry (for assistance with figures), and Fiona Stapleton (for data regarding microbiota and cases of microbial keratitis).

REFERENCES

1. van Cranenburgh B. What do practitioners think about continuous-wear lenses? *Optician* 1999;217:36–37.
2. Holden BA. The Glenn A. Fry award lecture 1988: The ocular response to contact lens wear. *Optom Vis Sci* 1989;66:717–733.
3. Sweeney DF, Keay L, Jalbert I, et al. Clinical performance of silicone hydrogel lenses. In: Sweeney DF, ed. *Silicone hydrogels: the rebirth of continuous wear contact lenses.* Oxford: Butterworth Heinemann, 2000:90–149.
4. de Carle J. Developing hydrophilic lenses for continuous wearing. *Aust J Optom* 1972;55:343–346.
5. Ruben M. Acute eye disease secondary to contact-lens wear. *Lancet* 1976;1:138–140.
6. Cooper R, Constable I. Infective keratitis in soft contact lens wearers. *Br J Ophthalmol* 1977;61:250–254.
7. Zantos SG, Holden BA. Ocular changes associated with continuous wear of contact lenses. *Aust J Optom* 1978;61:418–426.
8. Chalupa E, Swarbrick H, Holden B, et al. Severe corneal infections associated with contact lens wear. *Ophthalmology* 1987;94:17–22.
9. Adams C Jr, Cohen E, Laibson P, et al. Corneal ulcers in patients with cosmetic extended-wear contact lenses. *Am J Ophthalmol* 1983;96:705–709.
10. Donnenfeld E, Cohen E, Arentsen J, et al. Changing trends in contact lens associated corneal ulcers: an overview of 116 cases. *CLAO J* 1986;12:145–149.
11. Patrinely J, Wilhelmus K, Rubin J, et al. Bacterial keratitis associated with extended wear soft contact lenses. *CLAO J* 1985;11:234–236.
12. Spring TF. Reaction to hydrophilic lenses. *Med J Aust* 1974;1:449–450.
13. Lamer L. Extended wear contact lenses for myopes: a follow up study of 400 cases. *Ophthalmology* 1983;90:156–161.
14. Holden BA, Sweeney DF, Vannas A, et al. Effects of long-term extended contact lens wear on the human cornea. *Invest Ophthalmol Vis Sci* 1985;26:1489–1501.
15. Holden BA, Sweeney DF, Swarbrick HA, et al. The vascular response to long-term extended contact lens wear. *Clin Exp Optom* 1986;69:112–119.
16. Mondino B, Weissman B, Farb M, et al. Corneal ulcers associated with daily wear and extended wear contact lenses. *Am J Ophthalmol* 1986;102:58–65.
17. Allegretti D. Extended wear lens: blessing or public peril. *Capital Times* 1985.
18. Anon. A sceptic eye on contacts. *Time* 1986;57.
19. MacAlister G, Young G. Flexible wear—an answer to extended wear complications? *Trans BCLA Int Conference* 1988;5(Suppl):19–22.
20. Kame R. Disposability: an alternative to problems with hydrogel contact lenses. *Int Contact Lens Clin* 1988;12:371–376.
21. Driebe WJ. Disposable soft contact lenses. *Surv Ophthalmol* 1989;34:44–46.
22. Kotow M, Holden BA, Grant T. The value of regular replacement of low water content contact lenses for extended wear. *J Am Optom Assoc* 1987;58:461–464.
23. Grant T. Clinical aspects of planned replacement and disposable lenses. In: Kerr C, ed. *The contact lens year book.* Hythe, Kent: Medical and Scientific Publishing, 1991:15–25.
24. Grant T, Chong MS, Vajdic C, et al. Contact lens induced peripheral ulcer during hydrogel contact lens wear. *CLAO J* 1998;24:145–151.
25. Sankaridurg PR, Sweeney DS, Sharma S, et al. Adverse events with extended wear of disposable hydrogels: results for the first 13 months of lens wear. *Ophthalmology* 1999;106:1671–1680.
26. Schein OD, Glynn RJ, Seddon JM, et al. The relative risk of ulcerative keratitis among users of daily-wear and extended-wear soft contact lenses. *New Engl J Med* 1989;321:773–778.
27. Polse K, Mandell R. Critical oxygen tension at the corneal surface. *Arch Ophthalmol* 1970;84:505–508.
28. Mandell R, Farrell R. Corneal swelling at low atmospheric oxygen pressures. *Invest Ophthalmol Vis Sci* 1980;19:697–702.
29. Holden BA, Mertz GW, McNally JJ. Corneal swelling response to contact lenses worn under extended wear conditions. *Invest Ophthalmol Vis Sci* 1983;24:218–226.
30. Hamano H, Hori M, Hamano T, et al. Effects of contact lens wear on mitosis of corneal epithelium and lactate content of aqueous humor of rabbits. *Jpn J Ophthalmol* 1983;27:451–458.
31. Mizutani Y, Matsunaka H, Takemoto N, et al. The effect of anoxia on the human cornea. *Jpn Ophth Soc Acta* 1983;87:644–649.
32. Bonanno J, Polse K. Corneal acidosis during contact lens wear: effects of hypoxia and CO_2. *Invest Ophthalmol Vis Sci* 1987;28:522–530.
33. Holden BA, Mertz GW. Critical oxygen levels to avoid corneal edema for daily and extended wear contact lenses. *Invest Ophthalmol Vis Sci* 1984;25:1161–1167.
34. Mertz GW. Overnight swelling of the living human cornea. *J Am Optom Assoc* 1980;51:211–213.
35. La Hood D, Sweeney DF, Holden BA. Overnight corneal edema with hydrogel, rigid gas permeable and silicone elastomer lenses. *Int Contact Lens Clin* 1988;15:149–154.
36. Harvitt DM, Bonanno JA. Re-evaluation of the oxygen diffusion model for predicting minimum contact lens Dk/t values needed to avoid corneal anoxia. *Optom Vis Sci* 1999;76:712–719.
37. Papas E. On the relationship between soft contact lens oxygen transmissibility and induced limbal hyperaemia. *Exp Eye Res* 1998;67:125–131.
38. Sweeney D, Holden B. Silicone elastomer lens wear induces less overnight corneal edema than sleep without lens wear. *Curr Eye Res* 1987;6:1391–1394.
39. Tighe B. Silicone hydrogel materials: how do they work? In:

Sweeney D, ed. *Silicone hydrogels: the rebirth of extended wear contact lenses.* Oxford: Butterworth-Heineman, 2000:1–21.

40. Morgan P, Efron N. Comparative clinical performance of two silicone hydrogel contact lenses for continuous wear. *Clin Exp Optom* 2002;85:183–192.

41. Efron N, Brennan N, Sek B. Wearing patterns with HEMA contact lenses. *Int Contact Lens Clin* 1988;15:344–350.

42. Dumbleton K, Chalmers R, McNally J, et al. Effect of lens base curve on subjective comfort and assessment of fit with silicone hydrogel continuous wear contact lenses. *Optom Vis Sci* 2002; 79:633–637.

43. Fonn D, Situ P, Simpson T. Hydrogel lens dehydration and subjective comfort and dryness ratings in symptomatic and asymptomatic contact lens wearers. *Optom Vis Sci* 1999;76: 700–704.

44. Cox N. Contact lens drop outs. *J Br Contact Lens Assoc* 1985; 8:6–10.

45. Weed KH, Fonn D, Potvin R. Discontinuation from contact lens wear [AAO Abstract]. *Optom Vis Sci* 1993;70:S140(abst).

46. Fonn D, Pritchard N, Brazeau D, et al. Discontinuation of contact lens wear: the numbers, reasons and patient profiles [ARVO Abstract]. *Invest Ophthalmol Vis Sci* 1995;36:S312(abst 1455).

47. Chalmers R, McNally J, McKenney C, et al. The role of dryness symptoms in discontinuation of wear and unscheduled lens removals in extended wear of silicone hydrogel lenses [ARVO Abstract]. *Invest Ophthalmol Vis Sci* 2002;43:E(abst 3088).

48. McNally J, McKenney C. A clinical look at a silicone hydrogel extended wear lens. *Contact Lens Spectr* 2002;17:38–41.

49. Lam D, Houang E, Fan D, et al. Incidence and risk factors for microbial keratitis in Hong Kong: comparison with Europe and North America. *Eye* 2002;16:608–618.

50. Stapleton F, Dart JKG, Minassian D. Risk factors with contact lens related suppurative keratitis. *CLAO J* 1993;19:204–10.

51. Brennan NA, Chantal Coles M-L, Jaworski A, et al. Proposed practice guidelines for continuous contact lens wear. *Clin Exp Optom* 2001;84:71–77.

52. Solomon O. Corneal stress test for extended wear. *CLAO J* 1996;22:75–78.

53. Norn M. Vital staining of cornea and conjunctiva. *Contact Lens J* 1972;3:19–22.

54. Jalbert I, Sweeney DF, Holden BA. The characteristics of corneal staining in successful daily and extended disposable contact lens wearers. *Clin Exp Optom* 1999;82:4–10.

55. Young G, Holden BA, Cooke G. Influence of soft contact lens design on clinical performance. *Optom Vis Sci* 1993;70: 394–403.

56. Dumbleton KA, Chalmers RL, Richter DB, et al. Changes in myopic refractive error in nine months' extended wear of hydrogel lenses with high and low oxygen permeability. *Optom Vis Sci* 1999;76:845–849.

57. Jalbert I, Holden B, Keay L, et al. Refractive and corneal power changes associated with overnight lens wear: differences between low Dk/t hydrogel and high Dk/t silicone hydrogel lenses [AAO Abstract]. *Optom Vis Sci* 1999;76:S234.

58. Terry RL, Schnider CM, Holden BA, et al. CCLRU standard for success of daily and extended wear contact lenses. *Optom Vis Sci* 1993;70:234–243.

59. Brennan NA, Chantal Coles M-L. Where do silicone hydrogels fit into everyday practice? In: Sweeney DF, ed. *Silicone hydrogels: the rebirth of continuous wear contact lenses.* Oxford: Butterworth Heinemann, 2000:235–270.

60. Yamane SJ, Kuwabara DM. Ensuring compliance in patients wearing contact lenses on an extended-wear basis. *Int Contact Lens Clin* 1987;14:108–12.

61. Sankaridurg PR, Willcox MDP, Sharma S, et al. *Haemophilus influenzae* adherent to contact lenses associated with the production of acute ocular inflammation. *J Clin Microbiol* 1996;34: 2426–2431.

62. Efron N. Efron grading scales for contact lens complications (millennium edition). Appendix K. In: Efron N, ed. *Contact lens practice.* Oxford: Butterworth-Heinemann, 2002:487–489.

63. MacDonald K, Fonn D, Richter D, et al. Comparison of the physiological response to extended wear of an experimental high Dk soft lens versus a 38% HEMA lens [ARVO Abstract]. *Invest Ophthalmol Vis Sci* 1995;36:S310(abst).

64. Bullimore M, Nguyen M, Bozic J, et al. Overnight corneal swelling with 7-day continuous wear of soft contact lenses [ARVO Abstract]. *Invest Ophthalmol Vis Sci* 2002;43:E(abst 3100).

65. Comstock T, Robboy M, Cox I, et al. Presented at: British Contact Lens Association Conference, Birmingham, AL, May 1999. Poster available at: http://www.siliconehydrogels.com/. Accessed February 2003.

66. Fonn D, du Toit R, Situ P, et al. Apparent sympathetic response of contralateral nonlens wearing eyes after overnight lens wear in the fellow eye [ARVO Abstract]. *Invest Ophthalmol Vis Sci* 1998;39:S336(abst).

67. Mueller N, Caroline P, Smythe J, et al. A comparison of overnight swelling response with two high Dk silicone hydrogels. [AAO Abstract]. *Optom Vis Sci* 2001;78:S199(abst 126).

68. Rivera RK, Polse KA. Corneal response to different oxygen levels during extended wear. *CLAO J* 1991;17:96–101.

69. Holden BA, Grant T, Kotow M, et al. Epithelial microcysts with daily and extended wear of hydrogel and rigid gas permeable contact lenses [ARVO Abstract]. *Invest Ophthalmol Vis Sci* 1987;28:S372(abst).

70. Keay L, Sweeney DF, Jalbert I, et al. Microcyst response to high Dk/t silicone hydrogel contact lenses. *Optom Vis Sci* 2000;77: 582–585.

71. Keay L, Jalbert I, Sweeney DF, et al. Microcysts: clinical significance and differential diagnosis. *J Am Optom Assoc* 2001;72: 452–560.

72. Covey M, Sweeney DF, Terry RL, et al. Hypoxic effects on the anterior eye of high Dk soft contact lens wearers are negligible. *Optom Vis Sci* 2001;78:95–99.

73. Dumbleton KA, Chalmers RL, Richter DB, et al. Vascular response to extended wear of hydrogel lenses with high and low oxygen permeability. *Optom Vis Sci* 2001;78:147–151.

74. Papas EB, Vajdic CM, Austen R, et al. High-oxygen-transmissibility soft contact lenses do not induce limbal hyperaemia. *Curr Eye Res* 1997;16:942–948.

75. Du Toit R, Simpson T, Fonn D, et al. Recovery from hyperemia after overnight wear of low and high transmissibility hydrogel lenses. *Curr Eye Res* 2001;22:68–73.

76. Caroline P, Campbell R. Long term effects of hydrophilic contact lenses on myopia. *Contact Lens Spectr* 1991;16:68.

77. Edmonds C. Myopia reduction with frequent replacement of Acuvue lenses. *Int Contact Lens Clin* 1993;20:195–199.

78. Brennan N, Chantal Coles M, Comstock T, et al. A 1-year prospective clinical trial of Balafilcon A (PureVision) silicone hydrogel contact lenses used on a 30-day continuous wear schedule. *Ophthalmology* 2002;109:1172–1177.

79. Fonn D, Pritchard N, Dumbleton K. Factors affecting the success of silicone hydrogels. In: Sweeney D, ed. *Silicone hydrogels: the rebirth of extended wear contact lenses.* Oxford: Butterworth Heinemann, 2000:214–234.

80. McKenney C, Becker N, Thomas S, et al. Lens deposits with a high Dk hydrophilic soft lens [AAO Abstract]. *Optom Vis Sci* 1998;75:S276(abst).

81. Montero Iruzubieta J, Nebot Ripoll J, Chiva J, et al. Practical

experience with a high Dk lotrafilcon A fluorosilicone hydrogel extended wear contact lens in Spain. *CLAO J* 2001;27:41–46.

82. Long B, Robird S, Grant T. Six months of in-practice experience with a high Dk lotrafilcon A soft contact lens. *Contact Lens Anterior Eye* 2000;23:112–118.

83. Jones L, Senchyna M, Glasier M-A, et al. Lysozyme and lipid deposition on silicone hydrogel contact lens materials. *Eye Contact Lens* 2002;29:S75.

84. Tan J, Keay L, Jalbert I, et al. Mucin balls with wear of conventional and silicone hydrogel contact lenses. *Optom Vis Sci* 2003; 80:291–297.

85. Dumbleton K, Jones L, Chalmers R, et al. Clinical characterization of spherical post-lens debris associated with lotrafilcon high-Dk silicone lenses. *CLAO J* 2000;26:186–192.

86. Jalbert I, Stapleton F, Papas E, et al. In vivo confocal microscopy of the human cornea. *Br J Ophthalmol* 2003;87:225–236.

87. Pritchard N, Jones L, Dumbleton K, et al. Epithelial inclusions in association with mucin ball development in high-oxygen permeability hydrogel lenses. *Optom Vis Sci* 2000;77:68–72.

88. Jones L, MacDougall N, Sorbara L. Asymptomatic corneal staining associated with the use of balafilcon silicone hydrogel contact lenses disinfected with a polyaminopropyl biguanide-preserved care regimen. *Optom Vis Sci* 2002;79:753–761.

89. Morgan P, Maldonado-Codina C, Efron N. Comfort response to rigid and soft hyper-transmissible contact lenses used for continuous wear. *Eye Contact Lens* 2003;29(IS):S127–130.

90. Fonn D, Dumbleton K. Dryness and discomfort with silicone hydrogel contact lenses. *Eye Contact Lens* 2003;29(IS): S101–204.

91. Skotnitsky C, Sweeney DF, Keay L, et al. Patient responses and attitudes to 30 night continuous wear of high Dk silicone hydrogel lenses and attitudes to refractive surgery [AAO Abstract]. *Optom Vis Sci* 1999;76:S214.

92. Sweeney D, Keay L, Carnt N, et al. Practitioner guidelines for continuous wear with high Dk silicone hydrogel contact lenses. *Clin Exp Optom* 2002;85:161–167.

93. Schein OD, Ormerod LD, Barraquer E, et al. Microbiology of contact lens-related keratitis. *Cornea* 1989;8:281–285.

94. Sankaridurg PR, Sharma S, Willcox MDP, et al. Colonization of hydrogel lenses with *Streptococcus pneumoniae*: risk of development of corneal infiltrates. *Cornea* 1999;18:289–95.

95. Jalbert I, Willcox MDP, Sweeney DF. Isolation of *Staphylococcus aureus* from a contact lens at the time of a contact lens induced peripheral ulcer: case report. *Cornea* 2000;19:116–20.

96. Willcox MDP, Sweeney DF, Sharma S, et al. Contact lens induced peripheral ulcers are associated with increased bacterial contamination of contact lenses [ARVO Abstract]. *Invest Ophthalmol Vis Sci* 1995;36:S152(abst).

97. Willcox M, Harmis N, Holden B. Bacterial populations on high-Dk silicone hydrogel contact lenses: effect of length of wear in asymptomatic patients. *Clin Exp Optom* 2002;85:172–175.

98. Keay L, Willcox MDP, Sweeney DF, et al. Bacterial populations of 30-night extended wear silicone hydrogel lenses. *CLAO J* 2001;27:30–34.

99. MacRae S, Herman C, Stulting R, et al. Corneal ulcer and adverse reaction rates in pre-market contact lens studies. *Am J Ophthalmol* 1991;111:457–465.

100. Poggio EC, Glynn RJ, Schein OD, et al. The incidence of ulcerative keratitis among users of daily-wear and extended-wear soft contact lenses. *New Eng J Med* 1989;321:779–783.

101. Seal D, Kirkness C, Bennet H. Population-based cohort study of microbial keratitis in Scotland: incidence and features. *Contact Lens Anterior Eye* 1999;1999:49–57.

102. Cheng KH, Leung SL, Hoekman HW, et al. Incidence of con-

tact-lens associated microbial keratitis and its related morbidity. *Lancet* 1999;354:181–5.

103. Nilsson S, Montan P. The annualized incidence of contact lens induced keratitis in Sweden and its relation to lens type and wear schedule: results of a 3-month prospective study. *CLAO J* 1994;20:225–230.

104. Barr J. The 1998 annual report on contact lenses. *Contact Lens Spectr* 1999;15:1–5.

105. Cockington CD, Hyndiuk RA. Bacterial keratitis. In: Tabbara K, Hyndiuk R, eds. *Infections in the eye,* 2nd ed. Boston: Little, Brown and Company, 1996:323–347.

106. Ren D, Yamamoto K, Ladage P, et al. Adaptive effects of 30-night wear of hyper-O$_2$ transmissible contact lenses on bacterial binding and corneal epithelium: a 1-year clinical trial. *Ophthalmology* 2002;109:27–40.

107. Holden B, Sweeney D, Sankaridurg P, et al. Microbial keratitis and vision loss with contact lenses. *Eye Contact Lens* 2003; 29(IS):S131–134.

108. Sweeney D, Jalbert I, Covery M, et al. Clinical characterisation of corneal infiltrative events observed with soft contact lens wear. *Cornea* 2003;22:435-442.

109. Skotnitsky C, Jalbert I, O'Hare N, et al. Case reports of three atypical infiltrative events with high DK soft contact lens wear. *Cornea* 2002;21:318–324.

110. Sweeney DF, Grant T, Chong MS, et al. Recurrence and acute inflammatory conditions with hydrogel extended wear [ARVO Abstract]. *Invest Ophthalmol Vis Sci* 1993;34:S1008(abst).

111. Bates AK, Morris RJ, Stapleton F, et al. 'Sterile' infiltrates in contact lens wearers. *Eye* 1989;3:803–10.

112. O'Hare NA, Naduvilath TJ, Sweeney DF, et al. A clinical comparison of limbal and paralimbal superior epithelial arcuate lesions (SEALs) in high Dk EW [ARVO Abstract]. *Invest Ophthalmol Vis Sci* 2001;42:S595(abst 3195).

113. Holden BA, Stephenson A, Stretton S, et al. Superior epithelial arcuate lesions with soft contact lens wear. *Optom Vis Sci* 2001; 78:9–12.

114. O'Hare N, Stapleton F, Naduvilath T, et al. Interaction between the contact lens and the ocular surface in superior epithelial arcuate lesions. In: Sullivan D, Stern M, Tsubota K, Dartt D, Sullivan R, Bromberg B, eds. *Lacrimal gland, tear film, and dry eye syndromes 3,* Vol 506. New York: Kluwer Academic / Plenum Publishers, 2002:973–980.

115. Sankaridurg PR, Skotnitsky C, Pearce D, et al. Contact lens papillary conjunctivitis: a review. *Optom Pract* 2001;2:19–28.

116. Hart DE, Schkolnick JA, Bernstein S, et al. Contact lens induced giant papillary conjunctivitis: A retrospective study. *J Am Optom Assoc* 1989;60:195–204.

117. Allansmith MR. Giant papillary conjunctivitis. *J Am Optom Assoc* 1990;61:S41–S46.

118. Skotnitsky C, Kalliris A, Sankaridurg P, et al. Contact lens-induced papillary conjunctivitis is either local or general. *Int Contact Lens Clin* 2000;27:193–195.

119. Dumbleton K. Adverse events with silicone hydrogel continuous wear. *Contact Lens Anterior Eye* 2002;25:137–146.

120. Bergmanson J. Contact lens induced epithelial pathology. In: Bennett E, Weissman B, eds. *Clinical contact lens practice.* Philadelphia: LB Lippincott Company, 1992.

121. Clemons C, Cohen E, Arentsen J, et al. Pseudomonas ulcers following patching of corneal abrasions associated with contact lens wear. *CLAO J* 1987;13:161–164.

122. Fonn D, du Toit R, Simpson T, et al. Sympathetic swelling response of the control eye to soft lenses in the other eye. *Invest Ophthalmol Vis Sci* 1999;40:3116–3121.

C H A P T E R

37

CORNEAL VASCULARIZATION

ERIC B. PAPAS

INTRODUCTION

Physiologically, the process of corneal vascularization (CV) occurs in response to some form of tissue threat. When new vessels arrive at the injured site, a link with the general circulation is created that gives damaged cells access to essential nutrients as well as all the blood-borne elements of the immune system. When viewed from this perspective, the vascularization response can be considered an event that is fundamentally beneficial in that it acts to contain the potential for further damage and promote repair.

Unfortunately, the presence of infiltrating blood vessels in the cornea has additional consequences that, because of its role as the initial optical element of the eye, are distinctly undesirable. A primary consequence is the tendency for vessel tracks to scatter incident light and reduce corneal transparency. The resulting potential for severe visual interference is a major reason for the view of CV as a significant corneal disease and one of the more serious complications associated with contact lens wear.

While it is unusual for contact lens–related CV to be so severe as to seriously threaten the visual axis, the appearance of new corneal vessels is an important event because it serves to indicate that the tissue is under stress and, as a result, its health has been compromised. A particularly disturbing aspect of this situation is that vessel growth is accompanied by a rapid and persistent loss of immune privilege within the anterior chamber (1). In the short term this increases the risk of a devastating infection or inflammatory reaction, as well as increasing the likelihood of rejection for any corneal grafts that may be required in the longer term (2). The vigilant clinician thus views any level of corneal vascular development as a suspicious sign and an indication of the need to improve the interaction between the lens and the ocular environment.

PREVALENCE

The prevalence of CV in the general population is not precisely known. In a study looking at individuals consecutively presenting for eye examinations at a hospital outpatient department, Colby and Adamis (3) found that 4.14% of the sample of 845 were affected (3). This figure has been used as the basis for an estimate of up to 1.4 million episodes of CV occurring annually in the United States (4), although this is likely to overstate the true value and should probably be regarded as indicating the "worst-case" scenario.

Whatever the true figure, contact lens wear is recognized as being a major risk factor associated with the development of CV. The magnitude of that risk is not the same for all lens types, however. For rigid lenses and, in particular, gas-permeable (GP) examples, prevalence of CV appears to be low. Indeed several studies have reported no episodes of vascularization even when lenses were worn on an extended basis (5–7). It would not be reasonable to expect CV rates among the general GP-wearing population to be precisely zero, however, as new vessel growth has regularly been found in accompaniment to GP-related conditions such as 3- and 9-o'clock staining (8). Nevertheless, when Keech et al. (9) monitored 566 consecutive GP consultations to determine complications rates for various conditions, only about 1% of visits involved CV (9).

Several studies have considered the occurrence of CV among soft lens wearers, both in daily and extended wear. The resulting prevalence estimates vary widely, making it difficult to arrive at a consensus. For example, in daily wear, Grimmer (10) recorded no instance of vascularization in any of his group of 99 wearers (10), and Roth (11) reported a low prevalence of 1.3% (11). However, in Cunha et al.'s study, a figure of 16% was found (12). Keech et al. (9) observed CV at 18% of the 897 soft lens consultations they monitored, and Rapkin noted that 24% of a group of new wearers were affected (13). During extended wear, Lamer (14) reported a prevalence of 0.2%, Binder (15) 7%, and Stark and Martin (16) 8.7%.

This diversity is, no doubt, a reflection of the fact that the various investigators would have used different lenses, study designs, and populations during the conduct of each study. Particularly important in this respect is that they would also have employed a range of criteria to assess vessel encroachment onto the cornea. Although there are exceptions (10), these criteria are rarely stated, rendering it difficult to make meaningful inter-study comparisons. In these circumstances, studies such as those of Cunha et al. (12) and Keech et al. (9), where two or more modalities are assessed within the same design framework, are especially beneficial as the methodology and observational criteria are presumably consistently applied across all groups.

Prevalence rates among subjects wearing lenses for therapeutic reasons generally appear to be higher than in cosmetic cases. Schecter et al. recorded a prevalence of 35% among a group of subjects with a variety of corneal afflictions (17). Also working with a sample containing a high proportion of therapeutic wearers, Cunha et al. (12) found that 47% had corneal vascularization, while Sarver et al. (18) reported CV in 65% of all eyes in their group of aphakic subjects.

It is apparent from the foregoing that soft contact lenses in particular, represent a major risk factor for vessel growth within the cornea. Lee et al. (4) used a 1989 estimate of 13 million US soft contact lens wearers, together with reported prevalence rates for CV, to conjecture that between 128,000 and 470,000 individuals were affected at any one time. This would imply that between 9% and 34% of all cases of CV in the United States were associated with soft contact lens wear.

The use of contact lenses has increased substantially over the last decade so that there are currently around 100 million wearers worldwide (19). In 2001, approximately 35 million of these were in the United States and 87% used soft lenses (20). While it might have been expected that this rise would precipitate a corresponding increase in the number of individuals experiencing CV, it is probable that this has been offset to some extent by changes in prescribing habits. During this period, soft contact lens usage has tended toward thinner and more highly oxygen-permeable designs with disposable, daily disposable and, recently, silicone hydrogel (SiH) lenses becoming commonplace.

All of the soft lens studies mentioned to this point have involved subjects who were using conventional hydrogel lenses. Few data relating to the impact of either disposable or SiH lenses on CV prevalence have been published so far. Two studies have compared vascular changes in subjects wearing conventional and SiH lenses on an extended wear basis. In the first of these, Dumbleton et al. (21) reported significant vessel progression over the 9-month observation period for eyes wearing conventional lenses. SiH-wearing eyes, conversely, either did not change or showed some vascular regression (21). This result was not entirely replicated by Brennan et al. (22), who conducted a 1-year study during which subjects wore the same control lens as used by Dumbleton et al. but a different silicone hydrogel. While again no significant changes in CV were found in the SiH group, there was also no alteration in the status of the control group relative to baseline. These differing findings indicate the need for further data in this area but tend to support the proposition that prevalence rates for CV among wearers of modern soft lens designs are likely to be lower than with previous iterations.

TERMINOLOGY

For the purpose of describing changes in blood flow characteristics during this chapter, the term *perfusion* will be taken to refer to the presence of blood within a vessel or vessels and *erythema* to the appearance of redness in a tissue due to the presence of blood within it. *Hyperaemia* is, therefore, increased perfusion above some previously observed level and is typically indicated by the observation of increased erythema.

A variety of terms have been used to describe the appearance of blood vessels in the region of the limbus and peripheral cornea. Clinically, an important distinction needs to be made regarding whether the observed blood flow, whatever its level, is within existing normal vessels or new, pathological ones. In the former case, terms that have been applied to describe observed vascular changes include vessel filling, injection, engorgement, and vessel prominence. None of these descriptors is associated with any implication that structural alterations have occurred, either to the vessels themselves or the surrounding tissue. As this kind of change is fundamental to the process of true vasogenesis, the use of these terms should be limited to vascular events that do not involve new growth, although they may, of course, be appropriately used to describe phenomena that accompany or precede such growth.

The terms *vascularization* and *neovascularization* have usually been used to refer to the appearance of new vessels within a tissue. Despite attempts to establish guidelines for the appropriate use of these terms (23), they are commonly regarded as synonyms (8); however, *vascularization* will be used in the present text.

DEVELOPMENT OF NEW VESSELS

The visible sequence of events leading to the penetration of new vessels into the cornea has recently been closely observed in rabbits with the confocal microscope (24). Around 6 hours after injury, the first sign of a response is the beginning of inflammatory cell infiltration from the nearest group of limbal vessels. This is followed over the next 12 hours by dilation of the limbal veins in particular, such that the region of involvement covers an arc extending approximately 60 degrees on either side of the injury. It is about this time when the first indications of altered vessel structure become apparent as short, pointed protrusions (25) that emerge from the tops of capillary vessels and venules. These buds extend in the direction of the injury and initially are mostly associated with stromal nerves. It may be that this connection provides newly formed vascular tissue with a relatively easy route into the tightly packed corneal matrix, although the link is generally lost after about 3 days of vessel growth. By about 4 days after the injury, capillary budding has increased significantly with some sprouts starting to develop into tubular configurations. Movement of blood cells within the lumen of these rudimentary vessels can occur as early as 72 hours after the first bud forms. From this point, the new vessels proceed to grow in the direction of the injury site at a rate of about 0.5 mm per day.

MOLECULAR BASIS FOR CORNEAL ANGIOGENESIS

The series of observable events characterizing the appearance of new vessels in the cornea is associated with an array of mediators that interact with, and control the behavior of, various groups of cells that may be local to the site of tissue damage or relatively remote from it. While the full nature of these mediators and their range of activity has not been established, the fact that the cornea has been widely used as a model to study the phenomenon of angiogenesis in general has resulted in a greater understanding of its particular response characteristics.

It is commonly believed that the normal avascularity of the cornea is the result of an equilibrium maintained between two groups of molecules that are, respectively, angiogenic and antiangiogenic or angiostatic (26). This must of necessity be a dynamic equilibrium as corneal clarity is preserved even under conditions such as sleep, that are accompanied by the up-regulation of factors with potent angiogenic potential (e.g., IL-8) (27).

The precise characteristics required of a stimulus in order for it to be able to disturb the system sufficiently to precipitate vessel growth are not fully understood. When corneal tissue perceives that it has become appropriately disturbed, however, its cells respond by producing chemical signals that communicate with the nearest cells of the immune system. This typically occurs via the limbal capillaries at the closest point to the affected region of the cornea. What follows is a complex series of processes controlled by an array of molecules called chemokines and cytokines, which are able to modify cellular behavior in a variety of ways depending on their type.

Many of the known cytokines have angiogenic activity and one of these, vascular endothelial growth factor (VEGF), appears to play a particularly important role in CV. Studies using a rat model of vascularization have shown that VEGF is required for new vessel growth in response to a wound or an inflammatory stimulus (28), and considerable evidence exists suggesting that it also has a key role in human corneal angiogenesis. For example, VEGF is normally found at low levels in keratocytes, corneal epithelium and endothelium, as well as limbal vascular endothelial cells (29). When vascularization is present, however, its concentration increases substantially (29,30). This is significant because, among its range of effects, VEGF possesses the ability to induce mitogenic activity in vascular endothelial cells, apparently by directly interacting with receptor sites on their surfaces (28). Under normal circumstances, adult vascular endothelium cells have turnover rates that are typically of the order of a few years (i.e., they are very low). The effect of upregulating VEGF is to alter this stable state to one of active proliferation, creating a supply of vascular endothelial cells that are available for incorporation into newly forming vessels.

In addition to its direct mitogenic action, VEGF possesses other properties that are influential in the process of vasogenesis. The key to this process is its chemotactic activity with respect to monocytes. These cells, which are a type of leukocyte, appear to be centrally involved during new vessel growth. Studies of the vascularization process show not only that leukocyte infiltration constitutes the earliest observable activity following vasogenic injury (24), but also that the pattern of infiltration closely corresponds to the site and depth at which new vessels begin to form and to the direction they subsequently take (31–33).

Under the influence of chemotactic agents like VEGF, leukocytes in the blood stream are attracted to the injury site, their access being facilitated by the locally increased blood flow (hyperemia). On arrival, their progress is delayed due to an up-regulation of the intercellular adhesion molecule (ICAM-1). This acts to tether the leukocyte to the vascular endothelium, from where it can pass out of the vessels and into the surrounding tissue, a process known as extravasation.

Leukocytes, and in particular macrophages, are capable of producing a variety of potent angiogenic mediators and as a consequence are viewed as important factors in the angiogenic response. The significance of their presence is clearly demonstrated by the observation that preventing leukocyte extravasation substantially inhibits angiogenesis, even though the stimulating agent remains (34,35).

Once the cells of the vascular endothelium have been induced to proliferate under the action of substances like VEGF or basic fibroblast growth factor (bFGF), if they are to become organized into vessels they must be persuaded to migrate away from their origins in existing capillaries and penetrate into corneal tissue. Under normal circumstances, this movement is prevented by the dual anatomical constraints of basement membrane attachment and the surrounding extracellular matrix. Mathematical analysis of the configuration of new vessel tracks in the cornea suggests that progression of new vessels follows a percolation model (36) (i.e., they proceed along the line of least resistance). While in the early stages, vascular endothelial cells may conveniently follow the paths forged by local nerve trunks (24), in general, they require some other adjacent space into which they can easily move. Calculation of the minimum size requirement for these voids indicates that the existing interstitial spaces within corneal tissue are not large enough to permit this motion, even though they may have become expanded by edematous swelling. The movement of proliferating vascular endothelial cells thus appears to require some active assistance in creating convenient spaces.

Evidence from studies of the rat cornea suggests a role for the proteolytic enzymes known as matrix metalloproteinases (MMP) in this respect. MMPs are a family of proteases with a range of activities and MMP-2, in particular, has the ability to digest type IV collagen. Consequently it is also known as gelatinase A. When vascularization occurs in a rat model, MMP-2 becomes up-regulated (37,38), probably under the influence of angiogenic molecules such as VEGF or bFGF (39). The importance of this system can be seen from the observation that when it is inoperative, as occurs in animals that are deficient in the gene for gelatinase A, responses to angiogenic stimuli are substantially reduced (40).

Interestingly, heightened MMP activity seems to be accompanied by complementary changes in another group of endogenous substances called tissue inhibitors of metalloproteinases (TIMPs) (38). As their name suggests, these molecules are antagonistic to MMPs and control their activity such that the degree of tissue modification occurring is limited. This elegant interplay has the overall effect of preventing the occurrence of gross tissue changes, such as corneal melting, that might otherwise continue unchecked.

Alternative methods of facilitating vessel penetration through the remodelling of corneal tissue have been observed in other animal models. In the rabbit, macrophages have been found to be associated with producing local tissue changes during CV that precede the appearance of new vessels (41). The suggestion here is that extracellular matrix modification may proceed through mechanisms other than that provided by the action of MMPs. It is also further evidence that leukocytes play an important, and diverse role in the angiogenic process.

ASSESSMENT OF NEW VESSEL GROWTH

Clinical assessment of vascular progression in the region of the peripheral cornea is complicated by the absence of a well-defined anatomical reference point. The limbus is recognized to be a transition zone whose boundaries vary with corneal position and depth. This is most obvious superiorly where a region of vascularized transitional conjunctival and subconjunctival tissue overlying transparent corneal stroma can typically be observed. Sometimes referred to as a conjunctival wedge (42), this tissue is translucent rather than transparent because conjunctival epithelium is thicker and less regular than the corneal epithelium (43). The width of the translucent overlay varies around the limbus and is greatest superiorly, less inferiorly, and least at the nasal and temporal positions. Considerable individual variation also occurs. Taken together these factors mean that the point at which full corneal transparency is established can vary by as much as 2 mm from the limit of opaque sclera or visible iris. This does not constitute a particularly reliable reference point for gauging the extent of vessel progression and so it is not surprising that estimates made by different observers can differ substantially.

Superficial conjunctival and subconjunctival vessels are also commonly found within the translucent region (Fig. 37.1; see Color Plate 37.1). These are not corneal vessels but may be incorrectly categorized as vascularization unless localized to the translucent region using the biomicroscope and marginal retroillumination.

A further important factor is the capacity for vascular activity within normal vessels at the limbus. The limbal capillaries form part of the microcirculation. As such, the extent to which they are perfused is under exceptionally fine control. Local blood flow within small groups of capillaries can be altered in a variety of ways depending on conditions in the immediate vicinity (44). This behavior occurs continuously as a consequence of normal function, hence the observation of blood filled vessels where none had been previously evident would not necessarily be cause for concern.

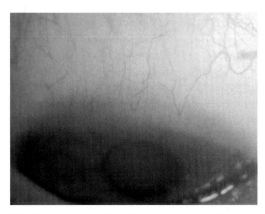

FIG. 37.1. Translucent conjunctiva and associated normal vessels encroaching onto the superior cornea. (See Color Plate 37.1.)

Likewise, the general level of erythema varies with position around the limbus such that the nasal quadrant typically has the reddest appearance and the inferior quadrant the least (45). Similar stimuli may thus produce different observed responses depending on their location. For example, the relative hyperemia induced by conventional hydrogel contact lens wear will usually be greater for inferior vessels than for those located nasally. This does not mean that the inferior limbus will necessarily appear redder than elsewhere, just that it will have changed from its starting appearance by a greater amount.

These factors must be taken into account when interpreting limbal vascular appearance. All hyperemic events should prompt careful consideration as potential indicators of acute or chronic problems. Warning signs that new vessel growth may be imminent include indications that local structural changes are occurring. The appearance of exudate from vessels, for example, is suggestive of the extravasation of inflammatory cells, while the emergence of vessel buds or spikes is evidence that vascular endothelial cells have begun to proliferate. It must be noted, however, that abruptly terminating vessels may also be observed in normal corneas (46).

In using the biomicroscope to observe vascular development, superficial corneal vessels can generally be seen to make connections with the limbal circulation. Where vessel growth is associated with tissue opacification, observation is relatively straightforward using direct focal illumination. Due to the lack of contrast, vessels without a blood column are likely to be more difficult to distinguish from the underlying tissue. Vessels that are very superficially sited may raise the epithelium so that a glistening specular reflex is visible when using a direct focal beam.

In the absence of opacification, the observation of vessels in, or over the transparent cornea is best achieved using direct retroillumination when there is a blood column. The detection of empty or ghost vessels usually will require the use of marginal retroillumination.

New corneal vessels invade at the level of the stimulating pathology. Deeper vessels can be observed emerging from,

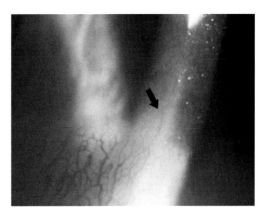

FIG. 37.3. A single straight superficial vessel (*arrow*) penetrating into the cornea of a 46-year-old woman who is a 38%-water content conventional hydrogel wearer. (See Color Plate 37.3.)

and disappearing into the sclera from the transparent stroma. Observation of nerve trunks entering the cornea may occasionally reveal the presence of an accompanying vessel sprout, as the nerve track appears to offer assistance in penetrating the compact corneal tissue during the early stage of vessel development (24).

Superficial vessels are usually tortuous, irregular, and arborescent, frequently exhibiting disorderly anastomoses (42) (Fig. 37.2; see Color Plate 37.2). Occasionally, superficial vessels do not form arcades and are more or less straight (Fig. 37.3; see Color Plate 37.3). At low magnification, arterial and venous vascular segments may be indistinguishable. At higher magnification, however, the two portions can generally be resolved. Under these conditions the arterial section may be seen to reflect sharply backward to form the returning venous portion, which then often follows an almost parallel course (Fig. 37.4; see Color Plate 37.4). These types are more likely to be new vessels, in contrast with more gently curving normal limbal loops that form arcades.

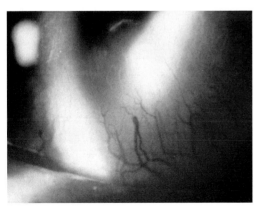

FIG. 37.2. Corneal vascularization. (See Color Plate 37.2.)

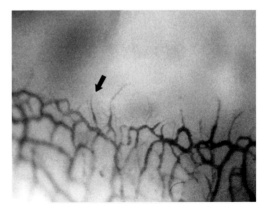

FIG. 37.4. High-magnification view of the limbus showing general hyperaemia and parallel tracked arterial and venous sections (*arrow*). (See Color Plate 37.4.)

Clinical Recording

Consistent assessment of vascular status requires the production of detailed clinical records, a task that traditionally has meant making accurate drawings of vessel position and extent relative to suitable landmarks. Obviously, imaging the region of interest provides a vastly preferable alternative, both in terms of accuracy and permanence. Recent advances in digital imaging technology permit high-quality results to be easily and quickly obtained, at reasonable cost, and with only relatively minor modifications to existing biomicroscopic equipment. It is thus feasible for clinicians to digitally capture images recording the vascular status of their contact lens wearers, and to maintain these along with the more conventional details of each case.

Apart from the opportunity this affords for direct visual comparison over time, it is also possible to apply analytical methods to these images to enhance the view that they present. While these techniques should be applied sparingly, and only after the original image has been saved and duplicated, they are capable of revealing aspects of vascular organization that might otherwise go unappreciated.

In addition to providing visual enhancement, several authors have applied image-processing techniques to extract objective measurement data that is representative of the vascular status, either for the individual as a whole, or for specific regions of the eye (47,48). This opens the possibility of more consistent comparisons, either over time or between clinical sites. Software suitable for this task is widely available. While specialized image analysis packages can be used, adequate results for the majority of applications can be achieved using standard image manipulation software such as Adobe Photoshop or Corel Photopaint. Routine use of digital imaging and analytical techniques should provide considerable benefits for the consistency of clinical assessment.

RISK FACTORS ASSOCIATED WITH CONTACT LENS WEAR

Because the stimulus and response characteristics of the process leading to corneal vascularization are not fully understood, it is difficult to accurately determine the particular aspects of contact lens wear that are likely to cause angiogenesis. However, because vascularization is essentially a protective response to tissue stress, we can focus our attention on those aspects of contact lenses that have the potential to interfere with corneal integrity.

Hypoxia

There is considerable circumstantial evidence linking contact lens-induced CV with hypoxia. As previously noted, much lower rates of CV are experienced during GP wear than soft lens wear. The suggestion that this is due to exposure of the peripheral cornea to the atmosphere is supported by the observation that the vascularization displayed in a group of soft lens wearers regressed when subjects either were refitted with GP lenses or ceased wear entirely (49). Taken alone, this result does not rule out the possibility that vascular changes occurred as a consequence of the lens mechanically interacting with the underlying ocular surface rather than by interfering with access to atmospheric oxygen. However, regression of CV has also been observed in polymethylmethacrylate (PMMA) scleral lens wearers after their lenses were refabricated using GP polymers (50), and rabbits showed less CV when wearing GP corneal lenses than in PMMA alternatives (51). In both these circumstances, the mechanical interactions are likely to have been either substantially unchanged or absent, leaving increased oxygen tension at the ocular surface as the likely reason for improvement.

Metabolic disturbances due to hypoxia cause corneal cells to generate a number of mediators with potentially angiogenic properties. Epithelial cells, for example, produce 12(R)-hydroxy-5,8,14-eicosatrienoic acid [12 (R)-HETrE] during arachidonic acid metabolism (52). This is an interesting molecule because it possesses the ability to promote vasodilation and vascular endothelial cell mitosis as well as being chemotactic for leukocytes. All of these are key elements in the process of new vessel formation, and 12(R)-HETrE does indeed appear to promote the growth of capillary like formations during *in vitro* experiments (53). Hypoxia-induced 12(R)-HETrE involvement has thus become implicated in the vascularization response occurring with closed eye contact lens wear, at least in rabbit models (62).

Despite these evidential links between hypoxia and angiogenesis, most individuals experience corneal swelling every night during sleep, and many contact lens users, especially hydrogel extended wearers, have corneas that are chronically hypoxic. While some of these eyes do develop CV, it is evident that the majority do not. This clearly points to a greater complexity in the process of CV than simply the occurrence of an hypoxic event. Thus, if the concept of a critical hypoxic load for vascularization is at all meaningful, it is likely to be a function of several factors. These would include both individual and tissue related elements and perhaps, integrative processes involving temporal or other locally acting agents that together modulate the vascularization response.

Epithelial Injury

Although epithelial damage occurs frequently during contact lens wear, it is usually not associated with corneal vascularization. The reason for this is presumably that the typical contact lens-related injury is neither sufficiently severe nor prolonged to generate a sustained chemokine/cytokine reaction. Severe corneal lesions destroy the barrier function of

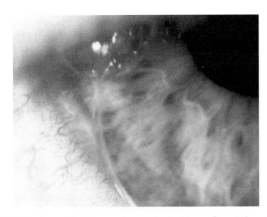

FIG. 37.5. Opacification and vascularization of peripheral cornea due to a poorly fitting rigid gas-permeable contact lens. (See Color Plate 37.5.)

the epithelium and cause the release of an array of mediators that ultimately initiate the cascade of wound healing responses (54). Minor episodes of superficial punctate epitheliopathy, conversely, are well tolerated and not greatly concerning from the point of view of CV.

Situations do arise, however, in which the behavior of the lens creates conditions in which sustained cellular damage occurs. Usually this will be the result of an inadequate fit that either causes the lens itself to directly impinge upon the ocular surface (Fig. 37.5; see Color Plate 37.5), or sufficiently disturbs the tear film to precipitate a localized region of poor wetting. The vascularization sometimes seen in association with 3- and 9-o'clock staining in rigid lens wear is one such example. A key factor is the maintenance of tear film integrity over the epithelial surface, as prolonged desiccation appears to be a potent initiator of corneal vessel growth.

It is intriguing that some episodes of epithelial injury do not cause vascularization even though they are apparently quite dramatic and sustained. The phenomenon of superior epithelial arcuate lesions (SEALs) is a particular case in point. Why the immune system does not appear unduly responsive to these deep epithelial splits is unclear and probably offers clues to the nature of the tissue damage in that condition.

Wearing Time

As far as hydrogel contact lenses are concerned, longer wearing times appear to be associated with increased prevalence of CV. In Rapkin's study (13), subjects were divided into two groups according to whether they wore lenses for less than, or more than, 12 hours per day. Among individuals with shorter wearing times, the prevalence of CV was 24%. However, for those wearing lenses for longer periods the rate more than doubled to 53%.

Lengthening wearing times even further, Cunha et al. (12) found that three times as many extended wearers in

their study were affected by CV as were daily wearers. Obviously, the fact that eye closure with lenses *in situ* occurred regularly for those on extended wear schedules was a confounding factor. Nevertheless, the overall length of time lenses are worn does appear to exert an overriding effect. This was evident in Binder's (15) sample of extended wearers, in which increasing numbers of patients developed CV as the study progressed.

It appears reasonably obvious that longer wearing times themselves do not directly cause corneal vascular changes. The likely mechanism is that the prolonged interaction with the contact lens potentiates the effects of other factors that have intrinsic vasogenic properties. Both hypoxia and the potential for epithelial damage would be possible candidates in this respect.

Significance of Limbal Hyperemia

Over half a century ago, Cogan (55) noted that local engorgement of the limbal capillaries occurred at a very early stage in the sequence of events leading to corneal vascularization. This observation has since been replicated by several other groups (24,56–58), prompting speculation, notably by McMonnies et al. (59) that the presence of chronic limbal hyperemia may be a risk factor for CV. Although little direct evidence exists that this is the case, by virtue of the known events leading to angiogenesis in the cornea, it is clear that any stimulus ultimately capable of producing new vessel growth must also be able to create a more immediate increase in limbal blood flow. Thus, the induction of limbal hyperemia is a necessary property for a suitable CV stimulus while, obviously, not being an entirely sufficient one.

Given that the remaining characteristics required for an effective vasogenic stimulus are unclear, and that many stimuli can cause hyperemia, it is probably prudent practice for clinicians to attempt to limit factors that exacerbate this latter phenomenon. Conventional soft contact lenses are an example of an agent that can cause both limbal hyperemia and CV. As their tendency to increase limbal vascular perfusion appears to be associated with their interference with oxygen levels in that region (60,61), it is tempting to suggest that hypoxia is the reason they can also cause CV. Such a proposal does not appear to be unreasonable in view of the increased prevalence of CV in circumstances of greater hypoxic load; e.g., longer wearing schedules (12,13), extended wear (9,15,18), or thicker lens designs (1,2,17,18). Additionally, contact lens-induced hypoxia is known to be associated with the production of potent angiogenic factors such as VEGF and 12 (R)-HETrE (62).

Clearly, not all soft lens wearers who have limbal hyperemia ultimately develop CV. Nevertheless, in the absence of other factors, the general level of limbal vascular activity can be viewed as a useful indicator of the hypoxic status beneath the contact lens. Thus, where strategies to reduce hypoxic stress on the cornea are successful they will generally result in quieter limbal vessels. As well as being desirable from a physiologic and cosmetic point of view, this situation carries the additional diagnostic advantage that any hyperemia occurring in response to other, potentially pathologic, stimuli will be easier to identify.

For similar reasons, it is important to recognize factors that may confound the ability to monitor the vascular status of the limbus and peripheral cornea. Thus, individuals suffering from allergies, tear deficiency, blepharitis or other conditions associated with conjunctival hyperemia, need to be appropriately treated and managed. Likewise, harsh conditions caused by wind, dust, glare, smoke, or air-borne pollutants should be avoided when possible. A further consideration, especially for soft lens wearers, is the possibility that the chemicals contained within the components of routinely used lens care products or cosmetics may stimulate toxic or allergic responses. Exposure to these should be eliminated or minimized. Finally the use of "over the counter" vasoconstrictor medications should be avoided or at least restricted, as they alter the normal appearance of the bulbar conjunctiva. Significant signs may thus be masked, leading to delays in treatment.

Limbal hyperemia can, of course, occur for reasons other than hypoxia. Thus, any activity of the limbal vessels that is persistent or prolonged may potentially indicate conditions that are conducive to vascular outgrowth. For example, a poorly fitting lens, decentered to the extent that its edge impinges upon the limbus and peripheral cornea, may cause tissue stress either through mechanical rubbing or tear film disruption. Hyperemia accompanying this situation may foreshadow a vascularization response if remedial steps are unduly delayed.

MANAGEMENT

Successful management of contact lens-induced CV is characterized by the withdrawal of blood columns from new vessels. What remains are generally referred to as ghost vessels and these may quickly refill if tissue stress returns. The prevention of ghost vessel formation requires that the vascularization process be detected at a very early stage. Theoretically this means taking action at about the time new vessel buds begin to sprout from existing capillaries. Even for eyes that are carefully evaluated on a regular basis, it is probably unrealistic to expect that this activity will, in fact, be observed as it happens. Rather more likely is that the clinician will be called upon to respond to a more advanced presentation where some vessel growth has already occurred. Therefore, from a strategic viewpoint, the institution of prophylactic measures that minimize the risk of exposure to vasogenic stimuli is highly desirable.

When CV is observed, the most important step in managing the condition is to remove the causative element responsible for tissue damage. Due to the incomplete under-

standing of the vascularization process, this factor might not always be obvious. Observation of the configuration of new vessels may be beneficial, as they tend to take the shortest route from the limbus to the injury site. Thus a single vessel or localized group penetrating some distance from the limbus probably indicates that the problem is located at or near to the termination of the new growth. A generalized sectorial or circumlimbal sprouting of vessels would be more likely to have origins that were relatively diffuse and sited peripherally within the cornea.

Although the lens itself is a likely culprit during contact lens wear, this is not inevitable. A number of pathologies exist that may be associated with CV irrespective of the presence of a contact lens. The origins of these conditions may be immunologic (Stevens-Johnson syndrome, cicatricial pemphigoid, graft rejection), infective (microbial keratitis), degenerative (pterygium, Terrien's marginal dystrophy), or traumatic (alkali burns, penetrating injury, postsurgical, etc.) (4,63). Many of these are serious conditions in their own right with significant visual consequences. The possibility of their presence should thus be eliminated at an early stage by taking a detailed history, conducting careful observations, and making an accurate differential diagnosis. Appropriate treatment measures can then be initiated in a timely fashion, minimizing the risk of severe consequences. This is particularly important when it is suspected that a corneal infection may be in progress.

Having established that the contact lens is the probable cause, consideration should be given to its performance and behavior. An evaluation of the material properties, fitting characteristics, dimensions, cleanliness, and general condition of the lens is indicated, together with a review of the circumstances of wear. The aim of this assessment should be to identify factors that may be responsible for inducing tissue stress.

In some cases the condition of the ocular surface and configuration of vessel growth will indicate a specific problem. For example, CV associated with desiccation staining in the 3- and 9-o'clock or 4- and 8-o'clock positions is characteristic of a poorly fitting rigid lens. Refitting to alleviate the problem is the obvious solution in such cases. Remedial steps include improving centration and optimizing the edge interaction with the epithelial surface in terms of both its clearance and thickness. Other possible problems are that the lens wets poorly as a result of deposition, polymer incompatibility or inefficient blink dynamics. If attention to these specific causes is not successful, it may be necessary to consider reducing wearing time or refitting with a soft lens design.

Whatever the lens type being worn, potential sources of epithelial injury should be eliminated. Replacement of lenses that are poorly manufactured or damaged is an obvious necessity and regular cleaning and replacement routines should be encouraged.

During soft lens wear, where hypoxia is suspected, the

strategy should be to improve oxygen availability in the postlens space and particularly in the region of the corneal periphery. Traditionally the options for achieving this end have included increasing lens oxygen transmissibility by reducing thickness or using higher water content materials, and improving the efficiency of tear exchange beneath the lens. Achieving this latter effect involves manipulating the fitting characteristics to increase the relative movement between the lens and ocular surface. Enhanced movement may be obtained by employing a flatter base curve or smaller diameter (64), and recent studies indicate that using stiffer materials (65) or fenestrating the lens (66,67) may also be beneficial strategies.

The task of improving oxygen availability at the ocular surface has now been greatly aided by the introduction of SiH materials. The oxygen transmissibilities achievable with these polymers can exceed the Holden-Mertz criterion of 87×10^{-9} (cm $\times$ mL O$_2$)/(sec $\times$ mL $\times$ mm Hg) needed to mimic no-lens levels of overnight corneal swelling (68). With appropriate lens designs, they also have the potential to meet the more stringent transmissibility criterion of 125×10^{-9} (cm $\times$ mL O$_2$)/(sec $\times$ mL $\times$ mm Hg) proposed by Harvitt and Bonnano to avoid anoxia throughout the cornea during eye closure (69). This means that hypoxic stress can effectively be eliminated from the corneas of many lens wearers even during sleep.

An additional advantage of high oxygen transmissibility is that it reduces the limbal hyperemia generally associated with soft lens wear (Fig. 37.6; see Color Plate 37.6). The amount of hyperemia induced by a lens is closely related to its peripheral oxygen transmissibility and it is interesting that the transmissibility estimated to be needed to completely avoid vascular changes (60) is very similar to that which induces minimal hypoxic response in the cornea (69). For many individuals, the use of SiH lenses can effectively eliminate both the corneal hypoxia and limbal hyperemia traditionally associated with soft lens wear. Because of this, refitting with SiH materials is the treatment of choice when

faced with soft lens induced vascular changes presumed to have an hypoxic etiology.

Inevitably however, circumstances will arise in which the use of SiH lenses will not be appropriate. Restrictions on parameters, for example, or the unavailability of a suitable refractive correction may render it unrealistic to satisfy the needs of particular individuals. In these cases it will be necessary to utilize the aforementioned traditional methods of improving lens performance.

Whatever the nature of the lens material, if efforts to optimize oxygen transmissibility prove unsuccessful, consideration should be given to adjusting the wearing schedule. Once again the aim is to reduce the impact of the lens on the ocular environment. Thus, reducing from extended to daily wear would be a particularly beneficial approach. Where the wearer is already routinely in daily wear, reducing the number of hours for which lenses are worn should be advised. Limiting exposure to the lens not only directly reduces the contact time between ocular tissue and potential angiogenic stimuli, but also increases, by a similar amount, the period during which the eye can recover from such stimuli. Thus, each extra hour without lenses can be expected to confer approximately 2 hours benefit in reduced contact lens effects.

If it becomes necessary to advise wearers to interrupt contact lens wear for regular periods, appropriate spectacles should be available. Ensuring that these make maximum use of current optical technology and are of contemporary styling will improve the likelihood of acceptance and thus reduce the risk of poor compliance with the altered contact lens schedule.

Should reducing wearing time not have the desired outcome, a period during which wear ceases completely may be advisable. Abstinence is more strongly indicated when vascularization is stromal or in more advanced cases of superficial growth. After resolution occurs, careful consideration should be given to the manner in which contact lens wear might be resumed, as neglecting to significantly improve the overall situation will invariably result in a recurrence of the original problem. While the availability of SiH lenses is likely to make this an easier task in the future than it has previously been, a particularly beneficial strategy is to consider refitting intractable soft lens cases with the GP lenses. Although it will often be necessary to carefully manage wearer concerns about discomfort, adaptation and handling, the low rates of CV associated with GP lenses together with the scope for handling a wide range of refractive conditions, make this a valuable alternative to soft lens wear as well as a powerful corrective modality in its own right.

The search for therapeutic agents beneficial in the treatment of CV began some time ago, and a variety of substances investigated for potential inhibitory activity. Recently, these have included cyclosporine (70), thalidomide (71), caffeic acid phenethyly ester (derived from bee-propolis) (72), flavonoids (derived from plant sources) (73), naked

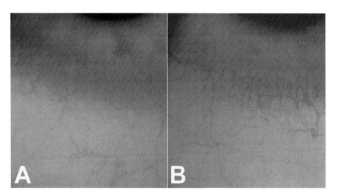

FIG. 37.6. Red-free image of right and left eyes of the same subject wearing a silicone hydrogel lens **(A)** and a 38% pHEMA lens **(B)**. Note relative hyperaemia of the limbal vessels. (See Color Plate 37.6.)

DNA (74), amniotic cell culture supernatant (75), and angiostatin (76), among others. While many of these entities have demonstrated potential efficacy in the animal models on which they have been evaluated, none so far, have progressed to clinical utility. Currently, the most commonly applied treatment for corneal vascularization in general remains topical corticosteroids (77). The levels of vascular involvement that are necessary to require use of this type of drug are typically relatively severe however, and it is unusual for this approach to be used in contact lens-related cases of CV.

It has recently been shown that the consumption of green tea inhibits the development of corneal angiogenesis (78). This suggests that nutrition has a role in ocular neovascular disease and, in particular, that diets rich in antioxidants may be beneficial. Further support for this view is provided by the observation that plant derived compounds, specifically the isoflavonoids and flavonoids, inhibit angiogenesis when applied topically to the rabbit cornea (73). The effective antiangiogenic concentrations for these substances in topical doses are, however, higher than those that typically occur due to oral intake, and it remains to be determined whether foods rich in isoflavonoids, such as soybeans, are able to offer significant protection against the development of CV.

Undoubtedly the potential for using dietary adjustment in managing corneal vascular disease will be an attractive proposition in some quarters. Whatever benefits this approach may ultimately turn out to possess, it is unlikely to be more than an adjunct to management strategies directly related to the contact lens itself. The primary avenues for preventing and alleviating CV should continue to involve the provision of an optimally fitted and maintained contact lens, constructed from the best available materials, supported by the regular and careful observation of the eye on which it is placed.

ACKNOWLEDGMENT

The author gratefully acknowledges the contribution of Charles McMonnies. Partial support during the preparation of this work was provided by the Cooperative Research Centre for Eye Research and Technology and the Australian Federal Government through the Cooperative Research Centres Program.

REFERENCES

1. Dana MR, Streilein JW. Loss and restoration of immune privilege in eyes with corneal neovascularization. *Invest Ophthalmol Vis Sci* 1996;37:2485–2494.
2. Maguire MG, Stark WJ, Gottsch JD, et al. Risk factors for corneal graft failure and rejection in the Collaborative Corneal Transplantation Studies. *Ophthalmology* 1994;101:1536–1547.
3. Colby KA, Adamis AP. Prevalence of corneal neovascularisation in a general eye service population. *Invest Ophthalmol Vis Sci* 1996;37:S593(abst) .
4. Lee P, Wang CC, Adamis AP. Ocular neovascularization: an epidemiologic review. *Surv Ophthalmology* 1998;43:245–269.
5. Kamiya C. Cosmetic extended wear of oxygen permeable hard contact lenses: one year follow up. *J Am Optom Assoc* 1986;57: 182–184.
6. Levy B. Rigid gas permeable lenses for extended wear: a 1-year clinical evaluation. *Am J Optom Physiol Opt* 1985;62:889–894.
7. Polse KA, Graham AD, Fusaro RE, et al. The Berkeley Contact Lens Extended Wear Study. Part II: clinical results. *Ophthalmology* 2001;108:1389–99.
8. Weissman BA. Corneal vascularisation: the superficial and the deep. *Contact Lens Anterior Eye* 2001;24:3–8.
9. Keech PM, Ichikawa L, Barlow W. A prospective study of contact lens complications in a managed care setting. *Optom Vis Sci* 1996; 73:653–658.
10. Grimmer PR. Soft contact lens water content and five common post fitting complications. Are there relationships? *Clin Exp Optom* 1992;75:182–187.
11. Roth HW. The etiology of ocular irritation in soft lens wearers: distribution in a large clinical sample. *Contact Intraocul Lens Med J* 1978;4:38–47.
12. Cunha MC, Thomassen TS, Cohen EJ, et al. Complications associated with soft contact lens use. *CLAO J* 1987;13:107–111.
13. Rapkin JS. The effect of daily wear time on contact lens complications. *CLAO J* 1988;14:139–142.
14. Lamer L. Extended wear contact lenses for myopes. A follow up study of 400 cases. *Ophthalmology* 1983;90:156–161.
15. Binder PS. Myopic extended wear with Hydrocurve II soft contact lenses. *Ophthalmology* 1983;90:623–626.
16. Starck WJ, Martin NF. Extended wear contact lenses for myopic correction. *Arch Ophthalmology* 1981;99:1963–1966.
17. Schecter DR, Emery JM, Soper JW. Corneal vascularization in therapeutic soft lens wear. *Contact Intraocul Lens Med J* 1975;1: 141–145.
18. Sarver MD, Sarver DS, Sarver LA. Aphakic patient responses to extended wear contact lenses. *J Am Optom Assoc* 1983;54: 249–254.
19. Holden BA, Stretton S, Evans K, Sweeney D. Contact lenses, where now and where to? *Contact Lens Spectr* 2003;Jan:18.
20. Health Products Research Inc. Whitehouse, NJ, 2002.
21. Dumbleton KA, Chalmers RL, Richter DB, et al. Vascular response to extended wear of hydrogel lenses with high and low oxygen permeability. *Optom Vis Sci* 2001;78:147–51.
22. Brennan NA, Coles ML, Comstock TL, et al. A 1-year prospective clinical trial of Balafilcon A (PureVision) silicone-hydrogel contact lenses used on a 30-day continuous wear schedule. *Ophthalmology* 2002;109:1172–7.
23. McMonnies CW, Chapman-Davies A, Holden BA. The vascular response to contact lens wear. *Am J Optom Physiol Opt*1982;59: 795–799.
24. Yaylali V, Ohta T, Kaufmann SC, et al. In vivo confocal imaging of corneal neovascularisation. *Cornea* 1998;17:646–653.
25. Burger PC, Chandler DB, Klintworth GK. Corneal neovascularisation as studied by scanning electron microscopy of vascular casts. *Lab Invest* 1983;48:169–180.
26. Polverini PJ. The pathophysiology of angiogenesis. *Crit Rev Oral Biol Med* 1995;6:230–247.
27. Thakur A, Willcox MD, Stapleton F. The pro-inflammatory cytokines and arachidonic acid metabolites in human overnight tears: homeostatic mechanisms. *J Clin Immunol* 1998;18:61–70.
28. Amano S, Rohan R, Kuroki M, et al. Requirement for vascular endothelial growth factor in wound- and inflammation-related corneal neovascularization. *Invest Ophthalmol Vis Sci* 1998;39: 18–22.

29. Philipp W, Speicher L, Humpel C. Expression of vascular endothelial growth factor and its receptors in inflamed and vascularized human corneas. *Invest Ophthalmol Vis Sci* 2000;41:2514–2522.

30. Cursiefen C, Rummelt C, Kuchle M. Immunohistochemical localization of vascular endothelial growth factor, transforming growth factor alpha, and transforming growth factor beta1 in human corneas with neovascularization. *Cornea* 2000;19:526–533.

31. Fromer CH, Klintworth GK. An evaluation of the role of leukocytes in the pathogenesis of experimental induced corneal neovascularization, I: comparison of experimental models of corneal vascularization. *Am J Pathol* 1975;79:537–554.

32. Fromer CH, Klintworth GK. An evaluation of the role of leukocytes in the pathogenesis of experimental induced corneal neovascularization, II: studies on the effect of leukocytic elimination on corneal vascularization. *Am J Pathol* 1975;81:531–544.

33. Fromer CH, Klintworth GK. An evaluation of the role of leukocytes in the pathogenesis of experimental induced corneal neovascularization, III: studies related to the vasoproliferative capability of polymorphonuclear leukocytes and lymphocytes. *Am J Pathol* 1976;82:157–170.

34. Becker MD, Kruse FE, Azzam L, et al. In vivo significance of ICAM-1–dependent leukocyte adhesion in early corneal angiogenesis. *Invest Ophthalmol Vis Sci* 1999;40:612–618.

35. Zhu SN, Dana MR. Expression of cell adhesion molecules on limbal and neovascular endothelium in corneal inflammatory neovascularization. *Invest Ophthalmol Vis Sci* 1999;40:1427–1434.

36. Daxer A, Ettl A. Corneal vascularisation and its relation to the physical properties of the tissue: a fractal analysis. *Curr Eye Res* 1995;14:263–268.

37. Kvanta A, Sarman S, Fagerholm P, et al. Expression of matrix metalloproteinase-2 (MMP-2) and vascular endothelial growth factor (VEGF) in inflammation-associated corneal neovascularization. *Exp Eye Res* 2000;70:419–428.

38. Ma DH, Chen JK, Kim WS, et al. Expression of matrix metalloproteinases 2 and 9 and tissue inhibitors of metalloproteinase 1 and 2 in inflammation-induced corneal neovascularization. *Ophthal Res* 2001;33:353–362.

39. Wang H, Keiser JA. Vascular endothelial growth factor upregulates the expression of matrix metalloproteinases in vascular smooth muscle cells. *Circ Res* 1998;83:832–840.

40. Kato T, Kure T, Chang JH, et al. Diminished corneal angiogenesis in gelatinase A-deficient mice. *FEBS Lett* 2001;508 :187–190.

41. Gan L, Fagerholm P. Leukocytes in the early events of corneal neovascularization. *Cornea* 2001;20:96–99.

42. Duke-Elder S, Leigh AG. Diseases of the outer eye. In: Duke-Elder S, ed. *System of ophthalmology,* Vol 8. London: Henry Kimpton, 1977:676.

43. Bergmanson JPG. Clinical anatomy of the external eye. *J Am Optom Assoc* 1990;61(Suppl):S7–S15.

44. Papas EB. The limbal blood supply *Contact Lens Anterior Eye* 2003;17:1–6.

45. Papas EB, Vajdic CM, Austen R, Holden BA. High-oxygen-transmissibility soft contact lenses do not induce limbal hyperaemia. *Curr Eye Res* 1997;16:942–948.

46. Lawrenson JG, Doshi S, Ruskell GL. Slit-lamp and histological observations of the normal limbal vasculature and their significance for contact lens wear. *J Br Contact Lens Assoc* 1991;14:169–172.

47. Papas EB. Key factors in the objective and subjective assessment of conjunctival erythema. *Invest Ophthalmol Vis Sci* 2000;41:687–691.

48. Fieguth P, Simpson TL. Automated measurement of bulbar redness. *Invest Ophthalmol Vis Sci* 2002;43:340–347.

49. Chan WK Weissman BA. Corneal pannus associated with contact lens wear. *Am J Ophthalmol* 1996;122:540–546.

50. Tan DTH, Pullum KW, Bukley RJ. Medical applications of scleral contact lenses, 2: gas permeable scleral contact lenses. *Cornea* 1995;14:130–137.

51. Duffin RM, Weissman BA, Ueda J. Complications of extended wear hard contact lenses on rabbits. *Int Contact Lens Clin* 1982;9:101–105.

52. Mieyal PA, Bonazzi A, Jiang H, et al. The effect of hypoxia on endogenous corneal epithelial eicosanoids. *Invest Ophthalmol Vis Sci* 2000;41:2170–2176.

53. Stoltz RA, Conners MS, Gerritsen ME, et al. Direct stimulation of limbal microvessel endothelial cell proliferation and capillary formation in vitro by a corneal-derived eicosanoid. *Am J Pathol* 1996;148:129–139.

54. Wilson SE, Mohan RR, Mohan RR, et al. The corneal wound healing response: cytokine mediated interaction of the epithelium, stroma and inflammatory cells. *Prog Retinal Eye Res* 2001;20:625–637.

55. Cogan DG. Vascularisation of the cornea: Its experimental induction by small lesions and a new theory of its pathogenesis. *Arch Ophthalmol* 1949;41:406–416.

56. Collin HB. Limbal vascular response prior to corneal vascularization. *Exp Eye Res* 1973;16:443–455.

57. McCracken JS, Burger PC, Klintworth GK. Morphologic observations on experimental corneal vascularisation in the rat. *Lab Invest* 1979;41:519–530.

58. Junghans BM, Collin HB. The limbal vascular response to corneal injury. An autoradiographic study. *Cornea* 1989;8:141–149.

59. McMonnies CW, Chapman-Davies A, Holden BA. The vascular response to contact lens wear. *Am J Optom Physiol Opt* 1982;59:795–799.

60. Papas EB. On the relationship between soft contact lens oxygen transmissibility and induced limbal hyperaemia. *Exp Eye Res* 1998;67:125–131.

61. Papas EB. The role of hypoxia in the limbal vascular response to soft contact lens wear. *Eye and Contact Lens* 2003;29(1Suppl):S72-4.

62. Mastuygin V, Mosaed S, Bonazzi A, et al. Corneal epithelial VEGF and cytochrome P450 4B1 expression in a rabbit model of closed eye contact lens wear. *Curr Eye Res* 2001;23:1–10.

63. Chang JH, Gabison EE, Kato T, et al. Corneal neovascularization. *Current Opinion in Ophthalmology,* 2001;12:242–249.

64. McNamara NA, Polse KA, Brand RJ, et al. Tear mixing under a soft contact lens: effects of lens diameter. *Am J Ophthalmol* 1999;127:659–665.

65. Paugh JR, Stapleton F, Keay L, et al. Tear exchange under hydrogel contact lenses: methodological considerations. *Invest Ophthalmol Vis Sci* 2001;42:2813–2820.

66. Chauhan A, Radke CJ. The role of fenestrations and channels on the transverse motion of a soft contact lens. *Optom Vis Sci* 2001;78:732–43.

67. Miller KL, Polse KA, Radke CJ. Fenestrations enhance tear mixing under silicone-hydrogel contact lenses. *Invest Ophthalmol Vis Sci* 2003;44:60–67.

68. Holden BA, Mertz GW. Critical oxygen levels to avoid corneal edema for daily and extended wear contact lenses. *Invest Ophthalmol Vis Sci* 1984;25:1161–1167.

69. Harvitt DM, Bonanno JA. Re-evaluation of the oxygen diffusion model for predicting minimum contact lens Dk/t values needed to avoid corneal anoxia. *Optom Vis Sci* 1999;76:712–719.

70. Lipman RM, Epstein RJ, Hendricks RL. Suppression of corneal neovascularisation with cyclosporin. *Arch Ophthalmol* 1992;110:405–407.

71. Kruse FE, Joussen AM, Rohrschneider K, et al. Thalidomide inhibits corneal angiogenesis induced by vascular endothelial

growth factor. *Graefes Arch Clin Exp Ophthalmol* 1998;236: 461–466.

72. Totan Y, Aydin E, Cekic O, et al. Effect of caffeic acid phenethyl ester on corneal neovascularization in rats. *Curr Eye Res* 2001; 23:291–297.

73. Joussen AM, Rohrschneider K, Reichling J, et al. Treatment of corneal neovascularization with dietary isoflavonoids and flavonoids. *Exp Eye Res* 2000;71:483–487.

74. Stechschulte SU, Joussen AM, von Recum HA, et al. Rapid ocular angiogenic control via naked DNA delivery to cornea. *Invest Ophthalmol Vis Sci* 2001;42:1975–1979.

75. Kobayashi N, Kabuyama Y, Sasaki S, et al. Suppression of corneal neovascularization by culture supernatant of human amniotic cells. *Cornea* 2002;21:62–67.

76. Ambati BK, Joussen AM, Ambati J, et al. Angiostatin inhibits and regresses corneal neovascularization. *Arch Ophthalmol* 2002; 120:1063–1068.

77. Stonecipher KG. Corneal neovascularization. In: Fraunfelder FT, Roy FH, eds. *Current ocular therapy,* 4th ed. Philadelphia: WB Saunders, 1995:484–485.

78. Cao Y, Cao R. Angiogenesis inhibited by drinking tea. *Nature* 1999;398:381.

CLINICAL MANAGEMENT OF IMMUNOLOGIC COMPLICATIONS

**KAREN K. YEUNG AND
BARRY A. WEISSMAN**

Ocular inflammation is common in both general ophthalmic and contact lens practices. It may be a result of infection, trauma (e.g., toxicity to chemicals), or hypersensitivity reactions (the body's inappropriate activation of defense mechanisms). Severe ocular hypersensitivity reactions may lead to tissue damage and, in some cases, visual impairment. A review of the basic mechanisms of inflammation and immunology is presented in Chapter 4.

The contact lens practitioner should be able to recognize and address ocular immunologic complications, both those caused directly by contact lens wear as well as others not caused by, but that may compromise, contact lens wear. The purpose of this chapter is to address these reactions (Table 38.1.) and their management.

Immune responses were originally classified by Gell and Coombs's into type I "immediate," type II, type III, and type IV "delayed" hypersensitivity, respectively. It must be understood that classification schemes can become outdated as mechanisms of disease unravel and the Gell-Coombs system has been updated to reflect the changes in disease pathogenesis (1). Type I [immunoglobulin E (IgE) mast-cell related] is essentially unchanged, but types II and III have been combined and are now considered "antibody-mediated" inflammatory responses. Type IV reactions are now considered "T-cell–mediated" responses, as the tissue damage produced is antibody independent.

This chapter will concentrate on two groups of ocular hypersensitivity reactions: (a) non–sight-threatening diseases that cause ocular discomfort [e.g., seasonal allergic conjunctivitis (SAC), perennial allergic conjunctivitis (PAC), giant papillary conjunctivitis (GPC), contact dermatitis, and marginal sterile keratitis] and; (b) potentially vision-threatening diseases [e.g., phlyctenular conjunctivitis, vernal keratoconjunctivitis (VKC), and atopic keratoconjunctivitis (AKC)] (Table 38.2.)

Classic "allergies" are type I hypersensitivity, exaggerated or inappropriate IgE mast-cell–related inflammatory reaction (2). Systemic allergy affects more than 15% of the world population—and 30% of the population in western-

ized industrial countries (3,4). *Atopy* refers to an inherited predisposition to develop allergic reactions. First described in 1923 by Cocoa and Cooke (5), atopic patients develop IgE hypersensitivities when exposed to normally harmless antigens, such as pollen, molds, animal dander, and dust mites. The first treatment of allergy is avoidance or prompt removal of the antigen when possible. Both systemic and topical antihistamines and steroids are treatment options.

Allergic symptoms and signs range from local to systemic, from mild irritation to death. Vasodilation appears as erythema at the site of antigen exposure. Increased vasopermeability can lead to local edema, wheals (soft-tissue swelling), and flare (a red ring surrounding a wheal). Widespread severe vasodilation can lead to a sudden drop in blood pressure and ultimately shock from the decreased organ perfusion. Mucous secretion leads to congested air passageways. Bronchial airway constriction causes coughing and wheezing (asthma). Stimulation of nerve endings causes itching and pain.

Seasonal allergic conjunctivitis and PAC, as well as GPC, are examples of ocular hypersensitivity reactions. Ocular symptoms include watery, itchy, eyes with mucous discharge, conjunctival injection and chemosis. About 15% of

TABLE 38.1. OCULAR IMMUNOLOGIC COMPLICATIONS: CL AND NON-CL RELATED

CL Related	Non-CL Related
Giant papillary conjunctivitis	Seasonal allergic conjunctivitis
Sterile central and peripheral subepithelial infiltrates (nummular and pseudodendritic)	Perennial allergic conjunctivitis
	Contact dermatitis
	Marginal sterile keratitis
	Phlyctenular keratoconjunctivitis
Care solution–related conjunctivitis and keratitis	Vernal keratoconjunctivitis
	Atopic keratoconjunctivitis
	Dry eye

CL, contact lens.

TABLE 38.2. OCULAR IMMUNOLOGIC COMPLICATIONS: SIGHT AND NON-SIGHT THREATENING

Non-sight threatening	Possible sight threatening
Seasonal allergic conjunctivitis	Phlyctenular keratoconjunctivitis
Perennial allergic conjunctivitis	Vernal keratoconjunctivitis
Contact dermatitis	Atopic keratoconjunctivitis
Sterile keratitis (central and peripheral)	
Giant papillary conjunctivitis	

the population (6) is affected by ocular allergies, with a higher predilection in males than females (7). Such patients often have concomitant asthma, hay fever, and atopic dermatitis.

T-cell–mediated ocular hypersensitivities, conversely, include marginal sterile keratitis, contact dermatitis, and phlyctenular keratoconjunctivitis. Corneal transplant rejection is considered primarily a T-cell–mediated process. T-cell–mediated hypersensitivities may be involved in some forms of dry eyes (8,9) (see Chapter 23). These hypersensitivities are "delayed" (as opposed to "immediate" IgE mediated) because it takes time for the cells (macrophages and various classes of T cells) to be recruited to the site of reaction. Patients usually develop cell-mediated hypersensitivity reactions within 24 to 48 hours of exposure (see Chapter 4).

Some ocular inflammations, such as AKC and VKC, share characteristics of both IgE- and T-cell–mediated hypersensitivities.

SEASONAL ALLERGIC CONJUNCTIVITIS/ PERENNIAL ALLERGIC CONJUNCTIVITIS

Allergic conjunctivitis caused by environmental antigens can be differentiated into SAC and PAC. Seasonal allergic conjunctivitis, the most common ocular allergy, represents about half of all cases of ocular allergy (10) and often accompanies hayfever. Perennial allergic conjunctivitis is caused by year-round allergens such as dust mites, animal dander, and mold. There is no age predilection for PAC, but SAC usually appears between ages 20 and 40 years (11). Both SAC and PAC increase IgE levels in tears and serum (12). Mast cells increase (60%) in the lamina propria during pollen season in SAC patients (13).

Signs/Symptoms

Ocular symptoms include low-grade itching, stinging, photophobia, and watery eyes (14). Whereas "dry" eyes often present with "burning" rather than itching as a symptom, SAC and PAC present more itching than burning. Occa-

sionally, more severe disease causes a mild watery to a ropy mucous discharge. This conjunctivitis usually recurs, but may vary with weather changes and contact with irritants. Perennial allergic conjunctivitis symptoms are generally milder than SAC symptoms.

Ocular signs are usually minimal but may include fine papillary hypertrophy of the superior palpebral conjunctiva (15). Bulbar and tarsal conjunctiva may be mildly or moderately hyperemic and chemotic, in severe cases appearing translucent, bluish, and thickened. Allergic "shiners," or dark circles in the periorbital area (16), may form from venous congestion around the skin and subcutaneous tissue. Corneal involvement is rare.

Treatment and Management

Seasonal allergic conjunctivitis and PAC have excellent prognoses. An allergist can provide skin testing (skin pricking and intradermal tests) to often identify specific allergen(s) as well as provide desensitization treatments.

Avoidance of antigens is extremely helpful, although not always possible. Some patients relocate or use air filters to minimize exposure to airborne allergens. Keeping windows closed at night and car windows closed during driving may also help. Frequent lavage with unpreserved unit dose artificial tear products and use of warm or cool compresses and lid hygiene may similarly relieve symptoms by limiting antigen exposure.

Over-the-counter decongestant ocular medications (e.g., naphazoline, tetrahydrozoline, phenylephrine, and oxymetazoline) used up to four times per day can temporarily relieve symptoms of SAC and PAC. Chronic use should be avoided, however, because these pharmaceuticals may mask symptoms of more serious ocular problems. Prolonged use may also cause rebound conjunctival hyperemia (17), decreased responsiveness and tolerance (11), and perhaps aggravate narrow-angle-closure glaucoma. Decongestants can be found in combination with antihistamine products (e.g., naphazoline/pheniramine, naphazoline/antazoline).

Topical antihistamines (H1 receptor antagonists such as emedastine difumarate or levocabastine) are effective therapy for SAC and PAC. Such antihistamines reversibly bind to histamine receptors to preclude histamine-receptor reactions, thereby providing temporary relief from conjunctival congestion and itching. Topical antihistamines are safely and effectively used four times a day for 1 or 2 weeks, then once to three times a day thereafter as needed for itching. Topical antihistamines are preferable to systemic antihistamines because of local effectiveness, faster action, and decreased side effects (18), especially (for contact lens wearers) dry eyes.

Mast-cell stabilizers, such as sodium cromolyn, are the oldest nonsteroid drugs for the treatment of SAC and PAC. Topical mast-cell stabilizers are benign, effective in the long-term care of PAC patients, and can be used prophylactically for SAC. They should be prescribed 1 month before known allergy seasons to preclude ocular symptoms.

Antihistamine/mast-cell stabilizer combinations (e.g., olopatadine hydrochloride and ketotifen fumarate) have become popular. Berdy et al. (19) reported that olopatadine hydrochloride was even more efficacious than loteprednol for the treatment of SAC. Ocular symptoms (itch) were found to be better treated with a topical antihistamine/mast-cell stabilizer combination when coupled with a systemic antihistamine than by either drug on its own (20,21).

In severe cases, nonsteroidal antiinflammatory drugs (NSAIDs; e.g., ketorolac) and topical steroids (e.g., loteprednol) may become necessary. Topical NSAIDs relieve itch through inhibition of prostaglandin production, but may lead to rare corneal defects and melts (22). Because of risk of severe side effects (cataract, glaucoma, reduced resistance to infection), steroids should be used judiciously (23) (Table 38.3).

Treatment/Management of Contact Lens Patients

Although contact lens wear can be difficult to tolerate during the allergy season, (24,25) an antihistamine/mast-cell stabilizer combination can be used to improve contact lens tolerance. Agents can be instilled 10 minutes prior to contact lens insertion and immediately upon removal of the contact lenses at night. Frequent replacement of contact lenses (even daily disposable contact lenses) and frequent use of unpreserved artificial tears can also minimize ocular

irritation. Systemic antihistamines, however, may dry out the eye and make contact lens wear less comfortable. Cosmetic contact lens wear should be discontinued when steroids are used; it may be necessary to continue noncosmetic wear (e.g., aphakia, keratoconus) but with caution.

GIANT PAPILLARY CONJUNCTIVITIS

First described by Spring in 1974 (26), GPC is a noninfectious superior conjunctival IgE-mediated inflammation specifically associated with hydrogel and gas permeable contact lens wear (27), prosthetic device wear (28–30), exposed sutures (31,32), glaucoma filtering blebs (33), and even corneal scars (34).

Giant papillary conjunctivitis occurs more frequently in hydrogel than gas-permeable (GP) contact lens wearers (35): 1% to 5% in hydrogel [reported at 21% in one study (36)] and 1% in GP contact lens wearers. The average presentation times of GPC are following 8 months and 8 years of use in hydrogel and rigid contact lens wearers, respectively. GPC occurs more frequently in high-water, high-ionic, "extended-wear" hydrogel contact lenses. The small diameter of rigid GP lenses stimulates GPC to develop from the lid margin to the more superior areas of the palpebral conjunctiva, opposite to hydrogel contact lenses that induces GPC in the reverse direction. The papillae of rigid GP lens GPC tend to be fewer in number, wider spaced, and flatter than those associated with hydrogel contact lens wear.

TABLE 38.3. ANTIINFLAMMATORY MEDICATIONS

Drug Class	Drug Name	Possible Adverse Effects
Decongestants	Naphazoline (Naphcon, Vasocon), Visine AC	Rebound vasodilation, increased ocular redness, narrow-angle glaucoma
Combinations: decongestant and antihistamine	Naphazoline (Naphcon A, Vasocon A, Opcon A)	Rebound vasodilation, increased ocular redness, narrow-angle glaucoma
Antihistamines	Levocabastine (Livostin), emedastine (Emadine)	Conjunctival injection, headaches, rhinitis, keratitis, narrow-angle glaucoma
Mast cell stabilizer	Cromolyn (Crolom), ketotifen (Zaditor), Iodoxamidec (Alomide), nedocromil (Alocril), pemirolast (Alamast)	Headaches
Combinations: mast cell stabilizer/antihistamine	Olopatadine (Patanol), ozelastine (Optivar)	Transient eye burning, headaches, bitter taste
NSAIDs	Diclofenac (Voltaren), flurbiprofen (Ocufen), ketorolac tromethamne (Acular)	Delay wound healing, epithelial defects, corneal melts, sterile infiltrates
Corticosteroids	Loteprednol (Alrex, Lotemax), FML, prednisolone (Pred-Forte), rimexolane (Vexol), etc.	Glaucoma, cataracts, secondary ocular infections
Oral antihistamines	Lotadine (Claritin), Cetirizine (Zyrtec), fexofenadine (Allegra)	CL intolerance, dry eyes, drowsiness, dry mouth
Oral NSAIDs	Aspirin, ibuprofen, naproxen	Kidney damage, abdominal bleeding, bruising, peptic ulcers
Oral steroids	Prednisone, methylprednisolone, etc.	Many secondary complications
Immunosuppressive	Cyclosporine (Restasis)	Conjunctival hyperemia, discharge, epiphora, eye pain, blurriness of vision

NSAIDs, nonsteroidal antiinflammatory drugs; CL, contact lens.

Signs and Symptoms

Giant papillary conjunctivitis causes symptoms of itch, mucous discharge, and increased contact lens awareness. In its early stages, symptoms are undetected or mild. Contact lens tolerance decreases with disease progression, including foreign body sensations, excessive contact lens movement, blurring from mucous and protein-coated lenses, and increased itching. Contact lenses also displace higher under the eyelids from the mechanical nature of GPC.

Continual exposure to the antigens and mechanical stimulation of the contact lenses causes superior tarsal conjunctival hyperemia, epithelium thickening, and macropapillae (0.3 to 1.0 mm) enlarge into "giant" papillae (1.0 to 2.0 mm). Trantas' dots and gelatinous nodules may even develop at the limbus (37). Ropy mucous strands concentrated in the inferior fornix are evident. Mechanical blepharoptosis has been reported in severe GPC (38) (Figs. 38.1–38.3.)

Treatment and Management

Treatment and management goals for GPC are to reduce and eventually eliminate the signs and symptoms of hyperemia, itch, mucous discharge and contact lens intolerance, and to ultimately restore the conjunctiva to its normal state. Discontinuing contact lens wear will generally resolve the inflammation although contact lens patients would typically prefer to maintain their contact lens wear.

Diligently removing contact lens debris and protein deposits with surfactant cleaners and enhanced enzyme cleaning can usually treat GPC. Unfortunately, even after combination of both surfactant and enzyme cleaning (39), deposits still may not be totally removed. Nonionic low water content lenses have less tendency to accumulate protein deposits compared to ionic hydrogel lenses (40); hence, switching contact lens materials (using rigid GP lenses as well) may also help GPC-prone patients.

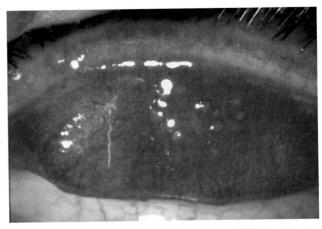

FIG. 38.2. Moderate giant papillary conjunctivitis induced by hydrogel contact lens wear. (Courtesy of Joseph Barr, OD.)

In moderate to advanced stages, ophthalmic preparations of antihistamine/mast-cell stabilizer combination medications (e.g., olopatadine, ketotifen) are additionally helpful. Twice-a-day dosage enhances convenience since ocular medications should be applied both 10 minutes prior to and after contact lenses are removed. During long-term treatment, enhanced cleaning regimens can be combined with use of topical mast-cell stabilizers (e.g., cromolyn sodium 2% or 4% four times a day, or emedastine difumarate) after acute symptoms are relieved. Kruger et al. (41) found that 70% of patients with moderate-to-severe GPC were able to continue wearing contact lenses with concomitant use of topical 4% cromolyn sodium solution.

The prognosis for treatment of GPC is quite good. With various frequent replacement schedules (even daily disposable, which eliminates the need for cleaning), alternate contact lens materials (perhaps rigid GP lenses), enhanced cleaning regimens (especially increased use of enzyme), and

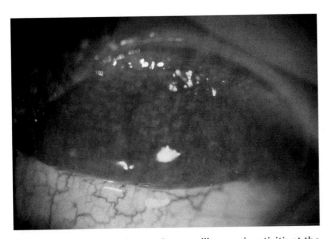

FIG. 38.1. Mild to moderate giant papillary conjunctivitis at the lid margin induced by rigid gas-permeable contact lens wear. (Courtesy of Joseph Barr, OD.)

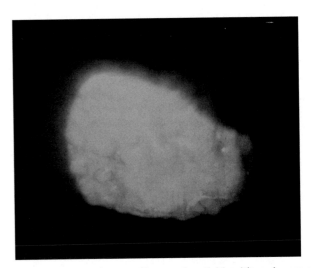

FIG. 38.3. Severe giant papillary conjunctivitis with copious mucous discharge. (Courtesy of Joseph Barr, OD.)

topical antiinflammatory medications, GPC can be controlled and patients return to contact lens tolerance in over 90% of all cases (42). There are no reported incidences of permanent visual loss from GPC. All patients will show symptomatic improvement once the inciting agent (e.g., contact lenses) is removed.

CONTACT DERMATITIS

Ocular contact dermatitis is a cell-mediated hypersensitivity reaction involving the eyelid, cornea, and conjunctiva (43). Contact dermatitis is one of the most frequent of hypersensitivity reactions seen by eyecare professionals.

Virtually any substance or medication can lead to contact dermatitis, although some substances are more commonly antigenic. Ocular preparations known to cause contact dermatitis include those containing benzalkonium chloride, thimerosal and chlorhexidine (both often found in older contact lens solutions), polyamino propyl biguanide, neomycin sulfate, gentamycin, idoxuridine, tobramycin, bacitracin, phenylephrine, gentamycin, idoxuridine, penicillin, brimonidine, and atropine (43). Severe, although extremely uncommon, responses have been associated with topical ester group anesthetics. Chronic reactions occur with some glaucoma medications (44). Other stimuli to contact dermatitis may occur from plastics, animal or vegetable products, rubber, or industrial chemicals (45). Parabens (a preservative in many cosmetics and facial creams) is frequently a cause contact dermatitis (46). Nickel sulfate is a common sensitizer found in jewelry and undergarments. Chromate, another common sensitizer, is used in costume jewelry, leather products, and automobile products (47).

Signs and Symptoms

Contact dermatitis from hands (rubbing the eyes after contact with soaps, detergents, or other chemicals) can cause severe itching, erythema, edema, and scaling in the skin area of contact, typically on the eyelids (48). The conjunctiva is often involved when the sensitizing agent enters the eye as from topically administered ocular medications (49). In the acute phase, the lower conjunctiva develops a follicular reaction accompanied by vasodilation, hyperemia, chemosis, and a watery discharge. The skin of the lower eyelids and canthal area may be red, edematous, and even ulcerate. In severe or chronic phases, lid dermatitis and eventual edema and stenosis of the puncta can occur (Fig. 38.4).

Both cell-mediated hypersensitivity and toxic reactions can lead to superficial punctate keratitis, conjunctival injection, and ocular discomfort, leading to confusion of these etiologies. Cell-mediated reactions also cause follicular conjunctivitis and/or corneal infiltrates (similar to viral infections). Either may be triggered by a change in contact lens care solution with different preservatives (especially those with thimerosal or chlorhexidine) and other ingredients. Thimerosal, in particular, has been shown to cause cell-mediated hypersensitivities and sterile corneal infiltrates as well as photophobia, conjunctival injection, edema, and, in some atypical cases, superior limbal keratitis and pseudodendritic corneal lesions (50–52). Mondino and Groden (53,54) confirmed by dermal patch testing that thimerosal can cause nummular subepithelial corneal infiltrates. Benzalkonium chloride (BAK)-preserved solutions (found in many GP lens solutions as well as pharmaceutical drops) can cause immediate red eyes and superficial punctate keratitis over the entire affected cornea (53); BAK reactions are to be primarily toxic. Antimicrobials in newer contact lens solutions have been designed as larger positive molecules to limit impregnating hydrogel materials and thereby limit corneal toxicity (55). Sterile corneal infiltrates (both nummular and pseudodendritic), and corneal epithelial staining, however, have both been found in association with contact lens "cold" disinfection systems preserved with thimerosal, Polyquad, chlorhexidine, and polyaminopropyl biguanide (56), most likely representing a form of cell-mediated contact keratitis (57) (Figs. 38.5 and 38.6).

Treatment and Management

Sensitivity can sometimes be proven by skin patch testing or interdermal injections. Treatment consists of treating the

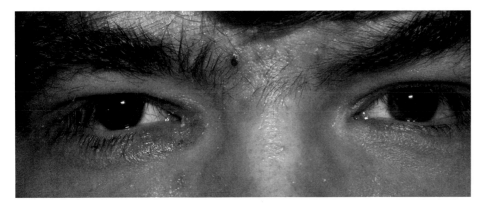

FIG. 38.4. Contact dermatitis from a topically administered ocular medication. Note the skin of the lower eyelids and canthal area is red, edematous, and ulcerating. (Courtesy of Bartley Mondino, MD.)

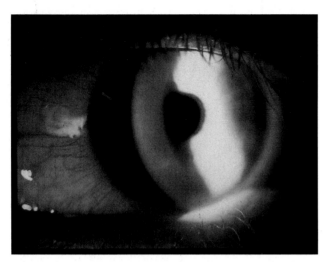

FIG. 38.5. Subepithelial infiltrate caused by contact lens solution hypersensitivity. (Courtesy of Joseph Barr, OD.)

ocular symptoms and removing the offending antigen (substituting with a nonoffending medication, contact lens solution, make-up, etc.). Treatment of mild acute cases includes unpreserved artificial tears and cool compresses, and occasionally topical vasoconstrictors. More severe reactions are treated with topical corticosteroids.

Treatment/Management of Contact Lens Patients

Rinsing contact lenses with sterile unpreserved saline prior to application should decrease ocular reactions in contact lens solution–hypersensitive patients. Safe and effective preservative-free cleaning systems include ultrasound/ultraviolet radiation cleaners (58) and hydrogen peroxide cleaning solutions (that neutralize into water and hydrogen) are alternatives. Use of 1-day disposable contact lenses eliminates all solution reactions.

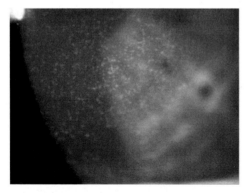

FIG. 38.6. Diffuse epithelial keratitis (possibly T-cell–mediated reaction) caused by polyamino biguanide toxicity. (Courtesy of Art Epstein, OD.)

MARGINAL STERILE KERATITIS

Signs and Symptoms

Marginal sterile keratitis is a cell-mediated hypersensitivity reaction associated with chronic (*Staphylococcus*) blepharitis. Patients present with sectorial conjunctival infection, minimal conjunctival chemosis, acute photophobia, pain, and itching. Patients may have a history of dry eyes, chronic blepharitis, acne rosacea, or collagen vascular diseases. Vision is not affected.

Multiple, sterile corneal infiltrates are typically observed at 3 or 4 and 8 or 9 o'clock in the peripheral cornea (about 1 mm inward from the limbus) where the lower eyelid is in proximity with the corneal surface. There is minimal to no sodium fluorescein staining of the cornea initially, since the epithelium is intact, and usually no anterior chamber reaction. Infiltrates may later ulcerate, however, creating peripheral scarring. There may also be associated phlyctenules and corneal neovascularization. Bacterial cultures of the corneal lesions are negative.

Treatment and Management

The prognosis of marginal sterile keratitis after managing both blepharitis and infiltrates is excellent with treatment. The keratitis can be initially controlled with topical antibiotics used four times a day. Long-term treatment of blepharitis is accomplished with warm compresses and lid scrubs, and courses of antibiotic ointments at bedtime in severe and stubborn cases. Oral antibiotics (e.g., tetracycline, doxycycline, or erythromycin) are often prescribed weeks or months at a time for severe meibomitis/blepharitis. Topical steroid/antibiotic combination drops or ointments can be used to treat the infiltrates with limited courses and as long as the corneal epithelium is intact. Intraocular pressures should be monitored during any steroid use.

Treatment/Management of Contact Lens Patients

Contact lens wear should be discontinued until the marginal sterile keratitis is resolved, especially if steroids are to be used for treatment.

PHLYCTENULAR KERATOCONJUNCTIVITIS

Phlyctenular keratoconjunctivitis is typically a cell-mediated hypersensitivity reaction. Tuberculosis has been a primary consideration in areas of poor sanitation and healthcare, affecting primarily children and young adults.

Staphylococcus is the leading cause of phlyctenular keratoconjunctivitis in areas where tuberculosis is more rare, affecting predominately adults and females (60% to 70%)

more than males. Other associations include acne rosacea, and other infectious agents such as fungi (*Candida albicans, Coccidioides immitis*) (59), other bacteria (*Bacillus, Staphylococcus aureus, Neisseria gonorrhoeae*), viruses (herpes simplex virus) (60), parasites (*Ascaris lumbricoides, Hymenolepis nana*) (61), and lymphogranuloma venereum. Idiopathic cases are extremely rare.

Signs and Symptoms

Symptoms include recurrent episodes of lacrimation, pruritus, foreign body sensation, and photophobia: similar to symptoms of a mild to moderate conjunctivitis. Symptom severity is greater with phlyctenules on the cornea and may include blepharospasm as opposed to less severe symptoms with conjunctival phlyctenules. Symptoms may persist from 1 or 2 weeks.

Phlyctenules may present on the conjunctiva, limbus, or cornea. Conjunctival phlyctenules present as slightly raised (1 or 2 mm in diameter), pinkish white or yellow nodules in the center of a hyperemic area. Conjunctival phlyctenules may appear anywhere on the bulbar conjunctiva, although they typically appear near the limbus, within the interpalpebral aperture. They are generally self-limiting; in 2 to 5 days, the center of the nodule becomes soft and less hyperemic, then sloughs and heals occasionally without any scarring.

More commonly occurring phlyctenules start at the limbus and either spontaneously resolve or migrate to clear cornea or conjunctiva (62). Limbal phlyctenules usually present on the inferior portion of the limbal cornea near the lower lid margin. Phlyctenules at the limbus may migrate onto the cornea leaving wedge-shaped trails of superficial corneal neovascularization behind their leading edges. Corneal phlyctenules, similar to conjunctival phlyctenules, are small, white nodules surrounded by dilated blood vessels at the limbus. Ulceration occurs but will heal over a course of 10 to 14 days, resulting in a triangular limbal-based anterior stromal scar. Corneal phlyctenules first appearing in the central cornea are rare but have been reported (63) (Fig. 38.7).

Phlyctenules should be differentiated from nodular episcleritis/scleritis, inflamed pingueculae, Salzmann's nodules, and the limbal papillae of vernal keratoconjunctivitis. Nodular episcleritis and inflamed pinguecula, unlike phlyctenules, do not migrate or ulcerate. Inflamed pingueculae are also typically located at the 3- and 9-o'clock position but by definition only on the conjunctiva. Salzmann's nodules are typically not inflamed. Trantas' dots in limbal VKC are smaller than phlyctenules, and VKC is also characterized by severe itching, cobblestone papillae, and thick ropy mucous discharge.

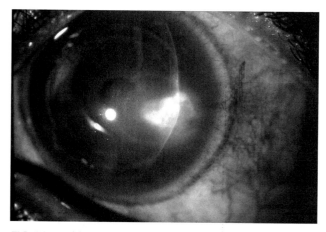

FIG. 38.7. Phlyctenule migrating to the cornea with a wedge-shaped trail of superficial corneal neovascularization and surrounding dilated blood vessels at the limbus. (Courtesy of Bartley Mondino, MD.)

Treatment and Management

Treatment should first include identifying and treating the organism causing the phlyctenule. If tuberculosis is the suspecting agent, comanagement and appropriate systemic therapy with an infectious disease physician after confirmation by purified protein derivative skin test, chest x-ray, and/or sputum cultures are recommended. Concurrent with antituberculosis treatment, topical corticosteroids can be used. Prednisolone acetate 1% can be topically administered every 3 to 6 hours and tapered as the condition improves. Topical antibiotics should be combined with corticosteroids if an epithelial defect is present.

Staphylococcal phlyctenulosis is often accompanied with concurrent blepharitis or meibomitis. Lid hygiene with lid scrubs two to three times per day is helpful. Topical antibiotic ointments or topical antibiotic/steroid combinations can be combined with the lid hygiene in moderate cases. Unless contraindicated, oral tetracycline, doxycycline, or erythromycin may be used for chronic or severe cases of blepharitis or meibomitis. In both staphylococcal and chlamydial phlyctenulosis, 250 mg tetracycline or 250 mg erythromycin four times a day orally for 2 to 4 weeks is considered effective (64). For phlyctenules of unknown etiology, a broad-spectrum antibiotic should be used initially to address a possible bacterial agent before treating the phlyctenule with corticosteroids. When unusually severe ulcerations lead to corneal perforation, cyanoacrylate glue may be initially used to seal small areas, but patch corneal grafts may be needed.

Treatment/Management of Contact Lens Patients

Contact lenses should not be used while phlyctenules are active. Patients who present with chronic disease are poor cosmetic contact lens candidates.

VERNAL KERATOCONJUNCTIVITIS

Vernal keratoconjunctivitis is a chronic, usually bilateral, rare but severe form of IgE- and cell-mediated hypersensitivity conjunctivitis. It affects males primarily from the age range of 1 to 22 years (65), with a peak incidence between 11 and 13 years. Boys are affected earlier (66) with twice the frequency of girls (65,67), although the male-to-female ratio decreases with age (66). The disease is self-limiting, but occasionally very severe in children. The average duration lasts 4 to 10 years and resolves following puberty. Adult onset of the disease, though rare, is typically more severe and can occur indefinitely. VKC is common in dry, hot climates (especially Africa, Japan, India, South America, and the Mediterranean area). There is a seasonal predilection for spring and summer, but 60% of patients may have symptoms all year round (66), especially those living in warm and subtropical and desert environments. Leonardi's case series of 221 patients showed that 35% of VKC patients have atopy (seasonal allergies, asthma, atopic dermatitis, and eczema) (65,68). Sixty-six percent of his patients had a familial history of atopy.

Signs and Symptoms

The primary symptom with VKC is extreme ocular itching. Patients may also have severe photophobia, foreign body sensation, blepharospasm, ptosis, burning, tearing, and blurry vision. Thick, ropy, yellow mucous discharge accompanies the disease. Compared to atopic keratoconjunctivitis, which affects the surrounding ocular adnexa, signs of VKC are limited to the ocular conjunctiva and cornea.

Clinically, there are three forms of VKC: palpebral, limbal, and mixed (69). Palpebral VKC is characterized by marked cobblestone papillae of the superior conjunctiva. The lower conjunctiva has few or no granulations. Cobblestone papillae, characteristically pale pink to gray and, at minimum, 1 mm in size, are often square in form, hard, closely packed, and flattened. Bonini et al. (66) noted that larger giant papillae correlated with poorer prognosis in chronic disease. Growth of the papillae involves conjunctival thickening, neovascularization, mucous hypersecretion, as well as tissue scarring. A milky-appearing film coats the upper tarsus and conjunctival folds. Conjunctival smears contain numerous eosinophils (Fig. 38.8).

Limbal conjunctivitis is characterized by a broad, thickened, gelatinous opacification of the limbus that can overlap the cornea. Though typically superior, this change can circumscribe the entire cornea. It presents with the same pink or gray color as the palpebral conjunctiva. Grossly visible papillae do not occur, but the tissue is elevated over the limbal area. Like palpebral vernal conjunctivitis, tiny blood vessels arise in the center of the nodular elevations. The tissue is infiltrated by lymphocytes, plasma cells, macrophages, basophils, and eosinophils. Horner-Trantas dots

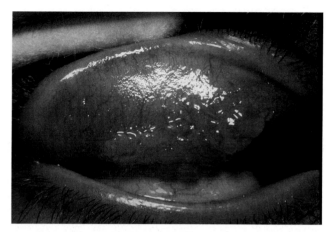

FIG. 38.8. Marked cobblestone papillae of the superior conjunctiva characteristic of palpebral VKC. (Courtesy of Bartley Mondino, MD.)

(white, chalklike dots composed of eosinophils and epithelial debris) are characteristic of limbal vernal conjunctivitis (Fig. 38.9).

Mixed VKC is a combination of both palpebral and limbal types. Fifty percent of patients with VKC have corneal involvement and the disease can be sight threatening. Corneal manifestations include punctate epithelial keratitis, epithelial erosions, superficial pannus, plaques, and subepithelial scarring. Punctate keratopathy can progress to coalesced epithelial erosions. A plaque containing fibrin and mucous can deposit over the epithelial defect to impair epithelial healing. A superficial pannus can grow in the area. "Shield" ulcers present (usually in the superior two thirds of the cornea) as horizontally oval, shallow, and nonvascularized epithelial/stromal defects. The edges have been described as "shaggy and gray," and infiltration of the underlying superficial stroma occurs. After ulcers heal, mild corneal opacities/scaring may persist (70) (Fig. 38.10).

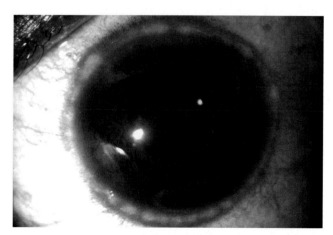

FIG. 38.9. Trantas dots in limbal vernal conjunctivitis circumscribing the entire cornea. (Courtesy of Bartley Mondino, MD.)

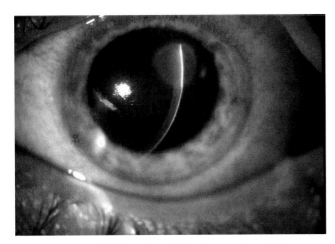

FIG. 38.10. Shield ulcer situated in the superior of the cornea with epithelial and stromal defects. (Courtesy of Bartley Mondino, MD).

Although the disease has a generally good prognosis, long-standing inflammation may cause severe visual impairment due to corneal complications, corneal scars, astigmatism, keratoconus, and steroid-induced cataract and glaucoma complications. Bonnini et al. (66) reported decreased visual acuities from corneal scarring in 6% of their patients ($n = 195$). Tabbara (71) reported that 21% of 58 patients had best-corrected visual acuities in one or both eyes less than 20/200; 34% had 20/50 to 20/200 vision, and 45% had 20/20 to 20/50 vision (Fig. 38.11).

Treatment and Management

Treatment and management of patients with VKC involves managing both ocular signs and symptoms. Environmental changes (moving to cooler climates and avoiding triggering antigens) can provide some relief, but is often impractical. In acute stages, cool compresses, artificial tears, and pulses

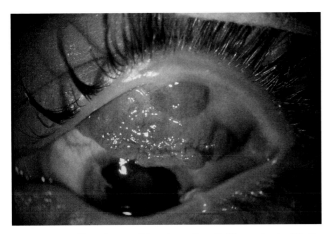

FIG. 38.11. Chronic vernal keratoconjunctivitis marked with tissue scarring. Note the shield ulcer on the cornea. (Courtesy of Bartley Mondino, MD).

of corticosteroids provide significant relief. Mast-cell stabilizers and antihistamines can be added concurrently to control inflammation as steroids are tapered. Appropriate antibiotics should be used to treat any corneal epithelial defects and shield ulcers that occur.

Topical mast-cell stabilizers (e.g., cromolyn sodium, lodoxamide tromethamine, nedocromil sodium) are approved by the US Food and Drug Administration (FDA) for management of VKC. Topical mast-cell stabilizers are extremely effective (by inhibiting mast-cell degranulation) when used four to six times a day until signs and symptoms resolve. Mast-cell stabilization often requires sustained treatment. Newer second-generation mast-cell stabilizers (e.g., nedocromil sodium) are reported to reduce ocular allergy symptoms in 2 to 15 minutes with twice-a-day dosing. (72) Combination mast-cell stabilizers/antihistamines (e.g., olopatadine) may be more effective than traditional mast-cell stabilizers alone.

Due to the chronic course of the disease, second-generation steroids (e.g., loteprednol etabonate) with "site specific" action may be helpful in decreasing use of classical steroids with attendant complications. Second-generation steroids are thought to remain in the target tissue long enough to render a therapeutic effect, but not long enough to cause as much increase in intraocular pressure and posterior subcapsular cataracts as traditional steroids. Novack et al. (73) showed that loteprednol etabonate has a lower propensity to cause significant intraocular pressure elevation than prednisolone acetate. Intraocular pressure elevation may occur as late as 6 weeks after the start of steroid use in susceptible patients, and usually reverses with termination of the steroid drug. Caution for infectious keratitis, glaucoma, and cataracts should still be maintained when using any steroids. Steroids can mask the infection and suppress the inflammatory symptoms, but the underlying disease remains the same. Steroids may be used up to eight times a day for a week and then tapered to as little as needed to maintain patient comfort. Mast-cell stabilizers applied concurrently with the steroid pulse will sustain decreased inflammation after the acute phase has been managed.

Short courses (several days) of oral antihistamines (e.g., cetirizine, loratadine, and ketotifen) are effective for mild-to-moderate VKC, especially those with concurrent systemic allergic symptoms. Side effects of systemic antihistamines include xerostomia and drowsiness.

Cyclosporin A, now FDA approved only for topical treatment of dry eye, suppresses T cells and is thought to be particularly helpful in treatment of all cell-mediated diseases (74) by decreasing clonal expansion of T-helper lymphocytes through inhibition of interleukin-2 production (75–77). Cyclosporin A reduces the number of T cells, normalizes CD4:CD8 ratios, decreases T-cell activation, and reduces T-cell cytokine expression (74). It has been found to be highly effective in patients with severe atopic dermatitis (78), AKC, and VKC (65,79–82). Bleik and Tabbara

(71) noted a statistically significant decrease in conjunctival hyperemia, papillary hypertrophy, punctate keratitis, and Trantas dots in 20 VKC patients using cyclosporin A compared to a placebo.

One study advocated aspirin therapy (0.5 to 1.0 g/d) utilized in conjunction with conventional VKC therapy to decrease the production of prostaglandins (83). Orally administered dosages of aspirin (maximum of 2,400 mg daily) may provide relief to patients unmanageable with steroids or mast-cell stabilizers (83). Another study utilized topical mitomycin C to treat VKC (84). Akpek et al. (84) noted that a 2-week course of mitomycin C decreased signs and symptoms of mucous discharge, photophobia, conjunctival hyperemia, and limbal edema without any adverse reactions. Surgical removal of corneal plaques is also useful to allow for corneal reepithelization and for decreasing VKC symptoms. Sridhar et al. (85) transplanted amniotic membranes to manage severe shield ulcers. Nishiwaki-Dantas et al. (86) proposed surgical resection of giant papillae and autologous conjunctival graft to treat severe cases of VKC with shield ulcers.

Treatment/Management of Contact Lens Patients

Vernal keratoconjunctivitis is a relative contraindication for cosmetic contact lens wear. Contact lens use can continue but with caution, concomitant treatment, and professional supervision while managing patients who have milder cases of VKC but also need to maintain contact lens wear (e.g., keratoconus, aphakia). Brodsky (87) found that topical olopatadine improved subjective tolerance, allowing such patients to continue wearing contact lenses.

ATOPIC KERATOCONJUNCTIVITIS

First described by Hogan in 1953 (88), AKC is a severe, bilateral, chronic inflammation of the conjunctiva and lids found in a subset of patients with atopic dermatitis. Atopic dermatitis affects approximately 3% of the population (88), yet 15% to 40% of patients with atopic dermatitis have AKC (89,90). AKC primarily affects males approximately twice as frequently as females (91), with an onset in the early teens or early 20s (rarely before puberty), though it may persist until the fourth or fifth decade of life (91). Incidence peaks in patients between age 30 and 50 years. These patients have a history of dermatitis (eczema is found in 95% of the patients), asthma (87% prevalence), and hay fever. Patients also have a family history of atopic disease. Sensitivity to typical allergens is quite high; 90% of patients are skin-prick positive to dust and house mites. Unlike VKC, AKC symptoms are perennial although there may be seasons when the symptoms are worse. There is no racial or geographical predilection for AKC.

Signs and Symptoms

Primary symptoms affect the eyelid skin and lid margin, conjunctiva, cornea, and lens. These include extreme itching, burning, redness, photophobia, and blurry vision. Dennie-Morgan folds (linear lid folds secondary to chronic eye rubbing) and Hertoghe's sign (absence of lateral eyebrows) may occur in the periorbital area. Unlike VKC, the eyelid margin may show meibomian gland dysfunction and keratinization resulting in eyelid thickening, tylosis, cilia loss, ptosis, cicatricial ectropion, and lagophthalmos. Staphylococcal colonization of eyelid margins is common and may result in a secondary blepharitis. The conjunctiva may be chemotic and erythematous, and copious mucous discharge may "glue" the eyelids together upon awakening. Differentiating itself from VKC, AKC has a prominent papillary hypertrophy of the inferior fornix. In severe cases, this may lead to symblepharon formation and fornical shortening. Lateral canthal ulceration, cracking, and madarosis may be present.

Corneal involvement ranges from minimal punctate epithelial keratopathy with persistent epithelial defects early in the course of the disease to corneal neovascularization, anterior stromal scarring, and shield shaped ulcers. There is a strong association with herpes simplex viral keratitis, occurring in 14% to 17.8% of patients with AKC (91,92). Keratoconus occurs in 6.7& to 16.2% of AKC patients (91). Fifty-three percent of keratoconic patients have a history of atopy (93). Lenticular changes, including anterior and posterior subcapsular cataract formation often in the configuration of a Maltese cross, have also been established, but it is uncertain whether the cataracts may be the result of chronic use of steroids. Slow-progressing cataracts are usually bilateral and present in the second generation of life. Degenerative vitreous changes and retinal detachments with or without cataract surgery have also been reported with AKC (94).

Treatment and Management

The goal of AKC treatment and management is to remove the allergen responsible for the disease as well as to provide symptomatic therapy. The combination of a systemic disease with ocular symptoms emphasizes the importance of comanaging the patient with an allergist who can provide both skin testing to identify any specific allergens and systemic treatment.

For mild cases of AKC, topical antihistamines with vasoconstrictors may be sufficient to provide some relief, but this does not treat the underlying immunologic disease. Topical mast-cell stabilizers have been effective in the long-term management of AKC (95). Topical steroids used eight times a day for a week will provide significant relief in lid disease or in the case of vision-threatening corneal involvement. The chronic nature of AKC, however, may encourage the prolonged use of topical and/or oral steroids that have possible undesirable side effects of increased intraocular pressures and cataracts. In patients with significant skin findings or asthma, oral antihistamines and NSAIDs may be used. Cyclosporin A was found highly effective in patients with severe atopic dermatitis. Interleukin-2 has also been found to be successful in treatment of atopic dermatitis, but it has not been specifically used for AKC. Concomitant herpes simplex virus infection should be treated with either topical or oral antiviral agents as needed. A subset of patients with recalcitrant and debilitating AKC may benefit from plasmapheresis (96).

Treatment/Management of Contact Lens Patients

Many AKC patients require contact lens care for optical treatment of secondary keratoconus and/or aphakia. Symptomatic ocular treatment may be occasionally achieved with topical or systemic steroid-sparing agents such as antihistamine and/or mast-cell stabilizers. Olopadatine, in particular, has shown to be effective in allowing patients suffering from mild disease to continue contact lens wear (86). As in VKC, cosmetic contact lens wear should probably cease while AKC is being actively treated with steroids, but noncosmetic wear may need to cautiously proceed in the absence of frank microbial infection when such lenses are required for visual function.

CONCLUSIONS

There are many different presentations of ocular immunologic complications, ranging from subclinical or mild to sight threatening. Diligent history taking and clinical examination are keys for recognition and diagnosis in order to properly diagnose and manage contact lens care with these often clinically similar yet etiologically very different entities. Treatment strategy is often straightforward in non–sight-threatening SAC, PAC, GPC, contact dermatitis, and both central and marginal sterile corneal infiltrates. The use of artificial tears, topical and oral vasoconstrictors, antihistamines, mast-cell stabilizers, and occasional NSAIDS or steroids usually proves effective. Contact lens wear can often be continued once the disease is under control. Sight-threatening disease (e.g., phlyctenular conjunctivitis, VKC, and AKC), however, requires extra clinical care to maintain and control both ocular and adnexal inflammation and often discontinuation of cosmetic contact lens use. Comanagement with other specialists is often appropriate in an effort to best manage both ocular and especially systemic manifestations during patient care.

ACKNOWLEDGMENT

The authors wish to extend acknowledgment to Joseph Barr, OD, Arthur Epstein, OD, and Bartley Mondino, MD, for the use of their clinical photos as indicated. They also thank Michael Giese, OD, PhD, for his help in preparing this chapter.

REFERENCES

1. Desotes J, Choquet-Kastylevsky G. Gell and Coombs's classification: is it still valid? *Toxicology* 2001;158:43–49.
2. Coombs RA, Gell PH. Classification of allergic reactions responsible for clinical hypersensitivity and disease. In: Gell PGH, Coombs RRA, Lachmann PJ, eds. *Clinical aspects of immunology*, 3rd ed. Oxford: Blackwell Scientific Publications, 1975: 761–782.
3. Bielory L. Update on ocular allergy treatment. *Expert Opin Pharmacother* 2002;3:541–553.
4. Bielory L. allergic and immunologic disorders of the eye. Part II: Ocular allergy. *J Allergy Clin Immunol* 2000;106:1019–1032.
5. Cocoa AF, Cooke RA. On the classification of the phenomena of hypersensitivities. *J Immunol* 1923;8:163–182.
6. Weeke ER. Epidemiology of hay fever and perennial allergic rhinitis. *Monogr Allergy* 1987;21:1–20.
7. Braude LS, Chandler JW. Atopic corneal disease. *Int Ophthalmol Clin* 1984;24:145–156.
8. Toda I, Shimazaki J, Tsubota K. Dry eye with only decreased tear break-up time is sometimes associated with allergic conjunctivitis. *Ophthalmology* 1995;102:302–309.
9. Fujishima H, Toda I, Shimazaki J, et al. Allergic conjunctivitis and dry eye. *Br J Ophthalmol* 1996;80:994–997.
10. Friedlaender MH, Okumoto M, Kelley J. Diagnosis of allergic conjunctivitis. *Arch Ophthalmol* 1984;102:1198–1199.
11. Ciprandi G, Buscaglia S, Cerqueti PM, et al. Drug allergic conjunctivitis. A review of the evidence. *Drugs* 1992;43:154–176.
12. Sainte Laudy J, Couturier P, Basset-Stheme D. Importance of lacrymal levels (total IgE, specific IgE and albumin) for the study of allergic conjunctivitis. *Allergy Immunol* 1994;26:95–96.
13. Anderson DF, MacLeod JD, Baddeley SM, et al. Seasonal allergic conjunctivitis is accompanied by increased mast cell number in the absence of leucocyte infiltration. *Clin Exp Allergy* 1997;27: 1060–1066.
14. Allansmith MR, Ross RN. Ocular allergy. *Clin Allergy* 1988;18: 1–13.
15. Donshik PC. Allergic conjunctivitis. *Int Ophthalmol Clin* 1988; 28:294–302.
16. Carlson RE, Hering PJ. Allergic shiners. *JAMA* 1981;246:835.
17. Opcon A [package insert]. Rochester, NY: Bausch & Lomb, 1998.
18. Abelson MB, Kaplan AP. A randomized, double blind, placebo-controlled comparison of emadastine 0.05% ophthalmic solution with loratadine 10 mg and their combination in the human conjunctival allergen challenge model. *Clin Ther* 2002;24:445–456.
19. Berdy GJ, Stoppel JO, Epstein AB. Comparison of the clinical efficacy and tolerability of olopatadine hydrochloride 0.1% ophthalmic solution and loteprednol etabonate 0.2% ophthalmic suspension in the conjunctival allergen challenge model. *Clin Ther* 2002;24:918–929.
20. Abelson MB, Lanier RQ. The added benefit of local Patanol therapy when combined with systemic Claritin for the inhibition of ocular itching in the conjunctival antigen challenge model. *Acta Ophthalmol Scand Suppl* 1999;228:53–56.
21. Lanier BQ, Gross RD, Marks BB. Olopatadine ophthalmic solution adjunctive to loratadine compared with loratadine alone in patients with active seasonal allergic conjunctivitis symptoms. *Ann Allergy Asthma Immunol* 2001;86:641–648.
22. Guidera AC, Luchs JI, Udell IJ. Keratitis, ulceration, and perfora-

tion associated with topical nonsteroidal anti-inflammatory drugs. *Ophthalmology* 2001;108:936–944.

23. Rentro L, Snow JS. Ocular effects of topical and systemic steroids. *Dermatol Clin* 1992;10:505–512.

24. Kari O, Haahtela T. Is atopy a risk factor for the use of contact lenses? *Allergy* 1992;47(Pt 1):295–298.

25. Kumar P, Elston R, Black D. et al. Allergic conjunctivitis and contact lens intolerance. *CLAO J* 1991;17:31–34.

26. Spring TF. Reaction to hydrophilic lenses. *Med J Aust* 1974;1:449–450.

27. Douglas JP, Lowder CY, Lazorik R, et al. Giant papillary conjunctivitis with rigid gas permeable contact lenses. *CLAO J* 1988;14:143–147.

28. MacIvor J: Contact allergy to plastic artificial eyes: preliminary report. *Can Med Assoc J* 1950;62:164–165.

29. Friedlaender MH. Conjunctivitis of allergic origin: clinical presentation and differential diagnosis. *Surv Ophthalmol* 1993;38(Suppl):105–114.

30. Srinivasan BD, Jakobiec FA, Iwamoto T, et al. Giant papillary conjunctivitis with ocular prostheses. *Arch Ophthalmol* 1979;97:892–895.

31. Sugar A, Meyer RF: Giant papillary conjunctivitis after keratoplasty. *Am J Ophthalmol* 1981;92:368–371.

32. Jolson AS, Jolson SC: Suture barb giant papillary conjunctivitis. *Ophthalmic Surg* 1984;15:139–140.

33. Heidemann DG, Dunn SP: Unusual causes of giant papillary conjunctivitis. *Cornea* 1993;12:78–80.

34. Dunn JP Jr, Weissman BA, Mondino BJ, et al. Giant papillary conjunctivitis associated with elevated corneal deposits. *Cornea* 1990;9:357–358.

35. Binder PS. The physiologic effects of extended wear soft contact lenses. *Ophthalmology* 1980;87:745–749.

36. Porazinski AD, Donshik PC. Giant papillary conjunctivitis in frequent-replacement contact lens wearers: a retrospective study. *CLAO J* 1999;25:142–147.

37. Meisler DM, Zaret CR, Stock EL. Trantas dots and limbal inflammation associated with soft contact lens wear. *Am J Ophthalmol* 1980;89:66–69.

38. Sheldon L, Beidner B, Geltman C et al. Giant papillary conjunctivitis and ptosis in a contact lens wearer. *J Pediatr Ophthalmol Strabismus* 1979;16:136–137.

39. Fowler SA, Allansmith MR. The effect of cleaning soft contact lenses. A scanning electron microscopic study. *Arch Ophthalmol* 1981;99:1382–1386.

40. Maissa C, Franklin V, Guillon M, et al. Influence of contact lens material surface characteristics and replacement frequency on protein and lipid deposition. *Optom Vis Sci* 1998.75:697–705.

41. Kruger CJ, Ehlers WH, Luistro AE, et al. Treatment of giant papillary conjunctivitis with cromolyn sodium. *CLAO J* 1992;18:46–48.

42. Donshik PC. Giant papillary conjunctivitis. *Trans Am Ophthalmol Soc* 1994;92:687–744.

43. Wilson FM 2nd. Adverse external ocular effects of topical ophthalmic medications. *Surv Ophthalmol* 1979;24:57–88.

44. Mathias CG, Mailbach HI, Irvine A, et al. Allergic contact dermatitis to echothiophate iodide and phenylephrine. *Arch Ophthalmol* 1979;97;286–287.

45. Rheinstrom SD. The conjunctiva. In: Chandler JW, Sugar J, Edelhauseer HF, eds. *Textbook of ophthalmology, Vol 8: External diseases.* London:Mosby,1994:2.8–2.9.

46. Sher MA. Contact dermatitis of the eyelids. *S Afr Med J* 1979;55:511–513.

47. Friedlaender MH. *Allergy and immunology of the eye.* New York: Raven Press, 1933.

48. Rich LF, Hanifin JM. Ocular complications of atopic dermatitis and other eczemas. *Int Ophthalmol Clin* 1985;25:61–76.

49. Theodore FH, Schlossman A. *Ocular allergy.* Baltimore: Williams and Wilkans,1958:64–77.

50. Stenson S. Superior limbic keratoconjunctivitis associated with soft contact lens wear. *Arch Ophthalmol* 1983;101:402–404.

51. Wilson-Holt N, Dart JK. Thiomerosal keratoconjunctivitis, frequency, clinical spectrum, and diagnosis. *Eye* 1989;3(Pt 5):581–587.

52. Sendele DD, Kenyon KR, Mobilia EF, et al. Superior limbic keratoconjunctivitis in contact lens wearers. *Ophthalmology* 1983;90:616–622.

53. Mondino BJ, Groden LR. Conjunctival hyperemia and corneal infiltrates with chemically disinfected soft contact lenses. *Arch Ophthalmol* 1980;98:1767–1770.

54. Mondino BJ, Salamon SM, Zaidman GW. Allergic and toxic reactions of soft contact lens wearers. *Surv Ophthalmol* 1982;26:337–344.

55. Christie C, Meyler J. Contemporary contact lens care products. *Contact lens and Anterior Eye* 1997;20:S11–S17.

56. Jones L, MacDougall N, Sorbara LG. Asymptomatic corneal staining associated with the use of balafilcon silicone-hydrogel contact lenses disinfected with polyaminopropyl biguanide-preserved care regimen. *Optom Vis Sci* 2002;79:753–7561.

57. Yeung KK, Weissman BA. Presumed sterile corneal infiltrates and hydrogel lens wear: a case series. *Int Contact Lens Clin* 1997;24:213–217.

58. Choate W, Fontana F, Potter J, et al. Evaluation of PuriLens contact lens care system: an automatic care system incorporating UV disinfection and hydrodynamic shear cleaning. *CLAO J* 2000;26:134–140.

59. Thygeson P. The etiology and treatment of phlyctenular keratoconjunctivitis. *Am J Ophthalmol* 1951;34:1217–1236.

60. Holland EJ et al. Ocular involvement in an outbreak of herpes gladiatorum. *Am J Ophthalmol* 1992;114:680–684.

61. Hussein AA, Nasr ME. The role of parasitic infetion in the aetiology of phlyctenular eye disease. *J Egypt Soc Parasitol* 1991;21:865–868.

62. Mondino BJ. Inflammatory disease of the peripheral cornea. *Ophthalmology* 1988;95:463–472.

63. Beauchamp GR, Gillette TE, Friendly DS. Phlyctenular keratoconjunctivitis. *J Pediatr Ophthalmol Strabismus* 1981;18:22–28.

64. Culbertson WW, Huang AJ, Mandelbaum SH. Effective treatment of phlyctenular keratoconjunctivitis with oral tetracycline. *Ophthalmology* 1993;100:1358–1366.

65. Leonardi A. Vernal keratoconjunctivitis: pathogenesis and treatment. *Prog Retin Eye Res* 2002;21:319–339.

66. Bonini S, Bonini S, Lambiase A, et al. Vernal keratoconjunctivitis revisited: a case series of 195 patients with long-term followup. *Ophthalmology* 2000;107:1157–1163.

67. Neumann E, Gutmann MJ, Blumenkrantz N, et al. A review of four hundred cases of vernal conjunctivitis. *Am J Ophthalmol* 1959;47:166–172.

68. Buckley RJ. Long-term experience with sodium cromoglycate in the management of vernal keratoconjunctivitis. In: Pepys J, Edward Am, eds. *The mast cell.* London: Pitman Medical, 1980:518–523.

69. Stock EL, Meisler DM. Vernal conjunctivitis. In: Tassman W, Jaeger EA, eds. *Duane's clinical ophthalmology,* Vol 4. Philadelphia: JB Lippincott, 1995:9.1–9.5.

70. Buckley RJ: Vernal keratoconjunctivitis. *Int Ophthalmol Clin* 1988;28(4):303–308.

71. Tabbara KF. Ocular complications of vernal keratoconjunctivitis. *Can J Ophthalmol* 1999;34:88–92.

72. Tauber J. Nedocromil sodium ophthalmic solution 2% twice daily in patients with allergic conjunctivitis. *Adv Ther* 2002;19;73–84.

73. Novack GD, Howes J, Crockett RS, et al. Change in intraocular

pressure during long-term use of loteprednol etabonate. *J Glaucoma* 1998;7:266–269.

74. Hingorani M, Calder VL, Buckley RJ, et al. The immunomodulatory effect of topical cyclosporine A in atopic keratoconjunctivitis. *Invest Ophthalmol Vis Sci* 1999;40:392–399.

75. Ben Ezra D, Matamoros N, Cohen E. Treatment of severe vernal keratoconjunctivitis with cyclosporine A eyedrops. *Transplant Proc* 1988;20(Suppl 2):644–649.

76. Secchi AG, Tognon MS, Leonardi A. Topical use of cyclosporine in the treatment of viral keratoconjunctivitis. *Am J Ophthalmol* 1990;110:641–645.

77. Bleik JH, Tabbara KF. Topical cyclosporine in vernal keratoconjunctivitis. *Ophthalmol* 1991;98(11):1679–1684.

78. Sowden JM, Berth-Jones J, Ross JS, et al. Double blind, controlled, crossover study of cyclosporine in adults with severe refractory atopic dermatitis. *Lancet* 1991;338(8760):137–140.

79. Fujishima H, Fukagawa K, Satake Y, et al. Combined medical and surgical treatment of severe vernal keratoconjunctivitis. *Jpn J Ophthalmol* 2000;44:511–515.

80. Gupta V, Sahu PK. Topical cyclosporine A in the management of vernal keratoconjunctivitis. *Eye* 2001;15(Pt 1):39–41.

81. Avunduk AM, Avunduk MC, Erdol H, et al. Cyclosporine effects on clinical findings and impression cytology specimens in severe vernal keratoconjunctivitis. *Ophthalmologica* 2001;215:290–293.

82. Holland EJ, Olsen TW, Ketcham JM, et al. Topical cyclosporine A in the treatment of anterior segment inflammatory disease. *Cornea* 1993;12:413–419.

83. Abelson MB, Butrus SI, Weston JH. Aspirin therapy in vernal conjunctivitis. *Am J Ophthalmol* 1983;95:502–505.

84. Akpek EK, Hasiripi H, Christen WG, et al. A randomized trial of low-dose, topical mitomycin-C in the treatment of severe vernal keratoconjunctivitis. *Ophthalmology* 2000;107:263–269.

85. Sridhar MS, Sangwan VS, Bansal A, et al. Amniotic membrane transplantation in the management of shield ulcers of vernal keratoconjunctivitis. *Ophthalmology* 2001;108:1218–1222.

86. Nishiwaki-Dantas MC, Dantas PE, Pezzutti S, et al. Surgical resection of giant papillae and autologous conjunctival graft in patients with severe vernal keratoconjunctivitis and giant papillae. *Ophthalmol Plast Reconstr Surg* 2000;16:438–442.

87. Brodsky M. Allergic conjunctivitis with contact lenses: experience with olopatadine hydrochloride 0.1% therapy. *Acta Ophthalmol Scand Suppl* 2000;230:56–59.

88. Hogan MJ. Atopic keratoconjunctivitis. *Am J Ophthalmol* 1953;36:937–947.

89. Garrity JA, Liesegang TJ. Ocular complications of atopic dermatitis. *Can J Ophthalmol* 1984;19:21–24.

90. Rich LF, Hanifin JM. Ocular complications of atopic dermatitis and other eczemas. *Int Ophthalmol Clin* 1985;25:61–76.

91. Tuft SJ, Kemeny DM, Dart JK, Buckley RJ. Clinical features of atopic keratoconjunctivitis. *Ophthalmology* 1991;98:150–158.

92. Foster CS, Calogne M. Atopic keratoconjunctivitis. *Ophthalmology* 1990;97:992–1000.

93. Zadnik K, Barr JT, Edrington TB et al. Baseline findings in the collaborative longitudinal evaluation of keratoconus (CLEK) study. *Invest Ophthalmol Vis Sci* 1998;39:2537–2346.

94. Hurlbut WB, Damonkos AN. Cataract and retinal detachment associated with atopic dermatitis. *Arch Ophthalmol* 1961;52:852–857.

95. Jay JL. Clinical features and diagnosis of adult atopic keratoconjunctivitis and the effect of treatment with sodium cromoglycate. *Br J Ophthalmol* 1981;65:335–340.

96. Aswad MI, Tauber J, Baum J. Plasmapheresis treatment in patients with severe atopic keratoconjunctivitis. *Ophthalmology* 1988;95:444–447.

INFECTIOUS KERATITIS IN CONTACT LENS WEARERS

ANTHONY J. ALDAVE
JAMES P. DUNN, JR.
MANOJ SHARMA
BARTLY J. MONDINO AND
BARRY A. WEISSMAN

Corneal ulcers are the most serious complication of contact lens wear. This chapter will review the epidemiology, clinical presentations, diagnosis, treatment, and prevention of this problem.

Keratitis simply denotes inflammation of the cornea. Any or all layers of corneal tissue may be involved. Keratitis may be either infectious or noninfectious. Causes of infectious keratitis include bacteria, protozoa, fungi, and viruses. Causes of noninfectious keratitis include tear-film abnormalities, exposure, immune reactions, denervation, dystrophies, photic and chemical injuries, mechanical trauma, and reactions to topical or systemic medications. Ulcerative keratitis (corneal ulcer) implies both inflammation and loss of corneal tissue. This may be associated with microbial keratitis as well as noninfectious immune and hypersensitivity reactions.

INCIDENCE

For several reasons, it is difficult to assess precisely the incidence of infectious keratitis in contact lens wearers. Most studies of contact lens–related ulcers are retrospective, not prospective, and do not involve a well-defined group of patients. Even in these times of expanded optometry practice, ophthalmologists treat most patients with contact lens–related ulcers, but they fit only about one fifth of the contact lenses that are dispensed (1) distorting their impressions. Since many patients are not referred to institutions where statistics are kept, there may be a substantial number of unreported ulcers. Different studies also use different definitions of "corneal ulceration." Some cases reported as culture-negative infectious keratitis may, in fact, represent noninfectious keratitis, such as the overwear syndrome with epithelial defects, or corneal infiltrates due to thimerosal. Finally, there is no uniformly accepted definition of "incidence," such as ulcers per patient-year.

An early study of nearly 50,000 hard contact lens wearers document only 14 cases of "lost or blinded" eyes, 8 of which were clearly associated with deficiencies in lens care (2). With the development of the cosmetic soft contact lens, and especially the cosmetic extended-wear soft contact lens, bacterial keratitis has been reported more frequently. The first report of a culture-proven bacterial corneal ulcer in a cosmetic soft contact lens wearer appeared in 1976 (3), with several other reports in the next several years (4–6). In several studies published in the 1980s, the percentages of cases of infectious keratitis that were contact lens–related had increased, with most studies demonstrating that about 25% to 30% of corneal ulcers were associated with contact lens wear (7–9). However, a study published in 2001 demonstrated a significant decrease in the number of contact lens–related corneal ulcers from 1988 to 1999 at a single institution (10). Even though the total number of non–contact lens–related ulcers remained constant during this period, the percentage of all ulcers related to contact lens wear decreased from 30% (1992–1995) to 12% (1996–1999). The authors suggested that this trend could be related to fewer ulcers being referred to their tertiary care practice, a secondary effect of improved treatment of smaller ulcers by community ophthalmologists and optometrists following the introduction of topical fluoroquinolones in 1995 (10).

Most studies indicate a higher incidence of infectious keratitis in patients using extended-wear lenses (EWSCL) than in those using daily-wear soft lenses (DWSCL) (11–19). Estimates of the incidence of infection during use of soft contact lenses range from 0.04% (17) to 1% (20), with an even higher figure in certain groups of aphakic patients using EWSCL (21–23). Weissman and associates (15,24) found an infection rate of 0.5% for cosmetic daily-wear hydrogel contact lens wearers and about 3% for extended-wear hydrogel lens wearers over a 2-year period. This six-fold increased risk of infection associated with EWSCLs vs DWSCLs is similar to the five-fold increased risk found by Chalupa and colleagues (12), who described an incidence rate of 1/15,000 for DWSCL and 1/3,000 for hydrogel EWSCLs. A subsequent large, prospective study performed in the United States again found a five-fold increased rate, with an incidence of 0.04% associated with the use of daily-wear hydrogel and rigid gas-permeable (GP) contact lenses and 0.2% with the use of extended-wear hydrogel lenses (17). Another prospective study, performed in Europe and published 10 years later, found similar results, with an estimated annualized incidence of microbial keratitis in 1.1 per 10,000 rigid GP wearers, 3.5 per 10,000 DWSCL wearers, and 20.0 per 10,000 EWSCL wearers (18). A US Food and Drug Administration survey, which reported on over 22,000 contact lens wearers, found an incidence in ulcers per patient-year to be 1 per 2,000 in cosmetic daily-wear soft and 1 per 1,500 in GP contact lenses, a rate two to four times higher in cosmetic EWSCL wearers compared with DWSCL wearers, and a rate nine times higher in aphakic EWSCL wearers compared with DWSCL wearers (25). While bacterial keratitis associated with extended wear of silicone hydrogel contact lenses has been reported in the form of small case series (26), no report of the incidence in these newer SCLs, with significantly higher oxygen transmissibility than hydrogel SCLs, has been published.

Debate continues as to whether the lens material or lens-wearing habits is more closely correlated with the risk of infectious keratitis. While a case–control study published in the early 1990s suggested that both disposable extended- and daily-wear lenses were associated with a higher risk of infectious keratitis than conventional extended- and daily-wear lenses (27), a study published 2 years later found that the wearing schedule, specifically if the lenses were worn overnight, was the primary risk factor for infection, as opposed to lens material (28).

Fungal keratitis (keratomycosis) associated with cosmetic contact lens wear is uncommon. A review of the world literature suggested that fungal keratitis accounts for only 3% of the infections associated with cosmetic contact lenses or contact lenses for aphakia, and 12% of infections associated with therapeutic lenses (29). The incidence of viral keratitis does not appear to be increased among contact lens wearers, but may occur incidentally.

DIFFERENTIAL DIAGNOSIS OF NONINFECTIOUS KERATITIS

A number of contact lens complications may mimic infectious keratitis. These include mechanical, hypoxic, immunologic, and hypersensitivity reactions.

Corneal abrasions that occur following overwear of a contact lens or poor lens fit are not uncommon, and may manifest with epithelial staining, conjunctival injection, pain, and cells and flare in the anterior chamber. Vision will be decreased if the visual axis is involved. If these find-

ings alone are present in a patient with a clear history of an abrasion, it is reasonable to treat this patient with a broad-spectrum antibiotic and perhaps a cycloplegic agent. Neither patching nor use of corticosteroids should be considered in contact lens–related abrasions because of the potential risk of rapid onset of *Pseudomonas* infections (30). The patient should be evaluated daily until healing occurs.

Corneal hypoxia may induce epithelial staining and defects, infiltrates, neovascularization, and cells and flare in the anterior chamber. Symptoms may be identical to those that are present in infectious keratitis. Hypopyon iridocyclitis may occur in extreme cases of tight lenses, or of large central epithelial defects, and hypopyon without corneal infiltrates may be present in an acutely red eye (31). This condition has been considered noninfectious because of negative cultures, a positive response to steroid treatment, and improvement upon discontinuation of lens wear.

Hypersensitivity reactions to contact lens solutions, especially thimerosal, include conjunctival injection, corneal infiltrates, possibly corneal dendrites, and a form of superior limbic keratoconjunctivitis. Finally, peripheral corneal infiltrates or epithelial defects due to chlamydial or herpetic infection or staphylococcal hypersensitivity reactions may occur incidentally in contact lens wearers. Appropriate cultures and relevant slit-lamp findings, such as follicles in chlamydial and herpetic conjunctivitis, corneal anesthesia in herpetic keratitis, and blepharitis in staphylococcal marginal keratitis, will help establish the diagnosis.

RISK FACTORS IN INFECTIOUS KERATITIS

Infectious keratitis in contact lens wearers is usually due to pathogens that are present in the conjunctival flora or contaminate lenses or lens care solutions. The common pathway in infectious keratitis, therefore, is the ability of the infectious agent to penetrate host defense and gain access to the corneal stroma.

Alteration of the Normal Ocular Flora

Organisms that constitute the normal ocular surface flora are felt to inhibit the proliferation of organisms of greater virulence. Therefore, any alteration of the normal flora, as in patients with ocular cicatricial pemphigoid or following chemical injuries may disrupt this natural balance and increase the risk of corneal infection.

Contact lens wearers comprise a diverse group that manifest different baseline flora. Normal conjunctival flora in the healthy adult, which probably reflects that of the eyelid skin (32), consists of both aerobic bacteria, predominately *Staphylococcus epidermidis, S aureus,* and the diphtheroids, and anaerobic bacteria, predominately *Propionibacterium acnes.* The presence of other bacteria, including *Pneumococcus, Streptococcus viridans,* and gram-negative rods, such as

Pseudomonas, is much less frequent. Nonbacterial flora includes *Pityrosporon ovale* and the arthropod *Demodex.* Fungi are not usually considered part of the ocular flora (33) even during contact lens wear (34,35). Protozoa such as *Acanthamoeba* as well as viruses also are not considered normal flora. Age is an uncertain factor; one study showed no age-related change in flora (36), while another indicated both a higher incidence of anaerobes and a greater number of species per eye in adults, with a higher incidence of *Streptococcus* species noted in children (37).

The conjunctival flora may be altered in patients with ocular surface disease in whom soft contact lenses may be necessary for therapeutic purposes. The conjunctival flora does not appear to be altered in immunosuppressed patients (38), but the incidence of fungi may be greater in patients using topical steroids (39).

Studies in both therapeutic and cosmetic EWSCL have not shown an increase or alteration in the conjunctival flora (34,35,40). These studies suggest that factors other than alteration of conjunctival flora are responsible for the increased risk of keratitis in contact lens wearers, and that prophylactic antibiotics are not indicated in cosmetic lens wearers (40).

Noncompliance with Standard Contact Lens Disinfection and Storage

Infectious keratitis may be related to lens contamination or the effect of the contact lens on the corneal epithelium. Wilson and colleagues (6) demonstrated that poor contact lens hygiene may directly lead to corneal infection by isolating the same serotype of *Pseudomonas* in corneal ulcers as in the lens case and solutions of these patients (6). Contamination of lenses and lens care systems is a well-documented phenomenon, especially with poor compliance. One study found that 40% of patients using daily-wear lenses were noncompliant by history (41). Noncompliance occurred more frequently among younger patients, after lenses had been worn for more than 2 years, and in those patients whose initial contact lens fitting and lens care instructions had been obtained elsewhere. Noncompliance rates as high as 82% have been reported among randomly selected patients (42).

A study of the lens care systems of 100 asymptomatic cosmetic contact lens wearers showed that over 50% were using contaminated care systems, with a similar incidence among rigid and soft lens wearers (43). There was no significant difference in contamination rates between 64% of patients who had reported that they handled, cleaned, and disinfected their lenses properly, and 36% who admitted they had not. A wide variety of organisms were recovered from the contaminated care systems, including such pathogenic organisms as gram-positive bacteria (*Staphylococcus, Streptococcus,* and *Bacillus* species), gram-negative bacteria (*Pseudomonas* and *Serratia*), fungi, and protozoa (*Acantha-*

moeba). Thirteen percent of commercial solutions were contaminated, as compared to a 100% contamination rate of bottles containing homemade saline solution. Although all but one bottle of commercial solution was used before its expiration date, the mean time of use was significantly higher for contaminated solutions than for uncontaminated solutions. Contamination was not found in preserved solutions that were used for fewer than 21 days, whereas large nonaerosol bottles of unpreserved saline were contaminated as early as 5 days after opening. No contamination was found in 48 bottles of commercial eyedrops, perhaps because of higher concentrations of preservatives.

Virulent Organisms

Several organisms were noted that deserved special comment. *Serratia,* an uncommon cause of corneal ulcers in contact lens wearers, was found only in the chlorhexidine- and benzalkonium chloride–preserved hard contact lens care systems (13). Resistant strains of *Serratia* may develop during exposure to chlorhexidine, with some resistance to benzalkonium chloride as well (44). *Bacillus* species were found in seven lens care systems. *Bacillus,* which has been found in up to 3% of contact lens–associated corneal ulcers (45), forms spores that are resistant to heat and many types of chemical disinfection (46) and may require prolonged exposure to 3% hydrogen peroxide for eradication (47). Another study suggested an additional source of contamination: a breach in the integrity of the contact lens case, noting defects that ranged from small linear cracks to large holes (48).

Biofilm Formation and Lens Polymer

Microbes such as bacteria (49) and fungi (50) adhere to contact lens surfaces, most likely by formation of biofilms. The contaminated contact lens, acting as a vector, transfers pathogenic organisms from contaminated cases or solutions to the ocular surface. Bacteria appear able to attach to unworn lenses, but show a 12-fold increase in adherence to lenses with a mucin coating (51). In contrast, fungal adherence to contact lens surfaces may depend upon degradation of the lens surface, resulting in an increase in the pore size. Both surface and enzyme cleaners are designed to remove such contaminates, but they do not disinfect the lens and are ineffective in totally eliminating mucin deposits (52). Commercially available enzyme cleaners, however, have been shown to reduce the adherence of *Pseudomonas* to mucin-coated soft contact lenses (51). The question remains, however, whether bacteria incorporated into a biofilm on a contact lens surface are able to leave the biofilm and infect the ocular surface.

While the presence of a bacterial biofilm on a silicone hydrogel contact lens has been demonstrated to increase adherence of other microbes, such as *Acanthamoeba,* a recent study (53) has demonstrated that the presence of a bacterial biofilm on silicon hydrogel contact lenses does not have an effect on the attachment of *Acanthamoeba* organisms. However, the primary finding of this study was that acanthamoebal attachment to the silicone hydrogel lenses was significantly greater than to the conventional hydrogel lenses. The authors hypothesized that the increased attachment found with the silicone hydrogel lens may be an inherent characteristic of the lens polymer or a result of the surface treatment procedure to which the lenses are exposed.

Diabetes Mellitus

Patients with diabetes may be at higher risk for corneal ulcerations, and merit particularly close attention in follow-up care (21,22).

Altered Ocular Defense Factors

Tears

Tears contain multiple factors with antibacterial properties, such as lactoferrin, lysozyme, betalysin, and antibodies such as immunoglobulin A. Therefore, any condition associated with a tear deficiency or a tear composition abnormality, such as Sjögren's syndrome or Stevens-Johnson syndrome, is associated with a predisposition to ocular surface infection.

Epithelium

An intact corneal epithelium serves as a barrier preventing the penetration of all but a very few bacteria (54). Therefore, an epithelial defect must typically be present before an organism can penetrate into the cornea. Experimental studies have shown increased adherence of *P aeruginosa* to injured or exposed basal epithelial cells compared with exposed corneal stroma or an intact epithelial surface (55). Additionally, the induction of a corneal epithelial defect followed by experimental bacterial inoculation has been shown to increase bacterial adherence to the cornea as well as produce corneal ulceration (56–58). Corneal epithelial defects may of course be the result of minor epithelial trauma associated with the insertion, wearing, or removal of a contact lens. However, other contact lens–related factors, such as induced corneal hypoxia, may also promote bacterial adherence to the ocular surface (59).

SPECIAL CONSIDERATIONS

Therapeutic Contact Lenses

Therapeutic soft contact lenses are employed for multiple indications, including symptomatic relief of filamentary keratitis or bullous keratopathy, to facilitate reepithelializa-

tion of persistent epithelial defects, etc. As most of these indications involve transient or persistent epithelial defects, and are often associated with coexisting disorders of the ocular surface, the risk for infection in this group is certainly higher than among cosmetic contact lens wearers (60,61). Brown and colleagues (62) described six corneal ulcers that developed in 38 eyes treated with therapeutic soft contact lenses for severely diseased epithelium caused by Stevens-Johnson syndrome, Sjögren's syndrome, ocular pemphigoid, neurotrophic keratitis, herpes simplex keratitis, or alkali burns. The infections, which included both bacterial and fungal keratitis, were attributed to several factors, including concurrent dry-eye states and the use of antibiotics and steroids that may have altered the conjunctival flora. Dohlman and colleagues (61) have also reported an increased rate of infectious keratitis in therapeutic soft lenses wearers. The investigators felt that prophylactic antibiotics were indicated in any therapeutic lens wearer with an epithelial defect, but the antibiotics were of questionable value in long-term wearers without epithelial defects (for example, patients with dry eye). They recommended nightly removal of the therapeutic lenses for patients with good vision, as is the case in many dry-eye states, in order to allow optimal oxygenation.

After Penetrating Keratoplasty

Contact lenses worn after penetrating keratoplasty, whether for refractive or therapeutic purposes, may pose special risks. Many of these contact lens wearers are on maintenance topical corticosteroids (12); they also may have epithelial defects and exposed sutures. A review of 68 bacterial and fungal corneal ulcers that developed after penetrating keratoplasty showed that 18 (26%) were associated with the use of soft contact lenses (63). Ten patients had worn a therapeutic bandage lens and the remaining eight patients had worn cosmetic hydrogel lenses; gram-positive infections predominated in the former and gram-negative infections in the latter.

Persistent Epithelial Defects

Sterile, nonhealing ulcers from rheumatoid arthritis or neurotrophic keratitis are often treated with bandage soft contact lenses to promote reepithelialization. Serial examinations and knowledge of the patient's history are necessary in such cases to avoid treating the patient with unnecessary and toxic antibiotics. It must be kept in mind, however, that concurrent infectious keratitis may develop in these patients.

The spectrum of infectious keratitis in therapeutic contact lens wear may be distinguished from that of cosmetic contact lens wear; there is a much higher relative incidence of gram-positive infection in the former (7), as well as a higher prevalence of polymicrobial keratitis or infection with quasicommensal organisms, such as α-hemolytic streptococci *(45)*. Corneal ulcers are particularly common when bandage contact lenses are used in patients with mucosal scarring disorders, such as ocular cicatricial pemphigoid, or dry-eye states (64).

Orthokeratology

While orthokeratology fell out of popularity in the 1980s, largely because of published reports of the limited efficacy and predictability of the procedure (65) the evolution of reverse-geometry GP lenses and material oxygen transmissibility has brought renewed interest to this procedure. Recent reports have suggested a possible association of nocturnal orthokeratology lens wear with risk of corneal infection (66–69). Predisposition to infection is thought to be secondary to compromise of the epithelial barrier function (70), from direct central epithelial trauma in the region of compressive point of contact, thinning of the central corneal epithelium, and altered epithelial cell desquamation and size (70).

MICROORGANISMS

Bacterial Keratitis

Reports of infectious keratitis in cosmetic hydrogel contact lens wearers consistently show a predominance of gram-negative organisms, particularly *P aeruginosa* and other *Pseudomonas* species; *Proteus* and *Serratia* are seen less frequently (7,11–14,17,71). *S aureus* is the most common gram-positive pathogen (5,7,11,12,14,44). This is contrast to most reports of non–contact lens–related infectious keratitis, in which gram-positive organisms predominate (9).

Gram-positive Organisms

Staphylococcus
Both *S epidermidis* and *S aureus* are part of the normal flora of the eyelid and conjunctiva. *S aureus* is associated with many of the most common external diseases, such as infectious blepharitis, conjunctivitis, marginal keratitis and phlyctenulosis. Both *Staphylococcus* species are also common causes of infectious keratitis, in cases both with and without a history of contact lens wear.

Streptococcus
Streptococcus pneumoniae and *S pyogenes* are also commonly implicated as the causative agents in bacterial corneal ulcers. *S pneumoniae* is part of the normal human adult flora of the upper respiratory tract, which may predispose to chronic recurrent conjunctivitis in colonized patients. Streptococcal keratitis is commonly associated with the development of a hypopyon, often displaying a more aggres-

sive course than *S aureus,* which in turn typically is associated with a more aggressive course than *S epidermidis.* Infectious crystalline keratopathy is commonly associated with corneal infection with streptococcal species (especially *S viridans,* another common normal inhabitant of the upper respiratory tract), where unchallenged stromal proliferation of the bacterium produces a crystalline infiltrate without evidence of an inflammatory response (72,73).

Gram-negative Organisms

Pseudomonas
Because of the high incidence of *P aeruginosa* in contact lens–related infections, it is this organism that has been most extensively studied. It survives well in the moist environment offered by contact lens cases and solutions (7). Surface hydrophobicity of different isolates of *P aeruginosa* appears to affect adherence to soft lenses (74). Furthermore, contact lens coatings, particularly mucin, facilitate the adherence of *P aeruginosa* to soft contact lenses (51).

Epithelial trauma related to corneal hypoxia or contact lens manipulation may allow the development of an infection if the contact lens is contaminated. *Pseudomonas* adheres to the edges of injured epithelium and stroma (55), especially partial-thickness epithelial injury (75). Although *Pseudomonas* species are not able to invade an intact epithelium, the release of endotoxins, exotoxins, and proteolytic enzymes can result in rapidly progressive corneal ulceration (Fig. 39.1).

Serratia
Another Gram negative rod, *Serratia,* is capable of releasing endotoxin, although associated corneal infections are typically not as rapidly developing or as severe as those associated with pseudomonal infection. Endotoxin is immuno-

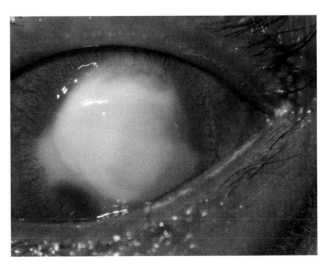

FIG. 39.1. Pseudomonal corneal ulcer with a large hypopyon (cosmetic soft contact lens wearer).

genic itself, and has been associated with annular corneal infiltrates, even in the absence of viable bacteria (76). *Serratia* has been reported to develop resistance to preservatives often used in contact lens care systems, including chlorhexidine and benzalkonium chloride.

Moraxella

While *Moraxella* species are well-recognized ocular pathogens, they are an uncommon cause of corneal ulceration in otherwise healthy hosts. Typically associated with ulcerative keratitis in immunocompromised patients or those with a debilitated ocular surface (Fig. 39.2), *Moraxella* species have only occasionally been associated with contact lens–related corneal ulceration.

Other Organisms

While the aforementioned bacteria are most commonly encountered in cases of culture-proven bacterial keratitis, a number of reports document contact lens–related corneal ulcers secondary to unusual organisms (77–81). As organisms such as *Comamonas acidovorans*, *Bacillus cereus*, and *Nocardia* species may demonstrate a clinical course and clinical appearance that is atypical for a bacterial keratitis, it is important to perform corneal scrapings for smears and cultures in any patient with an atypical contact lens–related infiltrate so that appropriate antimicrobial therapy may be instituted.

Protozoal Keratitis

Acanthamoeba

Acanthamoebae are free-living protozoa found in soil, water, and air. They exist in two forms, trophozoites and cysts,

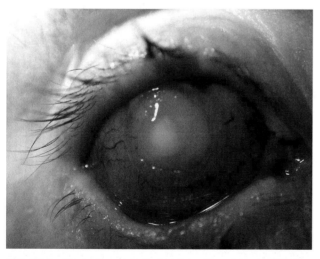

FIG. 39.2. Moraxella corneal ulcer in a corneal transplant. The transplant was performed for a corneal perforation, and the postoperative course was complicated by a persistent epithelial defect.

the latter of which is double-walled and, therefore, responsible for the organism's impressive resistance. *Acanthamoebae* have been found in air, soil, salt water, fresh water, chlorinated water, hot tubs, and in the water in frozen lakes. *Acanthamoebae* tolerate a pH range of 3.9 to 9.75 (82) and temperature ranges from –20°C (83) to 42°C (84,85). *A castellani*, *A polyphaga*, and *A culbertsoni* appear to be the most common pathogenic strains. Subclinical human infection appears to be more common than overt infection, and it has been suggested that exposure to nonpathogenic species stimulates both humoral and cell-mediated immunity against infection by pathogenic strains.

Acanthamoeba keratitis was first reported in 1973; (86) only a small number of cases were reported until 1981 (none in contact lens wearers). A dramatic increase in reported cases began in 1984; 62 cases were reported over the next 3 years, of which 82% occurred in contact lens wearers (29). The increased incidence appears partly as a result of better recognition of the disease, since a retrospective histopathologic study of eight penetrating keratoplasties performed for idiopathic corneal ulceration revealed two cases in which *Acanthamoeba* keratitis has been missed (87). Other retrospective studies of corneal buttons or whole eyes removed for keratitis or endophthalmitis before 1978, however, found no cases reporting *Acanthamoeba* (88,89).

Acanthamoeba is an infrequent cause of both nonocular (most notably granulomatous amoebic meningoencephalitis) and ocular disease, including a single case of uveitis in association with fatal meningitis (86). The emergence of *Acanthamoeba* keratitis has attracted popular and scientific attention and, according to Moore, "single-handedly changed our approach to contact lens–associated keratitis and our recommendations regarding contact lens disinfection" (90).

Most of the earliest cases that were reported were related to trauma, chronic herpetic keratitis (91), and exposure in contact lens wearers to contaminated water from hot tubs, swimming pools, or lakes (92). The association of *Acanthamoeba* keratitis in healthy wearers of soft contact lenses who use homemade saline for disinfection was first reported in 1985 (93). Infection was subsequently attributed to the use of a tap water rinse, intravenous saline, well water, and water from a home purification kit for lens care (90). Saliva also has been implicated (94). Daily-wear lenses, EWSCL, hard lenses, GP lenses, and combined hard-soft (e.g., SoftPerm) lenses all have been associated with the disease (95,96), although daily-wear use of soft lenses appears to be the principal predisposing factor (29).

The presumed etiology is through amoebic lens contamination during cleaning and storage, or contact with water. It is important to keep in mind that coinfection with bacterial pathogens such as *P aeruginosa* is possible, as many of the risk factors for infection with the two organisms, such as poor contact lens care habits, are the same (97). Additional evidence supports a possible synergistic effect between *Acan-*

thamoeba and bacterial species that are capable of supporting amoebic growth (98). Epithelial trauma may also be involved, but there are patients with superficial punctate keratopathy, corneal abrasions, and *Acanthamoeba* contamination of both contact lenses and cases who do not develop clinical infection (95). The development of infection may therefore depend on several factors, including the size and virulence of the inoculum, the frequency of contact with the cornea, and the host response (95). It is important to recognize that *Acanthamoeba* contamination of lens care systems occurs only when bacterial or, in many cases, fungal contamination also is present.

An epidemiologic review of *Acanthamoeba* keratitis in the United States confirmed many of the aforementioned risk factors for infection (99). Of nearly 200 cases of confirmed *Acanthamoeba* keratitis, 85% of affected patients had a history of contact lenses wear (all contact lens types were included, most commonly DWSCL and EWSCL). Sixty-four percent of the contact lens wearers gave a history of using saline prepared from distilled water and salt tablets. Patients age 50 years and older were more likely to have had a history of trauma than younger patients. Forty-nine percent of the cases occurred in males, although nationwide only 28% of soft contact lens wearers are male; the author suggested that this may be due to the higher incidence of trauma in males.

Microsporidiosis

While a rare cause of corneal infection, microsporidia may cause a stromal keratitis in immunocompetent patients and a chronic epithelial keratitis in immunocompromised patients (100). Microsporidial keratoconjunctivitis presenting as a multifocal diffuse epithelial keratitis and associated papillary conjunctivitis has been reported in an immunocompetent contact lens wearer (101).

Fungal Keratitis

Fungi are not part of the normal ocular flora, even in contact lens wearers. Fungi are, however, frequent contaminates of contact lens paraphernalia. Fungal growth has been found in up to 14% of soft contact lens cases belonging to asymptomatic patients (48), 3% of cases for rigid contact lenses (43), and in up to 50% of homemade saline solutions (43). Fungi also have been recovered from contact lenses themselves. One report noted 18 cases of fungal invasion in the contact lenses of asymptomatic patients (102). Eleven cases of fungal contamination were found in a group of approximately 450 extended-wear hydrogel soft contact lens users, which suggested an incidence of contamination between 2% and 5% (50). Geographic considerations may play a role in the extent of contamination, because there is clearly a higher incidence of fungal keratitis in non–contact lens

wearers in the southeastern United States compared more northern regions (103).

Laboratory studies show that fungi are able to adhere to and penetrate soft contact lens materials, especially those with a high water content (104,105). After adherence, fungal enzymes appear able to degrade hydrophilic lens polymers, permitting invasion and proliferation within the lens matrix (105). Deep fungal penetration of the contact lens may be present even in the absence of positive surface cultures (50).

Fungal keratitis has been associated with the use of frequent replacement (106), disposable (107), and daily disposable contact lenses (108). How fungal keratitis develops in patients whose contact lenses harbor fungi is not known. Grossly visible lens spots, resistant to cleaning and identified as fungi by slit-lamp examination, have been found in patients whose only clinical finding was blurred vision (50). Contact lenses of other patients who noted pain, blurred vision, conjunctival hyperemia, and corneal punctate staining, yielded fungi on culture. In each case, the keratoconjunctivitis disappeared within a few days without treatment after the patient stopped wearing the lenses. It was theorized that the findings were the result of fungal toxins (50).

The diseased epithelial surface may play a role in therapeutic contact lens wearers. Such patients often are being treated with topical corticosteroids, which contribute to additional risk factors for the development of fungal keratitis (109). As in non–contact lens wearers, patients with preexisting corneal disease have a higher incidence of yeast infections, such as *Candida,* than do other patients (109).

While fungal keratitis associated with contact lens wear may display characteristic features of corneal fungal infections such as pseudopod formation (108), infiltrate location in the deep stroma and the presence of feathery borders (106), features associated with other infecting organisms, such as a ring-shaped infiltrate (107), have been reported in cases of culture-proven fungal keratitis.

Viral Keratitis

There is no evidence to suggest that wearing contact lenses by healthy individuals increases the risk of viral infections, such as adenovirus or herpes simplex keratitis. Of greater concern is the fact that patients who wear therapeutic soft contact lenses for corneal surface disease secondary to viral disease may be at an increased risk for other types of microbial keratitis, particularly if topical steroids also are used in treatment.

A special note should be made about the human immunodeficiency virus (HIV). This virus has been isolated from human tears, conjunctiva, and cornea (110–112). Although there have been no cases reported in which the disease was spread through ocular contact, HIV-positive patients may be asymptomatic, or may deny or be unaware that they are infected. It is appropriate, therefore, to take reasonable precautions when fitting any patient for contact lenses. Fortunately, a number of different cleansing solutions for both soft and rigid contact lenses appear effective against the virus (113).

DIAGNOSIS

It is important to realize that not all epithelial loss is ulcerative, not all ulcerative keratitis is infectious, and not all infectious keratitis is bacterial. A systematic evaluation of keratitis, with appropriate laboratory workup, is essential for accurate diagnosis and appropriate management.

Regardless of keratitis type, common symptoms include pain, photophobia, tearing, blepharospasm, and decreased vision. Patients may complain of halos or floaters and morning lid crusting; a purulent discharge is highly suggestive of an infectious process. However, none of these symptoms are diagnostic, and, conversely, characteristic signs and symptoms may be mild or absent.

A proper history should record onset and duration of symptoms, prior treatment (if any), clinical response, and a careful review of the patient's contact lens wear and cleaning regimen, if appropriate.

Examination of the patient should begin with measurement of visual acuity. If a patient cannot wear contact lenses because of the keratitis, acuity should be measured while the patient is wearing glasses. If glasses are not available, a pinhole occluder is helpful, keeping in mind that patients with aphakia, high myopia, and those with high astigmatism require optical correction to within 5 D of the spherical equivalent for optimal accuracy. Some patients undergoing vision testing are unable to cooperate because of pain and tearing; topical anesthesia can be very helpful in these instances. Proparacaine 0.5% is the agent of choice because it has the least corneal toxicity and inhibition of subsequent cultures (114). (Corneal sensitivity should always be tested using a sterile cotton swab drawn to a fine point or dental floss before topical anesthesia is applied when evaluating suspected herpetic keratitis.)

Careful documentation of initial slit-lamp findings is important both medically and legally. A thorough evaluation includes: the lids for edema, vesicles, blepharitis, or discharge; the conjunctiva for hyperemia, chemosis, follicles, papillae, or foreign bodies; the cornea for infiltrates, ulceration, punctate keratopathy, thinning, vascularization, immune rings, endothelial plaques, or keratic precipitates; the anterior chamber for flare due to protein leak, cells, hypopyon, or peripheral anterior synechiae; the iris and the pupil for posterior synechiae, or pupillary reactivity; and the lens for cataract. In particular, the dimensions and depth of any stromal infiltrate and an overlying epithelial defect should be documented.

Contact lenses should be evaluated for fit on the eye(s) and any structural abnormalities. If an infection is suspected, the lens should be removed as aseptically as possible and appropriate cultures obtained. In a recently published series (115) an 84% concordance rate was found between cultures obtained from corneal scrapings and contact lenses. In the 16% of cases with discordant results, the contact lens culture was more likely to yield a microorganism, underscoring the importance of obtaining contact lens cultures in addition to corneal cultures. Patients should be advised to discontinue contact lens wear in the fellow eye if one eye is suspected of having an active infection.

A thorough discussion of culture techniques and antimicrobial therapy is beyond the scope of this chapter. The following is intended as an overview, and the reader is referred elsewhere for a more complete review (116).

Slit-lamp examination should be performed and all findings carefully noted prior to taking scrapings and cultures. If an exudate is present on the ulcer surface, it should be gently removed with a moistened sterile swab and cultured. This often can be done without the need for a topical anesthetic that may inhibit microbial growth. Cultures taken from the lid margins and inferior fornices are useful for comparative purposes. Moistened, rather than dry, swabs should be used, as the yield may be up to 50% higher (117). Calcium alginate swabs are preferable to cotton swabs, which contain fatty acids that may inhibit growth. Cultures plated directly on the various media have a higher yield than those in which a carrier medium is used initially.

Topical proparacaine 0.5% is then applied. A sterile platinum spatula is used to scrape material from the bed and leading edge of the ulcer. Successive scrapings should be taken to directly inoculate blood and chocolate agar, Sabouraud's agar and thioglycolate broth. These media will allow the growth of aerobic and anaerobic bacteria and fungi.

Other scrapings should be spread on a clean glass slide for bacterial and fungal stains, including Gram's and Giemsa or Gomori methenamine silver stain. These may provide the only clue to the cause of the ulcer in cases where a brief period of prior antibiotic treatment has rendered cultures negative. However, Gram's stain is reliable diagnostically in only 70% of untreated corneal ulcers (118).

Clinical suspicion may warrant additional cultures and scrapings to rule out *Mycobacterium* or *Acanthamoeba* infections under some circumstances. The former requires acid-fast stains and special media, such as Middlebrook or Lowenstein-Jensen.

Although endophthalmitis is a potential risk in infectious keratitis, it is rarely present at the time of diagnosis; any hypopyon that is present is typically inflammatory. For this reason, and to avoid unnecessarily seeding the inside of the eye, anterior chamber paracentesis for detection of possible organisms usually is not indicated.

There are no pathognomonic slit-lamp features of bacterial keratitis. In general, however, *Pseudomonas aeruginosa* tends to progress rapidly, with severe anterior chamber inflammation and hypopyon formation. Extension of the infiltrate is enhanced by the release of destructive enzymes by both bacteria and host polymorphonuclear leukocytes. Characteristically, diffuse epithelial edema, dramatic mucopurulent discharge, a soupy, or elevated, gelatinous ulcer appearance, and a ring infiltrate may be seen (Fig. 39.3). Untreated infections may develop corneal perforations within a few days. Other gram-negative organisms, such as *Serratia, Klebsiella,* and *Proteus,* usually cause more indolent ulcerations with fewer striking findings (114).

Gram-positive infections caused by *Staphylococcus* tend to remain localized with fairly distinct borders and relatively clear surrounding stroma. Satellite lesions (adjacent stromal infiltrates) are sometimes seen and may resemble those found in fungal infections (114). Ulcers caused by *S pneumococcus* may spread more rapidly, with corneal perforation much more likely than with *Staphylococcus.*

Because it often is difficult to determine whether corneal infiltrates are infectious or sterile, it is probably best to overtreat suspicious cases as infectious rather than risk delaying treatment or applying inappropriate treatment, such as corticosteroids. In one study, culture-positive corneal ulcers were correlated significantly with four variables: increased pain, discharge, epithelial staining, and anterior chamber reaction (119). Culture-negative infiltrates usually were less than 1 mm wide, multiple or arcuate, and without significant pain, epithelial staining, or anterior chamber reaction. The sterile infiltrates may be treated with lens removal, administration of regular-strength antibiotics for several days, and close follow-up. Patients' eyes should not be patched, because of the risk of infection that results from the creation of a warm, moist environment.

The diagnosis of *Acanthamoeba* keratitis often is difficult, and in many cases made only after a failure of treatment for suspected bacterial, fungal, or viral infection, especially herpes simplex. In one report, 90% of cases were presumed

at first to have been herpes simplex keratitis (94). However, failure to consider this diagnosis has important implications, because there is clearly a better prognosis when the disease is treated early in its course (91,93,120). The onset of the disease is variable, ranging from a few days to a few months, but typically involves a gradually worsening course over several months (121). Symptoms include foreign body sensation, epiphora, photophobia, and blepharospasm. Severe ocular pain out of proportion to the degree of inflammation is also characteristic.

Clinical findings include a relatively mild nongranulomatous anterior uveitis, severe chemosis, fluctuating epithelial defect, and decreased corneal sensation. Intraocular pressure may be elevated. An annular infiltrate together with radial keratoneuritis may be helpful features when distinguishing *Acanthamoeba* keratitis from herpes simplex and fungal keratitis (121). A wide variety of epithelial defects have been reported, including superficial punctate keratopathy, dendriform and pseudodendriform lesions, and scattered epithelial and subepithelial opacities. Elevated corneal epithelial lines found to contain *Acanthamoeba* have been noted (122). The epithelium may, however, be intact (95). Although scleritis has been reported in a relatively small number of cases, two cases were reported in which a severe nodular anterior scleritis was present adjacent to the area of inflamed cornea (posterior scleritis was present in one) (123). Both patients were infected with the same species, and both had used a hot tub at the same health club. It was suggested that scleritis might account for the severe pain in a greater number of patients. Koenig and colleagues (96) reported a patient with peripheral corneal hyperesthesia along with central hypoesthesia, and suggested that the former might serve as a helpful sign in differentiating *Acanthamoeba* keratitis from herpetic keratitis (96). Criteria that can be used to distinguish establish the diagnosis of *Acanthamoeba* keratitis are listed in Table 39.1.

In many cases, it remains difficult to diagnose *Acanthamoeba* on clinical examination alone. A high index of suspicion is essential, because there are several laboratory aids

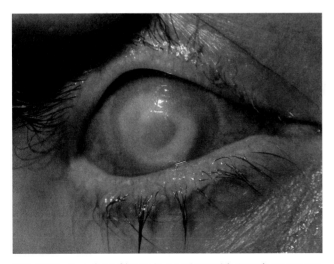

FIG. 39.3. Annular infiltrate in a patient with *Pseudomonas aeruginosa* corneal ulcer.

TABLE 39.1. CLINICAL FEATURES OF *ACANTHAMOEBA* KERATITIS (140)

Early findings
    Severe ocular pain, out of proportion to clinical findings
    Epitheliopathy (microerosions, scattered opacities, or dendriti-form keratitis)
    Subepithelial infiltrates (multiple, diffuse)
    Perineural infiltrates (radial keratoneuritis)
    Limbitis (limbal hyperemia and edema)
    Hypopyon in severe cases
    Slow progression of clinical findings
Late findings
    Limbitis
    Ring infiltrate
    Marked stromal opacification or thinning

that may identify the organism. These include impression cytology (122), indirect fluorescent antibody staining (124), and staining with calcofluor white (125). Gram and Giemsa stains have been reported to identify cysts or trophozoites, but may not distinguish them effectively from mononuclear cells or degenerated epithelium (125). The Gomori methenamine silver and Mallory trichrome stains also have been used (126). Air-drying of slides, however, might cause rupture of the trophozoites (127) or allow the cysts to become airborne and lost to examination (126). Instead, all specimens should be fixed immediately in 95% ethanol (126). Acid-fast stains may be necessary to undertake to rule out keratitis produced by mycobacteria, the most likely bacterial pathogen to be confused with *Acanthamoeba* infection (123). *Acanthamoeba* may be cultured using nonnutrient agar with *Escherichia coli* overlay (126).

Corneal biopsy may be required to obtain adequate tissue if scrapings do not yield a pathogen (127). Page's amoeba saline in a sterile glass vial, pretreated with a siliconizing agent, provides an excellent transport medium; the specimen should be kept at room temperature, and never frozen or refrigerated (126). Specular and confocal microscopy have been used to identify amoebic cysts *in vivo* in the stroma and may obviate the need for a biopsy (128–130).

Findings in patients with fungal keratitis may mimic those in other types of microbial keratitis. Certain features that have been attributed largely to fungal infection, such as satellite lesions, immune rings, and endothelial plaques, are not absolutely specific (103) (Fig. 39.4). As with *Acanthamoeba* keratitis, the most common condition simulating fungal keratitis is herpes simplex keratouveitis. However, there are several findings that are particularly suggestive of fungal keratitis, including a stromal infiltrate with feathery, hyphate edges, or an infiltrate that is elevated somewhat above the corneal surface and has a "gritty" appearance (Fig.

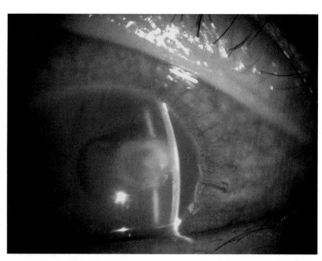

FIG. 39.5. Contact lens–related fungal ulcer in a patient secondary to *Aspergillus fumigatus.*

39.5). The course of fungal keratitis may be indolent in contrast to the rapid progression of a bacterial infection. Deterioration may be rapid if the patient is treated with topical steroids, which enhance fungal replication.

Laboratory diagnosis of fungal keratitis is made by positive cultures and scrapings. Sabouraud's agar's the culture medium of choice and should be inoculated with material taken from the ulcer base and leading edge with a sterile platinum spatula. Most fungi, however, also will grow well in blood agar. Ocular fungal isolates usually will grow out within 48 to 72 hours, but one should wait a week before declaring a culture negative (131). There are several stains that are helpful; the best are Gomori methenamine-silver and periodic acid-Schiff. Potassium hydroxide preparations, Giemsa stain, and Gram stain are less helpful. Because it is rare for fungal keratitis to progress to endophthalmitis, or for the hypopyon sometimes seen in fungal keratitis to be infectious, most authors do not recommend anterior chamber paracentesis as part of the initial workup.

TREATMENT

Appropriate management of contact lens–related corneal ulcers requires prompt attention on the part of both the patient and the eye care professional. Patients should know the warning signs of complications, such as discomfort, red eye, decreased vision, or even a visible white spot on the cornea, immediately remove both lenses, and contact the clinician. All contact lens wearers should have a backup pair of glasses so that discontinuation of contact lens wear is not functionally debilitating. The clinician, in turn, must treat potential corneal ulcers as ocular emergencies—the patient should be seen immediately.

Once the patient is seen and the tentative diagnosis made, the patient is best managed by a cornea specialist.

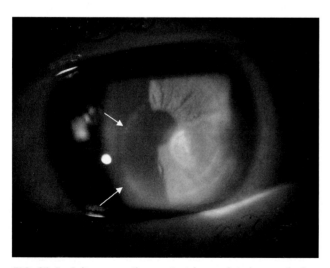

FIG. 39.4. Culture-negative contact lens–related corneal ulcer that resolved with topical antibiotic therapy. Arrows designate immune ring.

Bacterial Keratitis

Most contact lens–related corneal ulcers should be cultured prior to the institution of antibiotic therapy. If a practitioner does not have appropriate culture materials in his or her office, timely referral to a corneal specialist before institution of antibiotic therapy that may render subsequent cultures negative should be considered. While a positive scraping may allow identification of the causative organism, it does not allow *in vitro* confirmation of antibiotic efficacy.

Treatment of bacterial keratitis should involve broad-spectrum fortified antibiotics. One initial topical regimen is 50-mg/mL cefazolin and 15-mg/mL tobramycin, each applied every 30 minutes to 1 hour. High corneal antibiotic levels, above the minimal inhibitory concentration for bacteria producing keratitis, can be achieved by applying an initial series of five drops of each antibiotic over 5 minutes (132). With the advent of third- and fourth-generation fluoroquinolones with excellent gram-positive and gram-negative coverage (133), many practitioners are choosing monotherapy with these agents to treat contact lens–related ulcers. Others, such as the authors, are using these newer fluoroquinolones as monotherapy for non–sight-threatening corneal ulcers, but are still combining these agents with fortified cefazolin for sight-threatening ulcers. Vancomycin (25 to 50 mg/mL) should be substituted for cefazolin in patients with a penicillin allergy because of the risk of cross-reaction with cephalosporins. Vancomycin also is indicated in some cases of coagulase-negative staphylococcal keratitis in which a resistance to methicillin and cephalosporins is demonstrated. Cycloplegic agents may be used to relieve pain due to ciliary spasm and to prevent the formation of posterior synechiae.

The use of corticosteroids is controversial, but certainly never should be used initially, used without antibiotics, or used by anyone other than a corneal specialist. We have seen several cases in which topical corticosteroids, used to decrease stromal scarring, have caused recurrence of *Pseudomonas* infection in corneas that had appeared free of active disease.

Few patients require hospitalization, as the vast majority of patients are able to administer the antibiotic drops as requested by their practitioner. Patients who may benefit from hospital admission are those who have limited vision in the uninvolved eye, patients without a potential caregiver who require assistance with drop administration, and patients who are at high risk of noncompliance with the treatment regimen because of homelessness, poor understanding of the severity of the corneal infection, or social/geographic factors that would make it very difficult for them to return for frequent follow-up examinations.

The antibiotic drops are tapered according to clinical response. In some cases, this may take weeks. Clinical improvement is manifested by a decrease in pain and the size and density of the infiltrate, clearing of the anterior chamber inflammation, and healing of the epithelial defect. It must be remembered that many antibiotics are toxic to the epithelium so that epithelial defects, conjunctival injection, and superficial punctate keratopathy may persist until the drops are tapered.

Protozoal Keratitis

The treatment of *Acanthamoeba* keratitis may be medical or surgical. Increased awareness and understanding of the disease have led to slightly earlier diagnosis, more appropriate treatment, and improved outcomes (121). Early epithelial debridement may prove helpful in debulking the infectious load of *Acanthamoeba* (120,134).

Antiseptic Agents: Propamidine (Brolene) and Hexamidine

Medical treatment formerly was abysmal, because most commercially available antibiotics are ineffective in concentrations tolerated by the cornea. The first medical cure was reported in 1985, using propamidine isethionate (Brolene) (135), an over-the-counter drug in the United Kingdom, but typically available only through compounding pharmacies in the United States. Propamidine 0.1% appears to be both amoebicidal and cysticidal in *in vitro* studies (136). One side effect is epithelial toxicity that may result in recurrent epithelial defects, which may mimic a disease recurrence (91). Propamidine has been combined with a number of different agents with reported success, including either miconazole nitrate 1% (93,137) or clotrimazole 1% to 2% (138) with neomycin sulfate-polymyxin B sulfate-gramicidin. Hexamidine is another diamidine derivative that appears to have greater cysticidal activity than propamidine (139,140).

Polyhexamethylene Biguanide and Chlorhexidine

These cationic disinfectants have been demonstrated to be highly effective in killing both cysts and trophozoites (141, 142) although polyhexamethylene biguanide has a higher cysticidal activity against a number of strains when compared to other compounds, including chlorhexidine (143).

Antifungal Agents

Various topically and orally administered antifungal agents have been found to be effective against *Acanthamoeba,* including oral itraconazole and topical miconazole 0.1% (144) and oral and topical ketoconazole (145). Miconazole is amoebicidal and cysticidal as well at levels reached by topical application (146).

Clotrimazole 1% has been reported effective in several cases, two of which had developed recurrences while on propamidine, miconazole, and neomycin-polymyxin B gramicidin (Neosporin solution) (147). This medication generally is better tolerated than miconazole. It may be used either as a commercially available cream or as a 1% suspension formulated in artificial tears.

Antibacterial Agents

Although neomycin-polymyxin B gramicidin is commonly used in combination with the amoebicidal diamidines and cationic antiseptics, *in vitro* studies indicate the effect of antibacterials is only inhibitory (146).

Steroids

Topical steroids should be avoided because of the suppression of host response (90,95,138).

Penetrating Keratoplasty

In cases of medical failure, penetrating keratoplasty may be required. Although early corneal transplantation was at one time advocated to remove the bulk of the infected tissue (148), graft rejection or failure occurs 50% or more of the time when the transplant is done in the face of an active, progressive, and unresponsive infection (121,149,150). Recurrence in the graft is not uncommon and may be complicated by uncontrolled glaucoma, cataracts, wound leak, wound dehiscence, persistent epithelial defects, stromal melting, and phthisis (90).

The chance for a successful graft is increased if medical treatment can be maintained for 1 year prior to surgery (90). Medical management must be aggressive in order to saturate the cornea with propamidine and neomycin-polymyxin B gramicidin to kill the trophozoites, encourage encystment, and maintain drug levels high enough to kill any emerging trophozoites should the cysts survive (90). Some suggest that antiamoebic therapy be continued through the time of, and for months after, surgery to reduce recurrence (121).

Fungal Keratitis

A full description of the treatment of keratomycosis is beyond the scope of this chapter. The reader is referred to an excellent review for a more thorough discussion (151). It is rarely helpful to obtain fungal sensitivities. They may determine the most appropriate regimen, but they take much longer to obtain and are less reliable than antibiotic sensitivities. In general, treatment usually is started with topical pimaricin 5% (Natamycin) on an hourly basis. Other agents include the imidazoles (particularly miconazole, clotrimazole, and oral ketoconazole), which are most effective against filamentous fungi, and the polyene antibiotic amphotericin B, which is most effective against *Candida*

and other yeasts. The two groups of patients with fungal keratitis who respond least to medical therapy are those with deep corneal infection and those who had been treated with topical corticosteroids before the diagnosis was made. Steroids have no place in the management of fungal keratitis, even when combined with antifungal medications. If, however, steroids were used before the diagnosis was made, abrupt cessation may increase the inflammation and lead to rapid corneal thinning so that some authors suggest a tapered withdrawal (152).

Surgical management of fungal keratitis should be deferred as long as possible to allow the antifungal medication to render the organism nonviable; this seems to improve the general prognosis (103). Because viable fungi often remain deep in corneal tissue, lamellar keratoplasty or conjunctival flaps are generally not therapeutic options. Penetrating keratoplasty is indicated in the 10% to 20% of cases in which either medical management fails or the inflammatory response induces descemetocele formation or frank perforation (103). Topical corticosteroids should be withheld in the early postoperative period because of the risk of recurrence. Cyclosporin A has been shown to have antifungal activity, and is a better choice for prophylaxis against graft rejection (153,154).

PREVENTION OF INFECTION

While it is unrealistic to think that all contact lens–related corneal ulcers can be prevented, there is good reason to think that the incidence can be substantially reduced. Periodic professional examinations should be performed to ensure that damaged lenses are recognized and discarded, that early problems are detected and addressed prior to becoming symptomatic, and that compliance with good contact lens care is encouraged. The clinician must recognize early signs of corneal hypoxia, such as neovascularization, microcysts, or striate keratopathy, and address lens wear or type accordingly. Examination should be carried out every 6 to 9 months in the asymptomatic patient.

Because of its increased incidence and limited treatment efficacy, prevention of *Acanthamoeba* keratitis is critical. The single most important factor in this regard is proper contact lens care. By one estimate, over 90% of contact lens–related cases might be avoided by eliminating the use of homemade saline solutions and tap-water rinsing (95). Unfortunately, strict adherence to lens sterilization occasionally may be inadequate. One study found hydrogen peroxide ineffective against *A castellani* and *A polyphaga* (155), although another found hydrogen peroxide without a catalyst effective against *A castellani* (156). Other forms of cold disinfection appear variably effective. A conditioning solution preserved with polyaminopropyl biguanide for rigid gas permeable lenses is effective against both species (157).

Chlorhexidine-thimerosal and chlorhexidine-edetate have been shown effective against *A castellani* but not against *A polyphaga* (155,156), whereas alkyltriethanol ammonium chloride-thimerosal has been ineffective against both (155). Sorbic acid, potassium sorbate, and edetate disodium-thimerosal are ineffective against *A castellani* (156). Based on these findings, the following recommendations have been made: care must be taken not to expose contact lenses to contaminated solutions or tap water after sterilization. Storage of lenses may be in either preserved of nonpreserved saline, but if the latter is used, it should be dispensed from a single-dose unit container or an aerosol container. Tap water, intravenous saline, distilled water, or homemade saline solution should never be used for rinsing or storage of contact lenses.

A recent *in vitro* study demonstrated sodium salicylate inhibition of *Acanthamoeba* attachment to hydrogel contact lenses (158). The proposed mechanism is through alteration of *Acanthamoeba* attachment to biofilm-coated hydrogel lenses, indicating a possible benefit of adding salicylate to contact lens solutions (158). Contact lens cases may be effectively sterilized with exposure to microwave irradiation for only 3 minutes, providing an easy means for prevention of *Acanthamoeba* transmission through infected storage cases (159).

CONCLUSION

Infectious keratitis is a relatively rare but potentially devastating complication of contact lens wear. Bacterial corneal ulcers remain the most common type of infections, but *Acanthamoeba* keratitis has become a focus of attention. Fungal and viral keratitis are rare in contact lens wearers. Regardless of the cause of infection, prevention is easier and less costly than treatment. Strict attention to proper lens care hygiene should reduce, but probably not eliminate, infection, particularly in users of extended-wear contact lenses. It is, therefore, essential that patients recognize the early manifestations of corneal infections, discontinue lens wear, and seek immediate treatment. At the same time, eyecare professionals must manage such patients aggressively to reduce morbidity.

REFERENCES

1. Schwartz CA. Contact lens update. *Contact Lens Forum* 1986; 11:31–36.
2. Dixon JM, Young CA Jr, Baldone JA, Halberg GP, Sampson W, Stone W Jr. Complications associated with the wearing of contact lenses. *JAMA* 1966;195:901–903.
3. Freedman J. *Pseudomonas* keratitis following cosmetic soft contact lens wear. *Contact Lens J* 1976;10:21–25.
4. Krachmer JH, Purcell JJ Jr. Bacterial corneal ulcers in cosmetic soft contact lens wearers. *Arch Ophthalmol* 1978;96:57–61.
5. Weissman BA, Mondino BJ, Pettit TH, Hofbauer JD. Corneal ulcers associated with extended-wear soft contact lenses. *Am J Ophthalmol* 1984;97:476–481.
6. Wilson LA, Schlitzer RL, Ahearn DG. *Pseudomonas* corneal ulcers associated with soft contact-lens wear. *Am J Ophthalmol* 1981;92:546–554.
7. Alfonso E, Mandelbaum S, Fox MJ, Forster RK. Ulcerative keratitis associated with contact lens wear. *Am J Ophthalmol* 1986;101:429–433.
8. Dart JK. Predisposing factors in microbial keratitis: the significance of contact lens wear. *Br J Ophthalmol* 1988;72:926–930.
9. Gudmundsson OG, Ormerod LD, Kenyon KR, et al. Factors influencing predilection and outcome in bacterial keratitis. *Cornea* 1989;8:115–121.
10. Rattanatam T, Heng WJ, Rapuano CJ, Laibson PR, Cohen EJ. Trends in contact lens-related corneal ulcers. *Cornea* 2001;20:290–294.
11. Adams CP Jr, Cohen EJ, Laibson PR, Galentine P, Arentsen JJ. Corneal ulcers in patients with cosmetic extended-wear contact lenses. *Am J Ophthalmol* 1983;96:705–709.
12. Chalupa E, Swarbrick HA, Holden BA, Sjostrand J. Severe corneal infections associated with contact lens wear. *Ophthalmology* 1987;94:17–22.
13. Cohen EJ, Laibson PR, Arentsen JJ, Clemons CS. Corneal ulcers associated with cosmetic extended wear soft contact lenses. *Ophthalmology* 1987;94:109–114.
14. Mondino BJ, Weissman BA, Farb MD, Pettit TH. Corneal ulcers associated with daily-wear and extended-wear contact lenses. *Am J Ophthalmol* 1986;102:58–65.
15. Weissman BA, Remba MJ, Fugedy E. Results of the extended wear contact lens survey of the Contact Lens Section of the American Optometric Association. *J Am Optom Assoc* 1987;58:166–171.
16. Schein OD, Glynn RJ, Poggio EC, Seddon JM, Kenyon KR. The relative risk of ulcerative keratitis among users of daily-wear and extended-wear soft contact lenses. A case-control study. Microbial Keratitis Study Group. *N Engl J Med* 1989;321:773–778.
17. Poggio EC, Glynn RJ, Schein OD, et al. The incidence of ulcerative keratitis among users of daily-wear and extended-wear soft contact lenses. *N Engl J Med* 1989;321:779–783.
18. Cheng KH, Leung SL, Hoekman HW, et al. Incidence of contact-lens-associated microbial keratitis and its related morbidity. *Lancet* 1999;354:181–185.
19. Lam DSC, Houang E, Fan DSP, Lyon D, Seal D, Wong E. Incidence and risk factors for microbial keratitis in Hong Kong: comparison with Europe and North America. *Eye* 2002;16:608–618.
20. Holden BA, Kotow M, Grant T, et al. The CCLRU position on hydrogel extended wear, Unpublished data, CCLRV, New South Wales, Australia 1986.
21. Eichenbaum JW, Feldstein M, Podos SM. Extended-wear aphakic soft contact lenses and corneal ulcers. *Br J Ophthalmol* 1982; 66:663–666.
22. Spoor TC, Hartel WC, Wynn P, Spoor DK. Complications of continuous-wear soft contact lenses in a nonreferral population. *Arch Ophthalmol* 1984;102:1312–1313.
23. Salz JJ, Schlanger JL. Complications of aphakic extended wear lenses encountered during a seven-year period in 100 eyes. *CLAO J* 1983;9:241–244.
24. Weissman BA, Donzis PB, Hoft RH. Keratitis and contact lens wear: a review. *J Am Optom Assoc* 1987;58:799–803.
25. MacRae S, Herman C, Stulting RD, et al. Corneal ulcer and adverse reaction rates in premarket contact lens studies. *Am J Ophthalmol* 1991;111:457–465.
26. Lim L, Loughnan MS, Sullivan LJ. Microbial keratitis associated

with extended wear of silicone hydrogel contact lenses. *Br J Ophthalmol* 2002;86:355–357.

27. Matthews TD, Frazer DG, Minassian DC, Radford CF, Dart JK. Risks of keratitis and patterns of use with disposable contact lenses. *Arch Ophthalmol* 1992;110:1559–1562.

28. Schein OD, Buehler PO, Stamler JF, Verdier DD, Katz J. The impact of overnight wear on the risk of contact lens-associated ulcerative keratitis. *Arch Ophthalmol* 1994;112:186–190.

29. Wilhelmus KR. Review of clinical experience with microbial keratitis associated with contact lenses. *CLAO J* 1987;13:211–214.

30. Clemons CS, Cohen EJ, Arentsen JJ, Donnenfeld ED, Laibson PR. Pseudomonas ulcers following patching of corneal abrasions associated with contact lens wear. *CLAO J* 1987;13:161–164.

31. Snyder DA, Litinsky SM, Gelender H. Hypopyon iridocyclitis associated with extended-wear soft contact lenses. *Am J Ophthalmol* 1982;93:519–520.

32. McNatt J, Allen SD, Wilson LA, Dowell VR Jr. Anaerobic flora of the normal human conjunctival sac. *Arch Ophthalmol* 1978;96:1448–1450.

33. Ando N, Takatori K. Fungal flora of the conjunctival sac. *Am J Ophthalmol* 1982;94:67–74.

34. Smolin G, Okumoto M, Nozik RA. The microbial flora in extended-wear soft contact-lens wearers. *Am J Ophthalmol* 1979;88:543–547.

35. Tragakis MP, Brown SI, Pearce DB. Bacteriologic studies of contamination associated with soft contact lenses. *Am J Ophthalmol* 1973;75:496–499.

36. Locatcher-Khorazo D, Gutierrez EH. The bacterial flora of the healthy eye. In: Locatcher-Khorazo D, Seegal BC, eds. *Microbiology of the eye.* St. Louis: CV Mosby, 1972:13–23.

37. Singer TR, Isenberg SJ, Apt L. Conjunctival anaerobic and aerobic bacterial flora in pediatric versus adult subjects. *Br J Ophthalmol* 1988;72:448–451.

38. Miller B, Ellis PP. Conjunctival flora in patients receiving immunosuppressive drugs. *Arch Ophthalmol* 1977;95:2012–2014.

39. Nema HV, Ahuja OP, Bal A, Mohapatra LN. Effects of topical corticosteroids and antibiotics on mycotic flora of conjunctiva. *Am J Ophthalmol* 1968;65:747–750.

40. Binder PS, Worthen DM. A continuous-wear hydrophilic lens. Prophylactic topical antibiotics. *Arch Ophthalmol* 1976;94:2109–2111.

41. Chun MW, Weissman BA. Compliance in contact lens care. *Am J Optom Physiol Opt* 1987;64:274–276.

42. Roth HW. The etiology of ocular irritation in soft lens wearers. Distribution in a large clinical sample. *CLAO J* 1978;4:38–43.

43. Donzis PB, Mondino BJ, Weissman BA, Bruckner DA. Microbial contamination of contact lens care systems. *Am J Ophthalmol* 1987;104:325–333.

44. Prince HN, Nonemaker WS, Norgard RC, Prince DL. Drug resistance studies with topical antiseptics. *J Pharm Sci* 1978;67:1629–1631.

45. Ormerod LD, Smith RE. Contact lens-associated microbial keratitis. *Arch Ophthalmol* 1986;104:79–83.

46. Joslyn L. Sterilization by heat. In: Block SS, editor. *Disinfection, preservation, and sterilization.* Philadelphia: Lea & Febiger, 1983:3–46.

47. Donzis PB, Mondino BJ, Weissman BA. *Bacillus* keratitis associated with contaminated contact lens care systems. *Am J Ophthalmol* 1988;105:195–197.

48. Pitts RE, Krachmer JH. Evaluation of soft contact lens disinfection in the home environment. *Arch Ophthalmol* 1979;97:470–472.

49. Fowler SA, Greiner JV, Allansmith MR. Attachment of bacteria to soft contact lenses. *Arch Ophthalmol* 1979;97:659–660.

50. Wilson LA, Ahearn DG. Association of fungi with extended-wear soft contact lenses. *Am J Ophthalmol* 1986;101:434–436.

51. Stern GA, Zam ZS. The effect of enzymatic contact lens cleaning on adherence of *Pseudomonas aeruginosa* to soft contact lenses. *Ophthalmology* 1987;94:115–119.

52. Fowler SA, Allansmith MR. The effect of cleaning soft contact lenses. A scanning electron microscopic study. *Arch Ophthalmol* 1981;99:1382–1386.

53. Beattie TK, Tomlinson A, McFadyen AK, Seal DV, Grimason AM. Enhanced attachment of acanthamoeba to extended-wear silicone hydrogel contact lenses: a new risk factor for infection? *Ophthalmology* 2003;110:765–771.

54. Jones DB. Pathogenesis of bacterial and fungal keratitis. *Trans Ophthalmol Soc U K* 1978;98:367–371.

55. Stern GA, Weitzenkorn D, Valenti J. Adherence of *Pseudomonas aeruginosa* to the mouse cornea. Epithelial v stromal adherence. *Arch Ophthalmol* 1982;100:1956–1958.

56. Ramphal R, McNiece MT, Polack FM. Adherence of *Pseudomonas aeruginosa* to the injured cornea: a step in the pathogenesis of corneal infections. *Ann Ophthalmol* 1981;13:421–425.

57. Hyndiuk RA. Experimental *Pseudomonas* keratitis. *Trans Am Ophthalmol Soc* 1981;79:540–624.

58. Stern GA, Lubniewski A, Allen C. The interaction between *Pseudomonas aeruginosa* and the corneal epithelium. An electron microscopic study. *Arch Ophthalmol* 1985;103:1221–1225.

59. Imayasu M, Petroll WM, Jester JV, Patel SK, Ohashi J, Cavanagh HD. The relation between contact lens oxygen transmissibility and binding of *Pseudomonas aeruginosa* to the cornea after overnight wear. *Ophthalmology* 1994;101:371–388.

60. Kent HD, Cohen EJ, Laibson PR, Arentsen JJ. Microbial keratitis and corneal ulceration associated with therapeutic soft contact lenses. *CLAO J* 1990;16:49–52.

61. Dohlman CH, Boruchoff A, Mobilia EF. Complications in use of soft contact lenses in corneal disease. *Arch Ophthalmol* 1973;90:367–371.

62. Brown SI, Bloomfield S, Pearce DB, Tragakis M. Infections with the therapeutic soft lens. *Arch Ophthalmol* 1974;91:275–277.

63. Fong LP, Ormerod LD, Kenyon KR, Foster CS. Microbial keratitis complicating penetrating keratoplasty. *Ophthalmology* 1988;95:1269–1275.

64. Ormerod LD, Fong LP, Foster CS. Corneal infection in mucosal scarring disorders and Sjögren's syndrome. *Am J Ophthalmol* 1988;105:512–518.

65. Polse KA, Brand RJ, Vastine DW, Schwalbe JS. Corneal change accompanying orthokeratology. Plastic or elastic? Results of a randomized controlled clinical trial. *Arch Ophthalmol* 1983;101:1873–1878.

66. Hutchinson K, Apel A. Infectious keratitis in orthokeratology. *Clin Exp Ophthalmol* 2002;30:49–51.

67. Chen KH, Kuang TM, Hsu WM. *Serratia marcescens* corneal ulcer as a complication of orthokeratology. *Am J Ophthalmol* 2001;132:257–258.

68. Lau LI, Wu CC, Lee SM, Hsu WM. *Pseudomonas* corneal ulcer related to overnight orthokeratology. *Cornea* 2003;22:262–264.

69. Young AL, Leung AT, Cheung EY, Cheng LL, Wong AK, Lam DS. Orthokeratology lens-related *Pseudomonas aeruginosa* infectious keratitis. *Cornea* 2003;22:265–266.

70. Lin MC, Graham AD, Fusaro RE, Polse KA. Impact of rigid gas-permeable contact lens extended wear on corneal epithelial barrier function. *Invest Ophthalmol Vis Sci* 2002;43:1019–1024.

71. Sharma S, Gopalakrishnan S, Aasuri MK, Garg P, Rao GN. Trends in contact lens-associated microbial keratitis in Southern India. *Ophthalmology* 2003;110:138–143.

72. Meisler DM, Langston RH, Naab TJ, Aaby AA, McMahon JT,

Tubbs RR. Infectious crystalline keratopathy. *Am J Ophthalmol* 1984;97:337–343.

73. Reiss GR, Campbell RJ, Bourne WM. Infectious crystalline keratopathy. *Surv Ophthalmol* 1986;31:69–72.

74. Klotz SA, Butrus SI, Misra RP, Osato MS. The contribution of bacterial surface hydrophobicity to the process of adherence of *Pseudomonas aeruginosa* to hydrophilic contact lenses. *Curr Eye Res* 1989;8:195–202.

75. Klotz SA, Au YK, Misra RP. A partial-thickness epithelial defect increases the adherence of *Pseudomonas aeruginosa* to the cornea. *Invest Ophthalmol Vis Sci* 1989;30:1069–1074.

76. Belmont JB, Ostler HB, Dawson CR, Schwab I, Dulay D. Noninfectious ring-shaped keratitis associated with *Pseudomonas aeruginosa*. *Am J Ophthalmol* 1982;93:338–341.

77. Lema I, Gomez-Torreiro M, Rodriguez-Ares MT. Comamonas acidovorans keratitis in a hydrogel contact lens wearer. *CLAO J* 2001;27:55–56.

78. Sridhar MS, Cohen EJ, Rapuano CJ, Lister MA, Laibson PR. *Nocardia asteroides* sclerokeratitis in a contact lens wearer. *CLAO J* 2002;28:66–68.

79. Corrigan KM, Harmis NY, Willcox MD. Association of acinetobacter species with contact lens-induced adverse responses. *Cornea* 2001;20:463–466.

80. Keay L, Harmis N, Corrigan K, Sweeney D, Willcox M. Infiltrative keratitis associated with extended wear of hydrogel lenses and *Abiotrophia defectiva*. *Cornea* 2000;19:864–869.

81. Pinna A, Sechi LA, Zanetti S, Usai D, Delogu G. *Bacillus cereus* keratitis associated with contact lens wear. *Ophthalmology* 2001; 108:1830–1834.

82. Singh BN. *Pathogenic and non-pathogenic amoebae*. New York: Halsted Press, 1975.

83. Culbertson CG. The pathogenicity of soil amebas. *Annu Rev Microbiol* 1971;25:231–254.

84. Griffin JL. Temperature tolerance of pathogenic and nonpathogenic free-living amoebae. *Science* 1972;178:869–870.

85. Visvesvara GS. Free-living pathogenic amoeba. In: Lennette EH, Balows A, Hausler WJ, Truant JP, eds. *Manual of clinical microbiology*, 3rd ed. Washington, DC: American Society for Microbiology, 1980:704–708.

86. Jones DB, Visvesvara GS, Robinson NM. *Acanthamoeba polyphaga* keratitis and *Acanthamoeba uveitis* associated with fatal meningoencephalitis. *Trans Ophthalmol Soc U K* 1975;95: 221–232.

87. Cohen EJ, Buchanan HW, Laughrea PA, et al. Diagnosis and management of *Acanthamoeba keratitis*. *Am J Ophthalmol* 1985; 100:389–395.

88. Ashton N, Stamm W. Amoebic infection of the eye. A pathological report. *Trans Ophthalmol Soc U K* 1975;95:214–220.

89. Lund OE, Stefani FH, Dechant W. Amoebic keratitis: a clinicopathological case report. *Br J Ophthalmol* 1978;62:373–375.

90. Moore MB. *Acanthamoeba* keratitis. *Arch Ophthalmol* 1988; 106:1181–1183.

91. Yeoh R, Warhurst DC, Falcon MG. *Acanthamoeba* keratitis. *Br J Ophthalmol* 1987;71:500–503.

92. Samples JR, Binder PS, Luibel FJ, Font RL, Visvesvara GS, Peter CR. *Acanthamoeba* keratitis possibly acquired from a hot tub. *Arch Ophthalmol* 1984;102:707–710.

93. Moore MB, McCulley JP, Luckenbach M, et al. *Acanthamoeba* keratitis associated with soft contact lenses. *Am J Ophthalmol* 1985;100:396–403.

94. *Acanthamoeba* keratitis associated with contact lenses—United States. *MMWR Morb Mortal Wkly Rep* 1986;35:405–408.

95. Moore MB, McCulley JP, Newton C, et al. *Acanthamoeba* keratitis. A growing problem in soft and hard contact lens wearers. *Ophthalmology* 1987;94:1654–1661.

96. Koenig SB, Solomon JM, Hyndiuk RA, Sucher RA, Gradus

MS. *Acanthamoeba* keratitis associated with gas-permeable contact lens wear. *Am J Ophthalmol* 1987;103:832.

97. Dini LA, Cockinos C, Frean JA, Niszl IA, Markus MB. Unusual case of *Acanthamoeba polyphaga* and *Pseudomonas aeruginosa* keratitis in a contact lens wearer from Gauteng, South Africa. *J Clin Microbiol* 2000;38:826–829.

98. Bottone EJ, Madayag RM, Qureshi MN. *Acanthamoeba* keratitis: synergy between amebic and bacterial cocontaminants in contact lens care systems as a prelude to infection. *J Clin Microbiol* 1992;30:2447–2450.

99. Stehr-Green JK, Bailey TM, Visvesvara GS. The epidemiology of *Acanthamoeba keratitis* in the United States. *Am J Ophthalmol* 1989;107:331–336.

100. Weber R, Bryan RT, Schwartz DA, Owen RL. Human microsporidial infections. *Clin Microbiol Rev* 1994;7:426–461.

101. Theng J, Chan C, Ling ML, Tan D. Microsporidial keratoconjunctivitis in a healthy contact lens wearer without human immunodeficiency virus infection. *Ophthalmology* 2001;108: 976–978.

102. Berger RO, Streeten BW. Fungal growth in aphakic soft contact lenses. *Am J Ophthalmol* 1981;91:630–633.

103. Forster RK. Fungal diseases, 2nd ed. In: Smolin G, Thoft RA, eds. *The cornea*. Boston: Little, Brown and Company, 1987: 228–240.

104. Yamaguchi T, Hubbard A, Fukushima A, Kimura T, Kaufman HE. Fungus growth on soft contact lenses with different water contents. *CLAO J* 1984;10:166–171.

105. Simmons RB, Buffington JR, Ward M, Wilson LA, Ahearn DG. Morphology and ultrastructure of fungi in extended-wear soft contact lenses. *J Clin Microbiol* 1986;24:21–25.

106. Foroozan R, Eagle RC Jr, Cohen EJ. Fungal keratitis in a soft contact lens wearer. *CLAO J* 2000;26:166–168.

107. Salierno AL, Goldstein MH, Driebe WT. Fungal ring infiltrates in disposable contact lens wearers. *CLAO J* 2001;27:166–168.

108. Choi DM, Goldstein MH, Salierno A, Driebe WT. Fungal keratitis in a daily disposable soft contact lens wearer. *CLAO J* 2001;27:111–112.

109. Wilhelmus KR, Robinson NM, Font RA, Hamill MB, Jones DB. Fungal keratitis in contact lens wearers. *Am J Ophthalmol* 1988;106:708–714.

110. Fujikawa LS, Salahuddin SZ, Ablashi D, et al. HTLV-III in the tears of AIDS patients. *Ophthalmology* 1986;93:1479–1481.

111. Fujikawa LS, Salahuddin SZ, Ablashi D, et al. Human T-cell leukemia/lymphotropic virus type III in the conjunctival epithelium of a patient with AIDS. *Am J Ophthalmol* 1985;100: 507–509.

112. Salahuddin SZ, Palestine AG, Heck E, et al. Isolation of the human T-cell leukemia/lymphotropic virus type III from the cornea. *Am J Ophthalmol* 1986;101:149–152.

113. Vogt MW, Ho DD, Bakar SR, Gilbard JP, Schooley RT, Hirsch MS. Safe disinfection of contact lenses after contamination with HTLV-III. *Ophthalmology* 1986;93:771–774.

114. Hyndiuk RA, Synder RW. Infectious diseases. In: Smolin G, Thoft RA, eds. *The cornea*. Boston: Little, Brown and Company, 1987:147–229.

115. Martins EN, Farah ME, Alvarenga LS, Yu MCZ, Hofling-Lima AL. Infectious keratitis: correlation between corneal and contact lens cultures. *CLAO J* 2002;28:146–148.

116. Rao NA. A laboratory approach to rapid diagnosis of ocular infections and prospects for the future. *Am J Ophthalmol* 1989; 107:283–291.

117. Ostler HB, Dawson CR, Okumoto M. *Color atlas of infectious and inflammatory diseases of the external eye*. Baltimore: Urban & Schwarzenberg, 1987:2.

118. Jones DB. A plan for antimicrobial therapy in bacterial keratitis. *Trans Am Acad Ophthalmol Otolaryngol* 1975;79:95.

119. Stein RM, Clinch TE, Cohen EJ, Genvert GI, Arentsen JJ, Laibson PR. Infected vs sterile corneal infiltrates in contact lens wearers. *Am J Ophthalmol* 1988;105:632–636.

120. Holland GN, Donzis PB. Rapid resolution of early *Acanthamoeba* keratitis after epithelial debridement. *Am J Ophthalmol* 1987;104:87–89.

121. Auran JD, Starr MB, Jakobiec FA. *Acanthamoeba* keratitis: a review of the literature. *Cornea* 1987;6:2–26.

122. Florakis GJ, Folberg R, Krachmer JH, Tse DT, Roussel TJ, Vrabec MP. Elevated corneal epithelial lines in *Acanthamoeba* keratitis. *Arch Ophthalmol* 1988;106:1202–1206.

123. Mannis MJ, Tamaru R, Roth AM, Burns M, Thirkill C. *Acanthamoeba* sclerokeratitis. Determining diagnostic criteria. *Arch Ophthalmol* 1986;104:1313–1317.

124. Epstein RJ, Wilson LA, Visvesvara GS, Plourde EG Jr. Rapid diagnosis of *Acanthamoeba* keratitis from corneal scrapings using indirect fluorescent antibody staining. *Arch Ophthalmol* 1986;104:1318–1321.

125. Wilhelmus KR, Osato MS, Font RL, Robinson NM, Jones DB. Rapid diagnosis of *Acanthamoeba* keratitis using calcofluor white. *Arch Ophthalmol* 1986;104:1309–1312.

126. Johns KJ, Head WS, Elliot JH, O'Day DM. Isolation and identification of *Acanthamoeba* in corneal tissue. *CLAO J* 1987;13:272–276.

127. Newton C, Moore MB, Kaufman HE. Corneal biopsy in chronic keratitis. *Arch Ophthalmol* 1987;105:577–578.

128. Pfister DR, Cameron JD, Krachmer JH, Holland EJ. Confocal microscopy findings of *Acanthamoeba* keratitis. *Am J Ophthalmol* 1996;121:119–128.

129. Cavanagh HD, McCulley JP. In vivo confocal microscopy and *Acanthamoeba* keratitis. *Am J Ophthalmol* 1996;121:207–208.

130. Petroll WM, Cavanagh HD, Jester JV. Clinical confocal microscopy. *Curr Opin Ophthalmol* 1998;9:59–65.

131. Forster RK, Rebell G. The diagnosis and management of keratomycoses. I. Cause and diagnosis. *Arch Ophthalmol* 1975;93:975–978.

132. Glasser DB, Gardner S, Ellis JG, Pettit TH. Loading doses and extended dosing intervals in topical gentamicin therapy. *Am J Ophthalmol* 1985;99:329–332.

133. Mather R, Karenchak LM, Romanowski EG, Kowalski RP. Fourth generation fluoroquinolones: new weapons in the arsenal of ophthalmic antibiotics. *Am J Ophthalmol* 2002;133:463–466.

134. Brooks JG Jr, Coster DJ, Badenoch PR. *Acanthamoeba* keratitis. Resolution after epithelial debridement. *Cornea* 1994;13:186–189.

135. Wright P, Warhurst D, Jones BR. *Acanthamoeba* keratitis successfully treated medically. *Br J Ophthalmol* 1985;69:778–782.

136. Ferrante A, Rowan-Kelly B, Thong YH. In vitro sensitivity of virulent *Acanthamoeba culbertsoni* to a variety of drugs and antibiotics. *Int J Parasitol* 1984;14:53–56.

137. Berger ST, Mondino BJ, Hoft RH, et al. Successful medical management of *Acanthamoeba* keratitis. *Am J Ophthalmol* 1990;110:395–403.

138. D'Aversa G, Stern GA, Driebe WT Jr. Diagnosis and successful medical treatment of *Acanthamoeba* keratitis. *Arch Ophthalmol* 1995;113:1120–1123.

139. Brasseur G, Favennec L, Perrine D, Chenu JP, Brasseur P. Successful treatment of *Acanthamoeba* keratitis by hexamidine. *Cornea* 1994;13:459–462.

140. Illingworth CD, Cook SD. *Acanthamoeba* keratitis. *Surv Ophthalmol* 1998;42:493–508.

141. Larkin DF, Kilvington S, Dart JK. Treatment of *Acanthamoeba* keratitis with polyhexamethylene biguanide. *Ophthalmology* 1992;99:185–191.

142. Illingworth CD, Cook SD, Karabatsas CH, Easty DL. *Acanthamoeba* keratitis: risk factors and outcome. *Br J Ophthalmol* 1995;79:1078–1082.

143. Elder MJ, Kilvington S, Dart JK. A clinicopathologic study of in vitro sensitivity testing and *Acanthamoeba* keratitis. *Invest Ophthalmol Vis Sci* 1994;35:1059–1064.

144. Ishibashi Y, Matsumoto Y, Kabata T, et al. Oral itraconazole and topical miconazole with debridement for *Acanthamoeba* keratitis. *Am J Ophthalmol* 1990;109:121–126.

145. Kita Y, Nishizawa H, Takenobu J. A case of *Acanthamoeba* keratitis. *Jpn J Clin Ophthalmol* 1996;50:1513–156.

146. Nagington J, Richards JE. Chemotherapeutic compounds and *Acanthamoebae* from eye infections. *J Clin Pathol* 1976;29:648–651.

147. Driebe WT Jr, Stern GA, Epstein RJ, Visvesvara GS, Adi M, Komadina T. *Acanthamoeba* keratitis. Potential role for topical clotrimazole in combination chemotherapy. *Arch Ophthalmol* 1988;106:1196–1201.

148. Hirst LW, Green WR, Merz W, et al. Management of *Acanthamoeba* keratitis. A case report and review of the literature. *Ophthalmology* 1984;91:1105–1111.

149. Cohen EJ, Parlato CJ, Arentsen JJ, et al. Medical and surgical treatment of *Acanthamoeba* keratitis. *Am J Ophthalmol* 1987;103:615–625.

150. Ficker LA, Kirkness C, Wright P. Prognosis for keratoplasty in *Acanthamoeba* keratitis. *Ophthalmology* 1993;100:105–110.

151. Johns KJ, O'Day DM. Pharmacologic management of keratomycoses. *Surv Ophthalmol* 1988;33:178–188.

152. Wood TO. Fungal keratitis. *Clin Decisions Ophthalmol* 1983;7:3.

153. Bell NP, Karp CL, Alfonso EC, Schiffman J, Miller D. Effects of methylprednisolone and cyclosporine A on fungal growth in vitro. *Cornea* 1999;18:306–313.

154. Perry HD, Doshi SJ, Donnenfeld ED, Bai GS. Topical cyclosporin A in the management of therapeutic keratoplasty for mycotic keratitis. *Cornea* 2002;21:161–163.

155. Ludwig IH, Meisler DM, Rutherford I, Bican FE, Langston RH, Visvesvara GS. Susceptibility of *Acanthamoeba* to soft contact lens disinfection systems. *Invest Ophthalmol Vis Sci* 1986;27:626–628.

156. Silvany RE, Wood TS, Bowman RW, McCulley JP. The effect of preservatives in contact lens solutions on two species of *Acanthamoeba*. *Invest Ophthalmol Vis Sci* 1987;28:371.

157. Sly KS, Chou MH, Herskowitz R et al. The effect of polyaminopropyl biguanide in the Boston conditioning solution on two species of *Acanthamoeba*. Paper presented at: Contact Lens Association of *Ophthalmology* Annual Meeting, New Orleans, LA, January 1989.

158. Tomlinson A, Simmons PA, Seal DV, McFadyen AK. Salicylate inhibition of *Acanthamoeba* attachment to contact lenses: a model to reduce risk of infection. *Ophthalmology* 2000;107:112–117.

159. Hiti K, Walochnik J, Faschinger C, Haller-Schober EM, Aspock H. Microwave treatment of contact lens cases contaminated with *Acanthamoeba*. *Cornea* 2001;20:467–470.

4 0

MECHANICAL COMPLICATIONS OF CONTACT LENS WEAR

URS BUSINGER

INTRODUCTION

Mechanical complications include all problems caused physically by the presence of a contact lens, its surfaces, and its edges (and perhaps attached debris) that occur during contact lens use. An *in vivo* contact lens is an optical device embedded in a tear layer. It is unusual for the lens to physically touch the anterior surface of the eye. Due to its proximity to the tissues, however, interactions take place between the eye and the lens. No matter how oxygen permeable or biocompatible the lens may be, it undoubtedly creates microtrauma to the tissue from time to time. Severity of mechanically induced trauma can vary from almost invisible to severe scarring of the corneal tissue if the trauma is not interrupted and/or treated. The contact lens not only acts as any foreign object to damage the surface, but it also triggers both appropriate and inappropriate reactions of the host body.

Practitioners as well as patients naively believe that they quickly and easily, subjectively and objectively, recognize the signs and symptoms of mechanically driven contact lens problems. Unfortunately, not all mechanical problems due to contact lens wear will result in early subjective patient complaints. Many problems will, sooner or later, lead to some form of complaint, but it is the job of a good clinician to diagnose problems and prescribe solutions even before the patient achieves subjective awareness. Contact lens-induced trauma can vary in location and severity. Subjective awareness also can vary from unnoticeable to extreme discomfort. Subjective perception does not, therefore, always correspond with objective signs. Another misconception is that only gas permeable (GP) lenses induce mechanical complications. Daily contact lens practice indicates that hydrogel lenses are quite capable of causing such complications as well (1).

With refractive surgery gaining in popularity, we should also note that even minor and asymptomatic mechanically induced corneal shape changes may have adverse effects on surgical outcomes. If for no reason than because contact lens wearers often become refractive surgery candidates, cli-

nicians should take appropriate action to minimize these effects and especially to prevent any permanent damage to the eye (2).

This chapter considers the results of mechanical changes due to contact lens wear. Broadly, mechanical problems can lead to subjective complaints, surface defects of the anterior segment, and corneal shape change. More problems are created during GP rather than soft lens wear in general, but each specific lens type creates typical changes. These changes are discussed here, not just based on the type of patient subjective complains and anterior segment signs but also on the type of lenses worn.

CLINICAL TOOLS

The tools that clinicians use to diagnose mechanical complications include a comprehensive case history with careful attention to patient symptoms; conscientious observation of contact lenses both *in situ* and off the eye; ocular tissues and adnexa, observed both grossly and with the biomicroscope; and modern corneal topography.

Patient subjective visual reports and complaints, and both subjective refraction without lenses and associated corrected visual acuity, often provide a first indication of the existence of a mechanical problem. Corneal warpage and other corneal shape problems, even if the lesions are in the far corneal periphery, may have effects that reach the visual axis, changing the original refraction or reducing best-corrected visual acuity.

Vital stains (e.g., fluorescein, rose bengal, or lissamine green) all adjunctively help clinicians identify mechanical problems during slit-lamp biomicroscopy of the anterior segment, whether the patient is symptomatic and asymptomatic. Devitalized cells are observed using these stains. Fluorescein probably is the most common and arguably the most important; it assists with identification of corneal surface problems. Use of both cobalt blue excitement and yellow (barrier) observation filters enhance observation with fluorescein stain. Rose bengal or lissamine green stains can

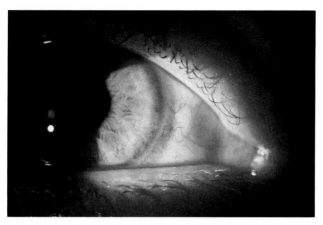

FIG. 40.1. Conjunctival staining seen with use of lissamine green stain. The staining is visible due to wear of a soft disposable lens with a rough edge.

be easily observed, even on the conjunctival surface. When slight conjunctival hyperemia accompanies staining, which is often the case, lissamine green is the stain of choice because it improves contrast with such hyperemia and is better tolerated (Fig. 40.1) (3).

The corneal topographer is especially helpful in visualizing corneal shape changes to detect early contact lens-associated corneal warpage. When no topographer is available, a diagnostic GP lens (with an overall diameter of 10 mm or more) of known back-surface design used with fluorescein ophthalmic dye can help to visualize corneal shape. The disadvantage of such a system is the lack of physical documentation.

SUBJECTIVE COMPLAINTS

Beginning Contact Lens Wearers

To discuss subjective complaints of contact lens wearers, one must first differentiate between experienced and neophyte contact lens wearers. The most typical problem of the new contact lens-wearing patient is simply the difficulty of subjective adaptation to the initial awareness of GP lenses. This remains a major limitation to increased use of GP lenses despite the substantial advantages, both optical and physiologic, such lenses often offer patients. For that reason, it is important that the initial lens design create as little subjective discomfort as possible. To this end, practitioners occasionally prescribe initial lens designs that optimize tolerance at the expense of other aspects of lens care.

From research considering which GP parameters affect initial tolerance, lens total diameter, edge shape (thickness and apex location), and lens centration have been perceived to be most important (4–6). Most patients perceive that a lens of overall diameter 9.5 mm is more comfortable than a lens of similar design but of overall diameter 9.0 mm or smaller. This does not mean that increasing lens overall

diameter alone will make GP lenses as comfortable as soft lenses, but comfort can be enhanced, hopefully to a level favorable for adaptation. Special attention should be devoted to other aspects of lens design, especially edge shape, optical zone radius and diameter, peripheral curve radii and widths, lens thickness, and selection of lens material (7).

A GP lens will always be noticeable, just by its pressure on the cornea. The interested reader may convince himself or herself of this by using a soft lens as a carrier lens underneath an GP lens. The wearer will immediately notice an increase in comfort, no matter how large the overall diameter of the GP lens.

Contact lens edges specifically play an important role in lens awareness. If the edge is too thin, less than about 0.08 mm, the apex is not easily made round and smooth, and comfort suffers. Optimal unfinished edge thickness should be about 0.12 mm (8). Because achieving such ideal edge thickness becomes more difficult with higher optical powers, lenticular designs should be considered. Lenticularization not only helps to create a more comfortable edge profile but also a more even thickness distribution over the entire lens. The apex of the edge also should be pointed one third the distance from the posterior aspect of the edge and two thirds the distance from the anterior aspect of the unfinished edge thickness for optimum tolerance. The edge should have the same thickness all around.

Clinicians should judge the appropriateness of the lens' edges during verification procedures. When a poor edge is recognized, the lens should be rejected. A good way to inspect a lens edge is to observe the reflex of a fluorescent tube on the lens' back surface while turning the lens slowly. One can easily judge both the location of the edge apex and the smoothness of the curves. Another technique is to place the lens under inspection on your hand, concave side toward the palm. Push the lens with a finger over the palm surface. If the lens slides smoothly over your sensitive palm, the apex has a good location and is round enough. If the lens digs into your skin, however, the edge may be too rough or the apex should be polished into better shape. Alternately, the lens edge can be inspected under high magnification with a light projector, with the lens immersed in an oil with a refractive index similar to that of the lens material. The lens apex and its relative location and smoothness are all then easily visualized (Fig. 40.2) (9).

Inadequately blended GP posterior curve junctions and poorly wetting surfaces both can lead to poor lens tolerance. Both can usually be addressed with in-office lens cleaning and modification.

Initial comfort problems with soft lenses usually are unrelated to size, as soft lenses generally are 13.8 mm or greater in overall diameter. Edge shape also does not have the same effect on comfort with soft as with GP lenses. Whereas the GP edge apex should be round and smooth for optimum tolerance, with soft lenses the shape of the apex seems not to have any effect on comfort as long as its apex is closer

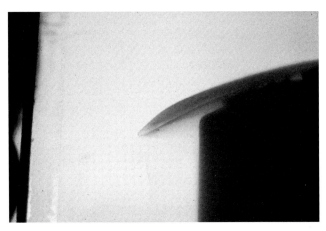

FIG. 40.2. Lens edge inspection by immersing the lens in an oil with a refractive index similar to that of the lens material.

to the conjunctiva than to the lid. Even smoothly polished soft lens edges will create discomfort, however, if the apex is more toward the outer third of the lens thickness. It is a common belief among practitioners that a thin soft lens that shows initial reasonable movement will be judged to be comfortable by patients. Research suggests that this is not necessarily the case; initial movement has no effect on comfort rating by patients (10,11). Thickness also does not appear to have an effect unless it is excessive (perhaps with toric lenses). If a foreign body (eyelash or small amount of debris) is trapped underneath an *in vivo* soft lens, it will create a strong reaction whether or not the patient has adapted to lens wear (Fig. 40.3). Cracked, chipped, or torn

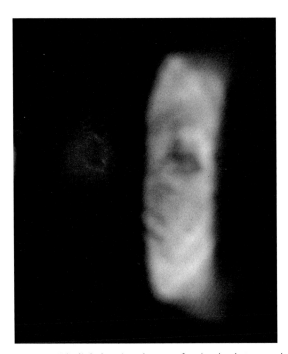

FIG. 40.3. Epithelial abrasion due to a foreign body trapped underneath a soft contact lens.

soft lenses also may create symptoms and signs but often surprisingly do neither. Patients should be advised to replace any damaged lens, whether or not it causes symptoms.

Adapted Contact Lens Wearers

When an adapted GP contact lens wearer complains of a discomfort problem, the clinician must first determine if a new lens has been just dispensed or if the problem has occurred with use of a worn lens. In the first case, most of the time it is an edge issue that commonly occurs when old GP lenses are replaced. The new GP lens will create discomfort because the patient is not adapted to the new lens edge or its slightly different apex location. Such problems often resolve without treatment by adaptation to the new lens, provided the clinician has ruled out lens defects and physiologic problems such as abrasion. In cases where adaptation fails or is protracted, a slight in-office polish and/or edge modification often will resolve the issue.

If a lens was well tolerated for some time and then suddenly changed, the clinician should inspect the lens, and especially its edge. These problems often are created by edge defects, especially chips, that require polishing. The lens also may be warped. Lens replacement is the common solution.

When soft lens wearers complain about sudden comfort decrease, torn or chipped lenses are usually the cause. These lenses may be initially tolerated on insertion, or they may create only slight irritation that worsens after a few minutes of wear and progresses as the day passes. Perceived comfort changes as the torn part of the lens varies in position with lid force and hydration.

Another reason for acute decrease in comfort with both GP and soft lens wear is soilage/deposit formation. If deposits are observed in the center of the back surface of a GP lens, they often are due to inefficient cleaning by the patient (e.g., cleaning the lens between thumb and finger, which also can warp the lens). The inside of the lens has not been cleaned sufficiently, as occurs when the patient uses one finger and the inside of the hand. If deposits are observed all over the lens, it often is due to an inefficient cleaner, poor tear layers, or both. If the clinician cannot resolve these issues with stronger cleaners, adding routine (e.g., 1/week) enzymatic cleaning may help.

Plaque formation/severe lens soilage is seldom observed with soft lenses today. Patients usually discard lenses before or once they begin to become uncomfortable. Practitioners may still encounter such issues, however, when patients complain about decreasing disposable soft lens lifespan or when patients use nondisposable custom toric lenses. Deposits do not necessarily look the same on soft and GP lenses. Whereas flat layers/plaques of material are observed on GP lenses, wartlike elevations, called *jelly bumps,* appear on soft lenses (Fig. 40.4). These jelly bumps are not easily removed without leaving a permanent mark on the surface of the lens.

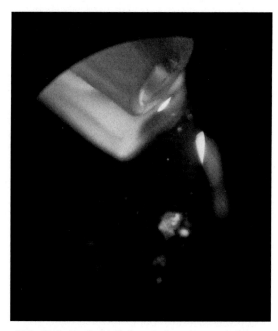

FIG. 40.4. Typical jelly bump deposit on a soft lens.

Because jelly bumps are known to consist of both lipid and protein (12), some can be at least partially removed using techniques not approved by the US Food and Drug Administration (FDA), if the practitioner elects such "heroic" procedures in these days of disposable soft lenses. Because lipids may be dissolved by heat, lenses can be boiled in small glass vials of saline. Several added drops of POLYCLENS cleaner will help because the polymer beads in the cleaner bind lipids. Boiling the lens in 3% hydrogen peroxide with a dissolved enzymatic tablet (e.g., subtilisin a) will then address proteins. One should take care that the particular soft lens material can be heated with hydrogen peroxide. Most soft lenses can be heated in peroxide, however, provided the temperature remains below 55°C (130°F); otherwise, the lens will break very easily. By repeating these procedures, one can end with an almost clean lens, or at least a lens without an elevated deposit; however, a permanent mark often remains on the surface of the lens. To decrease the future buildup of jelly bumps, the clinician can add an alcohol-based daily cleaner to the patient's care regimen.

Both soft and GP lens wearers can present with foreign material embedded in their lenses. Foreign bodies embedded in the front surfaces of lenses cause minimal subjective complaints. Embedded foreign objects on the lens back surfaces, however, often create an immediate decline in patient comfort that is alleviated only when the lens is removed but reoccurs when the lens is reinserted. How foreign bodies become embedded on lens back surfaces remains a mystery to the author, but it has been observed in daily practice. Soft lenses should be replaced. Polishing the back surface of an affected GP lens often is insufficient. Use of a small-grade injection needle often will dislodge the foreign body, however, and occasionally the lens back surface can then be satisfactorily polished to save the GP lens.

Rust spots are occasionally observed on soft lenses, but because the spots are flat they rarely create any symptoms. Such rust spots can often be observed on the lenses of wearers who commute by train to work daily and possibly are caused by the train metal brakes creating small iron particles. Patients who shower with their lenses *in situ* also develop rust spots, perhaps from small bits of iron liberated from their plumbing. These patients may benefit from advice to discontinue this practice due to the infectious hazards of exposure to fresh water (see Chapter 39, specifically the section on *Acanthamoeba* corneal infection).

GP lens edges that have small defects can be polished into better condition, but it might be better to replace the lens. Chipped soft disposable lenses are discarded. Damaged custom-made fairly new toric lenses are a particular problem because of their expense. Clinicians occasionally, can "recondition" such lenses, again without benefit of FDA approval, by cutting off the small torn edge while the lens is still in the wet stage. Before the soft lens can be repolished, it must be dried by putting it underneath an upside down glass. This prevents air flow (which would cause the lens to shrink in an uneven manner, leading to a very irregular surface that cannot be polished) to retain the shape of the lens. After a drying period of about 1 day, one can use a velvet cloth with a soft lens polishing solution and polish the edge of the lens manually. Because the material is rather soft, it will take only 2 to 3 minutes of manual polishing. The lens should be rehydrated and disinfected before use.

It is important to emphasize that not all comfort problems are mechanically caused by the lens itself. Tear deficiency or anterior segment complications, such as blepharitis or keratoconjunctivitis, also will lead to comfort problems even if there is no direct connection to a mechanical lens issue.

ANTERIOR SEGMENT SURFACE DAMAGE

Abnormal changes observed with the biomicroscope (or grossly) on the surface of the eye with or without the use of a vital stain such as fluorescein, rose bengal, or lissamine green are considered evidence of contact lens-related surface damage. No conclusions can be made concerning etiology from this simple statement.

3- and 9-O'Clock Staining

Representative of such a finding is the common peripheral cornea desiccation staining associated with GP lens wear called *3- to 9-o'clock* or *juxtapositional* staining. It has been studied for 50 years and remains the most prevalent complication of rigid corneal contact lens wear. Even moderate-to-severe 3- to 9-o'clock staining deserves attention to decrease the potential for this complication to advance to infection, dellen, or pseudopterygium/vascularized limbal keratitis (VLK) (Fig. 40.5) (13).

There is a suggestion in the literature that 3- to 9-o'clock staining may be more patient than lens design dependent (14). Why then should we discuss peripheral corneal desiccation as a mechanical problem?

Clearly this complication only occurs with lenses that do not fully cover the corneal surface, primarily corneal GP lenses (it should be noted that decentered 12.5-mm overall diameter soft lenses also cause a form of this stain). The reasoning is that any lens will have a certain edge thickness and, depending on this thickness and the uncovered corneal portion, a gap may be created between the lid, the lens edge, and the ocular surface where neither lid nor lens covers or wets that surface. Poor wetting of this gap leads to the complication. Therefore, this is, at least in part, a lens-related mechanical problem that should be addressed by optimizing lens design and fit (15,16).

Superficial microerosions of the corneal epithelium just lateral to contact lens edges are the primary sign of 3- to 9-o'clock staining. Acceptance of staining by the corneal epithelium can be minimal, mild, or (unusually) advanced to the point that the clinician considers abrasion as the more proper diagnosis. Conjunctival injection lateral to the corneal staining is an associated common sign and increases in prevalence and severity with the severity of the corneal erosions. Chronic and severe cases often develop an accompanying vascular pannus or pseudopterygium, or dellen.

The principal cause of 3- to 9-o'clock staining is a low-riding GP contact lens. Effort should be made to optimize the position of the low-riding contact lens by increasing its overall diameter and/or flattening its base curve to achieve

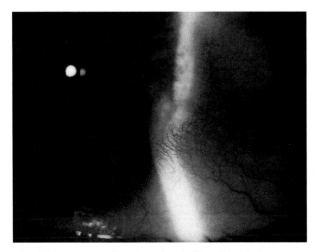

FIG. 40.5. Long-standing 3- to 9-o'clock staining led to a vascularized limbal keratitis. Cessation of lens wear was needed before the patient could be refitted.

"lid attachment." Occasionally, especially with a plus-powered lens, a peripheral minus carrier may bring the lens up so that its edge is under the upper lid. The clinician should maintain a moderately wide peripheral tear reservoir. The lens edge should be as thin as possible by minimizing center thickness (also reducing lens mass) and by reducing the optical diameter of the anterior surface of the lens. Choosing a material with a low specific gravity may be beneficial. For cases of substantial corneal astigmatism, bitoric GP lens designs should be considered. When the contact lens is seen to center well, however, the clinician should consider modifying the edge lift associated with the peripheral curve design and the edge thickness, as well as the overall diameter. The clinician also should consider whether contact lens binding is playing a role in the development of this corneal epitheliopathy (17).

The condition of the patient's lids/meibomian glands and tear layers is believed to contribute to 3- to 9-o'clock staining (18,19). Clinicians should screen potential and continuing GP lens patients for lid and anterior segment tear problems, and lid disease should be addressed (as discussed elsewhere in this text). Blink training may be helpful because it increases the number of complete blinks (20). Wear time is another factor that can be managed. If all attempts to solve the problem with GP contact lenses are unsuccessful and if there are no contraindications, prescription of soft contact lenses should be considered. Adapted GP lens-wearing patients who develop this complication usually do not wish to be refitted with soft contact lenses, however, because they know that visual acuity will suffer.

Symptoms of mild-to-moderate 3- to 9-o'clock staining usually are nonexistent to minimal. Experienced GP contact lens wearers often do not consider mild irritation worth mentioning. Such patients may be more bothered by the cosmetic appearance of accompanying horizontal conjunctival hyperemia. Practitioners can exploit this gross observation to explain the rationale of treatment, which may be inconvenient even if of minimal expense, so that patients comply with improvements in their care. The long-term complications of 3- to 9-o'clock staining include corneal neovascularization, epithelial hypertrophy, and reduced wearing time.

The common soft lens analogy to GP lens-related 3- to 9-o'clock staining is soft contact lens surface drying leading to underlying corneal desiccation (Fig. 40.6). This has long been believed a lens-related dehydration and thickness issue. Clinicians have been advised to use thicker soft lenses to resolve the complication when it is observed (21). With new soft lens materials, however, we find that dehydration may not be solely related to lens thickness. We now can achieve increased water binding by prescribing low dehydration polymers, such as hioxifilcon A, which lose minimal water content during wear (Fig. 40.7) (22,23).

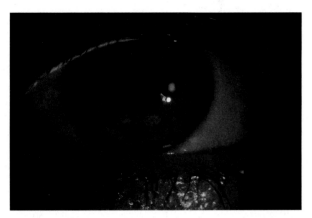

FIG. 40.6. Corneal desiccation due to dehydration of the contact lens while it was being worn.

Foreign Bodies

Experienced clinicians know that foreign bodies are easily trapped behind GP lenses. It appears that the length of time a particle remains trapped behind the lens can depend on the contact lens fit. Lenses fitted slightly flat allow foreign bodies to both enter and exit the post-lens tear pool faster than if a lens is slightly steep. Soft lenses rarely, if ever, cause this problem.

A special subset of this issue arises with the keratoconic patient who works or plays in a dusty environment. Practitioners often decline to specifically deal with this problem by only recommending protective goggles. Patients seldom follow this advice because goggles are bothersome or do not protect well enough. It may be more beneficial to prescribe a thin soft disposable lens as a carrier lens underneath the GP lens. This often decreases the problem of foreign bodies becoming trapped underneath the lens. The GP lens does not need to have a special design, except that it should not be fitted too steep and care should be taken that the lens has a nice smooth edge lift. The bottom soft lens should be of relatively steep base curve to fit the keratoconic corneal sagittal depth, of minimal thickness to allow oxygen supply, and of low power for even thickness distribution. Patients should be informed about the reduced oxygen delivery through these "piggyback" lens systems, and the two lenses should be worn together only when really needed (24,25). Another option in cases where only a GP lens can be worn but the environment is dusty is to fit a GP lens with an overall diameter 13 mm or more. Depending on lid positioning, large overall diameters not only prevent foreign bodies from becoming trapped underneath the lens but also decrease initial lens awareness, which is a common problem (26).

Pressure-Related Problems

An etiologically obscure problem seen in soft lens wear has been called *superior epithelial arcuate staining* (SEALs) (27). An arc of corneal staining is observed about 1 mm inward from and parallel to the superior corneal limbus (Fig. 40.8). Patients may be symptomatic, but not necessarily so. Although no claims of secondary infection or scarring have been reported, such sequelae are major concerns. Some believe this complication is caused by pressure transmitted to the corneal surface from the superior lid pushes down on the lens. Alternative proposed etiologies include the stiffness of the lens material and/or rough junctions either from the front or the back surface of the lens (28). There also appears to be a patient-dependent factor. Proposed schemes to treat or avoid SEALs include improved lens cleaning, a new lens of the same design, disposable lenses (even 1 day), or refitting with a different soft lens design, commonly with a thicker profile, perhaps using custom-made soft lenses in which thickness and diameter can be chosen independently (27,29,30).

If we see a similar appearance with GP lens wear, it usually is due to a rough back surface or a harsh junction from one to another curve. This problem usually is treated by polishing the back surface of the lens.

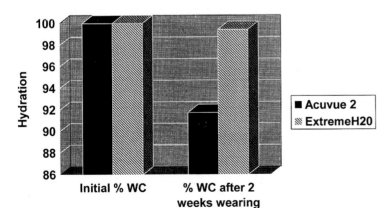

FIG. 40.7. Water content expressed in percent hydration. Lenses made of hioxifilcon A (ExtremH20) dropped from 100% to 99.43%, and the control lens made of etafilcon A (Acuvue2) dropped from 100% to 91.74% after a 2-week daily wear period (23).

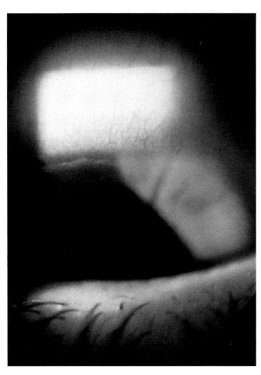

FIG. 40.8. Superior epithelial arcuate lesion (SEAL), also known as epithelial splitting. The patient had to be fitted with another lens design to eliminate the lesion.

SHAPE CHANGE

It is important that practitioners diagnose corneal shape changes and predict the time course for resolution. This becomes even more important with the increasing popularity of refractive surgeries to ensure a predictable and stable postsurgical result (2).

Corneal Warpage or Naturally Occurring Irregular Astigmatism?

Corneal shape changes are not commonly noted by patients unless lens wear is discontinued in favor of spectacles. They then can become aware of changes and quite concerned. Clinicians should evaluate cornea shape on a regular base to diagnose and treat early changes. Corneal topography is not the best tool to make this diagnosis because of its poor sensitivity. Instrument variability makes decisions only possible after sequential measurements. Routine keratometry and refraction, perhaps once a year, are more beneficial. Refraction has an advantage in that it is both highly repeatable and very sensitive. Corneal topography, however, will help quantify and document these changes.

Once shape change has been diagnosed, the clinician should try to determine the etiology so as to prevent continuing changes and perhaps restore the original shape of the cornea and allow the patient use of appropriate spectacles.

It is important to differentiate between more benign cor-

neal shape changes and corneal warpage. In the context of the following discussion, the term *corneal shape change* will be used to describe *regular* shape changes of the cornea for which appropriate refraction will restore optimum visual acuity. Conversely, *corneal warpage* refers to *irregular* astigmatic corneal shape changes that are not compensated by simple refractive change to restore original visual acuity. Corneal warpage may even be a precursor to keratoconus (31–34). Because some patients wear lenses for long periods before corneal warpage is detected, differentiating mechanically induced corneal warpage from the beginning keratoconus is difficult (Fig. 40.9; see Color Plate 40.9). Note that early keratoconus often shows no classic signs, such as Fleischer ring segments, Vogt striae, or obvious central corneal thinning. Lebow and Grohe (35) attempted to differentiate keratoconus from contact lens-induced corneal warpage. They found that keratoconic eyes showed statistically steeper simulated K readings, greater corneal toricity, a more variable shape factor, and greater elevation compared to a reference sphere than did warped corneas. Clinical decisions on the diagnosis of individual corneas still remain difficult. Definite diagnosis often can only be provided well after the patient has been fitted with new lenses made of a material with higher oxygen transmissibility and better shape congruity. Corneas that regularize over time with treatment (improved lens design or after lens discontinuation) are most likely to be warped by lens wear, whereas corneas that maintain irregular shapes or even progress may deserve the diagnosis of keratoconus.

Shape Changes Induced by Gas Permeable Lens Wear

Both corneal shape change and warpage usually are GP lens-induced problems thought due to oxygen deprivation, the rigidity of the lens materials, and inaccurate lens fitting.

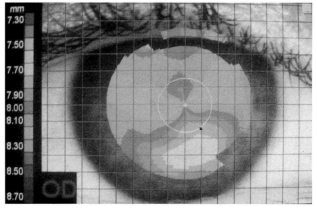

FIG. 40.9. Topography of the cornea shows inferior steepening, a sign that also can be seen in early keratoconic eyes. If no other classic signs of keratoconus can be found, then only time will tell if refitting was justified or if the finding was an indication of early keratoconus. (See Color Plate 40.9.)

Because it is relatively easy to optimize visual acuity with GP lenses, almost irrelevant of the mechanical fit, practitioners often have a tendency to be too easily pleased with their work.

Corneal curvature change and warpage once were considered primarily part of the oxygen problem associated with use of nonpermeable polymethyl methacrylate (PMMA) lenses (36). Most modern GP lenses allow sufficient oxygen to reach the underlying cornea, especially when the lenses are used only for daily wear and there is reasonable tear exchange (37,38), but clinicians may continue to observe unintentional or accepted cornea molding.

Use of flat base curves may minimize lens flexure to enhance stable visual acuity (39). It is important that clinicians differentiate between a *toric cornea,* which refers to corneal shape, and *astigmatism,* which refers to refractive optics (40). Astigmatism often can be corrected by a spherical lens on a toric cornea, but the shape of the spherical lens may not match the underlying corneal shape. Using a spherical back-surface GP lens, even of high Dk/t, on a toric cornea may push the tissue enough over time to substantially change the eye's optics, variably if only temporarily. The practitioner's goal, however, should be not only to enhance visual acuity with contact lens design but also to give his or her patient the option of using spectacles whenever desired, and for whatever time period, without necessarily requiring a protracted deadaptation process. To achieve this more complete contact lens goal, clinicians and patients should understand that more expensive and difficult toric GP lens designs might be required (Fig. 40.10; see Color Plate 40.10).

Multifocal GP design lenses (with highly aspheric back surfaces) used on corneas with low rigidities also distort corneal shape, regularly and irregularly (41). Backup spectacles often must be adjusted up to 1 D. Even "normal" corneas fitted with aspheric lenses undergo changes in corneal asphericity (42). The resultant shape change often has no observable effect on the refraction but rather on the image quality, fortunately at a level that that most patients will not notice.

Corneal Warpage Due to Poorly Centered Lenses

Mechanically induced corneal shape changes are found least with well-centered GP lenses. Sometimes such a position is easily achieved, whereas other times it is not. Corneal topography shows flattening in areas where GP lenses stabilize (43). If the lens rests superiorly, a flattening of the superior cornea, midperipheral corneal steepening, and inferior cornea flattening typically are observed (6). This pattern usually is referred to as an *inferior smile* pattern (Figs. 40.11 and 40.12; see Color Plates 40.11 and 40.12). Refraction without a lens often will show a reduction in minus power and an inverse astigmatism. The eye still can be corrected to 20/20 in early stages, but a long-standing high-riding lens often will cause slightly reduced spectacle best-corrected visual acuity, perhaps to 20/25.

Reasons that GP lenses ride high include the relatively thick lens edge of high-minus optically powered lenses leading to the "watermelon seed effect," with-the-rule astigmatism corrected with a spherical lens, and an inferiorly decentered corneal apex.

GP lens-induced corneal warpage often can be treated and reversed by discontinuing lens wear or by using soft

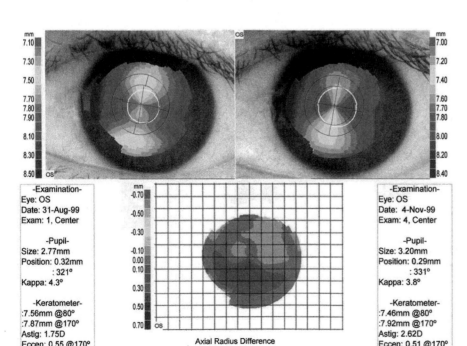

FIG. 40.10. Corneal topographies of a patient who complained that her vision decreased when wearing glasses instead of GP lenses for several days. **Left:** Topography after wearing a spherical GP lens that gave 20/20 acuity, refraction was −7.25 −1.00 × 170 degrees. **Right:** Topography after fitting the patient with a toric GP lens (20/20 acuity); refraction changed to −7.75 −3.00 × 170 degrees, and the patient could switch between glasses and contact lenses without a perceptible decrease in vision. (See Color Plate 40.10.)

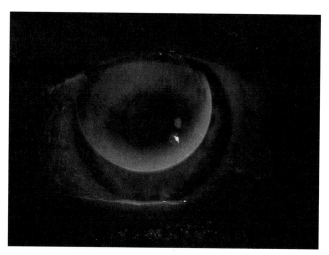

FIG. 40.11. Fluorescein pattern of a high-riding lens. (See Color Plate 40.11.)

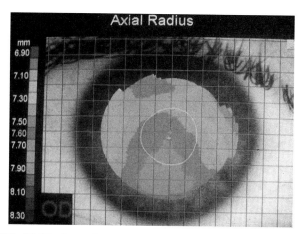

FIG. 40.13. Corneal topography after wearing a lens that rides constantly low. (See Color Plate 40.13.)

lenses with appropriate oxygen transmissibilities (44). Sometimes refitting with GP lenses of increased oxygen transmissibility, improved centration, and toric surfaces, as appropriate, may be beneficial as well.

For example, to avoid a high-riding lens (in case of a toric cornea), one could fit a toric back-surface lens or, at minimum, a lens that has a toric periphery. Alternatively, high-riding GP lenses can be addressed by use of lenticularization. If the lens is still too thick or the lens apex too high, modification (thinning) of the edge by use of a 120-degree diamond cone tool with polishing afterward may be helpful. Sometimes decreasing or increasing overall diameter may prove successful. Use of a prism-ballasted lens may achieve the desired effect of pulling the lens down.

Corneal warpage can occur if a GP lens rides constantly at the lower corneal limbus, leading to a flattened inferior corneal surface (Fig. 40.13; see Color Plate 40.13) (45). Low-riding GP lenses also will lead to 3- to 9-o'clock staining, which should be treated to prevent excessive conjunctival hyperemia, dellen, limbal hypertrophy, or corneal neo-

vascularization. Such low-riding GP lenses often are heavy due to excessive optical power (usually nonlenticulated plus power) or a material with a high specific gravity index. Use of GP lenses with relatively flat peripheral curves on corneas of low eccentricity will lead to lenses that ride low on the cornea. Corneas with inferiorly displaced apices (e.g., keratoconus) also are difficult to fit properly. Prefit corneal topography will assist in detection/diagnosis of many corneas with inferiorly positioned apices and keratoconus, but designing GP lenses to ride higher is not always easy.

It has been shown that the three most important factors for achieving successful lid attachment fit are high edge lift, sufficient edge thickness, and a minus front-surface carrier (46).

Techniques of raising the position of a GP lens include increased overall diameters, use of minus carrier edges, and GP materials of low specific gravity (most often lens materials of limited fluorine).

A warped lens can be the reason for a corneal shape change. This factor should always be considered during an evaluation. High oxygen permeable materials or lenses with high power often show base curve changes over time. Sometimes this can only be observed in the periphery of the lens.

Long-standing PMMA lens wear often leads to corneal shape changes or warpage. Before refitting a patient with a GP lens, it is important to inform him or her about the time course and the changes needed (47). Previous PMMA wearers often find that handling GP lenses results in repeatedly warped lenses because they are not familiar with lenses that damage as easily as current GP lenses. These patients must be reeducated on lens handling and lens care to minimize this problem *a priori.*

Shape Changes Induced by Soft Lens Wear

Corneal shape changes and warpage were initially believed to be complications only of GP lens wear, but several studies

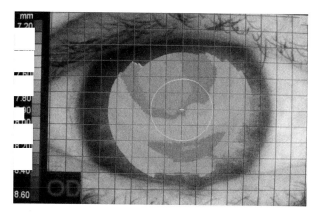

FIG. 40.12. Corneal topography after the lens was taken off the eye shown in Figure 40.11. (See Color Plate 40.12.)

suggest that soft lenses can create similar problems, especially when chronic corneal edema is generated (specifically after low-oxygen transmissibility soft lenses have been worn for many years) (48–52).

Corneal wrinkling is another mechanical corneal change observed following wear of very thin soft lenses (53–55). To resolve this problem, the patient must be fitted with another lens type that has a greater center thickness.

Decreased Visual Acuity

Decrease in contact lens corrected visual acuity can be a mechanical lens problem. The clinician must first rule out an organic cause of vision loss. Best refraction, use of pinhole, and biomicroscopy should assist with this decision. Then one must consider the contact lens causes, first soilage of either soft or GP lenses.

Use of large overall diameter hydrogel lenses can lead to decreased vision in patients who have pingueculae on both sides of the limbus. Vision initially may be good, as long as the hydrogel lens is fully hydrated. As soon as the lens starts to dehydrate, however, optics may distort, leading to a drop in visual acuity. Overkeratometry is beneficial diagnostically. The corneal curvature should be measured without the lens and repeated with the lens on the cornea. Toricity changes (amount and/or direction) indicate a soft lens that does not drape well.

Decreased visual acuity during GP lens wear may follow lens warpage (56,57). Patients can cause this when they squeeze the lens between fingers during care or "catch" the lens between the lens cap and the lens case during storage. It is important to verify GP base curves if a corneal shape change or a symptomatic drop in visual acuity is observed during contact lens consultation, as well as periodically while caring for asymptomatic patients. Another reason for a decrease in visual acuity with a GP lens is an unintended lens optical power change due to cleaning the lens with an abrasive cleaner and putting too much pressure on the lens (58).

CONCLUSION

Because a GP or hydrogel contact lens is, by its nature, a foreign body on the eye, both types of lenses can create many mechanical problems. These problems may be asymptomatic or they may lead to symptoms, especially reduced vision or comfort. The practitioner must consider all measurements and observations made during professional evaluation to determine if a mechanical problem exists and, if so, establish its cause so that proper treatment can be instituted.

REFERENCES

1. Ruiz-Montenegro J, Marfa CH, Wilson SE, et al. Corneal topography alterations in normal contact lens wearers. *Ophthalmology* 1993;100:128–134.
2. Wang X, McCulley JP, Bowman RW, et al. Time to resolution of contact lens-induced corneal warpage prior to refractive surgery. *CLAO J* 2002;28:169–171.
3. Manning FJ, Wehrly SR, Foulks GN. Patient tolerance and ocular surface staining characteristics of lissamine green versus rose Bengal. *Ophthalmology* 1995;102:1953 -1957.
4. Williams-Lyn D, MacNeil K, Fonn D. The effect of rigid lens back optic zone radius and diameter changes on comfort. *Int Contact Lens Clin* 1993;20:223–229.
5. La Hood D. Edge shape and comfort of rigid lenses. *Am J Optom Physiol Opt* 1988;65:613–618.
6. Sorbara L, Fonn D, Holden BA, et al. Centrally fitted versus upper lid attached rigid gas permeable lenses. Part II . A comparison of the clinical performance. *Int Contact Lens Clin* 1996;23:121–127.
7. Hazlett RD. Custom designing large-diameter rigid gas permeable contact lenses: a clinical approach intended to optimise lens comfort. *Int Contact Lens Clin* 1997;24:5–9.
8. Bussacker H. Der Einfluss der Randgestalt auf die Verträglichkeit von Corneallinsen. *Die Contactlinse* 1974;6:4–13.
9. Wilms KH. Zur Vorgeschichte der Betrachtung des Kontaktlinsenprofils in Immersion. *Neues Optiker J* 1972;14:329–331.
10. Young G. Evaluation of soft contact lens fitting characteristics. *Optom Vis Sci* 1996;73:247–254.
11. Businger U. Clinical performance of ExtremeH20 lenses versus Acuvue lenses in a cross over study. Study data on file at Benz R&D, Sarasota, Florida, 2001.
12. Brennan NA, Coles Ch M-L. Deposits and symptomatology with soft contact lens wear. *Int Contact Lens Clin* 2000;27:75–100.
13. Grohe RM, Lebow KA. Vascularized limbal keratitis. *Int Contact Lens Clin* 1989;16:197–207.
14. Schnider CM, Terry RL, Holden BA. Effect of patient and lens performance characteristics on peripheral corneal desiccation. *J Am Optom Assoc* 1996;67:144–150.
15. Businger U, Treiber A, Flury C. The etiology and management of three and nine o'clock staining. *Int Contact Lens Clin* 1989;16:136–139.
16. Schnider CM, Terry RL, Holden BA. Effect of lens design on peripheral corneal desiccation. *J Am Optom Assoc* 1997;68:163–167.
17. Swarbrick HA, Holden BA. Rigid gas permeable lens binding: significance and contributing factors. *Am J Optom Physiol Opt* 1987;64:815–823.
18. Korb DR, Henriquez AS. Meibomian gland dysfunction and contact lens intolerance. *Am J Optom Assoc* 1980;51:243–251.
19. Paugh JP, Knapp RL, Martinson JR, et al. Meibomian therapy in problematic contact lens wear. *Optom Vis Sci* 1990;67:803–806.
20. Collins M, Heron H, Larsen R, et al. Blinking patterns in soft contact lens wearers can be altered with training. *Am J Optom Physiol Opt* 1987;64:100–103.
21. Bennett ES, Gordon JM. The borderline dry eye patient and contact lens wear. *Contact Lens Forum* 1989;14:52–73.
22. Businger U. GMA/HEMA first report on a clinical trial. *Contact Lens Spectrum* 1995;10:19–25.
23. Businger U. A new material on the block of frequent replacement lenses. *Contact Lens Spectrum* 2000;15:49–51.
24. Yeung K, Eghbali F, Weissmann BA. Clinical experience with piggyback contact lens systems on keratoconic eyes. *J Am Optom Assoc* 1995;66:539–543.
25. Giasson CJ, Perreault N, Brazeau D. Oxygen tension beneath piggyback contact lenses and clinical outcomes of users. *CLAO J* 2001;27:144–150.
26. Pullum KW, Buckley RJ. A study of 530 patients referred for rigid gas permeable scleral contact lens assessment. *Cornea* 1997;16:612–622.
27. Malinovsky V, Pole J, Pence NA. Epithelial splits of the superior

cornea in hydrogel contact lens patients. *Int Cont Lens Clin* 1989; 16:252–255.

28. Young G, Mirejovsky D. A hypothesis for the aetiology of soft contact lens-induced superior arcuate keratopathy. *Int Contact Lens Clin* 1993;20:177–179.

29. Josephson JE. A corneal irritation uniquely produced by hydrogel lathed lenses and its resolution. *J Am Optom Assoc* 1978;49: 869–870.

30. Jalbert I, Sweeney DF, Holden BA. Epithelial split associated with wear of a silicone hydrogel contact lens. *CLAO J* 2001;27: 231–233.

31. Gritz DC, McDonnell PJ. Keratoconus and ocular massage. *Am J Ophthalmol* 1988;106:757–758.

32. Ing MR. The development of corneal astigmatism in contact lens wear as an environmental risk in keratoconus. *Ann Ophthalmol* 1976;8:309–314.

33. Steahly LP. Keratoconus following contact lens wear. *Ann Ophthalmol* 1978;10:1177–1179.

34. Gasset AR, Houde WL, Garcia-Bengochea M. Hard contact lens wear as en environmental risk in keratoconus. *Am J Ophthalmol* 1978;85:339–341.

35. Lebow KA, Grohe RM. Differentiating contact lens induced warpage from true keratoconus using corneal topography. *CLAO J* 1999;25:114–122.

36. Rengstorff RH. The Fort Dix report: longitudinal study of the effects of contact lenses. *Am J Optom Arch Am Acad Optom* 1965; 42:153–163.

37. Holden BA, Sweeney DF, Sanderson G. The minimum precorneal oxygen tension to avoid corneal oedema. *Invest Ophthalmol Vis Sci* 1984;25:476–480.

38. Brennan NA, Efron N, Holden BA. Oxygen permeability of hard gas permeable contact lens materials. *Clin Exp Optom* 1986;69: 82–89.

39. Herman JP. Flexure of rigid contact lenses on toric corneas as a function of base curve fitting relationship. *J Am Optom Assoc* 1983;54:209–213.

40. Sarver MD. Astigmatism. In: Mandell RB, ed. *Contact lens practice,* 3rd ed. Springfield, IL: Charles C. Thomas Publisher, 1981: 244–275.

41. Woods C, Ruston D, Hough T, et al. Clinical performance of an innovative back surface multifocal contact lens in correcting presbyopia. *CLAO J* 1999;25:176–181.

42. Maeda N, Klyce SD, Hamano H. Alteration of corneal asphericity in rigid gas permeable contact lens induced warpage. *CLAO J* 1994;20:27–31.

43. Wilson SE, Lin DT, Klyce SD, et al. Rigid contact lens decentration: a risk factor for corneal warpage. *CLAO J* 1990;16: 177–182.

44. Calossi A, Verzella F, Zanella SG. Corneal warpage resolution after refitting an RGP contact lens wearer into hydrophilic high water content material. *CLAO J* 1996;22:242–244.

45. Wilson SE, Lin DTC, Klyce SD, et al. Topographic changes in contact lens induced corneal warpage. *Ophthalmol* 1980;97: 734–44.

46. Sorbara L, Fonn D, Holden BA, et al. Centrally fitted versus upper lid-attached rigid gas permeable lenses. Part I. Design parameters affecting vertical decentration. *Int Contact Lens Clin* 1996;23:99–103.

47. Novo AG, Pavlopoulos G, Feldman ST. Corneal topographic changes after refitting polymethylmethacrylate contact lens wearers into rigid gas permeable materials. *CLAO J* 1995;21: 47–51.

48. Lee JR, Refojo MF, Leong FL. Tinted hydrogel lenses for cosmetic and optical problems. *Cont Lens Intraocul Med J* 1977;3: 22–26.

49. Grosvenor T. Changes in corneal curvature and subjective refraction of soft contact lens wearers. *Am J Optom Physiol Opt* 1975; 52:405–413.

50. Harris MG, Sarver MD, Polse KA. Corneal curvature and refractive error changes associate with wearing hydrogel contact lenses. *Am J Optom Physiol Opt* 1975;52:313.

51. Miller JP, Coon LJ, Meier RF. Extended wear of Hydrocurve II 55 soft contact lenses. *J Am Optom Assoc* 1980;51:225–233.

52. Schanzer MC, Mehta RS, Arnold TP, et al. Irregular astigmatism induced by annular tinted contact lenses. *CLAO J* 1989;15: 207–211.

53. Mobilia EF, Yamamoto GK, Dohlman CH. Corneal wrinkling induced by ultrathin soft contact lenses. *Ann Ophthalmol* 1980; 12:371–375.

54. Quinn T. Epithelial folds. *Int Contact Lens Clin* 1982;9:365.

55. Lowe R, Brennan N. Corneal wrinkling caused by a thin medium water content lens. *Int Contact Lens Clin* 1987;14:403–406.

56. Henry VA, Bennett ES, Forrest JF. Clinical investigation of the Paraperm EW rigid gas permeable contact lens. *Am J Optom Physiol Opt* 1987;64:728–729.

57. Henry VA, Bennett ES, Sevigny J. Rigid extended wear problem solving. *Int Contact Lens Clin* 1990;17:121–133.

58. O'Donnell JJ. Patient-induced power changes in rigid gas permeable contact lenses: a case report and literature review. *J Am Optom Assoc* 1994;65:772–773.

DIAGNOSTIC AND THERAPEUTIC PHARMACEUTICAL AGENTS RELEVANT TO CONTACT LENS PRACTICE

MICHAEL J. DOUGHTY

INTRODUCTION

Overall Perspective on Contact Lens Wear and Pharmaceutical Use

Topical ocular pharmaceutical agents will be commonly used during contact lens wear for many reasons. Drugs are used during procedures associated with contact lens selection and evaluation and then during follow-up evaluations. Diagnostic pharmaceutical agents include dyes and stains, as well as topical ocular anesthetics. Pharmaceuticals also are used for management of non–contact lens-related systemic diseases that affect contact lens comfort or tolerability, which include a range of dry eye conditions, and management of allergies in contact lens wearers. Lastly, pharmaceuticals are used for treatment of various types of contact lens or non–contact lens wear-related ophthalmic complications or disease encountered during contact lens wear. This last category includes conditions such as blepharitis, corneal abrasions, giant papillary conjunctivitis (GPC), various forms of noninfectious and infectious keratitis, and various inflammatory conditions affecting the anterior segment of the eye (1). Over the years, there have been considerable changes in contact lens types, ranging from polymethyl methacrylate (PMMA) to gas permeable (GP) lenses, and from early types of hydrogel (soft) lenses to the development of hydrogel lenses for extended wear and now continuous wear. Use of various pharmaceutical agents, as outlined in this chapter, generally apply to all types of contact lens wear;

however, some important distinctions must be made and are highlighted where appropriate.

Knowledge of the ingredients of ophthalmic pharmaceuticals and other products relevant to contact lens wear and the modes of action of the drugs in any of these products is important to facilitate optimum product selection and appropriate patient care. In this chapter, emphasis is placed on the action and use of drugs and products available in the United States. However, where appropriate, information is provided on similar drugs and products in Canada, the United Kingdom, and Australia.

Contact Lens Care Products for Cleaning and Disinfection

Successful contact lens wear requires the regular use of various care solutions. For compliant patients adapted to contact lens wear, the wearing and care of their lenses can be expected to be a relatively uncomplicated and trouble-free activity, especially with the continued evolution of care systems (2–11).

Full details of these products can be found elsewhere, but there is one issue that is highly relevant to the general use of pharmaceuticals or other ophthalmic products in contact lens wearers, namely, the development of adverse reactions or intolerance to these products. For the patient being evaluated for contact lens wear for the first time or for patients being switched to a different type of care system, intolerance to any of the ingredients of the solution may present itself acutely. Patients also may develop a definite or apparent intolerance to the ingredients of a contact lens care solution over time, rather than acutely (12–14). A previously known or expected sensitivity to any ingredient of a care system is a sufficient reason not to use that solution (15). Although the chemistry and physiochemical characteristics of such solutions can be complex, the actual mode(s) of action of the ingredients rarely need be a concern of the practitioner. If a care regimen is unacceptable to a patient or practitioner for comfort or convenience reasons, the "problem" often can be reduced or eliminated by switching to an alternative system or contact lens. There is rarely any simple "drug"-related or medical reason for changing a contact lens care regimen (12), except for a genuine hypersensitivity or toxic reaction (12–14).

Diagnostic Pharmaceutical Agents

A number of diagnostic pharmaceutical agents, especially the ophthalmic dyes, are routinely used during contact lens fitting. When contact lens discomfort or intolerance progressively develops, a practitioner's ability to define the cause of the problems and symptoms may be enhanced or facilitated with the adjunct use of diagnostic pharmaceutical agents such as dyes and stains. Other diagnostic drugs, such as topical ocular anesthetics (e.g., proparacaine), can be used during the initial fitting and adaptation to hard contact lenses, which has been usual for scleral lenses and PMMA lenses, and still can be applied to rigid gas permeable (RGP) lenses.

Palliative Agents

If a contact lens wearer has some degree of ocular discomfort and/or develops discomfort due to mild intolerance to lens wear, then a range of products are available to counter this discomfort. These include rewetting solutions, eye comfort drops, eye washes, and eyelid hygiene products. All of these pharmaceuticals and products are designed to counter the effects of drying (desiccation) of the contact lens or ocular surface usually associated with tear film instability. Use of palliative agents also should make the eye more comfortable, as well as quiet the external eye. Finally, if the discomfort is associated with the development of clinically significant desiccation of the ocular surface, the adjunct use of artificial tears may be appropriate to further offset the impact of tear film instability.

Therapeutic Pharmaceutical Agents

A contact lens wearer may have, or develop, discomfort that is more associated with genuine irritation of the eye (by the environment or workplace). This includes ocular surface inflammation associated with allergies (e.g., seasonal allergic conjunctivitis). Irritation of the ocular surface, especially the palpebral conjunctiva, also may be caused by the contact lens itself, in which case a slightly different form of inflammatory reaction develops, namely, contact lens papillary conjunctivitis (CLPC, once more commonly referred to as giant papillary conjunctivitis). In rare cases, the extent of inflammation will be severe. A range of pharmaceutical agents are available to manage everything from irritation-related hyperemia to the various grades of inflammation. A more recent perspective is that an important aspect of development of the use of therapeutic pharmaceutical agents by optometric practitioners involves being proactive, i.e., aggressive management of conjunctivitis in contact lens wearers with systemic allergies (16) or management of dry eye in established contact lens wearers who develop rheumatoid arthritis (17). Systemic medications are widely cited as causes of an abnormal tear film (18–27). A survey of 13,517 patients visiting optometry offices across Canada (including 3,285 contact lens wearers) provided data showing that significant risk factors for experiencing symptoms of dry eye included the use of medications for high blood pressure (including diuretics), birth control, stomach ailments, and menopause (28). Many dry eye treatments can be prescribed without discontinuing contact lens wear, albeit with perhaps slightly shorter lens wearing times. This should be accompanied by extra attention to hygiene and lens disinfection. If signs are present and/or develop, however, then contact lens wear should be discontinued, at least temporarily.

In rare cases, significant ocular surface disease (e.g., severe conjunctivitis or keratitis) may develop in the contact lens wearer as a result of either lack of compliance with wear or care regimens (resulting in contamination of the contact lens, lens case, or solutions) and/or inadvertent exposure of the eye to opportunistic pathogens (29–38). The risks of such serious complications of contact lens wear have changed slightly with the use of different contact lens materials, and especially with the type of wearing routine (e.g., daily wear, extended wear, continuous wear). If severe disease develops, contact lens wear should be discontinued and treatment initiated. Prompt discontinuation of contact lens wear and aggressive use of therapeutic pharmaceutical agents are necessary to manage the infection and associated inflammation. With the exception of special cases where a bandage lens is being used, contact lens wear should not be resumed until the eye is very quiet. Understanding the available therapeutic options and the actual selection and use of such therapeutic agents is important, even if the patient is simply being referred to an ophthalmologist. If the contact lens wear-related eye disease is being managed by the optometrist, then the importance of accurate diagnosis and provision of appropriate follow-up care are just as important as knowledge of the ophthalmic pharmaceuticals.

PRINCIPLES OF DRUG ACTION ON THE EYE

Time Base of Actions of Drugs on the Eye (Ocular Pharmacokinetics)

Most drugs used in ophthalmic products can be expected to have a specific action on the eye and periocular tissues. Most of these drugs specifically bind to discrete receptor sites distributed throughout the eye. A receptor-mediated action generally means that drug administration will elicit a defined response from ocular blood vessels, intraocular muscles, etc., or will have a selective action on pathogens compared to the ocular tissues. Furthermore, as a consequence of receptor specificity, two or more drugs can often be effectively and safely combined in a single eyedrop, e.g., combinations of vasoconstrictors with antihistamines, or corticosteroids with antiinfective drugs. For most diagnostic or therapeutic ocular pharmaceuticals, the concentration of the drug(s) in the pharmaceutical is such that there is sufficient quantity of drug to bind to most, if not all, of the available receptors. The concentrations selected are designed to essentially saturate the specific receptors with the drug for a finite period of time so as to produce a maximal response at the receptor level. In vivo, however, a certain time period is generally required for drug penetration to the receptor sites, especially the intraocular sites. As soon as the drug has penetrated to the appropriate receptor sites, bioelimination (or drug washout) starts. Such saturation of the receptor sites, therefore, may last for only a relatively brief period of time, e.g., 30 minutes. The clinical effects then will increase or decrease again. Therefore, when using ocular pharmaceuticals in practice, the overall clinical efficacy will be determined more by the frequency of administration of the pharmaceutical rather than the concentration of the drug (39–42).

Diagnostic, palliative, and therapeutic products are most commonly applied to the external eye as either solutions or suspensions. In the non–contact lens-wearing eye, the active drugs (and other ingredients of pharmaceuticals) disperse from a pharmaceutical form into the precorneal tear film prior to penetrating the corneal and conjunctival epithelia, which are the principal barriers to intraocular absorption (40–43). In addition to being absorbed into the corneal and conjunctival tissues, some of the drugs will pass into the anterior chamber and anterior uveal tissue of the eye.

As indicated, the effect of ophthalmic drugs on the ocular tissues can be expected to be very time dependent and is very much related to normal washout from the ocular surface. Within 1 to 2 minutes of instillation, about half of the drug contained in simple eyedrops can be expected to be eliminated from the ocular surface (44–50). To control the rate of washout, measures should be taken to reduce the rate of nasolacrimal drainage. This can be accomplished by eyelid closure for 30 seconds or application of gentle pressure over the puncta (51). The rate of drug washout will be dependent upon both the drop size and the volume of the tears present at the ocular surface. A topical anesthetic (e.g., proparacaine 0.5% as used as part of the examination of the eye) may substantially reduce the rate of washout by reducing reflex tearing (49), although repeated use of a topical ocular anesthetic also may increase drug penetration as a result of compromise of the epithelial barriers (see section III.C.2). Inclusion of any viscosity-enhancing polymer (a viscolizer, such as hydroxypropyl-methylcellulose or polyvinyl alcohol) will similarly reduce the rate of washout, perhaps by a factor of two (44,48,50,52–55). As a result, both the time period for which the drug is in contact with the ocular surface (50,53,54,56,57) and the quantity of drug entering the eye tissues should increase, so greater clinical effects likely will be observed (52,53,56–59).

Contact lens wear may mechanically compromise the barrier functions of the corneal epithelium and so facilitate enhanced penetration of drugs into the corneal tissue and the rest of the eye (33,60,61). Clinical data in this regard, however, are rather sparse and contradictory. One study suggested a slight, statistically insignificant, increase in the magnitude of mydriasis, produced by eyedrops containing the cholinergic-blocking drug tropicamide (62), in contact lens wearers. In another study, a small but statistically significant decrease was observed in the magnitude of mydriasis that could be produced by the adrenergic drug phenylephrine (63). However, in a case report, an unexpected pupillary dilation was noted in a contact lens wearer who had used an eyedrop containing low concentrations of another adrenergic drug (64). It was concluded that the modest mydriasis had occurred as a result of contact lens wear increasing drug penetration into the eye. Differences in the pH of pharmaceuticals can be expected to alter the transcorneal transfer of ionizable (charged) drugs (40,43). Therefore, contact lens-related hypoxia, either short or long term, and associated changes in the pH of the tear film, cornea, and aqueous humor may modify drug penetration and action. However, any such effects do not appear to be clinically significant.

A similar sequence of events occurs if drugs such as oral antihistamines are systemically administered to manage ocular disease, except that the barriers that need to be crossed are different, i.e., the blood–ocular barriers at the level of the retina, ciliary epithelium, and conjunctiva. Systemically administered drugs ultimately will enter the circulation and reach the eye via the ophthalmic artery and ciliary arteries. After crossing the blood–ocular barrier, drugs can reach the conjunctiva, eyelid tissue, and lacrimal glands. As a result, systemic medication use can affect the tear film and contact lens wear.

The pharmacokinetics discussed earlier primarily apply to the use and action of drugs on the eye when there is no contact lens in place, i.e., the contact lens wearer either is not wearing the lenses or has taken them out prior to the examination. When diagnostic drug use is indicated, contact lenses should be removed prior to eyedrop instillation for several reasons. Prior removal of a contact lens will expedite the examination and prevent unnecessary interruptions later. In the unlikely event of any adverse reaction developing in the period immediately after diagnostic drug instillation (65), delivery of patient care will not be complicated by the presence of a contact lens in the eye. As a general guideline, contact lenses should not be inserted after the use of a topical anesthetic until full corneal contact sensitivity has returned (although there are some special cases to be considered).

For drugs intended for intraocular action (mydriatics, cycloplegics, antiinflammatory drugs), lower anterior chamber drug concentrations may be realized if topical drugs are instilled into an eye with a contact lens in place because, in terms of ocular pharmacokinetics, a very different situation exists when a contact lens is on the eye. There are a number of important issues to be considered, namely, whether the tear-related pharmacokinetics will be different, whether the presence of a contact lens on the eye will alter drug delivery to the ocular tissues, and whether a soft contact lens will absorb the ingredients of eyedrops and be a useful delivery device. Lacrimation kinetics may be different when a contact lens is present on the ocular surface due to subtle alterations in corneal sensitivity with subsequent reductions in reflex lacrimation (which is an important determinant of ocular pharmacokinetics) (66–68). Hydrogel contact lenses absorb the ingredients of eyedrops if they already are in place on the eye, and decreased drug delivery can be expected if eyedrops then are applied over the contact lens surface (69–71). Such types of "on-eye" delivery can be used in the management of contact lens-related dryness, conjunctival hyperemia, and mild papillary reactions (72–80). An issue that also needs to be considered here is whether the presence of preservatives in eyedrops constitutes a risk for contact lens wearers (see section II.B.2).

That a hydrogel lens will readily absorb various drugs can be used advantageously to promote drug delivery to the external eye tissues; this is the premedicated bandage lens principle (81,82). Management of sterile peripheral corneal ulcers with general epitheliopathy could require that eyedrops be instilled over the soft contact lens (83,84) or that a medicated bandage lens be used in early stages. This is slightly different than the situation in which eyedrops are instilled onto a contact lens-wearing eye in that the drug is deliberately absorbed into the contact lens matrix before the lens is placed on the eye. Most hydrogel contact lenses will readily absorb drug from an aqueous solution. If a drug-presoaked contact lens is placed on the cornea, it will act as a reservoir for that drug (85). The drug should wash out of the contact lens matrix, principally by first-order kinetics, mix with the tear film, and then penetrate the cornea (69–71,86,87). Thus, the drug-soaked contact lens can be considered an extended-release device acting for a period of many minutes to prolong drug contact time with the ocular

surface. As a result, higher intraocular drug concentrations result compared to the use of eyedrops containing the same concentration of drug (69,87).

The medicated bandage lens can be selected for therapy of infectious or noninfectious ulcers of the epithelium in which there is the additional complication of rehealing difficulties. The hydrogel lens can be used to provide a protective covering for the corneal surface (60,72,83,88–90). Disposable contact lenses also can be used as bandage lenses (82, 91). A similar protective effect can be achieved with the slowly dissolving "collagen shield"; this too can be soaked in antibiotics prior to placement on the cornea (81,82,92). Although vision is obviously impaired when severe corneal infections are present, better vision may be achieved when a soft contact lens rather than a collagen shield is used as a bandage lens (92).

Principles of Preparation and Use of Ophthalmic Pharmaceuticals and Other Products

General Properties of Ophthalmic Products and Their Use

As a general principle, all ophthalmic products are formulated to meet specific stability requirements (42). Most products should be stored between 15° and 30°C (55°–77°F) and protected from light. By following manufacturers' guidelines on storage, drugs should exhibit the expected efficacy until the printed expiration date. A few products (e.g., topical ocular anesthetics) should best be stored in a 4°C refrigerator both before and after opening and often carry a note to this effect on the packaging, e.g., "refrigerate after opening." It has been established in animal studies that the efficacy of the topical ocular anesthetic proparacaine, which is recommended for refrigeration, deteriorates substantially if the product is kept at room temperature after opening (93). Deterioration is indicated by discoloration of the eyedrops or the appearance of dark-colored deposits around the dropper tip or cap of the bottle (14). As a general rule, however, refrigeration of ophthalmic products provides no extension of product stability unless this is actually stated on the manufacturers guidelines for use (e.g., with some topical ocular anesthetic products). Some diagnostic products even carry the specific warning: "Do not refrigerate." Similarly, some ophthalmic corticosteroid product labels also advise that "Refrigeration may produce harmful products." A practice, advocated by some, of refrigerating eyedrops prior to use is not recommended. Such practices are promoted to decrease the likelihood that eyedrop instillation will be uncomfortable. Notwithstanding such merits of cold eyedrops, such a practice is not recommended because it contradicts the manufacturer's guidelines for use of the product.

For unopened products, shelf life (storage) periods of 1

to 3 years are common for both ophthalmic pharmaceuticals and other products. The primary responsibility of the practitioner is to rotate stocks to ensure that products are used or dispensed prior to the expiration date. Such recommendations should be strictly observed because these products undergo a relatively rapid deterioration once the bottle is opened; product efficacy may decline significantly after this 30-day limit. Some manufacturers have provided a clear blank space on the bottle label where the opening date can be written in by the patient. Other products require specially sealed foil packaging and should be used on the day of opening if the pharmaceutical characteristics are to be those stated on the packaging.

Characteristics of Ophthalmic Solutions in Relation to the Preocular Tear Film

The preocular tear film in a contact lens wearer can be expected to have certain physicochemical characteristics, such as osmolality, electrolytes, pH, and protein and lipid content. Over the years, and especially with changes in contact lens materials and wearing schedules, increasing attention has been given to the composition of ophthalmic solutions so as to match the tears with respect to the first three characteristics.

Many ophthalmic solutions are labeled simply as isotonic. Numerous studies on the tears and lacrimal system of human subjects were performed many years ago to determine the acceptability or tolerance to solutions of differing osmolality (5,94–96). A simple context of equivalents of sodium chloride as a reference was used, with isotonic sodium chloride (NaCl) being between 0.9% and 1.0% weight to volume (w/v). Recent research confirms the 1950s estimates that, from a simple osmotic perspective, the external eye will tolerate occasional exposure to 0.6% and 1.3% NaCl (or its equivalent). Perhaps even 2% NaCl will be tolerated without significant consequence (97). It should be noted, however, that even slightly hypertonic solutions (363 mOsm/kg, about 1.2%) may promote mucin discharge (98). In addition, the overall rate of nasolacrimal drainage has been reported to increase following instillation of hypertonic saline (1.8%) by anywhere from 20% to 100% compared to baseline values (45,99). With either hypertonic or hypotonic saline eyedrops, however, tear film secretion should be return to initial values within about 30 minutes (100).

The tears are a mixture of electrolytes, cations, and anions (61,101). In more recent times, compatibility, if considered from a perspective of maintenance of epithelial physiology in vivo by appropriate electrolytes, probably can be improved by including other salts into artificial tears in addition to sodium chloride (102,103). As a result, a number of rewetting solutions and artificial tears have added electrolytes, namely, KCl, $CaCl_2$, $MgCl_2$, and even bicarbonate. In many cases, such electrolytes also can be added to saline

solutions, but this may not be possible with polymers used in ophthalmic products or with some therapeutic drugs. The electrolytes may alter the physical properties of the polymers (104,105), or insoluble complexes may form.

The pH of ophthalmic products is a different issue. A range of pharmaceutical and psychophysical studies indicate that eyedrop comfort can depend on pH, so this is important. Tear film pH is at least as dynamic as tear film osmolality. An acceptable subjective comfort range of 6.5 to 8.0 is a minimal one, and a slightly wider range likely will be tolerated but there will be a little "sting" to the eyedrops (45,106–108). Although the pH of some ophthalmic products might be outside the range of "normal" tear film pH, clinical measurements indicate that precorneal tear film pH will return to normal values within 10 minutes or less, even when such low pH solutions are used (106,109–111). From a contact lens-wearing perspective, "physiologic" pH seems to be slightly acidic at between pH 6.5 and 7.0, i.e., this is the pH of the post-lens tear film (33,107,112). From a pharmaceutical perspective, acid solutions may sting more than some neutral pH or slightly alkaline solutions, but further research is needed to define the cause of these effects. Solutions with different pH values may elicit different sensations, but it is not a simple matter to formulate ophthalmic products within an ideal pH range in terms of comfort. Factors such as drug solubility and stability in aqueous solutions will generally take priority in the formulation of ophthalmic pharmaceuticals (42,94,113,114). Whereas most eyedrops are likely to be formulated between pH 6.0 and 8.5, a topical ophthalmic anesthetic solution may have a pH that is lower than 6.0 and even close to 4.0 (109), and a topical antihistamine solution might have a pH of around 5.0 (115). This is simply because the optimum stability of some diagnostic and therapeutic drugs is in acidic aqueous solutions. If they were to be formulated at a higher pH, then the solutions would have an unacceptably short shelf life. Equally, if solutions are formulated on the alkaline side and include bicarbonate, special packaging is needed to provide a reasonable shelf life. Eyedrops often contain buffer compounds such as borate, phosphate, acetate, and citrate (42,94,113,114,116). Overall, the concentrations of these buffers usually are modest and unlikely to alter the secretion of the natural tear film buffering agents (bicarbonate, phosphate, etc.). However, the buffer type and its concentration in the eyedrops may determine the rate of recovery of the tear film pH after the eyedrops are instilled (117). In addition, and perhaps due to differences in pH and/or buffering compounds, different buffer ingredients may be tolerated differently. For example, use of a phosphate versus a borate buffer in an eyedrop may be noticed by some individuals (118).

Most ophthalmic pharmaceuticals do not contain proteinaceous or lipid material (119). With increasing interest in biologic peptides for ophthalmic use or the use of lipid-containing artificial tears, consideration of the compatibility of such ingredients with normal tear film proteins and lipids is likely to be a future issue, especially in product marketing.

Characteristics of Ophthalmic Solutions in Relation to Contact Lens Materials

There are several issues here, principally hydration of the lens, uptake of toxic substances (including preservatives) into a contact lens, and possible spoilation of a contact lens by pharmaceuticals.

The wettability and hydration level of a contact lens are important factors in determining comfort and tolerance. A hydrogel lens, on the eye, is likely to dehydrate slightly when the tear film is disrupted (66,85,89,120–124). Desiccation of the contact lens surface is more likely to be significant if the hydrogel lens has a high water content, but this does not mean that wearers of lower-water-content hydrogel lenses will have a more stable tear film! The impact of the osmolality of rewetting drops or artificial tears on such hydrogel lens dehydration in situ has been considered. Initial on-eye responses to soft lens wear with the concurrent use of hypertonic (670 mOsm/kg; 2% NaCl equivalents) or hypotonic (224 mOsm/kg; 0.6% NaCl) rewetting drops indicated no difference in lens hydration, with a 20% lens dehydration found in each case (125). Adapted lens wearers, however, may show a different sensitivity, especially because slight (but statistically significant) lens rehydration on eye has been reported with the use of a series of rewetting eyedrops formulated to 273 to 274 mOsm/kg (121). A slightly different effect would be expected for the newer and lower-water-content silicone hydrogel lenses.

Another issue in terms of ophthalmic solutions and contact lens use is whether a hydrogel contact lens will absorb the ingredients of eyedrops or whether the ingredients of a solution with be adsorbed onto the surface of a rigid lens. Overall, by current perspectives, practitioners should be cautious about generally recommending the use of any eyedrops while a patient is wearing hydrogel contact lenses. The obvious and special exception to this is the use of contact lens rewetting eyedrops that have been specially formulated for this purpose. The reason for this caution relates to the possible absorption of potentially toxic chemicals into the hydrogel contact lens, e.g., benzalkonium chloride, a preservative considered by many as being incompatible with hydrogel lens use. Currently, rewetting eyedrops generally contain other preservatives (see section IV.B). Current manufacturers recommend that contact lenses not be worn when eyedrops containing these drug-preservative mixtures are instilled. Concern has been expressed for a risk of progressive accumulation of preservative in the hydrogel contact lens with such "on-eye" use, and current manufacturer's guidelines for use stipulate that hydrogel contact lenses should not be worn while these products are being used.

The availability of preservative-free artificial tear products is due, in part, to a concern related to the possible interaction between hydrogel contact lenses and preservatives. Use of preservative-containing solutions to manage ocular symptoms in hydrogel contact lens wearers has been considered to result in unacceptable accumulation of preservatives in the contact lens matrix and possible episodes of toxic chemical keratitis (126–128), but this idea of sorption and/or binding of preservatives by hydrogel or GP lenses is not universally agreed upon (73,75,129,130). In the absence of reasonable epidemiologic data, it probably will remain the opinion of the practitioner as to whether or not this is clinically relevant.

These risks have not been considered as either proven or important by some (73,75,129), even with bandage lens use (72,131). Notwithstanding, when a patient who is using various eyedrops (other than rewetting solutions) over a hydrogel contact lens shows any signs of worsening corneal or conjunctival epithelial disease concurrent with the continued lens wear, both contact lens wear and eyedrop use should be discontinued and further investigations initiated. A practitioner should always be on the lookout for any eyedrop use-related (or induced) worsening of comfort or cosmesis in a contact lens wearer, and three studies help put this whole issue into perspective. First, in a deliberate but conservative challenge study, hydrogel contact lens wearers were asked to use a decongestant eyedrop twice daily (b.i.d.) over a period of 4 months (78). The eyedrops were preserved with benzalkonium chloride. Overall, no significant adverse reactions were noted that could be obviously attributed to the use of preservative-containing eyedrops. Other studies, based on measures of the preservative in soft contact lenses, have concluded that, although trace amounts can be detected, the impact should be minimal. For example, with b.i.d. use of an antihistamine eyedrop preserved with benzalkonium chloride, substantial accumulation of the preservative in the hydrogel contact lens would not be expected based on laboratory measures, i.e., a significant "reservoir" effect does not occur with such use (80). However, combinations of preservative-containing drugs, used as eyedrops, may form precipitates in hydrogel lenses (132). Similarly, in a study where another decongestant eyedrop (also preserved with benzalkonium chloride) was used, it was concluded that trace amounts of the preservative could be measured if eyedrops were used while a contact lens was in place (133). Far more importantly, it was noted that an interval of just 5 minutes between instillation of the eyedrops and insertion of hydrogel contact lenses all but eliminated detection of even these trace amounts of preservative in the hydrogel lens. A reasonable guideline appears to be "do not use preservative-containing eyedrops while—or immediately before—wearing soft contact lenses." The remaining issues are whether this can be occasionally ignored and whether the interpretation of "immediately" should be 5 or 15 minutes. A conservative manufacturer or distributor of ophthalmic products may well recommend an interval of 15 minutes, but others would likely argue that this is completely impractical from a clinical perspective.

Pharmaceutical use could cause discoloration of a hydrogel contact lens matrix on the eye. Although lens discoloration can develop, especially over the long term with lenses that are not replaced, it is a minor issue today. An often cited example is that of a black-brown color imparted to hydrogel lenses by use of epinephrine eyedrops (134, 135). The photo-oxidation product causing the discoloration may be removable with extended soaking in 3% hydrogen peroxide. This effect is most unlikely to be encountered today because there is little use of epinephrine eyedrops. This type of lens discoloration is distinct from that observed following certain types of disinfection, sterilization, or cleaning regimens (136,137), or the sorption or (bio)chemical transformation of systemic drugs (138). A hydrogel lens matrix may readily absorb the fluorescein dye used as a diagnostic drug (139), and so a polymer form of the dye is available (see section III.B.2). Common therapeutic drugs, such as prednisolone or dexamethasone-neomycin-polymyxin B combinations, are not expected to be able to stain (discolor) hydrogel lenses (139,140), although white precipitates may form within a hydrogel matrix with repeated clinical use in combination with such therapeutic drugs (132).

DIAGNOSTIC DRUGS USED IN CONTACT LENS PRACTICE

Historical Perspective

The scope of optometric practice now includes the routine use of diagnostic drugs as aids to fitting contact lenses or ocular health examination in general. In the United States, Canada, United Kingdom, and Australia, legislation generally permits the use of diagnostic drugs in all states and all provinces, although their use is restricted to a few designated drugs in some of the Canadian provinces.

Dyes and Stains

Chemical Properties of Dyes and Stains for Ophthalmic Use

Dyes and stains used during examination of the external eye consist of water-soluble organic compounds that will provide greater definition of the precorneal tear film, epithelial cells, or conjunctival cells (Table 41.1).

The terminology (i.e., dyes and stains) is obscure because, according to the mode of usage and the condition of the external eye, these substances may be dyes (i.e., "impart a new [and often permanent] color to [a solution or tissue] especially by impregnating with a dye," Webster's Dictionary) or stains ("a dye or mixture of dyes used in [bio]microscopy to make visible minute and transparent

structures, to differentiate tissue elements . . . ," Webster's Dictionary). Furthermore, even compounds labeled as "vital dyes" by their exponents have been reviewed for their mechanism of action (141–146), making the terminology even more uncertain. Notwithstanding, for now the terms dyes and staining agents probably will continue to be used for ophthalmic products.

Mechanisms of Action and Use of Dyes and Stains for Topical Ophthalmic Use

Three dyes and stains are routinely available for use, namely, fluorescein, rose bengal, and lissamine green. Fluorescein sodium is likely the most widely used dye in routine contact lens practice, but both rose bengal and lissamine green are used for evaluation of ocular surface disorders.

A number of different types of fluorescein sodium are available (Table 41.1). The strips should be stored in a dry place at room temperature. If the outer packaging of the fluorescein strip is damaged in any way, the strip should be discarded (147). The same applies for strips containing rose bengal or lissamine green (see later). For some contact lens fitting procedures, a high-molecular-weight form of fluorescein is available. A sterile solution (e.g., a sterile contact lens saline product) can be used to prewet the strip for patients with aqueous tear deficiencies, and options with three different amounts of fluorescein/strip are available (Table 41.1). A microsized fluorescein strip (with a specially tapered end) has been made available recently because it has been argued that a microdose volume of fluorescein provides the practitioner with a superior diagnostic aid (148). In contrast, should abundant amounts of color or very substantial fluorescence be required, fluorescein 1% or 2% solutions can be used.

The sodium salt of fluorescein is extremely soluble in aqueous solutions at physiologic pH and thus readily mixes with the precorneal tear film. Regardless of the reason for using fluorescein, continued tear production and drainage will wash the fluorescein from the ocular surface within a few minutes (48,58). Some of the dye can be expected to penetrate the cornea and enter the eye rather than simply be washed away (52,58,149). However, any interaction of fluorescein with the corneal or conjunctival tissue is not permanent, and any discoloration of the lid margins and other structures likely will disappear within 15 minutes. Mixing of the dye with the tear film and availability to interact with the ocular surface will occur following either application of a sterile fluorescein-impregnated strip to the bulbar conjunctiva or instillation of drops of fluorescein-containing solutions into the lower cul-de-sac (147, 150–152). For convenience and safety, the use of sterile strips is preferable. Two basic types of phenomena can be visualized with the use of fluorescein, namely, characteristics of the tear film (and its interface with the ocular surface)

TABLE 41.1. OPHTHALMIC DYES AND STAINS FOR TOPICAL OCULAR USE

Compound	Examples of Commercial Products	Pharmaceutical Details	Size
Fluorescein	Ful-Glo	0.6-mg strips, sterile	Pkg 300
Fluorescein	Flurets, Fluor-I-Strip-A.T.	1-mg strips, sterile	Pkg 100, 300
Fluorescein	Fluor-I-Strip	9-mg strips, sterile	Pkg 300
Fluorescein	DET strips	0.1-mg strips with special tip, sterile	
Fluorescein	Fluorescein (generic)[a]	2% solution	1, 2 mL
Fluorexon	Fluoresoft	0.35% solution, unit dose	0.5 mL
High-molecular-weight fluorescein (fluorexon)	Soft-Glo	0.5-mg strips	Pkg 50
Rose bengal	Rose bengal strips, Rosets	1.3-mg strips, sterile	Pkg 100
Rose bengal	Rose bengal 1%	1.0% solution[b]	5 mL
Lissamine green	Lissamine green strips	1.5-mg strips	Pkg 100

[a] Minims fluorescein (0.3 mL) is available in Canada, the United Kingdom, and Australia.
[b] No commercial products listed for the United States, but a Minims rose bengal is available in Canada, the United Kingdom and Australia.

and the integrity of the ocular surface (where the dye highlights or stains aspects of the ocular surface).

For assessment of tear film volume, the dye will produce a dull orange-yellow color if viewed under normal lighting or a brilliant green-yellow color if viewed under long wavelength ultraviolet light via a cobalt blue-yellow filter combination (153). When viewed under either lighting condition, fluorescein may be observed as a shallow crescent along the lower eyelid margin, usually referred to as the tear meniscus or tear prism (154). Some investigators have ventured an opinion that a normal tear meniscus height (TMH) of less than 0.3 mm is an indicator of aqueous tear deficiency (155–157). Evaluation of a range of studies, however, indicates that the normal TMH is actually close to 0.2 mm, with a "normal" value expected to be between 0.1 and 0.25 mm (154). If fluorescein is applied, especially as a solution, the tear prism will be full, and 2 to 3 minutes should be allowed to elapse before an assessment is made (158). The full tear prism stained with fluorescein may persist for many minutes if there is any significant obstruction of the puncta or nasolacrimal ducts or other impairment of the normal nasolacrimal drainage (e.g., poor eyelid–globe contact) (159–161). Use of fluorescein in this way provides a simple and quick assessment of the patency of nasolacrimal drainage.

Fluorescein highlights irregularities in the bulbar conjunctival surface within the palpebral aperture. Such irregularities can be observed with the slit lamp under white light, but after fluorescein instillation and viewing under cobalt blue light these microcreases, microridges, or folds can be readily observed. These irregularities have been referred to as lid-parallel conjunctival folds (LIPCOF), and their presence has been considered, at least by some, as an indicator of dry eye (162). Similarly, fluorescein can be used to highlight patterns across the tarsal conjunctiva following the development of mild-to-severe papillary hypertrophy in contact lens wearers (163,164). Fluorescein assists visualization of the

normal spreading of the tear film. When the eye is viewed under cobalt blue light, a uniformly fluorescent, but dull, film will be briefly evident. This is the thin film of the tear layer on the corneal surface and will persist until the tear film spontaneously disrupts in the absence of blinking. Assessment of the time required for this disruption to occur is the tear breakup time (TBUT) (165). Studies have shown that breakup of the tear film can occur anywhere across the corneal surface, but there can be a tendency for this occur in the inferior or superior aspects of the cornea (166,167) or what have been termed parameniscal zones (167). If tear film breakup occurs in the same location (within probably 0.1 mm or less), then the TBUT not only is likely to be extremely short but is the result of "dry" spot on the corneal surface, a dellen (168).

Fluorescein staining of the tear film is used as a method to accentuate the epithelial surface to improve the reproducibility of corneal thickness measurements by optical pachometry or intraocular pressure (IOP) measurements by applanation tonometry (169–172). Fluorescein is used as a means to detect any defects in the ocular surface, e.g., punctate or localized staining of the corneal epithelium. After the initial film of fluorescein has dispersed, any physical defects on the epithelial surface will tend to serve as local reservoirs for the fluorescein. The result is that any such lesions will continue to exhibit significant fluorescence intensity for several minutes after the fluorescein has been presented to the ocular surface (123,159,173–182). Some cells may actually stain with fluorescein (183,184) or at least adsorb significant quantities of fluorescein (185), especially if the cells are repeatedly exposed to the dye and/or compromised. The position and extent of staining across the cornea and bulbar conjunctiva can be used as an aid in the diagnosis of patient tolerance of contact lens wear. Staining is more likely to occur across the inferior and superior aspects of the cornea (186,187), i.e., in locations similar to where tear breakup is more likely to be observed. A 3- and 9-o'clock staining pattern, across or just inferior to the horizontal meridian and extending across onto the bulbar conjunctiva, has long been considered as an indicator of contact lens wear-related tear film destabilization (173,178,179). For detection of subtle corneal surface lesions, repeated application of fluorescein has been advocated as beneficial (186,188, 189), but it has been found that repeated use of the dye may be mildly toxic and so induce some mild staining in itself (187). As an alternative, a high-molecular-weight fluorescein polymer (see later) also can be used to highlight epithelial defects (190). As noted earlier, it also has been argued that optimum detection of surface staining is best achieved with the minimum amount of fluorescein (148).

A fluorescein-dyed tear film is used to determine the position, alignment, and movement of a rigid (GP) contact lens with the epithelial surface, and, for this purpose, the ordinary fluorescein strips can be used. For the same fitting assessment with a soft (hydrophilic) lens, ordinary fluorescein strips can be used, but the contact lens matrix will be stained if it is in contact with fluorescein for too long. Fluorescein will define the tear meniscus, both at the eyelid margin and around the lens edges. Its presence can serve to highlight whether there are any problems with the apposition of the lens edge and the ocular surface, especially with larger overall diameter lenses. Two forms of a high-molecular-weight fluorescein polymer are available. As originally introduced, this high-molecular-weight fluorescein is called fluorexon, and this polymer of fluorescein is absorbed into soft contact lenses but at a rate some 20 times slower than for ordinary low-molecular-weight fluorescein (191). Fluorescein staining of the contact lens material itself should be minimal, yet the polymer should still be able to define corneal surface lesions (190). Some practitioners advocate that use of high-molecular-weight fluorescein is unnecessary for evaluation of regular soft lens or silicone-hydrogel lens wearers because the contact time of the fluorescein with the lens is short. If the lens is removed, rinsed, and reinserted 5 minutes later, then the chance of significant lens matrix staining is very small. A high-molecular-weight fluorescein strip has been introduced, but no literature is available on either its sorption into soft lenses or its ocular surface staining characteristics.

Rose bengal is a fluorescein derivative that is very soluble in water but is nonfluorescent. It will not commonly be used in contact lens practice simply because patients with a positive outcome from a rose bengal test are not very likely to be contact lens wearers. Like fluorescein, rose bengal can be presented to the eye in the form of impregnated strips (192) or eyedrops (193) (Table 41.1). As with sodium fluorescein strips, the rose bengal strips can be wetted with sterile nonpreserved saline just before use. Providing 1 to 2 minutes is allowed to elapse after dye presentation to the ocular surface, rose bengal will color the tear film meniscus crimson and, unlike fluorescein, will fairly readily stain the eyelid margins (142,143). Part of the reason for this staining is

that rose bengal stains devitalized cells, and our skin is covered with these keratinized squamous cells. For the eye, rose bengal traditionally has been viewed as a vital stain in that it will be taken up by devitalized cells (141,143,180, 194–197). The crimson color is best visualized across the bulbar conjunctiva and is generally well visible across the cornea of individuals with blue irides. Rose bengal also will bind strongly to mucus, so any mucus drops or strands on the ocular surface will be stained crimson.

Some practitioners are reluctant to use rose bengal because it produces ocular discomfort. However, this really should be considered a relatively minor issue and steps can be taken to minimize it. There is a tendency for rose bengal, especially if the solutions are used, to initially produce a some stinging sensation, but this is not always the case. For patients with severe dry eyes, the degree of stinging with instillation of the rose bengal solution has been considered an indicator of the degree of epitheliopathy (197). Although systematic studies of such an effect do not appear to have been published, it can be anecdotally reported that eye closure after rose bengal instillation, and keeping the eyes closed for 30 to 60 seconds, will likely improve staining as well as increase patient comfort. A delay of 1 or 2 minutes after presentation of the dye to the ocular surface usually is required to obtain optimum staining and, if the patient is left with the eyes open, reflex tearing may reduce the probability of obtaining optimum staining. Irrigation of the eye, after this initial interval, may help in optimizing visualization of stained areas and improve patient comfort. After this time, slit-lamp examination should reveal discrete areas that are stained crimson. The extent of punctate or generalized staining on the cornea and bulbar conjunctiva is indicative of the degree of compromise of the ocular surface and can be used diagnostically in dry eye conditions. In borderline cases, the vital staining of cells in the corneal epithelium may not be that evident when grossly viewed against dark irides or when there is hyperemia, chemosis, injection, or even pigmentation of the bulbar conjunctiva; therefore, slit-lamp examination is necessary. The position and/or nature of the vitally stained regions can be documented with simple sketches placed in a patient's record or by photography. Rose bengal staining traditionally has been associated with devitalized tissue (or mucus) and is not readily removed by reflex tear action, or even by irrigation with saline or balanced salt solutions. It has been proposed recently that rose bengal staining of cells can be attributed to loss of a protective mucus coat from the cell surfaces. Without such a protective coat, rose bengal may actually devitalize the cells (146). Similarly, it has been reported, especially in patients with some sort of ocular surface disease, that instillation of rose bengal results in enhanced punctate staining of the corneal epithelium with fluorescein, indicating mild toxicity (198). Regardless of the actual mechanism of action, rose bengal staining still is indicative of compromised cells and so is a vital stain.

A particular aspect of the staining that does not often receive much attention is that affecting the oculomucocutaneous junction. As noted earlier, the use of rose bengal can readily stain the eyelid margins a crimson lake color, which may be particularly noticeable and cosmetically unsatisfactory for those with pale skin color. In addition to this, there may be staining just inside the lid margin. That a strip of conjunctiva, about 1 mm wide and just along the eyelid margin distal to the orifices of the meibomian glands, can be highlighted with various dyes and stains was noted by Marx (199). The phenomenon was confirmed by Norn (142,143), who proposed that this strip of tissue should be called Marx's line.

An alternative to rose bengal, namely, lissamine green, is available in strip form (Table 41.1) but also sometimes as a solution. The overall mechanism of action is likely to be very similar to that of rose bengal (180,193,200). Lissamine green can be used to detect devitalized cells across the bulbar conjunctiva, i.e., so that green-stained punctate lesions will be observed instead of crimson red-stained lesions that would be seen with rose bengal (193,201–203). Lissamine green may be particularly beneficial in staining Marx's line (204) because the green staining likely will be easier to visualize than rose bengal. Use of lissamine green may be better tolerated than rose bengal (193).

Other alternative chemicals include methylene blue and Alcian blue, which have occasionally been advocated for use as vital stains and can be considered possible alternatives to rose bengal (119).

Topical Ocular Anesthetics

Mechanism of Action of Topical Ocular Anesthetics

Topical ocular anesthetics reduce sensations to a range of stimuli (and so allow for contact to the surface of the eye to be made without reflex blinking) and reduce reflex tearing. Local anesthetics, for injection, will produce the same but more substantial and prolonged effects.

The clinical effect of topical ocular anesthetics is limited to the site of application. They have an ability to attenuate the frequency of spontaneous electrical discharges recorded from efferent corneal and conjunctival nerves (205). Studies with nonocular nerve preparations in vivo indicate that these anesthetics block corneal and conjunctival nerve conduction by preventing voltage-dependent activation of nerve ion channels, principally those for Na^+ and K^+ ions (206–208). Nerve conduction blockade usually is considered as nonspecific in that no specific receptor or drug-binding moiety for these drugs has been unambiguously identified in biochemical studies. Nonspecific actions are, most likely, partially responsible for the ability of these drugs (at least in vitro) to reduce or eliminate transcorneal potential difference properties (209,210). Such nonspecific actions also can explain a mild bacteriostatic action that is attributed to topical anesthetics (211–213).

Clinical Effects and Use of Topical Ocular Anesthetics

Topical ocular anesthetics are currently available in concentrations of 0.4% to 0.5% in solution form, although ointment forms have been available. Combinations with fluorescein dye also are available (Table 41.2).

All commercial products containing topical ocular anesthetics may be considered clinically equivalent, even though they may have slightly different anesthetic concentrations (214–219). Lower concentrations of anesthetics have occasionally been advocated, but the currently available commercial products all are suitable for routine use, and practitioners should not consider preparing their own diluted eyedrops. Following the instillation of one or two drops, anesthesia should be effective within 60 to 90 seconds and sometimes in shorter times (211,214,218,220). For 5 to 10 minutes, essentially a complete loss of sensitivity should be present, thus allowing for various contact procedures to be undertaken. Slow recovery then will occur. Typical average times for recovery of some contact sensitivity have been reported to be around 15 minutes (218–220), although the sensitivity to other stimuli (e.g., thermal) may take a little longer to return. Overall, however, as significant sensitivity to stimuli likely will return only 20 to 30 minutes following instillation of anesthetic drops, it is important that all patients be specifically informed of this. Patients should be instructed to avoid rubbing their eyes and not to reinsert contact lenses for, at minimum, 30 minutes after anesthetics have been instilled. These instructions are important so as to minimize the chance of inadvertent ocular surface damage because sensory detection is impaired, e.g., to a foreign body.

Some other effects of topical ocular anesthetics should be considered. Immediately following the instillation of topical anesthetics (with or without fluorescein), some stinging and reflex lacrimation may occur (214,219–222). Substantial reflex tearing can be expected to reduce the efficacy of the topical anesthesia. In cases of eyes with moderate irritation and accompanying lacrimation, two to three drops (separated by, at minimum, 90 seconds) (211) of anesthetic may be necessary to provide sufficient surface anesthesia within a reasonable time period (i.e., 4–5 minutes). The topical anesthesia may reduce the reflex tearing as well (50,160). Overall, any differences in patient reaction to the instillation of ophthalmic anesthetic solutions likely are due to the vehicles in which the anesthetics are dissolved rather than the anesthetic drugs themselves, e.g., tetracaine per se does not sting more than proparacaine, but some tetracaine-containing eyedrops may sting more compared to some proparacaine-containing eyedrops (219,220,223). Similarly, some proparacaine-fluorescein eyedrops may elicit less initial dis-

TABLE 41.2. TOPICAL OCULAR ANESTHETIC AND ANESTHETIC/DYE COMBINATIONS

Drugs	Commercial Products[a]	Pharmaceutical Details	Size
Proparacaine	Proparacaine HCl (generic)	0.5% solution	1, 2, 15 mL or 1 mL UD
Proparacaine	Ak-Taine, Alcaine, Ophthetic	0.5% solution	15 mL
Proparacaine c. fluorescein	Proparacaine HCl and fluorescein sodium (generic)	0.5%/0.25% solution	5 mL
Proparacaine c. fluorescein	Fluorocaine	0.5%/0.25% solution	5 mL
Tetracaine	Tetracaine (generic)	0.5% solution	1, 2, 15 mL
Tetracaine	AK-T-Caine PF	0.5% solution	15 mL
Benoxinate c. fluorescein	Fluress, Fluorox	0.4%/0.25% solution	5 mL

[a] Minims lidocaine 4% – fluorescein 0.25% product is available in Canada and the United Kingdom. Minims Benoxinate (as oxybuprocaine) also is available in the United Kingdom, as are Minims products of proparacaine (proxymetacaine), tetracaine (amethocaine), and proparacaine (proxymetacaine) with fluorescein.
UD, unit dose = single-dose unit (SDU).

comfort than other products containing the same active ingredients (222).

A number of different procedures can be performed with the patient under topical anesthesia. Routine ocular examination procedures include applanation tonometry (169, 224–226) and contact (ultrasound) pachometry (227). Anesthesia of the corneal surface and the presence of fluorescein is generally required for any form of contact applanation tonometry (169,226). The combination of an anesthetic with fluorescein can be produced by instilling a drop of anesthetic onto the cornea and then touching the conjunctival surface with a moistened fluorescein-impregnated strip or by using an anesthetic drop to moisten the fluorescein strip. Combination pharmaceuticals that contain anesthetic and fluorescein are available (Table 41.2), with little difference in their clinical efficacy. The combination products provide the practitioner with both convenience and assurance of fluorescein stability and sterility (228). Anesthetics, usually with fluorescein present, should be used when examination of an irritated eye is performed, e.g., examination for a reported foreign body or an ocular surface laceration. Patients with any form of external eye infection may fail to respond to a single drop of topical anesthetic solution. If extended examination of such an irritated eye is expected, more than one drop may be required. Repeated instillations of ophthalmic anesthetic solutions during the course of an eye examination may, however, produce punctate fluorescein staining of the epithelium (188,211,220), with mild residual conjunctival hyperemia or irritation occurring in some patients after the anesthetic effects wear off (214,221). Such mild effects are very distinct from allergic reaction to the topical anesthetic solution (e.g., tetracaine 0.5%, 2 gtt) in which the epithelium shows intense "spotty, splotchy, confluent or diffuse staining" after a single drop has been instilled (224). It should be noted, however, that this is not excessive use or abuse of anesthetics.

Procedures such as removal of an embedded contact lens require deeper anesthesia; a specially formulated lidocaine 2% solution for injection into the lid tissue has been used

by physicians (229). For fitting of scleral or PMMA lenses, a topical anesthetic usually was indicated (29). Past practices also included the prescribing of tetracaine eyedrops for domiciliary use to ease the discomfort associated with scleral or PMMA lenses (211). It is currently accepted that these products are not indicated for self-use. A long record of clinical reports has established that there is an unacceptable risk of precipitating secondary disease of the cornea or conjunctiva with excessive use of topical anesthetic, especially when abrasive trauma has occurred (230–238). Use of a topical anesthetic during the fitting of hard lenses was considered to allow for more rapid evaluation of the lens-to-cornea fitting relationship and can ease the apprehension of some patients about initial discomfort associated with the wearing of such a lens. The same perspective has been adopted more recently for initial evaluation and the first fitting (dispensing) of GP lenses as well, i.e., a single drop of topical ocular anesthetic (e.g., proparacaine 0.5%) will aid patients in the initial adaptation (239). No side effects were reported in these recent studies. Obviously, such patients need to be informed that there will be a reduced awareness of lens presence if they keep wearing their lenses after the fitting session. If the question arises, they should be advised that the topical anesthetic is not for routine use. If patients were to rub their eyes after such anesthetic application, subjective awareness of the subsequent corneal damage will likely be lessened or even absent and the resultant damage could be substantial.

A closing comment on patient-related factors pertaining to topical ocular sensitivity is appropriate. There is a dearth of useful clinical information on the efficacy of topical anesthetics for contact lens-wearing patients. A reduction in corneal sensitivity in PMMA or GP lens wearers can expected (68,240), and even hydrogel lens wearers may have slight reductions in corneal sensitivity (240). It is not known, however, whether less anesthetic then is required for ocular examination procedures or a different period of effective anesthesia will be observed in patients who already have altered corneal sensitivity.

PALLIATIVE DRUGS USED IN CONTACT LENS PRACTICE

Historical Perspective and the Tear Film in Contact Lens Wear

The preocular tear film plays an extremely important role in the wearing of contact lenses (67). Many contact lens-wearing patients can be expected to experience some type of dry eye symptoms (18,27,28,67,89,120,122,241). With a progressively aging population, tear film compatibility with contact lens wear is likely to become more important, and recent surveys clearly reveal that such patients can still be wearing contacts lenses (28). Older patients (50 years and above) once would have not been considered as candidates for contact lens wear. Similarly, patients with mild-to-moderate dry eye disease (e.g., as associated with rheumatoid arthritis) can still be contact lens wearers with appropriate management of the tear film (17).

There has been considerable interest and research on the physiology and biochemistry of the tears and cornea in both contact lens wearers and nonwearers (67,242–244). However, relatively little is known about how contact lens wear affects the tear film and thus potentially alters drug delivery to the cornea, conjunctiva, and anterior segment. Changes in the tear film following contact lens wear include considerations of tear flow, tear film evaporation, tear film osmolality, tear film pH, tear film buffering capacity, and ion content. Quantities of various proteins usually found in the tear film also may change in contact lens wearers. What is not well understood, however, is how these various factors fail to properly interact and thus produce a tear film that is no longer compatible with comfortable contact lens wear.

Contact Lens Rewetting Solutions and Their Clinical Use

Contact lens wear, in itself, may exacerbate symptoms of discomfort and/or dryness (18,27,89,120,122,241,245, 246). Tired or irritated eyes may require more than just a brief period of discontinuation from contact lens wear (89, 247). Finally, concurrent irritation and minor allergic or inflammatory diseases of the eyelids may destabilize the tear film such that it proves to be very difficult to establish reasonable contact lens wearing times (18,67,89,120,122,241, 248).

There are a number of reasons why a contact lens wearer may develop some discomfort or dryness symptoms while wearing their contact lenses, namely, drying of the lens, destabilization of the tear film, or both. Drying of a lens matrix is a characteristic of hydrogel lenses. A case can also be made that patient-oriented questionnaires can be most beneficial in the diagnosis of symptoms of dry eye in that systemic medication use can be readily identified as a causative factor (27,124,241,249,250). Overall, regardless of the cause of a "dry eye" in a contact lens wearer, symptomatic

relief often can be provided with the use of a rewetting solution or comfort drop (123,251). It really does not matter that the relief may only be brief, for the provision of some relief is better than none at all. It should be noted that patients using rewetting drops may still have some discomfort and some corneal staining (with fluorescein) (123). The important issue is not that either symptoms or signs are present, but that neither is moderate to severe in intensity (severity). A contact lens has an inherent capacity to adsorb various ingredients of the natural tear film (252). A badly soiled contact lens (i.e., one with significant deposits on it) may not wet well and so contribute to destabilization of the tear film. From this perspective, palliative treatment with rewetting drops should be considered as likely to be successful in many patients. Modern-day contact lens rewetting solutions likely will contain ingredients (i.e., surfactants) to reduce this buildup of deposits (251,252). It should be noted that the chronic instability of the tear film likely will lead to the development of ocular surface disease. Similarly, ocular discomfort, associated with tear film destabilization, will likely also be present when there is significant compromise or disease of the ocular surface (see section IV.F).

Regardless of the contact lens type, the first approach to management of the dryness and discomfort associated with contact lens wear is the use of some form of rewetting solution (18,89,120,241). This distinction should be made, compared to what might be labeled an artificial tear or ocular lubricant (251). This distinction is important because, by definition, the patient is still wearing contact lenses, and destabilization of the pre-lens tear film (for hydrogel and GP lenses) and/or desiccation of the lens surface (for hydrogel lenses) likely are initiating ocular discomfort. Numerous contact lens rewetting products are available (Table 41.3).

The impact of various solutions on the wettability of the corneal surface has been considered in detail (168,253,254), but it is still not possible to claim that a particular solution has better wetting properties. Therefore, use of such solutions will still primarily be on a trial-and-error basis.

Based on the rationale that significant dry eye symptoms are associated with tear film evaporation and development of a hypertonic tear film, the rewetting products (or artificial tears) should not be "hypertonic." Overall, it does not appear to be important that rewetting solutions (or artificial tears) range in osmolality from 0.9% to 1.27% equivalents of NaCl, and some artificial tears have an even lower value (94,255–257). In fact, nonviscous salines may prove to be more comfortable to some contact lens wearers (120) or those with dry eyes (258). This is because the use of more viscous solutions may result in faster spoilation of the contact lens surface, and a soiled contact lens is less likely to be comfortable.

Contact lens rewetting solutions are generally equivalent to 0.93% to 1.23% w/v NaCl (255–257,259) but still may be hypotonic to an unstable post-lens tear film and promote

TABLE 41.3. REWETTING SOLUTIONS AND CONTACT LENS COMFORT DROPS[a]

Ingredients	Use	Commercial Products	Size
Hydroxyethylcellulose, polyvinyl alcohol, EDTA, chlorhexidine	RGP	Boston Rewetting Drops	10 mL
Hydroxyethylcellulose, polixetonium	RGP	Claris Rewetting Drops	15 mL
Carbamide, Poloxamer 407, NaCl, EDTA, sorbic acid	RGP SL	Lens Drops	15 mL
Hydroxypropylmethylcellulose, dextran, NaCl, KCl, EDTA, polidronium	RGP SL	Opti-Tears Soothing Drops	15 mL
Hydroxyethylcellulose, NaCl, KCl, poloxamer 407, EDTA, sorbic acid	SL	Clerz 2 Lubricating and Rewetting Drops	15 mL
Hydroxymethylcellulose, NaCl, tyloxapol, EDTA, polyhexamethylene biguanide	SL	Complete Lubricating and Rewetting Drops	15 mL
Polyoxyethylene-propylene copolymers, NaCl, EDTA, sorbic acid	SL	Focus Lens Drops	5, 15 mL
Polyvinyl alcohol, NaCl, KCl, EDTA, benzalkonium chloride	SL	Just Tears Lubricant Eye drops	15 mL
NaCl, EDTA, polidronium	SL	Opti-Free Rewetting Drops, Opti-One Rewetting Drops	10 mL
NaCl, EDTA, sorbic acid	SL	ReNu Lubricating Rewetting Drops	15 mL
NaCl, KCl, EDTA, povidone	SL	ReNu Multiplus Lubricating Rewetting Drops	8 mL
NaCl, EDTA, sorbic acid	SL	Sensitive Eyes Drops	30 mL
NaCl	SL	Lens Plus Rewetting Drops	0.35 mL UD

RGP, for use with rigid gas permeable lenses; SL, for use with soft (hydrogel) lenses; UD, unit dose = single-dose unit (SDU).
[a] All products are available over the counter in the United States and Canada. Similar products are marketed in the United Kingdom (251) and Australia.

contact lens rehydration. Fluid alone is not necessarily sufficient to counteract problems, however, and predicting which eyes or lenses will respond favorably to on-eye use of a rewetting solution remains a process of clinical trial-and-error (120,260,261).

Moisturizers and Other Comfort Eyedrops

Use of a contact lens rewetting drop should both increase the likelihood of the lens surface remaining wettable and provide symptomatic relief; therefore, these products sometimes are called comfort drops (251). A number of other products that may be listed as moisturizers or comfort drops are available, but it is important to distinguish such products from "artificial tears." As with rewetting solutions, it is likely that patients will prefer low-viscosity "salines" (121, 258). The very concept of a rewetting solution for concurrent use with contact lens wear implies that such solutions should be very similar to the natural tears, serving to rewet the ocular surface and provide symptomatic relief. There has also long been an interest in "exotic" (i.e., strange, exciting or glamorous, Webster's Dictionary) eyedrops and the potential beneficial effects of bodily health, diet, and dietary supplements on the eye. This extends into the category products containing various vitamins and natural ingredients (119,251). Some of these are indicated for concurrent use with contact lenses, whereas others are not for use "while

or immediately before" wearing contact lenses. Because no medicinal claims are made for the exotic ingredients, however, the basic formulation (i.e., a form of buffered saline) should be considered as the basis for any patient liking or even having a preference for such products (121,260,261).

Eyewashes and Astringents

Use of a rewetting drop, comfort drop, or moisturizer, in itself, may serve as what might be called a mini eyewash. This is because the volume of the eyedrop generally exceeds the capacity of the cul-de-sac. Instillation of even a drop or two of these products will tend to wash any debris or irritants from the ocular surface and off the surface of the contact lens. Something more substantial is required in some patients in whom the eye needs an eyewash or astringent. For those electing to continue with contact lens wear despite an adverse environment (e.g., smoke, dust, pollutants, smog, allergens), a regular (and even daily) "eyewash" may provide symptomatic relief to allow continuation of contact lens wear and can be expected to improve contact lens wearing times (262).

Eyewashes of saline or borate (or borate-buffered saline) have long been considered beneficial in reducing the symptoms of allergy sufferers (see later), and such individuals obviously can include contact lens wearers. Currently, a range of eyewash products are available, including saline, borate-buffered saline, and phosphate-buffered saline

(Table 41.4). As a general guideline, contact lenses should be removed and the eyewash performed. Because these products can contain preservatives such as benzalkonium chloride, contact lens wear can be resumed later (see section on Characteristics of Ophthalmic Solutions in Relation to Contact Lens Materials).

Use of astringents (defined in Webster's Dictionary as an agent "able to draw together the soft organic tissues) follows from herbal or medicinal remedies for ailments of the eye, including chemicals such as borate (263). Legislation (e.g., from the US Food and Drug Administration [FDA]) is designed to limit the number and types of actions that can be accredited to such products (264). The Federal Register lists zinc sulfate as an approved astringent and indicates that products containing ingredients such as rose petal extract may have mild astringent properties. It needs to be recognized, however, that numerous other "inactive ingredients" can be included in pharmaceuticals that may or may not augment an astringent action (264,265). For both the United States and United Kingdom, such inactive ingredients include extracts of witch hazel, geranium, peppermint, eucalyptus, and camphor. Some of these ingredients also can be found in moisturizer products (see section on Moisturizers and Other Comfort Eyedrops).

The ophthalmic astringents are considered to be extremely mild in action. Unlike topical skin astringents, they are not intended to precipitate proteins but rather simply to provide a soothing and washing effect. The action of ocular astringents might be considered as one such that surface mucus on the corneal or conjunctival surface is modified so as to make its removal easier. Such ideas are a little speculative, as contemporary research studies on the actions of any of these compounds on the cornea or conjunctiva do not appear to have been published. Beyond toxicity testing (e.g., 20 days, 0.25% $ZnSO_4$, q.i.d.) (264), it can only be noted that excessive use of zinc sulfate may retard corneal healing (264) or otherwise alter corneal epithelial integrity

(266). Zinc sulfate is not considered to act as a vasoconstrictor, although it can provide relief for minor eye irritations (264,267). Zinc sulfate has been considered to have a mild bacteriostatic action, although zinc sulfate solutions still generally contain a preservative (268,269). Witch hazel-containing eyedrops have been noted as being able to provide symptomatic relief in allergy sufferers, presumably by removing the allergen (270).

Lid Scrub (Eyelid Hygiene) Products

Individuals with blepharitis are more likely to have substantial bacterial colonization of their eyelid margins (271,272). Any form of meibomian gland dysfunction may result in higher levels of deposits on hydrogel contact lens (273). Mild-to-moderate blepharitis may develop in contact lens wearers and cause tear film destabilization and so result in some ocular discomfort (37,248).

It has long been accepted that if an individual is observed to have clinically significant blepharitis during the prefitting evaluation, then this condition should be successfully treated prior to initiating contact lens wear (29,37,274, 275). Whether it is observed prior to or during contact lens wear, blepharitis can be associated with seborrheic dermatitis and dandruff; therefore, these conditions should be managed as well with suitable shampoo products (276). Scales or greasy accumulations along the eyelid margin are readily removed with a course of twice-daily "lid scrubs" over a few weeks, but they can leave small ulcerative lesions along the lid margin if the scrubbings are performed too aggressively. The use of lid scrubs, along with massage of the eyelid margins, also can be beneficial when there is mild meibomian gland dysfunction in contact lens wearers (277). The ongoing use of such products should improve ocular comfort as well as increase contact lens wearing time. A limited number of products are available (Table 41.5). These commercial lid scrub products are designed to replace

TABLE 41.4. TOPICAL OCULAR WASH AND ASTRINGENT SOLUTIONS

Ingredients	Commercial Products	Size
Saline (NaCl), preservative-free	Oxysept 2, Unisol	15 mL SDU
Borate buffer, benzalkonium chloride	Collyrium for Fresh Eyes Wash	120 mL
Phosphate buffer, NaCl, benzalkonium chloride	Eye Wash, Optgene	118, 180 mL
Phosphate buffer, NaCl, KCl, benzalkonium chloride	Dacriose	15, 118, 120 mL
Borate buffer, sodium carbonate, KCl, EDTA, benzalkonium chloride	AK-Rinse, Eye Wash	30, 118 mL
Borate buffer, sodium carbonate, KCl, EDTA, sorbic acid	Eye Irrigating Solution	188 mL
Acetate-citrate buffer, NaCl, KCl, $MgCl_2$, $CaCl_2$, benzalkonium chloride	BSS, Eye-Stream	18, 30, 118 mL
Zinc sulfate	a	
Witch hazel	b	

All products are available over the counter.
[a] No commercial products listed for the United States, but zinc sulfate eyedrops are marketed in the United Kingdom, and decongestant-zinc sulfate eyedrops are marketed in the United States (Table 41.8).
[b] Also known as *Hamamelis* water. No commercial products currently are available as astringents in the United States, but products containing witch hazel (e.g., Optrex) are marketed in Canada, the United Kingdom, and Australia.
SDU, single-dose unit.

TABLE 41.5. LID SCRUBS (EYELID HYGIENE PRODUCTS)

Ingredients	Commercial Products	Size
PEG-200 glyceryl tallowate, PEG-78 glyceryl cocoate, sodium lauryl sulfosuccinate, cocoamido-propylamine oxide, EDTA, benzyl alcohol	Eye-Scrub	Individual pads 30s and 120-mL bottle
PEG-80, PEG-150 distearate, PEG-15 tallow polyamine, sodium laureth-13 carboxylate, sodium trideceth sulfate, lauroamphocarboxyglycinate, cocoamidopropyl hydroxy-sultaine, quaternium-15	OCuSoft	Individual pads 30s and 120-mL bottle
PEG-200 glyceryl tallowate, PEG-78 glyceryl cocoate, sodium laureth-23, NaCl, glycerin, cocoamidopropylamine oxide, phosphate buffer	Lid Wipes-SPF	Individual pads 30s

the use of diluted baby shampoo (262,278), although such shampoos are still available and can be used at a dilution of around 1:5 in warm water.

Lid scrubs usually are sufficient to control blepharitis; however, a brief course of topical antibiotic therapy may be considered appropriate in moderate-to-severe cases (275). A mild keratitis may develop in chronic cases of blepharitis, perhaps due to sensitivity to staphylococcal exotoxins; therefore, use of topical antibiotic should reduce the likelihood of corneal infection development. External hordeola (styes) are commonly associated with poor hygiene and an underlying blepharitis. Management, in addition to hygiene, requires the external application of hot compresses for several minutes on a daily basis to prompt pointing and eventual discharge of the affected gland. Aggressive management also could include the use of a seborrhetic shampoo containing selenium sulfide at the 1% concentration (276) or 0.5% v/v (275) as a lid scrub. The diluted shampoo should be carefully worked into the eyelid margin with a cotton-tipped applicator. Because selenium is toxic to the ocular surface, direct contact with other parts of the ocular surface should be avoided.

Artificial Tears as Substitutes for Natural Tears

For the majority of contact lens wearers, minor-to-moderate symptoms of discomfort and dryness may be effectively managed with a rewetting solution (see section on Contact Lens Rewetting Solutions and Their Clinical Use). It can be assumed that most contact lens wearers do not have a "dry eye" per se but simply are suffering from symptoms of dryness (27,28). However, a contact lens wearer may develop a dry eye-like condition in which there is clinically significant ocular surface damage, i.e., as visible with fluorescein staining. Such a condition might develop from overwear of contact lenses without the use of rewetting solutions and/or a poorly fitting contact lens. In either case, the pre-lens tear film or that immediately surrounding the contact lens can be considered as simply inadequate (i.e., unstable) to maintain a wetted surface. Similarly, progressive changes in tear secretion and/or stability may result from hormonal changes or the use of systemic medications (27,28).

In such cases, the patient may need something more substantial than a rewetting solution, such as artificial tears or even an ocular lubricant. These generally will not be for use concurrent with contact lens wear (see later). Numerous types of products are available, both in multidose presentation (Table 41.7) and in preservative-free unit-dose options (Table 41.6). Because many of these products contain preservatives (Table 41.7), they should not be routinely used while, or immediately before, the wearing of contact lenses (see section on Characteristics of Ophthalmic Products in Relation to Contact Lens Materials). In addition, it should be noted that although most preservative-free artificial tears would be suitable for use as temporary rewetting agents for

TABLE 41.6. UNIT-DOSE, PRESERVATIVE-FREE ARTIFICIAL TEAR PRODUCTS

Ingredients	Commercial Products	Size
Hydroxypropylmethylcellulose 2910, dextran 70	Tears Naturale Free	0.6 mL UD
Hydroxypropylmethylcellulose 2910, dextran 70, $NaHCO_3$	Bion Tears	0.45 mL UD
Hydroxypropylmethylclelulose, dextran, dextrose, NaCl, KCl	Ocucoat PF	0.5 mL UD
Carboxymethylcellulose, NaCl, KCl, $CaCl_2$, $MgCl_2$, sodium lactate	Refresh Plus	0.3 mL UD
Carboxymethylcellulose, NaCl, KCl, $CaCl_2$, $MgCl_2$, $NaHCO_3$	Thera Tears	0.6 mL UD
Polyvinyl alcohol, polyvinylpyrrolidone, NaCl	Refresh	0.3 mL UD
Polyvinyl alcohol, PEG-400, dextrose, EDTA	Hypoteras PF	0.5 mL UD
PEG-400, dextran 70, polycarbophil, NaCl, EDTA	Aquasite	6 mL UD
Glycerin, NaCl, KCl	Dry Eye Therapy	3 mL UD
Propylene glycol, glycerin, NaCl, KCl, EDTA	Moisture Eyes Preservative Free	

UD, unit dose.

TABLE 41.7. MULTIDOSE ARTIFICIAL TEAR PRODUCTS

Ingredients	Commercial Products	Size
Hydroxypropylmethylcellulose 2910, NaCl, benzalkonium chloride	Isopto Plain, Isopto Tears, Ultra Tears	15, 30 mL
Hydroxypropylmethylcellulose 2910, NaCl, KCl, benzalkonium chloride	Teargen II	15 mL
Hydroxypropylmethylcellulose, KCl, Na$_2$CO$_3$, EDTA, benzalkonium chloride	Tearisol	15 mL
Hydroxypropylmethylcellulose, NaCl, sodium perborate	Genteal	15, 25 mL
Hydroxypropylmethylcellulose, dextran 70, NaCl, KCl, EDTA, benzalkonium chloride	Tears Naturale, Tears Renewed	15, 30 mL
Hydroxypropylmethylcellulose, dextran 70, NaCl, KCl, polyquaternium-1	Tears Naturale II	15, 30 mL
Hydroxypropylmethylcellulose, dextran, dextrose, NaCl, KCl, benzalkonium chloride	Ocucoat	15 mL
Hydroxypropylmethylcellulose, PEG-400, dextrose, glycerin, NaCl, KCl, MgCl$_2$, sodium lactate, ascorbic acid, benzalkonium chloride	Visine Tears	15 mL
Carboxymethylcellulose, NaCl, KCl, CaCl$_2$, MgCl$_2$, stabilized oxychloro complex	Refresh Tears	15 mL
Methylcellulose, propylene glycol, NaCl, methylparaben, propylparaben	Murocel	15 mL
Polyvinyl alcohol, NaCl, chlorobutanol	Liquifilm Tears	15, 30 mL
Polyvinyl alcohol, NaCl, EDTA, benzalkonium chloride	Akwa Tears, Artificial Tears (generic), Teargen	15 mL
Polyvinyl alcohol, NaCl, KCl, EDTA, benzalkonium chloride	20/20 Tears, Just Tears	15 mL
Polyvinyl alcohol, PEG-400, dextrose, EDTA, benzalkonium chloride	Hypotears, Nu-Tears II, Puralube Tears	15, 30 mL
Polyvinyl alcohol, polyvinylpyrrolidone, chlorobutanol	Tears Plus	15, 30 mL
Polyvinyl alcohol, polyvinylpyrrolidone, dextrose, NaCl, KCl, NaHCO$_3$, EDTA, benzalkonium chloride	Murine Tears	15, 30 mL
Propylene glycol, glycerin, benzalkonium chloride	Moisture Tears	15, 30 mL

a contact lens wearer, they are generally not marketed for this purpose.

A variety of polymers are included in these types of artificial tear products and they are not unique; similar polymers are found in rewetting solutions (Table 41.3). It is arguable as to whether one particular polymer is preferable to another, but patient comfort and preference are likely to the be the principal reasons for selection and use of a product.

If an artificial tear is used to facilitate contact lens wear, it has been suggested that several characteristics are ideal (18). There is still, however, little consensus on which, if any, of these characteristics are either more important or essential. A number of issues are worthy of consideration, namely, the interaction of artificial tears with the ocular surface and tear film, the prevention of desiccation of the ocular surface, and the viscosity characteristics of the various products.

On the first issue, an artificial tear should be able to replace the natural tear film (279) and be able to form an optically transparent, smooth, nonirritating coat across the corneal and conjunctival surfaces. This requires an effective wetting action of the artificial tears. For example, mucomimetic action traditionally was considered important because the preocular mucus layer was believed to facilitate "wetting" of the epithelial surfaces (168,253). Thus, polymers such as povidone (polyvinylpyrrolidone) have been considered wetting or "mucomimetic" agents (244). However, even if they were good mucomimetic agents, this does not necessarily mean that their use would result in an adequate

tear film. For example, povidone has not been found to be a good stabilizer of artificial tear films (280,281).

On the issue of desiccation in "dry eyes," the supplying of adequate water to both the lenses and the ocular surface also can be considered important. The normal human corneal epithelium is able to respond rapidly to exposure to hypotonic (or hypertonic) saline solutions (282), but how a stressed corneal epithelium will respond is unknown. It has been argued that hypotonic artificial tears could serve to rehydrate the surface cells and increase the volume of the tear film (61,283). Such products can clearly provide clinical relief, yet there is still an absence of clear clinical evidence indicating either that the corneal epithelial squamous cells are dehydrated in a "dry eye" (caused by tear hyposecretion) or that hypotonic artificial formulations actually serve to rehydrate these cells (284).

The appropriate viscosity for artificial tears is a complex issue. For contact time and duration of effect, it is still generally considered that for artificial tears (or rewetting solutions) to be clinically effective, then prolonged contact with the ocular surface is important. The viscosity of normal tears can be considered as low because nasolacrimal drainage via the puncta is rapid (46). Although it is still unclear whether the viscosity of the pre-lens tear film changes in patients with tear film aqueous deficiency, many artificial tears (and rewetting solutions) contain various polymers to increase viscosity. If of suitable molecular size and in sufficient concentration, they should raise the viscosity of the solutions by around fourfold (44,54,104,285). The amount of time that such solutions can be in contact with the surface of the eye increases, because the rate of drainage slows down (44,56). As a result of this slowed elimination, the bulk volume of the tear film at the surface of the eye may increase and tear film stability generally should increase (107,286, 287). Such an increase in stability may be sufficiently large that the measurable TBUT will increase. Although generally beneficial, there is a limit to the use of some viscolizers, especially the older ones. Prolonged retention of a more viscous polymer solution may not only fail to provide relief but can exacerbate symptoms. Furthermore, different polymers and various strengths of these polymeric viscolizers may generally prove to be unacceptable to some patients (288).

Artificial tears should have minimal toxicity to ocular surface cells because they are likely to be frequently used. From an overall perspective, rewetting solutions and artificial tears should present a minimal toxic risk to the epithelial cells of the cornea and conjunctiva, as well as the rest of the eye. Most of these solutions, directly or indirectly, will have been assessed by a Draize test or its equivalent for a 21-day regimen of use (264,289). Notwithstanding, there is still a commonplace adverse press toward some ingredients of these solutions, such as the preservatives (290,291). If a patient reports intolerance (which could be due to the presence of a preservative) (14,15,291,292), the eyedrops or solutions should be changed. Similarly, a case can be made that, in cases of where a long-standing epitheliopathy already is present, nonpreserved saline or other nonpreserved eyedrops should be used (including when a bandage lens is being used) (83). A sensible approach would be to consider the use of unit-dose, preservative-free products when there is either a chronic history of ocular surface compromise or an acute episode of the same. Such preservative-free products are available (Table 41.6). The majority of patients, including contact lens wearers, can be adequately managed with a preservative-containing artificial tear. A number of multidose products are available (Table 41.7).

In summary, for artificial tears and contact lens wear, many issues can be raised concerning patient acceptability and the physiologic consequences of the use of rewetting solutions or simple artificial tears on the ocular surfaces, especially when a contact lens is in place. All of these issues (mucomimetic effects, osmolality, viscosity, compatibility, pH) probably contribute to patient tolerance and comfort and limit the potential impact of desiccation of the ocular surfaces. However, the ideal solution has yet to be realized, and it is perhaps for this reason that a number of other alternatives periodically receive significant attention. A number of alternatives to simple saline/polymer-containing artificial tears have been advocated (119) and usually presented as being more natural and/or more compatible with the ocular surface. As with the moisturizers (see section IV.C), ingredients have included various vitamins, lipids, blood extracts, and herbal ingredients. Within an overall context of health and medications, one also can consider nutritional balance and the potential effects of malnutrition in the tear film. No unequivocal association has been established between diet and remission of dry-eye states in a well-nourished population, regardless of whether or not they wear contact lenses (293).

THERAPEUTIC DRUGS USED IN CONTACT LENS PRACTICE

Overall Perspective

Topical ocular pharmaceuticals and some orally administered medicines can be used for treatment of various types of contact lens or non–contact lens-related ophthalmic complications or ocular disease encountered during contact lens wear. Conditions such as blepharitis, corneal abrasions, GPC, various forms of noninfectious and infectious keratitis, and various inflammatory conditions affecting the anterior segment of the eye can be encountered during routine contact lens wear. The goal of therapeutic intervention is to keep any adverse reaction to contact lens wear to a minimum or to maximize comfort in a contact lens wearer. In rare situations, urgent intervention is needed to combat severe disease that has developed as a result of contact lens wear, e.g., an infected corneal ulcer.

The involvement of optometrists in the use of therapeutic drugs for contact lens wearers will much depend on their training. Without full training (e.g., the Treatment and Management of Ocular Disease [TMOD] in the United States), the use of therapeutics likely will be limited to the use of over-the-counter (OTC) preparations, whereas with full training many contact lens specialists will manage most conditions, including just about anything an ophthalmologist specializing in cornea would manage. In the following sections, the various levels of intervention are considered.

Direct-Acting Decongestants

General Utility and Use of Topical Ocular Decongestants

The conjunctival vessels dilate in response to any form of stress or trauma (294–297). An eye may already have some background level of mild response (e.g., hyperemia) or develop this condition during contact lens wear. The hyperemia may be cosmetically unappealing, and a certain degree of discomfort may be associated with the condition. Such vasodilation is distinct from neovascularization, which must be treated as a chronic inflammatory condition (see sections V.E. and V.F.). Decongestants are designed to improve the appearance of the eye, and their use also can make the eye feel more comfortable. As a general rule, topical ocular decongestants are not for use during or immediately before wearing hydrogel lenses, but occasional use by contact lens wearers is not unlikely.

Conjunctival vasodilation may be general and involve only the finer vessels (hyperemia) or be more localized and affect only the major vessels (injection). In some cases, the nature of the irritant stimulus may be such that all vessels are involved and a distinct "red eye" develops. If the cause can be established as essentially a minor irritant, then the use of decongestants is appropriate. There are also some special cases where decongestants can be used to promote comfort in infected eyes (see section on Management of Viral Infections in Contact Lens Wear).

Many ophthalmic decongestants are available for treatment of minor-to-moderate hyperemia and injection (Table 41.8). These products are designed to attenuate mild reactions to irritant stimuli regardless of the actual nature of the stimuli. These pharmaceuticals are intended "for the relief of redness of the eye due to minor eye irritations" and generally carry a warning of the type: "Do not use for more than 72 hours except under the advice and supervision of a physician. If symptoms persist or worsen, discontinue use of this product and consult a physician" (264). Decongestants are not for use in acute-onset red eyes that result from bacterial infections (298) or toxic insult (e.g., hydrogen peroxide) (14).

These ophthalmic decongestants contain drugs that primarily act as agonists at α_1-adrenergic receptors, e.g., phenylephrine, naphazoline, tetrahydrozoline, or oxymetazoline (Table 41.8). The introduction of these α_1-adrenergic drugs in the 1950s replaced the use of nonspecific remedies such as boric acid (299) or a range of other drugs such as hydroxyamphetamine 1% eyedrops (300) or epinephrine 1:1,000 eyedrops (299,267,301) used as vasoconstrictors (decongestants). Oxymetazoline, a drug with both α_1- and α_2-adrenergic action, was introduced in the late 1970s (302,303). At the concentrations used, all of these adrenergic drugs act as vasoconstrictors on the more superficial vessels (veins) to whiten the eye (304–307); they often are referred to as eye whiteners. The effect of these products should be rapid in onset (i.e., within 1 minute) and should last for, at minimum, 1 hour. If slightly higher concentrations or perhaps multiple drops are used, tetrahydrozoline 0.1% should have some effect on conjunctival vasodilation within 30 seconds, with the effect lasting from 3 to 4 hours (306).

Most current products contain somewhat lower concentrations of vasoconstrictors (Table 41.8), perhaps because of concerns over possible ocular or systemic side effects (see later).

Clinical Actions and Efficacy of Topical Ocular Decongestants

The various decongestant-containing products can be expected to promptly reduce vasodilation (hyperemia) (118, 302,306,308–313). Appropriate use of these decongestants also should help relieve symptoms such as irritation, mild burning, and photophobia (304,305,313). Some studies indicate that reflex lacrimation (watery eyes) also may be reduced after the use of topical decongestants (304,305, 309–311,314).

All of the presently marketed OTC solutions containing decongestants can be considered as having similar efficacy in simple cases of irritant-related conjunctivitis (309,310, 311,314–316). Their combination with antihistamine (see section on Combination Products of Decongestants with Antihistamines), an astringent such as zinc sulfate (267), or a chemical such as methylene blue (317) or brilliant blue (278), may provide extra relief and added cosmesis. Combination products with antihistamines were introduced to provide relief from dryness symptoms and to produce a

TABLE 41.8. TOPICAL OCULAR DECONGESTANTS

Ingredients	Commercial Products	Size
Phenylephrine 0.12%[a]	AK-Nefrin, Prefrin Liquifilm	15, 20 mL
Phenylephrine 0.12%	Relief	0.3 mL UD
Naphazoline 0.012%	Allergy Drops, Clear Eyes, Naphcon	15 mL
Naphazoline 0.02%	Vasoclear	15 mL
Naphazoline 0.03%	Allergy Drops Maximum Strength	15 mL
Naphazoline 0.1%	Naphazoline Eye drops (generic)	15 mL[b]
Naphazoline	AK-Con, Albalon, Nafazair, Naphcon Forte, Vascon Regular	15 mL[b]
Tetrahydrozoline 0.05%	Tetrahydrozoline (generic)	15, 30 mL
Tetrahydrozoline 0.05%	Colyrium Fresh, Eyesine, Geneye, Murine Tears Plus, Optigene 3, Tetrasine, Tetrasine Extra, Visine, Visine Advanced Relief	15 mL (some 22.5, 30 mL)
Oxymetazoline 0.025%	Ocuclear, Visine L.R.	15, 30 mL
Phenylephrine 0.12%, zinc sulfate 0.25%	Zincfrin	15 mL
Naphazoline, zinc sulfate 0.25%	20/20 Eye Drops, Clear Eyes ACR Eye Drops, Vasoclear A Eye Drops	15, 30 mL
Tetrahydrozoline, zinc sulfate 0.25%	Visine AC	15 mL

[a] Phenylephrine 0.125 also is found in combination with the antibacterial drug sulfacetamide (Table 41.14).
[b] Prescription-only product in the United States; over the counter elsewhere.
[c] Combination products with antihistamines also are available (Table 41.9).

"calming effect on blepharospasm" following application (304). It has not been established if any particular drug (or combination) displays a greater efficacy in contact lens wear-related conjunctivitis, either in management of the condition or as prophylactic agents.

The recommended doses for symptomatic relief and cosmesis (i.e., whitening of the eye) vary widely, ranging from 1 to 8 drops per day in each eye. Such products should not be used p.r.n. for long periods. This is a current perspective and differs from optimistic ideas on the general utility of these types of products, i.e., they were once advocated for p.r.n. use (304). However, with professional supervision there is no reason why the use cannot be intensive, providing the patient tolerates this and there are no medical contraindications to intensive use.

Despite the vagueness regarding suitable dosing, the regular use of topical ocular vasoconstrictors and/or antihistamines in contact lens wearers probably dates back to the introduction of glass scleral lenses, when improved tolerance to these lenses was noted following use of such pharmaceuticals (295). The routine use of vasoconstrictor-containing (rewetting) solutions during adaptation to contact lens wear has been advocated (74) and most likely is commonly performed with OTC product use. For hydrogel contact lens-wearing eyes, the extended use of tetrahydrozoline (2 gtt, b.i.d. for 4 months) was reported to have no obvious beneficial effects on contact lens-related mild conjunctival changes (superficial punctuate keratitis [SPK], follicles, vasodilation) (78). No substantial complications were found to develop with this chronic use of a decongestant in contact lens wearers. Use of decongestants (with or without antihistamines) can be combined with astringents, and their actions have long been considered superior to the use of astringents such as zinc sulfate (304,305). Contemporary and objective evaluations to support such ideas are largely lacking and would be beneficial.

A recurrent issue with the use of topical ocular decongestants is whether there is rebound vasodilation with overuse. Such considerations arise from the rebound congestion that can follow nasal application of vasoconstrictors (318). For the most part, the evidence supporting such a specific effect on conjunctival vasculature is lacking, even though there are warnings on some product packaging that this can occur. For example, the intensive use of topical decongestants in both animal eyes (319) and human eyes (304,309) not subjected to a specific irritant solution has not been found to produce a rebound effect. No rebound vasodilation was observed in human eyes following acute irritant testing and subsequent use of decongestants even as frequently as eight times per day (320). It is possible that vasodilation noted in studies assessing the medium-term use of decongestants, however, reflect a rebound effect, i.e., the blood vessels dilated to a greater degree to that observed in the absence of decongestant use (78). Similarly, pharmaco-vigilance studies of the long-term use of ocular decongestants clearly indi-cate that overuse of these products can produce significant hyperemia (321), and that this can be part of a general irritation response of the conjunctiva that included a follicular reaction. The question that must be asked is whether there was a rebound vasodilation or whether the abuse of such products produced a general irritation (a medicamentosa) that included hyperemia and injection (14). Overall, specific rebound effects and/or general hyperemia are possible outcomes of the use of ocular decongestants. Thus, as part of the assessment of an irritated eye, patients could be asked to refrain from use of these OTC medications for 1 day prior to reexamination.

Although some ocular irritation can develop with overuse, these topical ocular decongestant/antihistamine drugs (Tables 41.8 and 41.9) have an excellent safety record. This is why they usually, but not always, are available OTC. Excessive use of such adrenergic vasoconstrictors or antihistamines can result in complications, however, and it is only with supervised use that these complications can be prevented. Alternatively, the practitioner needs to be alert to the signs and symptoms that could indicate inappropriate use. There will always be individuals, including contact lens wearers, who will attempt to alleviate the symptoms of any acute red eye with these products (64,322). In addition to potentially allowing an infectious conjunctivitis to progress, dilute solutions of phenylephrine may produce a slight pupillary dilation (118). The same can be expected with overuse of naphazoline (64,304,305) and tetrahydrozoline eyedrops (301). An enhanced effect might be observed in a contact lens wearer (64), even without overuse of the products. However, the use of one or two drops of tetrahydrozoline has been found to produce either no mydriasis (313) or only a just-measurable mydriasis (323). Repeated use oxymetazoline eyedrops has not been found to produce measurable pupillary dilation (118,302,313,324). Whereas a just-measurable mydriasis was found with drops of xylometazoline with the antihistamine antazoline (325), a single challenge with tetrahydrozoline with the antihistamine chlorpheniramine was found to produce slight pupillary dilation (323). The additive effect of the antihistamine was attributed to its mild cholinergic blocking actions. One has to conclude that some pupillary dilation could occur with the use of these products. This is important because, in at-risk (susceptible) individuals, the mydriasis may be associated with acute-onset angle-closure "glaucoma" (322). This is the reason for the small-print warning on some of these products that they should not be used in individuals with "glaucoma." All such decongestants should be used with caution and should not be recommended for use in patients who are known to have an extremely narrow anterior chamber angle or active glaucoma. Pupillary dilation is more likely to be evident under lower levels of illumination and in blue-eyed individuals and probably is more likely when there is some significant compromise of the corneal epithelial barrier (322,326).

Antihistamines with Ocular Effects

Combination Products of Decongestants with Antihistamines

One aspect of the vasodilation of the conjunctival vasculature is regulated by histamine. Histamine is a well-known vasodilator (294) released by mast cells and white blood cells within the conjunctiva as part of the inflammatory response. It is generally accepted that contact lens wear per se can precipitate an inflammatory (allergic-type) reaction suggestive of histamine release (327–331). There is a special case for contact lens wearers in that the allergic reaction could be due to bacterial antigens or toxins in cases with blepharitis or due to low-grade chronic infection of the eyelid margins without substantial signs of blepharitis (330, 332). A logical approach to management of these types of ocular irritation is use of an antihistamine, i.e., a drug with histamine H_1-receptor blocking activity.

As noted earlier, ocular decongestants should produce vasoconstriction and help relieve symptoms (e.g., irritation, mild burning, photophobia, reflex lacrimation) (304,305, 309,310,314). From a cosmetic effect, an antihistamine such as antazoline would not be expected to produce substantial vasoconstriction (333). However, in both animal (298,334) and human eyes (310,333), use of topical decongestants (e.g., naphazoline, tetrahydrozoline, oxymetazoline) has been shown to be able to attenuate histamine-induced conjunctival vasodilation. Therefore, a topical ocular antihistamine could be used in combination with a decongestant (see section on Antihistamine Eyedrops). With the addition of an antihistamine to a decongestant, significant relief from itching should be provided (309,314, 335).

Ophthalmic products containing histamine H_1 blockers (e.g., chlorpheniramine, pheniramine, and, much later, antazoline) have been evaluated (295,304,309,336). The currently marketed products contain combinations of vasoconstrictors and histamine H_1 blockers (Table 41.9). Other antihistamines, such as pyrilamine and pheniramine, have been used as adjuncts to decongestants (314). Overall, these combination products were once widely used and will still have a general use as OTC products, but they likely have been superseded given the higher-efficacy topical histamine H_1 blockers (see section on Antihistamine Eyedrops).

Antihistamine Eyedrops

A number of other direct-acting topical ocular antihistamines (H_1-blocking drugs) have been introduced in recent years for the management of seasonal allergic conjunctivitis. All should be suitable for management of this condition in contact lens wearers.

Levocabastine (337–342) was introduced in 1994, followed by azelastine (343–346) and emedastine (347). The latest additions are olopatadine (348,349) and ketotifen (349,350) (Table 41.10). The last two drugs, olopatadine and ketotifen, should be considered special antihistamines because both drugs have secondary actions as mast cell stabilizers (see section on Indirect-Acting Antihistamines with Mast Cell Stabilizer Actions).

The efficacy of topical ocular antihistamines has been assessed in several ways, largely in non–contact lens wear-related situations. Older reports on the clinical action of products containing these drugs simply noted whether there was improvement of ocular symptoms in patients suffering from typical allergic reactions as a means to comparing drugs and products. Such general efficacy, tolerance, and safety studies have been reported for some of the current topical ocular antihistamines. However, in more recent studies, it has become commonplace to use a conjunctival challenge test. This is an important development because it is now the standard by which products are compared. When using data from such challenge tests to make comparisons, however, it is important to note that the particular challenge tests can be very different.

The conjunctival challenge test was developed in an attempt to provide an objective means of comparing a wide range of decongestant drugs with or without antihistamines (307). The challenge test has two components. The first component is assessment of the extent of the reaction. The second component is use of the decongestant/antihistamine and assessment of the extent of the recovery from the challenge (or attenuation of the reaction). Differences in the protocols should be carefully considered before concluding that one drug or product is superior to another.

TABLE 41.9. COMBINATION TOPICAL OCULAR ANTIHISTAMINES WITH DECONGESTANTS

Drugs	Commercial Products	Size
Pheniramine 0.3%, naphazoline 0.025%	Naphcon-A Solution	15 mL
Pheniramine 0.315%, naphazoline 0.027%	Opcon-A Solution	15 mL
Antazoline 0.5%, naphazoline 0.05%	Vascon-A Solution	15 mL

All of these products are available without prescription as over-the-counter medications in the United States and Canada. In the United Kingdom, a combination of oxymetazoline with antazoline (Otrivin-Antistine) is available.

TABLE 41.10. TOPICAL OCULAR ANTIHISTAMINES

Drugs	Commercial Products	Size
Levocabastine 0.05%	Livostin	2.5, 5, 10 mL
Azelastine 0.05%	Optivar	10 mL
Emedastine 0.05%	Emadine	5 mL
Olopatadine 0.1%	Patanol[a]	5 mL
Ketotifen 0.025%	Zaditor[a]	5, 7 mL

[a] Products have some mast cell stabilizer activity as well (see section on *Indirect-Acting Antihistamines with Mast Cell Stabilizer Actions* and Table 41.11).

For example, with histamine being part of the reaction, some challenges have involved the instillation of eyedrops containing histamine salts, usually 50 to 75 µg/mL. The resultant reaction is graded on a four-point scale (0 to 3+) (314) or a five-point scale (0 to 4+) (303,310). Such grading schemes replace the older descriptive terms of as mild, moderate, and severe reactions (307). Assuming effective delivery of single drops, these types of histamine challenges should have resulted in actual histamine doses to the ocular surface of 4 µg or less. In some cases, much higher doses have been used, e.g., 10× (336) or even 100× this level (337). The eye can be alternatively challenged with a ragweed pollen extract (e.g., using a solution of 5,000 allergen units/mL) and the reaction graded on a four-point scale (0 to 3) (309). The outcome of challenges with various plant allergen or allergen mixtures (e.g., those containing ragweed and blue grass extracts at a concentration of 100,000 allergen units /mL) have been graded on four- or five-point scale in other cases (335,351). Cat allergen extract (dander) has been used in more recent studies (351). Different signs and symptoms may have been selected for assessments. Assessments might include just redness (hyperemia), but they can include redness, lid swelling, chemosis, tearing, and itching (335,343). Both the strength of the challenge agent and the nature of the grading scales can be different between studies, and the outcomes may seem different.

In most cases, challenges with single entities have involved the instillation of a decongestant and/or antihistamine drug 5 to 15 minutes after exposure to the allergen. With such test protocols, the degree of reversal of redness and itching can be assessed, perhaps over a period of 10 minutes, using the same set of subjective scales (303,309, 351). The protocols can, however, be very different. For example, the antihistamine might have been instilled just 1 minute after the histamine challenge, e.g., in some studies with levocabastine (341). In contrast, the efficacy of some topical ocular antihistamines has been assessed by instillation 20 to 30 minutes after a challenge with allergen extracts (343).

Greater emphasis appears to have been placed on a different type of challenge recently. The reverse scenario has been evaluated, i.e., how well will an eye be able to cope with an allergen if it was previously treated with an antihistamine.

Again there are substantial differences in the protocols used. For example, the efficacy of decongestants or antihistamines has been assessed by instilling the allergen 10 minutes after the decongestants or antihistamines (335,347,351,352), instilling the allergen 30 minutes after the drugs (348), or instilling the allergen 1 hour after the drugs (353). With this change of protocol, an even more realistic challenge is to assess the impact of exposure to airborne pollen grains in a special room as opposed to instilling eyedrops containing allergens (354). For example, the efficacy of azelastine eyedrops has been assessed by challenging subjects with airborne pollen 1 hour after instillation of azelastine drops (354).

These various types of challenge tests require that the appearance of the eye be graded, and such grading has been supported by an appropriate set of photographs in recent studies (351). In contrast, the symptoms of itching are graded by the test subjects, after they are presented with certain guidelines. Grading of the conjunctival response to irritants can be performed by using close-up photographs as opposed to slit-lamp evaluations (355).

In summary, a rather complex set of evaluation strategies have been used for antihistamine eyedrops. Beyond checking the details of the protocols used, it is beneficial to consider the overall clinical perspective of the challenge tests. As noted earlier, although histamine and vasodilation have long been associated (295), only some patients respond to even recognized allergens with a detectable increase in tear film histamine levels (333,356,357). Changes in the appearance of the eyes, as might be expected, are dose dependent for the allergen (351). In the studies that have been reported, the histamine levels in the tears do not appear to exceed 50 ng/mL in either allergen- or contact lens-related reactions (333,356–359). The challenge tests may actually produce a moderate red eye, but the levels of histamine or allergen used usually are grossly in excess of irritant-related tear film levels. From a pharmacokinetic perspective, it is possible that a hydrogel contact lens may provide a reservoir effect such that there will be a sustained elevation of tear film histamine (or other inflammatory mediators) at the ocular surface. Even with such effects, however, the resultant levels of inflammatory mediators still would not be expected to be anywhere near those used in many of the challenge tests.

Any of these topical ocular antihistamines should be suitable for management of seasonal allergic conjunctivitis in contact lens wearers, but there are few specific studies on this. For example, use of olopatadine eyedrops b.i.d. over a few weeks was found to reduce symptoms, redness, and papillary reactions in contact lens wearers (360). Notwithstanding, a wide range of efficacy and tolerance studies on these products (337,338,340–350) indicate that they should be effective in contact lens wearers.

Overall, two issues regarding the use of antihistamines have arisen, namely, efficacy and comfort. The comfort issue is simple, but assessment of efficacy is complicated by the fact that different tests have been used. On the comfort issue, bearing in mind that the ocular reaction to allergens can produce significant morbidity (e.g., ocular discomfort referred to as the awful itchy-burnies), it is somewhat surprising that patients can prefer different antihistamine eyedrops despite their overall ocular discomfort (115,349,361). The differences in acceptability of the antihistamine eyedrops, as with decongestants (118), unlikely are due to the antihistamines per se but rather to the vehicle. In the case of antihistamines, the pH of the vehicle appears to be a possible cause for the temporary discomfort experienced after the use of some products (115).

Oral Antihistamines

For some patients, including contact lens wearers, adjunct use of oral antihistamines may be beneficial to reduce the need to repeatedly instill eyedrops, as well as to manage nasal symptoms (rhinitis and congestion). Use of an oral antihistamine may reduce ocular signs and symptoms, although only some oral antihistamine-containing products have a documented ability to accomplish this goal. Therefore, whether it is the management of seasonal allergic conjunctivitis or perennial allergic conjunctivitis that is being considered, it seems logical to select those oral antihistamines that have been specifically evaluated (Table 41.11), such as chlorpheniramine (362), azelastine (363), loratadine (353,364,365), cetirizine (366–368), and fexofenadine (365,369–371).

Antihistamines are used to "dry up" secretions (i.e., a runny nose). For some patients, watery eyes might be reduced (i.e., antihistamines are beneficial). Use of oral antihistamines can reduce the ocular symptoms associated with allergic conditions, e.g., watery and itchy eyes (353, 362–371). A challenge test has been used for oral antihistamines, e.g., allergen eyedrops administered 1 hour after ingestion of the oral antihistamine loratadine (353).

Drugs such as chlorpheniramine have been classified as "sedating antihistamines" for many years (372). With the introduction of newer second-generation oral antihistamines, they then have been presented as "nonsedating" and superseded by even better lesser-sedating drug options, e.g., acrivastine (373,374), loratadine (353,364), terfenadine (375,376), astemizole (377,378), cetirizine (379), and fexofenadine (369–371).

Oral antihistamines are indicated for use on a q.i.d. (older antihistamines) to q.d. (newer antihistamines) basis. It should be noted, however, that an exaggerated response might indicate slight aqueous tear deficiency (380). Specific studies, supported by epidemiologic data, strongly indicate that use of oral antihistamines is associated with dry eye symptoms (27,28). This must be considered a minor response because relief from irritation and watery eyes often is beneficial to the patient. Notwithstanding, for contact lens wearers, the drying effect might prove occasionally problematic. Because tear hyposecretion likely is associated with the ability of these drugs to also block cholinergic receptors, it would be expected to be greater with the older sedating antihistamines. For contact lens wearers, therefore, it might be beneficial to simply avoid use of the older drugs and to recommend a second-generation drug, such as fexofenadine.

When oral antihistamines are to be recommended to patients, an issue that must be addressed is whether their use may cause systemic side effects. The side effect considered to be most important is that of sedation, with the older

TABLE 41.11. ORAL ANTIHISTAMINES WITH OCULAR EFFECTS

Drugs	Commercial Products	Size
Chlorpheniramine 2 mg	Chlo-Amine[a]	Pkg 96
Chlorpheniramine 4 mg	Chlorpheniramine (generic),[a] Aller-Chlor,[a] Allergy,[a] Chlor-Trimeton Allergy 4h[a]	Pkg 24, 48, 100
Chlorpheniramine 8 mg	Chlor-Trimeton Allergy 8 h[a]	Pkg 24
Chlorpheniramine 12 mg	Chlor-Trimeton Allergy 12 h[a]	Pkg 15
Brompheniramine 4 mg	Dimetapp Allergy[a]	Pkg 24
Phenindamine 25 mg	Nolahist[a]	Pkg 100
Clemastine 1.34 mg	Clemastine (generic)[a]	Pkg 100
Clemastine 2.68 mg	Clemastine (generic)2, Tavist[b,c]	Pkg 28, 100
Azelastine	c	
Acrivastine	c	
Azatadine 1 mg	Optimine[b]	Pkg 100
Loratadine 10 mg	Claritin[b,c]	Pkg 28, 100
Cetirizine 5 mg or 10 mg	Zytec[b,c]	Pkg 100
Fexofenadine 30 mg	Allegra[b]	Pkg 100
Tripelennamine 25 mg	PPZ[b]	Pkg 100

[a] Over-the-counter products in the United States.
[b] Prescription-only products in the United States.
[c] available as over-the-counter products in the United Kingdom.

antihistamines being are more likely to cause this effect. It should be borne in mind, however, that a condition such as seasonal allergic rhinitis (with congestion) may in itself cause a form of drowsiness (381), i.e., a "thick" or "stuffed" head feeling. Patients' lifestyles should be considered before recommending a particular oral antihistamine product.

Rare but important side effects have been found to develop with some oral antihistamines. Use of terfenadine and astemizole was found to be associated with very substantial morbidity and even mortality in very rare cases, if the drugs are coadministered with a range of common systemic medications (382). Both drugs have now been withdrawn from general use. As a result of the substantial adverse publicity associated with terfenadine, some practitioners may be wary of recommending any oral antihistamines to their patients.

Indirect-Acting Antihistamines with Mast Cell Stabilizer Actions

Mechanisms of Action of Mast Cell Stabilizers

For chronic and recurrent allergic conjunctivitis, the appropriate management is use of a special group of indirect-acting "antihistamines," namely, the mast cell stabilizers (35,328,330). This should be the first option considered and applies especially to contact lens wearers. This includes hydrogel lens wearers in whom the allergic reaction develops after an extended period of time, i.e., after 1 to 2 years, and leads to generalized discomfort, contact lens intolerance, and papillary reactions of the tarsal conjunctiva (383–390). Individuals with seasonal or perennial allergic conjunctivitis are perhaps more likely to develop contact lens wear-related papillary conjunctivitis (391). Development of the condition has not changed substantially over many years, even with the substantial changes in contact lens materials. However, when it does occur nowadays, it is generally milder (CLPC) rather than GPC.

In response to contact lens wear, an activation of conjunctival mast cells can occur. This likely will be followed by histamine release, along with other inflammatory mediators (327), and this reaction has similarities to other types of irritant- and allergen-related conjunctivitis. For management of CLPC, GPC, or papillary conjunctivitis of a seasonal nature in contact lens wearers, two medical options now are available. There are first-generation drugs that are considered to simply be mast cell stabilizers. There also are second-generation drugs with histamine H_1-blocking actions as well as mast cell stabilizer actions (see section on Antihistamine Eyedrops). In addition, there has been some debate as to what other actions these "mast cell stabilizers" can have, especially on eosinophils (392,393), i.e., these drugs also could antagonize any eosinophil migration into the conjunctival tissue, which might occur as part of the contact lens-related response (328).

The idea behind using a mast cell stabilizer is to attempt

to prevent the mast cells from discharging histamine. If this can be achieved, there should be a reduction in the tear film levels of inflammatory mediators despite the continued presence of the allergen, the chemical stimulus for mast cell degranulation, or the presence of the contact lens. Lens deposits, in themselves, may act as allergens. These mast cell stabilizers have been shown to reduce mast cell discharge (degranulation) in a dose-dependent fashion (394–398). In addition, this suppression of mediator release from the mast cells may reduce recruitment of white blood cells onto the ocular surface (399,400). The efficacy of mast cell stabilizers in ocular allergies and inflammation has generally been assessed by monitoring patient reactions after repeated usage (see later). Two types of challenge tests also have been used. In the first type, the efficacy of a mast cell stabilizer has been assessed by a challenge test performed 30 minutes after mast cell stabilizer use (401). A second type of challenge test has involved 1 week of treatment with a mast cell stabilizer before allergen (358,399). This variant of the challenge test used for topical decongestants and antihistamines (see section on Antihistamine eyedrops) recognizes the fact that the action of a mast cell stabilizer is not rapid in onset (343, 401); therefore, 1 week of treatment with drugs such as lodoxamide is required to demonstrate a real efficacy against an allergen challenge (358,399). Several mast cell stabilizer-containing eyedrops are available (Table 41.12).

Clinical Efficacy and Use of Topical Mast Cell Stabilizers

There are two types of contact lens conditions that might be treated with a mast cell stabilizer, namely, concurrent allergic conjunctivitis and inflammatory reaction to contact lens wear. It should be noted that the current product use information for these drugs in the United States indicates that these topical ocular mast cell stabilizers are indicated for treatment of vernal conjunctivitis, keratoconjunctivitis, and keratitis, but unlabeled uses include management of CLPC and seasonal allergic conjunctivitis. Elsewhere, the

TABLE 41.12. OPHTHALMIC MAST CELL STABILIZERS[a]

Drugs	Commercial Products	Size
Cromolyn sodium 4%	Cromolyn Sodium (generic)	10, 15 mL
Cromolyn sodium 4%	Crolom, Opticrom	2.5, 10 mL
Lodoxamide 0.1%	Alomide	10 mL
Nedocromil sodium 2%	Alocril	5 mL
Pemirolast sodium 0.1%	Alamast	10 mL
Ketotifen 0.025%	Zaditor[b]	5, 7 mL

[a] Prescription-only pharmaceuticals in the United States, but cromolyn 2% (generally known as sodium cromoglicate) and lodoxamide are available over the counter in the United Kingdom.
[b] Drug has histamine H_1-blocking activity as well (see section on *Antihistamine Eyedrops* and Table 41.10).

indications for use of mast cell stabilizers are for all of these conditions.

For contact lens wearers who have (or develop) seasonal allergic conjunctivitis or related conditions, it is logical to use a mast cell stabilizer. For CLPC, the logic of such a treatment might be questioned because cromolyn sodium is not considered to have any constitutive antiinflammatory activity. The principle of management of longer-term conditions such as CLPC is similar to that for any type I ocular allergies (35,328–330,392,402,403). A period of discontinuation of contact lens wear may be recommended as part of the management (34,35,262,330,331,389). Discontinuation should result in reduction in the severity of the condition over several days, often allowing resumption of contact lens wear within a few weeks. Discontinuation of cosmetic contact lens wear, if possible, is entirely equivalent to the first "law" of management of allergic conjunctivitis, i.e., "to isolate the eye from the offending agent(s)" (404). Some practitioners will, however, consider a course of action by which the use of mast cell stabilizer is aimed at maintaining a patient in contact lens wear (see later). Such treatments have been reported effective, including when there is continued contact lens wear (see later).

These drugs, especially cromolyn sodium, have a long track record of being able to effectively manage a range of types of allergic conjunctivitis (405–414). A similar track record is being established for lodoxamide (399,408,410, 412) and nedocromil sodium (378,407,413,414–416). Other mast cell stabilizers such as lodoxamide and nedocromil also should have some efficacy in CLPC, but long-term studies on the safety and efficacy of these newer drugs have yet to be reported. Conservative management of moderate/severe cases of CLPC (i.e., those that do not quickly respond to discontinuation of lens wear and lubricant/decongestant treatment) might include initiation of a regimen of a mast cell stabilizer after discontinuation of lens wear.

A q.i.d. regimen of the mast cell stabilizer (e.g., cromolyn sodium 4%) should be continued until the eyelid is quiet and staining of papillae with fluorescein is reversed (35,262, 417–418). Most resolution should take 2 to 4 weeks, after which the dosing could be reduced to t.i.d. or b.i.d. for an additional 2 to 3 weeks to ensure complete resolution of mild-to-moderate contact lens-related GPC (262).

A more controversial approach (but one admittedly once prompted by product advertising) has been to continue contact lens wear and instill cromolyn sodium drops q.i.d. (73, 75–77,79). Such an approach is logical in that it should provide continuous suppression of the conjunctival reaction to the continuous irritant, which, in this case, is a contact lens. Such therapy, while essentially continuing GP lens wear, has been reported to be effective and implied as being without side effects for up to 18 months (77). Presumably, lodoxamide eyedrops will be evaluated for similar use. This scenario also could be be considered for other mast cell stabilizer-containing solutions, although nedocromil so-

dium drops have a yellow color and, therefore, could stain a hydrogel lens matrix (415).

Some practitioners may consider a middle-of-the-road approach for daily lens wearers. This would entail instillation of the mast cell stabilizer prior to morning lens insertion, instillation of drops in the middle of the day with the lens in place, and then instilation of one or more sets of drops over the evening hours after the contact lenses have been removed. However, if a patient exhibits signs of worsening corneal epithelial disease concurrent with continued lens wear and cromolyn sodium or lodoxamide eyedrop use, both contact lens wear and eyedrops should be discontinued.

It should be noted that although the use of eyedrops containing drugs such as cromolyn sodium or lodoxamide may promptly alleviate symptoms such as itching and watery eyes, it can be argued that initial management should be with saline eyewashes, artificial tears, or decongestants simply because the major cause of the CLPC has been removed. A case can and should be made that if such eyes so readily respond to cromolyn sodium eyedrops (or another mast cell stabilizer) (419,420), then substantial activation of the mast cells has not occurred, and a little saline and decongestant treatment probably would prove adequate to manage the condition.

There are important caveats to the use of mast cell stabilizers (e.g., cromolyn sodium) as eyedrops, especially if dispensed to manage CLPC while contact lens wear is continued. As with use of decongestants, the patient may attempt to manage a more severe reaction—even a red eye due to infection—simply by increasing the dosing with the mast cell stabilizer. Overall, however, cromolyn sodium eyedrops have an extraordinary safety record in that adverse effects reports are rare (73,291,421). It should be noted that one report of adverse reactions involved the inappropriate ophthalmic use of nasal sodium cromoglycate solution (421). Some of the adverse effects appear to be related to reaction to the drug, i.e., hypersensitivity reaction, but some may simply be offset by reducing the frequency of use of the cromolyn sodium drops (73).

Topical Ocular Nonsteroidal Antiinflammatory Drugs

Mechanism of Action of Nonsteroidal Antiinflammatory Drugs

Long-term and/or extended wear of contact lenses may result in mild-to-moderate inflammatory responses that are refractory to treatment with frequent lens replacement, eyewashes, and decongestant use or even a 2- to 4-week period of therapy with eyedrops containing a mast cell stabilizer such as cromolyn sodium. Although the tarsal plate may not exhibit an exaggerated reaction, such inflammatory reactions now likely include a hardening of the palpebral conjunctival infiltrates. The appearance of peripheral corneal epithelial reactions (including superior limbic keratitis [SLK] and superior epithelial arcuate lesion [SEAL]) are well-known complications of extended wear and still a problem with modern-day continuous wear of silicone hydrogel lenses. Corneal infiltrates and even larger stromal infiltrates, as opposed to small and localized perilimbal infiltrates, also can develop (33,390,422,423). Such conditions are less likely to be acute in presentation but progressive. A further extension of such reactions may be the development of neovascularization or deeper infiltrates (in the palpebral conjunctiva, corneal epithelium, or stroma), both of which are the clear signs of extended recruitment of inflammatory cells in response to persistent irritation.

Vascular engorgement and some of the discomfort may be alleviated with use of decongestants (and cold water compresses). However, in terms of a "cure," the condition is unlikely to be successfully managed with either antihistamines and/or mast cell stabilizers. There is a need for antiinflammatory drugs that do more than just attenuate histamine release, calm the vasculature, and reduce symptoms of itching and discomfort. One of these options is to consider the use of nonsteroidal antiinflammatory drugs (NSAIDs).

The rationale for use of such drugs is that the underlying etiology is the specific recruitment of the immune system with resultant cell-based reactions and elaboration of leukocyte and eosinophil-originating inflammatory mediators (296,297,392). Although the pathophysiology of these mediators is still the subject of much research, different groups of mediators can be identified as targets of therapy. For the NSAIDs, these are the fatty acid type molecules, i.e., the prostaglandins and the related leukotrienes (297,424,425). The NSAIDs are a group of drugs that include the "aspirinlike" drugs (acetylsalicylic acid and diclofenac sodium), as well as a number of related drugs (e.g., oxyphenbutazone, piroxicam, naproxen, suprofen). The collective mechanism of action of NSAIDs is to inhibit a group of enzymes known as the prostaglandin synthetases. If these enzymes are blocked, then the amount of prostaglandins that are released is reduced. Prostaglandins have been detected in human tears in cases of chronic inflammatory conditions affecting the cornea and conjunctiva, e.g., vernal conjunctivitis (297). Gross cryodamage (426) or continuous wear of PMMA lenses (427) can produce significant corneal edema and neovascularization associated with elevated levels of a leukotriene metabolite, 5-HETE. Corneal edema could be caused by this inflammatory mediator rather than the prostaglandins. It also has been demonstrated that eyedrops containing prostaglandins can produce red eye and edema (428).

Clinical Use and Efficacy of Topical Ocular Nonsteroidal Antiinflammatory Drugs

Currently in the United States, only two NSAIDs are indicated for general ophthalmic use, which could include management of systemic allergies in contact lens wearers and management of contact lens wear-related allergic reactions. The two topical NSAIDs ketorolac tromethamine 0.5% and diclofenac sodium 1% have labeled or unlabeled uses in the management of seasonal allergic conjunctivitis and/or CLPC. Two products are marketed (Table 41.13). In terms of antiinflammatory activity, an older NSAID such as oxyphenbutazone was considered to be equivalent to moderate corticosteroid therapies (429), whereas diclofenac 0.1% has been considered to have a similar efficacy to stronger corticosteroids such as dexamethasone 0.1% q.i.d. (430). Other topical NSAIDs are marketed but are for use during intraocular operations and so are not included here.

There is a long history associated with the use of NSAIDs for management of inflammations of the conjunctiva and sclera, including those associated with contact lens wear. There also has been considerable interest in trying to establish if the corneal edema associated with contact wear is associated with the release of prostaglandins and/or leukotrienes. With the new therapeutic options now available, this history is relevant.

Oral acetylsalicylic acid therapy was advocated as a cureall for many inflammations of the anterior segment (including various types of keratitis), even at the turn of the century (263). Oral acetylsalicylic acid therapy (e.g., up to 325 mg, q2h) has been advocated as an adjunct medication to topical cromolyn sodium or other antiinflammatory drugs (431–433). Sodium salicylate eyedrops have been assessed in patients with allergic conjunctivitis, although in combination with cromolyn sodium or oxymetazoline (406). As combinations were used with oral or topical therapies, it still is not possible to assess whether sodium salicylate is indeed an efficacious antiinflammatory agent. Oxyphenbutazone, another NSAID, was used widely in Europe as Tanderil eye ointment. It was used as a postoperative antiinflammatory drug, but it also was used for the management of milder cases of conjunctivitis and keratitis (434–436) and of abrasions and foreign bodies (436,437).

The relationship between corneal edema and prostaglandins was investigated in several ways in the 1980s, and a variety of studies investigated whether corneal edema could be substantially reduced by NSAIDs. It was essentially argued that a contact lens wear-induced red eye should respond to blockade of prostaglandin synthesis, but mixed results have been obtained. Oral acetylsalicylic acid was not found to produce a thinner cornea in subjects without anterior segment inflammation (438), but preoperative and

TABLE 41.13. TOPICAL OCULAR NONSTEROIDAL ANTIINFLAMMATORY DRUGS

Drugs	Commercial Products[a]	Size
Diclofenac 0.1%	Voltaren	5 mL
Ketorolac 0.5%	Acular	5 mL

postoperative administration of oral naproxen (439,440) or oral tiaprofenic acid (441) have been reported to reduce cataract operation-related corneal edema. Such oral NSAIDs could have reduced the permeability of the blood–aqueous barrier (297,424,439), but it has been noted that active metabolites (e.g., salicylic acid) also can be secreted in the tears (442). Regardless of the mechanism, oral naproxen was not found to have any effect on acute corneal edema induced by thick hydrogel lenses (443), although the authors acknowledge that the level of edema produced may not have been sufficient to induce a significant prostanoid response.

From a topical perspective, indomethacin 1% eyedrops were reported to reduce postoperative corneal edema (444) and to improve patient comfort in cases of severe corneal disease (445). In animal models, flurbiprofen 0.03% eyedrops have been reported to reduce neovascularization that developed with continuous wear of rigid contact lenses (446.) Piroxicam 0.5% eyedrops (q.i.d.) have been reported to reduce the grade and extent of neovascularization associated with extended wear of hydrogel lenses (447); contact lens wear was continued during therapy. Similarly, suprofen 1% (q.i.d.) eyedrops were reported to reduce both acute conjunctival inflammation and any GPC developing with hydrogel lens use (448). However, preadministration of diclofenac sodium 0.1% eyedrops (q.i.d.) was found to have no effect (compared to artificial tears) on acute-onset corneal edema induced by wearing thick hydrogel lenses (449).

For allergic conjunctivitis, the efficacy of topical ocular NSAIDs has been assessed in challenge tests, this time with the allergen being instilled either 10 minutes (347) or 30 minutes (450) after the NSAID ketorolac. For ketorolac (347,450), such tests have found that topical NSAIDs may reduce inflammation and redness but have little impact on symptoms, such as itching, compared to an antihistamine. A similar effect has been noted for diclofenac in clinical studies where there is repeated use of these eyedrops (451, 452), and so a topical ocular antihistamine still may be required to control all symptoms (451). In general repeated use, topical ocular NSAIDs have been reported to be effective in managing seasonal allergic conjunctivitis. These include piroxicam 0.5% eyedrops (453), naproxen 0.5% eyedrops (454), ketorolac 0.5% eyedrops (455,456), and diclofenac sodium 0.1% eyedrops (430,451,452,456,457). Some topical NSAIDs may, however, be less comfortable compared to, at minimum, some topical ocular antihistamines (347).

The successful use of eyedrops containing diclofenac (458) or ketorolac (131) in the management of corneal abrasions has been reported, e.g., a fingernail abrasion or one caused by grit under a contact lens. The primary reason for use likely is to improve patient comfort, as these drugs have analgesic activity. However, topical diclofenac sodium drops were not found to improve comfort and adaptation to GP lenses (459). A special use of diclofenac eyedrops is for pa-

tient comfort and pain management after refractive surgery (460–462). Some of these patients may be fitted with a hydrophilic bandage lens immediately postoperatively.

Overall, the use of topical ocular NSAIDs, as antiinflammatory agents, has been associated with relatively few side effects compared to corticosteroids (see section V.F). The use of topical ocular NSAIDs is not considered to cause clinically significant increases in IOP (424,430,463). Recent attention has been given to the possibility that a form of toxic keratitis can develop after the use of topical ocular NSAIDs such as diclofenac and ketorolac (464,465). Such problems appear to be associated with intensive use, especially as a postoperative medicine, and, therefore, do not generally apply to the use of topical NSAIDs for management of allergies or abrasions in contact lens wearers. A side effect that must be considered with use of topical ocular NSAIDs is allergies, either local or systemic. Systemic allergies, leading to anaphylaxis and bronchoconstriction, are rare complications of topical ocular NSAID use but should not be ignored (466,467).

Topical Ocular Corticosteroids Drugs

Mechanisms of Action and Overall Effects of Topical Ocular Corticosteroids

For inflammatory conditions of the anterior segment that might develop with contact lens wear, the last option to be considered is the cautious use of topical ocular corticosteroids. The gross inflammatory response of the eye to contact lens wear can produce a grade IV GPC or an acute-onset "red eye" (the toxic lens syndrome), substantial perilimbal reaction, infiltrates, and an accompanying anterior chamber reaction (33,422,468). In addition to prompt discontinuation of lens wear, such eyes may need aggressive but carefully monitored treatment with topical ocular corticosteroids.

Topical corticosteroid therapy for the acute gross inflammatory response to contact lens wear should reduce conjunctival vessel leakiness within a few hours (469), reduce leukocyte and macrophage recruitment (470), and reduce any further elaboration and secretion of other inflammatory mediators by the leukocytes (471). The latter effects should reduce the risk of sequelae (such as stromal scarring, corneal distortion, or endothelial dysfunction) (425,472). Animal and human studies indicate that such a response includes substantial recruitment of leukocytes and macrophages following compromise of the conjunctival and anterior uveal vasculature and blood–ocular barrier (296,392,473,474). Although the prostaglandins may be responsible, in part, for compromise of the blood–aqueous barrier (296,424, 425), the current standard therapy for such a substantial red eye is not with NSAIDs but rather with topical ocular corticosteroids.

Corticosteroid therapy of the eye has traditionally been viewed as palliative in that it would "cover up" the signs of inflammation (475–477). The mechanism by which corticosteroids produced their clinical effects on the eye was unknown at that time. It now is known that a special aspect of the action of corticosteroids involves a group of peptide hormones (the lipocortins) (478). With the recognition that corticosteroids exert their effects by mediation lipocortin-induced inhibition of cell membrane-located phospholipase enzymes, corticosteroids must be considered as more than palliative therapy but a true treatment. Corticosteroids can bind to glucocorticoid receptors in the ocular tissues and counter the effects of inflammation-induced production of arachidonic acid (the precursor of prostanoids) via the action of the phospholipase A_2 enzyme activity (474). In addition to affecting the ocular tissue and vasculature, specific corticosteroid binding to leukocytes and macrophages apparently is involved (479). The corticosteroids will exert their antiinflammatory actions and produce a range of side effects, both ocular and systemic (see later). A new approach to ocular corticosteroid therapy has been the development of the "soft" steroids (480) in which the corticosteroid exerts its antiinflammatory actions and then is metabolized by ocular tissues to produce an inactive metabolite (480–482). Any side effects should be substantially depressed with the use of a "soft" steroid. Two slightly different types of corticosteroids are available for topical ocular use, namely, the older corticosteroids and the newer "soft" steroids such as loteprednol. These are listed in Table 41.14.

The clinician may care for patients who require contact lens correction (e.g., unilateral aphakia) with concomitant use of topical steroids to control collateral disease (e.g., uveitis). These patients should be approached cautiously, as discussed earlier, and provided with contact lenses only if a positive risk-to-benefit ratio exists.

Clinical Efficacy of Topical Ocular Corticosteroids

Topical ocular corticosteroids are generally selected for use based on their "strength," so this property needs to be taken into account before the overall efficacy is considered. The currently available ophthalmic corticosteroids differ somewhat in their inherent antiinflammatory activity. Hydrocortisone ophthalmic preparations (e.g., cortisone) were introduced in the 1950s (475) and remain the standard against which antiinflammatory activities are assessed. Current products are considered to have a relative potency of 1 to 58 on a rather undefined scale (425,472,474,483).

Prednisolone probably is the most widely used and the most important ophthalmic corticosteroid. It is considered to have 3.5× times greater antiinflammatory activity than hydrocortisone and is available as both solutions (as sodium phosphate salts) and as a suspension (acetate salts). Both low and high concentration products are available, thus providing the clinician with a mild and strong topical cortico-

TABLE 41.14. TOPICAL OCULAR CORTICOSTEROIDS[a]

Compound	Pharmaceuticals	Size[d]
Hydrocortisone		
Prednisolone 0.12%	Pred Mild	5, 10 mL
Prednisolone 0.125%	AK-Pred, Econopred, Inflamase Mild	3, 5, 10 mL
Loteprednol 0.2%	Alrex	5, 10 mL
Medrysone 1%	HMS	5, 10 mL
Clobetasone	b	
Dexamethasone 0.1%	Dexamethasone Sodium Phosphate (generic)	5 mL
Dexamethasone 0.1%	AK-Dex, Decadron Phosphate, Maxidex	5 mL
Fluorometholone 0.1%	Fluorometholone (generic)	5, 10, 15 mL
Fluorometholone 0.1%	Fluoro-Op, FML, Flarex, eFlone	Various to 15 mL
Betamethasone	c	
Loteprednol 0.5%	Lotemax	2.5, 5, 10, 15 mL
Fluorometholone 0.25%	FML Forte	2, 5, 10, 15 mL
Prednisolone acetate 1%	Econopred Plus, Pred Forte, Prednisolone Acetate Ophthalmic	1, 5, 10, 15 mL
Prednisolone phosphate 1%	Prednisolone Sodium Phosphate (generic)	5, 10, 15 mL
Prednisolone phosphate 1%	AK-Pred, Inflamase Forte	3, 5, 10, 15 mL
Rimexolone 1%	Vexol	5, 10 mL
Dexamethasone 0.05%	Dexamethasone Sodium Phosphate (generic)	3.5-g tubes
Dexamethasone 0.05%	AK-Dex	3.5-g tubes
Fluorometholone 0.1%	FML S.O.P.	3.5-g tubes

[a] Marketed in the United Kingdom as opthalmic ointments.
[b] Clobetasone eyedrops were marketed in the United Kingdom until recently.
[c] Betamethasone 0.1% ophthalmic products are marketed in Canada and the United Kingdom.
[d] Not all size options are available for all the products lists.
[e] Currently only indicated for management of postoperative inflammation.

steroid. There has been considerable controversy over the years as to whether the solutions or suspensions of prednisolone have a superior antiinflammatory action (484). Product selection or preferences based on patient comfort and convenience are defensible reasons for selecting the solutions, as they do not contain soft particulates and do not need to be shaken prior to instillation. Betamethasone has a relative antiinflammatory activity of 15 compared to hydrocortisone (472), and even low concentrations show good efficacy for management of lid and conjunctival inflammations (485, 486). Dexamethasone is considered to have 23 × the antiinflammatory activity of hydrocortisone (472). It also is available in solution (sodium phosphate salts) and in suspension (as the alcohol). Although generally considered more potent, it is only available at the 0.1% concentration, so an antiinflammatory effect equivalent to that of hydrocortisone 2.5% solution or suspension can be expected (430,451). Similar clinical efficacy has been reported for clobetasone (486,487). Fluorometholone is considered to have an even greater antiinflammatory effect (58X) compared to even dexamethasone (472), which allows it to have a high clinical efficacy comparable to higher concentrations of prednisolone in external eye inflammation when used at low concentrations (486,488,489). On equivalence to fluorometholone 0.1% is the new "soft" steroid loteprednol (490). When used at the 0.2% concentration, its principal application is for allergic conjunctivitis; therefore, it is relevant for management of contact lens wearers (481,491,492). An alternative use for the higher concentration of 0.5% is as a standard postoperative antiinflammatory drug (493). An ophthalmic corticosteroid with limited penetration into the eye is medrysone. This drug was widely used to manage mild inflammatory conditions of the cornea and conjunctiva (e.g., as associated with allergic conjunctivitis (494,495). It is still available but has probably been largely superseded by other corticosteroids (e.g., fluorometholone 0.1%) or even by the ophthalmic NSAIDs (ketorolac and diclofenac).

Topical ocular corticosteroid use for contact lens wear–related ocular inflammation requires making decisions as to whether the inflamed eye also is infected (see section on Overview of Bacterial Infections of the External Eye). If the eye is infected, then severe consequences could occur if topical corticosteroids are indiscriminately used at presentation (i.e., herpes simplex, *Pseudomonas*). Notwithstanding, there is a range of uses of topical ocular corticosteroids.

A short-term topical ocular corticosteroid regimen may be beneficial in well-developed cases of GPC compared to CLPC associated with hydrogel lens wear (73). By current perspectives, regular lens replacement, improved lens hygiene, and patient education are considered the mainstay of preventing GPC from developing in the first place. A brief course of topical ocular corticosteroids can be used simply to manage discomfort associated with persistent allergic conjunctivitis, including vernal keratoconjunctivitis (VKC) (488,494–496). Such a condition could be present in a contact lens wearer. These types of therapy are considered essential to quiet the eye (and thus provide patient comfort) and to improve appearance by reducing conjunctival hyperemia (495). Although some might argue that it would be illogical and risky to prescribe even milder corticosteroids (e.g., prednisolone 0.1% or fluorometholone 0.1%) concurrent with contact lens wear, such a practice is advocated by some. Bandage lenses also have been used concurrently with topical corticosteroid therapies (84,88), although such treatments must be monitored carefully (see later). Concurrent use of the newer corticosteroids (e.g. loteprednol) with ongoing contact lens wear for treatment of CLPC or GPC has been assessed (481). Although major side effects were not encountered in these studies, any use of topical ocular corticosteroids should be undertaken only when regular professional monitoring of the patient is available (88,481). For GP lenses, however, the argument for risks of altered epithelial healing must remain, so on-eye corticosteroid therapy concurrent with GP lens wear probably should be avoided.

Assuming a noninfectious etiology to the acute-onset palpebral or limbal conjunctivitis or corneal infiltrates, the corticosteroid of choice often will be prednisolone because of its long-established efficacy and the ready availability of a range of pharmaceuticals (Table 41.14). For acute severe conditions, aggressive therapy with prednisolone 1% solutions (e.g., q1h or q2h initially, and continued for 2–3 days) should be sufficient to quiet the eye and reduce sequelae. Effective management of the acute inflammatory response can be expected only if the corticosteroids are used in the initial stage of presentation. This treatment must begin as early as possible after an infectious etiology is ruled out (34, 83). Ideally, the minimum effective dosing should be used for the shortest period of time possible to secure the desired clinical response. This approach is conservative and is designed to minimize the probability of side effects developing (see later). For recurrent and moderate conditions, lower concentrations (e.g., 0.1%) of prednisolone or other corticosteroids should be adequate and used moderately aggressively (e.g., q3h to q4h). Following initial frequent dosing, the corticosteroid therapies can be progressively reduced by either reducing the regimen or reducing the concentration (e.g., dosing from q2h to q4h to q.i.d. to b.i.d. over several days, depending on the response of the eye).

In most cases, the course of corticosteroid treatment will be brief, i.e., no more than a maximum of a few weeks. The efficacy of topical corticosteroid therapy should be assessed with the expectation of reduced symptoms and biomicroscopy to confirm reduction of edema, quieting of the vasculature, and reduction in infiltrates and anterior chamber reaction (475,476). Biomicroscopy should be performed after the initial period of intensive therapy as a basis for subsequent continued regimen or tapering schedule. In cases presenting with an acute sterile corneal ulcer, fluorescein staining of the cornea is essential to assess epithelial status, because continued aggressive use of corticosteroids should be performed only if epithelial resurfacing is clearly ongoing (474). As long as there is an open "wound" (i.e., an epithelial defect), leukocyte recruitment is likely to continue (497), and the sooner a wound resurfaces, the faster the secondary recovery stage of the inflammation. It can be emphasized that removal of the offending contact lens, in itself, should reduce most of the exogenous inflammatory stimulus, so the aim of steroid therapy is to arrest further development of inflammatory cell recruitment and to promote recovery. Generally, cosmetic contact lens wear should not be resumed until the eye is completely quiet again, following successful management of the inflammation with corticosteroids. Lens wear might be reconsidered after a suitable abstention (e.g., a few weeks after cessation of corticosteroid therapy).

In addition to corticosteroids, cycloplegics (e.g., atropine 1% q.d./b.i.d. or homatropine 5% b.i.d.) and oral analgesics may be indicated. Additional symptomatic relief can be provided at any point through the adjunct use of topical ocular decongestants and/or cold water compresses (applied to the closed eye for 15 to 30 minutes).

Decisions to use topical ocular corticosteroids should always be made with a certain degree of caution, because most of these drugs may carry a somewhat higher risk of side effects or adverse drug reactions compared to other therapies (291). The main side effect to be considered for most corticosteroids is an elevation of IOP. Other side effects that often are listed include cataracts, opportunistic infections, and a delay in wound healing.

Unsupervised topical ocular corticosteroid use over extended periods, as was often performed in the 1950s, showed that it was possible to produce glaucomatous changes, e.g., substantial elevation of IOP, disc cupping, and visual field loss (472,474,498). Subsequent studies showed that only some individuals are especially susceptible to these types of unwanted and avoidable side effect. Based on the rationale that any sustained elevation in IOP ($\geq$30 mm Hg) is a risk factor for glaucomatous damage, substantial efforts have been made to identify individuals who are likely to show a significant elevation of IOP. This will occur after just 2 to 4 weeks of standard treatment (i.e., q.i.d.) with topical ocular corticosteroids. These susceptible individuals are known as corticosteroid responders and have a genetic predisposition that results in the response (472, 499–502). Unless a patient or practitioner is aware that this response occurs, there is no simple practical test that can be implemented to quickly identify those individuals who truly are at risk for the side effect.

Therefore, for the use of any ophthalmic corticosteroid, manufacturers guidelines clearly state that IOP should be monitored regularly. The key to effective management is to try to prevent any measurable increases in IOP (i.e. 5 mm Hg). In principle, manufacturers advise that topical ocular corticosteroid therapy should not be performed without obtaining initial measurements of IOP, even though this is

surely unlikely if the ocular inflammation was being managed by a general medical practitioner. Some manufacturers state these measurements should be taken every 10 days thereafter. Prospective and retrospective evaluations indicate that elevations in IOP rarely exceed 15 mm Hg and should reverse fairly quickly following cessation of (or reduction in) topical corticosteroid therapy (291,425,472, 474). The corticosteroid concentration as well as the frequency and duration of administration are important factors in development of ocular hypertension. Allowing for differences in the concentrations and normally indicated regimens for use, the different topical ocular corticosteroids appear to differ somewhat in their ability to produce ocular hypertension in susceptible individuals.

Early studies with topical hydrocortisone showed that substantial IOP increases could be produced over a few weeks (472,474). It has been argued that patients with open-angle glaucoma, or their relatives, would more likely be corticosteroid responders (500), and it can be logically argued that older patients perhaps are more likely to develop more substantial elevations in IOP than younger patients. However, there is a poor case to be made that an eye that develops mild-to-moderate increases in IOP (e.g., 10– 15 mm Hg) following a 2-week period of topical ocular corticosteroid therapy is in a worse state than the eye with uncontrolled intraocular inflammation that could proceed to develop secondary complications such as synechiae and secondary angle closure, as well as substantial corneal edema and scarring. More recent studies generally indicate that dexamethasone is more likely to produce a greater elevation in IOP compared to fluorometholone or prednisolone therapies (474,486,500,503.) For high-risk patients who needed corticosteroid therapy, a practitioner could elect to use a steroid for which the risk of development of ocular hypertension was considered less. However, such a selection should not mean that a check of IOP should not be performed prior to initiating therapy and that IOP monitoring still does not need to be performed. Recent developments with soft steroids (e.g., loteprednol) have been aimed at providing a topical ocular corticosteroid that has even lesser potential to elevate IOP (504). Long-term studies, including some with contact lens wearers, indicate that, compared to prednisolone 1%, the risk of ocular hypertension was less with loteprednol use but could still occur (502).

The hypertensive response of the eye to topical corticosteroid therapy is not unique to this mode of presentation. It has been estimated that the risk of developing ocular hypertension after oral corticosteroid use was substantially less than with topical corticosteroids (505). An adjusted odds ratio for topical therapy was 8.0 compared to 1.4 for oral corticosteroids. Notwithstanding, systemic corticosteroid therapies, such as oral prednisolone, can result in elevated IOP, especially in younger patients with arthritis (506) or chronic inflammatory bowel disease (507). Inhaled corticosteroids for asthma also have been implicated with steroid glaucoma (508). Even a few days of oral corticosteroid therapy for skin irritation has been reported to produce modest increases in IOP (509) without apparently affecting contact lens wear/comfort.

Before simply concluding that topical or systemic corticosteroid use can raise IOP and that such an effect can be readily assessed by tonometry, the effect of corticosteroids on the cornea must be considered. Many years ago, topical dexamethasone treatment was noted to be associated with a small increase in measured CCT and IOP (510). There could be considerable uncertainty in the interpretation of this finding because an elevation could compromise the corneal endothelium and lead to edema, or a higher IOP reading could be obtained if the steroids, per se, increased corneal thickness. The role of IOP in development and/or recovery from corneal edema is uncertain because it appears to be dependent on whether or not the corneal epithelium is compromised (511). In recent years, there has been renewed and substantial interest in whether CCT has a significant impact on measures of IOP (512). A thicker cornea can result in higher tonometry readings and vice versa. In generally healthy eyes, the magnitude of the effect is such that a 10% change in CCT could result in a 1- to 1.5-mm Hg difference in the outcome of clinical tonometry. It has been concluded that the routine correction for an effect of this magnitude is essentially impractical (512), especially because a 10% edema level is an unlikely finding in routine optometric practice. However, in the elderly and for those eyes with chronic disease, a 10% change in CCT could result in a 2.5-mm Hg difference in tonometry readings (512,513). This might well be considered worthy of correction (514). As a closing note, it remains to be established whether the reverse scenario is applicable, i.e., would small chronic elevations in IOP (>5 mm Hg) result in the development of corneal edema (512,513,515)?

Topical ocular corticosteroid therapy has been implicated in the premature development of posterior subcapsular cataracts in patients with concurrent systemic diseases such as kidney failure and/or advanced diabetes (516–518). Steroid cataracts are primarily associated with systemic corticosteroid therapy (519), with the corticosteroids (or their metabolites) reaching the eye via the posterior vasculature. Patients receiving chronic oral therapies with high doses of corticosteroids (e.g., those with severe rheumatoid arthritis or recipients of kidney transplants) (520,521) are considered to be at the highest risk for developing these unusual cataracts, which can lead to changes in refractive error and modest changes in visual acuity (519,522). Periodically, case reports of other associations between chronic corticosteroid therapy and the development of cataracts, e.g., when administered as aerosols for asthma, are published (519,523). These are all extremes, however, and have little relationship to the perspective of short-term use of topical ocular corticosteroids for management of inflammations of the external eye. The practitioner should consider whether a patient with arthritis and who is on corticosteroid therapy is more at risk for developing cataracts. This could have implications on whether cataract surgery is to be performed. However, for the average contact lens wearer, the benefits of successful management of ocular inflammation with a brief course of topical ocular corticosteroids far outweigh the risks of cataract development. For example, corneal scarring and corneal endothelial dysfunction can be expected to result in ocular morbidity at least as severe as posterior subcapsular cataracts.

Antibacterial Drugs for Conjunctivitis, Keratitis, and Infectious Corneal Ulcers

Overview of Bacterial Infections of the External Eye

It was established in the 1980s that extended wear of hydrogel contact lenses was accompanied by an unacceptable risk of developing severe corneal infections (31). Inappropriate contact lens care, inadvertent ocular or lens exposure to a heavily contaminated solution, or known abrasion of the ocular surface are other risk factors for the development of serious infectious ulcers (29–31,34,35,37). In short, if a contact lens wearer develops an acute red eye with signs of an ulcer, contact lens wear should be discontinued immediately and aggressive antibiotic therapy started (32,34,35). Alternatively, a contact lens wearer may develop bacterial conjunctivitis that may either be simply annoying (and a cause of some lens discomfort) or prompt him or her to seek emergency attention (and require immediate discontinuation of lens wear). In either ase, the development of significant ocular discomfort, a red eye, and concurrent mucopurulent discharge are the accepted hallmarks of bacterial conjunctivitis (32,524–528). All such eyes may not, however, prove to be culture positive (529–532).

Allowing for the huge number of successful contact lens wearers, the incidence of such infections is relatively low, and a number of predisposing factors usually are required before an infection actually develops. These include general consideration of ocular hygiene and, in cases of recurrent hordeola, blepharitis or blepharoconjunctivitis in the contact lens wearer. The introduction of suitable lid hygiene measures [see section on Lid Scrub (Eyelid Hygiene) Products] is important. Such measures should reduce the risk of infection.

Following corneal abrasions associated with contact lens wear, treatment with broad-spectrum antibiotic therapy should reduce the risk of an infection developing as a result of compromise of the epithelial barrier (88). Regardless of the type of bacterial infection, antibacterial drugs can be effectively used to manage the condition, providing the organisms are susceptible to the drugs. There is no guarantee of such susceptibility, but certain organisms are more commonly sensitive to certain antibacterial drugs or groups of drugs (533). Notwithstanding, if an acute-onset red eye develops with signs of mucopurulent discharge, bacterial infection should be assumed. When such an assumption is made of an acute (and possibly substantial) bacterial infection, special attention should be given to evaluate the ocular surface for any epithelial breaks (defects, ulcers) and their location to check for signs of ulcers. Some form of "shotgun" therapy should be initiated as soon as possible. The initial therapy should be much more aggressive if there are signs of a corneal ulcer (32,34,524,534,535).

Mechanisms of Action of Topical Ocular Antibacterial Drugs

Antibacterial drugs can kill bacteria (i.e., are bactericidal) or they can stop further replication of bacteria (i.e., are bacteriostatic). Ophthalmic products containing single antibacterial drugs are listed in Table 41.15. Products containing two or more combinations of antibacterial drugs are listed in Table 41.16. In general terms, the choice of antibacterial drug or combination of drugs for clinical use is based on the sort of coverage desired and the expected efficacy, not on whether the drugs are expected to be bacteriostatic or bactericidal. If a substantial effect is deemed necessary, then the frequency of administration is increased, i.e., q1h instead of q.i.d. The various antibacterial drugs have different mechanisms of action targeted at the mechanisms of protein synthesis in bacteria, DNA replication, the intermediate metabolism of the bacteria, the outer cell wall, or the inner cytoplasmic (cell) membrane of bacteria. Various products that contain single antibacterial drugs are available (Table 41.15).

The aminoglycoside antibiotics such as gentamicin and tobramycin are considered to be active against a broad spectrum of bacteria (providing resistance to the antibiotics has not developed), and so can be expected to have good efficacy against the more common Gram-negative bacteria (536–540). Gentamicin and tobramycin interfere with ribosome-based protein synthesis in bacteria and effect a bacteriostatic action, but at higher concentrations they can be bactericidal. This is because they can perturb the integrity of the cytoplasmic membrane of susceptible bacteria, especially Gram-negative organisms (541,542). The current expectations for occurrence of resistance to gentamicin is such that tobramycin should be considered the better drug if intensive shotgun therapy is needed. Neomycin, another aminoglycoside, has a mechanism of action similar to that of gentamicin and tobramycin (542). Neomycin was once widely used in ophthalmology (543,544) but, due to the development of both resistance and allergies, its current availability is limited to combination products (see later). Framycetin, which was introduced in the 1960s, is an aminoglycoside very similar to neomycin (542) and can be considered simply as an alternative to other aminoglycosides for mild-to-moderate bacterial infections of the external eye (545,546). Erythromycin

was introduced in the 1950s (547) and is a bacterial protein synthesis inhibitor with an action similar to that of the aminoglycosides (542).

Chloramphenicol, another protein synthesis inhibitor, was introduced in the 1950s and has a similar broad spectrum of activity to the aminoglycosides (542,548). There is no obvious evidence that its overall efficacy has declined in recent years. However, it now is recognized that, from a practical perspective, ophthalmic chloramphenicol is not for intensive use, should not be used on a chronic basis (including therapies for recurrent infections), and should be avoided if there is a patient or family history of bone marrow disorders of any type. Inappropriate chronic use and overuse of chloramphenicol eyedrops or ointments prompted a considerable degree of professional concern over its routine use for any ocular infections. This concern extended to the use of chloramphenicol as a short-term, all-purpose topical ocular antibacterial for conjunctivitis (mild-to-moderate bacterial "red eye") (549,550).

There is an important history pertaining to risks associated with use of topical ocular chloramphenicol. Even in the late 1970s, manufacturer's instructions on some ocular chloramphenicol products clearly noted that the drug was not intended for chronic use (551). The product listings stated the following: "Prolonged or frequent intermittent use of topical chloramphenicol should be avoided." The reason for this was that, at least as early as 1965, extraordinary cases of systemic toxicity—leading to development of a bone marrow aplasia—were reported following the chronic use of topical ocular chloramphenicol (552). For example, one report noted that a patient had a prescription for chloramphenicol eyedrops refilled about 25 times over a 23-month period! Other cases of fatal bone marrow aplasia apparently have followed the chronic use of topical ocular chloramphenicol. Although some might debate that the use of topical ocular chloramphenicol poses an unacceptable morbidity or mortality risk to patients (550), the probability of such systemic toxicity is extraordinarily rare (553,554). A contributing cause of what can be fatal adverse reaction to chloramphenicol pertains to the patient having a rare pharmacogenetic difference in the way the drug is metabolized. and it is these metabolic products that appear to be the cause of bone marrow destruction (555). If the risk of serious complications is associated with a predisposition to bone marrow aplasia, then such patients should not be treated with topical ocular chloramphenicol. One might desire to extend this to relatives of patients with bone marrow aplasia. However, it is impractical, cost ineffective, and of questionable value to subject "at-risk" patients to blood tests in an attempt to identify those patients with bone marrow disorders.

Fusidic acid is another broad-spectrum antibiotic that is directed at protein synthesis, is used as an ophthalmic gel, and has an efficacy equivalent to that of chloramphenicol eyedrops or ointment (546,556,557). As a gel, it can be

TABLE 41.15. ANTIBACTERIAL DRUGS COMMERCIALLY AVAILABLE FOR TOPICAL OPHTHALMIC USE

Compound	Pharmaceuticals	Size
Gentamicin 0.3%	Gentamicin Ophthalmic (generic)	5, 15 mL
Gentamicin 0.3%	Garamycin, Genoptic, Gentacidin, Gentak	1, 3, 5, 15 mL
Tobramycin 0.3%	Tobramycin (generic)	5 mL
Tobramycin 0.3%	Aktob, Tobrex	5 mL
Neomycin	a	
Framycetin	b	
Chloramphenicol 0.5%	Chloramphenicol (generic)[f]	7.5 mL
Chloramphenicol 0.5%	AK-Chlor, Chloromycetin, Chloroptic	2.5, 7.5, 15 mL
Sulfacetamide 1%	Sulster	5, 10 mL
Sulfacetamide 10%	Sulfacetamide Sodium (generic)	15 mL
Sulfacetamide 10%	AK-Sulf, Belph-10, Ocusulf-10, Sodium Sulamyd	2, 5, 15 mL
Sulfacetamide 10%	Sulf-10	1 mL UD
Sulfacetamide 30%	Sulfacetamide Sodium (generic)	15 mL
Sulfacetamide 30%	Sodium Sulamyd	15 mL
Sulfacetamide 0.15% with phenylephrine 0.125%	Vasosulf	1, 15 mL
Ciprofloxacin 0.3%	Ciloxan	2.5, 5, 10 mL
Norfloxacin 0.3%	Chibroxin	5 mL
Ofloxacin 0.3%	Ocuflox	1, 5, 10 mL
Levofloxacin 0.5%	Quixin	2.5, 5 mL
Polymyxin B fortified	Polymyxin B Sulfate Sterile	20-mL vials
Gentamicin 0.3%	Gentamicin Ophthalmic (generic)	3.5-g tubes
Gentamicin 0.3%	Garamycin, genoptic S.O.P., Gentacidin, Gentak	3.5-g tubes
Tobramycin 0.3%	Tobrex	3.5-g tubes
Erythromycin 0.5%	Erythromycin (generic)	3.5-g tubes
Erythromycin 0.5%	Ilotycin	3.5-g tubes
Chloramphenicol 1%	AK-Chlor, Chloroptic S.O.P., Chloromycetin	3.5-g tubes
Chlortetracycline	c	
Oxytetracycline	d	
Fusidic acid	e	
Sulfacetamide 10%	Sulfacetamide Sodium (generic)	3.5-g tubes
Sulfacetamide 10%	AK-Sulf, Bleph-10, Isoptocetamide, Sodium Sulamyd	3.5-g tubes
Ciprofloxacin 0.3%	Ciloxan	3.5-g tubes
Bacitracin 500 U	Bacitracin (generic)	3.5, 3.75-g tubes
Bacitracin 500 U	AK-Tracin	3.5-g tubes

[a] not usually used on its own (although a Minims Neomycin is marketed in Canada, the United Kingdom and Australia) but is widely used in combination products (Table 41.16).
[b] Framycetin ophthalmic solutions also are marketed in Canada and the United Kingdom.
[c] No ophthalmic products are currently listed for the United States; Aureomycin is still listed for Canada and the United Kingdom.
[d] No single products, but available in combination products (Table 41.16).
[e] No current products listed for the United States, but Fucithalmic is available in Canada, the United Kingdom, and Australia.
[f] Chloramphenicol solutions should be refrigerated until dispensed.

routinely used on a b.i.d. rather than q.i.d. basis. Fusidic acid is used in the United Kingdom and Australia.

The fluoroquinolone antibacterial drugs (ciprofloxacin, norfloxacin, ofloxacin, levofloxacin) are broad spectrum and have a mechanism of action directed at bacterial DNA replication rather than protein synthesis (558). They can be confidently used in cases of severe infections not susceptible to aminoglycosides (and vice versa). Some resistance has developed even though these drugs are relatively new (559).

"Sulfa drugs," typified by sulfacetamide sodium, were introduced in the late 1940s (560,561). With the mechanism of action linked to the bacterial utilization of p-aminobenzoic acid, the presence of substantial purulent discharge may limit the efficacy of topical ocular sulfonamides (526, 560,562). Utilization of p-aminobenzoic acid is linked to the action of these drugs as inhibitors of the intermediary metabolism of bacteria, which involves the synthesis of folic acid from p-aminobenzoic acid (542,562,563), especially in

TABLE 41.16. COMBINATIONS OF ANTIBACTERIAL DRUGS COMMERCIALLY AVAILABLE FOR TOPICAL OPHTHALMIC USE

Compound	Pharmaceuticals	Size
Neomycin + polymyxin B + gramicidin	Neomycin Sulfate-Polymyxin B Sulfate-Gramicidin Solution (generic)	2, 10 mL
Neomycin + polymyxin B + gramicidin	AK-Spore, Neosporin Ophthalmic Solution	2, 10 mL
Trimethoprim + polymyxin B	Polytrim Ophthalmic Solution, Trimethoprim Sulfate and Polymyxin B Ophthalmic Solution	5, 10 mL
Neomycin + polymyxin B + bacitracin	Triple Antibiotic Ophthalmic Ointment (generic)	3.5-g tubes
Neomycin + polymyxin B + bacitracin	Bacitracin Neomycin Polymyxin B Ointment (generic)	3.5-g tubes
Neomycin + polymyxin B + bacitracin	AK-Spore Ointment, Neosporin Ophthalmic Ointment	3.5-g tubes
Polymyxin B + bacitracin	AK-Poly-Bac Ointment, Bacitracin Zinc and Polymyxin B Ointment, Polysporin Ophthalmic Ointment	3.5-g tubes
Polymyxin B + oxytetracycline	Terramycin with Polymyxin B Ointment, Terak Ointment	3.5-g tubes

Gram-positive bacteria. For many minor-to-moderate cases of bacterial conjunctivitis, sulfa drugs may still prove to be very effective, but excessive discharge, if present, must be removed to improve the probability of obtaining an effect with the sulfa drug. Many years ago, this would have been a reasonable option to consider; however, today these drugs are far less likely used if there is much discharge. It should be noted that sulfacetamide and related drugs have the potential to precipitate a very severe oculocutaneous reaction known as Stevens-Johnson syndrome (291,542,564). As with the potential adverse reaction to chloramphenicol, this sulfonamide sensitivity is caused by a unique pharmacogenetic defect in drug metabolism (565). A number of other antibacterial drugs are available in combination products, i.e., containing two or more antibacterial or other drugs (Table 41.15).

Trimethoprim is a drug that is related to sulfacetamide but blocks a later stage in the synthesis of folic acid (542, 566,567). Polymyxin B and gramicidin nonspecifically perturb (disturb/disrupt) the inner cytoplasmic membrane of common Gram-negative and Gram-positive organisms (542,568,569). Bacitracin was introduced in the 1950s as a narrow-spectrum antibiotic that interferes with synthesis of the cell wall, especially in Gram-positive bacteria (542, 570). The tetracycline antibiotics (chlortetracycline, oxytetracycline, tetracycline) also are protein synthesis inhibitors (542). They were widely used and important ophthalmic antibacterial drugs in the 1950s and 1960s (571,572). This widespread use, usually as ointments at the 1% concentration, resulted from their broad spectrum of activity against most common Gram-positive and Gram-negative bacteria.

Clinical Use and Efficacy of Topical Ocular Antibacterial Drugs

Various types of bacterial infections can develop in the eye. These range from largely inconsequential conditions, such as blepharitis or a mild conjunctivitis, to keratitis and corneal ulcers. Many ophthalmic antibacterial products contain a single drug suitable for management of many of these conditions (Table 41.15).

There are many different ways in which a contact lens wearer may present with or develop a bacterial infection. Appropriate therapy can be developed from consideration of the risk factors for infection, the drug type, and the risk of side effects associated with use of these drugs.

Blepharitis [see section on Lid Scrub (Eyelid Hygiene) Products] should principally be managed with hygiene measures. Staphylococcal blepharitis, if observed during patient prefitting evaluation, should be managed prior to dispensing the lens (29,275). An antibiotic ointment, such as bacitracin or erythromycin (276,573,574) or even gentamicin (574–576), can be applied at bedtime for a few weeks, but lid scrubs usually are sufficient to control the condition after a course of antibiotic therapy (275). Because mild superficial keratitis may develop in chronic cases of blepharitis (perhaps due to sensitivity to staphylococcal exotoxins), use of the antibiotic also should reduce the risk of corneal infection.

External hordeola (styes) are commonly associated with poor hygiene and an underlying blepharitis. Management, in addition to hygiene, requires the external application of hot compresses for several minutes on a daily basis to prompt pointing and eventual discharge of the affected gland. Antibiotic ointments (bacitracin, erythromycin, or combinations) or solutions can be used several times a day as the stye matures. If prophylactic coverage is considerable, it is advisable to limit the spread of infection to both the adjacent glands and the conjunctiva. Use of erythromycin, largely as a result of its rather narrow spectrum of activity against Gram-positive bacteria, is generally restricted to eyelid infections caused by such bacteria (577), and it is generally only available in ointment form for this use. These eyelid infections, however, also include inclusion conjunctivitis caused by *Chlamydia* (578). Similarly, bacitracin can be used in specific cases of bacterial keratoconjunctivitis or conjunctivitis (573,579), but its use, in ointment form, is now generally restricted to management of Gram-positive eyelid infections (577). It can be effectively alternated with erythromycin ointment to limit the development of resistance in chronic conditions (275). Larger and usually more painful internal hordeola generally require the use of systemic antibiotics, and a brief course of erythromycin (e.g., 250 mg, q.i.d. for 2 weeks) often is effective.

Whenever patients present with conjunctival or corneal abrasions related to contact lens wear, prophylactic coverage with antibiotics is indicated. Contact lens wear should be discontinued and not resumed until the ocular surface and ocular defenses against infection are fully restored. For such coverage, combination antibiotic eyedrops t.i.d. or q.i.d. is generally advisable to minimize the risk of an infection developing. When bandage contact lenses are used, broad-spectrum antibiotic coverage also is advisable (83,84,88). Chloramphenicol once was the antibiotic of first choice for such uses but now has generally been superseded by an aminoglycoside (tobramycin) or a fluoroquinolone. Patching, after a corneal abrasion, is an option that can improve patient comfort and rehealing of the abrasion, but it should be performed only if a follow-up visit within 24 hours is probable (83,176,535). Acute bacterial conjunctivitis should be managed with discontinuation of contact lens wear, hygiene measures (including eyewashes), and, depending on the severity at presentation, single antibiotics (e.g., gentamicin, chloramphenicol, framycetin, ofloxacin) (524, 580,581) or combination antibacterial eyedrops (577). Various combinations are available (Table 41.16).

For acute-onset mild-to-moderate bacterial conjunctivitis, the first-choice therapy often will be an aminoglycoside, such as gentamicin or tobramycin. When used on a q.i.d. basis at the 0.3% concentration in eyedrops (or as ointments HS), the treatment should be needed for only 1 week. The most common limitation to use of these aminoglycoside antibiotics probably is the development of allergies or toxic keratitis (291,536,537,582). A toxic keratitis is more likely to occur if there is overuse of the antibiotics. The allergy risk is considered highest for neomycin; the allergy is a delayed hypersensitivity (type IV) reaction and can result in contact dermatitis of the eyelid margins or conjunctiva (291,544). Topical ocular sulfonamides are widely available in the United States and Canada for management of milder bacterial conjunctivitis and keratoconjunctivitis (577) but are no longer marketed in the United Kingdom. Sulfonamides, as general antiinfective drugs, have a higher potential for causing milder allergic reactions than newer drugs. These reactions include contact dermatitis of the eyelids and conjunctiva. For milder cases of conjunctivitis, use of sulfacetamide 10%, trimethoprim-polymyxin B (567), or other combination products (e.g., neomycin with gramicidin) q.i.d. for 7 to 10 days should resolve the discomfort and reduce the bacterial flora to background levels.

Special cases of conjunctivitis include those in infants and those associated with chlamydial infections. In addition to their use for conjunctivitis and keratoconjunctivitis, tetracyclines were popularized in the 1950s as an alternative

agent for infant conjunctivitis (583). Until recently, they would have been considered as an alternative to erythromycin for ocular chlamydial infections (inclusion conjunctivitis) where a 2- to 3-week course of therapy usually is sufficient (584,585); however, no individual ophthalmic products are currently listed for the United States.

The broad-spectrum drug chloramphenicol probably is still widely used (especially by physicians) for brief courses of treatment for common bacterial pathogens that cause conjunctivitis. Chloramphenicol remains an extremely effective (533) and safe drug (533,542,553,554,586). However, in the United States and Canada, current recommendations from pharmaceutical companies generally suggest that ophthalmic chloramphenicol should be used only if other suitable antibiotics are not available, especially for conditions such as bacterial conjunctivitis. Where its use is still considered appropriate, it may be effectively used over the short-term in the management of contact lens-related bacterial conjunctivitis on a q.i.d. basis (182,587).

Purulent or hyperacute bacterial conjunctivitis generally starts as mild-to-moderate bacterial conjunctivitis, but it can worsen substantially so that it involves the cornea as well. The risk of this occurrence must be established at the initial presentation and a clinical judgment made as to how aggressive the therapy should be. Milder nonulcerating bacterial conjunctivitis is likely to be self-limiting, providing ocular hygiene is reasonable, and may not even require antibiotic intervention (524). Conversely, others have argued that the failure to begin antibiotic therapy places the cornea at risk (588) and so should always be started regardless of the severity at initial presentation. In moderate-to-severe cases, the antibiotic therapy should be with a single broad-spectrum antibiotic (aminoglycoside, chloramphenicol, or a fluoroquinolone) q2h initially if there are no signs of ulceration and continued for 1 to 3 days before the dosing is reduced to q.i.d. Failure of the eye to improve probably indicates either a wrong diagnosis or a resistant strain of bacteria. Therapy must be continued for 7 to 10 days and then for several days after the eye is quiet to ensure that the condition has resolved (34,83,524). Nightly application of a broad-spectrum antibiotic ointment, either during the period of aggressive therapy or for a few days afterward, should improve the chance of ensuring eradication of the pathogen.

Contact lens wearers who present with very red and grossly uncomfortable eyes should be treated as ophthalmic emergencies. After culture samples are taken, the initial therapy should be at least q1h for the first 24 hours. Hospitalization should be considered to ensure that the eyedrops can be regularly administered if a corneal ulcer is clearly evident. Cultures should be taken immediately so that antibiotic sensitivity is already known if the condition does not show signs of improvement within 48 hours. Severe ulcerating lesions of the conjunctiva or cornea need aggressive therapy, preferably with aminoglycoside or fluoroquinolone antibiotics (32,524,589,590). The fluoroquinolone antibacterial drugs (ciprofloxacin, norfloxacin, ofloxacin, levofloxacin) display similar efficacy against most common bacteria causing eye infections when used on a q.i.d. basis (591–594). When used at the 0.3% concentration, they also are suitable for intensive use (i.e., q1h or more frequently) for bacterial corneal ulcers (595–597) given that they can be expected to be efficacious against *Pseudomonas*. This issue of sensitivity of *Pseudomonas* to antibacterial drugs is an important one, because it is a pathogen commonly associated with corneal ulcers. Both gentamicin and tobramycin antibiotics are suitable for use in corneal ulcers, especially if they are used at higher concentrations as fortified antibiotics (see later). Neomycin is not generally considered to be efficacious against *Pseudomonas* (533), and neither is chloramphenicol (533). Therefore, chloramphenicol is not indicated for use in corneal ulcers both because it should not be used intensively and because of poor efficacy. Ophthalmic tetracyclines are not considered efficacious against *Pseudomonas* (533). Although relatively concentrated solutions of polymyxin B and gramicidin can be used intensively in the management of corneal ulcers due to *Pseudomonas* (598), their use currently is usually in combination products indicated for mild-to-moderate bacterial infections of the eyelids and conjunctiva. Overall, therefore, the current choice of antibiotics for corneal ulcers is a fluoroquinolone, unless fortified preparations are used (see later).

For corneal ulcers, it is essential that both cultures be taken (to establish antibiotic sensitivity) and aggressive therapy initiated (e.g., a fluoroquinolone or an aminoglycoside q1h or q2h).There should be regular follow-up of the patient to ensure that the condition does not worsen. One commonly used strategy of applying antibiotic ointments under a pressure patch is no longer advisable (32,534). The discharge should abate within 48 hours; if it does not, the antibiotic should be changed, taking into consideration the culture (or reculture) results.

A number of other antibacterial drugs can be used for management of severe cases of ocular infection (e.g., central corneal ulcers) or infections not susceptible to commercially available antibacterial drugs, e.g., the penicillins, the cephalosporins, vancomycin, and other aminoglycosides (542, 577,589,597,599,600). The corneal ulcer may be of sufficient magnitude or due to a resistant organism so that fortified antibiotics are indicated (589,599). The principles of the use of fortified antibiotics originate from the once commonplace therapies of *Pseudomonas* ulcers with subconjunctival injections with penicillin or streptomycin (601). These fortified antibiotics must be formulated at a pharmacy, so their use is restricted to specialist eye clinics at hospitals. These eyedrops (e.g., those containing up to 1.4% aminoglycosides or cephalosporins) must be prepared on a daily basis by a hospital pharmacy. Follow-up cultures need to be performed regularly until the cultures are negative for the major pathogen. Slit-lamp examination of the cornea in severe infections probably requires the use of topical ocular

anesthetics. This poses a strategic problem because the anesthetics might interfere with cultures. If at all possible, cultures (at least from the lid margins) should be taken before the anesthetics are used to reduce the probability of interference of the anesthetics with culture tests (211–213,532).

Moderate-to-severe cases of nonulcerative conjunctivitis or keratitis require consideration of the careful use of corticosteroids at some stage of the therapy, both for patient comfort and to reduce the likelihood of conjunctival or corneal scarring (602). Eyedrops containing corticosteroids with gentamicin and tobramycin, as well as chloramphenicol, are available. For moderate conditions (e.g., a blepharoconjunctivitis), some argue that therapy should be started with an antibiotic-corticosteroid combination, whereas others prefer to first bring the infection under control before introducing corticosteroids. The palliative aspect of corticosteroid therapy (see section V.F.1) will mean that the signs and symptoms of worsening bacterial infection may be masked, i.e., the eye may look less red and feel more comfortable than it would be without the corticosteroids. Those who advocate the use of corticosteroids likely will argue that combination products should be routinely used at initial presentation because part of the treatment goals should be to make the eye quiet and comfortable as soon as possible. Overall, however, corticosteroid therapy should not be needed, but inflammation of the eyelid margins or conjunctiva may be managed by later supplementing the antibiotic therapy with a moderate-to-strong corticosteroid for a few days on a tapered schedule (275,495). Steroid use should be tapered as soon as the inflammatory sequelae to the infection are brought under control and the antibiotic eyedrops continued for a few more days.

For any corneal infection, ophthalmic corticosteroids probably are indicated at some stage, once the infection is under control (599,602). Such aggressive adjunct use of prednisolone 1% eyedrops q.i.d., along with the antibiotics, should be continued for as long as clear signs of tissue edema are evident because irreversible epithelial or stromal scarring could be the much unwanted sequela to corneal ulcers if judicious use of steroids is not implemented as early as possible (599,602). Corticosteroid therapy then should be tapered well before antibiotic therapy is discontinued (32, 524,527). Concurrent treatment with cycloplegics (e.g., homatropine 5% or atropine 1% b.i.d.) is generally required for patient comfort and to reduce sequelae of anterior segment inflammation (i.e., synechiae).

Antiviral Drugs for Ophthalmic Use

Overview of Viral Infections of the External Eye

Viral infections of the eye can develop in contact lens wearers. Instead of a red eye with mucopurulent discharge, patients may present with acute-onset watery eyes with a negative allergy history. They also may have a marked foreign body sensation (rather than itching or burning) and episodic pain. Biomicroscopy reveals no foreign body; therefore, a viral etiology should be considered. Three types of viral infection are considered here, and all three can be partially managed with ophthalmic therapeutic pharmaceutical agents.

Adenovirus infections such as epidemic keratoconjunctivitis (EKC) may cause a watery eye with follicular conjunctivitis and marked hyperemia and/or chemosis that may be accompanied by fever symptoms, a sore throat, and palpable preauricular lymph nodes (603–605). One eye may be affected several days before the other, before bilateral ocular involvement usually develops and follows a course of a few days. EKC often has a characteristic punctate infiltrative keratitis that begins within a day or so of the conjunctivitis (603,606). A similar presentation may be expected for oculopharyngeal fever.

Herpes simplex virus (HSV) infections of the eye also can cause a red watery eye with marked hyperemia and some chemosis. It can be unilateral and result in some foreign body sensation and some degree of ocular discomfort (607, 608). The hallmark signs of HSV infection include small periocular pustular (blisterlike) skin lesions and the ultimate development of dendritic lesions of the corneal epithelial surface. Marked follicular conjunctivitis or tarsal conjunctival ulcers can be present, especially in recurrent cases (608, 609).

Herpes zoster (varicella; shingles) infections can affect the eye. The condition usually is unilateral, and the accompanying skin lesions usually respect the midline. These skin lesions starts as small red spots but can quickly develop into open red sores with pigmented edges and/or scabs (because the patient cannot help irritating them). Any ocular involvement is generally characterized by considerable pain, and pseudodendritic lesions and intrastromal infiltrates of the cornea can develop (609). The ocular involvement usually will begin only after large periocular skin lesions have developed.

A few notes have appeared in the literature on the development of dendritic or fluorescein-positive branching patterns on the corneal epithelium in asymptomatic hydrogel contact lens wearers (32,610–612). The cause of these unusual superficial lesions is unknown and, because the patient is largely asymptomatic, the lesions rarely require treatment other than discontinuation of contact lens wear to allow for effective monitoring (32).

Mechanisms of Action of Antiviral Drugs for Ocular Use

Several drugs are available to combat viral infections of the eye. Topical drugs include trifluridine, idoxuridine, vidarabine, acyclovir, and ganciclovir. The mechanism of antiviral drugs used for eye infections involves their acting as competitive antagonists of viral DNA synthesis (613–615). A specificity for the viral nucleic acid replication usually is achieved by the unique action of phosphorylase enzymes of the virus-infected cell that convert the viral prodrugs into active phosphorylated derivatives.

The most commonly used ophthalmic antiviral in the United States is trifluridine, also known as trifluorothymidine or F3T (616,617). After topical application to the eye, the trifluridine is converted into its triphosphate, and this trifluridine triphosphate then blocks thymidine-requiring DNA synthesis. Virus replication and further spread of the virus to neighboring cells is thus substantially slowed. Trifluridine is primarily active against HSV, but it can have some activity against varicella zoster.

Idoxuridine (IDU) was introduced in the 1960s as the first commercially marketed ophthalmic antiviral (618). It differs from other currently used antiviral drugs in that it is not a prodrug but directly inhibits adenine-linked DNA replication. As a result, it is potentially highly toxic to corneal epithelial cells. Toxic keratitis can develop if idoxuridine is used excessively (either too frequently or for too long); thus, it has a narrow therapeutic index.

Vidarabine, also known as adenine arabinoside (Ara-A), is another prodrug and is converted to its phosphorylated form in virus-infected cells (619). The in vitro antiviral activity of vidarabine includes HSV, but it displays activity against varicella zoster as well. It is well tolerated.

Acyclovir is another prodrug, with acyclovir triphosphate as the active derivative (613,620), that displays good activity against herpes simplex and varicella zoster. It is very well tolerated. It is not marketed as an ophthalmic product in the United States or Canada, however, it is available in the United Kingdom and Australia as a 3% ophthalmic ointment for 5× per day application. Another topical ocular antiviral drug, recently available in the United Kingdom, is ganciclovir. It is used as a 0.15% ophthalmic gel and displays efficacy equivalent to that of acyclovir 3% ointment (621,622).

Management of Viral Infections in Contact Lens Wear

The different ocular viral infections require very different management and do not necessarily involve the use of antiviral drugs. All management options for viral infections in contact lens wearers require that contact lens wear be discontinued immediately.

EKC management requires three strategies. The most important is patient hygiene, with respect to face flannels and hand towels, to minimize spreading the virus to other family members. Equally important are hygiene measures that must be adopted by the practitioner so as to minimize the risk of cross-patient transfer of the virus (603,623–625). The patient's contact lenses might be disinfected with extended hydrogen peroxide treatment, but ideally the contact lens should simply be replaced. This will eliminate the risk of virus being transferred back to the eye in patients with hydrophilic lenses. Third, the question to be posed is whether the disease process can be controlled or its consequences reduced by any treatment.

There is no specific therapy for EKC, although cases have been treated with antibiotics and antiviral drugs (624). In recent years, both animal and clinical trials have been performed with topical ocular cidofovir (626). This is a possible specific antiviral drug for EKC. Even though no specific treatments currently being available, there are two management options. Patient comfort can be greatly improved with the use of cold compresses, general use of astringents, and judicious use of decongestants (623,627). Cold compresses are best applied with disposable pads (made of gauze or tissue). If a face flannel were to be used, it should be placed in boiling water immediately after use.

Additional therapeutic measures may include the use of corticosteroids, although this option must be used with great caution. Virus-related epithelial infiltrates, if present in significant amounts, can be managed with a brief course of topical ocular corticosteroid therapy (603,623,627), e.g., prednisolone 0.12%, q4h for 1 to 2 weeks. Any peripheral epithelial infiltrates in a contact lens wearer also may be due to staphylococcal toxins (rather than EKC), and these infiltrates may also respond well to a brief course of topical ocular corticosteroid therapy (83). For other virus infections (e.g., HSV and zoster), specific drug therapies are available. Topical ophthalmic products are listed in Table 41.17.

Adult cases of herpes simplex keratitis require aggressive therapy to minimize the risk of significant corneal morbidity (608). Such morbidity will occur if the virus causes deep ulcerating dendritic lesions in the corneal epithelium that then enter the corneal stroma. Most corneal damage results in some scarring with distortion of the cornea (leading to astigmatism). However, even a small scar right on the visual axis could cause substantial reduction in vision.

For HSV keratitis or conjunctivitis, contact lens wear must be discontinued, and the contact lenses sterilized or preferably discarded. Biomicroscopy should be performed with fluorescein to identify the position and extent of any corneal epithelial lesions. Even if the presenting lesions are small and nondendritic (e.g., Y-shaped and only 1 mm

TABLE 41.17. ANTIVIRAL DRUGS COMMERCIALLY AVAILABLE FOR TOPICAL OPHTHALMIC USE

Drugs	Commercial Products	Size
Trifluridine 1%	Viroptic	7.5 mL
Idoxuridine 0.1%	Herplex	15 mL
Vidarabine 3%	Vira-A	3.5 g
Acyclovir	a	
Ganciclovir	a	

[a] No products are listed for the United States and Canada, but they are available in the United Kingdom.

long), the treatment for first-time sufferers usually is antiviral eyedrops such as trifluridine (617,628–630). The alternatives, where available, are antiviral eye ointments or gels (acyclovir or ganciclovir). The dosage regimen should be at least q2h for eyedrops and at least q3h for ointments. The intensive topical therapy should be continued for at least 1 day for first-time cases. The subsequent course of therapy can be less frequent (e.g., $5\times$ per day) but should be dictated by clinical assessments to verify that the lesions are not becoming larger.

Overall, the treatment of HSV keratitis should be continued for up to 14 days on a q3h or q4h schedule (617,619, 631). A similar strategy should be adopted for suspected conjunctival HSV infections, with the intent to minimize the risk of significant corneal disease developing (630). Topical antiviral therapy should continue for several days after the cornea appears totally free of any surface anomalies and the patient is asymptomatic. This is to ensure that the virus has been eradicated from the superficial corneal cells as a result of their natural cycle of desquamation. However, care should be taken to avoid overdosing with topical ocular antivirals because there is a toxicity risk. Some have suggested a maximum of nine applications per day to limit the risk of a toxic keratitis developing. This risk is considered to be much greater for idoxuridine compared to trifluridine or acyclovir (291,616,617,632). The eye should generally not be patched, although an eye shield or pad may provide some relief from photophobia (629).

Recurrent milder cases of herpes simplex keratitis can be effectively managed from the initial presentation with 7 to 10 days of therapy with vidarabine 3% ophthalmic ointment q3h or q4h (619,631), but only if such therapy is clearly adequate to arrest further enlargement of the epithelial lesions (619). Successful therapeutic treatment of herpes simplex keratitis with acyclovir administered orally has been reported (632), and oral acyclovir also is considered beneficial for reducing the likelihood of herpetic keratitis recurrence. In initial or repeated case adult sufferers, more substantial lesions require not only intensive topical antiviral therapy but also consideration of the use of debridement, although this is not a frequent treatment today. The debridement is done with a cotton bud applicator (Q-Tip) or spear (Weck-Cel) or even the edge of a surgical blade. Such debridement should be carried out under extended topical anesthesia (i.e., multiple drops of tetracaine) and the intensive antiviral therapy continued.

If the epithelial lesions in HSV keratitis are deep and have resulted in subepithelial or anterior stromal infiltrates, topical corticosteroid therapy is essential to minimize resultant scarring (607,608,616,617). Despite patient discomfort, corticosteroid use should not be started until biomicroscopy and fluorescein staining clearly show that the epithelial lesions are healing (608). Thereafter, a short course of intensive corticosteroid therapy (e.g., prednisolone 1%, q4h for 1 week) should limit damage and scarring of the stromal tissue. Use of the corticosteroids should be followed by regular biomicroscopy to ensure that the steroid therapy has not exacerbated the epithelial viral infection (602,608,609,633,634). Antiviral therapy should be continued throughout the period of topical corticosteroid use.

Zoster infections require systemic antiviral drugs as well as strong systemic analgesics, including narcotic analgesics. The dendriform patterns or plaques in zoster corneal infections usually will be highlighted by rose bengal stain and may be removed under topical anesthesia using a cotton-tipped applicator to leave fluorescein-staining superficial lesions. Because of the dendriform patterns, therapy can be initiated with topical trifluridine or vidarabine, which may have some effect (616,635) and should follow a similar course and intensity as for herpes simplex lesions. However, a secondary inflammation and even infection of the cornea may be more likely to produce significant sequelae in zoster lesions, so additional treatment with a topical ocular corticosteroid such as prednisolone 1% q.i.d. can be considered (609,636). Topical ocular broad-spectrum antibiotic coverage (e.g., neomycin-polymyxin B, q.i.d.) also can be initiated throughout the course of the periocular skin lesions. The condition requires systemic treatment, and the current standard of therapy in the United States is oral acyclovir (Zovirax, 200 mg, 5× per day) for 1 to 2 weeks (637–639). Oral famciclovir (Famvir, up to 500 mg, t.i.d.) also can be used for the same purpose (640,641). Systemic therapy may include large doses of oral corticosteroids as well (636). Once the herpes simplex or zoster infections are under control, residual epitheliopathy and/or exposure keratitis can be managed with artificial tears or ocular lubricants, preferably nonpreserved, on at least a q.i.d. regimen.

Antifungal and Antiprotozoan Drugs for Ocular Use

Overview of Fungal and Viral Infections of the External Eye

Whenever a viral-like infection with severe keratitis and keratouveitis does not resolve after a few weeks of intensive therapy, a fungal or protozoan origin of the infections should be considered (589,642–645). There are a number of significant risk factors for such devastating infections, the most widely publicized of which perhaps is the use of homemade saline solutions for rinsing contact lenses.

Mechanisms of Action of Antifungal and Antiprotozoan Drugs for Eye Infections

Once diagnosed, these types of infections require extraordinary measures of topical and systemic therapy with general antiinfective (propamidine) and antifungal/antiprotozoan drugs (ketoconazole, amphotericin B) and narcotic analgesics. No standard therapy has been developed, and whatever

TABLE 41.18. ANTIFUNGAL AND ANTIPROTOZOAN DRUGS FOR TOPICAL OPHTHALMIC USE

Drugs	Commercial products	Size
Natamycin 5%	NATACYN	15 mL
Propamidine 0.1%	BROLENE, GOLDEN EYE[a]	10 mL
Polyhexamethylene biguanide (PHMB) 0.02%	b	
Chlorhexidine 0.2%	b	

[a] For the United States, propamidine eyedrops would need to be brought in from the United Kingdom.
[b] Will be prepared by a pharmacy at a major hospital or eye clinic.

therapies are attempted, they likely will be used over the course of many months (589,644,645). Considerable controversy exists on the concurrent use of local fortified antibiotics and strong corticosteroids for fungal or protozoan infections (589,602,646,647).

Management of Fungal and Protozoan Infections

Management of fungal and protozoan infections of the cornea and conjunctiva should be performed by a specialist. A number of drugs are available, but most will be formulated by a hospital pharmacy (Table 41.18).

For management of fungal infections in contact lens wearers, the principal drug is natamycin 5% ophthalmic solution (589,648–650). Oral antifungal drugs, including the azole antifungal drugs (e.g., niconazole, ketoconazole) also can be used (649).

Current options for the management of protozoan infections, such as those caused by *Acanthamoeba*, include the intensive use of propamidine 0.1% eyedrops q1h or more frequently (645,651–654). Other alternatives that have been developed include the use of polyhexamethylene biguanide (PHMB) 0.02% eyedrops (645,652,654,655) and chlorhexidine 0.2% eyedrops (653,646,656,657). All three can be used singly or concurrently, especially if signs of resistance become evident (656,658). In addition, a broad-spectrum antibacterial drug or drug combinations are used to limit protozoan replication (because they feed on bacteria) and reduce the chance of secondary infection by bacteria (646,651,652,655).

GENERAL RESOURCES

Bartlett JD, Fiscella RG, Bennett E, et al., eds. *Ophthalmic Drug Facts 2002*. St. Louis: Facts & Comparisons, 2002.

Doughty MJ. *Drugs, Medications and The Eye*, 12th ed. Helensburgh, Scotland: Smawcastellane Information Services, 2004.

Physician desk reference (PDR) ophthalmology. Oradell, NJ: Medical Economics, 2002.

Melton R, Thomas R. 2002 clinical guide to ophthalmic drugs. *Rev Optom* 2002;[Suppl]:1A– 56A.

REFERENCES

1. Dewart MR, Elliott LJ. Management of contact lens-associated or lens-induced pathology. In: Bennett ES, Henry VA, eds. *Clinical manual of contact lenses,* 2nd ed. Philadelphia: Lippincott Williams & Williams, 2000:582–610.
2. Dabezies OH. Contact lenses and their solutions: a review of basic principles. Eye Ear Nose Throat Monthly 1966;45:82–84.
3. Jenkin L, Tyler-Jones R, Jenkin L. Contact lens solutions and drugs. In: *Theory and practice of contact lens fitting.* London: The Hatton Press, 1969:101–105.
4. Cureton GL, Sibley MJ. Soft contact lens solutions. Past, present and future. *J Am Optom Assoc* 1974;45:285–291.
5. Phillips AJ. Contact lens solutions. *Contact Lens J* 1977;6:3–23.
6. Hopkins GA. Drugs and solutions used in contact lens practice. *Contact Lens J* 1979;16:161–167.
7. McLaughlin R, Barr JT. Contact lens solutions update. *Contact Lens Spectrum* 1989;4:21–25.
8. Egan DJ, Myers RI. CL care systems: from regulation to elimination. *Contact Lens Forum* 1990;15:27–43.
9. Barr JT, Bergmanson JPG, Hill RM, et al. The changing face of disinfection and care. *Contact Lens Spectrum* 1990;5:51–64.
10. Christie CL, Meyler JG. Contemporary contact lens care products. *Contact Lens Anterior Eye* 1997;20[Suppl.]:S11–S17.
11. Jones L. RGP contact lens care. In: Jones LW, ed. *Contact lens solutions.* Oxford: Butterworth-Heinemann, 2004, in press.
12. Coward BD, Neumann R, Callender M. Solution intolerance among users of four chemical soft lens care regimens. *Am J Optom Physiol Opt* 1984;61:523–527.
13. Wilson-Holt N, Dart JKG. Thimerosal keratoconjunctivitis, frequency, clinical spectrum and diagnosis. *Eye* 1989;3:581–587.
14. Doughty MJ. Local allergic and toxic responses to contact lens solutions and topical ocular drugs. In: Jones LW, ed. *Contact lens solutions.* Oxford: Butterworth-Heinemann, 2004, in press.
15. Gordon A. Prospective screening for thimerosal hypersensitivity: a pilot study. *Am J Optom Physiol Opt* 1988;65:147–150.
16. Ramsey WS. Allergies: the gateway to your TPA practice. *Optom Management* 2000;March:66–76.
17. O'Callaghan GJ, Phillips AJ. Rheumatoid arthritis and the contact lens wearer. *Clin Exp Optom* 1994;77:137–143.
18. Morrison RJ, Shovlin JP. The contact lens patient with dry eye symptoms. *Contemp Optom* 1985;4:7–11.
19. Crandall DC, Leopold IH. The influence of systemic drugs on tear constituents. *Ophthalmology* 1979;86:115–125.
20. Polak BCP. Side effects of drugs and tear secretion. *Doc Ophthalmol* 1979;67:115–117.
21. Polak BCP. Contact lens tolerance and ocular side effects of drugs. *Concepts Toxicol* 1987;4:56–58.
22. Buonfiglio R, Favini E, Berva C, et al. Rilievo statistico dell'alterazioni del film lacrimale, effettuato in ambiente ambulatoriale su in gruppo eterogeneo di 1179 pazienti. *Minerv Oftalmol* 1983;25:47–54.
23. Wartman RH. Contact lens-related side effects of systemic drugs. *Contact Lens Forum* 1987;12:42–44.
24. Sorbara L, Talsky C. Contact lens wear in the dry eye patient: predicting success and achieving it. *Can J Optom* 1988;50:234–242.
25. Baldi F, Rolando M, Rinaldi M, et al. Effetto del farmaci somminstrati per via sistemica sulla secrezione lacrimale. *Ann Ottalmol Clin Ocul* 1989;115:617–622.
26. Vale J. The effects of drugs on the tear film and contact lenses. *Trans Br Contact Lens Assoc Scientific Meetings* 1990:21–23.
27. Doughty MJ, Blades KA, Ibrahim N. Assessment of the number of eye symptoms, and the impact of some confounding variables, for office staff in non-air-conditioned buildings. *Ophthalmic Physiol Optics* 2002;22:143–155.
28. Doughty MJ, Fonn D, Richter D, et al. A patient questionnaire approach to estimating the prevalence of dry eye symptoms in patients presenting to optometric practices across Canada. *Optom Vis Sci* 1997;74:624–631.
29. Nadbath RP. Complications and troubles (of contact lens wear). *Trans Pacific Coast Oto-Ophthalmol Soc* 1961;42:117–121.
30. Spoor TC, Hartel WC, Wynn P, et al. Complications of continuous wear soft contact lenses in a nonreferral population. Arch *Ophthalmol* 1984;102:1312–1313.
31. Schein OD, Glynn RJ, Poggio EC, et al. The relative risk of ulcerative keratitis between extended and daily wear soft contact lens wearers: a case control study. *N Engl J Med* 1989;321:773–778.
32. Fisch B. Corneal ulcers and contact lens wear. *Contact Lens Spectrum* 1990;5:48–58.
33. Bruce AS, Brennan NA. Corneal pathology with contact lens wear. *Surv Ophthalmol* 1990;35:25–47.
34. Asbell PA, Torres MA. Therapeutic dilemmas in external eye diseases. *Drugs* 1991;42:606–615.
35. Shovlin JP. Contact lens pathology: how would you manage these conditions? *Rev Optom* 1991;128:31–37.
36. Cohen EJ, Gonzalez C, Leavitt KG, et al. Corneal ulcers associated with contact lenses including experience with disposable lenses. *Contact Lens Assoc Ophthalmol J* 1991;17:173–176.
37. Weissman BA, Mondino BJ. Risk factors for contact lens associated microbial keratitis. *Contact Lens Anterior Eye* 2002;25:3–9.
38. Brennan NA. Is there a question of safety with continuous wear? *Clin Exp Optom* 2002;85:127–140.
39. Mishima S, Nagataki S. Pharmacology of ophthalmic solutions. *Contact Intraocul Lens Med J* 1978;4:22–46.
40. Maurice DM, Mishima S. Ocular pharmacokinetics. In: Sears MD, ed. *Handbook of experimental pharmacology.* New York: Springer-Verlag, 1984:19–64.
41. Schoenwald RD. Ocular drug delivery. Pharmacokinetic considerations. *Clin Pharmacokinet* 1990;18:255–269.
42. Doughty MJ. General principles of pharmacology. In: Onofrey BE, ed. *Clinical optometric pharmacology and therapeutics.* Philadelphia: JB Lippincott, 1991:1–38.
43. Burstein NL, Anderson JA. Ocular penetration and ocular bioavailability of drugs. *J Ocul Pharmacol* 1985;1:309–326.
44. Sugaya M, Nagataki S. Drop size and viscosity of ophthalmic solution (In Japanese). *Jpn J Clin Ophthalmol* 1978;32:563–570.
45. Conrad JM, Reay WA, Polcyn RE, et al. Influence of tonicity and pH on lacrimation and ocular drug bioavailability. *J Parenter Drug Assoc* 1978;32:149–161.
46. Doane MG. Turnover and drainage of tears. *Ann Ophthalmol* (Chicago) 1984;16:111–114.
47. Barendsen H, Oosterhuis JA, Van Heringen NJ. Concentration of fluorescein in tear fluid after instillation as eye-drops. I. Isotonic eye-drops. *Ophthalmic Res* 1979;11:73–82.
48. Benedetto DA, Shah DO, Kaufman HE. The instilled fluid dynamics and surface chemistry of polymers in the preocular tear film. *Invest Ophthalmol Vis Sci* 1975;14:887–902.
49. Ludwig A, Van Ooteghem M. The influence of the dropsize on the elimination of an ophthalmic solution from the precorneal area of human eyes. *Pharm Acta Helvetica* 1987;62:56–60.

50. Ludwig A, Van Ooteghem M. Influence of viscolysers on the residence of ophthalmic solutions evaluated by slit lamp fluorophotometry. *STP Pharma Sci* 1992;2:81–87.

51. White WL, Glover T, Buckner AB. Effect of blinking on tear elimination as evaluated by dacryoscintigraphy. *Ophthalmology* 1991;98:367–369.

52. Waltman SR, Patrowicz TC. Effects of hydroxypropyl methylcellulose and polyvinyl alcohol on intraocular penetration of topical fluorescein in man. *Invest Ophthalmol Vis Sci* 1970;9:966–970.

53. Shrewsbury RP, Swarbrick J, Newton KS, et al. Influence of ophthalmic formulations on sodium cromoglycate disposition in the albino rabbit eye. *J Pharm Pharmacol* 1985;37:614–617.

54. Zaki I, Fitzgerald P, Hardy JG, et al. A comparison of the effect of viscosity on the precorneal residence of solutions in rabbit and man. *J Pharm Pharmacol* 1986;38:463–466.

55. Li VH-K, Robinson JR. Solution viscosity effects on the ocular disposition of cromolyn sodium in the albino rabbit. *Int J Pharm* 1989;53:219–225.

56. Bach FC, Adam JB, Mc Whirter HC, et al. Ocular retention of artificial tear solutions. *Ann Ophthalmol* (Chicago) 1972;4:116–119.

57. Tota G, La Marca F. Ulteriori indagini su alcuni colliri a base di prossimetacaina: correlazione tra il tempo di contatto corneale e l'effetto del farmaco. *Ann Ottalmol Clin Ocul* 1987;113:805–812.

58. Adler CA, Maurice DM, Paterson ME. The effect of viscosity of the vehicle on the penetration of fluorescein into the human eye. *Exp Eye Res* 1971;11:34–42.

59. Saettone MF, Giannaccini B, Teneggi A, et al. Vehicle effects on ophthalmic bioavailability: the influence of different polymers on the activity of pilocarpine in rabbit and man. *J Pharm Pharmacol* 1982;34:464–466.

60. Aquavella JV. Morphology of the epithelium in relation to contact lenses. *Contact Intraocul Lens Med J* 1982;8:147–151.

61. Tripathi RC, Tripathi BJ, Millard CB. Physicochemical changes in contact lenses and their interactions with cornea and tears: a review and personal observations. *Contact Lens Assoc Ophthalmol J* 1988;14:23–32.

62. Dillon JR, Tyhurst CW, Yolton RL. The mydriatic effect of tropicamide on light and dark irides. *J Am Optom Assoc* 1977;48:653–658.

63. Doughty MJ, Lyle W, Trevino R, et al. A study of mydriasis produced by topical phenylephrine 2.5% in young adults. *Can J Optom* 1980;50:40–60.

64. Williams TL, Williams AJ, Enzenauer RW. Unilateral mydriasis from topical Opcon-A and soft contact lens. *Aviat Space Environ Med* 1997;68:1035–1037.

65. Yolton DP, Kandel JS, Yolton RL. Diagnostic pharmaceutical agents: side effects encountered in a study of 15,000 applications. *J Am Optom Assoc* 1980;51:113–118.

66. Sorensen T, Taagehoj F, Christensen U. Tear flow and contact lenses. *Acta Ophthalmol* 1980;58:182–187.

67. Farris RL. Tear analysis in contact lens wearers. *Trans Am Ophthalmol Soc* 1985;83:501–545.

68. Draeger J. The influence of contact lenses on corneal sensitivity. In: Draeger J, ed. *Corneal sensitivity, measurement and clinical importance.* New York: Springer-Verlag, 1984:90–98.

69. Hull DS, Edelhauser HF, Hyndiuk RA. Ocular penetration of prednisolone and the hydrophilic contact lens. *Arch Ophthalmol* 1974;92:413–416.

70. Binder PS, Worthen DM. A continuous-wear hydrophilic lens. Prophylactic topical antibiotics. *Arch Ophthalmol* 1976;94:2109–2111.

71. Ellis PP, Matsumura M, Rendi MA. Pilocarpine concentrations in aqueous humor following single drop application. I. Effect of soft contact lenses. *Curr Eye Res* 1985;4:1041–1047.

72. Lemp MA. Bandage lenses and the use of topical solutions containing preservatives. *Ann Ophthalmol* (Chicago) 1978;10:1319–1321.

73. Kruger CJ, Ehlers WH, Luisrto AE, et al. Treatment of giant papillary conjunctivitis with cromolyn sodium. *Contact Lens Assoc Ophthalmol J* 1992;18:46–48.

74. Kemmetmuller H. Susceptibility of lacrimation to the application of contact lenses. *Contact Lens J* 1986;14:6–9.

75. Iwasaki W, Kosaka Y, Momose T, et al. Absorption of topical disodium cromoglycate and its preservatives by soft contact lenses. *Contact Lens Assoc Ophthalmol J* 1988;14:155–158.

76. Donshik PC, Ballow M, Luistro A, et al. Treatment of contact lens-induced giant papillary conjunctivitis. *Contact Lens Assoc Ophthalmol J* 1984;10:346–350.

77. Douglas JP, Lowder CY, Lazorik R, et al. Giant papillary conjunctivitis associated with rigid gas permeable contact lenses. *Contact Lens Assoc Ophthalmol* 1988;14:143–147.

78. Peyton SM, Joyce EG, Edrington TB. Soft contact lens and corneal changes associated with Visine use. *J Am Optom Assoc* 1989;60:207–210.

79. Lustine T, Bouchard CS, Cavanagh HD. Continued contact lens wear in patients with giant papillary conjunctivitis. *Contact Lens Assoc Ophthalmol* 1991;17:104–107.

80. Dassanayake NL, Carey TC, Owen GR. A laboratory model to determine the uptake and release of olopatadine by soft contact lenses. *Acta Ophthalmol Scand* 2000;78:16–17.

81. Friedberg ML, Pleyer U, Mondino BJ. Device drug delivery to the eye. Collagen shields, iontophoresis, and pumps. *Ophthalmology* 1991;98:725–732.

82. Lesher GA, Gunderson GG. Continuous drug delivery through the use of disposable contact lenses. *Optom Vis Sci* 1993;70:1012–1018.

83. Kenyon KR. Decision-making in the therapy of external eye disease. Noninfected corneal ulcers. *Ophthalmology* 1982;89:44–51.

84. Smiddy WE, Hamburg TR, Kracher GP, et al. Therapeutic contact lenses. *Ophthalmology* 1990;97:291–295.

85. Sorensen T, Taagehoj Jensen F, et al. A human and in vitro study on the exchange of water and solutes from soft contact lenses. *Acta Ophthalmol* 1980;58:576–587.

86. Brettschneider R, Praus R, Krejci, et al. Intraocular penetration of bacitracin and polymyxin B after administration by means of hydrophilic gel contact lenses. *Ophthalmic Res* 1975;7:296–302.

87. Jain MR. Drug delivery through soft contact lenses. *Br J Ophthalmol* 1988;72:150–154.

88. Cavanagh HD, Phlaja D, Thoft RA, et al. The pathogenesis and treatment of persistent epithelial defects. *Trans Am Acad Ophthalmol* 1976;81:OP754–OP769.

89. Mackie IA. Contact lenses in dry eyes. *Trans Ophthalmol Soc UK* 1985;104:477–483.

90. Alimgil ML, Erda N, Gonenc D. Unsere Ergebnisse mit Verbandlinsen. *Contactologia* 1990;12:168–170.

91. DePaolis MD. Can we really use hydrophilic disposable lenses for therapeutic purposes. *Contact Lens Spectrum* 1991;6:21–22.

92. Willoughby CE, Batterbury M, Kaye SB. Collagen corneal shields. *Surv Ophthalmol* 2002;47:174–182.

93. Stiles J, Krohne S, Rankin A, et al. The efficacy of 0.5% proparacaine stored at room temperature. *Vet Ophthalmol* 2001;4:205–207.

94. Lamy PP, Shangraw RF. Physico-chemical aspects of ophthalmic and contact lens solutions. *Am J Optom Am Acad Optom* 1971;48:37–51.

95. Schaeffer AJ. Osmotic pressure of the extraocular and intraocular fluids. *Arch Ophthalmol* 1950;43:1026–1035.

96. Trolle-Lassen C. Investigations into the sensitivity of the human eye to hypo- and hypertonic solutions as well as solutions with unphysiological hydrogen ion concentrations. *Pharm Weekblad* 1958;93:148–155.

97. Fletcher EL, Brennan NA. The effect of solution tonicity on the eye. *Clin Exp Optom* 1993;76:17–21.

98. Huang AJW, Belldegrin R, Hanninen L, et al. Effects of hypertonic solutions on conjunctival epithelium and mucinlike glycoprotein discharge. *Cornea* 1989;8:15–20.

99. Maurice DM. The tonicity of an eye drop and its dilution by tears. *Exp Eye Res* 1971;11:30–33.

100. Holly FJ, Lamberts DW. Effect of nonisotonic solutions on tear film osmolality. *Invest Ophthalmol Vis Sci* 1981;20:236–245.

101. Doughty MJ. The cornea and conjunctival surfaces in relation to the tear film. In: Korb DR, et al., ed. *The tear film.* Oxford: Butterworth-Heinemann, 2002:1–18.

102. Bachman WG, Wilson G. Essential ions for maintenance of the corneal epithelial surface. *Invest Ophthalmol Vis Sci* 1985; 26:1484–1488.

103. Doughty MJ. Evaluation of the effects of saline versus bicarbonate-containing mixed salts solutions on rabbit corneal epithelium in vitro. *Ophthalmic Physiol Optics* 1995;15:585–599.

104. Ünlü N, Ludwig A, Van Ooteghem M, et al. Formulation of Carbpol 940 ophthalmic vehicles, and their in vitro evaluation of the influence of simulated lacrimal fluid on their physicochemical properties. *Pharmazie* 1991;46:784–788.

105. Oechsner M, Keipert S. Polyacrylic acid/polyvinylpyrrolidone bipolymeric systems. I. Rheological and mucoadhesive properties of formulations potentially useful for the treatment of dry-eye-syndrome. *Eur J Pharm Biopharm* 1999;4:113–118.

106. Norn M. Tear pH after instillation of buffer in vivo. *Acta Ophthalmol* 1985;63[Suppl. 173]:32–34.

107. Norn MS, Opauski A. Effects of ophthalmic vehicles on the stability of the precorneal tear film. *Acta Ophthalmol* 1977;55: 23–34.

108. Raber I, Breslin CW. Toleration of artificial tears: the effect of pH. *Can J Ophthalmol* 1978;13:247–249.

109. Browning DJ. Tear studies on ocular rosacea. *Am J Ophthalmol* 1985;99:530–532.

110. Coles WH, Jaros PA. Dynamics of ocular surface pH. *Br J Ophthalmol* 1984;68:549–52.

111. Longwell A, Birss S, Keller N, et al. Effect of topically applied pilocarpine on tear film pH. *J Pharm Sci* 1976;65:1654–1657.

112. Efron N, Ang JHB. Corneal hypoxia and hypercapnia during contact lens wear. *Optom Vis Sci* 1990;67:512–521.

113. Riegelman S, Vaughan DG. A rational basis for the preparation of ophthalmic solutions. *Surv Ophthalmol* 1958;3:471–492.

114. Mullen W, Shepherd W, Labovitz J. Ophthalmic preservatives and vehicles. *Surv Ophthalmol* 1973;17:469–483.

115. Kurosawa A, Kuretake Y, Tachihara R, et al. Comparison of eye irritation caused by seven antiallergic eyedrops (in Japanese). *Folia Ophthalmol Jpn* 2001;52:220–223.

116. Lyle WM, Dean TW, Doughty M. Constituents of ophthalmic preparations. *Can J Optom* 1985;47:163–169.

117. Ahmed I, Chaudhuri B. Evaluation of buffer systems in ophthalmic product development. *Int J Pharm* 1988;44:97–105.

118. Samson CR, Danzig MR, Sasovetz D, et al. Safety and toleration of oxymetazoline solution. *Pharmatherapeutica* 1986;2: 347–350.

119. Doughty MJ. Diagnostic and therapeutic pharmaceutical agents for use in contact lens practice. In: Bennett E, Weissman BA, eds. *Clinical contact lens practice.* Philadelphia: Lippincott-Raven, 1996; chapter 9:1–38.

120. Efron N, Golding TR, Brennan NA. Do in-eye lubricants for contact lens wearers really work? *Trans Br Contact Lens Assoc* 1990:14–19.

121. Efron N, Golding TR, Brennan NA. The effect of soft lens lubricants on symptoms and lens dehydration. *Contact Lens Assoc Ophthalmol J* 1991;17:114–119.

122. Faber E, Golding TR, Lowe R, et al. Tear film stability. *Optom Vis Sci* 1991;68:380–384.

123. Nichols KK, Mitchell GL, Stonebraker KM, et al. Corneal staining in hydrogel lens wearers. *Optom Vis Sci* 2002;79:20–30.

124. Nichols JJ, Mitchell L, Nichols KK, et al. The performance of the contact lens dry eye questionnaire as a screening survey for contact lens-related dry eye. *Cornea* 2002;21:469–475.

125. Aiello JP, Insler MS. The effects of hypotonic and hypertonic solutions on the fluid content of hydrophilic contact lenses. *Am J Ophthalmol* 1985;99:521–523.

126. Ruben M. Chlorhexidine (CH) and the PHEMA soft lens. *Contact Lens J* 1980;13:3–14.

127. Papadimitrou JT. Complications of preservatives in contact lens solutions. *Aust J Optom* 1983;66:220–226.

128. Sterling JL, Hecht AS. BAK-induced chemical keratitis? *Contact Lens Spectrum* 1988;March:62–64.

129. Hoffman WC. Ending the BAK-RGP controversy. *Int Contact Lens Clin* 1987;14:31–35.

130. Chapman JM, Cheeks L, Green K. Interactions of benzalkonium chloride with soft and hard contact lenses. *Arch Ophthalmol* 1990;108:244–246.

131. Donnenfield ED, Selkin BA, Perry HD, et al. Controlled evaluation of a bandage contact lens and a non-steroidal anti-inflammatory drug in treating traumatic corneal abrasions. *Ophthalmology* 1995;102:979–984.

132. Macsai MS, Goel AK, Michael MM, et al. Deposition of ciprofloxacin, prednisolone phosphate, and prednisolone acetate in SeeQuence disposable contact lenses. *Contact Lens Assoc Ophthalmol J* 1993;19:166–168.

133. Christensen MT, Barry JR, Turner FD. Five-minute removal of soft lenses prevents most absorption of a topical ophthalmic solution. *Contact Lens Assoc Ophthalmol J* 1998;24:227–231.

134. Sugar J. Adrenochrome pigmentation of hydrophilic lenses. *Arch Ophthalmol* 1974;91:11–12.

135. Miller D, Brooks SM, Mobilia E. Adrenochrome staining of soft contact lenses. *Ann Ophthalmol* (Chicago) 1976;8:65–67.

136. Sibley MJ, Chu V. Understanding sorbic acid-preserved contact lens solutions. *Int Contact Lens Clin* 1984;11:531–542.

137. McKenney C. The effect of pH on hydrogel lens parameters and fitting characteristics after hydrogen peroxide disinfection. *Trans Br Contact Lens Assoc* 1991;13:46–51.

138. Shovlin JP. Systemic medications and their interaction with soft contact lenses. *Int Contact Lens Clinics* 1990;17:250–251.

139. Miranda MN, Garcia-Castineiras S. The effects of pH and some common topical ophthalmic medications on the contact lens Permalens. *Contact Lens Assoc Ophthalmol J* 1983;9:43–48.

140. Bergen G, Slonim CB. The effects of ophthalmic solutions on the transmission of light through hydrogel lenses. *Contact Lens Assoc Ophthalmol J* 1990;16:114–116.

141. Norn MS. Vital staining of cornea and conjunctiva. *Acta Ophthalmol* 1962;40:389–401.

142. Norn MS. Vital staining of the canaliculus lacrimalis and the palpebral border (Marx' line). *Acta Ophthalmol* 1966;44: 948–959.

143. Norn MS. Rose Bengal vital staining. Staining of the cornea and conjunctiva by 10% Rose Bengal, compared with 1%. *Acta Ophthalmol* 1970;48:546–559.

144. Norn MS. Vital staining of cornea in contact lens wearers-with fluorescein-rose bengal mixture. *Contacto* 1971;15:50–53.

145. Norn MS. Method of testing dyes for vital staining of the cornea and conjunctiva. *Acta Ophthalmol* 1972;50:809–814.

146. Feenstra RPG, Tseng SCG. What is actually stained by rose bengal? *Arch Ophthalmol* 1992;110:984–993.

147. Kimura SJ. Fluorescein paper. A simple means of ensuring the use of sterile fluorescein. *Am J Ophthalmol* 1951;34:446–447.

148. Korb DR, Greiner JV, Herman J. Comparison of fluorescein break-up time measurement reproducibility using standard fluorescein strips versus the Dry Eye Test (DET) method. *Cornea* 2001;20:811–815.

149. Reidy JJ, Limberg M, Kaufman HE. Delivery of fluorescein to the anterior chamber using the corneal collagen shield. *Ophthalmology* 1990;97:1201–1203.

150. Hausler HR. Fluorescein filter papers for corneal staining. *Bull Acad Med* 1956;29:227–230.

151. Brav SS, Feinstein RR. Fluorescein applicators: Fluor-I-Strips. *Trans Am Acad Ophthalmol Otolaryngol* 1956;6:487–488.

152. Dolezalova V, Zmolikova J. Fluoresceinovy prouzek. *Ceskegke Oftalmol* 1977;33:289–290.

153. Justice J, Soper JW. An improved method of viewing topical fluorescein. *Trans Am Acad Ophthalmol* 1976;81:OP927–OP928.

154. Doughty MJ, Laiquzzaman ML, Oblak E, et al. The tear (lacrimal) meniscus height in human eyes: a useful clinical measure or an unusable sign? *Contact Lens Anterior Eye* 2002;25:57–65.

155. Lithgow FW. Eloisin, tratamiento de eleccion de la hiposecrecion lagrimal. *An Inst Barraquer* (Barcelona) 1996;25:713–719.

156. Kinney KA. Detecting dry eye in contact lens wearers. *Contact Lens Spectrum* 1998;13:21–28.

157. Terry JE. Eye disease in the elderly. *J Am Optom Assoc* 1984;55:23–29.

158. Lim KJ, Lee JH. Measurement of the tear meniscus height using 0.25% fluorescein. *Korean J Ophthalmol* 1991;5:34–36.

159. Lupelli L. A review of lacrimal function tests in relation to contact lens practice. *Contact Lens J* 1986;14(7–8):4–17 and 14(10):8–19.

160. Lamberts DW, Foster CS, Perry HD. Schirmer test after topical anesthesia and the tear film meniscus height in normal eyes. *Arch Ophthalmol* 1979;97:1082–1085.

161. Meyer DR, Antonello A, Linberg JV. Assessment of tear drainage after canalicular obstruction using fluorescein dye disappearance. *Ophthalmology* 1990;97:1370–1374.

162. Höh H, Schirra F, Kienecker C, et al. Lid-parallel conjunctival fold (LIPCOF) and dry eye: a diagnostic tool for the contactologist. *Contactologia* 1995;17E:104–117.

163. Doughty MJ, Potvin R, Pritchard N, et al. Evaluation of the range of areas of the fluorescein staining patterns of the tarsal conjunctiva in man. *Doc Ophthalmol* 1995;89:355–371.

164. Potvin RJ, Doughty MJ, Fonn D. Tarsal conjunctival morphometry of asymptomatic soft contact lens wearers and non-lens wearers. *Int Contact Lens Clin* 1994;21:225–231.

165. Lemp MA, Hamill JR. Factors affecting tear break up in normal eyes. *Arch Ophthalmol* 1973;89:103–105.

166. Bitton E, Lovasik JV. Modelling the tear film rupture pattern using dynamic digital imaging techniques. *Can J Optom* 1994;56:94–98.

167. Bruce AS, Mainstone JC, Golding TR. Analysis of tear breakup on Etafilcon A hydrogel lenses. *Biomaterials* 2001;22:3249–3256.

168. Holly FJ. Tear film physiology and contact lens wear. I. Pertinent aspects of tear film physiology. II. Contact lens-tear film interaction. *Am J Optom Physiol Opt* 1981;58:324–330, 331–338.

169. Fenton PJ. Applanation tonometry using one drop of an anesthetic-fluorescein mixture. *Br J Ophthalmol* 1965;49:205–208.

170. Gloster J. The accuracy of tonometry. *Int Ophthalmol Clin* 1965;5:997–1005.

171. Crook TG. Fluorescein as an aid in pachometry. *Am J Optom Physiol Opt* 1979;56:124–127.

172. Roper DL. Applanation tonometry with and without fluorescein. *Am J Ophthalmol* 1980;90:668–671.

173. Koetting RA, Von Gunten T. The effect of polyvinylpyrrolidone with hydroxyethylcellulose on three o'clock and nine o'clock staining. *Contacto* 1971;15:30–33.

174. Hamano H, Hori M, Kawabe H, et al. Clinical examination criteria for fluorescein stainings of cornea caused by contact lenses. *Contacto* 1979;23:9–23.

175. Kline LN, DeLuca TJ, Fishberg GM. Corneal staining relating to contact lens wear. *J Am Optom Assoc* 1979;50:353–357.

176. Finley HM. Recurrent corneal erosions. *J Am Optom Assoc* 1986;57:392–396.

177. Dundas M, Walker A, Woods RL. Clinical grading of corneal staining of non-contact lens wearers. *Ophthalmic Physiol Optics* 2001;21:30–35.

178. Lakkis C, Brennan NA. Bulbar conjunctival fluorescein staining in hydrogel contact lens wearers. *Contact Lens Assoc Ophthalmol J* 1996;22:189–194.

179. Jalbert I, Sweeney DF, Holden BA. The characteristics of corneal staining in successful daily and extended disposable contact lens wearers. *Clin Exp Optom* 1999;82:4–10.

180. Creuzot-Garcher C. L'examen clinique du film lacrymal. *J Fr Ophtalmol* 1999;22:461–466.

181. Holden BA, Stephenson A, Stretton S, et al. Superior epithelial arcuate lesions with soft contact lens wear. *Optom Vis Sci* 2001;78:9–12.

182. Morgan PB, Efron N. Comparative clinical performance of two silicone hydrogel contact lenses for continuous wear. *Clin Exp Optom* 2002;85:183–192.

183. Wilson G, Ren H, Laurent J. Corneal epithelial fluorescein staining. *J Am Optom Assoc* 1995;66:435–441.

184. Thomas ML, Szeto VR, Gan CM, et al. Sequential staining: the effects of sodium fluorescein, osmolarity, and pH on human corneal epithelium. *Optom Vis Sci* 1997;74:207–210.

185. Tabery HM. Dual appearance of fluorescein staining in vivo of disease human corneal epithelium. A non-contact photomicrographic study. *Br J Ophthalmol* 1992;76:43–44.

186. Korb DR, Herman JP. Corneal staining subsequent to sequential fluorescein instillations. *J Am Optom Assoc* 1979;50:361–367.

187. Ueda K, Yamashiro K, Kurimoto S. Contact lens wear-associated 3 & 9 o'clock staining of the cornea (in Japanese). *J Jpn Contact Lens Soc* 1992;34:38–46.

188. Josephson JE, Caffery BE. Corneal staining after instillation of topical anesthetic (SSII). *Invest Ophthalmol Vis Sci* 1988;29:1096–1099.

189. Caffery BE, Josephson JE. Corneal staining after sequential instillations of fluorescein over 30 days. *Optom Vis Sci* 1991;68:467–469.

190. Norn MS. Fluorexon vital staining of the cornea and conjunctiva. *Acta Ophthalmol* 1973;51:670–673.

191. Holly FJ, Lamberts DW. Sorption of high molecular weight fluorescein by Polymacon hydrogel contact lenses. *Intraocul Lens Contact Lens J* 1979;5:160–174.

192. Snyder C, Paugh JR. Rose Bengal dye concentration and volume delivered via dye-impregnated paper strips. *Optom Vis Sci* 1998;75:339–341.

193. Manning FJ, Wehrly SR, Foulks GN. Patient tolerance and ocular surface staining characteristics of lissamine green versus rose bengal. *Ophthalmology* 1995;102:1953–1957.

194. Kronning E. Conjunctival and corneal stainability with rose bengal. *Am J Ophthalmol* 1954;38:351–361.

195. Sjögren H, Block KJ. Keratoconjunctivitis sicca and the Sjogren syndrome. *Surv Ophthalmol* 1971;16:145–159.

196. Josephson JE, Caffery BE, Tepperman CL, et al. Rose bengal

staining before and after anesthetic. *Optom Vis Sci* 1990;67: 659–660.

197. Laroche RR, Campbell RC. Quantitative rose bengal staining technique for external ocular disease. *Ann Ophthalmol* (Chicago) 1988;20:274–277.

198. Tabery HM. Toxic effect of rose bengal dye on the living human corneal epithelium. *Acta Ophthalmol Scand* 1998;76:142–145.

199. Marx E. Über vitale Färbung des Auges und der Augenlider. I. Über Anatomie, Physiologie und Pathologie des Augenlidrandes und der Tränenpunkte. *Graefes Arch Ophthalmol* 1924;114: 465–482.

200. Chodosh J, Dix RD, Howell RC, et al. Staining characteristics and antiviral activity of sulforhodamine B and lissamine green B. *Invest Ophthalmol Vis Sci* 1994;35:1046–1058.

201. Khurana AK, Chaudhary R, Ahluwalia BK, et al. Tear film profile in dry eye. *Acta Ophthalmol* 1991;69:79–86.

202. Franck C, Boge I. Break-up time and lissamine green epithelial damage in "office-eye syndrome." Six month and one-year follow-up investigations. *Acta Ophthalmol* 1993;71:62–64.

203. Amaki S, Ogata T, Konishi M, et al. Lissamine green B staining in the evaluating of keratoconjunctivitis sicca (in Japanese). *Folia Ophthalmol Jpn* 1999;50:536–539.

204. Doughty MJ, Naase T, Donald C, et al. Visualization of 'Marx's line' along the marginal eyelid conjunctiva of human subjects with lissamine green dye. *Ophthal Physiol Opt* 2004;24:1–7.

205. Bartsch W, Knopf K-W. Eine modifizierte Methode zur Prufung der Oberflachenanasthesie an der Kaninchen-Cornea. *Arzneimittelforschung* 1970;8:1140–1143.

206. Seeman P. The membrane actions of anesthetics and tranquilizers. *Pharmacol Rev* 1972;24:583–655.

207. Ohki S, Shinagawa Y, Graves C. Mode of action of tertiary amine local anesthetics on axon membrane excitability. *Biochim Biophys Acta* 1978;507:395–407.

208. Wildsmith JAW, Gissen AJ, Takman B, et al. Differential nerve blockade: esters v. amides and the influence of pK_a. *Br J Anaesthesiol* 1987;59:379–384.

209. Weekers J-F. Reserches experimentales sur la genese des lesions corneennes dues aux anesthesiques. *Arch Ophtalmol* (Paris) 1974;34:121–132.

210. Andermann G, Erhart M. Are local tolerance tests in animals always necessary? *Methods Findings Exp Clin Pharmacol* 1983; 5:321–333.

211. Schlegel HE, Swan KC. Benoxinate (Dorsacaine) for rapid corneal anesthesia. *Arch Ophthalmol* 1954;51:663–670.

212. Kleinfeld J, Ellis P. Effects of topical anesthetics on growth of microorganisms. *Arch Ophthalmol* 1966;76:712–716.

213. Vitale Brovarone F, Fea A, et al. The effect of NOVESINE and fluorescein instillation on the result of conjunctival cultures in course of experimentally-induced bacterial and mycotic infections. *New Trends Ophthalmol* 1989;4:319–327.

214. Linn JG, Vey EK. Topical anesthesia in ophthalmology. *Am J Ophthalmol* 1955;40:697–704.

215. Bryant JA. Local and topical anesthetics in ophthalmology. *Surv Ophthalmol* 1969;13:263–283.

216. Polse KA, Kenner RJ, Jauregui MJ. Dose-response effects of corneal anesthetics. *Am J Optom Physiol Opt* 1978;55:8–14.

217. Jauregui MJ, Sanders TL, Polse KA. Anesthetic effects from low concentrations of proparacaine and benoxinate. *J Am Optom Assoc* 1980;51:37–41.

218. Draeger J, Langenbucher H, Bannert C. Efficacy of topical anesthetics. *Ophthalmic Res* 1984;16:135–138.

219. Lawrenson JG, Edgar DF, Tanna GK, et al. Comparison of the tolerability and efficacy of unit-dose, preservative-free topical ocular anaesthetics. *Ophthalmic Physiol Optics* 1998;18: 393–400.

220. Boozan CW, Cohen IJ. Ophthaine. A new topical anesthetic for the eye. *Am J Ophthalmol* 1953;36:1619–1621.

221. Emmerich R, Carter GZ, Berens C. An experimental clinical evaluation of Dorsacaine hydrochloride (benoxinate Novesine). *Am J Ophthalmol* 1955;40:841–848.

222. Kernie MA, Proehl GA, Remington LA. A comparative study of Fluoracaine and Fluress in Goldman tonometry. *South J Optom* 1990;8:13–15.

223. Shafi T, Koay P. Randomised prospective masked study comparing patient comfort following the instillation of topical proxymetacaine and amethocaine. *Br J Ophthalmol* 1998;82: 1285–1287.

224. Jervey JW. Tonometry and the cornea. *Arch Ophthalmol* 1956; 56:109–127.

225. Tanton JH. Fluorescein-proparacaine hydrochloride. Combination drops for applanation tonometry. *Am J Ophthalmol* 1964; 58:1055–1056.

226. Perkins ES. Hand-held applanation tonometer. *Br J Ophthalmol* 1965;49:591–593.

227. Giasson C, Forthomme D. Etude comparative de deux methods de mesure de l'epasseur de la cornee humaine. *Can J Optom* 1988;50:176–181.

228. Yolton DP, German CJ. Fluress, fluorescein and benoxinate: recovery from bacterial contamination. *J Am Optom Assoc* 1980; 51:471–474.

229. Richter S, Sherman J, Horn D, et al. An embedded contact lens in the upper lid masquerading as a mass. *J Am Optom Assoc* 1979;50:372–373.

230. Henrotte J, Weekers J-F. Etude clinique des lesions corneenes due a l'application locale et prolongee d'anesthesiques. *Arch Ophtalmol* 1972;32:449–456.

231. Henkes HE, Waubke TN. Keratitis from abuse of corneal anaesthetics. *Br J Ophthalmol* 1978;62:62–65.

232. Adenis JP, Merle L, Dangoumau J, et al. Problèmes posés par l'utilisation des collyres et pommades anesthésiques en ophtalmologie. *Therapie* 1978;33:791–795.

233. Pau H. Anasthetikum-keratitis. *Klin Monatsbl Augenheilkd* 1980;176:885–892.

234. Offret G, Oger C. Du danger des anesthesiques de contact en ophtalmologie. *Bull Acad Nat Med* 1981;165:197–202.

235. Penna EP, Tabbara KF. Oxybuprocaine keratopathy: a preventable disease. *Br J Ophthalmol* 1986;70:202–204.

236. Brent MH, Slomovic AR, Easterbrook M. Keratitis associated with the use of proparacaine hydrochloride. *Can Med Assoc J* 1987;136:380–381.

237. Rosenwasser GOD, Holland S, Pflugfelder SC, et al. Topical anesthetic abuse. *Ophthalmology* 1990;97:967–972.

238. Rapuano CJ. Topical anesthetic abuse: a case report of bilateral corneal ring infiltrates. *J Ophthalmic Nursing Technol* 1990;9: 94–95.

239. Bennett ES, Smythe J, Henry VA, et al. Effect of topical anesthetic use on initial patient satisfaction and overall success with rigid gas permeable contact lenses. *Optom Vis Sci* 1998;75: 800–805.

240. Murphy PJ, Patel S, Marshall J. The effect of long-term, daily contact lens wear on corneal sensitivity. *Cornea* 2001;20: 264–269.

241. Robboy M, Orsborn G. The response of marginal dry eye lens wearers to a dry eye survey. *Contact Lens J* 1989;17:8–9.

242. Adler FH. Symposium on the theoretical and practical aspects of corneal contact lens application. *Trans Pacific Coast Oto-Ophthalmol Soc* 1961;42:101–113.

243. Grosvenor TP. Contact lens solutions. In: Grosvenor TP, ed. *Contact lens theory and practice.* Chicago: The Professional Press, 1961:236–246.

244. McKee MC, Keech PM. Some clinical aspects of tears. A review. *Int Contact Lens Clin* 1988;15:20–24.

245. Farris RL. Contact lens wear in the management of the dry eye. *Int Ophthalmol Clin* 1987;27:54–60.

246. Farris RL. Staged therapy for the dry eye. *Contact Lens Assoc Ophthalmol J* 1991;17:207–215.

247. Brown RA. Treatment of anterior segment inflammatory disorders. *Prob Optom* 1992;4:313–326.

248. Shimazaki J, Sakata M, Tsubota K. Ocular surface changes and discomfort in patients with Meibomian gland dysfunction. *Arch Ophthalmol* 1995;113:1266–1270.

249. McMonnies CW. Key questions in a dry eye history. *J Am Optom Assoc* 1986;57:512–517.

250. McMonnies CW, Ho A. Patient history in screening for dry eye conditions. *J Am Optom Assoc* 1987;58:296–301.

251. Doughty MJ. Re-wetting, comfort, lubricant and moisturizing solutions for the contact lens wearer. *Contact Lens Anterior Eye* 1999;22:116–126.

252. Rebeix V, Sommer F, Marchin B, et al. Artificial tear adsorption on soft contact lenses: methods to test surfactant efficacy. *Biomaterials* 2000;21:1197–1205.

253. Sharma A. Energetics of corneal epithelial cell-ocular mucus-tear film interactions: some surface-chemical pathways of corneal defense. *Biophys Chem* 1993;47:87–99.

254. Holly FJ, Lemp MA. Wettability and wetting of corneal epithelium. *Exp Eye Res* 1971;11:239–249.

255. Holly FJ, Esquivel ED. Colloid osmotic pressure of artificial tears. *J Ocul Pharmacol* 1985;1:327–336.

256. Ruben M, Hopkins G. Separation of eye solution deposits (in vitro study of wetting drops for eye and contact lens). *Contact Lens J* 1985;13:5–11.

257. Carney LG, Barr JT, Jochum J, et al. Contact lens lubricants. Part 1. *Contact Lens Spectrum* 1988;3:24–26.

258. Simon Castellvi JM, Verges C, Camins JL, et al. Tratamiento del sindrome de ojo seco analisis comparativo. *Arch Soc Esp Oftalmol* 1989;56:185–192.

259. Barr JT, Carney LG, Jochum K, et al. Contact lens lubricants. Part II. Clinical considerations. *Contact Lens Spectrum* 1988;3:44–52.

260. Golding TR, Brennan NA. Survey of optometric opinion on dry eye topics. *Clin Exp Optom* 1992;75:98–108.

261. Caffery BE, Josephson JE. Is there a better "comfort drop?" *J Am Optom Assoc* 1990;61:178–182.

262. Farkas P, Kassalow TW, Farkas B. Clinical management and control of giant papillary conjunctivitis secondary to contact lens wear. *J Am Optom Assoc* 1986;57:197–200.

263. Wood CA. *A system of ophthalmic therapeutics.* Chicago: Cleveland Press, 1909.

264. Department of Health, Education and Welfare. Ophthalmic drug products for over-the-counter human use. Part II. *Federal Register* 1980.

265. Brown JL. Incomplete labeling of pharmaceuticals: a list of "inactive ingredients." *N Engl J Med* 1984;309:439–441.

266. Taoka S. Studies on the permeability of the cornea. Part III. On the effect of some metals (astringent) (In Japanese). *Fol Ophthalmol Jpn* 1957;8:466–470.

267. Havener WH. Management of conjunctivitis. *Ohio State Med J* 1956;52:40–42.

268. Hogan MJ. The preparation and sterilization of ophthalmic solutions. *Calif Med* 1949;71:414–416.

269. Hart A. Antibacterial activity of phenylmercuric nitrate in zinc sulphate and adrenaline eye drops B.P.C. 1968. *J Pharm Pharmacol* 1973;25:507–508.

270. Clark MJ, Chapman ND, Noyella RM, et al. An open multiple dose study of Optrex Eye Lotion in eye irritation due to hay fever. *Br J Clin Pract* 1989;43:357–359.

271. Cagle GD, Abshire RL. Quantitative ocular bacteriology: a method for the enumeration and identification of bacteria from the skin-lash margin and conjunctiva. *Invest Ophthalmol Vis Sci* 1981;20:751–757.

272. Groden LR, Murphy B, Rodnite J, et al. Lid flora in blepharitis. *Cornea* 1991;10:50–53.

273. Robin JB, Nobe JR, Suarez E, et al. Meibomian gland evaluation in patients with extended wear soft contact lens deposits. *Contact Lens Assoc Ophthalmol J* 1986;12:95–98.

274. Henriquez AS, Korb DR. Meibomian glands and contact lens wear. *Br J Ophthalmol* 1981;65:108–111.

275. Fisch BM. Clinical management of eyelid disease. *Contact Lens Spectrum* 1991;6:40–50.

276. Smolin G, Okumoto M. Staphylococcal blepharitis. *Arch Ophthalmol* 1977;95:812–816.

277. Paugh JR, Knapp LL, Martinson JR, et al. Meibomian therapy in problematic contact lens wearers. *Optom Vis Sci* 1990;67:803–806.

278. Doughty MJ. A guide to ophthalmic pharmacy medicines in the United Kingdom. *Ophthalmic Physiol Optics* 1997;17[Suppl. 1]:S2–S8.

279. Bright AM, Tighe BJ. The composition and interfacial properties of tears, tear substitutes and tear models. *J Br Contact Lens Assoc* 1993;16:57–66.

280. Holly FJ. Surface chemical evaluation of artificial tears and their ingredients. I. Interfacial activity at equilibration. *Intraocul Lens Contact Lens J* 1978;4:14–31.

281. Holly FJ. Surface chemical evaluation of artificial tears and their ingredients. II. Interaction with a superficial lipid layer. *Intraocul Lens Contact Lens J* 1978;4:52–65.

282. Chan RS, Mandell RB. Corneal thickness changes from bathing solutions. *Am J Optom Physiol Opt* 1975;52:465–469.

283. Holly FJ, Lemp MA. Tear physiology and dry eyes. *Surv Ophthalmol* 1977;22:69–87.

284. Roberts DK. Keratoconjunctivitis sicca. *J Am Optom Assoc* 1991;62:187–199.

285. Hill RM, Terry JE. Viscosity: the "staying power" of ophthalmic solutions. *J Am Optom Assoc* 1975;46:239–241.

286. Lemp MA, Goldberg M, Roddy MR. The effect of tear substitutes on tear film break-up time. *Invest Ophthalmol Vis Sci* 1975;14:255–258.

287. Brezzo MV, Alitta P, Giordano G, et al. Effetto di una lacrima artificiale a base di alcool polivinilico 3% su alcune caratterische del film lacrimale. *Boll Oculist* 1989;68[Suppl.]:165–199.

288. Dudinski O, Finnin BC, Reed BL. Acceptability of thickened eye drops to human subjects. *Curr Ther Res* 1983;33:322–327.

289. Duprat P, Conquet P. Predictive value of ocular irritation tests. *Adv Vet Sci Comp Med* 1987;31:173–195.

290. Burstein NL. Corneal cytotoxicity of topically-applied drugs, vehicles and preservatives. *Surv Ophthalmol* 1980;25:15–30.

291. Wilson FM. Adverse external ocular effects of topical ophthalmic therapy: an epidemiologic, laboratory and clinical study. *Trans Am Ophthalmol Soc* 1983; LXXXI:854–965.

292. Fassihi AR, Naidoo NT. Irritation associated with tear-replacement ophthalmic drops. A pharmaceutical and subjective investigation. *South Afr Med J* 1989;75:233–235.

293. Caffery BE. Influence of diet on tear function. *Optom Vis Sci* 1991;68:58–72.

294. Shepherd EM. Histamine diphosphate used topically in the eye. *W V Med J* 1949;45:62–64.

295. Nemeth L. Antihistamines in ophthalmology. *Br J Ophthalmol* 1949;33:665–669.

296. Millichamp NJ, Dziezyc J. Mediators of ocular inflammation. *Prog Vet Comp Ophthalmol* 1991;1:41–58.

297. Bhattacherjee P. Prostaglandins and inflammatory reactions in the eye. *Methods Findings Exp Clin Pharmacol* 1980;2:17–31.

298. Xuan B, Chiou GCY. Efficacy of oxymetazoline eye drops in non-infectious conjunctivitis, the most common cause of acute red eyes. *J Ocul Pharmacol Ther* 1997;13:363–367.

299. Speas WP. Some allergic manifestations of the eye. *N C Med J* 8:364–367.

300. Lipsius EI. Paredrine hydrobromide in chronic conjunctivitis. *Am J Ophthalmol* 1956;39:1692–1694.

301. Muljiani RH. Clinical trials with a new ocular decongestant—Tyzine. *J Indian Med Prof* 1961;8:3600–3602.

302. Breakey AS, Cinotti AA, Hirshman M, et al. A double-blind, multi-centre controlled trial of 0.025% oxymetazoline ophthalmic solution in patients with allergic and non-infectious conjunctivitis. *Pharmatherapeutica 1980;2:353–356.*

303. Duzman E, Anderson J, Vita JB, et al. Topically applied oxymetazoline. Ocular vasoconstrictive activity, pharmacokinetics, and metabolism. *Arch Ophthalmol* 1983;101:1122–1126.

304. Daily RK, Daily L. Use of Privine-Antistine drops in ophthalmology. *Am J Ophthalmol* 1949;32:441–442.

305. Hurwitz P, Thompson JM. Uses of naphazoline (Privine) in ophthalmology. *Arch Ophthalmol* 1950;43:712–717.

306. Grossmann EE, Lehman RH. Ophthalmic use of Tyzine. A clinical study of this new vasoconstrictor. *Am J Ophthalmol* 1949;32:121–123.

307. Scheven H. Die Auslösbarkeit der allergischen Ophthalmoreaktion als klinisches Kriterium für die Wirksamkeit vasokonstriktorischer Substanzen. *Klin Monatsbl Augenheilkd* 1963;142:847–853.

308. Hurwitz P. Ophthalmic Otrivin solution. *Am J Ophthalmol* 1960;50:467–469.

309. Miller J, Wolf EH. Antazoline phosphate and naphazoline hydrochloride, singly and in combination for the treatment of allergic conjunctivitis: a controlled, double-blind clinical trial. *Ann Allergy* 1975;35:81–86.

310. Abelson MB, Yamamoto GK, Allansmith MR. Effects of ocular decongestants. *Arch Ophthalmol* 1980;98:856–858.

311. D'Esposito M, Cortese G, Brusorio S, et al. Validità terapeutica di un collirio a base di ossimetazolina cloridato 0,025% e polivinil alcooh 1,4% somministrato due volte al giorno. *Boll Ocul* 1991;70:303–308.

312. Nayak BK, Kishore K, Gupta SK. Evaluation of oxymetazoline and naphazoline in benign red eyes: a double blind comparative clinical trial. *Indian J Ophthalmol* 1987;35:190–193.

313. Duzman E, Warman A, Warman R. Efficacy and safety of topical oxymetazoline in treating allergic and environmental conjunctivitis. *Ann Ophthalmol* (Chicago) 1986;18:28–31.

314. Leon J, Charap A, Duzman E, et al. Efficacy of cimetidine/pyrilamine eyedrops. *Ophthalmology* 1986;93:120–123.

315. Smith JP, Lanier BQ, Tremblay N, et al. Treatment of allergic conjunctivitis with ocular decongestants. *Curr Eye Res* 1982/1983;2:141–148.

316. Lanier BQ, Tremblay N, Smith JP, et al. A double masked comparison of ocular decongestants as therapy for allergic conjunctivitis. *Ann Allergy* 1983;50:174–182.

317. Brownstein S, Liszauer AD, Jackson WB. Ocular complications of a topical methylene blue-vasoconstrictor-anesthetic preparation. *Can J Ophthalmol* 1989;24:317–324.

318. Graf P, Hallen H, Juto J-E. Four-week use of oxymetazoline nasal spray (Nezeril) once daily at night induces rebound swelling and nasal hyperreactivity. *Acta Otolaryngol* 1995;115:71–75.

319. Tanaka H, Fukunaga K, Miichi H. Absence of rebound vasodilation following continuous instillation of decongestants (in Japanese). *J Eye* 1991;8:1465–1467.

320. Abelson MB, Butrus SI, Weston JH, et al. Tolerance and absence of rebound vasodilation following topical ocular decongestant usage. *Ophthalmology* 1984;91:1364–1367.

321. Soparkar CNS, Wilhelmus KR, Koch DD, et al. Acute and chronic conjunctivitis due to over-the-counter ophthalmic decongestants. *Arch Ophthalmol* 1997;115:34–38.

322. Rumwelt MB. Blindness from misuse of over-the-counter eye medications. *Ann Ophthalmol* (Chicago) 1988;20:26–30.

323. Gelmi C, Ceccuzzi R. Mydriatic effects of ocular decongestants studied by pupillography. *Ophthalmologica* 1994;208:243–246.

324. Fox SL, Samson CR, Danzig MR. Oxymetazoline in the treatment of allergic and non-infectious conjunctivitis. *J Int Med Res* 1979;7:528–530.

325. Trew DR, Wright LA, Smith SE. Otrivine-Antistin: pupil, corneal and conjunctival responses to topical administration. *Eye* 1989;3:294–297.

326. Carli M, De Carli M. Variazioni pupillari indotte da comuni collirii decongestionanti o antibiotici contenenti sostanze simpaticomimetiche. *Boll Ocul* 1984;63:683–688.

327. Allansmith MR, Ross RN. Ocular allergy and mast cell stabilisers. *Surv Ophthalmol* 1986;30:229–244.

328. Allansmith MR, Baird RS. Percentage of degranulated mast cells in vernal conjunctivitis and giant papillary conjunctivitis associated with contact-lens wear. *Am J Ophthalmol* 1981;91:71–75.

329. Friedlaender MH. Conjunctivitis of allergic origin: clinical presentation and differential diagnosis. *Surv Ophthalmol* 1993;38[Suppl.]:105–114.

330. Mondino BJ, Salamon SM, Zaidman GW. Allergic and toxic reactions on soft contact lens wearers. *Surv Ophthalmol* 1982;26:337–344.

331. Trocme SD, Raizman MB, Bartley GB. Medical therapy for ocular allergy. *Mayo Clinic Proc* 1992;67:557–565.

332. Tuft SJ, Ramakrishnan M, Seal DV, et al. Role of Staphylococcus aureus in chronic allergic conjunctivitis. *Ophthalmology* 1992;99:180–184.

333. Abelson MB, Baird RS, Allansmith MR. Tear histamine levels in vernal conjunctivitis and other ocular inflammations. *Ophthalmology* 1980;87:812–814.

334. Tanaka H, Fukunaga K, Miichi H. Comparison of the decongestant effects of naphazoline and tetrahydrozoline (in Japanese). *J Eye* 1991;8:1269–1271.

335. Abelson MB, Paradis A, George MA, et al. Effects of Vasocon-A in the allergen challenge model of acute allergic conjunctivitis. *Arch Ophthalmol* 1990;108:520–524.

336. Kirkegaard J, Secher C, Mygind N. Effect of the H_1 antihistamine chlorpheniramine maleate on histamine-induced symptoms in the human conjunctiva. *Allergy* 1982;37:203–208.

337. Abelson MB, Smith LM. Levocabastine: evaluation in histamine and compound 48/80 models of ocular allergy in humans. *Ophthalmology* 1988;95:1494–1497.

338. Rimas M, Kjellman NIM, Blychert LO, et al. Topical levocabastine protects better than sodium cromoglycate and placebo in conjunctival provocation tests. *Allergy* 1990;45:18–21.

339. Dechant KL, Goa KL. Levocabastine. A review of its pharmacological properties and therapeutic potential as a topical antihistamine in allergic conjunctivitis. *Drugs* 1991;41:202–24.

340. Azevedo M, Castel-Branco MG, Ferraz Oliviera J, et al. Double-blind comparison of levocabastine eye drops with sodium cromoglycate and placebo in the treatment of seasonal allergic conjunctivitis. *Clin Exp Allergy* 1991;21:689–694.

341. Janssens M. Efficacy of levocabastine in conjunctival provocation studies. *Doc Ophthalmol* 1992;82:341–351.

342. Doughty MJ. Levocabastine, a topical ocular antihistamine available as a pharmacy medicine: a literature review. *Pharm J* 2002;268:367–370.

343. Ciprandi G, Buscaglia S, Catrullo A, et al. Azelastine eye drops reduce and prevent allergic conjunctival reaction and exert anti-allergic activity. *Clin Exp Allergy* 1996;27:182–191.

344. Lenhard G, Mivsek-Music E, Perrin-Fayolle M, et al. Double-blind, randomised, placebo-controlled study of two concentrations of azelastine eye drops in seasonal allergic conjunctivitis or rhinoconjunctivitis. *Curr Med Res Opin* 1997;14, 21–28.

345. Sabbah A, Marzetto M. Azelastine eyedrops in the treatment of seasonal allergic conjunctivitis or rhinoconjunctivitis in young children. *Curr Med Res Opin* 1998;14:161–170.

346. Giede-Tuch C, Westhoff M, Zarth A. Azelastine eye-drops in seasonal allergic conjunctivitis or rhinoconjunctivitis. *Allergy* 1998;53:857–862.

347. Discepola M, Deschenes J, Abelson M. Comparison of the topical ocular antiallergic efficacy of emedastine 0.05% ophthalmic solution to ketorolac 0.5% ophthalmic solution in a clinical model of allergic conjunctivitis. *Acta Ophthalmol Scand* 1999; 77:43–46.

348. Abelson MB, Spitalny L. Combined analysis of two studies using the conjunctival allergen challenge model to evaluate olopatadine hydrochloride, a new ophthalmic antiallergic agents with dual activity. *Am J Ophthalmol* 1998;125:797–804.

349. Aguilar AJ. Comparative study of clinical efficacy and tolerance in seasonal allergic conjunctivitis management with 0.1% olopatadine hydrochloride versus 0.05% ketotifen fumarate. *Acta Ophthalmol Scand* 2000;78:52–55.

350. Mikuni I, Fujiwara T, Togawa K, et al. Therapeutic effects of a new, anti-allergic ophthalmic preparation. *Tokai J Exp Clin Med* 1982;7:279–294.

351. Abelson MB, George MA, Smith BS. Evaluation of 0.05% levocabastine versus 4% sodium cromolyn in the allergen challenge model. *Ophthalmology* 1995;102:310–316.

352. Deschennes J, Discepola M, Abelson M. Comparative evaluation of olopatadine ophthalmic solution (0.1%) versus ketorolac ophthalmic solution (0.5%) using the provocative allergen challenge model. *Acta Ophthalmol Scand* 1999;228[Suppl.]:47–52.

353. Abelson MB, Welch DL. An evaluation of onset and duration of action of Patanol (olopatadine hydrochloride ophthalmic solution 0.1%) compared to Claritin (loratadine 10 mg) tablets in acute allergic conjunctivitis in the conjunctival allergen challenge model. *Acta Ophthalmol Scand* 2000;78:60–63.

354. Horak F, Berger UE, Menapace R, et al. Dose-dependent protection by azelastine eyedrops against pollen-induced allergic conjunctivitis. *Drug Res* 1998;48:379–384.

355. Kjaergaard SK, Pedersen OF, Taudorf E, et al. Assessment of changes in eye redness by a photographic method and the relation to sensory eye irritation. *Int Arch Occup Environ Health* 1990;62:133–137.

356. Kari O, Salo OR, Halmepuro L, et al. Tear histamine levels during allergic conjunctivitis challenge. *Graefes Arch Clin Exp Ophthalmol* 1985;223:60–62.

357. Montero Irubietta J, Linan Martinez R, Lopez Elorza F, et al. Test de liberacion de histamina (TLH) an las queratoconjuctivitis primaverales (QCP). Estudio de nuestra casuitica. *Arch Soc Esp Oftalmol* 1988;54:685–690.

358. Leonardi AA, Smith LM, Fregona IA, et al. Tear histamine and histaminase during the early (EPR) and late (LPR) phases of the allergic reaction and the effects of lodoxamide. *Eur J Ophthalmol* 1996;6:106–112.

359. Leonardi A. Role of histamine in allergic conjunctivitis. *Acta Ophthalmol Scand* 2000;78:18–21.

360. Brodsky M. Allergic conjunctivitis and contact lenses: experience with olopatadine hydrochloride 0.1% therapy. *Acta Ophthalmol Scand* 2000;78:56–59.

361. Artal MN, Luna JD, Discepola MA. Forced choice comfort study of olopatadine hydrochloride 0.1% verus ketotifen fumarate 0.05%. *Acta Ophthalmol Scand* 2000;78:64–65.

362. Wong L, Hendeles L, Weinberger M. Pharmacologic prophylaxis of allergic rhinitis: relative efficacy of hydroxyzine and chlorpheniramine. *J Allergy Clin Immunol* 1981;67:223–228.

363. Kramer B, Klimek L, Gülicher D, et al. Sequential therapy with azelastine in seasonal allergic conjunctivitis. *Drug Res* 1999;49: 912–919.

364. Olsen OT, Petersen LN, Høi L, et al. Comparison of loratidine and terfenadine in allergic seasonal rhinoconjunctivitis with emphasis on nasal stuffiness and peak flow. *Drug Res* 1992;42[II]: 1227–1231.

365. Van Cauwenberge P, Juniper EF, The STAR study investigating group. Comparison of the efficacy, safety and quality of life provided by fexofenadine hydrochloride 120 mg, loratidine 10 mg and placebo administered once daily for the treatment of seasonal allergic rhinitis. *Clin Exp Allergy* 2000;30:891–899.

366. Rihoux JP, Mariz S. Cetirizine. An updated review of its pharmacological properties and therapeutic efficacy. *Clin Exp Allergy* 1993;11:65–88.

367. Kantar A, Oggiano N, Coppa GV, et al. Cetirizine reduces the priming capacity on neutrophilic polymorphonuclear leukocytes of lacrimal fluid from subjects with allergic conjunctivitis after specific challenge. *Clin Drug Invest* 1997;4:346–352.

368. Katalin S, Margit V, Piroska F, et al. Cetirizine szerepe a szezonális alergiás conjunctivitis ambuláns kezalésében. *Szemészet* 1993;130:111–113.

369. Bernstein D, Schoenwetter WF, Nathan RA, et al. Efficacy and safety of fexofenadine hydrochloride for treatment of seasonal allergic rhinitis. *Ann Allergy Asthma Immunol* 1997;79: 443–448.

370. Bronsky EA, Falliers CJ, Kaiser HB, et al. Effectiveness and safety of fexofenadine, a new nonsedating H_1-receptor antagonist, in the treatment of fall allergies. *Allergy Asthma Proc* 1998; 19:135–141.

371. Mason J, Reynolds R, Rao N. The systemic safety of fexofenadine HCl. *Clin Exp Allergy* 1999;29[S-3]:163–170.

372. Mattila MJ, Paakkari I. Variations among non-sedating antihistamines: are there real differences? *Eur J Clin Pharmacol* 1999; 55:85–93.

373. Gervais P, Bruttman G, Pedrali P, et al. French multi-center double blind study to evaluate efficacy and safety of acrivastine as compared with terfenadine in seasonal allergic rhinitis. *J Int Med Res* 1989;17:47B-54B.

374. Nielsen L, Johnsen CR, Bindslev-Jensen C, et al. Efficacy of acrivastine in the treatment of allergic rhinitis during natural pollen exposure: onset of action. *Allergy* 1994;49:630–636.

375. Kemp JP, Buckley CE, Gershwin ME, et al. Multicenter, double-blind, placebo-controlled trial of terfenadine in seasonal allergic rhinitis and conjunctivitis. *Ann Allergy* 1985;54:502–509.

376. Leino M, Carlson C, Kikku O, et al. The effect of sodium cromoglycate eyedrops compared to the effect of terfenadine on acute symptoms of seasonal allergic conjunctivitis. *Acta Ophthalmol* 1992;70:341–345.

377. Hesse A, Reggiardo F, Satragno L, et al. Sperimentazione clinica con una nuova molecola antihistaminica nelle conguintiviti allergiche. *Minerv Med* 1988;79:883–886.

378. Miglior M, Scullica L, Secchi AG, et al. Nedocromil sodium and astemizole, alone or combined, in the treatment of seasonal allergic conjunctivitis. *Acta Ophthalmol* 1993;79:73–78.

379. Volkerts ER, Van Willigenburg APP, Van Laar MW, et al. Does cetirizine belong to the new generation of antihistamines? An investigation into its acute and subchronic effects on highway driving, psychometric test performance and daytime sleepiness. *Hum Psychopharmacol* 1992;7:227–238.

380. Koffler BH, Lemp MA. The effect of an antihistamine (chlorpheniramine maleate) on tear production in humans. *Ann Ophthalmol* (Chicago) 1980;12:217–219.

381. Spaeth J, Klimek L, Mösges R. Sedation in allergic rhinitis is

caused by the condition and not by antihistamine treatment. *Allergy* 1996;51:893–906.

382. González MA, Estes KS. Pharmacokinetic overview of oral second-generation H_1 antihistamines. *Int J Clin Pharmacol Ther* 1998;36:292–300.

383. Allansmith MR, Korb DR, Greiner JVW. Giant papillary conjunctivitis in contact lens wearers. *Am J Ophthalmol* 1977;83: 697–708.

384. Alemanny AL, Reedal P. Giant papillary conjunctivitis in soft and rigid lens wear. *Contactologica* 1991;13:14–17.

385. Meisler D, Keller W. Contact lens type, material and deposits and giant papillary conjunctivitis. *Contact Lens Assoc Ophthalmol J* 1995;21:77–80.

386. Katelaris CH. Giant papillary conjunctivitis: A review. *Acta Ophthalmol Scand* 1999;77:17–20.

387. Porazinski AD, Donshik PC. Giant papillary conjunctivitis in frequent replacement contact lens wearers: a retrospective study. *Contact Lens Assoc Ophthalmol J* 1999;25:142–147.

388. Sandaridurg PR, Sweeney DS, Sharma S, et al. Adverse events with extended wear of disposable hydrogels: results for the first 13 months of wear. *Ophthalmology* 1999;106:1671–1680.

389. Skotnitsky C, Sandaridurg PR, Sweeney DF, Holden BA. General and local contact lens induced papillary conjunctivitis (CLPC). *Clin Exp Optom* 2002;85:193–197.

390. Fonn D, MacDonald KE, Richter D, Pritchard N. The ocular response to extended wear of a high Dk silicone hydrogel contact lens. *Clin Exp Optom* 2002;85:176–182.

391. Begley CG, Riggle A, Tuel JA, Association of giant papillary conjunctivitis with seasonal allergies. *Optom Vis Sci* 1990;67: 192–195.

392. Ben Ezra D, Bonini S, Carreras B, et al. Guidelines on the diagnosis and treatment of conjunctivitis. *Ocul Immunol Inflam* 1994;2[Suppl.]:S1–S55.

393. E Silva PMR, Martins MA, Castra-Faria-Neto HC, et al. Nedocromil sodium prevents in vivo generation of the eiosinophilotactic substance induced by PAF but fails to antagonise its effects. *Br J Pharmacol* 1992;105:436–440.

394. Kusner EJ, Dubnick B, Herzig GJ. The inhibition by disodium cromoglycate in vitro of anaphylactically induced histamine release from rat peritoneal cells. *J Pharmacol Exp Ther* 1973;184: 41–49.

395. Theoharides TC, Siegart W, Greengard P, et al. Antiallergic drug cromolyn may inhibit histamine secretion by regulating phosphorylation of mast cell protein. *Science* 1980;207:80–82.

396. Tanaka H, Umento M, Miichi H, et al. Evaluation of an antiallergic agent (disodium cromoglycate) in rat conjunctiva using monoclonal IgE antibody. *Ophthalmic Res* 1987;19:240–244.

397. Pearce FL, Al-Laith M, Bosman L, et al. Effects of sodium cromoglycate and nedocromil sodium on histamine secretion from mast cells from various locations. *Drugs* 1989;37[Suppl 1]:37–43.

398. Yanni JM, Weimer LK, Glasser Rl, et al. Effect of lodoxamide on in vitro and in vivo conjunctival immediate hypersensitivity responses in rats. *Int Arch Allergy Immunol* 1993;101:102–106.

399. Bonini S, Schiavone M, Bonini S, et al. Efficacy of lodoxamide eyedrops on mast cells and eosinophils after allergen challenge in allergic conjunctivitis. *Ophthalmology* 1997;104:849–853.

400. Oguz H, Bitiren M, Aslan OS, et al. Efficacy of lodoxamide eye drops on tear fluid cytology of patients with vernal conjunctivitis. *Acta Med Okayama* 1999;53:123–126.

401. Ciprandi G, Buscaglia S, Catrullo A, et al. Antiallergic activity of topical lodoxamide on in vivo and in vitro models. *Allergy* 1996;51:946–951.

402. Oliver GE. How to manage allergic conjunctivitis. *Rev Optom* 1989;126:73–78.

403. Richmond PP. Giant papillary conjunctivitis: an overview. *J Am Optom Assoc* 1979;32:1457–1462.

404. Wood AC. The diagnosis and treatment of ocular allergy. *Am J Ophthalmol* 1949;32:1457–1478.

405. Van Bijsterveld OP. A double-blind crossover study comparing sodium cromoglycate eye drops with placebo in the treatment of chronic conjunctivitis. *Acta Ophthalmol* 1984;62:479–484.

406. Batra D, Mohan M, Sharma P, et al. Patterns of responses to alternative medicines in controlling allergic conjunctivitis. *Indian J Ophthalmol* 1988;36:17–21.

407. Blumenthal M, Casale T, Dockhorn R, et al. Efficacy and safety of nedocromil sodium ophthalmic solution in the treatment of seasonal allergic conjunctivitis. *Am J Ophthalmol* 1992;113: 56–63.

408. Caldwell DR, Verin P, Hartwich-Young R, et al. Efficacy and safety of lodoxamide 0.1% vs cromolyn sodium 4% in patients with vernal conjunctivitis. *Am J Ophthalmol* 1992;113: 632–637.

409. Leino M, Ennevaara K, Latvala A-L, et al. Double-blind group comparative study of 2% nedocromil sodium eyedrops with 2% sodium cromoglycate and placebo eye drops in the treatment of seasonal allergic conjunctivitis. *Clin Exp Allergy* 1992;22: 929–932.

410. Fahy GT, Easty DL, Collum LMT, et al. Randomised double-masked trial of lodoxamide and sodium cromoglycate in allergic eye disease. A multicentre study. *Eur J Ophthalmol* 1992;2: 144–149.

411. Frostad AB, Olsen AK. A comparison of topical levocabastine and sodium cromoglycate in the treatment of pollen-provoked allergic conjunctivitis. *Clin Exp Allergy* 1993;23:406–409.

412. Santos CI, Huang AJ, Abelson MB, et al. Efficacy of lodoxamide 0.1% ophthalmic solution in resolving corneal epitheliopathy associated with vernal conjunctivitis. *Am J Ophthalmol* 1994; 117:488–497.

413. Alexander M. Comparative therapeutic studies with Tilavist. *Allergy* 1995;50[Suppl. 21]:23–29.

414. Kjellman N-IM, Stevens MT. Clinical experience with Tilavist: an overview of efficacy and safety. *Allergy* 1995;50[Suppl. 21]: 14–22.

415. Bailey CS, Buckley RJ. Nedocromil sodium in contact lens associated papillary conjunctivitis. *Eye* 1993;7[Pt. 3, Suppl.]:29–33.

416. Möller C, Berg I-M, Berg T, et al. Nedocromil sodium 2% eyedrops for twice daily treatment of seasonal allergic conjunctivitis: a Swedish multicentre placebo-controlled study in children allergic to birch pollen. *Clin Exp Allergy* 1994;24:884–887.

417. Meisler DM, Berzius UJ, Krachmer JH, et al. Cromolyn treatment in giant papillary conjunctivitis. *Arch Ophthalmol* 1982; 100:1608–1610.

418. Vakil DV, Ayiomamitis A, Nizami RM. Treatment of seasonal conjunctivitis: comparison of 2% and 4% sodium cromoglycate ophthalmic solutions. *Can J Ophthalmol* 1984;19:207–211.

419. Juniper EF, Guyant GH, Ferrie P, et al. Sodium cromoglycate eyedrops: regular versus "as needed" use in the treatment of seasonal allergic conjunctivitis. *J Allergy Clin Immunol* 1994; 94:36–43.

420. Montan P, Zetterstrom O, Elliasson E, et al. Topical sodium cromoglycate (Opticrom) relieves ongoing symptoms of allergic conjunctivitis within 2 minutes. *Allergy* 1994;49:637–640.

421. Redfern DC, Serafin WE. Adverse reaction to ocular cromolyn sodium. *J Allergy Clin Immunol* 1992;90:866.

422. Aakre BM, Ystenaes AE, Doughty MJ, et al. A 6-month follow-up of successful refits from daily disposable soft contact lenses to continuous wear of high-Dk silicone hydrogel lenses. *Ophthal Physiol Opt* 2004;24:130–141.

423. Terry RL, Schnider CM, Holden BA, et al. CCLRU standards

for success of daily and extended wear contact lenses. *Optom Vis Sci* 1993;70:234–243.

424. Masuda K. Anti-inflammatory agents: nonsteroidal anti-inflammatory drugs. In: Sears ML, ed. *Ocular pharmacology.* Berlin: Springer-Verlag, 1984:539–551.

425. Leopold IH. Pharmacology of cellular elements of inflammation. *Biomed Found Ophthalmol* 1987;3:1–51.

426. Bazan HEP, Birkle DL, Beuerman RW, et al. Inflammation-induced stimulation of the synthesis of prostaglandins and lipoxygenase-reaction products in rabbit cornea. *Curr Eye Res* 1985; 4:175–179.

427. Davis KL, Conners MS, Dunn MW, et al. Induction of corneal epithelial cytochrome arachidonate metabolism by contact lens wear. *Invest Ophthalmol Vis Sci* 1992;33:291–297.

428. Eakins KE, Bhattacherjee P. Histamine, prostaglandins and ocular inflammation. *Exp Eye Res* 1977;24:299–305.

429. Watson PG, McKay DAR, Clemett RS, et al. Treatment of episcleritis. A double-blind trial comparing betamethasone 0.1 per cent., oxyphenbutazone 10 per cent., and placebo eye ointments. *Br J Ophthalmol* 1973;57:866–870.

430. Stodtmeister R, Marquardt R. Ein nichtsteroidaler Entzungshemmer bei chronischer Conjunctivitis. *Fortschr Ophthalmol* 1986;83:199–202.

431. Abelson MB, Butrus SI, Weston JH. Aspirin therapy in vernal conjunctivitis. *Am J Ophthalmol* 1983;95:502–505.

432. Meyer E, Kraus E, Zonis S. Efficacy of antiprostaglandin therapy in vernal conjunctivitis. *Br J Ophthalmol* 1987;71:497–499.

433. Srinvas C. Adjuvant therapy of aspirin and cromoglycate 2% eye drops in vernal conjunctivitis. *Korean J Ophthalmol* 1989; 3:42–46.

434. Nemetz U. Zur Behandlung ausserer Augenerkrankungen mit Tanderil-Augensalbe. *Klin Monatsbl Augenheilkd* 1972;160: 618–623.

435. Murphy JE. Tanderil eye ointment. *J Int Med Res* 1973;1: 136–141.

436. Orou F, Gnad HD. Erfahungen mit einer neuen antiphlogistischen Augensalbe (Tanderil-Augensalbe). *Wien Med Wochenschr* 1974;124:623–624.

437. Dyster-Aas K. Oxyphenbutazone eye-ointment in the treatment of foreign bodies in the cornea. *Acta Ophthalmol* 1973;51: 791–797.

438. Olsen T, Ehlers N, Bramsen T. Influence of tranexamic acid and acetylsalicylic acid on thickness of the normal cornea. *Acta Ophthalmol* 1980;58:767–772.

439. Nielsen CB. Prostaglandin inhibition and central corneal thickness after cataract extraction. *Acta Ophthalmol* 1982;60: 252–258.

440. Nissen JN, Ehlers N. No additive effect of tranexamic acid and naproxen on corneal deswelling. *Acta Ophthalmol* 1986;64: 291–294.

441. Massin M. Action anti-inflammatoire de l'acide tiaprofenique dans les suites de la chirugue oculaire. *J Fr Ophthalmol* 1985;8: 559–563.

442. Valentic JP, Leopold IH, Dea FJ. Excretion of salicylic acid into tears following oral administration of aspirin. *Ophthalmology* 1980;87:815–820.

443. Efron N, Holden BA, Vannas A. Effect of prostaglandin-inhibitor naproxen on the corneal swelling response to hydrogel contact lens wear. *Acta Ophthalmol* 1984;62:746–752.

444. Mochizuki M, Sawa M, Masuda K. Topical indomethacin in intracapsular extraction of senile cataract. *Jpn J Ophthalmol* 1977;21:215–226.

445. Frucht-Perry J, Levinger S, et al. The effect of topical administration of indomethacin on symptoms in corneal scars and edema. *Am J Ophthalmol* 1991;112:186–190.

446. Duffin RM, Weissman BA, Glasser DB, et al. Flurbiprofen in the treatment of corneal neovascularisation induced by contact lenses. *Am J Ophthalmol* 1982;93:607–614.

447. Pizzino A, Scorolli L, Martini E, et al. Trattamento topico con piroxicam della neovascolarizzazione corneale in portatori di lenti a contatto morbide. *Ann Ottalmol Clin Ocul* 1985;111: 116–125.

448. Wood TS, Stewart RH, Bowman RW, et al. Suprofen treatment of contact lens-associated giant papillary conjunctivitis. *Ophthalmology* 1988;95:822–826.

449. Goldberg MA, McNamara N, Nguyen NT, et al. Effect of diclofenac sodium (Voltaren™) on hypoxia-induced corneal edema in humans. *Contact Lens Assoc Ophthalmol J* 1995;21: 61–63.

450. Leonardi A, Busato F, Fregona I, et al. Anti-inflammatory and antiallergic effects of ketorolac tromethamine in the conjunctival provocation model. *Br J Ophthalmol* 2000;84:1228–1232.

451. Van Husen H. Lokale Behandlung mit Diclofenac-Na-Augentropfen bei Erkrankungen der vorderen Augenabschnitte. *Klin Monatsbl Augenheilkd* 1986;188:615–619.

452. Laibovitz RA, Koester J, Schaich L, et al. Safety and efficacy of diclofenac sodium 0.1% ophthalmic solution in acute seasonal allergic conjunctivitis. *J Ocul Pharmacol Ther* 1995;11: 361–368.

453. Iorio P, Mancini A, Baglioni L, et al. Efficacia clinica del piroxicam nel trattamento delle conjunctiviti allergiche. *Boll Ocul* 1988;67:181–188.

454. Berruto A, Bonini S, Centofanti M, et al. Conguintiviti allergiche: Effetto del naprossene dopo stimolazione conjunctivale specifica. *Ann Ottalmol Clin Ocul* 1990;116:443–448.

455. Ballas Z, Blumenthal M, Tinkelman DG, et al. Clinical evaluation of ketorolac tromethamine 0.5% ophthalmic solution for the treatment of seasonal allergic conjunctivitis. *Surv Ophthalmol* 1993;38[Suppl.]:141–148.

456. Tauber J, Raizman MB, Ostrov CS, et al. A multicenter comparison of the ocular efficacy and safety of diclofenac 0.1% solution with that of ketorolac 0.5% solution in patients with acute seasonal allergic conjunctivitis. *J Ocul Pharmacol Ther* 1998;14: 137–145.

457. Ilic S, Gigon S, Leuenberger PM. Comparaison de l'effet anti-inflammatoire des collyres de dexamethasone et de diclofenac. *Klin Monatsbl Augenheilkd* 1984;184:494–498.

458. Szucs PA, Nashed AH, Allegra JR, et al. Safety and efficacy of diclofenac ophthalmic solution in the treatment of corneal abrasions. *Ann Emerg Med* 2000;35:131–137.

459. Gordon A, Bartlett JD, Lin M. The effect of diclofenac sodium on the initial comfort of RGP contact lenses: a pilot study. *J Am Optom Assoc* 1999;70:509–513.

460. Frangouli A, Shah S, Chatterjee A, et al. Efficacy of topical nonsteroidal drops as pain relief after excimer laser photorefractive keratectomy. *J Refract Surg* 1998;267:S207-S208.

461. Vantesone DL, Luna JD, Muiño JC, et al. Effects of topical diclofenac and prednisolone eyedrops in laser in situ keratomileusis patients. *J Cataract Refract Surg* 1999;25:836–841.

462. Montard M, Chopin C, Delbosc B, et al. Tétracaïne versus diclofénac dans le traitement da la douleur après photokeratectomie réfractive. *J Fr Ophthalmol* 1999;22:14–20.

463. Draeger J, Kahleyss B, Huber H. Investigation into the influence of anti-inflammatory substances on intraocular pressure. *Ophthalmic Res* 1973;5:274–278.

464. Congdon NG, Schein OD, Von Kulajta P, et al. Corneal complications associated with topical ophthalmic use of nonsteroidal antiinflammatory drugs. *J Cataract Refract Surg* 2001;27: 622–631.

465. Gaynes BI, Fiscella R. Topical nonsteroidal anti-inflammatory drugs for ophthalmic use. A safety review. *Drug Saf* 2002;25: 233–250.

466. Polachek J, Shvertzman P. Acute bronchial asthma associated with the administration of ophthalmic indomethacin. *Israel J Med Sci* 1996;32:1107–1109.

467. Sharir M. Exacerbation of asthma by topical diclofenac. *Arch Ophthalmol* 1997;115:294–295.

468. Zantos S, Holden B. Guttae endothelial changes with anterior eye inflammation *Br J Ophthalmol* 1981;65:101–107.

469. Stegman R, Miller D. A human model of allergic conjunctivitis. *Am J Ophthalmol* 1975;93:1354–1356.

470. Basu PK, Avaria M, Jankie R. Effect of hydrocortisone on the mobilization of leukocytes in corneal wounds. *Br J Ophthalmol* 1981;65:694–697.

471. Smith RJ, Iden SS. Pharmacological modulation of chemotactic factor-elicited release of granule-associated enzymes from human neutrophils. Effects of prostaglandins, nonsteroidal anti-inflammatory agents and corticosteroids. *Bioch Pharmacol* 1980;29:2389–2395.

472. Nelson EL. Ophthalmic steroids. In: Kaufman HE, ed. *Symposium on ocular antiinflammatory therapy*. Springfield, IL: Charles C. Thomas, 1970:217–233.

473. Rowland FN, Donovon MJ, Lindsay M, et al. Demonstration of inflammatory mediator-induced inflammation and endothelial cell damage in the anterior segment of the eye. *Am J Pathol* 1983;110:1–9.

474. Polansky JR, Weinreb RN. Anti-inflammatory agents. Steroids as anti-inflammatory agents. In: Sears ML, ed. *Pharmacology of the eye*. New York: Springer-Verlag, 1984: 459–538.

475. Duke-Elder S. The clinical value of cortisone and ACTH in ocular disease. *Br J Ophthalmol* 1951;35:637–671.

476. Duke-Elder S, Duthie OM, Foster DJ, et al. A series of cases treated locally by cortisone. *Br J Ophthalmol* 1951;35:672–694.

477. Steffenson EH, Olson JA, Margulis RR, et al. The experimental use of cortisone in inflammatory eye disease. *Am J Ophthalmol* 1950;33:1033–10442.

478. Pepinsky RB, Tizard R, Mattaliano RJ et al. Five distinct calcium and phospholipid-binding proteins share homology with lipocortin 1. *J Biol Chem* 1988;263:10799–10811.

479. Simonsson B. Evidence for a glucocorticoid receptor in human leukocytes. *Acta Physiol Scand* 1976;98:131–135.

480. Visor GC. Drug design strategies for ocular therapeutics. *Adv Drug Deliv Rev* 1994;14:269–279.

481. Bartlett JD, Howes JF, Ghormley NR, et al. Safety and efficacy of loteprednol etabonate for treatment of papillae in contact lens-associated giant papillary conjunctivitis. *Curr Eye Res* 1993;12:313–321.

482. Howes J, Novack GD. Failure to detect systemic levels and effects of loteprednol etabonate and its metabolite, PJ-91, following chronic ocular administration. *J Ocul Pharmacol Ther* 1998;14:153–158.

483. Langham ME, Shalash BA. The relationship between the anti-inflammatory and the ocular hypertensive properties of glucocorticosteroids. In: Kaufman HE, ed. *Ocular anti-inflammatory therapy*. Springfield. IL: Charles C. Thomas, 1970: 69–87.

484. Sousa FJ. The bioavailability and therapeutic effectiveness of prednisolone acetate vs. prednisolone sodium phosphate: a 20-year review. *Contact Lens Assoc Ophthalmol J* 1991;17:282–283.

485. Maeda K, Sumie K, Nakatani H, et al. Clinical study of 0.01% betamethasone (In Japanese). *Folia Ophthalmol Jpn* 1979;30: 1173–1175.

486. Kadom AHM, Forrester JV, Williamson TH. Comparison of the anti-inflammatory activity and effect on intraocular pressure of fluorometholone, clobetasone butyrate and betamethasone phosphate eye drops. *Ophthalmic Physiol Opt* 1986;6:313–315.

487. Ramsell TG, Bartholomew RS, Walker SR. Clinical evaluation of clobetasone butyrate: a comparative study of its effects in postoperative inflammation and on intra-ocular pressure. *Br J Ophthalmol* 1980;64:43–45.

488. Fairbairn WD, Thorson JC. Fluorometholone. Anti-inflammatory and intraocular pressure effects. *Arch Ophthalmol* 1971;86: 138–141.

489. Ohara H, Hayashi K, Nishioka K, et al. A double-blind study of fluorometholone (in Japanese). *Folia Ophthalmol Jpn* 1977; 28:625–634.

490. Dell SJ, Lowry GM, Northcutt JA, et al. A randomized, double-masked, placebo-controlled parallel study of 0.2% loteprednol etabonate in patients with seasonal allergic conjunctivitis. *J Allergy Clin Immunol* 1998;102:251–255.

491. Asbell PA, Howes J, The loteprednol GPC study group II. A double-masked placebo-controlled, evaluation of the efficacy and safety of loteprednol etabonate in the treatment of contact-lens associated giant papillary conjunctivitis. *Contact Lens Assoc Ophthalmol J* 1997;23:31–36.

492. Friedlaender MH, Howes J. A double-masked, placebo-controlled evaluation of the efficacy and safety of loteprednol etabonate in the treatment of giant papillary conjunctivitis: the Loteprednol giant papillary conjunctivitis study group I. *Am J Ophthalmol* 1997;123:455–464.

493. Loteprednol Etabonate Postoperative Inflammation Study Group. A double-masked, placebo-controlled evaluation of 0.5% loteprednol etabonate in the treatment of postoperative inflammation. *Ophthalmology* 1998;105:1780–1786.

494. Bedrossian RH, Eriksen SP. The treatment of ocular inflammation with medrysone. *Arch Ophthalmol* 1969;81:184–189.

495. Donshik P, Kulvin SM, McKinley P, et al. Treatment of chronic staphylococcal blepharoconjunctivitis with a new topical steroid-antibacterial ophthalmic solution. *Ann Ophthalmol* (Chicago) 1983;15:162–167.

496. Neumann E, Gutmann MJ, Blumenkrantz N, et al. A review of 400 cases of vernal conjunctivitis. *Am J Ophthalmol* 1959; 47:166–172.

497. Ashton N, Cook C. Effect of cortisone on healing of corneal wounds. *Br J Ophthalmol* 1951;35:708–717.

498. Miller D, Peczon JD, Whitworth CG. Corticosteroids and functions in the anterior segment of the eye. *Am J Ophthalmol* 1965; 59:31–34.

499. Doughty MJ, Lyle WM. Ocular pharmacogenetics. In: Fatt HV, Griffin JR, Lyle WM, eds. Genetics for primary eye care practitioners, 2nd ed. Boston: Butterworth-Heinemann, 1992: 179–193.

500. Akingbehin T. Corticosteroid-induced ocular hypertension. *J Toxicol Cutan Ocul Toxicol* 1986;5:45–53.

501. Bartlett JD, Wooley TW, Adams CM. Identification of high intraocular pressure responders to topical ophthalmic corticosteroids. *J Ocul Pharmacol* 1993;9:35–45.

502. Novack GD, Howes J, Crockett S, Sherwood MB. Change in intraocular pressure during long-term use of loteprednol etabonate. *J Glaucoma* 1998;7:266–269.

503. Morrison E, Archer DB. Effect of fluorometholone (FML) on the intraocular pressure of corticosteroid responders. *Br J Ophthalmol* 1984;68:581–584.

504. Bartlett JD, Horowitz B, Laibovitz R, et al. Intraocular pressure response to loteprednol etabonate in known steroid responders. *J Ocul Pharmacol* 1993;9:157–65.

505. Garbe E, Boivin J-F, LeLorier J, et al. Selection of controls in database case-control studies: glucocorticoids and the risk of glaucoma. *J Clin Epidemiol* 1998;51:129–135.

506. Ohguchi M, Ohno S, Takeuchi T, et al. Intraocular pressure in children on systemic corticosteroid therapy (in Japanese). *Jpn J Clin Ophthalmol* 1977;31:781–785.

507. Goldman D. Ocular complications of steroid use in pediatric

patients: a lesson for gastroenterologists. *Gastroenterology* 1992; 102:2164–2165.

508. Derby L, Maier WC. Risk of cataract among users of intranasal corticosteroids. *J Allergy Clin Immunol* 2000;105:912–916.

509. Long WF. A case of elevated intraocular pressure associated with systemic steroid therapy. *Am J Optom Physiol Opt* 1977;54: 248–250.

510. Baum JL, Levene RZ. Corneal thickness after topical corticosteroid therapy. *Arch Ophthalmol* 1968;79:366–369.

511. Ytteborg J, Dohlman CH. Corneal edema and intraocular pressure. *Arch Ophthalmol* 1965;74:477–484.

512. Doughty MJ, Zaman ML. Human corneal thickness and its impact on intraocular pressure measures: a review and meta-analysis approach. *Surv Ophthalmol* 2000;44:367–408.

513. Doughty MJ, Laiquzzaman M, Muller A, et al. Central corneal thickness in European (white) individuals, especially children and the elderly, and assessment of its possible importance in clinical measures of intraocular pressure. *Ophthalmic Physiol Opt* 2002;22:491–604.

514. Stodtmeister R. Applanation tonometry and correction according to corneal thickness. *Acta Ophthalmol Scand* 1998;76: 319–324.

515. Skaff A, Cullen AP, Doughty MJ, et al. Corneal swelling and recovery following wear of thick hydrogel contact lenses in insulin-dependent diabetics. *Ophthalmic Physiol Opt* 1995;15: 287–297.

516. Jain JS, Gill MMS. Effect of topical steroids on intraocular pressure in young diabetics. *J All-India Ophthalmol Soc* 1969; 17:95–98.

517. Shin DH, Becker B, Koller AE. Topical corticosteroid response and retinopathy in juvenile-onset diabetes mellitus. *Diabetes* 1977;26:757–759.

518. Yablonski ME, Burde RM, Kolker AE, et al. Cataracts induced by topical dexamethasone in diabetics. *Arch Ophthalmol* 1978; 96:474–476.

519. Urban RC, Cotlier E. Corticosteroid-induced cataracts. *Surv Ophthalmol* 1986;31:102–110.

520. Ticho U, Durst A, Licht A, et al. Steroid-induced glaucoma and cataract in renal transplant recipients. *Isr J Med Sci* 1977; 13:871–874.

521. Linmaye SR, Pillai S, Tina L. Relationship of steroid dose to degree of posterior subcapsular cataracts in nephrotic syndrome. *Ann Ophthalmol* (Chicago) 1988;20:225–227.

522. Koch H-R, Siedek M. Linsenmyopie bei der Steroidkatarakt. *Klin Monatsbl Augenheilkd* 1977;171:620–622.

523. Fraunfelder FT, Meyer SM. Posterior subcapsular cataracts associated with nasal or inhalation corticosteroids. *Am J Ophthalmol* 1990;109:489–490.

524. Baum J. Therapy for ocular bacterial infection. *Trans Ophthalmol Soc UK* 1986;105:69–77.

525. Brook I, Petit TH, Martin WJ, et al. Anaerobic and aerobic bacteriology of acute conjunctivitis. *Ann Ophthalmol* (Chicago) 1979;11:389–393.

526. Cakanak C. What you should know about your antibiotics. Fine-tune your Rx's with this simple guide. *Rev Optom* 1990; April:95–99.

527. Limberg MB. A review of bacterial keratitis and bacterial conjunctivitis. *Am J Ophthalmol* 1991;112[Suppl.]:2S–9S.

528. Fitch CP, Rapoza PA, Owens S, et al. Epidemiology and diagnosis of acute conjunctivitis at an inner-city hospital. *Ophthalmology* 1989;96:1215–1220.

529. Hampton MJ, Edmondson W. Laboratory testing for ocular infections. *Int Eye Care* 1986;2:319–325.

530. Darougar S, Woodland RM, Walpita P. Value and cost effectiveness of double culture tests for diagnosis of ocular viral and chlamydial infections. *Br J Ophthalmol* 1987;71:673–675.

531. Ficker L, Kirkness C, McCartney A, et al. Microbial keratitis: the false negative. *Eye* 1991;5:549–559.

532. Perrigin J. Laboratory workup of microbial keratitis. *J Am Optom Assoc* 1992;63:243–248.

533. Kairys D, Smith MD. General principles of antibacterial agents. In: Onofrey BE, ed. *Clinical optometric pharmacology and therapeutics.* Philadelphia: JB Lippincott, 1991:1–25.

534. Callegan MC, O'Calleghan RJ, Hill JM. Pharmacokinetic considerations in the treatment of bacterial keratitis. *Clin Pharmaceut* 1994;27:129–149.

535. Clemons CS, Cohen EJ, Arentsen JJ, et al. Pseudomonas ulcers following patching of corneal abrasions associated with contact lens wear. *Contact Lens Assoc Ophthalmol J* 1987;13:161–164.

536. Bellizi M, Asciano F, Reibaldi A. La gentamicina-solfato collirio e pomata in alcune affezioni flogistiche oculai. *Ann Ottalmol* 1974;100:445–449.

537. Records RE. Gentamicin in ophthalmology. *Surv Ophthalmol* 1976;21:49–58.

538. Liabson P. A clinical comparison of tobramycin and gentamicin in the treatment of ocular infections. *Am J Ophthalmol* 1981; 92:836–840.

539. Cagle G Davis S, Rosenthal A, et al. Tobramycin and gentamicin in the treatment of ocular infections: a multicenter study. *Curr Eye Res* 1982;1:523–534.

540. Wilhelmus K, Gilbert M, Osato M. Tobramycin in ophthalmology. *Surv Ophthalmol* 1987;32:111–122.

541. Bryan LE, Kwan S. Roles of ribosomal binding, membrane potential, and electron transport in bacterial uptake of streptomycin and gentamicin. *Antimicrob Agents Chemother* 1983;23: 835–845.

542. Gale E. Mechanisms of antibiotic action. *Pharmacol Rev* 1963; 15:481–530.

543. Lopez S. Topical use of neomycin in ophthalmology. *Antibiotics Chemother* 1954;4:1189–1195.

544. Saraux H. Le collyre a la neomycine dan les conjunctivites. *Sem Hop Paris* 1956;32:1504–1506.

545. Mahajan VM, Angra SK. In vitro activity of framycetin and gentamycin against microbes producing ocular infections. *Indian J Ophthalmol* 1977;24:13–17.

546. Dirdal M. Fucithalmic in acute conjunctivitis. Open, randomized comparison of fusidic acid, chloramphenicol and framycetin eye drops. *Acta Ophthalmol* 1987;65:129–134.

547. Naib K. Observations on the ocular effects of erythromycin. *Am J Ophthalmol* 1955;39:395–398.

548. Roberts W. Topical use of chloramphenicol in external ocular infections. *Am J Ophthalmol* 1951;34:1081–1088.

549. Fraunfelder FT, Grover GC, Kelly DJ. Fatal aplastic anemia following topical administration of ophthalmic chloramphenicol. *Am J Ophthalmol* 1982;93:356–360.

550. Fraunfelder FT, Morgan RL, Yunis AA. Blood dyscrasias and topical ophthalmic chloramphenicol. *Am J Ophthalmol* 1994; 115:812–813.

551. Physicians Desk Reference, 33rd ed. Oradell, NJ: Medical Economics, 1979: 1312.

552. Rosenthal RL, Blackman A. Bone-marrow hypoplasia following use of chloramphenicol eye drops. *J Am Med Assoc* 1965;191: 148–149.

553. Besamusca FW, Bastiaensen LA. Blood dyscrasias and topically applied chloramphenicol in ophthalmology. *Doc Ophthalmol* 1986;64:87–95.

554. Laporte J-R, Vidal X, Ballarin E, et al. Possible association between ocular chloramphenicol and aplastic anaemia: the absolute risk is very low. *Br J Clin Pharmacol* 1998;46:181–184.

555. Yunis AA. Chloramphenicol. Relation of structure to activity and toxicity. *Annu Rev Pharmacol Toxicol* 1988;28:83–100.

556. Van Bijsterveld OP, el Batawi Y, Sobhi FS, et al. Fusidic acid in infections of the external eye. *Infection* 1987;15:16–19.

557. Horven I. Acute conjunctivitis. A comparison of fusidic acid viscous eye drops and chloramphenicol. *Acta Ophthalmol* 1993; 71:165–168.

558. Radl S. Structure-activity relationships in DNA gyrase inhibitors. *Pharmacol Ther* 1990;48:1–17.

559. Goldstein MH, Kowalski RP, Gordon J. Emerging fluoroquinolone resistance in bacterial keratitis. A 5-year review. *Ophthalmology* 1999,106:1313–1318.

560. Thygeson P. Sulfonamide compounds in treatment of ocular infections. *Arch Ophthalmol* 1943;29:1000–1009.

561. Mayer L. Sodium sulfacetamide in ophthalmology. *Arch Ophthalmol* 1948;39:232–237.

562. Brown GM. The biosynthesis of folic acid. II. Inhibition by sulfonamides. *J Biol Chem* 1962;237:536–540.

563. Woods DD. The biochemical mode of action of the sulphonamide drugs. *J Gen Microbiol* 1962;29:687–702.

564. Rubin R. Ophthalmic sulfonamide-induced Stevens-Johnson syndrome. *Arch Dermatol* 1977;113:235–237.

565. Wolkenstein P, Carriere V, Charue D, et al. A slow acetylator genotype is a risk factor for sulfonamide-induced toxic epidermal necrolysis and Stevens-Johnson syndrome. *Pharmacogenetics* 1995;5:255–258.

566. Bell TAG, Slack M, Harvey SG, et al. The effect of trimethoprim-polymyxin B sulphate ophthalmic ointment and chloramphenicol ophthalmic ointment on the bacterial flora of the eye when administered to the operated and unoperated eyes of patients undergoing cataract surgery. *Eye* 1988;2:324–329.

567. Saxby C, Samples JR. Polytrim. *J Toxicol Cutan Ocul Toxicol* 1991;10:249–252.

568. Hunter FE, Schwartz LS. Gramicidins. In: Gottlieb D, Shaw PD, eds. *Antibiotics. Volume I. Mechanism of action.* New York: Springer-Verlag, 1967: 642–648.

569. Storm DR, Rosenthal KS, Swanson PE. Polymyxin and related peptide antibiotics. *Annu Rev Biochem* 1977;46:723–763.

570. Weinberg ED. Bacitracin, gramicidin and tyrocidine. In: Gottlieb D, Shaw PD, eds. *Antibiotics. Volume II.* New York: Springer-Verlag, 1967: 244–247.

571. Trope RA. Topical Aureomycin (oily suspension) in ophthalmology. First reports on 47 cases. *South Afr Med J* 1951;25:53–54.

572. Thygeson P. Terramycin in ocular infections. *Trans Am Ophthalmol Soc* 1952;49:185–189.

573. Jones DB. A plan for antimicrobial therapy in bacterial keratitis. *Trans Am Acad Ophthalmol* 1975;79:OP95–OP103.

574. McCulley P. Blepharoconjunctivitis. *Int Ophthalmol Clin* 1984; 24:65–77.

575. Gordon DM. Gentamicin sulfate in external eye infections. *Am J Ophthalmol* 1970;69:300–306.

576. Seal DV, Barrett SP, McGill JI. Aetiology and treatment of acute bacterial infection of the external eye. *Br J Ophthalmol* 1982;66:357–360.

577. Steinert RF. Current therapy for bacterial keratitis and bacterial conjunctivitis. *Am J Ophthalmol* 1991;112:10S–14S.

578. Patamusucin P, Rettig PJ, Faust KL, et al. Oral versus topical erythromycin therapies for chlamydial conjunctivitis. *Am J Dis Child* 1982;136:817–821.

579. Bellows J, Farmer C. The use bacitracin in ocular infections. Part II. Bacitracin therapy in experimental and clinical ocular infections. *Am J Ophthalmol* 1948;31:1211–1214.

580. Halasa AH. Gentamicin in the treatment of bacterial conjunctivitis. *Am J Ophthalmol* 1967;63:1699–1702.

581. Bron AJ, Leber G, Rizk SNM, et al. Ofloxacin compared with chloramphenicol in the management of external ocular infection. *Br J Ophthalmol* 1991;75:675–79.

582. Stern GA, Kilingsworth DW. Complications of topical antimicrobial agents. *Int Ophthalmol Clin* 1989;29:137–142.

583. Clark S, Culler A. Aureomycin as prophylaxis against ophthalmia neonatorum. *Am J Ophthalmol* 1951;38:840–842.

584. Naccache R. Topical use of Terramycin ointment in trachoma. *Br J Ophthalmol* 1953;37:106–108.

585. Darougar S, Jones BR, Viswalingam N, et al. Topical therapy of hyperendemic trachoma with rifampicin, oxytetracycline, or spiramycin eye ointments. *Br J Ophthalmol* 1980;64:37–42.

586. Buckley RJK, Kirkness CM, Kanski JJ, et al. (Chloramphenicol) Safe in patients with no history of blood dyscrasia. *Br Med J* 1995;311:450.

587. McDonnell PJ. How do general practitioners manage eye disease in the community. *Br J Ophthalmol* 1988;72:733–736.

588. Leibowitz HM, Pratt MV, Flagstad IJ, et al. Human conjunctivitis. II. Treatment. *Arch Ophthalmol* 1976;94:1752–1756.

589. Lemp MA, Blackman J, Koffler BH. Therapy for bacterial and fungal infections. *Int Ophthalmol Clin* 1979;19:135–147.

590. Mikuni M, Oishi M. Treatment of Pseudomonas corneal ulcers. *Jpn J Clin Ophthalmol* 1971;25:256–258.

591. Grosset J. Norfloxacine: une quinalone a large spectre por les infections oculaires superficielles. *Pathol Biol* 1990;38:735–741.

592. Goldstein EJG, Citron DM, Bendon L, et al. Potential of topical norfloxacin therapy. Comparative in vitro activity against clinical ocular bacterial isolates. *Arch Ophthalmol* 1987;105: 991–994.

593. Tabbara KF, El-Sheikh HF, Monowarul Islam SM, et al. Treatment of acute bacterial conjunctivitis with topical lomefloxacin 0.3% compared to topical ofloxacin 0.3%. *Eur J Ophthalmol* 1999;9:269–275.

594. Zhang M, Hu Y, Chen F. Clinical investigation of 0.3% levofloxacin eyedrops on the treatment of cases with acute bacterial conjunctivitis and bacterial keratitis (in Chinese). *Eye Sci* 2000; 16146–148.

595. Parks DJ, Abrams DA, Sarfarzi F, et al. Comparison of topical ciprofloxacin to conventional antibiotic therapy in the treatment of ulcerative keratitis. *Am J Ophthalmol* 1993;115:471–477.

596. Honig MA, Cohen EJ, Rapuano CJ, et al. Corneal ulcers and the use of topical fluoroquinolones. *Contact Lens Assoc Ophthalmol J* 1999;25:200–203.

597. Gangopadhyay N, Daniell M, Weih L, et al. Fluoroquinolone and fortified antibiotics for treating bacterial corneal ulcers. *Br J Ophthalmol* 2000;84:378–384.

598. Lund MH. Colistin sulfate ophthalmic in the treatment of ocular infections. *Arch Ophthalmol* 1969;81:4–10.

599. Carmichael TR, Gelfand Y, Welsh NH. Topical steroids in the treatment of central and paracentral ulcers. *Br J Ophthalmol* 1990;74:528–531.

600. Hyndiuk RA, Eiferman RA, Caldwell DR, et al. Comparison of ciprofloxacin ophthalmic solution 0.3% to fortified tobramycin-cefazolin in treating bacterial corneal ulcers. *Ophthalmology* 1996;103:1854–1863.

601. Bignell JL. Infection of the cornea with B. pyocyaneus. *Br J Ophthalmol* 1951;35:419–423.

602. Stern GA, Butross M. Use of corticosteroids in combination with antimicrobial drugs in the treatment of infectious corneal disease. *Ophthalmology* 1991;98:847–853.

603. Pilat A, Coronini C, Moritsch H. Zur Klinik und Aetiologie der Keratoconjunctivitis epidemica. *Wien Klin Wochenschr* 1954;66: 798–801.

604. Dawson CR, Hanna L, Wood TR, et al. Adenovirus type 8 keratoconjunctivitis in the United States. Epidemiologic, clinical and microbiological features. *Am J Ophthalmol* 1970;69: 473–8.

605. Knopf HLS, Hierholzer JC. Clinical and immunological re-

sponses in patients with viral keratoconjunctivitis. *Am J Oph-thalmol* 1975;80:661–667.

606. Keenlyside RA, Hierholzer JC, D'Angelo LJ. Keratoconjunctivitis associated with adenovirus type 37: an extended outbreak in an ophthalmologist's office. *J Infect Dis* 1983;147:191–198.
607. Garber JM. Steroids' effects on the infectious corneal ulcer. *J Am Optom Assoc* 1980;51:477–483.
608. Liesegang TJ. Ocular herpes simplex infection: pathogenesis and current therapy. *Mayo Clin Proc* 1988;63:1092–1105.
609. Marsh RJ, Ffraunfelder FT, McGill JI. Herpetic corneal epithelial disease. *Arch Ophthalmol* 1976;94:1899–1902.
610. Seedor JA, Waring GO. Dendriform lesions of the cornea induced by soft contact lenses. *Arch Ophthalmol* 1987;105:1021.
611. Josephson JE. Contact lens-induced epithelial dendriform configurations. *Arch Ophthalmol* 1988;106:164.
612. DePaolis MD, Shovlin JP. Contact lenses and anterior segment disease: considerations in differential diagnosis. *Pract Optom* 1993;4:142–146.
613. Hutchinson DW. A biochemists view of antiviral agents. *IRCS Med Sci* 1986;14:965–968.
614. Kaufman HE. Treatment of viral disease of the cornea and external eye. *Prog Retinal Eye Res* 2000;19:69–85.
615. Gordon YJ. The evolution of antiviral therapy for external ocular viral infections over twenty-five years. *Cornea* 2000;19:673–680.
616. Pavan-Langston D. Ocular antiviral therapy. *Int Ophthalmol Clin* 1980;20:149–161.
617. Pavan-Langston D, Foster CS. Trifluorothymidine and idoxuridine therapy of ocular herpes. *Am J Ophthalmol* 1977;84:818–825.
618. Drance SM. Pharmacology and toxicology. *Arch Ophthalmol* 1963;70:261–280.
619. Pavan-Langston D, Buchannan RA. Vidarabine therapy of simple and IDU-complicated herpetic keratitis. *Trans Am Acad Ophthalmol Otolaryngol* 1976;81:OP813–OP825.
620. Wagstaff AJ, Faulds D, Goa KL. Acyclovir. *Drugs* 1994;47:153–205.
621. Hoh HB, Hurley C, Claoue C, et al. Randomised trial of ganciclovir and acyclovir in the treatment of herpes simplex dendritic keratitis: a multicentre study. *Br J Ophthalmol* 1996;80:140–143.
622. Colin J, Hoh HB, Easty DL, et al. Ganciclovir ophthalmic gel (Virgan, 0.15%) in the treatment of herpes simplex keratitis. *Cornea* 1997;16:393–399.
623. Muller-Jensen K. Behandlung und Prophylaxe der Keratoconjunctivitis epidemica. *Berische Deutsch Ophthalmol Gesamte* 1972;71:270–273.
624. Marmion VJ. Treatment of adenovirus type 8 kerato-conjunctivitis. *Trans Ophthalmol Soc UK* 1972;92:619–623.
625. Jernigan JA, Lowry BS, Hayden FG, et al. Adenovirus type 8 keratoconjunctivitis in an eye clinic: risk factors and control. *J Infect Dis* 1993;167:1307–1313.
626. Hillenkamp J, Reinard T, Ross RS, et al. The effects if cidofovir 1% with and without cyclosporin A 1% as a topical treatment of acute adenoviral keratoconjunctivitis. *Ophthalmology* 2002;109:845–850.
627. Hutter H. Keratoconjunctivitis epidemica: Therapiergebnisse wahrend einer Epidemie. *Klin Monatsbl Augenheilkd* 1990;197:214–247.
628. Patterson A, Jones BR. The management of ocular herpes. *Trans Ophthalmol Soc UK* 1967;87:59–72.
629. Wellings PC, Awdry PN, Bors FH, et al. Clinical evaluation of trifluorothymidine in the treatment of herpes simplex corneal ulcers. *Am J Ophthalmol* 1972;73:932–942.
630. Colin J, Chastel C. Traitement précoce de l'herpès oculaire. A propos de 6 cas de conjonctivites herpétiques. *J Fr Ophtalmol* 1985;8:801–802.
631. Jackson WB, Breslin CW, Lorenzetti DWC, et al. Treatment of herpes simplex keratitis: comparison of acyclovir and vidarabine. *Can J Ophthalmol* 1984;19:107–111.
632. Collum LMT, McGettrick P, Akhtar J, et al. Oral acyclovir (Zovirax) in herpes simplex dendritic corneal ulceration. *Br J Ophthalmol* 1986;70:435–438.
633. Mitsui Y. Corneal infections after cortisone therapy. *Br J Ophthalmol* 1955;39:244–253.
634. Power WJ, Hillery MP, Benedict-Smith A, et al. Acyclovir ointment plus topical betamethasone of placebo in first episode disciform keratitis. *Br J Ophthalmol* 1992;76:711–713.
635. Hyndiuk RA, Seideman S, Leibsohn JM. Treatment of vaccinial keratitis with trifluorothymidine. *Arch Ophthalmol* 1976;94:1785–1786.
636. Moffatt GH. Herpes zoster ophthalmicus. *Aust J Optom* 1979;62:214.
637. Cobo LM, Foulkes GN, Liesegang T, et al. Oral acyclovir in the treatment of acute herpes zoster. *Ophthalmology* 1985;92:1574–1583.
638. Buchi ER, Herbort CP, Ruffieux C. Oral acyclovir in the therapy of herpes zoster ophthalmicus. *Am J Ophthalmol* 1986;102:531–532.
639. Jackson JL, Gibbons R, Meyer G, et al. The effect of treating herpes zoster with oral acyclovir in preventing postherpetic neuralgia. *Arch Intern Med* 1997;157:909–912.
640. Tyring S, Barbarash RA, Nahlik JE, et al. Famciclovir for the treatment of acute herpes zoster: effects on acute disease and post herpetic neuralgia. *Ann Intern Med* 1995;123:89–96.
641. Saltman R, Boon R. The safety of famciclovir in patients with herpes zoster. *Curr Ther Res* 1995;56:219–225.
642. Johns KJ, O'Day DM, Head WS, et al. Herpes simplex masquerade syndrome: *Acanthamoeba* keratitis. *Curr Eye Res* 1987;6:207–211.
643. Shovlin JP, DePaolis MD, Edmonds SE, et al. *Acanthamoeba* keratitis: contact lenses as a risk factor. Case reports and review of the literature. *Int Contact Lens Clin* 1987;14:349–359.
644. Cohen EJ, Parlato CJ, Arentsen JJ, et al. Medical and surgical treatment of *Acanthamoeba* keratitis. *Am J Ophthalmol* 1987;103:615–625.
645. Azuara-Blanco A, Sadiq AS, Hussain M, et al. Successful medical treatment of *Acanthamoeba* keratitis. *Int Ophthalmol* 1998;21:223–227.
646. Parks DH, Palay DA, Daya SM, et al. The role of topical corticosteroids in the management of *Acanthamoeba* keratitis. *Cornea* 1997;16:277–283.
647. O'Day DM, Head WS. Advances in the management of keratomycosis and *Acanthamoeba* keratitis. *Cornea* 2000;19:681–687.
648. Abad JC, Foster CS. Fungal keratitis. *Int Ophthalmol Clin* 1996;36:1–15.
649. Foroozan R, Eagle RC, Cohen EJ. Fungal keratitis in a soft contact lens wearer. *Contact Lens Assoc Ophthalmol J* 2000;26:166–168.
650. Sridhar MS, Gopinathan U, Garg P, et al. *Aspergillus fumigatus* keratitis with wreath pattern infiltrates. *Cornea* 2001;20:534–535.
651. John T, Lin Jm Sahm, DF. *Acanthamoeba* keratitis successfully treated with prolonged propamidine isethionate and neomycin-polymyxin-gramicidin. *Ann Ophthalmol* (Chicago) 1990;22:20–23.
652. Varga JH, Wolf TC, Jensen HG, et al. Combined treatment of *Acanthamoeba* keratitis with propamidine, neomycin and polyhexamethylene biguanide. *Am J Ophthalmol* 1993;115:466–470.

653. Seal DV, Hay J, Kirkness C, et al. Successful medical therapy of *Acanthamoeba* keratitis with topical chlorhexidine and propamidine. *Eye* 1996;10:413–421.

654. Duguid IGM, Dart JKG, Morlet N, et al. Outcome of *Acanthamoeba* keratitis treated with polyhexamethylene biguanide and propamidine. *Ophthalmology* 1997;104:1587–1592.

655. Larkin DFP, Kilvington S, Dart JKG. Treatment of *Acanthamoeba* keratitis with polyhexamethylene biguanide. *Ophthalmology* 1992;99:185–191.

656. Murdoch D, Gray TB, Cursons R, et al. *Acanthamoeba* keratitis in New Zealand, including two cases with in vivo resistance to polyhexamethylene biguanide. *Aust N Z J Ophthalmol* 1998;26: 231–236.

657. Kosrirukvongs P, Wanachiwanawin D, Visvesvara GS. Treatment of *Acanthamoeba* keratitis with chlorhexidine. *Ophthalmology* 1999;106:798–802.

658. Lindquist TD. Treatment of *Acanthamoeba* keratitis. *Cornea* 1998;17:11–16.

PRACTICE MANAGEMENT

THOMAS QUINN
PATRICIA KEECH
ROBERT L. DAVIS
KEITH AMES
REX GHORMLEY
JACK J. YAGER
AND EDWARD S. BENNETT

Success in a contact lens practice depends on effective patient management and efficient practice administration. To accomplish these goals, the practice must have an education program, a trained and professional staff, a comprehensive fee policy, and a follow-up care system.

EDUCATION PROGRAM

For practice growth, a practitioner must have a strong education program. Those participating in this program should include the doctor, the staff, and the patient.

The Doctor

The education program starts with the doctor, who must stay updated on all new developments in contact lens materials, care system, and practice administration. An up-to-date clinician must read professional journals on a regular basis and attend local, regional, and national educational meetings. The Annual Meeting of the American Academy of Optometry is an excellent source for outstanding continuing education and the latest in clinical research. Publications such as *Contact Lens Spectrum (www.clspectrum.com)* and *Review of Contact Lenses (www.rcl@jobson.com)* are excellent sources of contact lens clinical articles, columns, and updates. In addition, *Contact Lens Today* is a weekly newsletter pertaining exclusively to updated contact lens developments. An online newsletter has been recently introduced by the Gas Permeable Lens Institute (GPLI). The knowledge gained from these sources can be shared with staff and patients.

Staff Education

Staff education is the second element necessary for an educational program. A patient's first and most frequent contact with any office is with a member of the staff. Staff personnel should have a comprehensive knowledge of contact lens care so that they can answer patients' questions properly, provide sound advice, and make intelligent recommendations for professional care. Likewise, it is important for them to have some understanding of corneal physiology, lens materials, and lens designs.

New employees in an office will come from varied backgrounds and training; some may be experienced in the optical field, some may be graduates of an optometric technician program, and some may have an absence of knowledge about contact lenses or vision care. For most representative practices, the latter is usually the case. Therefore, most practices need an organized training for all new employees. This can include textbooks, video tapes, and the Internet.

1. *Textbooks.* Several beneficial educational texts are available, including the following:

- *The Ophthalmic Assistant: Fundamentals and Clinical Practice* (Stein, Slatt, and Stein, Elsevier Publishing)
- *Home Study Course for Optometric Assistants* (American Optometric Association)
- *Contact Lenses* (Lowther and Snyder, Elsevier Publishing)

In addition, the American Optometric Association is in the process of developing a PowerPoint presentation on contact lenses for staff training purposes.

2. *Video tapes.* Video tapes on modification, verification, and patient education of gas permeable (GP) lenses are available from the GPLI *(www.rgpli.org).* They also have video tapes pertaining to use of the lensometer, the radiuscope, and the keratometer. Vistakon has developed an excellent series of educational modules for staff training developed by Sue Connelly and Ursula Lotzkat. The modules (to date) include the following:

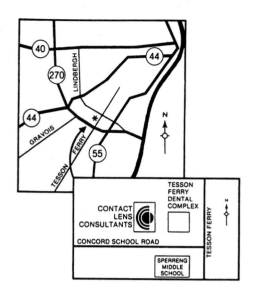

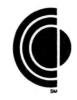

Contact Lens Consultants

Patient Information

"We always want to maintain good communication between our patients, doctors and staff. In order to efficiently provide quality vision care, it is important that all our patients understand our office procedures. If you have any ques-

Contact Lens Care
Visual Examinations
Ocular Health Care
Optical Dispensary

Our goal — to always provide our patients with the finest in vision and eye health care. With one of the fastest growing practices in the midwest, we feel our success results from a sincere interest in our patients. If you have questions, just ask!

FIG. 42.1. Informational brochure providing directions to the practice location.

- Defining moments
- Where did my day go?
- Speaking eye to eye

In addition, Harriett Stein & Associates (Baltimore, MD) has a video tape series that is quite comprehensive and includes a series of videos on staff training:

3. *Internet.* Wink Productions has a staff education Internet site that will be available in 2004. It will be a very comprehensive program in which the practice can subscribe to this service and new staff members can receive the training they deserve.

Staff members should be provided with the opportunity to update their education at state, regional, and national meetings that provide staff education. The staff members can report on what they have learned at the next scheduled staff meeting. Likewise, the practitioner can provide pertinent contact lens articles from professional publications and circulate them among the staff. Staff members also benefit from an enthusiastic practitioner who will bring them into the examination room to observe and discuss an interesting contact lens case.

The ongoing education of staff is benefited tremendously via regularly scheduled staff meetings. Often held 1 to 2 times per month (but sometimes held more frequently depending upon the length of the meeting), these meetings should be held during office hours, with much of the time devoted to new developments in the contact lens field. It is very important for practitioners to have personal involvement in the ongoing education of their staff, as well as providing constant reinforcement and feedback.

Patient Education

Patient education is the third element in a practice education program. This process begins when the patient first contacts the office. An educated assistant will always ask every new caller if he or she is currently wearing contact lenses and indicate that the practitioner fits lenses. Likewise, if the caller is not a contact lens wearer, the staff member will inquire as to his or her interest in contact lenses, presenting it as a viable corrective option and indicating that the office fits lenses. The patient can be informed of new contact lens designs and materials that may solve his or her visual problems. An informational brochure providing directions to the practice location can be given to the patient (Fig. 42.1).

Office brochures can be beneficial in describing different types of contact lens options, including general contact lens wear and benefits, as well as special designs (Fig. 42.2). Generic brochures are available from organizations such as the American Optometric Association and the GPLI (Fig. 42.3). After the eye examination, the practitioner can make recommendations to the patient. In most situations, the patient is looking to the eye care professional to make a recommendation and will comply with the type of lens suggested to him or her even if it contrasts with the patient's original inclination (i.e., patient heard soft lenses were more comfortable but practitioner finds that GP lenses would provide better vision). A laminated pocket card available from the GPLI shows the benefits and applications of GP lenses (for the patient) on one side and design, fitting, and troubleshooting pearls on the other side (for the practitioner) (Fig. 42.4).

It is important for the practitioner to explain why he or she has arrived at this recommendation so that the patient understands why this choice is a good match. It certainly is true that understanding breeds compliance. Such an explanation is as follows:

> A special design lens, called a *toric lens,* will correct your nearsightedness and astigmatism. Most contact lens complications are associated with dirty lenses, so I am recommending you be fit with toric lenses, which you will replace every 2 weeks. This will ensure you are wearing a clean lens, keeping you seeing well with a lens that is comfortable and safe to wear.

Whether the contact lenses are to be provided from inventory the same day or ordered for the patient to receive at a separate visit, sufficient time must be provided for the patient to feel comfortable with handling and care of the new lenses. It is highly desirable that the staff member(s) providing this education be contact lens wearers themselves. Ideally, they should have some experience with both GP and soft lenses to be able to both educate and troubleshoot contact lens care. One of the most common reasons for contact lens dropouts pertains to the results of inadequate patient education. The patients did not feel confident in handling the lenses; they were not properly informed of the proper care of their lenses; and perhaps they were not informed of the possible consequences if they failed to comply with the proper care and recommended wearing time with their contact lenses. Ideally, patient instruction should be comprehensive and consistent. A checklist can be used by staff members to ensure that this occurs (Table 42.1).

At this contact lens education class, the patient should be provided with a comprehensive contact lens instruction book, observe an educational video tape (available from several soft lens companies and the GPLI), and participate in a hands-on instruction session with a staff member. The instruction booklet can be developed by the office (Fig. 42.5), or standard booklets available from Anadem Publications (Columbus, OH) can be customized for an individual office. Whatever booklet is used, it should be of high print quality, with the most important instructions in bold or larger type. This booklet should provide information on the lens type, care products, replacement frequency, wearing schedule, and any other recommendations (Fig. 42.6).

It is important to recognize that patients should not be expected to read and retain all of the information provided in an educational booklet. Therefore, the most important component in patient education is the instructional session provided by the staff member. The patient should be able to successfully insert and remove the lenses several times prior to being allowed to leave the office with the lenses. In addition, the patient should be able to repeat the staff member's instructions on lens care, specifically, the routine upon lens removal at night through insertion of the lenses the next morning, what solution is used for what purpose, etc.

Repetition is important during the patient education process. An important component of the patient education program is to repeat important instructions and to ensure compliance at each follow-up visit, with the initial visit (typically at 1 week) being the most important. Patients should be asked, at minimum, the following:

- "How are you doing with the handling of your lenses?"
- "How many hours per day are you wearing the lenses?"

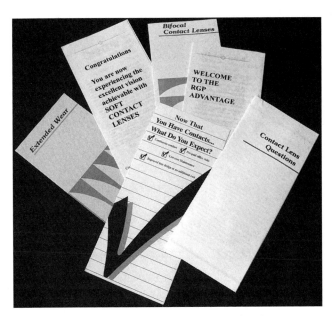

FIG. 42.2. Generic contact lens patient brochures.

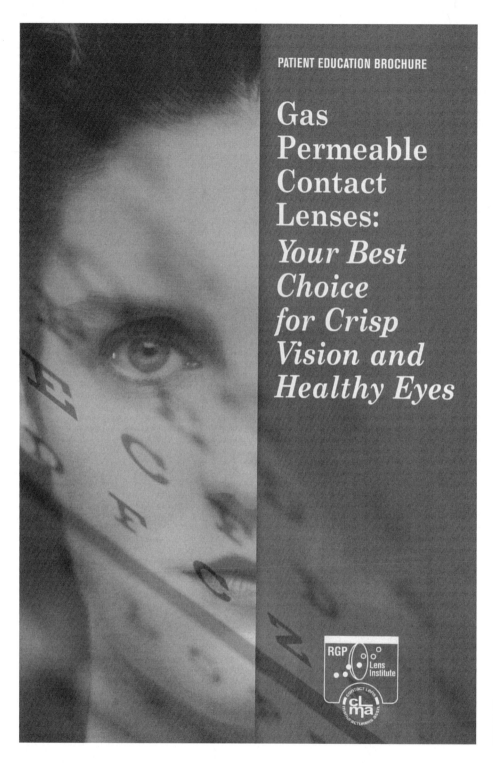

FIG. 42.3. Consumer brochure on gas permeable lens correction of myopia and presbyopia from the Gas Permeable Lens Institute.

RGP Lens Institue
Fluorescein Pattern Identification Card

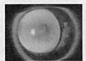

2D flatter than "K"
Excessive apical bearing, excessive inferior edge standoff

2D steeper than "K"
Excessive peripheral sealoff

1D flatter than "K"
Excessive apical bearing, excessive inferior edge standoff

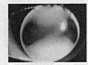

1D steeper than "K"
Mild peripheral sealoff

Alignment pattern
Even pattern centrally with slightly greater clearance peripherally

Spherical BCR on 3D WTR astigmatic cornea
Horizontal bearing and excessive vertical pooling is observed

FITTING PEARLS

- Use topical anesthetic during the fit
- Diagnostic lenses are available (contact CLMA member laboratory)
- Apply fluorescein and a yellow filter over observation system to evaluate fitting relationship
- Lens always moves along the steeper meridian
- Attempt to achieve alignment; alignment may occur with a BCR fit "on K" and often results with a BCR fit flatter than "K" due to the asphericity of the cornea

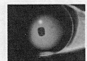

Pattern observed without the use of yellow filter over observation system

Identical pattern with the addition of yellow filter, notice greater fluorescence

MAKING LENS DESIGN CHANGES

To maintain the same fitting relationship:
- flatten BCR 0.25D for every 0.4-0.5mm increase in OZD
- steepen BCR 0.25D for every 0.4-0.5mm decrease in OZD

To improve the fitting relationship, make a large change in lens design:
- Change OAD/OZD at least 0.3mm
- Change BCR at least 0.50D
- Change CT at least 0.03mm
  - Decrease if lens decenters inferiorly
  - Increase if flexure is present
- Change PC radius at least 1.0mm
  - Flatten if peripheral sealoff
  - Steepen if excessive edge clearance
- Change PC width at least 0.2mm
  - Increase if peripheral sealoff
  - Decrease if excessive edge clearance

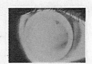

"On K" BCR with a 9.5mm Dia: 8.4mm OZ
Observe apical clearance and Insufficient peripheral clearance

"On K" BCR with a 9.5mm Dia: 7.6mm OZ
A more alignment fitting relationship with greater peripheral clearance

Bicurve design with a 10.0mm PCR: 0.5mm wide
Acceptable edge clearance, although narrow in width

Bicurve design with a 10.0mm PCR: 1.0mm wide
An increase in edge clearance can be observed

Bicurve design with a 9.0mm PCR: 0.8mm wide
Insufficient edge clearance can be observed

Bicurve design with a 12.0mm PCR: 0.8mm wide
Observe greater clearance

For a complete listing of lenses from CLMA member laboratories go to **www.rgpli.org**

FIG. 42.4. Laminated pocket card from the Gas Permeable Lens Institute giving the benefits and applications of gas permeable lenses on one side of the card for the patient and fitting pearls and fluorescein patterns of GP lenses on the other side of the card for the practitioner.

TABLE 42.1. CONTACT LENS DISPENSING CHECKLIST

Insertion and Removal
- Wash hands with nonoily soap
- Work over a flat surface with a bowl
- How to remove lens from case or package
- How to tell inside/out
- How to recenter lens
- How to store lenses
- Proper solutions for cleaning, storage, rinsing

Wearing Schedule/Replacement Schedule

What is it and why is it that way?

Hints:
- Never wear a lens that is uncomfortable
- Insert lenses before applying makeup and remove contact lens before removing makeup (use nonoily makeup removers and water-soluble mascara only)
- Avoid any aerosols (hair spray, PAM) while wearing contact lenses
- If you want to swim with your contact lenses, talk to your doctor
- If you experience persistent light sensitivity or tearing, please report that to your doctor the same day
- Be sure to wear your contact lenses for a few hours (at least) before your follow-up visits, and bring your glasses!!!
- If you can't wear your contact lenses, call us first!

- "What solutions are you using?"
- "How are you cleaning your lenses?"
- "How often are you replacing your lenses (if applicable)?"

The last question is particularly important. It becomes a simple matter of math to determine if the patient has been compliant. If the patient presents 1 year after dispensing of an annual supply and has 10 unopened pair of lenses at home or, conversely, if the patient is on the last pair but the annual supply was provided 18 months ago, compliance has been poor.

A comprehensive and repetitive patient education program benefits both patient and practice. Because education

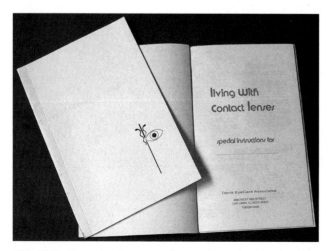

FIG. 42.5. Example of a contact lens patient education booklet.

and compliance go "hand in hand," every practitioner should review the commitment to patient education and continue to update the information provided by staff to patients. Staff meetings represent an excellent method for allowing practitioners and staff members to partner together in reviewing methods of patient education and compliance and how to improve and update this information.

FEES

Fee Schedule and Presentation

A contact lens fee system should be easy to understand. It also should be comprehensive so that the fee policy is applicable to as many situations as possible. The fee system should differentiate between new contact lens patients and standard or complex patients who are being refit. A printed fee schedule serves the purpose of indicating what services and materials are included in the fee. The fee system should not be totally inflexible, but exceptions or modifications to the established structure should not be routine. The fee can be all inclusive or a combined fee in which services and lens materials are included in one overall fee. Most practices separate or divide the services fees for professional care from the material fees. To compete effectively in today's consumer-based environment, it is important to price material fees competitively but to charge appropriately for services provided. It is the service that differentiates a practice that emphasizes contact lenses; the more specialized the service, the higher the fee. Patients often are quite willing to pay for high-quality care.

Often the contact lens fees are presented by staff members. It is important that the staff members be well qualified to both present the fees effectively and answer questions pertaining to the fees. For example: "Mrs. Jones, your contact lens fee includes a comprehensive vision examination, your contact lens preassessment and fitting examination, your contact lens materials, a 3-month supply of solutions, an educational visit to ensure that you will fee comfortable in handling and caring for your lenses, and 6 months of follow-up evaluations." The fees should be presented by the staff member (or the practitioner) after the practitioner has discussed the findings and made a recommendation. Fees should always be discussed prior to application of contact lenses.

Fee Policies and Agreements

Every fee system needs an established refund policy. The refund policy should be stated verbally to the patient and printed on the schedule. Ideally, this policy should be simple and easily understood. Many practices have a policy in which a full material refund is provided within a designated time period (often 60–90 days but may depend upon laboratory refund policies) after materials are returned. Certain

Thomas G. Quinn, O.D., M.S., F.A.A.O.
Susan G. Quinn, O.D., F.A.A.O.
Sherry Crawford, O.D., M.S.
416 West Union Street
Athens, Ohio 45701

DOCTORS of OPTOMETRY
• family practice
• contact lenses
• low vision
• vision therapy

Phone: (740) 594-2271 • Fax: (740) 594-2270 • www.athenseyecare.com

SOFT
CONTACT LENS INFORMATION

FOR: _John Doe_

DATE: _10-23-03_

YOUR LENSES ARE:

	SPHERICAL	_X_ DAILY WEAR _2wk REPL._
_____	TORIC	_____ FLEX WEAR
_X_	BIFOCAL	_____ EXTENDED WEAR

YOUR WEARING SCHEDULE IS:

DAY

| 1 | 2 | 3 | 4 | 5 | 6 | 7 | 8 | 9 | 10 |

HOURS
OF
WEAR _4 6 8 10 12 ⟶_

YOUR CARE PRODUCTS:

CLEANING _____

SOAKING _Clear Care_

WETTING _____

OTHER _Refresh Tears_

YOUR NEXT APPOINTMENT: _~/wk_

*Be sure to have worn your lenses at least 4 hours at the
time of your next visit unless specifically instructed
otherwise.

NOTE: We recommend all contact lens wearers have UV
protective **sunglasses** for enhanced visual comfort
and safety during lens wear.

FIG. 42.6. Soft contact lens information form.

professional fees, including the vision examination and contact lens fitting fees, should not be subject to refund. Information pertaining to the refund policy and other important
policy and care information can be included in an agreement that can be signed in duplicate (Fig. 42.7).

Some practices have agreements—essentially acting as
an informed consent—when patients are fit into extended
wear, monovision, and/or corneal reshaping. These agreements outline the benefits, risks, and other pertinent information patients need to know about their contact lens mo-

Contact Lens Service
(314) 516-5609

IN CASE OF EMERGENCY:

1. **During normal business hours**: please **remove** the contact lenses and call for an appointment at the Contact Lens Service, 516-5609 or Center for Eye Care, 516-5131 during clinic hours. You may leave a message at 516-5609 after clinic hours or if the phone is in use. We will return your call as soon as possible. If you have lost or damaged a contact lens, and need a replacement lens, please call the Contact Lens Service (516-5609).

2. **After hours**: if you remove the contact lens and the problem persists even after contact lens wear is discontinued, please contact us at 407-5375 or go to the nearest emergency service. This number is for <u>eye emergencies only</u> and is **not** for contact lens replacements. No one at this number will be able to provide you with a contact lens replacement.

REFUND POLICY:

It is our belief that most patients can be successfully fit with contact lenses. If we determine that a patient can not be successfully fit at the fitting examination, we inform the patient at that time and do not fit contact lenses. After a patient receives lenses, we try our best to work with a patient experiencing difficulty with lens wear, lens handling or vision, so that they may be successful. This may require ordering new or different lenses. If a patient is not happy with their contact lenses and wants to return their lenses within 60 days of the dispensing, we will refund a portion of their lens fees. Fitting fees are non-refundable. Please return for recommended follow-up visits so that potential lens wear difficulties may be addressed as early as possible. If you are experiencing any contact lens problems and do not have an appointment scheduled, please call to make a follow-up appointment as soon as possible.

REPLACEMENT POLICY:
Rigid Contact Lenses:
DW/EW Rigid lens*......................
*Keratoconic & High minus lenses
Toric Rigid lens...........................
Bifocal ....
Soft Contact Lenses:
DW SCL...................................
EW/Tinted SCL.........................
Toric.......................................
Bifocal ....
Prosthetic ....
FRP/Disposable........................

The fitting fee includes contact lenses, starter kit of solutions and 4 months of contact lens follow-up visits. Follow-up visits are suggested every 6 months after the initial period. The standard fee for a follow-up visit is   A comprehensive eye examination should be performed every year.

Please be advised that a contact lens is a FDA regulated medical device used in direct contact with the eye, and has potential to cause damage to the eye. Ongoing professional care is essential in maintaining the safe use of contact lenses. Missouri State law does not require the release of a contact lens prescription to an individual; therefore, the release of your contact lens prescription is conditional upon your identification of either a licensed optometrist or ophthalmologist that will monitor and be responsible for your eye health while wearing contact lenses. Your contact lens prescription is not final until the contact lenses have been dispensed and followed for a period of time to ensure that the lens fit and prescription is accurate. Your contact lens prescription expires one year from your fitting examination.

FEES AND COSTS ARE SUBJECT TO PERIODIC REVISIONS

STATEMENT BY PATIENT
This is to certify that I received instructions in the proper methods of insertion, removal, use and care of my contact lenses; and have reviewed the information on this page. Having proven myself to be competent enough to carry out these instructions, the contact lenses were given to me. I realize that success with contact lenses cannot be guaranteed and that any refund will be subject to the policy outlined on this page.

_____   _____
Patient's Signature   Student Intern's Signature

_____ _____   _____
Date   Clinical Instructor's Signature

FIG. 42.7. Representative patient agreement.

dality. An example of an agreement for a corneal refractive therapy patient is shown in Fig. 42.8.

Although service agreements are not as common as in the past due to the popularity of disposable lenses and the time involved in administering and explaining such an agreement, they still can benefit the contact lens practice.

Certainly, any practice that commonly provides GP lenses would benefit by providing patients with such an agreement. Replacement lenses can be provided at a reduced fee, services such as polishing can be included, and bulk packs of solutions can be provided at a reduced fee. An example of such an agreement is shown in Fig. 42.9.

Highland Vision Clinic, P.S.
721 North 182nd Street #302
Shoreline, WA 98133
206-542-7406

Corneal Refractive Therapy Fee Agreement

I request that Dr. Otto or Dr. Keech evaluate me for Corneal Refractive Therapy (CRT), which involves fitting rigid contact lenses for overnight wear for the purpose of altering the corneal shape to reduce myopia. This effect is not permanent, and requires the routine overnight wear of rigid contact lenses. The risks of this procedure are minor and may include: corneal abrasion and/or infection. The effect is reversible and has not resulted in permanent vision loss in clinical trials.

The initial evaluation is in addition to the routine visual examination and includes corneal topography, biomicroscopy, and trial contact lens fitting. *The fee for this evaluation is* ███*and is nonrefundable.*

If the procedure appears to be viable for you after the initial evaluation, *an additional* ███ *fee will be charged* as your fitting fee. This fee covers the cost of your CRT lenses, training, and all necessary follow up visits within a six-month period.

Lenses broken within sixty days of dispensing will be replaced at no charge, *if the pieces are returned to the clinic.* After sixty days from the date of this agreement, broken lenses are replaced at ███ each.

If, for any reason, you decide to terminate the treatment, ███ will be refunded to you within the first two weeks of receiving your CRT lenses. If the fitting process is terminated after two months of services, the refund is ███. The lenses must be returned for any refund to be processed. The full value of lost lenses (███ each) will be deducted from any refund.

Results are not guaranteed, and individual responses vary.

_____   _____
Print name   Signature

_____
Date

FIG. 42.8. Representative corneal refractive therapy fee agreement.

Dear Patient,

Your record indicates that the anniversary of your Contact Lens Service Agreement is near. This is really much more than lens replacement insurance. The reason for this agreement is just what the name implies — SERVICE.

More important, you'll be less likely to put off needed eyecare when you have prepaid protection. Please call if you have any questions. Thank you.

Davis EyeCare Associates

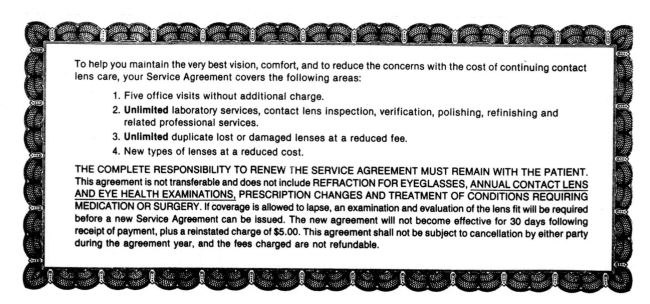

To help you maintain the very best vision, comfort, and to reduce the concerns with the cost of continuing contact lens care, your Service Agreement covers the following areas:

1. Five office visits without additional charge.
2. **Unlimited** laboratory services, contact lens inspection, verification, polishing, refinishing and related professional services.
3. **Unlimited** duplicate lost or damaged lenses at a reduced fee.
4. New types of lenses at a reduced cost.

THE COMPLETE RESPONSIBILITY TO RENEW THE SERVICE AGREEMENT MUST REMAIN WITH THE PATIENT. This agreement is not transferable and does not include REFRACTION FOR EYEGLASSES, <u>ANNUAL CONTACT LENS AND EYE HEALTH EXAMINATIONS,</u> PRESCRIPTION CHANGES AND TREATMENT OF CONDITIONS REQUIRING MEDICATION OR SURGERY. If coverage is allowed to lapse, an examination and evaluation of the lens fit will be required before a new Service Agreement can be issued. The new agreement will not become effective for 30 days following receipt of payment, plus a reinstated charge of $5.00. This agreement shall not be subject to cancellation by either party during the agreement year, and the fees charged are not refundable.

FIG. 42.9. Contact lens service agreement.

Third Party Plans

In recent years third party plans have had a large impact on how a contact lens practice is administered compared to the days when patients paid full fee for service. The down side to such plans is that there may be limitations to the amount of reimbursement and the lenses covered by the plan, and the patient may have a sense of entitlement, expecting the insurance to cover it all. In this way, these plans have changed the doctor–patient loyalty relationship. Practitioner selection can be dictated by the provider list as opposed to referrals and interpersonal relationships. The positive effect is that some patients may not come to the office for an examination and contact lens care if they did not have third party coverage. In addition, the insurance coverage of materials provides the practitioner with the opportunity to supply contact lens-wearing patients with spectacles and contact lenses. As some popular plans provide increased coverage on spectacles than contact lenses, it provides an incentive for the practice to provide backup spectacles.

An important factor is to let all new and established patients know what plans you accept in the practice. Patients should know that the practice will work with them such that they will receive maximum benefits. All benefits and deductibles should be explained to the patient. It can be made easy by promptly submitting all claims for the patient. Also, patients need to know that there are two types of insurance accepted by contact lens practitioners: vision insurance (i.e., VSP) and major medical (i.e., BC/BS). Major medical can be used to cover costs for certain patients (i.e., those with dry eyes, corneal scars, irregular cornea, keratoconus).

It is important to note that, for the most part, these plans do not affect the contact lens practice as much as they do other examination fees and materials. Most plans simply have an allowance and the practice can charge the patient the balance, which can generate business. When the fees and material charges are dictated by the plan, it is important to review the plan carefully prior to agreeing to be a provider because it may be difficult to profit from some plans. VSP is particularly good in compensation for medically necessary contact lenses, such as for keratoconus. An interim request for benefits form can be completed, the necessary information provided, and the topography maps attached. The appropriate fees typically are approved within 48 hours. Many other insurance companies are not as experienced with keratoconus to have a cogent, consistent policy. In those cases, it may be preferable to have the patient provide the fees up front and collect reimbursement from the insurance company. Regardless, whenever a practice agrees to sign up as a provider for any third party plan, it is important to follow the rules.

One method of counteracting the negative impact of third party plans on the practice is to emphasize specialty contact lenses (i.e., bifocals, corneal reshaping, high astigmatism, irregular cornea, postsurgical) within the practice. These lenses can result in an emphasis on fee for service, patient loyalty, and referrals.

Third party plans have affected all aspects of eye care practice, including contact lenses. By limiting fees-for-services and materials, practitioners have to adapt by becoming more efficient in their fitting and more selective in the types of materials offered.

Increasing Profitability

Certainly practice profitability from contact lenses can be optimized by several of the aforementioned methods (i.e., careful selection of third party plans, effective presentation of contact lenses as an option, service agreements). In addition, purchasing of contact lens solutions and materials (when applicable) can reduce costs and increase profit. In many contact lens practices, however, the fitting of special design lenses has had the single most significant impact on practice growth. Many of these patients have been told they are not good candidates for contact lenses due to their refractive error. Once they are successfully fit into contact lenses, they are likely to be enthusiastic and refer other patients. Those practitioners who fit specialty design contact lenses set themselves apart from their colleagues. The willingness to assume the risk of specialty fitting provides the opportunity for greater profits by charging a higher fee for assuming the risk. This is particularly true when fitting the presbyopic patient and the myope who desires corneal reshaping to reduce refractive error. It is important to charge a fee consistent with the amount of office time necessary to manage the patient. Presbyopic patients often are very excited about the fact that they can be successfully fit into contact lenses, and this is a group on individuals who typically are in control of their own finances. In addition, as with myopes desiring corneal reshaping, they will often willingly pay more for contact lenses and associated services if they perceive their quality of life is enhanced by lens wear. For myopes, this procedure has the benefits of a lower fee, being nonsurgical and temporary compared to refractive surgery.

PRACTICE PROMOTION

There are several methods of promoting the practice, including in-office brochures, newsletters and other mailings, the media, and—hopefully—word of mouth. A newsletter, often provided quarterly or semiannually, can provide new developments in the contact lens field, as well as new products and materials available from the practice (Fig. 42.10). If the practitioner has been involved in contact lens continuing education or clinical research or has contributed to publications, this can be highlighted in the newsletter. The newsletter can be edited by an interested staff member. The goal is to keep the newsletter simple and easy to read, being careful not to overwhelm the patient with too much detail, which likely would compromise comprehension of the material.

Having generic brochures, as discussed earlier, can be beneficial and can be presented to patients who may be good candidates for certain designs. A "visual needs assessment questionnaire" (Fig. 42.11) can be given to every patient who presents for a comprehensive vision examination.

The media can help with practice promotion. Contacting local radio and television stations, as well as newspapers, can result in interviews on contact lens topics. Practitioners who provide local media with a curriculum vitae in addition to a cover letter indicating contact lens topics with which they have expertise and which may be timely for consumers likely will be invited for interviews. This can be followed up with occasional news releases when appropriate (i.e., fitting a new specialty lens, serving as a clinical investigator for a new material or product, etc.). "Save Your Vision Week" is a good time to be available for interviews. One of the authors (TQ) sponsors public radio because this audience is consistent with the type of patients he finds desirable in his practice.

The most effective method of practice promotion, however, continues to be word of mouth. A satisfied patient, particularly a patient who could not be (or would not be) fit elsewhere and is successfully fit in a practice, likely will tell several other people about this positive experience.

PATIENT RETENTION

Patients often will return if they recognize that the fitting practice provides services as well as value that they may not receive elsewhere. This can include providing loaner lenses, replacing defective lenses, a fair warranty program, and willingness to take the time necessary to verify the lenses, educate the patient, and provide sufficient follow-up care. The process begins at the patient's initial visit when the importance of regular care can be emphasized. Without the patient's understanding of the health and vision benefits of regular care, all other forms of encouragement can appear to be solicitous and self-serving. The entire office staff must

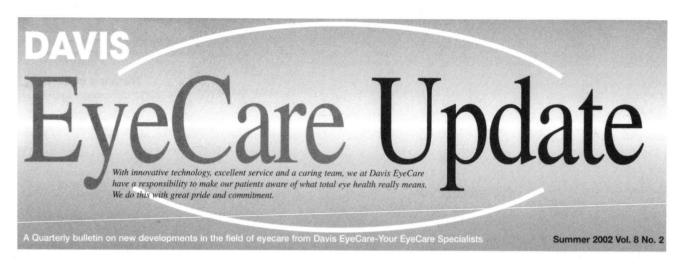

FIG. 42.10. Contact lens practice patient newsletter.

be on board with the "quality care requires regular care" philosophy.

The best time to make the recommendation for follow-up care is at the conclusion of the examination, and this recommendation should come from the doctor. "I want to see you in 6 months for a contact lens evaluation to make sure the lenses are fitting properly," or "I want to see you in 1 year for your annual eye examination to make sure your contact lenses are performing properly and to check the health of you eyes." It also would be recommended to make the appointment at that time, if possible. A phone call a few weeks in advance of this visit will remind the patient of the upcoming appointment. If the patient does not desire to schedule the appointment at that time, an active mail recall system is important. Whereas mailing the annual supply of lenses to the patient's home or workplace is a beneficial service, it will be important to evaluate the lenses on a regular basis to ensure they are fitting and performing properly.

LENS FITTING, STORAGE, AND DISINFECTION

Diagnostic Sets

It is important to have as many fitting sets and inventories as possible. Multiple disposable inventories, including toric and bifocal inventories, are important in order to provide same-day service for new patients, as well as for replacement lenses for established patients. If the 1-week follow-up visit shows a less than optimum fitting relationship, reduced vision, or both, a new lens can be provided immediately. As recommended in Chapter 13, several spherical GP fitting sets are recommended, including plus power, low-minus power, and high-minus power lenses. An inventory would be preferable and would offer several of the benefits of soft lenses. If the practitioner frequently fits GP lenses, discussing an inventory plan with the laboratory would be a viable idea. A bitoric fitting set and multiple bifocal fitting sets would be recommended. At a minimum, an aspheric mul-

Patient Visual Needs Assessment
Drs. Quinn, Quinn and Crawford

Your Name _____ Age _____ Today's Date _____

1. So we may best meet your visual needs, please list specific visual demands you have (work or recreation related):

   _____

2. What is your primary form of visual correction? (please circle)

   glasses   *soft contact lenses*   *gas permeable contact lenses*   *no correction*

3. How do you wear your current glasses? (please circle)

   all day   *distance tasks*   *near tasks*   *as needed*   *don't wear*

4. Are you interested in considering contact lenses? (please circle one)

   * *To wear daily*   * *To wear on occasion*   * ***NEW**: To wear continuously for up to 1 month*

   * *Haven't considered*   * *I already wear*   * *Not interested*

5. Are you interested in contact lenses that will change or enhance eye *color?*   **Y   N**

6. Have you worn contact lenses in the past? (please circle)

   Soft lenses   *Gas permeable lenses*   *Hard lenses*   *Haven't worn*

7. Are you interested in considering **C**orneal **R**efractive **T**herapy (wearing a gas permeable lens overnight to re-shape the eye, so when removed in the morning, uncorrected vision is clear)?
   Yes   No   Not sure

8. Are you interested in considering laser treatment to reduce your dependence on corrective lenses?
   Yes   No   Not sure

020102

Thank you! Please return this form to the receptionist.

FIG. 42.11. Patient "visual needs assessment questionnaire."

tifocal GP fitting set and a segmented translating set should be acquired; ultimately, more than one set in each of these two categories would increase the success rate in fitting bifocal lenses. Both plus power and minus power lenses should be included in the sets.

For fitting irregular cornea and postsurgical corneas, 1 to 2 keratoconic sets and a reverse geometry set for postsurgical cases is recommended. One of the large-diameter special design lenses discussed in Chapter 28 is recommended for fitting post-penetrating keratoplasty patients. The special design lenses should be ordered on a "per case" or warranted basis to allow for exchanges. An inventory of corneal refractive therapy (CRT) lenses (or other corneal reshaping design) is recommended for fitting myopic patients interested in this procedure.

Fitting Methods

Three fitting methods are often used: inventory, diagnostic, and empirical. The fitting approach is dictated by the patient's case presentation, the lenses available, and the practitioner's preferred approach. Regardless of the approach, the intent is to provide the patient with the most optimal lens design with minimal lens modification.

1. *Inventory.* As mentioned previously, most soft lenses (>75%) should be provided via inventory due to the limited lens parameter designs and availability of inventories. Certainly the inventory approach creates both patient and doctor satisfaction by fitting the patient with the appropriate contact lens at one visit, reducing time and increasing efficiency. This allows the patient the opportunity to go directly into lenses that provide good vision as opposed to waiting for lenses and possibly even changing his or her mind about contact lens wear in general during the interim period. One disadvantage of this fitting procedure is that it gives the perception that the design is not special and perhaps that anyone could fit this device. Having the patient wait a few days for the lenses to arrive can provide the perception that the lenses were made custom for his or her eyes only. In addition, office personnel need to be aware that sufficient time to properly educate the patient will become necessary if the practitioner makes the decision to fit directly from inventory.

One of the authors (PK) is a strong advocate of GP lens fitting from inventory. She has three overall diameters (8.5, 9.0, 9.5 mm), base curve radii in 0.1-mm steps from 7.4 to 8.2 mm, and powers from −1.00 D to −6.00 D in 0.50 D steps. In her experience, this will fit 80% of her patients. With GP lens patients, a large benefit of this fitting approach is that they can obtain the most important advantage from this modality immediately: good quality of vision. If a smaller inventory is desired, two diameters can be used: 8.8 and 9.3 mm. The diameter to be selected will depend on factors such as upper lid position and pupil size. The benefit of a multiple-diameter inventory is that one diameter lens can be fit to one eye and the other diameter to the other eye, and the lens-to-cornea fitting relationship can be compared.

2. *Diagnostic.* A diagnostic fitting approach has the advantage (vs empirical) of observing a GP contact lens on the eye and using fluorescein to define the best fitted contact lens. A diagnostic fitting process allows for fine tuning, which minimizes lens changes. It also provides the patient with the experience of wearing contact lenses. This is important with special design lenses in which inventories are essentially not possible (i.e., GP bifocals, keratoconus and postsurgical designs, bitorics, and oblique axis and high-cylinder soft toric lenses). However, it is important for the practitioner to use diagnostic lenses to arrive at the best lens-to-cornea fitting relationship, because empirical fitting may result in multiple reorders and greater time expended in these cases. The disadvantages of diagnostic fitting versus inventory are the need for multiple visits and the inability to immediately provide lenses that provide satisfactory vision. The latter is also a disadvantage compared to empirical fitting. Use of a topical anesthetic prior to diagnostic fitting should improve the initial experience if, in fact, the diagnostic lens has a power that differs greatly from that required for the patient. In addition, after the first several fits, practitioners should be able to achieve sufficient first-fit success to order the lenses on a "per lens" basis and save the higher cost of ordering warranted lenses.

3. *Empirical* fitting is a popular method of fitting spherical GP lenses, particularly in practices where an inventory is not available. The primary advantage of the empirical method (vs diagnostic) is that the patient's first experience is often a positive one as it pertains to quality of vision obtained. Therefore, any negative experiences from initial lens awareness should be reduced as a result of the vision obtained. This method has increased first-fit success in recent years due to factors such as excellent quality of manufacturing resulting in consistent edge quality, aspheric or aspheric-like peripheral designs, and ultrathin construction. In addition, the use of topography-based designs, which allow practitioners to better simulate the actual lens-to-cornea fitting relationship, also optimizes first-fit success. However, simply providing the laboratory with the refraction and keratometry readings is not as effective in achieving early success with GP lenses. The more "hands-on" the practitioner is in the process (i.e., use of a topographer, evaluating factors such as lid position, pupil size, and fissure size) while determining, at minimum, overall diameter, base curve radius, and power, the more likely empirical fitting will be successful.

Lens Storage and Disinfection

1. *Storage.* With the amount of storage room needed for disposable lenses, it is recommended—whenever possible—to have direct mail programs available for patients. With today's free shipping of annual lens supplies, it is not cost effective or space efficient to do otherwise. Manufacturers of disposable contact lenses offer mailing services to patients directly from their distribution sites. Although this is convenient, it creates a relationship with the manufacturer instead of the office. Doctors also can offer direct mail programs to their patients. Solutions also can be incorporated into the fitting package, thus providing an additional service to the patient.

If patients are encouraged to purchase an annual supply, they are both likely to adhere to the replacement schedule when they have a complete supply and less likely to look elsewhere to purchase lenses. It also is recommended that when the patient prefers a 3- or 6-month supply of lenses, the balance of the annual supply can be mailed to the patient's home or work place. It can be documented when the patient's prescription will expire so when the patient calls in, the front office staff will know it is acceptable to process the order without needing to schedule the patient for an examination.

2. *Disinfection.* The trend in recent years has been away from disinfecting diagnostic lenses and, in fact, to discarding all diagnostic lenses that have been used but not dispensed. This reduces the risk of ocular complications and the possibility for the diagnostic lenses to not perform optimally after disinfection. This philosophy also reinforces to the patient the importance of proper hygiene. When nondisposable specialty lenses are ordered, for example, highly astigmatic soft toric lenses, they can be provided directly to the patient or, if unsuccessful, returned to the laboratory to avoid reuse. If the lenses are disinfected in-office and reused, the use of either Opti-Free Express or ClearCare is recommended. GP lenses should be, at minimum, cleaned with Miraflow or a laboratory cleaner and stored dry. Use of a 10-minute hydrogen peroxide soak after cleaning and prior

to storage also would be recommended. Some lens materials are recommended to be stored in the wet state, however. Menicon lenses should be stored in either Claris or Optimum. Some laboratories provide specific Paragon Vision Sciences materials in the wet state, specifically using Unique pH for storage.

SUMMARY

It is evident that every practice is different, and some of the ideas presented in this chapter will be applicable to one given practice over others. The key to a successful contact lens practice is a comprehensive education program for the doctor, staff members, and patients. It also is evident that the highest earning potential lies with the fitting of specialty lenses such as torics, multifocals, and GP lenses. Many practitioners do not make such a commitment, so practitioners who fit the more challenging cases reap the benefits and rewards. These patients are often the most enthusiastic, helping build the practice through the best possible method: word of mouth. Professional satisfaction is one of many benefits derived from fitting the best lens for any given patient as opposed to not fitting lenses or fitting a simpler but perhaps less rewarding lens to the patient.

LEGAL ISSUES IN CONTACT LENS PRACTICE

MICHAEL G. HARRIS AND
ROBERT E. DISTER

INTRODUCTION

Legal issues have become an everyday part of contact lens practice. In today's society, it is as important for a contact lens practitioner to know about contracts, informed consent, and malpractice as it is to know about fluorescein patterns, contact lens design, and slit-lamp biomicroscopy findings. We live in a litigious society. This is evidenced by the recent increase in the number of lawsuits against health care practitioners. In optometric practice, no area of patient care leads to more law suits than contact lenses (1,2).

Prudent contact lens practitioners must understand the legal issues involved in contact lens practice. They must use sound judgment not only in what they do clinically for the patient but also in how they act from a legal perspective. If practitioners are technically wrong in their evaluation of a contact lens fit, the consequences may be the need to refit the patient or refund the fitting fee. These are relatively minor in comparison to the consequences if practitioners fail to properly document that they obtained the patient's informed consent to be fitted with an investigational contact lens. Here the practitioners could face a prolonged lawsuit, financial loss, and damage to their reputation.

By understanding the legal issues in contact lens practice and utilizing appropriate forms and procedures, contact lens practitioners can minimize the likelihood of being sued. They will be communicating more effectively with their patients and reducing the possibility of misunderstandings. They also will be doing a more effective job of providing for the patient's visual and physiologic well-being. This chapter discusses some of the major legal issues encountered in contact lens practice, including doctor–patient agreements, informed consent, contact lens prescription release, theories of liability, malpractice, and proper record keeping.

DOCTOR–PATIENT AGREEMENTS

Contracts are agreements we make with one other that are enforceable by law (3). Contracts are a part of everyday life.

In addition to the formal contracts we sign when closing a business deal or buying a house, we enter into contracts when we sell a car, get married, take a new job, or buy something at the local store. Contracts are a necessity of a civilized society.

Contracts have a useful and vital place in contact lens practice (4). They can be used to establish the obligations and responsibilities of the practitioner and the patient. In addition, they can be used to safeguard the rights of both parties. These contracts take the form of doctor–patient agreements that are used to clarify the relationship between the practitioner and the patient.

Contracts can be used in contact lens practice to formalize the contact lens fitting arrangements with the patient, to emphasize the importance of proper lens care and follow-up care, to establish a prepaid service agreement with the patient, to document the patient's "informed consent" to a specialized contact lens procedure, or to emphasize the patient's obligation to follow the instructions provided by the contact lens practitioner (5). As in any doctor–patient relationship, there are numerous opportunities for miscommunication in contact lens practice. Use of written contracts helps to reduce the possibility for misunderstanding or disagreement between the practitioner and patient.

Basics of Contract Law

Three elements are vital to the formation of any contract: (i) an appropriate offer, (ii) a proper acceptance, and (iii) an adequate consideration exchanged by the parties. In addition, there must be no legally recognized defense to the formation of the contract (6,7).

Formation of a contract requires two parties to mutually assent or agree to the same bargain at the same time without any misunderstandings. This mutual agreement takes the form of an offer and acceptance. When this mutual consent is communicated by written or oral words, an "expressed" contract has been formed (6). However, the law also recognizes contracts where the promises are "inferred" from the acts or conduct of the parties rather than from the communicated words (6). These "implied" contracts can be seen when a bidder signifies his or her desire to buy an item at auction or when a patient consults a health care practitioner. These acts imply the promise to pay the costs involved.

The first element of a contract is the *offer* (7). An offer is a proposal by one party (the *offeror*) that manifests a willingness to enter into a bargain with another party (the *offeree*). To qualify as an offer, the words or actions must (i) show a present intent to agree, (ii) have certain and definite terms, and (iii) be communicated to the offeree. This commitment must be more than just an indication of the intent to negotiate. It is evaluated objectively according to the actual language used, the customs of the industry, the course of normal business dealing, and the surrounding circumstances.

The offer must contain certain and definite terms. The four essential terms of a contract are (i) the parties, (ii) the subject matter, (iii) the time for performance, and (iii) the price. The courts will imply reasonable terms if the subject matter is delineated in the contract. Reasonable terms are those that are consistent with the intention of the parties and that can be logically implied from the surrounding circumstances.

An offer may be terminated prior to its acceptance by any of three means: (i) revocation of the offeror, (ii) rejection of the offeree, or (iii) operation of law (7). An offeror must terminate an offer by indicating this intention before the offeree accepts the offer. The offeree can terminate the offer by indicating his or her rejection by words or conduct that reasonably implies his or her refusing, modifying, or qualifying the offer.

The power to accept an offer also may be terminated by the operation of law. This occurs when the subject matter of the offer is destroyed, when one of the parties to the contract dies, or when the proposed contract has an illegal purpose.

If the offer has not been terminated prior to acceptance, the designated offeree can accept the offer by communicating to the offeror his or her present unequivocable consent to the terms of the offer (7). The *acceptance,* which is the second element needed to form a contract, must mirror the terms of the offer exactly. Any minor changes in terms are considered both a rejection and a counteroffer, which then must be accepted by the original offeror. Acceptance can be shown expressly by words of agreement or by conduct that indicates a commitment to enter into contract. Courts attempt to view the words and actions of the parties to make an enforceable contract provided this can be accomplished without "making the bargain for the parties" (7).

The third element needed to form a contract is *consideration* (8). Consideration has been defined as "the inducement to a contract" that leads to a legal liability to do or forbear from doing something (6). To have a binding bargain, each party must incur a legal liability in order to gain a legal right. The courts insist that the consideration be "adequate." Any valuable promise or item usually suffices. Without adequate

consideration, an agreement is not an enforceable contract. In some situations, however, there can be a substitute for consideration. This is called *promissory estoppel* (9). When the offeree relies reasonably and foreseeably to his or her detriment on the offeror's promise, promissory estoppel substitutes for consideration and an enforceable contract is formed.

If these three elements are present, a binding contract exists unless there is a legal defense to the contract. These defenses can be made to the formation of the contact or to the enforcement of certain contract terms. The law will not recognize a contract as legally binding if there is evidence that the parties never formed an agreement or if public policy prohibits enforcement of the agreement. Incapacity on the part of one of the parties can lead to an invalid contract because a contract is voidable by the incapacitated party. These include minors under the age of consent (18 years in most states), mentally incompetent individuals, and intoxicated persons.

A contract is invalid if the subject matter or purpose of the contract is illegal, or if there has been misrepresentation, fraud, or duress on the part of one of the parties to the contract. A contract also is invalid if there was a mutual mistake as to the terms of the contract or if the contract is deemed "unconscionable" in that is grossly unfair to one of the parties involved.

A major defense to the formation of a contract is the *Statute of Frauds* (10). The law recognizes that oral contracts generally have the same validity as written contracts. However, some oral contracts may be voidable under the Statute of Frauds unless there is tangible evidence that a contract exists. The tangible evidence must be some form of written manifestation of an intent to agree. As a general rule, however, oral contracts are valid and enforceable, but they are more difficult to interpret and enforce because there is no tangible evidence of their content.

The following section contains specific application of contracts in contact lens practice.

Contact Lens Fitting Agreements

Contact lens fitting agreements (4,5) are used to formalize the relationship between the doctor and the patient and to provide the patient with written details of what is involved in the contact lens fitting process. Although verbal descriptions of materials and services are necessary in order to assure complete patient understanding, written agreements formalize the relationship and gives the patient a printed expression of the details of the fitting arrangement to which the patient can refer to as necessary.

There are three basic reasons for utilizing a contact lens fitting agreement (5):

1. To provide a signed contract that serves as legal evidence of the agreement between the doctor and the patient

2. To ensure that the patient fully understands the policies, fees, and refund schedule of the practice and how the fees are to be paid
3. To educate the patient to recognize the fact that services are a major part of the contact lens fitting process

A well-drafted fitting agreement states the cost of the services and materials involved in the fitting and emphasizes the fact that the contact lens fitting is the joint responsibility of the patient and the doctor. It emphasizes the patient's responsibility by indicating that the patient is entering into a comprehensive treatment plan that requires the patient's ongoing cooperation. It should detail the types of follow-up examinations and the frequency of such examinations that are required of the patient. The formality of a written contractual agreement that emphasizes the importance of service and follow-up care can make a major impression on the patient. The contract reinforces the fact that the patient is not just purchasing a pair of contact lenses but is actually purchasing the practitioner's skill and time in providing proper care during the fitting and thereafter. A properly composed agreement can assist the practitioner in his or her effort to make the patient more cooperative and receptive in understanding the contact lens fitting and follow-up process.

All such agreements should contain a common minimum amount of information, including the patient's name, the cost and payment policy, the services supplied, the length of the fitting period, the progress evaluation program, the materials supplied, the refund policy, the lens replacement policy, the patient's signature, and the date of the agreement (4). A member of the doctor's staff can witness the signing of the agreement. It is best if this and other doctor–patient agreement forms are printed in duplicate so that one copy can be placed in the patient's record and the other can be taken home by the patient. Figure 43.1 shows an example of a contact lens fitting agreement.

Proper training by the practitioner or by the staff is essential to a successful patient response. To aid in enhancing patient compliance, the practitioner should augment the training and the instructions given to the patient in the office through the use of a printed form that lists key matters and individual requirements (5). This separate agreement form can be used to document the training and instructions given to the patient on the proper wear and care of contact lenses. This serves to establish the guidelines for the new patient and describes the contact lens care and handling regimen, the wearing schedule, the follow-up examination schedule, and any other specific information relevant to the patient's treatment plan.

Contact Lens Service Agreements

Another type of doctor–patient agreement that can be used in a contact lens practice is a prepaid contact lens service agreement (4,5). These agreements are designed to provide the patient with prepaid services for a period of time, usually 1 year, and for the replacement of contact lenses at a reduced fee. These agreements should delineate the services provided by the doctor and allow the patient to return for annual or semi-annual examinations, as well as emergency care.

If the practitioner's services have already been paid for, the patient is more likely to return to the doctor for assistance if difficulties arise. These forms need to emphasize that the practitioner offers a comprehensive plan for caring for his or her contact lens patients, including adequate follow-up care and prevention of future problems. Thus, the emphasis should be on services, with the replacement of contact lens materials being an incidental benefit of such an agreement.

These agreements should be drafted in such a fashion that they are service agreements and not merely insurance policies against lost contact lenses. Insurance policies can only be offered by a licensed insurance company, which must be bonded and supervised by an appropriate state agency. Without bonding and supervision, it would be possible for a practitioner to sell "contact lens insurance," collect the "premiums," and then close down the office, leaving the patient without appropriate recourse (11).

Contact lens service agreements are viewed differently in different states. Practitioners should check with their state agencies to determine if contact lens service agreements are legal in their state. If so, the contact lens service agreement should be offered to each original fitting patient at the end of the fitting process, with specific terms allowing for annual renewal if the patient returns at the end of the 1-year period for an evaluation. These prepaid service agreements should be limited to patients actually fitted in your office who return as required for their semi-annual or annual examination.

An appropriate prepaid service agreement must contain a statement of purpose. In addition, each agreement should contain information that specifies the services and materials covered, encourages the patient's return for appropriate follow-up care and services, the lens exchange policy, and the program for routine and emergency examinations (5). The cost of materials should be, at minimum, the actual laboratory cost of contact lenses or the agreement could be viewed as contact lens insurance. It should provide for semi-annual or annual follow-up examinations, appropriate lens cleaning and polishing, and state the fees for the various services involved. The patient and the practitioner should sign the agreement, with one copy being retained in the patient's record and the other being given to the patient. If desired, a member of the doctor's staff can witness the agreement. These forms can be modified to fit the needs of the individual practitioner. An example of a prepaid service agreement is shown in Figure 43.2.

Although the use of contracts such as the doctor–patient agreements discussed here may seem time consuming, they

Fitting you with contact lenses places a joint responsibility on both of us. Therefore, you must understand what our contact lens fitting program includes. Please read this over carefully, and if you have any questions, feel free to discuss them with us.

Our contact lens patients receive the following materials and services:
1. Examination of ocular health.
2. Vision analysis and spectacle prescription.
3. Examination for contact lenses.
4. Dispensing of contact lenses, patient care kit, and instructional materials; education and instruction in handling, care and maintenance of your contact lens.
5. Evaluation of lens fit with the lenses on the eye.
6. Progress evaluatuon and follow-up care for a period on ____ months.

Since there are many variables to contact lens fitting, there is no guarantee that you will become a successful contact lens wearer. However, we will use up to ____ lenses in the fitting procedure and will work with you and follow-up for __ months without additional charge.

Contact lenses are made by many laboratories employing various materials and designs. As a result, costs vary. And on occasion we will fit a patient with lenses from one laboratory and after several weeks or months will feel that better results might be obtained with lenses from another laboratory. Whenever this situatuon occurs, you will be advised, and the fee structure will be adjusted to reflect any differences in costs.

If the fitting of your lenses is discontinued within the __ month fitting period, a refund of ___% of all contact lens material fees paid will be made upon return of all lenses. After the __ month fitting period, no refunds will be made.

We agree to fit _____ with contact lenses as per above, using _____ lenses, for a fee of $_____, the fitting period commencing on the day the contact lenses are dispensed. Contact lenses are not dispensed until payment is received in full.

During the fitting period, lost lenses will be replaced at a cost of $_____ per lens, damaged lenses at a cost of $_____ per lens, when the damaged lens is returned to this office, and additional lenses, if required, at $_____ per lens. These prices are subject to purchase of our in office contact lens service agreement.

I have read and understood the above agreement.

_____   _____
Patient   Witness

_____
Parent or guardian (if patient is under 18)

FIG. 43.1. Contact lens fitting agreement.

can provide significant benefits for the practitioner and the patient. They will serve as legal evidence of the agreements between the doctor and the patient should a dispute ever arise.

INFORMED CONSENT

"It is the patient's right to refuse or consent to a proposed medical procedure and the doctor's duty to provide suffi-cient information so that the patient can make the decision in an intelligent, knowledgeable manner." This doctrine, known as *informed consent,* applies to all aspects of patient care and to contact lens practice in particular (12–15).

Under the informed consent doctrine, the practitioner who fails to warn a first-time bifocal wearer of the danger of navigating a staircase may be liable if the patient falls and suffers an injury. A contact lens practitioner may be liable for failure to warn an extended wear patient of the possible problems associated with this procedure. It makes

The routine care and regular maintenance of your contact lenses is very important to your continuing contact lens success. Even with proper care, changes of your lenses and eyes can occur gradually. Routine care for your eyes should include a complete eye examination each year and one or more doctor office visits for lens inspection and cleaning. It has been found that patients who are properly fit initially, and who regularly maintain their contact lenses and eye health, are those who enjoy their contact lenses the best.

In order to care properly for your contact lenses and eye health, we offer four contact lens service agreements (CLSA). We recommend that you choose the one that suits you best.

Our CLSA offers	CLSA-1	CLSA-2	No CLSA (Approx. fees)
1) Contact lens inspection, cleaning and polishing	no charge	no charge	$20 per visit
2) Contact lens modification	no charge	no charge	$20 per visit
3) Contact lens office visits 1 daily; 3 extended	no charge	no charge	$25 per visit
4) Complete eye examination	no charge	$70	$70
5) Reduced fee for contact lens replacements	_____	_____	_____
Yearly fee for CLSA	$85	$28	
The yearly fee for CLSA for extended wear lenses	$110	$75	

The CLSA-1 is an annual service agreement which offers contact lens professional service plus your yearly comprehensive eye examination and replacement lenses at a reduced fee. The cost is $85 per year.

The CLSA-2 is an annual service agreement designed to provide contact lens professional service and lens replacement at a reduced fee, excluding the comprehensive eye examination. The cost is $28 per year.

CLSA 1 & 2 are also offered for extended wear patients. The cost is slightly higher because it is imperative that the ocular health and contact lenses themselves are inspected more regularly to insure successful wear.

PATIENT:_____   DATE:_____

OFFICE REPRESENTATIVE:_____

FIG. 43.2. Contact lens service agreement.

no difference that the procedure was clinically sound; the failure to warn is sufficient to create liability (12).

The contact lens practitioner should take the time to obtain an informed consent for three reasons. First, the patient will be better educated and less likely to be displeased with the course of treatment because of unrealistic expectations. Second, the doctor will comply with state law requiring that the patient be given the information necessary for an informed consent. Third, the doctor will be better able to mount a legal defense to malpractice charges, if necessary.

The informed consent doctrine almost always applies to the contact lens practitioner. However, practitioners do not always abide by its rules, with potentially disastrous consequences. It is the purpose of this section to explain the informed consent doctrine—including its origins and modern-day application—so that the contact lens practitioner can avoid its possible pitfalls (12).

Origins

The law of informed consent has its origins in the common law intentional tort of battery, which is legally defined as a "harmful or offensive touching" (16). The courts considered touching a person without his or her consent a legal wrong for which damages could be awarded. With certain exceptions, this rule applies to the doctor–patient relationship. Although informed consent traditionally was applied to medical doctors, today it is applicable to all health care practitioners, including contact lens practitioners. This should not be surprising because contact lens practitioners frequently touch their patients and, like surgeons, may actually alter the body tissues. Early consent cases usually were concerned with whether the patient gave express consent to a medical procedure rather than whether the consent was informed. As the consent doctrine evolved, the courts put greater emphasis on whether the doctor was negligent in informing the patient as to the risks and consequences of a given procedure. The burden was placed on the doctor to disclose enough information for the patient to make an "informed consent."

Modern Case Law

There is no "bright line" demarcating what the doctor must tell the patient, but two standards have evolved as to what will be considered an adequate disclose (17). Under the earlier "subjective" standard, the doctor was not negligent if he or she disclosed the information that an average "reasonable practitioner" would have disclosed (18). The problem with this rule was that a patient was not protected if an entire profession was routinely failing to disclose sufficient information to allow a patient to make an informed decision. The subjective standard currently is followed in only a few states.

The modern rule is the "patient-based" or "objective" standard under which the doctor must disclose enough information for the "reasonable patient" to decide whether to undergo a procedure (19). This rule is based on the belief that "respect for the patient's right of self-determination on particular therapy demands a standard set by law for physicians rather then one which physicians may or may not impose upon themselves" (19). It reflects a modern-day distrust of institutional control over the ultimate decisions affecting the patient. The rule helps the litigating patient because expert testimony is not necessary to establish the

prevailing community standard of care or to show that the patient would not have undergone treatment had an adequate disclosure been made.

Some California cases have adopted a mixed standard under which an informed consent disclosure must meet both the subjective and objective standards (20,21). Under this line of reasoning, a practitioner could be held liable for failure to disclose information that either professional practice or reasonable patient needs would deem material to an informed consent.

Informed Consent as Applied in the Eye Care Setting

Gates v Jensen (22) illustrates the modern trend in the law of informed consent as applied in a case involving an eye care professional. In *Gates v Jensen,* an ophthalmologist determined that the 54-year-old Mrs. Gates had intraocular pressures of 23.8 mm Hg by Schiotz tonometry. The doctor performed undilated ophthalmoscopy using a direct ophthalmoscope and found no abnormality. No other tests were performed.

Mrs. Gates inquired about the intraocular pressure test, and the doctor responded that he had tested for glaucoma and had found none. The doctor diagnosed that her visual problems were caused by her contact lenses and treated her accordingly. Mrs. Gates visited the doctor 12 more times in the next year, complaining of blurred and foggy vision and reduced visual acuity. The doctor tested her intraocular pressures during the first of three visits and found them to be in the high end of the normal range.

The Supreme Court of the State of Washington held that the informed consent doctrine required the doctor to advise Mrs. Gates that her intraocular pressures were borderline high and that additional diagnostic procedures, namely, dilated ophthalmoscopy and a visual field test, were available to determine whether or not she had glaucoma. The court stated the following:

> Important decisions must frequently be made in many non-treatment situations in which medical care is given, including procedures leading to a diagnosis, as in this case. These decisions must all be taken with the full knowledge and participation of the patient. The physician's duty is to tell the patient what he or she needs to know in order to make them. (22)

The court agreed with Mrs. Gates' contention that had she been given the necessary information, she might have undergone additional testing and may have saved her sight.

The court also found that although the doctor apparently had "complied with the applicable professional standard of care by examining Mrs. Gates' optic nerve discs with a direct ophthalmoscope, . . . where the risk of glaucoma was high and the pressure tests arguably inclusive, . . . reasonable prudence may require a higher standard of care applies" (22). Thus, as the Gates case held, the practitioner cannot rely on an existing professional standard as a shield against liability for negligence and presumably cannot rely on an existing professional standard of disclosure in meeting the informed consent requirement.

Disclosure of Practitioner-Specific Information

Recent cases have addressed the duty to disclose practitioner-specific information as part of informed consent. In *Johnson v Kokemoor* (23), a patient sued her surgeon following brain aneurysm surgery that resulted in partial quadriplegia. In addition to alleging failure to disclose the specific risks of the procedure, the patient alleged that the surgeon failed to reveal his relative inexperience in performing the procedure. The Supreme Court of the State of Wisconsin in effect held that the patient could proceed with litigation based on the doctor's failure to provide for adequate informed consent. The court found that a doctor's own experience level in performing a particular procedure, as well as success rates when the procedure was performed by doctors with more experience, were relevant to an adequate informed consent agreement. In addition, the court found that the surgeon's failure to refer the patient to a more experienced physician was potentially actionable.

Similarly, in *Hidding v Williams* (24), the Louisiana Court of Appeals held that a doctor's failure to disclose his history of alcoholism had negated a patient's consent to a medical procedure that was performed unsuccessfully, even though there was no evidence of a connection between the doctor's alcoholism and the patient's injury. *Moore v Regents of the University of California* involved a physician who stood to potentially profit from the removal of a patient's spleen and body tissues by using them in pursuit of a commercial patent (25). The California Supreme Court ruled that an informed consent cause of action was created by the doctors' failure to inform his patient of research and economic interests that could affect his medical judgment.

These cases indicate that in some jurisdictions, it may be necessary for the doctor to disclose particular information about himself or herself as part of the informed consent procedure. Potentially relevant information could include the doctor's own medical history, lack of experience in the procedure, or possible financial benefit from the patient's willingness to undergo the procedure

In *Arato v Avedon* (26), the California Supreme Court took a more restrained approach as to the necessity of disclosing specific information as part of an informed consent procedure. In *Arato,* the family of a pancreatic cancer victim claimed that the doctor failed in his informed consent duty by not disclosing specific information such as the patient's statistical life expectancy. The family argued that the patient would have spent his final days with friends and family rather than undergoing a painful medical procedure. Citing the unreliability of statistical information in the context of

individual cases, the court held that as a matter of law, a physician was not required to disclose medical information such as mortality rates that might be material to a patient's nonmedical needs; however, the materiality of life expectancy information was deemed an appropriate issue for a jury to decide.

In *Kaskie v Wright* (27), the Pennsylvania Superior Court rejected the proposition that personal information about the treating doctor was relevant to informed consent, holding that disclosure should be restricted to medical information specifically related to the proposed treatment. Similarly, the Georgia Supreme Court recently held that it was not necessary for a practitioner to disclose life factors such as drug use "which might be subjectively considered to adversely affect the professional's performance" unless specifically asked to do so by the patient (28).

These cases indicate that the law is as yet unsettled as to what types of information must be included in an adequate informed consent procedure. This situation probably is to be expected, given the inherent difficulty of creating a coherent doctrine from cases with unique fact patterns occurring in many different legal jurisdictions. As one author recommended: " . . . [C]linicians are probably best advised to fall back on the spirit of the informed consent doctrine for guidance. Sufficient information should be disclosed to provide a patient with a genuine opportunity to consider risks and benefits and to participate fully in the selection among appropriate options" (29).

Informed Consent and Malpractice

It should be pointed out that although an action for negligent nondisclosure under the informed consent doctrine is similar to one for malpractice, the two actually are different and usually will be pleaded as separate counts within a single complaint. In some circumstances, a practitioner might be liable for failure to disclose but not liable for malpractice. A properly fitted and instructed contact lens patient who loses vision due to a corneal ulcer might lose a malpractice action but prevail on a negligent nondisclosure action under the theory that he or she would not have opted for contact lenses if informed of the risk of ulcers.

State Laws

The law governing informed consent in a particular state will be found in either the court opinions or the statutes of that state. Although other state courts may choose to follow the precedent of cases such as *Gates v Jensen,* they are not obligated to do so. Some states have enacted statutes that deal specifically with informed consent, whereas others are parts of larger, comprehensive malpractice reform acts or state medical practice acts (30,31). In general, the law of an individual state will be based on either the "professional community" or "reasonable patient" standard (32).

State Medical Acts frequently contain language requiring that physicians disclose information necessary for a valid informed consent, but these generally do not apply to other contact lens practitioners. For example, Wisconsin Statute Sec. 448.30 states the following:

Any physician who treats a patient shall inform the patient about the availability of all alternate, viable medical modes of treatment and about the benefits and risks of these treatments. The physician's duty to inform the patient under this section does not require disclosure of

1. Information beyond what a reasonably well-qualified physician in a similar medical classification would know
2. Detailed technical information that in all probability a patient would not understand
3. Risks apparent or known to the patient
4. Extremely remote possibilities that might falsely or detrimentally alarm the patient
5. Information in emergencies where failure to provide treatment would be more harmful to the patient than treatment
6. Information in cases where the patient is incapable of consenting

Informed consent concerns, however, caused the State Optometry Examining Board of Wisconsin in 1985 to promulgate an emergency administrative rule requiring disclosure of potential problems related to extended wear contact lenses. This rule, now adopted as Wisconsin Administrative Code Sec. Opt. 5.14, requires an optometrist to provide the extended wear contact lens patient with a written disclosure form that warns of possible side effects. A copy of the original required form is reproduced in Figure 43.3.

The disclosure must indicate that a regular schedule of cleaning and disinfection is necessary and provide a recommended schedule of follow-up appointments for evaluation and adaptation to contact lens wear. Business items such as service agreements, warranties, refunds, and information about replacement lenses are not permitted on the disclosure form; neither are instructions regarding proper solutions or lens care. The disclosure must be signed by the patient or the patient's guardian prior to the patient's receipt of the lenses, and a copy of the signed disclosure must be placed in the patient's file.

In other states with less specific regulations, some general rules have evolved. The courts at various times have determined that a health care practitioner must discuss the following items before a patient can give a valid informed consent (29,33):

1. Diagnosis
2. Nature, purpose, and benefits of treatment
3. Risk, consequences, and side effects of treatment
4. Feasible alternative treatments
5. Probability of success
6. Prognosis in the absence of treatment

The relative importance of these items depends upon the procedure involved. For a nontherapeutic contact lens fitting, a discussion of the diagnosis, nature of treatment, probability of success, and prognosis in absence of treatment is a relatively straightforward affair, and none of these items is a likely source of informed consent liability. However, the risk, consequences, and side effects are of major concern. A discussion of feasible alternatives will often be important, especially when fitting extended wear contact lenses, because daily wear lenses are a less risky alternative (15).

There is no set rule as to which risks must be disclosed, but it often is beneficial to look at the seriousness of a risk and the probability of its occurrence. An important risk with serious consequences should be disclosed, e.g., the risk of *Acanthamoeba* keratitis to a patient making homemade saline (15). Less common risks also should be disclosed, both to minimize the possibility of lawsuits and to ensure that the patient has realistic expectations about the eventual course of treatment. A patient who suffers a temporary red eye condition due to initial overwear of a contact lens may not sue, but he or she will not likely return or refer new patients.

Third Parties

The doctor may be liable to third parties with whom he or she has no special relationship and whom he or she has never met. For example, a pedestrian who is injured by an inadequately informed monovision contact lens wearer driving with compromised vision may sue the contact lens fitter. If the patient has no liability insurance, the doctor and malpractice carrier offer a convenient "deep-pocket" target for the injured third party.

Elements of Claim

A patient who brings an informed consent suit must prove that the doctor failed to adequately inform him or her about the risks and benefits of the treatment, that he or she was unaware of these risks and benefits, and that he or she suffered damages because of the treatment. The doctor in turn may offer defenses showing why informed consent was unnecessary. The courts generally have recognized that informed consent need not be given in the following situations (34,35):

1. The risk is too commonly known to warrant disclosure or the patient already had sufficient knowledge of the risk
2. The patient assured the doctor that he or she did not want to be warned of the risks, or that he or she would undergo the procedure regardless of the risks (waiver exception)
3. Consent by or on behalf of the patient was not reasonably possible (e.g., an ocular emergency or patient incompetence in the absence of a legal guardianship)

```
        Wisconsin Administrative Code sec. Opt 6.14 requires that this disclosure
be provided by optometrists to patients receiving contact lenses for use on an
extended wear basis.  This statement must be signed by the patient (or his or
her guardian) prior to receipt of extended wear lenses.

        As with any other drug or device, the use of extended wear contact lenses
is not without risk.  A small, but significant, percentage of individuals
wearing extended wear lenses develop potentially serious complications which
can lead to permanent eye damage.

        If you have any unexplained
• Eye pain or redness
• Watering of the eye or discharge
• Cloudy or foggy vision
• Decrease in vision, or
• Sensitivity to light

Remove your lenses and make arrangements to see your eye care professional
before wearing your lenses again.

        Regular inspection by a licensed eye care professional is important to
evaluate your eyes' tolerance to extended wear lenses.  Your apointment
schedule for follow-up care is:


_____

_____

_____

_____


It is important to the health of your eyes that you carefully follow the
schedule recommended by your optometrist for cleaning and disinfecting your
lenses.

        By my signature, I acknowledge that 1 have received a copy of this
document.



_____
Patient (or Guardian)



_____
Date
```

FIG. 43.3. Wisconsin extended wear disclosure form.

4. The doctor reasonably believed that full disclosure would substantially affect the patient in an adverse way and so used reasonable discretion in limiting the manner and extent of disclosure (therapeutic privilege)
5. Treatment legally compelled by court order (compulsory treatment exception)

With limited exceptions, a valid informed consent can only be given by an adult who is competent to understand the proposed treatment and its risks and benefits. If the patient is a minor (usually defined by state law as someone less than 18 years of age), a parent or the minor's court-appointed guardian normally must give the informed consent, although some jurisdictions recognize an exception for treatment of mental illness, substance abuse, venereal disease, or pregnancy, issues that are usually not relevant in the contact lens setting (36). In an emergency, an informed consent need not be obtained if a parent or guardian cannot be contacted. A minor may give a valid informed consent if he or she is "emancipated," a legal condition usually requiring that the minor be married or that the parents have voluntarily relinquished control (37,38).

If the patient is a legally incompetent adult, the legal guardian must obtain an informed consent unless emergency treatment is involved. Examples of legal incompetency in an informed consent procedure include (i) inability to render a decision, (ii) inability to understand the informed consent disclosures, (iii) inability to understand the nature and consequences of the treatment options, and (iv) inability to engage in a proper decision-making process (36). If the patient giving the consent is under the influence of alcohol or another intoxicant, the prudent course is to delay treatment until the person can competently give consent. Regardless of who gives it, an informed consent is invalid if the proposed treatment is illegal or contrary to public policy.

Informed Consent Documentation

Although there is no legal requirement that an informed consent be in written or taped form, it is in the doctor's interest to have a permanent record of the consent (39,40), otherwise the patient's word will be weighed against the doctor's word, and juries often are inclined to favor a sympathetic injured patient over a seemingly wealthy doctor and his or her insurance company.

A written or taped record also serves to emphasize the importance of the doctor's warnings to the patient. Studies have shown that patients often remember only a small percentage of what the doctor tells them (41,42). Likewise, the doctor's recall of what was said may be be faulty. A written record prevents this difficulty.

Printed forms probably the most common means of documenting warnings. However, printed forms are not conclusive proof of an informed consent, because the patient can always assert that the warning was not explained in a manner that engendered true understanding.

Some clinicians and investigators have used video presentations and videotaping as means to present information and to document the obtaining of an informed consent (40). Because some patients may have difficulty reading and understanding a printed form due to limited education or visual impairment, there are some advantages to using video documentation (39). The doctor should be sure to obtain the patient's permission for taping, either in writing or on the tape itself.

The consent form should be written in plain language and free of optometric terminology (e.g., you should tell the monovision patient that "you may have trouble judging how far apart things are" rather than "your stereoacuity may be reduced"). The consent language cannot be too broad. It should be limited to matters pertinent to the proposed treatment. It should not include clauses in which the patient appears to waive legal rights. It should avoid exculpatory language and other legal "boilerplate" that appear to relieve the doctor of liability. They have little or no legal effect and may bias a jury against the doctor.

The patient should be asked whether he or she understands everything that was discussed and whether he or she has any questions. The patient's permanent record should document this discussion. If written, the informed consent should be signed by the patient. A written record need not be witnessed, but it should be stored in a safe place until the applicable statute of limitations expires.

Application to Contact Lens Practice

There have been few, if any, published informed consent opinions involving contact lens practice. Nevertheless, the contact lens field historically has provided fertile ground for malpractice lawsuits, and the contact lens practitioner should be familiar with the rules governing informed consent.

Prefitting Evaluation

During the prefitting evaluation, the doctor must perform a comprehensive case history and discuss with the patient the general risks and benefits of contact lenses. The doctor also must discuss the possible alternatives and their likely prognosis. If the patient's chances of success are remote, the patient must be so advised so that he or she can intelligently decide whether to proceed with the contact lens fitting. The practitioner should document the discussion in the patient's record as previously indicated.

Based on the *Gates* case, the practitioner has a legal obligation to advise a patient of prefitting borderline findings even before contact lenses are placed on the patient's eyes. If any abnormalities or questionable results are discovered, the optometrist should advise the patient of the findings and their possible implications. The practitioner also should advise the patient of possible additional testing that could be used to rule out or confirm the tentative diagnosis.

Daily Wear Lenses

The patient interested in daily wear contact lenses should be advised of the relative advantages and disadvantages of soft and rigid contact lenses based on the patient's own individual situation. The prudent practitioner will consider the patient's vocation, avocation, refractive error, keratometer readings, and ocular health in determining the appropriate lens type. If several lens types seem appropriate, the patient should be so advised so that he or she and the practitioner can decide which of these options best suits the patient's needs. Figure 43.4 shows an example of a daily wear contact lens information and informed consent document.

Extended Wear Lenses

In no aspect of optometric practice is informed consent more important than in the fitting of extended wear contact lenses. Studies have shown that the possibilities of corneal infections and corneal ulcers are significantly greater in extended wear patients than in daily wear patients (43–45). Other corneal complications also are more likely when lenses are worn on a 24-hour-a-day basis (46–48).

The practitioner must thoroughly advise the patient of these potential risks prior to fitting extended wear lenses. The patient should be advised that the actual period of wear

---

UNIVERSITY OF CALIFORNIA
School of Optometry

Contact Lens Services, Meredith W. Morgan University Eye Center, Berkeley, CA 94720-2020
(510) 642-2020

Contact Lens Services, Tang Center Eye Clinic, Berkeley, CA 94720-2020
(510) 643-2020

www.caleyecare.org

Contact Lens Services
Information and Policy

March 2000 ©

INFORMATION ON CONTACT LENS SERVICES

The University of California School of Optometry provides contact lens services for University students, faculty, employees, and the general public. Our primary emphasis is proper patient care and instruction. *All services are provided by optometry students under the supervision of the attending clinical faculty.*

The School provides two categories of contact lens services: (1) Examinations and fitting services, and (2) Extended care services for patients currently wearing contact lenses.

1. **Examination and Fitting Services**
   A. *Patient Eligibility:* The patient must have had a primary care eye examination within one year prior to obtaining a contact lens examination and fitting. This eye examination can be performed in our Eye Center as part of the contact lens fitting or by an outside eye doctor.
   B. *Services included in the examination and fitting:* A contact lens examination and evaluation will be performed by an optometry student clinician at the time of the first appointment in the Eye Center. Final acceptance as a patient will depend upon the results of this examination. If contact lenses are advisable, tentative lenses will be prescribed and ordered upon the payment of the necessary fee. After the patient's response to the contact lenses has been properly evaluated, the lens prescription will be finalized. If either the attending doctor or the patient decides that the fitting should not be completed, a portion of the fee may be refunded. The following services specific to a contact lens evaluation and fitting are included in the contact lens examination:
      1. Consultation and history
      2. Refraction and vision analysis
      3. Examination for ocular disease or abnormalities
      4. Measurement of eye dimensions
      5. Prediction of lens type and dimensions
      6. Diagnostic lens fitting
      7. Design of lenses
      8. Tentative prognosis
      9. Prescribing and ordering of appropriate tentative lenses
      10. Dispensing and evaluation of tentative lenses
      11. Instructions in lens care and handling
      12. Initial supply of contact lens care products
      13. Evaluation of patient response
      14. Follow-up visits for a period not exceeding 3-6 months
      15. Necessary lens changes in the 3-6 month fitting period
      16. Final contact lenses.

   C. *Fitting Schedule:* Contact lenses are fitted throughout the year. The examination takes about 1-1/2 to 2 hours. Subsequent visits may be scheduled for the same day of the week as the original appointment. The time required for these subsequent visits is from 1/2 to 1-1/2 hours. A minimum of 3 follow-up visits are usually required over a 3 month period. Because of the thoroughness of our examination and fitting process, the time involved until dismissal may be longer than that encountered in some private practices.
   D. *Request for Fitting:* Persons who want to be fitted with contact lenses can make an appointment at the University Eye Center Appointment Desk [(510)642-2020] or the Tang Center [(510)643-2020] in person or by telephone. Patient scheduling will be based upon the nature of the patient's visual needs. Patients are generally scheduled within 1 - 2 weeks for an appointment.

2. **Extended Care Services**
   A. *Patient eligibility:* Extended care services are available for patients fitted at the Eye Center who have passed the 3-6 month fitting period and for patients fitted elsewhere. To be eligible for extended care contact lens services, the patient should have (1) had a primary care eye examination within the past year, and (2) adequate contact lens examination and fitting information on file at the Eye Center. Patients fitted elsewhere should have a referral report sent to the Eye Center by the original practitioner or have a primary care eye examination and a contact lens evaluation at the Eye Center. Referral report forms are available at the Appointment Desk. Emergency services are available without referral reports.
   B. *Extended Care Services Available:*
      1. Examination and evaluation of contact lens patients
      2. Post-fitting examinations and evaluation
      3. Replacement of current contact lens (may be ordered by mail, phone, fax, etc.) Applies only to patients examined at the University Eye Center within the past year who have a successful response to their current contact lenses. Some patients may need to be examined before lenses are ordered. The lens replacement fee includes the required dispensing appointment and one follow-up appointment but does not include the examination or fitting if needed.
      4. Lens adjustments, refinishing, repolishing, inspection, cleaning
      5. Prescription changes (for patients examined at the Eye Center)
      6. Contact lens refitting

FIG. 43.4. Daily wear contact lens information and informed consent document.

7. Advice and instruction
8. Additional examination and fitting procedures.
9. Emergency Services

C. *Fees:* $25 to $52 per examination (depending on services required). An additional charge will be made for any special services or materials required. Fees must be paid at the time of the visit and before any materials are ordered.

D. *Appointments:* Appointments are available throughout the year. They can be made in person at the Appointment Desk, by calling the University Eye Center at (510) 642-2020, or the Tang Center at 643-2020.

3. **Additional Information**
A. *Parking:* Parking is available on-campus with shuttle service to the University Eye Center. Street parking is available at the Tang Center.
B. *Vision Care Plans:* Many vision care plans and insurance programs provide partial coverage for contact lens services. Contact your individual plan for information.
C. *Contact Lens Prescriptions:* A contact lens prescription can be released only to patients we have fitted after the contact lens examination and fitting have been completed and the patient is wearing contact lenses successfully. Patients who have not been examined in the Eye Center within the past six months may need to be re-examined before a contact lens prescription can be released.

4. **Policy**
The fee for the contact lens examination and fitting depends on the nature of the patient's visual needs and the type of lenses ordered The exact fee will be quoted before lenses are ordered. The contact lens examination and fitting fees generally range from $150 - $340, similar to or lower than those encountered in private practice for similar services and materials. Fees may be higher for specialty fittings and lenses. Payment will be expected on the day of the first appointment. If lenses are not prescribed, there is a $52 fee for the examination and evaluation. Additional fees are charged for duplicate or replacement contact lenses and other supplies or services. Fees must be paid in full prior to the ordering of any materials. The $52 evaluation and examination fee is non-refundable.

Most patients are able to wear contact lenses successfully; however, a successful fit cannot be guaranteed. Those who are not successful with the initial pair of lenses ordered may be refitted with additional lenses. Additional fees will apply if additional services or more expensive lenses are needed. Patients who cannot be fitted successfully may be eligible for a partial refund.

If contact lens wear is discontinued for any reason within the initial 60 day fitting period, the refund will not exceed 50% of material and fitting fees. Any refund will be reduced by the cost of additional materials used in an attempt to complete the fitting. No refund is available after the initial 60 day fitting period has ended.

PATIENT INFORMED CONSENT

I am requesting contact lens services at the University of California Berkeley School of Optometry. These services may include a primary care examination, a contact lens examination, evaluation and fitting, and/or extended care services. I will be able to ask any questions I have about the Eye Center's policies and contact lenses prior to the ordering of the lenses. I give my permission to the School of Optometry to perform all the tests involved in a primary care eye examination, a contact lens examination, evaluation and fitting, and/or extended care services. I understand that contact lenses have many benefits, but as with any other drug or device, they are not without possible risks. A small percentage (less than 1%) of wearers develop potentially serious complications which can lead to permanent eye damage and vision loss.

I agree to follow the advice and instructions given to me by the Eye Center. I will remove my lenses and seek care immediately from the Eye Center, an eye doctor, or a hospital emergency room if I experience any unexplained eye pain, redness, discharge or vision change.

I have read and received a copy of the Information on Contact Lens Services. I understand the current policies,

Signed _____
(Patient)

Signed _____ : Date _____
(Parent or guardian if patient is a minor)

FIG. 43.4. *Continued.*

may be significantly less than the wearing period approved by the US Food and Drug Administration (FDA) for that particular lens. Furthermore, the patient must be informed of the necessity or regular follow-up evaluations. The doctor should emphasize the importance of proper cleaning and disinfection when the lenses are removed and the possibility of frequent lens replacement. Only when the patient has this vital information can he or she give informed consent to be fitted with extended wear contact lenses.

Failure to give this information and obtain an informed consent resulted in one of the most publicized suits in contact lens practice (1).

A 15-year-old Wisconsin boy had been fitted with extended wear lens at an optical outlet without parental permission. Because the patient was a minor and could not legally give informed consent, it was the responsibility of the practitioner to obtain an informed consent from a parent or legal guardian. Within 1 week of receiving and wearing the lenses, the youngster developed a corneal ulcer that led to severe loss of vision in one eye. He and his parents sued the optical outlet, claiming the lenses had been sold to him without his parents' consent and without any warning as to the risks inherent in extended wear contact lenses. The family sought $5.3 million in damages.

Disposable and Frequent-Replacement Lenses

Patients interested in single-use disposable lenses should be advised in the same manner as patients wearing standard daily wear lenses, in addition to the advantages and disadvantages of this particular modality. The practitioner should advise the patient that the lenses are approved only for a single use, and that the lenses should not be cleaned, disinfected, stored overnight, and reused. Recommending reuse of such lenses in contradiction of their FDA-approved use could be considered evidence of *"negligence per se,"* under which the violation of a statute, rule, or regulation itself can be considered to constitute negligence (see section of Malpractice).

Patients interested in frequent-replacement lenses should be advised of the risks and benefits of standard daily wear lenses or extended wear lenses, depending upon whether the lenses will be removed each day or worn overnight. In addition, the practitioner should discuss the advantages and disadvantages of replacing the lenses on a more frequent basis. The patient should be advised that the lenses must be replaced at the recommended time. Recommending that such lenses be kept for a longer period than specified in the packaging instructions could be considered evidence of negligence *per se* on the part of the practitioner.

Therapeutic Lenses

The need for informed consent is apparent when fitting a patient with therapeutic contact lenses. Keratoconics,

aphakes, and others with corneal pathology generally have compromised corneas and need to be thoroughly advised as to the risks and benefits of contact lenses, as well as the alternatives to contact lens therapy.

A keratoconic patient should be advised of the potential adverse effects of contact lenses. He or she also should be told of the possible vision problems with spectacles. Many contact lens specialists believe that keratoconic patients should not be fitted with contact lenses until the vision has deteriorated with spectacle correction to a point that it is unsatisfactory for the patient, or until the cornea has undergone significant corneal thinning and protrusion to necessitate the fitting of a contact lens. Such patients should be advised of the potential for a corneal transplant and the ramifications if a transplant is necessary.

Patients with corneal pathologies, such as bullous keratopathy and recurrent corneal erosion, often obtain improved vision and comfort with therapeutic soft contact lenses. Before such lenses are fitted, however, the patient needs to be advised of the possibility of adverse effects and what to do if such effects do occur.

Specialty Lenses

Specialty contact lens fitting provide another area where informed consent can play an important role. Presbyopes seeking a contact lens correction for their refractive condition must be counseled as to the risks and benefits of the various types of contact lenses suitable for their needs (15, 49). These include monovision, bifocal contact lenses, distance contact lenses and reading glasses, modified monovision correction, or bifocal spectacles.

Patients fitted with monovision or bifocal contact lenses need to be warned of the potential vision problems associated with wearing these lenses compared to spectacle bifocal correction. Because monovision and bifocal contact lens correction compromises binocular vision, patients need to be advised that depth perception and peripheral vision may be reduced. These types of vision reductions can be especially dangerous when driving or operating industrial equipment where acute binocular vision is important.

Before dispensing a monovision or bifocal contact lens correction to a patient, the prudent practitioner should allow the patient to wear the lenses in the controlled environment of the doctor's office to determine how well the patient responds to this vision correction. Any significant adverse response would indicate that the patient is not as appropriate candidate for monovision contact lenses.

When fitting toric and bitoric lenses, the practitioner should advise the patient of the additional cost and time involved with these types of correction. The patient needs to know what alternatives are available so that he or she can help choose the appropriate lens modality.

Tinted contact lenses pose another area of concern, especially where the color portion of the lens covers the pupil.

These lenses can cause a decrease in night vision, thus affecting the patient's ability to drive and walk safely. Patients fitted with such lenses need to be advised of this problem so that they can choose whether to wear lenses under dark illumination conditions.

Investigational Lenses

Many practitioners are active investigators for contact lens companies. It is imperative that the lenses being fitted are FDA investigational lenses and that the practitioner is a registered clinical investigator for that lens type. When fitting FDA investigational lenses, the practitioner must follow certain guidelines to ensure that the patient has given proper informed consent.

The Department of Health and Human Services has issued regulations outlining the informed consent requirement for clinical investigators. These regulations, known as the *Common Rule,* are followed by nearly all federal agencies funding research and must be provided to either the subject or the subject's legally authorized representative. The elements of this informed consent are as follows (50):

1. A statement that the study involves research, an explanation of the purposes of the research and the expected duration of the subject's participation, a description of the procedures to be followed, and identification of any procedures which are experimental
2. A description of any reasonably foreseeable risks or discomforts to the subject
3. A description of any benefits to the subject or to others that may reasonably be expected from the research
4. A disclosure of appropriate alternative procedures or courses of treatment, if any, that might be advantageous to the subject
5. A statement describing the extent, if any, to which confidentiality of records identifying the subject will be maintained
6. For research involving more than minimal risk, an explanation as to whether any compensation and an explanation as to whether any medical treatments are available if injury occurs and, if so, what they consist of, or where further information may be obtained
7. An explanation of whom to contact for answers to pertinent questions about the research and research subjects' rights, and whom to contact in the event of a research-related injury to the subject, and
8. A statement that participation is voluntary, refusal to participate will involve no penalty or loss of benefits to which the subject is otherwise entitled, and the subject may discontinue participation at any time without penalty or loss of benefits to which the subject is otherwise entitled

These regulations also provide that, when appropriate, one or more of the following elements of information shall be provided to each subject:

1. A statement that the particular treatment or procedure may involve risks to the subject (or to the embryo or fetus, if the subject is or may become pregnant) that are currently unforeseeable
2. Anticipated circumstances under which the subject's participation may be terminated by the investigator without regard to the subject's consent
3. Any additional costs to the subject that may result from participation in the research
4. The consequences of a subject's decision to withdraw from the research and procedures for orderly termination of participation by the subject
5. A statement that significant new findings developed during the course of the research that may relate to the subject's willingness to continue participation will be provided to the subject, and
6. The approximate number of subjects involved in the study

An Institutional Review Board (IRB) may change or waive the above informed consent requirements if it finds and documents that

1. The research involves no more than minimal risk to the subjects
2. The waiver or alteration will not adversely affect the rights and welfare of the subjects
3. The research could not practically be carried out without the waiver or alteration, and
4. Whenever appropriate, the subjects will be provided with additional pertinent information after participation

The informed consent must be in writing and signed by the patient or the patient's legally authorized representative (51).

It must be remembered that the agreement with the patient cannot contain exculpatory language in which the patient waives legal rights for recourse against the doctor. Furthermore, it is important that the practitioner follow the protocol approved for these lenses. Proper follow-up care is important. Proper record-keeping procedures should be followed, including documentation in the patient's record and a report of findings to the manufacturer.

Solutions and Lens Care

The practitioner must be aware of the patient's allergies and sensitivities, as well as previous problems with particular solutions. Only by knowing this information and advising the patient adequately can the practitioner choose appropriate FDA-approved contact lens solutions and procedures. The doctor should advise the patient orally and in writing about proper lens care and handling. It is best if both the practitioner and the patient sign a form indicating what solutions, procedures, and instructions have been given. One copy of this form should be retained in the patient's record; the other should be given to the patient.

If the practitioner uses special in-office procedures to clean or disinfect the lenses, the patient should be advised as to the nature of these procedures and their possible adverse effects. The practitioner should utilize these procedures only with the patient's informed consent.

All practitioners should be cautious about using or recommending any unusual or unapproved lens care solutions or procedures. Recommending such procedures leaves the practitioner vulnerable to a malpractice suit should the patient suffer any discomfort or harm to the eye or lenses. Investigators for solution manufacturers should use the same informed consent guidelines that are recommended for contact lens investigators when providing patients with investigational solutions.

Follow-Up Care

All contact lens patients should be advised of the need for regular and routine follow-up care. The practitioner has a duty to the patient to provide a reasonable wearing schedule and adequate follow-up examinations to ensure that the patient has been informed of this necessity and has given consent to routine and regular follow-up care should the practitioner proceed with a contact lens fitting.

Conclusion

The legal doctrine of informed consent is extremely important in contact lens practice, but unfortunately, many practitioners overlook it. Such oversights can be detrimental to both the patient and the practitioner. The procedures for informed consent are straightforward and relatively simple to apply. When the practitioner has the patient's best interest in mind, informed consent is a natural part of contact lens practice. Only by careful attention to the requirements of informed consent can a practitioner provide the patient with the information needed to make an intelligent decision about being fitted with contact lenses. Failure to comply with informed consent requirements will undoubtedly be a major source of culpability for contact lens practitioners in the future.

RELEASE OF CONTACT LENS PRESCRIPTIONS

Federal Requirements

Until recently, practitioners who fit patients with contact lenses faced a difficult clinical and legal issue regarding con-

tact lens prescription release (52,53). A ruling of the Federal Trade Commission (FTC), popularly referred to as the "Eyeglasses I" rule (54), required practitioners to give patients a copy of the spectacle prescription at the conclusion of the examination. This prescription release requirement was generally reaffirmed by the FTC in "Eyeglasses II," and in its 1997 "Spectacle Prescription Release Rule" (54), which clarified that the requirement was not applicable to contact lens prescriptions. Thus, under these prior FTC rules, contact lens patients were entitled only to spectacle refractive data; contact lens parameters did not have to be included unless required by state law (Table 43.1) (55). However, the Federal Fairness to Contact Lens Consumers Act (FCLCA) of 2003 mandates new rules for the release of contact lens prescription information nationwide (56).

The FCLCA requires the practitioner to provide the patient with a copy of the contact lens prescription at the completion of the contact lens fitting, whether or not requested to do so by the patient. For the purposes of the FCLCA, a contact lens fitting is defined as the process that begins with the initial eye examination and ends when a successful fit has been achieved; in the case of a renewal prescription, the fitting ends when the practitioner determines that no change in prescription is required. The practitioner may not charge the patient or require a release or waiver from the patient for providing a copy of the contact lens prescription. The patient cannot be required to purchases lenses from the practitioner or a third party as a condition of prescription release (56).

The FCLCA specifies a 1-year expiration date for contact lens prescriptions, unless state law provides for a longer expiration date. An expiration date shorter than 1 year is permitted if based on medical judgment regarding the ocular health of the patient. The reasons for the shorter expiration date must be documented in the patient's record (56).

The FCLCA provides that a contact lens seller cannot provide contact lenses to a patient unless the patient or prescriber presents the prescription or a facsimile of the prescription to the seller, or unless the prescription is verified by direct communication between the prescriber and seller. A prescription is considered verified if, after the seller communicates to the prescriber the prescription information, the prescriber (1) confirms that the prescription is accurate, (2) informs the seller that the prescription is inaccurate and provides the accurate prescription, or (3) fails to communicate with the seller within 8 business hours, or a similar time as defined by the Federal Trade Commission (56).

The FCLCA forbids a contact lens seller from making any changes to the prescription other than substituting identical lenses from the same manufacturer marketed under a different label (56). The FCLCA does not impose liability

TABLE 43.1. SPECIFIC STATE CONTACT LENS PRESCRIPTION REQUIREMENTS

Alabama: Information sufficient to order replacement lenses; reasonable expiration date.

Arizona: Lens brand name; type, tint, and all other specifications necessary to accurately dispense the prescription. One year or earlier expiration.

Arkansas: Rx written in accordance with state law and rules promulgated by State Board of Optometry. One year or earlier expiration.

California: Including, but not limited to, power, material or manufacturer or both, base curve or appropriate designation, diameter when appropriate, and appropriate expiration date.

Colorado: Patient's full name; the date; all usual and customary specifications; manufacturer's name and manufacturer's trade or brand name necessary for an exact replacement contact lens; the statement, "No Substitution Without Doctor Approval"; the doctor's signature, name, license number, address, and phone number; a reasonable limit on refills; a reasonable expiration date not to exceed 1 year.

Delaware: Lens curvature, diameter, power, material, manufacturer; an expiration date not to exceed 1 year; appropriate instructions for the care and handling of the lenses.

Florida: Sphere power; cylinder power, if necessary; cylinder axis, if necessary; range of specific contact lens type/brand; range of base curve, if not included in type/brand; range of diameter, if not included in type/brand; follow-up care requirements, if any. Two-year expiration.

Georgia: Name, address, and state licensure number of a prescribing practitioner; explicitly states an expiration date of not more than 12 months from the date of the last prescribing contact lens examination, unless a medical or refractive problem affecting vision requires an earlier expiration date; explicitly states the number of refills; explicitly states that it is for contact lenses and indicates the lens brand name and type, including all specifications necessary for the ordering or fabrication of lenses; and the information is kept on file by the person selling or dispensing the replacement contact lenses for at least 24 months after the prescription is filled; all parameters for fabrication of the lenses must be included.

Idaho: All prescriptions for rigid contact lenses must contain at least the following information: base curve; peripheral curve(s) including width; overall diameter; optical zone diameter; power; center thickness; color; expiration date of the prescription. All prescriptions for soft contact lenses must contain at least the following information: lens manufacturer or "brand" name; series or base curve; power; diameter, if applicable; color, if applicable; and expiration date of the prescription.

Illinois: "Contact lens prescription" means a written order bearing the original signature of a duly licensed optometrist or physician or an oral or electronic order issued directly by an optometrist or physician that authorizes the dispensing of contact lenses to a patient.

Indiana: All information required to properly duplicate the contact lenses, including an expiration date of not more than 1 year; number of refills permitted. Instructions for use must be consistent with recommendations of the contact lens manufacturer, clinical practice guidelines, and the professional judgment of the prescribing optometrist or physician.

Iowa: Date of issuance; name and address of patient for whom the contact lens is prescribed; name, address, and signature of the practitioner; all parameters required to duplicate properly the original contact lens; a specific date of expiration, not to exceed 18 months, the quantity of lenses allowed, and the number of refills allowed; at the option of the prescribing practitioner, the prescription may contain fitting and material guidelines and specific instructions for use by the patient.

Kansas: Rigid contact lens prescriptions shall include lens material, base curve, back vertex power, prism power, overall diameter, optic zone diameter, peripheral curve radii and widths, center thickness, tint, and edge shape. Flexible contact lens prescriptions shall include base curve; power; diameter, when necessary; manufacturer; water content, where necessary; type, spherical, toric, or extended wear; color; and manufacturer's suggested sterilization method. The following information shall be included on any prescription issued by a licensee for any ophthalmic lenses: printed name and license registration number of the prescribing licensee; address and telephone number at which the patient's records are maintained and at which the prescribing licensee can be reached for consultation; name of the patient; signature of the prescribing licensee; date the prescription was issued, date of the examination, and expiration date, if appropriate; any instructions necessary for the fabrication or use of the ophthalmic lenses; and any special instructions. Twelve-month or less expiration.

Kentucky: (a) The ophthalmic information necessary to accurately fabricate or dispense the lenses including the lens manufacturer, lens series, and the lens material if applicable; (b) Power and base curve; (c) Name, license number, telephone number, and for written orders, the signature of the prescribing optometrist, osteopath, or physician; (d) Patient's name and address, expiration date of the prescription, and number of refills or lenses permitted; and (e) The date of issuance. The prescription may also include the diameter, axis, add power, cylinder, peripheral curve, optical zone, and center thickness. Twelve-month or less expiration.

Louisiana: Information specifying the physical design, material type, curvatures, diameters, pertinent measurements, refractive power; expiration date not to exceed 18 months.

Maine: Prescription must contain all the information necessary to be properly dispensed and must specify whether it is for contact lenses or ophthalmic lenses. All prescriptions must include the name of the patient, date of prescription, name and office location of prescriber, and an expiration date. Contact lens prescription must contain an expiration date not to exceed 24 months from the date of issue; the prescription may contain fitting guidelines and may contain specific instructions for use by the patient.

Maryland: Including but not limited to the lens manufacturer, type of lens, power of the lens, base curve, lens size, name of the patient, date the prescription was given to the patient, name and office location of the licensed optometrist who writes the replacement contact lens prescription, and expiration date of the replacement contact lens prescription. Expiration date not to exceed 24 months from the time the patient was first examined.

Massachusetts: Prescription for rigid contact lenses at minimum must contain the name, office address, telephone number, and license number of the optometrist issuing the prescription; name of the patient; date on which the patient was examined; date of issuance of the prescription (if different) and the expiration date; power; diameter; optic zone diameter, if applicable; inside base curve radius; center thickness, if applicable; lens manufacturer and material, if applicable; tint and/or any other special design features, if applicable; and any applicable notations as to when the lenses are to be worn. A prescription for soft contact lenses at minimum must contain the name, office address, telephone number, and license number of the optometrist issuing the prescription; name of the patient; date on which the patient was examined, date of issuance of the prescription (if different) and the expiration date; power; diameter; optic zone diameter, if applicable; inside base curve radius, if applicable; lens manufacturer and material, or trade name; series of the lens to be provided, if applicable; tint, water content, and/or any other special design features that may be applicable; and any applicable notations as to when the lenses are to be worn.

Minnesota: Manufacturer's brand name, power, base curve, the name and telephone number of the prescribing optometrist or physician, patient's name, and the expiration date of the prescription. If applicable, the prescription may include diameter, axis, add power, cylinder, peripheral curve, optical zone, or center thickness. Two-year or less expiration.

Mississippi: Written prescription for hard contact lenses must include base curve, power, diameter, optical zone size, secondary curve-radius and width, lens size, material to be used, degree of blend (light, medium, heavy). Written prescription for soft contact lens must include base curve, power, diameter, manufacturer's name, lens size, type lens, material to be used, and tint of lens. Contact lens prescription is valid for 1 year.

Nebraska: All the parameters needed to describe the lens so that it can be correctly provided to the patient and can be precisely duplicated in the future. These parameters can include lens material, power, base curve, overall diameter, color; manufacturer; series; optical zone; peripheral curve radii, widths, and blends; and edge treatment. Each contact lens prescription shall be valid for the duration of the prescription as indicated by the optometrist or physican or for a period of 12 months from the date of issuance, whichever period expires first. Upon expiration, an optometrist or physican may extend the prescription without further examination.

Nevada: Prescription issued for ophthalmic lens by optometrist must contain lines or boxes in substantially the following form:
Approved for contact lenses
Not approved for contact lenses
If the prescription is for a contact lens, the form must include expiration date of the prescription; number of refills; and any other information necessary for the prescription to be filled properly. A prescription for polymethylmethacrylate (hydrophobic) contact lenses must specify the base curve, diameter, and refractive power of the lenses. A prescription for rigid gas permeable contact lenses must specify the base curve, diameter, and refractive power of the lenses; the brand name and type of lens, or the actual materials along with their ability to transmit oxygen; and whether the prescription is for daily wear or for a stated maximum number of 24-hour periods. A prescription for soft (hydrophilic) contact lenses must specify the base curve or equivalent, diameter, and refractive power of the lenses; the brand name and type of lens, or the actual materials desired along with their percentage of water content and thickness; and whether the prescription is for daily wear or for a stated maximum number of 24-hour periods.

TABLE 43.1. *(Continued)*

New Hampshire: Power, size, curvature, color, and material composition of the contact lenses. Other parameters or instructions, including but not limited to lens manufacturer, prescription expiration date, number of permitted refills, and a statement prohibiting substitutions, may be included at the prescriber's professional discretion. Unless otherwise specified by the prescriber for health reasons, a contact lens prescription shall expire 1 year from the date of issue.

New Jersey: All prescriptions must include the prescriber's full name, address, telephone number, license number, and academic degree, or identification of professional practice; this information shall be preprinted on all prescriptions. The prescription also must include the full name, age, and address of the patient; the date of issuance of prescription; and the hand-written signature of the prescriber. If an optometrist releases a contact lens prescription directly to a patient, the optometrist must provide the patient with a written warning, which includes the following language: *You should be aware that the physical measurements of your eyes may change over time. Using contact lenses that are not properly fitted can endanger your eye health. If you wish to obtain replacement lenses, you should see your eye doctor to assure that your lenses are fitting properly.* Two-year or less expiration.

New Mexico: New Mexico Statutes Annotated 61-2-10.4 provides that a contact lens prescription shall:
1. Explicitly state that it is for contact lenses
2. Specify the lens type
3. Include all specifications for the ordering and fabrication of the lenses
4. Include the date of issue, the name and address of the patient, and the name and address of the prescriber
5. Indicate a specific date of expiration, which shall be 24 months from the date of the prescription, unless in the professional opinion of the prescriber, a longer or shorter expiration date is in the best interests of the patient.

New Mexico Statutes Annotated 61-2-10.5 provides that a replacement contact lens prescription must contain all the information necessary for the replacement contact lens prescription to be properly dispensed, including:
a. Lens manufacturer
b. Type of lens
c. Power of the lens
d. Base curve
e. Lens size
f. Name of the patient
g. Date the prescription was given to the patient
h. Name and office location of the licensed optometrist who writes the replacement contact lens prescription
i. Expiration date of the replacement contact lens prescription

Code of New Mexico Rules 16.16.19.11 provides that a contact or corneal lens prescription release, upon patient request, shall contain the following:
A. Date of issue;
B. Name and address of the patient;
C. Name, professional designation, address, and signature of the prescribing optometrist;
D. All parameters including, but not limited to, base curve, power, diameter, brand name, materials type, required to properly duplicate or replace the contact lens supply;
E. A specific date of expiration, not to exceed 12 months;
F. Any limitation on refills and notification of scheduled follow-up visits and recommended lens replacement interval;
G. An explicit statement that the prescription is a contact or corneal lens prescription;
H. A specific statement noting that any person, firm, or corporation that dispenses or sells contact or corneal lenses from the prescription should inform the patient in writing of the following:
   1. That the patient should return to the prescribing optometrist to ascertain the accuracy and suitability of the contact or corneal lenses;
   2. That the prescribing optometrist or physician shall not be responsible for any damage or injury resulting from negligence of third parties to include, but not be limited to, negligence in packaging, manufacturing, substitution, improper care regimen, recommendations (cleaning, disinfection, and wetting), or instructions provided by the seller that lead to overwearing of the contact or corneal lenses; improper care of contact or corneal lenses that results in damage to the lenses or the visual system; change of the parameters of the contact lens; or filling the prescription after the expiration date.
I. Notice that the contact or corneal lens dispenser shall not adapt, substitute, or change the contact lens prescription, including brand name or specific material types, without prior authorization from the prescribing optometrist or physician, because to do so would constitute the practice of optometry;
J. The words "OK for contact lens," "fit with contact or corneal lenses," or similar wording do not constitute a contact lens prescription.

New York: Name, address, and signature of the prescriber and date of the prescription.

North Carolina: A prescription for contact lenses shall explicitly state that it is for contact lenses and specify the lens type and all specifications necessary for the ordering and fabrication of the lenses. Expiration date of not less than 1 year.

North Dakota: Every contact lens prescription shall have noted thereon an expiration date not to exceed 12 months and may only be released in written form.

Ohio: Rigid contact lens prescriptions must include base curve; peripheral curve(s), including curvature and width; overall diameter; optical zone diameter; power; center thickness; color; and material. Hydrophilic contact lens prescriptions must include manufacturer and lens type; power; base curve; overall diameter; and color. The examining optometrist may expire a contact lens prescription at the end of 1 year after the eye examination under normal circumstances. The prescription shall continue to be issued on request for a minimum of 2 years unless medical reasons would prohibit the release of the prescription.

Oklahoma: Date of issue; name and address of patient; name, address, and signature of the prescribing optometrist; all parameters required to properly supply the contact lenses, including brand names and materials types; specific date of expiration, not to exceed 12 months; any limitation on refills and notification of scheduled follow-up visits; explicit statement that it is a contact lens prescription; specific notation that any person, firm, or corporation that dispenses or sells contact lenses from the prescription should inform the patient in writing that they should return to the prescribing optometrist to ascertain the accuracy and suitability of the contact lenses and that the prescribing optometrist shall not be responsible for any damage or injury resulting from negligence of third parties to include, but not limited to, negligence in packaging, manufacturing, improper care regimen, recommendations (cleaning, disaffection, and wetting), or instructions provided by the seller that lead to overwearing of lenses or improper care of lenses that results in damage to lenses or visual system, and that the prescribing doctor shall not be responsible for contact lens damage, eye injury, or damage occurring during the time that lenses are provided by another dispenser.

Oregon: Patient's name, doctor's name, address, and phone number; sphere, cylinder, axis, and/or add; lens base curve or series; lens diameter; lens material and/or brand name; any special features that may include, but are not limited to, type of bifocal, trifocal, or progressive lens style, prism, material, tints, coatings or edge polish; a reasonable and clinically prudent expiration date; the maximum number of refills; and any limitations, including wearing schedule and follow-up care. If a patient has not completed a reasonable and clinically prudent trial period, the prescription released need only meet the spectacle prescription requirements.

Tennessee: All information necessary for the accurate fabrication and/or supply of the contact lens, including, but not limited to, the following: base curve, power, diameter, lens material or manufacturer's name, date of expiration, doctor's signature, and doctor's license number.

Texas: Ophthalmic lens prescription must include the signature of the optometrist or therapeutic optometrist, and information and parameters the optometrist or therapeutic optometrist considers relevant or necessary. Contact lens prescription must be written and must contain the patient's name; the date the prescription was issued; the manufacturer of the contact lens to be dispensed, if needed; the expiration date of the prescription; the original signature of the physician, optometrist, or therapeutic optometrist; if the prescription is for disposable contact lenses, the total number of lenses authorized to be issued under the prescription and the recommended lens replacement interval; if the prescription is issued by an optometrist, specification information required by Texas Optometry Board rule; and if the prescription is issued by a physician, specification information required by Texas State Board of Medical Examiners rule. Rigid contact lens prescription must include base curve, unless set by manufacturer; power; diameter, unless

(Continued)

TABLE 43.1. *(Continued)*

set by manufacturer; optical zone, unless set by manufacturer; peripheral curve, unless set by manufacturer; peripheral curve width, unless set by manufacturer; secondary curve, unless set by manufacturer; secondary curve width, unless set by manufacturer; blend, unless set by manufacturer; thickness, unless set by manufacturer; color, unless set by manufacturer; brand name; material, unless set by manufacturer; prescription date; expiration date; optometrist's signature or authorized signature; number of lenses; and substitution language. Soft contact lens prescription must include base curve, unless set by manufacturer; power; diameter, unless set by manufacturer; color, if needed; brand name; prescription date; expiration date; optometrist's signature or authorized signature; number of lenses; and substitution language. A physician, optometrist, or therapeutic optometrist may not issue a contact lens prescription that expires before the first anniversary of the date the patient's prescription parameters are determined, unless a shorter prescription period is warranted by the patient's ocular health or by potential harm to the patient's ocular health.

Utah: Commencement date of the prescription; base curve, power, diameter, material, or brand name; expiration date; for a written order, the signature of the prescribing optometrist or physician; for a verbal order, a record maintained by the recipient of the name of the prescribing optometrist or physician and the date the prescription was issued or ordered. A prescription may include a limit on the quantity of lenses that may be ordered under the prescription if required for medical reasons documented in the patient's files, and the expiration date of the prescription, which shall be 2 years from the commencement date, unless documented medical reasons require otherwise. When a provider prescribes a private label contact lens for a patient the prescription shall include the name of the manufacturer, the trade name of the private label brand, and if applicable, the trade name of the equivalent national brand.

Vermont: Expiration date, which shall be no earlier than 1 year after the examination date unless a medical or refractive problem affecting vision requires an earlier expiration date.

Virginia: Including, but not limited to, power, material or manufacturer, or both; base curve or appropriate designation; diameter when appropriate; and medically appropriate expiration date. The following information must appear on all prescription for ophthalmic goods: printed name of the prescribing optometrist; address and telephone number at which the patient's records are maintained and the optometrist can be reached for consultation; name of the patient; signature of the optometrist; date of the examination and an expiration date, if medically appropriate; and any special instructions.

Washington: Prescription must be in writing. At a minimum, the following specifications for a contact lens prescription must be retained in the records of the licensed optometrist who writes the prescription: dioptric power; base curve (inside radius of curvature); thickness, when applicable; secondary/peripheral curve, when applicable; diameter; color, if used; type of material used; special features equivalent to variable curves, fenestration, or coating. If the patient requests contact lenses and has received an eye examination for contact lenses, the prescription also must include the notation "OK for Contacts" or similar language indicating there are no contraindications for contacts. All optical prescriptions must include expiration date, not more than 2 years for contact lenses.

Wisconsin: Specifications needed to adequately duplicate the contact lens; name, signature, and license number of the prescribing optometrist; date of the prescription; date of expiration; and provision for a reasonable number of refills.

Wyoming: Expiration date, wearing schedule, care regimen, and all parameters necessary in order to fabricate a contact lens.

Source: American Optometric Association, 2003.

on a prescriber for ophthalmic goods and services dispensed by a seller pursuant to a correctly verified prescription. In the past, a contact lens prescriber potentially could have been found liable if a patient was injured by inappropriate lenses substituted by a contact lens seller (57). Under the FCLCA, there is little compelling legal reason to include wording such as "no substitutions" on a contact lens prescription, although such language might be desirable to remind the contact lens seller of the duty not to substitute. State laws permitting a seller or dispenser of contact lens to make substitutions would be preempted by the FLCLA.

State Requirements

The FCLCA provides that a patient has a right to his or her contact lens prescription. Around the time of enactment of the FCLCA, there were 34 states that had their own laws or rules regarding the release of contact lens prescriptions, and these may place additional requirements on the practitioner (58) (Table 43.2). Some states have requirements that may obligate a practitioner to allow patients access to additional information in their records: for example, freedom-of-information acts, professional practice acts, or rules and regulations of boards of medicine and optometry may affect the release of records (53).

Definition of a "Contact Lens Prescription"

A prescription is a written, signed order from one health care practitioner to another that describes the drug or medi-cal device to be dispensed by the practitioner. The FCLCA requires that a contact lens prescription must be written in accordance with state and federal law, and must contain sufficient information for the complete and accurate filling of the prescription, including:

1. Name of the patient
2. Date of the examination
3. Issue date and expiration date of the prescription
4. Name, address, telephone number, and fax number of the prescriber
5. Lens powers and the material or manufacturer, or both
6. Base curves or appropriate designation
7. Lens diameters, when appropriate
8. In the case of a private label contact lens, the name of the manufacturer, the trade name of the private label brand, and, if applicable, the trade name of the equivalent brand name (56).

The elements of a contact lens prescription also appear in the state optometry laws and board regulations of 38 states (Table 43-1). When confronted with a request for a prescription, optometrists in these jurisdictions must comply with any state requirements that are in addition to those imposed by the FCLCA.

Although not required by FCLCA, it is desirable to include information such as the lens care regiment and directions for wearing, such as "daily wear only." In the case of disposable or frequent replacement lenses, it is also desirable to include the number of permissible refills to prevent the

TABLE 43.2. STATES THAT HAVE EXISTING CONTACT LENS PRESCRIPTION RELEASE LAWS AND RULES

	State	Citation	Effective Date
mlm	AL	ADC §630-X-12-.03	Adopted 12/14/91, Effective 1/20/92
2	AZ	ADC §R4-21-305	Adopted Effective 4/1/91
3	AR	§17-90-108(a)(2)(A)	Enacted 3/31/03, Effective _____
4	CA	§2541.2	Enacted 9/23/02, Effective 1/1/03
5	CO	§12-40-117(3), ADC §9.00.01	Effective 7/1/92
6	DE	ADC §4.02 [Renumbered ADC §8.02 in 1998]	Readopted 12/27/90 (May have been in effect earlier—Board office had no way to know.)
7	Fl	§463.012(b), ADC §21Q-3.012(3)	1986
8	GA	§31-12-12	Effective 7/1/95
9	IN	§16-39-1-1(c)	1993 (Revised in 1996 to be more specific regading content of Rx.)
10	IA	§§147.108, 147.109	1994
11	KS	ADC §65-8-5	Adopted May 24, 2000
		§65-4966	Enacted May 16, 2002, Effective January 1, 2003
12	KY	Citation pending	Enacted March 6, 2003, Effective June 24, 2003
13	LA	§1299.97	1995
14	ME	Chapter 34-A §2417 4-A	1993
15	MD	§11-404.4	Enacted 5/21/98, Effective 10/1/98
16	MA	ADC §§5.02(4)(5)(6)(7)	10/8/93
17	MN	§145.712	Enacted March 22, 2002, Effective august 1, 2002
18	NE	§69-303(3)	Enacted 4/30/01, Effective 4/30/01
19	NH	§327:25-a1	Effective 7/22/94
20	NJ	§§52:17B-41.26–41.31	1991, Effective 4/17/92
21	NM	§16.16.19	June 8, 2001
		Citation pending	Enacted 4/7/03, Effective July 1, 2003
22	NY	ADC Part 29.8(a)(3)	Several decisions made in 1976 regarding glasses and lenses probably required release, however, release has been required for sure at least since 1981.
23	NC	§90-127.3, ADC §42E.0103(b)	1981
24	OH	§4725.17(A)	1978
25	OK	ADC §505:10-5-14	June 13, 1996
26	OR	§683.190(3), ADC §852-01-002(8)(k)	Amendment in 1989 required release of an appropriate written prescription for correcting refractive errors immediately upon completion of the necessary visual exam. A January 1991 AG opinion interpreted this requirement to include Cl Rxs. The optometry Board by policy satement (and later by regulation) began enforcing this provision that same month.
27	SD	ADC §20:50:10:02	Effective 1/1/95
28	TX	Art. 4552-A, §3(a)(b)(c), [recodified eff. Sept. 1, 1999 as Chap. 353, Subchap. D, §353.156(a)(b)(c)]	Enacted 6/20/97, Effective 1/1/98
29	UT	§58-16a-306(c)(d), §58-16a-502(7)	Enacted 3/13/00, Effective 5/5/00
30	VT	Chapter 30§§1719, 1727	1993
31	VA	ADC VR510-01-1 Part III §§3.1(3)(4)(5)(6)	7/20/88. Revised effective 7/26/95 to further specify the content of the Rx.
32	WA	§§18.195.010, 18.195.030, ADC §§246-852-101(1)(5), ADC §246-852-030	1994
33	WI	ADC Opt 5.16	Effective 1-1-02
34	WY	§33-23-101	1995

Source: American Optometric Association, 2003.

patient from "stockpiling" lenses that may not be appropriate for future wear.

All contact lens prescriptions must be signed by a licensed optometrist, physician, or other person authorized by state law to issue the prescription. A sample contact lens prescription containing these elements is included in this chapter (Fig. 43.5).

Refractive data, examination findings, or record summaries are not prescriptions and such information is not sufficient to constitute a contact lens prescription. Specific testing procedures are necessary to determine the prescription, including measurement of corneal curvatures and a detailed examination of the health of the eye.

Even with this added information, a contact lens pre-

John O. Doe, O.D.
123 Main Street
Anytown, US 12345
(555) 555-1234
(555) 555-4321 (FAX)[1]

Name[2] _____   Date of Rx[3] _____

Soft Contact Lens Specifications:[4]

	Manufacturer	Material	Axis	Lens Diameter	BC or Series	Sphere Power	Cylinder Power	Add/ Prism	Color
O.D.									
O.S.									

Gas Permeable Contact Lens Specifications:[4]

	Lab or manuf	Base Curve	Lens Diam	O.Z. Diam	2nd curve radius	2nd curve width	3rd curve radius	3rd curve width	Sph Pwr	Cyl. Pwr	Axis	Edge	Add/ Prism	Color
O.D.														
O.S.														

Examination Date:[5]_____   Special Instructions:[9]

Expiration Date:[6]_____

Number of Refills:[7]_____

Lens wear:[8]   daily wear only
daily wear and extended wear

_____[10]
John O. Doe, O.D.   License # 1234

FIG. 43.5. Sample contact lens prescription form. 1, Practitioner name, address phone and fax numbers. 2, Patient name. 3, Date of issue. 4, Lens parameters and manufacturer. 5, Examination date. 6, Expiration date. 7, Prescription refills. 8, Lens wear (daily wear only or daily wear and extended wear). 9, Special instructions (e.g., lens care regimen, wearing schedule, instructions for wear, required follow-up care). 10, Practitioner signature line and other identifying information. © University of California School of Optometry.

scription cannot be formulated until lenses are fitted on a patient's eyes to determine what lens type and dimensions fit best and are likely to give the patient the optimal visual and physiological response. Diagnostic contact lenses must be evaluated on the patient's eyes to determine what specific lens dimensions are appropriate for that particular patient.

Once the initial fitting is completed and the tentative lens dimensions are chosen, the contact lens prescription is still not finalized until the patient has demonstrated that the vision, comfort, and physiological response to the lenses are satisfactory. Only then can it be stated that the examina-

tion has been concluded and the contact lens prescription obtained (59).

A contact lens prescription differs significantly from a spectacle prescription. A contact lens prescription is not a copy or summary of the patient's record, the contact lens itself, the spectacle lens itself, the spectacle lens prescription, the optometrist's notes, the old contact lens container, or the prescription wall.

The contact lens prescription provides the information necessary to fabricate the contact lenses that will provide the patient with a proper visual, physical, and physiological response. Thus, the prescription for contact lenses does not exist until these factors have been determined. Furthermore, these factors can't be determined properly until lenses are fitted and the patient's response to them is evaluated. While a contact lens prescription may contain additional information such as the lens care regimen, wearing schedule, instructions for wear, and scheduled follow-up, this information may be more appropriate in the contact lens fitting agreement than in the prescription.

Conclusion

Prescriptions for contact lenses must include the elements specified in the FCLCA of 2003 as well as any additional information required by state law. A contact lens prescription must include a reasonable expiration date in accordance with the FCLCA and state law and should include the number of permissible refills. An expiration date shorter than 1 year must have a sound medical reason that is documented in the patient's record.

OPTOMETRIC MALPRACTICE

Theories of Liability

In all aspects of patient care, the practitioner is liable to the patient for the practitioner's conduct. Malpractice has been defined as "any professional misconduct, unreasonable lack of skill or fidelity in professional or fiduciary duties, evil practice, or illegal or immoral conduct" (6). The practitioner can help avoid conflicts with patients and the possibility of a malpractice suit by proper management of this potential liability.

Negligence

In order to establish a case of negligence, the plaintiff must prove each of the following four elements of negligence, and the defendant must not be able to establish any legally recognized defense (60).

1. The existence of a duty or obligation requiring the defendant (doctor) to conform to a certain standard of conduct for the protection of the plaintiff (patient) against an unreasonable risk of injury

A general duty of care is imposed on all human activity. When a person engages in any activity, he or she has a legal duty to act as an ordinary, reasonable, prudent person would under the same or similar circumstances. Some people are held to a higher standard of conduct in certain situations. A health care professional, such as a contact lens practitioner with special skills and training, is required to possess and exercise the knowledge and skill of a member of his or her profession in good standing in the same or similar locality.

2. Breach of that duty by the defendant

When the defendant's conduct is less than the level required by the applicable standard of care owed to the plaintiff, the defendant has breached his or her duty. This is a question of fact for either the jury or the judge if he or she sits without a jury.

3. The breach of the duty by the defendant must be the actual and legal cause of the plaintiff's injury

The defendant's conduct must be a cause in fact of the plaintiff's injury. An act is the cause in fact of an injury when the injury would not have occurred "but for" that act by the defendant. Where several causes concur to initiate the injury and any one would have been sufficient to cause the injury, it must be shown that the defendant's conduct was a "substantial factor" in causing the injury.

In addition, the defendant's act must be the legal or proximate cause of the plaintiff's injury. This legal doctrine requires a certain or reasonable closeness between the defendant's act and the plaintiff's subsequent injury and is a method of limiting liability in unforeseeable or unusual circumstances (61).

4. Damages to the plaintiff or his or her property

Damages are an essential element of the plaintiff's case for negligence. This means that the plaintiff must suffer actual harm or injury. The plaintiff is to be compensated for his or her actual damages and for prospective future damages.

Punitive damages also are available if the defendant was willfully or grossly negligent. They are designed to punish the defendant and deter him or her and others from similar behavior in the future.

There are three generally accepted defenses to charges of negligence (62). Any negligence on the part of the defendant relieves the plaintiff of liability in jurisdictions that accept the defense of "contributory negligence." In jurisdictions that accept the defense of "comparative negligence," the relative contributions of the parties' negligent acts are compared (weighed) and the defendant is liable for his or her portion of the damages. The third defense is "assumption of risk." Here the defendant is relieved of liability for his or her negligent act if the defendant knowingly and willingly assumed responsibility for the risks involved.

Practitioners are not only liable for their own acts and omissions, but they also may be liable for those of their employees and partners. Under the doctrine of "respondeat superior" or vicarious liability, liability is imputed to the employer for his or her employees' negligent acts performed in the course of employment (15,63). Because vicarious liability depends only upon the relationship between the employer and the employee, the employer can be liable even if he or she was not physically present when the employee performed the negligent act (64).

Liability may be imputed even though the defendant claims he or he never intended to form an employer–employee relationship. Liability may be imposed regardless of the intentions if, in fact, an employer–employee relationship exists (64). Even if the nonnegligent defendant claims that the negligent individual is an "independent contractor" (a legal status that would otherwise exclude the nonnegligent defendant from liability), the nonnegligent defendant may be vicariously liable if the actual relationship was that of employer and employee (64).

In many practices, the care and handling of contact lenses and accessory solutions, the verification of contact lens prescriptions and parameters, the training of contact lens patients, and other duties are delegated to contact lens assistants or technicians. An inadequately trained staff or poorly organized office may contribute to the opportunity for liability (2).

To be vicariously liable, the negligent individual must be acting within the line and scope of his or her employment (63). Thus, the employing practitioner would be vicariously liable for the injury to a patient whose contact lenses were soaked in a cleaning solution instead of a saline solution by the contact lens technician, but not for the injury caused when the employee struck the patient while driving home from work (2,65).

Partners are liable for the professional negligence of their partners when done within the scope of the partnership (63). Partnership liability, often referred to as "joint and several liability," is based on the concept that each partner is the agent of the other and that each partner will be regarded as being responsible for the acts or omissions of the other (64).

Thus, one should exercise due care in selecting employees and partners, because he or she might find himself or herself liable for their negligent acts. The degree of supervision required in contact lens practice may be determined by state laws or state board regulations (2).

Sources of Negligence Claims in Contact Lens Practice

By agreeing to fit a patient with contact lenses, an optometrist assumes a legal responsibility to conform to certain standards of conduct intended to protect the patient from the risk of injury. Failure to measure up to this "standard of care" is negligence and subjects the practitioner to a claim for damages (see Appendix, point f).

Negligence claims against contact lens practitioners are the most common source of professional liability claims within optometry (2,32). Although the fitting process and the wear of lenses are cited as the causes of many claims, the most significant liability cases usually arise out of inadequate follow-up or failure to monitor ocular health (15).

All contact lens patients should be given an initial eye health examination. Failure to detect disease, especially open-angle glaucoma, retinal detachment, and ocular tumors, is the leading cause of large malpractice claims against

optometrists (1,15). For this reason, contact lens patients should undergo periodic eye health assessment to rule out the presence of disease.

The risk of complications in extended wear cases can be minimized by proper communication with the patient, with emphasis on the use of a proper wearing schedule, appropriate lens care regimen, and a suitable recall program. Should complications ensue, patients should recognize the need to be seen promptly, and optometrists must be prepared to institute the appropriate therapy or to refer the patient to another practitioner as necessary. Failure to observe these rules creates the opportunity for litigation.

A frequent complication of contact lens wear is corneal abrasion, with its potential for subsequent infection, ulceration, and permanent loss of acuity. Optometrists must conform to recognized standards of care in the detection, management, and follow-up of contact lens complications, or they must be prepared to refer patient in a timely manner to other practitioners.

Extended Wear Lenses

The development of the extended wear contact lens has ushered in a new era of liability in contact lens practice (66). This additional source of liability claims can hardly be welcome news to contact lens practitioners. Contact lens-related claims jumped from 10% of all claims filed against optometrists in 1960 to nearly 50% of claims in the 1980s (1,67). Although the great majority of these claims involve daily wear lenses, minor injuries, and small damages, the claims arising from the use of extended wear lenses may involve significant injuries and substantial damages.

Careful monitoring of ocular health is especially important when extended wear is involved:

> A young female attorney was fitted with extended wear contact lenses by an optometrist. She returned as scheduled the day after the fitting, and the practitioner found no complications or contraindications, so she was scheduled for another appointment 3 days later. She did not return until a week had passed, at which time the optometrist found the lenses were not clean and that there was a small area of epithelial loss in one eye, causing the patient to complain of irritation. He prescribed a typical antibiotic and instructed the patient to return the next day, but she failed to keep the appointment. However, she did consult an ophthalmologist about a week later. The physician discovered a corneal ulcer about 2 to 3 mm in size, hospitalized the patient, and took cultures, which revealed the ulcer to be due to *Pseudomonas*. The patient sued the optometrist for negligence in the management of her case (2).

Studies have indicated that the risk of complications with extended wear lenses is greater than the risk with daily wear lenses. These complications include acute red eye, giant papillary conjunctivitis, superior limbic keratoconjunctivitis, conjunctival hyperemia, corneal infiltrates, corneal edema, vertical striae, and transient endothelial changes (68–81).

More serious complications, such as epithelial microcysts, neovascularization, and endothelial polymegethism, also have been reported (68,69,82–84). Holden and colleagues (84) found that extended wear of hydrogel lenses could cause significant changes in all layers of the cornea, which might suppress aerobic epithelial metabolism and thus compromise the epithelial barrier to infection.

Severe corneal infections and corneal ulcers have been well documented in extended wear soft contact lens patients (43,85–94). These infections, which include severe microbial keratitis, fungal infections, and *Pseudomonas* ulcers, occurred at a significantly greater incidence than among daily soft contact lens wearers (94). In many situations, the infections were associated with patient error or lack of compliance; however, some seemingly compliant patients also had complications with extended wear contact lenses regardless of the wearing schedule (68).

A survey by Weissman and associates (95) indicated that these severe complications are not limited to situations where patients fail to receive appropriate contact lens fitting and follow-up care. This increased risk requires the conscientious practitioner to regard patients seeking extended wear contact lenses differently than those seeking daily wear lenses. When prescribing extended wear lenses, one of the most important considerations is the selection of the patient (15). The patient should be prepared for the responsibilities of extended wear, and extended wear lenses should not be fitted on patients for whom there are physiologic or psychological contraindications. There are several clinical considerations of importance as well: selection of the appropriate lenses; determination of an adequate lens fit; use of the appropriate care system; institution of a reasonable wearing schedule; and frequent evaluation of the eyes and lenses.

Although a practitioner is under no duty to seek out a patient who has failed to keep a recall appointment, in some cases—such as a complication related to extended wear of contact lenses—it may be advisable to do so. When negligence is at issue, the conduct of both parties will be subjected to legal scrutiny, and in most states the negligence of the patient will not be a complete bar to recovery (see Appendix, point g). For this reason, it often is wise to follow up on patients who miss recall appointments. If patients fail to return as scheduled, this fact should be documented. Likewise, the failure of patients to comply with instructions, wearing schedules, or recommendations for cleaning should be noted in the patients' record.

Because employers are legally responsible for the acts or omissions of employees that occur while they are acting within the line and scope of their duties, contact lens practitioners should be certain that assistants or technicians are adequately skilled to undertake the tasks assigned them (15, 64). Furthermore, practitioners are obligated to supervise these individuals adequately if they clean, dispense, verify, or otherwise handle contact lenses.

As with other aspects of contact lens practice, it is beneficial to use written forms to describe the proper regimen for contact lens care and handling (4,5). These written instructions should include the proper cleaning and disinfection procedure, the appropriate wearing schedule, and the necessary follow-up care appointments. Such forms also should state that no substitutions in this routine should be made without first consulting the contact lens practitioner. They also can provide information about the normal and abnormal symptoms that occur while adapting to extended wear contact lenses.

The practitioner and the patient should sign the form. A copy should be given to the patient and the original retained in the patient's permanent record. It also is appropriate to retain a copy of the contact lens prescription tendered to the patient. Figure 43.6 shows an example of a comprehensive extended wear fitting, follow-up care, and informed consent agreement (see Appendix, point h).

In summary, extended wear lenses bring new requirements, both clinical and legal, to contact lens practice. Practitioners should carefully assess patients before considering them for extended wear and should regard these patients as being in a special category as far as clinical care is concerned. Extended wear patients must be monitored on a regular basis, and complications should be attended to promptly. Because communication is a vital aspect of reasonable care, the use of printed forms and instructions is advisable. Lastly, documentation of the care rendered to extended wear patients should not be neglected, because a comprehensive and contemporaneous account of the patient's care is the practitioner's best defense should litigation ensue.

Informed Consent

Communication is of vital importance when fitting patients with extended wear lenses, because patients must be prepared for the increased obligations required of them. This communication is necessary clinically in order to ensure that patients comply with instructions and thus minimize the risk of complications, or, if complications are encountered, that they are promptly diagnosed and managed. Communication also is necessary for legal reasons, the foremost of which is the doctrine of informed consent.

The concept of informed consent was discussed earlier. It can become a legal issue for contact lens practitioners in numerous ways, especially when fitting extended wear lenses, because it obliges the clinician to discuss the following aspects of the contact lens fitting process:

- Advising the patient about the feasibility of contact lens wear
- Determining if the patient is best suited for daily wear or extended wear lenses
- Notifying the patient of any special problems, such as keratoconus, aphakia, or pathologies such as recurrent corneal erosion or bullous keratopathy

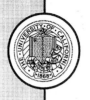

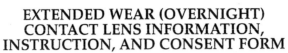

UNIVERSITY OF CALIFORNIA
SCHOOL OF OPTOMETRY

Contact Lens Services, Optometric Eye Center, Berkeley, CA 94720-2020
(510) 642-2020
Contact Lens Services, Tang Center, Berkeley, CA 94720-4300
(510) 643-2020

EXTENDED WEAR (OVERNIGHT) CONTACT LENS INFORMATION, INSTRUCTION, AND CONSENT FORM

DECEMBER 1, 1995©

EXTENDED WEAR MEANS EXTENDED CARE

The use of extended wear contact lenses has additional responsibilities and requirements. You must adhere to the recommended lens wear and care procedures, and you must return to the Clinic for periodic progress evaluations (see schedule).

We *require* the following Progress Evaluation Schedule:

- 24 hours after receiving extended wear contact lenses
- 3 days after receiving extended wear contact lenses
- 1 week after receiving extended wear contact lenses
- 2 weeks after receiving extended wear contact lenses
- 4 weeks after receiving extended wear contact lenses
- Each 12 week period after receiving extended wear contact lenses

It is impossible to determine in advance whether a patient will have a successful response to extended wear contact lenses. Certain personal, physiological, and environmental factors may adversely affect the success of extended wear contact lenses, and may necessitate a change in the recommended wearing schedule or termination of lens wear.
These factors include:

- Poor lens hygiene
- Inability or unwillingness to return for follow-up visits
- Manual dexterity problems which would prevent periodic lens removal and cleaning
- Severe emotional stress
- Use of certain medications
- Inability or unwillingness to follow instructions

The use of extended wear contact lenses is not without risk. A small, but significant, percentage of individuals wearing extended wear lenses develop potentially serious complications which can lead to permanent eye damage and vision loss.

IF YOU HAVE ANY OF THE FOLLOWING SYMPTOMS:

- EYE PAIN OR REDNESS
- WATERING OF THE EYE OR DISCHARGE
- CLOUDY OR FOGGY VISION
- DECREASE IN VISION
- SENSITIVITY TO LIGHT

REMOVE YOUR LENSES AND CALL THE CLINIC IMMEDIATELY. WE WILL ARRANGE TO HAVE YOUR EYES EXAMINED AS NEEDED. DO NOT RESUME WEAR UNTIL ADVISED TO DO SO BY US. IF YOU ARE UNABLE TO REACH THE CLINIC, CALL AN EYE DOCTOR OR GO TO THE NEAREST EMERGENCY HOSPITAL IMMEDIATELY.

PATIENT RESPONSIBILITY

You understand that your cooperation is vital to successful usage of extended wear contact lenses.

You have been instructed in the proper methods of lens care and handling. You understand the importance of adhering to proper lens care procedures and the need for periodic follow-up examinations. You agree to follow the recommended wearing schedule and to keep scheduled appointments. You agree to follow the Clinic's advice for safe extended wear as indicated on this form and in your record. You will notify the Clinic immediately if any eye or vision problem occurs. If you are unable to reach the Clinic you will call an eye doctor or the nearest emergency hospital immediately.

You understand that extended wear contact lenses have many benefits, but as with any other drug or medical device they entail possible risks. The risks of complication with extended wear lenses are 5 to 15 times greater than those with daily wear. Even one night of overnight wear may carry the risk of serious injuries. A percentage of wearers develop serious complications including corneal ulcers which can lead to permanent eye damage and vision loss. You agree to follow the advice and instructions given to you by the Clinic. You will remove your lenses and seek care immediately if you experience any unexplained eye pain, redness, or vision change.

You have been told the nature, purpose and benefits of extended wear contact lenses. You have also been told the possible risks, consequences, and side effects of extended wear contact lenses which are greater than those of daily wear contact lenses. You know there are feasible alternatives, including daily wear contact lenses and spectacles. You understand your chances of success with extended wear contact lenses. You will be able to ask any questions you have about the Clinic's policies and contact lenses prior to the ordering of lenses.

FIG. 43.6. Comprehensive extended wear fitting, follow-up care, and informed consent agreement.

LENS CARE INSTRUCTIONS

Proper care is necessary for successful wear, proper vision, good eye health and normal lens life. You have been instructed in the proper methods of lens care and handling. You have been provided with products to clean, disinfect and store your extended wear lenses. Use them as instructed. You have been fitted with the following kind of extended wear contact lenses:

Type   *Manufacturer/Brand*

☐   soft contact lenses _____

☐   rigid gas permeable contact lenses _____

☐   disposable soft contact lenses _____

Your lens cleaner is _____

Your lens disinfectant is _____

Your soaking solution is _____

Your rinsing solution is _____

Eyedrops to use before sleep and upon waking _____

Other _____

NOTE: **1)** These products have been prescribed specifically for your eyes and lenses. Do not change or substitute brands unless you check with us first. Use of improper solutions may result in eye irritation or lens damage.

2) Patients should wear their lenses no longer than advised. Patients should never wear extended wear lenses for more than 6 consecutive days. Lenses must be left off overnight before lens wear can be resumed. We are advising you to follow the wearing schedule listed below.

WEARING SCHEDULE

_____

_____

_____

_____

_____

Like any medical device contact lenses must be monitored on a regular basis. Professional follow-up care is the most important element in successful long term lens wear. Regular examination by a licensed eye care professional is necessary to evaluate your eyes' response to extended wear lenses. Your appointment schedule for follow-up progress examination is:

First _____

Second _____

Third _____

Fourth _____

Fifth _____

Sixth _____

Additional examinations will be scheduled as needed and in accordance with the "Progress Evaluation Schedule." It is important for the health of your eyes that you carefully follow the schedule recommended by the Clinic for wearing, cleaning, and disinfecting your lenses.

If a lens accumulates deposits such as protein, calcium, nicotine, etc., which cannot be removed, that lens must be replaced. In some instances a lens may become displaced from the eye and get lost or damaged, requiring a replacement.

DISPOSABLE EXTENDED WEAR LENSES

If you are wearing disposable contact lenses, you must remove your lenses and discard them according to the following schedule. Only new lenses should be worn during the next wearing period. Disposable lenses should not be replaced on the eyes after removal. Patients should not wear disposable extended wear lenses for more than 6 consecutive days. We are advising you to follow the wearing schedule listed below:

Remove lenses after _____ days of wear.

Keep lenses off eyes for _____ hours.

Replacement lenses can be worn for _____ days.

You must inspect each new lens carefully and not wear any lens that looks defective. Further you should not wear any lens that doesn't provide proper vision and comfort. If no problems are encountered, repeat the above schedule for _____ weeks at which time a progress evaluation will be scheduled and a new supply of lenses will be dispensed.

PATIENT INFORMED CONSENT

By signing this consent form, I acknowledge that I have read, understood, and received a copy of the "Information on Extended Wear (Overnight) Contact Lenses." I have also read, understood, and received a copy of the "Information on Contact Lens Services." I understand the Clinic's current policies, fees and refund schedule. I understand my responsibilities as stated on this form and by the Clinic. I agree to follow the instructions given to me by the Clinic.

Signature _____
              Patient

Signature _____
              Parent or Guardian if patient is a minor

Contact Lenses Dispensed by _____ Date _____

FIG. 43.6. *Continued.*

- Advising the patient concerning the need for special contact lens designs, such as bifocals, toric or bitoric lenses, or monovision fit
- Prescribing the appropriate care regimen and solutions for the patient's lenses
- Informing the patient if investigational or nonapproved lenses are to be prescribed

The doctrine of informed consent is why clinical investigators must sort through reams of paperwork whenever nonapproved lenses or solutions are undergoing clinical trials. Failure to disclose the experimental nature of lenses or materials can lead to liability if the patient sustains an injury (15,96). Similarly, the use of approved materials for nonapproved purposes, especially if extended wear is involved, may become a source of legal woes:

> An ophthalmologist prescribed rigid gas permeable contact lenses for a young patient, and although the lens material was approved only for daily wear at the time, the physician recommended that the lenses be used for extended wear. The patient's mother subsequently discovered that the lenses had been prescribed for use in a nonapproved manner, and although the child suffered no ocular injury, field a complaint with the state board of medicine and with FDA (2).

Patients who are being fitted with extended wear lenses should be managed differently than daily wear patients. Practitioners should inform these patients of the increased risks of extended wear; should emphasize that the responsibility for care is a joint undertaking, and should incorporate follow-up appointments into the clinical regimen. Documentation of instructions and the use of written materials to increase patient understanding are desirable, and practitioners may find that written agreements specifying these matters can improve patient compliance (see earlier discussion).

Although the specific matters to be included in written agreements will differ among practitioners, there are certain provisions that all practitioners will probably find to be desirable. Statements that should be used in such a written agreement include the following:

- Extended wear patients incur additional responsibilities that are a part of the contractual agreement
- Recommended lens care procedures must be adhered to
- Periodic progress evaluations are required
- Return to daily wear may be necessary
- Certain specified symptoms will require clinical evaluation or removal of the lenses
- Extended wear lens life is unpredictable
- The patient understands and agrees to abide by the requirements of the contract
- The patient's dated signature represents agreement to the above

The original agreement is retained in the record, and a copy is given to the patient. Should the patient fail to comply with the provisions of the contract, the practitioner should document this fact in the patient record. Pertinent aspects of patient care, such as changes in the wearing schedule or the lens care regimen, complications or contraindications to extended wear, or instructions to discontinue extended wear, should always be documented. Adequate records are of invaluable help if a legal dispute results from the practitioner's management of the patient's case.

Product Liability

Another potential source of liability in contact lens practice is based on product liability law. This legal doctrine can hold the designer, manufacturer, or seller (including a contact lens practitioner) of a "defective" product liable for any injury suffered when that product is being used for its customary and intended purpose and the injury resulted from poor design, improper manufacture, or any other defective condition (97). Classic product liability cases involve products such as spectacle lenses that break upon impact and cause eye injuries (98).

The product liability doctrine holds a practitioner to absolute or strict liability for the consequences regardless of how careful he or she was. Thus, even if the practitioner is acting in an appropriate fashion and is not at fault, he can be held liable as a matter of law if the product (e.g., a contact lens or solution) causes injuries to the patient because it was "defective."

In order to establish that a product (e.g., a contact lens or solution) is "defective," it must be proven that the product is unreasonably dangerous or unsuitable for the purpose for which it was sold. Thus, the designer, manufacturer, or seller is legally responsible if the following are true (99):

1. The product reaches the consumer without substantial change in the condition in which it is sold
2. The product is used in a reasonably foreseeable and intended manner
3. The product is "defective," i.e., it is unreasonably dangerous for the purpose sold or does not meet the reasonable expectation of an ordinary consumer as to its safety

Product liability cases involving rigid contact lenses are potentially complex because these lenses are custom made (100). A patient who was fitted with rigid contact lenses by an optometrist employed by an optical chain suffered pain, discomfort, and corneal scarring as a result of the poor lens fit. He sued under product liability law and was awarded $10,000 after a jury trial, but the judgment was appealed. The appellate court reversed, holding that there could not be liability under product liability law where there was no claim that the lenses were defective in themselves and where the lenses were not a finished product offered to the public in regular channels of trade. The jury award was disallowed.

It should be noted that this case involved PMMA lenses

and is more than 30 years old. With the advent of gas permeable and soft lenses, especially extended wear and disposable lenses sold as a prepackaged finished product out of stock, the opportunity to apply product liability theory to contact lens practice appears to have been given new life (66). Not surprisingly, lawsuits have been filed seeking to test this application of the law:

> An optical outlet sold a 15-year-old male extended wear soft lenses, which were advertised as usable for up to 30 days of wear without removal. While wearing the lenses "in accordance with the instructions given," the youngster developed a corneal ulcer in one eye and ultimately suffered a loss of visual acuity. He sued the contact lens manufacturer and the optical shop under product liability law, alleging that the lenses were "unreasonably dangerous and defective," and that they had been sold to him without any warning of "the risks inherent in extended wear of contact lenses." The case was resolved out of court with a six-figure settlement for the patient (101).

If product liability law is applied to soft contact lenses, a new source of litigation will be opened up against contact lens practitioners, although the primary defendant in these cases probably will be the contact lens manufacturer (see Appendix, point e). Therefore, prospects are good for contact lens practice to remain a leading source of professional liability claims.

Ocular Health Assessment

A large number of claims in contact lens practice arise from the failure to detect ocular disease in a contact lens patient (2,102). The most significant allegations of misdiagnosis include failure to detect glaucoma, ocular tumors, or retinal detachment, with failure to detect glaucoma the most common source of claims (103). Claims of this type result from the fact that some practitioners do not routinely evaluate the ocular health of their contact lens patients.

Before contact lenses are fitted, every potential contact lens patient must be given a comprehensive eye examination to rule out the presence of ocular disease. All contact lens patients should undergo routine, regular, periodic eye health examinations, including tonometry, ophthalmoscopy, biomicroscopy, and visual field analysis (2).

These should be performed, at minimum, on a yearly basis. A leading ocular malpractice case, *Helling v Carey*, was based on the failure to evaluate a contact lens patient's ocular health on a routine basis (104). Ms. Helling had been fitted with PMMA lenses by Dr. Carey, an ophthalmologist. She was 23 years old and myopic. During the next 9 years, she was seen numerous times with various symptoms of vision problems that seemed to be associated with contact lens wear. Her intraocular pressure and visual field were not tested until she was 32 years old, when she was found to have glaucoma. Her visual field was reduced to 5 degrees vertical and 10 degrees horizontal. She filed

suit, alleging negligence on the part of the defendants for failing to test her for glaucoma in more timely fashion.

At trial, evidence offered by the defendant physicians and by expert witnesses testifying on their behalf established that glaucoma was a relatively rare disease in the population below age 40, with an incidence of approximately 1 in 25,000. For this reason, it was not the standard of care to test routinely in this age bracket for the disease. Consequently, the trial court awarded a judgment in favor of the doctors.

Ms. Helling appealed the decision, arguing that the standard of care was inadequate to protect her from injury, and the Washington State Supreme Court, in reversing the trial court, made the following observation:

> "The incidence of glaucoma in one out of 25,000 persons under the age of 40 may appear quite minimal. However, that one person, the plaintiff in this instance, is entitled to the same protection as afforded persons over 40, essential for timely detection of the evidence of glaucoma where it can be arrested to avoid the grave and devastating result of this disease. The test is a simple pressure test, relatively inexpensive. There is not judgment factor involved, and there is no doubt that by giving the test the evidence of glaucoma can be detected. The giving of the test is harmless if the physical condition of the eye permits. The testimony indicates that although the condition of the plaintiff's eyes might at times have prevented the defendants from administering the pressure test, there is an absence of evidence in the record that the test could not have been timely given" (104).

In particular, it should be noted that reduced visual acuity or other vague complaints may erroneously be attributed to the contact lenses, thereby permitting the underlying disease to go undetected. This failure to detect and diagnose will create the basis upon which liability will be imposed against the practitioner. The importance of periodic evaluations of ocular health in all contact lens patients cannot be overemphasized.

PRESBYOPIC CONTACT LENSES

One of the major problems facing contact lens practitioners is caring for presbyopic patients (105). As the contact lens wearing population ages and the presbyopic population grows in size, finding a successful way to fit presbyopes with contact lenses has become a popular pastime for both practitioners and researchers. Among the alternatives that have been used to correct presbyopes are pinhole contact lenses, zonal bifocal contact lenses, simultaneous vision bifocal contact lenses, aspheric or multifocal contact lenses (all commonly referred to as "bifocal"), and monovision contact lenses.

Monovision contact lenses, which achieve simultaneous vision by correcting one eye for distance and the other eye for near, require no more fitting skill than traditional contact lenses and provide an expected and usually satisfactory corneal response. Success with monovision contact lenses has been reported to be significantly greater than with bifocal contact lenses. Although bifocal contact lenses have achieved wide practitioner acceptance in the past decade, they have yet to achieve the popularity of monovision as a modality for presbyopic patients (106–111).

Effects on Vision

Contact lens practitioners should consider the potentially adverse effects of monovision and bifocal contact lenses on the patient's visual performance.

Previous studies have found that overall visual performance, contrast sensitivity, glare, stereopsis, and task performance were reduced with both bifocal soft contact lenses and monovision compared to spectacle bifocals. For example, Brenner (112) found that contrast sensitivity was reduced with the use of certain diffractive and front aspheric soft bifocal contact lens designs. McGill and Erickson (113) reported a reduction in stereopsis with the use of a simultaneous vision bifocal contact lens. Back et al. (114) found that their subjects had better stereopsis but decreased binocular visual acuity with a concentric design bifocal contact lens correction compared to monovision correction.

A series of studies by Sheedy, Harris, and colleagues (115–117) found that visual acuity and stereoacuity both were reduced in patients wearing concentric bifocal contact lenses, diffractive bifocal contact lenses, and monovision compared to distance contact lenses and reading spectacles. Other researchers have found that monovision contact lenses do compromise vision to some extent, but they do not disrupt stereopsis as much as originally thought (118–127).

Thus, special consideration must be given to the fact that monovision and bifocal contact lens wear is a situation created by the contact lens practitioner that may compromise vision to some extent. The practitioner is legally and clinically responsible for the effects of these lenses; therefore, legal considerations must be taken into account when fitting patients with them.

Legal Considerations

The obligation to provide warnings to patients is a legal obligation, and the fitting of monovision or bifocal contact lenses incurs other legal responsibilities as well. Because the monovision or bifocal fit reduces visual acuity and may impair stereopsis, there is some potential for injury if the lenses are improperly fitted or their limitations are inadequately represented. The legal theory upon which liability rests is negligence.

Negligence in contact lens practice has been the object of various commentaries (2,68,128). Underlying negligence law is the concept of duty. The relationship between a practitioner and a patient creates a duty on the part of the practitioner to adhere to a course of conduct that minimizes the risk of injury to the patient while the patient is under the practitioner's care. This duty often is referred to as the doctor's obligation to provide "due care," which may be defined as care that a reasonable practitioner would provide under the same or similar circumstances. If the doctor fails to provide due care and as a proximate consequence the patient is injured, then the doctor is legally responsible for the patient's damages.

Proof of negligence inevitably requires the testimony of an expert, one who is familiar with the standard of care expected of the practitioner and who can link together the practitioner's actions (or failure to act) and the injury suffered by the patient. In a case involving monovision or bifocal contact lenses, the expert witness would have to be a contact lens practitioner familiar with the prescribing, fitting, dispensing. and follow-up necessary to satisfy the standard of care for patients wearing lenses fit in this manner. Some of the clinical factors that would be considered by such an expert have already been described.

Failure to satisfy the standard of care may result from any of the following:

- Negligently prescribing monovision or bifocal lenses (e.g., prescribing a monovision or bifocal fit when it is contraindicated or without a proper description or demonstration of its limitations)
- Negligently fitting the lenses prescribed (e.g., inadequate or improper lens fit, inappropriate lens power)
- Negligently dispensing the lenses (e.g., dispensing the incorrect lenses, failing to instruct the patient concerning insertion or removal techniques, recommending an inappropriate lens care regimen)
- Negligently failing to monitor the patient (e.g., neglecting to follow-up after dispensing to ensure that the patient is using the lenses appropriately and is not experiencing any unanticipated difficulties).

The practitioner should discuss with the patient the risks of the proposed therapy—in this case, monovision or bifocal contact lenses—so that the patient's consent can be obtained prior to the institution of treatment (49). Because the effects of monovision or bifocal fits are best demonstrated by wearing the lenses, a trial fitting is advisable. Failure to describe or demonstrate the effects of a monovision or bifocal fit, if this breach of the duty to warn is proximately related to an injury suffered by the patient, can lead to liability being imposed upon the contact lens practitioner.

Failure to warn of the side effects of treatment not only subjects an practitioner to liability for injuries experienced by the patient but also raises the possibility that third parties injured by the patient may themselves bring an action against the practitioner (129,130). Because monovision or bifocal contact lenses may impair a patient's ability to operate a motor vehicle safely, the appropriate warning or demonstration should always be given to patients who drive.

Warnings or demonstrations also are necessary for patients who plan to wear their lenses while operating dangerous machinery or performing other potentially hazardous activities. Because of these risks, it may be necessary to provide the patient with alternative means of correction, such as spectacles for wear while performing critical tasks (e.g., driving a car).

If a patient is involved in an accident and injuries himself or herself (or others), the doctor must establish that he or she gave an adequate warning or he or she will be held liable (131). The legal criterion for satisfying the doctrine of informed consent, however, varies from state to state. Regardless of the state, a practitioner's defense to a claim of failure to warn or negligence depends in large measure upon the documentation that he or she can offer to support his or her assertion that the proper warning was given.

UNAPPROVED OR UNUSUAL CONTACT LENS CARE

Introduction

Contact lens cleaning regimens have been improved and simplified in the last decade, and the use of homemade saline and other non-FDA approved care regimens has decreased (132). However, some practitioners and patients continue to use unusual or unapproved lens care procedures (133). These procedures include those not specifically recommended by the manufacturer or approved by the FDA for use in the United States, and FDA-approved procedures that are used in an unusual or unapproved manner. It is possible that such care regimens could have adverse effects on the patient's eyes and contact lenses. Equally important, the use of unapproved or unusual lens care procedures has legal implications that practitioners should consider before implementing such procedures (15). For these reasons, practitioners and their patients should use FDA-approved solutions in accordance with manufacturers guidelines.

What are the legal implications and ramifications if a practitioner or a patient is using unusual or unapproved soft lens care procedures in the office or at home? There are a number of legal doctrines that apply to these situations.

Malpractice

The first legal concept that applies is malpractice. Malpractice can be considered to be professional misconduct toward a patient. In legal terms, malpractice is negligence in the practice of one's profession. The elements of negligence were discussed earlier.

An individual can avoid acting in a negligent fashion by acting as a reasonable, ordinary, prudent person would under the same or similar circumstances. As contact lens practitioners are held to a higher standard, we must ask ourselves, "What would a reasonable contact lens practitioner do?" If that practitioner would not have used an unusual technique for cleaning or disinfecting contact lenses or would not have recommended that patients use an unapproved procedure at home, then such use and recommendations are likely to be outside of what an ordinary, reasonable, prudent person would do.

In addition to acting as a prudent professional, the practitioner must follow FDA rules and regulations, which have essentially the same authority as laws enacted by Congress. Even though other practitioners in the community are using unusual procedures without ill effects, the FDA rules and regulations indicate that a conscientious, prudent practitioner should not do the same. Failure to follow FDA rules and regulations could be considered negligence *per se,* as could failure to follow a manufacturer's package insert or labeling guidelines for contact lens care. This legal doctrine establishes negligence regardless of the standard of care provided by the practitioner if his or her performance specifically violates rules and regulations established by government enactment (60,134).

Product Liability

Another potential source of liability when using contact lens care products is based on product liability law as discussed earlier. Specifically, contact lens practitioners face liability if they use or recommend products that may injure the patient's eyes or lenses because the product is "defective." This has been interpreted to mean that it "subjects persons or property to an unreasonable risk of harm" (97). For example, recommending a baking soda slurry for soft lens cleaning could fit this definition. In order to establish that a solution or lens is defective, it must simply be proven that the product is unusually dangerous or unsuitable for the purpose for which it was sold. Thus, even though baking soda is suitable for many cooking uses, it has not been found suitable by the FDA for cleaning soft contact lenses.

Informed Consent

Another legal doctrine with implications for the practitioner who uses or recommends unapproved or unusual lens care procedures is the doctrine of informed consent (see earlier discussion). This concept makes the doctor liable in negligence to patients for failing to disclose to patients significant known risk of the procedure being used.

Clinical investigators must comply with the Department of Health and Human Services guidelines on informing their patients about investigative or experimental products or procedures as discussed earlier (50). This includes the use of unapproved or unusual lens care procedures that have not been approved by the FDA.

In a case involving soft contact lenses, a practitioner provided a young boy with an experimental contact lens solution but failed to inform the boy's parents that the fluids were experimental (128). The boy's eye became inflamed and blurred vision resulted from chemical burns. The patient suffered for several months. Suit was filed seeking damages for injury to the boy, recovery of medical expenses, and punitive damages against the doctor. The doctor involved was confronted with using experimental products not approved by the FDA, which constitutes an illegal act in the practice of his profession. This was aggravated by the fact that the patient was a minor and the practitioner had not disclosed the experimental nature of his work or obtained parental consent or a written release. He also faced possible criminal action for battery, which is an unlawful touching of another person, and questionable malpractice insurance coverage because his policy only protects him for actions legally performed within his license. The use of nonapproved products was not within the statutory definition of his profession.

Even though the practitioner's liability may be mitigated or discharged in some instances by patient noncompliance or failure to keep progress appointments, it is best to avoid these potential legal problems in the first place. One of the easiest and most effective ways to avoid legal complications for using contact lens solutions is by giving patients proper instructions and advice on the use and care of contact lenses and the adjunct solutions. These instructions can be given orally and should be supplemented by written brochures that specifically indicate the instructions and advice for that patient. Demonstration of the appropriate procedures in the doctor's office is an excellent way to provide proper instructions for the patient.

Use of specific forms with printed information on lens care and handling, as discussed earlier, is a valuable means of ensuring that patients have proper advice on lens care and handling. This also provides for proper documentation of the prescribed care regimen in the patient's record. Practitioners can tailor these forms to indicate the specific solutions and care techniques, wearing schedule, and follow-up schedule that the patient is supposed to follow. The patient should be advised not to change solutions or techniques without first discussing such changes with the practitioner.

Proper documentation of everything that occurred in the examination and training session, along with the names of all solutions and devices given the patient, should be noted in the patient's record. The patient should be advised of any potential adverse effects from the recommended solutions or care regimen. This also should be noted in the patient's record. This information, along with advice and instruction of lens care, constitutes an appropriate informed consent, which should be signed by both the patient and the practitioner.

On follow-up visits, the practitioner should discuss with the patient the lens care procedures currently being used. This helps ensure that the patient is following the doctor's instructions appropriately. Any discrepancy from what was prescribed should be noted in the patient's record. The patient then should be advised again of the appropriate procedures to follow. When working with minors, the practitioners should advise both the patient and the parent of the proper procedures and have both individuals sign the forms involved (135).

By being aware of the unapproved and unusual soft contact lens care procedures that can be used and understanding their potential legal implications, practitioners can avoid problems and help ensure that patients are using the proper solutions in an appropriate manner. Thus, the practitioner can avoid the possible adverse effects of inappropriate procedures on the patient's eyes and lenses, and their potential legal ramifications.

RECORD KEEPING

Documentation

Patient records are essential to provide patients with appropriate health care and to preserve patients' rights (136–139). The following are reasons for maintaining patient records (140,141):

1. To aid medical science, and to facilitate the care of a particular patient who requires treatment or hospitalization at a later time
2. To provide a record for assisting a patient in enforcing his or her claim for injuries against parties other than a physician, hospital, or member of their respective staffs
3. To assist a physician, hospital, or member of a medical or nursing staff or other personnel in defending against an allegation of negligence made by or on behalf of a patient
4. To assist a physician or hospital in collecting an unpaid debt due from a patient

In determining liability for malpractice, the jury will ultimately ask, "What did the practitioner do or fail to do?" As the testimony of the practitioner and the patient may be inaccurate or biased, the most conclusive evidence will be drawn from the practitioner's records. Two often quoted truisms indicate the importance of good records and documentation: "In the courtroom, work not written is work not done," and "Records are witnesses that never lie" (137).

Because of time constraints, practitioners often do not make lengthy record entries that attempt to summarize communications with patients. Time will be well spent, however, if pertinent entries, such as those noting that a warning was given, are routinely placed in patient's records. If a legal action ensues, this entry then may be explained by the doctor in terms of the routine warning that was issued. Assuming that the warning satisfies the appropriate legal criterion (i.e., professional community or reasonable patient rule), the practitioner will be able to defend his or her conduct, even if the entry is a succinct one. The problem-oriented record system allows practitioners to make necessary entries (such as warnings) in an efficient and orderly manner and should be utilized by practitioners who provide episodic care, such as is found in contact lens practice (142).

Many practitioners only record abnormalities, but this does not show the extent of the examination given. Practitioners should always record each and every examination procedure performed, normal and abnormal findings, instructions given to the patient, referrals made, and any other relevant data to show they rendered prudent care, including advise and recommendations for future care. Recordings such as "Neg. O.K." or "clear" do not adequately describe the scope of the examination or what was found (138). The most thorough practitioner may be found liable even if he or she met the appropriate standard of care if he or she did not properly document the care and findings in the patient's record with no record to support his or her contention (143).

Content

Twelve states (Alaska, Kansas, Kentucky, Louisiana, Massachusetts, New Jersey, New Mexico, Rhode Island, Tennessee, Texas, Virginia, and Wisconsin) have statutory requirements as to the minimum requirements for a contact lens examination and therefore a contact lens record (144). However, common sense and the standard of care dictate a certain minimum amount of testing and recording at any contact lens examination regardless of statutory requirements. Absent any such requirements, each practitioner will have to decide what and how to record in a patient's record. This may be based on past experience and office routine. However, it is best if each record contains all the relevant information gathered as part of the patient examination. With contact lens patients, each record should contain at least the following (136,137):

1. Case history. This should be obtained and updated in detail at each visit. It should indicate the reason for the patient's visit, the symptoms and complaints, previous problems, general health history, ocular health history, allergies, current medications, family health history, occupation and avocation, type of lenses worn, wearing schedule, past experiences with contact lenses, lens care procedures, and the names of prior practitioners.
2. Visual acuity, especially the corrected acuity with contact lenses for each eye, should be recorded. Entrance acuity should be recorded after taking the history but before any other tests are performed. The refraction over the contact lenses and best-corrected acuity should be noted.
3. Examination of the external eye and adnexa, including evaluation of the lids, lashes, conjunctiva, and corneas.
4. Detailed corneal examination using the slit-lamp biomicroscope with fluorescein. This is especially impor-

tant before fitting contact lenses and should be done at each and every examination visit. The practitioner should note and grade any edema, staining, vascularization, striae, opacities, or other abnormalities. All findings should be recorded in detail.
5. Keratometry, including the measurement of corneal curvature and the clarity of the mires.
6. Postwear refraction and the best attainable visual acuity with that spectacle prescription.
7. Contact lens inspection and measurement, including all measurable parameters and inspection for defects.
8. Any instructions, precaution, service agreements, or warranties regarding contact lenses should be stated in written or printed handouts. The recommended lens care regimen should be recorded in detail.
9. Advise and treatment given should be recorded in detail, including what the patient was told about any problems, abnormal findings, referrals, recall, risks, or other advise or recommendations. The wearing schedule and next appointment time should be noted.
10. Date and time of all office visits, including missed or canceled appointments.
11. All entries should be signed and dated by the practitioner.
12. When a patient asks that records be sent to another practitioner or for a copy of his or her prescription, a copy of the patient's written consent to release that information should be kept in the record.
13. All communications with the patient (e.g., letters, phone conversations) should be documented in the record.

Ownership

Who owns the patients' records? The practitioner owns the records and has the right to possess and control them. However, the patient has a right to the information they contain (58,137,145). In a legal action, the patient can demand a complete copy of his or her record. Therefore, it is best not to include comments in the record that might embarrass the practitioner or the patient (137).

The practitioner must keep the records for a reasonable time. How long depends upon the patient's need for continuous care and the state statute of limitations regulations regarding malpractice, contracts, and tax law. Records should be kept for a minimum of 10 years after the patient was last seen; ideally they should be retained forever (141)

The statute of limitations on contracts is normally about 8 years. This might apply if the patient claims the practitioner promised a successful result and breached that warranty.

The statute of limitations for malpractice is generally 1 or 2 years after the incident occurred or the act of malpractice was discovered. However, a number of court decisions have weakened statute of limitations protection for medical practitioners. In *Calle v Kazerian* (146), the California Court of Appeals suspended the statute of limitations in a lawsuit against an obstetrician who failed to diagnose Down's syndrome until the time when the parents learned that the abnormality could have been discovered by amniocentesis. In *Brown v Bleiberg* (147), the California Supreme Court permitted a patient to sue 12 years after surgery because of uncertainty as to whether the physician had explained the procedure sufficiently for the patient to discover whether negligence had occurred. In *Borderlon v Peck* (148), the Texas Supreme Court held that a lawsuit could be brought after the 2-year statute of limitations had lapsed if it could be shown that the physician fraudulently concealed the existence of a potential cause of the patient's injury.

There is a 3-year statute of limitations from the due date of the return for federal taxes, unless there was a gross (25% or greater) underreporting of income, in which case the limitation is 6 years. There is no statute of limitations if the return is fraudulent (137,149).

It is important to note that the statute of limitations for a minor does not begin to run until he or she reaches the age of majority or discovers an injury that might have been due to malpractice. These laws may be different in different jurisdictions.

Confidentiality

The doctrine of "privileged communication" requires a doctor to keep private patient information confidential (143). Information from a patient's record should never be released without prior authorization from the patient. This authorization should be in the form of a written consent, which should be kept in the patient's record. Patient information, including contact lens prescription data, should not be given over the phone unless written permission has been obtained previously or an emergency exists. Although a patient can request a complete copy of his or her record, it is preferable to have the relevant information extracted from the record and provided in the form of a letter, a copy of which remains in the record along with the written signed request form. Information not requested should not be released.

Health Insurance Portability and Accountability Act Privacy Standards

Federal regulations promulgated under the Health Insurance Portability and Accountability Act of 1996 (HIPAA) (150,151) have established privacy standards that health care providers who electronically transmit data must comply with by April 14, 2003 (152). These regulations require that a Notice of Privacy Practices form must be given to each patient, outlining the practitioner's possible uses and disclosures of protected health information (PHI). A patient must sign a Patient Consent Form before the practitioner may use PHI as part of treatment, "health care operations,"

or to obtain payment for services. The patient must also sign an Authorization for Release of Identifying Health Information appropriate for the planned use or disclosure (153). Copies of model forms have been made available by the American Optometric Association, but these forms will likely have to be customized to a particular practitioner's mode of practice (154).

Modifications to the HIPAA privacy rules proposed by the Department of Health and Human Services were adopted on August 14, 2002. These modifications served to simplify practitioner compliance in a number of areas, such as permitting treatment of a patient who refused to sign a consent form, and allowing the use of a single type of authorization form (155). It undoubtedly will require some learning and adjustment before compliance with these new regulations and proposed changes can become a routine part of practice.

Computerized Records

Optometrists traditionally relied on handwritten records as a means of documenting and storing business and patient information. With the advent of cost-effective computer systems, the electronic collection and storage of patient data has become more commonplace (156). At present, the majority of computerized optometric records are likely to contain financial and business data rather than examination information. This is largely due to the perceived cost and inconvenience of computerized data collection in the examination room. However, as optometric software and hardware becomes more user friendly and inexpensive, it is only a matter of time before computerized examination records become the norm.

One of the most important reasons for maintaining complete and accurate records is as a defense to a malpractice liability action. However, before a record can be admitted into evidence it must be authenticated. Traditionally, authentication was by accomplished by handwritten signature; however, as computer use has become more widespread, regulatory entities and accrediting organizations increasingly are contemplating the authentication of medical records by computer entry (157).

A record usually will be authenticated and admissible into evidence if it was compiled routinely at the time of the examination and if the data can be proven trustworthy by the custodian of the records, who usually is the practitioner or an employee (158). Such authentication is relatively straightforward for a handwritten record, because handwriting provides information as to authorship and whether the record has been altered. For example, an expert witness may use microscopic analysis of papers and inks to determine whether an entry was obliterated, written over, or made subsequent to the original entry (159).

A computerized record is a printed or electronic document rather than a handwritten one. Its author cannot be recognized from handwriting. Because a computerized record often is created by transferring data from a handwritten examination form to a computer disk to a paper printout, authentication is more difficult and falsification is easier because of the added steps and persons involved. It is more complicated to create a computer analogue to the lining out, initialization, and dating of an addition or modification to a handwritten record. Furthermore, in a system without individual computer access keys, it is nearly impossible to determine the author of an entry, deletion, or modification. The best systems are those that identify the author by individual access keys and use an internal calendar-clock to automatically indicate the date and time of data entry.

Although state medical and hospital record requirements are not binding on optometrists, they are indicative of the attempts that have been made to solve authentication problems. Most states still require that a medical record contain a written signature, thereby precluding the use of computerized records without a written backup (157).

At least two states authorize computerized medical records. Indiana law specifically states that computerized hospital records are to be considered original records for purposes of admissibility into evidence. Such records may be authenticated by showing that the computer equipment used is standard at the hospital and secure from unauthorized access, that records of entries and modifications are maintained, and that entries were made during the regular course of business and in a timely manner (160). In California, a hospital physician may authenticate a hospital record by means of a signature stamp or computer key only if he or she places a signed statement in the hospital administrative office to the effect that he or she is the only person who has possession of the stamp or key and is the only person who will use it (161). Other states permit authentication by nonsignature means such as rubber stamps or handwritten initials (157). Each practitioner should check the laws of his or her own state for guidance. If there is any doubt, the doctor should save the handwritten original records for at least as long as the applicable statute of limitations period.

Regardless, the practitioner should not be tempted to alter a record without clearly indicating the change. Courts may attach severe penalties in the case of falsified records. For example, a New Jersey court held that a physician's falsification of a medical record was gross malpractice and a basis for license revocation (162). A Florida court held that intentional destruction of medical records gave rise to an irrebuttable presumption of malpractice (163), Thus, a computerized record system should retain any modified or deleted entries within the files in order to protect the practitioner from allegations of record falsification.

Policies and Procedures

Regardless of the size of the system involved, policies and procedures should be made clear to those having access to the computerized records. Rules pertaining to confidentiality should be carefully discussed with staff members. Abbreviations commonly used by the doctors and staff when recording examination data should be listed. For the sake of smooth office operation and legal documentation, this information should be outlined in a policies and procedures manual.

The American Medical Association has published the following guidelines regarding confidentiality of computer records (164):

5.07 Confidentiality: Computers.

The utmost effort and care must be taken to protect the confidentiality of all medical records, including computerized medical records

The guidelines following are offered to assist physicians and computer service organizations in maintaining the confidentiality of information in medical records when that information is stored in computerized databases:

1. Confidential medical information should be entered into the computer-based patient record only by authorized personnel. Additions to the record should be time and date stamped, and the person making the additions should be identified in the record.
2. The patient and physician should be advised about the existence of computerized databases in which medical information concerning the patient is stored. Such information should be communicated to the physician and patient prior to the physician's release of the medical information to the entity or entities maintaining the computer databases. All individuals and organizations with some form of access to the computerized databases, and the level of access permitted, should be specifically identified in advance. Full disclosure of this information to the patient is necessary in obtaining informed consent to treatment. Patient data should be assigned a security level appropriate for the data's degree of sensitivity, which should be used to control who has access to the information.
3. The physician and patient should be notified of the distribution of all reports reflecting identifiable patient data prior to distribution of the reports by the computer facility. There should be approval by the patient and notification of the physician prior to the release of patient-identifiable clinical and administrative data to individuals or organizations external to the medical care environment. Such information should not be released without the express permission of the patient.
4. The dissemination of confidential medical data should be limited to only those individuals or agencies with a *bona fide* use for the data. Only the data necessary for the bona fide use should be released. Patient identifiers should be omitted when appropriate. Release of confidential medical information from the database should be confined to the specific purpose for which the infor-

mation is requested and limited to the specific time frame requested. All such organizations or individuals should be advised that authorized release of data to them does not authorize their further release of the data to additional individuals or organizations, or subsequent use of the data for other purposes.

5. Procedures for adding to or changing data on the computerized data base should indicate individuals authorized to make changes, time periods in which changes take place, and those individuals who will be informed about changes in the data from the medical records.

6. Procedures for purging the computerized database of archaic or inaccurate data should be established, and the patient and physician should be notified before and after the data has been purged. There should be no commingling of a physician's computerized patient records with those of other computer service bureau clients. In addition, procedures should be developed to protect against inadvertent mixing of individual reports or segments thereof.

7. The computerized medical database should be online to the computer terminal only when authorized computer programs requiring the medical data are being used. Individuals and organizations external to the clinical facility should not be provided online access to a computerized data base containing identifiable data from medical records concerning patients. Access to the computerized data base should be controlled through security measures such as passwords, encryption (encoding) of information, and scannable badges or other user identification.

8. Backup systems and other mechanisms should be in place to prevent data loss and downtime as a result of hardware or software failure.

9. Security:

A. Stringent security procedures should be in place to prevent unauthorized access to computer-based patient records. Personnel audit procedures should be developed to establish a record in the event of unauthorized disclosure of medical data. Terminated or former employees in the data processing environment should have no access to data from the medical records concerning patients.

B. Upon termination of computer services for a physician, those computer files maintained for the physician should be physically turned over to the physician. They may be destroyed (erased) only if it is established that the physician has another copy (in some form). In the event of file erasure, the computer service bureau should verify in writing to the physician that the erasure has taken place.

There are many advantages to computerized optometric records. They permit easy manipulation and recall of data. They are compact and durable. They are becoming less ex-

pensive and more convenient to implement. The practitioner must, however, be aware of the need to make computerized records a reliable and authenticatable documentation of the course of patient treatment. Thus, the records should conform to state law controlling admissibility into evidence at trial.

In addition to containing information that normally would be included in a handwritten record, the computerized record system should utilize individual access keys and automatic date/time entry to indicate when an entry was made and by whom. The contents of any entries that were altered and corrected should be retained in the file. Confidentiality of data should be safeguarded, and backup files should be created as often as necessary to prevent loss of data. Files should be retained for at least the applicable statute of limitations period. Office staff should be informed of and understand procedures regarding office records, and these procedures should be stated in writing.

DISCHARGING LIABILITY

The practitioner rendering care remains responsible for the patient until liability is discharged. Liability can be discharged by proper referral, termination of practice, or failure of the patient to cooperate or follow instructions.

Proper referral when necessary is a duty of all practitioners (136). All referrals should be duly recorded in the patient's record. The referring practitioner should make the appointment for the patient. This avoids any miscommunication or misperception on the part of the patient.

Malpractice cases often involve questions of credibility between the practitioner and the patient. The practitioner may claim he or she referred the patient to a specialist, whereas the patient denies any such referral. Under no circumstances should a practitioner alter records at a later date to note that a referral was made (136,137,143). Such alterations, which can be detected easily by handwriting experts, are seen as "admissions of guilt" and can lead to criminal charges for fraud. The following guidelines should be followed when making a referral (137):

1. The patient must understand why the referral is being made. The patient should be told about any problems or abnormalities found.

2. The referral appointment should be made by the referring practitioner or his or her staff while the patient is in the office. The name, address, and phone number of the consulting specialist, along with the date and time of the referral appointment, should be given to the patient and recorded in detail in the patient's record, along with the reason for referral.

3. A letter should be sent to the specialist detailing the examination findings and the reason for the referral. A copy should be kept in the patient's record.

4. Every referral should be followed to ensure that the patient saw the specialist. Letters and phone conversations from the specialist should be documented in the patient's record.

There is an important distinction between referral and patient abandonment. Patient abandonment occurs when there is a unilateral severance by a professional of the relationship between the professional and the patient without reasonable notice and at a time when there is still a necessity for continuing attention to the condition of the patient or an emergent condition (136).

A doctor–patient relationship ceases and there is no abandonment when the relationship is ended by the mutual consent of both parties, when the professional service is no longer needed, or when the professional gives the patient reasonable notice so as to provide the patient an opportunity to secure other professional services.

When a practitioner is engaged for a specific occasion or service, the practitioner is under no duty to continue treatment after the specific occasion or service has been rendered. Furthermore, the failure of a patient to cooperate with the practitioner or follow instructions generally justifies the practitioner in terminating the relationship unilaterally.

To avoid charges of negligence or abandonment, practitioners must provide for emergency care for their contact lens patients. This means they must have an answering service that can contact them in emergencies, provide patients with their home phone numbers, or provide instructions on how to obtain care from another practitioner if necessary.

MINIMIZING THE POSSIBILITY OF A MALPRACTICE SUIT

Many malpractice actions arise because of a lack of effective communication with the patient. The patient who perceives the practitioner as unresponsive to his or her needs and too busy to discuss that patient's particular problem is a prospective plaintiff. A patient who has received a detailed explanation of the possible risks, complications, side effects, expected benefits, and alternative treatments is less likely to file suit even if the results are less than optimal (136).

There is no way to guarantee that a practitioner will never be sued for malpractice. However, there are guidelines that, if followed, can reduce the likelihood that a practitioner will be sued for malpractice. These guidelines should be followed at each and every office visit (136).

1. Keep clear, accurate, timely records.
2. Once you accept a patient, be sure to adhere to generally accepted standard of practices.
3. If the case is one you do not wish to handle, refer it to another competent practitioner.
4. Be available to your patients 24 hours a day, 7 days

a week, or make suitable arrangements for coverage by a competent colleague.
5. Respect patients' time by providing convenient scheduling. Do npt keep patients waiting for their scheduled appointment.
6. Communicate with patients as friends.
7. Listen to your patients. Good communication is a key to avoiding malpractice suits.
8. Always inform the patient of any hazards related to a treatment plan if the possibility of risk is not remote and discuss reasonable alternatives.
9. Never guarantee a cure or results.
10. Do not hesitate to consult with another practitioner about your treatment plan.
11. Telephone the specialist to whom you are referring a patient and always note any referral in the patient's records.
12. Get written permission (i.e., informed consent) before starting any experimental, controversial, or unusual procedure on a patient.
13. Supervise employees closely and do not permit them to perform duties that they are not qualified to perform.
14. Make friends with your patients. A practitioner who maintains good rapport with his or her patients lessens the chances of being sued. Patients do not want to sue people they like.
15. Remember "the golden rule" in minimizing the likelihood of malpractice claims. Do to your patients as you would like have done to you. Always do what is in the best interests of your patient's visual and general well-being.

CONCLUSION

The legal issues in contact lens practice are numerous and often complicated. By being aware of the importance of the legal ramification of contact lens patient care, the practitioner can initiate appropriate procedures to minimize the possibility of a legal dispute. The use of doctor–patient agreements, informed consent documents, prudent practice procedures, proper record keeping, and conformance to accepted legal standards will help avoid legal disputes with patients. Equally important, following these procedures will provide better patient care.

REFERENCES

1. Scholles JR. Malpractice: watch your step. *Rev Optom* 1986; 123:26.
2. Classe' JG. Optometrist's liability for contact lenses. *South J Optom* 1986;4:52–57.
3. Calamari JD, Perillo JM. *The law of contracts,* 4th ed. St. Paul, MN: West Publishing, 1998:1–21.
4. Classe' JG. Contractual considerations in contact lens practice. *J Am Optom Assoc* 1986;57:220–226.
5. Harris MG, Classe' JG. Contracts for contact lens patients. *Optom Manage* 1988;12:48–59.

6. Gardner BA, ed. *Black's law dictionary,* 7th ed. St. Paul, MN: West Publishing 1999:318–327.

7. Calamari JD, Perillo JM. *The law of contracts,* 4th ed. St. Paul, MN: West Publishing, 1998:23–118.

8. Calamari JD, Perillo JM. *The law of contracts,* 4th ed. St. Paul, MN: West Publishing, 1998:165–221.

9. Calamari JD, Perillo JM. *The law of contracts,* 4th ed. St. Paul, MN: West Publishing, 1998:247–267.

10. Calamari JD, Perillo JM. *The law of contracts,* 4th ed. St. Paul, MN: West Publishing, 1998:710–778.

11. Bailey NJ. The "service contract" debate. *Contact Lens Spectrum* 1988;10:17–21.

12. Harris MG, Dister RE. Informed consent in contact lens practice. *J Am Optom Assoc* 1987;58:230–236.

13. *Schloendorff v Society of New York Hospital,* 105 NE 92, 93 (NY 1914).

14. Classe' JG. Informed consent and contact lens practices. *J Am Optom Assoc* 1996;67:132–133.

15. Classe' JG. Avoiding liability in contact lens practice. *Optom Clin* 1994;4:1–12.

16. Keeton WP, Dobbs DB, Keeton RE, et al. *Prosser and Keeton on torts,* 5th ed. St. Paul, MN: West Publishing, 1984:33–66.

17. Schultz MM. From informed consent to patient choice: a new protected interest. *Yale Law J* 1985;95:219.

18. *Natanson v Kline,* 350 P2d 1093 (Kan 1960).

19. *Canterbury v Spence,* 464 F2d 772 (DC Cir 1972).

20. *Daum v Spinecare Medical Group,* 52 Cal App 4th 1285 (1997).

21. *Jambazian v Borden,* 25 Cal App 4th 835 (1994).

22. *Gates v Jensen,* 595 P2d 919 (Wash 1979).

23. *Johnson v Kokemoor,* 545 NW2d 495 (1996).

24. *Hidding v Williams,* 578 So2d 1192 (La Ct App 1991).

25. *Moore v Regents of the University of California,* 793 P2d 479 (Cal 1990).

26. *Arato v Avedon,* 858 P2d 598 (1993).

27. *Kaskie v Wright,* 589 A2d 213 (Pa Super Ct 1991).

28. *Albany Urology Clinic PC v Cleveland,* 528 SE2d 777 (2000).

29. Berg JW, Applebaum PS, Lidz CW, et al. *Informed consent: legal theory and clinical practice.* New York: Oxford University Press, 2001:41–74.

30. Rosoff AJ. *Informed consent: a guide for health care providers.* London: Aspen Systems Corp., 1981:75–185.

31. Rozovsky F. *Consent to treatment, a practical guide,* 3rd ed. Gaithersburg, MD: Aspen, 2000;1:1–2:41.

32. Classe' JG, Harris MG. Medico-legal complications of contact lens wear. In: Silbert J, ed. *Anterior segment complications of contact lens wear,* 2nd ed. Boston: Butterworth-Heinemann, 2000:511–533.

33. Rosoff AJ. *Informed consent: a guide for health care providers.* London: Aspen Systems Corp., 1981:33–63.

34. Kraushar M, Steinberg J. Informed consent: surrender or salvation. *Arch Ophthalmol* 1986;104:352–353.

35. Berg JW, Applebaum PS, Lidz CW, et al. *Informed consent: legal theory and clinical practice.* New York: Oxford University Press, 2001:75–129.

36. Berg JW, Applebaum PS, Lidz CW, et al. *Informed consent: legal theory and clinical practice.* New York: Oxford University Press, 2001:94–129.

37. Harris MG. Legal responsibilities when fitting minors with contact lenses. *Optometry* 2000;71:118–121.

38. Rozovsky F. *Consent to treatment, a practical guide,* 3rd ed. Gaithersburg, MD: Aspen, 2000;5:1–5:17.

39. Berg JW, Applebaum PS, Lidz CW, et al. *Informed consent: legal theory and clinical practice.* New York: Oxford University Press, 2001:188–207.

40. Rozovsky F. *Consent to treatment, a practical guide,* 3rd ed. Gaithersburg, MD: Aspen, 2000;12:1–12:16.

41. Morgan LW, Schwab IR. Informed consent in senile cataract extraction. *Arch Ophthalmol* 1986;104:4245.

42. Priluck IA, Robertson DM, Buettner H. What patients recall of the preoperative discussion after retinal detachment surgery. *Am J Ophthalmol* 1979;87:620–623.

43. Weissman BA, Mondino BJ, Pettit TH, et al. Corneal ulcers associated with extended wear soft contact lenses. *Am J Ophthalmol* 1984;97:476–481.

44. Wilson LA, Schilitzer RL, Ahearn DG. *Pseudomonas* corneal ulcers associated with soft contact lens wear. *Am J Ophthalmol* 1981;92:546–554.

45. Hassman G, Sugar J. *Pseudomonas* corneal ulcer with extended wear soft contact lenses for myopia. *Arch Ophthalmol* 1983;101:1549–1550.

46. Holden BA, Sweeney DF, Vannas A, et al. The effect of long-term extended wear contact lenses on the human cornea. *Invest Ophthalmol Vis Sci (Suppl)* 1984;25:192.

47. Weissman BA, Mondino B. Complications of extended wear contact lenses. *Int Eye Care* 1985;1:230–240.

48. McMahon T. Comments on the incidence of ocular complications from contact lens wear. *Int Eye Care* 1985;1:304–305.

49. Harris MG. Informed consent for presbyopic contact lens patients. *J Am Optom Assoc* 1990;61:717–723.

50. 45 CFR 46.116. 56 *Federal Register* 28012, 28022, June 18, 1991.

51. 21 CFR 50.27(a). 49 *Federal Register* 8951, January 27, 1981, as amended 61 *Federal Register* 57280, November 5, 1996.

52. Classe' JG. Release of contact lens prescriptions: an update. *J Am Optom Assoc* 1997;68:125–129.

53. Classe JG. Management of contact lens prescriptions. *Optom Clin* 1994;4:93–102.

54. Trade regulations rule on the advertising of ophthalmic goods and services. 16 CFR §456. 57 *Federal Register* 18822, May 1, 1992.

55. Fairness to Contact Lens Consumers Act, 15 U.S.C.: 7601–7610 (Dec. 4, 2003).

56. Contact Lens Prescription Release Act of 2001, HR 2663 IH (May 16, 2001).

57. Classe' JG. The impact of Eyeglasses II on contact lens practitioners. *Contact Lens Forum* 1987;12:26–29.

58. Classe' JG. Clinicolegal aspects of practice: optometrist's duty to release patient information. *South J Optom* 1987;5:9–15.

59. Sarver MD, Harris MG. A standard for success in wearing contact lenses. *J Am Optom Assoc* 1971;48:382–385.

60. Keeton WP, Dobbs DB, Keeton RE, et al. *Prosser and Keeton on torts,* 5th ed. St. Paul, MN: West Publishing, 1984:160–234.

61. Harris MG. Failure to advise. *J Am Optom Assoc* 1991 62:867–869.

62. Keeton WP, Dobbs DB, Keeton RE, et al. *Prosser and Keeton on torts,* 5th ed. St. Paul, MN: West Publishing, 1984:451–498.

63. Keeton WP, Dobbs DB, Keeton RE, et al. *Prosser and Keeton on torts,* 5th ed. St. Paul, MN: West Publishing, 1984:499–533.

64. Gabel W. Vicarious liability. *J Am Optom Assoc* 1987;58:599–601.

65. Reported in the *AOA News,* June 15, 1976.

66. Classe' JG, Harris MG. Liability and extended wear contact lenses. *J Am Optom Assoc* 1987;58:848–854.

67. Scholles JR. A review of professional liability claims in optometry. *J Am Optom Assoc* 1986;57:764.

68. Kenyon E, Polse KA, Seger RG. Influence of wearing schedule on extended-wear complications. *Ophthalmology* 1986;93:231–236.

69. Allansmith MR, Baird RS, Greiner JV. Vernal conjunctivitis and contact lens associated giant papillary conjunctivitis compared and contrasted. *Am J Ophthalmol* 1979;87:544.

70. Fichman S, Baker VV, Horton HR. Iatrogenic red eyes in soft contact lens wearers. *Int Contact Lens Clin* 1978;15:202.

71. Allansmith MR, Korb DR, Greiner JV, et al. Giant papillary conjunctivitis in contact lens wearers. *Am J Ophthalmol* 1977; 83:697.

72. Korb DR, Greiner JV, Allansmith MR, et al. Biomicroscopy of papillae associated with wearing of soft contact lenses. *Br J Ophthalmol* 1983;67:733.

73. Miller RA, Brightbill FS, Slama S. Superior limbic kerato-conjunctivitis in soft contact lens wearers. *Cornea* 1982;1:293.

74. Mondino BJ, Groden LR. Conjunctival hyperemia and corneal infiltrates with chemically disinfected soft contact lenses. *Arch Ophthalmol* 1980;98:1767.

75. Sendele DD, Kenyon K, Mobilia EF, et al. Superior limbic keratoconjunctivitis in contact lens wearers. *Ophthalmology* 1983;90:616.

76. Josephson JE, Caffery BE. Infiltrative keratitis in hydrogel lens wearers. *Int Contact Lens Clin* 1979;16:223.

77. Crook T. Corneal infiltrates with red eye related to duration of extended wear. *J Am Optom Assoc* 1985;56:698–700.

78. Polse KA, Sarver MD, Harris MG. Corneal edema and vertical striae accompanying the wearing of hydrogel lenses. *Am J Optom Physiol Opt* 1975;52:185.

79. Zantos SG, Holden BA. Transient endothelial changes soon after wearing soft contact lenses. *Am J Optom Physiol Opt* 1977; 54:856.

80. Swarbrick HA, Holden BA. Complications of hydrogel extended-wear lenses. In: Silbert J, ed. *Anterior segment complications of contact lens wear,* 2nd ed. Boston: Butterworth-Heinemann, 2000:273–308.

81. Schnider C. Rigid gas-permeable extended-wear lenses. In: Silbert J, ed. *Anterior segment complications of contact lens wear,* 2nd ed. Boston: Butterworth-Heinemann, 2000:309–328.

82. Sweeney DF, Holden BA, Vannas A, et al. The clinical significance of corneal endothelial polymegathism. *Invest Ophthalmol Vis Sci* 1985;23[Suppl]:53.

83. Zantos SG, Holden BA. Ocular changes associated with continuous wear of contact lenses. *Aust J Optom* 1978;61:418–426.

84. Holden BA, Sweeney DF, Vanna A, et al. Effects of long-term extended contact lens wear on the human cornea. *Invest Ophthalmol Vis Sci* 1985;26:1489–1501.

85. Adams CP, Cohen EJ, Laibson PR, et al. Corneal ulcers in patients with cosmetic extended wear contact lenses. *Am J Ophthalmol* 1983;96:705–709.

86. Hassman G, Sugar J. *Pseudomonas* corneal ulcer associated with extended soft contact lenses for myopia. *Arch Ophthalmol* 1983; 101:1549–1550.

87. Cohen EJ, Laibson PR, Arentsen JJ, et al. Corneal ulcers associated with cosmetic extended wear soft contact lenses. *Ophthalmology* 1987;94:109–114.

88. Wilson LA, Schlitzer RL, Ahern DG. *Pseudomonas* corneal ulcers associated with soft contact lens wear. *Am J Ophthalmol* 1981;92:546.

89. Krachmer JH, Purcell JJ Jr. Bacterial corneal ulcers in cosmetic soft contact lens wearers. *Arch Ophthalmol* 1978;96:57.

90. Lemp MA, Blackman J, Wilson LA. Gram-negative corneal ulcers in elderly aphakic eyes with extended wear lenses. *Ophthalmology* 1984;91:60.

91. Berger RO, Streeten BW. Fungal growth in aphakic soft contact lenses. *Am J Ophthalmol* 1981;91:630.

92. Margolies LJ, Mannis MJ. Dendritic corneal lesions associated with soft contact lens wear. *Arch Ophthalmol* 1983;101:1551.

93. Chalupa E, Swarbrick HA, Holden BA, et al. Severe corneal infections associated with contact lens wear. *Ophthalmology* 1987;94:17–22.

94. Mondino BJ, Weissman BA, Farb MD, et al. Corneal ulcers associated with daily wear and extended wear contact lenses. *Am J Ophthalmol* 1986;102:58–65.

95. Weissman BA, Remba MJ, Fugedy E. Results of the extended wear contact lens survey of the Contact Lens Section of the American Optometric Association. *J Am Optom Assoc* 1987;58: 166–171.

96. Classe' JG. Legal problems in contact lens practice. *South J Optom* 1980;22:28–35.

97. Keeton WP, Dobbs DB, Keeton RE, et al. *Prosser and Keeton on torts,* 5th ed. St. Paul, MN: West Publishing, 1984: 677–724.

98. Classe' JG. Clinicolegal aspects of practice: optometrist's liability for ophthalmic lenses: the law after polycarbonate. *South J Optom* 1986;4:36–43.

99. Based upon Sec 204 (a) of the Restatement of Torts, which may not be applicable in all jurisdictions. The various Restatements of the law, including the Restatement of Torts, are authored and published by the American Law Institute, an organization of judges, lawyers, and law scholars. The Restatements attempt to outline a particular field of the law in a clear and systematic way, and they may include what are essentially proposed changes to current legal doctrine that the drafting committee determines to be appropriate. A particular jurisdiction is under no obligation to follow the law as set forth in the Restatements, although some jurisdictions may incorporate all or part of a particular Restatement into their statutes.

100. *Barbee v Rogers,* 425 SW2d 342 (Tex 1968).

101. New review: patient sues Sterling. *B & L. Rev Optom* 1985; 122:3.

102. Classe' JG. A review of 50 malpractice claims. *J Am Optom Assoc* 1989;60:694.

103. Classe' JG. *Standards of practice for primary eyecare.* Columbus, OH: Anadem, 1998.

104. *Helling v Carey,* 83 Wash 2d 514, 519 P2d 981 (1974).

105. Harris MG, Classe' JG. Clinicolegal considerations of monovision. *J Am Optom Assoc* 1988;59:491–495.

106. Mandell RB. *Contact lens practice,* 4th ed. Springfield, IL: Charles C. Thomas, 1988:785–823.

107. Wood WW. Monovision does work. *Optom Manage* 1985;21: 49–50.

108. Back AP, Holden BA. Why aren't we prescribing contact lenses for the presbyope? Presented at the 6th International Contact Lens Congress, Broadbeach Gold Coast, Queenlands, Australia, October 9, 1987.

109. Sheedy JE, Harris MG, Busby L, et al. Monocular contact lenses and occupational task performance. *Am J Optom Physiol Opt* 1988;65:14–18.

110. Westin E, Wick B, Harrist RB. Factors influencing success of monovision contact lens fitting: survey of contact lens diplomates. *Optometry* 2000;71:757–763.

111. Multifocal use increases, practitioners confident. *Contact Lens Spectrum* 2001;17:7.

112. Brenner MB. An objective and subjective comparative analysis of diffractive and front surface aspheric contact lens designs used to correct presbyopia. *Contact Lens Assoc Ophthalmol J* 1994;20:19–22.

113. McGill, E, Erickson P. Stereopsis in presbyopes wearing monovision and simultaneous vision bifocal contact lenses. *Am J Optom Physiol Opt* 1988;658:619-626.

114. Back A, Woods R, Holden BA. The comparative visual performance of monovision various concentric bifocals. American Academy of Optometry Meeting Abstracts. *Am J Optom Physiol Opt* 1986;63:104P.

115. Sheedy JE, Harris MG, Busby L, et al. Monovision contact lens wear and occupational task performance. *Am J Optom Physiol Opt* 1988;65:14–18.

116. Sheedy JE, Harris MG, Bronge MR, et al. Task and visual performance with concentric bifocal contact lenses. *Optom Vis Sci* 1991;68:537–541.

117. Harris MG, Sheedy JE, Gan CM. Vision and task performance with monovision and diffractive bifocal contact lenses. *Optom Vis Sci* 1992;69:609–614.

118. McLendon JH, Burcham JO, Pheiffer CH. Presbyopic patterns and single vision contact lenses: II. *South J Optom* 1968;10:7–36.

119. Beddow RD, Martin JS, Pheiffer CH. Presbyopic patients and single vision contact lenses. *South J Optom* 1966;8:9–11.

120. Koetting RA. Stereopsis in presbyopes fitted with single vision contact lenses. *Am J Optom Arch Am Acad Optom* 1970;47:557–561.

121. Slaton P. Alternating vision system [Letter]. *Optom Weekly* 1973;64:255.

122. Christie N, Sarver MD. The effect on stereopsis of a unilateral contact lens add for presbyopes. In: *O.D. research reports.* Berkeley, CA: University of California, 1971.

123. Fonda G. Presbyopia corrected with single vision corneal lenses. In: Girard LJ, ed. *Corneal and scleral contact lenses.* St. Louis: CV Mosby, 1967:276–279.

124. Koetting RA. Monocular fitting: a viable alternative for the presbyope. *J Am Optom Assoc* 1982;53:134–135.

125. Wirt SE. A new near-point stereopsis test. *Optom Weekly* 1947;38:647–649.

126. Lebow KA, Goldberg JB. Characteristics of binocular vision found for presbyopic patients wearing single vision contact lenses. *J Am Optom Assoc* 1975;46:1116–1123.

127. Loshin DS, Loshin MS, Comer G. Binocular summation with monovision contact lens correction for presbyopia. *Int Contact Lens Clin* 1982;9:161–165.

128. Scholles JR. A review of professional liability claims in optometry. *J Am Optom Assoc* 1986;57:764–766.

129. Gold AR. Failure to warn. *J Am Optom Assoc* 1987;58:230–237.

130. Classe' JG. Optometrist's duty to warn of vision impairment. *South J Optom* 1986;4:66–69.

131. Holder AR. *Medical malpractice law.* New York: Wiley and Sons, 1975:132–174.

132. Harris MG. Legal implications of unapproved or unusual soft contact lens care. *Int Contact Clin* 1967;14:232–236.

133. Gower LA, Stein JM, Turner FD. Compliance: a comparison of three lens care systems. *Optom Vis Sci* 1994;71:629–634.

134. Dister RE, Harris MG. Legal consequences of the FDA's 7-day extended wear letter. *J Am Optom Assoc* 1980;61:212–214.

135. Harris MG. Legal responsibilities when fitting minors with contact lenses. *Optometry* 2000;71:118–121.

136. Classe' JG, Harris MG. Clinicolegal issues in contact lens practice. Presented at Optifair '87, New York, New York, March 17, 1987.

137. Scholles JR. Documentation and record keeping in clinical practice. *J Am Optom Assoc* 1986;57:141–143.

138. Classe' JG. Recordkeeping and contact lens practice. *Optom Clin* 1994;4:69–91.

139. AOA Eyecare Benefits Center. Good patient records: your keys to successful practice. *Optometry* 2001;72:7.

140. Medical records: retention and release. *Texas Med* 1981;77:78–80.

141. Harris MG, Thal LS. Retention of patient records. *J Am Optom Assoc* 1992;63:430–435.

142. Classe' JG. The impact of Eyeglasses II on contact lens practitioners. *Contact Lens Forum* 1987;12:26–29.

143. Classe' JG. Record-keeping and documentation in clinical practice. *South J Optom* 1987;5:11–25.

144. American Optometric Association. State statute and board rule reference to minimum patient examination requirements, April 15, 2002.

145. Classe' JG. Malpractice and optometry: a personal commentary. *South J Optom* 1987;5:26–31.

146. *Balle v Kazerian,* 135 Cal App 3d 426 (1982).

147. *Brown v Bleiberg,* 32 Cal 3d 426 (1982).

148. *Borderlon v Peck,* 661 SW2d 907 (Tex 1983).

149. Internal Revenue Code sec 6501; Income Tax Regulations sec 301.6501.

150. Health Insurance Portability and Accountability Act of 1996 (also known as the Kassebaum-Kennedy Act), Pub L No. 104–191, 110 Stat 1936 (1996) (codified in scattered sections of U.S.C.).

151. Mazlin R. The complexities of HIPAA and administration simplification. *Optometry* 2000;71:727–732.

152. Standards for the Privacy of Individually Identifiable Health Information; Final Rule. 45 CFR 160–164. 65 *Federal Register,* no. 250, December 28, 2000.

153. Sax JR. HIPAA privacy rules: what they are and what they mean for optometrists. *Optometry* 2001;72:529–530.

154. Sax JR, A question of privacy. *Optometry* 2001;72:531–540.

155. Standards for Privacy of Individually Identifiable Health Information, 45 CFR Parts 160 through 164.

156. Dister RE, Harris MG, Computerized optometric records and the law. *J Am Optom Assoc* 1989;60:56–58.

157. Roach WH, The Aspen Health Law and Compliance Center. *Medical records and the law,* 3rd ed. Rockville, MD: Aspen Systems Corp., 1998:44–59.

158. Berenato M. Keeping your patients' medical records—how long, O Lord? *Legal Aspects Med Pract* 1984;12:5–7.

159. Gage S. Alteration, falsification, and fabrication of records in medical malpractice actions. *Medical Trial Technique Quarterly 1981 Annual* 1981:476–488.

160. Ind Code Ann §§34–3-15.5–1 et seq (West Supp 1983).

161. 22 Cal Adm Code §70751(g).

162. *In re Jascalevich,* 182 NJ Super 455, 442 A2d 635 (App Div 1981).

163. *Valcin v Public Health Trust of Dade County,* 473 So2d 1297 (Fla 3d DCA 1984).

164. AMA Standards and Opinions 5.07.

ENVIRONMENT AND CONTACT LENS WEAR

ANTHONY P. CULLEN

THE OCULAR ENVIRONMENT

From birth, and even prior to birth, the eye finds itself in a potentially hostile environment. Hazards range from mechanical and physical to chemical and biologic. Fortunately, a number of natural defense mechanisms avert damage, and most eyes endure the siege and escape from being in a constant state of trauma or disease. The physical location of the globe within the orbit ensures that some protection is provided from larger, relatively slow-moving foreign bodies, while the overhang of the brow provides a natural shade from overhead solar radiation. The blink reflex, which is initiated by bright light, loud noise, or contact with the cilia, cornea, or conjunctiva, protects the cornea from many acute hazards. Spontaneous blinking, with its sweeping action toward the inner canthus coupled with the multifunction attributes of the normal tears, serves to maintain an optically uniform corneal surface, free from excessive debris, foreign matter, and pathogens. The corneal surface epithelium undergoes constant replenishment as old or damaged cells are sloughed into the tear film. Some stressful stimuli result in a partial closure of the palpebral fissure, whereas others result in excessive tearing; the former response serves to restrict access to the globe while the latter assists in the flushing of the conjunctival sac.

EFFECTS OF CONTACT LENS WEAR

Contact lens wear and associated solutions can adversely affect most of the structures of the anterior eye (1,2). The eyelids may develop blepharitis, abnormal blink patterns, an induced ptosis, or tarsal (meibomian) gland dysfunction. Conjunctival and limbal injection may occur, and variety or benign and more serious corneal responses may be observed.

The contact lens is an extraocular foreign body, whether its haptic is resting on the bulbar conjunctiva with the optic vaulting the cornea, it is clinging to the cornea and limbal conjunctiva, or it is floating in the precorneal tear layer. Its presence on the eye may induce a variety of changes in the ocular environment (3) that, in turn, produce the physiologic and in some cases pathophysiologic responses in the ocular tissues. The changes and responses include the following:

- Hypoxia (4–6)
- Tear chemistry and flow disturbance
- Hypoesthesia (7)
- Edema
- Altered immune response
- Increased susceptibility to infection

Although the initial manifestations may be asymptomatic and considered clinically insignificant, the possibility of infection always exists (as in a non–contact lens-wearing eye). The effects of relative hypoxia are well established, and some are reversible. These may be observed as conjunctival hyperemia and, in the cornea, as epithelial edema and microcysts; stromal edema and striae; and endothelial guttae, bedewing, blebs, and folds. Effects that may resolve only partially are hypoesthesia, stromal thinning, and polymegathism and pleomorphism. Neovascularization is irreversible because ghost vessels remain even when a normal oxygen environment is reestablished.

The presence of a contact lens, more commonly a soft lens with deposits, in contact with the tarsal conjunctiva can induce a hypersensitivity reaction (8) in the form of giant papillary conjunctivitis (GPC) (9,10). More specifically, the conjunctival response is termed *contact lens-associated papillary conjunctivitis* (CLPC).

All of the cornea's normal defense mechanisms against microbial invasion can be altered by contact lens wear, but this does not *per se* increase susceptibility to infection. The key factor contributing to infection in contact lens wearers appears to be corneal epithelial damage or disturbance produced by trauma, hypoxia, or toxicity.

RISK VERSUS PERCEIVED RISK

Because both contact lenses and certain environments or situations may produce adverse ocular effects, it is tempting to assume that a contact lens wearer is at greater risk in a hazardous environment because of presumed additive and/or synergistic effects. A simplistic approach has been to ban contact lenses in any situation where there is a perceived or actual risk to the eye without regard to all factors involved.

In risk assessment and management it is necessary to balance risk with benefits and to differentiate objectively a perceived risk from the actual risk. Obsessive and unrealistic risk avoidance with its accompanying overregulation and bans may reduce quality of life and productivity while contributing little to safety.

When considering the advisability of wearing contact lenses in a given environment or for a particular activity, a number of questions must be addressed (11):

- Is there an actual ocular hazard?
- Does the wearing of a contact lens place the eye at greater risk than a naked eye?
- Does the removal of a contact lens increase the risk to the eye or increase its susceptibility to insult?
- Is the risk different for various contact lens designs and materials?
- Are there associated risks for the contact lens wearer who removes lenses?
- Do contact lenses decrease other safety strategies?

MEDIA REPORTS, SAFETY BULLETINS, AND PARANOIA

A hazardous environmental situation in which there is limited well-documented research provides an ideal circumstance for the generation and dissemination of misinformation. In addition, zealous modification and embellishment of subsequent reports and bulletins frustrate the efforts of those attempting to defuse the resulting paranoia. The most widely circulated example of this phenomenon concerns the presumed "welding" of a contact lens onto the cornea of a contact lens wearer by an arc flash. Cordrey's excellent review of the history of this incident concluded with the hope that his "lengthy quotation will finally put this myth to bed" (12). Perhaps due to the limited circulation of his article and despite reiteration in the *British Medical Journal* by Kersley in 1977, his hope has not been fulfilled. Cordrey's investigations revealed a case in July 1967 in which a Baltimore shipyard steelworker reported sick with "corneal ulcerations." These were treated and vision returned to normal within 2 weeks, with no corneal scarring. Cordrey (12) provides more details of the story as follows. A welder at the Bethlehem Steel Corporation was plugging welding units into a 440-V service line when the electrical switch box "exploded." He was wearing contact lenses *and* industrial safety glasses. He had no immediate complaints following the incident and did not remove his contact lenses for at least 17 to 18 hours. The next day he was found to have large corneal "ulcerations." The two ophthalmologists who treated him were of the opinion (in retrospect) that the

electric flash played no part in the corneal injuries, which were due to contact lens overwear.

This appears to be the case cited by Novak and Saul in 1971 when they described the following scenario. "A steelworker opened a circuit breaker while wearing safety glasses over his contact lenses. The breaker arced and flashed. When the worker removed his contact lenses he took part of the corneas with them. Apparently the lenses concentrated the heat of the flash and burned the corneas." In August 1973, the case was elaborated in the *Journal of Occupational Safety and Health* (15) by the statement that the contact lens had conducted the heat of the arc flash to the cornea of the eye. The next month, *Oil and Gas Journal* (16) repeated the story with the additional comment that "electric arc flashes from short circuit can cause contact lenses to adhere to the cornea."

In 1975, an engineer with the Metropolitan Water Division (England) circulated a notice that described "a shipyard worker wearing safety glasses over his contact lenses when he opened a 240 volt box . . . the breaker arced and a flash occurred . . . . When he tried to take out his contact lenses large areas of dried cornea came off his eyes with them. Doctors were unable to save his sight. They found that the contact lenses had served to concentrate the heat of the arc flash on the cornea of the eye which was subsequently damaged" (17).

In 1982, an inquiry from Cullen et al. (18) to the National Safety Council (NSC) in Chicago concerning their frequently quoted publication drew the following response from the NSC's Supervisor of Industrial Hygiene: " . . . I must agree with you that some of the statements in the cited article may be inappropriate . . . our librarian failed to retrieve this particular article, possibly published by our editorial staff without consulting our technical personnel (many of our publications are written by outside volunteers) . . . . "

Cullen et al. (18) concluded that the condensing effect cited by Novak and Saul could not occur without a violation of a fundamental principle of physics. Heat generated in the contact lens would be dissipated by conduction, convection, and radiation; therefore, the residual heat absorbed by the corneal epithelium would be less than if no contact lens were worn.

Furthermore, the corneal damage of the type described by Novak and Saul is more characteristic of ultraviolet (UV) radiation exposure, and for this to occur the worker could not have been wearing UV-absorbing safety lenses. An infrared (IR) corneal burn produces symptoms and signs immediately. Regardless of repeated discreditation (19–22) of this "safety alert," based on one misquoted incident, it continues to resurface with ever increasing augmentation (Fig. 44.1) and with the addition of two "recent incidents" at Duquesne Electric and United Parcel Service (these incidents were circulated without verification that they actually occurred). More recent alerts are further expanded to claim

CASE HISTORY 2

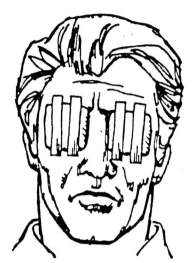

A MAN was wearing safety glasses over his contact lenses when he opened a 440-volt box to connect a welding cable. When the circuit breaker was opened, the breaker arced and a flash occurred. Later, when the man tried to remove his contact lenses, large amounts of dried cornea came off with each lens.

The contacts evidently served to concentrate the heat of the arc flash on the cornea of the eye.

Contact lenses should never be worn under safety glasses or in any area where an arc flash could occur.

FIG. 44.1. Typical example of an overstated safety bulletin.

that "the cornea of the eye was removed along with the lens resulting in PERMANENT BLINDNESS!" and that "the electric arc generates microwaves that instantly dry up the fluid between the eye and the lens, causing the cornea to be bonded to the lens, this trauma is painless." This claim is incredible and not physically, anatomically, or physiologically possible (23). Electric arcs do not generate significant levels of microwaves, and were they to do so they would not selectively heat the precorneal tear film. The work of Chou and Cullen (24) with Ontario Hydro measuring the output and ocular effects of arcing switches up to 27 kV and 340 A supports this statement. Additionally, our laboratory studies confirm that a contact lens-wearing eye is at no greater risk than a non–contact lens-wearing eye when exposed to suprathreshold levels of UV (25).

Although Cordrey thought that there was a mischievous element to the story, we have found that recirculation of the "Contact Lens Alert" usually is motivated by a genuine concern for worker safety, and retractions usually are issued when factual information is provided (26).

ENVIRONMENTAL FACTORS AND CONTACT LENS WEAR

In the assessment of the potential hazard of wearing contact lenses in a specific environment, it is useful to consider the effect of the various risk factors encountered, both on the eye and on the individual who is not wearing contact lenses. Once this is determined, the situation can be evaluated theoretically using the known physical parameters and physiologic effects of the contact lens. There may or may not be laboratory studies, epidemiologic data, or well-documented case reports to support or refute the theoretical conclusions.

CHEMICAL

The direct toxic effects on the eye of thousands of chemical substances and the secondary effects on the eye and visual system following ingestion, inhalation, or absorption through the skin and/or mucous membranes are readily located in textbooks of ocular toxicology (27,28) and general toxicology (29–31), agency publications (32–35), surveys in the literature (36), and relevant sites on the World Wide Web. The danger, when assessing an incident, is to assume that simply because the victim was wearing contact lenses that they were the causative or a contributing factor. There is a perception that chemicals may be trapped behind hard contact lenses or may be absorbed, concentrated, and released by soft contact lenses onto an already compromised cornea. Some safety bulletins actually claim, without providing documented evidence in support of their assertions, that contact lenses cause worse than normal burns from chemicals by holding the agent against the eye. In addition, it has been suggested that the presence of a lens in the eye would prevent adequate irrigation following a chemical injury. The basis for this appears to be a case report by Hedwig Kuhn (cited by Novak and Saul without a reference) in which a process engineer was conducting an experiment in an eye hazardous area wearing both contact lenses and safety goggles. Some 50% caustic splashed into his "eyes and face." The emergency bath was reported to have flushed the chemical from his face and partially from his eyes. It was claimed that some of the chemical pooled beneath the contact lens, causing "severe burns of the eye" before the contact lenses could be removed. The possibility of such an occurrence while a person is wearing safety goggles is highly questionable, yet cases such as this form the basis for claims that contact lenses have no place in any chemical laboratory.

TABLE 44.1. FORMS OF AIRBORNE MATTER

Substance	Distribution
Aerosol	Liquid droplets or solid particles dispersed in air that are so fine they remain dispersed for a period of time
Dust	Airborne solid particles 0.1–25 µm. Particles >5 µm do not remain airborne except in windy or turbulent environments
Fumes	Solid particles of material (~1 µm) formed by condensation from the gaseous state; fumes may flocculate and coalesce
Gas	Aeriform material that does not become liquid or solid at ordinary environmental temperatures
Mist	Liquid droplets 0.5 to <10 µm formed by condensation from gaseous or liquid state, by atomizing, foaming, or splashing (includes sprays)
Smoke	Carbon or soot particles <0.1 to 0.25 µm formed by the incomplete combustion of carbonaceous materials; also may contain other airborne materials
Vapor	Gaseous form of a solid or liquid substance formed following evaporation or volatilization

Fumes and Vapors

Noxious gases, vapors, fumes, aerosols, and smokes (Table 44.1) have the ability to seep behind inappropriate protective devices and directly affect the outer coats of the eye. The ocular response, as with other types of chemical injury, varies with the concentration and the physical chemical properties of the agent (Table 44.2). Highly toxic substances stimulate the protective mechanisms of blepharospasm and lacrimation, which limit access to the eye and dilute the concentration of the chemical, respectively. Avoidance may be initiated by a characteristic odor or stimulation of other parts of the respiratory tract. Insidious long-term exposure may produce a chronic conjunctivitis, possibly with a mild superficial keratitis, and it is unlikely that individuals subjected to such environments would wear contact lenses comfortably or would even have had them prescribed. A number of chemicals, which are inert toward ocular tissues, may act as lacrimogens while producing little or no detectable changes in the cornea or conjunctiva. Other vapors may produce a delayed response that manifests several hours after a symptomless exposure; the clinical signs include loss of epithelial cells, edema, and epithelial vacuoles. The ocular nasolacrimal route is insignificant relative to the respiratory route when considering systemic absorption of airborne toxins.

Many soft contact lens wearers have reported that they are able to peel onions without the usual excessive tearing, thus demonstrating protection by the lenses against the lacrimonogenic action of the allyl disulfides present in onions. Tear gases also tend to be insoluble in water, and soft contact lenses have been found to be effective in protecting the eye from the tear gas CS (ortho chlorobenzylidine malonitrile). Following their studies of the protection afforded by soft lenses against tear gas, Rengstorff (37) and Kok-van Alphen et al. (38) reported that the Special Patrol Guard of the Dutch Police (who are no longer required to wear gas masks) permitted the wearing of soft contact lenses during action with tear gas involvement.

It is improbable that the corneal response to volatile sub-

TABLE 44.2. CHEMICAL AND PHYSICAL PROPERTIES OF TOXIC AGENTS

Chemical	Exposure Limits (ppm)	MW	Solubility (%)	External Ocular Effects Reported
Acetone	750	58	Miscible	Rare
Ammonia	25	17	25	Irritation, corneal clouding, conjunctivitis
Bromine	0.1	160	3.5	Intense irritation
Carbon dioxide	5000	68	0.8	Corneal edema
Carbon disulfide	10	76	0.2	Rare
Chlorine	1	71	0.7	Stinging and burning
Chlorine dioxide	0.1	68	0.8	Possible corneal edema
Chloroacetophenone (MACE)	0.05	154	Insoluble	Stinging, involuntary lid closure, corneal exfoliation, scarring
Ethyl acetate	400	88	8.7	Conjunctivitis
Formaldehyde	1	30	Miscible	Irritation, lacrimation
Hexane	500	86	0.014	Rare
Hydrogen sulfide	10	34	2.9	Keratitis, haloes
Osmium tetroxide	0.0002	254	7	Keratitis, pain, photophobia, blepharospasm
Oxygen	10^6	32	3.16	None
Ozone	0.1	49	0.00003	Irritation
Sulfur dioxide	5	64	10	Rare
Trichloroethylene	100	131	0.1	Rare, conjunctivitis
Turpentine	100	136	Insoluble	Irritation
Xylene	1,000	106	0.00003	Keratopathy (?)

MW, Molecular Weight.

stances would be significantly affected by the wearing of a rigid contact lens, because these substances would be eliminated rapidly by tear flow; on the other hand, water-soluble gases and fumes and substances capable of binding to or being absorbed into soft lens materials would be expected to produce prolonged exposure, with the resulting more severe or chronic response.

Nilsson and Andersson (39) found that the uptake of trichloroethylene and xylene by high plus soft lenses, when suspended in 640 ppm and 700 ppm, respectively, was up to 90 times the uptake of physiologic saline. However, the release of the solvents into simulated tears was far less than the release into the air. They concluded that the absorption of these solvents by soft contact lenses is not as dangerous as previously thought and that the "vacuum cleaner" effect of the lenses would result in a lower concentration at the corneal surface than if exposed directly. LaMotte et al. (40) found similar results using ammonia.

Cerulli et al. (41) studied the effects of isopropanol and ethanol vapor, at the maximum levels recommended by the American Conference of Governmental Industrial Hygienists (ACGIH® International), on 38% water content hydroxyethyl methacrylate (HEMA) lenses. From their results, they extrapolated that these two vapors could pass through or bind to the contact lens surface, to be released later into the tear film. This was not confirmed *in situ*. They suggested that workers should "take care" when wearing hydrophilic contact lenses in such environments.

Using human subjects wearing "impermeable" contact lenses, Coe and Douglas (42) found that exposure to 50 ppm SO_2 produced no significant change in the level of tear production, whereas the production in unshielded control subjects increased by 83%. They reemphasized that although their results did not contraindicate the wearing of contact lenses in certain occupations, the necessity for stringent restrictions is less pressing if protective eyewear is worn.

Oily mist in the air can be adsorbed onto soft contact lenses and cause them permanent damage but can be washed off hard lenses (43). Actual chemical reaction of fumes with contact lens does not appear to be a major problem. Jenks (44) reported a case of an operating room nurse exposed to methylmethacrylate polymerization materials while wearing soft contact lenses who experienced discomfort and watering that necessitated the removal of her lenses. Sometime after removal, the lenses became hard, and one was so brittle that it cracked. It was assumed that the lenses had undergone a "chemical reaction." No mention was made of whether the lenses were in solution or left to dry out. Of more importance in this report is the fact that the discomfort, presumably caused by the fumes, forced the nurse to remove her lenses and no injury was suffered.

Chemical Splash

The accidental splashing of toxic chemicals into the eye is one of the most frequent causes of serious eye injury in the workplace and in other environments. More severe injury results from immersion or from spills of large volumes of liquid. Most commonly used organic solvents react only physically with external ocular tissues. Although this may result in the loss of corneal epithelium with accompanying severe discomfort, the stroma is unaffected other than by transient edema until reepithelialization is complete (Table 44.3). Detergents and surfactants may produce a similar response with far fewer symptoms. Prolonged exposure to hypertonic solutions or some volatile solvents may produce corneal epithelial desiccation (Fig. 44.2).

In 1966 Wesley (45) studied the effect of corrosive substances on eyes wearing polymethyl methacrylate (PMMA) lenses. The technique involved spraying and squirting 0.25 mL of varying percentages of H_2SO_4, NaOH, and creosol into the eyes of rabbits. The animals had been injected with an analgesic that spared the protective reflexes in order to permit protection by blinking. The results indicated that an eye without a contact lens was 1.8 times more likely to suffer total corneal opacity than an eye with a contact lens, and that the eye with a contact lens is more likely to be damaged if the lens is dislodged during the splash or subsequent irrigation. Similar protection by PMMA lenses

TABLE 44.3. INJURY RATING OF CHEMICAL SPLASH ON RABBIT CORNEA 24 HOURS AFTER SPLASH

Solvent	Injury Rating	Use(s)
Acetone	4	Solvent (pharmaceutical)
Alcohol (ethyl alcohol, anhydrous)	4	Solvent, disinfectant
Benzene	3	Solvent (resins), chemical manufacturing
Butyl alcohol (α-butanol)	7	Same as benzene
Cresols	5	Disinfectant, solvent
Dioxane	4	Solvent
Ether	2	Solvent, inhalation anesthetic
Ethyl acetate	2	Solvent
Ethylene glycol	1	Antifreeze
Gasoline	2	Fuel
Isopropyl alcohol	4	Antifreeze ingredient, solvent, after-shave lotions
Kerosene	0	Fuel, degreasing agent
Methanol (wood alcohol)	3	Solvent
Methyl acetate	5	Solvent
Sodium hydroxide (>1 molar)	10	Chemical manufacturing, petroleum refining, drain cleaner
Toluene	3	Chemical manufacturing
Turpentine	4	Solvent, polish base
Xylene	4	Solvent, chemical manufacturing

Most severe injuries are rated.
Ten rating values from Smyth et al. cited by Grant WM. *Toxicology of the eye,* 3rd ed. Springfield, MA: Charles C. Thomas, 1986, and Doughty MJ, *personal communication,* 1989.

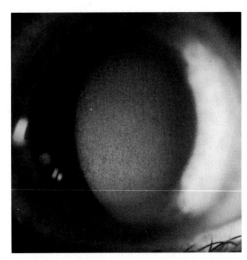

FIG. 44.2. Corneal epithelial desiccation due to prolonged exposure to a hypertonic solution.

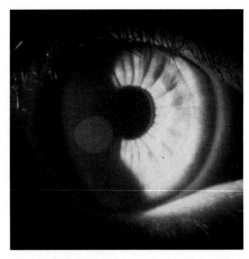

FIG. 44.3. Superficial corneal scar caused by and acid splash. Had the eye been wearing a contact lens, the drop of acid would have been diluted by the tears prior to reaching the cornea, and the scar would not have occurred.

against splashed 5% acetic acid, 0.5% n-butylamine, and 50% acetone was reported by Guthrie and Seitz (46). They found that the chemicals were not trapped behind the lenses; rather, the blepharospasm induced by the chemical irritation acted to tighten the lens against the cornea, creating a "barrier" effect.

These results do not suggest that contact lenses can be used as a substitute for protective eyewear, but they do emphasize that a contact lens wearer with appropriate protection is at no greater risk than a non–contact lens-wearing colleague. It is essential that workers in such situations be reminded that even the seemingly most trivial eye injury has the potential for disastrous results and that emergency procedures must be followed. Kingston (47) described an unfortunate incident where a worker did not irrigate his eyes after a chemical splash for fear of losing his contact lenses.

Caustic Substances

When splashed into the eye, concentrated acids and alkalis—with their extremes of pH—result in a rapid destructive response in the extraocular tissues and adnexa. If prompt emergency irrigation is not initiated, severe and permanent damage will result. Acids tend to be self-limiting (Fig. 44.3), whereas alkalis may rapidly disrupt, soften, and penetrate the cornea to involve the intraocular elements including the lens, retina, and uvea.

Nilsson and Andersson (39) evaluated the effect of strong alkalis and acids on the corneas of anesthetized rabbits wearing soft contact lenses. Neither type of soft lens provided any protection against 20% or 40% NaOH, but the lenses did not worsen the condition either. Leaving the lens on the eye for a minute or two did not make any significant difference. The protection provided by high plus lenses against the effects of 20% and 40% HCl was definite, reduc-

ing the corneal damage by about 75%. Dickinson (48) reported a case in which splashed boiling acid from a test tube produced a punctate burn on the cheek and presumably "pit marked" a corneal lens with no effects to the cornea.

MECHANICAL

Mechanical injuries to the eye result from contusion and concussion, foreign bodies (which may be superficial or perforating), exposure to atmospheric dust and particles, and wounds (which includes abrasions, cuts, and lacerations). These may occur as isolated incidents or in combination.

The incidence of different injuries depends largely on location, time, and circumstances. For instance, comparing Birmingham (United Kingdom) and Belfast (North Ireland), Roper-Hall (49) found that in both cities the major group of perforating eye injuries was classified as "childhood and domestic," with incidences that corresponded to similar data for major cities worldwide. On the other hand, probably due to the civil strife in Belfast, the assault injury group increased to 15% compared with 8% in Birmingham. It also could be derived from the data that an industrial worker in Birmingham had a similar chance of receiving a perforating eye injury to the "man in the street" in Belfast.

Contusion and Concussion

Contusion and concussion injuries to the eye can be classified into three groups (50): contusion, concussion due to tissue conduction, and concussion due to air conduction. Contusion injuries are caused by the direct impact of blows from blunt objects to external ocular tissues. Kicks, punches, and being struck in the eye by bats, sticks, racquets, balls, and a variety of other projectiles can result in ecchymosis, subconjunctival hemorrhage, corneal abrasion, epithelial and stromal edema, hyphema, angle recession, dislocated lens, rupture of various intraocular tissues, and retinal detachment. Rupture of the entire cornea is rare.

Concussion injuries are due to shock waves transmitted through the ocular or orbital tissues to a structure distant from the point of impact (the contra-coup effect). For example, a blow to the apex of the cornea may cause a posterior subcapsular cataract and damage the macular region. Explosions, such as may occur in the mining industry or from bombs, shells, or grenades, produce shock waves with wave velocities up to 7.5 k/ms at a pressure of 20,000 kPa; it is not surprising that the globe may be ruptured by such impact (51). It is reasonable to speculate that a haptic (scleral) contact lens would provide considerable protection from both contusion and concussion injury, whereas a thin high water content soft lens would offer little protection.

There are numerous cases in the literature describing the protection from blunt trauma provided by contact lenses. A patient fitted with PMMA microcorneal lenses was struck in the eye with a field hockey stick that fractured the lens. Despite ecchymosis, there was only slight staining of the cornea, and the patient was able to continue contact lens wear as soon as the replacement lens was available (52).

Brown (53) reported three instances of punches resulting in fracture of PPMA lenses in the eye where, despite severe lid lacerations, the minor trauma to the eye had recovered in days. No damage to deeper ocular structures was reported. Similarly, a school teacher wearing a fluid-type haptic lens was struck in the eye with such force that the lens was fractured into two pieces; the concussion from the impact was sufficient to produce conjunctival and internal hemorrhage. It was evident that the eye would have been lost but for the haptic lens (54).

Foreign Bodies

A superficial corneal foreign body is one of the most common minor ocular injuries. The symptoms of pain, foreign body sensation, and lacrimation are readily alleviated by simple removal of the offending particle. If a foreign body of suitable size, shape, and velocity impinges on the eye, it may penetrate into the cornea or sclera or actually perforate the globe. The energy levels of various missiles are given in Table 44.4. The protection of the cornea by a contact lens depends on the thickness and rigidity of the lens. Although foreign bodies may be trapped beneath rigid lenses (Fig. 44.4), this does not happen with soft lenses unless the speck is inserted with the lens.

Nilsson et al. (55) exposed the eyes of anesthetized rabbits wearing contact lens to showers of burning grit particles. They found that all particles rebounded from the surface of hard lenses, effectively protecting the covered part of the cornea. High and low water content soft lenses also offered

TABLE 44.4. APPROXIMATE IMPACT ENERGY LEVELS OF MISSILE INJURIES

Missile	Energy (J)
6.5-mm steel ball fired at 14 m/s (CSA)	0.11
15.9-mm (5/8-inch) steel ball, 127-cm(50-inch) drop (FDA)	0.20
25.4-mm (1-inch) steel ball, 127-cm (50-inch) drop (Z-87)	0.85
Pitched baseball (hard ball)	28.47
Thrown softball (home plate to second base)	23.05
Medium apple tossed 2 m	1.02
Volleyball (spike)	4.08–8.13
Human fist (punch)	2.71–5.42
Head to car dashboard, in 32 km/h crash	90.83
Gravel (4.5 g) 50 km/h	0.43
Gravel (4.5 g) 100 km/h[1]	1.74
Grinding wheel chips at 60 cm	1.0–40.0

From data supplied by John Davis and B. Ralph Chou.

some protection, but the lenses themselves were severely damaged. An occasional particle perforated a soft lens and damaged the epithelium superficially. Because their study simulated the use of a grinding wheel, the operation of which is usually brief, they believed that with normal eye protection the use of contact lenses would hardly involve any additional risk. Rather, the wearing of contact lenses under these conditions would provide additional protection for the cornea. Ritzmann et al. (56) confirmed that both rigid and hydrogel lenses provided additional protection of a porcine cornea from air-propelled iron particles (Fig. 44.5).

In order to approximate the condition of an eye hit by a larger sharp projectile, Nilsson et al. (55) fired a 22-mm-long, 1-mm-diameter metal projectile from an air gun. Their results for high water content lenses confirmed the opinion of Highgate (57) that a soft lens offers no protec-

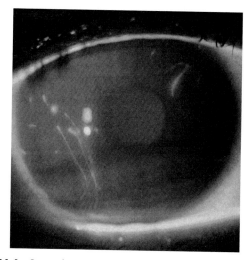

FIG. 44.4. Corneal scratches due to a foreign body trapped beneath a rigid contact lens. (Courtesy of Dr. Debbie Jones.)

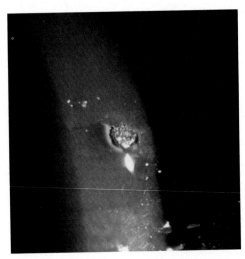

FIG. 44.5. Airborne iron foreign body embedded in a hydrogel contact lens. The underlying cornea was undamaged.

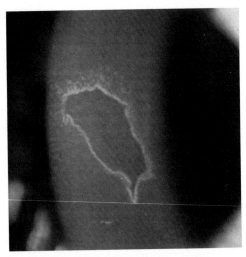

FIG. 44.6. Corneal abrasion caused by the edge of a sheet of paper. A contact lens would have provided some protection.

tion. Surprisingly, low water content lenses significantly increased the energy required for corneal perforation (32 mJ vs 21 mJ for an eye without a contact lens). Hard lenses shattered when energy levels reached 8.3 mJ; splinters of plastic entered the cornea, thereby introducing a complicating factor. In this study the muzzle of the gun was placed only 6 mm from the contact lens, and the incidence was normal to the surface. Thus, 16 mm of the projectile remained in the barrel at time of contact, ensuring constant force yet preventing deflection. It is improbable that trauma such as this could occur frequently. Although corneal laceration by a contact lens is rare, O'Rourke (58) reported a case in which fragments of a PMMA lens became embedded in the corneal stroma following a shattered windshield impacting the eye. It was concluded that the stress broke the lens before the cornea was perforated.

Cohen (59) describes a case where a corneal lens patient was attempting to reduce the length of a screw using a hammer and chisel. The screw broke and flew into his right eye. The lens was badly fractured, but the eye sustained only a slight central abrasion. Had the lens not been present, the eye probably would have been perforated. In a similar accident, an aircraft riveter was struck in the eye with a rivet. There was a gouge out of the lens with no damage to the eye (E.J. Fisher, *personal communication*, 1989).

Atmospheric Dust and Particles

Subjects wearing soft contact lenses, who worked in an environment moderately contaminated with metal particles and oil droplets, were followed for a period of 2 years (60). At no time were there any signs of damage to the eye, and there were no subjective complaints. It is evident that soft contact lenses can be worn safely in environments that may appear hazardous on cursory inspection and may still contraindicate the use of hard lenses.

Abrasions and Lacerations

Grazing the corneal surface with a finger nail, sheet of paper (Fig. 44.6), or other small object results in loss of the epithelium down to the basement membrane. Contact lens overwear and lens manipulation by less than dexterous patients also may result in abrasions. Penetration deeper than this may be considered a laceration. Lacerations of the cornea may be partially penetrating or penetrating, with the latter frequently complicated by iris prolapse and/or ocular lens damage. These injuries usually are caused by accidents or assaults involving sharp objects such as knives, scissors, chisels, glass, or flying metal.

The presence of a rigid lens could be expected to provide some protection, depending upon the direction of the offending impact, whereas a soft lens would offer little resistance to a sharp object. Dickinson (48) described a road traffic accident that resulted in an incision by broken windshield across the brow and cheek. Corneal lenses were removed in the emergency department. He speculated that spectacles would have increased the risk to the eye in this case.

HYPERTHERMIA

High environmental temperatures such as those encountered in smelting industries have both systemic and local effects that tend to be reversible. Severe disfiguring and debilitating burns result from direct contact with flashes, plasma, flames, hot bodies, or liquids. The response of the cornea and conjunctiva to exposure to, or direct application of, heat varies with temperature and duration (61). Mild superficial burns, with only epithelial clouding or possibly some erosion, heal without scarring within 48 hours (62). Hoffman and Krug (63) heated rabbit corneas in hot water for 1 to 2 minutes and found that 47°C produced corneal clouding, stromal edema occurred at 65°C, and the endothelium was involved at 80°C. Such exposures are unlikely to be encountered by the worker or in the home. Temperatures in excess of 1,000°C produced immediate tissue destruction with loss of the eye (64). Sequelae to less devastating burns include corneal leukomata, traumatic keratopathies, anterior staphylomata, and pseudopterygia. It is evident that no type of contact lens would have any effect on the severity of high temperature burns; haptic or soft lenses may offer slight protection to the critical limbal region in moderate burns.

The air temperature in a sauna may rise as high as 80°C to 100°C without affecting contact lens wear (65). If the sauna is the dry type, evaporation of the tear film and drying of soft contact lenses may be partially avoided by increasing the blink rate.

HYPOTHERMIA

Exposure to low environmental temperatures may be experienced at extreme northern or southern latitudes, at high altitudes, or in occupations associated with refrigeration. The presence of highly vascular adnexa and uvea have a warming effect that protects the cornea from freezing in most situations. Even following severe chilling, superficial corneal damage has been found to be reversible (66). Laboratory studies (67) using temperatures as low as −190°C produced disruption of the cornea, including Descemet membrane, yet the cornea returned to clinical normality within weeks. Local damage to the cornea caused by a liquid nitrogen splash has shown a similar pattern of recovery. Rapid cooling, such as may occur at high altitudes, coupled with wind chill, may result in dry gangrene followed by necrotic sloughing of the lids and globe. Temperature falls of about 10°C per 1,500-m increase in altitude to a minimum of −50°C.

Corneal epithelial damage has been reported in cross-country skiers in still conditions with a temperature of −16°C. Sédan (68) described interpalpebral striae, "needles," and epithelial blisters following 8 hours of exposure to cold and wind. There is an anecdotal report that Zeiss contact lenses (glass) used by German pilots in World War I did not become iced (69). A Royal Air Force test pilot, exposed to wind and a temperature of −20°C noticed no visual impairment, wearing haptic contact lenses. Modern contact lenses, which are much thinner and in closer proximity to the cornea, would be expected to provide less protection than sealed haptic lenses.

Socks (70) fitted rabbits with rigid (PMMA) contact lenses and exposed them to temperatures of −28.9°C with winds up to 125 km/h (78 mph) for 3-hour periods. He found no effects of cold or contact lenses in 85% of the eyes; the remainder showed only a mild keratitis that cleared

within a few hours. No histologic abnormalities attributable to the cold were detected. Socks concluded that rabbits wearing contact lenses in extreme cold suffered no acute deleterious effects to the eye and believed that contact lenses may be acceptable and even offer protection to eyes from wind-driven ice and snow in cold environments.

RADIATIONAL

Electromagnetic radiation (EMR) is composed of oscillating magnetic and electrical fields with a spectrum (Fig. 44.7) extending from extremely low frequency (1–10 Hz), through radio frequencies, microwaves, optical radiation, and γ radiation to cosmic radiation with frequencies in excess of 10 Hz. For a given waveband of EMR to exert an effect on a given tissue, it must be absorbed by the tissue or, in some instances, adjacent tissues. The effects occur by three mechanisms: thermal, photochemical, and ionizing. The final response may be a combination of more than one effect. The thermal effect occurs when sufficient radiant energy is absorbed at a rate quicker than it is dissipated in the tissue, resulting in temperature rise above a physiologically acceptable level. Very rapid absorption of high radiant energy levels may result in photomechanical, photoacoustic, or photoablative effects. Photochemical damage is wavelength dependent and occurs when incident photons are absorbed and alter molecular structure; in the cornea, photochemical effects have a latency period of less than 24 hours. Ionizing damage occurs when the incident radiant energy has a frequency capable of splitting the constituent molecules in a cell into ions.

The absorption characteristics of a contact lens will determine whether the lens will provide any protection. These have been thoroughly examined for the optical wavebands (71–74), and it has been assumed that contact lens materials are radiotransparent outside of these and immediately adjacent (extremely high frequency [EHF] and soft x-ray) bands. There is no scientific rationale supporting the notion that a contact lens is capable of concentrating any waveband of EMR onto the cornea.

Infrared

IR radiation occupies that band of the EM spectrum between 780 nm (the upper limit of the visible spectrum) and 1 mm. It is divided into three regions: infrared-A (URA) (780–1,400 nm), infrared-B (IRB) (1,400–3,000 nm), and infrared-C (IRC) (3 μm–1 mm). The apparent arbitrary division between URA and IRB was chosen because 1,400 nm is the limit of IR reaching the retina in the normal eye (75). When absorbed by a tissue, IR is converted into heat and the response is nonspecific. The effect of IR absorption in the skin ranges from the feeling of warmth to third-degree burns. The ocular effects of IR irradiation are due

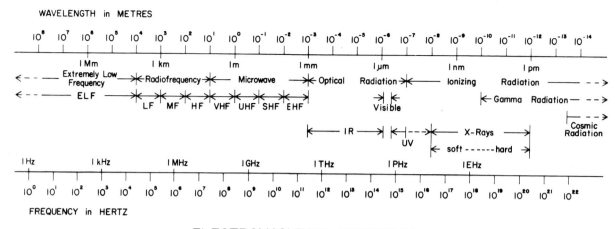

FIG. 44.7. Electromagnetic spectrum indicating the location of the various wavebands by wavelength and frequency. EHF, extremely high frequency; ELF, extremely low frequency; HF, high frequency; IR, infrared; LF, low frequency; MF, medium or moderate frequency; SHF, super high frequency; UHF, ultrahigh frequency; UV, ultraviolet; VHF, very high frequency.

to either direct heating of a structure or indirect heating from adjacent structures or fluids. The high prevalence of cataracts in blacksmiths and glass blowers was recognized in the 17th century, and the literature on this subject has been reviewed by Lydahl (76). The historical description of these cataracts was that of a posterior subcapsular variety (77) and was attributed to the direct effect of the IR on the lens, although a possibility of a systemic hydration contribution also was recognized. Laboratory studies produced anterior subcapsular opacities, and Goldmann (78) believed that these were secondary to heating of the posterior iris in apposition to the anterior lens capsule. More recent investigators have been unable to produce damage to the lens with incoherent IR and have supported Goldmann's hypothesis (79).

In the workplace, irradiance levels range from essentially zero to 100 to 600 mWcm^2 in the glass industries to 250 to 1,000 mWcm^2 in the steel industries. Direct solar IR irradiance is approximately 60 mWcm^2. Pitts and Cullen (79) found that at IRA irradiance levels greater than 3.5 Wcm^2, acute damage was related to the rate of delivery. During this study, they reported that IR caused drying of the outer eye with a reflex lid closure. Corneal damage increased with radiant exposure from epithelial haze to epithelial exfoliation with stromal involvement. Aqueous flare and miosis were noted before there was any biomicroscopic evidence of epithelial damage. Their damage threshold data are given in Table 44.5 and may be compared to the estimated maximum daily doses for glass and steel workers of 2.25 kJcm^2 and 1.75 kJcm^2, respectively (76). Lydahl (76) concluded that the effect (i.e., cataract) of chronic exposure to IR was not apparent until after age 60 years. It is clear that rapid drying of the corneal surface will result in immediate discomfort or pain, closure of the eyelids, and evasive eye and head movements, prior to any serious damage occurring.

IR heaters used in the motor industry for drying paint produce very little or no visible light. Lövsund et al. (80) found that the unanesthetized eye of a conscious rabbit shut or partially closed when exposed to an IR heater. If the eye was kept open, the temperature of the corneal surface rose to approximately 44°C whether or not a soft HEMA-type lens was worn. In experiments in which the eyes were kept open, they found that the lenses dried completely, became deformed, and fell from the eye. We have observed the same phenomenon. No epithelial lesions resulted from exposure to the IR heater while individuals wore contact lenses. Similar results were found in other studies involving welding arcs (81); complete protection from this effect was provided by the use of an appropriate welding filter.

Welders, furnace workers, and other personnel in environments rich in IR (and UV) often are exposed to arcs while they are not using protective equipment. If soft contact lenses are worn, they dry and become more adherent to the cornea. Instillation of a few drops of wetting solution will accelerate rehydration. This must occur before any attempt is made to remove the lenses.

Visible Radiation (Light)

Visible levels that are hazardous to the retina and particularly the fovea are uncomfortable to look at, and the blink

TABLE 44.5. INFRARED RADIANT EXPOSURE FOR ACUTE DAMAGE (kJ/cm^2)

	Cornea		
Rabbit (2.3–2.9 W/cm)	5.5	4	4
Monkey (4.2–4.9 W/cm^2)	8	8	10

Derived from Pitts DG, Cullen AP. Determination of infrared radiation levels for acute ocular cataractogenesis. *Graefes Arch Clin Exp Ophthalmol* 1981;217:285–297.

reflex (~0.1 s) and other aversion responses act to protect the normal eye. However, individuals do look at hazardous sources such as the sun (especially at the time of an eclipse), arcs, and lasers. Regardless of whether such exposures are accidental or intentional, the result may be transient or permanent loss of function in the region exposed. The hypothesis that visible light damage to the retina is always thermal has been shown to be erroneous by Harwerth and Sperling (82), Lawwill et al. (83), and Ham et al. (84,85). Blue light is several orders of magnitude more hazardous to the retina than IR. Pitts et al. (86) exposed rabbits for extended periods of time to light from "cool white" fluorescent tubes at a distance of 20 cm. They found mild damage to the corneal epithelium and endothelium and the lens. Eight hours of exposure produced mild retinal edema, whereas 20 hours resulted in photoreceptor damage. However, when their findings are placed in perspective, it can be concluded that fluorescent lights as used in the office and other workplaces are not hazardous.

Contact lens wearers frequently complain of increased photophobia when wearing their lenses. The reasons for this are evasive. The light incident on the cornea can be calculated, using the Fresnel equation, to be only approximately 8% higher than with spectacle lenses. This increase is insignificant when the dynamics of retinal adaptation are considered and is unlikely to be the causative factor.

Most contact lens wearers suffer from a slight increase in corneal thickness, presumably due to edema. Is this edema sufficient to create sufficient scatter to degrade the retinal image sufficiently to produce veiling glare? Results of contrast sensitivity function studies (87–94) are inconclusive. Dumbleton (95) and Cullen found no significant differences in contrast sensitivity among wearers of spectacle lenses, UV-absorbing contact lenses, and non–UV-absorbing contact lenses under laboratory conditions. However, subjects wearing UV-absorbing lenses reported a significant ($p < 0.05$) increase in visual comfort and a decrease in glare in snowy conditions on sunny days. This suggests that when the ratio of ambient UVA to visible light is high, ocular lenticular fluorescence is sufficient to produce veiling glare and photophobia.

Ultraviolet

UV radiation usually is divided by photobiologists into three bands: UVA, which extends from 315 to 400 nm and is less likely to produce acute ocular damage; UVB, which ranges from 280 to 315 nm and is responsible for sunburn and photokeratoconjunctivitis; and UVC, which ranges from 200 to 280 nm and is even more damaging to the corneal epithelium. UV below 200 nm bridges the gap between the ionizing and nonionizing regions of the EM spectrum. Most UV below 200 nm is absorbed by oxygen to form ozone, which in turn absorbs UV up to 280 nm. This accounts for the absence of the more hazardous UV wavebands from the solar spectrum as measured at terrestrial altitudes (Fig. 44.8). Exposure levels of UV from industrial

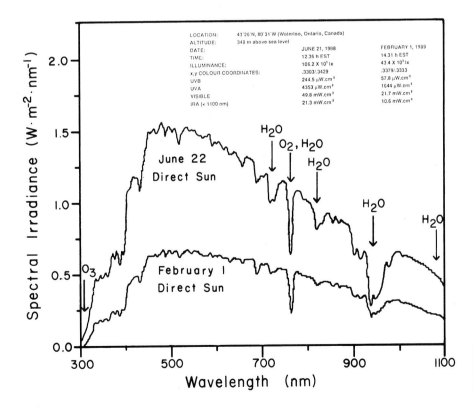

FIG. 44.8. Solar spectral irradiance as measured at Waterloo, Ontario, Canada in winter and summer. Principal atmospheric absorption bands are indicated.

arcs and other manmade sources may be orders of magnitude greater than solar UV.

In recent years, it has become increasingly apparent that the effects of UV are much more insidious and detrimental to the eye and vision than had been suspected previously. The effects may be acute (usually after a latent period), long term after an acute exposure, or chronic following long-term exposure to levels of UV below those required for acute effects.

Exposure of the eye to suprathreshold levels of UV (Fig. 44.9) (96) results in photokeratoconjunctivitis (photokeratitis, snow blindness, arc eye, photophthalmia). The symptoms of extreme pain, photophobia, blepharospasm, profuse tearing, and reduced visual acuity usually are far more dramatic than the actual corneal damage, which consists of loss of superficial corneal epithelial cells, autolysis of wing cells (97), and total desquamation of the central corneal epithelium at higher radiant exposures. Cullen observed that vision appeared clearer during the latent period, possibly due to reduced epithelial scatter as superficial cells are lost.

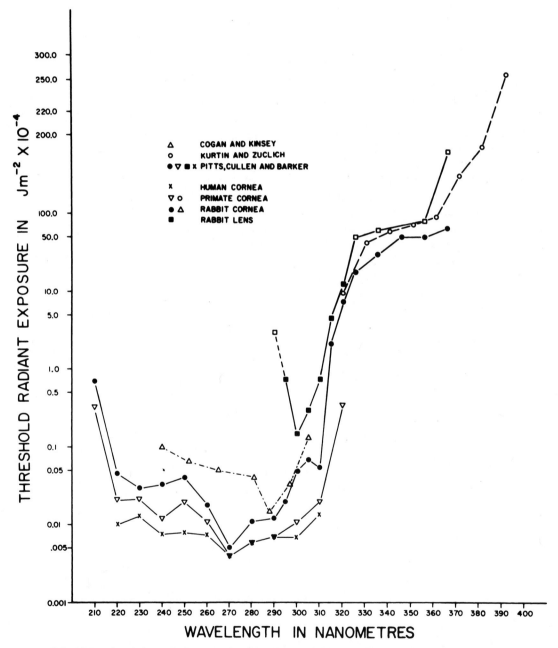

FIG. 44.9. Ultraviolet action spectra for the rabbit, monkey, and human cornea and the action spectrum for acute cataractogenesis in the rabbit. (Modified from Pitts DG. Ocular effects of radiant energy. In: Pitts DG, Kleinstein, RN, eds. *Environmental vision: interactions of the eye vision, and the environment.* Boston: Butterworth-Heinemann, 1993:151–220, with permission.)

Within the same time frame, corneal sensitivity decreases (98). Damage to the epithelium and endothelium (99,100) results in corneal swelling and loss of transparency. In common with other types of corneal insult, there is a secondary response in the anterior uvea with resulting aqueous flare. Electron microscopic studies have revealed that the keratocytes also are damaged but the basement membrane of the corneal epithelium and Descemet membrane are spared (97, 101). The cornea appears resilient to this type of damage and returns to clinical normality within days. Some patients complain of photophobia following the resolution of photokeratitis, and this may be related to endothelial damage. Laboratory studies have indicated that even a single just-suprathreshold dose of UVB may produce structural and functional damage to the endothelium, which is evident at 1 year and probably longer after exposure (102).

Chronic exposure to environmental UV is believed to be a major factor in the etiology of droplet keratopathy (103–108) and may be responsible for early onset of some other age-related changes in the cornea. Other retrospective epidemiologic studies suggest that UV is a major factor in the development of pterygium (109). It has been found that the prevalence of pterygium increases more than 10% in equatorial regions. In more temperate zones, the prevalence appears to correspond to outdoor exposure to sunshine coupled with certain occupations (e.g., farming). Pingueculae show some similar pathologic changes to pterygia (110, 111), and because they occur in exposed areas of the conjunctiva, UV may be a factor in their development (112).

Pitts et al. (96) were able to produce acute anterior subcapsular cataracts with single exposures as low as 0.75 Jcm^2 of narrow-band UV between 295 and 320 nm (Fig. 44.6),

providing support to the earlier work of Bachem (113). He found that repeated high doses of UV between 293 and 313 nm were cumulative and cataractogenic. Studies using UV lasers have demonstrated that permanent cataracts can result from a single high radiant exposure to coherent UV longer than 290 nm at exposure levels comparable to those used for incoherent (nonlaser) studies (114–116).

The effects of chronic exposure to UVA (and perhaps UVB) at ambient environmental levels have been implicated in the development of age-related cataracts. Geographic and interoccupational epidemiologic studies have shown that cataracts occur more frequently in individuals exposed to higher levels of solar UV (117–120).

Fortunately, very little UV radiation reaches the retina of the phakic eye except in the very young. However, aphakes and babies are potentially susceptible to the damaging effects of UV on the retina.

The need to protect ocular tissues from excessive exposure to UV using appropriate ophthalmic and industrial absorptive glass and plastic materials is generally accepted and well understood (121–123). The recurrent warning of the hazard of wearing contact lenses in the workplace prompted evaluation of the absorptive properties of contact lenses (18,71,72), and it was found that most contact lens materials provided little protection from UV (Fig. 44.10). As a result, rigid and soft contact lenses were developed that offer various levels of protection from UV according to the absorption characteristics of the incorporated UV absorber and the thickness of the lens (Fig. 44.11). Chou et al. (124) derived protection factors for a number a UV-absorbing contact lenses that exhibited transmittance windows within the UV spectrum.

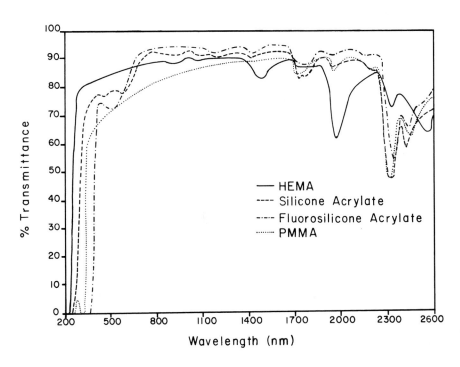

FIG. 44.10. Spectral transmittance of contact lenses.

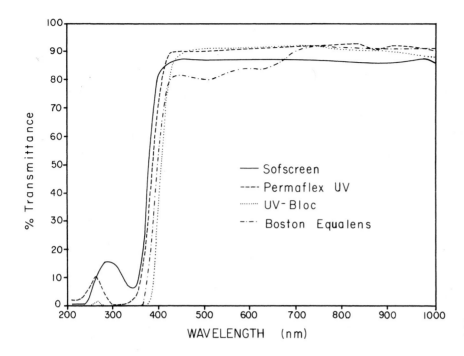

FIG. 44.11. Spectral transmittance of ultraviolet-absorbing contact lenses.

Pitts and Lattimore (125) showed empirically that when a soft contact lens, which absorbed all incident radiation of the experimental waveband, was placed on the eye, it provided complete protection of the cornea. These clinical findings were confirmed histologically (126). Cullen et al. (127) confirmed that consideration of the optical absorption characteristics of a given lens, and the related protection factors, may be used to predict the protection offered by a given

lens. They also found that a UV-transmitting soft lens increased the UVB threshold (of the rabbit cornea) minimally, but at suprathreshold radiant exposures there was no difference in the clinical response between a cornea wearing the lens and that without a lens. This strongly suggests that an individual who is accidentally exposed to UV while wearing soft contact lens is at no greater risk than the non-contact lens wearer. Evaluation of the protection afforded by a UV-

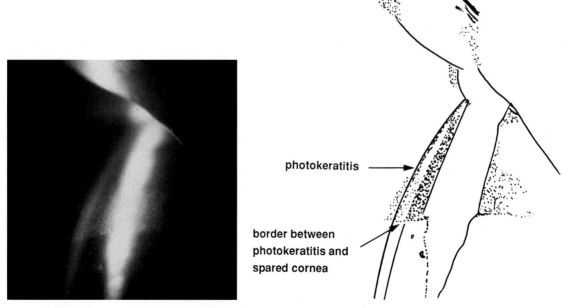

photokeratitis

border between photokeratitis and spared cornea

FIG. 44.12. Rabbit cornea 24 hours after exposure to 0.75 J/cm² of UVB while wearing a rigid gas permeable UV-absorbing contact lens. Epithelial granules and haze can be seen above an arc of demarcation indicating the position of the contact lens during irradiation.

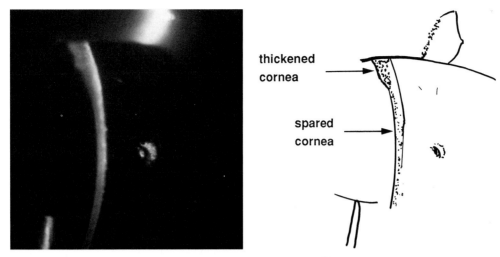

FIG. 44.13. Rabbit cornea 24 hours after exposure to 1.00 J/cm² of UVB. Local edema and corneal thickening result from epithelial and endothelial damage to region not of UVB protected by the rigid gas-permeable UV-absorbing contact lens.

absorbing rigid gas-permeable (RGP) lens revealed that the area of the cornea covered by the lens during irradiation was spared while the exposed areas of the cornea and conjunctiva were damaged (Figs. 44.12 and 44.13) (128).

Ahmedbhai and Cullen (129) found that there was a dramatic difference in the nature of the response to UVB between eyes adapted to RGP lenses and control eyes. The adapted eyes showed less superficial damage and more "granules." They argued that because adapted eyes may have lost fragile superficial squamous epithelial cells (130,131), the deeper wing cells were subjected to more radiant exposure (Fig. 44.14). They also found that corneal swelling was less after irradiation in eyes that had been wearing contact lenses. Despite these differences, the rates of recovery and recovery times were similar for both groups, suggesting that

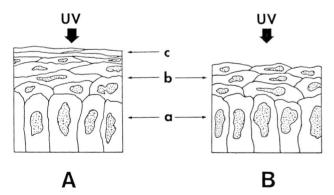

FIG. 44.14. A: Rabbit corneal epithelium of a non–contact lens-wearing eye. Because the superficial epithelium is present, UV energy is absorbed by these cells, as well as by the wing cells, resulting in more stippling and less granules. **B:** Rabbit eye corneal epithelium of a contact lens-wearing eye. UV energy is absorbed mainly in the wing cells because no superficial epithelium is present. This resulted in less stippling and more granules. a, basal cells; b, wing cells; c, superficial epithelium.

a worker exposed to UV irradiation after removing contact lenses would be incapacitated no longer than a similarly exposed non-contact lens wearer.

Microwaves

The principal effects of microwaves on ocular tissues *in situ* are vibrational and rotational at the molecular level, thereby producing a thermal response. Distribution and absorption of microwave radiation is dependent on its wavelength, the size and shape of the total structure (or subject), and the chemical nature of the tissue irradiated. EHF and super high frequency (SHF) produce superficial injury to the cornea and adnexa, and even ultrahigh frequency (UHF) damage is confined to the anterior segment. For cataractogenic effects in the anesthetized rabbit, radiant exposures of 90 to 720 Jcm² are required (132). In alert animals or humans, the heating effect of EHF to UHF radiation produces an avoidance response prior to the occurrence of serious damage. Aurell and Tengroth (133) reported retinal damage due to microwaves, but this has not been substantiated by other researchers. In other retrospective studies of microwave workers and age-matched controls, no correlation between cataract and occupational exposure has been confirmed (134). No microwave damage to the eye has been reported in workers wearing contact lenses. One may reasonably speculate that the superficial heating effect on high water contact lenses would result in drying similar to that produced by IR. Theoretical considerations also negate the possibility of microwaves welding a contact lens to the cornea or selectively evaporating the precorneal/sublens tear layer.

Lasers

It has been demonstrated that the transmittance of laser light by ocular media corresponds to the transmittance of

TABLE 44.6. LASERS INCLUDING THOSE USED FOR LASER COAGULATION AND ABLATION

Laser	Wavelength (nm)
Argon (Ar)	477,488,515
Carbon dioxide(CO$_2$)	10,600
Carbon monoxide (CO)	4,800–800^2 (many lines)
Excimer	
ArFl	193
KrFl	248
XeFl	350
Gallium arsenide (GaAs)	850,905
Helium neon (HeNe)	633
Krypton (Kr)	647, 676, 867
Neodymium:yttrium aluminum garnet (Nd:YAG)	1,065
Ruby	695–1,100

incoherent light of the same wavelength (135). Thus, transmittance (absorptance) studies of the human eye can be used to predict the action of a laser on a given ocular tissue or if it reaches the structure (136–138). Similarly, the absorptance data for contact lenses can be used to determine whether a given lens contributes to eye protection.

The high absorption by the anterior corneal structures of UV shorter than 290 nm and IR beyond 1,400 nm results in lasers of sufficient power, e.g., excimers, CO, and CO$_2$, photoablating or burning the cornea. Neodymium:yttrium aluminum garnet (Nd:YAG) and argon lasers have the ability to damage intraocular structures, intentionally or unintentionally (139). Argon, krypton, HeNe, and ruby laser light will reach the retina (Table 44.6 and Fig. 44.15), and some are used for laser coagulation of the retina and other structures. Intraocular lenses have been damaged during laser capsulotomy. Most contact lens materials will absorb incident excimer, CO, or CO$_2$ laser radiation, but the power would disintegrate the lens.

Ionizing Radiation

Ionizing EM radiation, so called because of its ability to split molecular bonds to form ions or charged particles, extends from 100 nm down to 3×10^{-14} m and includes all types of x-ray and γ radiation. Due to high energy levels, the effects of ionizing radiation are best considered using quantum field theory. Ionizing radiation also exists in particulate forms, including electrons, protons, fast and slow neutrons, and α particles. The effects of ionizing EM radiation and ionizing particulate matter are similar for given energy levels and tissue penetrance. Due to the variety of radiation units and the unreliability, and in some cases irrelevance of dosimetric methods, the Health Protection Branch of Health and Welfare Canada recommended in 1979, when practical, an immediate conversion to the International System of Units (SI) radiation units. Unfortunately, many publications and regulations still use non-SI units. The obsolete but commonly used unit of biologic

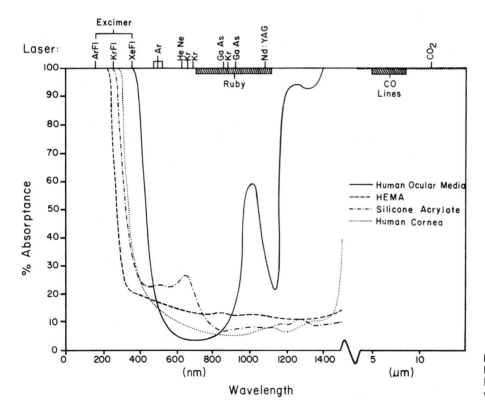

FIG. 44.15. Absorptance curves for human ocular media and contact lenses showing their relationship to various clinical and other lasers.

effect of radiation is the "rem" (radiation equivalent in man), which represents the effect of one rad (0.01 J/kg) of x-ray or γ radiation at 200 keV in human tissue; the SI unit is the sievert (Sv) or the biologic effect produced by one gray (Gy) (1 J/kg) of absorbed dose of 200 keV of x-ray or γ radiation. The former unit of irradiance, the roentgen (R), is replaced by the coulomb per kilogram (C/kg), where 1 C/kg ~ 3,876 R.

Soft x-rays and α particles have low penetrance, producing damage to the superficial corneal and conjunctival epithelia with associated hypoesthesia, hyperemia, and edema similar to the response to UVC but with a longer latent period. Any contact lens would provide some protection against such irradiation and against low-energy β radiation. Higher-energy β radiation may damage corneal epithelium and endothelium, resulting in corneal edema. This radiation requires more than 1 cm of lucite or 1.5 mm of lead for protection. X-rays, γ radiation, β radiation, and neutrons are potentially cataractogenic with a characteristic long latent period (6 months to several years), which is inversely proportional to dose yet inversely proportional to age. The typical ionizing cataract is posterior, subcapsular, and peripheral; it may or may not progress to involve the whole lens. Radiation exposure as low as 5 Gy or 0.15 C/kg of certain ionizing radiation may produce damage. Because of cumulative somatic and genetic effects, exposure guidelines usually are expressed on the basis of weekly or annual exposure ranging from 50 mSv/year for workers to 1 mSv/year for school children. Therapeutic γ radiation and x-rays used in and around the eye require appropriate protection for the lens; this may be in the form of a lead haptic lens or a molded shell with a lead button glued to the front surface. Although at 25 KeV only 1-mm thickness of lead is adequate, a 5-mm button usually is used.

BAROMETRIC PRESSURE

The interest in the effects of hypobaric, hyperbaric, and rapidly changing atmospheric pressure environments has increased with the desire of many to wear their contact lenses at high altitudes, when flying, and during a variety of underwater activities.

Bennett (140) concluded that soft hydrogel lenses are preferable for divers and that they can be used "with care" by experienced divers for sports and commercial diving. Because of the potential hazard from *Pseudomonas aeruginosa,* which apparently thrives on the inside walls of pressure chambers, contact lenses should not be permitted for saturation diving(140).

It has been suggested for some time that the reason for discomfort among some air travelers wearing contact lenses is the effect of low atmospheric pressure resulting in relative hypoxia (141–143), although the pressure in a modern commercial aircraft corresponds to a modest 2,000 to 3,000

m of altitude. In decompression chamber experiments, Castrén (144) noted corneal changes in soft contact lens wearers that were not seen in control subjects after 3 hours. Habitual (haptic type) contact lenses wearers have been reported to consistently develop bubbles under their lenses when they are subjected to simulated altitudes in excess of 5,400 m (145).

Five climbers on the British 1975 assault on Mount Everest were fitted with continuous wear soft lenses (146). Two wore their lenses for more than 50 days up to an altitude of 7,925 m with no observed corneal problems. The other three reverted to their glasses for reasons other than discomfort or corneal problems. It should be noted that in an avocation such as mountain climbing, the rate of decompression is, of necessity, slow. On the other hand, despite adherence to standard decompression schedules, it is not unusual for divers wearing hard contact lenses to complain of ocular discomfort, halos, and decreased acuity immediately after decompression. These symptoms may persist for several hours. Simon and Bradley (147) evaluated the effects of decompression on two divers wearing PMMA lenses exposed to a depth of 45.5 m (150 ft) in a hyperbaric chamber for 30 minutes. They noticed the formation of small bubbles beneath the hard lenses at 21 m (70 ft) en route to the stop point of 9 m (30 ft); these coalesced as the "surface" was approached. No bubbles formed in the precorneal tear film if no contact lenses were worn, if soft lenses were worn, or if the PMMA lenses were fenestrated centrally. The bubbles disappeared after 30 minutes at sea level, leaving "nummular patches of corneal epithelial edema." These lesions, presumed secondary to the trapping of nitrogen (148) between the epithelium and the hard lens, persisted for up to 2 hours. In a study of the effect of altitude, Simon and Bradley (149) noted no bubble formation in an ascent to a simulated 11,277 m (37,000 ft). At this altitude, a few minute bubbles appeared in the tear layer. These did not coalesce and disappeared within 10 minutes without inducing any symptoms.

Similar studies have shown that bubbles also occur under hydrogel lenses and RGP lenses during decompression from a hyperbaric environment (Fig. 44.16) (150–152). The degree of bubble formation and subsequent corneal insult was less than with PMMA lenses. Some subjects reported that the lenses were more comfortable after reaching the bottom and during decompression than on the surface. Socks et al. (151) found that no type of lens was displaced during dives and suggested that it is relatively safe for military and sport divers to wear contact lenses in lieu of the cumbersome modifications otherwise necessary to the diving mask.

Brennan and Girvin (153) reported that rapid decompression of subjects (2,438–11,582 m) produced no bubble formation in either soft contact lenses or the cornea. Although recognizing the potential hazards for the aircrew, they believed that soft contact lenses would be beneficial to young myopes flying fast jet aircrafts. This opinion is

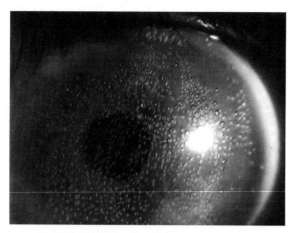

FIG. 44.16. Nitrogen bubbles trapped between the cornea and contact lens following decompression. (Courtesy of Dr. Robert Straff.)

supported by the results of Eng et al. (154), whose tests at simulated altitudes of 6,096 and 9,144 m used supplementary oxygen. No lenses were dislodged. No bubbles formed in or under the soft lenses. Some subjects did report that their eyes were dry and tired. Their findings are contradicted by Castrén et al. (155), who concluded that the additive effect of hypoxia and low atmospheric pressure produced ocular symptoms. Although their studies were conducted at a simulated altitude of 4,000 m, their soft contact lens subjects suffered from corneal erosions and stromal opacities. It is interesting and perhaps relevant that their experiments were carried out at a relatively high humidity.

Flynn et al. (156) and Strath (*personal communication, 2002*) have verified that the physiologic responses of the cornea to soft contact lens wear (e.g., corneal thickening) are greater at high altitudes. Despite this, the former researchers concluded that soft contact lenses can be worn while individuals fly military aircraft, thus supporting the 25 years or more of experience of pilots in the Swedish and other air forces (157).

VIBRATIONAL STRESS

Vibrational stress may be encountered while operating machinery such as pneumatic drills or chain saws, or while traveling in or on modes of transportation ranging from low-capacity motor cycles to aerospace vehicles. Whereas the symptoms associated with low-frequency oscillation usually are attributed to vestibular disturbance, more rapid vibration will reduce acuity depending on frequency and compensatory or associated involuntary head and eye movements. Coermann (158) found variation among subjects for ranges of frequency producing maximums in the reduction of visual acuity with frequencies beyond 140 Hz having no influence on vision. Byrnes (159) claimed that vibrations

of approximately 40 Hz caused resonance of the eyeball producing severe visual impairment. Based on an evaluation of many published studies, Hornick (160) concluded that 10- to 25-Hz vibration is most detrimental to overall visual performance. It is evident from these early studies that the nature, waveform, direction, and magnitude of vibration are contributing factors to visual degradation. Other factors that also must be considered are illumination, type of visual task, and whether it is also vibrating at the same or another frequency. Considering the relative stability of a contact lens and its closer proximity to the nodal points of the eye, one might anticipate less visual disturbance for the contact lens wearer than the spectacle lens wearer, especially for higher refractive corrections. Brennan and Girvin (153) vibrated subjects, who were wearing conventional flying spectacles or soft contact lenses, sinusoidally at frequencies from 2 to 32 Hz. Snellen acuity was impaired at 6 and 8 Hz, but no significant difference between the two methods of correction occurred. No contact lens was dislodged during these experiments.

ACCELERATION STRESS

When stationary, the body is subjected to a gravitational force (G) that would produce a downward acceleration of 9.8 ms. Linear acceleration and centrifugal (radial acceleration) stresses usually are expressed in terms of G. The direction of the force is designated relative to the principal axes of the body; a force from head to feet is positive ($+G_z$). Positive G_z forces produce ptosis and sagging of soft tissues coupled with blanching of the face and conjunctiva. A similar vascular draining response affects the retina and brain, resulting in peripheral field loss, loss of vision ("grayout"), and ultimately unconsciousness. Conversely, negative G_z forces produce increased cranial vascular pressure and an associated throbbing headache, confusion, and coordination problems. Conjunctival hemorrhages may be produced but, despite the possibility of visual "redout," consciousness is retained.

It has been speculated that high G forces would cause a contact lens to dislodge from the cornea. To evaluate this hypothesis, Brennan and Girvin (153) subjected volunteer Royal Air Force (RAF) aircrew to $+4 G_z$ and $+6 G_z$ for 20-second periods while wearing two types of soft lens (50% and 75% water content). They found that the maximum downward displacement of any lens was only 1.5 mm at $+4 G_z$ and 1.75 mm at $+6 G_z$. Tightly fitted lenses remained central regardless of the G forces. Any reduction in vision observed during these studies were due to retinal ischemia rather than displacement of the contact lenses. Similar results for RGP lenses have been reported by Dennis et al. (161); positive G_z forces of $+3$, $+4$, $+6$, and $+9$ caused all lenses to decenter downward along the z-axis with a maximum decentration of 2 to 3 mm at the highest $+G_z$.

Acuity was not affected adversely. Jet fighter pilots may be exposed to acceleration forces of up to +12G for brief periods during combat maneuvers, yet soft contact lenses have been worn successfully under these circumstances. Hart (162) speculated that the zero gravity of space flight would have little negative effect on the cornea-to-contact lens relationship and proposed that continuous wear contact lenses would be suitable for ametropic mission specialists. During long-term flight on Solyut-7 and on the Mir orbital stations, an ametropic crew member wore a soft contact lens for 5-hour periods without problems, thus confirming that contact lenses can be used during space flight (163).

ULTRASOUND

Ultrasonic irradiation of the cornea at 3 W·cm^2 produces transient corneal haze and swelling, whereas higher levels of irradiance result in corneal leukomata formation (164) and chorioretinal burns (165). It is doubtful that an individual would be subjected to these levels of ultrasound accidentally, because such levels are achieved by direct application of a transducer to the cornea or via a coupling medium. Clinical ophthalmic ultrasound in the frequency range from 8 to 10 MHz produces an irradiance level of approximately 5 mW·cm^2. The presence of a contact lens on the eye will affect the ultrasonogram in accordance with the acoustic impedance and absorption of the lens material. No increased risk is created. There have been no reports of corneal damage resulting from airborne ultrasound (166).

COMPUTERS AND VIDEO DISPLAY TERMINALS

The introduction of the computer into the workplace in the form of the video display terminal (VDT) or video display unit (VDU) created problems and concerns. In addition to the expected visual and other symptoms associated with prolonged visual tasks and concentration, the initial lack of consideration of the overall working conditions, design of workstations, lighting, characteristics of the display, and task scheduling aggravated the symptoms and concerns. Attention to a variety of psychological, physical, and ergonomic factors (Table 44.7) has aided in alleviating many of the problems associated with VDT use.

Initially there was considerable concern that, based on perceived radiation hazards, the VDT was a health hazard. Cataracts, recurrent corneal erosions, miscarriages, birth defects, and skin rashes all have been attributed to VDT use. In common with many electrical and electronic conveniences of modern life, the computer is capable of producing a broad spectrum of EMR (Fig. 44.17). Extensive and repeated measurements have shown that the emission levels are far below international safety limits (Table 44.8) (167–177). There has not been one substantiated report of any type of radiation damage among millions of VDT workers (178). The levels of UV emitted by VDTs has been a specific concern of some workers; our measurements (Table 44.9) indicate that, in an average office, a VDT will increase UVA irradiance of the user by only 20%, and the provision of UV protection is not necessary. Banning of smoking in the workplace is far more appropriate for the protection of VDT workers (and their fetuses) than shields, screens, and lead aprons.

It also is evident that the level of UVA is so low, relative to overall illuminance, that it would not produce sufficient lenticular fluorescence to induce veiling glare or visual discomfort (179). The consensus among most VDT researchers is that tinted lenses are neither indicated nor contraindicated for use with VDTs, and that any subjective improvement probably is due to the placebo effect (180).

The VDT user who wears contact lenses has less surface reflections and perhaps fewer of certain spectacle lens aberrations. These advantages are offset by a number of potential disadvantages. Myopic wearers require a presbyopic addition earlier. Some practitioners are willing to ignore residual refractive errors, especially low levels of astigmatism, despite findings that they may contribute to VDT user discomfort (181–185). Similarly, problems of binocularity may be con-

TABLE 44.7. FACTORS AFFECTING COMFORT AND EFFICIENCY WHILE USING A VIDEO DISPLAY TERMINAL

Psychological	Ergonomic	Physical
Adaptation stress	Working position	Fatigue
Motivations and interest	Heights	Musculoskeletal
Monotony	Viewing angles/distances	Refractive status
Familiarity with task	Workload	Binocular status
Change in routine	Lighting	Pregnancy
Job satisfaction	Heat levels	
Machine authority	Humidity levels	
Irritability	Noise	
Anxiety	Terminal design	

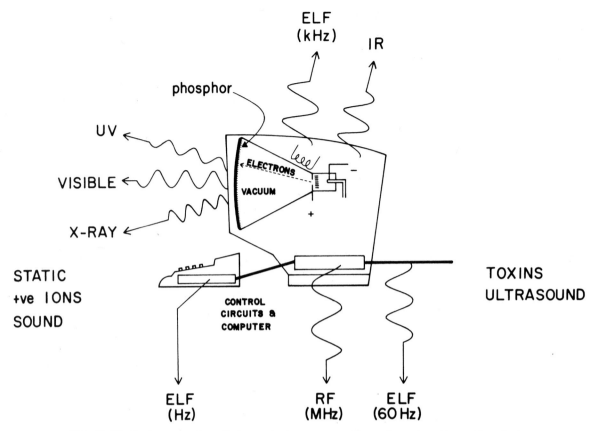

FIG. 44.17. Electromagnetic radiation and other suggested hazards produced by a video display terminal.

TABLE 44.8. RADIATION GENERATED BY VIDEO DISPLAY TERMINALS

Waveband	Occupational Exposure Standard	
	Emission	Recommendation or Guideline
X-ray (> 10 keV)	0.003 mR.h^{-1}	0.5 mR.h^{-1} [a]
Far UV (200–320 nm)	1.25 × 10^{-4}μ W.cm^{-2}	0.1 μ W.cm^{-2} [b]
Near UV (320–400 nm)	1.8 × 10^{-2}μ W.cm^{-2}	1 mW.cm^{-2} [b]
IR (700 nm–4.1 μm)	2 × 10^{-3}mW.cm^{-2}	10 mW.cm^{-2} [b]
Microwave, E-field (10 MHz–10 GHz)	7.26 × 10^{-9}mW.cm^{-2}	1.5 mW.cm^{-2c}
RF and LF, E-Field (1 kHz–10 MHz)	1.3 × 10^{-5}mW.cm^{-2}	(10,000; 100; 1 mW.cm^{-2})[b]
HF and LF, H-field (1 kHz–10 MHz)	3.03 × 10^{-5}mW.cm^{-2}	(10,000; 100; 1 mW.cm^{-2})[b]
RF and microwave, E-field (10 MHz–2.45 GHz)	<0.5 mW.cm^{-2}	(5; 1 mW.cm^{-2})[c]
RF, H-field (10–300 MHz)	<0.05 mW.cm^{-2}	1 mW.cm^{-2} [c]
LF and RF, E-field (10 kHz–200 MHz)	<1 V.m^{-1}	(600; 60 V.m^{-1})[b]
Static, E-field (<1 Hz)	<1 kV.m^{-1}	10 kV.m^{-1b}

[a] Federal Regulation
[b] Provincial Recommendation (Ontario)
[c] Federal Safety Code
( ), Two or more values indicated change of guideline within range given at left.
<, Emission too small to be measured with instrument with sensitivity limit indicated.
HF, high frequency; IR, infrared; UV, ultraviolet.[3]
Adapted from Wohlbarsht ML, O'Foghludah FA, Sliney DH, et al. Electromagnetic emission from visual display units: a non-hazard. In: Non-ionizing radiation. Proceedings of an AC-GIH Topical Symposium, Washington, DC, November 26–28, 1979, pp 193–201; and Muc AM. Video display terminals: do they emit dangerous levels of radiation. *Occup Health Ontario* 1987;8:182–199, with permission.

TABLE 44.9. TYPICAL ULTRAVIOLET IRRADIANCE LEVELS

Type of Source	UVB (280–315 nm)	UVA (315–400 nm)
Video display terminal	<1 pW.cm^{-2}	6×10^{-7} mW.cm^{-2}
Ambient in office (fluorescent lighting)	0.1×10^{-5} mW.cm^{-2}	3×10^{-6} mW.cm^{-2}
Direct sunlight (midday June, Waterloo, Ontario)	0.2 mW.cm^{-2}	4.4 mW.cm^{-2}
Recommended standard	<1 µW.cm^{-2}	1 mW.cm^{-2} [a]

[a] *2002 TLVs® and BEIs® threshold limit values for chemical substances and physical agents. Biological Exposure Indices. Cincinnati, OH: ACGIH International, 2002.*

veniently considered insignificant. VDT tasks requiring concentration may reduce the blink rate, which in turn will reduce lens movement and increase drying effects.

COMMERCIAL BUILDING ENVIRONMENT

In offices where the poor quality of the air is contributing to the *sick building syndrome,* it is logical to anticipate that some of the factors involved, such as temperature, relative humidity, air movement, CO_2 levels, and airborne pollutants (Table 44.10), would adversely affect contact lens wear.

HUMIDITY

Based on climatic chamber experiments, Lövsund et al. (186) concluded that there are no risks for contact lens users in environments with high relative humidity. They also found no differences in adhesion for either hard or soft lenses between environments with relative humidities of 21% and 97%, respectively. The work of Andrasko and Schoessler (187) and Brennan et al. (188) indicates that temperature and humidity are not important factors for contact lens wearers, except in situations where the environment is very dry.

However, the comfort and performance of very thin high water content contact lenses are susceptible to changes in humidity. This type of lens dries and distorts, thereby contributing to corneal desiccation in conditions of low relative humidity(189). Hood (190) reported on a high water content (67.5%) lens that was not as affected by high altitude and low humidity as other high water content lenses. It should not be overlooked that non-contact lens wearers, especially those with dry eye syndromes, also experience increased symptoms under conditions of low humidity.

TABLE 44.10. POTENTIAL FACTORS CONTRIBUTING TO POOR INDOOR AIR QUALITY

Ventilation	Plants
Improper exchange rate	Pollen
Contaminated intake/ductwork (dust, pollen, bacteria, fungi)	Fungi
Poor filtration	Insects
Temperature extremes	Insecticides/fungicides/herbicides
Humidity extremes	Standing water
Carbon dioxide buildup	People
Low oxygen levels	Body odor
Odors	Perfume/cologne
Flooring/Carpeting/Furniture	Tobacco smoke
Potential microbial or chemical reservoir	Skin particulates
Volatile organic chemicals	Transmittable diseases
Asbestos tiles	Computers/Copiers/Printers
Poorly sealed concrete	Ozone
Ceilings	Volatile chemicals
Fiberglass	Particulates
Asbestos	Electromagnetic fields
Vermiculite	Heat buildup
Mold	Miscellaneous
Bacteria	Air freshners
Dust	Cleaning products
Paints/Stains	Sewage gas
Volatile chemicals	Water leaks (mold, mycotoxins, fungi, bacteria)
Lead (pre- 1978 paint)	Carbon monoxide
Preservatives/fungicides	Exhaust fumes
Flaking	Rodents/insects/avians (byproducts, odors, pathogens)
Aerosols	

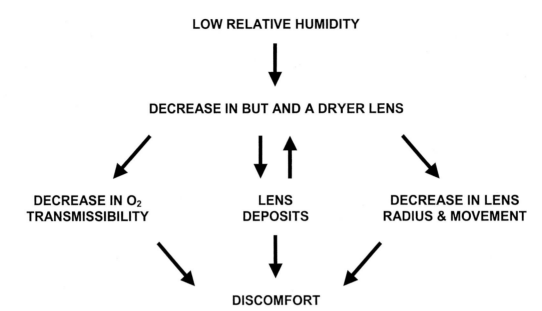

FIG. 44.18. Possible scheme for the relationship between low relative humidity and ocular discomfort in contact lens wear. (Suggested by Nilsson SEG, Andersson L. Contact lens wear in dry environments. *Acta Ophthalmol* 1986;64:221–225.)

The optimum humidity range for comfort is between 40% and 60%. Eng et al. (191) suggest that, during air travel, where cabin humidity may drop to 11% within 30 minutes of takeoff, humidity is possibly more significant than other environmental factors in contributing to the discomfort of soft contact lenses while flying.

Nilsson and Andersson (192) noted a relationship between discomfort, tear breakup time (TBUT), lens deposits, and low relative humidity (Fig. 44.18). They concluded that the discomfort was more prominent in a relative humidity less than 25% or when lens deposits were present in a relative humidity of greater than 40%. Subjects with lens deposits and a short TBUT on a soft contact lens were particularly sensitive to low relative humidities. Factors that may be responsible for the discomfort include decreased hydration of the surface of the lens, which decreases TBUT and oxygen transmissibility (193), an increase in lens deposits, and a tightening of the lens with decreased movement. Useful strategies in improving comfort in dry environment are frequent lens replacement, "loose " fitting techniques, and use of enzymatic cleaners (194).

FLYING

The environment encountered while flying varies with the type of aircraft, from relatively low-altitude recreational craft through commercial to high-performance combat planes.

The main environmental factors that influence contact lens wear, for passengers and crew alike, include low humidity, hypobaria, low partial pressure of oxygen in the cabin,

and the possibility of pathogens recirculating in the air. The symptoms produced vary from a sensation of dryness to red, uncomfortable, and possibly infected eyes.

Beverages containing alcohol or caffeine exacerbate dryness, as do certain medications (195). Soft lenses, especially high water contact lenses, tend to create more dryness, and the lens dehydration may reduce oxygen supply to the cornea. Appropriate lens care may not be used because of the lack of suitable facilities. If lenses are worn while flying, factors that may aggravate or create discomfort should be avoided. Practical advice can be given to air travelers wearing contact lenses who experience symptoms (Table 44.11).

Civilian pilots were not allowed to fly with contact lenses until 1976. Dille and Booze (196) determined that civil aviation airmen wearing contact lenses had less than average accident involvement. Since that time, contact lens materials and designs have evolved significantly while aircraft cockpits have enjoyed even more sophisticated advances. How-

TABLE 44.11. ADVICE FOR CONTACT LENS WEARERS IN DRY PRESSURIZED CABINS

Thoroughly cleans lenses before commencing air travel
Be aware of reduced tear production due to alcohol and coffee
  consumption
Read only in intervals and remember to blink
Do not sleep or nap in the lenses (unless extended wear)
Use lubricating drops during the flight
Remember that long flights increase the possibility of lens
  dehydration
If discomfort persists, remove the lenses
Carry an up-to-date pair of spectacles

ever, many of these have increased the complexity of the visual tasks involved. Nakagawara et al. (197) found that the prevalence of contact lens use by civilian airmen was about 3% in 1997 and that the vast majority of aviators find contact lenses beneficial in the cockpit environment. They concluded that, applied appropriately, contact lens use can continue as a safe alternative for pilots but caution that some types of lens, including bifocals and monovision, may be prohibited. Therefore, prescribers and dispensers should be aware of current regulations in their jurisdiction.

The use of contact lenses is particularly attractive to military pilots because of their many advantages over spectacles when contact lenses are worn with breathing systems and communication devices. Lenses have been found to be operationally superior to spectacles under combat conditions (198).

WIND

Wind can be expected to have two effects in the eye: drying and stimulation of tearing. Following a study of military helicopter pilots, Crosley et al. (199) found that 61% of their subjects experienced a drying effect of direct air currents on their soft contact lenses. Similarly, some firefighters have experienced no drying of their extended wear contact lenses while riding the tailboard at speeds up to 80 km/h (200), whereas others noticed that their lenses dried out.

AIR POLLUTION

Manmade atmospheric pollutants are increasingly added to the list of naturally occurring gases and particulate matter (Table 44.12). As a result, the poetic fogs and mists of the countryside and seashore yield to the smog (*smoke + fog*, a term coined by Des Veux in 1905) of major cities. Even on "clear" days, the smoke and fumes in the atmosphere of large cities may produce irritative conjunctivitis, hyperemia, punctate epithelial erosions (PEE). Gasoline and oil byproducts may produce follicular conjunctivitis (201) or marginal corneal ulcers.

The possibility of adaptation by the millions of people exposed to smog has been suggested by Jacobson (202). He found that residents of the San Gabriel Valley (just east of Los Angeles, California) were symptomatic in the summer. Their complaints ranged from burning to foreign body sensation. Artificial tears generally alleviated these symptoms. It was his experience that longtime residents of smoggy areas suffered less than recent arrivals or visitors, suggesting that some mechanism plays a role in the development of tolerance to air pollution in inhabitants of smoggy areas. Exposure to even low levels of pollution may result in stinging symptoms, increased blinking, and lacrimation. Jaffe (203) found that eye irritation correlated well with total oxidant

TABLE 44.12. NATURAL AND MANMADE ATMOSPHERIC CONSTITUENTS

Gaseous	Particulate
Natural	
Argon	Ash
CO_2	Dust
H_2O	Microorganisms
Methane	Pollen
N_2	Salt
O_2	Water droplets
O_3 (stratospheric)	
Manmade	
Acrolein	Ash
Aldehydes	Grit
Aromatic olefins	Soot
Chlorofluorocarbons	Tar
CO	
CO_2?	
HFI[4]	
Methane	
Nitrous oxides	
O_3	
Peroxylacetyl nitrate	
Peroxylbenzoyl nitrate	
SO_2	
SO_3	
Volatile organic peroxides	
Volatile unsaturated hydrocarbons	
Volatile sulfides/mercaptans	

concentration in the atmosphere. Others have determined that there is a reduction of the concentration of tear lysozyme in eyes exposed to smog (204–207).

Andrés et al. (208) confirmed that changes in the pH of the surface of the cornea due to absorption of atmospheric SO_2 produced varying effects. They found that ultrathin lens wearers showed smaller changes in pH, with corresponding increased tolerance. They also concluded that artificial tears served to counter the increased acidity, with an increased tolerance to contact lens wear.

COSMETICS

Cosmetics, soaps, perfumes, lotions, and even nicotine may adhere to the skin of the hands or lids. It has been suggested that written instructions be given to patients to alert them to the possible untoward effects of such substances, along with recommendations for suitable alternate products (209). Depending on the type of ingredients involved, the unwanted material may tarry for more than a day. We frequently observe particles of mascara floating in the conjunctival sac or other substances adherent to the surface of the skin. Skin pH is less than 6, yet the pH of soaps is rarely less than 7. It is evident that chemicals on the insertion finger of a patient probably are transferred onto or into

TABLE 44.13. ADVICE ON THE USE OF EYE COSMETICS BY CONTACT LENS WEARERS

Do Not	Do
Apply cosmetic to an infected, red, or swollen eye	Wash hands in oil- and fragrance-free soap before handling lenses
Share cosmetics	
Reuse applicators	Remove makeup daily using hypoallergic remover
Lubricate applicator with saliva	Remove mascara and cyeliner regularly
Apply eyeliner inside lashes	
Apply makeup when in motion	Apply makeup sparingly
Use aerosols with eyes open	Apply cosmetics *after* inserting lenses
Use nail polish (varnish) or remover after inserting lenses	Remove lenses *before* removing makeup
Allow makeup to touch lenses	Use water-resistant mascara
Use makeup without preservatives	Use oil- and fragrance-free makeup
Expose cosmetics to heat	Consult contact lens prescriber if redness, swelling, pain, or irritation occurs
Leave cosmetics exposed to the atmosphere	Replace cosmetics regularly
Use oil-based removers	
Use makeup with mercurial preservatives	

Modified from Baldwin JS. Cosmetics: too long concealed as culprit in eye problems. *Contact Lens Forum* 1986;11:34–41, with permission.

the contact lens, with resulting decrease in comfort. Other hazards to the contact lens wearer are awaiting the unwary in beautician and hairdresser establishments, including fumes such as ammonia and hair spray, which may produce superficial punctate keratitis or adhere to the surface of a contact lens, resulting in damage to the lens and ocular irritation.

In addition, Baldwin (210) reminds us of the following: the pigments, oils, and solvents in cosmetics may not only be irritative but also allergenic; labels such as "hypoallergenic" mean that no known severe allergen is contained; "natural" and "organic" products are perhaps more likely to be allergenic; and claims such as "allergy tested" and "dermatologist tested" give no information as to the nature of the testing or the results. She provides a list of guidelines on the use of cosmetics by contact lens wearers (Table 44.13).

It has long been recognized that eye cosmetics are potential reservoirs for microbial contamination that is not limited to the normal flora of the skin of the face and fingers (211).

Most commonly, *Staphylococcus epidermidis* is associated with the development of blepharitis or conjunctivitis that readily responds to good hygiene practices and topical antibiotics. More serious infections (mainly corneal ulcers) and their complications have been caused by mascara contaminated with *Pseudomonas aeruginosa* (212). The usual mode of transmission is by inoculation (scratch) with a mascara

bush. The presence of a contact lens on the eye would reduce the chance of infection.

CONTACT LENSES IN THE WORKPLACE

As the number of successful contact lens wearers continues to increase, it is inevitable that most will wish to wear their lenses constantly, including in the workplace. Occupational health and safety personnel find themselves in a dilemma due to conflicting and sometimes controversial information circulated by various agencies concerning the advisability of wearing contact lenses in the workplace. Contact lenses add a complicating factor to eye safety considerations. When decisions on whether to permit contact lens wear in particular environments are the responsibility of those with little knowledge of contact lenses and how their wear may affect the level of risk for eye injury or how contact lens removal may adversely affect the wearer, then unreasonable and discriminatory policies may result.

A survey conducted by the National Safety Council (USA) in conjunction with its Industrial Division's Chemical Section Executive Committee revealed that only 53% of members who replied to the survey had formal policies on contact lenses in their companies (213). The variability of policies from one company to the next emphasizes the arbitrary manner in which contact lens policies have been generated and enforced. An example of this is a 38-year-old steel worker who had a traumatic cataract removed, was advised by a safety director that he was not allowed to return to work wearing a contact lens, nor could he return to his job with monocular vision (214).

Responsibilities

The Canadian Centre for Occupational Health and Safety (CCOHS) suggests that both the employer and the worker share the responsibility to ensure the safe use of contact lenses in the work environment and believe that the following steps should be followed *(http://www.ccohs. ca/oshanswers/preventin/contact__len.html)*.

The employer should perform the following:

- Ensure that proper health and safety practices and procedures are followed.
- Provide training and education about eye hazards, particularly those specific to contact lens use, and training on the proper use of eyewash stations and procedures for rinsing the eyes.
- Clearly identify contact lens wearers. The information should be on the employee's medical file and, at least, the personnel who provide first aid should know who wears contact lenses. It is important that workers wearing contact lenses be clearly identified (especially for first aid). To assist the setup and maintenance of an eye protection

program, identification methods such as the Medic-Alert insignia may be helpful.

- Have personnel available who are knowledgeable in the removal of contact lenses in case of an emergency. If removal of contact lenses is necessary, personnel should be available to provide assistance. In some situations, an ophthalmologist or optometrist may be required to remove contact lenses.
- Provide access to a clean place for regular maintenance and periodic cleaning of personal protective eyewear (PPE) and contact lenses (for example, removal of dust particles).

The worker should perform the following:

- Take special care to keep the contact lenses clean. Follow the advice of you eye care specialist.
- Discuss your work environment and any possible hazards with your eye care specialist.
- Make sure that your fellow employees and employers know that you are wearing contact lenses.
- Be alert for changes in the workplace and changes to environmental conditions that may be hazardous to you.
- Keep eye glasses available for unforeseen circumstances.
- Wear personal protective equipment when required.
- Learn about eye hazards and encourage your employer and joint health and safety committee members to do the same.

Assessment of Hazards

Identification, evaluation, measurement, and control of potential problems, factors, and stresses in the workplace are the functions of the industrial hygienist, in cooperation with industrial health and safety personnel, management, unions, and workers. Radiation and chemical hazards should be classified as stochastic (having a threshold) or nonstochastic; population differences should be considered and the actual risk characterized based on scientific evidence and experience. Decisions may be made to minimize an industrial environmental hazard by the following:

- Substitution of a hazardous agent
- Modification of a process
- Isolation of a hazardous operation
- Improved ventilation and cooling/heating systems
- Use of "wet" methods to reduce dust
- Control of worker exposure to the hazard
- Provision of personal protective equipment (eyes, ears, face, body)
- Provision of protective masks, screens, and shields
- Provision of showers, eyewashes
- Reduction of chemicals to *de minimus* levels

Ocular hazards are greater in some occupations than others. Clearly, optometrists and ophthalmologists who prescribe contact lenses for industrial workers should be concerned about the advisability of wearing the lenses in a given environment. The type of work involved may influence the selection of lens type. In making the decision *if* and *what* to prescribe, an expansion of the case history may be useful in determining the following:

- Toxic chemicals and physical agents that may be encountered
- Raw material and byproducts involved
- Potential for exposure
- Protective equipment available and used
- Other protective measures available
- Hygiene facilities available
- Presence or absence of health personnel
- Factors that may influence compliance with cleaning and wearing schedules

Patients with hazardous avocations and lifestyles place an even greater responsibility on the prescribing practitioner. In evaluating an incident, it is essential to be familiar with all of the possible signs of trauma and/or toxicity (Table 44.14), the mechanisms by which they occur, and the diverse alternatives to the claimed etiology of the injury or toxic response.

Advantages of Contact Lenses

The contact lens is a prosthetic device (215), yet there is still a tendency for nontherapeutic use for correction of refractive errors to be described as cosmetic. For some, spectacle lens wear has become a status symbol rather than a stigma. For authorities and insurance companies to classify contact lenses, used to correct a refractive error, as a fashion device while reimbursing the cost of designer spectacles is illogical and discriminatory.

Contact lenses offer a number of advantages over spectacle lenses and include the following:

- Improved performance in rain or mist
- Fewer broken or lost spectacles
- No fogging with changing temperatures or humidity
- Elimination of spectacle lens reflections
- No mechanical interference when using instruments such as microscopes
- Elimination of the broken spectacle lens hazard
- No spectacle lens greasing or smearing or dust accumulation when performing tasks in unclean environments
- Reduced perspiration problems
- More compatible with gas masks and other safety equipment
- Increased visual field
- No "jack in the box" effect
- No ring scotomata
- Improved visual acuity in some cases, e.g., high myopes/keratoconics

In a study of police officers, Good and Augsberger (216) found that 52% who routinely wore prescription spectacles

TABLE 44.14. ANTERIOR SEGMENT SIGNS OF TRAUMA OR TOXICITY

Lids	Cornea	Conjunctiva	Anterior Chamber	Lens
Blepharitis	Abrasion	Chemosis	Angle recession	Anterior subcapsular
Dermatitis	Central cornea clouding	Follicular response	Cells	Opacities
Ecchymosis	Chalcosis	Foreign body	Engorged iris	Capsular exfoliation
Ectropion	Corneal decomposition	Giant papillary	Flare	Dislocation
		conjunctivitis		
Edema	Debris	Hyperemia	Foreign body	Foreign body
Entropion	Endothelial changes	Ischemia	Hyphema	Loss of anterior clear zone
Foreign body	Epithelial desiccation	Lacerations	Hypopyon	Nuclear brunescens
Laceration	Epithelial edema (bedewing)	Limbal injection	Iridodialysis	Posterior subcapsular
Scarring	Epithelial erosion	Mucous strands	Iridodonesis	Opacities
	Epithelial granules	Papillary response	Iris prolapse	Radiation cataract
	Erosion	Phlyctenule	KP[5]	Rupture of capsule
	Foreign body	Pinguecula	Pupil anomalies	Subluxation
	Hyposensitivity	Pseudopterygium	Shallow anterior chamber	Traumatic cataract
	Infiltrates	Pterygiuposterior[6]	Synechiae (anterior,	Vossius ring
			posterior)	
	Laceration	Scarring		
	Microcysts	Staining (rose bengal)		
	Micropannus	Subconjunctival		
		hemorrhage		
	Neovascularization	Symblepharon		
	Opacification	Tatooing		
	Pannus	Xerosis		
	Perforation			
	Ruptured membranes			
	Scarring			
	Siderosis			
	Staining (rose bengal)			
	Stippling			
	Stromal edema (swelling)			
	Striae			
	Superficial punctate keratitis			
	Ulceration			
	Vacuoles			
	Whorl-type dystrophy			

while on duty had their glasses dislodged while performing police duties. Officers who wore contact lenses on duty had their contact lenses dislodged as follows: hard 31%, RGP 10.5%, and soft 19%. They noted that 56% had needed to remove their glasses in order to see because of fogging and rain or snow. They also reported that 56% of hard lens wearers, 58% RGP lens wearers, and 47% of soft lens wearers had removed their lenses while on duty because of irritation due to environmental factors (dust, smoke, wind). Following a similar study of Royal Canadian Mounted Police (RCMP) constables, in 1997 the Canadian Ophthalmological Society recommended the following (217):

"1. Owing to the possibility that contact lens users may not always be wearing their lenses on duty or given the high probability of spectacles becoming dislodged or obscured, there is a considerable chance that the constables who are contact lens wearers will be requested to function in an uncorrected state at some time while on duty. Therefore, we recommend that the RCMP should not grant a waiver to applicants who do not meet the uncorrected visual standards required by the force.

2. In recent years disposable and continuous wear soft contact lenses have become available. Although new materials in lenses are available, it is our opinion that there is no new lens technology that would allow the use of contact lenses as a reasonable accommodation to the uncorrected standard."

On the other hand, Kartchner (200) found that extended wear contact lenses are ideal for firefighters. All of his subjects commented that the self-contained breathing apparatus was much easier to use while wearing the contact lenses.

Reasons for Not Removing Contact Lenses

There are many explanations for why an individual would elect not to remove his or her contact lenses in the workplace or in an environment perceived to contraindicate contact lens wear. These reasons may be optical, therapeutic, hygienic, or cosmetic, or simply that the individual does not accept or recognize the risk (Table 44.15).

Contact Lens Emergencies and First Aid

The management of any industrial injury involving contact lenses is enhanced by the existence of proactive policies and operating procedures that involve responsibilities for employer and employee.

Contact lens wearers in the workplace should ensure that appropriate management and health personnel are aware that contact lenses are being worn in case emergency removal is required. Preferably, contact lenses should be removed by the wearer when the situation warrants. A spare pair of contact lenses, alternate spectacles, and appropriate cleaning solutions should be available on site. Adherence to existing policies governing the wearing of personal protective equipment is presumed.

Health and safety personnel should record on the employee's health record the type of lenses worn (rigid or hydrophilic) and the name, address, and telephone number of the prescribing optometrist. Ocular first aid procedures for the contact lens wearer are essentially the same as those for any similar incident not involving contact lenses. All

TABLE 44.15. REASONS WHY A CONTACT LENS MAY NOT BE TEMPORARILY REMOVED IN A HAZARDOUS ENVIRONMENT

Optical
  No alternate spectacle correction
  Spectacle blur with long-term wear of polymethyl methacrylate
    lenses
  Oblique astigmatism
  Irregular astigmatism
  Change in depth perception
  Change in spatial adaptation
Therapeutic
  Albinism
  Aniridia
  Aphakia, monocular and binocular
  Keratoconus
  Nystagmus
  Bandage lens
  Ptosis
Cosmetic
  Prosthesis
  Cosmetic shells
  Scars
Hygiene
  No access to clean facilities
  No case
  No solutions
Other
  Rigid adherence to wearing schedule
  Lens used to aid color discrimination
  Unable to remove lens due to poor instruction
  Ignorance of hazard

personnel should be familiar with the procedures likely to be encountered in a given workplace. Emergency removal of contact lenses by a person other than the wearer is rarely indicated. The exception is when the victim is unconscious and a chemical or other foreign material has entered the eye. Another contact lens wearer is typically the best qualified to carry out this procedure.

Suggested first aid management, by wearer or safety personnel, for emergency and other contact lens-related problems is given in Table 44.16. The same procedures are appropriate for similar problems encountered in leisure or home environments.

CASE HISTORIES

In addition to the legend of the contact lens welded to the cornea by an arc flash, other case reports surface and resurface from time to time, sometimes with augmentation and elaboration from the original report. An example of a report circulated by a Canadian chemical company and reprinted by a number of publications, including one produced at the University of Waterloo for high school chemistry teachers (218), is as follows.

Injury due to the wearing of contact lenses in inappropriate conditions involved a second-year undergraduate student working in a university laboratory. He suffered acute optic neuritis due to solvent fumes absorbed into soft contact lenses during chromatography work, despite reasonably well-ventilated conditions.

The student, who had been working with ethyl acetate and/or hexanes, had to undergo intensive corticosteroid therapy for 6 weeks. He had several episodes of temporary total blindness, severe episodes of color hallucinations, and severe headaches as a result of the absorption.

Action taken:

1. Attempts were made to minimize the escape of solvent fumes, where practical, with a fume hood.
2. It was stressed to technicians that they avoid using contact lenses when working with volatile chemicals.

Note: In general, the wearing of contact lenses in a chemical environment should be avoided.

In order to evaluate reports such as this, it is essential to obtain a copy of the original report, preferably with any clinical records that may be available. There is a tendency for terms such as "presumed," "perhaps," "possibly," and "maybe" to be lost in the story telling. Second, knowledge of the response of the non-contact lens wearer exposed to similar circumstances would be of value. Third, access to materials that provide physical, chemical, toxicologic, and other data pertinent to the actual or perceived environmental hazard will aid in the assessment of the report. Additionally, because the signs and symptoms may be unrelated to either the circumstances described or contact lens wear,

TABLE 44.16. FIRST AID FOR CONTACT LENS EMERGENCIES

Exposure to Fumes or Vapors

Remove lenses for cleaning and rinsing. If no eye irritation is experienced, then the lenses can be reinserted.

Chemical Splash

Copiously irrigate the eye with water while holding the lids apart. Do not worry about losing the contact lens. If the lens remains after initial flushing, remove it or slide it onto the conjunctiva and reirrigate, then refer for emergency professional management. For caustic splash, irrigation should be continued during transportation.

Foreign Bodies

Remove the lens and irrigate the eye if indicated. If the eye remains uncomfortable, it seems that the foreign body has remained in the eye or vision is blurred, the eye should be examined by an eye care practitioner prior to reinserting lenses. All cases of high-speed flying particles should be professionally evaluated.

Dust in Eyes

Remove the contact lenses and irrigate eyes. Clean lenses and reinsert if eyes are not red or uncomfortable. If eyes are red or reinsertion causes discomfort, consult practitioner before wearing lenses.

Blunt Trauma

Swelling or lacerations may make lens (or pieces of lens) removal difficult. Professional evaluation of whole eye is indicated.

Uncomfortable Lenses, or Red or Sore Eyes

Do not wear the lenses. Seek advice from prescribing practitioner.

Adherent Lenses

If due to drying of hydrogel material by hyperthermia, infrared radiation, wind, or low humidity environments, do not attempt to remove the lenses until they have rehydrated. This may be accelerated by appropriate eye drops.

Dry Eyes or Environments

Increase humidity if possible. Request practitioner to prescribe suitable lubricating eye drops.

Exposure to Welding or Other Arc

If protective filters were not in place, then remove lenses prior to the onset of photokeratitis. If there are no symptoms, resume contact lens wear in 24 hours; otherwise, consult practitioner before wearing lenses again.

Blurred Vision

Remove and clean the lenses. If vision remains blurred on reinsertion (after ensuring that lenses are in the appropriate eyes), consult prescribing practitioner.

Lost Lens(es)

Check that lens is not displaced onto the conjunctiva. If it is, carefully recenter the lens. Check clothing and surrounding floor. If the lens is found clean, evaluate it for damage. If undamaged, reinsert. If this causes discomfort or if the lens is damaged, consult practitioner.

Modified from Cullen AP. Contact lenses in the work environment. In: Pitts DG, Weissman BA, eds. *Environmental vision.* Boston: Butterworth-Heinemann, 1992:315–331, with permission.

knowledge of other possible causes of the general and ocular responses described is essential.

An evaluation of "Case History 5" was published in a later edition of the journal (219), as follows.

Case History 5 represents a typical example of anecdotal evidence that ultimately will find its way into the literature as established fact. The inference that soft contact lenses absorb solvents to cause optic neuritis because a student working with volatile chemicals who developed acute optic neuritis was wearing soft contact lenses is a *non sequitur.* The original report to BDH Chemicals Canada Limited states the following: "solvent fumes presumed to have sorbed into soft contact lenses . . . . " Apparently no uptake studies were performed on the lenses.

Hexanes, which are virtually insoluble in water and have a low affinity for the plastic material of soft contact lenses, are used to extract other organic solvents (e.g., trichloroethylene and xylene) from soft contact lenses during uptake studies. Ethyl acetate is soluble in water and, therefore, could be taken up by the lenses; however, recent studies have shown that uptake of solvents by soft contact lenses does not worsen the ocular response to the chemicals over direct exposure of the eye and, in some cases, protection is provided to the eye. The known ocular effect of ethyl acetate is an insidious and chronic conjunctivitis with a superficial keratitis building up over days of exposure. The victim would experience extremely irritated eyes and, if the fumes were also inhaled, there would be a similar response in the mucosa of the nose, throat, and even lungs. No effects have been reported on the peripheral or central nervous systems. Hexanes, when inhaled, produce light-headedness, nausea and headache, numbness, muscle weakness, and external ocular irritation.

Penetration of chemicals into the eye is not a matter of simple diffusion because the outer coats of the eye are relatively impermeable to electrolytes but are freely permeable to fat-soluble substances, whereas the stroma of the cornea and sclera require ionization for free transversal. If a lipid- and water-soluble toxin does manage to penetrate into the eye, a severe inflammatory response would be anticipated in the anterior internal structures of the eye rather than the remote optic nerve.

The majority of cases of optic neuritis are of unknown etiology, although there have been suggestions that they follow nonspecific viral infections of the upper respiratory or gastrointestinal tract. In cases where a definitive etiology is detected, it most commonly is due to a demyelinating disease such as multiple sclerosis; other less common causes include infectious mononucleosis, inflammations of the sinuses, orbit, or meninges, and granulomatous inflammatory diseases such as syphilis, tuberculosis, and sarcoidosis. For optic neuritis to be caused by an organic toxin, the route of entry would be either inhalation or ingestion.

Ideally, it would be better if unsubstantiated case reports

were not published until they were scientifically and clinically verified. Anecdotes have a tendency to be cited as fact.

If we are not willing to evaluate carefully a particular case involving a problem with contact lenses in a particular environment, perhaps it would be better for all concerned if the response to the common question, "Could it be due to my work?," is "I don't know," rather than a vague "possibly."

PROTECTION BY CONTACT LENSES

The question of whether or not contact lenses cause a greater risk of more severe ocular trauma in the event of an accident involving the eyes has been posed since contact lenses became available for general use. Girard (220) stated that one of the most common misconceptions expressed by patients is that if a patient is injured while wearing contact lenses, the lens will contribute to the extent of the injury. When one examines the situation, however, it becomes evident that, in many cases, contact lenses are far safer than spectacles. Over the years, surveys of optometrists and ophthalmologists have been conducted by a variety of organizations, including the National Eye Research Foundation, the Z-80 Subcommittee on Contact Lenses of the American National Standards Institute (ANSI), and the College and University Safety Council of Ontario. The results of these surveys provide no evidence to support the claim that contact lenses increase the risks.

A number of review articles (221–223) and reports (224–229) also confirm that, in most instances, contact

lenses provide some degree of protection. The nature of the injury and the type of contact lens worn govern the extent of protection (Table 44.17).

Girard (220) reminds us that the eye is greatly protected by the brow, cheek, and nose. Most blows falling about the eye cause injuries to these structures rather than to the eye itself. These are natural body defenses of the eye. When lenses are worn, these defenses are always in operation. When ordinary spectacles are worn, all of these defenses are rendered less effective by the fact that the spectacles extend beyond the defenses. Any blow about the face is liable to strike the spectacles and break the lenses, which may injure the eye. This is particularly true of missiles flying toward the eye.

There is a striking paucity in the refereed scientific literature of documented cases where a contact lens increased the severity of an injury when compared with the hundreds of instances in which a contact lens provided protection (Table 44.18). A skeptical individual could suggest that those reporting the injuries are biased; however, laboratory research supports the clinical findings.

REGULATIONS

Following the evaluation of 55 employees who successfully wore rigid contact lenses in a heavy industry (San Francisco Federal Naval Shipyard), Silberstein (230), a pioneer industrial optometrist, tentatively concluded in 1962 "(a) That contact lens wearers in industry should not be permitted to work in certain jobs and particular environments that are

TABLE 44.17. MODIFYING EFFECT OF CONTACT LENS WEAR ON ENVIRONMENTAL HAZARDS OR STRESS

	Type of Lens	
Nature of Hazard/Stress	Hard	Soft
Large flying objects	Safer then glasses	Safer than glasses
Flying particles, dust	Contraindicated	Some protection, lens replacement required
Abrasive blasting materials	Contraindicated	Some protection
Alkali splash	Some protection	Some protection
Molten metal splash	No difference	No difference
Wind	No difference	May dry out
Fumes, vapors	Some short term protection	Protection from insoluble vapors More research needed: *caution* indicated
Heat, infrared	No difference	May dry out
Cold	Some protection	Some protection
Ultraviolet	No protection, unless UV blocking	No protection, unless UV blocking
Chemical burns	Some protection	Some protection
Glare (visible light)	Worse than glasses, unless tinted	Worse than glasses, unless tinted
Barometric stress	Bubble formation, not contraindicated	Bubble formation, not contraindicated
Vibration	No difference	No difference
Acceleration	No difference	No difference
Humidity	No difference	Low relative humidity; lens may dry out
Lacerations	Some protection	No difference

UV, ultraviolet.

TABLE 44.18. EYE HAZARDS AGAINST WHICH CONTACT LENSES HAVE PROVIDED PROTECTION

Acetone	Fist with ring	Metal clip	Pencil point	Screwdriver	Tear gas (CS)
Acid	Flame	Metal particles	Plastic	Shell casing	Thumb
Acid fumes	Flour	Metal piece	Plastic comb	Ski pole	Tip of fishing pole
Baton tip	Football shoe	Metal shaving	Popgun	Solvents	Toy rocket
Broomstick	Foreign body	Metal sliver	Radiator contents	Squash ball	Tree
Bullwhip	Glass	Metal splinter	Rattail comb	Stairs	Tree limb
Cardboard box	Grease	Molten slag	Rear view mirror	Staple	Truck wheel
Caustic soda	Hair spray	Nail	Religious medal	Steel-tipped dart	Ultraviolet
Chlorox[7]	Hot metal	Needle	Rivet	Steel pellet	Umbrella rib
Cleaning fluid	Hydrochloric acid	Orange	Rope	Stick	Varnish
Electric plug	Hypothermia	Oven cleaner	Rosin	Stone	Varnish remover
End mill	Kitchen knife	Paint	Rugby boot	Sulfur vapors	Wind
Field hockey stick	Lacrosse stick	Paint fumes	Scissors	Sulfuric acid	Windshield glass
Fingernail	Metal buckle	Pea	Screw	Sun visor	Wood chip
Fist	Metal chip				

specifically and peculiarly hazardous to them. (b) That in the field of visual rehabilitation, contact lenses have unique advantages to the industrially employed as well as to others and they can be successfully used in full time unrestricted industrial employment providing administrative, medical and safety supervision is exercised. (c) That contact lens wearers can be employed in a wide variety of industrial positions safely and efficiently provided they are adequately trained in the use of their lenses and they observe normal industrial eye-safety practices."

Since that time, numerous industries, educational authorities, and other organizations have arbitrarily restricted the use of contact lens within their administrative domains. In support of these policies there is reference to the early articles of Novak and Saul and others. In addition, exhaustive lists of chemicals with which the use of contact lenses is contraindicated have been generated (231) with no supporting evidence and, in some instances, include chemicals that are innocuous or less traumatic than substances used therapeutically.

Many authorities, such as Dixon (232), have been opposed to a universal ban of contact lenses in the workplace. The need to wear eye protection in eye hazardous areas is self-evident, and this should be enforced in accordance with regulation. Thus, the answer to industrial eye safety is to enforce safety regulations in the workplace rather than indiscriminately banning the wearing of contact lenses on the job (233). Education and voluntary action tend to be more effective than a regulation that is perceived to be unjustified or unreasonable. The fact that those formulating the regulation may be unfamiliar with the nature and performance of contact lenses in different environments is not an indictment of contact lenses; rather, it indicates a need for ongoing education in this area.

The US Occupational Safety and Health Administration prohibited the wearing of contact lenses with any respirator. These regulations have been challenged by users of self-contained breathing apparatus (SCBA). Following a study of firefighters, da Roza and Weaver (234) found that safety-related problems caused by spectacles were proportionately higher than those caused by contact lenses. Their investigations indicated that the contact lens-related problems were not hazardous and that the use of contact lens with respirators should not be prohibited. Stones and Spencer (235) agreed that, based on their extensive evaluation of the scientific literature, a ban of contact lenses in the workplace was unjustified and that the British Columbia regulation might be considered a model in providing a realistic approach. The British Columbia Industrial Health and Safety Regulation states that no worker shall wear contact lenses where gases, vapors, or other materials are present that, when absorbed by contact lenses, may harm the eyes, or dusts or other materials are present that may harm the eyes or cause distraction that may expose the worker to other injury. Recommendations and regulations governing the use of contact lenses in the workplace are continuing to be relaxed in compliance with scientific research and clinical experience. Unfortunately, it seems that regulations are easier to create than repeal.

CONCLUSION

An evaluation of the preceding material indicates that contact lenses can be worn safely under a variety of environmental situations, including those that, from a superficial evaluation, might appear hazardous (Table 44.17). Indeed, some types of contact lenses may give added protection to spectacle lens and nonspectacle lens wearers in instances of chemical splash, dust, flying particles, and nonionizing radiation. The evidence also refutes the claims that contact lenses negate the protection provided by safety equipment or make the cornea more susceptible to damage by nonionizing radiation, particularly arc flashes. Thus, a universal ban of contact lenses in the workplace or other environments is unwarranted.

Regulations limiting the wearing of contact lenses in any given circumstance must be scientifically defensible and effectively enforceable; they should not be based on perceived hazards, random experience, isolated unverified case histories, or unsubstantiated personal opinions. Conversely, it would be imprudent for a practitioner to prescribe contact lenses in order to circumvent uncorrected visual acuity standards in those occupations where individuals may be required to function without correction on some occasions or in environments contraindicated for the type of lens prescribed.

In conclusion, optometrists and ophthalmologists who prescribe contact lenses should be concerned about the advisability of their patients wearing lenses in any particular environment. All practitioners must stress that personal protective equipment, including safety eyewear, is not replaced by contact lenses. Where circumstances create the necessity, eye protection must be worn.

REFERENCES

1. Jones LW, Jone DA. *Common contact lens complications: their recognition and management.* Oxford: Butterworth-Heinemann, 2000.
2. Efron N. Complications. In: Efron N, ed. *Contact lens practice.* Oxford: Butterworth Heinemann, 2002:405–437.
3. Woodward G. The effect of contact lens wear on the ocular environment. *Optom Today* July 2, 1999;27–32.
4. Bonanno JA, Polse KA. Hypoxic changes in the corneal epithelium and stroma. In: Tomlinson A, ed. *Complications of contact lens wear.* St. Louis: Mosby Year Book, 1992:21–36.
5. Bergmanson JPG, Weissman, BA. Hypoxic changes in corneal endothelium. In: Tomlinson A, ed. *Complications of contact lens wear.* St. Louis: Mosby Year Book, 1992:37–67.
6. Brennon NA, Coles M-LC. Continuous wear. In: Efron N, ed. *Contact lens practice.* Oxford: Butterworth Heinemann, 2002: 275–294.
7. Millodot M. Corneal anesthesia following contact lens wear. In: Tomlinson A, ed. *Complications of contact lens wear.* St. Louis: Mosby Year Book, 1992:89–101.
8. Allansmith MF, Ross RN. Ocular allergy and mast cell stabilizers. *Surv Ophthalmol* 1986;30:229–244.
9. Spring TF. Reaction to hydrophilic lenses. *Med J Aust* 1974;1: 499–503.
10. Allansmith MF, Korb DR, Greiner JV, et al. Giant papillary conjunctivitis in contact lens wearers. *Am J Ophthalmol* 1977; 83:697–708.
11. Cullen AP. Contact lenses in the work environment. In: Pitts DG, Weissman BA, eds. *Environmental vision.* Boston: Butterworth-Heinemann, 1992:315–331.
12. Cordrey P. Arc flash and the contact lens wearer: a modern myth. *Eye* 1977;4:3–4.
13. Kersley HJ. Arc flash and the contact lens wearer. *Br Med J* 1977;2:639–640.
14. Novak JF, Saul RW. Contact lenses in industry. *J Occup Med* 1971;13:175–181.
15. Occupational Safety Health. October 1973, cited by Cordrey P. Arc flash and the contact lens wearer: a modern myth. *Eye* 1977;4:3–4.
16. Ewing RC. New and improved safety programs challenge refiners. *Oil Gas J* 1973;71:72–76.
17. Circular to employees of Thames Valley Water Authority from the Senior Resident Engineer, July 16, 1975, cited by Kersley HJ. Arc flash and the contact lens wearer. *Br Med J* 1977;2: 639–640.
18. Cullen AP, Chou BR, Egan DJ. Industrial non-ionizing radiation and contact lenses. *Can J Pub Health* 1982;73:251–2519.
19. Authorities deny contact lenses fused to workers' eyes. *Occupational Health and Safety Letter,* August 22, 1983, p. 20.
20. Contact lens rumour cleared up. *Accident Prevention* 1984; Jan:3.
21. Warning on blindness from arc welding found erroneous; hazard/alert withdrawn. *Occup Safety Health Reporter* 1983;12:926.
22. Gould D. Cambridge eyewash. *New Scientist* 1984;101:44.
23. Cullen AP. Contact lenses and electric arcs. *Can J Optom* 1990; 52:100–101.
24. Chou BR, Cullen AP. Ocular hazards associated with operating in-line switches at high voltage. *Health Phys* 1991;61:473–479.
25. Ahmedbhai N, Cullen AP. The influence of contact lens wear on the corneal response to ultraviolet radiation. *Ophthalmic Physiol Opt* 1988;8:183–189.
26. Contact lens alert is unfounded. *The Maintainer* 1988;4:3.
27. Grant WM. *Toxicology of the eye,* 3rd ed. Springfield, IL: Charles C. Thomas, 1986.
28. Duke-Elder S. *System of ophthalmology, vol. XIV, injuries, part II non-mechanic injuries.* London: Henry Kimpton, 1972.
29. Reeves AL, ed. *Toxicology: principles and practice.* New York: John Wiley & Sons, 1981.
30. Deichman WB, ed. *Toxicology and occupational medicine.* New York: Elsevier/North Holland, 1979.
31. Gad SC, ed. *Product safety evaluation handbook.* New York: Marcel Dekker, 1988.
32. *NIOSH pocket guide to chemical hazards (NPG).* NIOSH publication no. 97-140. NIOSH Publications Office, 1997.
33. Regulations respecting control of exposure to biological or chemical agents made under the occupational health and safety act. Toronto: Queen's Printer for Ontario, 1987.
34. *2002 TLVs® and BEIs® threshold limit values for chemical substances and physical agents. Biological exposure indices.* Cincinnati, OH: ACGIH International, 2002.
35. *NIOSH pocket guide to chemical hazards and other databases.* DHHS (NIOSH) publication no. 2001-145. Cincinnati, OH: Department of Health and Human Services, Centers for Disease Control and Prevention, National Institute for Occupational Safety and Health, 2001.
36. Hrynchak PK. Ocular toxicity of common household agents. *Can J Optom* 1984;46:185–195.
37. Rengstorff RH. The effects of riot control agent CS on visual acuity. *Military Med* 1969;134:219–221.
38. Kok-van Alphen CC, van der Linden JW, et al. Protection of the police against tear gas with soft contact lenses. *Military Med* 1985;150:451–454.
39. Nilsson SEG, Andersson L. The use of contact lenses in environments with organic solvents, acids or alkalis. *Acta Ophthalmol* 1982;60:599–608.
40. LaMotte J, Smith G, Chang-Smith A. Absorption of ammonia by high water content hydrogel lenses: an inexpensive method of analysis. *Optom Vis Sci* 1995;72:605–607.
41. Cerulli L, Tria M, Bacaloni A, et al. Lenti a contatto idrofile ed inquinamento in ambiente di lavoro. *Boll Ocul* 1985;64: 299–305.
42. Coe JE, Douglas RB. The effect of contact lenses of ocular responses to sulphur dioxide. *J Soc Occup Med* 1982;32:92–94.
43. Mäkitie J. Contact lenses in the work environment. *Acta Ophthalmol* 1984;[Suppl. 161]:151–122.
44. Jenks C Jr. Letter to the editor. *J Am Assoc Nurse Anesth* 1984; 52:262.

45. Wesley NK. Chemical injury and contact lenses. *Contacto* 1966; 10:15–20.

46. Guthrie JW, Seitz G. An investigation of the contact lens problem. *J Occup Med* 1975;17:163–166.

47. Kingston DW. Contact lenses in the laboratory. *J Chem Ed* 1981;58:A289–A290, A293.

48. Dickinson F. Contact lenses: the safety factor. *Optician* 1969; 158:355.

49. Roper-Hall MJ. The changing pattern of injury. In: Tengroth B, ed. *Current concepts in ergophthalmology.* Stockholm: Karolinska Institute, 1977:225–229.

50. Gombos GM. Trauma: part I. In: Gombos GM, ed. *Handbook of ophthalmologic emergencies,* 2nd ed. Flushing, NY: Medical Examination Publishing Company, 1977:105.

51. Zorab EC. War surgery of the eye in forward areas. *Br J Ophthalmol* 1945;29:579–593.

52. Blackstone MR. Contact lenses as eye protectors. *Optician* 1967; 154:469.

53. Brown DVL. Traumatic fracture of plastic contact lenses. *Arch Ophthalmol* 1964;72:319–322.

54. Dickinson F. An eye saved by a contact lens. *Optician* 1957; 134:266.

55. Nilsson SEG, Lövsund P, Øberg PA. Contact lenses and mechanical trauma to the eye: an experimental study. *Acta Ophthalmol (Copenh)* 1981;59:402–408.

56. Ritzmann KE, Chou BR, Cullen AP. Ocular protection by contact lenses from mechanical trauma. *Int Contact Lens Clin* 1992; 19:162–166.

57. Highgate DJ. Contact lenses at work. *Occup Health Safety* 1974; 3:8–11.

58. O'Rourke PJ. Traumatic fracture of contact lens with corneal injury. *Br J Ophthalmol* 1971;55:125–127.

59. Cohen JM. Corneal protection through contact lenses. *Optom Weekly* 1964;55:30–31.

60. Nilsson SEG, Lindh H, Andersson L. Contact lens wear in an environment contaminated with metal particles. *Acta Ophthalmol (Copenh)* 1983;61:882–888.

61. Roper-Hall MJ. Thermal and chemical burns. *Trans Ophthalmol Soc UK* 1965;85:631–653.

62. Campbell FW, Michaelson IC. Blood vessel formation in the cornea. *Br J Ophthalmol* 1949;33:248–255.

63. Hoffman W, Krug E. Ber Wärmeschädigungen des Auges. *Graefes Arch Ophthalmol* 1934;132:155–181.

64. Duke-Elder S. Thermal injuries. *System of ophthalmology, vol. XIV, part II.* London: Henry Kimpton, 1972:767.

65. Mäkitie J. Contact lenses and the work environment. Presented at the Ergophthalmology Symposium, Tampere, Finland, August 6–7, 1983.

66. Carroll F. Frostbite of the cornea. *Am J Ophthalmol* 1933;16: 994.

67. Maumenee AE, Kornblueth W. Regeneration of the corneal stromal cells II. Review of the literature and histologic study. *Am J Ophthalmol* 1949;32:1051–1064.

68. Sédan J. De la gelure cornéene des aviateurs. *Méd Aéronautique* 1947;2:27–35.

69. Mercier A, Dugnet J. *Physiopathology of the flyer's eye.* Translated by the United States Air Force, 1950:83.

70. Socks JF. Contact lenses in extreme cold environments: response of rabbit corneas. *Am J Optom Physiol Opt* 1982;59:297–300.

71. Nilsson SEG, Lövsund P, Øberg PA, et al. The transmittance and absorption properties of contact lenses. *Scand J Work Environ Health* 1979;5:262–270.

72. Chou BR, Cullen AP, Egan DJ. Spectral transmittance of contact lens materials. *Int Contact Lens Clin* 1982;11:106–114.

73. Chou BR, Cullen AP, Dumbleton KA. Protection factors of ultraviolet-blocking contact lenses. *Int Contact Lens Clin* 1988; 15:244–250.

74. Parker JH. A qualitative evaluation of some commercially available UV filtering soft contact lenses. *Contact Lens J* 1988;16: 61–63.

75. Boettner EA, Wolter JR. Transmission of the ocular media. *Invest Ophthalmol Vis Sci* 1962;1:766–783.

76. Lydahl E. Infrared radiation and cataract. *Acta Ophthalmol* 1984;[Suppl. 166]:1–63.

77. Meyhöfer W. Zur Aetiologie des grauen Staars Jugendliche Katarakten bei Glasmachern. *Klin Monatsbl Augenheilkd* 1886;24: 49–67.

78. Goldmann H. Genesis of heat cataract. *Arch Ophthalmol* 1933; 9:314.

79. Pitts DG, Cullen AP. Determination of infrared radiation levels for acute ocular cataractogenesis. *Graefes Arch Ophthalmol* 1981; 217:285–297.

80. Lövsund P, Nilsson SEG, Lindh H, et al. Temperature changes in contact lenses in connection with radiation from infrared heaters. *Scand J Work Environ Health* 1979;5:280–285.

81. Lövsund P, Nilsson SEG, Lindh H, et al. Temperature changes in contact lenses in connection with radiation from welding arcs. *Scand J Work Environ Health* 1979;5:271–279.

82. Harwerth RS, Sperling HG. Effects of intense visible radiation on the increment threshold spectral sensitivity of the Rhesus monkey eye. *Vision Res* 1975;15:1193–1204.

83. Lawwill T, Crockett S, Currier G. Retinal damage secondary to chronic light exposure thresholds and mechanisms. *Doc Ophthalmol* 1977;44:379–402.

84. Ham WT Jr, Muller HA, Ruffolo JJ Jr, et al. Sensitivity of the retina to radiation damage as a function of wavelength. *Photochem Photobiol* 1979;29:735–743.

85. Ham WT Jr, Mueller HA, Ruffolo JJ Jr, et al. Action spectrum for retinal injury from near-ultraviolet radiation in the aphakic monkey. *Am J Ophthalmol* 1982;93:299–306.

86. Pitts DG, Bergmanson JPG, Chu LW-F. Rabbit eye exposure to broad-spectrum fluorescent light. *Acta Ophthalmol Suppl* 1983; 159:1–54.

87. Applegate RA, Massoff RW. Changes in contrast sensitivity function induced by contact lens wear. *Am J Optom Physiol Opt* 1975;52:840–846.

88. Hess RF, Garner LF. The effect of corneal edema on visual function. *Invest Ophthalmol Vis Sci* 1977;16:5–13.

89. Woo G, Hess R. Contrast sensitivity function and soft contact lenses. *Int Contact Lens Clin* 1979;6:37–42.

90. Mitra S, Lamberts DW. Contrast sensitivity in soft lens wearers. *Contact Intraocul Lens Med J* 1981;7:315–322.

91. Bernstein IH, Brodrick J. Contrast sensitivity through spectacles and soft contact lenses. *Am J Optom Physiol Opt* 1981;58: 309–313.

92. Tomlinson A, Mann G. An analysis of visual performance with soft contact lens and spectacle correction. *Ophthalmic Physiol Opt* 1985;5:53–57.

93. Kirkpatrick DL, Roggenkamp JR. Effects of soft contact lenses on contrast sensitivity. *Am J Optom Physiol Opt* 1985;62: 407–412.

94. Teitelbaum BA, Kelly SA, Gemoules G. Contrast sensitivity through spectacles and hydrogel lenses of different polymers. *Int Contact Lens Clin* 1985;12:162–166.

95. Dumbleton KA. The effects of UV-A induced lenticular fluorescence on visual function. M.Sc. Thesis, University of Waterloo, 1988.

96. Pitts DG, Cullen AP, Hacker PD. Ocular effects of ultraviolet radiation from 295 to 365 nm. *Invest Ophthalmol Vis Sci* 1977; 16:932–939.

97. Cullen AP. Ultraviolet induced lysosome activity in corneal epithelium. *Graefes Arch Clin Exp Ophthalmol* 1980;214:107–118.

98. Millodot M, Earlam RA. Sensitivity of the cornea after exposure to ultraviolet light. *Ophthalmic Res* 1984;16:325–328.

99. Cullen, Chou BR, Hall MG, et al. Ultraviolet-B damages corneal endothelium. *Am J Optom Physiol Opt* 1984;61:473–478.

100. Karai I, Matsumara S, Takise S, et al. Morphological changes in the corneal endothelium due to ultraviolet radiation in welders. *Br J Ophthalmol* 1984;68:544–548.

101. Pitts DG, Bergmanson JPG, Chu LW-F, et al. Ultrastructural analysis of corneal exposure to UV radiation. *Acta Ophthalmol* 1987;65:263–273.

102. Doughty MJ, Cullen AP. Long-term effects of a single dose of ultraviolet-B on albino rabbit cornea—I. in vivo analysis. *Photochem Photobiol* 1989;49:185–196.

103. Bietti GB, Guerra P, Ferraris de Glasspare PF. La dystrophie corneene nodulaire en ceinture des pays tropicau a sol aride. *Bull Soc Fr Ophthalmol* 1955;68:101–129.

104. Freedman A. Labrador keratopathy. *Arch Ophthalmol* 1965;74: 198–20105. Forsius H. Climatic changes in the eyes of Eskimos, Lapps and Cheremisses. *Acta Ophthalmol (Kbh)* 1972;51: 532–539.

106. Freedman A. Climatic droplet keratopathy. *Arch Ophthalmol* 1973;89:193–197.

107. Fraunfelder FT, Hanbna C. Spheroidal degeneration of the cornea and conjunctiva. 3. Incidences, classification and etiology. *Am J Ophthalmol* 1973;76:41–50.

108. Johnson GJ, Green JS, Patterson GD, et al. Aetiology of sphaeroidal degeneration of the cornea in Labrador. *Br J Ophthalmol* 1983;65:270–283.

109. Clear AS, Chirambo MC, Hung MSR. Solar keratosis, pterygium, and squamous cell carcinoma of the conjunctiva in Malawi. *Br J Ophthalmol* 1979;63:102–109.

110. Hogan MJ, Alvardo J. Pterygium and pinguecula: electron microscopic study. *Arch Ophthalmol* 1967;78:174–186.

111. Austin P, Jakobiec FA, Iwamoto T. Elastodysplasia and elastodystrophy as the pathologic bases of ocular pterygia and pinguecula. *Ophthalmology* 1983;90:96–109.

112. Hill JC, Maske R. Pathogenesis of pterygium. *Eye* 1989;3: 218–226.

113. Bachem A. Ophthalmic ultraviolet action spectra. *Am J Ophthalmol* 1956;41:969–975.

114. MacKeen D, Fine S, Fine BS. Production of cataracts in rabbits with an ultraviolet laser. *Ophthalmic Res* 1973;5:317–324.

115. Ebber RW, Sears D. Ocular effects of 325 nm ultraviolet laser. *Am J Optom Physiol Opt* 1975;52:216–223.

116. Zuclich JA, Connolly JS. Ocular damage induced by near-ultraviolet laser radiation. *Invest Ophthalmol Vis Sci* 1976;15: 760–764.

117. Zigman S, Datiles M, Torczynski G. Sunlight and human cataracts. *Invest Ophthalmol Vis Sci* 1979;18:462–467.

118. Hollows F, Moran D. Cataract: the ultraviolet risk factor. *Lancet* 1981;8259:1249–1250.

119. Weale RA. The age variations of senile cataract in various parts of the world. *Br J Ophthalmol* 1982;66:31–34.

120. Taylor HR, West SK, Rosenthal FS, et al. Effect of ultraviolet radiation on cataract formation. *N Engl J Med* 1988;319: 1429–1433.

121. Chou BR, Cullen AP. Spectral transmittance of selected tinted ophthalmic lenses. *Can J Optom* 1983;45:192–198.

122. Pitts DG. Threat of ultraviolet radiation to the eye: how to protect against it. *J Am Optom Assoc* 1981;52:949–957.

123. Gies P, Colin CR. Ocular protection from ultraviolet radiation. *Clin Exp Optom* 1988;71:27–7.

124. Chou BR, Cullen AP, Dumbleton KA. Protection factors of ultraviolet-blocking contact lenses. *Int Contact Lens Clin* 1988; 15:244–250.

125. Pitts DG, Lattimore MR. Protection against UVR using the Vistakon UV-Block soft contact lens. *Int Contact Lens Clin* 1987;14:22–29.

126. Bergmanson JPG, Pitts DG, Chu LWF. The efficacy of a UV-blocking soft contact lens in protecting cornea against UV radiation. *Acta Ophthalmol (Copenh)* 1987;65:279–286.

127. Cullen AP, Dumbleton KA, Chou BR. Contact lenses and acute exposure to ultraviolet radiation. *Optom Vis Sci* 1989;30: 407–411.

128. Dumbleton KA, Cullen AP, Doughty MJ. Protection from acute exposure to ultraviolet radiation by ultraviolet absorbing RGP contact lenses. *Ophthalmic Physiol Opt* 1991;11:232–238.

129. Ahmedbhai N, Cullen AP. The influence of contact lens wear on the corneal response to ultraviolet radiation. *Ophthalmic Physiol Opt* 1988;8:183–189.

130. Bergmanson JPG, Chu LWF. Epithelial morphological response to soft hydrogel contact lenses. *Br J Ophthalmol* 1985;69: 373–379.

131. Francois J. The rabbit corneal epithelium after wearing hard and soft contact lenses. *CLAO J* 1983;9:267–274.

132. Appleton B, Hirsch S. Investigation of single-exposure microwave ocular effects at 3000 MHz. *Ann NY Acad Sci* 1975;247: 125.

133. Aurell E, Tengroth B. Lenticular and retinal changes secondary to microwave exposure. *Acta Ophthalmol (Copenh)* 1973;51: 764–771.

134. Appleton B, Hirsch S, Kinion RO, et al. Microwave lens effects in humans: II. Results of five-year survey. *Arch Ophthalmol* 1975;93:257–258.

135. Elkington AR, Watts GH. Ruby laser transmission and the lens. *Br J Ophthalmol* 1970;54:423–427.

136. Geeraets WJ, Williams RC, Chen C, et al. The loss of light energy in the retina and choroid. *Arch Ophthalmol* 1960;64: 606–615.

137. Geeraets WJ, Berry ER. Ocular spectral characteristics as related to hazards from lasers and other light sources. *Am J Ophthalmol* 1968;66:15–20.

138. Boetner EA, Wolter JR. Transmission of the ocular media. *Invest Ophthalmol Vis Sci* 1962;1:766–783.

139. McCanna P, Chandra SR, Stevens TS, et al. Argon laser-induced cataract as a complication of retinal photocoagulation. *Arch Ophthalmol* 1982;100:1071–1073.

140. Bennett TQM. The use of contact lenses for diving (sport and commercial). *Contact Lens J* 1988;16:171–172.

141. Polse KA, Mandell RB. Critical oxygen tension at the corneal surface. *Arch Ophthalmol* 1970;84:505–508.

142. Hapnes R. Soft contact lenses worn at a simulated altitude of 18,000 feet. *Acta Ophthalmol* 1980;58:90–95.

143. Millodot M, O'Leary DJ. Effect of oxygen deprivation on corneal sensitivity. *Acta Ophthalmol* 1980;58:434–439.

144. Castrén J. The significance of low atmospheric pressure on the eyes with reference to soft contact lenses. *Acta Ophthalmol Suppl* 1984;161:123–127.

145. Jaeckle C. Practicability of the use of contact lenses at low atmospheric pressures. *Arch Ophthalmol* 1944;31:326–328.

146. Clarke C. Contact lenses at high altitude: experience on Everest south-west face 1975. *Br J Ophthalmol* 1976;60:479–480.

147. Simon DR, Bradley ME. Corneal edema in divers wearing hard contact lenses. *Am J Ophthalmol* 1978;85:462–464.

148. Strath RA, Morariu GI, Lepawsky M. Effects of oxygen on gas bubbles entrapped in tear film. In: Gennser M, ed. Collection of manuscripts for the XXIV annual meeting of the Underwater and Baromedical Society. Stockholm Sweden, 1998;212–215. (FAO Report FAO-B-98-00342-721-SE).

149. Simon DR, Bradley ME. Adverse effects of contact lens wear during decompression. *JAMA* 1980;244:1213–1214.

150. Molinari JF, Socks JF. Effects of hyperbaric conditions on cornea physiology with hydrogel contact lenses. *Br Contact Lens Assoc J* 1986;9:3–7.

151. Socks JF, Molinari JF, Rowey JL. Rigid gas permeable contact lenses in hyperbaric environments. *Am J Optom Physiol Opt* 1988;65:942–945.

152. Strath RA, Morario GI, Mekjavic. Tear film bubble formation after decompression. *Optom Vis Sci* 1992;69:973–975.

153. Brennan DH, Girvin JK. The flight acceptability of soft contact lenses: an environmental trial. *Aviat Space Environ Med* 1985; 56:43–48.

154. Eng WG, Rasco JL, Marano JA. Low atmospheric pressure effects on wearing soft contact lenses. *Aviat Space Environ Med* 1978;49:73–75.

155. Castrén J, Tuovinen E, Länsimies E, et al. Contact lenses in hypoxia. *Acta Ophthalmol* 1985;63:439–442.

156. Flynn WJ, Miller RE, Tredici TJ, et al. Soft contact lens wear at altitude: effects of hypoxia. *Aviat Space Environ Med* 1988; 59:44–48.

157. Nilsson K, Rengstorff RH. Continuous wearing of Duragel contact lenses by Swedish Air Force pilots. *Am J Optom Physiol Opt* 1979;56:356–358.

158. Coermann R. Untersuchungen uber die einwetkung von Schwingungen Organismus. *Luftfartmed* 1939–1940;4:73–17.

159. Byrnes VA. Visual problems of supersonic speeds. *Am J Ophthalmol* 1951;34:169–177.

160. Hornick RJ. Vibration. In: Parker JF, West VR eds. *Bioastronautics data book,* 2nd ed. Washington DC: NASA, 1973:312.

161. Dennis RJ, Woessner WM, Miller RE, et al. The effect of fluctuating + Gz exposure on rigid gas permeable contact lens wear. *Optom Vis Sci Suppl* 1989;66:167.

162. Hart LG. Wearing contact lenses in space shuttle operations. *Aviat Space Environ Med* 1985;56:1224–1225.

163. Plyasova-Bakunina A, Volkov VV, Kiraev A, et al. Soft contact lenses in prolonged space flight: first use (in Russian). *Kosm Biol Aviak Med* 1989;23:32–34.

164. Baum G. The effect of ultrasonic radiation upon the eye and ocular adnexa. *Am J Ophthalmol* 1956;42:696–706.

165. Pernell EW, Sokollo A, Holasek E. The production of focal chorioretinitis by ultrasound. *Am J Ophthalmol* 1964;58: 953–957.

166. Repacholi MH. *Ultrasound: characteristics and biological action.* Publication no. NRCC 19244. Ottawa, Ontario: National Research Council, 1981.

167. Moss CE, Murray WE, Parr WH, et al. A report on electromagnetic radiation surveys of video display terminals. DHEW (NIOSH) publication no. 78-29, 1977.

168. Wolbarsht ML, O'Foghludah FA, Sliney DH, et al. Electromagnetic emission from visual display units: a non-hazard. In: *Nonionizing radiation.* Proceedings of an ACGIH Topical Symposium, Washington, DC, November 26-28, 1979; pp. 193–201.

169. Weiss MM, Petersen RC. Electromagnetic radiation emitted from video computer terminals. *Am Indust Hygiene Assoc J* 1979; 40:300–309.

170. Bureau of Radiological Health. An evaluation of radiation emission from video display terminals. HHS Publication. US Food and Drug Administration 81-8153, February 1981.

171. Butler GC. Radioactivity in the Canadian environment. Publication no. NRCC 18134. Ottawa, Ontario: National Research Council of Canada, 1980.

172. Murray WE, Moss CE, Parr WH, et al. Potential health hazards of video display terminals. NIOSH Research Report. DHHS (NIOSH) publication no. 81-129, June 1981.

173. Dutt GC. Bureau of Radiological Health. An evaluation of radiation emission from video display terminals. HHS Publication FDA 81-8153, February 1981.

174. Health and Welfare Canada. Investigation of radiation emissions from video display terminals. Report no. 83-EHD-91, 1983.

175. Stuchly MA, Lecuyer DW, Mann RD. Extremely low frequency electromagnetic emissions from video display terminals and other devices. *Health Phys* 1984;43:713–722.

176. Suess MJ. Visual display terminals and radiation. Proceedings of International Scientific Conference: Work with Display Units, Part 2. Stockholm, Sweden, 1986, pp. 76–79.

177. Elliott G, Gies P, Joyner KH, et al. Electromagnetic radiation emissions from video display terminals (VDTs). *Clin Exp Optom* 1986;69:53–61.

178. Muc AM. Video display terminals: do they emit dangerous levels of radiation. *Occup Health Ontario* 1987;8:182–199.

179. Elliott DB, Yang KCH, Dumbleton KA, et al. UV-induced lenticular fluorescence: intraocular straylight affecting visual function. *Vision Res* 1993;33:1827–1833.

180. Obstfeld H, Thompson D. Visual display units, visual discomfort and VDU spectacles. *Optometry Today* 1985;25:732–733.

181. Cakir A, Hart DJ, Stewart TFM. *Visual display terminals.* Chichester: John Wiley and Sons, 1979:208–214.

182. Cole BL. VDUs: not a new disease: a new challenge. *Aust J Optom* 1981;64:24–27.

183. Dain S, Chan T, Williams L. Visual and ocular changes in VDU operators. *Publ Health Lond* 1985;99:275–287.

184. Woo GC, Strong G, Irving E, et al. Are there subtle changes in vision after use of VDT's. In: Knave B, Widebäck PG, eds. *Work with display units 86.* North Holland: Elsevier Science Publishers, 1987:490–503.

185. Daum KM, Good G, Tijerina L. Symptoms in video display terminal operators and the presence of small refractive errors. *J Am Optom Assoc* 1988;59:691–697.

186. Lövsund P, Nilsson SEG, Öberg PA. The use of contact lenses in wet or damp environments. *Acta Ophthalmol* 1980;58, 794–804.

187. Andrasko G, Schoessler JP. The effect of humidity on the dehydration of soft contact lenses on the eye. *Int Contact Lens Clin* 1980;7:210–213.

188. Brennan NA, Efron N, Bruce AS, et al. Dehydration of hydrogel lenses: environmental influences during normal wear. *Am J Optom Physiol Opt* 1988;65:277–281.

189. Orsborn GN, Zantos SG. Corneal desiccation staining with thin high water content contact lenses. *CLAO J* 1988;14:81–85.

190. Hood DA. Sof-form 67 CL's in the high-altitude environment. *Contact Lens Spectrum* 1988;3:71–72.

191. Eng WG, Harada LK, Jagerman LS. The wearing of hydrophilic contact lenses aboard a commercial jet aircraft: I. Humidity effects on fit. *Aviat Space Environ Med* 1982;53 235–238.

192. Nilsson SEG, Andersson L. Contact lens wear in dry environments. *Acta Ophthalmol* 1986;64:221–225.

193. Hill RM. Dehydration deficits. *Int Contact Lens Clin* 1983;10: 364–365.

194. Nilsson SEG. Contact lenses in relation to work environment. *J Br Contact Lens Assoc* 1989;12:15–19.

195. Garston M. When meds disrupt contact lens wear. *Rev Optom* 1993;130:49–50.

196. Dille JR, Booze CF. The prevalence of visual deficiencies among 1979 general aviation accident airmen. Report no. FAA-AM-81-14. Washington DC: Department of Transport/Federal Aviation Administration, 1981.

197. Nakagawara VB, Wood KJ, Montgomery RW. Contact lens use in the civil airman population. Report no. DOT/FAA/AM-2/6. Washington DC: Federal Aviation Administration, 2002.

198. Moore RJ, Green RP. A survey of U.S. air force flyers regarding their use of extended wear contact lenses. *Aviat Space Environ Med* 194;65:1025–1031.

199. Crosley JK, Braun EG, Bailey RW. Soft (hydrophilic) contact lenses in U.S. Army aviation: an investigative study of the Bausch and Lomb Soflens. *Am J Optom Physiol Opt* 1974;51: 470–477.

200. Kartchner MN: Fight fires with contacts? *Contact Lens Forum* 1985;10:13, 21, 23–25, 27–30.

201. Sédan J, Bauby S. Reactions conjonctivales aux fum,es de gax-oil degagees par les poids lourds sur le voie publique. *Ann Oculist (Paris)* 1951;184:168.

202. Jacobson A. Letter to the editor. *Ann Ophthalmol (Chicago)* 1985;17:371.

203. Jaffe LS. Photochemical air pollutants and their effects on men and animals II. Adverse effects. *Arch Environ Health* 1968;16: 241–254.

204. Sapse AT, Bonavida B, Stone W, et al. Human tear Lysozyme III. Preliminary study on lysozyme levels in subjects with smog eye irritation. *Am J Ophthalmol* 1968;66:76–80.

205. Sapse AT, Bonavida B, Kadin M, et al. Smog eye irritation: effect of air pollution on the tear protein pattern. *Ophthalmol Addit Ad* 1969;158:421–428.

206. Okawada N, Iwamura Y, Ichikawa H, et al. Effects of photochemical smog on the human eye. *Folia Ophthalmol* 1977;Jpn 28:561 (English summary).

207. Shimizu K, Ishikawa S, Miyata M, et al. Effects of photochemical smog on the human eye. *Jpn J Ophthalmol* 1979;23:174–18.

208. Andrés S, Garcia ML, Espina M, et al. Tear pH, air pollution, and contact lenses. *Am J Optom Physiol Opt* 1988;65: 627–631.

209. Backman HA. Soaps, cosmetics and contact lenses. *Contact Lens Spectrum* 1988;3:70–72.

210. Baldwin JS. Cosmetics: too long concealed as culprit in eye problems. *Contact Lens Forum* 1986;11:34–4211. Wilson LA, Kuehne DG, Hall SW, et al. Microbial contamination in ocular cosmetics. *Am J Ophthalmol* 1971;71:1298–1302.

212. Wilson LA, Ahearn DG. Pseudomonas-induced corneal ulcers associated with contaminated eye mascaras. *Am J Ophthalmol* 1977;84:112–119.

213. Nejmeh G Jr. To keep them in or keep them out, on the job—that is the question. *Natl Safety News* June 1982;58–61.

214. Crossen RJ. Safety of contact lenses in industry. *Contact Intraocul Lens Med J* 1977;3:28–29.

215. Bergmanson JPG. Are you so vain. *Contact Lens Spectrum* 1989; 4:68.

216. Good GW, Augsberger AR. Uncorrected visual acuity standards for police applicants. *J Police Sci Admin* 1987;15:18–23.

217. Wells G A, Brown JJ, Casson EJ, et al. To wear or not to wear: current contact lens use in the Royal Canadian Mounted Police. *Can J Ophthalmol* 1997;32:158–162.

218. Case history 5. *Chem 13 News* March 1983;140:8.

219. Cullen AP. Comments on case history 5. *Chem 13 News* September 1983;142:10.

220. Girard LJ. Indications and contraindications for the use of corneal contact lenses. In: *Corneal contact lenses.* St. Louis: CV Mosby, 1964:118.

221. Pearson RM. Ocular injury and contact lens wear. *Contact Lens* 1972;3:6, 8, 19.

222. Robinson L. Contact lenses are eye savers. *Contacto* 1966;10: 7–14.

223. Rengstorff RH, Black CJ. Eye protection from contact lenses. *J Am Optom Assoc* 1974;45:270–275.

224. Von Györffy ST. Das Verhalten der Kontaktschale bei Augenverletzungen. *Ophthalmologica* 1951;122:344–347.

225. Ellison LB. Protection afforded corneal contact lenses. *Contacto* 1960;4:101–102.

226. Schwartz A, Glatt LD. Contact lenses for children and adolescents—a survey. *J Am Optom Assoc* 1960;32:143–146.

227. Samland HL. Wie eine Korneallinse eine perforierende Verletzung verhinderte. *Klin Monatsbl Augenheilkd* 1966;148: 897–898.

228. Shindo S. Selective traumatic retinal damage while wearing a contact lens (in Japanese with English summary). *Jpn J Clin Ophthalmol* 1968;22:1297–1299.

229. Nathan J. Clinical note: traumatic damage prevented by contact lens wear. *Aust J Optom* 1981;64:79–80.

230. Silberstein IW. Contact lenses in industry. *Am J Optom Arch Am Acad Optom* 1962;39:111–129.

231. Curtis JB. Hazardline chemicals which indicate a hazard for contact lens wearers. Document 9056Q. Canadian Centre for Occupational Health Safety, Hamilton, Ontario, 1985.

232. Dixon WS. Contact lenses: do they belong in the workplace? *Occup Health Safety* May 1978;36–39.

233. Koetting R. Contact lenses and welding, myth or fact (interview by CR Metzgar). *Safety Manage* 1977;3:24–29.

234. da Roza RA, Weaver C. Is it safe to wear contact lenses with a full-face respirator? Report UCRL-53653. Livermore, CA: Lawrence Livermore National Laboratory. 1985.

235. Stones I, Spencer G. Contact lenses in the workplace: the pros and cons. Document P85–1E. Canadian Centre for Occupational Health and Safety, Hamilton, Ontario, 1985.

CLINICAL RESEARCH METHODOLOGY AND STATISTICS

ALAN TOMLINSON AND
PAUL N. DE LAND

INTRODUCTION

This chapter attempts to describe, in an ophthalmic context, the design, analysis, and interpretation (application) of clinical research. This is meant to be a selective and not a comprehensive description. It is hoped that it makes a small contribution to the general literature in the field (1–12).

In the first section of this chapter, the basic designs applicable to clinical research are discussed. This approach is adopted in order to provide readers with methodologies suitable for contact lens research; therefore, designs for laboratory research and epidemiology will not be described in any detail. This chapter intends to provide an overview of the major clinical research designs, the circumstances in which they are used, and the mechanisms by which they provide investigators with answers to clinical questions. The following clinical research designs are listed in order of this discussion and, to some degree, complexity and cost:

1. Case reports
2. Case series
3. Surveys
4. Case-control (retrospective) studies
5. Cross-sectional studies
6. Cohort (prospective) studies
7. Clinical trials (experimental)
8. Single-subject studies
9. Other clinical research designs

RESEARCH DESIGN

Case Reports

This is the simplest form of clinical research design used in contact lens research. The description of a single patient may be used to indicate the complications of lens fitting (13), new procedures (14,15), problems in fitting (16), and manifestations of conditions that may be helpful in their diagnosis (17–22). Case reports are beneficial in generating hypotheses and ideas that may be tested in later studies involving series of patients or other research designs.

Case Series

When more than one case is included in a report, this constitutes a case series and provides additional information on how the cases vary. In contact lens research, the case series design is applied most commonly in major studies. The clinical investigations required for United States Food and Drug Administration (FDA) approval of new contact lenses and solutions are large case series or prospective evaluations of patients over a specified period of time. Because these investigations do not include a control group of patients who are not wearing lenses or using solutions, they cannot be thought of as true prospective or cohort studies (see later).

The literature includes case series that illustrate the effectiveness of new lens fitting procedures (23), care regimens (24), and the complications of contact lens wear (25). The insights provided by case series may establish the effectiveness of the techniques on the patient population reported. Unfortunately, the results obtained on carefully selected populations by experienced practitioners do not always translate to the same levels of success on patients fitted in routine contact lens practice. The most dramatic example of this has been the comparative failure of bifocal soft lenses when fitted to the general population of contact lens patients (26). This is an example of the concern that is expressed in the contact lens community when extrapolating from the results of FDA clinical investigations to general clinical practice.

Even though case reports or case series designs are, in some ways, less scientific than the designs to be described later, they have implicit, if not actual, control groups. In making judgments that a particular type of contact lens has resulted in problems in fitting, the clinician is basing the patient's signs or symptoms on a comparison with his or her recollection of normalcy in other forms of contact lens wear. These are known as *historic controls*.

Surveys

The survey attempts to determine the prevalence of a particular condition in a specified population. This may be the incidence of amblyopia in school-aged children (27), of polymegethism in an extended wear contact lens population (28), and of ulceration in the contact lens population (29). It also could include surveys of the changing views of contact lens wear (30). Although surveys can provide interesting estimates of the incidence of conditions, they are rarely definitive, because the exact parameters of the population from which they are drawn are difficult to determine.

In the next four sections of the chapter, the principal designs for clinical research are discussed.

Case-Control (Retrospective) Studies

This is a study design that has been used infrequently in ophthalmic (31) and only occasionally in contact lens research (32–34). As with the aforementioned designs, both case-control and cohort studies can be described as observational in distinction from experimental designs (e.g., clinical trials). Both case-control and cohort studies are designed to investigate causal relationships between a condition and the factors that produce that condition. The two basic approaches differ in the direction in which the association between cause and effect is determined. In a cohort study, the direction is from postulated cause to effect; in a case-control study, an attempt is made to work back from effect to cause. In both designs, however, the etiology of the condition is the focus of attention.

In the case-control study, two groups of individuals are selected. These include *cases,* or individuals who have developed the condition under investigation prior to the start of the study. The controls in this study design are individuals who have not developed the condition. Both cases and controls are compared for existing or past attributes or exposures that are thought by investigators to be relevant to the development of the condition under study.

It is sometimes necessary to make a distinction among the sources from which cases and controls are selected (23). In population-based case-control studies, all of the cases in the study are from a defined geographic area. Both cases and controls are selected on a random basis from the large available population in the geographic region. In hospital-based or practice-based case-control studies, all cases of the condition entering a hospital or practice during a specified period of time may be selected for the study. In this more limited population, controls also must be selected appropriately (e.g., from the same hospital or practice from individuals admitted for conditions other than that under study).

To illustrate the various designs being discussed, an example of a hypothetic study is chosen from the contact lens field. The ways in which this study may be carried out according to the different designs is described.

Example: Case-Control Study

Microcystic edema has been found to occur in extended contact lens wear (35). A case-control study of microcystic edema and contact lens wear is carried out to determine if the epithelial appearance is associated with extended lens wear.

One hundred patients from a large contact lens practice are chosen in whom epithelial microcysts, greater in number than 50, are observed under slit-lamp examination. A control group of patients is chosen from the same practice in whom microcysts are absent or do not exceed 10 in each eye. To determine the influence of extended contact tens wear on the development of microcysts, it is necessary to determine how many patients in the control and case groups regularly sleep wearing the contact tenses.

It then is possible to compare the case and control populations by using the results to estimate the proportions of patients from each group who wore their lenses on an extended basis. In view of the observed association between the incidence of epithelial microcysts and chronic edema found in extended wear, it is likely that a larger number will have had extended wear experience in the case than in the control group (35). Such a finding would allow conclusions to be drawn about a possible mechanism of chronic edema in extended wear leading to the development of the epithelial microcysts. From this conclusion, extrapolations may be made concerning the fate of other patients from other practices who wear contact lenses on an extended wear basis.

This is an example of how a case-control, or retrospective, study can be carried out in contact lens research and helps to illustrate how the methodology enables a conclusion to be made about the association between the cause (extended contact lens wear) and the effect (the development of epithelial microcysts) or, because causal relationships are so difficult to establish, between the risk factor (extended wear) and the outcome (epithelial microcysts).

The advantage of the case-control, or retrospective, study is that it provides a design that is well suited to the study of rare diseases or conditions or those with long latency (1, 2). It is a quick and easy study to perform and, therefore, is relatively inexpensive (12). It is likely to give meaningful results with comparatively fewer subjects than would be required in other designs. As in the example, existing records from a practice may be used. Also, because the condition previously developed, there is no additional risk to subjects. Another significant benefit is that it allows study of multiple potential causes of a condition in addition to the cause targeted by the study.

Case-control studies, however, have significant methodologic failings. Many of these errors involve the accuracy of the data about the prior characteristics of the patients studied. Specifically, this information is dependent on patient recall or clinic records and is difficult to validate. It is almost impossible to control extraneous variables that may have some effect on the results of a retrospective study. Also, it is very difficult to select an appropriate comparison or control group, and the technique does not allow a detailed study of the mechanism between cause and effect (12).

Cross-Sectional Studies

A cross-sectional study is one in which a proportion of the study population is chosen without regard to, or prior knowledge of, either the subject's outcome or risk factor status. Except in the measurement of the outcome, these are identical to case-control, or retrospective, studies (2). The difference, for instance, in the previous example, is that the study characteristic (extended contact lens wear) and the outcome (epithelial microcysts) are measured at the same point in time.

Cross-sectional studies are useful for examining networks of causal links (12) and where a researcher is in the ethical dilemma of requiring continued exposure to a potentially dangerous cause right up to the time that an effect is seen. For example, in a study to determine the effect of heavily contaminated soft contact lenses on the development of corneal ulceration, a group of patients is identified in whom some have developed corneal ulceration. It is determined whether patients with ulceration are more likely to have heavily contaminated lenses at the time of the ulceration than is a comparable group without infection. Cross-sectional studies are occasionally found in the contact lens literature (36–38).

Case-control studies, described earlier, also may be called *analytic studies* because the investigation is designed to test an hypothesis concerning the cause of the condition under study. For instance, an hypothesis that epithelial microcysts are caused by relative hypoxia during extended contact lens wear is very clear and amenable to investigation in this way. An alternative form of case-control study, called an *exploratory study* or *fishing expedition,* is one in which multiple hypotheses are proposed for investigation (1). The purpose of such a study is to learn enough about possible causes of a condition so that a specific hypothesis can be suggested for later detailed investigation.

Example: Exploratory Study

A recent study of the causes of lens binding in extended wear of rigid gas permeable contact lenses evaluates the effect of several factors on this problem (39). No specific hypothesis is advanced prior to the study regarding the effect of any of these factors on binding. However, as a result of the study, it is possible to advance a hypothesis that thinning of the post-lens tear film during sleep results in a very thin, highly viscous layer of mucus-rich tears between the lens and the cornea. This layer has the effect of binding the lens to the cornea and rendering it nonmoving on the eye opening. This hypothesis should be tested by a further case-control, analytic study.

Cohort (Prospective) Studies

The other major form of observational study is the cohort, or prospective, study. In this type of study, the investigation proceeds from cause to effect, or in the opposite direction to that of a case-control study. Therefore, the unique feature of this type of cohort study is that it begins before a group of individuals have developed a condition under investigation. This group is followed forward in time to determine who subsequently develops the condition. In such a study, two cohorts or groups of individuals who share common experiences are chosen. The subject group, or cohort, possesses the characteristic under study; the other cohort does not possess this particular characteristic. Therefore, the individuals are selected for observation and followed forward in time depending on the presence or absence of certain characteristics that are thought to influence the development of the condition.

Returning to our proposed study of the relationship between epithelial microcysts and extended soft contact lens wear, it is possible to investigate this problem using a cohort, or prospective, study design. In such a design, the intention of the study is to follow a group of extended contact lens wearers to determine the proportion of patients who develop the epithelial microcysts. This number is compared to the number of patients demonstrating the effect (microcysts) in a control group of daily wear, soft lens patients. The number of patients in each group who develop epithelial microcysts provides a measure of the relative risk of developing the condition. *Relative risk* is defined as the risk of the outcome (microcysts) if the risk factor is present (i.e., extended wear) divided by the risk of the outcome (microcysts) if the risk factor (extended wear) is absent.

Example: Cohort (Prospective) Study

A group of soft lens patients beginning extended soft lens wear is chosen, and a similar group, or cohort, of daily soft lens wearers also is selected. During the course of the study, these two groups are monitored to determine how many patients demonstrate clinically significant (>10 per cornea) epithelial microcysts when observed at follow-up contact lens assessment. In the analysis of data, it is possible to compare the risk of developing epithelial microcysts for the patients in extended wear and daily wear soft lenses. Therefore, the risk of microcysts in extended wear can be compared to the risk in daily wear. From these extrapolations, the risk to other extended wear patients outside the study who develop epithelial microcysts can be assessed.

The major advantage of cohort, or prospective, studies over case-control, or retrospective, studies is the greater assurance that the characteristic under study precedes the outcome (2,12). In our contact lens example, a cohort study is more likely to provide assurance to the investigator that extended soft lens wear precedes the development of epithelial microcysts than a case-control study because of the measurement of the presence of microcysts before and after development. In determining a cause-and-effect relationship, this assurance of cause preceding effect is essential. Other advantages of the cohort study is that, in principle, it provides a complete description of the experience of a patient prior to exposure to the cause under consideration (1). This may include the progression through the stages of the condition and its natural history. Also, it permits multiple potential effects of a given exposure to be determined and for the estimation of rates of the condition in exposed and unexposed individuals.

There are, however, significant disadvantages to this study design. Generally, cohort studies require large numbers of subjects in order to study rare conditions. In addition, they often require long duration for follow-up. As a consequence, cohort studies are expensive to conduct, and it is difficult to maintain follow-up (12). They also do not provide a detailed study of the mechanism relating cause and effect. Cohort studies produce more in-depth understanding of the effect of an etiologic factor. However, they are much less likely than retrospective studies to uncover new etiologic factors.

As stated earlier, the conventional or concurrent cohort studies are expensive and time consuming. However, it is possible to conduct a cohort study without lengthy time involvement if reliable data on the presence or absence of the study characteristic (in the earlier examples, extended contact lens wear) are available from an earlier time. If this is the case, it is possible to carry out a *nonconcurrent cohort study*. In such a study, the placing of individuals into particular groups is made based on this past information. The time needed for follow-up in this case is only from the point of assignment of individuals to the development of the condition. In a contact lens practice in which a cohort study of the relationship between epithelial microcysts and extended soft lens wear is being undertaken, it should be possible to have reliable information about the patients who have been on extended wear prior to the start of the study. If this is the case, it is easy to allocate an individual to the extended or daily wear group and then monitor the incidence of microcysts.

Another form of cohort study in which even less time is required for follow-up is in the case of the historic cohort study. This is the study in which the outcome has occurred before the start of the investigation, cohorts established, and their experience assessed from existing records (40). Historic cohort studies are similar to retrospective studies, except that subjects are chosen based on exposure or nonexposure to the risk factor.

There are clearly advantages and disadvantages to both major forms of observational study. The benefits and limitations of case-control and cohort studies have been described. In order to derive the greatest amount of information on the causative factors for a condition, ideally both case-con-

trol and cohort studies should be carried out simultaneously. Such a study of ulceration secondary to contact lens wear has been funded by the Contact Lens Institute (41). This study adopts both case-control and cohort designs to derive the maximum information. It has obtained information about the causative factors in this relatively low-incidence condition and determined, with the greatest degree of assurance, which factors are responsible for the condition.

Clinical Trial (Experimental) Studies

Experimental studies performed in clinical research are called *clinical trials*. This is a design widely used in medical research and, over the past 30 years, has been used to evaluate treatments in ophthalmology (11). Unlike the observational studies described earlier, a clinical trial is one in which a planned intervention on factors suspected of altering the phenomenon under study is performed (1). However, the intention of this experimental study is still the same as for an observational study, which is to clarify cause-and-effect relationships.

As is true with cohort studies, clinical trials monitor patients over a period of time to determine if they develop a particular condition under investigation. They are different, however, in the method by which individuals are assigned to the treatment and control groups. This assignment is always random and often blindly determined or determined in a masked manner. *Random assignment* means that any individual has an equal probability of being in the study or control group. *Blind* or *masked assignment* means that neither the participants nor the investigators know to which group the individual has been assigned.

Example: Clinical Trial

To continue with the universal example of a hypothetical contact lens study problem, it is possible to perform a clinical trial to determine the relationship between epithelial microcysts and extended soft contact lens wear. In this design, patients are randomly assigned to either the extended wear (treatment) group or the daily wear (control) group. In this example, it is not possible to assign the patients blindly because they must be aware of whether or not they should sleep wearing their contact lenses. The two groups are then monitored to determine who develops clinically significant epithelial microcysts. The probability of developing microcysts in patients with daily and extended wear lenses is estimated. From this information, conclusions can be drawn about the meaning of the difference for patients in daily and extended wear groups and their likelihood of developing epithelial microcysts.

The randomized clinical trial has emerged as the most effective design for evaluating the safety and efficacy of a procedure or technique in ophthalmic research (42,43). Simplified variations of this design have appeared in the contact lens literature (44).

The principal advantage of the clinical trial is the ability to impose an intervention on the study group that helps to establish the cause-and-effect relationship by determining that altering the cause alters the effect. By this means it is possible to untangle a complex causal problem in a stepwise fashion by breaking the main problem down into subproblems and exploring each by a series of separate experiments (1). There are, however, some significant disadvantages to this design. The experimental approach may not be feasible for certain problems. The limitations of the number of human subjects who may be available may prevent the resolution of a question by direct experimentation. For example, it is possible that the incidence of corneal ulceration secondary to contact lens wear (particularly daily wear) is so low that a large enough sample of patients could not be obtained to describe the relative incidence adequately. Another problem of such a study would be that it may require a considerable duration of time before the ulceration develops. Long studies are extremely expensive to maintain, particularly as a high rate of loss of patients to follow-up can occur, thus reducing the validity of the results obtained. Obviously, there is an ethical consideration about continuing a procedure that is known to cause a serious effect, such as corneal ulceration. It is an abiding ethical problem in clinical trials whether to continue the trial when it becomes clear that a large proportion of the study group is afflicted by a serious condition (effect). Clinical trials also can provide significant public relation problems for practitioners. The involvement of practitioners in clinical trials may require the tacit acknowledgment to patients that they are uncertain about which method or technique is preferable. This may shatter the illusion that the practitioner is fully knowledgeable regarding the effect of all techniques that he or she adopts. Patients may have prejudices against being subjects in research studies. They also may have a preference for one particular technique or type of contact lens wear over another. For these reasons, randomized clinical trials can be difficult to perform in clinical practice.

An early classic study using the technique of clinical trials was performed by Lind (45), who showed the efficacy of a citrus diet in overcoming scurvy on British naval ships in the mid-eighteenth century. The basic clinical trial technique of randomization was introduced by Box and Fisher (3) and first applied to agricultural research. The first clinical trial using a form of random assignment of subjects to form a study group was reported in 1933. The classic study of the effect of streptomycin therapy on patients with tuberculosis performed by Bradford Hill (46) in 1948 was the first to use random numbers in allocating subjects to experimental and control groups.

Clinical trials now represent the most powerful tool in the researcher's armamentarium of research designs, but the technique was not widely used before 1950. Since that time, however, it has been used in medical research, in pharmacology (11), and in optometry to determine the efficacy of new procedures and techniques. In recent time, comprehensive texts describing the design have been published (4,5,47).

The timing of clinical trials in the development of a new technique or therapy is a difficult question. Often a much needed therapy gains widespread use before effective testing on a controlled trial basis is possible. An example of this is the use of anticoagulants after myocardial infarction. Whether or not the clinical use of anticoagulants in people who have suffered myocardial infarction is beneficial is unclear. Widespread use of the drug therapy makes it impossible to resolve the issue at this time because of the lack of availability of suitable sample groups for study (5).

Another important issue for timing of clinical trials is the point of development of a therapy or technique at which the trial is instituted. Many techniques continue to develop over a period of years. A question arises at what point they should be tested for efficacy. Certainly, during long-term clinical trials, it is possible that advancements may make the technique being studied obsolete before the end of the trial, but evaluating a technique of several years may not reflect the current status of advancement in the technique. An example of this is the Prospective Evaluation of Radial Keratotomy (PERK) study (48). Evaluation of the eight-cut incision technique may not represent the current state of knowledge in the field of refractive surgery 4 to 5 years after the onset of study. The PERK study is not strictly a clinical trial because it does not have a control group; however, it does serve as an illustration from the ophthalmic field of the problems of timing with clinical trials.

Another important dilemma in clinical trials is the ethics of continuing the trials after trends in the data have indicated that a particular intervention is effective in treating a serious condition. One way in which this is overcome is by advance agreement by subjects and investigators that they will not be told interim results until the study is over. However, in situations where there is a conflict between the investigator's perception of what is good for the subject and the needs of a trial, it is usually what is good for the subject that predominates. In all cases, however, proper informed consent is essential.

As in all research designs, a complete protocol for the clinical trial is required. In view of the nature of the study, its length, and the need for understanding among the investigators and the subjects concerning the aims of the trial, a full and complete protocol is essential. The outlines of clinical trial protocols are described in the literature (4,5,47).

Although the use of randomized clinical trials has been attempted in the determination of the efficacy of techniques in the ophthalmic field (42,43), it is in the field of clinical pharmacology and toxicology that the technique is used most frequently.

These drug trials often are classified into four phases of experimentation. The first experiments are primarily concerned with drug safety, not efficacy. These phase 1 trials have, as an objective, the determination of the acceptable single-drug dosage. The phase 2 trial is the initial clinical investigation for treatment effect to determine the effectiveness and safety of the drug. The third phase, the full scale evaluation and treatment, is preferred after the drug has been found to be reasonably effective. In this phase, the drug is compared with the current standard method of treatment for the same condition in a large-trial population. It is this third phase that is the most commonly recognized when discussing clinical trials. There is also a fourth phase, postmarketing surveillance, after approval for marketing of a new drug. In this phase, the further assessment of adverse effects and additional large-scale, long-term studies are performed.

Of the large amount of funding expended by the pharmaceutical industry in the research and development of new drugs, approximately one fourth is devoted to clinical trials (46). It takes about 7 to 10 years for completion of an entire research program for a new drug, and approximately half of that time is spent in clinical trials.

In optometric research, limited clinical trials have been performed to determine the efficacy of contact lens cleaning systems (44,49), to evaluate cromolyn sodium in the treatment of keratoconjunctivitis (50), to determine the physiologic response to new contact lens materials (51), to determine the efficacy of various techniques in refitting long-term polymethyl methacrylate (PMMA) lens wearers (52), and to compare new with established techniques of fitting gas permeable (53) and toric soft lenses (54).

Single-Subject Designs

Another form of experimental study that lends itself well to the clinical situation is the single-subject design (55). In this design, data are collected from a single subject under various test conditions. This technique can provide the researcher with a mechanism for systematically evaluating the interventions used in clinical practice. It is used frequently in pilot studies from which research hypotheses are formulated. These hypotheses are then investigated in later, more extensive studies.

The single-subject design requires graphical presentation of data with the dependent variable expressed on the vertical axis and time expressed on the horizontal axis. Changes in the independent variable are indicated by vertical lines separating data obtained during different phases of the study. Although this design may involve measurements on multiple subjects, it is the effect of the independent variable that is monitored for each subject separately.

Example: Single-Subject Design

Examples of this design may be found in the contact lens literature (56) and in the study shown in Fig. 45.1. In this figure, the tear film evaporation rate before and after the instillation of a drop of saline into the eye was measured. In all single-subject designs, a baseline condition must be determined. The baseline observations of the dependent variable (tear evaporation rate) were noted before introduction of the experimental

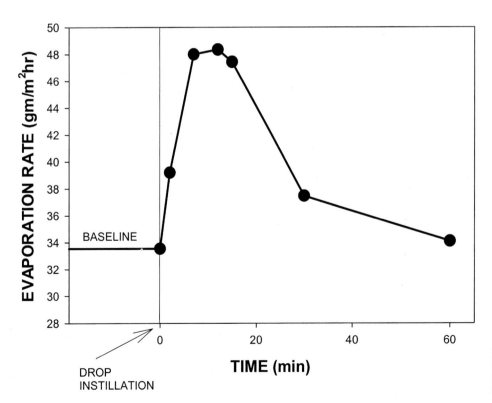

FIG. 45.1. Plot of the time course of evaporation rate following hypromellose administration from a single-subject design study.

intervention (insertion of the fluid drop). The purpose of the baseline is to provide reference data for determining whether the dependent variable is affected by introduction of the independent variable (saline drop).

A design in which a single intervention takes place is referred to as an AB design, where A is the baseline and B is the condition in which the intervention is introduced. To verify the effect of the intervention on the dependent variable, an ABA design can be used. In this design, the intervention is removed and the return to baseline of the dependent variable monitored (the return to baseline observed in Fig. 45.1). This allows a demonstration that changes observed during the intervention were attributable to the intervention rather than to extraneous random factors associated with the passage of time.

In the past 15 to 20 years, a new type of clinical trial has been developed based on a single-subject research design known as a *single-patient clinical trial* (10). These experiments using the AB or BA design for treatment intervention or placebo are double blind and prospective.

In some single-subject designs, a multiple-baseline design is used. This provides an alternative method for demonstrating the effects of an intervention in an experimentally controlled manner. This technique requires collecting baseline data in two or more dimensions simultaneously (55). For example, data could be collected simultaneously for the same independent variable in two or more subjects, for the same subject in two or more settings, or for two or more different dependent variables in the same subject.

Another single-subject design variant is that of the changing criterion design. This is particularly beneficial when the dependent variable is a behavior or skill that will be acquired gradually by the subject (57). The experimenter sets an initial criterion goal for the subject's behavior (dependent variable). This criterion is gradually changed as the subject reliably attains that criterion.

There are several advantages to the single-subject design over the more traditional research designs. First, many clinical researchers have ethical concerns about the use of placebo or no treatment control conditions. This concern is minimized in single-subject designs because treatment can be provided to every subject in a systematic manner. Second, with group designs it often is difficult to obtain a sample large enough to provide adequate statistical power for evaluating the effects of an intervention, particularly if the disorder is rare. With single-subject designs, few subjects are needed. Third, group designs focus on demonstrations of differences among groups. The implication is that patients who appear similar to those in the randomized study will respond similarly. However, in all group designs, some patients in the treatment group do not benefit. Thus, it becomes difficult for the clinician to predict the effectiveness of a particular treatment for an individual case. More important, it is difficult to know how long to continue with the treatment or whether to try an alternative if the patient does

not appear to be responding. Thus, extrapolating from the research literature to clinical practice is hampered. In the single-subject design, however, the effect of the intervention on the patient can be observed. Finally, group designs emphasize between-subject variability and attempt to minimize within-subject variability. This latter variability typically is referred to as a *measurement error* and considered a problem. However, in single-subject designs, within-subject variability is, in fact, very important because it provides a real description of the course of treatment.

Other Clinical Research Designs

Not all clinical research studies fall neatly into the categories just outlined. Looking at the contact lens literature, it is not possible in all cases to categorize a particular study as a case-control study, a cohort study, a clinical trial, or a survey. In an attempt to include in this review more of the designs that are found in the literature, the following other designs are described.

Cross-over (Prospective) Study

This study has some of the features of prospective studies and some of clinical trials. The design incorporates the evaluation of the effect of two or more treatments on a particular feature of, for example, contact lens wear or corneal physiology. The characteristic of this type of study is that the patient experiences first the wear of a contact lens or treatment applied to the test eye for a period of time to determine its effect. This is followed by the test eye being fitted with a second contact lens or exposed to a new form of treatment. A comparison of contact lenses or treatments then can be made under highly controlled conditions in the same test eyes of the same group of patients. This allows a within-patient, as distinct from a between-patient, comparison found in other designs. Because each subject is observed twice, variability is reduced because the measured effect of the intervention is the difference in an individual subject's response. This reduction in variability allows smaller sample sizes to be used in cross-over studies (4). This design is often used in the early clinical trials of new drug therapies (5).

The design has, therefore, the advantage of avoiding the effect of variability between patients in the evaluation of two contact lens modalities or treatments (58). However, it does have the disadvantage that in those situations where the initial contact lens or treatment radically changes the response of the patient, this can affect the results obtained for the second contact lens or treatment (this is known as a *carryover effect*) (12). This disadvantage can be alleviated by randomizing the order in which patients are exposed to the two test conditions, by the use of a washout period between exposures (5), or by the use of a statistical method developed by Grizzle (59) to check the assumption of no interaction between period and treatment. This test lacks sensitivity, however, and the cross-over design is discouraged by Brown (58), Hills and Armitage (60), and by the FDA (5). Examples of this type of study in the contact lens literature include investigations of the effectiveness of monovision and bifocal contact lenses in the correction of presbyopia (61) and studies of the deposit resistance of various hydrogel lens polymers (62,63).

Simultaneous Comparison Study

In vision research, another type of within-patient study is possible. This is the comparison of different treatments applied to the two eyes of the same patient simultaneously. This design has been used in ophthalmology to examine the effect of new photocoagulation techniques in diabetic retinopathy (64) and in contact lenses to evaluate the effect of different materials on overnight corneal swelling response (51). The design has the advantage of testing an intervention on a subject group simultaneously, without any concern for the period–treatment interaction of cross-over studies. Simultaneous comparison studies require only the smaller sample sizes that are possible when considering within-patient variability. The simultaneous comparison study may, however, be susceptible to errors from sympathetic reactions between fellow eyes (65). For example, a rigid lens worn in one eye may cause tearing in both eyes and thereby affect the data from a hydrogel lens worn in the contralateral eye.

Factorial Designs

This design allows comparison of the effect of two interventions or conditions on a single control in one experiment (10); thus, the time and expense of two separate experiments is saved without major increases in the sample size. However, in the event of significant interactions between interventions, the design should be treated with caution.

Experiments in Clinical Research

Another form of clinical research is described in the literature in which experiments are performed in a manner somewhat analogous to the *bench-type* research of the pure sciences. Examples of this type of study include measurement of the effect of induced changes in human corneal thickness on limbal vascularization (66). This experimental design has been applied extensively in contact lens research to the determination of the effect of fitting relationship and lens design on contact lens performance on the eye (67–72). The technique also is applied in clinically related bench experiments, such as preliminary studies of new experimental procedures for measuring hard lens flexure (73) and the effect of reducing agents on the enzymatic cleaning of in *vitro* deposited hydrogel contact lenses (74).

The benefit of experimental clinical research studies are

that they provide immediate information on the effect of varying measurements or cleaning techniques on a group of lenses from a particular patient population. They also allow fine control of the variations in technique or procedure to determine critical levels of change. However, they have the disadvantage of being susceptible to the methodologic errors found in all experimental research (69,70). In this type of study, the patient sample size is rarely large enough to allow for compensation for these errors. Another significant disadvantage of this research design is the inability to extrapolate data obtained from the small sample and apply it to the general population.

Meta-analyses of Multiple Studies

The objective analysis, through the statistical synthesis of the results of previous studies, is referred to as *pooling*, meta-analysis, or systematic review (75). It can provide a means of reducing biases inherent in the studies and enhancing the precision of treatment effects. The approach can lead to reductions in false-negative results and more rapid introduction of effective treatments and definition of new study problems. The approach must be adopted continuously with due regard to the appropriate methodology so that the results of the analyses are valid (75).

Conclusion

This description of different clinical research designs should provide the reader with an overview of the methods that can be applied in designing a clinical research study. Depending on the intentions of the study, a particular design may be preferable to others. The design chosen should maximize the information obtained given the restrictions imposed by the feasibility of performing many measurement procedures on only limited patient groups. Generally, the principal research designs described in this section may be ranked in the following descending order of strength: randomized clinical trials, cohort studies, case-control studies, and case series (76). It is desirable in each case to select the strongest design feasible.

ORGANIZING A RESEARCH STUDY

Before organizing a study, it is important to state clearly the hypothesis to be investigated. This must include specific and concrete objectives that appear to be achievable in the study (77). At first, a research question may be suggested in a broad and ambitious way. In due course, however, this is refined to a more succinct statement of the question to be investigated (2). This refinement comes from a careful review of the populations available for study, the ability to obtain the information required, and the time and cost of certain types of investigations. It is essential that the research question, or the study hypothesis, be fully defined within the constraints of the eventual design used. If this precise definition is not achieved, the answer to the question may not be obtained with sufficient clarity to attain an adequate result from the study.

It is important to state hypotheses and objectives in such a way that they are testable; generalized statements should be avoided. In stating the research hypothesis, some authors favor a statement in a positive form rather than in the form of a null hypothesis (77). For example, the statement "patients wearing extended wear hydrogel soft lenses are more likely to show microcystic edema than those with daily wear lenses" is preferable to, "both extended and daily wear soft lens wearers will experience the same degree of microcystic edema." An advantage of a positively stated hypothesis is that it allows the use of a one-sided statistical testing procedure in the analysis of results and thereby increases the power of the experiment without the need for an increase in sample size. The organization of a clinical research study will now be reviewed.

Irrespective of the type of design chosen for a study, its organization falls into five separate phases: *selection* (assignment) of individuals for a study or a control group, *measurement* (assessment) of the results for the study and control groups, *analysis* or comparison of the results obtained for study and control groups, *interpretation* of the results obtained from the study and control groups to draw conclusions about the differences among these groups, and *application* (extrapolation) of the results from the study and control groups to a wider population.

Selection (Assignment) of Patients

In any study involving measurements on human subjects, a number of ethical and regulatory guidelines apply to protect the patient's right to informed consent before undergoing measurement and therapy (10). The nature of informed consent is captured in the Helsinki Doctrine of the World Medical Association (1964) and the legislation in the US regarding Institutional Review Boards (Volume 46, *Federal Register* 8975, 1/27/81, 21 Code of Federal Regulations 56 and HS FR 3C390 5/30/80, 21 CFR 50). These rights are ensured by the requirement for research study protocols to be submitted to the Ethics Committee in the Review Board of the institution overseeing the investigation.

In the principal designs in clinical research (case-control, cohort, and clinical trials), the careful selection of individuals for both the study and control groups is essential. The study and control groups should be identical in all respects, except for that which is the focus of the study (2).

Unfortunately, in most clinical research designs, limitations in the very designs themselves can result in an error being introduced during the selection of patients. This is known as *selection bias.* This problem applies particularly to case-control and cohort studies. In case-control studies,

investigators can observe only that individuals have, or do not have, a particular condition and in cohort studies that individuals have, or do not have, a particular characteristic. The introduction of selection bias during the selection of patients for groups can unintentionally introduce factors that may predetermine the outcome of the study.

Among the factors that may lead to this type of bias are the differential surveillance, diagnosis, and referral (or selection) of individuals for these studies (1). If a condition under study is relatively mild or asymptomatic and, therefore, is less likely to be observed at a routine examination, study subjects are more likely to have the condition observed than controls because of more frequent observation. This is particularly so in case-control studies (e.g., in the study of epithelial microcysts in extended contact lens wear, a more frequent observation of extended wearers, the study group, may lead to a greater likelihood of observations of the asymptomatic epithelial microcysts in that group).

In other cases, the validity of the diagnosis of a condition may be called into question because it may lead to bias. For example, low-grade giant papillary conjunctivitis (GPC) secondary to contact lens wear is more likely to be diagnosed in patients wearing extended wear hydrogel contact lenses, as it is known that GPC occurs frequently in patients with heavily deposited lenses. Therefore, in a study that evaluates GPC in extended contact lens wear, the mere knowledge of exposure may alter the diagnosis of the condition. This is more likely to occur for lower grades of GPC in which the diagnosis is more questionable.

Differential referral patterns are another source of potential bias in hospital- or clinic-based, case-control studies (1). The differential rates of hospitalization or clinic visits, for exposed and unexposed cases, can distort the apparent incidence of the condition when the assessment is based on results from selective practices. An example of this is found in the contact lens literature in which the incidence of corneal ulceration secondary to contact lens wear has been attempted from case-control studies performed in hospitals (78). A case-control study based on cases derived from a major hospital eye clinic, which is the referral center for such cases, would tend to overestimate the relative risk in the general population. In the selection of patients for a case-control or cross-sectional study, it is important that investigators do not key in on cases exposed to the study factor. Any practice that selects even a fraction of potential cases may introduce this form of bias into the sample.

Another factor that may introduce selection bias is derived from potential patients' refusals or nonresponses to invitations to participate in a study. Different rates of response among cases and controls may not introduce bias in those situations in which the proportion of patients exhibiting a particular condition is equal between refusing and participating individuals in both groups. However, in many cases this cannot be guaranteed, and similar rates or responses among cases and controls are desirable.

Example: Selection Bias in a Cohort Study

A cohort study is proposed. Two new extended wear, rigid gas-permeable contact lens materials are to be compared by the number of patients achieving long-term overnight wear and by the swelling response produced in the cornea. For material A, a group is chosen that includes previously successful extended contact lens wear patients. In the choice of subjects for material B, only new contact lens wearers are selected.

The results of the study indicate that material A is more successful for extended wear than material B, with a greater proportion of patients remaining in extended wear with the first material. Also, the average overnight corneal swelling response with material A is significantly less than with that of material B.

Material A might be better than material B, but there is a significant selection bias introduced into the study by the inclusion in the group wearing material A of previously successful extended contact lens wearers. Previous success indicates that the corneal physiology of these patients is more suited to the relative hypoxia of extended wear. Studies with gas goggles in which various hypoxic environments are presented to the cornea indicate widely varying minimum oxygen tension levels required to maintain a normal corneal deturgescence in different persons (79).

This example illustrates important features of selection bias. The study and control groups were not representative of all individuals who could have been included, and the factor making the two groups different could have affected the results.

The last example illustrated selection bias in the assignment of individuals to study and control groups of a prospective or cohort study. Case-control, or retrospect, studies also may suffer from the same form of bias, which can be observed from the next hypothetical example.

Example: Selection Bias in Case-Control Study

A retrospective study of the causes of neovascularization compares the past use of extended wear contact lenses among 100 patients with neovascularization (study group) with a control group of 100 contact lens patients selected from those with GPC. It is found that 30% of the study group had used extended-wear contact lenses during the past 5 years, whereas only 3% of those with GPC (control group) attempted extended wear. It is concluded that there is a strong association between the use of extended wear lenses and the development of neovascularization.

This may or may not be the case, but it must be asked whether selection bias exists in the choice of patients in the control group. To determine this, it is important to know whether the patients in the control group are representative of all patients without neovascularization. This is unlikely to be true, because those patients are unique in being chosen on the basis of having GPC. This uniqueness is likely to affect the probability of developing neovascularization because extended wear is known to exacerbate GPC and is less likely to be recommended. Thus, the uniqueness of the GPC in these patients contributes to the lower-than-expected use of extended wear lenses and thus incorporates possible selection bias into the assignment of patients to the control group.

In both case-control and cohort studies, proper study design often can eliminate selection bias. In clinical trials, selection bias is avoided by randomly and blindly assigning the persons to study and control groups (80). Unfortunately, even careful study design cannot guarantee that groups are actually similar; chance alone may result in important differences. To determine whether chance differences have occurred, investigators should attempt to define a broad range of potentially relevant characteristics of the study and control groups, particularly those that might be related to the outcome. Where the study and control groups differ by chance in a factor that affects the results of the study, there is said to be a lack of comparability between the groups.

As an example of a lack of comparability between the study and control groups, the following hypothetical clinical trial is described.

Example: Lack of Comparability

This study was intended to determine the effect of a new extended wear contact lens material on the incidence of polymegethism secondary to extended wear. To evaluate its effectiveness, a clinical trial was conducted in which 100 patients were randomly and blindly assigned to either the study group wearing the new material or to the control group wearing a conventional mid-water-content soft lens. The average age of the study group was 27 years versus 55 years in the control group. The investigators found that during the next 5 years, the control group had an average coefficient of variation (a measure of polymegethism) of 0.45, whereas the study group had an average of 0.30. As the former coefficient of variation was closer to the normal noncontact lens wearers value of 0.25, it was concluded that the new material was safer and more effective for an extended wear modality than the conventional lens.

However, the investigators had not considered the effect of the age difference between the two study groups. An increase in polymegethism is found with age; thus, the difference found in the study could have been accounted for by the lack of comparability between the study and control groups. A factor that differs between the study and control groups and is likely to affect the outcome is known as a *confounding variable*. The existence of a confounding variable does not necessarily invalidate an investigation. If the lack of comparability between the groups is recognized, the difference frequently can be taken into account in the analysis. In the example, subsets of patients from the control and study groups could be selected that were matched for age and the coefficient of variation between these subsets compared (discussed later).

Measurement (Assessment) of Results

To assess the results of a study, researchers must define the result or outcome they intend to measure. This will depend, to some extent, on the type of study performed and, therefore, is a little confusing. Both cohort and clinical trials begin with a study group that possesses the characteristic under study and a control group that is free from the characteristic. For instance, in our example of epithelial microcysts in extended contact lens wear, the characteristic under study is extended contact lens wear. Individuals in the study group are monitored to determine whether they will develop the condition of epithelial microcysts. In both studies, the hypothesized condition (i.e., the development of microcysts) is known as the outcome. Case-control studies, conversely, begin with the patient having developed the condition, epithelial microcysts, and these patients (case group) are compared to others who have not developed the condition (controls). Investigators review the history of both the case and the control groups to determine whether these individuals have been exposed to, or are in possession of, the hypothesized prior characteristic (i.e., extended contact lens wear).

To constitute a valid result or outcome for a study, the following criteria must be satisfied (2). Measurement of a result or outcome must be appropriate, precise, complete, and not affected by the process of observation.

Appropriateness of the Measure of Results

It is important in clinical studies that measurements are taken with an appropriate technique.

Example: Inappropriate Measurement Technique

A clinical trial of two new contact lens materials is performed in which it is desired to measure the loss in corneal transparency during extended wear of contact lenses made from the materials. Patients are blindly and randomly assigned to wear one of the two materials, and their corneal thickness is monitored by corneal pachometry during a 1-year period. It is found that the patients wearing material A show approximately twice the overnight corneal swelling response of those wearing material B. The investigators conclude that loss in corneal transparency with material A is significantly greater than that with material B.

Unfortunately, measurement of corneal thickness by pachometry does not evaluate the loss in corneal transparency. There is a relationship between increase in corneal thickness and loss of corneal transparency, but the relationship is not direct, and at lower levels of corneal swelling no loss of corneal transparency is detectable. The investigators have

not measured what they thought they were measuring; therefore, the technique of measurement is inappropriate and invalid as a measurement of corneal transparency.

Precision of Measurement

Imprecise measurements may be obtained in clinical research studies as a result of incorrect reports by study patients, reading from test instruments, or measurements by the study investigator.

Reports from Study Patients

Lack of precision in measurement may come from recall or reporting errors in information provided by study patients. Recall errors imply defects in memory in those situations in which one group is more likely to recall events than the other (31). Reporting errors occur when one group of subjects is more accurate than the other in reporting information.

Example: Recall Errors and Imprecise Measurement

A case-control study of ulceration and extended contact lens wear is performed. One hundred patients who had ulcers secondary to extended lens wear are studied; 100 patients without ulceration, but with extended contact lens wear, are the control group. Of the patients who developed ulceration, 50% reported that they cleaned their contact lenses with enzymatic cleaner once a month, whereas only 5% of those without ulceration performed such infrequent enzymatic cleaning. Investigators concluded that they had found an association between infrequent cleaning with enzymes and the development of corneal ulceration secondary to extended contact lens wear.

Before accepting this conclusion, it must be determined whether recall errors explain the findings. It is likely that patients who experienced the trauma of ulceration may well have searched their memories more carefully than those without this complication. It is in situations like this that inconsequential prior events may be recalled. Therefore, the results of this study may be attributable, in part, to recall errors and doubt is cast on the alleged association.

Reporting errors also may impair the precision of experimental data.

Example: Reporting Error and Imprecise Measurement

A study is performed to determine the relationship between deposits on soft contact lenses and patient diet. A study group of 100 patients with large amounts of deposit on lenses is selected from a large contact lens practice. This study group is required to complete for 1 month, on a daily basis, questionnaires describing their dietary habits. A control group of 100 patients, who show little or no deposits with soft lenses, also is selected. This group is interviewed at the end of a 1-month period to determine their dietary habits. The study group reports an average of twice as much intake of dairy products than the control group. It is concluded that patients with heavy lens deposits have dietary habits that influence their ability to wear contact lenses.

It can be argued that patients with lens deposits who have experienced the need to change lenses on a frequent basis would be under greater pressure to report, in detail, their dietary habits. In addition, this group is required to complete extensive questionnaires requiring daily descriptions of their meals. The other group is not required to provide such extensive information. It is likely in the situation in which one group experiences more pressure to report information and where the problem (lens deposits) has resulted in greater financial investment in lens wear that this group is more likely to report previous events accurately. Such inequities between the groups may result in reporting errors.

Recall or reporting errors also may occur as a result of interviewer bias (1). This occurs in the situation where the interviewer stimulates or encourages a particular answer to questions as a result of knowing the hypothesis under consideration. For example, interviewers may probe patients in the treatment category more intensely for history or exposure than they do the comparison or control subjects.

Unfortunately, it is never possible to avoid the natural human inclination for people, including researchers, to see what they want to see or expect to see. One method of avoiding this problem is to keep investigators, those who make the assessment of the results, from knowing the group to which an individual patient is assigned. Masked or blind assessment may be used in both case-control and cohort studies, as well as in clinical trials. However, it may be impossible to mask information from an experienced observer, even if a subject has removed contact lenses before examination. It also should be noted that an investigator who thinks he or she can carry out a masked study alone probably is fooling himself or herself.

Completeness of the Assessment
If, during a study, all the follow-up visits for both groups of patients are incomplete, the possibility exists that those not included in the final data collection had a different result from those that were included.

Instrument Error

Errors in measurement may occur as a result of imprecise measurement by testing instruments.

Example: Instrument Errors and Imprecise Measurement

A study is performed to determine the amount of corneal edema produced by a new daily wear contact lens material. A clinical trial is performed to compare the effect of the new material on a group of patients blindly and randomly selected from a contact lens clinic population. The control subjects, from the same clinic population, are given a standard low-water-content soft lens to wear. To determine the amount of edema produced by the new material and by the standard lens, the investigators observed all patients with a slit-lamp biomicroscope to detect the presence of corneal striae. Investigators found no difference in the number of striae observed between the new and the old contact lens materials. They concluded that the new material did not produce a significant decrease in edema during daily wear.

The investigators did not recognize that the observation of corneal striae, particularly in daily wear patients in whom corneal thickness change is likely to be less than 6% of total corneal thickness, is a poor measurement of edema. Even if the new material did produce significantly less edema than found with existing materials, the slit-lamp biomicroscope would not be adequate to identify its presence; therefore, any conclusion based on this measurement is invalid.

Investigator Error

When the measurement of the results of a study depend on subjective interpretation of data, the possibility of misinterpretation is very real. Unfortunately, it is never possible to avoid the natural human inclination for people, including researchers, to see what they want to see or expect to see. One method of avoiding this problem is to keep investigators, those who make the assessment of the results, from knowing the group to which an individual patient is assigned. Masked or blind assessment may be used in both case-control and cohort studies, as well as in clinical trials. However, it may be impossible to mask information from an experienced observer, even if a subject has removed contact lenses before examination. It also should be noted that an investigator who thinks he or she can carry out a masked study alone probably is fooling himself or herself.

In the example just cited, in addition to improving measurement procedures by using different instrumentation, an electronic pachometer, for instance, the investigator performing the assessment of corneal edema should be unaware of which contact lens each patient is wearing.

Completeness of the Assessment

If, during a study, all the follow-up visits for both groups of patients are incomplete, the possibility exists that those not included in the final data collection had a different result from those that were included.

Example: Incompleteness of Assessment and Imprecise Measurement

An FDA clinical investigation of a new contact lens material for 30-day extended wear is initiated on 250 patients. Patients *are required to be seen at 1 week, 2 weeks, 1 month, 2 months, 3 months, 4 months, 5 months, and 6 months after dispensing of lenses. The results from this case series are recorded in tabular form; the slit-lamp complications experienced are listed at each visit. Of the initial 250 patients, only 150 attend all follow-up visits throughout the study. The results for all patients completing 6 months of wear indicate minimal slit-lamp complications observed during the study. It is concluded by the sponsors, in the report to the FDA, that the material is safe and effective for extended contact lens wear.*

Unfortunately, the results of this study may be affected by the incompleteness of the data. It is possible that the 100 patients who did not complete the study and on whom data are not reported had significant slit-lamp complications. This may explain why they did not complete the study. It is not possible to maintain that a material is safe for extended wear if a significant number of patients did not complete the required number of follow-up visits. The effect of dropout of patients from a study is to introduce bias into the results, which makes it difficult to extrapolate the results to a larger patient group (10).

In addition to incomplete data, unequal numbers of follow-up visits in studies involving study and control groups of patients may lead to invalid results. For example, a new extended wear contact lens material was fitted to a study group of patients, as described earlier, and the results compared with a control group of patients wearing another approved extended wear lens on which only one follow-up report was completed. In such a situation, a greater incidence of reports of symptoms of lens discomfort in the study group of patients may not indicate a problem with the new material because there was a greater number of opportunities for such a report to be made.

Effect of Observation

Even if the three criteria discussed are avoided in the measurements of the results of study, it still is possible that the very process of observation itself may have an effect.

Example: Effect of Observation on Imprecise Measurement

A study is designed to assess the effect of the frequency of contact lens replacement on the comfort of a new disposable soft contact lens. In this study, a study group is instructed to replace the lenses on a weekly basis. A control group of subjects is allowed to change the lenses whenever they choose and with whatever frequency they desire. Over a period of 6 months, both the study and control groups are questioned, on a weekly basis, about lens replacement. The comfort is graded on a subjective scale. At the end of the 6-month period, no difference was found in the comfort with lenses in the study and control groups. Investigators concluded that the frequency of lens replacement did not affect the comfort with the lens.

This conclusion may be invalid because it is possible that continual questioning of patients in the control group about the frequency of replacement may have resulted in these subjects replacing lenses more frequently. In this situation, the control subjects could switch voluntarily from the control to the study group. In this way, the process of observation would affect the results of the study. This influence on patient behavior of the process of evaluation is the Hawthorne effect in the context of biomedical research (10).

Analysis of Study Results

When comparing the results obtained from the study and control groups of patients, it may be necessary to adjust for, or to take account of, factors other than those studied that may have affected the results. This is accomplished by adjusting the data or the prior matching of subjects.

Adjustment of Data

Most clinical research designs compare study and control groups for individual characteristics that may affect the measurements obtained in the study. If the two groups differ, the question must be asked whether the difference could affect the results. Differences between the groups, which affect results, are called *confounding variables.* It may be possible to avoid problems arising from confounding variables by adjustment of the data obtained from the study.

Adjustment is performed by separating the subjects into subgroups, with the subgroups presenting different levels of the confounding variable. Groups with the same level of confounding variable are then compared to see if the differences persist. Perhaps the most common example of a variable that can confound data is the age of the patient group. By subdividing the two patient groups into subgroups of the same age, it can be determined whether the difference persists when the affect of age is eliminated.

Example: Confounding Variables

A clinical comparison study of the subjective comfort of thin and thick low-water lenses is performed. Two groups of patients are selected, one to wear each type of lens. Both groups are asked to report the subjective comfort of each lens on a five-point scale. The group wearing the thin hydrogel lens reports significantly more discomfort than the group wearing the thicker lens. It is concluded that the thinness of the low-water content soft lens results in lens dehydration, corneal drying, and patient discomfort.

Unfortunately, in comparing the individual characteristics of each study group, it is found that the group wearing the thin lens included a large number of postmenopausal women. It is possible that this group had a greater predisposition to dry eyes that may have biased the data, with menopause and the consequent dry eyes being the confounding variable in the study.

A way in which this confounding variable could have been adjusted for was by singling out from the low-water-content lens group those patients who were premenopausal and comparing them with a similar group wearing the high-water-content lens. By this means, a more reliable conclusion can be made about the patient preference for thin low-water-content or thick high-water-content lenses. Alternatively, confounding may be avoided by stratification or adjustment of data during analysis (12) by a similar process of matching.

Prior Matching

Another method by which the problem of confounding variables can be avoided is to match individuals prior to the start of the study. Investigators choose persons for both the study and control groups who are similar with respect to any possible confounding variable.

In a previous example, the presence of GPC, a known contraindication to extended contact lens wear, was a potential confounding variable when comparing the incidence of neovascularization in a study group of patients wearing extended wear lenses to a control group of subjects selected from contact lens wearers with GPC. In this case, the presence of the GPC would have affected the proportion of the control group patients who developed neovascularization as a result of extended wear. In such a situation, the presence or absence of GPC in a certain patient group could be a confounding variable on which investigators might desire to match the groups. The disadvantage of matching groups prior to the initiation of an investigation is that it precludes the study of the effects of the factor on which the two study groups are matched.

Prior matching of treatment and control subjects for a particular feature that may affect the results of the study is only the first of a two-step process often used to control for confounding variables (1). This process includes the prior matching of subjects or a matched design followed by the appropriate statistical analysis of data. Alternatives to matching to control confounding variables, include stratified sampling, frequency matching, poststudy stratification, and regression analysis (1).

Statistical Principles and Procedures

Study of a Population Using Random Sampling

In a typical contact lens study, the issue of interest can be posed in terms that refer to some population. For example, a patient might ask the question, "How long can I expect to wear my new contact lenses each day once I become accustomed to them?" A definitive answer to this question may be difficult to give, but information about the popula-

tion of daily wearing times for such lenses in similar patients offers a means to predict this patient's daily wearing time, that is, a helpful response might be, "For patients in your age group with your type of lens, the mean and median daily wear times are 10.5 hours, but 99% of these patients wear lenses for times ranging from 5 to 16 hours."

Such useful and precise information is rarely available, because it is impossible or impractical to accumulate the totality of all population values. In this example, the population of average daily wear times of these lenses for all current and future patients who have approximately the same ocular health profile as the original patient probably is not accessible. The usual strategy is then to collect a subset of the population values, termed a *sample,* and use it to extrapolate to the population. The accuracy and reliability of this extrapolation procedure are largely dependent on the quality of the sample. The ideal sample, termed a *random sample,* has two features: every population member has an equal chance of being included, and any particular selection for inclusion is independent of any other such selection (81).

There are two fundamental advantages to having a random sample. First, by selecting a random sample, the researcher greatly reduces the potential for selecting a biased sample, that is, a random sample is more likely to be representative of the entire population and hence an appropriate basis from which to draw inferences about the population. Second, most of the fundamental statistical procedures that might be applied to this sample have a theoretic foundation built on the notion of a random sample. Hence, attempting to extrapolate statistically to the population on the basis of some other sample may lead to inappropriate conclusions.

A random sample is an ideal that is fairly difficult to achieve in practice. One can argue that a perfectly random sample is impossible; however, the integrity of a study can be enhanced greatly by the researcher's demonstrated commitment to implement a sampling strategy that eliminates selection bias.

Example: Comparison of Two Sampling Schemes

Consideration will be given to two possible sampling procedures for a contact lens study designed to assess the duration of daily wear. The first researcher, Dr. Bonnett, recognizes that this study requires access to the subjects over a period of several months and, hence, a high level of commitment from them. Consequently, Dr. Bonnett, who teaches at the ABC School of Optometry, chooses to utilize first-year ABC optometry students as his subjects. Another researcher, Dr. Wiseman, proposes a considerably more involved sampling scheme. Dr. Wiseman has enlisted the cooperation and participation of 10 randomly selected optometric clinics that are geographically dispersed across the United States. Each clinic has agreed to compile a list of their next 100 patients who fit the designated profile and to whom the lenses in question will be dispensed. Wiseman then selects a set number of patients, say 20, from each list using 10 different computer-generated lists of random numbers. These 10 lists are compiled to give a total subject sample size of 200.

It is evident that Dr. Wiseman's sampling scheme requires a greater expenditure of resources when compared to Bonnett's. Bonnett's sample has the potential to introduce biases with regard to such factors as age, socioeconomic background, educational level, commitment to successful contact lens wear, and perhaps others. Such a sample runs a high risk of being unrepresentative of the population. Although one might argue that Wiseman's sample is also not perfectly random, the biases built into it are considerably more subtle than those suggested for Bonnett's sample. Consequently, although the quality of the population information that Bonnett's scheme gives is questionable, a more reliable estimate of daily wear time is likely to result from Wiseman's scheme.

Samples of convenience are often fraught with danger (6). Many of those dangers can be avoided by pursuing a sampling scheme that reflects a commitment to random selection, a process enhanced by the planned introduction of chance (e.g., use of random number tables or computer-generated lists of random numbers).

In ophthalmic research, there is always a strong temptation to increase sample size by viewing each eye from the same patient as a separate subject. Unfortunately, any variable measured on the eyes of one patient will tend to result in highly correlated values; hence, those values will not be independently determined. This, of course, injects a bias into the sample and renders it unusable as a random sample. Careful planning of a study at the design stage is necessary in those studies that include the use of both eyes from some or all patients.

Random Allocation of Subjects to Treatment Groups

A common feature of many contact lens studies is the comparison of different, but parallel, protocols (62). For example, low-water-content hydroxyethyl methacrylate (HEMA) contact lenses are the accepted clinical standard for patients who have a particular ocular profile. A new product, a mid-water-content non-HEMA contact lens, comes on the market as a competitor, and, naturally, clinicians are interested to know if it compares favorably with the standard lens. An investigation is proposed in which two groups of patients, who would be candidates for the standard lens, will be selected. The first group will have the standard lens dispensed to them; the second group will be given the new lens. In such a study, the principle of randomization is an important feature. By randomization one means that not only is the totality of subjects in the two treatment groups a random sample from the population of potential standard lens patients, but also the assignment of each patient to one of the treatment groups is performed by chance. Randomization serves as an important safeguard against selection bias and

other accidental biases, as well as a foundation for the statistical techniques that will be used to analyze the data.

In a study like the proposed comparison of the standard HEMA contact lenses and the new non-HEMA lenses, the temptation is great to compromise on randomization. For example, researchers frequently have ready access to subjects who are optometry students, so, as a matter of convenience, one or both treatment groups might consist of such student subjects. Again, such a sample is not likely to be representative of the population of all potential standard lens patients. A compromise design might feature using a random selection of patients for the experimental group (subjects who would be fitted with the new lens) and a group of students as the control group (subjects who would be fitted with the standard lens). Any differences between the performance of the standard lens and the new lens are likely to be confounded with the initial heterogeneity of two such groups. An explicit design assumption is the homogeneity of the two groups with respect to all factors except the type of contact lens used.

A more subtle, and virtually undetectable, randomization flaw occurs when assignment to treatment groups is affected by the preference of the researcher. For example, in the comparison study of the accepted standard lens with the new competitor, an experienced clinician who has had good success with the standard lens may have a tendency to prescribe it to subjects whose profile indicates future clinical problems, feeling that the patient will be better served. Such selection bias can dramatically affect a study's conclusion. Two safeguards should be observed here. Any subject who is evidently a stronger candidate for one treatment over all others should, of course, be given that treatment, but then the subject must be excluded from the study. Also, no clinician or researcher who has a strong preference for one treatment should be involved in the assignment of subjects to treatment groups.

Another common problem in the methodology of studies testing the efficacy of new contact lenses is to fit them to a patient sample of previous contact lens dropouts. Such a sample will reflect selection bias and violate all random allocation to treatment guidelines. Studying a lens as a lens of last resort provides very little information about its value to the general population of contact lens patients.

Even after a random sample has been apportioned randomly into treatment groups, it is prudent to compare those groups for potential confounding factors, especially when the sample size is small and the probability of a biased allocation with respect to such a factor is appreciable. For example, in the study comparing the standard and new lenses, once the treatment groups have been established through a random allocation and before any contact lens protocol has begun, the groups should be compared with respect to factors such as age, sex, refractive error, and the usual fitting parameters. If the groups differ substantially on any one of these factors, the random allocation process should be repeated until a more suitable homogeneity of the groups is obtained.

Statistical Inference

The two fundamental components of applied statistics are descriptive statistics and inferential statistics. *Descriptive statistics* pertain to characterizing and describing sample information. Such familiar tools as histograms, scatter plots, sample mean, sample median, standard deviation, range, and correlation are frequently used to describe graphically and summarize numerically a data set.

Inferential statistics use such sample information as the basis for generalization to characteristics of the population from which the sample was drawn. Statistical inference has two basic subcategories: estimation and hypothesis testing. Estimation uses sample information to approximate unknown numerical population characteristics or parameters. For example, the sample mean is a frequently used estimator for the population mean. Hypothesis testing is used when a study is concerned with the validity of conjecture about a population. The fundamental issue is to determine the extent to which the sample information is consistent with the conjecture.

Statistical Estimation

Most research studies use hypothesis testing, but the use of estimation also is prevalent although often inappropriately overlooked. Estimation should be the primary tool in the initial study of a population.

Simple Case of Estimation

An investigation is mounted in which the incidence of epithelial microcysts among patients wearing a new extended wear soft contact lens is studied. The primary issue in this study is the estimation of the population proportion (p) of patients who develop microcysts. In such a study, a random sample of patients would be assembled and monitored over a specified time period. The most straightforward estimate of p is given by:

$$\hat{p} = \frac{\text{No. of patients in the sample who develop microcysts}}{\text{Sample size}}$$

Such a sample proportion $\hat{p}$ is an example of a point estimate for a population parameter (p). Other common examples of point estimates for population parameters are the sample mean, which estimates the population mean and the sample standard deviation, which estimates the population standard deviation. In order to assess the reliability of any point estimate, the issues of accuracy and precision are considered. *Accuracy* in this context refers to the absence of systematic error, that is, a point estimate is accurate if it arises from a sample that is entirely free of bias and, hence, is representative of the population. *Precision* refers to the extent to which

the estimate is free of random error. Random error is quantified using knowledge of the sample distribution of the estimate, that is, different samples from the same population will result in different estimates of the same parameter. This sampling variability is frequently measured using the standard error, which is simply the standard deviation of the population of all possible values of the estimator (81).

Standard Error of the Mean

The most commonly encountered example of a standard error is the standard error of the mean. Suppose a population having mean μ and standard deviation σ is being studied. The usual estimate for μ from a data set x_1, x_2, x_3, x_n, which is a random sample from this population, is the sample mean.

$$\bar{x} = \frac{1}{n} \sum_{k=1}^{n} x_k \text{ (sample mean)}$$

Also, the usual estimator for σ is the sample standard deviation.

$$s = \sqrt{\frac{1}{n-1} \sum_{k=1}^{n} (x_k - \bar{x})^2} \text{ (Sample standard deviation)}$$

The standard deviation of the sampling distribution of $\bar{x}$ is $s/\sqrt{n}$, which is then the standard error of the mean. The sample standard error of the mean $s/\sqrt{n}$ serves as the estimator of the standard error of the mean.

The standard error of an estimator provides quantitative information about its precision: the smaller the standard error, the greater the precision of the estimate. A very useful technique for conveying this precision is through the use of confidence intervals. A confidence interval for a parameter is determined from a data set (a random sample, of course), and it provides an interval of possible parameter values that are compatible with that sample (75).

Example: Interpreting a Confidence Interval

In a study designed to investigate the time of daily wear of a particular contact lens, it is reported that the sample mean wearing time is 9 hours, and a 95% confidence interval for the population mean is from 6 to 12 hours. We interpret this to indicate that the observed mean of 9 hours is a reasonably likely result for any actual population mean value from 6 to 12. The notion of reasonability is quantified by the 95% confidence level, which is a measure of the success rate of the confidence interval estimation process (81). If we were to repeat the sampling process and calculation, which resulted in the confidence interval (6, 12) 1,000 times, we would obtain 1,000 different confidence interval estimates for the population mean. However, about 950 of those 1,000 intervals (95%) would contain the actual population mean value. It is in this sense that we have 95% confidence in our original interval.

Confidence intervals for population means are frequently utilized and, for at least moderately sized samples, a 95% confidence interval for a mean is approximately given by:

$$\bar{x} \pm 2 \frac{s}{\sqrt{n}} \text{ (Approximate 95\% confidence interval for a population mean)}$$

That is, half the length of the confidence interval, termed the *margin of error,* is actually two times the sample estimate of the standard of error of the mean. Suppose in this example daily wearing time study, from a sample of size 16, we obtain $\bar{x} = 9$ and $s = 6$. The estimated standard error of the mean is $s/\sqrt{16} = 1.5$. Then the 95% confidence interval for the mean is $9 \pm 2 \cdot (1.5)$ or $(6, 12)$.

Sample size determination in this population mean estimation context depends on the level of precision that is desired. The larger the sample size, the greater the level of precision. In estimating the mean of a population that has standard deviation σ, sample size is determined with a specification of a desired margin of error. As the margin of error is about $2\sigma/\sqrt{n}$ (at the 95% confidence level), for a specified margin of error m, n should be chosen so that $2\sigma/\sqrt{n} \leq m$ or $n \geq 4\sigma^2/m^2$.

Suppose in our mean daily wear time example it is specified that the population mean be estimated at the 95% confidence level with a margin of error of no more than 0.5 hour. Using the preliminary study described, it is assumed that $\sigma = 6$, and so $n \geq 4(6^2)/(0.5)^2 = 576$. It can be observed that the demand for increased precision can dramatically increase sample size.

Statistical Hypothesis Testing

Many investigational studies in the health sciences are designed to assess the validity of a particular proposition of interest or conjecture regarding a population, termed a *research hypothesis*. If this research hypothesis can be translated into a statement about population parameters, then the tools of statistics may provide the method of assessment.

Example: Translating a Research Hypothesis into a Statistical Hypothesis

It is well established that 7% of patients with extended wear of conventional hydrogel contact lenses will develop sufficiently serious clinical problems within 3 months of their initial fitting such that use must be discontinued. A new extended wear contact lens is introduced on the market, which is claimed by its manufacturer to be superior to existing materials. In particular, this manufacturer claims that the new material reduces the rate of contact lens dropouts. A study is proposed to test that claim. A random sample of patients wearing the new material is to be monitored for 3 months and the proportion of patients who are discontinue wear is to be observed.

The population parameter of interest here is p, the proportion of all patients with the new lens who discontinue wear within 3 months. In weighing the relative merits of the lens types, the researchers ask, "Is p less than 7%?" They set up two competing statistical hypotheses:

1. The null hypothesis states that the new lens is as good as the old material with respect to short-term acceptability allowing for continued wear (i.e., p = 7%).

2. The alternate hypothesis states that the new lens is superior to the old in this same regard (i.e., p < 7%).

These null and alternative hypotheses are frequently denoted by H_0 and H_1, respectively, and in this case the following standard notation would be used:

H_0: p = 0.07
H_1: p < 0.07.

In general, a statistical hypothesis test is designed to assess the validity of two competing and mutually exclusive hypotheses pertaining to a population parameter or parameters. The first of the hypotheses, the null hypothesis, is, in most cases, an assertion of equality between a parameter and a specified value (as in the example) or between two or more parameters, perhaps from separate populations. For example, the null hypothesis might be that two different population means μ_1 and μ_2 are equal or H_0: $\mu_1 = \mu_2$. The alternate hypothesis is the claim that the equality stated in the null hypothesis is not true. The null hypothesis is the "no difference" or "no effect" option, whereas the alternate hypothesis asserts that a difference or effect exists. Hence, it is frequently the case that the research hypothesis for a study is translated into the alternate hypothesis within the statistical test (82). The actual statistical test will focus on a value computed from the data, termed a *test statistic*. When the proper assumptions for this test statistic are met, the distribution of its values is completely specified by assuming the null hypothesis to be true. The strength of the evidence against a null hypothesis from a data set is then measured in terms of a probability computed using this distribution of the test statistic. This probability, termed the *p* value, gives the likelihood of obtaining a value of the test statistic, at least as far away as the actual obtained value, from what is expected if H_0 were true. Hence, the smaller the *p* value, the less the likelihood that the observed value of the test statistic represents a reasonable chance occurrence when H_0 is true, and so the greater is the weight of the evidence against H_0 and in favor of H_1.

The decision to reject or not reject H_0 in favor of H_1 is made by comparing the *p* value to a designated probability threshold termed the *significance level* and denoted by α. The usual convention is to select $\alpha = 0.05$ or $\alpha = 0.01$. With *P* denoting the *p* value, the decision rule is:

1. If $P \leq \alpha$, then reject H_0;
2. If $P > \alpha$, then do not reject H_0.

In a case where $\alpha = 0.01$ and it is obtained that $P \leq 0.01$, then a value of the test statistic has been obtained that would be as extreme in only about 1 of 100 repetitions of the same experiment. Because this is a fairly remote possibility, it is concluded that the difference between the obtained value of the test statistic and that expected, if H_0 is true, is not convincingly explained by chance. It is then said that the difference is statistically significant at $\alpha = 0.01$. Thus, statistical significance is equivalent to having results that differ from what is expected when H_0 is true, and that difference is not reasonably explained by chance.

Testing a Statistical Hypothesis

It is conjectured that no more than 80% of all contact lens patients will be sufficiently satisfied with their lenses so that 6 months after initial dispensing they will wear the lenses for more than 8 hours per day. If p is the corresponding population proportion, a study is initiated with the purpose of testing:

H_0: $p = 0.80$
H_1: $p < 0.80$.

A random sample of 10 patients is monitored for 6 months, after which it is reported that 5 of the 10 are still successfully wearing their lenses, at a minimum of 8 hours per day.

The test statistic in this case is the number of successful contact lens patients. In this study, with a sample size of 10 and assuming $p = 0.80$, the probability of observing any given number of successful patients, 0 through 10, is given in Table 45.1 (8). This listing is one way of completely describing the test statistic's theoretic distribution. Under the null hypothesis, eight patients would be expected to be successful, so the interpretation of the results should focus on the extent to which the observed number of successful patients falls below eight. The p value in this case is the

TABLE 45.1. PROBABILITY OF OBSERVING A NUMBER OF SUCCESSFUL PATIENTS FROM A SAMPLE OF SIZE 10

Successful Patients	Probability (p)
0	0.0000
1	0.0000
7	0.0001
3	0.0008
4	0.0055
5	0.0264
6	0.0881
7	0.2013
8	0.3020
9	0.2684
10	0.1074

probability of observing five or fewer successful patients. From the table, we obtained that

$P = 0.264 + 0.0055 + 0.0008 + 0.0001 = 0.0328.$

So if y = 0.05, then $P \leq \alpha$ and, hence, H_0 is rejected in favor of H_1, and it is concluded that the data do support the claim that fewer than 80% of contact lens patients will be successful after 6 months of wear.

In making this statistical decision, two different errors are possible. H_0 could be rejected when it is really true; this is the *type I error*. An alternative interpretation of the significance level α is that it is the probability of the type I error, and hence it is always chosen to be small. Another error, the *type II error,* occurs when H_1 is really true, and H_0 is not rejected.

It is desirable to keep the chances of a type II error small. Unfortunately, the probability of a type II error is not one single value, as is the probability of the type I error. Rather, this probability, denoted by β, varies with the actual difference of the quantities that are claimed to be equal within the null hypothesis. If a minimum difference between these quantities that is clinically meaningful can be established (δ), then β is the probability that H_0 is not rejected given that this difference is δ; so β depends on δ. The ideal approach in setting up a statistical test is first to select a, β, and δ, and then use them to determine the sample size n. Unfortunately, if these values are selected to be too small, the necessary sample size frequently becomes unrealistically large. The usual compromise is to increase β. The *power of a test* is the probability of correctly rejecting a false null hypothesis and hence equals $1 - \beta$. It measures a test's sensitivity in detecting clinically meaningful differences. Increases in β reduce this sensitivity or power.

Effect of β on Sample Size

Suppose the study in which the following hypotheses are to be tested is considered once again:

H_0: $p = 0.80$
H_1: $p < 0.80$,

where p is the proportion of successful extended wear contact lens patients wearing the new material who succeed in the first 3 months. If it is specified that $\alpha = 0.01$ and the test should have a good chance of rejection if p is 0.70 (so $\delta = 0.80 - 0.70 = 0.10$) or less, then Table 45.2 provides the necessary sample size for specified values of β.

TABLE 45.2. REQUIRED SAMPLE SIZE FOR VARIOUS VALUES OF β

β	Sample Size
0.001	554
0.01	400
0.05	285
0.10	230
0.20	174

This example demonstrates that the cost (or high statistical power, that is, a low β) can be considerable, so it is not unusual to design studies with β set at 0.10 or even 0.20. In the previous example in which the sample size was set at 10, β was 0.91 (again with α = 0.01 and δ = 0.10), which means the test would be grossly insensitive to clinically meaningful differences in the proportion of successful contact lens patients.

Tools of Statistical Inference

As a vehicle for illustrating some of the most important and useful statistical techniques for ophthalmic clinical research, a hypothetical, composite experimental study from the contact lens literature is described. This study is designed to address several different clinical questions. The responses to these questions will provide applications of the ideas of statistical estimation and testing that were presented in the previous section.

The results of this study may provide the answers to several clinical questions. What follows is a discussion of some of those questions, including examples of some of the statistical techniques that are most likely to be used in answering these questions. These same techniques are among those most frequently applied in ophthalmic clinical research.

Example: Complex Clinical Study to Determine the Comparative Physiologic Effect of Silicone Hydrogel Contact Lenses

The principal objective of this study was to determine the comparative physiologic impact of a new generation of contact lens materials when used for continuous (extended) wear. In the study, the physiologic effects of an approved and an experimental silicone hydrogel lens material were referred to the effect of existing (conventional) hydrogel lenses. There was two phases to this study.

Phase 1. An initial study was carried out to determine the physiologic impact of lens design measured by the change in the number of epithelial microcysts in the extended wear of lenses of different thicknesses. The presence of epithelial microcysts in a cornea can indicate the presence of hypoxia during extended contact lens wear (83).

Two groups of 40 patients were randomly selected from a pool of new volunteers at a major contact lens research institute. All patients were ametropes aged 20 to 40 years who had no previous experience of contact lens wear, history of anterior ocular surface disease, or current systemic disease. One group was assigned to wear conventional hydrogel lenses and the other group to the newly approved silicone hydrogel lens. Both groups were fitted with lenses in the appropriate material with center thicknesses of 0.035, 0.09, and 0.20 mm. These thicknesses were selected because they represented the design of lenses previously used for extended wear (the 0.035-mm thickness for the

conventional hydrogel), the design anticipated for use in extended wear of the silicone hydrogel (0.09-mm thickness), and the "thicker lens" intended to give greater durability during lens wear (0.20-mm thickness).

Before any lenses were dispensed to either group, a slit-lamp examination of the cornea of the right eye of each patient was carried out to determine the number of microcysts present. Patients then were assigned in random order to pairs of lenses in each thickness. Each pair of lenses was worn on an extended wear basis, for 6 nights in the eye and 1 night out, for a 3-month period. At the end of that period, following 6 nights of extended wear, lenses were removed and the number of microcysts present in the cornea of the right eye of each patient was recorded. In this way, the number of microcysts induced by the extended wear of each lens could be observed. Between the wear of each thickness of lens, the patients discontinued all contact lens wear for a period of 4 months to ensure that any induced microcysts had been eliminated (84). An additional "experimental" silicone hydrogel was also tested on a third group of 40 patients. This experimental material was developed to give a more flexible polymer in the attempt to reduce some of the adverse mechanical effects observed with approved silicone hydrogel material (85). The new lens was cut in a 0.09-mm thickness, which provided an oxygen transmission of 70% of that of the approved silicone hydrogel lens. After the wear of the experimental material for 3 months, the change in the number of microcysts (from baseline) was recorded (Tables 45.3 and 45.4).

At the end of the third month of extended wear with the 0.035-mm thick hydrogel and the 0.09-mm thick approved silicone contact lenses, patients in each group had their central corneal thickness measured with an electronic pachometer in the right eye. This thickness measurement was taken before resuming lens wear after 1 night of nonwear in their 6 days on–1 day off cycle, and following the first overnight wear of the lens in the next cycle. The overnight swelling response of the cornea to the wear of contact lenses is a measure of the corneal hypoxia during lens wear (86). Also at this latter time point the corneal epithelial cell shedding or desquamation rate was measured by the contact lens cytology techniques of Wilson (87). Epithelial shedding rate provides a surrogate measure for the rate of epithelial cell mitosis, which can be affected (reduced) by the corneal hypoxia occurring during extended contact lens wear (88–90). The data obtained in the first phase of this study are given in Tables 45.3 and 45.4.

Phase 2. In the second phase of the study, two new groups of patients wore the optimum design in each lens type (0.035 mm for the conventional and 0.09 mm for the approved silicone hydrogel). Each group consisted of 1,000 patients. Lenses were worn on an extended wear basis (6 nights on–1 night off) for 12 months. At the end of the year, the patients were evaluated for the presence of inflammatory responses (contact lens acute red eye) and the symptoms of contact lens-induced dry eye (CLDE). Prior to the beginning of this 1-year, extended wear experience, all patients had been given a new dry eye question-

TABLE 45.3. DATA FOR PATIENTS WEARING ONE OF THREE CONVENTIONAL HYDROGEL LENSES

Patient	NIM 0.035	0.09	0.20	ONS	EDR
1	22	21	44	13.12	8
2	55	70	91	15.23	19
3	45	57	75	12.53	18
4	67	116	113	15.67	26
5	14	16	12	7.55	8
6	50	66	74	16.41	19
7	56	60	73	16.90	18
8	48	76	84	13.69	28
9	38	66	87	13.20	15
10	45	75	87	11.91	26
11	15	38	47	10.98	4
12	43	54	87	10.91	20
13	25	42	66	12.70	14
14	27	42	57	11.81	21
15	36	62	77	14.55	17
16	46	71	82	16.84	16
17	34	44	61	15.23	14
18	42	58	81	13.67	23
19	30	42	60	13.57	18
20	12	17	34	11.64	7
21	15	38	45	11.77	11
22	24	41	50	9.43	19
23	28	42	40	13.30	19
24	11	13	33	9.78	13
25	53	84	96	13.61	20
26	24	37	44	13.49	12
27	39	65	63	15.52	18
28	40	90	69	12.89	17
29	17	45	31	12.10	8
30	21	71	55	12.35	19
31	10	22	34	9.11	14
32	28	52	80	9.04	17
33	26	64	58	12.67	15
34	22	23	55	7.29	17
35	34	43	48	13.47	13
36	9	19	19	10.75	8
37	59	80	97	16.38	16
38	18	24	21	8.44	14
39	10	7	16	9.74	11
40	22	58	58	10.75	11

For each of the three lens thicknesses (0.035 mm, 0.09 mm, and 0.20 mm), the number of induced microcysts (NIM) is given. ONS is the percentage of overnight swelling and EDR is the epithelial desquamation rate (cells/min), both for wear of the 0.035-mm lens.

TABLE 45.4. DATA FOR PATIENTS WEARING ONE OF THREE SILICONE HYDROGEL LENSES

Patient	NIM 0.035	0.09	0.20	ONS	EDR
1	2	4	13	5.73	14
2	7	6	15	5.48	22
3	2	5	14	4.76	13
4	5	10	23	3.63	10
5	1	9	22	3.07	17
6	4	7	19	2.11	5
7	6	14	23	4.09	5
8	2	4	11	4.06	18
9	3	1	12	4.68	7
10	2	4	12	5.15	20
11	7	6	17	3.48	19
12	2	5	14	7.11	8
13	4	10	23	6.28	8
14	1	2	12	3.69	8
15	1	0	7	4.53	11
16	1	1	10	4.53	14
17	3	5	16	5.34	7
18	5	9	19	5.73	17
19	3	1	11	1.92	16
20	2	5	15	3.40	14
21	4	2	13	3.41	12
22	3	4	14	5.15	5
23	4	9	20	4.25	4
24	5	4	14	6.35	18
25	4	9	21	2.38	13
26	1	5	13	4.14	10
27	3	6	15	4.79	15
28	1	2	11	3.08	20
29	2	1	10	4.36	20
30	3	3	13	6.06	16
31	2	4	11	6.73	1
32	2	5	14	5.16	16
33	3	6	14	4.69	13
34	3	10	21	3.43	12
35	3	4	13	4.08	9
36	4	7	19	5.98	8
37	4	7	19	4.56	9
38	1	4	15	5.71	12
39	2	5	15	2.94	12
40	2	0	10	3.76	10

For each of the three lens thicknesses (0.035 mm, 0.09 mm, and 0.20 mm), the number of induced microcysts (NIM) is given. ONS is the percentage of overnight swelling and EDR is the epithelial desquamation rate (cells/min), both for wear of the 0.09-mm lens.

naire based on the comparison of morning and evening sensations of dryness during contact lens wear, which had shown potential as a predictive tests for CLDE (91).

Question 1a. To substantiate the relationship between corneal hypoxia and epithelial microcysts, the researchers were interested in determining if, for the conventional hydrogel lens, the number of induced microcysts (NIM) was affected by the thickness of the contact lens. In particular, were there more induced microcysts for the standard lens having a thickness of 0.035 mm compared to the 0.09-mm thick lens?

TABLE 45.5. SUMMARY OF INDUCED MICROCYST DATA FOR THE GROUP OF PATIENTS WHO WORE THE CONVENTIONAL 0.035-MM AND 0.09-MM THICK HYDROGEL LENSES

Lens Thickness (mm)	Induced Microcysts Mean	Standard Deviation	Median
0.035	31.5	15.49	28.0
0.09	50.3	23.93	48.5
Difference	18.8	13.53	16.0

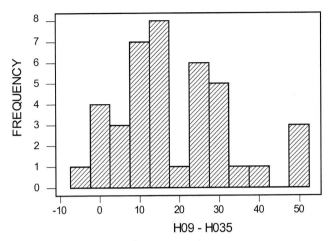

FIG. 45.2. Frequency histogram of the differences between the number of induced microcysts when patients wore the 0.035-mm thick conventional hydrogel lens (H035) and when they wore the 0.09-mm thick lens (H09).

A numerical summary of the pertinent data is given in Table 45.5. It appears that the distribution of induced microcysts for the 0.09-mm lens fit is shifted to the right of that for the 0.035-mm lens.

In Fig. 45.2, the histogram of the differences between the two conventional hydrogel lens thicknesses provides graphical evidence that NIM with the 0.09-mm lens tends to exceed that with the 0.035-mm lens. The differences range from −3 to 50, but 95% (38/40) of the patients have differences >0. The question that should be asked is, "If there really is no essential difference in the NIM with the 0.035-mm and 0.09-mm lenses, can the observed differ-

ences be reasonably explained by chance?" The most frequently used statistical approach to answer questions like this is to carry out a *paired sample t test.*

In this study, the procedure will test the null hypothesis that the population mean of induced microcysts for the 0.035 lens (denoted μ_{035}) is equal to the population mean for the 0.09 lens (denoted μ_{09}). The alternate hypothesis is that these two population means are not equal. These hypotheses are abbreviated as follows:

H_0: $\mu_{035} = \mu_{09}$ (or $\mu_D = 0$) (HI)

H_1: $\mu_{035} \neq \mu_{09}$ (or $\mu_D \neq 0$),

where μ_D is the population difference of means for the 0.035 and 0.09 populations of NIM ($\mu_D = \mu_{09} - \mu_{035}$). The test statistic is

$$T_{n-1} = \frac{\bar{X}_D - \mu_D}{S_n/\sqrt{n}}$$ (t statistic for the paired sample *t*-test)

where n is the number of differences (40 in this case), $\bar{X}$ is the sample mean of the differences, and S_D is the sample standard deviation of the differences. Under assumptions that are not too restrictive, T_{n-1} has what is known as a *t* distribution, which, when graphically depicted, is a bell-shaped curve centered at 0. As n changes, the distribution of T_{n-1} changes. In fact, as n becomes larger, the bell-shaped curve corresponding to the distribution of T_{n-1} approaches the standard normal or gaussian bell-shaped curve (Fig. 45.3).

This distribution can be used to estimate μ_D with a 95% confidence interval, which, in general, is given by

$$\bar{X}_D \pm t_{n-1} S_D/\sqrt{n},$$ (Confidence interval for μ_D)

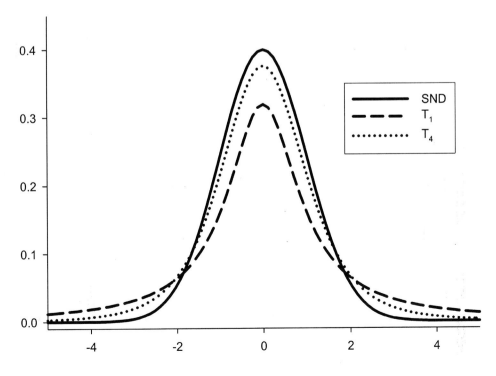

FIG. 45.3. Comparison of two t distributions, one with 1 degree of freedom (T_1) and the other with 4 degrees of freedom (T_4), with the standard normal distribution (SND).

where t_{n-1} is the 97.5% percentile of the t distribution corresponding to n − 1 (frequently referred to as *degrees of freedom*). t_{n-1} is a value that T_{n-1} will exceed with probability 0.025 (92).

The *confidence interval estimate for the mean difference* in NIM for the 0.035-mm and 0.09-mm hydrogel lenses (μ_D) and the paired sample t test[iii] is illustrated below.

Using the data summary in Table 45.5, the confidence interval estimate for μ_D can be made, and the paired sample t-test of hypothesis H_1 can be carried out. In this case, $\bar{X}_D = 18.8$, $S_D = 13.53$, n = 40, and $t_{39} = 2.02$, so the 95% confidence interval for μ_D is

$$18.8 \pm 2.02 \cdot 13.53/\sqrt{40} \text{ or } (14.5, 23.1).$$

Hence, the data are consistent (at the 95% confidence level) with values of μ_D between 14.5 and 23.1, which suggests that on the average there are more induced microcysts with the 0.09-mm lens than the 0.035-mm lens.

This result is supported by the outcome of the significance test of the hypothesis H_1. The obtained value of the test statistics (see the boxed display of the t statistic) in this situation is

$$T_{39} = \frac{18.8 - 0}{13.53/\sqrt{40}} = 8.79$$

(under H_0 it is assumed that $\mu_D = 0$), so the p value is $P = [|T_{39}| \geq 8.79] < 0.001$. Hence, at one of the standard significance levels α (0.01 or 0.05) $P \leq \alpha$, so H_0 is rejected in favor of H_1.

It is useful to expand on the implication of the obtained p value, $P < 0.001$. Assuming that the mean NIM for the 0.09-mm and 0.035-mm lenses is equal, in 1,000 repetitions of this study, it would be expected that a mean absolute difference of 18.8 or greater would occur at most once, that is, assuming the null hypothesis is true, the obtained result is a very unlikely outcome.

This casts a high level of doubt on the null hypothesis, so it is rejected in favor of the alternate hypothesis that the two means are different. The conclusion is that the obtained difference is not reasonably explained by chance, assuming H_0 is true, so H_1 is viewed to be consistent with the data. In this case where H_1 is rejected, the result is said to be statistically significant. To present this statement in clinical terms, the data support the claim that *the NIM with the 0.09-mm thick lens exceeds that with the 0.035-mm thick lens on the average; or, the thickness of a hydrogel lens affects the hypoxic reaction of the typical patient, with the thicker lens engendering a more extreme response.*

Clinical Implication of Result The number of microcysts induced by a 0.09-mm thick hydrogel lens exceeds that with the thinner (0.035-mm) lens as a result of the increased hypoxia with the thicker lens.

A retrospective look at the power of this test also can be instructive.

Power in a Paired Sample t Test Using the standard power calculation procedure (92), if the minimum desired (clinically) detectable mean difference in the test of H_1 is set at $\delta = 10$ microcysts and $\alpha = 0.05$, then with n = 40, the power of this test $1 - \beta$ is 0.995 (or $\beta = 0.005$). This power is quite high, indicating a high level of sensitivity of this procedure to detect statistically a mean difference as low as 10. However, if δ is set at 5, then β becomes 0.375, which is considered unacceptable. This emphasizes the importance of the clinical decision about what constitutes a minimum clinically important difference.

Another way to view this issue of power or sensitivity is to calculate the minimum mean difference that would have given statistical significance. In this case, the p value would have been <0.05, so statistical significance would have been achieved if

$$|T_{39}| \geq 2.02 \text{ or } \frac{|X_D|}{13.53/\sqrt{40}} \geq 2.02$$

This implies that $X_D \geq 4.3$, which means that with the same sample size and amount of variation in the data, any absolute difference in the 0.09-mm and 0.035-mm means exceeding 4.4 would have given statistical significance at $\alpha = 0.05$.

This type of calculation is interesting here, but it is more important to do when a result does not give statistical significance. It conveys whether all clinically important differences would have had a reasonable chance of being statistically detected.

Nonparametric Approaches

One assumption that is made in conducting this t-test is that the underlying population of differences has a normal or gaussian distribution or, absent that, the population distribution is not so unusual (e.g., radically skewed or multimodal). As long as the population distribution of interest is reasonably well behaved, the distribution of the sample mean will approximate a gaussian distribution when the sample size is sufficiently large, usually 30 or more (82). This is a sufficient basis on which to conduct the t-test. In situations in which these assumptions are in doubt, researchers can use a vast collection of nonparametric tests. With these techniques, much less stringent assumptions are made regarding the population distribution; however, these nonparametric tests are generally less powerful than their parametric counterparts. A standard nonparametric test that could be used in this context is the Wilcoxon matched pairs signed rank test (93). This procedure would test the null hypothesis that the population median difference M_D between induced microcysts for the 0.09-mm lens and the 0.035-mm lens is zero, versus the alternative hypothesis that it is not zero; this is denoted by

$H_0: M_D = 0$ (H2)

$H_1: M_D \neq 0$.

To use this procedure, the 40 differences are ranked in order of absolute size (i.e., the sign of the difference is ignored). These ranks are then partitioned into two groups, those that correspond to negative differences and those that correspond to positive differences. The sum of the ranks in each group is determined, and the test statistic T is the minimum of those two sums. Intuitively, when the null hypothesis is true, the sums of the ranks within each group should be about the same, or about half the total sum of all the ranks.

Hence, small values of T cast doubt on the validity of H_0. For small values of n, critical values of T are tabled, but for larger n, T has a distribution that approximates a gaussian distribution (94).

Wilcoxon Matched Pairs Signed Rank Test. In order to test the hypothesis H_2, the value of the test statistic W must be calculated. The steps outlined earlier are given in Table 45.6. In the second and third columns are the NIM for the

TABLE 45.6. APPLICATION OF WILCOXON MATCHED PAIRS SIGNED RANK TEST TO THE NUMBER OF INDUCED MICROCYSTS DATA FOR PATIENTS WHO WORE THE 0.035-MM AND THE 0.09-MM THICK CONVENTIONAL HYDROGEL LENSES

	NIM			Ranks		
Patient	0.035 mm	0.09 mm	Difference	Absolute Difference	Positive Difference	Negative Difference
1	22	21	−1	1.5		1.5
2	55	70	15	18.5	18.5	
3	45	57	12	14	14	
4	67	116	49	38	38	
5	14	16	2	3.5	3.5	
6	50	66	16	20.5	20.5	
7	56	60	4	6	6	
8	48	76	28	32	32	
9	38	66	28	32	32	
10	45	75	30	34	34	
11	15	38	23	25.5	25.5	
12	43	54	11	12	12	
13	25	42	17	22.5	22.5	
14	27	42	15	18.5	18.5	
15	36	62	26	29.5	29.5	
16	46	71	25	28	28	
17	34	44	10	10.5	10.5	
18	42	58	16	20.5	20.5	
19	30	42	12	14	14	
20	12	17	5	7	7	
21	15	38	23	25.5	25.5	
22	24	41	17	22.5	22.5	
23	28	42	14	17	17	
24	11	13	2	3.5	3.5	
25	53	84	31	35	35	
26	24	37	13	16	16	
27	39	65	26	29.5	29.5	
28	40	90	50	39.5	39.5	
29	17	45	28	32	32	
30	21	71	50	39.5	39.5	
31	10	22	12	14	14	
32	28	52	24	27	27	
33	26	64	38	37	37	
34	22	23	1	1.5	1.5	
35	34	43	9	9	9	
36	9	19	10	10.5	10.5	
37	59	80	21	24	24	
38	18	24	6	8	8	
39	10	7	−3	5		5
40	22	58	36	36	36	
	Rank Totals			820	813.5	6.5

NIM, number of induced microcysts.

0.035-mm and 0.09-mm lenses for each subject, and in the fourth column are their differences. The fifth column provides the ranking of the absolute value of the differences in the third column. Where there are equal absolute differences, the corresponding ranks are averaged. For example, in Table 45.6, the two smallest differences are -1 and 1, so their absolute differences are both 1. Thus, they are both assigned a rank of 1.5, the average of ranks 1 and 2. The sixth and seventh columns give the rankings corresponding to the positive and negative differences in the third column, respectively. The totals for the sixth and seventh columns are 813.5 and 6.5, respectively, so W is the minimum of those two totals, or $W = 6.5$, which is small relative to the expected value of 410 if the null hypothesis were true (410 is half the sum, 820, of the ranks of 1–40). The p value is $P = \text{Prob}(T \le 6.5) < 0.001$. As with the t test, statistical significance is obtained, and this procedure also supports the claim that the NIM tends to be greater with the 0.09-mm lens than with the 0.035-mm lens.

The success of every clinical study depends, in part, on the reliability of the measurements that are taken. In the analysis, the reliability of the counting of microcysts is fundamental to the comparison of the H035 and H09 lenses. In order to assess the quality of this microcyst count data, the researchers sought to answer the following:

Question 1b. What is the reliability of the microcyst count process on the H035 lens?, that is, will a second count of the microcysts on a particular patient made in close time proximity to the first give a result that is essentially the same as the first?

After the first group of subjects wore the H035 lens for 3 months, microcysts were counted as part of a slit examination. A second clinician, without knowledge of the first result, then performed a second count. The results for both counts are given in Table 45.7.

The standard index of reliability is the intraclass correlation coefficient (ICC) (95–98). It is the ratio of between-subject variability to total variability, which is the sum of between-subject and within-subject variability. A small within-subject variability corresponds to a high level of reliability, so large values of the ICC indicate high reliability and low values indicate low reliability. ICC ranges from 0 to 1, with the following common standard of interpretation:

$0 \le \text{ICC} < 0.4$ indicates poor reliability

$0.4 \le \text{ICC} < 0.75$ indicates fair to good reliability

$0.75 \le \text{ICC} \le 1$ indicates good to excellent reliability.

ICC for the microcyst count data in Table 45.7 is 0.94 [95% confidence interval (0.89, 0.97)], so the reliability is considered excellent.

Interpretation of the ICC is given additional context with an analysis of the distribution of the differences between the first and second microcyst counts. The methods of Bland and Altman (97,99) can be applied here. Figure

TABLE 45.7.

Patient	MC1	MC2
1	25	25
2	56	66
3	49	53
4	68	63
5	17	18
6	54	58
7	62	60
8	54	64
9	43	35
10	49	52
11	20	17
12	48	57
13	30	28
14	28	33
15	40	42
16	52	46
17	37	34
18	49	48
19	33	31
20	16	18
21	19	21
22	27	30
23	32	39
24	17	16
25	59	59
26	27	24
27	44	44
28	44	34
29	21	28
30	28	40
31	14	14
32	33	33
33	30	26
34	28	31
35	39	35
36	13	19
37	62	56
38	22	33
39	17	20
40	25	22

For the patients who wore the 0.035-mm thick conventional hydrogel lens, MC1 is the actual microcyst count obtained by the first clinician and MC2 is that obtained by the second clinician.

45.4 shows a scatter plot of the difference between these two counts (second count minus first count) and the average of the two. The pattern of this plot is somewhat horizontal. These pairs have a correlation of $r = -0.003$, indicating the difference of the two counts does not depend on the magnitude of the counts. Three horizontal lines are shown on this plot, one at the mean difference of 1.03. A paired sample t-test shows that this mean is not significantly different from zero ($P = 0.23$), which indicates that the second count does not have a significant bias, that is, that it does not tend to be either consistently larger or consistently smaller than the first count.

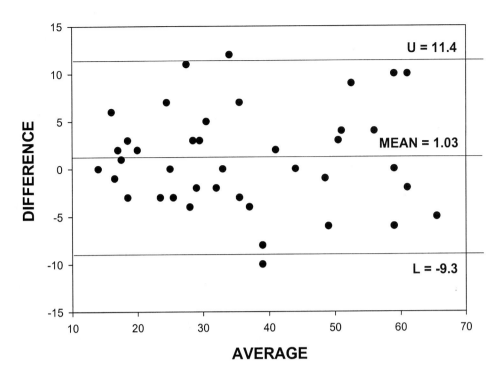

FIG. 45.4. Scatter-plot of the difference between the first and second microcyst counts and their average. The mean difference is 1.03 and the 95% limits of agreement are L = 9.3 and U = 11.4.

The variability of the differences between the two counts is the central reliability quantity. A large variability would indicate low reliability, and vice versa. In cases where the differences follow a normal distribution, the standard deviation, the most common measure of variability, can be used to give simple estimates for upper and lower bounds for most differences between counts. Bland and Altman have termed these bounds the *95% limits of agreement,* and they are given by

$$\bar{x}_D \pm 1.96 \cdot s_D$$

where $\bar{x}_D$ and s_D are the sample mean and sample standard deviation for the differences. The differences for the microcyst count data roughly follow a normal distribution as seen informally in Fig. 45.5, where the shape of the plot is essentially unimodal and symmetric. More formally, the Shapiro-Wilk test, which tests the hypothesis that the distribution of differences is normal, did not yield significance ($P = 0.68$). The 95% limits of agreement are $1.03 \pm 1.96 \cdot 5.28$ or $(-9.3, 11.4)$. The other two horizontal lines in Fig. 45.4 are at these limits of agreement values. Hence, from these data, it is estimated that 95% of the differences of microcyst counts will be between -9.3 and 11.4. Using 10 as the threshold value for an important clinical difference, one concludes that nearly all patients will have repeated counts of microcysts that are clinically interchangeable. In fact, in this sample, 38 (95%) of 40 subjects had differences in the two counts that were 10 or less.

Clinical Implication of the Result. For patients who wear the H035 lens, the count of microcysts is a highly reliable

measurement that we expect close proximity repeated counts to be within 11 microcysts of each other, with the vast majority within 10 and, hence, clinically equivalent.

Question 2a. The researchers were interested in finding if the approved silicone hydrogel contact lens offered a better physiologic environment to the cornea in extended wear. They compared the relative hypoxia in extended wear of the silicone hydrogel lens with that of a conventional hydrogel by the number of microcysts induced. They asked the question: "Is there a difference in the NIM when wearing the standard hydrogel 0.035-mm thick lens (H035) compared to the number when wearing the approved silicone hydrogel 0.09-mm thick lens (SH09)?

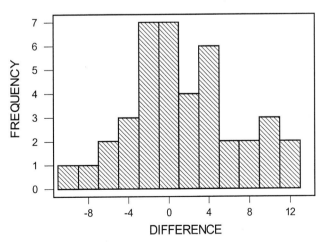

FIG. 45.5. Frequency histogram showing the distribution of the differences between the microcyst counts from two different clinicians.

TABLE 45.8. NUMERICAL SUMMARY OF THE NUMBER OF INDUCED MICROCYST DATA FOR THE H035 AND SH09 LENSES

| Lens | Induced Microcysts | | |
	Mean	Standard Deviation	Median
H035	31.5	15.49	28.0
SH09	5.1	3.16	5.0

Table 45.8 summarizes the induced microcyst data for the group of patients who wore H035 lens and for the group who wore SH09 lens. In Fig. 45.6, the parallel box plots give a graphical comparison of the distributions of induced microcysts for each group. Both of these data summaries indicate that the H035 group tended to have larger increases in microcysts than the SH09 group.

A *t* statistic,

$$T_k = \frac{(\bar{X}_H - \bar{X}_S) - (\mu_H - \mu_S)}{S_D} \text{ (test statistic for the two-sample } t \text{ test)}$$

can be used to test hypotheses concerning $\mu_H - \mu_S$, where X_H, X_S, μ_H, and μ_S are the corresponding sample and population means for H035 and SH09, and S_D is an estimator for the standard error of $X_H - X_S$ in which the data from both samples are used. The degrees of freedom k is determined by the method of computation of S_D. The resulting 95% confidence interval for $\mu_1 - \mu_2$ is (21.3, 31.4). This interval excludes zero, which indicates that the data are consistent with a difference between the actual means, a differ-ence that on the average exceeds 20 microcysts. A two-sample *t* test can be used to test

H$_0$: $\mu_H = \mu_{SH}$ (H3)
H$_1$: $\mu_H \neq \mu_{SH}$.

Two-Sample t Test Using the information in Table 45.8, the value of the test statistic (see earlier), which is used in testing H3, can be calculated. The obtained value of the test statistic is

$$T_{42} = \frac{31.5 - 5.1}{\sqrt{\dfrac{15.50^2}{40} + \dfrac{3.16^2}{40}}} = 10.55.$$

The degrees of freedom k = 42 is determined from the use of the "separate variance"approach to computing S_D as shown, which was used because the sample variances for the two groups were quite different. From the above calculation we obtain $P = \text{Prob}(|T_{42}| \geq 10.55) < 0.001$. Again, statistical significance is obtained, indicating that the data provide strong evidence for a difference between the means μ_H and μ_S.

Clinical Implication of the Result The approved silicone hydrogel contact lens offers a better physiologic environment in extended wear than the 0.035-mm thick hydrogel lens, as evidenced by the significantly lower number of microcysts induced.

Question 2b. A new (experimental) silicone hydrogel lens has been developed that offers a less rigid material than the approved silicone hydrogel. It is hoped that this new

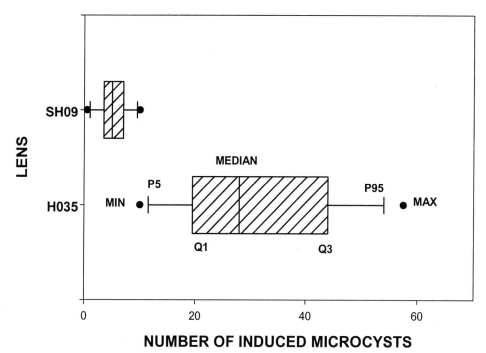

FIG. 45.6. Parallel box plots comparing the distributions of the number of induced microcysts for those patients who wore the conventional hydrogel 0.035-mm thick lens (S035) and those who wore the 0.090mm thick silicone hydrogel lens (SH09). Each plot shows the sample minimum (MIN), the 5th percentile (P5), the first quartile (Q1), the median, the third quartile (Q3), the 95th percentile (P95), and the maximum (MAX).

material will reduce adverse reactions (superior epithelial arcuate lesions [SEALs]) observed with the approved lens (85). The new lens is designed with a center thickness of 0.09 mm, which reduces the oxygen transmission of the material to about two thirds that of the approved silicone hydrogel. Researchers were interested in determining if there was a difference in the NIM when wearing the approved silicone hydrogel 0.09-mm thick lens (SH09) compared to wearing an experimental silicone hydrogel lens 0.09-mm thick (ESH09).

Table 45.9 and Fig. 45.7 give numerical and graphical summaries of the distributions of induced microcysts for two groups of subjects, one who wore the SH09 and the other ESH09. The ESH09 group tends to have more microcysts. A two-sample *t*-test can be used to test the hypothesis that the actual means for the corresponding populations are equal. The observed value of the test statistic is

$$T_{78} = \frac{7.1 - 5.1}{S_p\sqrt{\frac{1}{40}+\frac{1}{40}}} = 2.57,$$

where S_p is the pooled estimate for the common standard deviation for the two populations. This pooling of information from the two samples is used when the sample standard deviations are comparable, as in this case. For this data,

$$S_p = \sqrt{\frac{39 \cdot 3.16^2 + 39 \cdot 3.69^2}{78}} = 3.43.$$

It follows that $P = \mathrm{Prob}(|T_{78}| \geq 2.57) = 0.012$ and, hence,

TABLE 45.9. NUMERICAL SUMMARY OF NUMBER OF INDUCED MICROCYST DATA FOR ESH09 AND SH09 LENSES

Lens	Induced Microcysts		
	Mean	Standard Deviation	Median
ESH09	7.1	3.69	7.0
SH09	5.1	3.16	5.0

that the observed means are (statistically) significantly different. The corresponding 95% confidence interval for $\mu_{ESH} - \mu_{SH}$ is (0.4, 3.5), indicating that the observed means are statistically different but clinically interchangeable because the minimum threshold for clinical significance is 10 microcysts.

The Mann-Whitney test provides a nonparametric alternative to the two-sample *t* test (93). It is a test on the medians M_{SH} and M_{ESH} corresponding to SH09 and ESH09, respectively. Specifically, it tests

H_0: $M_{SH} = M_{ESH}$ (H4)

H_1: $M_{SH} \neq M_{ESH}$.

As in the Wilcoxon one-sample test, the Mann-Whitney test statistic depends on ranks. In this case, all 80 values of induced microcysts observed from both groups would be pooled and put in rank order. The ranks of the observations from the ESH09 sample are summed. Assuming that H_0 is true, one would expect this total S to be about half of the total of all ranks from 1 to 80, or 1,620. (The total of the

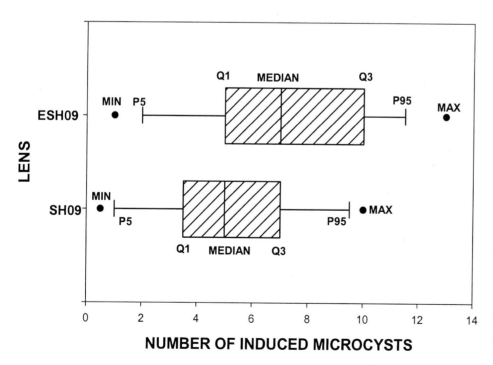

FIG. 45.7. Parallel box plots comparing the distributions of the number of induced microcysts for those patients who wore the experimental silicone hydrogel 0.09-mm thick lens (ESH09) and those who wore the 0.09-mm thick silicone hydrogel lens (SH09). Each plot shows the sample minimum (MIN), the 5th percentile (P5), the first quartile (Q1), the median, the third quartile (Q3), the 95th percentile (P95), and the maximum (MAX).

ranks from 1 to 80 is 3,240, so half of that total is 1,620.) Hence, if S is considerably different from 1,620, H_0 is cast in doubt. Tables of critical values for the Mann-Whitney test are available for small samples (94); for large samples, an approximation to the gaussian distribution is used.

Mann-Whitney Test The steps, which were described earlier and involved in determining the value of the test statistic S in this case where the hypothesis (H4) is to be tested, are detailed in Table 45.10. The second and sixth columns indicate which lens the patient wore; the third and seventh columns list the number of SH09-induced microcysts. The fourth and eighth columns give the rank order of the numbers in the second and sixth columns, respectively. The total of the ranks in column 4 corresponding to patients who wore ESH09 is the value of the test statistic S. For this case, S = 1,889.5 (fractional ranks occur when there are tied observations). Using the large sample approximation, one obtains

$$P = \text{Prob}(|S - 1,620| \geq 1,889.5 - 1,620 = 269.5) = 0.0093.$$

This result is consistent with the two-sample *t*-test results of statistically significant differences of 5 (SH09) and 7 (ESH09).

Clinical Implications of Result The experimental silicone hydrogel induces more microcysts than the approved silicone hydrogel lens. However, this result is not of clinical significance because the number of microcysts induced with both lenses, 5 (SH09) and 7 (ESH09), are below the 10 thought to be of clinical importance (100).

One-Sided Versus Two-Sided Tests In each of the earlier procedures, the two-sample *t* test and the Mann-Whitney test, a two-sided test has been conducted, that is, each test was concerned with any shifts in the distributions of numbers of induced microcysts for SH09 and ESH09, whether it indicated a tendency for ESH09 to result in higher values than SH09, or *vice versa*. Suppose the original research question had been, "Do patients wearing SH09 have fewer induced microcysts than patients wearing ESH09?" Implicit in this question is the clinical assumption that SH09 will perform at least as well as ESH09 and, hence, that it will not induce more microcysts than ESH09. In this circumstance, a one-sided test can be performed. For example, the hypotheses tested with the two-sample *t*-tests would be:

$H_0: \mu_{SH} = \mu_{ESH}$ (H5)

$H_1: \mu_{SH} < \mu_{ESH}$.

Because the concern is only with a shift in the NIM, indicating that it tends to be greater for ESH09 than SH09, H_0 would be rejected only if $\bar{X}_{ESH}$ is substantially greater than $\bar{X}_{SH}$. The p value calculation reflects this one-sided focus

TABLE 45.10. APPLICATION OF MANN-WHITNEY TEST TO INDUCED MICROCYST DATA FROM PATIENTS WHO WORE THE SILICONE HYDROGEL 0.09-MM THICK LENS (SH09) AND THOSE WHO WORE THE EXPERIMENTAL SILICONE HYDROGEL 0.09-MM THICK LENS (ESH09)

	SH09			ESH09	
Patient	NIM	Rank	Patient	NIM	Rank
1	4	23	41	11	73.5
2	6	42.5	42	9	61.5
3	5	32.5	43	9	61.5
4	10	68.5	44	11	73.5
5	9	61.5	45	11	73.5
6	7	52	46	13	77.5
7	14	79	47	16	80
8	4	23	48	6	42.5
9	1	6.5	49	6	42.5
10	4	23	50	0	2
11	6	42.5	51	5	32.5
12	5	32.5	52	8	57
13	10	68.5	53	9	61.5
14	2	12	54	3	16.5
15	0	2	55	3	16.5
16	1	6.5	56	7	52
17	5	32.5	57	10	68.5
18	9	61.5	58	10	68.5
19	1	6.5	59	1	6.5
20	5	32.5	60	6	42.5
21	2	12	61	4	23
22	4	23	62	9	61.5
23	9	61.5	63	11	73.5
24	4	23	64	6	42.5
25	9	61.5	65	12	76
26	5	32.5	66	7	52
27	6	42.5	67	6	42.5
28	2	12	68	3	16.5
29	1	6.5	69	2	12
30	3	16.5	70	5	32.5
31	4	23	71	5	32.5
32	5	32.5	72	7	52
33	6	42.5	73	10	68.5
34	10	68.5	74	13	77.5
35	4	23	75	7	52
36	7	52	76	7	52
37	7	52	77	6	42.5
38	4	23	78	2	12
39	5	32.5	79	7	52
40	0	2	80	1	6.5
Total		1889.5			1350.5

NIM, number of induced microcysts.

by removing the absolute value (see earlier) from the test statistic; consequently, $P = \text{Prob}(T_{78} \geq 2.57) = 0.006$. In this case, the decision on whether this test should be one or two sided would be especially important if $\alpha = 0.01$ had been set as the significance threshold, because the one-sided test gives statistical significance at this level, whereas the two-sided test does not. This is a clinical and practical decision that must be made in the design phase of a study,

TABLE 45.11. MEAN NUMBER OF INDUCED MICROCYSTS FOR EACH LENS THICKNESS FOR THE CONVENTIONAL HYDROGEL AND SILICONE HYDROGEL GROUPS

Lens Material	Thickness			All Thicknesses
	0.035 mm	0.09 mm	0.20 mm	
Conventional hydrogel	31.5 (15.49)	50.3 (23.93)	60.1 (24.55)	47.3
Silicone hydrogel	3.0 (1.59)	5.1 (3.16)	15.1 (4.12)	7.7
Both materials	17.5	27.7	37.6	27.5

Values in parentheses are standard deviations.

not *after the results have been obtained.* In most studies in the biologic and health sciences, two-sided tests are preferred (7). Effects of new treatments or, as in this case, new materials can be varied and complex, which can result in either improvement or decline from the performance of the standard. For example, ESH09 has the potential to surpass SH09 in microcyst induction performance, but it also may fall short of SH09 in this regard. The two-sided test allows for both possibilities and is appropriate, unless there is substantial clinical information that virtually precludes the possibility that ESH09 could perform below the SH09 level.

Question 3. To confirm the general relationship between NIM and corneal hypoxia during extended wear of the approved silicone hydrogel lens and the conventional hydrogel lens, the researchers asked the question, "Is there a difference in the number of microcysts induced between the conventional and silicone hydrogel lenses for all three lens thicknesses, 0.035 mm, 0.09 mm, and 0.20 mm?"

All of the induced microcyst data are summarized in Table 45.11, where the sample mean (and sample standard

deviations) for each material at each thickness are given. These same means are plotted by material against thickness in Fig. 45.8. This preliminary inspection of the results indicates that the conventional hydrogel lenses, on the average, have greater numbers of induced microcysts than silicone hydrogel lenses for all three thicknesses, and these numbers tend to increase with lens thickness for both materials. Furthermore, this difference between the materials is more pronounced for the 0.09-mm and 0.20-mm lenses as compared to the 0.035-mm lenses.

In order to determine if these observed differences in means can be explained by chance, a procedure is needed that will take into consideration more than two population means (in this case, six means). A family of such techniques is commonly referred to as *analysis of variance* (ANOVA). ANOVA is applied to a large variety of experimental designs, but a fundamental idea is used in all of these designs. The total variation in a set of data is partitioned into component parts, which are attributed to factors, such as lens material and lens thickness, combinations of those factors,

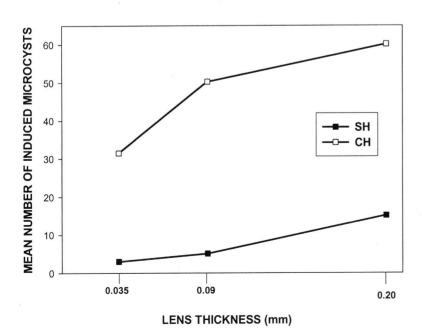

FIG. 45.8. Plots of mean number of induced microcysts versus lens thickness for each lens material.

TABLE 45.12. ANOVA TABLE FOR TWO-FACTOR (LENS MATERIAL AND LENS THICKNESS) REPEATED-MEASURES ANALYSIS OF VARIANCE PROCEDURE APPLIED TO THE INDUCED MICROCYST DATA

Source	SS	Df	MS	F	P
Lens material	357.7	1	357.7	3147.3	<0.0005
Error1	8.865	78	0.114		
Thickness	8.438	2	4.219	316.1	<0.0005
Mat*Thk	1.784	2	0.892	66.8	<0.0005
Error2	2.082	156	0.0134		

df, degrees of freedom; F, value of the F statistic; MS, mean sum of squares; P, P value; SS, sum of squares.

termed *interaction effects,* and residual or random variation. Under particular null hypotheses (H_0) concerning population means, one expects certain pairs of these components of variation, properly adjusted, to be equal. The test statistic in these cases is the appropriate quotient of these two adjusted components of variation, which has an F distribution when the null hypothesis is valid (101). Such F-tests are one sided, so a rejection of the null hypothesis will occur when the F statistic is sufficiently >1, the value of the quotient expected under H_0.

In this particular study, because the same variable, NIM, was measured on each patient in the three fitting modes, a fairly involved ANOVA procedure, termed a *repeated measures design* (101), is necessary. Repeated measures designs are frequently used in the health sciences when measurements are taken from the same subjects under different treatment conditions or over time. In this design there are two factors or effects: lens material, which is a group factor, and lens thickness, which is a within-group factor, that is, lens material was used as the basis for subject allocation

to groups, but within each group each patient has NIM determined for all three lens thicknesses.

Analysis of Variance: A Repeated Measures Design The ANOVA results for this study are summarized in Table 45.12. In this table, the column headed "Source" lists the factors to which components of the total variation are associated. The SS (sum of squares) column provides the actual components of variation for each of those factors; the df (degrees of freedom) column provides parameter values corresponding to each factor. The MS (mean sum of squares) column provides the adjusted component of variation for each factor, which is simply the SS entry divided by its corresponding df entry. The F and P columns provide the values of the F statistics and their corresponding p values for the specific tests of significance.

Each of these tests results in statistical significance. Whereas the main effects, lens material and lens thickness, are the central clinical considerations in this ANOVA, it is also important to determine if the effects of material and

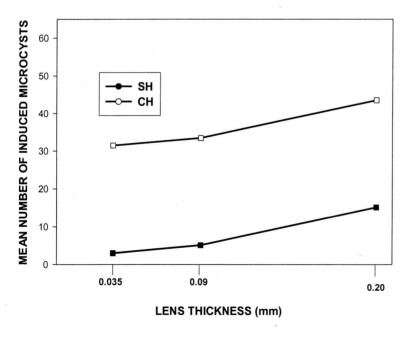

FIG. 45.9. Hypothetical plots of mean number of induced microcysts versus lens thickness for each lens material in which one plot is a vertical shift of the other, indicating that there is no interaction effect between the effects of lens material and lens thickness.

fit interact with each other. The interaction question can be posed as, "Is the effect of lens material uniform across the three thicknesses?" A positive response to this question would imply that the two main effects are not interacting. However, Figure 45.8 suggests that the response may be negative. The conventional hydrogel plot shows a greater increase in mean induced microcysts between the 0.035-mm and 0.09-mm thicknesses than does the silicone hydrogel. If there were this uniformity of lens material effect across thicknesses, the two plots would appear to be more parallel, as in the hypothetical plot shown in Fig. 45.9.

The results of the test of the null hypothesis that there are no interaction effects is shown in Table 12 under Mat*Thk (material by thickness) and Error2, where F(2, 156) = 66.8 and P < 0.0005. Hence, the data statistically support the notion that the two main effects are interacting. In the presence of such interaction effects, one should be cautious in interpreting the tests on the main effects (material and thickness). We will proceed to the results on those main effects with this background on interaction in mind.

A central issue in this study is the comparison of the conventional hydrogel (CH) and silicone hydrogel (SH) lens materials. It may be asked, when inspecting Table 45.11, if the overall sample means for NIM for the two materials (47.3 for CH and 7.7 for SH) are significantly different. Therefore, the following hypotheses are tested:

H_0: μ_{CH} = μ_{SH} (H6)
H_1: μ_{CH} ≠ μ_{SH},

where μ_{SH} and μ_{CH} are the population means across all three thicknesses for each material. For this test, referring to Table 45.12, F(1, 78) = 357.7/0.114 = 3147.3, and P = Prob(F(1, 78) ≥ 3147.3) < 0.0005, so H_0 is rejected. In the presence of the material by thickness interaction effect, there is uncertainty regarding this material effect at all three thickness levels. Table 45.13 gives for each thickness the means, standard deviations, and results of the two-sample *t* tests, which test for the equality of the lens material-induced microcyst means. Because each of these results is both statistically and clinically significant, the data support the conclusion that, at all three thicknesses, the conventional hydrogel lens will tend to induce more microcysts than the silicone hydrogel lens.

TABLE 45.14. RESULTS OF ONE-WAY ANALYSIS OF VARIANCE TESTING THE SIGNIFICANCE IN DIFFERENCES OF OBSERVED MEAN NUMBER OF INDUCED MICROCYSTS FOR THE THREE THICKNESSES OF THE TWO LENS MATERIALS

Lens Material	F(2, 117)	P Value
Conventional hydrogel	17.91	<0.0005
Silicone hydrogel	169.57	<0.0005

A second main issue is the effect of lens thickness on NIM, irrespective of lens material. The sample means for each thickness across both materials are 17.5, 27.7, and 37.6 for the 0.035-mm, 0.09-mm, and 0.20-mm thicknesses, respectively (Table 45.11). To determine if these results represent a reasonable chance occurrence, assuming that thickness has no effect on NIM, the following hypotheses are tested:

H_0: μ_{035} = μ_{09} = μ_{20} (H7)
H_1: H_0 is not true,

where μ_{035}, μ_{09}, and μ_{02} are the corresponding lens thickness population means. The results of this test are detailed in Table 45.12 under Thickness and Error2, where F(2, 156) = 316.1 and P < 0.0005. Again, the presence of the interaction effect complicates the interpretation of this result, as the thickness effect may not be uniform across both lens materials. An ANOVA procedure can be applied to the CH and SH data separately in order to test the hypothesis that there is no difference among the population means for induced microcysts for the three thicknesses. Table 45.14 summarizes the results, which show significance for both lens materials. Hence, we conclude that for both materials, NIM tends to increase with lens thickness in both the conventional and silicone hydrogel lenses.

Clinical Implication of the Result As lenses get thicker, the degree of corneal hypoxia during extended wear becomes greater, resulting in more microcyst formation. This is true for both lens materials, but the number of microcysts is clinically acceptable for the 0.035- and 0.09-mm silicone hydrogel lenses.

TABLE 45.13. RESULTS OF TWO-SAMPLE T-TESTS COMPARING MEAN NUMBER OF INDUCED MICROCYSTS BETWEEN SUBJECTS WHO WORE THE CONVENTIONAL AND SILICONE HYDROGEL LENSES FOR EACH OF THE THREE LENS THICKNESSES

Thickness (mm)	Conventional Hydrogel	Silicone Hydrogel	Observed t	P Value
0.035	31.5	3.0	11.59	<0.0005
0.09	50.3	5.1	11.83	<0.0005
0.20	60.1	15.1	11.44	<0.0005

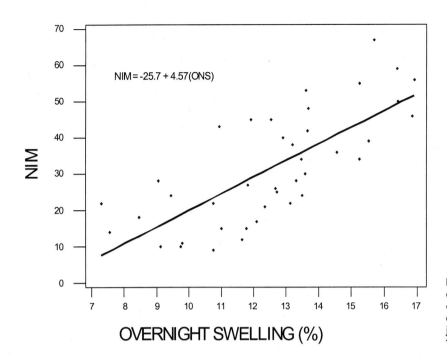

FIG. 45.10. Scatter-plot of the number of induced microcysts (NIM) versus the percentage of overnight swelling with the superimposed estimated regression line for the data from subjects who wore the 0.035-mm thick conventional hydrogel lens.

Question 4a. The phenomenon of microcyst formation is thought to be due to corneal hypoxia during extended wear of contact lenses (100); therefore, it might be expected to be related to other hypoxic events, such as the overnight swelling response (ONS). Thus, the researchers asked the question, "For the conventional hydrogel 0.035-mm thick lens, does ONS provide a useful predictor of NIM?"

Figure 45.10 shows a scatter-plot of NIM versus ONS for those patients who used the 0.035-mm thick hydrogel lenses. There appears to be a positive relationship between these two variables, and the plot suggests that it will be reasonable to view that relationship as a linear one, that is, the plot suggests that NIM may be a linear function of ONS, or NIM = α + β(ONS), termed a *regression line*. Here, β is the amount of change in NIM for every unit change in ONS. In this context, α and β are population parameters that can be estimated from the data. The usual method of estimation is a least-squares technique in which the estimates of α and β, denoted a and b, respectively, correspond to a line y = a + bx in which the total of the squares of the vertical distance from each point to the line is minimized. This line is referred to as the *estimated regression line* (101,102).

In this case the estimated regression line is given as

NIM = -25.7 + 4.57 (ONS),

and its graph has been superimposed over the scatter plot shown in Fig. 45.10.

This estimated regression line specifies a linear relationship between the variables NIM and ONS, but it does not indicate how strong that linear relationship is. For that purpose, a numerical index, termed the *coefficient of determina-*

tion and denoted by r^2, is used. The r^2 can be viewed as the estimated proportion of the total variation in the dependent variable (NIM in this case) that can be accounted for by the linear relationship with the independent variable (ONS in this case). The r^2 varies between 0 and 1, with values close to 1 indicating a strong linear relationship between the dependent and independent variables. As an approximate guideline, $r^2 \geq 0.6$ would be considered high, $0.25 \leq r^2 \leq 0.6$ moderate, and $r^2 \leq 0.25$ negligible to low (9).

The usual assumption in the significance testing (discussed later) is that for every fixed value of the independent variable, the population values of the dependent variable have a gaussian distribution. If, for each fixed value of the dependent variable, the population values of the independent variable also have a gaussian distribution, then the concept of correlation can be considered. The correlation coefficient ρ is a parameter that measures the actual strength of the linear relationship between the independent and dependent variables. The ρ varies between -1 and 1, with values close to -1 and 1 indicating a stronger linear relationship, and the sign indicating whether the relationship is direct (positive) or indirect (negative). The estimator for ρ is the product moment correlation coefficient $r = \pm \sqrt{r^2}$, where the sign is the same as the sign of b, the estimated regression line slope (102). From the ONS versus PCS data, r = 0.74 and r^2 = 0.55, indicating that the sample values of NIM and ONS are exhibiting a moderately strong linear relationship. In fact, 55% of the variation in NIM values is explained by the linear relationship between NIM and ONS.

To assess whether this observed linear relationship can be attributed to chance, the following hypotheses are tested:

$H_0: \beta = 0$ (H8)
$H_1: \beta \neq 0$.

If the regression line slope β is zero, then the line is horizontal; therefore, NIM would not be linearly dependent on ONS. Hence, this is actually a test of the hypothesis that a useful linear relationship exists between NIM and ONS. In cases in which correlation is considered, the test of the hypotheses H8 is equivalent to testing:

$H_0: \rho = 0$ (H9)
$H_0: \rho \neq 0$.

If $\rho = 0$, then NIM and ONS would be uncorrelated and, in fact, independently determined quantities, so no linear relationship between them would be useful. The test statistic for either of these formulations has a t distribution and, under the null hypothesis, can be given by

$$T_{n-2} = \frac{b}{S_b} \text{ or } T_{n-2} = \frac{r\sqrt{n-2}}{\sqrt{1-r^2}} \text{ (Test statistic in simple linear regression)}$$

where S_b, is the standard error for b. In this study,

$$T_{38} = 4.57/0.67 = 6.8 \text{ or, } T_{38} = \frac{0.74\sqrt{38}}{\sqrt{1-(0.74)^2}} = 6.8,$$

so $P = \text{Prob}(|T_{38}| \geq 6.8) < 0.0001$. It can be concluded that a significant linear relationship exists between NIM and ONS.

Clinical Implications of Results Given the strength of that linear relationship (recall $r^2 = 0.54$), it is reasonable to infer that ONS is a useful predictor of NIM for patients using the conventional 0.035-mm thick hydrogel lens.

Question 4b. The researchers were interested to see if the "hypoxic" relationship between microcysts and ONS applied to the approved silicone hydrogel 0.09-mm thick lens.

Figure 45.11 shows a scatter-plot of NIM versus ONS for the approved silicone hydrogel lens. No relationship between the variables is apparent in this plot; in fact, for these data, $r = -0.017$ (which gives $P = 0.92$) and $r^2 = 0.0002$. From these data there is no evidence that ONS is a predictor of NIM for the approved silicone hydrogel lens.

Clinical Implications of Result The absence of a relationship between microcysts and corneal swelling during extended wear of the approved silicone hydrogel lens indicates that the degree of hypoxia was sufficiently limited to give minimal microcyst formation or corneal swelling.

Question 5a. A hypoxic mechanism is proposed for microcyst development (100). Corneal hypoxia with extended contact lens wear leads to a reduction in epithelial mitosis and an increase in the regeneration time for corneal epithelial cells (103); therefore, ONS and mitotic rate may be predictors of the level of microcysts observed during extended wear. Mitotic rate is difficult to measure, but an analogue is the epithelial desquamation rate (EDR). Ren et al. (90) have shown that short-term precorneal hypoxia down-regulates epithelial cell desquamation in humans who show a concurrent increase in corneal swelling. The researchers in the studies described earlier desired to determine, for the conventional 0.035-mm thick hydrogel lens, if the combination of ONS and the decrease in EDR is a useful predictor of NIM.

In the response to Question 4a, ONS was established as a useful predictor of NIM using simple linear regression. In applying the same techniques to the prediction of NIM

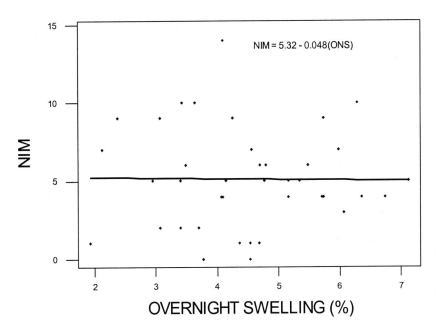

FIG. 45.11. Scatter-plot of the number of induced microcysts (NIM) versus the percentage of overnight swelling with the superimposed estimated regression line for the data from subjects who wore the 0.09-mm thick silicone hydrogel lens.

from the decrease from baseline of EDR, one obtains the estimated regression line NIM $= -0.93 + 2.06$ (EDR), $r = 0.71$, $r^2 = 0.51$, and statistical significance ($P < 0.0001$) in the test of the main hypotheses. Hence, the data support the characterization of EDR as a useful linear predictor of NIM.

In comparing these results to those obtained for the regression NIM on ONS, ONS would be preferred over EDR as a linear prediction of ONS. Not only is the coefficient of determination higher when ONS is the predictor (0.55 vs 0.51), but comparison of the standard errors of estimation also indicates that ONS is the better linear indicator of NIM. This standard error is interpreted as the typical amount by which the predicted values of NIM differ from the observed values. It is given in the units of the dependent variable (NIM in this case) and is denoted by S_e. When ONS is used as the predictor variable, $S_e = 10.55$, but with EDR, $S_e = 11.02$. Hence, there is less variation in the observed points from the estimated regression line when ONS is the predictor than when EDR is, indicating that there is a better fit of the regression line to the observed points in the ONS case (101).

The decrease in EDR may still be a useful predictor, especially if it has predictive value that goes beyond that of ONS alone. This predictive value can be used in a procedure, termed *multiple linear regression* (101), in which ONS and EDR are used together as predictors of NIM. As an extension of the simple linear regression model, the prediction equation is assumed to have form:

NIM $= \beta_0 + \beta_1$(ONS) $+ \beta_2$(EDR).

Here, β_1 is the amount of change in NIM for each unit change in ONS with EDR fixed, and β_2 is the amount of change in NIM for each unit change in EDR, with ONS fixed. The parameters β_0, β_1, and β_2 are estimated using the least-squares idea; in this case, the estimated regression equation is

NIM $= -35.5 + 3.47$(ONS) $+ 1.50$(EDR).

The coefficient of multiple determination, denoted as R^2, measures the strength of the linear dependence of NIM on ONS and EDR together. Analogous with the single predictor case, R^2 is interpreted as an estimate of the proportion of the total variability in NIM, which is explained by its joint linear dependence on ONS and EDR (102). In this case, $R^2 = 0.77$, so it would appear that ONS and EDR together are very useful linear predictors of NIM and that EDR contributes additional predictive value to ONS in predicting NIM.

To assess whether these results can be attributed to chance, the following main hypotheses are tested:

H_0: $\beta_1 = \beta_2 = 0$ (H10)
H_1: $\beta_1 \neq 0$ or $\beta_2 \neq 0$.

The test statistic has an F distribution and in this case is given by

$$F(2,37) = \frac{R^2/2}{(1 - R^2)\cdot 37} = 67.51.$$

So $P = $ Prob(F(2, 37) $\geq$ 67.51) < 0.0001, indicating that the observed multiple regression equation is statistically significant. Because the data support H_1, it is also useful to conduct tests to determine which of the regression coefficients β_1 and β_2 are significant. In each case (i $= 1$ or 2),

H_0: $\beta_i = 0$ (H11)
H_1: $\beta_i \neq 0$.

are being tested. The test statistic has a t distribution and is $T = b_i/s_{b_i}$ where b_i is the estimated regression coefficient for β_i, and s_{b_i} is the estimated standard deviation for b_i. Table 45.15 summarizes the results. Because both tests give statistical significance, the data strongly indicate that each of the independent variables (ONS and EDR) is a useful linear predictor of ONS, and that the prediction process will be improved significantly if both are used together.

Clinical Implication of the Result The result suggests that microcysts, ONS, and EDR are all consequences of contact lens-induced hypoxia with the 0.035-mm thick hydrogel lens worn for extended periods and supports the hypothesis that ONS and EDS can be used to predict microcyst formation.

Question 5b. The researchers were interested to determine if the same relationship held for the approved 0.09-mm thick silicone hydrogel lens, i.e., does the combination of ONS response and the decrease in EDR provide a useful predictor of NIM when the amount of hypoxia (and microcyst number) is less?

TABLE 45.15. RESULTS OBTAINED BY MULTIPLE REGRESSION ANALYSIS OF THE NUMBER OF INDUCED MICROCYST DATA FOR SUBJECTS WHO WORE THE 0.035-MM THICK CONVENTIONAL HYDROGEL LENS USING OVERNIGHT SWELLING AND EPITHELIAL DESQUAMATION RATE AS PREDICTORS

Predictor	Estimated Coefficient (b_i)	SE of b_i	t	P Value
ONS	3.47	0.502	6.92	<0.0005
EDR	1.50	0.235	6.39	<0.0005

EDR, epithelial desquamation rate; ONS, overnight swelling.

TABLE 45.16. OBSERVED FREQUENCIES OF CONTACT LENS ACUTE RED EYE AMONG PATIENTS WHO WORE THE 0.035-MM THICK CONVENTIONAL HYDROGEL LENS (H035) AND THOSE WHO WORE THE 0.09-MM THICK SILICONE HYDROGEL LENS (SH09)

Lens	Normal	Clare
H035	972	28
SH09	984	16

CLARE, contact lens acute red eye.

The same multiple regression analysis can be applied to the data in which ONS, EDR, and NIM are measured for the subjects who wore the silicone hydrogel 0.09-mm thick lens. In this case, the estimated regression equation is

$$NIM = 3.93 - 0.055(ONS) + 0.092(EDR).$$

However, $R^2 = 0.024$ and $P = 0.63$. Furthermore, neither of the regression coefficients was significantly different from zero, that is, for this lens, the combination of ONS and EDR is not a useful predictor of NIM.

Clinical Implications of the Result In this case, ONS and EDR are not found to be good predictors of the induced microcyst number in corneas of patients wearing the 0.09-mm thick approved silicone hydrogel lens. In these patients, the amount of hypoxia is limited (shown by the small increase in microcysts and ONS), but epithelial desquamation is significantly reduced. A similar result has been found by Ren et al. (104) with the extended wear of silicone hydrogel lens. Although EDR is reduced by hypoxia with some lenses, it is also clearly affected by other factors in contact lens wear. Wear of all lenses reduces the ability of cells to shed from the cornea by exfoliative irrigation, suggesting a lens-induced decrease in normal epithelial desquamation (104). Therefore, as the highly oxygen transmitting silicone hydrogel lens appears to have least effect on basal layer proliferation (105), the resultant effect will be of a clinical stagnation of the ocular surface (104).

Question 6. The silicone hydrogel material provides more oxygen to the cornea in extended wear, but a question exists about the inflammatory reactions to the new lenses. After 12 months of extended wear of the new lens, the incidence of contact lens acute red eye (CLARE) is compared with that for conventional hydrogels. The question is asked, "Do the patients wearing the approved silicone hydrogel 0.09-mm thick lenses (SH09) have a comparable prevalence of CLARE to those patients wearing the conventional hydrogel 0.035-mm thick lens (H035)?"

Table 45.16 provides the observed frequencies of the occurrences of CLARE for both lenses. The observed rate of success for patients wearing the SH09 lenses is 1.6% versus 2.8% for patients wearing the H035 lenses. The Chi-square test provides a means for determining if this difference in prevalences could be explained by chance. The hypotheses to be tested are

$$H_0: p_{H035} = p_{SH09}$$
$$H_0: p_{H035} \neq p_{SH09},$$

where p_{H035} and p_{SH09} are the respective prevalence for the two populations.

Chi-square tests are applied more generally to frequency data that have been cross-categorized using two sets of categories. For example, suppose four different lens materials were used in this study, and each patient was randomly assigned to wear one of the four materials and then graded his or her satisfaction with the lens. A two-way table summarizing the observed frequencies might look like Table 45.17. n_{ij} denotes the number of patients who wore a material i (where i is 1, 2, 3, or 4) and who were satisfied with it at level j (j ranges from grades 1–5 and corresponds to *very satisfied* to *unsatisfied*, respectively). n_i is the total number of patients who used the lenses with material i, and n_j is the total number of patients who were satisfied at level j. The question that would be addressed here is whether the distribution of satisfaction levels varied by lens material.

The null hypothesis would be that these distributions are the same for all four materials. This would be equivalent to claiming that the level of satisfaction does not depend on which lens material was worn.

TABLE 45.17. HYPOTHETICAL FREQUENCIES OF RATINGS FOR FOUR TYPES OF LENS MATERIAL

Lens Material	Rating					Total
	Very Satisfied	**Satisfied**	**Not Sure**	**Unsatisfied**	**Very Unsatisfied**	
A	n_{11}	n_{12}	n_{13}	n_{14}	n_{15}	$n_{1.}$
B	n_{21}	n_{22}	n_{23}	n_{24}	n_{25}	$n_{2.}$
C	n_{31}	n_{32}	n_{33}	n_{34}	n_{35}	$n_{3.}$
D	n_{41}	n_{42}	n_{43}	n_{44}	n_{45}	$n_{4.}$
Total	$n_{.1}$	$n_{.2}$	$n_{.3}$	$n_{.4}$	$n_{.5}$	n

The test statistic used here is

$$X = \sum_{i=1}^{4} \sum_{j=1}^{5} \frac{(n_{ij} - e_{ij})^2}{e_{ij}} \text{ (Test statistic for a Chi-square test)}$$

where e_{ij} is the estimated expected frequency in the ijth cell assuming the null hypothesis is true. e_{ij} is determined by

$$e_{ij} = \frac{n_{i\cdot} \cdot n_{\cdot j}}{n} \text{ (Estimated expected frequencies for a Chi-square test)}.$$

If the null hypothesis is true, then each observed frequency n_{ij} should be reasonably close to its corresponding expected frequency e_{ij}. So when H_0 is valid, X should be a *small* positive value. Hence, large values of X are not consistent with the null hypothesis, so the p value for this test is $P = \text{Prob}(X \geq x)$, where x is the observed value of the test statistic X.

In order to compute *P*, the distribution of X must be specified. Under the conservative requirement that each $e_{ij} \geq 5$ for each combination of i and j, X has an approximate Chi-square distribution. There are detailed guidelines for relaxing this requirement in situations in which the sample size is insufficient. Also, in the case where the contingency table is 2 by 2 (as in Table 45.16), the exact p value can be calculated using the Fisher exact test (102). Other computationally intensive exact methods also are available (106).

Chi-Square Test Table 45.18 replicates the observed frequency information in Table 45.16 and, in addition, provides the estimated expected frequencies in parentheses (calculated as described earlier). For example, $n_{12} = 28$, $\mu_1 = 1,000$, $n_2 = 44$, and $n = 2,000$, so

$$e_{12} = \frac{1000 \cdot 44}{2000} = 22.$$

The observed value x of the test statistic is

$$x = \frac{(972 - 978)^2}{978} + \frac{(28 - 22)^2}{22} + \frac{(984 - 978)^2}{978} + \frac{(16 - 22)^2}{22} = 3.346,$$

so $P = \text{Prob}(X \geq 3.346) = 0.067$. Using the Fisher exact

test, $P = 0.093$. Consequently, the observed difference in prevalence for patients wearing the two lens materials is not statistically significant, that is, the observed data are not inconsistent with the hypothesis that success of contact lens patients is independent of whether they wear either extended wear lens.

The clinical significance of the prevalence difference is still problematical. It is quite likely that a contact lens with a prevalence of 1.6% would be viewed substantially more positively than a lens with a 2.8% prevalence by the clinician, because this suggests that a H035 patient is 75% more likely to have CLARE than a SH09 patient. In that case, a retrospective look at power and the type II error considerations is important (i.e., the failure to recognize that the performance of the two lenses was in fact different). With the current study design, there was only a 45% power to detect as statistically significant (at $\alpha = 0.05$) the observed proportions of 0.016 and 0.028. In order to have a power of 80% to detect as significant such a small difference, it would have required that the sample size of each group be 2,345. This is a recurring issue in studies that focus on rates or proportions, as Chi-square tests typically require large samples. In these situations, investigators are frequently left with uninformative null results.

Clinical Implications of the Results At the present level of wear of the approved silicone hydrogel lenses, the incidence of inflammatory reactions of the eye (CLARE) appears to be similar to that for conventional hydrogel extended wear. Further study on larger samples may show an increased incidence with the new material.

Question 7. The silicone hydrogel lens is surface treated to improve wettability and retains most of its water content during wear because it is not susceptible to dehydration on the eye (107). Therefore, it may be suitable as a lens for patients with marginal dry eye. A new dry eye questionnaire is developed that asks patients to compare morning with afternoon sensations of dryness (91). The results from the questionnaire given to all patients prior to the 12-month (phase 2) wear study are compared with the actual reports of dry eye problems reported during wear to determine if the questionnaire offers a screening test sufficiently sensitive and specific to detect problem cases before fitting.

The 1,000 patients who wore the H035 lens were administered the dry eye questionnaire and assessed for dry eye (CLDE). The questionnaire results were scored on a scale from 1 to 9, with the higher scores indicating greater potential for dry eye. The results, using a cutoff score of 6 on the questionnaire, are given in Table 45.19.

The questionnaire is a diagnostic test for dry eye, and the proportions of sensitivity and specificity can be used to assess the effectiveness of this test. *Sensitivity* is the proportion of subjects who test positive for the condition under consideration among those who have the condition. It is a

TABLE 45.18. EXPANDED VERSION OF TABLE 45.16² SHOWING OBSERVED FREQUENCIES, EXPECTED FREQUENCIES IN EACH CELL, AND ROW AND COLUMN TOTALS

Lens	Normal	CLARE	Total
H035	972 (978)	28 (22)	1,000
SH09	984 (978)	16 (22)	1,000
Total	1,956	44	2,000

Values in parentheses are expected frequencies in each cell.
CLARE, contact lens acute red eye.

TABLE 45.19. CROSS-CLASSIFIED FREQUENCIES OF H035 PATIENTS BASED ON THE OCCURRENCE OF DRY EYE AND THE QUESTIONNAIRE SCORE USING A CUTOFF OF 6

Questionnaire Score Q	Dry Eye Status		
	Dry Eye	No Dry Eye	Total
Q > 6	197	107	304
Q ≤ 6	109	587	696

measure of how well the test it detects the condition. In this study, we have

$$Specificity = \frac{197}{304} = 0.65.$$

These data suggest that 65% of H035 patients who will experience dry eye score above 6 on the questionnaire.

Specificity is the proportion of subjects who test negative for the condition among those who do not have the condition. It measures how well the test detects absence of the condition. From Table 45.19 we have

$$Specificity = \frac{587}{696} = 0.85.$$

These data suggest that 85% of H035 patients who will not experience dry eye score no higher than 6 on the questionnaire.

The choice of 6 as the cutoff score is somewhat arbitrary and may not be optimal. As the cutoff score is increased, the sensitivity of the test will tend to increase, whereas the specificity will tend to decrease. This inverse relationship between sensitivity and specificity is sometimes graphically displayed in a receiver-operating characteristic (ROC)

curve. It is a line plot of sensitivity versus 1 − specificity determined by using different cutoff points for the diagnostic test. The ROC curve for the questionnaire/dry eye data from patients who wore the H035 lens is shown in Fig. 45.12. Note that using the cutoff of 7, the sensitivity is 0.82 and the specificity is 0.79, which gives the optimal balance between the two, indicating that 7 provides the preferred cutoff value.

The ROC curve for the patients who wore the approved silicone hydrogel 0.09-mm thick lens (SH09) is shown in Fig. 45.13. Here the optimal balance between sensitivity and specificity occurs when the cutoff score of 6 is used. Here the sensitivity is 0.72 and the specificity is 0.81. These lower values compared to those for H035 indicate that the questionnaire has somewhat more diagnostic value for CLDE for conventional hydrogel lens wearers.

Clinical Implications The new dry eye questionnaire using a cutoff value of 7.0 is found to have good sensitivity and specificity for a group of extended wear patients with a conventional hydrogel lens (H035). A similar dry eye questionnaire cutoff value for patients wearing the approved silicone hydrogel lens shows less specificity and sensitivity. This possibly is due to the different properties of the silicone hydrogel lens (it is surface treated to improve wettability and does not display dehydration on the eye), which makes it more suitable for marginal dry eye patients. Improved sensitivity and specificity with the dry eye test for the silicone hydrogel lens wearers is shown with a cutoff value of 6.0.

Note on Statistical Software Packages

A wide variety of general purpose statistical software is available for data analysis and data management. Statisticians

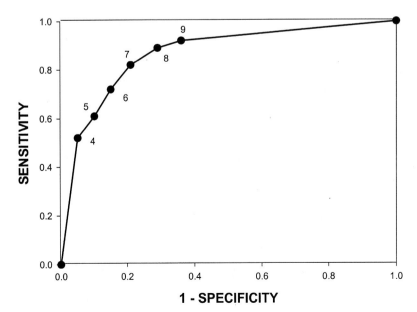

FIG. 45.12. Receiver-operating characteristic curve for the H035 data.

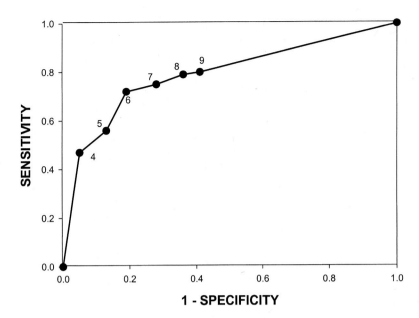

FIG. 45.13. Receiver-operating characteristic curve for the SH09 data.

tend to use SAS (108), S-Plus (109), Stata (110), and SPSS (111), although individuals have other personal preferences, which include Systat (112), Statistica (113), Minitab (114), Data Desk (115), NCSS (116), and JMP (117). Many of these packages have a "point-and-click" user interface, which makes them easy to use for basic statistical techniques. Others require the use of a package-specific programming language in order to take advantage of their full power and flexibility. SAS and S-Plus are widely regarded as state of the art with regard to statistical procedures, and Stata users have the same high regard for its capabilities. These three packages are among those that require programming input and, consequently, are viewed as more challenging to learn.

Minitab originally was designed as a teaching tool and has maintained its popularity over time among statistics instructors. However, Minitab has matured as an analytic tool and is sufficiently powerful so that its use in analyzing research data is common. Its user-friendly interactive interface is easy to learn. SPSS is also relatively accessible to the user and provides powerful statistical analysis and data management capabilities.

The choice of package is largely an individual decision based on statistical needs, access, and state of current familiarity. Each of these packages will serve the user well on the basic statistical procedures. For nonstandard applications, the flexibility and power of packages such as SAS, S-Plus, or Stata may be required. For the statistical novice, it may be advisable to start with user-friendly, yet powerful, packages such as Minitab and SPSS.

Interpretation of Results

After the collection and analysis of the results of a study, it is necessary to interpret the meaning. Investigators apply criteria, or information, from outside the study to draw a conclusion about the meaning of the results (2). In performing that interpretation, it is usual to decide the clinical usefulness, or importance, of the results and determine whether cause-and-effect relationships have been established.

Clinical Importance

When considering the results from research studies, questions must be asked about the statistically significant differences found. Is the difference large enough to be clinically useful, and what is the degree of overlap between the groups?

It is possible that a statistically significant difference exists between results obtained from study and control groups of patients when this difference is clinically of no importance. This is particularly the case in a large study that has the power to demonstrate statistical significance for a small and clinically unimportant difference. An example of such a case is given in the main study described in Question 2b.

Example: Clinical Importance

In the complete study described on page 935, a group of patients wore a commercially available and an "experimental" silicone hydrogel contact lens with center thicknesses of 0.09 mm. The mean changes in microcyst number with each of these lens designs were 5.1 ± 3.16 and 7.1 ± 3.69 (Table 45. 9). A statistically significant difference in microcyst number was found between these lenses. Investigators conclude that the wear of the commercially available lens offers a better physiologic response of the cornea.

It must be asked, however, whether the difference in induced microcysts between these two lenses is of clinical importance. As clinical significance usually is determined from surveying the opinion of key practitioners in the field (10), a level of less than 10 microcysts in a cornea is not thought to indicate a clinically significant level of corneal hypoxia (100,118). It is unlikely that the difference found for the commercial lens offers a clinical advantage over the experimental design. In this example, the large number of patients in the group allows investigators to detect a small difference statistically between the groups but which has no importance clinically.

Example: Clinical Importance

Studies are performed to determine the usefulness of a predictive test for the overnight corneal swelling response to soft contact lens wear. In this test, 200 successful and 200 unsuccessful extended contact lens wearers are subjected to 3 hours of wear of a thick (0.3-mm) low-water-content hydrogel lens. Measurements of corneal thickness are taken before and after the wearing of this lens. The average corneal swelling response obtained in the group of successful extended contact lens wearers is 6.5% and in the unsuccessful wearers 7.3%. A statistically significant difference between these averages for the two groups is found (P < 0.05). Investigators conclude that the wear of the thick low-water-content hydrogel lens is predictive of the ability of patients to wear hydrogel contact lenses for extended wear.

It must be asked, however, whether the difference between the successful and unsuccessful patient groups is, in addition to being statistically significant, of clinical importance. The large number of patients in each group allowed the investigators to detect a very small difference between the groups. It is unlikely, however, that this difference, less than 1%, would allow clinicians to differentiate between those who are likely to be successful and those likely to be unsuccessful with extended wear.

In this example, the difference between the groups is described by the average corneal swelling response for each group. The use of averages is the most frequent way in which group data are described. However, it is insufficient as a description of the data because it fails to describe how values in each group vary about the mean. This is important because values for any individual patient in one group may overlap the values for patients in the other group, despite a statistically significant difference between the averages. In considering overlap between patient groups, statistical theory assumes that the populations are in bell-shaped or gaussian distributions. Even if this is not the case, statistical theory has shown that at least 75% of all values will be within 2 SD of the average and at least 88% will lie within 3 SD. To illustrate the importance of the degree of overlap between populations of patients, the example can be considered again.

Example: Overlap of Data

The dispersion of data obtained for the successful and unsuccessful extended contact lens wearers in the previous example is as follows: clinical importance can be described in terms of the standard deviation for the successful (± 3.0%) and for the unsuccessful wearers (± 4.0%). The overlap can be found by considering the corneal swelling response contained within 2 SD on either side of the mean for each study group. Irrespective of the form of the distribution, 75% of the corneal swelling responses for the successful extended wearers will lie between 0.5% to 12.5% and for the unsuccessful wearers between 0.7% and 15.3%. Therefore, a substantial group of both study populations will fall between 0.5% and 12.5% corneal swelling. Consequently, it will be very difficult to determine the clinical significance of results obtained for any subject falling within this degree of corneal swelling response.

This further illustrates the problem of attributing clinical importance to data obtained from two groups of subjects, even when they are statistically significantly different from each other. For emphasis, it should be said that not all statistically significant differences are important and not all important differences are statistically significant (2). The conventional significance levels, 5%, 1%, or 0.1% are useful, but only as guides to interpretation, not as strict rules (119).

Contributory Cause

The second part of the requirement in interpreting the data from a study is to determine whether a cause-and-effect relationship has been established. The clinical concept of cause, called *contributory cause,* is an empiric definition that requires fulfillment of the following criteria. First, the characteristic referred to as the cause must be shown to precede the effect; and second, altering only the cause must be shown to alter the effect.

It often is difficult to establish, by a case-control study, that the cause occurs prior to the effect. A much better way of establishing that cause precedes effect is by a prospective study, and the most convincing evidence is from a randomized clinical trial (10f). An example of a case-control study that fails to establish adequately that cause precedes the supposed effect is given.

Example: Establishing Cause Precedes Effect

Clinicians conduct a case-control study of the clinical signs reported by extended wear lens patients with GPC in the days immediately preceding the development of the condition. They were looking for the precipitating cause of the condition. Patients who developed GPC were compared to patients returning to the practice for routine contact lens follow-up examinations. The investigators found that the GPC patients were 20 times as likely to have reported a need for increased lens cleaning as the controls during the days preceding the return for examination. The clinicians concluded that an increase in lens cleaning was associated with subsequent GPC.

These investigators believed that they had established the

first condition demonstrating causation (i.e., that cause precedes effect). Unfortunately, this is not the case. If patients have discomfort resulting from a developing corneal ulcer, they may misinterpret the discomfort and try to alleviate it by increased lens cleaning. The increase in lens cleaning is performed to help the discomfort caused by ulceration and does not truly precede the condition. Therefore, this study fails to establish a prior or antecedent cause because it does not clarify whether the condition (ulceration) resulted in patients increasing their rate of lens cleaning or whether the lens cleaning precipitated the development of the condition. Prospective studies are much more efficient in establishing that cause precedes effect than case-control studies. The ability of the prospective study to establish that cause precedes effect is enhanced when the time interval between cause and effect is long.

Even if cause is definitely established as preceding effect, it is necessary to establish that altering the cause alters the effect.

Example: Altering Cause Alters Effect

A prospective study was performed to determine the effect of wearing ultrathin and standard thickness hydrogel soft lenses on corneal desiccation. This was a cross-over study in which two groups of patients first wore the thin hydrogel lens and then the standard thickness hydrogel lens or vice versa. Patients wore lenses for a period of 1 month and were observed at weekly intervals to determine the amount of corneal desiccation occurring. Prior to the start of the study, all patients were established as having no corneal staining. At the end of 2 months, the data from all patients were collected and the incidence of corneal desiccation compared after the wearing of thin and standard thickness lenses. Desiccation was found with both soft lenses, but the incidence was 10 times higher with the wearing of the thin hydrogel lens.

In this situation, both criteria for establishing cause and effect have been met. First, the corneal desiccation is observed to occur after the wearing of hydrogel soft lenses. The second criterion, altering the cause alters the effect, can be illustrated by comparing slit-lamp findings in the patients in whom corneal desiccation was observed after wearing thin and standard thickness lenses. A much smaller incidence of desiccation was found after the wearing of standard thickness lenses than was demonstrated with thin hydrogel lenses, indicating that altering the cause (lens dehydration, which varies with lens thickness) alters the effect (amount of corneal desiccation).

In this example, a prospective cross-over study is described that shows that altering the contributory cause can alter the effect. Generally, clinical trials in which patients are blindly and randomly assigned to study groups and only one of the study groups is exposed to the possible cause are the most powerful tool for demonstrating the criteria necessary for establishment of contributory cause.

It should be remembered that in establishing contributory cause in this way, it is not necessary to elucidate the intermediate mechanism by which contributory cause brings about the effect. In our example, it is not necessary to describe completely the mechanism of corneal desiccation secondary to thin hydrogel lens wear. It may be possible, however, in subsequent experimental studies to determine the mechanism by which contributory cause brings about its effect. Thus, most observational studies (case-control or prospective) or clinical trials end with an opinion or judgment about causality, not a claim of proof (120). In the current scientific environment, however, it is usual to attempt to elucidate the mechanism linking cause and effect by later experimental studies.

Other experimental criteria to determine the etiology of diseases or conditions have been postulated. In the last century, Koch developed a series of conditions that needed to be fulfilled before a microorganism could be considered to cause a disease. The conditions, known as *Koch's Postulate*, included requirements that the organism always be found with the disease and that the organism was not found with any other disease.

These conditions represent additional requirements found to be beneficial in studies of infectious disease, particularly where the disease is acute and resulting from a single agent. However, it is difficult to satisfy Koch's Postulate for chronic disease or conditions. For example, the chronic edema experienced under extended wear contact lenses has been determined to be a contributory cause in the increased incidence of microcysts. However, microcysts are not always associated with contact lens extended wear, and, in addition, extended lens wear may contribute to polymegethistic changes in the corneal endothelium. Therefore, the conditions of Koch's Postulate are not met by this example, even though there is a cause-and-effect relationship between corneal edema and epithelial microcysts.

Even with infectious conditions, Koch's Postulate may be too strict to be clinically useful. For example, corneal ulcers often are shown to have the bacterium *Pseudomonas aeruginosa* as a contributory cause. However, other bacteria and viruses also may be shown to cause corneal ulceration. Again, Koch's Postulate is not fulfilled.

Consequently, new criteria have been derived to explain causation, particularly in observational studies (1). Described previously is the temporal sequence relating cause and effect (cause preceding effect) and the specificity of the effect (altering the cause alters the effect). In addition, the criteria of consistency, strength of association, biologic gradient, and collateral and biologic plausibility may be applied. To reinforce any causal relationship established in a study, repeated consistent observations of the association under slightly different conditions of study increase the evidence for a cause-and-effect relationship. The strength of association also can be demonstrated. In this situation, the larger the value of the relative risk, the less likely is the association to be spurious (1). In addition, the existence of a biologic gradient or a dose–response curve makes a causal relationship more plausible. This is more likely to be demonstrable in cause-and-effect relationships in physics and biochemistry or in the use of medical treatment for therapy.

In practice, collateral evidence and biologic plausibility are used extensively to support or refute a hypothesis of cause and effect. Altman (119) has observed that the deduction of a causal relationship from an observed (statistical) association can rarely be justified from data alone. For example, the association between extended hydrogel contact lens wear and the increased incidence of corneal ulceration was developed from reports by individual clinics (78) and by evidence of the comparative incidence of corneal ulcers in daily and extended contact lens wear given at the May 1986 meeting of the FDA's Ophthalmic Advisory Panel. At this meeting, evidence of the relative risk in the two forms of wear was found from data obtained from FDA approval studies, from the number of cases per million lenses distributed by manufacturers, and from the Contact Lens Institute's collation of adverse reaction reports. The weight of evidence from these three sources showed the increased risk of ulceration with extended wear to be approximately 10 times that with daily wear.

Use of these additional criteria for determination of contributory cause is well established in clinical research. The satisfaction of all of these requirements is desirable but not always possible, so the minimum criterion of cause preceding effect, and alterations in cause altering effect, is acceptable.

Application of the Results (Extrapolation)

In most studies it is desirable to apply the meaning of a study to a larger (outside) population. To do this, it is necessary to extrapolate the results of the study to a new and potentially different situation. This can be fraught with difficulty.

A number of possible errors can occur in extrapolating results to larger populations (10). We review four errors here: extrapolating beyond the range of data, errors in extrapolating from population data to a conclusion about individuals, errors resulting from unappreciated factors in the new population, and errors in extrapolating from the study to general populations.

Extrapolating Beyond the Range of Data

In clinical studies, individuals or patients are exposed to factors thought to be associated with the outcome for only a limited amount of time or at a limited range of exposure. In generalizing the results from study samples to wider populations, it is important that researchers do not stray too far from the restrictions of time and exposure placed on the data by the parameters of the original investigation.

As an example, let us return to the consideration of the effect of varying hydrogel lens thickness on corneal desiccation.

Example: Extrapolating Beyond the Range of the Data

A group of patients in a prospective case series are fitted with ultrathin soft lenses with a center thickness of 0.06 mm. After 1 month of lens wear, they exhibited an incidence of corneal drying of 25%. Patients discontinued lens wear, and their corneal epithelium was allowed to regenerate. They then were fitted with a second lens of the same hydrogel material with a center thickness of 0.1 mm. With this lens, only 5% of patients showed corneal desiccation staining.

The investigators concluded that, by increasing the center thickness of the lens to 0.14 mm, they would be able to eliminate all desiccation staining in patients. Although this is possible, it may be that the changes in lens design had reached the maximum effectiveness at the 0.1-mm center thickness and that increases in center thickness would not reduce further the number of patients with corneal drying. Therefore, to conclude, without experimental evidence, that greater contact lens center thicknesses would reduce corneal drying is to extrapolate beyond the range of the data.

Another type of error associated with extrapolation beyond the range of data pertains to potential side effects experienced as a result of increased time of exposure to a causative agent.

Example: Extrapolation Beyond the Range of Data

An example of this problem is found in the FDA's early preapproval studies of conventional hydrogel extended wear lenses in the 1980s. The first of these studies required 2 years of follow-up on 500 patients (23). Many of the initial studies showed little or no incidence of corneal ulceration secondary to 30 days of extended wear of hydrogel lenses. The conclusion was reached from these studies that hydrogel contact lenses were safe and effective in extended wear. As a result, clinicians have fitted these lenses to larger numbers of patients who have worn them now for several years.

Subsequent reports in the literature indicate that the original predictions of safety were not correct and that there is a significant increase in risk of ulceration with this type of contact lens(29,78). Investigators and the FDA had extrapolated from the 2-year study to allow long-term, extended wear of hydrogel lenses. This is clearly an example of extrapolation beyond the range of the original data.

Extrapolation from Population Data to Individuals

A second error can arise from extrapolating from population data to conclusions about individual patients. Studies that elicit population data are known as *ecologic studies*. When using group population data, the problem is that investigators frequently have little information about the individuals making up the population. This absence of individual data may lead to investigators committing extrapolation errors or ecologic fallacies (2).

Example: Extrapolation from Population Data to Individuals

A population study demonstrates that the rate of GPC in soft lens patients is five times that of those individuals wearing gas permeable hard lenses. The study data also demonstrate that clinically detectable lens debris on soft lenses is five times that observed on gas permeable lenses. The authors of the study conclude that debris is associated with GPC.

This conclusion may be true, but in order to establish an association, the authors must show that those patients with heavy debris are the ones more likely to develop GPC. Relying on population figures alone does not provide enough information about the cause-and-effect relationship experienced by individuals. For instance, it is possible that among the soft lens-wearing population, it is the patients with low accumulations of debris on lenses who develop GPC. It may be something about the lens design, perhaps the larger diameter of soft lenses, that precipitates the GPC response in the upper lid. Establishment of an association between lens debris and the development of GPC requires demonstrating that the relationship holds on an individual level. This is an example of an error created in extrapolating from population data to conclusions about individuals.

Another example of a similar type of error is illustrated next.

Example: Extrapolation from Population Data to Individuals

In a study of two populations of gas-permeable lens extended wearers, the first wore lenses with an oxygen transmissibility value of 40. The second wore lenses with an oxygen transmissibility of 60. Although the available oxygen to the corneas in the second population was almost 1.5 times that in the first population, the average overnight swelling response of the second group was found to be 14% compared to the 8% for the first group. The authors of the study concluded that higher oxygen transmissibility did not reduce the corneal swelling response during overnight wear of the lenses.

The authors had extrapolated from data based on a study population to conclusions about individual patients' swelling responses. Other explanations for the observed data, other than the oxygen transmissibility of the lens material, are possible. It has been found that individual patient response to hypoxia varies enormously; some individuals require an equivalent oxygen percentage of almost 21%, whereas others can avoid corneal edema with as low as 7%

(79). It is possible that the results in this hypothetical study originated (or developed) from patients in the first population having lower individual requirements for corneal oxygenation than those in the second population.

Extrapolation Error due to Unappreciated Factors in a New Population

A third type of extrapolation error occurs when data from one study are extrapolated to a different population in which unappreciated factors are operative. In performing this extrapolation, many authors assume that the new population is identical to their study group. This can result in the considerable problems shown in the following hypothetical study.

Example: Extrapolation to a Population Possessing Unappreciated Factors

A study is undertaken of the therapeutic effect of prescribing extended wear soft lenses with high oxygen transmissibility for those patients demonstrating marginal corneal infiltration. The population studied had a prevalence of marginal corneal infiltration of 40%. By switching to the new silicone hydrogel lenses with much greater oxygen availability, the incidence of infiltration dropped to less than 5%. A report of the decrease in corneal infiltration was read by a clinician who decided to apply this technique to all his patients exhibiting corneal infiltration.

In extrapolating to a second patient population, this clinician had assumed that the presence of corneal infiltration meant the same among his patients as among the original study group. However, in many cases, corneal infiltration can result from necrotic material trapped beneath a contact lens. Instead of indicating the need for more corneal oxygenation, this indicates the need for a loose-fitting lens to allow flushing of debris from beneath the lens. In such a case, the application of another lens with higher oxygen transmissibility would not reduce corneal infiltration. The second clinician had ignored the fact that the presence of corneal infiltration had different causes in different groups.

Errors in Extrapolation from Study to General Populations

When valid results from a study population are applied directly to a general population without considering the frequency of the condition in the general population, another extrapolation error can occur. This results from lack of knowledge of the degree of risk observed in the study population and its differentiation from the degree of risk in the general population.

The risk among the study population is known as *relative risk;* this measures the risk in the treatment group versus the risk in the control group. When applying this risk to the general population, researchers ask what proportion of the disease in the general population is attributable to the factor under study. This proportion is known as the *attributable risk* (2).

A large relative risk for a rare condition may account for only a small attributable risk in the general population. Conversely, if a study factor is very common in the general population, a small relative risk in the study population may result in a large attributable risk in the general population. This need to distinguish between relative risk and attributable risk is emphasized in these examples.

Example: Extrapolation from a Study to the General Population

A study of the incidence of Acanthamoeba keratitis secondary to daily soft lens wear finds the incidence to be reduced significantly by the use of multipurpose chemical disinfection systems (121). The researchers conclude that the widespread use of multipurpose solutions would significantly reduce the incidence of microbial keratitis in the general contact lens-wearing population.

In this example, the investigators had studied only keratitis caused by the protozoan *Acanthamoeba* in daily wearers and extrapolated their data to all contact lens wearers. Even the complete elimination of all *Acanthamoeba* keratitis in daily soft lens wearers does not mean that the incidence of corneal infections from other organisms secondary to other forms of lens wear, involving other materials, would be similarly affected. Indeed, many more infections occur as a result of bacterial invasion of the cornea following extended wear of hydrogels than occur with the organism or form of wear in the study. This example illustrates that the occurrence of a large relative risk in a study population may result only in a small attributable risk when applied to the general population.

Example: Extrapolation from Study to General Populations

A clinical trial is carried out of a new soft contact lens material that is reported to have greater surface biocompatibility and wettability. The trial randomly assigns patients to a group wearing either a conventional hydrogel material or the new biocompatible material. All patients wear lenses on a daily basis for 1 year and replace them at monthly intervals. After 1 year, the incidence of CLDE with the new material is reported as 20% and with the conventional hydrogel as 30%.

In this case, the reduction in CLDE is only 10% less with the new lens material; however, if it were dispensed to the daily soft lens-wearing population, a very large number of patients would be saved the misery of dry eye. Consequently, the absolute number of patients who could continue to wear lenses in comfort would be very large. In the United States alone this could represent 2.5 million wearers. In extrapolating the results of their study to a general popu-

lation, it is important that the authors consider not only the relative reduction in risk in their study population but also the effect of applying their results to a general population. This example illustrates how a small decrease in relative risk can result in a large reduction in occurrence of a condition in the general population.

CONCLUSION

The five-part organization of clinical research described in this chapter represents a uniform format that can be applied to most clinical research designs. If correctly implemented, a study should yield results that are valid and from which interpretations can be drawn that can be applied to the larger universe of patients wearing contact lenses.

This chapter has attempted to give the reader an overview of the clinical research designs for the organization of a contact lens research study. This overview necessarily has been superficial, and readers are encouraged to gain more information by consulting the references and by applying the principles and techniques described to a critical reading of the contact lens literature and to the conduct of research studies in their own clinical practices.

REFERENCES

1. Schlesselman JJ. *Case control studies.* Oxford: Oxford University Press, 1982.
2. Riegelman RK. *Studying a study and testing a test.* Boston: Little, Brown and Company, 1981.
3. Box JF, Fisher RA. Design of experiments: 1922–1926. *Arc Stat* 1980;34:1–7.
4. Friedman LM, Furberg CD, DeMets DL. *Fundamentals for clinical trials.* Littleton, MA: PSG Publishing Company, 1981.
5. Pocock SJ. *Clinical trials: a practical approach.* New York: Wiley Chichester, 1983.
6. Harnett DJ. *Statistical methods,* 3rd ed. Menlo Park, CA: Addison-Wesley Publishing, 1982.
7. Bland M. *An introduction to medical statistics.* Oxford: Oxford University Press, 1987.
8. Dixon WJ, Massey FJ. *Introduction to statistical analysis,* 3rd ed. New York: McGraw-Hill Book Company, 1969.
9. Schmidt MJ. *Understanding and using statistics: basic concepts.* Lexington, MA: DC Hath & Co., 1975.
10. Spilker B. *Guide to clinical trials.* New York: Raven Press, 1991: 39, 203, 277, 530, 536, 699, 694, 700.
11. Kertes PJ, Conway MD. *Clinical trials in ophthalmology.* Baltimore: Williams & Wilkins, Baltimore, 1998.
12. Hulley SB, Cummings SR, Brownen WS, et al. *Designing clinical research.* Philadelphia: Lippincott, Williams & Wilkins, 2001:97, 109, 119, 133, 169.
13. Zadnik KA. Case of dimple veiling/staining. *Contact Lens Forum* 1988;4:69.
14. Seger RG, Grant SS. Alternative contact lens cleaning approaches. *Int Contact Lens Clin* 1987;14:202–203.
15. Weiner B. Contact lenses for post-surgery patients. *Contact Lens Spectrum* 1987;2:24–32.
16. McLaughlin WR, Schoessler JP. Manufacturing defect in a rigid gas permeable lens. *Int Contact Lens Clin* 1987;14:167.

17. Hart D. Calcium deposits: an incorrect diagnosis. *Contact Lens Forum* 1988;13:54–59.

18. Wallace WA. The SLACH syndrome. *Int EyeCare* 1985;1:220.

19. Wallace WA. Soft contact lens associated superior limbic keratoconjunctivitis. *Int EyeCare* 1985;1:302–303.

20. Wallace WA. Marginal corneal infiltrates. *Int EyeCare* 1985;1:427–428.

21. Wallace WA. Soft contact lens associated infectious corneal ulcer. *Int EyeCare* 1986;2:171–172.

22. Gero G. Superficial punctate keratitis with CSI contact lenses dispensed with the Allergan Hydrocare Cold Kit. *Int Contact Lens Clin* 1984;11:674–676.

23. Zuccaro V, Thayer TO, Poland OD. Hydrocurve II extended wear: a five year study. *Int EyeCare* 1985;1:379–385.

24. Blackhurst R, Brotherman D, Fetch D, et al. Optisoft: a one-year study with thermal disinfection. *Contact Lens Forum* 1988;13:61–63.

25. Moore MB, McCulley JP, Newton C, et al. Acanthamoeba keratitis: a growing problem in soft and hard contact lens wearers. *Ophthalmology* 1987;94:1654–1661.

26. Gwinn L. Clinical experience with bifocal soft contact lenses. *Contacto Miniabstracts* 1984;28: 19–22.

27. Flom MC, Neumaier RW. Presence of amblyopia. *US Public Health Report* 1966;1:329–341.

28. Holden BA, Sweeney DF, Vannas A, et al. Effects of long-term extended wear on the human cornea. *Invest Ophthalmol Vis Sci* 1985;26:1489–1501.

29. Weissman BA, Remba MJ, Fujedy E. Results of the extended wear contact lens survey of Contact Lens Section of the American Optometric Association. *J Am Optom Assoc* 1987;58:166–172.

30. Kennedy JR. Changing views on contact lens wear. *Contact Lens Spectrum* 1986;1191:45–51.

31. Segal D. Designs for clinical research. *Arch Ophthalmol* 1987;105:1647–1649.

32. Stehr-Green JK, Bailey TM, Brandt FH, et al. Acanthamoebic keratitis in soft contact lens wearers. *JAMA* 1987;258:57–60.

33. Tomlinson A, Schwartz CA. Position of the corneal apex in keratoconus. *Am J Optom Physiol Opt* 1980;57:29–32.

34. Kastl PR, Donzis PB, Cole HP, et al. A 20-year retrospective study of the use of contact lenses in keratoconus. *CLAO J* 1987;13:107–111.

35. Zantos S. Cystic formations in the corneal epithelium during extended wear of contact lenses. *Int Contact Lens Clin* 1983;10:128–148.

36. Chen-Ling T, Curmi J. Changes in corneal endothelial morphology in cats as a function of age. *Curr Eye Res* 1988;7387–392.

37. Donenfeld ED, Cohen EJ, Arentson JJ, et al. Changing trends in contact lens associated corneal ulcers: an overview of 116 cases. *CLAO J* 1986;12:145–150.

38. Robin JB, Nobe JR, Suarez E, et al. Meibomian gland evaluation in patients with extended wear soft contact lens deposits. *CLAO J* 1986;12:95–98.

39. Swarbrick HA. A possible etiology for RGP lens binding (adherence). *Int Contact Lens Clin* 1988;15:13–19.

40. McMahon B, Cue TF. *Epidemiology: principles and methods.* Boston: Little, Brown and Company, 1970.

41. Schein OD, Glynn RJ, Poggio EC, et al. The relative risk of ulcerative keratitis among users of daily-wear and extended-wear soft contact lenses. *N Engl J Med* 1989;321:773–783.

42. Early Treatment Diabetic Study Research Group. Photocoagulation for diabetic macular edema: early treatment diabetic retinopathy study report No. 1. *Arch Ophthalmol* 1985;103:1796–1806.

43. Diabetic Retinopathy Vitrectomy Research Group. Early vitrectomy for severe vitreous hemorrhage in diabetic retinopathy: two year results of a randomized trial: Diabetic Retinopathy Vitrectomy Study Report No. 2. *Arch Ophthalmol* 1985;103:1644–1652.

44. Kotow M, Grant T, Holden BA. Avoiding ocular complications during hydrogel extended wear. *Int Contact Lens Clin* 1987;14:95–99.

45. Lind J. *A treatise of the scurvy.* Edinburgh: Sands, Murray and Cochran, 1753.

46. Hill AB. The clinical trial. *Br Med Bull* 1951;7:278–282.

47. Meinert CL. *Clinical trials: design, conduct and analysis.* Oxford: Oxford University Press, 1986.

48. Waring GO, Moffitt SD, Gilander H, et al. Rationale for and design of the National Eye Institute Prospective Evaluation of Radial Keratotomy (PERK) study. *Ophthalmology* 1983;90:40–58.

49. Lasswell LA, Tarantino N, Kono D. Enzymatic cleaning of extended wear lenses: papain vs. pancreatin. *Int Contact Lens Clin* 1986;2:101–105.

50. Foster S. The Cromolyn Sodium Collaborative Study Group: evaluation of topical cromolyn sodium in the treatment of vernal keratoconjunctivitis. *Ophthalmology* 1988;95:195–201.

51. Bennett ES, Tomlinson A, Mirowitz MC, et al. Comparison of overnight swelling and lens performance in RGP extended wear. *CLAO J* 1988;14:94–100.

52. Bennett ES, Tomlinson A. Comparison of two techniques of refitting long-term polymethyl methylacrylate contact lens wearers. *Am J Optom Physiol Opt* 1983;60:139–145.

53. Bennett ES, Henry V, Davis L, et al. A clinical comparison of empirical and diagnostic fitting of daily wear fluorosilicone acrylate lenses. *Contact Lens Forum* 1989;14:320–323.

54. Tomlinson A. Evaluation of methods of fitting a toric soft contact lens. *Int Contact Lens Clin* 1980;17:201–209.

55. Collins FL, Baer RA, Blount RL. Single-subject research designs for optometry. *Am J Optom Physiol Opt* 1985;62:516–522.

56. Cedarstaff TH, Tomlinson A. Comparative study of tear evaporation rates and water content of soft contact lenses. *Am J Optom Physiol Opt* 1983;60:167–174.

57. Hartmann DP, Hall RV. The changing criterion design. *J Appl Behav Anal* 1976;9:527–532.

58. Brown BW. Statistical controversies in the design of clinical trials: some personal views. *Control Clin Trials* 1980;1:13–27.

59. Grizzle JF. The two period change-over design and its use in clinical trials. *Biometrics* 1965;21:467–480.

60. Hills M, Armitage P. The two-period cross-over clinical trial. *Br J Clin Pharmacol* 1979;8:7–20.

61. Josephson J, Caffery B. Monovision versus bifocal contact lenses: a crossover study. *J Am Optom Assoc* 1987;64:38–40.

62. Tomlinson A, Caroline PJ. Comparison of the contamination resistance of HEMA, modified HEMA and non-HEMA hydrogel lenses. *J Br Contact Lens Soc* 1989;12:9–14.

63. Tomlinson A, Caroline PJ. Comparative evaluation of the surface deposits on high water content hydrogel contact lens polymers. *CLAO J* 1990;16:121–127.

64. Diabetic Retinopathy Study Research Group. Preliminary report on effects of photocoagulation therapy. *Am J Ophthalmol* 1976;18:383–396.

65. Tomlinson A, Soni PS. The effect of the design and fitting of soft lenses on corneal physiology. *J Br Contact Lens Assoc* 1980;3:161–167.

66. Tomlinson A, Haas DD. Changes in corneal thickness and limbal vascularization with contact lens wear. *Int Contact Lens Clin* 1980;17:26–37.

67. Tomlinson A, Bibby MM. Movement and rotation of soft con-

tact lenses: effect of fit and lens design. *Am J Optom Physiol Opt* 1980;57:275–279.

68. Tomlinson A, Soni PS. Peripheral curve design and the tear pump mechanism. *Am J Optom Physiol Opt* 1980;57:356–359.

69. Tomlinson A, Schoessler JP, Andrasko G. The effect of varying prism and truncation on the performance of soft contact lenses. *Am J Optom Physiol Opt* 1980;57:714–720.

70. Lowther GE, Tomlinson A. Critical base curve and diameter interval in the fitting of spherical soft contact lenses. *Am J Optom Physiol Opt* 1981;58:355–360.

71. Tomlinson A, Cedarstaff TH, Bibby MM. Validation of a model describing soft lens movement as a function of lens specification. *Am J Optom Physiol Opt* 1983;60:292–296.

72. Tomlinson A, Bibby MM. Determination of the effective diameter for the calculation of equivalent thickness of soft contact lenses. *Am J Optom Physiol Opt* 1985;62:398–401.

73. Fatt I. Hard contact lens flexing: a preliminary study of a new experimental procedure. *Int Contact Lens Clin* 1987;14:360–367.

74. Dea D, Huth S. The effect of reducing agents on enzymatic cleaning efficacy. *Int Contact Lens Clin* 1988;15:256–259.

75. Egger M, Smith GD, Altman DG. *Systematic reviews in health care.* London: BMJ Publishing Group, 2001.

76. Department of Clinical Epidemiology and Biostatistics, McMaster's University Health Sciences Center. How to read the clinical journals: IV: to determine etiology or causation. *Can Med Assoc J* 1981;124:985–990.

77. Krathwohl BR. How to prepare a research proposal. Syracuse, NY: Syracuse University Bookstore, Syracuse University, 1965.

78. Mondino BJ, Weissman BA, Farb MD, et al. Corneal ulcers associated with daily wear and extended wear contact lenses. *Am J Ophthalmol* 1986;102:58–65.

79. Holden BA, Sweeney DE, Sanderson G. The minimum precorneal oxygen tension to avoid corneal edema. *Invest Ophthalmol Vis Sci* 1984;25:476–480.

80. Altman DG. Statistics and ethics in medical research part 4. *Br Med J* 1980;281:1399–1401.

81. Rosner BA. *Fundamentals of biostatistics,* 5th ed. United States: Duxbury Pacific Grove, California, 2000.

82. Moore DS. *Statistics: concepts and controversies,* 5th ed. San Francisco: WH Freeman and Company, 2000.

83. Holden BA, Sweeney DF, Vomnas A, et al. Effects of long term extended contact lens wear in the human cornea. *Invest Ophthalmol Vis Sci* 1985;26:1489–1451.

84. Holden BA. The Glenn A Fry Award Lecture 1988. The ocular response to contact lens wear. *Optom Vis Sci* 1989;66:717–733.

85. Holden BA, Sankaridurg PR, Jalbert I. Adverse events and infections: which ones and how many? In: Sweeney DR, ed. *Silicone hydrogels: the rebirth of continuous wear contact lenses.* Oxford: Butterworth Heinemann, 2000:150–213.

86. Holden BA, Mertz GW, McNally JJ. Corneal swelling response to contact lenses worn under extended wear conditions. *Invest Ophthalmol Vis Sci* 1983;24:218–226.

87. Laurant J, Wilson G. Size of cells collected from normal subjects using contact lens cytology. *Optom Vis Sci* 1997;74:280–287.

88. Hamano H, Hori M, Hamano T, et al. Effects of contact lens wear on the mitosis of corneal epithelium and lactate content in aqueous human of rabbit. *Jpn J Ophthalmol* 1983;27:451–458.

89. Ladage PM, Yakamolo K, Petroll WM, et al. Effects of RGP contact lens extended wear on epithelial mitosis in the rabbit. *Invest Ophthalmol Vis Sci* 1999;40:S908.

90. Ren DH, Petroll WH, Jester JV, et al. Short term hypoxia down regulates epithelial cell desquamation in vivo, but does not increase Pseudomonas aeruginosa adherence to exfoliated human corneal epithelial cells. *CLAO J* 1999;25:73–79.

91. Chalmers RL, McNally JJ, McKinney CD, et al. The role of dryness symptoms in the discontinuation of wear and the scheduled lens removals in extended wear of silicone hydrogel lenses. *Invest Ophthalmol Vis Sci* 2002;43:S124.

92. Snedecor GW, Cochran WG. *Statistical methods,* 7th ed. Ames, IA: The Iowa State University Press, 1980.

93. Sprent P, Smeeton NC. *Applied nonparametric statistical methods,* 3rd ed. London: Chapman & Hall/CRC, 2001.

94. Daniel WW. *Applied nonparametric statistics.* Boston: Houghton Mifflin Company, 1978.

95. Fleiss JL. *The design and analysis of clinical experiments.* New York: Wiley, 1986.

96. Dunn G. *Design and analysis of reliability studies: the statistical evaluation of measurement errors.* New York: Oxford University Press, 1989.

97. Bland JM, Altman DG. A note on the use of the intraclass correlation coefficient in the evaluation of agreement between two methods of measurement. *Comput Biol Med* 1990;20:337–340.

98. Shoukri MM, Pause CA. *Statistical methods for health sciences,* 2nd ed. New York: CRC Press, 1999.

99. Bland JM, Altman DG. Statistical methods for assessing agreement between two methods of clinical measurement. *Lancet* 1986;1:307–310.

100. Holden BA, Sweeney DF. The significance of the microcyst response: a review. *Optom Vis Sci* 1991;68:703–707.

101. Glantz SA, Slinker BK. *Primer of applied regression and analysis of variance.* New York: McGraw-Hill, 1990.

102. Zar JH. *Biostatistical analysis,* 4th ed. Upper Saddle River, NJ: Prentice-Hall, 1999.

103. Wilson G. The epithelium in extended wear. In: Sweeney DF, ed. *Silicone hydrogels: the rebirth of continuous wear contact lenses.* Oxford: Butterworth Heinemann, 2000:22–44.

104. Ren DH, Petroll WH, Jester JV, et al. The relation between contact lens oxygen permeability and binding of Pseudomonas aeruginosa to human corneal epithelial cells after overnight and extended wear. *CLAO J* 1999;25:80–100.

105. Ren DH, Petroll WM, Jester JV, et al. Preliminary studies into the effects of extended contact lens wear on proliferation of rabbit corneal epithelial cells using bromodeoxyuridine labelling. *Invest Ophthalmol Vis Sci* 1998;39:47–49.

106. Mehta CR, Patel NR. *StatXact 4 for Windows user manual.* Cambridge, MA: Cytel Software Corporation, 1999.

107. Tighe B. Silicone hydrogel materials: how do they work? In: Sweeney DF, ed. *Silicone hydrogels: the rebirth of continuous wear contact lenses.* Oxford: Butterworth Heinemann, 2000:1–21.

108. SAS System 8.2 (computer software). Cary, NC: SAS Institute, 2002.

109. S-Plus 6 (computer software). Seattle, WA: Insightful Corporation, 2002.

110. Stata 7 (computer software). College Station, TX: Stata Corporation, 2002.

111. SPSS 11.0 (computer software). Chicago, IL: SPSS Science, 2002.

112. Systat 10.2 (computer software). Richmond, CA: Systat Statistical Software, 2002.

113. Statistica 6 (computer Software). Tulsa, OK: StatSoft Inc., 2002.

114. Ryan BE, Joiner BL, Ryan TA. Minitab Data Analysis Software, release 13.3 (computer software). State College, PA: Minitab, 2002.

115. Data Desk 6.1 (computer software). Ithaca, NY: Data Description, 2002.

116. NCSS 2001 Statistical Analysis System (computer software). Kaysville, UT: NCSS Statistical Software, 2001.

117. JMP 5 (computer software). Cary, NC: SAS Institute, 2002.

118. Hickson S, Papas E. Prevalence of radiopathic corneal abnormalities in a non-contact lens wearing population. *Optom Vis Sci* 1997;74:293–297.

119. Altman DG. Statistics and ethics in medical research, part 7. *Br Med J* 1980;281:1612–1614.

120. Cochran WG. Planning of observation studies of human populations. *J Roy Stat Assoc* 1965;128:234–265.

121. Beattie T, Tomlinson A, McFadyen AK, et al. Enhanced attachment of Acanthamoeba to extended wear silicone hydrogel contact lenses: a new risk factor for infection? *Ophthalmology* 2003; 110:765–771.

4 6

CONTACT LENS APPLICATIONS AND THE INTERNET

MILTON M. HOM

INTRODUCTION

Gerald Lowther remarked some years ago that an Internet search under "contact lenses" revealed a preponderance of mail-order web sites. It has not changed much since that time. In April 2002, a Google search *(www.google.com)* yielded an interesting result in the first 20 sites. The majority of sites were still mail order related (60%). The major contact lens companies and company related sites have increased their share to 25%. Other assorted sites made up the last 10%.

In an *International Contact Lens Clinic* commentary dated 1996, Lowther (1) predicted much of what contact lens fitters are doing today on the Internet. He wrote, "you can . . . take educational courses (including sound, pictures and movies), consult through your system concerning your patient's condition and care, view photos of ocular conditions, do library searches on any topic, find information about and register for meetings, find information on products, purchase products . . . talk with colleagues, and more at any time of the day or night you desire."

EDUCATIONAL CLASSES

The ability to take contact-related classes over the Internet is largely limited by bandwidth. With a 56k modem, a text-based site is fast and efficient. Even with properly compressed photos, a site can load effectively with a slow connection. However, when multimedia elements are added, a 56k modem can really bog down and result in slow loading times. There are two continuing education sites that incorporate some multimedia elements. They are *visioncarece.com* and *SECOinternational.com*.

Visioncarece.com

Visioncarece.com is a self-standing site devoted to online continuing education (CE). Boucher Communications, Inc. (BCI), the publisher of Optometric Management and Con-

tact Lens Spectrum, sponsors the site. The site is updated by the addition of classes regularly. All of the optometry classes are Council on Practitioner Education (COPE) approved. An online test is offered at the end of each course. The CE certificate is e-mailed within minutes of completing the online test. The site features many contact lens classes. Some classes have online video segments. Recent classes include subjects such as bifocal contact lenses, back and bitoric rigid gas-permeable (GP) lenses, and four-zone orthokeratology.

SECOinternational.com

A part of the SECOinternational *(www.secointernational.com)* site, the CE section, offers lecture-based classes. At the time of this writing, a few of these classes were related to contact lenses. About half of the classes are COPE-approved. An audio track with corresponding slides is shown for each course. After taking the test, a transcript is mailed to the participant. Many of the classes on this site are industry sponsored.

Another site worthy of mention is *www.sightstreet.com*. *Sightstreet.com* offers CE classes in a text-based format. Most of the classes are disease-based.

jnjvision.com

The movement toward greater visibility for contact lens companies and sponsored sites on the web is both refreshing and positive for contact lens practitioners. Vistakon sponsors a library of CE classes on their site *(www.jnjvision.com)*. The classes are all contact lens related. There is an audio track available with a VOX audio plug-in. The classes pertain to many soft lens topics. Some of the topics are monovision, torics, contact lenses for teens and kids, and practice management.

CONSULTATIVE RESOURCES

Because of the immediacy of the Internet, it is a wonderful resource to consult with colleagues about patients. For information access, the Internet is unmatched because of its availability, speed, and capacity. Chat rooms and e-mail lists are popular among online contact lens fitters.

Online Symposia

If one seeks help with a GP lens patient, there is no better source than the RGP Lens Institute (RGPLI) monthly online symposium. This monthly session is held on the second or third Tuesday of every month at 9:00 P.M. eastern time. Formerly in the "Review Online" chat room of America Online, it has since moved to its own web site *(www.rgpli. org)*. One advantage of moving to the web site was the capability of viewing cases online. The speaker can write up the pertinent information about the case for review by the participants. Images such as fluorescein patterns and topographies can be displayed and archived. Ed Bennett, O.D., M.S.Ed., moderates the chat.

The format for the online symposium is divided into two sections. The first hour is dedicated to the topic. The remaining time becomes an open forum. The participants can present cases, ask questions, or introduce a new topic. Benefits of the online symposium are uninhibited exchange of information and speed. One optometric expert has compared the online symposium to one big conference because of the spontaneity and instantaneous feel. Another expert likened the chat experience to "going out for coffee with an expert after the lecture. It's great for face-to-face learning, but it's much more relaxed" (2).

Practitioners log into the system and are able to see the names of the other participants on the screen. Online participants type in their questions or comments, and the text appears on everyone's screen (2). The time it takes for comments to be observed by others depends upon connection speed and Internet traffic. Many of the speakers are well known and offer great information.

Optcom List

The Optcom list is another way to interact with colleagues. Although the forums encompass a variety of topics, many times contact lens cases are up for open discussion. If one has any clinical questions about a particular patient, there is no faster way of getting great advice than the Optcom list.

The Optcom list was originally a mailing list. It can be said that it represents the very essence of online optometry. It is offered through the Optometric Computing site *(www.optcom.com)*, which is associated with the Southern Council of Optometrists *(SECOinternational.com)*. The list is moderated by Walt Mayo, O.D., a pioneer in the field of technology for optometrists (3).

Before the Internet became commonplace, Dr. Mayo founded the Optnet Bulletin Board System in the 1980s and early 1990s. A handful of ODs would log onto the system and exchange ideas and news. Much of the same networking and sharing of information occurs today on the Optcom list. The Optnet system subsequently evolved and found a place on the Internet. The Optcom list has a membership of approximately 1,500 optometrists. The advantage of the Internet is the worldwide access. Optometrists all over the world are forming the optometric online community created by Dr. Mayo.

One problem Mayo encountered in the beginning was an absence of sponsorship. At the outset, Dr. Mayo financed the Optcom list himself. He devoted a great deal of time and money to develop online optometry (3). Since that time, SECOinternational has gained ownership.

The Optcom list has evolved and became available in four forms: mailing list, digest, newsgroup, and web board. The mailing list is the original format. Messages are sent to the subscribers as e-mail as they are posted. The digest format sends the subscriber a packet of messages. There is also an option to have the digest sent in a compressed (zip) format. There are numerous conferences on different topics available. The conference that has been written about in many journals is called the *main conference.*

The Optcom list has a new community system in place called *Optcom Central.* Still located at the same URL *(www.optcom.com)*, Optcom Central is the latest incantation of the Optcom list. It features forums, free e-mail, chat rooms, clubs, upload/download file libraries, and polls. One of the more notable forums for contact lens practitioners is the orthokeratology forum. Many reverse geometry lens designers frequent this forum.

One site worth noting as a discussion forum for optometrists is *seniordoc.org.* It is devoted to the retired or senior doctor. Although it is not a contact lens site, it sometimes offers limited discussion on contact lenses. The site requires registration as a new user to access many of its message forums.

Toric Calculators

Many years ago, contact lens fitters relied on phone calls to the consultation lines for help with soft torics. Fitters had to stay on the phone line while the consultant entered in the numbers to give the proper resultants. The Internet has made the toric calculator available without the need for a consultant or calculator. A few sites offer online toric calculators. The calculator is very beneficial in fitting toric lenses. One site with a calculator is CooperVision *(www.coopervision.com)*.

CooperVision's calculator is called *ToriTrack.* One can select the type of calculation needed, either Hydrasoft or other. The calculator has two calculations: spectacle and overrefraction. Spectacle calculation provides the proper power from the spectacle Rx (prescription) and vertex distance. The overrefraction calculator comes up with the

CooperVision lens using the spectacle Rx, contact lens Rx, and overrefraction.

CONTACT LENS INFORMATION SEARCH

If one prefers a less interactive source for consultation help, there is a wealth of archived information available on the Internet. One author likens it to a library with one billion books. The most significant problem may be finding where the information is located. All of the books in the virtual library are piled on the floor. Many books will disappear within months, and thousands of new ones appear daily (4).

Search Engines

The method most people use for searches is search engines for web pages. The problem with search engines is that even the best ones document only 20% of all the pages on the Internet (4). Search engines also have a hard time discerning the meaning of the keyword. Another disadvantage is the ability only to search hypertext markup language (HTML). If the pages have built-in security, it is likely the search will miss the pages. A commonly used search engine such as AltaVista *(www.altavista.com)* indexes medium-sized sites more completely than large or small sites (4).

One method to avoid the bias of one search engine is to use several engines. The Big Seven search engines are AltaVista *(www.altavista.com)*, Excite *(www.excite.com)*, HotBot *(www.hotbot.com)*, Infoseek *(infoseek.go.com)*, Lycos *(www.lycos.com)*, Northern Light *(www.northernlight.com)*, and Yahoo *(www.yahoo.com)* (5).

Yahoo is the most popular search engine on the Internet. At the same time, it has one of the smallest databases for a search engine. In 1997, Yahoo had an estimated one million pages in its database. In contrast, Excite and Lycos have 50 million pages. AltaVista, HotBot, and Northern Light search over 100 million pages (5).

Yahoo is essentially a large web directory. There are fewer "bad" or duplicative pages than on the other Big Seven engines. The engine is easy to use and generates quality results. Yahoo is an acronym for Yet Another Hierarchical Officious Oracle (5).

In the past, my personal preference has been Dogpile *(www.dogpile.com)*. Dogpile enlists the help of several search engines. It is known as a *meta-search engine*. The problem with the different search engines is that their databases are different. This can be easily demonstrated by searching a particular keyword on several different engines. The number one match on one engine usually is different than that on another engine. A meta-search engine searches several engines with a single query. When a keyword is entered, Dogpile gives the top results of several of the most commonly

used search engines. It uses multiple engines with only one stop.

Most recently, my search patterns have changed. The search engine I prefer to use is Google *(www.google.com)*. Google is known as one of the "next-generation" search engines. Google rates a site according to how many sites link to it. The more sites that link to it, the higher up on the page it appears. Google is excellent for finding the "official site." Usually, the official site is listed first because it has the most links to it. In some ways, Google is actually a popularity contest. If no one links to a site, it would have a low rating (5). I like Google for contact lens information searches because many times I am seeking the official site for a particular brand or type of contact lenses. Currently, I prefer Google over Dogpile because Dogpile usually provides too many duplication of sites for someone to have to review. However, one drawback of Google is the inability to locate obscure information. Because it is a popularity contest, unknown sites do not register very well. For these types of searches, Dogpile is preferable.

Usenet

Usenet or the newsgroups are other areas of the Internet that can be searched. Newsgroups are messages posted by users pertaining to a particular topic or interest area. One newsgroup open to everyone is *sci.med.vision*. Some practitioners do not like *sci.med.vision* because the members display an anti–eye care practitioner stance. Most participants are patients honestly seeking information about their eyes. However, there are several vocal members who can be very argumentative and abrasive. The numbers of these disenfranchised members are few; however, they sometimes post the majority of the messages. I personally find *sci.med.vision* an interesting forum to occasionally read. It provides a pulse on what patients are thinking today.

Newsgroups themselves are difficult to read. They are somewhat organized by thread (message subject), but many times the thread wanders away from the original topic. However, the newest information can be found first in the newsgroups. It sometimes can be bewildering to find information because of the inherent disorganization. Web pages are more organized, but the information needs to be processed before it appears on the site. Newsgroups are almost spontaneous in its ability to post information. Searching Usenet can be accomplished with a search engine such as Dogpile or Google (under groups).

PubMed

Another more conventional search engine is PubMed *(http://www.ncbi.nlm.nih.gov/PubMed/)*. This engine searches the medical literature and is very current. Formerly, literature searches were only available in libraries or on expensive CD-ROM collections. PubMed makes literature searches accessible from the Internet. The US-based optometric journals that PubMed searches are peer reviewed: *Optometry and Vision Science* and *Optometry* (formerly *Journal of the American Optometric Association*). PubMed is the best search engine for leading someone to peer-reviewed studies related to contact lenses. Because the vast majority of contact lens information has been written in non–peer-reviewed journals, PubMed has limited use.

Archive by Archive

A journal-by-journal archive search is very effective in finding valuable contact lens information. Contact Lens Spectrum *(www.clspectrum.com)*, *Optometric Management (www.optometric.com)*, *Primary Care Optometry News (www.slackinc.com)*, and *Review of Optometry and Review of Contact Lenses (www.revoptom.com)* all have archives on their web sites. The major disadvantage of the archives is that only recent years are available. Finding older issues still requires a trip to an ophthalmic library. Another disadvantage is the lack of viewable pictures that appear in the article. Despite these disadvantages, an archive-by-archive search is a very useful tool.

WEB PAGES

Manufacturers' Web Pages

Web pages of manufacturers are highly useful for information about contact lenses. Depending upon the site, many manufacturers have fitting guides, lens parameters, and educational resources on their web sites. In the past, the primary purpose was to offer information. Many manufacturers have shifted the focus of their sites to e-commerce for the practitioner. As mentioned in the Introduction, the e-commerce sites allow the contact lens fitter to purchase products over the Internet. Some of company sites are Vistakon *(www.jnjvision.com)*, CibaVision *(www.cibavision.com)*, Bausch and Lomb *(www.bausch.com)*, CooperVision *(www.coopervision.com)*, Ocular Sciences, Alcon *(www.alconlabs.com)*, and Allergan *(www.allergan.com)*.

Educational Web Pages

Separating educational web sites from manufacturers' pages may not be entirely accurate. Contact lens companies sponsor many of these web sites/newsletters in some way. Sites such as *Allaboutvision.com* and newsletters such as *CL Today* gain their support through advertising.

Sometimes, the site requires registration to access the information. Registration for a site offers the sponsor better security measures and more statistical information. Many users find registration an annoyance and a way to harvest their personal information, such as e-mail addresses.

Contact Lens Council

The Contact Lens Council (CLC) is supported by professional organizations and industry. The CLC has a consumer-oriented web site, *www.contactlenscouncil.org*. Advisory members of the CLC include The American Optometric Association, Contact Lens Association of Ophthalmologists, and the Contact Lens Society of America. The CLC is sponsored by, and works closely with, the Contact Lens Institute (CLI), a trade association that includes as members Alcon Laboratories, Allergan Optical, Bausch & Lomb, Biocompatibles, CIBA Vision, Coopervision, Vistakon (a division of Johnson & Johnson Vision Products, Inc.), and Wesley Jessen.

The CLC states that its primary goal is to promote the safe use of contact lenses. Their web site answers questions such as "Are contacts for you?," "Is it difficult to wear contact lenses?," and "Are contact lenses right for teenagers?" There is also an online video on how to insert contact lenses.

RGPLI.org

The Rigid Gas Permeable Lens Institute (RGPLI) offers a many resources on their web site *(www.rgpli.org)*. The RGPLI is the educational division of the Contact Lens Manufacturers Association (CLMA). A database of GP lenses is available in searchable form. There is a directory of GP laboratories and a listing of GP materials. The RGPLI online symposia schedule and symposia content summaries can be found here. The resources described in the GP educational resources chapter are available on the web site. The optometry schools and colleges workshop schedule is listed, as well as areas to sign up for both the student and practitioner newsletters. Links to the RGPLI consumer site *(www.contactlenses.org)* and other sites also are listed.

Allaboutvision.com

Allaboutvision.com is a consumer site with many articles on contact lenses. It is a product of Access Media. Other topics such as laser *in situ* keratomileusis (LASIK), computer vision, nutrition, and eyeglasses are covered. Personally, I find this site helpful as a literature resource for patients. I use the site to help explain more complicated procedures, such as orthokeratology. Unfortunately, the manufacturer sites tend to provide biased viewpoints toward many procedures or products. Although indirectly sponsored by industry, *allaboutvision.com* offers a little more generic perspective perhaps as to not favor one company.

Siliconehydrogels.org

Siliconehydrogels.org is sponsored by the Centre for Contact Lens Research (CCLR) of the University of Waterloo, and the Cooperative Research Centre for Eye Research and Technology (CRCERT) and Cornea and Contact Lens Research Unit (CCLRU) at the University of New South Wales. The site is for the benefit of practitioners, colleagues, and students. The three sponsoring organizations directly or indirectly benefit from large research monies from the contact lens manufacturers. The site requires registration as a new user to access the information.

Contact Lens Newsletters

Contact Lens Today (CL Today; www.cltoday.com/) is the weekly Internet newsletter devoted to contact lenses. The subscription is free. Although an archive search is not offered at this time, the best fitting tips on *CL Today* can be found here.

E-Commerce for Patients

As mentioned before, mail-order contact lens sites ranked the highest and most often on virtually any search engine. The Internet accounted for millions of ophthalmic e-commerce (electronic commerce) in 1999 (5). Much of it was the Internet sales of contact lenses to patients. 1-800-Contacts had total sales of almost $100 million, with the Internet accounting for $18.7 million (6). Half of the contact lens wearers obtain their lenses from nontraditional sources such as mail order. Two of every five patients obtain their lenses from a practitioner other than the doctor who prescribed them (5). Buying online offers convenience, one-stop shopping, and, many times, lower costs.

Manufacturers state that selling to Internet and mail-order companies is not in their policy. Through the tracing of bar codes, the manufacturers have shut down accounts that resell the product. Over the years, companies have claimed to have closed down dozens of accounts. Some have adopted a "no slit-lamp, no product" policy. However, companies such as 1-800-Contacts have huge inventories. The mail-order and online companies are thought to receive their lenses from the gray market, overseas sales, and diverted products from eye care professionals who chose to resell their product. 1-800-Contacts purchased 38% of its contact lens inventory from a single source in 1999, and its top three suppliers accounted for 68% of that inventory (6).

In 2001, 1-800-Contacts purchased contact lenses directly from CIBA Vision and Bausch & Lomb as a result of prior legal settlements. Vistakon (Johnson & Johnson) continues not to sell to 1-800-Contacts. In late 2001, Vistakon filed suit against 1-800-Contacts and asked the judge to force the Internet company to stop misleading advertising. Johnson & Johnson claimed that 1-800-Contacts was promoting Vistakon lenses to lure customers to the site, only to sell them lenses from Johnson & Johnson's rivals.

In late November 2001, federal judge John Schlesinger (Florida) said 1-800-Contacts was using deceptive advertising and ordered the company to discontinue the practice. The judge told 1-800-Contacts it could not use a study comparing the modalities of two lenses as if it were comparing the quality of the lenses.

The Vistakon suit also claims that contact lens practitioners received recorded messages, often during times when their offices were closed, from 1-800-Contacts requesting patients' contact lens prescriptions and threatening to list the practitioners as not compliant if they did not produce the prescription. The suit also claims that 1-800-Contacts prompted patients to see a different practitioner to obtain a prescription for a lens other than an Acuvue lens and then paid that practitioner for switching the consumer to the other brand, typically CIBA Vision lenses. CIBA Vision said it did not cooperate with this approach (7).

Ocular Sciences (OSI) stopped the sales of its lenses from unauthorized wholesale distributors such as JG Optical in New York and *Weblens.net* in Canada. OSI claimed *Weblens.net* changed labels and sent its customers an e-mail saying another company's lens was "virtually" the same as the OSI lens. OSI also resolved a legal dispute with *G02Contacts.com,* another Internet seller of contact lenses. The Internet company agreed not to purchase, distribute, advertise, or sell any OSI lenses, not to substitute other companies' lenses when a customer wanted to order an OSI product, and to remove all references about OSI from the *G02Contacts.com* web site (7).

SUMMARY

The Internet continues to be an important source of practitioner information on contact lens availability, parameter information, and clinical resources. It would be worth any practitioner's effort to frequently review the sites listed in this chapter, as well as new sites as they are introduced.

REFERENCES

1. Lowther GE. Internet and the world wide web. *Int Contact Lens Clin* 1996;23:40–41.
2. Gilfor M. Contact lenses in cyberspace. *Contact Lens Spectrum* 1997;12:30.
3. Top 10 ODs of the decade. *Optom Manage* 34:9.
4. Maino DM. It's all on the web . . . if you can find it. *Rev Optom* 134;5.
5. Miller M. *The complete idiot's guide to online search secrets.* Indianapolis, IN: Que, 1999.
6. Goodwin J. Mail order: public benefit or public health threat? *Optom Manage* 35;9:30.
7. Barr JT. Contact lenses 2001. *Contact Lens Spectrum* 2002;17.

TORIC GRAND ROUNDS

**EDWARD S. BENNETT AND
ROBERT L. DAVIS**

INTRODUCTION

Astigmatism is the most ignored factor when fitting contact lenses. In gas-permeable (GP) contact lenses, residual astigmatism is corrected by placing the correction on the front surface of the contact lenses. Back-surface toric or bitoric GP lenses are used when the corneal astigmatism compromises the fitting of a spherical lens on a toric corneal surface. In soft lens fittings, toric lenses can improve vision by correcting as little as 0.75 D of astigmatism. Assuming 0.75 D to be the maximum acceptable level of uncorrected astigmatism, 40% of prospective contact lens patients would require toric soft lenses. Practitioners need to acknowledge the fact that correcting astigmatism enhances the patient's optical properties and physical relationship of the contact lens.

The purpose of this chapter is to present a variety of clinical presentations and the methods of managing the astigmatic patient. Lens designs, material changes, and fitting pearls to toric contact lens fitting difficulties are illustrated by the following case presentations. Both GP and soft toric lens designs will be used to solve common contact lens challenges you see in everyday practice.

The primary focus in a toric lens fitting is lens rotational stability. All toric lenses have spherocylindrical powers that are kept at the proper orientation by rotational stabilizers. Prism ballast, truncation, periballast, thin zones, or eccentric lenticulation are integrated into the lens design to counteract the forces created by the blink and lid. Corneas with higher surface toricity utilize back-toric designs in addition to one of the rotational stabilizers to align the meridians for greater consistency.

The ocular structure must be adequate to receive a contact lens for a precise fit to generate a predicted and reliable prescription. Lid configuration, tear quality and quantity, lens cleanliness, and corneal topography are the ingredients that must be taken in consideration when designing a contact lens. Patient motivation, occupational requirements, and leisure pursuit are the unknowns that must be defined in order to achieve a successful outcome.

Regular astigmatism is defined by the major meridians of the refractive curvatures 90 degrees away from each other. With-the-rule astigmatism is defined by the minus cylinder axis at or near the 180-degree meridian. Against-the-rule astigmatism is where the minus cylinder axis is at or near 90-degree meridian. Against-the-rule powers are more stable because the horizontal meridian of the lens is thickest and tends to orientate between the lids. With-the-rule powers are thickest in the vertical meridian, which causes the upper lid to rotate the lens downward. Irregular astigmatism is where the major astigmatic meridians are not 90 degrees away. Irregular astigmatic patients cannot be fitted in soft lenses or spectacles and have their best visual outcomes in GP lens designs.

A GP lens with a spherical front and back surface is the most consistent method of neutralizing corneal astigmatism. An aspheric lens design will neutralize the same corneal astigmatism in addition to providing better centration and a uniform flow of tears. Residual astigmatism results when the contact lens/tear/cornea combination fails to neutralize the total ametropia of the eye. This can be internal or corneal depending on the type of contact lens placed on the eye. Residual astigmatism is often attributed by the crystalline lens and can be corrected by fitting a front-surface toric GP lens or a toric soft lens. The residual astigmatism of a soft hydrogel lens is the refractive cylinder uncorrected. Lens warpage, lens flexure, lens decentration, and the result of fitting GP toric lenses can induce residual astigmatism that must be corrected by a front-toric GP lens. Residual astigmatism is the astigmatic power not neutralized by placing a contact lens on the cornea surface

Front-toric GP lenses are used to improve the optical quality of the image by neutralizing the residual astigmatism. The spherical back surface, prism base down, and a toric front surface generates fitting design, stability, and astigmatic correction. The toric back-surface GP lens serves to obtain the optimal fitting relationship while stabilizing the lens design on a corneal surface with toricity. It is important to understand that even when a GP lens exhibits good centration in a patient with high astigmatism, the absence of alignment caused by excessive regions of bearing and clearance can have undesirable effects on both corneal topography and blink quality. The beauty of fitting a spherical power effect bitoric is in the fluorescein pattern. The bitoric lens design on a toric cornea appears as if you are fitting a spherical lens on a spherical cornea. Patients discover that the bitoric designs are very comfortable with good acuity and without corneal compromise.

The presence of astigmatism, whether great or small, should certainly not be a contraindication to contact lens wear. Notably, the quality of vision as well as the fitting benefits of toric lenses make them the logical option in many cases. It is the perceived difficulties in the application, design, and fitting of these specialty lenses that provide the most significant obstacle to their use. A false impression is that the greater the cylinder, the greater your chair time and the lower your success rate. These case presentations will demonstrate that the use of toric lenses will become an easy solution to your patient's ametropia with a very good rate of success.

SOFT TORIC LENSES

Monthly Fresh Lens Toric Lens Design

Initial Summary

A 32-year-old man who is part owner of a very busy 24-hour restaurant was interested in contact lenses because of the inconvenience of glasses at work. His intense work habits create tremendous physical stress on his eyes and body. He operates a restaurant between the hours of 4:00 p.m. to 1:00 a.m. and 10:00 a.m. to 1:00 p.m. His sleep habits are very erratic. S.D.'s free time is spent with his family. He enjoys watching sporting events as time permits. He came into the office as an unsuccessful polymethylmethacrylate (PMMA) lens wearer due to intolerance, asking for soft contact lenses. His immediate goals were to wear contact lenses comfortably with good vision.

During the case history he reported that eyeglasses are very troublesome, especially when the weather is hot. "I have always wanted the convenience of soft extended-wear lenses," he said. "My life does not permit me to spend the time nor do I have the patience to deal with the contact lenses on a daily-wear basis." This patient had no genetic history of systemic diseases. He was not taking any medications and had no allergies. His primary reason for requesting an eye examination was to investigate the possibility of wearing soft hydrogel extended wear lenses.

Ocular Evaluation

The results of the examination included normal lateral and up Bell's phenomenon. Lid eversion revealed normal satin appearance of tarsal conjunctiva without papillae or follicles.

There existed two or three clogged meibomian glands on the lid margin. Upon pressure normal contents were expressed. Lid appearance was not flaccid or tight, typical for a 32-year-old man. Lids exhibited no swelling, injection, congestion, or granulations. Conjunctiva and sclera exhibited no inflammation or congestion. Pupils were equal, round, and reactive to direct, consensual, and accommodative reflexes. There was no sign of an afferent pupil defect in either eye. Extraocular muscle movements were full and smooth in all directions of gaze in both eyes. Lenticular evaluation illustrated clear media with a distinct Mittendorf dot bilaterally. The palpebral aperture heights measured 11.0 mm. The tear meniscus was approximately 1 mm wide at the base and 3 mm high.

Keratometry:
Right eye (OD): 40.00 @ 180; 41.75 @ 090

Left eye (OS): 40.00 @ 180; 41.50 @ 090

Distance visual acuity (VA) uncorrected:
OD: 20/100 near J1
OS: 20/80 near J1

Retinoscopy:
OD: $-3.00 -1.50 \times 180$ 20/20 -2
OS: $-2.50 -1.00 \times 180$ 20/20

Subjective:
OD: $-3.25 -1.75 \times 165$ 20/20
OS: $-2.50 -1.25 \times 180$ 20/20

Calculated residual cylinder:
OD: $-1.75 -(1.75) =$ plano
OS: $-1.25 -(1.50) = -0.25 \times 90$

Schirmer I without anesthetic:
OD: 32 mm in 5 minutes
OS: 30 mm in 5 minutes

Tear break-up time:
OD: 18 seconds
Invasive method:
OS: 17 seconds

Biomicroscopy

The anterior chamber was clear in both eyes. The anterior chamber depth 4+ where the distance between the posterior cornea and iris is equal to the corneal thickness. Iris shape, color, and size were free of pathology and abnormalities. Fluorescein staining revealed intact corneas without defects. Lenticular evaluation illustrated clear crystalline surface with a distinct Mittendorf dot in each eye (OU). Neither eye exhibited any signs of neovascularization or edema. There existed a slight inflammation of the meibomian gland margins for which the use of scrubs and warm compresses was demonstrated and prescribed.

Material Selection

The patient requires a correction for his compound myopic astigmatism. A discussion was held addressing the advantages of GP lenses. Due to his visual demands, erratic work habits, and his extended-wear criteria, the Ciba monthly replacement Focus toric contact lens was prescribed. New lenses usually do not cause complications. Filmy and coated lenses initiate the classic red eye phenomenon. Reusable extended-wear soft lenses do not practice preventive vision care. Reusable extended-wear lenses force us to react to an already risky situation. With the proliferation of disposables and fresh lens toric lens modalities, it was suggested to fit this patient with a monthly frequent-replacement toric extended-wear lens. This lens replacement regimen is more preventive. Replacement of lenses prior to complications arising maintains a healthy ocular environment.

Lens Specifications	OD	OS
Base curve	8.9 mm	8.9 mm
Diameter	14.0 mm	14.0 mm
Power	$-3.00 - 1.75 \times 180$	$-2.50 - 1.00 \times 180$
Visual acuity distance	20/20	20/20
Visual acuity near	J1	J1
Overrefraction	Plano	Plano

The lenses were dispensed and instructions were given explaining application/removal, lens care regimen, and wearing schedule. The cleaning/disinfecting regimen included chemical multipurpose solution, surfactant, and liquid enzyme. The toric marking at 3 and 9 o'clock on each lens showed slight nasal rotation with rapid recovery. A wearing schedule was given to include all waking hours with no overnight wear. A return appointment was scheduled 1 week later.

Fitting/Troubleshooting

Clinical success with toric hydrogel lenses includes the standard criteria of good physical and physiologic performance. Patients who have failed to adapt to GP lenses because of discomfort or edge awareness are motivated by the comfort of hydrogel lenses. A trial fit gains confidence for both patient and doctor to reach their visual and comfort goals for a usable prescription.

The various lens-stabilization methods available in soft hydrogel contact lenses include prism ballast, thin zones, periballast, truncation, eccentric lenticulation, and combinations of these designs. The Ciba Focus Toric lens is a 55% Vifilcon A molded back-surface toric lens design. Re-

gardless of lens designs, orientation is achieved as a result of thickness differential among the superior, central, and inferior portions of the lens, with edge configuration playing a significant role (1).

The dynamic stabilization is created by removing material from the upper and lower regions of the lens leaving the thickest portion in the center. The lids cover portions of the thin zones and exert sufficient forces on the lens to stabilize rotation. The design is most successful when there is a thickness differential across the surface of the lens, such as in higher myopic corrections or against-the-rule cylinders maximizing the wedge effect. This technique produces a comfortable lens wear and maintains good stability due to the thin edges. Back- or front-surface toric lens designs do not significantly add to the stability or optical characteristics of the lens (2). Both are single toric lenses and assume bitoric characteristics and configuration when placed on a toric cornea.

A loose lens may show excessive movement with each blink and decenter superiorly or laterally exposing the limbus. A loose lens can also exhibit inferior edge lift or vaulting. A tight lens will center well with little or no postblink movement. A tight lens will initially feel comfortable because of decreased lens movement. Physiologic complications will result when tears debris and metabolic by products cannot flush from under the lens. Excessive tight toric lenses will mislocate and orientate at an unpredictable axis. The mnemonic LARS (left add, right subtract) helps compensate the axis when prescribing toric hydrogel lenses when they do not orientate properly. The LARS rule is compensated to the clinician's left perspective.

S.D. returned 1 week later for his first follow-up visit. He was very satisfied with his vision and comfort. He was pleased that for the first time he was able to wear contact lenses comfortably throughout his waking hours. He asked when he could start sleeping with his lenses. He had worn lenses 6 hours prior to this office visit.

Distance visual acuity:
OD: 20/20
OS: 20/20

Near visual acuity:
OD: J1
OS: J1

Overrefraction:
OD: plano -0.25×180
OS: plano

It was explained to S.D. that the extended-wear toric lenses require less handling and maintenance, although less cleaning and disinfection usually means a shorter lens life. It was also explained that wearing lenses overnight is associated with an increased risk for infections, abrasions, and corneal ulceration compared with daily wear. Ocular physiologic stress can results in increased edema, neovascularization, and corneal ulcers. So if he experiences any change in vision, increased lens awareness or ocular hyperemia the lenses should be removed and discarded. It is misleading for the patient to think the symptoms might go away in the morning. Typically this is not the case and the symptoms will only increase in severity. The follow-up care is very important in extended wear. Visual performance, corneal physiology changes, and lens condition will be evaluated every 3 months. This is where a service agreement policy is important. S.D. should not think about coming into the office because of the costs associated with an office visit. They are all prepaid. These policies will reduce unwanted complications. Extended-wear patients must be educated and rechecked on the maintenance of their lens hygiene. Corneal oxygen demand and debris removal are important for extended wear. In a clinical setting we have found this can be patient dependent. Long-term oxygen deprivation and carbon dioxide accumulation can place the cornea tissue at risk. Debris removal and limiting tear stasis has been implicated in acute inflammatory episodes and needs to be maintained for proper corneal function (2). Extended wear is a modality that needs close control, and we offer our patients the necessary service to maintain a healthy clinical strategy.

A discussion was held pertaining to leaving the lenses in for a maximum of 6 days. However, he was told that if the lenses became uncomfortable or if it was convenient to take the lenses out, they should be removed. He was satisfied with his vision and comfort.

Summary

Factors influencing the decision to fit an astigmatic patient with soft toric lenses rather than a GP lens include: previous lens-wearing history, occupational and recreational needs and immediate comfort. Patients who experience physiologic problems or poor tolerance with GP lenses are prime candidates for soft toric lenses. Frequent replacement of extended-wear toric lenses represents an important niche. The problems with coated lenses, which include dry eye, giant papillary conjunctivitis (GPC), acute red eye syndrome (ARES), blurred vision, and axis misalignment can be solved with a replacement of lenses every week to a month.

Hydrogel Toric Multifocal Lens Design

Initial Summary

A 50-year-old gemologist wearing soft toric lenses for 16 years has become disillusioned with contact lens due to the limitations of acuity. At work she has increasingly had to grab a jewelers loop in order to look at precious stones. Monovision has been acceptable, although she is no longer willing to compromise distance or near vision. The visual demands at work and at home require distance, intermediate, and near visual requirements. A spectacle prescription is not an option due to the cosmetic appearance and the aberrations her present prescription provides. She has been replacing her contact lenses every 18 months due to deposit buildup. The patient has been on a daily wearing schedule using Aosept chemical disinfection regimen to clean and disinfect her lenses. She was not taking any medications and was allergic to streptomycin. Her primary reason for requesting an eye examination was to investigate the possibility of improving her distant and near vision with soft hydrogel toric daily-wear lenses.

Ocular Evaluation

Lid eversion revealed slightly hyperemic appearance of tarsal conjunctiva without papillae or follicles as a result of the condition of the contact lens surface characteristics. Upon pressure to the meibomian glands on the lid margin, normal contents were expressed. Lid appearance was slightly flaccid, typical for a 50-year-old woman. Lids exhibited no swelling, injection, congestion, or granulations. The palpebral aperture heights measured 11.5 mm. The inferior tear meniscus was adequate in height to support contact lens wear.

Keratometry:
OD: 42.87 @ 180; 44.62 @ 090
OS: 42.62 @ 180; 44.37 @ 090

Distance VA uncorrected:
OD: 20/60 near J4
OS: 20/60 near J4

Subjective:
OD: +1.75 −2.50 × 100 20/20 add +1.75 D J1
OS: +1.75 −2.00 × 070 20/20 add +1.75 D J1

Schirmer I without anesthetic:
OD: 26 mm in 5 minutes
OS: 24 mm in 5 minutes

Tear break-up time:
OD: 15 seconds

Invasive method:
OS: 16 seconds

Biomicroscopy
Anterior chamber was clear in both eyes. Fluorescein staining revealed intact corneas without defects. Neither eye exhibited any signs of neovascularization or edema. Grade 1 bulbar conjunctival injection was present. There existed a mild inflammation, grade 1 injection, of the tarsal conjunctiva for which the use of warm compresses was demonstrated

and prescribed. The ocular reaction most likely was due to the poor surface characteristics of the hydrogel lenses. Meibomian glands excreted clear fluid upon gentle expression.

Material Selection

The patient received a diagnosis of hyperopic astigmatic presbyope. The astigmatism was against-the-rule. All other findings confirmed that she was a good candidate for contact lens wear. The options discussed with the patient included toric contact lenses for distance and a reading prescription over the contact lenses, monovision correction with soft toric lenses, monovision with GP lenses, GP bifocals, and soft toric bifocal contact lenses. Soft toric lenses with a reading prescription were not acceptable due to the unacceptable age stigma that reading glasses possess. Monovision was not an acceptable option due to her previous contact lens experience. The summation of two eyes would be less of a compromise than with the monovision technique. GP lenses were not an acceptable option due to discomfort. The soft toric bifocal lens modality offers a multifocal aspheric design and an annular configuration in the patient's prescription. A discussion with the patient emphasized the desire not to return to a spectacle prescription. The aspheric multifocal toric bifocal lens was fitted and ordered empirically due to the multiple visual demands at work and at home. If the multifocal toric lens design does not meet the patients goal's and expectations then the annular toric lens design would be attempted.

The contact lens specifications from United Contact lens Company were as follows:

Base curve:
8.7 mm (OD); 8.7 mm (OS)

Diameter:
14.7 mm (OD); 14.7 mm (OS)

Power:
+2.00 −2.00 × 100 add + 2.00 D (OD)
+2.00 −2.00 × 70 add + 2.00 D (OS)

Fitting/Troubleshooting

Prism-ballast lens design incorporates a 0.75- to 2.0-prism base down resisting rotation forces. In hydrogel lenses with base down prism, the upper lid exerts the force to stabilize the prism of the lens in a downward direction. Gravity plays a minimal role stabilizing toric hydrogel lens rotation. The "watermelon seed principle" relates to a wedge that is squeezed, it is propelled away from the apex. Toric lenses usually do not rotate on patients' eyes while lying on their side. This is an example as to why gravity plays an insignifi-

cant role in contrast to the lens–cornea adherence and lid forces. Prism-ballasted lenses require inferior chamfering or a slab-off for good comfort.

The optimal patient includes wide aperture, complete lid closure during the blink, a lower lid margin on line with the limbus, no raised conjunctival tissue, and a normal stable precorneal tear film. The amount of visual disruption resulting from a nonstable lens depends on the power of the cylinder, the degree of rotation, and the speed and recovery as the lens regains its resting position following a blink or change of gaze.

An important consideration when evaluating the physical lens fit is to determine the draping and flexure characteristics. These terms quantify the degree in which the lens wraps itself over the cornea. A lens that properly drapes the cornea will not grab the conjunctiva and produce conjunctival drag. Thicker lenses flex incompletely. Irregular flexure results in poor optical quality and symptoms of blur haziness, ghosting, and fluctuating acuity. Flexure and draping qualities can be assessed by keratometry and retinoscopy observations over the contact lens. The optimal fit will have a clear regular keratometric or retinoscopic image. A flat lens will have clear keratometry mires except after the blink when the mires will be blurry. A steep fit will have blurry mires except after the blink when the mire image will be clear.

Annular and progressives soft lenses operate on a simultaneous vision principle. The simultaneous vision design focuses both far and near targets on the retina without a change in lens position. The annular simultaneous lens design has distinct borders between the two powers creating a prismatic effect, which may result in the patient experiencing diplopia. When this occurs, if the divided border is slightly blended, this effect can be neutralized. Changes in pupil size will affect vision due to better near vision with dilation and enhanced distant vision with pupillary constriction. Success depends on proper distance-to-near ratio within the optic zone to avoid confusion from overlapping images. Another design problem is created when accommodative effort is engaged at near point and pupil constriction occurs. A design change can solve this problem with near power centrally and distant zone surrounding (reverse central).

The progressive bifocal lens is constructed with aspheric curves ground from the center towards the periphery of the lens. The aspheric curve provides a varying amount of additive plus power towards the periphery dependent on eccentricity. The eccentricity defines the rate at which the radius flattens towards the periphery. If the lens does not center, distance vision is reduced because the distance zone is small and greater plus power is progressively increased towards the periphery.

Problems in fitting simultaneous annular or progressive designs are created by the distance image degraded by the out-of-focus near image and near vision degraded by the out-of-focus distant image. Another problem is created during low levels of illumination when the pupil dilates, accessing further into the near zones degrading distance vision. Flare, halos, or ghosting may be associated with lights obscuring the vision around them. Acceptance is patient specific. Not all patients are able to adapt to their vision equally. These lens designs are pupil dependent both for vision under normal illumination and under low levels of illumination.

The patient was dispensed the soft toric multifocal contact lenses and educated about deposit buildup. The patient was told that if any discomfort was experienced the lens should be removed and an appointment be made to evaluate the surface characteristics of the lens. The Aosept disinfecting regimen was chosen so that a preservative-free care system could eliminate the source of lid complication. These lenses were evaluated after 1 hour to allow sufficient time for the lenses to stabilize. Visual acuity and overrefraction were as follows: OD 20/20 plano − 0.50 × 100; OS: 20/25 −0.25 − 0.50 × 70.

Biomicroscopy

The lenses centered well and revealed a 0.5-mm lag with the blink. Both toric markings were positioned at 6:00 with slight temporal rotation with the blink although recovery was rapid. The lens surface appeared to be clean and wet evenly. A wearing schedule was given to include all waking hours. A 1-week follow-up appointment was scheduled to discuss the acceptability of this lens design. The left lens was reordered to attempt to achieve better acuity.

The patient returned 1 week later for her follow-up visit. She was satisfied with her vision and comfort. The left lens acuity was not as good as the right lens. She also experienced fireworks and halos at night around lights out of the left lens. She was pleased that during the week there was no need for the jewelers loop to adequately accomplish near point work. The left lens was exchanged and the vision seemed to immediately improve.

Summary

This case is a good example of attempting to fit a toric-bifocal lens modality in a patient who requires multiple visual working distant requirements. Success is accomplished by matching the patient's visual needs with the contact lens modality. The lens design decision is attained by educating the patient about the various possibilities that would achieve his or her visual expectations. The doctor's job is to describe the various advantages and disadvantages of each lens design and proceed with the patient, problem solving along the way until the patient's goals have been reached.

Dry Eye Toric Lens Design

Initial Summary

A 39-year-old sales representative has been wearing soft toric contact lenses since 1980. He presented himself to the office with the complaint of dry eye. He has been experiencing a reduction in wearing time and a gritty feeling while wearing his lenses. He has been replacing his contact lenses every 12 months due to the lenses not feeling as comfortable as when they are new. The patient wears his lenses on a daily wearing schedule and disinfects with the Opti-Free surfactant cleaning, enzyme treatment, and disinfection system nightly. His mother has systemic lupus with signs and symptoms of extreme dry eye. His primary reason for requesting an eye examination was to investigate the possibility of improving his comfort with a replacement of soft hydrogel toric daily-wear lenses.

Ocular Evaluation

Upper lid eversion revealed that the tarsal conjunctivae were pink and smooth in appearance without any signs of papillae or follicles. Upon gentle pressure to the meibomian glands on the lid margin, normal contents were expressed. Lid tensions were average, typical for a 39-year-old man. The lids exhibited no swelling, injection, congestion, or granulations. The palpebral aperture heights measured 11.0 mm. The inferior tear meniscus was adequate in height to support contact lens wear.

Keratometry:
OD: 42.50 @ 180; 43.87 @ 090
OS: 42.25 @ 180; 44.00 @ 090

Distance VA uncorrected:
OD: 20/300 near J2
OS: 20/300 near J2

Subjective:
OD: −5.50 − 1.25 × 180 20/20 J1
OS: −6.00 − 1.25 × 70 20/20 J1

Schirmer I without anesthetic:
OD: 18 mm in 5 minutes
OS: 16 mm in 5 minutes

Tear break-up time:
OD: 8 seconds

Invasive method:
OS: 9 seconds

Biomicroscopy

Anterior chamber was clear in both eyes. Fluorescein staining revealed superficial corneal stain smattered throughout the corneas. Neither eye exhibited any signs of neovascularization or edema. Grade 1 bulbar conjunctival injection was present. There existed a mild inflammation. The ocular reaction was due to fragile corneal epithelium from dry eye syndrome and poor surface characteristics of the hydrophilic lenses.

Localized dehydration of nonrotating toric lenses causes a mild superficial punctate stain. Flushing tear debris from under the contact lens may be impaired, with toric lenses developing epithelial stain and stippling. Dryness and related staining are more common in patients with incomplete blinking and a deficient tear lipid layer. Epithelial edema can develop because of deficient corneal epithelium metabolism and increased inferior lens bulk and thickness. Advanced corneal edema is characterized by vertical striae related to hypoxia conditions. The patient perceives spectacle blur when lenses are removed at the end of the day. Conjunctival or scleral indentation from the pressure of impinging edge configurations is observed with larger and/or steeper fitting lenses. If perilimbal congestion, limbal swelling, or acute red eye response develops, a thinner or smaller, looser fitting lens is needed to eliminate the complications.

Contact lenses with higher water content will dehydrate an already dry eye. The negative charged monomer allows the increase in water content with a side effect of protein binding and lens dehydration. Superior arcuate corneal staining (SEALS) is commonly a sign of high water dehydration and corneal desiccation. Thicker lenses are optimal for dry eye syndrome because the lens mass is increased. This has an effect of increasing lens movement and minimizing adherence. Lower-water thicker lenses, due to their mass, will also reduce the effects of dehydration. Hydroxyethylmethacrylate (HEMA) has long been known as a material that would deposit and soil. The formations of lens deposits create nonwettable areas, poor optics, and a lack of surface smoothness leading to corneal staining and ARES. The spoiling factor of contact lenses results in faster surface drying, poor visual acuity, and changes in lens parameters especially important in toric lens wear. This has been the primary force behind frequent-replacement lens systems. The limitations on hydrogel lens wear are directly related to the materials available.

Material Selection

This patient was experiencing dry eye symptoms with clinical signs resulting from a deficient lipid tear layer These symptoms were further aggravated by the poor contact lens surface characteristics. Biocompatibles has developed a synthetic material that is analogue of phospholipid called phosphatidylcholine. The Proclear material, omafilcon A, is a new material that will change the way hydrogels react on the eye. The material is a zwitterion, having both a negative and positive charge rendering the molecule electrically neutral. This resists protein and lipid deposits on the lens material. The neutral molecule at water content 59% has less dehydration than other ionic materials at similar water content. The patient was refitted into Proclear toric soft lens for oxygen transmissibility and low dehydration characteris-

tics to achieve comfort and stable vision from his dry eye syndrome.

The contact lens specifications from Biocompatibles were as follows:

Base curve:
8.5 mm (OD); 8.5 mm (OS)

Diameter:
14.5 mm (OD); 14.5 mm (OS)

Power:
$-5.50 - 1.00 \times 180$ (OD)
$-6.00 - 1.00 \times 180$ (OS)

The lenses were fit with a 6-month replacement strategy. Unpreserved single-dose Lens Plus rewetting drops were given for tear lubrication.

Fitting/Troubleshooting

Dry eye syndrome is a condition in which the tear film does not adequately coat the conjunctiva and cornea. It may result from a decreased quantity of otherwise normal tears or an abnormal quality of the tear film. The primary symptoms include ocular burning, drying, and foreign-body sensation. The symptoms are usually exacerbated by prolonged use of the eyes and by environmental factors such as wind, heat, smoke, and low humidity (3). Paradoxically, patients may complain of excess tearing if the eye becomes so irritated that reflex tearing mechanisms are activated. A decreased tear lake and a decreased tear film breakup time are common. Other signs include punctate fluorescein or rose bengal staining of the cornea and conjunctiva, typically inferiorly or in the interpalpebral zone. Excess mucus, filaments, or both may be seen. A Schirmer's test will typically reveal reduced baseline tear secretion. Tear break-up time illustrates the adequacy of the lipid component of the tear film layer. Rose bengal gives us insight into the severity of the disease as well as the mucin continuity. A deficiency in any one of the layers allows an unprotected cornea subject to the 16-hour blinking action of the lids. A contact lens on top of a deficient tear layer only aggravates an already potential chaffing action coupled with the increased friction from the lack of lubricant. The symptom is then defined by the patient as dry eye.

The numerous underlying causes that should be considered include systemic medications, such as antihistamines and oral contraceptives; collagen vascular diseases, such as Sjögren's syndrome and rheumatoid arthritis; ocular cicatricial pemphigoid; Stevens-Johnson syndrome; lupus; and vitamin A deficiency. A stepwise approach to treatment is appropriate, beginning with regular artificial tears several times a day for mildly dry eyes. For moderate dry eye syndrome, preservative-free tears are used up to every 1 or 2 hours during the day, with artificial tear ointment used at night. In severe cases, more viscous drops and more frequent applications of ointment are used. Punctal occlusion, sustained-release gels, or lateral tarsorrhaphy may be required if less aggressive therapy fails.

Summary

This case illustrates that toric lens fitting associated with dry eye syndrome requires proper diagnostic testing to properly select the appropriate lens therapy and treatment. The treatment for an aqueous tear deficiency problem is different from that for a lipid tear deficiency problem. Toric lenses usually are thicker than their spherical lens counterpart, which will reduce contact lens dehydration. Environmental factors are important to uncover since they might exacerbate the condition. New materials, such as Proclear, can potentially convert contact lens dropouts into successful contact lens wearers.

High Cylinder Hydrogel Toric Lens Design

Initial Summary

A 23-year-old police cadet came into the office seeking better vision with soft lenses in order to pass a entrance examination. With glasses, best-corrected visual acuity monocularly was 20/40 OU. With the use of a pinhole, no further visual improvement could be obtained. He was told that he would not pass the physical requirements unless he could attain better-corrected visual acuity. He has failed to adapt previously with GP lenses due to intolerance. The only possible contact lens modality included SoftPerm lenses or toric lenses. A discussion with the patient pertained to explaining the difficulties with soft lenses achieving better acuity than with a spectacles prescription. It was demonstrated to him how a toric lens neutralizes the prescription of the eye and the possible variable vision from the rotation of the lens on the eye caused by the blinking action of the lid. The patient had no genetic history of systemic diseases. He was not on any medications and had no allergies. He had never experienced any eye surgeries or injuries. His primary reason for requesting a contact lens fitting was to investigate the possibility of improving his vision with contact lenses.

Ocular Evaluation

Upon pressure to the meibomian glands on the lid margin, normal contents were expressed. Lid appearance was tight, typical for a 23-year-old man. Lids exhibited no swelling, injection, congestion, or granulations. Lid eversion revealed smooth satin appearance of tarsal conjunctiva without hyperemia, papillae, or follicles. The palpebral aperture heights measured 11.5 mm. The inferior tear meniscus was adequate in height to support contact lens wear.

Keratometry:
OD: 40.12 @ 180; 47.50 @ 090
OS: 39.25 @ 180; 47.25 @ 090

Corneal topography (Fig. 47.1)

Distance VA uncorrected:
OD: 20/200 near J5
OS: 20/200 near J5

Subjective:
OD: $+2.75 - 6.50 \times 15$ 20/40 J3
OS: $+3.00 - 6.50 \times 165$ 20/40 J3

Schirmer I without anesthetic:
OD: 33 mm in 5 minutes
OS: 34 mm in 5 minutes

Tear break-up time:
OD: 22 seconds

Invasive method:
OS: 24 seconds

Biomicroscopy
Anterior chamber was clear in both eyes. Fluorescein staining revealed intact corneas without defects. Neither eye exhibited any signs of neovascularization or edema. Meibomian glands excreted clear fluid upon gentle expression. Iris shape, color, and size were free of pathology and abnormalities.

Material Selection

He has difficulty visually through a spectacle correction because of his high with-the-rule prescription. The spectacle lenses need constant adjustment to keep the orientation of the meridians in alignment. A discussion of the advantages and disadvantages of SoftPerm lenses and toric lenses was explained. The overall diameter of a SoftPerm lens is 14.3 mm with a 8.0-mm rigid center. Conceptually the SoftPerm lens should be fitted with an alignment philosophy in order to distribute the bearing evenly across the cornea. A toric lens would be initial lens of choice due to the physiologic restrictions of SoftPerm lenses and the frequent separation between the transition rigid portion and the soft skirt. The Coast Hydrasoft toric lens made of methafilcon 55% water content with a lathe-cut eccentric lenticulation lens design incorporating 2.1 prism base down was empirically ordered. When there is no axis mislocation and no power compensation is necessary, empirical fitting has a good chance of success. The patient was told that if the toric soft lens did not meet his visual expectations, then a SoftPerm lens fitting would be attempted.

Optical Cross

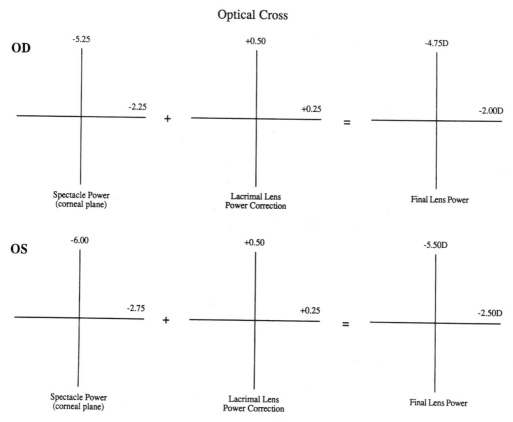

FIG. 47.1. The optical cross method of determining bitoric lens powers.

Lens Specifications	OD	OS
Base curve	8.9 mm	8.9 mm
Diameter	15.0 mm	15.0 mm
Power	+3.00 −6.50 × 180	+3.25 −6.50 × 180
Visual acuity distant	20/20	20/20
Visual acuity near	J1	J1
Overrefraction	Plano	Plano

Eccentric lenticulation is created by removing lens material from the anterior lenticular surface in the direction of the base of the prism. The removal of excess material on the anterior surface reduces the differential edge thickness that increases both stability and comfort creates better limbal-sclera draping and minimizes compression on the sclera conjunctiva. This design has upper and lower thin zones of equal thickness and reduced lens mass. The prism is in only the center two-thirds of the lens. The increased stability is especially evident in oblique cylinder corrections when the lid margin closure first meets the thicker part of the lens at an oblique angle and often results in torsional mislocation. The anatomy of eyelids and lid closure has a significant effect on lens axis location and rotation. The upper lid has the greatest influence on lens rotation in a nasodownward direction. Tight lids and narrow palpebral apertures often produce excessive force on the lens initiating lens rotation. He was told that special attention should be directed if the lens rotated and to correct the poor vision by looking up and forcefully blinking.

Fitting/Troubleshooting

The lenses were applied on the eye and the patient immediately reported that his vision was clear, although it appeared hazy. It was explained to him that vision is different through a 55%-water lens than through spectacles. He is looking through water, and adaptation will occur while he gets adjusted to the hydrogel lens. Biomicroscopy exhibited central positioning with good movement with a lag of 0.5 mm OU with straight-ahead gaze. Both toric markings were positioned at 6 o'clock with slight temporal rotation with the blink, although recovery was rapid. The lenses were dispensed and instructions were given explaining application/removal, lens care regimen, and wearing schedule. The cleaning/disinfecting regimen included Aosept, MiraFlow surfactant cleaner, and Ultrazyme enzyme. The patient watched a video presentation on contact lens wear and was provided with an instructional manual on lens handling and care. He felt that his vision appeared quite good. A return appointment was scheduled 1 week later to discuss the acceptability of his vision at work. One week later, the patient returned for a follow-up appointment and reported his vision was excellent and the comfort was better than he could imagine. Biomicroscopy showed that the lenses exhibited central positioning with good movement with a lag of 0.5 mm OU with straight-ahead gaze. Both toric markings were positioned at 6 o'clock and torqued a few degrees temporally with the blink, although recovery was rapid. The patient occasionally experienced that each lens appeared blurry, although vision came back after the blink. He indicated that his vision appeared quite good, and he was ecstatic that he could finally pass the vision portion of the police cadet entrance examination.

Summary

This case demonstrates the importance of attempting a soft toric lens fitting even when the prescription is better suited in a GP lens design. Patients need to be informed of the complications of each lens design and partner with the practitioner to determine the best alternative. As long as the patient is informed of the complexities and understands how the lens might fail, the patient can make an educated decision to proceed. This custom toric soft hydrogel lens case proved satisfactory, although problems with this lens modality include increased fragility, short lens life, rotational problems, and reduced optical qualities. Custom soft toric lenses have all of the astigmatism correction on one surface. When the lens rotates a few degrees with the blink, vision can be reduced dramatically. The Becherer Twist test indicates the patient's tolerance for axis rotation with a toric soft lens by twisting the axis knob on the phoropter a few degrees clockwise and counterclockwise (4). Another version of this test involves having the toric lens in place and has the practitioner spin the lens a few degrees off axis and check the patient's response to the vision while he or she is looking at an acuity chart. Even when the perfect fit is realized and the vision is excellent, lens deposits and lens fragility can cause patient and doctor frustration.

Custom Toric Lens

Initial Summary

A corneal specialist referred a 48-year-old stockbroker to our practice for a contact lens refitting. The patient had a bilateral corneal graft with mixed results. M.B. was having visual difficulties both at near and at distance. M.B.'s immediate goal was to pass a driver's license visual acuity test and to successfully read the trade board at the stock exchange. Her contact lens history included unsuccessful GP lens wear due to intolerance as well as unsuccessful SoftPerm contact lens wear due to lens seal off that created ARES. Presently she is wearing a piggyback soft/hard combination that is very cumbersome and requires significant amount of lens care. M.B.'s expectation is to limit the amount of personal

energy required to successfully wear and maintain contact lenses.

Biomicroscopy

Upper lid eversion exhibited normal tarsal conjunctival appearance without hyperemia or papillae activity. Lid tension was typical for the age of the patient and would not significantly affect contact lens wear. The tear quantity and quality was adequate to support contact lens wear. There did exist a paracentral midstromal corneal opacity in the right eye that did not interfere with vision. Fluorescein staining revealed negative staining on top of the scar location demonstrating the tissue's inability to adequately receive tears and maintain the small area wettable.

Manifest refraction:
OD: $-12.25 - 3.50 \times 70$ add $+0.75$ D
OS: $-7.50 - 1.75 \times 150$ add $+0.75$ D

Keratometry:
OD: 59.25 @ 171; 56.25 @ 81
OS: 48.12 @ 025; 47.00 @ 115

Assessment/Plan

M.B. represents a group of patients that has attempted contact lens wear many times without success. These patients reach out to practitioners with the hope that their expectations can be met. Edge lift off was exhibited upon trial fitting many soft toric lens designs. The left lens appeared to have 20% more edge lift off than the right. A search of the steepest soft toric contact lens design resulted in an unsuccessful lens–corneal fitting relationship. A discussion has held with the patient addressing the options of contact lens wear. The Macro lens or Dyna-Intralimbal GP lens was discussed with the advantage of using the peripheral cornea as the landing zone while vaulting over the central cornea. A custom-designed soft toric lens was discussed, explaining that trial lenses would be ordered and adjusted to reach a proper fitting design. The patient understood the time commitment and office time required if multiple lens orders were necessary to arrive at an appropriate contact lens–corneal relationship. The patient preferred a soft toric fitting design, although if unsuccessful would opt for a large GP lens if this modality would meet her contact lens goals.

Material Selection

The specification for the Eycon toric contact lens were as follows:

	OD	OS
Base curve	8.45 mm	8.2 mm
Diameter	14.5 mm	14.5 mm
Power	$-11.00 -2.25$	$-7.25 -1.75$
	$\times 70$	$\times 150$

Upon applying the contact lenses onto the eye, the right lens centered well with the markings positioning at 7 o'clock with very little lens movement with the blink. The left lens demonstrated edge lift off. The patient was instructed to allow the lens to settle on the eye for about 20 minutes and then a reevaluation would be performed. After approximately 20 minutes, the right eye exhibited capillary blanching and conjunctival drag due to a tight lens while the left eye still demonstrated severe lens liftoff. The right lens did not move with upward gaze and could not recenter itself after the blink. The left lens markings were moving temporally without any consistency. The lenses were removed and modifications of the fitting characteristics were reordered.

	OD	OS
Base curve	8.6 mm	7.9 mm
Diameter	14.5 mm	14.5 mm
Power	−11.00 −2.25 × 70	−7.25 −1.75 × 150

Lenses arrived at the office in approximately 2 weeks and the patient was called to make an appointment. The lenses were applied to the eyes and a biomicroscopy evaluation revealed properly centering lenses binocularly with upper movement with the blink approximately 0.5 mm with rapid centering of the lens markings at 6 o'clock. The Aosept Clear Care peroxide disinfection system was utilized to avoid lens contamination and allergic complications. The lenses were reevaluated 30 minutes later to allow sufficient time for the lens design to stabilize. Visual acuity and overrefraction revealed the following:

OD: plano −0.50 × 70 20/25
OS: plano −0.50 × 150 20/25

Summary

This case demonstrates the principal lens fit characteristics affecting lens orientation were postblink movement and lens tightness (5). Very loose toric lenses exhibit no consistency in lens movement and cannot influence axis determination. Lens movement influence axis location through recovery after the blink. Without any lens movement, proper axis alignment is not possible unless the lens is properly orientated from initial lens placement. A properly fitted toric lens will induce some postblink movement associated with stable lens orientation.

To determine the proper fitting characteristics in a complex astigmatic case, a trial lens fitting will lead you to the proper custom soft contact lens fitting relationship. Some of the complex toric cases will not lend themselves to an empirical fitting. The custom toric fitting option allows for flexibility in ordering base curve and diameter selection. The anatomy of the lids and the effects of the blink will have a significant effect on lens location and rotation. In-

complete lid closure may cause lens dehydration and increase deposit formation inferiorly, affecting lens positioning and wearing time. Smaller palpebral apertures exert less influence on the rotation characteristics of the lens and create a more stable lens orientation. The mnemonic LARS is used to determine the axis compensation when the marking of the lens drifts away from their proper orientation. Poor centration can also cause a degrading visual effect that can be compensated by ordering a larger or steeper lens design. Retinoscopy or corneal topography over the soft toric lens will demonstrate poor draping characteristics of the soft lens resulting in irregularities in the optical zone producing unstable and poor vision. Flattening the base curve or using a thinner lens design will cause the lens to drape over the cornea more smoothly resulting in improved vision.

The soft toric lens option does not have to be abandoned because the patient fitting characteristics fall outside the normal stock toric lens parameters. Trial fitting will lead you to the appropriate fitting parameters if you utilize some of the normal soft toric fitting rules. Many practitioners abandon the soft toric contact lens modality when stock lenses do not fulfill the fitting criteria. This case represents how a customized soft toric lens can be a last fitting option.

Low Refractive Cylinder

Initial Summary

An out-of-state practitioner called my office concerned about one of his patients performing a 3-month intern project in Chicago under the guidance of Duke University. The patient called the practitioner complaining that something was wrong with her vision. The left eye was blurred with her glasses and her contact lenses. The practitioner wanted me to rule out any retinal involvement. L.G. is on no medications, although does have allergies to amoxicillin and Septra. L.G. has no family history of glaucoma, macular degeneration, hypertension, or diabetes.

Present Rx:
OD: −3.00 DS
OS: −3.00 DS

Present contact lens specification: Biomedics 55 Ocufilcon

	Base Curve	Diameter	Power
OD	8.6 mm	14.2 mm	−2.75 D
OS	8.6 mm	14.2 mm	−3.00 D

L.G. has been wearing Biomedics 55 for 3 years and uses Opti-Free disinfection system. Visual acuity with contact lenses and spectacles were 20/20 monocularly although the left eye vision was more distorted than the right.

Ocular Evaluation

Pupils were equal round and reactive to direct, consensual, and accommodative reflexes. There was no sign of an afferent pupil defect in either eye. Extraocular muscle movements were full and smooth in all directions of gaze in both eyes. Lid appearance was tight and exhibited no swelling, injection, congestion, or granulations. Upon pressure to the meibomian glands on the lid margin, normal contents were expressed. The sclera exhibited no inflammation or congestion. Lenticular evaluation illustrated clear media. The inferior tear meniscus was adequate in height to support contact lens wear.

Keratometry:
OD: 43.75 @ 180; 44.87 @ 090
OS: 44.12 @ 180; 45.25 @ 090

Corneal topography (Fig. 47.2)

Distance VA uncorrected:
OD: 20/200 near J1
OS: 20/200 near J1

Subjective:
OD: $-3.25 - 0.75 \times 175 \ 20/15 \ J1$
OS: $-3.50 - 0.75 \times 005 \ 20/15 \ J1$

Tear break-up time:
OD: 22 seconds
OS: 24 seconds

Biomicroscopy

The anterior chamber was clear in both eyes. Fluorescein staining revealed intact corneas without defects. Neither eye exhibited any signs of neovascularization or edema. Iris shape, color, and size were free of pathology and abnormalities. Lid eversion revealed smooth satin appearance of tarsal conjunctiva without hyperemia, papillae, or follicles.

Retinal Evaluation

Dilated pupil examination performed utilizing binocular indirect ophthalmoscopy and slit-lamp examination with the Volk 90-D lens. This examination revealed normal maculae free of atrophic changes; a positive macular reflex; no drusen, exudates or hemorrhages; and healthy peripheral retinal structures. The retinal vasculature was normal and consistent with age. The vasculature did not show hemorrhages or exudates. No lesions, breaks, tears, or degeneration were noted. Optic nerve exhibited normal color, size, and shape with intact neuroretinal rims 360 degrees. Flat and sharp borders were noted, as well as a normal appearance of nerve fiber layer OU. The vitreous body was clear and fully attached

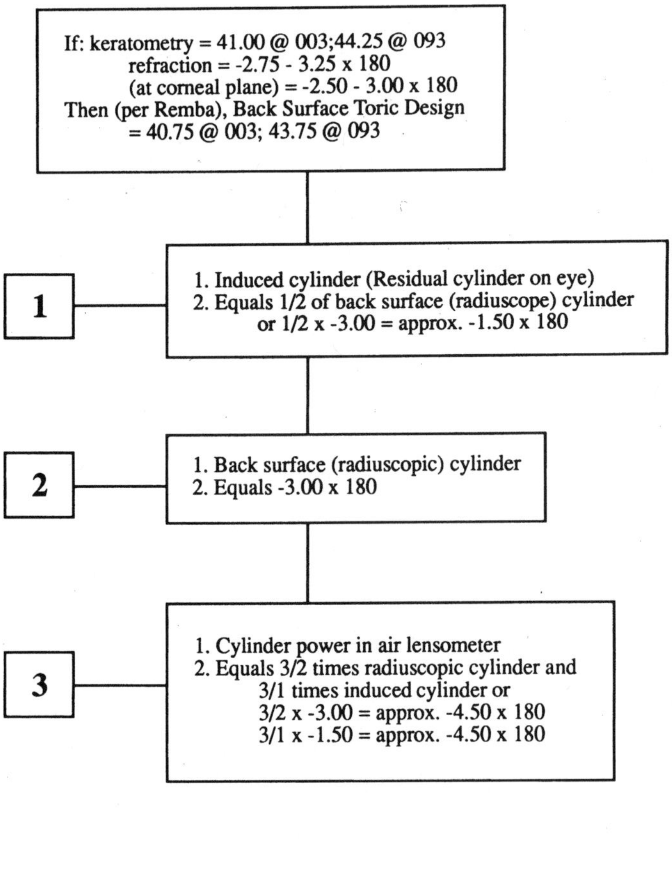

FIG. 47.2. The 1:2:3 Principle. (From Bennett ES, Blaze P, Remba MR. Correction of astigmatism. In: Bennett ES, Henry VA, eds. Clinical manual of contact lenses, 2nd ed. Philadelphia: Lippincott Williams & Wilkins, 2000:351–409, with permission.)

Material Selection

L.G. has a low degree of astigmatism in her present prescription. The spectacle lenses and contact lenses do not correct for the astigmatism found in her present refraction. Undetected prior to the realization of the blur, L.G. thought there was something pathologically wrong with her eyes. L.G. was going back home in 1 week, so we decided to provide a disposable toric soft lenses until her previous doctor could evaluate her.

Lens Specifica-tions Biomedics	OD	OS
Base curve	8.7 mm	8.7 mm
Diameter	14.5 mm	14.5 mm
Power	−3.00 −0.75 × 180	−3.25 −0.75 × 180
Visual acuity distance	20/15	20/15
Visual acuity near	J1	J1
Overrefraction	Plano	Plano

I decided to provide the same material that she was wearing successfully to avoid any material complication while she is finishing her intern project in Chicago. Upon applying the new prescription, L.G. commented that the vision in her left eye was pristine and that the pressure above her eyes had been relieved. We discussed that since she will not be coming back to Chicago it seems reasonable that her previous doctor finish the fitting process. We allowed the lenses to settle on her eyes for approximately 30 minutes and reevaluated the lens positioning and subjective opinion of the vision. After the trial lens had an opportunity to stabilize, the lens marker had remained at the 6-o'clock position with less than 1 mm of movement. The patient's subjective response was consistent with the resolution of the visual complaint.

Summary

This case demonstrates the importance of correcting astigmatism equal to 0.75 D or greater. These astigmatic patients, often through a routine examination, have vague complaints that can be resolved by correcting the astigmatism. Patients can accept an uncorrected amount of astigmatism although asthenopia may exist. A small degree of uncorrected astigmatism will perceptually change sight although it will not render vision distorted. These patients often have symptoms of fatigue, accommodative spasms, convergence excess, or variable vision. Compensatory reactions to the uncorrected astigmatic error will often lead to accommodative dysfunction.

Toric soft lenses in the ametropic market fail to be represented when correcting 0.75 D of astigmatism or greater.

The soft toric market should account for 35% of the lenses instead of approximately 16%. Practitioners perceive that soft toric lenses are more difficult to fit, require more chair time, and create more variable vision. With advances in the lens design, repeatable performance, and frequent replacement, practitioners have greater choices to find the optimal lens modality for their patients. Patients deserve the right to choose between the advantages of toric lenses versus the advantages of spherical lenses. Disposable lenses have improved our ability to challenge our patients with new and improved designs.

Soft Lens and Keratoconus

Initial Summary

S.D. has seen four different practitioners attempting to obtain a prescription that will allow him to see. He has no preference between contact lenses or spectacles. Previous practitioners have told S.D. that he has keratoconus. S.D. has unsuccessfully worn GP spherical lenses, GP bitorics, SoftPerm, and spectacles in an effort to improve his visual acuity. Contact lenses have been unsuccessful because of discomfort, and spectacles have not provided adequate vision. S.D. complained of glare, ghosting, and doubling of vision with glasses. S.D. is a 29-year-old man who owns a car wash business. He is frequently wet and dirty at the end of the day. His environment is prime for an ocular infection with contact lenses if cleaning and disinfection instructions are not carefully followed. He has no ocular history, and S.D. takes no medication. His father has a history of heart disease. S.D. commented that practitioners do not listen to his problems of obtaining a usable prescription. None of the attempts to provide adequate vision have been successful because the doctors provide devices without partnering with the patient to develop an action plan.

Unaided visual acuity:
OD: 20/300
OS: 20/400

Manifest refraction:
OD: −6.00 −8.00 × 085 20/30
OS: −8.00 −8.00 × 070 20/25

Keratometry:
OD: 47.75 @170 51.75 @ 080
OS: 45.75 @ 160 51.75 @ 070

Biomicroscopy

Eyelids and adnexa were free of pathology. Munson sign was evident on downward gaze. Cilia were free of debris. Lid eversion exhibited normal satin appearance of the palpebral conjunctiva without hyperemia or staining. Epithelial edema was noted with a loss of corneal luster observed.

Bulbar conjunctiva was slightly hyperemic (1+) without signs of inflammation. Cornea exhibited normal tear film, adequate to support contact lenses. Cornea demonstrated stromal thinning, vertical Vogt's striae, and a brownish Fleischer's ring was observed at the base of the cone. Anterior chambers were deep and without signs of cells and flare.

Ophthalmoscopy

Abnormal red oil droplet reflex was observed typical of keratoconus.

Phenol red thread test:
OD: 19 mm
OS: 18 mm

Tear break-up time:
OD: 22 seconds
OS: 21 seconds

Assessment/Plan

Previously S.D. has been unsuccessful seeking contact lens wear. S.D. requires a prescription to correct his compound myopic astigmatic correction. Keratoconus is usually defined as a deformity of the cornea in which it becomes cone shaped due to a thinning and stretching of the tissue in its central area. Since the cornea thins centrally and presents an irregular shape, an unusual light reflex or teary appearance will be the result of the corneal distortion. Eyeglasses are unable to provide adequate vision because of the irregular surface topography. Keratoconus is suspected when frequent changes in glass prescription, requiring more correction for nearsightedness with a marked increase in astigmatism. Keratoconus patients may complain of poor vision through their spectacles, such as monocular diplopia, photophobia asthenopia, headaches, halos around lights, and reduced contrast sensitivity. The only nonsurgical method to provide effective vision is the wearing of contact lenses. Historically it is thought that contact lenses may either stop or slow the progression of keratoconus, but there has never been a definitive study to substantiate this belief.

The treatment plan centers on the fitting of this anomaly with contact lenses replacing the irregular corneal surface with uniform contact lens-tear film-cornea sandwich. Applying a contact lens on the irregular keratoconic cornea surface can lead to problems associated with reduced visual acuity, fluctuating visual acuity, lens discomfort, corneal staining, and scarring. Haptic lenses and penetrating keratoplasty are treatment options reserved for the most problematic cases.

Spherical lenses are usually perfectly acceptable on large amounts of cornea toricity due to the toricity confined to a small region of the cone. The superior peripheral corneal portion of the keratoconus patient is relatively regular and often appears flatter than normal. As keratoconus progresses, the cornea steepens and the apex decenters inferi-

orly. When spherical GP lenses are fit on a highly toric cornea, flexure can create visual difficulties. The difficulty always exists with steep corneal topography accompanying high amounts of irregular corneal astigmatism with a decentered inferior temporal or inferior nasal cone. Specially designed GP lenses can neutralize the power differential across the cornea. Therefore, a GP contact lens will counteract the distortion and irregularity of the corneal surface, resulting in improved visual acuity compared to spectacle or hydrogel modalities.

Several contact lens designs have been commonly used for the treatment of this corneal anomaly. The various fitting philosophies include soft toric lenses, aspheric GP lenses, three point touch GP lenses, large flat GP lenses, apical clearance GP lenses, piggyback lenses, and SoftPerm lenses. S.D. had tried them all with the exception of soft toric hydrophilic lenses. A discussion was held with the patient explaining the time commitment and office time required to achieve a successful conclusion with the use of soft toric lenses. I had the advantage of listening to all of S.D.'s failures with contact lenses. We discussed that a new option would be tried. To avoid further frustration with contact lenses, we decided to proceed with a soft toric contact lens fitting.

In order to meet S.D.'s goals, a modality that included low risk for ocular complications and the acknowledgment that his hygiene is not meticulous directed us to fit a frequent-replacement lens. A frequent-replacement daily-wear soft toric lens will provide him a margin of safety by replacing the lenses every 3 months. The strategy of replacing the lenses every 3 months will help avert the risk of ocular complications. A decision was made to fit S.D. with Coopers Option Hydrasoft frequent-replacement lens.

	Base Curve	Diameter	Power	Visual Acuity
OD	8.9 mm	15.0 mm	−6.00 −8.00 × 090	20/25
OS	8.9 mm	15.0 mm	−7.00 −8.00 × 070	20/40

At the dispensing visit, the lenses were applied and allowed to settle on the eye for approximately 20 minutes. S.D. was instructed to clean and disinfect the lenses with the Aosept method because of his work environment and questionable hygiene. This method included an enzyme treatment as well as a daily rub regimen with a surfactant cleaner. Slit-lamp biomicroscopy was performed to observe the fit and rotational characteristics of the lens design. The lenses moved 1 mm with the blink although the left lens 10 degrees to the left. The LARS method was applied and the lenses were reordered. The lenses were dispensed and a reappointment was scheduled to dispense the corrected left lens axis.

	Base Curve	Diameter	Power
OS:	8.9 mm	15.0 mm	−7.00 −8.00 × 080

Visual acuity: 20/25

Summary

The treatment plan centers on fitting this patient with soft toric contact lenses. Problems created by placing a soft toric contact lens on this irregular cornea surface range from reduced and/or fluctuating visual acuity from a improper corneal contact lens fitting relationship. The conservative approach would be to fit this patient with a GP lens. It was actually an advantage to have four previous doctors failing to reach an acceptable fit. Therefore, it was decided to employ a lens design not used previously and incorporate basic soft toric lens fitting rules to reach an acceptable outcome. Managing the patient's attitude towards contact lenses is as important as the fit and the design. Fitting this patient with a soft toric lens design improved his motivation by attempting to fit a lens he had not yet experienced.

Keratoconus is a noninflammatory progressive conical deformity of the central portion of the cornea. In advanced cases, spectacles cannot adequately correct the astigmatism. A GP contact lens in effect replaces the cones irregularity with a smooth, regular optical surface. However, due to mechanical trauma and poor centration caused by the GP contact lens, central trauma and discomfort can occur. Occasionally treatment with soft toric lenses can be the lens of choice. Utilizing the basic soft toric fitting rules will provide a successful outcome.

GAS-PERMEABLE TORIC CORRECTION

The first section pertains to correction of residual astigmatism. As emphasized elsewhere in this volume, there are many options of correction of residual astigmatism. If the patient has minimal to no refractive cylinder, spherical soft lenses are indicated. Likewise, if the patient is motivated for soft lenses and has 0.75 to 2.00 D of with-the-rule or against-the-rule refractive astigmatism, soft toric lenses are a viable option. Nevertheless, a need still exists for rigid lens correction of residual astigmatism with front-surface toric lenses for persons who are satisfied spherical GP lens wearers but could benefit by correction of their residual astigmatism and for persons who are good soft lens candidates. In addition, there are a small, but significant, number of patients in whom residual astigmatism can be corrected, at least in part, by a flexing spherical rigid lens.

Most of this section will pertain to correction of high corneal astigmatism. Traditionally, it has been the opinion of many practitioners that spherical GP lenses should be used to correct as much corneal astigmatism as possible because of the simplicity of the design and the lesser expense involved. However, when spherical lenses are fit on high corneal astigmatism (typically >2.50 D), several problems occur, such as flexure (6), decentration (7), and corneal curvature changes, including warpage (7,8). It is important to understand that even when the lens is exhibiting good centration in a patient with high astigmatism, the absence of alignment caused by excessive regions of bearing and clearance can have undesirable effects on both corneal topography and blink quality. A bitoric lens is the optimum correction option in these cases and typically involves a design and fit similar to those required for a spherical GP lens.

Case 1: Residual Astigmatism—Flexure

Initial Summary

A 32-year-old male teacher was interested in new contact lenses. He was a 12-year GP lens wearer who was satisfied with the comfort and wettability of his lenses. However, his vision was slightly blurry and he experienced symptoms of eyestrain after prolonged reading. Pertinent examination information was as follows:

Visual acuity with contact lenses:
OD: 20/25–2 Overrefraction: $+0.25 - 1.00 \times 095$ 20/20 + 2
OS: 20/25–1 Overrefraction: $+0.50 - 1.00 \times 090$ 20/20 + 2

Biomicroscopy with contact lenses:
OD: inferior decentration; mild with-the-rule astigmatic fluorescein pattern
OS: identical to OD

Manifest refraction:
OD: $-2.25 - 1.00 \times 003$ 20/15–2
OS: $-2.00 - 0.75 \times 180$ 20/15–2

Keratometry:
OD: 41.75 @180; 43.75 @090
OS: 42.00 @180; 44.00 @090

Current lens parameters:

	OD	OS
Material	Paraperm 02	Paraperm 02
Power	−2.25 D	−2.00 D
Overall/optical zone diameter	9.0/7.6 mm	9.0/7.6 mm
Base curve radius	8.04 mm	8.08 mm
Secondary curve radius/width	9.4/0.3 mm	9.4/0.3 mm
Peripheral curve radius/width	12.25/0.4 mm	12.25/0.4 mm
Center thickness	0.16 mm	0.15 mm

Assessment/Plan

The blurred vision is the result of residual astigmatism. Because residual astigmatism with rigid contact lens wear is obtained by subtracting the keratometric astigmatism from the refractive astigmatism, the predicted residual astigmatism would equal:

* OD $-1.00 - (-)2.00 \times 180 = +1.00 \times 180$ or $+1.00 - 1.00 \times 090$
* OS: $-0.75 - (-)2.00 \times 180 = +1.25 \times 180$ or $+1.00 - 1.25 \times 090$

These results are comparable to the overrefraction (i.e., OD $= -1.00 \times 095$; OS $= -1.00 \times 090$). Another possible cause is warpage; however, the base curve radii were verified as spherical. The following diagnostic lenses were used:

	OD	OS
Material	Fluorocon	Fluorocon
Power	−3.00 D	−3.00 D
Overall/optical zone diameter	9.5/8.4 mm	9.5/8.4 mm
Base curve radius	7.99 mm	7.94 mm
Center thickness	0.10 mm	0.10 mm

Biomicroscopy with contact lenses:
OD: good centration; slight apical clearance
OS: similar to OD

Overrefraction:
OD: $+0.50 - 0.25 \times 090$ 20/20+2 $+0.50$ DS 20/20+1
OS: $+0.50 - 0.25 \times 085$ 20/20 +1 $+0.50$ DS 20/20

Overkeratometry:
OD: 39.25 @ 180: 40.00 @ 090
OS: 39.50 @ 180: 40.50 @ 090

Contact lenses ordered:

	OD	OS
Material	Fluorocon	Fluorocon
Power	−2.50 D	−2.50 D
Overall/optical zone diameter	9.5/8.4 mm	9.5/8.4 mm
Base curve radius	7.99 mm	7.94 mm
Center thickness	0.12 mm	0.12 mm

Alternative Management/Summary

This lens design was able to provide improved visual acuity relative to the previous lenses because of the ability of lens flexure to correct most of the residual astigmatism. Flexure is present when both the overrefraction and overkeratometry exhibit cylinder but no warpage is present via the radiuscope. It has been found that when the corneal toricity is with-the-rule and the residual astigmatism is against-the-rule, a thin spherical lens will flex and reduce the amount of residual astigmatism (9). Not only is center thickness

important, but selecting a steeper than "K" base curve radius will induce flexure on a with-the-rule astigmatic cornea. Likewise, selection of a large optical zone diameter (OZD) is more likely to induce flexure (10). The Fluorocon 9.5-mm-diameter lens is optimum in these cases because of its thin lens design, large OZD, and high [60] oxygen permeability. When this lens is fit steeper than "K" on a with-the-rule astigmatic cornea, flexure is very likely the result.

Although these cases are relatively uncommon, if this form of residual astigmatism is present (especially with an otherwise successful rigid lens wearer), a spherical lens is most likely to provide good vision and an optimum lens-to-cornea fitting relationship. A soft toric lens is another good option; however, in an otherwise successful GP wearer, it is often preferable to continue wear of a similar material. A front-surface toric GP lens is another option, but the increased mass due to the prism ballast can create a series of other problems, including blurred vision, discomfort, poor optics, corneal desiccation, and asthenopia (11).

Case 2: Residual Astigmatism—Front-surface Toric

Initial Summary

A 26-year-old woman wanted to be refit with a new pair of contact lenses. She previously wore disposable soft extended-wear lenses and had a history of complications, including GPC, neovascularization, and, most recently, a peripheral corneal ulcer. She discontinued contact lens wear 4 weeks earlier for treatment of the corneal ulcer. Once it had resolved, resulting in a small scar in that region, she was receptive to a refit into daily-wear GP lenses.

Manifest refraction:
OD: $+2.50 - 1.75 \times 173$ 20/20
OS: $+3.00 - 2.00 \times 010$ 20/20

Keratometry:
OD: 41.25 @180; 42.00 @090
OS: 41.50 @180; 42.50 @090

Lid-to-cornea relationship:
OU: upper lid positioned approximately 1 mm over superior limbus; lower lid positioned at lower limbus

Assessment/Plan

The following residual astigmatism would be predicted in this case:

OD: $-1.75 - (-)0.75 \times 180 = -1.00 \times 180$
OS: $-2.00 - (-)1.00 \times 180 = -1.00 \times 180$

Although this amount of residual astigmatism with spherical GP lens application should result in compromised vision, it is recommended that one apply diagnostic lenses to determine if the predicted amount of residual astigmatism equals the actual amount. Because this amount of residual astigmatism is uncommon, it is important to rule out other factors. If diagnostic fitting of a spherical GP lens results in little or no residual astigmatism, it is likely that the refraction and/or keratometry values were inaccurate.

The following diagnostic lenses were used:

	OD	OS
Material	Fluoroperm 60	Fluoroperm 60
Power	+3.00 D	+3.00 D
Overall/optical zone diameter	9.4/8.0 mm	9.4/8.0 mm
Base curve radius	8.18 mm	8.13 mm

Biomicroscopy with contact lenses:
OU: both lenses moved excessively and decentered interiorly.

Overrefraction:
OD: $-0.25 - 1.00 \times 175$ 20/20+1
OS: $+0.25 - 1.00 \times 180$ 20/20+2

As a result of the residual astigmatism with contact lens wear, it was decided to order front-surface toric GP lenses. Because no diagnostic fitting set was available, the following lenses were ordered empirically (letters in parentheses refer to information in paragraphs that follow):

	OD	OS
Material(a)	Fluoroperm 60	Fluoroperm 60
Power(b)	$+1.75 + 1.00 \times 070$	$+2.25 + 1.00 \times 105$
Overall diameter (OAD)(c)	9.4/9.0 mm	9.4/9.0 mm
Base curve radius	8.18 mm	8.13 mm
Secondary curve radius/width	9.2/0.3 mm	9.2/0.3 mm
Peripheral curve radius/width	11.2/0.3 mm	11.2/0.3 mm
Center thickness:	0.36 mm	0.36 mm
Prism(c)	1.25 PD	1.25 PD

Double dot OD

(a) All plus power and/or prism-ballast lenses require a high-Dk (i.e., >50) GP material to allow sufficient oxygen transmission to meet the Holden-Mertz criteria for an edema-free corneal environment (12).

(b) The overrefraction was added to the diagnostic lens power to obtain the lens power:

OD: $+3.00 + (-0.25 - 1.00 \times 175) = +2.75 - 1.00 \times 175$

Transpose to plus cylinder form because plus cylinder will be added to the front surface of the lens:
$= +1.75 + 1.00 \times 085$

Compensate for approximate 15 degrees excyclorotation (by way of LARS [rotation to the left, add; rotation to the right, subtract] principle):

$= +1.75 + 1.00 \times 070$

OS: $+3.00 + (+0.25 - 1.00 \times 180)$
$= +3.25 - 1.00 \times 180$
$= +2.25 + 1.00 \times 090$
$= +2.25 + 1.00 \times 105$

(c) A truncated design should add stability, and a lower lid positioned at the lower limbus or above should allow the truncation to align with the lower lid. Because truncating a plus lens actually increases the ballast of a GP lens, less prism is required than with a minus lens. Therefore, 1 to 1.25 PD should be sufficient to provide adequate pupil coverage. A 9.4-mm horizontal and a 9.0-mm vertical diameter were selected. The OZD should be slightly decentered superiorly for optimum visual performance.

(d) Determination of center thickness can also be calculated with the following formula (13):

* Center thickness $\times$ 100 = prismatic power $\times$ OAD

In this case, the center thickness of a +2.00-D spherical lens is approximately 0.25 mm; therefore:

* (Center thickness added to 0.25 mm) $\times$ 100
$= 1.25$ PD $\times$ 9.0 mm
* $= 0.1125$ mm $\times$ 100 $= 11.25$

Therefore, adding 0.11 to 0.25 mm equals 0.36 mm

In addition, the base of the prism of the right lens should be double dotted; the left prism base could be identified by a single dot. A minus lenticular can be considered if the lens does not exhibit movement with the blink.

Approximately 1 mm of movement is recommended.

Alternative Management/Summary

Although the applications of front-surface toric lenses are few (as a result of improvements in soft toric quality and parameter availability), this option should be considered in a patient exhibiting residual astigmatism who has experienced soft lens–induced complications. The aforementioned limitations of front-surface toric lens designs also limit their use. However, in this case, the reduced oxygen transmission of a soft toric lens as compared with a high-Dk GP lens material could result in further complications. In addition, if a spherical lens is used and flexes, the induced astigmatism would add to the residual astigmatism already present.

Case 3: Residual Astigmatism—Front-surface Toric

Initial Summary

A 17-year-old female patient who was a 2-year wearer of a low-Dk GP lens material had symptoms of blur while driving at night. In addition, she mentioned that her eyes were tired after prolonged reading.

Visual acuity with contact lenses:
OD: 20/25–2 overrefraction: $+0.25 -1.25 \times 175$ 20/15–2
OS: 20/25 overrefraction: plano -1.00×180 20/20

Biomicroscopy with contact lenses:
OU: good centration with an alignment lens-to cornea fitting relationship.

Manifest refraction (spectacle plane):
OD: $-4.75 -2.00 \times 180$ 20/15–1
OS: $-5.00 -1.75 \times 005$ 20/20+2

Manifest refraction (corneal plane):
OD: $-4.50 -1.75 \times 180$
OS: $-4.75 -1.50 \times 005$

Keratometry:
OD: 43.00 @180; 43.50 @090
OS: 43.25 @180; 43.75 @090

Lid-to-cornea relationship:
OU: The lower lid was positioned approximately 1 mm below the lower limbus. The lids also appeared to be rather flaccid or loose.

Current contact lens specifications:

	OD	OS
Material	Fluorex 300	Fluorex 300
Power:	-5.00 D	-5.00 D
Overall/optical zone diameter	9.2/7.8 mm	9.2/7.8 mm
Base curve radius	7.89 mm	7.85 mm

Assessment/Plan

Because the patient was satisfied with GP lens wear, other than for critical vision needs, front-toric lenses were prescribed. The astigmatic overrefraction appeared to be the result of residual astigmatism because no base curve toricity was present with verification. Because this patient exhibited

a good fitting relationship with her present lenses and a front-surface toric fitting set was not available, these lenses were used as a starting point for empirically designing the front-toric lenses. The following lenses were ordered (letters in parentheses refer to paragraphs that follow):

	OD	OS
Material	Fluorex 700	Fluorex 700
Power(a)	$-6.00 +1.25$ $\times 070$	$-6.00 +1.00$ $\times 105$
Overall diameter (OAD)	9.4 mm	9.4 mm
Base curve radius	7.89 mm	7.85 mm
Secondary curve radius/width	9.00 mm	9.00 mm
Peripheral curve radius/width	11.00 mm	11.00 mm
Center thickness(b)	0.24 mm	0.24 mm
Prism (c)	1 PD	1 PD

(a) Similar to Case 2, once the overrefraction is added to the patient's contact lens power, the values are:

OD: $-5.00 + (+0.25 - 1.25 \times 175) = -4.75 -1.25 \times 175$
OS: $-5.00 + (\text{plano} -1.00 \times 180) = -5.00 -1.00 \times 180$

Once these values have been transposed and allowance for probable rotation has occurred, the aforementioned powers are derived.

(b) Using the Borish equation:

* Center thickness $\times 100 =$ prismatic power $\times$ OAD
*100 $\times = 1 \times 9.4 = 0.094$ mm

If the center thickness of a -5.00-D spherical lens is 0.15 mm, the predicted center thickness of the lenses should equal:
0.15 + 0.09 = 0.24 mm

(c) Because a high-minus lens already has a relatively thick edge, a lower amount of prism is necessary than with either a plus-powered prism-ballast-only design or a high-minus prism-ballast/truncated design. A prism-ballast-only method for stabilization was selected as a result of the position of the lower lid. It is unlikely that a truncated lens would exhibit sufficient inferior decentration to rest on the lower lid.

Alternative Management/Summary

If a truncated lens design is not indicated because of a low lower lid position and/or loose lids, the use of a prism-ballast-only design should be successful. If this lens rotates excessively, the use of a flatter base curve radius and an increase in the amount of prism should provided greater stability. As with the previous case, a spherical GP lens (designed to flex) will only increase the amount of uncorrected astigmatism. A soft toric lens is a viable alternative if a front-surface toric lens does not provide satisfactory vision or comfort.

Case 4: High Astigmatism—Aspheric Lens Design

Initial Summary

A 14-year-old female student desired to wear contact lenses. She was a spectacle wearer for 4 years and desired contact lenses for cosmesis and because she was tired of wearing sports goggles for basketball and soccer. Her refractive findings were as follows:

Manifest refraction:
OD: −2.50 −1.75 × 095 20/20
OS: −2.00 −2.00 × 080 20/20

Keratometry:
OD: 42.25 @090; 44.00 @180
OS: 42.50 @085; 44.50 @175

Biomicroscopy

No signs of ocular disease were present. Tear volume and quality were normal.

Assessment/Plan

As a result of the degree of myopia and the probable trend to wear decreasing refractive error, diagnostic fitting with rigid lenses was attempted. The first diagnostic lenses were as follows:

OD: base curve radius (BCR): 7.95 mm; OAD: 9.2 mm; power −3.00 D; material: Boston ES
OS: BCR: 7.85 mm; OAD: 9.2 mm; power: −3.00 D; material: Boston ES

Biomicroscopy with Contact Lenses

Both lenses decentered temporally and provided poor pupillary coverage. A second diagnostic fitting was performed with the Boston Envision biaspheric lens design. The following lenses were selected:

OD: BCR: 8.00 mm; OAD: 9.6 mm; power: −3.00 D
OS: BCR: 7.90 mm; OAD: 9.6 mm; power: −3.00 D

Both lenses provided good vertical centration with the blink. A slight temporal decentration was still evident; however, this was less than with the spherical design and was considered acceptable. A very mild against-the-rule astig-matic pattern was present with greater pooling of fluorescein in the horizontal than in the vertical meridian. Approximately 1 mm of movement was present with straight-ahead gaze in both eyes.

Overrefraction:
OD: −0.50 DS 20/20
OS: −0.75 DS 20/20

The following lenses were ordered:

	OD	OS
Material/design	Boston XO/ Boston Envision	Boston XO Boston Envision
Power	−2.50 D	−2.25 D
OAD	9.6 mm	9.6 mm
Base curve radius	8.0 mm	7.9 mm

Alternative Management/Summary

It may be difficult in moderate against-the-rule astigmatic patients to obtain a successful lens-to-cornea fitting relationship. A soft toric lens would be an acceptable option, especially if the patient is motivated for soft lenses or if good centration cannot be achieved with a GP lens. The benefits of astigmatic correction and slowing down the progression of myopia make a GP lens a very desirable option for young people. Although lens dislodgement and loss are possible with young athletes, the selection of a large-diameter lens with a uniform (not high) edge clearance and limited movement with the blink minimizes this problem.

An aspheric lens design was indicated because GP lenses tend to follow the steeper corneal meridian. In with-the-rule astigmatic corneas, the lenses follow the vertical meridian. However, in against-the-rule astigmatism, they follow the horizontal meridian, sometimes resulting in symptoms of flare. An aspheric design can sometimes minimize this problem by providing better alignment of lens-to-cornea with less horizontal displacement. Likewise, in patients exhibiting a moderate amount (but less than 2.5 D) of corneal astigmatism, an aspheric lens will often result in closer alignment than will a spherical design.

Case 5: Gas-permeable Bitoric—Empirical Fitting

Initial Summary

A 19-year-old female patient had a history of lens awareness and intermittent adherence with spherical GP lenses. At the time of this visit, she had been wearing spectacles for the past 3 months.

The following refractive findings were recorded:

Manifest refraction (spectacle plane):
OD: −2.25 −3.50 × 175 20/20
OS: −2.75 −3.75 × 180 20/20

Manifest refraction (corneal plane):
OD: $-2.25 -3.00 \times 175$
OS: $-2.75 -3.25 \times 180$

Keratometry (sim K values from topography):
OD: 40.75 @178; 43.75 @088
OS: 41.00 @003; 44.25 @093

Biomicroscopy with Contact Lenses

The cornea, conjunctivae, tear film, and external findings were unremarkable.

Assessment/Plan

As a result of the high refractive cylinder with essential no residual component, it was decided to fit this patient with bitoric GP lenses. Because no diagnostic fitting set was available, empirical determination of the lens design was performed.

1. Base curve radii

   The base curve radii were selected using Remba's philosophy (1,14) (Table 47.1). With this system the following base curve radii were selected:

   OD: 40.50/43.25   OS: 40.75/43.75

2. Power

   There are three methods that can be used to determine the desired bitoric powers. These include the use of optical crosses, computational using Sarver's formula (15), and computational considering this design as two spherical designs.

   a. Optical cross. This is illustrated in Figure 47.1.
   b. Sarver's formula: $Fs = Ff + (Kf - Ks)$, where:
      - Fs = back vertex power (BVP) in steep meridian
      - Ff = BVP in flat meridian
      - Ks = BCR in steep medidian
      - Kf = BCR in flat meridian

   Right eye:
   $$BCR = 40.50(8.33 \text{ mm})/43.25(7.80 \text{ mm})$$
   $$Ff = -2.25 + \text{tear lens correction}$$
   $$= -2.25 + (+)0.25$$
   $$= -2.00 \text{ D}$$
   $$Fs = Ff + (Kf - Ks)$$
   $$= -2.00 + (40.50 - 43.25)$$
   $$= -2.00 + (-)2.75$$
   $$= -4.75 \text{ D}$$

TABLE 47.1. REMBA BASE CURVE SELECTION FOR BACK AND BITORIC RIGID DESIGNS (14)

Corneal Astigmatism	Flat Meridian	Steep Meridian
2 D	Fit 0.25 D flat	Fit 0.25 D flat
3 D	Fit 0.25 D flat	Fit 0.50 D flat
4 D	Fit 0.25 D flat	Fit 0.75 D flat
5 D	Fit 0.50 D flat	Fit 0.75 D flat

Left eye:
$$BCR = 40.75(8.28 \text{ mm})/43.75(7.71 \text{ mm})$$
$$Ff = -2.75 + \text{tear lens correction}$$
$$= -2.75 + (+0.25)$$
$$= -2.50 \text{ D}$$
$$Fs = Ff + (Kf - Ks)$$
$$= -2.50 + (40.75 - 43.75)$$
$$= -2.50 + (-3.00)$$
$$= -5.50 \text{ D}$$

   c. Consider as two spherical lenses:
      Essentially, a bitoric lens can be considered as two separate spherical designs With tear lens calculations in the horizontal and vertical meridians.

   Right eye:
   BCR: 40.50(8.33 mm)/43.25(7.80 mm)
   Using "SAM/FAP" (i.e., steep add minus/flat add plus), the powers become 0.25 D more plus in the horizontal meridian and 0.75 D more plus in the vertical meridian:
   $$-2.25 + (+)0.25 = -2.00 \text{ D}$$
   $$-5.25 + (+)0.50 = -4.75 \text{ D}$$

   Left eye:
   BCR: 40.75(8.28 mm)/43.75(7.71 mm)

   Using "SAM/FAP," the powers become 0.25 D more plus in the horizontal meridian and 0.50 D more plus in the vertical meridian:
   $$-2.75 + (+)0.25 = -2.50 \text{ D}$$
   $$-6.00 + (+)0.50 = -5.50 \text{ D}$$

To obtain these powers, plus cylinder will have to be provided on the front surface of the lens. A back-surface toric only lens design in situ induces a cylinder in the optical system (contact lens-fluid lens) designed to correct the ametropia. The minus cylinder is the result of the difference between the refractive index of the contact lens (n = 1.47 − 1.49 in most cases; 1.49 will be used here) and the index of the tear lens (n = 1.336) The amount would equal 0.456 (or approximately 0.5) times the back-surface toricity. The minus cylinder axis will lie along the flatter principle meridian of the toric back surface of the contact lens. The amount of cylinder power measured with the lensometer is slightly greater than three times the induced cylinder or 3/2 the back-surface toricity of the lens. This is termed the "1:2:3 Principle" (ref). As "2" (the back-surface toricity) can easily be determined through selection of the base curve radii, "1" (induced cylinder) is approximately one-half of this value, and "3" (lensometer cylinder) is approximately 3/2 this value. An example, using the left eye of this patient, is given in Figure 47.2 (1).

In this case, the amount of induced astigmatism would equal approximately one-half of -3.00×180 or -1.50×180. If a plus correcting power cylinder of the same amount and axis is applied to the front surface, in this case +1.50 × 180, a bitoric lens is created. In addition, as no residual astigmatic correction is necessary—only induced—this lens will have a spherical power effect; it can rotate on the eye without affecting vision.

3. Peripheral Curves

Either spherical or toric peripheral curves can be applied. In this particular case, as less than 4 D of corneal cylinder was present, a tricurve spherical peripheral curve system was used. This was arrived at by adding 1 mm to the mean base curve value for the secondary curve radius (SCR) and 2 mm to the SCR to arrive at the peripheral curve radius (PCR).

Right Eye	Left Eye
Mean BCR: $\frac{40.50 + 43.25}{2}$	$\frac{40.75 + 43.75}{2}$
= 42.00D (8.04 mm)	= 42.25D (7.99 mm)
SCR = 8.04 + 1 mm	SCR = 7.99 + 1 mm
= 9.04 (or 9 mm)	= 8.99 (or 9 mm)
PCR = SCR + 2 mm	PCR = SCR + 2 mm
= 9 + 2 = 11 mm	= 9 + 2 = 11 mm

4. Center Thickness

A bitoric lens is essentially a thin lens design; therefore, the center thickness should equal the thickness of the more plus-power meridian.

If, for example, a 30-Dk fluorosilicone/acrylate lens material was used and the most plus-power meridian was −2.00D OD and −2.50D OS, a center thickness of approximately 0.16 mm OD and 0.15 mm OS should be feasible.

5. Diameter

The overall diameter and optical zone diameters can be determined as with any other patient based on such factors as pupil size, vertical fissure size, corneal diameter, and corneal curvatures. In this case, average diameter and optical zone diameters of 9.4/8.2 mm were selected. The final order would therefore be:

	Material	BCR	Power
OD	FP 30	8.33/7.80 mm	−2.00/−4.75 D
OS	FP 30	8.28/7.71 mm	−2.50/−5.25 D

	OAD/OZD	SCR/W	PCR/W
	9.4/8.2 mm	9/0.3 mm	11/0.3 mm
	9.4/8.2 mm	9/0.3 mm	11/0.3 mm

Alternative Management/Summary

Other options for this patient would include soft toric lenses, back-surface toric GPs, or spherical GPs. In high refractive astigmatism, any rotation or instability of a soft toric lens can have a significant impact on vision. Unless the patient is strongly motivated for soft lens wear and understands the possibility of vision compromise, a GP lens should be selected. Back-surface toric lenses are not a viable option due to the amount of astigmatism induced by this lens design. Spherical GP lenses had already resulted in lens adherence and subjective discomfort and would not be indicated due to the high amount of corneal cylinder.

A bitoric lens design in patients with regular (not oblique) astigmatism should result in both good vision and an optimum lens-to-cornea fitting relationship. A lens material with good dimensional stability that results in undistorted optics is desired. One of the most important factors that differentiates a laboratory from its competition is the ability to manufacture a bitoric lens with good optical quality. Typically, the low-Dk (i.e., 25–50) materials are easier to fabricate in these designs. However, when higher-Dk materials are indicated, as in plus-power prescriptions, the increasing quality of toric lens manufacturing should result in little if any optical compromise.

Case 6: Bitoric Empirical Fitting—Mandell-Moore Method

Initial Summary

A 19-year-old male college student presented with the primary symptoms of lens awareness and redness resulting from rigid contact lens wear. He has been wearing GP lenses for 5 years and typically wears them during all of his waking hours.

Visual acuity (with contact lenses):
OD: 20/25 overrefraction: −0.25 − 0.75 × 163 20/20

OS: 20/25−2 overrefraction: −0.50 − 0.50 × 024 20/20

Biomicroscopy with Contact Lenses

Both contact lenses presented with a bowtie or astigmatic fluorescein pattern with horizontal bearing and vertical clearance. Both lenses were also decentered inferiorly after every blink.

His refractive findings were as follows:

Manifest refraction:
OD: −3.00 − 3.75 × 006 20/20 − 2
OS: −2.75 − 4.25 × 175 20/20 + 1
Keratometry:
OD: 42.00 @ 005; 46.25 @ 095
OS: 41.75 @ 175; 46.25 @ 085

Biomicroscopy after Lens Removal

Mildly coalesced punctate staining was present in the 3- and 9-o'clock regions of both eyes.

Contact lens parameters:

	OD	OS
BCR	7.81 × 7.90 mm	7.83 × 7.87 mm
Power	−3.50 D	−3.00 D
OAD/OZD	9.0/7.8 mm	9.0/7.8 mm
Corneal thickness (CT)	0.14 mm	0.15 mm
Material	Unknown	

RIGHT EYE

| KERATOMETRY | 42.00 | @ 005 | | 46.25 | @ 095 |
| SPECTACLE Rx (MINUS CYL FORM) | | -3.00 -3.75 | | X 006 | |

		FLATTEST K	SPHERE POWER		STEEPEST K	SPH + CYL POWER
1	ENTER K	42.00	XXXXXXXX		46.25	XXXXXXXX
2	ENTER SPECTACLE POWER		-3.00			-6.75
3	VERTEX CORRECTED		-3.00			-6.25
4	FIT FACTOR	(-) 0.25	(+) 0.25		(-) 1.00	(+) 1.00
	ADD LINES	1 & 4	3 & 4		1 & 4	3 & 4
5	FINAL C.L. Rx	41.75	-2.75		45.25	-5.25
		BASECURVE	POWER		BASECURVE	POWER

LEFT EYE

| KERATOMETRY | 41.75 | @ 175 | | 46.25 | @ 085 |
| SPECTACLE Rx (MINUS CYL FORM) | | -2.75 -4.25 | | X 175 | |

		FLATTEST K	SPHERE POWER		STEEPEST K	SPH + CYL POWER
1	ENTER K	41.75	XXXXXXXX		46.25	XXXXXXXX
2	ENTER SPECTACLE POWER		-2.75			-7.00
3	VERTEX CORRECTED		-2.75			-6.50
4	FIT FACTOR	(-) 0.25	(+) 0.25		(-) 1.00	(+) 1.00
	ADD LINES	1 & 4	3 & 4		1 & 4	3 & 4
5	FINAL C.L. Rx	41.50	-2.50		45.25	-5.50
		BASECURVE	POWER		BASECURVE	POWER

VERTEX DISTANCE CORRECTION

4.00	3.75	8.00	7.25	12.00	10.50	16.00	13.25
4.25	4.00	8.25	7.50	12.25	10.75	16.25	13.50
4.50	4.25	8.50	7.75	12.50	10.75	16.50	13.75
4.75	4.50	8.75	8.00	12.75	11.00	16.75	13.75
5.00	4.75	9.00	8.00	13.00	11.25	17.00	14.00
5.25	5.00	9.25	8.25	13.25	11.25	17.25	14.00
5.50	5.25	9.50	8.50	13.50	11.50	17.50	14.25
5.75	5.50	9.75	8.75	13.75	11.75	17.75	14.50
6.00	5.50	10.00	9.00	14.00	12.00	18.00	14.50
6.25	5.75	10.25	9.00	14.25	12.00	18.25	14.75
6.50	6.00	10.50	9.25	14.50	12.25	18.50	15.00
6.75	6.25	10.75	9.50	14.75	12.50	18.75	15.00
7.00	6.50	11.00	9.75	15.00	12.50	19.00	15.25
7.25	6.75	11.25	10.00	15.25	12.75	19.25	15.50
7.50	7.00	11.50	10.00	15.50	13.00	19.75	15.75
7.75	7.00	11.75	10.25	15.75	13.00	20.00	16.00

FIT FACTOR

CORNEAL CYL	FLAT MERIDIAN	STEEP MERIDIAN
2.0 DIOP	ON K	.50 FLATTER
2.5 "	.25 FLATTER	.50 "
3.0 "	.25 "	.75 "
3.5 "	.25 "	.75 "
4.0 "	.25 "	1.00 "
5.0 "	.25 "	1.25 "

If the spectacle lens power is less than 4.00 diopters then line 5 = line 4. Otherwise: For minus power spectacle lenses find the power in the left side of the column and convert to the power in the right side, but retain the minus sign. For plus power spectacle lenses find the power in the right side of the column and convert to the power in the left side, but retain the plus sign.

FIG. 47.3. An example of the Mandell-Moore Guide.

Assessment/Plan

The clinical signs of corneal desiccation and a poor lens-to-cornea fitting relationship in combination with the patient's symptoms of lens awareness and dryness resulted in the decision to refit the patient into a bitoric GP lens design. The moderate corneal astigmatism resulted in poor alignment of lens to cornea with a spherical design. As no diagnostic fitting set was available, the Mandell-Moore guide (16) was used to determine the lens parameters. This is an empirical fitting method that uses a simple step-by-step method to determine the bitoric base curve radii and powers. As shown in Figure 47.3, if the keratometry and refraction values are provided, the powers at the corneal plane are then determined. Next, the so-called fit factor or tear lens compensation for fitting each meridian flatter than "K" according to their table is listed. Finally, simple addition of the powers and curvature values results in the recommended

bitoric base curve radii and powers. As with Case 5, these are the powers that should be verified with a lensometer. To result in these powers, the laboratory will need to place plus cylinder power on the front surface to correct for residual and induced cylinder.

Due to the high corneal cylinder, toric peripheral curves were ordered for this patient. They were determined by simply adding 1 mm to the base curve radii to obtain the secondary curve radii and adding 2 mm to the secondary curve radii to obtain the peripheral curve radii. In this case the following parameters were ordered:

OD: BCR = 41.75 D(8.08 mm)/45.25 D(7.46 mm)
SCR = 8.08 + 1 ≅ 9.1 mm/7.46 + 1 ≅ 8.5 mm
PCR = 9.1 + 2 = 11.1 mm/8.5 + 2 = 10.5 mm

OS: BCR = 41.50 D(8.13 mm)/45.25 D(7.46 mm)
SCR = 8.13 + 1 ≅ 9.1 mm/7.46 + 1 ≅ 8.5 mm
PCR = 9.1 + 2 = 11.1 mm/8.5 + 2 = 10.5 mm

The following lenses were ordered:

	OD	OS
Material	Boston ES	Boston ES
BCR	8.08/7.46 mm	8.13/7.46 mm
Power	$-2.75/-5.25$ D	$-2.50/-5.50$ D
OAD/OZD	9.4/7.8 mm	9.4/7.8 mm
SCR/W	9.1/8.5 @ 0.4 mm	9.1/8.5 @ 0.4 mm
PCR/W	11.1/10.5 @ 0.4 mm	11.1/10.5 @ 0.4 mm
CT	0.15 mm	0.15 mm

The patient was also educated about careful cleaning of the lenses in the palm of the hand upon removal at night to minimize warpage. He admitted to cleaning them digitally between the fingers.

Alternative Management/Summary

As in Case 5, soft toric lenses could have been considered with this patient. However, if the problems induced by spherical GP lenses can be managed by a bitoric design, the benefits can be greater with GP lenses. As a college student has definite critical visual demands, any rotational instability of a soft toric lens can cause asthenopic symptoms. This case was simply a matter of improving the lens-to-cornea fitting relationship via the use of a bitoric design.

The Mandell-Moore guide is a very beneficial method for empirical determination of bitoric lens powers and base curve radii. Although the applications are limited, practitioners often perceive the determination of powers and base curve radii as complex, resulting in the use of spherical GP or soft toric lens designs. This method confirms that the calculation of these parameters should be little different than with a spherical GP lens design.

Case 7: SPE Bitoric Diagnostic Fitting

Initial Summary

A 25-year-old female teacher presented with symptoms of constant blurred vision from her contact lenses. She had been a spherical rigid lens wearer for 6 years but was refit 1 year previously into soft torics as a result of a gradual onset of lens awareness. However, she indicated that her previous practitioner only fit soft lenses and, therefore, soft torics were selected. Over the past 12 months she was refit several times but was never satisfied with her vision.

Visual acuity with contact lenses:
OD: 20/30−2 Overrefraction: $+0.50 - 1.25 \times 158$
OS: 20/25−2 Overrefraction: $+0.25 - 1.00 \times 027$

Biomicroscopy with Contact Lenses

Both lenses rotated slightly temporally; however, the amount of rotation varied with the blink. The rotational stability was poor as the resting position of the lenses varied after each blink.

Biomicroscopy after Lens Removal

The cornea, conjunctivae, and lids were unremarkable except for very mild (grade 1) papillary hypertrophy of the superior tarsal conjunctiva OU.

The refractive findings were as follows:

Manifest refraction:
OD: $-6.00 - 3.75 \times 180 \ 20/20 + 1$
OS: $-5.50 - 3.75 \times 004 \ 20/20 - 1$

Manifest Refraction (at corneal plane):
OD: $-5.50 - 3.25 \times 180$
OS: $-5.25 - 3.00 \times 004$

Keratometry:
OD: 43.00 @ 180; 46.25 @ 090
OS: 43.25 @ 180; 46.25 @ 090

Assessment/Plan

As a result of the high corneal and refractive astigmatism in combination with the soft toric lens rotational instability, GP bitoric lenses were fit. Diagnostic fitting was performed with the Polycon 3D SPE Bitoric (Ciba Vision) fitting set. This 10-lens diagnostic fitting set is available in the following base curve radii: 40.50/43.50 D to 45/48 D in 0.50-D steps. All lenses are 9.0 mm in diameter with powers equal to plano/-3.00 D. As the induced astigmatism is corrected on the front surface, these are bitoric lenses that have a spherical power effect on the eye.

The fitting philosophy for these lenses is to fit the diagnostic lens, which is $0.12 - 0.50$ D flatter than "K." Therefore, the following lenses were selected:

OD: BCR = 42.50/45.50 plano/-3.00 D
OS: BCR = 43/46 plano/-3.00 D

As with a spherical base curve rigid lens, a spherical overrefraction is then performed. In this case, the following powers were obtained and ordered:

OD	OS
Overrefraction: -5.00 DS 20/20	Overrefraction: -5.00 DS 20/20
Final powers = Dx lens + OR	Final powers = Dx lens + OR
= Plano + $(-)5.00$	= Plano + $(-)5.00$
= -5.00 D/-3.00	= -5.00 D/-3.00
+ $(-)5.00$ =	+ $(-)5.00$ =
-8.00 D	-8.00 D

Biomicroscopy with Contact Lenses

Both lenses resulted in an alignment lens-to-cornea fitting relationship and good centration.

The following lenses were ordered:

	OD	OS
Material	Fluorex 300	Fluorex 300
BCR	7.94/7.42 mm	7.85/7.34 mm
Power	$-5.00/-8.00$ D	$-5.00/-8.00$ D
OAD/OZD	9.0/7.8 mm	9.0/7.8 mm
SCR/W	8.7/0.3 mm	8.6/0.3 mm
PCR/W	10.7/0.3 mm	10.6/0.3 mm
CT	0.13 mm	0.13 mm

Alternative Management/Summary

This is a good example of a patient who should have been fit into bitoric lenses at an earlier interval. It is also a beneficial case for emphasizing how routine a GP bitoric fitting can be. When diagnostic lenses are used and minimum or no residual astigmatism is present—as in this case—the final powers are obtained just as with spherical designs, adding the overrefraction to the diagnostic lens power. The only difference in this case is the overrefraction is added to both diagnostic lens powers.

The other benefit of using bitoric diagnostic lenses is the ability to evaluate the fitting relationship and achieve an optimum fit prior to ordering. The Polycon SPE fitting set is very useful in such cases and is also available in both 2 D and 4 D of base curve toricity. As the oxygen permeability of this lens material is quite low, it would be recommended to order the final lens design in a higher-Dk material. In addition, most contact lens laboratories would be able to fabricate a similar diagnostic set in any desired GP lens material.

Case 8: SPE Bitoric Fitting with both Residual and High Astigmatism

Initial Summary

A 29-year-old female housewife presented with blurred vision from her rigid contact lenses. She had been wearing these same lenses for a period of 6 years without need for replacement. However, she indicated that they have always been slightly blurry and it was not uncommon for her to experience a headache after prolonged reading. Pertinent examination information was as follows:

Visual acuity with contact lenses:
OD: 20/30 − 2   Overrefraction: +0.25
(fluctuates)   −1.50 × 175 20/20
OS: 20/30 + 1   Overrefraction: plano −
(fluctuates)   1.25 × 180 20/20

Biomicroscopy with contact lenses:
OU: Both lenses decentered inferiorly and exhibited a mild with-the-rule fluorescein pattern.

Manifest refraction (spectacle plane)
OD: −4.00 − 6.00 × 172 20/20 + 1
OS: −4.25 − 5.00 × 005 20/20 + 2

Manifest refraction (corneal plane)
OD: −3.75 − 5.25 × 172
OS: −4.00 − 4.25 × 005

Keratometry:
OD: 41.50 @ 175; 46.00 @ 085
OS: 41.75 @ 180; 45.25 @ 090

Biomicroscopy

The only significant findings were the presence of grade 1 papillary hypertrophy of the upper tarsal conjunctiva OU, and grade 1+ 3- and 9-o'clock staining OU.

Lens Verification

The lens parameters as provided by her previous eyecare practitioner and confirmed via in-office verification were as follows:

	OD	OS
Material	Polycon II	Polycon II
Powers	−4.25/−6.25 D	−4.00/−6.00 D
Overall diameter	9.0 mm	9.0 mm
Base curve radius	8.08/7.71 mm	8.08/7.71 mm

Assessment/Plan

As a result of the poor visual acuity and lens-to-cornea fitting relationship, bitoric diagnostic fitting was indicated. However, the plan would be to attempt to achieve an improved lens-to-cornea fitting relationship while providing better visual acuity. As this patient is a 4- to 5-D astigmat with only a 2-D (i.e., 41.75/43.75) back-toricity design, the mild astigmatic fluorescein, in addition to a poor lens-to-cornea fitting relationship, would not be unexpected. As the difference in refractive and keratometric cylinder would be predictive that the overrefractive cylinder is residual in nature, this would be determined as well.

Diagnostic fitting was performed with the Polycon 3D SPE Bitoric (Ciba Vision) fitting set. As indicated in Case 7, this is a 10-lens diagnostic fitting set available in the following base curve radii: 40.50/43.50 D to 45/48 D in 0.50-D steps, a 9.0-mm diameter, and powers equal to plano/−3.00 D. As the fitting philosophy for these lenses is to fit the diagnostic lens, which is 0.12 to 0.50 D flatter than "K," the following lenses were selected:

OD: BCR = 41/44 plano/−3.00 D
OS: BCR = 41.50/44.50 plano/−3.00 D

As with a spherical base curve rigid lens, a spherical overrefraction is then performed. In this case, the following powers were obtained:

OD: −3.50 DS 20/25−2
OS: −4.00 DS 20/25

If a spherical overrefraction results in reduced visual acuity, the cause is most likely residual astigmatism and, as with a spherical rigid lens, a spherocylindrical overrefraction is indicated. This resulted in the following:

OD: −3.25 − 1.00 × 177 20/20
OS: −3.75 − 0.75 × 004 20/20 + 1

To obtain the final lens powers is essentially the same as with a spherical lens; that is, add the power of the overrefraction to the power of the diagnostic lens. However, in this case it should be performed per meridian (17). The power in the flat meridian should be added to the overrefractive power in that same meridian; the power in the steep meridian should be added to the overrefractive power in that meridian. In this case, the following powers were derived:

OD: Diagnostic power (flat or horizontal meridian) = Plano

Overrefraction (flat or horizontal meridian) = −3.25 D

Final power = Dx power + OR
= Plano + (−)3.25 = −3.25 D

Diagnostic power (steep or vertical meridian) = −3.00 D

Overrefraction (steep or vertical meridian) = −4.25 D

Final power = Dx power + OR
= −3.00 + (−)4.25 = −7.25 D

OS: Diagnostic power (flat or horizontal meridian) = Plano

Overrefraction (flat or horizontal meridian) = −3.75 D

Final power = Dx power + OR
= Plano + (−)3.75 = −3.75 D

Diagnostic power (steep or vertical meridian) = −3.00 D

Overrefraction (steep or vertical meridian) = −4.50 D

Final power = Dx power + OR
= −3.00 + (−)4.50 = −7.50 D

Biomicroscopy with Contact Lenses

The right lens demonstrated good centration but a slight with-the-rule astigmatic pattern. The left lens resulted in an alignment lens-to-cornea fitting relationship and good centration.

The following lenses were ordered:

	OD	OS
Material(a)	Fluoroperm 30	Fluoroperm 30
BCR(b)	8.23/7.50 mm	8.13/7.58 mm
Power(c)	−3.25/−8.25 D	−3.75/−7.50 D
OAD/OZD	9.4/7.8 mm	9.4/7.8 mm
SCR/W(d)	9.2/8.5 mm @ 0.4 mm	9.1/8.6 mm @ 0.4 mm
PCR/W(d)	11.2/10.5 mm @ 0.4 mm	11.1/10.6 mm @ 0.4 mm
CT(e)	0.14 mm	0.13 mm

(a) A low-Dk fluorosilicone/acrylate lens material was selected for wettability and stability reasons. Polycon II is a very-low-Dk silicone/acrylate material.

(b) As the fluorescein pattern was slightly astigmatic via the use of a lens with 3 D of back-surface toricity on a cornea having 4.5 D, the steep meridian was changed from 44 D to 45 D to create a better-alignment fitting relationship.

(c) Because the steep meridian was increased by 1 D, the power needs to change accordingly; therefore, instead of −7.25 D, a −8.25-D lens power is ordered. The flat meridian remains unchanged.

(d) Due to the high corneal astigmatism, toric peripheral curves were selected with the SCR equal to 1 mm flatter than the base curve radii, and the PCR equal to 2 mm flatter than the SCR.

(e) The center thickness was selected by referring to a spherical lens center thickness chart and selecting the recommended power for the most plus power meridian (i.e. OD = −3.25 D; OS = −3.75 D)

Alternative Management/Summary

Several other options could have been considered in this case. If the patient was very motivated for soft lenses, a soft toric lens could have been considered. However, with over 5 D of refractive cylinder, fluctuating or constant blurred vision was certainly possible. A spherical GP lens may provide adequate centration—even with high corneal toricity—but the poor lens-to-cornea fitting relationship could result in undesirable corneal topography changes over time. Although the temptation to avoid a bitoric lens design is understandable due to the reduced vision and poor fitting relationship experienced with the previous lenses, it is important to determine the causes of the problems. In this case, uncorrected residual cylinder in combination with insufficient back-surface cylinder correction were the causative factors. Fitting a bitoric with greater back-surface toricity and incorporating the residual astigmatism into the correction should solve both problems. If the corneal toricity is much greater than the toricity of the diagnostic lens, resulting in a slight dumbbell or astigmatic pattern, all that is required is to steepen the steep meridian of the lens and add the corresponding amount of minus power to the same meridian.

Whenever residual astigmatism is corrected in a bitoric lens design, the spherical power effect is not present. In other words, if the lens rotates on the eye, the patient's vision may fluctuate. However, as even 0.50 D to 0.75 D of residual astigmatism can result in symptoms of blurred vision, this should be corrected. As the lenses tend to align with the corresponding corneal meridians, such rotation on the eye is rare.

Case 9: Back-surface Toric Lens

Initial Summary

A 25-year-old male attorney enters with symptoms of blurred vision through his GP contact lenses. He has been a rigid contact lens wearer for the past 12 months and has noticed symptoms of blur and eyestrain after prolonged reading. His examination revealed the following:

Visual acuity (with contact lenses):
OD: 20/25–2 Overrefraction: $+0.25 - 1.00 \times 090$ 20/20
OS: 20/25–1 Overrefraction: $+0.25 - 1.00 \times 090$ 20/20

Biomicroscopy with Contact Lenses

Both lenses tended to decenter inferotemporally with the blink. The fluorescein pattern revealed an against-the-rule astigmatic pattern with mild clearance horizontally and bearing vertically.

Biomicroscopy after Lens Removal

Mild (grade 1) 3- and 9-o'clock staining was present OU and very mild papillary hypertrophy was present on the superior tarsal conjunctiva of both eyes. All other findings were normal with a tear break-up time of greater than 10 seconds OU.

Manifest refraction:
OD: $-1.50 - 3.25 \times 090$ 20/20
OS: $-0.75 - 3.00 \times 090$ 20/20

Manifest refraction (at corneal plane):
OD: $-1.50 - 3.00 \times 090$
OS: $-0.75 - 3.00 \times 090$

Keratometry:
OD: 42.50 @ 090; 44.50 @ 180
OS: 42.75 @ 090; 44.75 @ 180

Current lens specifications:

	OD	OS
BCR	7.85 mm	7.85 mm
Power	-2.00 D	-1.25 D
OAD/OZD	9.0 mm	9.0 mm
CT	0.16 mm	0.18 mm

Assessment/Plan

In this case, the patient's refractive against-the-rule astigmatism is much greater than the corneal against-the-rule cylinder. The predicted residual astigmatism equals -1.00 D $\times$ 090 OU. If a back toric lens is designed to have 2 D of back-surface toricity [for example in this case, base curve radii of OD: 42 D(8.04 mm)/44 D(7.67 mm); OS: 42.25 D(7.99 mm)/44.25 D(7.63 mm) were empirically selected], the residual astigmatism induced by the back-surface toricity would be approximately 0.5×2 D or $-1.00 \times$ 090. Therefore, if a back toric lens is selected for this patient, the induced astigmatism will correct the physiologic residual astigmatism. The lens design parameters were selected as follows:

Right eye:
BCR: 42(8.04 mm)/44(7.67 mm)

Using "SAM/FAP" (i.e., steep add minus/flat add plus), the power becomes 0.50 D more plus in the vertical meridian:

$$* -1.50 + (+)0.50 = -1.00D$$

Using the aforementioned 1:2:3 Principle, the induced astigmatism [1] = 1 D; the back-surface toricity = 2 D (or 2×1); therefore, the amount of lensometer cylinder should equal 3 D (i.e., "3×1" or "$3/2 \times 2$"). Therefore, if the flat meridian measures -1.00 D, the steep meridian should equal $-1.00 + (-)3.00$ or -4.00 D.

Left eye:
BCR: 42.25(7.99 mm)/44.25(7.67 mm)

Using "SAM/FAP," the power becomes 0.50 D more plus in the vertical meridian:

$$* -0.75 + (+)0.50 = -0.25 \text{ D}$$

Using the aforementioned 1:2:3 Principle, the induced astigmatism [1] = 1 D; the back-surface toricity = 2 D (or 2×1); therefore, the amount of lensometer cylinder should equal 3 D (i.e., "3×1" or "$3/2 \times 2$"). Therefore, if the flat meridian measures -0.25D, the steep meridian should equal -0.25 + (−)3.00 or -3.25 D.

The following back toric lenses were ordered:

	OD	OS
Material	Fluoroperm 30	Fluoroperm 30
BCR	8.04/7.67 mm	7.99/7.63 mm
Power(a)	-1.00 D	-0.25 D
OAD/OZD	9.4/7.8 mm	9.4/7.8 mm
SCR/W	9.0 mm @ 0.4 mm	9.0 mm @ 0.4 mm
PCR/W	11.0 mm @ 0.4 mm	11.0 mm @ 0.4 mm
CT	0.17 mm	0.19 mm

(a) Typically, with a back-surface only toric lens design, only the power in the flat meridian is specified.

Alternative Management/Summary

This patient could have been fit into either soft toric lenses or a GP bitoric lens design. Certainly if the back toric lens design did not provide good centration or vision, a soft toric lens could be considered. However, this patient has critical vision demands and has been accustomed to rigid lens wear. Likewise, a bitoric rigid lens could have been considered; however, if it is apparent that a less complicated lens design should result in both good vision and a well-centered lens-to-cornea fitting relationship, this should be considered. According to Silbert (17), two cases in which a back toric lens is indicated due to the induced correcting the physiologic residual astigmatism are the following:

1. A patient whose refractive with-the-rule cylinder is much greater than the corneal with-the-rule cylinder.
2. The previous example in which the patient's refractive

against-the-rule astigmatism is much greater than the corneal against-the-rule cylinder.

SUMMARY

The astigmatic patient, notably the high-astigmatic patient, benefits greatly from contact lens correction. The specific correction depends on several factors. Often a GP or GP toric correction will provide better quality of vision. However, for patients who are not good candidates or who are not motivated for GP lenses, the introduction of more-custom soft toric lens parameters complemented by higher-quality manufacturing has made these designs more competitive. Likewise, more consistent and higher quality GP bitoric designs have resulted in high success rates with these designs. These cases show the many applications of GP and soft—both custom and disposable—for the contact lens correction of the astigmatic patient.

REFERENCES

1. Bennett ES, Blaze P, Remba MR. Correction of astigmatism. In: Bennett ES, Henry VA, eds. *Clinical manual of contact lenses, 2nd ed.* Philadelphia: Lippincott Williams & Wilkins, 2000: 351–409.
2. Hanks AJ, Weisbarth RE, McNally JJ. Clinical performance comparisons of a toric contact lens design. *Int Contact Lens Clin* 1987; 14:16.
3. Bennett ES, Gordon JM. The borderline dry-eye patient and contact lens wear. *Contact Lens Forum* 1989;14:52.
4. Becherer PD. Soft torics: a viable modality. *Contact Lens Update* 1990;9:17.
5. Young G, Hunt C, Covey M. Clinical evaluation of factors influencing toric soft contact lens fit. *Optom Vis Sci* 2002;79:11–19.
6. Herman JP. Flexure. In Bennett ES, Grohe RM (eds.). *Rigid gas-permeable contact lenses.* New York: Professional Press, 1986: 137–150.
7. Wilson SE, Lin DTC, Klyce SD, et al. Topographic changes in contact lens-induced corneal warpage. *Ophthalmology* 1990;97: 734.
8. Wilson SE, Lin DTC, Klyce SD, et al. RGP decentration: a risk factor for corneal warpage. *CLAO J* 1990;16:177.
9. Harris MG, Chu CS. The effect of contact lens thickness and corneal toricity on flexure and residual astigmatism. *Am J Optom* 1972;49:304.
10. Brown S, Kochanny L, Pole J, et al. Effect of optic zone diameter on lens flexure and residual astigmatism. *Int Contact Lens Clin* 1984;11:759.
11. Bennett ES. Astigmatic correction. In Bennett ES, Grohe RM, eds. *Rigid gas-permeable contact lenses.* New York: Professional Press, 1986:345–380.
12. Holden B, Mertz GW. Critical oxygen levels to avoid corneal edema for daily and extended wear contact lenses. *Invest Ophthalmol Vis Sci* 1984;25:1161.
13. Borish IM. Vision correction with contact lenses. In: Borish IM, ed. *Clinical refraction, 3rd ed.* Chicago: Professional Press, 1970: 971–1005.
14. Remba MJ. Contact lenses and the astigmatic cornea. *Contacto* 1967;11:38.
15. Sarver MD, Mandell RB. Toric lenses. In: Mandell RB, ed. *Contact lens practice, 4th ed.* Springfield, IL: Charles C. Thomas, 1988:284–309.
16. Mandell RB, Moore CF. A bitoric lens guide that really is simple. *Contact Lens Spectr* 1988;3:83.
17. Silbert JA. Rigid lens correction of astigmatism. In: Bennett ES, Weissman BA, eds. *Clinical contact lens practice.* Philadelphia: JB Lippincott, 1991:1–24.

4 8

BIFOCAL GRAND ROUNDS

ROBERT L. DAVIS
EDWARD S. BENNETT
AND DAVID W. HANSEN

INTRODUCTION

One of the most important and beneficial applications of contact lenses is also one of the most underutilized, and that is for presbyopic correction. Presbyopic patients are often among the most motivated and also very likely to refer others. However, it is not uncommon for the presbyope to comment that (s)he has never been told about bifocal contact lenses or, if told, that they "don't work" or "have not been perfected." The low usage of gas-permeable (GP) bifocal and multifocal lens designs and contact lens presbyopic designs in general is most likely the result of several factors. These designs are perceived as being complicated or challenging to fit. As a result of this practitioner apprehension, patients are often offered an easier and often less satisfactory correction such as monovision, single-vision contact lenses in combination with reading glasses, or spectacles only. The purpose of this chapter is to provide clinical cases that will show the applications, lens design, fitting, and troubleshooting of bifocal contact lenses and hopefully increase the comfort zone for practitioners interested in benefiting their presbyopic patients interested in contact lenses.

GAS-PERMEABLE LENS DESIGNS

Aspheric Multifocal

Initial Summary

A 44-year-old woman (L.F.) presented for a complete eye examination and a refit from her GP lenses into soft toric lenses. She was a previous long-term polymethylmethacrylate (PMMA) wearer who had been wearing Polycon II lenses for 4 years. She was experiencing headaches after several hours of lens wear, and she believed that they were caused by her contact lenses.

Visual acuity (with contact lenses):
Right eye (OD): 20/20 − 2
Left eye (OS): 20/20

The contact lens parameters were as follows:

Material: Polycon II (OD); Polycon II (OS)
Base curve radius: 7.55 mm (OD); 7.55 mm (OS)
Overall diameter: 9.0 mm (OD); 9.0 mm (OS)
Power: −2.62 D (OD); −2.00 D (OS)

Biomicroscopy

Both contact lenses were heavily scratched, and tended to be picked up by the lids and then bumped inferiorly. After contact lens removal, the lids and lashes were healthy in each eye (OU). Pingueculae were present at the nasal and temporal bulbar conjunctiva OS. The cornea was clear and quiet OU. The tear break-up time was greater than 10 seconds OU.

Manifest refraction:
−3.00−1.00 × 172 20/20 (OD)
−2.75−0.75 × 178 20/20−1 (OS)

She was advised to discontinue Polycon lens wear for 1 week to obtain refractive stability. At her next visit, her manifest refraction had changed to the following:

−2.75−2.25 × 172 20/20−2 (OD)
−2.25−1.50 × 008 20/20−1 (OS)

After diagnostic fitting with the Optima Toric (Bausch & Lomb), the following lenses were ordered:

Base curve radius: 8.6 mm (OD); 8.6 mm (OS)
Power: −2.75−1.75 × 180 (OD); −2.25−1.25 × 170 (OS)

L.F. experienced blurred vision at near with these lenses, and I decided to try monovision. The left lens power was changed to −1.25 − 1.25 × 170. After 1 month of monovision lens wear, she was still dissatisfied with her near vision and was interested in pursuing other options. The right lens tended to rotate in a variable manner with the blink.

Material Selection

The following corrective options were presented to L.F.:

1. Two distance-power soft lenses with reading spectacles
2. Multifocal GP lenses
3. Spectacle wear only

She was interested in bifocal contact lenses. She was initially prescribed Tangent Streak lenses (Fused Kontacts). However, at diagnostic fitting, it was observed that, although her lid tension appears to be normal, her upper lid contour appears to induce excessive lens rotation. Therefore, the decision was made to fit her into a rigid aspheric bifocal lens. The Lifestyle GP (Permeable Technologies) was selected because it was a newly introduced design that has much potential. For optimum vision at both distance and near, a superior lens-to-cornea fitting relationship was important.

Fitting/Troubleshooting

Keratometry:
44.25 @ 168: 44.37 @ 078 (OD)
43.75 @ 010: 44.75 @ 100 (OS)

The Lifestyle GP uses an equivalent (EQ) base curve radius for diagnostic fitting. The EQ selected for fitting is typically similar to the base curve radius selected when fitting a spherical GP. The actual base curve radius is approximately 1.00 D steeper than the EQ value.

The following diagnostic lenses were fit:

Design: Lifestyle GP (OD); Lifestyle GP (OS)
Base curve radius: 7.60 EQ (OD); 7.50 EQ (OS)
Power: −2.12 D (OD); −2.37 D (OS)
Overrefraction: −1.00 DS 20/20− (distance) 20/20 (near) (OD); −0.75 DS 20/20 (distance) 20/20 (near) (OS)

Biomicroscopy

The right lens provided a slightly superior lens-to-cornea fitting relationship as recommended by the manufacturer (Fig. 48.1). The left lens resulted in an interpalpebral fitting relationship.

Therefore, a 7.6-mm EQ lens was fit. This lens provided an optimum fitting relationship, and the aforementioned overrefraction was performed over this lens.

The following lenses were ordered:

Design: Lifestyle GP (OD); Lifestyle GP (OS)
EQ: 7.60 mm (OD); 7.60 mm (OS)
Power: −3.00 D (OD); −2.75 D (OS)

A +1.50-D effective bifocal add was desired with these lenses. The actual base curve radius was 7.44 mm, providing an actual fitting relationship equal to 1.0 to 1.5 D steeper than K.

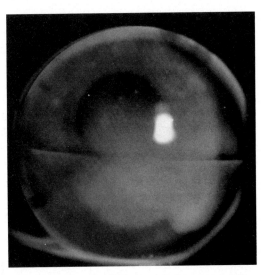

FIG. 48.1. A Tangent Streak lens with the segment line at the lower pupil margin.

At the dispensing visit, her visual acuity was 20/30 (OD) and 20/30+ (OS).

Overrefraction:
−0.50 D 20/20 (distance): 0.25 D 20/25 (near) (OD)
−0.05 D 20/20 (distance); −0.50 D 20/25 (near) (OS)

Biomicroscopy

A slightly superior fitting relationship with about 1 mm movement with the blink was present.

At the 1-week progress visit, the patient complained of slight blur at distance. The lens powers were changed to: −3.50 D (OD) and −3.00 D (OS).

After 3 months of lens wear, she was very pleased with both comfort and vision at distance and near.

Visual acuity (with contact lenses):
20/20 (distance); 20/20 (near) (OD)
20/20 (distance); 20/20 (near) (OS)
Biomicroscopy: unchanged from previous visits.

Summary

This case demonstrates the importance of having several options available when fitting patients with bifocal contact lenses. Initially, the patient did not have near complaints and desired a distance-only correction. However, at her age, near testing should have been performed initially and the options for near correction explained at that time. Monovision was unsuccessful due, in part, to lens rotation caused by an upper lid contour that tended to shift the lens in a variable manner. In addition, because she was a long-term PMMA and then a very-low Dk-GP lens wearer, excessive refractive changes occurred when she was refit into soft lenses. If a patient is a long-term rigid lens wearer (and not very displeased with his or her lenses), it is preferable, in most cases, to keep the patient in GP lens wear.

Eventually, the patient was prescribed GP bifocal lenses, initially Tangent Streak and then Lifestyle GP. Bifocal GP fitting is not all that complicated or unsuccessful if diagnostic fitting is performed and, at minimum, two different types of lens designs (typically one simultaneous vision and one segmented translating) are available. In her case, it was evident that the segmented-translating design was rotating excessively; therefore, an aspheric design could promptly be fit and ultimately resulted in a satisfied and successful patient.

One-Piece Segmented Translating Bifocal

Initial Summary

M.L. is a 48-year-old woman who presented with symptoms of blur while reading. She was currently wearing Acuvue disposable lenses in combination with reading glasses. She was interested in bifocal contact lenses.

Visual acuity (VA) (with current contact lenses):
20/30+2 (distance) 20/20−1 (near) (OD)
20/40 (distance) 20/20−1 (near) (OS)

Overrefraction:
Plano 20/30+2 (OD)
−.50 DS 20/30−1 (OS)

Biomicroscopy: Both lenses exhibited good centration with acceptable movement with the blink.

Manifest refraction:
−3.50 DS (OD)
−5.00 DS (OS)
+1.50 D add OU

Keratometry:
45.00 @ 180; 45.50 @ 090 (OD)
45.75 @ 180; 46.00 @ 090 (OS)

Because she indicated a desire to maintain soft lens wear, she was diagnostically fit with the Hydron Echelon diffractive bifocal lens. This is a simultaneous-vision lens, which has the advantage of being pupil independent as incoming light is either diffracted (for near vision) or refracted (for distance vision) in equal amounts. The following lenses were diagnostically fit:

Design: Echelon (OD); Echelon (OS)
Base curve: 8.70 mm
Overall diameter: 14.0 mm
Power: −3.50 D (OD); −3.75 D (OS)
Add: +1.50 D (OD); +2.00 D (OS)
Visual acuity (with contact lenses): 20/40 (distance) (OD); 20/40 (distance) (OS)

Biomicroscopy: The right lens provided good centration; however, the left lens exhibited excessive inferior edge lift.

Material Selection

As a result of the poor distance vision in both eyes and excessive edge lift of the left lens, it was decided to refit her with the Tangent Streak one-piece segmented lens design. It was our intention that, if properly fitted, this lens could provide good vision at both distance and near due to translation.

Fitting/Troubleshooting

Before fitting, the following measurements were performed:

Pupil size: 4 mm (normal, illumination)
Vertical fissure size: 10 mm
Lower lid position: adjacent to inferior limbus
Distance from lower lid to pupil center: 5.5 mm

All measurements were OU.
Because a flatter-than-K fitting philosophy is very successful with low astigmatic patients being fit with this design, the following diagnostic lenses were used:

Lens design/material: Tangent Streak/Fluorex 700 (OU)
Base curve radius: 7.50 mm (OD); 7.42 mm (OS)
Overall diameter: 9.40/9 mm (OD); 9.40/9 mm (OS)
Power/add: −2.00/+2.00 D (OD); −2.00/+2.00 D (OS)
Seg height: 4.2 mm (OD); 4.2 mm (OS)
Prism: 2Δ (OD); 2Δ (OS)
Seg height: 4.6 mm (OD); 4.4 mm (OS)

At the dispensing visit, the following vision and fit information was obtained for visual acuity:

20/20 (distance with some fluctuation), 20/30 (near (OD)
20/20+ (distance), 20/20 (near with some ghost vision) (OS)

Biomicroscopy

The seg height appeared to be slightly high (i.e., 0.5 to 1 mm above lower lid margin) OU. Good translation was present with downward gaze.

She was provided with an adaptation schedule (4 hours the first day, increasing 1 hour per day). She was also provided with realistic expectations of what to expect with lens wear and was scheduled for a follow-up evaluation in 1 week.

At her first follow-up evaluation, she reported fluctuating vision at distance out of her right lens, which she believed was caused by the bifocal line being too high. Otherwise, both lenses were comfortable and her left lens was performing very well.

Visual acuity:
20/20−2 (distance); 20/25+ (near) (OD)
20/20 (distance); 20/25 (near) (OS)

Biomicroscopy

The right lens appeared to move excessively with the blink on straight-ahead gaze. Approximately 2 to 3 mm of lag was present; 1 mm would be considered optimum. Both lenses translated well with near gaze.

The right lens was recorded with the following parameters: prism 2.5∆ and seg height 4.4 mm.

At subsequent follow-up visits, she indicated her vision at distance out of the right lens was slightly better but that she has to tilt her head down slightly to see without ghost images. A new right lens with an even smaller seg height (4 mm) was ordered, and she reported good comfort and vision at all subsequent visits.

Summary

This case is a good example of the benefits of a segmented translating bifocal design in providing good vision at distance and near. The importance of performing careful anatomic measurements in combination with accurate seg height determination is critical to successful fitting. The patient needs to be fixating straight-ahead when evaluating seg height (Fig. 48.2). Any deviation, even slight, can result in a misleading seg height position. If in doubt about the seg height position, the patient can be asked to tilt his or her head forward or backward to determine if the vision improves. Likewise, the patient should be given realistic expectations about bifocal lens wear. They should understand that these small pieces of plastic on the eye function in a more dynamic manner than spectacles; therefore, the fitting is more complex and slight compromise may result. In addition, it may take more than one lens to result in success. If the fitting is approached in this manner, these patients are generally successful.

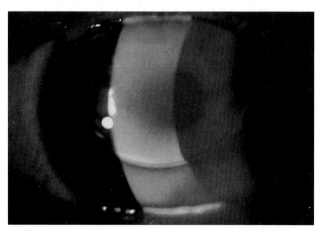

FIG. 48.2. An optimum-fitting Lifestyle GP lens.

Solitaire Translating Gas-permeable Bifocal

Initial Summary

A 49-year-old female homemaker was seen routinely for years, and wore spectacles. Approximately 10 years previously she wore PMMA lenses for about 1 year but they were very uncomfortable. Her eyes were dry and the doctor fenestrated the contact lenses in an effort to improve comfort

She was tired of wearing glasses, especially with her presbyopic changes, and requested bifocal contact lenses. There were no significant intermediate demands; therefore, it was decided that a translating GP lens would be the best choice. Her manifest refraction was as follows:

−3.00 + 1.00 × 100 20/20 +1.75 D add (OD)
−2.25 + 1.25 × 075 20/20 +1.75 add (OS)

Auto keratometry:
40.12 @ 162; 40.62 @ 0072 (OD)
40.37 @ 177; 41.50 @ 087 (OS)

The analytical examination revealed 11 esophoria for distance, and reduced binocular performance with lower fusion duction ranges. The esophoric condition produced asthenopia and visual headaches. Visual acuity with habitual prescription was 20/30 in each eye. The external examination indicated the pupils were equal, round, and responsive to light and accommodation. Mesopic conditions revealed 5 mm OU, and scotopic illumination exhibited 6 mm OU. The horizontal visible iris diameter was 11.5 mm OU and the palpebral aperture size was 10 mm OU. There was normal lid tension superiorly and inferiorly, with the inferior lid position tangent to the inferior limbus. Biomicroscopy with fluorescein application resulted in a tear break-up time of 30 seconds OU. The inferior tear meniscus revealed 1 + normal tear meniscus OU, and the cornea was clear OU and absent of pathology with sodium fluorescein application.

Material Selection

Due to the flat corneal curvature readings, and her lessened intermediate needs, a translating bifocal lens design was selected. The Solitaire lens (Tru-Form Optics) is basically a prismatic reading lens with a monocentric distance segment cut on the superior lens surface. The near segment extends across the lower half of the lens. This lens is inherently bottom heavy, and requires less prism to achieve proper orientation because of the removal of weight in the distance viewing area. The top of the bifocal segment is fit at inferior position of the lower papillary margin under normal mesopic conditions. This style of lens is ideal for flat corneas because there is less overall mass.

Fitting/Troubleshooting

A diagnostic examination was administered, and the following lens parameters were used (Solitaire translating bifocal contact lens parameters):

Base curve radius: 8.30 mm (OD); 8.18 mm (OS)
Power: −2.25 D (OD); −2.24 D (OS)
Overall diameters: 9.5/9.2 mm (OD); 9.5/9.2 mm (OS)
Optical zone diameter: 8.1 mm (OD); 8.1 mm (OS)
Seg height: 3.5 mm (OD); 3.5 mm (OS)
Prism: 2.00 PD (OD); 2.00 PD (OS)
Material: Fluoroperm 30 (Paragon Vision Sciences) blue tint (OU)

After instruction regarding all aspects of lens care, lens handling, and so on was given, Sereine Wetting and Soaking Solution with Lobob cleaner was prescribed. The patient presented two weeks later seeing 20/20 in each eye at distance, and J1 (20/15) in each eye at near. She was having minor filming problems; therefore, an enzymatic cleaner was added to the care regimen. This lens, manufactured by Tru-Form Optics, can be produced from a variety of GP lens materials. Patients with ptosis or blepharochalasis are poor candidates because of the insufficient clearance needed for superior displacement of the lens when the patient looks through the reading segment. Also, patients with flaccid lids are not ideal candidates for this lens.

Summary

This case demonstrates the importance of matching occupational needs with anatomic and physiologic conditions. With this patient, the flatness of the overall central curvature of the cornea contraindicated an aspheric or other simultaneous vision design. Also, many of the translating lenses produce excessive prism and mass, making it difficult to reposition the lens for distance and near viewing. Additional comfort was achieved with weekly enzyming and polishing of the edges in my laboratory with a procedure known as "fingerlishing." This is an edge treatment technique in which the contact lens is spun in the modification unit, and the index finger of the technician is used as the polishing pad. By working from the inside edge out and back and forth, the lens edge design and comfort can be improved. Due to the thickness and mass of many translating lenses, it is difficult to use standard polishing techniques. Corneal topography also indicated that the corneas were relatively uniform with no exaggerated apex. This corneal topography greatly assisted in lens design selection.

Front-surface Toric, Prism-ballasted Tangent Streak No-Line Multifocal

Initial Summary

A 52-year-old preschool teacher presented herself to our office complaining about her vision both at distance and at near. Her previous doctor had fit her with Tangent Streak No-Line aspheric bifocals about 1 year ago. Her goals with contact lenses included reading comfortably as well as walking around the room looking at the students work at their desk. The patient's visual needs included distance, intermediate, and near vision in a one-lens design system. As a preschool teacher, her nearpoint visual demands incorporate many different working distances. She was not interested in supplementing her contact lens prescription with reading glasses. She did not understand why her vision with contact lenses was not as good as with eyeglasses.

Previous contact lens specifications:

OD, OS	Tangent Streak	Aspheric Bifocal Design
Fitting base curve	7.60 mm	7.60 mm
Base curve	7.44 mm	7.44 mm
Overall diameter	9.0 mm	9.0 mm
Optical zone	7.8 mm	7.8 mm
Power	−0.25 D	+0.25 D
Material	Boston ES	
Visual acuity distance	20/30	20/30
Visual acuity near	J3	J3

Overcorrection:
OD: plano − 1.00 × 120
OS: plano − 1.00 × 60

Distance visual acuity uncorrected:
OD: 20/100 near J5
OS: 20/100 near J5

Refraction:
OD: +2.00 −3.00 × 110 +1.75 add
OS: +1.25 −2.50 × 75 +1.75 add

Keratometry:
OD: 46.75 @ 90 45.00 @ 100
OS: 46.75 @ 90 45.25 @ 80

* Calculated residual astigmatism = keratometric astigmatism − total refractive astigmatism
* OD: 1.25 = 3.00 − 1.75
* OS: 1.00 = 2.50 − 1.50

Tear break-up time:
OD: 22 seconds
OS: 21 seconds
Palpebral aperture: 11.5 mm
Pupil size: 4.2 mm
Lower lid position: 2 mm below limbus

Ocular Evaluation

Eyelids and adnexa were free of pathology. Cilia were free of debris. Lids exhibited no swelling, injection, congestion, or granulations. Lid eversion revealed normal satin appearance of tarsal conjunctiva without papillae or follicles. Conjunctiva and sclera exhibited no inflammation or congestion.

Biomicroscopy

Tear film layer was adequate to support contact lens wear. Anterior chambers are deep and without signs of cells and flare. Neither eye exhibited any signs of neovascularization or edema. Iris shape, color, and size were free of pathology and abnormalities.

Material/Design

The actual amount of residual astigmatism is the amount of astigmatism measured after a spherical GP lens is applied to the eye and approximates the calculated residual astigmatism. In this case, the overrefraction with the Tangent Streak No-Line exhibited:

    OD: plano −1.00 × 120 20/20
    OS: plano −1.00 × 60 20/20

The reduction in visual acuity is a result of uncorrected residual astigmatism. The methods of correcting residual astigmatism include spherical rigid lens, soft toric lens, and front-surface toric lens. If the corneal toricity is with-the-rule and the residual astigmatism is against-the-rule, a thin spherical lens can flex and reduce the amount of residual astigmatism. Soft toric lenses are rapidly replacing the front-surface toric GP rigid lens because of the ease of fit, available parameters, quality of optics, and patient comfort. This case presentation exemplifies its requirement when the optimal design is a GP lens.

The fitting of a front-surface toric, prism-ballasted lens is similar to a spherical back-surface GP lens with a prism incorporated into the lens design for rotational stability. The purpose of the prism is to stabilize the lens from possible rotational movements induced by the action of the lids. As the myopia increases less amounts of prism are required to counteract the greater thickness of the superior aspect of the lens. To determine lens rotational characteristics, vertical positioning, and lens dynamics, the use of prism-ballasted spherical diagnostic lenses is optimal because it allows greater accuracy. Usually 1 D of prism integrated into the lens provides stability. In plus powers and low minus, the thinness of edge profiles requires greater amounts of prism. The increase in lens thickness associated with prism ballasting necessitates greater-oxygen-transmissibility materials.

Contact lens specifications: Tangent Streak aspheric bifocal design

	OD	OS
Fitting base curve	7.60 mm	7.60 mm
Base curve	7.44 mm	7.44 mm
Overall diameter	9.0 mm	9.0 mm
Optical zone	7.8 mm	7.8 mm
Power	+1.75 − 1.00 × 120	+1.75 − 1.00 × 60
Prism	1Δ BD	1Δ BD
Material	Boston XO Blue	
Visual acuity distance	20/20	20/20
Visual acuity near	J1	J1
Visible dot	Dot	Double dot

Assessment/Plan

Although the patient's previous Tangent Streak No-Line prescription was adequate for most visual tasks, when she needed detail acuity the lens prescription could not perform adequately. The patient did not have any comfort problems and the lens design utilized an alignment fitting philosophy. The previous lens design was treated as a diagnostic lens and the overrefraction resulted in residual astigmatism that correlated well with the calculated amount. A front-surface toric, prism-ballasted, GP Tangent Streak No-Line bifocal was the lens of choice to meet the patients visual acuity and range of vision. The lens was ordered in a Boston XO material because of the superior oxygen transmissibility needed to counteract the increase thickness caused by the ballasting prism. Dotting the base of the prism is desired for fit evaluation. Visible dots were incorporated into the base of the prism at axis 90 to observe the rotational characteristics of the lens and to allow the patient to differentiate between the left and right lens. If the lens did not exhibit good lens movement into the bifocal portion of the lens, a minus lenticular design would improve the lens translation. A soft toric lens could have provided adequate distance acuity although the patient would have had to incorporate the near prescription into the lens design. The prism-ballast method for lens stability was used because of the improved comfort, lower lid position and tight lids, and availability of bifocal parameters.

After the lens was delivered, the slit-lamp evaluation exhibited a nasal rotation of each lens on the eye about 10 degrees. The upper lid exerts a torque on the lens that the power axis must be compensated for pristine vision. Using the LARS (left add, right subtract) method, the lenses were reordered OD axis 110 and OS axis 60. Degrading the acuity from rotational effects of the lens is variable according to the blur interpretation of the patient. Five degrees and less rarely has an effect on vision.

Summary

Residual astigmatism can be induced by lens warpage, flexure, or internal characteristics of the eye. The only options available include a soft toric lens or a front-surface toric, prism-ballasted lens. Certain situations necessitate a GP lens design including complications from soft lenses, giant papillary conjunctivitis (GPC), soft lens edema, GP bifocal and specialty GP designs such as MacroLens, keratoconus lenses, and post–refractive surgery designs. If there exists a high amount of corneal toricity with residual astigmatism, a bitoric lens would be the lens of choice to improve the fitting and visual characteristics. If the lens rotates during the blink then the LARS principal needs to be executed in order to prescribe the correct axis. Most lenses tend to rotate on the eye 10 to 15 degrees nasally. The final contact lens prescription would be modified according to the amount of rotation.

"Modified Multifocal"

Initial Summary

A 53-year-old woman presented with symptoms of blurred vision from her soft concentric bifocals. She had worn PMMA spherical lenses for 15 years followed by 13 years of spherical GP lens wear. She was then fit into an aspheric GP multifocal, which she wore for 8 years. When she eventually experienced symptoms of blur at near from these lenses, her practitioner persuaded her to use soft bifocals. Despite numerous lens changes, she was never satisfied with her vision at distance and near. In addition, in her position as an administrative assistant, her intermediate vision was important for her frequent computer use. She experiences mild seasonal allergies and was not taking any medications.

Subjective:
OD: −5.75−1.00 × 005
OS: −6.00−1.00 × 176
Add: +2.00 D OU

Keratometry:
OD: 43.00 @ 180; 44.00 @ 090
OS: 43.75 @ 180; 44.75 @ 090

Ocular Evaluation

The lid position in the both eyes was 1.5 mm below the lower limbus and the lid tension was normal. Complete blinking was exhibited

Dominance: right eye
Pupil Diameter: 3.5 mm in normal illumination
Tear break-up time: 13 seconds OD; 14 seconds OS
Biomicroscopy: The anterior segment was healthy and the upper lid exhibited a grade 1 papillary appearance OU.

Diagnostic Fitting

This patient was fitted into the Essentials aspheric multifocal GP lens (Blanchard Contact Lens). A segmented translating design was deemed unacceptable due to the position of the low lower lid. In addition, this design is available in a series of three add powers.

She was fit into the following lenses:

	OD	OS
Base curve	7.70 mm	7.60 mm
Diameter	9.5 mm	9.5 mm
Power	−4.00 D	−4.00 D
Add	Series II OU	
Material	Boston ES OU	

Both lenses tended to move excessively on the eye and decenter inferiorly. She was then refit into a 7.60-mm base curve radius in the right eye and a 7.50-mm base curve radius in the left eye. Centration was much improved and only 1 mm of lens lag with the blink was present. An overrefraction of −2.75D OU resulted in distance visual acuity of 20/20 + 2 OD and 20/20 OS. However, the near acuity was 20/30 + 2 OU. Therefore, the following lenses were ordered:

	OD	OS
Base curve	7.60 mm	7.50 mm
Diameter	9.5 mm	9.5 mm
Power	−6.75 D	−6.50 D
Add	Series II	Series III
Material	Boston ES OU	

At dispensing, the lens-to-cornea fitting relationship was similar to the diagnostic fitting. The distance visual acuity was 20/20 + 1 OD; 20/20 + 2 OS; 20/15−2 OU. The near visual acuity was 20/30 + 1 OD; 20/25 + 2 OS; 20/20−2 OU. Subsequent follow-up visits resulted in excellent patient satisfaction and ocular integrity.

Summary

Aspheric multifocal lenses are now a viable option for patients of any add-power requirement. Several newer designs, often via adding near power in a concentric manner on the front surface, are able to provide higher add powers than previous generation designs. Although the effective optical zone for distance often decreases therefore impacting distance vision, it has allowed for patients with advanced presbyopia to be successful in aspheric GP lens designs. Nevertheless, patients with +2.00 D or greater add demand often require a "modified multifocal" approach in which one eye has a stronger add than the other eye and/or the nondominant eye is slightly "overplussed" (in this case by only 0.25 D). This will typically result in good distance, good intermediate, and acceptable near vision from the dominant eye and acceptable distance, and good intermediate and good near vision from the nondominant eye. This case also demonstrates how an undesirable fitting relationship, excessive lens lag with the blink, can often be remediated by refitting with a steeper base curve radius.

Crescent Bifocal for Optimum Distance and Near Vision

Initial Summary

A 47-year-old male attorney inquired into the possibility of wearing contact lenses. He wore hard lenses when he was in his teens but discontinued when he entered law school due, in part, to dryness symptoms. He has been wearing spectacles since that time; for the last 4 years he has been wearing a progressive addition correction. He had inquired about contact lenses with his previous practitioner but was told that bifocal contact lenses would not be a good option for him. He indicated that he was motivated to discontinue spectacle wear but also wanted to maintain good distance and near vision. He was not currently taking any medications.

Subjective:
OD: −4.75−1.25 × 175
OS: −4.50−1.50 × 002
Add: + 1.50 D OU

Keratometry:
OD: 42.00 @ 180; 43.00 @ 090
OS: 41.75 @ 180; 43.00 @ 090

Ocular Evaluation

The lid position in the both eyes was at the lower limbus and the lid tension was normal. Complete blinking was exhibited.

Pupil diameter: 5 mm in normal illumination
Tear break-up time: 11 seconds OD; 12 seconds OS
Biomicroscopy: The anterior segment was healthy and the upper lid was satin in appearance OU.

Diagnostic Fitting

This patient was diagnostically fit with the Solutions Bifocal (X-Cel Contact Lens Laboratory), a segmented crescent translating lens design that provides correction at distance and near. This design is available in low, medium, and high prism and in five seg heights (standard, 0.5 mm smaller, 1 mm smaller, 0.5 mm larger, and 1 mm larger). As per the fitting guide, the lenses were fit "on K" to slightly flatter. The following diagnostic lenses were fit:

	OD	OS
Base curve	8.08 mm	8.08 mm
Diameter	9.60 mm	9.60 mm
Power	−3.00 D	−3.00 D
Prism	Medium OU	
Add	+ 2.00 D OU	
Material:	Paragon HDS OU	

Both lenses appeared to position well, although the seg line was positioned about 1 mm below the lower pupil mar-gin. Translation was adequate although only intermittent OS. The overrefraction was−1.25 DS OD 20/20 + 2; −1.25 D OS 20/15−2. With an additional−0.50-D trial lenses, the near acuity was J1 OD, OS, OU. The following lenses were ordered:

	OD	OS
Base curve	8.08 mm	8.08 mm
Diameter	9.60 mm	9.60 mm
Power	−4.25 D	−4.25 D
Prism	Medium OU	
Add	+ 1.50 D OU	
Seg height	0.5 mm above geometric center	
Material:	Paragon HDS OU	

At dispensing, the vision was similar to the diagnostic fitting, although it appeared that both lenses were being picked up too high with the blink with both lenses and a note was made to reevaluate this at the 1-week visit. Translation was consistent OD but intermittent OS.

At the 1-week visit, the patient was able to increase his wearing time to 10 hours and overall was surprised at the comfort achieved. He did comment, however, that his vision was variable at distance and he felt that the lenses "had not settled."

Visual acuity (distance): OD: 20/20 (with difficulty); OS: 20/20 + 1 (with difficulty)
(near): OD: J1; OS: J1 (with difficulty)

Biomicroscopy
Both lenses appeared to be picked up, at minimum, 2 mm with the blink such that the seg line was well within the pupil. In addition, the left lens only translated on approximately one-third of his blinks. Therefore, the prism was increased OU and a flatter base curve was selected OS to increase the edge clearance and, hopefully, to ensure that the lower edge would be in greater contact with the lower lid. The following changes were made:

	OD	OS
Base curve	8.08 mm	8.18 mm
Power	−4.25 D	−3.75 D
Prism	Heavy OU	

The patient was able to continue to wear the first pair of lenses while waiting for the new lenses to arrive. After dispensing of theses lenses, the patient observed an immediate improvement in his vision. Both lenses were only lifted approximately 1 mm with the blink. Translation—although not occurring every time the patient viewed inferiorly—was much more consistent. Subsequent follow-up visits confirmed that this design was successful and the patient was very pleased with his lenses.

Summary

Assuming a proper lower lid position, the best option for a presbyopic patient desiring good unaided vision with contact lenses at both distance and near is via a translating design. Often practitioners will be hesitant to fit a non-wearer into GP bifocal lenses, fearing that initial comfort will be a problem, not to mention how complicated segmented bifocal designs appear to be. In this case, the Solutions Bifocal, a user-friendly lens design with limited choices for prism and seg height, was successful in optimizing vision at both distances. The initial comfort, as with many GP bifocal and multifocal lens designs, was not a problem. This was, in part, because these lenses move little with the blink, and also because a topical anesthetic was applied immediately before the initial diagnostic lenses were inserted. This case also exhibited two of the common problems that can occur with segmented translating designs and how these problems can be easily remedied. Whenever segmented lenses are lifted such that the seg line goes well into the pupil (i.e., >1 mm), increasing the prism will often reduce or eliminate this problem. Likewise, if a lens does not translate or only translates intermittently, flattening the base curve radius by, at minimum, 0.50 D will increase the edge clearance, often allowing the lid to provide a positive stop to the lens edge on downward gaze.

Annular for Midrange Vision

Initial Summary

A 57-year-old woman was interested in bifocal contact lenses. She is employed as a banker and works at a computer a minimum of 3 hours per day. She previously wore spherical GP lenses for 10 years. She experiences difficulty reading but does not enjoy using reading glasses. She has been unable to wear contact lenses since being treated for Bell's palsy 2 years ago. She has mild ptosis of the left eye and marginal dry eye symptoms.

Previous contact lens specifications:

	OD	OS
Base curve	7.50 mm	
	7.34 mm	
Overall diameter	8.80 mm	8.80 mm
Power	−4.25 D	−3.25 D
Optical zone	7.50 mm	7.80 mm
Center thickness	0.14 mm	0.14 mm
Material	Paraperm 02 OU	

Subjective:
OD: −3.75−0.75 × 055
OS: −3.50−0.75 × 110
Add: +2.00D OU

Keratometry:
OD: 45.00 @ 164; 46.00 @ 074
OS: 45.75 @ 030; 46.62 @ 120

Ocular Evaluation

The lid position in the left eye demonstrated a moderate amount of ptosis as a result of the inflammatory disorder related to Bell's palsy, and the left vertical aperture measured 1.5 mm smaller.

Pupil diameter: 4 mm in normal illumination
Tear break-up time: 8 seconds OU; however, the blink was complete OU
Lens performance: near vision was unacceptable OU; left lens decentered inferiorly

Diagnostic Fitting

This patient was fit with the Mandell Seamless bifocal (Concise Contact Lens Laboratory), a front-surface concentric translating lens design that provides correction at distance, intermediate, and near. The final lens design was the following:

	OD	OS
Base curve	7.54 mm	7.42 mm
Overall diameter	9.80 mm	9.60 mm
Power	−3.50 D	−2.50 D
Optical zone	8.00 mm	
	7.80 mm	
Distance zone	3.80 mm	3.80 mm
Prism	0.75Δ OU	
Add	+2.25D OU	
Material	Boston ES OU	

Both lenses utilized a 1-mm intermediate zone and the distance visual acuity was 20/20 OD and OS with J1 at near OD and OS.

Summary

This patient presented with a great desire to wear multifocal contact lenses. She also had a problematic situation as a result of her episode of Bell's palsy, which resulted in left upper lid ptosis and a marginal dry eye condition. The reduction of the diameter in the left lens, as well as the inclusion of prism, provided the centration and stability to provide good distance vision; however, it did not interfere with the need for the lens to translate for mid- and near-vision tasks. The Mandell Seamless bifocal is a good example of a new generation of translating bifocals that are able to provide an intermediate correction. This case also demonstrates how a well-designed multifocal GP lens can provide a good range of vision for a patient with an eyelid dysfunction and marginal dry eye.

Gas-permeable Aspheric X-chrome Bifocal

Initial Summary

A 50-year-old printer came into the office inquiring about the possibility of using a visual device to improve his color vision. In the past, J.F. has had extreme difficulties matching colors and distinguishing shades of colors. The patient is a previous spherical rigid lens wearer of 16 years. Recently J.F. has had visual problems with his nearpoint work. In order to proof his client's work, J.F. has had to go to the drug store and purchase reading glasses. J.F. has to take his glasses off when he is on the computer. The inconvenience of pulling the glasses off and on is one of J.F.'s goals at this annual visit. I explained to the patient the X-chrome lens does not produce the perception of color. The X-chrome lens creates shades that allow discrimination of colors. The X-chrome lens is a monocular filter that allows the patient to match colors and distinguish between colors. One lens is designed with a magenta tinted lens whereas the other lens is a clear lens without tint. This lens could be designed in a bifocal modality where reading glasses were no longer necessary.

Present contact lens specifications:

	OD	OS
Base curve	7.80 mm	7.80 mm
Overall diameter	9.0 mm	9.0 mm
Power	−5.50 D	−5.50 D
Optical zone	7.8 mm	7.8 mm
Color	Blue	
Visual acuity distance	20/20	20/20
Visual acuity near	J1	J1
Overrefraction	Pl	Pl

Distance VA uncorrected:
OD: 20/300 near J1
OS: 20/300 near J1

Refraction:
OD: −4.50 DS +1.50 D add
OS: −4.50 DS +1.50 D add

Keratometry:
OD: 42.87 @175 43.62 @ 85
OS: 42.87 @005 43.37 @ 95

Tear break-up time:
OD: 18 seconds
OS: 17 seconds

Ishihara plate color vision test: 2 out of 24—red/green color deficiencies
Palpebral aperture: 11 mm
Horizontal visible iris diameter: 11.5 mm
Pupil size: 3.5 mm
Lower lid position: 1 mm below limbus

Ocular Evaluation

The results of the examination included normal lateral and up Bell's phenomenon. Eyelids and adnexa were free of pathology. Cilia were free of debris. Lid eversion revealed normal satin appearance of tarsal conjunctiva without papillae or follicles. Lids exhibited no swelling, injection, congestion, or granulations. Extraocular muscle movements were full and smooth in all directions of gaze in both eyes. Conjunctiva and sclera exhibited no inflammation or congestion. Pupils were equal round and reactive to direct, consensual, and accommodative reflexes. There was no sign of an afferent pupil defect in either eye.

Biomicroscopy

Anterior chambers are deep and without signs of cells and flare. Iris shape, color, and size were free of pathology and abnormalities. Fluorescein staining revealed intact corneas without defects. Cornea exhibited normal tear film, adequate to support contact lenses. Neither eye exhibited any signs of neovascularization or edema. Lenticular evaluation illustrated a clear crystalline surface.

Material Selection

J.F. requires a correction for his myopia. The most appropriate bifocal design was discussed, addressing the patient's work environment and hobbies. Due to his various visual demands, working distances, and multiple head orientations, an aspheric lens incorporating the X-chrome design was mutually decided.

Lens specifications: Tangent Streak No-Line

	OD	OS
Base curve	7.80	7.80
Overall diameter	9.5	9.5
Optical zone	8.4	8.4
Power	−6.25 D	−6.25 D
Add	+1.75 D	+1.75 D
Color	Clear	Magenta
Visual acuity distance	20/20	20/20
Visual acuity near	J1	J1
Overrefraction	Plano	Plano

The Tangent Streak No-Line is an aspheric lens design. In fitting this lens, the true base curve is approximately 16 mm steeper than the fitting base curve. A well-fitted GP aspheric multifocal will exhibit apical clearance with mid-peripheral alignment and wide peripheral clearance.

J.F. picked up his contact lenses and instructions regarding application/removal, lens care regime, and wearing schedule were provided. The cleaning/disinfecting regime included the Optimum cleaning, disinfection, and surfactant solution. A wearing schedule was given to include all waking hours with no overnight wear because the patient was a previous rigid lens wearer.

Biomicroscopy

The lens position was slightly superior and moved with the blink, creating a good tear pump. Observation with fluorescein exhibited apical clearance with midperipheral alignment and peripheral edge clearance. The lenses displayed a lag of approximately 1.5 mm with slightly superior positioning after the blink

The Ishihara test was given and J.F. scored 20 out of 24. He noticed that when he closed one eye at times the images would be more apparent.

Fitting/Troubleshooting

Multifocal aspheric GP lenses move vertically across the cornea into a reading zone during translation and downward gaze. This controlled feature during the fitting process delivers sharp vision both at distance and at near. GP aspheric bifocal lenses generally have eccentricities greater than one. Good centration and lens movement is necessary for visual success. A decentered lens will need to be steepened or increased in diameter to improve centration. This lens modality is pupil sensitive, giving better distance vision with small pupils and better near vision with larger pupils. Changing the eccentricity will control the improvement of vision. Lowering the eccentricity will improve distance vision with large pupils. Increasing the eccentricity will improve near vision with small pupils. Typically the base curve is slightly steeper (0.75 D to 1.25 D) than the central keratometry readings. This will position the midperiphery of the lens to align with the cornea. Increasing the overall diameter of the lens will produce stability as well as good centration.

Lens movement is the next critical characteristic that will ensure the patient a successful outcome. Movement with the blink and translation on downward gaze should be smooth and efficient. The lens should glide back to a central location after the blink to provide for a good tear exchange. Lens translation will help the bifocal patient to move into the periphery to improve near point visual acuity. Little movement indicates a steep fit and can be corrected by flattening the base curve. Excessive movement indicates that the lens is too flat, and steepening the base curve or increasing the lens diameter will improve lens movement. Multifocal aspheric lenses require careful fitting to guarantee the proper power is on the visual axis during straight-ahead positioning. Patients need to be cautioned about the corneal molding effect of these lenses. The corneal flattening characteristics of the lens fit will reduce the spectacle Rx when the lens is removed. In the morning, the spectacle Rx will increase in minus after the lens is off the cornea during sleep as the cornea will resume its original shape.

Summary

This case demonstrates the ability to meet the patient's visual expectations by choosing the proper bifocal design. Incorporating a solution to the patient's color deficiency matches the patient's needs with contact lenses. Using GP fitting philosophies, creating the proper cornea/contact lens relationship will increase success. In order to reach a successful outcome, the patient needs to be a good bifocal contact lens candidate. Motivation is the key. If a patient can persevere through the fitting process, the outcome is usually positive. Next, the ocular structure and health must be adequate to support contact lens wear. Age has a tendency to reduce the effectiveness of the cornea, lids, and tear film. A bifocal patient tends to be your patient for life because every few years the degrading of the accommodative system creates a need for a stronger reading prescription

Macro Front Annular Bifocal

Initial Summary

A 41-year-old man complained of poor vision 5 years after undergoing a radial keratotomy (RK) procedure. S.C. claimed that each year after the RK procedure, his vision seemed to get worse. He especially had problems at night with glare and halos around lights. During the day vision seems to be better, although close work becomes problematic. His family history includes paternal father with hypertension and diabetes. S.C. has a history of allergies to thimerosal as well as hay fever. S.C.'s goals with contact lenses were to reduce the vision fluctuations and to improve his near point acuity.

Distance VA uncorrected:
OD: 20/60 near J4
OS: 20/50 near J4

Refraction:
OD: $+2.00 -2.50 \times 155 +1.50$ D add
OS: $+1.50 -2.75 \times 025 +1.50$ D add

Keratometry:
OD: 29.50 @ 025; 38.87 @ 115
OS: 38.50 @ 165; 41.12 @ 15

Tear break-up time:
OD: 12 seconds
OS: 11 seconds

Palpebral aperture: 11.5 mm
Horizontal visible iris diameter: 12.0 mm
Pupil size: 3.8 mm
Lower lid position: at limbus

Ocular Evaluation

Eyelids and adnexa were free of pathology. Cilia were free of debris. The lids exhibited no swelling, injection, congestion, or granulations. Lid eversion revealed normal satin appearance of tarsal conjunctiva without papillae or follicles. Extraocular muscle movements were full and smooth in all directions of gaze in both eyes. Conjunctiva and sclera exhibited no inflammation or congestion. Pupils were equal round and reactive to direct, consensual, and accommodative reflexes. There was no sign of an afferent pupil defect in either eye.

Biomicroscopy

Negative fluorescein staining along the incisional lines was observed. Anterior chambers were deep and without signs of cells and flare. Neither eye exhibited any signs of neovascularization or edema. Iris shape, color and size free from pathology and abnormalities. Lenticular evaluation illustrated clear crystalline surface.

Material Selection

S.C.'s objectives were to have stable vision at all visual ranges and to improve near vision. S.C. especially wanted to reduce the problems he encountered with the headlights of oncoming cars. A discussion with the patient was held describing the visual advantages of the various bifocal lens designs and the advantages of large lens designs. The most appropriate lens design to reduce the glare and variable vision in combination was the MacroLens design. The MacroLens bifocal would have to incorporate a simultaneous vision lens design because the lens would not translate into a near zone. The aspheric lens design or a front-surface annular lens design would give S.C. the best chance of success. Due to his various visual demands, working distances and multiple head orientations an aspheric bifocal lens design was ordered.

Lens specifications: macro front-surface aspheric bifocal design

	OD	OS
Base curve	7.85 mm	7.67 mm
Overall diameter	14.8 mm	14.8 mm
Optical zone	9.0 mm	9.0 mm
Power	−3.75 D	−4.25 D
Add	+1.25 D	+1.25 D
Color	Clear	Clear
Visual acuity distance	20/20	20/20
Visual acuity near	J1	J1
Overrefraction	Plano	Plano

The large-diameter scleral lens is a specialized type of GP rigid contact lens used in applications such as advanced keratoconus, irregular corneas, corneal transplants, post–refractive surgical therapies, peripheral corneal desiccation syndrome, athletes who have special visual requirements, pristine visual requirements, and for contact lens–sensitive patients. The MacroLens, Epicon lens, and Dyna Inter-Limbal Lens have the comfort of a hydrogel and the optics of a GP lens utilizing a large-diameter scleral fitting philosophy. These large-diameter lenses are fitted in cases where the lens needs to vault over the cornea, inhibit debris underneath the contact lens, create little vertical movement, and develop confidence in no lens displacement. Our fitting

goals for S.C. were the same as for any other patient. A consequence of this lens design, which incorporates a relatively large lens diameter compared to conventional GP lenses, is an increased sagittal depth. This results in vaulting over the central cornea, assuming a cornea with relatively normal eccentricity. Philosophically the lens must clear the cornea centrally and have alignment in the midperiphery. Thus, the fitting is controlled between the cornea eccentricity and the sag of the lens. As the vaulting of the lens changes so does the angle of the lens edge as it meets the sclera. Generally the center 3 mm of the cornea has the greatest amount of toricity. The peripheral cornea as it approaches the limbus has a more spherical configuration. The intermediate portion of the cornea has a varied eccentricity as it approaches the limbus (Fig. 48.3). In order to start with basic alignment, the initial base curve should be 0.50 D flatter than "K." Our objective was to have pooling in the secondary that acts as the primer for the tear pump. The tear pump for the MacroLens is not the conventional rocking motion but more of an in-and-out motion. The peripheral zone has a basic edge-clearance fitting philosophy. Patients with regular or irregular corneal astigmatism derive excellent visual rehabilitation, as with any GP lens, but with the added benefit of vaulting the central cornea, which may exhibit significant corneal toricity or corneal pathology.

The MacroLens bifocal would have to incorporate a simultaneous-vision lens design because the lens would not translate into a near zone. An aspheric lens design or a front-surface annular lens design would give S.C. the best chance of success.

Biomicroscopy revealed a centered large-diameter lens with minimum lens movement with apical clearance leading to a parallel fit in the intermediate zone. The lens exhibited an even flow of fluorescein centrally with pooling in the secondary curve area and good peripheral pooling exhibiting an adequate edge lift in the right eye and some seal-off in the left. The lenses were ordered and a lens-dispensing visit was scheduled. It was decided that if the lenses appeared to

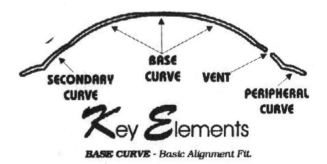

BASE CURVE - Basic Alignment Fit.

SECONDARY CURVE - Area for Tear Pooling.

VENT - A large hole for Anti-Adhesion and Tear Exchange.

PERIPHERAL CURVE - Basic Alignment Fit.

FIG. 48.3. Key elements of the MacroLens.

fit tight after an initial settling period, a reduction in the overall diameter would be performed in the office to loosen the overall fitting relationship.

S.C. picked up his contact lenses 1 week later and instructions regarding application/removal, lens care procedures, and wearing schedule were given. All MacroLens patients are given a suction cup to be used if problems exist during lens removal. The MacroLens incorporates a 1.0-mm fenestration in order to break up the negative pressure underneath the lens, which aids in tear exchange and lens removal. The antiadhesion characteristic of this large vent hole helps in lens removal. The cleaning/disinfecting regimen included the Optimum cleaning, disinfection, and surfactant solution. Celluvisc is used as a wetting solution to be placed on the concave part of the lens and should not be rinsed off. Because the patient was a previous rigid lens wearer, the wearing schedule given was to start at 4 hours and increase 2 hours each day with no overnight wear. An appointment was rescheduled for 1 week.

At the follow-up appointment S.C. described continued flare and glare, although he said it was different than the visual distortions from his normal vision. It was explained to the patient that using 0.5% pilocarpine can significantly reduce the flare and glare. S.C. was willing to attempt the pupillary constriction if the treatment would eliminate the visual distortions. The prescription was written and a follow-up appointment was made for 1 week.

At the 1-week appointment, S.C. said that his visual field was constricted although the symptoms of flare and glare had been eliminated. He expressed concern that his field of view was restricted, which presented a dangerous situation when driving a car. He also experienced problems reading with the contact lenses when the pilocarpine was administered. S.C. stopped the application of 0.5% pilocarpine after 3 days and continued to wear the aspheric MacroLens.

The visual acuity of the aspheric bifocal MacroLens seemed to go in and out of focus with the blink although it was perfect if he opened his eyes wide and did not blink. At night S.C. also experienced halos around lights as well as ghosting of images. The fitting options with the aspheric MacroLens did not seem to be able to satisfy his visual requirements, and a refit with the front-surface annular simultaneous-vision MacroLens was initiated.

The annular bifocal lens design change was made with an adjustment in base curve and overall diameter. The parameter modification allowed for a slightly flatter fitting relationship and a shallower sagittal height. This parameter adjustment would allow for some additional lens movement and greater edge lift. The annular design incorporates two distinct focal points to reduce some of the flare and glare generated by an aspheric lens design. A distance zone size of 4.0 mm was selected from the photopic pupil size of 3.8 mm. The remaining portion of the optical zone incorporated the near-add prescription.

Lens specifications: macro front-surface annular bifocal design

	OD	OS
Base curve	7.85 mm	7.58 mm
Overall diameter	14.5 mm	14.2 mm
Optical zone	9.0 mm	9.0 mm
Distance zone	4.0 mm	4.0 mm
Power	−3.75 D	−4.50 D
Add	+1.50 D	+1.50 D
Color	Clear	Clear
Visual acuity distance	20/20	20/20
Visual acuity near	J1	J1
Overrefraction	Plano	Plano

S.C. returned for a lens-dispensing visit 2 weeks later and the bifocal designs were exchanged. Visual acuity exhibited 20/20 monocularly for distance and J2 monocularly for near vision. Initially S.C. experienced less distortion in the periphery and the near vision seemed to be adequate to read. Biomicroscopy with the installation of fluorescein revealed a well-centered lens with apical clearance centrally moving to a parallel fit in the intermediate and pooling of tears within the secondary curve. The eccentricity of the lens exhibited basic alignment in the peripheral curve zone.

Summary

Recognizing the distinctive differences between bifocal lens designs can assist in contact lens selection. Each lens selection is based on the visual requirements and expected patient adaptation response. Extensive case histories will lead you to the pitfalls needed to be resolved before success can be achieved. It is the delicate balance of distant and near vision that enables the patient to succeed with bifocal contact lenses. Successes in fitting bifocal contact lenses require a motivated patient and a lens design appropriate to the patient's visual requirement. Communication is the basis of your partnership with the patient. The patient's visual needs and history should guide the selection to the most appropriate bifocal lens type. Patients want clarity, comfort, and convenience without visual distortions. Many times the only scenario to solve the visual dilemma is to attempt a lens design in order to determine the visual difficulties experienced. The fitting process allows for modifications and refitting. Patients who need to be fitted after refractive surgery represent just another category that tests your creativity with all the available tools.

SOFT BIFOCAL LENSES

Advanced Presbyopia Requiring Lens Change

Initial Summary

M.M. had been successfully wearing Ciba progressive soft disposable bifocal contact lens for the past 2.5 years. Recently she has had to purchase reading glasses to wear over her contact lenses to read fine detail materials at near point. M.M.'s lenses work perfectly for the computer and distance, although when she has to perform nearpoint work, the bifocal does not provide enough power as before due to the aging of her accommodative system. M.M. has no family history of glaucoma, macular degeneration, or diabetes. Her maternal mother does have a history of hypertension. M.M. takes levothyroxine (Synthroid) due to a thyroid disorder, although she does not have any seasonal allergies.

Ocular Evaluation

Extraocular muscle movements were full and smooth in all directions of gaze in both eyes. Bell's phenomenon exhibited a normal lateral and up. Lid eversion revealed normal appearance of tarsal conjunctiva without papillae or follicles. Upon pressure to the meibomian glands on the lid margin, normal contents were expressed. Lid appearance was tight, typical for a 46-year-old woman. Lids exhibited no swelling, injection, congestion, or granulations. The inferior tear meniscus was adequate in height to support contact lens wear. The sclera exhibited no inflammation or congestion. Pupils were equal, round, and reactive to direct, consensual, and accommodative reflexes. There was no sign of an afferent pupil defect in either eye. Lenticular evaluation illustrated clear media. Tear break-up time and the Schirmer tear test results were within normal limits.

Keratometry:
OD: 42.37 @ 170; 43.12 @ 080
OS: 43.25 @ 020; 43.00 @ 110

Distance VA uncorrected:
OD: 20/100 near J3
OS: 20/100 near J3

Subjective:
OD: −1.00DS 20/20 add +1.50 D J1
OS: −1.00DS 20/20 add +1.50 D J1

Schirmer I without anesthetic:
OD: 19 mm in 5 minutes
OS: 21 mm in 5 minutes

Tear break-up time: OD 17 seconds
Invasive method: OS 16 seconds

Biomicroscopy

The anterior chamber was clear in both eyes. Fluorescein staining revealed intact corneas without defects. Neither eye exhibited any signs of neovascularization or edema. Grade 1 bulbar conjunctival injection was present.

Material Selection

M.M.'s visual anomaly incorporated both a distance myopic prescription as well as a prescription at near for presbyopia.

All other findings confirmed that she was a good candidate for contact lens wear. The contact lens options discussed with the patient included fitting a spherical disposable for distance and a reading prescription over the contact lenses, monovision correction with soft disposable lenses, monovision with GP lenses, GP bifocals, and soft bifocal contact lenses. A soft distance disposable lens in conjunction with a reading prescription was not acceptable due to the "age stigma" and the inconvenience that reading glasses possess. Monovision was not an acceptable option due to her previous contact lens experience. The summation of two eyes would be less of a compromise than with the monovision technique. GP lenses were not an acceptable option due to discomfort. The soft bifocal lens modality offers a multifocal annular/aspheric design. A discussion with the patient emphasized the desire not to return to a spectacle prescription. The office time commitment and possible multiple lens orders were discussed to make the patient aware the difficulties in achieving the visual requirement.

Fitting/Troubleshooting

Previous contact lens design:
Focus Progressive:
OD: −0.75 D
OS: −0.75 D

The annular/aspheric Cooper Frequency multifocal was trial fitted using −1.00D spherical lens with a +1.50D near prescription. Both lens designs incorporated the D variety with distance in the center and near in the periphery.

The contact lens specifications from CooperVision were as follows:

Base curve: 8.7 mm (OD); 8.7 mm (OS)
Diameter: 14.4 mm (OD); 14.4 mm (OS)
Power: −1.00 D add + 1.50D (OD); −1.00 D add + 1.50D (OS)

The Ciba Vision Focus Progressive is a near-center aspheric lens design with a add prescription (+ 1.25 D). Usually, a + 0.50 D must be added to the manifest spheroequivalent prescription to arrive at the appropriate distance prescription. This prescription alteration will take advantage of the full bifocal power but won't degrade far vision. This lens design can also be fit by offsetting the distance prescription by another 0.5 D to integrate additional add power in a modified monovision technique.

The CooperVision Frequency Bifocal incorporates a spherical center zone surrounded by an aspheric intermediate zone with an additional spherical zone in the periphery. The primary advantage to this lens design involves the integration of a distance-centered lens for the dominant eye and near-centered lens for the nondominant eye. The distance-centered lens integrates a 2.3-mm spherical distance prescription whereas the near-centered lens has a 1.7-mm spherical near prescription in the center (Fig. 48.4). The

D lens

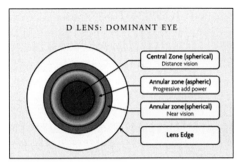

Central Spherical Zone: 2.3mm
Aspheric Annular Zone: 5.0mm
Spherical Annular Zone: 8.5mm

N lens

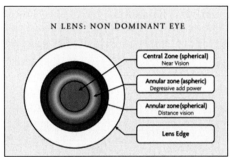

Central Spherical Zone: 1.7mm
Aspheric Annular Zone: 5.0mm
Spherical Annular Zone: 8.5mm

FIG. 48.4. The CooperVision Frequency Bifocal D Lens and N Lens.

distance center lens design usually needs a + 0.25 D added to the distance prescription while the near-centered lens requires −0.50 D added to the distance prescription.

The manufacturer suggests an initial lens selection of a D lens for the dominant eye and an N lens for the nondominant eye. Initially, two D lenses were selected and the quality of the near vision evaluated. If the patient requires improvement in the near vision, replacing the nondominant lens with the N lens usually solves the inadequacy. If the patient still needs improvement in the near vision, the D lens in the dominant eye can be replaced with an additional N lens. The higher-add prescriptions usually have a deteriorating effect on the quality of the distance vision. The primary advantage of this lens design is the flexibility to fit a majority of patients with this one lens modality due to the many options.

M.M. required an additional reading power over the Ciba progressive lens. The two D lenses of CooperVision's Frequency Bifocal provided adequate distance and near vision. It was discussed with the patient that in the future we would have to change the lenses again because the near prescription would progressively get worse. In this lens design we have the option of increasing the bifocal add or changing to an N lens, near center, to enhance the visual range and visual acuity at near.

Summary

A trial lens fitting is used to define the best lens design. Adding or subtracting 0.5 D allows for investigating acceptable visual ranges monocularly. Visual acuity should always be checked under binocular conditions. Trial lens fittings give the patient the visual experience of the lens design, but more importantly gives the practitioner the ability to refine the prescription, the fitting parameters, and the patient's subjective response. The trial lens procedure allows the prac-

titioner to gain insight into the patient's ability to process visual information through the lens design.

Pupil size can be an ally or an enemy in these annular zone lens designs. During the day, when the pupil is constricted, the center zone prescription will be enhanced. During scotopic conditions, when the pupil is dilated, the surround prescription may degrade the center prescription. The real advantage of these lens designs is the ability of the visual system to decipher multiple prescriptions in a relative small annular space. Flare and glare at night can destroy the image quality at night. Some patients experience halos or streaks around lights. Investigating different bifocal designs will change the annular size and configuration minimizing the flare and glare effect. Investigating scotopic and photopic conditions will reduce chair time and narrow the lens selection.

This case demonstrates the need to manage the presbyopic patients throughout their progressive loss of the accommodative power. The management of these cases reflects the need for a design change every 4 to 5 years. Listening to the patients as they define their visual difficulties and acknowledge the need for a lens change is important. Generally pushing plus on the distance prescription or aspheric lens designs will evolve to annular lens designs or translating lens modalities. Adequately meeting your presbyopic patient's goals and expectations will result in a patient for life.

Hydrogel Aspheric Multifocal Fitting

Initial Summary

A 47-year-old policeman (B.W.) had been successfully wearing soft spherical hydrogel lenses for 7 years. While driving, he noticed that the speedometer was beginning to blur and double. The computer in his car was also difficult to see without moving around to find a clear zone. B.W. also described difficulties in reading and writing reports at work. During practice rounds at the gun range, B.W. could no longer keep his gun sight clear while looking at the target. His distance vision remained unchanged and he also explained that his arms were "just not long enough" when reading the newspaper.

Present contact lens specifications:

	OD	OS
Base curve	8.6 mm	8.6 mm
Diameter	14.8 mm	14.8 mm
Power	−2.00 D	−2.25 D
Material	Crofilcon A	Crofilcon A

Manifest refraction:
OD: −2.00 DS 20/20
OS: −3.25 − 0.50 × 045 20/20
Add: + 1.50 D J1 OD, OS, OU

Keratometry:
OD: 47.37 @ 080; 47.87 @ 170
OS: 48.25 @ 070; 49.25 @ 160

Pupil size: 3.6 mm (mesopic conditions); 4.2 mm (scotopic conditions)

Biomicroscopy

The tarsal conjunctiva exhibited a normal satin appearance with an absence of papillae and follicles. The Meibomian glands excreted clear fluid upon gentle expression. The tear break-up time was 14 seconds OD and 15 seconds OS. No corneal staining was present with fluorescein instillation.

It was explained to the patient that he has been wearing nonbifocal lenses fit in a monovision approach. This technique will slightly blur the distance image in one eye by increasing the plus in the prescription to improve near vision. With intense distance demands this technique eventually will not be tolerated. Monovision incorporates both simultaneous and alternating vision philosophies when fitting this technique. The patient receives distance and near images simultaneously from both eyes, and cortically the patient will selectively alternate his attention to the necessary image. Monovision allows for a full aperture viewing without aberrations from a bifocal arrangement. Monovision also is not dependent on lens position or head orientation. The advantage of this technique is that each eye individually will see a clear image at the prescribed focal point. Bifocals allow for the summation of binocular images to improve stereopsis and an increase range of vision. Improved intermediate vision is an important criterion for patients whose occupations and hobbies mandate clear and concise vision.

Material Selection

B.W. wanted to wear bifocal contact lenses due to the visual demands of his occupation. Chasing criminals is very diffi-

cult when wearing spectacles in an environment with abrupt temperature changes and high physical demands. A flexible wear schedule was also preferred due to his long working hours. The Hydrocurve II Bifocal (Ciba Vision) aspheric design was selected to meet the patient's needs. This variable aspheric lens has a maximum eccentricity of 1.3 on the posterior surface near the optical center and decreases to below 1.0 in the periphery. This typically results in a reduction in flare during pupil dilation. This lens moves very little with the blink so the pupil diameter controls the available add power for near point work. If the lens movement is excessive, the distance vision is degraded from the spreading of the focused light caused by the varying focal power of the lens.

Fitting/Troubleshooting

The Hydrocurve II posterior aspheric multifocal lens was applied to test acceptability of vision and lens-to-cornea fitting relationship. The lens parameters were base curve: 9.0 mm OU, diameter 14.8 mm, and power −2.25D OD and −3.25D OS The patient responded with acceptable distance vision with good comfort. The near vision, however, was still similar to the spherical hydrogel lens haze the patient was presently experiencing. The complete distance prescription did not satisfy the near demands; therefore, the left Hydrocurve II multifocal prescription was changed to −2.75 D, improving the distance vision of his present soft lens prescription. The modified monovision design improved near vision significantly without degrading the distance vision. These lenses exhibited good centration and moved 0.5 mm with the blink.

Lens parameters:

	OD	OS
Base curve	9.0 mm	9.0 mm
Diameter	4.8 mm	14.8 mm
Power	−2.25 D	−2.75 D

The patient was dispensed these multifocal lenses with the Aosept care regimen. A daily-wear schedule was prescribed for one week and an appointment was made for a follow-up visit. The patient was instructed to test the acceptability of vision in his work environment. At the 1-week follow-up appointment, the patient responded that the lens design was comfortable and the vision at near, intermediate, and distance was significantly better than the previously worn spherical lenses. The patient also confessed that during his 24-hour shift, he did not remove his lenses. In the morning he instilled saline for lubrication without experiencing any adverse effects. The patient was told that foggy vision in the morning or halos around lights is indicative of corneal swelling.

A schedule of 3-month follow-up visits was discussed with the patient to maintain lens hygiene, promote corneal health, and sustain clear and concise vision while driving.

A discussion with the patient emphasized the risk of extended wear and the necessary benefits of this type of lens demanded by his occupation.

Summary

Gas-permeable bifocal lenses had also been considered for this patient. However as a result of the dangerous nature of his job and the possibility of lens dislocation or debris underneath the lens, a decision was made to only consider soft lens options. In his case, the compatibility of the lens modality with the patient's occupation was an important criterion. The lens design option was further narrowed due to the long working hours. The Acuvue Bifocal, Ciba Vision Focus Progressive bifocal, Frequency 55 Multifocal, or Sunsoft Additions lenses could have been an option if vision was not acceptable. The patient did not want to go into a disposable lens due to his contact lens history. Monovision did not give the patient the quality of vision required, especially with the loss of binocularity and limited intermediate vision range.

Hydrogel Near-centered Annular Bifocal Fitting

Initial Summary

A 45-year-old television producer (T.G.), experiencing difficulty at near point, recently observed that his distance vision was beginning to blur. T.G. especially had problems reading the monitors and news copy during a broadcast. He realized that a full-time vision correction might be required and he desired to investigate options with contact lenses. He has never worn a prescription to satisfy his visual needs. He also indicated a preference for soft disposable lenses because of convenience and his fast-paced lifestyle.

Unaided distance visual acuity:
OD: 20/40
OS : 20/40
OU: 20/30

Manifest refraction:
OD: + 1.25 DS 20/20
OS : +1.00 DS 20/20
Add: +1.25 DS J1

Keratometry:
OD: 42.37 @ 015; 44.25 @ 105
OS: 42.25 @ 010; 43.87 @ 100

Pupil size: 3.8 mm (mesopic conditions); 4.5 mm (scotopic conditions)

Biomicroscopy

The inferior tear meniscus appeared to be clear and adequate in height to allow successful contact lens wear. His tear break-up time was 16 seconds OD and 15 seconds OS. Lid eversion revealed a normal satin appearance of the tarsal conjunctiva without papillae or follicle formation. Fluorescein application revealed an absence of staining.

Material Selection

T.G. was psychologically ready for a correction of his hyperopia and presbyopia. Contact lenses were his only avenue to correct for his ametropia because of the stigma of glasses. Having the flexibility of either sleeping with his contact lenses or wearing them daily was consistent with his unpredictable lifestyle. Due to the hyperopic prescription pushing plus at distance always increases the probability of success in soft bifocal lens patients. The convenience of having the prescription in place instead of placing on and removing glasses is an added benefit contact lenses provide.

The first option considered for this patient was disposable monovision lenses. This option would fulfill his flexible wearing criteria. A + 1.50 D Frequency lens was fit on the right eye and a + 2.50 D lens was fit on the left eye. The 8.7-mm base curve radius and the 14.2-mm diameter were chosen as the most optimum initial design for diagnostic fitting. Any additional plus power in the left eye adversely affected distance visual acuity. The vision was adequate at far and intermediate distances, although the near vision was inadequate.

The second option considered was the Unilens (Unilens). This soft posterior aspheric multifocal design was fitted to determine quality of vision. A 9.0-mm base curve radius, 14.5-mm overall diameter, and a + 2.00 D power was applied to the right eye and a + 1.75 D lens was fitted to the left eye. The Unilens design is usually + 0.50 D to + 0.75 D over the distance prescription. The patient's initial reaction was that distance and intermediate vision was adequate. However, the near vision resulted in shadows surrounding the letters and glare when viewing lights at night.

Next the Acuvue simultaneous bifocal was considered to test visual acceptability of the distance-center annular lens design. The distance-center annular design utilizes concentric rings alternating distance and near refractive zones. The Acuvue Bifocal disposable lens is a flexible design that is replaced every 2 weeks. The bifocal add powers can be configured with + 1.00 D, + 1.50 D, + 2.00 D, or + 2.50 D add powers. This two-power lens design can be fitted either in a bifocal arrangement or a multifocal lens design by offsetting the add powers. The alternating distance and near concentric annular power strategy reduces the problems that are encountered at night or in dim illumination. In low levels of light, when the pupil dilates, light falls upon an adjacent zone of distance power, aiding the ability for distance vision in conditions such as night driving. Typically the distance prescription needs to be increased by −0.50 D for optimal distance viewing. This simultaneous lens design incorporates alternating distance and near powers inside the pupillary zone. Increasing the bifocal power reduces the quality of vision in the distance due to the near prescription affecting alternating power separation within the pupil. Offsetting the bifocal powers creates a multifocal approach resulting in an improved distance, near and intermediate visual range as compared to the straight bifocal fitting strategy.

Fitting/Troubleshooting

The Acuvue Bifocal has an 8.5-mm base curve with a diameter of 14.2 mm. The lens is approved for extended wear and has a Dk/1 value of 37. The higher adds create distortion in the patient's distance visual acuity. Reducing the add in the dominant eye will improve the distance acuity in a modified bifocal approach. The distance prescription, especially in plus power, can be changed by ± 0.25 to improve the range of vision. Adding these two fitting philosophies together, the patient was trailed with the following lenses:

Lens parameters:

	OD	OS
Power	+ 1.25 D/ + 1.00 D add	+ 1.25 D/ + 1.50 D add
Base curve	8.5 mm	8.5 mm
Diameter	14.2 mm	14.2 mm

Visual acuity:
OD: 20/20 J3
OS : 20/20 J3

Adaptation to the lenses was rapid and the patient was comfortable after 15 minutes. The lenses exhibited good centration and had 0.5-mm lag with straight-ahead gaze after the blink.

The lenses were dispensed to the patient. In addition, he was provided with Opti-Free (Alcon) solution regimen instructions and care and handling information. Due to the oxygen permeability of the 58% etafilcon material, the flexible wear concept was explained. A 1-week follow-up appointment was scheduled to discuss the acceptability of this lens design in his own visual environment. After 1 week of lens wear, his vision was adequate at all working ranges. The lenses were worn comfortably at all waking hours, and occasionally the patient took naps while wearing the lenses without any adverse effects. The lenses centered well and moved well with the blink. It was explained to the patient that soft lenses degrade over time and need to be replaced if they become coated or deposited. Abrupt changes in vision, comfort, wearing time, or eye redness need to be investigated to maintain soft bifocal lens success.

The patient was instructed to reschedule in 1 month to reevaluate the prescription and to assess any problem areas that might be encountered. The lens was prescribed in a 2-week replacement schedule with a quarterly progress visit schedule to evaluate lens surface integrity, prescription changes, corneal health, and lens cleaning. Preventative maintenance serves to ensure compliance.

Summary

Other hydrogel and rigid bifocal contact lens designs could have been considered in this case. Such options as the hydrogel MV2, Ciba Focus Progressive, Frequency 55 Multifocal, high-Dk flexible-wear rigid aspherics, or high-Dk flexible-wear rigid annular designs would have been considered if the Acuvue Bifocal was unsuccessful. However, based upon the patient's motivation and visual needs, the Acuvue Bifocal fulfilled the patient's criteria of visual acuity, comfort, and flexible wear.

Annular Lens Design

Initial Summary

A 51-year-old schoolteacher (S.T.) wearing soft bifocal contact lenses at her annual visit described her frustrations after replacing six lenses during the past year. Her previous bifocal contact lens experience included Tangent Streak one-piece alternating GP lens bifocals and a soft monovision design. Presently S.T. is wearing a daily-wear reusable annular center-near bifocal design. The patient wears her lenses all her waking hours and does not have a pair of glasses as a backup. S.T. uses Opti-Free cleaning and disinfection regimen every night before she goes to bed. She is very happy with the comfort and vision through her contact lenses, although the lenses tear frequently and deposited easily.

Contact lens specifications:

	OD	OS.
Base curve	8.6 mm	8.6 mm
Diameter	14.0 mm	14.0 mm
Power	−4.75 D	−4.00 D
Add	+ 2.50 D	+ 2.50 D
Near zone	2.3 mm	2.3 mm
Distance visual acuity	20/25	20/25
Near visual acuity	J3	J3

Manifest refraction:
OD: −4.50 DS 20/20
OS: −4.25 −0.50 × 180 20/20

Keratometry:
OD: 42.37 @ 030; 43.87 @ 120
OS: 42.50 @ 170; 43.37 @ 080

Pupil size: 3.5 mm (mesopic conditions); 4.2 mm (scotopic conditions)

Biomicroscopy

Upon lid eversion, the tarsal conjunctiva exhibited a mild grade 1 injection with grade 1 papillary hypertrophy. The inferior tear meniscus appeared to be clear and adequate in the height to support contact lens wear. The tear break-up time was 13 seconds OD and 14 seconds OS. The Meibomian glands excreted clear fluid upon gentle expression. No corneal staining was evident with fluorescein application.

Material

The patient had been pleased with the comfort and vision provided by the Annular Bifocal near-center soft contact lens. The durability problems experienced with this bifocal frustrated the patient and, due to the expense of replacing numerous lenses, the patient was interested in another bifocal contact lens alternative. Overall, the patient had enjoyed the benefits of having near and distance correction in contact lenses and for the most part had been successful. Spectacles were not an option because of the visual differences and aberrations between contact lenses and spectacles. It was explained that it would not be possible to simply refit her into a more durable lens design with the same existing contact lens specifications because manufacturers have a patent on each lens and material design. However, an effort would be made to fit a more durable lens in a lens design that was not radically different. The other option would be to refit S.T. into a disposable bifocal modality. This lens design has the advantage of replacing the lens every 2 weeks to 1 month; in the event a lens became torn or deposited, a new lens would not have to be purchased as well as no interruption of lens wear. The SimulVue reusable lens (Unilens Corporation) design was selected because it is a concentric near center made out of a durable material polymacon. The Unilens aspheric lens is manufactured with a 45% hefilcon material. It is a center-near front aspheric design with three base curves (8.4 mm, 8.7 mm, and 9.0 mm) and a 14.5-mm diameter. The SimulVue is a concentric near-center lens design also made with a 45% hefilcon material. The center add zone is available in widths of 2.35 and 2.55 mm. The 2.35-mm near-center zone provides better distance vision whereas the 2.55-mm near-center zone provides better near vision.

The Lifestyle 4-Vue Hi-Add (Permeable Technologies) lens design was also selected as a result of our experience its durability. This is a posterior aspheric annular design with two distinct aspheric zones with a central spherical distance zone, made from a polymacon (Fig. 48.5). The first aspheric zone surrounding the distance zone has a +1.75 D bifocal prescription at its lowest position in the lens. A distance vision aspheric zone surrounds the bifocal portion for when the pupil dilates at night to increase the quality of distance vision. The conventional Lifestyle 4-Vue lens has the same lens design with a lower add equal to +1.00 D.

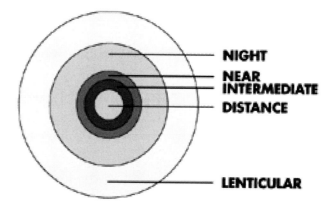

FIG. 48.5. The Lifestyle 4-Vue Lens design.

These daily-wear materials are less fragile than other bifocal lenses in the marketplace. The Acuvue 2-week disposable or the Frequency 55 monthly replacement multifocal lens designs were selected because of their annular configuration. Replacing soft lenses at regular intervals will maintain a clean lens, provide stable vision, ensure continued comfort, and improve ocular safety. Practitioners need to be proactive and ask patients to replace lenses before an adverse reaction occurs. The goal is to have a lens that is less likely to soil in an environment where lens coating is more likely to occur with loss of tear quality and quantity. Frequent-replacement lenses have shorter lens life and require less care to maintain good performance. Frequent-replacement lenses also guarantee a spare lens available in the unexpected scenarios of torn or damaged lenses.

Fitting/Troubleshooting

The Lifestyle 4-Vue Hi-Add was applied to both eyes and an assessment of comfort and visual acuity was made. A series I (8.80) lens was placed on the right eye and a series II (8.50) lens was placed on the left eye. The diameter of both lenses was 14.5 mm; the power of the right lens was −4.25 D and the left lens power was −4.00 D. The lenses were allowed to equilibrate for a period of 10 minutes prior to evaluation. With biomicroscopy both lenses exhibited good centration and, upon both upward and straight-ahead gaze, 1 mm of lens movement was present. Both lenses were also perceived as comfortable by the patient. The quality of vision was evaluated with both the Snellen Acuity Chart and the Stereo Optical "Optec 3000" Vision Tester contrast sensitivity chart. The resultant distance vision was equivalent to her spectacles (i.e., 20/20 OU). Her reading at near point was blurry; therefore, the prescription in both lenses was reduced. The second set of diagnostic Lifestyle 4-Vue lenses had lens powers of −4.00 D OD and −3.75 D OS. This prescription improved near vision without compromising distance vision. Further reducing the left lens distance prescription to −3.50 D improved near vision with little effect on distance vision.

The final contact lens specifications were as follows:

	OD	OS
Base curve	Series I	Series II
Diameter	14.5 mm	14.5 mm
Power	−4.00 D	−3.50 D
Material	Polymacon	Polymacon
Distance visual acuity	20/20	20/20
Near visual acuity	J3	J2

The Lifestyle 4-Vue lenses were dispensed and a patient reeducation program was instituted. In addition, GPC was explained to the patient. Our goal was to discuss the importance of lens hygiene and the direct cause of GPC from soiled lenses. The patient was instructed to instill a drop of olopatadine (Patanol) in both eyes twice a day and Aosept was selected as the solution regimen to eliminate the possible source of lid complication from a presolution. Handling and cleaning techniques were demonstrated to minimize the potential of lens damage. Digital cleaning was illustrated to avoid frustration from lens damage and tarsal reactivity from soiled lenses. At the follow-up visit, the second phase of the reeducation program demonstrated the patient's confidence in manipulating and handling the lens. The positive experience of the reeducation program turned a potential contact lens dropout into a successful contact lens patient. Comprehensive patient education communicates the proper methods to avoid misunderstanding and failure.

Summary

Each bifocal modality has a variety of parameter modifications that can turn bifocal contact lens failure into success. Every presbyopic patient has specific visual demands and visual goals that translate to lens success when they are met. Monitoring a patient's expectations while they are wearing bifocal lenses is a key for bifocal lens acceptability. Adaptation and cortical interpretation occurs when the patient integrates the vision presented by the bifocal into everyday actions. The final stage of adaptation is when the patient can rely on the information coming in through their eyes. Other bifocal lenses including the Unilens (Unilens), Hydrocurve II (Ciba Vision), or UltraVue (Lifestyle) could have been applied. GP lenses in either the annular, segmented, or aspheric lens designs probably could have fulfilled the patient's criteria of acceptability. Likewise, monovision in either the soft or GP version could have been attempted. However, based upon our experience with the Lifestyle 4-Vue bifocal and the specific lens design, power availability and durability resulted in patient satisfaction and success. In addition, reeducation on compliance with lens handling, cleaning, and disinfection was performed to ensure that compliance would be present with the Lifestyle 4-Vue lens.

Frequency Multifocal

Initial Summary

B.B. a is 47-year-old female CEO who travels to Europe frequently. She presented to our office with red irritated eyes and complained of reduced contact lens wearing time. More specifically, she said her Acuvue bifocals did not feel as comfortable during the second week of wear as they did during the first week. B.B. also complained that during airplane flights her contact lenses became very dry and lubricating drops were necessary every 30 minutes. She also felt that her near vision was not good as with her bifocal spectacle lenses. When she was at work on the computer and reading from a manuscript, the vision seemed to go in and out of focus. She also had trouble driving on the expressway. The overhead exit signs seemed to be out of focus until her car was a few feet away. The patient has been a soft contact lens wearer for 23 years, and has a history of lens deposits. The protein buildup on her lenses apparently led to superficial punctate keratitis (SPK) diagnosed via fluorescein staining. We instructed the patient to discontinue lens wear, use ciprofloxacin (Ciloxan) antibiotic drops four times daily for 3 days, and then return for a follow-up appointment.

Present contact lens specifications: Acuvue disposable lens

	OD	OS
Power	+3.75 D	+3.75 D
Add	+1.00 D	+1.50 D
Base curve	8.5 mm	8.5 mm
Diameter	14.2 mm	14.2 mm
Distance visual acuity	20/25	20/25
Near visual acuity	J2	J2

Manifest refraction:
OD: +3.75 −1.00 × 180 20/20
OS: +3.75 −1.00 × 180 20/20

Add:
OD: +1.75 D
OS: +1.75 D

Keratometry:
OD: 43.75 @ 180; 44.25 @ 090
OS: 43.87 @ 180; 44.37 @ 090

At the follow-up visit, I (R.L.D) discussed with the patient other bifocal options to improve the quality of vision and wear ability. Contact lens cleaning and disinfection was discussed as well as the importance of routine 2-week lens replacement. It was decided to refit the patient in the Frequency 55 Multifocal (CooperVision), a monthly replacement multifocal lens. Supraclean enzyme treatment will be used in the lens case when the lenses are removed for nightly disinfection. Ketotifen (Zaditor) was prescribed twice a day to reduce the GPC and lid involvement.

Ocular Evaluation

Extraocular muscle movements were full and smooth in all directions of gaze in both eyes. Bell's phenomenon exhibited a normal lateral and up. Upon lid eversion the tarsal conjunctiva exhibited a mild grade 1 injection with grade 1 papillary hypertrophy. Upon pressure to the meibomian glands on the lid margin, normal contents were expressed. The lids exhibited slight swelling but no injection, congestion, or granulations. The inferior tear meniscus was adequate in height to support contact lens wear. Sclera exhibited no inflammation or congestion. Pupils were equal, round, and reactive to direct, consensual, and accommodative reflexes. There was no sign of an afferent pupil defect in either eye. Lenticular evaluation illustrated clear media. Both tear break-up time and Schirmer tear test results were within normal limits. No corneal staining was evident with fluorescein application.

Lens Material

Frequency 55 is a patented inverse-geometry lens system with two different annular lens designs: one intended for the dominant eye, the other for the nondominant eye. Both have a spherical central zone surrounded by an aspheric annular zone followed by spherical peripheral annular zone. The central zone sizes are different between the D lens (2.3 mm) and N lens (1.7 mm) so as to maximize both the visual performance at the centralized vision demand zone and also the complimentary peripheral vision demand zone. Patients are provided with one distance-center and one near-center lens, two distance-center lenses, or two near-center lenses. We initially fit this patient in a distance-center lens for the dominant eye and a near-center lens with a surrounding distance zone for the nondominant eye, but she reported distance blur. Next, two distance-center lenses were prescribed with unequal adds of + 1.50 D OD and + 2.00 D OS, which gave her adequate distant and near vision. The results of the lens change produced 20/20 at distance and near, and no further problems with lens deposits or red eyes.

Summary

A thorough history is essential to develop a treatment plan. The patient's visual needs must be considered, including occupation and hobbies, as well as the patient's preferred wearing schedule. It is important to determine if the patient has had a history of any problems with contact lens wear. Although the Frequency 55 Multifocal Contact Lens was more appropriate for this patient, other patients might benefit from features offered by different brands of bifocal contact lenses. The Ciba Focus Progressive, MV2 Bifocal, Acuvue Bifocal, or Sunsoft Additions are frequent-replacement lenses that could have been used with positive results. With bifocal lenses, trial fitting is essential (and sometimes time consuming). Frequency 55 bifocal offers a choice of a distance center or near center. It is recommended to start the patient with one distance and one near lens. If that combination provides satisfactory vision, the lenses can be dispensed. If the patient's vision is inadequate, he or she can be refit in two distant or two near lenses, depending on what visual needs the patient stated during the case history.

Some patients are unable to interpret the information that the lens focuses on the retina. For example, two near-center lenses and distance peripheries were initially attempted on this patient, but she could not tolerate any distant blur; therefore, this was resolved by switching her lenses to two distance-center designs. The patient's pupil size can be beneficial in making this decision. If the patient has smaller pupils (less than 3.5 mm), he or she will have difficulty seeing the surrounding portion of the lens, whether its distance or near. With small-pupil patients, the selection of one distance-center and one near-center lens is recommended. If the patient has larger pupils, he or she will be able to see the surrounding zone well, so two near lenses should be successful. Finally, it is important to ensure that the lens centers well on the eye and let your patients guide you towards the optimal fitting design.

Multiple Bifocal Designs to Satisfy Visual Needs

Initial Summary

A 51-year-old insurance salesman who is having problems reading at work came into the office for an annual examination. Distance vision has never been a problem with contact lenses or spectacles. He is an avid hiker, who spends all of his free time camping out in the backcountry. He enjoys mountain climbing, shooting rapids, hunting, and snowshoeing. He has worn soft contact lenses for 28 years and does not want to contend with spectacles. Previously he had worn CSI spheres, Softmate spheres, MV2, Acuvue Bifocals, LifeStyle Xtra, and Seequence disposables. His present contact lens prescription is as follows:

Lens specifications: Ciba Focus Progressive

	OD	OS
Base curve	8.6 mm	8.6 mm
Diameter	14.0 mm	14.0 mm
Power	−4.75 D	−4.50 D
Visual acuity distance	20/25	20/25
Visual acuity near	J2	J2
Overrefraction	Plano	Plano

At this annual visit, the patient's goal was to improve near vision so that he does not have to find the sweet spot of his gun without degrading the distance visual acuity. The Ciba Focus Progressive lens is a comfortable wearing lens that is adequate for general viewing. This bifocal design is especially helpful when hunting because the gun sight and distance object is clear. Problems arise when the patient has to read for any length of time. The patient likes the disposability of the lens and the convenience of the no-rub cleaning and disinfection. The patient also asked if distance vision could be improved.

Ocular Evaluation

Upper lid eversion revealed tarsal conjunctiva grade 1 hyperemia and small papillae lining zone 3. Upon gentle pressure to the meibomian glands on the lid margin, normal contents were expressed. The cilia were free of debris. The lids exhibited no swelling, injection, congestion, or granulations. The palpebral aperture heights measured 11.5 mm. The inferior tear meniscus was adequate in height to support contact lens wear.

Biomicroscopy

Anterior chamber was clear in both eyes. Fluorescein staining revealed intact corneas without defects. Neither eye exhibited any signs of neovascularization or edema. The tear film layer was adequate to support contact lens wear.

Keratometry:
OD: 43.25 @ 180; 44.25 @ 090
OS: 43.75 @ 180; 44.25 @ 090

Distance VA uncorrected:
OD: 20/300 near J2
OS: 20/300 near J2

Subjective:
OD: −5.00 DS 20/20
OS: −4.75 DS 20/20

Add:
OD: +1.75 D J1
OS: +1.75 D J1

Schirmer I:
OD: 24 mm in 5 minutes
OS: 26 mm in 5 minutes

Tear break-up time:
OD: 15 seconds
OS: 16 seconds

Pupil size: 4.0 mm (photopic); 4.5 mm (scotopic)

Material Selection

The Sunsoft Bifocal lens strategy uses three aspheric design profiles to optimize the visual acuity as presbyopia progresses. The 55% methafilcon A material is molded on the front-surface design and lathe cut on the posterior surface.

The A profile is for patients who are emerging presbyopes. The A add near zone has a power rating of +1.25 D. The B profile is for confirmed presbyope with an add power rating of +2.00 D. The C profile is for the mature presbyope with an add power rating of +2.50 D. The near-center aspheric lens design can be best fit using different add powers for each eye to achieve optimal vision in a modified bifocal strategy.

Pupil size will affect the success of a simultaneous bifocal arrangement. Patients with small pupils will never view into the peripheral portion of the lens. These patients are very sensitive to lens movement and perform much better in a monovision lens design. Large pupils have blurring from the periphery that can distort the center prescription. It is the patient's ability to suppress areas in the lens prescription that will help him or her experience success.

The Sunsoft Bifocals were applied to the patient's eyes to compare the improvement in the patient's range of vision. The trial lens selection were as follows:

Lens specifications: Sunsoft Bifocals

	OD	OS
Base curve	8.7 mm	8.7 mm
Diameter	14.2 mm	14.2 mm
Power	−5.25 D	−4.25 D
Add design	B	C
Visual acuity distance	20/20	20/25
Visual acuity near	J2	J1
Overrefraction	Plano	−0.50

The patient was satisfied with his distance vision as well as his near vision, although he felt his intermediate vision was better in the Focus Progressive design. He had brought one of his guns into the examination room to test his ability to view simultaneously the gun sight and distance. He could not adjust to the bifocal design when shooting his gun. The vision at the computer and reading a newspaper seemed to be adequate. The left lens was changed to the following specifications in attempt to improve his vision when using his gun:

Lens specifications: Sunsoft Bifocals

	OS
Base curve	8.7 mm
Diameter	14.2 mm
Power	−4.50 D
Add design	B
Visual acuity distance	20/20
Visual acuity near	J2
Overrefraction	−0.25

This change in prescription improved both distance vision and intermediate vision, although it did make near vision worse. The patient still preferred the Focus Progressive lens to the Sunsoft lens for hunting and outdoor activities. The difference in lens design and not the prescription provided a better solution when viewing the gun sight.

Many times, a presbyope's experience with one bifocal design will not satisfy the spectrum of visual needs when performing occupational tasks and hobbies. Spectacles and contact lenses will create clear vision for a specific range, which may not be the same for all visual tasks. The options are then to have two types of bifocal designs or supplement the one bifocal design with spectacles. A discussion describing the visual limitations of the various bifocal contact lens designs and the different options to supplement the range of vision was discussed with the patient. The patient did not want the inconvenience of spectacles, especially in the outside environment when the spectacles might fog or become wet or dirty. The patient also did not want to wear additional spectacles over his contact lenses in the work environment when communicating with clients. An option was given to wear the Ciba Focus Progressive single-use daily-wear bifocals when engaged with outside sports and the Sunsoft Additions lens during occupational tasks. The single-use Focus Progressive Bifocal lens appeared to be the correct solution for this patient because of his visual demands of his hobbies.

Lens specifications: Ciba single-use Focus Progressive Bifocals

	OD	OS
Base curve	8.6 mm	8.6 mm
Diameter	14.0 mm	14.0 mm
Power	−5.00 D	−4.50 D
Visual acuity distance	20/20	20/25
Visual acuity near	J2	J2
Overrefraction	Plano	Plano

The Sunsoft Addition Quarterly replacement Bifocal improved his distance vision as well as his near vision when performing occupational-related work.

Lens specifications: Sunsoft Bifocals

	OD	OS
Base curve	8.7 mm	8.7 mm
Diameter	14.2 mm	14.2 mm
Power	−5.25 D	−4.25 D
Add design	B	C
Visual acuity distance	20/20	20/25
Visual acuity near	J2	J1
Overrefraction	Plano	−0.50

Summary

Fitting presbyopic patients with contact lenses is defined by developing a bifocal design that satisfies each patient's visual needs. The case history is an important fitting tool to lead you to the bifocal design. That is where you obtain the information to match the most appropriate bifocal design to satisfy the patient's goals. At times the patient's visual expectations cannot be satisfied by one bifocal design because the range of vision is too extensive to fulfill the pa-

tient's visual requirements. This case demonstrates the option of offering the patient's two different contact lens bifocals to satisfy occupational tasks and hobbies.

For everyday occupational requirements, the Sunsoft Bifocal Additions lens in a quarterly-replacement modality provides the necessary visual ranges to perform work related activities. On those occasions where the patient is engaged in sporting activities, the single-use Focus Progressive Dailies Bifocal delivers the convenience and visual ranges to perform with confidence. The single-use Focus Progressive Dailies Bifocals are used in his sporting activities where cleaning and disinfection is not convenient, and they offer a margin of safety when proper hygiene is not possible. The 90-day packaging will offer the patient enough lenses to deliver a cost-effective solution to his unique situation.

Presbyopia demands your continued commitment to a long-term relationship with your presbyopic patients seeking out solutions from their ever-changing accommodation system. The longer a presbyope wears contact lenses, the more you must fine-tune the bifocal design to maintain pristine vision.

Monovision

Initial Summary

A practitioner close to my (R.L.D.) office retired from optometry after 52 years of private practice. One of his former patients came into the office complaining of having to wear spectacle lenses in order to read at near. This 49-year-old fourth grade teacher had to carry a pair of reading glasses in order to perform her work at school or at home. She had numerous pairs of reading glasses scattered around her house and at school to wear over her contact lenses. Her frustration with the reading glasses developed because she could never find a pair when she needed them. She refused to wear one of those chains attached to the glasses around her neck. A discussion took place talking about the various bifocal options. She has been wearing GP lenses for 26 years and the specifications are as follows:

Lens specifications: Boston Equalens

	OD	OS
Base curve	7.22 mm	7.46 mm
Peripheral curve	10.50/0.4 mm	10.50/0.4 mm
Power	−3.00 D	−3.00 D
Center thickness	0.14 mm	0.14 mm
Diameter	9.2 mm	9.2 mm

The patient has hay fever and is allergic to animal dander and pollen. She complains that when the lenses are removed the eyelids itch moderately for a few minutes. At times the lenses seem to get filmy for no apparent reason, and the contact lenses must be removed and cleaned to provide clear vision. The patient is taking valsartan (Diovan) and Disogen medications.

Manifest refraction:
OD: −4.25 − 2.75 × 045 add +1.75 D
OS: −3.00 − 1.50 × 150 add +1.75 D

Visual acuity:
OD: 20/50
OS: 20/25

Keratometry:
OD: 46.25 @ 040; 49.25 @ 130 grade 2 distortion
OS: 45.12 @ 150; 46.25 @ 060 grade 1 distortion

Pupil size: 2.5 mm (mesopic conditions); 2.0 mm (scotopic conditions)
Horizontal visible iris diameter: 11 mm
Palpebral aperture size: 9 mm

Biomicroscopy

Upon lid eversion, the tarsal conjunctiva exhibited a mild grade 1 injection with grade 2 follicles. Lid tension was typical for the age of the patient and would not significantly affect contact lens wear. The inferior tear meniscus appeared to be clear and adequate in the height to support contact lens wear. The tear break-up time was 18 seconds OD and 19 seconds OS. The Meibomian glands excreted clear fluid upon gentle expression. The lower lid margin in each eye exhibited a few plugged glands. Slight 3- and 9-o'clock staining was evident with fluorescein application.

Material Selection and Treatment

The patient's primary objective was to provide a greater range of vision without the use of spectacle lenses for her work in the classroom. Secondarily, the patient wanted to improve her comfort and eliminate the development of film on her lenses. To eliminate the necessity of spectacle lenses for near point work, bifocal contact lenses was discussed as the optimal solution. The Presbylite (Lens Dynamics) bifocal lens was selected to provide the best intermediate vision in an alternative design. The Tangent Streak No-Line aspheric design was selected in the simultaneous fitting philosophy.

The itching and film was related to the lid pathology. Both GPC and the plugged meibomian glands contributed to the patient's symptoms of lens film, itch, and 3- and 9-o'clock stain. A treatment was immediately instituted of lid scrubs, saline flushes, and the installation of olopatadine (Patanol) twice a day.

Fitting/Troubleshooting

The major obstacle in fitting a bifocal lens in this case is the pupil size. In the alternating lens design the pupillary margin would have to reside as close as possible to the seg line in order for the pupil to progress sufficiently into the reading zone. The Presbylite was selected because of the aspheric zone dividing the upper distance zone and lower near zone for enhanced intermediate vision. The Presbylite GP bifocal is manufactured by Pro Cornea in The Netherlands and imported into the United States by Lens Dynamics, Inc. The bifocal design has a triangle-shaped near segment that is cut spherically for near vision, a spherical zone that encompasses 70% of the front optics for distance vision, and a small aspheric area at the top of the triangle for intermediate tasks. The Presbylite does not use truncation in its design. The lens has monocentric optics, with all optical cuts on the front surface.

The aspheric zone will satisfy the patient's goal for improved intermediate vision but will also make it more difficult to translate into the reading zone over a two-zone alternating bifocal design. A trial lens fitting resulted in adequate distance vision with good intermediate vision and poor near vision. Because of the patient's physical structure and pupil size, the alternating lens design was abandoned for an aspheric lens design.

The Tangent Streak No-Line multifocal lens was then trialed incorporating a simultaneous vision fitting philosophy. The small pupil creates difficulty in placing both distance and near prescriptions into a small area. Many times, patients with a small pupil will receive conflicting visual information when the lens design focuses light onto the retina. This effect will create unclear vision both at distance and near as well as variable vision with the blink.

Lens specifications:

	OD	OS
Fitting curve	7.50 mm	7.70 mm
Base curve	7.34 mm	7.54 mm
Power	−3.25 D	−1.50 D
Center thickness	0.14 mm	0.14 mm
Diameter	9.5 mm	9.5 mm

To provide improved near vision the Tangent Streak No-Line was ordered with a +0.50 D placed on the front surface of the lens. The Tangent Streak No-Line multifocal design provides natural-like distance, intermediate, and near correction simultaneously, so the lens performance is not dependent on its orientation

At the follow-up appointment, the patient complained of poor distance vision although more disconcerting was the vision coming in and out of focus with the blink. An overrefraction of OD − 0.75 DS and OS −0.50 DS revealed improved distance vision, although it did not eliminate the variable vision through the lens design.

A monovision design was then applied without describing the lens design to the patient in order to elicit an unbiased response from the patient.

Lens specifications: Menicon Z

	OD	OS
Base curve	7.30 mm	7.40 mm
Power	−2.00 D	−3.00 D
Center thickness	0.14 mm	0.14 mm
Diameter	9.6 mm	9.6 mm

The patient immediately responded that the vision was much clearer and the variable vision was eliminated. Unlike the other two lens designs, the patient did not experience any distortion in her peripheral visual field.

Summary

Monovision is the practitioner's creation of anisometropia with contact lenses to achieve adequate vision at near and far without the use of spectacles. The advantages of monovision include lower patient expense and ease of fitting single-vision lenses compared to bifocal contact lenses. Monovision provides a full aperture viewing by one eye both at distance and near. Monovision wearers commonly complain of decreased visual abilities in low-light situations, especially during night driving. Monovision patients also have reduced stereoacuity. Many factors can influence the success of monovision, including ocular dominance, unilateral suppression of blur, reduced contrast sensitivity, and reduced stereoacuity. Monovision creates both distance and near vision in a simultaneous philosophy while the brain alternates attention between the two images using alternating vision principles.

SUMMARY

Bifocals contact lenses—both GP and soft—can build your practice. As these cases show, there are many patients who can benefit, numerous options are available, and the lens design selected may vary among individual patients. The most important factor is to utilize these options as the primary contact lens correction option for interested presbyopes. In doing so, a very satisfied patient base is created who, in turn, will refer others to a practice emphasizing bifocal contact lenses.

CHAPTER
49

IRREGULAR CORNEAS GRAND ROUNDS

TIMOTHY B. EDRINGTON
LORETTA B. SZCZOTKA-FLYNN
JULIE A. YU
AND HARUE J. MARSDEN

INTRODUCTION

Patients with irregular astigmatism provide eye care practitioners with their most challenging, but rewarding, contact lens fits. Irregular astigmatism may be induced by trauma, corneal disease, corneal surgery, or rigid contact lens wear.

Patients with irregular astigmatism secondary to trauma often present with corneal scarring that may additionally decrease vision. Even if the scarring is central and severe, the resulting visual acuity obtained through a gas-permeable (GP) contact lens may be surprisingly good. Although keratometry readings or videokeratography values may be used as a starting point for base curve selection, trial lens fitting is necessary to prescribe the appropriate fitting parameters. Using sodium fluorescein to interpret the fit, the goal is to avoid localized areas of harsh lens bearing or excessive clearance and to provide adequate tear exchange. It is also important to assess lens position: a larger overall diameter might be necessary to achieve adequate lens centration. Corneal staining patterns at follow-up visits are important to monitor the appropriateness of the lens fit. Also, the patient's manifest refraction should not be used to determine contact lens power; instead, an overrefraction should be performed through the best-fitting diagnostic contact lens.

This area of contact lens care is more completely discussed in Chapter 28. The current chapter provides several case reports illustrating clinical care of patients with irregular astigmatism secondary to corneal disease and surgery. Included are cases involving keratoconus, pellucid marginal degeneration, and patients who have undergone penetrating keratoplasty (PKP), radial keratotomy (RK), photorefractive keratectomy (PRK) and laser in situ keratomileusis (LASIK).

Even when keratometry and videokeratography indicate large amounts of irregular astigmatism, spherical base curve lenses are usually the GP lens design of choice. Toric back-surface GP lens designs are seldom necessary to optimize fitting characteristics. If an undesirable amount of residual astigmatism is present in the overrefraction through the spherical design, toric lens designs may be considered, or the cylinder may be corrected in a spectacle overcorrection.

Long-term rigid contact lens wear may lead to corneal warpage with accompanying corneal distortion and/or irregular astigmatism. GP lenses not fitted "alignment"—that is, with localized areas of lens bearing—may contribute to focal areas of corneal distortion. Long-term wear of polymethylmethacrylate (PMMA) or low-Dk (oxygen permeability) GP as well as "lid-attached" or superior positioning GP fits may induce corneal warpage and lead to a corneal topography pattern with inferior steepening similar in appearance to a map of keratoconus (Fig. 49.1).

Patients with corneal warpage secondary to contact lens wear should be refitted with lenses that provide a more appropriate mechanical fit, e.g., without harsh areas of localized bearing. Higher-Dk materials should be prescribed. It is not necessary to deprive the patient of lens wear during this process, however, unless the integrity of the corneal surface is compromised.

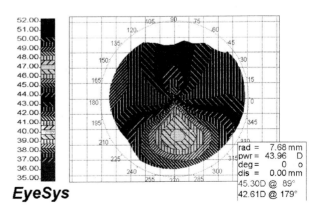

FIG. 49.1. Videokeratography map of cornea after long-term wear of a superior-positioning rigid gas-permeable contact lens.

CORNEAL DISEASE–INDUCED IRREGULAR ASTIGMATISM CASES

Keratoconus

Initial Summary

A 25-year-old man was referred for a contact lens evaluation and fitting. The patient was wearing a spectacle prescription, but he had not previously worn contact lenses. The referring doctor suspected keratoconus based on steep keratometry readings (left eye > right eye). The patient's personal medical history was unremarkable, but his father was being medically managed for diabetes mellitus. There was no known family history of keratoconus and no positive history of atopic disease, connective tissue disorders, or eye rubbing. The following data were obtained:

Keratometry:
Right eye (OD): 46.75 @ 020 / 50.00 @ 110; 2+ mire distortion
Left eye (OS): 52.87 @ 015 / 54.75 @ 120; 3+ mire distortion

The range of the keratometer was extended with a +1.25 D spectacle trial lens for the left eye measurements.

Manifest refraction:
OD: +3.25 −3.00 × 095 20/40 +2/5
OS: +2.50 −3.50 × 085 20/40 −2/5

Biomicroscopy

Eyelids, eyelashes, and conjunctivae were clear. Fleischer's ring and Vogt's striae were present in both corneas. There was no corneal staining or scarring. The tear film and tear break-up times were normal. Anterior chambers were deep and quiet and the crystalline lenses and vitreous were clear in both eyes.

Videokeratography

The patient's corneal topography revealed a localized area of steepening displaced slightly inferior and pathognomonic of keratoconus (Fig. 49.2).

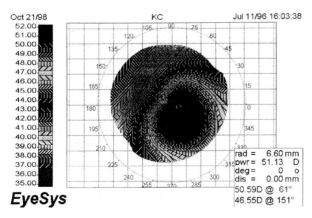

FIG. 49.2. Videokeratography map of keratoconus.

The referring doctor's diagnosis of keratoconus was confirmed based on the distorted keratometric mires, the presence of Fleischer's ring and Vogt's striae, and videokeratography results. There were no contraindications to GP contact lens wear. The patient was further educated regarding keratoconus and its prognosis. After his questions were answered and his options discussed, a GP contact lens fitting was performed.

Material Selection

Gas-permeable lenses are the contact lens option of first choice for keratoconus patients with reduced vision due to corneal distortion. The tear lens, combined with the smooth anterior surface of the GP contact lens, serves to reduce the optical distortion. Spectacles and soft contact lenses are appropriate vision correction modalities for patients with mild forms of keratoconus.

Fitting

The following initial pair of diagnostic GP contact lenses was applied and fluorescein patterns were evaluated:

Base curve: OD 49.62 D (6.80 mm); OS 53.62 D (6.30 mm)
Power: OD −6.00 D; OS −9.00 D
Overall diameter: OD and OS 8.6 mm
Optic zone diameter: OD 7.0 mm; OS 6.8 mm

The fluorescein pattern for the right eye revealed three-point touch with light central bearing. A wide band of pooling was observed beneath the optic zone around the area of central touch. Average peripheral clearance was noted. The left eye's fluorescein pattern was evaluated as heavy apical touch resulting in poor lens centration.

A second pair of diagnostic contact lenses with steeper base curves was applied:

Base curve: OD 50.37 D (6.70 mm); OS 55.37 D (6.10 mm)
Power: OD −7.00 D; OS −9.00 D
Overall diameter: OD and OS 8.6 mm
Optic zone diameter: OD 7.0 mm; OS 6.8 mm

The fluorescein patterns revealed apical clearance with minimal peripheral clearance in the right eye and apical touch with excessive peripheral clearance in the left eye.

A third diagnostic lens was applied to the patient's left eye:

Base curve: OS 57.25 D (5.90 mm)
Power: OS −9.00 D
Overall diameter: OS 8.6 mm
Optic zone diameter: OS 6.5 mm

The fluorescein pattern revealed apical clearance with minimal peripheral clearance. Overrefractions were performed through the following diagnostic contact lenses:

Base curve: OD 49.62 D (6.80 mm); OS 55.37 D (6.10 mm)

Power: OD –6.00 D; OS –9.00 D
Overall diameter: OD and OS 8.6 mm
Optic zone diameter: OD 7.0 mm; OS 6.8 mm
Overrefractions: OD: plano –1.25 × 160; 20/20; OS: –2.50 –050 × 075; 20/25

Based on these findings, the following Fluoroperm 30 (Dk = 30) GP contact lenses were ordered:

Base curve: OD 49.62 D (6.80 mm); OS 56.00 D (6.03 mm)

Power: OD –6.62 D; OS –12.37 D
Overall diameter: OD and OS 8.6 mm
Optic zone diameter: OD 6.7 mm; OS 6.5 mm
Secondary curve radius: OD and OS 8.50 mm
Peripheral curve radius: OD and OS 11.00 mm
Peripheral curve width: OD and OS 0.2 mm
Center thickness: OD and OS 0.13 mm
Blend: OD and OS medium

Prescribed base curves were determined by evaluating the fluorescein patterns of diagnostic contact lenses. Initial trial lens base curves were selected to approximate the steep keratometry readings. The resulting fluorescein patterns were interpreted to be apical touch or flat relative to the apex of the cone. The goal of base curve selection was to determine that base curve that would lightly touch the apex of the cone—that is, be slightly flatter than the first apical clearance diagnostic lens (1). Steeper base curves were applied until apical clearance was observed (Figs. 49.3 and 49.4).

The left lens power was determined by adding the equivalent sphere of the overrefraction (–2.75 D) to the diagnostic lens power (–9.00 D) and compensating for any change of tear lens resulting from the difference between the base curves of diagnostic and ordered lenses (–0.62 D). The diameter of the optic zone of the right lens was ordered smaller than that of the diagnostic lens due to the wide band of fluorescein pooling around the base of the cone. Because the left cornea exhibited a more advanced presenta-

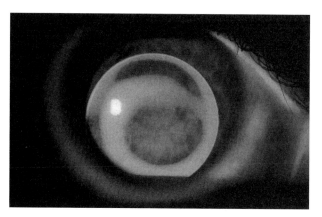

FIG. 49.3. Apical touch fluorescein pattern in keratoconus.

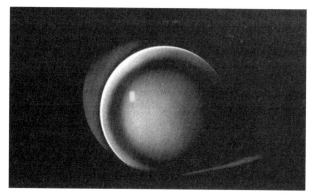

FIG. 49.4. Apical clearance fluorescein pattern in keratoconus.

tion of keratoconus, a slightly smaller optic zone diameter (6.5 mm) was ordered. A secondary curve radius in the 8.00 to 9.00 mm range was indicated because when the lens centers over the apex of the cone, the secondary curve will position over a portion of the cornea that is generally not topographically affected by the disease. Therefore, normal secondary curve radii are appropriate. The amount of peripheral clearance will be assessed by fluorescein pattern evaluation at the dispensing visit. If the amount of peripheral clearance is insufficient the secondary curve will be flattened by in-office modification.

Summary

The goal in fitting keratoconus patients with GP contact lenses is to improve vision without increasing corneal damage, not to alter the progression of the disease. To determine the base curve, diagnostic rigid lenses are applied, starting with a lens with a base curve approximately equal to the steep keratometry reading. Generally, the fluorescein pattern of the first lens applied will be apical touch. Additional diagnostic lenses are applied until the fluorescein pattern reveals apical clearance. When apical clearance is achieved, the next flattest lens should be reapplied and a spherocylinder overrefraction performed. The goal is to achieve a "feather" three-point touch apical fitting relationship.

The peripheral curve system must provide sufficient tear exchange. If peripheral clearance is inadequate, tolerance and wear time will probably be reduced. Flattening the peripheral curves and reblending often alleviates reduced wearing time.

If stipple staining or dimple veil staining is observed around the base of the cone, the probable cause is excessive midperipheral pooling of tear debris. The optic zone diameter should be reduced and the junction between the base curve and secondary curve reblended.

Keratoconus

Initial Summary

A 28-year-old man was referred for an eye examination after failing the visual acuity test at the Department of Motor

Vehicles. He was diagnosed with keratoconus and evaluated for GP contact lenses.

Entering visual acuities (unaided): OD: 2/200, PH 20/200; OS: 20/70, PH 20/40

Keratometry:
OD: 56.75 @ 100 / 58.50 @ 020; 3+ mire distortion
OS: 45.37 @ 125 / 49.00 @ 049; 2+ mire distortion

Manifest refraction:
OD: −7.00 − 7.50 × 110 20/200
OS: +2.00 − 4.00 × 140 20/30

Biomicroscopy

The eyelids and eyelashes were clear in both eyes. Grade 1+ bulbar injection was observed in both eyes. Vogt's striae and Fleischer's ring were present in the right cornea. The left cornea was clear. There was no corneal staining or scarring in either eye.

Material Selection

There are several different management options for keratoconus patients, including spectacles, soft spherical and toric contact lenses, GP contact lenses, hybrid and piggyback contact lens designs, and PKP. Disease severity usually dictates which type of correction is prescribed. In mild cases, either hydrogel lenses or spectacles may be effective. As the disease progresses, and irregular astigmatism becomes more problematic, GP contact lenses are commonly prescribed as they "correct" irregular astigmatism more effectively by optically neutralizing the corneal irregularity using the tear layer. In this case, GP lenses were indicated due to significant keratometric mire distortion and the poor visual acuities obtained with the manifest refraction.

Fitting

Proposed GP fitting philosophies for keratoconus patients include apical clearance, apical touch, three-point touch or divided support, and high riding (or lid attached). With the exception of the lid-attached fitting philosophy, lenses are designed to position primarily over the apex of the cone. A lens that bears too heavily on the cone can compromise the anterior corneal surface, resulting in punctate keratopathy and potential corneal scarring. Conversely, a lens fitted apical clearance may lead to compromised integrity of the peripheral cornea because the bearing portion of the contact lens is entirely on the midperipheral cornea.

A GP trial lens set containing spherical tricurve lenses with steep base curves appropriate for keratoconus patients was used for the diagnostic fitting. The base curve of the initial diagnostic lens should approximate the steep keratometry reading. The fitting strategy for keratoconus is as follows: if the first diagnostic lens is too steep, successive

lenses with flatter base curves (in approximately 0.1-mm increments) are applied until three-point touch is achieved. Conversely, if the first diagnostic lens is too flat, lenses with successively steeper base curves are applied until definite apical clearance is achieved. An overrefraction is subsequently performed over the steepest lens that exhibits an apical touch fitting relationship. The following lenses were applied and the fluorescein patterns were evaluated:

Base curve: OD: 58.00 D (5.82 mm); OS: 48.50 D (6.96 mm)
Power: OD: −8.00 D; OS: −4.00 D
Overall diameter: OD: 8.6 mm; OS: 8.6 mm
Optic zone diameter: OD: 6.8 mm; OS: 7.0 mm

Evaluation with sodium fluorescein revealed apical clearance, good centration, and minimal peripheral clearance in the right eye; the left lens demonstrated light apical three-point touch with good centration and minimal peripheral clearance. Based on these findings, a second pair of diagnostic GPs was applied to the patient's eyes:

Base curve: OD 57.00 D (5.92 mm); OS 49.25 (6.85 mm)
Power: OD −8.00 D; OS −5.00 D
Overall diameter: OD 8.6 mm; OS 8.6 mm
Optic zone diameter: OD 6.8 mm; OS 7.0 mm

The fluorescein pattern revealed light three-point apical touch, good centration, and average peripheral clearance in the right eye; the left lens showed apical clearance with good centration and minimal peripheral clearance. A spherocylinder overrefraction was performed through the lenses with the base curves of 57.00 D and 48.50 D for the right and left eye, respectively.

Overrefraction: OD −3.75 DS (20/20), OS −1.00 − 0.25 × 062 (20/20)

The following lenses were ordered:

Base curve: OD 57.00 D (5.92 mm); OS 48.50 D (6.96 mm)
Power: OD −11.75 D; OS −5.12 D
Overall diameter: OD 8.6 mm; OS 8.6 mm
Optic zone diameter: OD 6.8 mm; OS 7.0 mm
Secondary curve radius: OD 8.80 mm; OS 9.00 mm
Peripheral curve radius: OD and OS 12.00 mm
Peripheral curve width: OD and OS 0.2 mm
Blend: medium OD and OS
Material: Fluoroperm 30 (Dk = 30) OD and OS

These base curves were prescribed because they lightly touched the apex of the cone. To determine contact lens power, the spherical equivalent of the spherocylinder overrefraction was added to the power of the diagnostic contact lenses. The peripheral curves must have sufficiently flat radii to allow the tears that collect under the optic zone of a keratoconic lens to adequately flush out and exchange into the periphery. Corneal topography adjacent to the base of the cone has been shown to be similar in curvature to that of nonkeratoconic corneas. If a selected secondary curve radius is too steep in relation to the peripheral cornea, a midperipheral seal could be established, trapping tears and metabolic waste products beneath the contact lens and leading to stagnation and ultimately physiologic insult. However, if this problem were to occur, in-office modification could be performed to flatten and/or blend the peripheral curve system to enhance tear exchange.

At the dispensing visit, the in situ visual acuities were OD 20/20, OS 20/20.

Overrefraction:
OD: +0.25 − 0.50 × 090 (20/20)
OS: plano −0.50 × 050 (20/20)

The lenses exhibited light apical three-point touch with good centration and average peripheral clearance. The lenses were dispensed after the patient was instructed on lens application, removal, recentering, and care. He was instructed to start with 4 hours of lens wear and increase his wearing time by 2 hours per day with a maximum daily wearing time of 8 hours.

At his first follow-up visit, he indicated that the comfort of the lenses had consistently improved since dispensing. His wearing time at this visit was 6 hours. His maximum wearing time was 8 hours.

Entering visual acuities with his contact lenses were OD 20/20, OS 20/20.

Overrefraction:
OD: +0.25 − 0.75 × 105 (20/20)
OS: plano −0.50 × 060 (20/20)

The lenses exhibited light three-point touch with good centration and average peripheral clearance. Upon lens removal, trace 3- and 9-o'clock staining was noted in both eyes. He was advised to use rewetting drops four times a day to remedy this problem. Because ocular health was virtually unaffected by contact lens wear and the patient seemed to be adapting well, he was instructed to increase his wearing time to a maximum of 12 to 14 hours per day and return for follow-up care in 2 weeks. If the rewetting drops were unsuccessful, the lens edge would be reevaluated and thinned as much as possible to increase apposition of the eyelid against the globe. If the 3- and 9-o'clock staining increased, a piggyback lens design could be considered. In a piggyback system, the soft lens acts as a bandage by protecting the cornea. Fortunately, in this patient's case, his subsequent follow-up visits were unremarkable for corneal staining.

Summary

The diagnosis of keratoconus is made based on the presence of corneal distortion observed with keratometry mires or retinoscopy reflex and biomicroscopic signs such as Fleischer's ring, Vogt's striae, or corneal scarring. Localized corneal steepening, as viewed with computer-assisted topography, assists in confirming the diagnosis. GP contact lenses are the primary clinical management for keratoconus due to their ability to optically smooth an irregular refracting surface using the tear lens. Although keratoconus patients generally appreciate the improved vision with GP contact lenses, careful follow-up is necessary to ensure that the lens fit remains optimal. Although corneal scarring may be a natural result of keratoconus, care must be taken not to exacerbate it with a poor lens fit (2).

Keratoconus

Initial Summary

A 34-year-old woman presented with a chief complaint of moderate irritation with her left GP contact lens for the past 4 months. This irritation prevented her from achieving adequate lens wearing time due to lens discomfort, tearing, and photophobia. On the days she wore her left contact lens, she reported that the irritation would begin within a few hours after lens application. She had been diagnosed with keratoconus at 22 years of age. A previous PMMA lens wearer, she was refitted into GP contact lenses 8 years ago. Her last examination was 2 years prior; her right contact lens was 3 years old and her left lens was 10 months old. Her current wearing time for her right contact lens was 12 hours per day. She presented to the examination wearing both of her contact lenses.

Entering visual acuities: OD 20/30; OS 20/60 (PH 20/50)

Habitual contact lenses:
Base curve: OD 49.00 D (6.88 mm); OS 55.50 D (6.08 mm)
Power: OD −8.75 D; OS −10.75 D
Overall diameter: OD 8.6 mm; OS 8.6 mm
Optic zone diameter: OD 6.5 mm; OS 6.5 mm
Overrefraction: OD −0.25 − 0.50 × 145 (20/25); OS +3.50 DS (20/50)

Fluorescein patterns:
OD: light apical touch, good centration with average peripheral clearance
OS: heavy apical touch, good centration with excessive peripheral clearance

Biomicroscopy

The eyelids and eyelashes were clear in both eyes. Grade 1+ bulbar injection was observed in the right eye; grade 2+ bulbar injection was observed in the left eye. Vogt's striae and Fleischer's ring were present in both eyes. Faint central corneal scarring was observed in the left eye. Significant corneal staining (grade 2+) was noted over the apex of the cone and near the limbus at 3 and 9 o'clock in the left eye.

Because the patient's left eye was irritated and stained significantly with sodium fluorescein, she was asked to discontinue lens wear in that eye and return in 3 days for refitting. Artificial tears were prescribed on an as-needed basis.

Fitting/Troubleshooting

At the refitting visit, the patient reported that the comfort in her left eye had improved.

Biomicroscopic evaluation revealed resolved keratitis in the left cornea.

Keratometry:
OD: 50.75 @ 170 / 51.50 @ 080; 2+ mire distortion
OS: 56.00 @ 145 / 61.25 @ 055; 3+ mire distortion

The following diagnostic lens was applied to the patient's left eye:

Base curve: OS 60.00 D (5.62 mm)
Power: OS −8.00 D
Overall diameter: OS 8.6 mm
Optic zone diameter: OS 6.5 mm

Evaluation with sodium fluorescein revealed apical clearance, good centration, and minimal peripheral clearance. Based on these findings, a second diagnostic GP contact lens was applied to the patient's left eye:

Base curve: OS 59.00 D (5.72 mm)
Power: OS −8.00 D
Overall diameter: OS 8.6 mm
Optic zone diameter: OS 6.5 mm

The fluorescein pattern revealed light three-point touch, good lens centration, and average peripheral clearance. An overrefraction was performed with this lens in place:

Overrefraction: OS −2.25 − 0.75 × 125 (20/30)

Evaluation of the patient's right lens revealed significant scratches and protein deposition. Because the fit and contact lens power were determined to be appropriate at the previous visit, a lens with similar parameters was prescribed. The following GP contact lenses were ordered:

Base curve: OD 49.00 D (6.88 mm); OS 59.00 D (5.72 mm)
Power: OD −9.25 D; OS −10.62 D
Overall diameter: OD 8.6 mm; OS 8.6 mm
Optic zone diameter: OD 7.0 mm; OS 6.5 mm
Secondary curve radius: OD 8.50 mm; OS 8.25 mm
Peripheral curve radius: OD and OS 11.00 mm
Peripheral curve width: OD and OS 0.2 mm
Blend: Medium OD and OS
Material: Fluoroperm 30 (Dk = 30) each eye (OU)

At the contact lens dispensing visit, the in situ distance visual acuities were:

OD: 20/25; OS 20/40
Overrefraction: OD +0.50 − 1.00 × 060 (20/25); OS +0.50 − 1.00 × 115 (20/30)

Both lenses exhibited light three-point touch with good lens centration and average peripheral clearance. Our patient complained that her vision fluctuated when she blinked. To remedy this symptom, the junction between the optic zone and the secondary curve was reblended. Subsequently, the patient stated that vision improved.

At the next follow-up visit, the patient indicated good vision and comfort with her new lenses. Wearing time at this visit was 14 hours per day.

Entering visual acuities: OD 20/25, OS 20/40
Overrefraction: OD +0.25 − 0.25 × 075 (20/25), OS +0.25 − 0.75 × 130 (20/40)

Both lenses exhibited light three-point touch with good centration and average peripheral clearance. Upon lens removal, very mild arc-shaped superficial punctate staining was noted in the left eye; no staining was present in the right eye. Further blending of the peripheral curves was performed, and the patient was subsequently dismissed for 6 months.

Summary

This case illustrates the importance of regular follow-up care for keratoconus patients. An evaluation for a contact lens refitting may be indicated as frequently as every 6 months if the disease is progressing at a rapid rate. Although it is difficult to predict how quickly keratoconus will progress for each individual patient, only 10% to 20% of cases progress to a point where a corneal transplant is indicated (3). In this case, the patient needed to be refitted with a steeper base curve to prevent excessive bearing on the cone.

Pellucid Marginal Corneal Degeneration

Initial Summary

A 38-year-old man presented with a chief complaint of poor vision through his habitual soft contact lenses. His keratoconus had been diagnosed 7 years previously and he was unsuccessful in GP contact lens wear at that time. He was wearing disposable spherical soft contact lenses on a 2-week extended-wear basis. Entering distance visual acuities through his habitual spherical soft contact lenses were 20/30+ each eye.

Keratometry:
OD: 45.25 @ 180 / 45.50 @ 090; no mire distortion
OS: 44.50 @ 090 / 47.50 @ 180; no mire distortion

Both mires were vertically oval (OS>OD).

Manifest refraction:
OD: −4.75 −2.00 × 035 (20/20)
OS: −4.25 −1.25 × 105 (20/25)

Biomicroscopy

Eyelids and eyelashes were clear. Fleischer's ring, Vogt's striae, and corneal scarring were not observed in either cornea. Optic sections did not reveal any thinning of the central cornea, but both corneas exhibited thinning inferiorly near the limbus. There was limbal vascularization present superiorly and inferiorly OU. Both anterior chambers were quiet and both crystalline lenses were clear.

Videokeratography

The computerized corneal map (Fig. 49.5; see Color Plate 49.5) showed areas of inferior steepening in a winged pattern pathognomonic of pellucid marginal degeneration. There was no central area of corneal steepening.

The diagnosis of keratoconus was rejected based on the absence of corneal distortion on keratometry, the appearance of the videokeratography maps, and the lack of biomicroscopic signs (i.e., no Fleischer's ring or Vogt's striae). A diagnosis of pellucid marginal corneal degeneration (PMD) was made based upon the slit-lamp observation of inferior corneal thinning near the limbus, oval but not distorted keratometry mires, and videokeratography results (4).

Material Selection

Typically, manifest refraction visual acuity is acceptable for patients with mild and moderate presentations of PMD. This is due to the small degree of central corneal distortion and/or irregular astigmatism. Many patients with pellucid have high amounts of against-the-rule astigmatism. Several contact lens options may be considered:

- Spherical GP contact lenses
- Toric GP contact lenses
- Toric soft contact lenses
- Flexlens or piggyback combination soft/GP contact lens designs
- SoftPerm or hybrid contact lens designs

Spherical GP contact lenses were not considered a viable option for this patient due to the predicted overrefraction cylinder and the anticipated inferior lens position on the cornea. To rule out this lens design the practitioner would need to apply a spherical diagnostic GP contact lens, perform a spherocylinder overrefraction, and evaluate the lens fit and position. In this case, corneal toricity as measured by keratometry does not correlate well with the manifest refraction cylinder; therefore, an unacceptable amount of residual cylinder could be anticipated in the overrefraction. However, with irregular astigmatism (as found in both keratoconus and pellucid marginal degeneration), it is important not to rely on this refractive data, but to apply a diagnostic lens and perform an overrefraction. Since spherical and toric base curve GP contact lenses often position too inferiorly PMD corneas, a larger overall diameter is necessary to position the optic zone over the pupil or to achieve a lid-attached fitting relationship.

A toric soft contact lens is an option because the manifest refraction provides acceptable vision. If the corneal surface is too distorted or if a moderate amount of irregular astigmatism is present, then the resulting vision might not be acceptable. The cornea should be regularly monitored for neovascularization if a toric soft contact lens is prescribed for a PMD patient.

Both soft/GP and hybrid lens designs are not necessary for this patient due to simpler acceptable contact lens options but these designs would improve on the lens centration achieved with a GP lens alone. A primary concern with either the soft/GP or hybrid design is compromised corneal physiology due to decreased oxygen provided to the cornea and minimized tear exchange to remove metabolic debris.

Fitting/Troubleshooting

CooperVision Hydrasoft XW toric soft contact lenses were ordered empirically. The Hydrasoft toric is a back-surface soft toric design manufactured in a Food and Drug Administration group 4 material. Many practitioners prescribe back-surface toric soft contact lens designs for patients with moderate to high amounts of corneal toricity. This is the case for this patient's left eye, but not for his right eye. Hydrasoft toric lenses were selected because of their clinical reputation for good rotational stability, not because of the back-surface toric design. The thinner profile XW design was ordered because of the patient's history of extended wear and preexisting limbal vascularization of the cornea. After patient education regarding extended wear, the patient

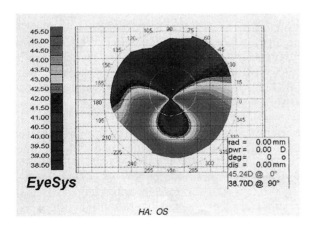

FIG. 49.5. Videokeratography map of pellucid marginal corneal degeneration. (See Color Plate 49.5.)

was instructed to remove his lenses nightly. To determine the powers and axes for the order, the manifest refraction was vertex distance corrected to the corneal plane as follows:

Manifest refraction vertex distance corrected to the corneal plane:
(13 mm vertex distance)
OD: −4.50 −1.75 × 035
OS: −4.00 −1.12 × 105

The following CooperVision Hydrasoft XW toric soft contact lenses were ordered:

Base curve: OD and OS 8.3 mm
Power: OD −4.25 −1.75 × 035; OS −3.75 −1.00 × 105
Overall diameter: OD and OS 14.2 mm

The sphere powers were ordered a 0.25 D more plus to compensate for on-eye flexure effects.

At the dispensing visit, the distance in situ visual acuities were OD 20/20+; OS 20/20−.

Overrefraction:
OD: plano −0.25 × 125 (20/20+)
OS: +0.50 −0.50 × 85 (20/20)

Biomicroscopy

The lenses moved 0.75 mm on a blink, lateral and vertical movement was 0.5 mm, coverage was complete, and the lenses were centered on the corneas. The base-down marking on the right lens was at 6 o'clock and stable. The base-down marking on the left lens was stable and located 10 degrees temporally.

The visual acuity obtained with the right contact lens in place was two letters better than the manifest refraction visual acuity. This could either be explained by the repeatability of the visual acuity measurement or by an improvement of the anterior refracting surface created by the firmness of a toric soft contact lens. Perhaps the vision of the left eye could have been improved by reordering the axis at 95 degrees to compensate for the temporal orientation of the prism base. This was not deemed necessary, and the lenses were dispensed.

At follow-up visits the patient reported satisfaction with vision and comfort through the toric soft contact lenses. He was also compliant with the prescribed daily-wear wearing schedule and the prescribed lens care system. The lenses were judged to be fitting well and the corneas were clear except for the existing limbal vascularization, which had not increased in encroachment.

Summary

This case illustrates the importance of a proper diagnosis in providing the most appropriate contact lens care for a patient. Understanding the patient's corneal topography al-

lowed us to prescribe a simple but appropriate lens design. Pellucid marginal degeneration is a rare but underdiagnosed corneal condition. Many cases are initially misdiagnosed as keratoconus. GP contact lenses fitted on keratoconic corneas tend to position centrally or slightly inferiorly over the apex of the cone. If the rigid lens positions too inferiorly after exhausting trial fitting options, pellucid marginal degeneration of the cornea should be suspected. Videokeratography, as well as a careful reevaluation of slit-lamp findings, should be performed to assist in the diagnosis.

Pellucid Marginal Corneal Degeneration

Initial Summary

A 22-year-old man presented with a chief complaint of poor vision through his spectacles. Although his keratoconus had been diagnosed 10 years previously, he had not been fitted with contact lenses. There was no other significant ocular or medical history.

Habitual spectacle prescription:
OD: plano −10.75 × 090 20/50
OS: +2.50 −5.50 × 090 20/30

Keratometry:
OD: 39.50 @ 090 / 50.00 @180; 2+ mire distortion
OS: 38.87 @ 090 / 45.50 @ 180; 1+ mire distortion
Mires were vertically oval OU.

Manifest refraction:
OD: plano −11.00 × 090 20/50
OS: +2.25 −6.00 × 090 20/30+

Manifest refraction vertex distance corrected (13 mm vertex distance):
OD: plano −9.62 × 090
OS: +2.25 −6.00 × 090

Biomicroscopy

Eyelids and eyelashes were clear both eyes. Optic sections revealed inferior corneal thinning near the limbus (OD> OS). Fleischer's ring, Vogt's striae, and corneal scarring were not present in either eye. Both anterior chambers were quiet. Inferior cortical cataracts were present OU.

Videokeratography

Corneal maps showed areas of inferior steepening in a winged pattern pathognomonic of PMD. There was no central area of corneal steepening.

The diagnosis of keratoconus was rejected based on the appearance of the videokeratography maps and the absence of biomicroscopic signs (i.e., no Fleischer's ring or Vogt's striae). A diagnosis of PMD was made based upon the slit-lamp observation of inferior corneal thinning near the limbus and the videokeratography results.

The cause of the cortical cataracts could not be determined.

Material Selection

Spherical GP contact lenses were applied to the patient's corneas to determine how much of his reduced vision was caused by corneal surface irregularity (distortion and/or irregular astigmatism) versus cortical cataracts. Diagnostic GP contact lenses plus a spherocylinder overrefraction showed that an improvement of visual acuity to 20/25 (OD and OS) could be achieved. This confirmed that corneal irregularities contributed largely to the patient's reduced vision. Therefore, soft contact lens options would not achieve our vision goals. The GP lens options for this patient included:

- Spherical GP contact lenses
- Toric GP contact lenses
- Flexlens or piggyback combination soft/GP contact lens designs
- SoftPerm or hybrid contact lens designs

The spherical diagnostic GP contact lenses were positioned very inferiorly and the overrefraction cylinder was unacceptable (Fig. 49.6). It is possible that the inferior lens position could have been successfully managed with a spherical design by using other base curves, increasing the overall diameter, or fitting lid-attachment. However, a toric GP lens design would be needed to correct the residual cylinder. The combination soft/GP and hybrid designs are prescribed when GP contact lens options have been exhausted.

Fitting

A pair of bitoric GP contact lenses was ordered empirically using the keratometry and manifest refraction data. The "diagnostic" order follows:

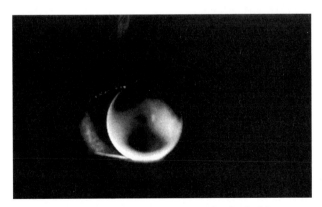

FIG. 49.6. Keyhole fluorescein pattern of spherical base curve rigid contact lens on a cornea with pellucid marginal degeneration. (Photograph courtesy of Dr. Jessica Chen.)

	OD	OS
Base curves	48.50 D (6.96 mm)	44.00 D (7.67 mm)
	39.50 D (8.54 mm)	38.87 D (8.68 mm)
Powers	−8.12 D / plano D	−2.25 D / +2.25 D
Overall diameter	9.8 mm	9.8 mm
Optic zone diameter	8.4 mm	8.4 mm
Secondary curve radius	9.25 mm toric by 9.00 D	9.50 mm toric by 5.12 D
Peripheral curve radius	12.00 mm	12.00 mm
Peripheral curve width	0.2 mm	0.2 mm
Center thickness	0.20 mm	0.25 mm
Material	Fluoroperm 60 (Dk = 60)	Fluoroperm 60 (Dk = 60)

A bitoric lens design was selected due to the high degree of corneal toricity as measured by keratometry and the large amount of astigmatism measured in the manifest refraction. The bitoric lens design was also selected to optimize lens centration because the spherical diagnostic contact lens positioned too inferiorly, but bitoric designs do not always improve lens mechanical characteristics for corneas with irregular astigmatism. Additionally, if cylinder power effect design (CPE) bitoric lenses are not rotationally stable, the correcting cylinder will not properly align to the eye's refractive astigmatism and unwanted resultant cylinder will occur (note spherical power effect design lenses due not have this problem).

The base curves were ordered such that the flat meridian "aligned" with the flat keratometry reading (on K) and the steep meridian was ordered 1.50 D flatter than the steep keratometry reading. Lens powers were ordered by adding the resultant tear lens values to each meridian of the vertex distance corrected manifest refraction. Therefore, the contact lens powers in the flat meridians were the same as the spherical component of the vertex distance corrected manifest refraction (tear lens power of plano) and the contact lens powers in the steep meridians were 1.50 D more plus than the vertex distance corrected manifest refraction values in the steep meridians (tear lens power of −1.50 D). Large overall diameters were ordered to assist in lens centration. Similarly large optic zone diameters were ordered to ensure coverage of the pupil even if the lenses positioned inferiorly. The secondary curve radii were ordered toric by the same amount as the base curve toricity to enhance lens centration and to obtain a round optic zone. The center thicknesses were ordered based on the power of the most plus meridian. A Dk 60 material was prescribed to maintain lens stability while providing the cornea with adequate oxygen transmission.

At the dispensing and follow-up visits, the lenses positioned slightly inferior but were adequately centered for the optic zones to cover the patient's pupils. The lenses were also rotationally stable such that vision did not fluctuate on a blink. Follow-up care revealed no clinically significant corneal staining.

Summary

This case of PMD again illustrates the importance of proper diagnosis and of understanding corneal topography. Spherical GP contact lenses are the first choice in fitting corneas with irregular astigmatism. Even though the cornea as measured by keratometry is highly toric, toric back-surface GP lens designs are not generally necessary to position the lens properly. As spherical GP diagnostic lenses positioned inferiorly in this case, however, bitoric lenses were ordered to determine if they would improve lens centration. A lid-attachment design was not indicated due to the high position of the upper eyelid relative to the superior limbus. If adequate lens position had not been achieved with bitoric rigid contact lenses, a semiscleral (large overall diameter GP), a soft/GP, or a hybrid design could have been considered.

Pellucid Marginal Corneal Degeneration

Initial Summary

A 50-year-old female hand surgeon was diagnosed with PMD by a corneal specialist and referred for specialty contact lens fitting. Soft toric contact lens wear had been discontinued 6 weeks prior to the diagnosis of PMD. The diagnosis was based on an irregular corneal surface, decreased best-corrected spectacle acuities, high against-the-rule astigmatism, inferior corneal thinning, and corneal topography displaying the classic butterfly appearance of inferior corneal steepening, superior corneal flattening,

and high against-the-rule toricity (Fig. 49.7; see Color Plate 49.7).

Manifest refraction:
OD: − 4.00 − 3.50 × 095 (20/40)
OS: − 1.00 − 3.75 × 075 (20/40)

Central pachometry:
OD: 556, 553, 555 μm
OS: 555, 555, 555 μm

Inferior pachometry:
OD: 524, 517, 513 μm
OS: 540, 538, 537 μm
Pupils 6 mm in normal illumination OD, OS

Material Selection

Corneal GP contact lenses were initially recommended to address irregular astigmatism. A large overall diameter was selected to reduce edge-related glare. A moderate-Dk material [Paragon HDS (paflufocon B; Dk 58)] was prescribed to allow sufficient oxygen transmissibility without encouraging lens flexure in a large-diameter design on a patient with a high amount of corneal toricity. PMD patients can often be fitted with larger-diameter lenses (compared to keratoconus patients) since the area of ectasia is generally larger and displaced more inferiorly compared to keratoconus. (In keratoconus, the ectasia is limited to a smaller central portion of the cornea.)

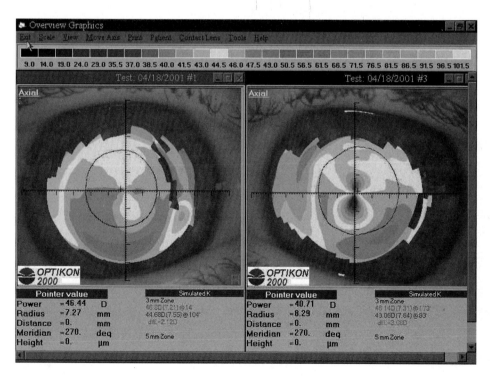

FIG. 49.7. Classic butterfly appearance of pellucid marginal degeneration showing inferior corneal steepening, superior corneal flattening, and high against-the-rule toricity. (See Color Plate 49.7.)

The following parameters were ordered and dispensed:

	OD	OS
Base curve	45.00 D (7.50 mm)	45.62 D (7.40 mm)
Power	−6.37 D	−6.12 D
Overall diameter	9.9 mm	9.9 mm
Optic zone diameter	8.5 mm	8.5 mm
Secondary curve radius	8.50 mm	8.50 mm
Third curve radius	11.50 mm	11.50 mm
Third curve width	0.2 mm	0.2 mm

A spherocylinder overrefraction revealed:

OD: +1.00 − 1.25 × 068 (20/25)
OS: +0.75 −0.75 × 018 (20/25)

While the lenses provided improved vision for her daily living activities, the patient noticed intolerable glare through both lenses. She also complained of decreased vision after lens removal. Slit-lamp evaluation revealed a lid-attached lens fit with mild apical touch over the inferior cornea, minimal lens movement in the right eye, and good movement in the left. The lenses were removed and an adherence ring was noted inferiorly on the right cornea. Corneal topography was repeated and prominent impression rings were noted in both eyes which explained the patient's significant spectacle blur when lenses were removed (Fig. 49.8; see Color Plate 49.8).

In an attempt to limit inferior corneal impingement and impression rings yet still provide a large optical zone size to allow full pupillary coverage, the sagittal depth of the lenses were decreased by flattening the base curves 0.15 mm (0.87 D) in each eye. The new lenses ordered were as follows:

	OD	OS
Base curve	44.12 D (7.65 mm)	44.75 D (7.55 mm)
Power	−5.25 D	−5.25 D
Overall diameter	9.9 mm	9.9 mm
Optic zone diameter	8.4 mm	8.4 mm
Secondary curve radius	8.90 mm	8.90 mm
Peripheral curve radius	13.00 mm	13.00 mm
Peripheral curve width	0.3 mm	0.3 mm

These lenses exhibited a high-riding lid-attachment fitting relationship, apical touch with average peripheral clearance, and sufficient movement with each blink. The patient reported a significant improvement in symptoms compared to the previous lens design; however, she was still bothered by glare and spectacle blur. Because her profession requires distinct visual acuity, such symptoms were not tolerable to her. The glare was assumed to be secondary to large pupils and a decentered optical zone from the flat, high-riding lid-attachment fit. Improving the centration would require increasing the sagittal depth, but steeper lenses had been already tried and resulted in lens adherence. Ultimately, a semiscleral lens was recommended.

Fitting/Troubleshooting

The patient was refit in Macrolens A Semiscleral GP lenses. The Macrolens A is a large-diameter (13.9 to 15.0 mm) GP lens. The basic lens design is the same as a corneal GP lens, in that it has a base curve and secondary and peripheral curves. The difference is the large overall diameter requiring the lens to rest on the sclera, and therefore the lens exhibits minimal or no vertical movement. These features were selected for the patient to improve lens centration, to elimi-

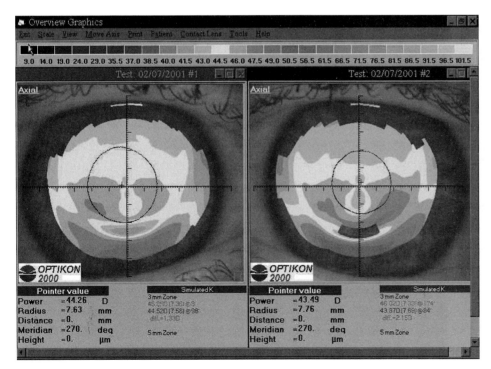

FIG. 49.8. Epithelial impression ring noted on topography of patient in this case and in Fig. 49.7, after wearing corneal gas-permeable lenses of diameter 9.9 mm OU. This explains the patient's spectacle blur upon lens removal. (See Color Plate 49.8.)

nate glare, and to limit corneal molding by distributing the bearing pressure onto the sclera. The Macrolens A is fenestrated to enhance tear exchange. With each blink, pressure is exerted on the lens pressing it to the ocular surface squeezing out tears from the lens edge and out through the fenestration. As the lid opens, pressure is relieved and tears are drawn under the lens as well as through the fenestration.

The following are the Macrolens parameters prescribed in Boston XO material (Dk = 100):

	OD	OS
Base curve	47.25 D (7.14 mm)	47.25 D (7.14 mm)
Power	−8.37 D	−7.75 D
Overall diameter	14.2 mm	14.2 mm
"E value" (peripheral eccentricity)	0.8	0.8

Macrolens base curves are prescribed as close to corneal "alignment" as possible and independent of lens peripheral curves. Expect a 270- to 360-degree band of tear pooling and adjust the peripheral fitting relationship with the E (peripheral eccentricity) value and curve widths. Recall that an E value describes the rate of peripheral flattening of a curve. The higher the E value, the greater the rate of peripheral flattening. With this lens design, a 0.60 E value is typically tight, a 0.80 E is described as a medium edge, and a 1.0 E is described as loose. Expect a scleral edge lift with an alignment central fluorescein pattern, and adjust this by expanding or decreasing the peripheral curve width as you would do in standard GP lenses.

These lenses provided acceptable visual acuity and no symptoms of glare. However, the patient complained of "pinching" inferiorly right eye only. At the 5-o'clock position, the edge lift was assessed as tight, with no fluorescein pooling, leaving a mild conjunctival imprint. This was alleviated by ordering a lens with a flatter secondary curve: a 1.0 "E value," which is the loosest E value available (Fig. 49.9; see Color Plate 49.9).

Summary

Customizing a lens to a patient's needs is the role of every specialty contact lens practitioner. Although this patient had mild corneal disease, she proved to be a challenging case due to her professional and visual requirements, and large pupils. Semiscleral and ultra-large corneal GP lenses are problem solvers that are rapidly gaining popularity. With the introduction of high-Dk GP materials, corneal hypoxia associated with the PMMA scleral lenses of the past is less of a clinical concern. Large-diameter GP lenses may also be beneficial for patients with extremely distorted corneas that cannot support a small GP lens, GP lens–intolerant patients, or those with lid deficiencies that cannot support a corneal lens.

POSTSURGICAL-INDUCED IRREGULAR ASTIGMATISM CASES

Post–Penetrating Keratoplasty

Initial Summary

A 30-year-old man was referred for a contact lens evaluation 2 years after receiving a PKP secondary to advanced keratoconus in his right eye. His left keratoconic cornea had not been grafted.

Entering visual acuities (no correction OD, GP contact lens OS) were OD 5/400, OS 20/40.

Keratometry:
OD: 38.00 @ 030 / 44.50 @113; 2+ mire distortion
OS: 58.75 @ 050 / 61.00 @170; 3+ mire distortion

Manifest refraction:
OD: −1.00 − 1.00 × 135 (20/200)
OS: −28.00 DS (20/400)

Biomicroscopy OD

Eyelids and eyelashes were clear. Mild bulbar injection was present. The graft was approximately 6 mm round and clear. A running suture was present. No corneal staining with sodium fluorescein was noted.

Videokeratography OD

Corneal topography revealed a central flat astigmatic island with midperipheral and peripheral steepening (Fig. 49.10).

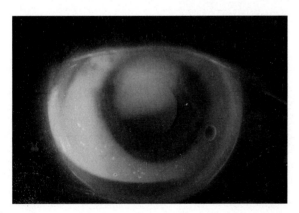

FIG. 49.9. Final Macrolens fluorescein pattern of the patient shown in Fig. 49.7. (See Color Plate 49.9.)

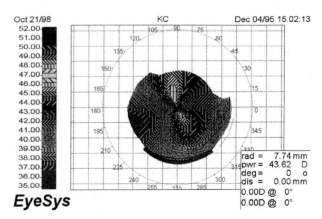

FIG. 49.10. Videokeratography map after penetrating keratoplasty.

Material Selection

Contact lens fitting may be performed as soon as 4 months after PKP. The decision to proceed with contact lenses depends on factors such as the condition of the host cornea and donor button, the suturing technique, and individual healing factors. GP contact lenses are often indicated due to irregular astigmatism that results following corneal transplant surgery. As with keratoconus patients, GP lenses effectively neutralize a majority of the cornea's surface irregularity, thus allowing a smoother refracting surface and improved vision. Although hydrogel lenses may be used in some cases, they increase the risk of neovascularization and graft rejection.

Fitting/Troubleshooting

Due to the irregular topography of the cornea after a corneal transplant, fitting usually involves multiple diagnostic contact lenses. Corneal topography is helpful in determining which base curve to use first. Lenses fit excessively flat may cause excessive corneal staining, whereas lenses fitted too steep may induce lens adherence and an acute red eye, corneal edema, and neovascularization. Care must be taken in determining which GP lens provides the most even distribution of bearing across the entire cornea. Lens centration is usually improved with large overall diameter lenses. A conventional spherical tricurve GP trial lens set was used for this diagnostic fitting. The following lens was applied to the patient's right post-PKP eye:

Base curve: 41.00 D (8.23 mm)
Power: −2.00 D
Overall diameter: 9.5 mm
Optic zone diameter: 8.0 mm

Fluorescein pattern evaluation revealed an irregular area of central pooling and bearing to the midperiphery, temporal lens positioning relative to the graft, and excessive peripheral clearance.

Overrefraction (vertex distance corrected): −7.62 DS (20/50)

Because the lens positioned temporally, a lens with a larger overall diameter was ordered. To compensate for this increase in sagittal height, a 0.25 D flatter base curve was prescribed:

Base curve: 40.75 D (8.28 mm)
Power: −9.37 D
Overall diameter: 10.0 mm
Optic zone diameter: 8.0 mm
Secondary curve radius: 9.00 mm
Third curve radius: 11.00 mm
Third curve width: 0.2 mm
Blend: medium
Material: Fluoroperm 60 (Dk = 60)

At the dispensing visit, the in situ distance visual acuity for the right eye was 20/40.

Overrefraction: plano DS (20/40)

This lens exhibited both bearing and pooling beneath the optic zone, good centration, and average peripheral clearance. The lens was dispensed and the patient was instructed to begin with 4 hours of lens wear and to increase his wearing time by 2 hours per day up to a maximum of 8 hours per day.

At the 1-week follow-up visit, the patient indicated that lens comfort had improved. His wearing time at this visit was 6 hours with a maximum wearing time of 8 hours.

Entering distance visual acuity through his right contact lens was 20/40.

Overrefraction: +0.25 − 0.50 × 105 (20/40)

The fluorescein pattern was unchanged. On lens removal, mild superficial corneal staining was noted nasally at the junction between the host and the graft. However, this small amount of mild staining was not considered significant enough to warrant a refit. He was dismissed for 3 months.

Summary

Localized corneal staining in areas of heavy lens bearing or excessive clearance are common. Ideally, the lens fit allows even distribution of bearing across the cornea. However, with patients who have undergone PKP, the irregularity of the cornea may be so great that small areas of heavier bearing are observed even with an optimal lens design. When indicated, lens parameters should be altered to minimize corneal staining. Large overall diameters are indicated when lens centration is poor. Reverse-geometry designs may be indicated.

Post–Penetrating Keratoplasty

Initial Summary

A 62-year-old woman presented with a chief complaint of constant contact lens irritation while wearing her GP contact lenses. Her ocular history included PKP secondary to keratoconus in both eyes performed 25 years prior to this visit and a repeat PKP of the right eye 3 years later secondary to corneal graft rejection. Intracapsular cataract extractions had been performed 20 and 19 years previously for the right and left eye, respectively, and wedge resection surgery of the right eye for high corneal astigmatism was performed 16 years previously. Ocular medications at the time of the examination included medrysone four times daily OU, prednisolone acetate 0.125% as needed OU, and artificial tears as needed OU.

Testing revealed the following habitual contact lens corrected distance visual acuities: OD 20/50; OS 20/30−1

The patient's habitual GP contact lens parameters follow:

	OD	OS
Base curve(s)	53.62 D (6.30 mm)/	
	54.50 D (6.20 mm)	
	49.62 D (6.80 mm)	
Power(s)	−6.50 D / −2.50 D	−6.50 D
Overall diameter	9.0 mm	9.0 mm
Optic zone diameter	7.4 mm	7.2 mm
Peripheral curves	7.60 /8.10 mm @	7.00 mm @ 0.4mm
	0.6mm	
	11.00 mm @ 0.2mm	7.80 mm @ 0.3mm
		9.50 mm @ 0.2mm
Material	Fluorex 700	Fluorex 700
	(Dk = 70)	(Dk = 70)

Overrefraction:
OD: −1.00 DS (20/30); OS −0.50 DS (20/30)

Manifest refraction:
OD: +5.00 −4.00 × 156 (20/200)
OS: +0.25 −5.50 × 062 (20/100)

Keratometry:
OD: 43.00 @ 170 / 56.00 @ 080, 2+ mire distortion
OS: 48.00 @ 080 / 54.00 @ 170, 2+ mire distortion

Biomicroscopy

The contact lenses adhered to the cornea and positioned superonasally OD and inferonasally OS. Upon lens mobilization, fluorescein pattern evaluation revealed heavy central bearing with paracentral dimple veiling OD, and heavy paracentral bearing with minimum edge clearance OS. Stromal neovascularization was seen, extending from the limbus but not crossing the graft–host junction, and 2+ epithelial erosive keratitis were noted in both eyes.

The patient was instructed to discontinue contact lens wear for 1 week and to return for corneal topography. At the return visit, videokeratography maps were obtained with the 31-ring cone of the Topographic Modeling System (TMS-1; Tomey Technology, Cambridge, MA), and the resultant maps are displayed for the left eye in Figure 49.11 (see Color Plate 49.11).

Material Selection

Although standard keratometry readings suggested a high degree of corneal toricity, topographic analysis revealed asymmetric irregular astigmatism in each eye. The right eye's topography is best described as an asymmetric oblate bow-tie pattern, flatter in the center and steeper in the periphery. Although keratometry may initially suggest fitting a bitoric lens design for the right eye to align with the steep and flat meridians, a bitoric design was contraindicated due to the asymmetry of the astigmatism and the uneven distribution of curvature along a given meridian. Thus, the videokeratoscopic data contributed to the decision of discontinuing the toric back-surface design and using a spherical lens design for the right eye to hopefully optimize both centration and movement.

Topographic analysis of the left cornea revealed a steep to flat graft tilt. Review of the patient's original left lens fit revealed a low-riding adhered lens that settled inferiorly over the steepest portion of the graft. Goals in refitting this eye were to enhance lens movement, increase lid attachment, and improve centration. The corneal map provided guidance to flatten the posterior lens curvature, allowing better

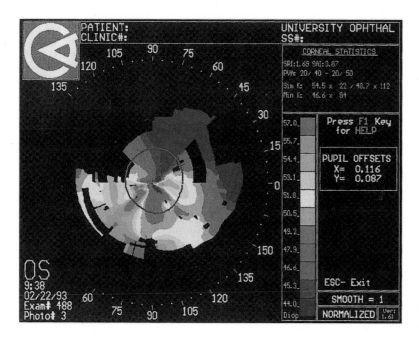

FIG. 49.11. Irregular corneal topography after penetrating keratoplasty. (See Color Plate 49.11)

alignment with the flatter superior corneal curvature for a potential superior lid-attachment fitting relationship.

Fitting/Troubleshooting

The optimal lens base curve-to-cornea fitting relationship desired for this patient was one which would provide minimal central and midperipheral surface bearing with adequate corneal clearance to create a sufficient tear layer, but not excessively steep as to cause bubble formation. The patient's habitual lenses were used as diagnostic lenses in refitting. A change of at least 0.2 mm in the average base curve radius is generally required to significantly alter tear layer patterns and GP lens fitting characteristics for the majority of patients who have undergone PKP. Also, the overall and optic zone diameters were reduced to limit peripheral seal-off and wider peripheral curve systems were prescribed to promote sufficient tear exchange. Final lens powers were calculated by adding the additional minus power found in the initial overrefraction to the patient's habitual lens powers, as well as additional plus power to compensate for the minus-power tear lens induced by refitting to flatter base curves.

The following lenses were prescribed:

	OD	OS
Base curve	50.37 D (6.70 mm)	51.87 D (6.50 mm)
Power	−4.25 D	−4.37 D
Overall diameter	8.6 mm	8.6 mm
Optic zone diameter	6.7 mm	6.7 mm
Peripheral curves	7.50 mm @ 0.75mm	7.20 mm @ 0.75mm
	10.50 mm @ 0.2mm	10.50 mm @ 0.2mm
Material	Fluoroperm 60 (Dk = 60)	Fluoroperm 60 (Dk = 60)

Visual acuities through the new lenses: 20/30 (OD); 20/30 (OS)

Overrefraction: +0.50 DS (OD); plano DS (OS)

Biomicroscopy

Both lenses were lid-attached and moved approximately 1 mm on a blink. The left lens positioned slightly nasal. The fluorescein pattern is displayed in Figure 49.12 (see Color Plate 49.12) for the left eye. Both fluorescein patterns and contact lens fits were considered clinically acceptable.

At 3 months after dispensing, both grafts were clear and compact, with no superficial staining, and neovascularization was unchanged. The lenses moved and centered well, considering the irregular corneal shape. The patient was able to wear the lenses all waking hours, and her complaint of dryness was managed with ocular lubricants or lens rewetting drops on an as-needed basis

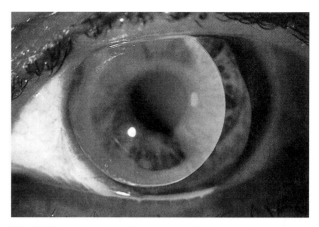

FIG. 49.12. Spherical rigid gas-permeable fluorescein pattern on cornea in Figure 49.11. (See Color Plate 49.12)

Summary

Despite advances in surgical techniques, many corneal surfaces remain irregular and/or have high amounts of astigmatism after PKP. Furthermore, significant anisometropia may result, requiring contact lens correction to achieve binocularity. GP contact lenses are usually the correction of choice for postkeratoplasty patients because of the need to correct regular and irregular astigmatism and modern GP lenses offer enhanced oxygen transmission. Computer assisted topographic analysis is advantageous in assessing the baseline topography of irregular corneas and can assist in fitting postsurgical GP lenses.

For this patient, corneal videokeratoscopy guided the GP lens design for each eye through the selection of a qualitative global fitting philosophy based on topographic analysis. The central graft contour and the shape and asymmetry induced at the midperipheral transitions of the wound with the host cornea were crucial variables in determining contact lens selection. Computerized videokeratoscopy provides additional data, as compared to keratometry, that assist in fitting and managing contact lenses for patients with irregular corneal surfaces.

Post–Penetrating Keratoplasty "Contact Lens Problem"

Initial Summary

A 57-year-old woman presented with a chief complaint of recent-onset contact lens irritation soon after lens application. Penetrating keratoplasty surgery had been performed in her left eye for Fuchs' endothelial corneal dystrophy 18 months prior to this examination. Her surgery was uneventful and there were no unusual postoperative complications. She had discontinued all medications and had been successfully fitted with a GP contact lens, which she typically wore for 12 to 14 hours per day.

The clinical examination revealed the following:

Contact lens corrected visual acuity: 20/25 (OS)
Overrefraction: plano DS (OS)

Biomicroscopy OS

Her lids and lashes had 1+ dried mucous debris. The conjunctiva was sectorially injected from 6 to 8 o'clock and minimally injected elsewhere. The cornea revealed a clear graft with a running suture and four interrupted sutures still present around the graft-host circumference. The GP contact lens moved 1 to 2 mm on a blink and was fitted lid-attachment. The lens had mucous accumulation on the front surface. With each blink, the lens was observed to drag an exposed loop of the running suture at the 7-o'clock position. The suture also accumulated mucous debris. Fluorescein staining revealed moderate epithelial disruption, predominantly on the host cornea at 7 o'clock. There were no infiltrates and no associated neovascularization, and the anterior chamber was clear and quiet.

The diagnosis of an exposed/loose running corneal suture was made, and the patient was referred to her corneal surgeon for prompt treatment and probable suture removal. The corneal surgeon removed the entire running suture without complication. The patient was able to resume contact lens wear 4 weeks after suture removal with her habitual GP contact lens.

Troubleshooting

Because contact lens management can begin as early as 4 months postoperatively, sutures are often present when the first lens is dispensed. Most surgeons believe that remaining sutures are not a contraindication to GP lens wear unless suture removal is soon planned. GP lenses can be safely fitted after PKP as long as sutures are completely covered by epithelium and all knots are buried.

It is surprising how many patients do not know if they have any remaining sutures. Informing the patient that sutures are still present is critical so that possible suture complications may be detected early. Often the first symptom may be contact lens intolerance, which the patient usually attributes to a faulty lens. The patient might also delay reporting the problem and discontinue lens wear until the problem worsens. Classical signs and symptoms of exposed sutures include foreign-body sensation, pain, photophobia, giant papillary hypertrophy, conjunctival injection, epithelial erosion, dellen formation, corneal vascularization, and occasionally iritis, which may lead to graft rejection (5).

If a loose or broken suture is discovered, prompt removal is required to avoid a target for mucous accumulation, a nidus of infection, and/or a stimulus to neovascularization and secondary rejection. Additionally, if any intact/buried suture stimulates vascularization along the suture tract or the recipient stroma, referral to the corneal surgeon is necessary. The surgeon may remove some or all of the sutures, depending on the suturing technique, time elapsed after surgery, and the ocular status. Common suturing techniques include single or double running sutures, combination interrupted and running sutures, and interrupted sutures alone. If a continuous suture is affected, removal is based on wound healing and whether additional sutures are present to support the wound. If exposed loops or knots occur but the wound is not completely healed, the surgeon may remove the exposed portion alone, with the remaining suture taken out as it unravels during subsequent patient visits.

Summary

Even many years after PKP, patients may still be at risk for surgical complications, which can be difficult to distinguish from contact lens–related problems. In fact, patients often first present to the contact lens practitioner with new ocular complaints, such as recent-onset GP intolerance, decreased visual acuity, or ocular pain and redness, which they attribute to contact lens wear. However, the underlying condition may be a surgical complication such as a broken suture, a suture abscess, or early graft rejection.

Removal of a suture and subsequent healing may disturb corneal topography necessitating a contact lens refit. This is more likely with the removal of a running suture, or multiple interrupted sutures, and less likely with the removal of one single interrupted suture. Patients should therefore be reevaluated after healing prior to the resumption of contact lens wear.

If appropriately managed, such patients should enjoy many years of successful contact lens wear.

Post–Radial Keratotomy Refractive Surgery

Initial Summary

A 37-year-old woman presented 3 years after undergoing bilateral RK. She noticed difficulty with her near work. She also noticed symptoms of haloes and glare with fluctuation of vision throughout the day. Her general health was excellent and she reported using no medication at the time of the examination. Prior to RK she wore extended-wear soft contact lenses for 7 years.

Visual acuity (unaided):
OD: 20/30 distance, 20/60 near
OS: 20/30 distance, 20/60 near

Manifest refraction:
OD: +1.75 − 0.75 × 175, 20/25 distance and near
OS: +2.00 − 1.00 × 10, 20/25 distance and near

Keratometry:
OD: 37.75 @ 180 / 38.50 @ 090; 1+ mire distortion
OS: 36.25 @ 180 / 37.75 @ 090; 1+ mire distortion

Biomicroscopy

Eight radial incisions extending from a central clear zone approximately 3.0 mm in diameter to a point 2.0 mm from the limbus were observed. There was vascular encroachment extending 1.5 mm from the limbus, probably secondary to previous wear of soft extended wear contact lenses. No corneal staining was present upon sodium fluorescein instillation.

Material Selection

Postoperative compound hyperopic astigmatism, probably due to surgical overcorrection or postsurgical hyperopic "creep," was diagnosed. By correcting the hyperopia and astigmatism, improvement in both distance and near visual acuity was anticipated. The following contact lens options are available for post-RK patients:

- Soft spherical lenses
- Soft toric lenses
- Conventional GP lenses
- Reverse-geometry GP lenses

If the RK incisions extend to the limbus, avoid prescribing soft contact lenses because of the increased possibility of corneal vascularization. More recent RK techniques use shorter and shallower incisions, generally allowing successful soft lens wear with fewer complications of corneal vascularization along the incisions. If soft contact lenses are being considered, prescribe high-Dk silicone hydrogels. Because this patient already had preexisting corneal vascular encroachment, soft lens options were excluded. Also, due to corneal distortion secondary to the RK surgery, a GP contact lens might provide improved vision.

Fitting/Troubleshooting

It has been suggested that presurgical corneal curvature data are beneficial in determining diagnostic lens selection; however, these data are not always available. Corneal topography provides greater information over a larger area of the cornea (Fig. 49.13). Despite limitations, corneal curvature values generated by topography are beneficial in describing the area of central flattening and the area of midperipheral steepening. In addition to corneal curvature values, the size of the surgical optic zone is important in prescribing the appropriate contact lens optic zone size.

Numerical topography maps provide "curvature" values at various diameters from the center. These values can generate an average curvature to use for the selection of an initial diagnostic lens base curve. It is important to remember that axial values should be viewed only as estimates of curvature.

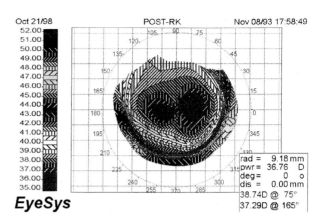

FIG. 49.13. Videokeratography map of post–radial keratotomy.

Therefore, diagnostic lens fitting is necessary to determine the optimal base curve and lens design.

Reverse-geometry GP lens designs allow the practitioner to better "align" the central flat zone while maintaining an adequate peripheral fitting relationship over the steeper midperiphery of the post–refractive surgery cornea. The steeper secondary curve also assists in the centration of the lens. When prescribing a reverse-geometry lens design, the optic zone diameter should approximate the area of central corneal flattening, which when viewed on an axial map is generally 5 to 7 mm. The base curve radius should be the average value over the area of flattening.

For this patient, reverse-geometry diagnostic lenses were selected. The initial diagnostic lenses were:

Base curve: OD and OS 38.12 D (8.85 mm)
Power: OD and OS plano
Overall diameter: OD and OS 9.5 mm
Optic zone diameter: OD and OS 6.0 mm
Secondary curve radius: OD and OS 8.20 mm (41.12 D, 3.00 D steeper than the base curve)

With diagnostic lenses in place, the fluorescein patterns revealed an area of light central pooling and moderate bearing inferonasal on the right eye and inferotemporal on the left eye, consistent with the location of the steeper areas of the cornea. Both lenses positioned superiorly. Overrefraction was OD –1.00 DS (20/20) and OS – 2.00 DS (20/20). Overall diameters were ordered at 10.0 mm to improve lens centration. Ordered optical lens powers were determined by adding the equivalent sphere over refractions to the powers of the diagnostic contact lenses.

The following reverse-geometry GP contact lenses were prescribed (Menicon SF-P Plateau design):

Base curve: OD 38.12 D (8.85 mm); OS 38.12 (8.85 mm)
Power: OD –1.00; OS –2.00
Overall diameter: OD and OS 10.0 mm
Optic zone diameter: OD and OS 6.0 mm

Secondary curve radius: OD and OS 8.20 mm (41.12 D, 3.00 D steeper than the base curve)

No adjustment was made in the base curve to compensate for the change in sagittal height induced by increasing the overall diameter.

At the dispensing visit, increased overall lens diameters indeed resulted in improved lens centration and decreased bearing along inferior steeper corneal areas both eyes. By improving lens centrations, the steeper secondary curves were also better aligned over the steeper corneal midperipheries. The patient's in situ visual acuities were 20/20 at distance and near.

Summary

Some patients who have undergone RK exhibit continued hyperopic shifts years after surgery. A reverse-geometry GP contact lens design was prescribed for this post-RK patient to optimize lens fit and enhance vision. As often occurs with postsurgical GP lens fitting, visual acuity improves since the tear lens assists in optically "smoothing" the irregular corneal surface. The contact lens power required additional minus power to compensate for the steep plus tear lens over the central cornea.

Unfortunately, fitting patients who have undergone RK may require numerous lens changes to optimize the base curve-to-cornea fitting relationship (no excessive central tear pooling) and to enhance lens centration. The reverse-geometry lens should be prescribed with a secondary curve steep enough and wide enough to prevent excessive bearing at the "knee" (or flattened junction of the midperipheral cornea). Reverse-geometry rigid contact lenses may not be warranted by GP contact lens laboratories; therefore, diagnostic fitting assists in minimizing the number of lens reorders.

Post–Radial Keratotomy Refractive Surgery

Initial Summary

A 33-year-old man presented with a chief complaint of fluctuating vision. He reported undergoing bilateral RK 2 years previously. His general health was excellent and he was taking no medications. Before undergoing RK, he wore daily-wear soft contact lenses for 9 years. As a competitive marksman, he noticed some difficulty sighting subsequent to the RK surgery.

Visual acuity (unaided):
OD: 20/25 distance, 20/20 near
OS: 20/40 distance, 20/20 near

Manifest refraction:
OD: −0.50 DS, 20/25 distance, 20/20 near
OS: −1.00 − 0.50 × 165, 20/25 distance, 20/20 near

Keratometry:
OD: 38.37 @ 180 / 38.87 @ 090; 1+ mire distortion
OS: 39.50 @ 165 / 40.62 @ 075; 1+ mire distortion

Biomicroscopy

Four corneal radial incisions extending from a central clear zone approximately 3.5 mm in diameter to a point 2.5 mm from the limbus were observed bilaterally. There were two astigmatic incisions on the vertical meridian of the left eye. No corneal staining was present with sodium fluorescein instillation.

Data from 3 years prior to the RK surgery follow:

Visual acuity (unaided):
OD: 20/200 distance, 20/20 near
OS: 20/200 distance, 20/20 near

Manifest refraction:
OD: −3.00 DS (20/20 distance, 20/20 near)
OS: −2.75 − 1.75 × 160 (20/20 distance, 20/20 near)

Keratometry:
OD: 41.00 @ 180 / 41.50 @ 090; no mire distortion
OS: 41.00 @ 160 / 42.50 @ 070; no mire distortion

Because the patient presented with a chief complaint of fluctuating vision, he was reexamined 1 week later. His refractive findings at that visit were:

Visual acuity (unaided):
OD: 20/30 distance, 20/20 near
OS: 20/50 distance, 20/20 near

Manifest refraction:
OD: −0.75 DS (20/25 distance, 20/20 near)
OS: −1.00 − 1.00 × 160 (20/25 distance, 20/20 near)

Keratometry:
OD: 38.62 @ 180 / 39.12 @ 090; 1+ mire distortion
OS: 39.00 @ 160 / 40.62 @ 070; 1+ mire distortion

Material Selection

This patient had undercorrected postrefractive (RK) surgery myopia in the right eye and compound myopic astigmatism in the left eye. Contact lens options available are the same as those listed in the previous case. Because the post-RK scars are short (not reaching the limbus) and shallow, soft lenses were considered—spherical for the right eye and possibly toric for the left. However, because of the patient's complaints of fluctuating vision and his dissatisfaction with his vision during competitive shooting, GP contact lenses were the best option.

Fitting/Troubleshooting

Postoperative fluctuation of vision is often reported after RK. In this case, the patient's keratometric values fluctuated, altering spherical and astigmatic refractive findings. GP contact lenses can minimize the effect of this fluctuation by allowing the tear lens to adjust for these diurnal variations. The post–contact lens tear lens also "smooths" corneal surface irregularities to enhance vision. Because presurgical data were available, the initial diagnostic lenses selected (39.50 D) were 1.50 D flatter than the presurgical flat-K readings (41.00 D). The diagnostic GP lenses selected were conventional tricurve designs. In the right eye there was central pooling with a few small bubbles present, minimal bearing at the junction between the flat, central cornea and the steep midperiphery (knee), and average peripheral edge clearance; the lens positioned centrally. To eliminate the bubbles beneath the optic zone, a lens with a 1.00 D flatter base curve was diagnostically fitted. The central pooling remained, but without any bubbles. There was slightly more bearing on the knee, although not excessive, and the lens positioned superiorly. The fluorescein pattern for the left lens exhibited central pooling with moderate lens bearing on the knee and average edge clearance, and the lens positioned slightly inferior. Since the patient had a low degree of central flattening, a conventional tricurve GP lens design was prescribed.

The patient's postoperative topography revealed the flattest axial values of 38.50 D in the right eye and 36.50 D in the left eye. This is representative of post-RK corneas. Because the GP contact lens base curve was steeper than the flattest corneal curvature, a final contact lens power with significant minus power was required. For this patient the final GP contact lens prescription was:

Base curve: OD 38.50 D (8.77 mm); OS 39.50 D (8.54 mm)
Power: OD –1.75 D; OS –2.50 D
Overall diameter: OD and OS 9.5 mm
Optic zone diameter: OD and OS 7.5 mm
Secondary curve radius: OD 9.50 mm; OS 9.25 mm
Peripheral curve radius: OD and OS 12.00 mm
Peripheral curve width: OD and OS 0.2 mm

Summary

The patient was disappointed at the prospect of wearing contact lenses; however, he reported that his vision was generally stable through his GP contact lenses and his visual performance was improved for sighting with his rifle. If lens centration had not been achieved with tricurve GP lenses, large overall diameter, aspheric or even reverse-geometry lens designs would have been considered (Figs. 49.14 and 49.15).

Post–Photorefractive Keratectomy

Initial Summary

A 41-year-old man presented 18 months after PRK surgery in which he was surgically corrected for monovision (dis-

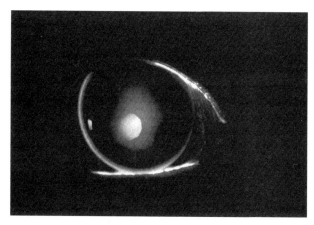

FIG. 49.14. Spherical tricurve rigid gas-permeable fluorescein pattern on post–radial keratotomy cornea.

tance viewing with his right eye and near viewing with his left eye). He complained of difficulty with near work and with adapting to monovision. He was employed as a real estate broker and noticed difficulty reading residential listings. His general health was excellent and he reported using no medication at the time of examination. The patient had no prior contact lens history.

Visual acuity (unaided):
OD: 20/25 distance, 20/70 near
OS: 20/50 distance, 20/20 near

Manifest refraction:
OD: +1.50 – 0.25 × 170 20/20 distance; +1.00 add, 20/20 near
OS: –1.00 – 0.50 × 180 20/20 distance, +1.00 add, 20/20 near

Keratometry:
OD: 40.12 @ 170 / 41.25 @ 90; no mire distortion
OS: 39.75 @ 180 / 42.00 @ 75; no mire distortion

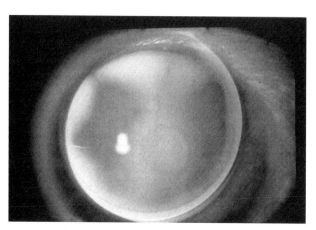

FIG. 49.15. Reverse-geometry rigid gas-permeable fluorescein pattern on post–radial keratotomy cornea.

Biomicroscopy

Examination of both corneas revealed slight stromal haze. No corneal staining was present in either eye with sodium fluorescein instillation. All other anterior segment structures were clear and quiet.

Videokeratography

Corneal topography revealed a central area of flattening approximately 5 to 6 mm in diameter, with a very gradual area of peripheral steepening (Fig. 49.16; see Color Plate 49.16). Corneal topography axial "curvatures" were 40.25 D centrally, 41.62 D at 2.5 mm from center, 43.25 D at 3.5 mm from center, and 44.62 D at 4 mm from the central cornea.

Material Selection

The smooth transition of the post-PRK cornea allows the following contact lens options:

- Spherical soft contact lenses
- Toric soft contact lenses
- Spherical GP contact lenses
- Aspheric GP contact lenses
- Reverse-geometry GP contact lenses

Fitting/Troubleshooting

By improving the overcorrected (hyperopic) right eye, the patient's vision at near should be enhanced. A spherical disposable soft contact lens with a +1.25-D power was selected for demonstration. The patient reported immediate improvement in visual comfort with no compromise of distance vision (20/20). The lens provided good movement, centration and comfort. The following lens was dispensed to the patient for use in the right eye:

Ciba Vision Precision UV 8.7 mm / +1.25 / 14.4 mm

The patient reported improved tolerance to monovision with the contact lens for the distance eye.

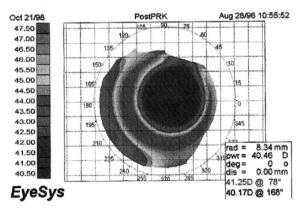

FIG. 49.16. Videokeratography map of post–photorefractive keratectomy. (See Color Plate 49.16.)

Summary

Post-PRK as well as post-LASIK corneas are relatively simple to fit with soft or GP contact lenses. The junction between the flat, central cornea and the steeper midperiphery is generally a smooth transition that allows for adequate draping of a soft contact lens. Conventional sphere and aspheric GP lens designs are generally successful; rarely is a reverse-geometry design necessary. If an irregular corneal surface exists, GP contact lenses may improve vision.

The excimer laser has proven to be efficient in refractive error modification. When fitting contact lenses on the post-PRK eye, patient education and compliance are important. Spherical disposable soft contact lenses with a multipurpose solution care system were prescribed for this patient to assist in compliance. Because he had never worn contact lenses, a disposable lens that optimized handling characteristics and flex-wear capability for increased oxygen permeability was prescribed. High-Dk silicone hydrogel lenses would have been another option to optimize the available oxygen. It was emphasized to this patient that he may require a contact lens in the future for the left eye as his presbyopia progresses.

It is important to remember that corneal integrity has been compromised in PRK and LASIK, but not as dramatically as in RK. Careful follow-up is necessary to ensure that if infections occur, they are managed early enough to prevent serious corneal damage.

Post-LASIK Corneal Ectasia

Initial Summary

A 27-year-old woman was referred for a contact lens evaluation and fitting. The patient had undergone LASIK 2 years prior to the initial contact lens evaluation. She presented to the contact lens evaluation with symptoms of blurred vision when driving and reading for the past 3 months. Three pairs of spectacles had been prescribed within the past 3 months. GP contact lenses (post-LASIK) had previously been unsuccessful due to discomfort and redness. The referring practitioner suspected post-LASIK corneal ectasia. The patient's personal and family medical history was unremarkable. There was no known family history of keratoconus and no positive history of atopic disease, connective tissue disorders, or eye rubbing. The following data were obtained:

Habitual spectacles and entering visual acuities:

OD: plano −5.00 × 062 (20/40)
OS: −0.25 −5.50 × 098 (20/60)

Simulated keratometry (Dicon CT 200; Vismed, San Diego, CA):
OD: 48.87 @ 067 / 51.25 @ 157
OS: 48.25 @ 108 / 50.87 @ 018

Manifest refraction:
OD: plano −5.00 × 050 (20/40)
OS: −1.00 −5.50 × 105 (20/40)

Biomicroscopy

Eyelids, eyelashes, and conjunctivae were clear. There was no corneal staining. Fleischer's ring and Vogt's striae were not observed. The LASIK flap junctions were visible. The tear film and tear break-up times were normal. The anterior chambers were deep and quiet and the crystalline lens and vitreous were clear in both eyes.

Videokeratography

Corneal topography revealed an inferior area of steepening suggestive of keratoconus (Fig. 49.17; see Color Plate 49.17).

There were no contraindications to GP contact lens wear. The patient was educated regarding keratoconus, contact lens options, and her prognosis. A GP contact lens fitting was performed.

Material Selection

Gas-permeable contact lenses are indicated when patients present with decreased best-corrected vision due to an irregular corneal surface. The quality of this patient's vision through spectacles was not satisfactory or stable. Spherical soft contact lenses are not appropriate due to the high degree of refractive astigmatism. Currently available toric soft contact lenses are not an optimal choice due to their thicker profile reducing oxygen availability to the cornea and questionable vision when a significant astigmatism error needs to be corrected. Silicone hydrogels could be considered in the future if they become available in toric designs. However, even with the increased firmness of toric soft contact lenses, they generally do not provide sufficient masking of irregular astigmatism. GP contact lenses with a Dk of 50 or higher are indicated for this patient.

Fitting

The following initial pair of diagnostic rigid contact lenses was applied and fluorescein patterns were evaluated:

	OD	OS
Base curve	51.12 D (6.57 mm)	50.37 D (6.69 mm)
Overall diameter	8.6 mm	8.6 mm
Optic zone diameter	6.5 mm	6.5 mm

The fluorescein patterns revealed apical clearance (steep) with minimal peripheral clearance for both eyes.

A second pair of diagnostic lenses was applied:

	OD	OS
Base curve	50.37 D (6.69 mm)	49.62 D (6.80 mm)
Power	−9.00 D	−7.00 D
Overall diameter	8.6 mm	8.6 mm
Optic zone diameter	6.5 mm	6.5 mm

Contact lens fluorescein pattern analysis suggested light apical touch with average peripheral clearance both eyes. These fluorescein patterns were typical for keratoconus and the fit of this pair of lenses was judged to be good. A spherocylinder overrefraction was performed through the second pair of diagnostic lenses.

Overrefraction:
OD: +2.50 −1.00 × 075 (20/20)
OS: +1.50 −0.75 × 105 (20/20)

Based on these findings, the following Fluoroperm 60 (Dk = 60) GP contact lenses were ordered:

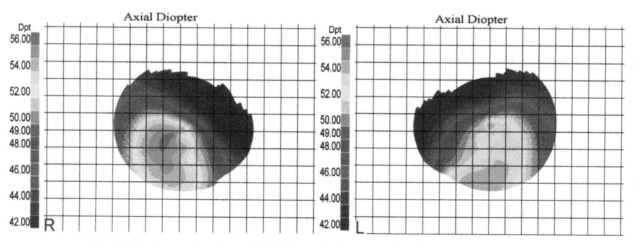

FIG. 49.17. Topography of a post-LASIK (laser *in situ* keratomileusis) patient revealing ectasia indicative of keratoconus. (See Color Plate 49.17.)

	OD	OS
Base curve	50.37 D (6.69 mm)	49.62 D (6.80 mm)
Power	−7.00 D	−5.87 D
Overall diameter	9.0 mm	9.0 mm
Optic zone diameter	7.4 mm	7.4 mm
Secondary curve radius	8.50 mm	8.50 mm
Peripheral curve radius	11.00 mm	11.00 mm
Peripheral curve width	0.2 mm	0.2 mm
Center thickness	0.14 mm	0.14 mm
Blend	Medium	Medium

Base curves were prescribed from fluorescein pattern evaluation. Initial diagnostic lens base curves were selected to approximate the steep keratometry values. Since the initial diagnostic lenses were judged to be steep, flatter lenses were applied and the fluorescein patterns were evaluated. The final base curve was determined by bracketing the fluorescein pattern to determine the "steepest" apical touch lens. The power was determined by adding the equivalent sphere of the overrefraction to the diagnostic lens power. If the diagnostic base curve is not the same base curve to be prescribed, optical power should be adjusted by the dioptric change in lens base curve.

Overall and optic zone diameters larger than standard for keratoconus patients were prescribed to optimize lens centration. Generally, smaller overall diameters (approximately 8.6 mm) and optic zone diameters (5.5 to 7.0 mm) are prescribed for keratoconus patients. Secondary curves are prescribed flat relative to the base curve for keratoconus. Eight to 9.00 mm is standard.

Follow-up Care

Two weeks following lens dispensing the patient reported intermittent blurred vision after approximately 2 hours of lens wear each day. The patient noticed the symptoms more frequently with the right lens. Entering visual acuities were 20/50 both OD and OS. Fluorescein pattern evaluation revealed bubbles beneath the optic zone superior to the area of apical touch. Slit-lamp biomicroscopy revealed corresponding areas of dimple veiling (Fig. 49.18). Flatter base

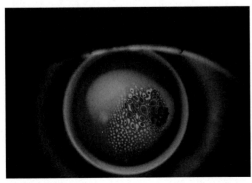

FIG. 49.18. Fluorescein pattern of post-LASIK (laser in situ keratomileusis) ectasia patient showing bubbles beneath optic zone leading to dimple veil staining.

curve lenses were ordered to reduce the space between the base curve of the lens and the cornea superior to the cone apex.

	OD	OS
Base curve	48.87 D (6.91 mm)	49.00 D (6.88 mm)
Power	−5.50 D	−5.25 D
Overall diameter	9.4 mm	9.4 mm
Optic zone diameter	7.8 mm	7.8 mm
Secondary curve radius	8.75 mm	8.75 mm
Third curve radius	11.00 mm	11.00 mm
Third curve width	0.2 mm	0.2 mm
Center thickness	0.14 mm	0.14 mm
Blend	Medium	Medium

Contact lens powers were adjusted to compensate for the flatter base curves. Overall diameters were ordered larger to improve lens centration.

Further follow-up care revealed an apical touch fluorescein pattern, good lens centration, and no evidence of dimple veiling. The patient was pleased with the vision (20/20 OD and OS) and comfort provided by the lenses. She was rescheduled for follow-up care in 6 months.

Summary

Post-LASIK keratectasia may be iatrogenic, resulting from a thin postsurgical corneal bed. LASIK surgery is also occasionally performed on patients with subclinical or formefruste keratoconus. Topographic and corneal signs and vision symptoms of keratoconus may occur months to years after the surgery (6,7).

Fitting contact lenses to post-LASIK patients who develop ectasia is extremely challenging (8). Prior to LASIK, the cornea is a prolate shape; after LASIK, the cornea is often an oblate shape in which the central cornea is less curved than the peripheral cornea. Sometimes it is advantageous to prescribe reverse-geometry contact lenses for post-LASIK patients needing additional vision correction. The contour within the treatment zone of a post-LASIK ectasia cornea is both oblate and protrudes. This makes it more challenging to "align" the central cornea. The goal is to minimize harsh bearing on the cone while minimizing areas of excessive clearance over the oblate portion of the cornea. These two objectives are contrary in that minimizing one will result in making the other worse. For example, if you prescribe a steeper base curve to minimize bearing on the cone, the area of clearance beneath the optic zone, but peripheral to the cone, may become excessive. In this case, bubbles formed within this area of excessive clearance resulting in reduced vision and dimple-veil staining. Assuming that the base curve touches the cone, prescribe the steepest base curve that does not result in bubble formation beneath the optic zone. This may be achieved by prescribing a spherical, aspheric, or reverse-geometry rigid contact lens.

CORNEAL TRAUMA–INDUCED IRREGULAR ASTIGMATISM CASES

Postcorneal Trauma

Initial Summary

A 5-year-old boy presented with a history of a full-thickness corneal laceration in his left eye secondary to an accident with a steak knife. Although his vision had improved after the accident from "count fingers" to 20/60, the referring eye care practitioner wanted to determine if the patient's vision could be further improved with a contact lens.

Entering distance visual acuities (with spectacles) were OD 20/25, OS 20/100 (Lighthouse cards).

Keratometry:
OD: 41.37 @ 107 / 42.25 @ 017; no mire distortion
OS: 46.00 @ 033 / 48.00 @ 115; 2+ mire distortion

Manifest refraction:
OD: plano −1.25 × 100 (20/20)
OS: −0.50 − 3.00 × 090 (20/80)

Biomicroscopy

Eyelids and lashes were clear both eyes. Grade 1+ bulbar injection was present both eyes. The right cornea was clear. An arc-shaped corneal scar just outside and almost congruent with the superior pupillary border from 8 to 4 o'clock was present in the left eye. There were areas of corneal thinning around the full thickness corneal scar. No positive or negative corneal staining with sodium fluorescein was noted in either eye.

Videokeratography

Corneal topography of the left eye revealed a localized area of steepening 1 mm temporal to the pupillary axis. This area was approximately 2 mm wide and 3 mm high (Fig. 49.19; see Color Plate 49.19).

Material Selection

Vision correction options available to this patient were limited due to the nature of his injury. Although soft contact

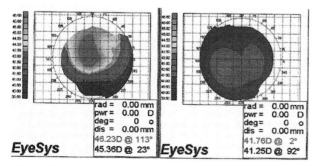

FIG. 49.19. Videokeratography maps of corneas after penetrating injury in the left eye. (See Color Plate 49.19)

lenses offer good initial comfort, they generally have a limited ability to mask irregular corneal astigmatism. A hybrid lens design, which has a GP lens center surrounded by a soft lens skirt, offers the initial comfort of a soft lens and the excellent optics of a GP contact lens. However, it was not ideal for this young patient due to its large overall diameter and its potential for splitting at the junction between the soft lens skirt and the GP center. Therefore, a GP contact lens was prescribed for this patient. Spherical GP lenses work well optically for patients with this type of injury because they optically "smooth" the corneal irregularity.

Fitting

Only the left eye was fitted with a GP contact lens to eliminate the risk of potential complications associated with contact lens wear in the "better" eye. The ametropia in his right eye was easily corrected with spectacles that also provided polycarbonate protection for both eyes. The importance of protective eyewear was emphasized to this patient and to his parents since he was young and had one eye with decreased corneal integrity secondary to trauma. A trial lens set containing conventional tricurve spherical GP contact lenses was selected for the diagnostic fitting. Due to the irregular astigmatism and scarring present secondary to the patient's injury, the base curve of the GP lens was chosen so that the lens lightly touched the steepest portion of the cornea, similar to a keratoconus fit. The following diagnostic GP contact lens was applied to the left eye:

Base curve: 47.00 D (7.18 mm)
Power: −2.00 D
Overall diameter: 9.0 mm
Optic zone diameter: 7.4 mm

Evaluation with sodium fluorescein revealed light bearing centrally with an arc of pooling inferiorly, good centration, and minimal peripheral clearance.

A spherocylinder overrefraction revealed −3.75 DS (20/30).

Because the base curve of the diagnostic GP lens lightly touched the steepest portion of the cornea, no change was indicated. The contact lens power of the prescribed contact lens was determined by combining the power of the diagnostic contact lens (−2.00 D) with the spherical equivalent of the overrefraction (−3.75 D). However, the peripheral clearance with this diagnostic contact lens was minimal because the periphery of the cornea remained relatively unaffected by the trauma. Therefore, the peripheral curves were prescribed to approximate those indicated for a "normal" cornea. The GP contact lens prescription follows:

Base curve: 47.00 D (7.18 mm)
Power: −5.75 D
Overall diameter: 9.0 mm
Optic zone diameter: 7.4 mm

Secondary curve radius: 8.50 mm
Peripheral curve radius: 12.00 mm
Peripheral curve width: 0.2 mm
Blend: medium
Material: Fluoroperm 30 (Dk = 30)

At the dispensing visit, in situ distance visual acuity was 20/25.

Overrefraction: +0.50 − 0.50 × 055 (20/25)

The lens exhibited light bearing centrally with an arc of pooling inferiorly, good centration, and average peripheral clearance. The contact lens was dispensed after the patient's mother was instructed on application, removal, recentering, and care of the lens. He was instructed to start with 4 hours of lens wear and increase his wearing time by 2 hours per day.

At his first follow-up visit, he indicated that the comfort of the lens was good. His wearing time at this visit was 2 hours. His maximum wearing time had been 8 hours.

Entering visual acuities with his contact lens: 20/25
Overrefraction: OS +0.25 − 0.50 × 090 (20/25)

The lens exhibited light bearing centrally with an arc of pooling inferiorly, superior–inferior lens positioning, and average peripheral clearance. Upon lens removal, biomicroscopy revealed no changes. At his 1-month follow-up visit, the patient was doing well and was subsequently rescheduled for follow-up in 6 months.

Summary

Irregular corneal astigmatism is commonly associated with corneal or corneoscleral lacerations and punctures. The extent to which corneal contour is altered depends on the severity of the injury. Most changes in corneal topography occur at the site of the wound and the area immediately surrounding it. This effect diminishes as one measures farther away from the damaged area.

In cases where irregular astigmatism is present after corneal trauma, spherical GP lenses are the lens of choice because of their ability to optically correct corneal surface distortion using the tear lens. To determine the contact lens prescription, a diagnostic fitting was performed. Due to the irregular astigmatism present secondary to the patient's injury, the base curve of the GP lens was chosen so that the lens lightly touched on the steepest portion of the cornea. However, the secondary curve was selected to approximate that of a "normal" cornea because the periphery of the cornea remained relatively unaffected. The secondary curve must have a sufficiently flat radius to allow tears that collect in the midperiphery to adequately flush and exchange into the periphery. If the secondary curve dispensed to a patient is too steep in relation to the peripheral cornea, a midperipheral seal could be established, trapping tear and metabolic waste products in the environment under the contact lens. This could potentially lead to physiologic insult. However, in-office modification can be used to flatten the peripheral curves and remedy this situation.

POSTCORNEAL TRAUMA

Initial Summary

A 45-year-old man who had extensive ocular trauma in the left eye secondary to a softball injury presented for a contact lens evaluation. The softball injury resulted in a superior corneal laceration as well as a blowout fracture of the left orbit. He developed secondary hyphema, glaucoma, and cystoid macular edema. The patient eventually underwent cataract extraction with secondary anterior chamber intraocular lens and trabeculectomy in his left eye.

The patient's main complaint was blurred vision and excessive glare in the left eye. His primary goal with contact lenses was to decrease glare with a secondary goal of improved cosmesis. The examination revealed:

Contact lens corrected distance visual acuity: OD 20/20
Uncorrected distance visual acuity: OS 20/100

Manifest refraction:
OD: −3.00 DS (20/20)
OS: −1.25 −2.75 × 175 (20/60); pinhole no improvement

Keratometry:
OD: 44.50 @ 180 / 45.00 @ 090; no mire distortion
OS: 43.75 @ 043 / 49.25 @ 133; 2+ mire distortion

Biomicroscopy
The left cornea had a peripheral arcuate scar extending from 10 o'clock to 1 o'clock superiorly. The iris was minimally present with small fragments peripherally extending 360 degrees. There was a well-positioned anterior chamber intraocular lens visible in its entirety through the iris fragments.

Material Selection

The anterior segment pathology requiring contact lens management included pseudophakia OS, secondary surgically induced anisometropia, aniridia OS, and irregular astigmatism OS. Treatment goals were to reduce glare utilizing a tinted prosthetic iris soft contact lens and to correct the irregular corneal astigmatism with a GP contact lens. Due to the patient's aniridia, an opaque painted iris lens was required. Thus, a piggyback contact lens system with a GP fitted over the prosthetic soft lens was the most likely combination to optimize vision and minimize glare.

Fitting/Troubleshooting

A trial lens fitting of the left eye was initiated with the following Ciba Vision prosthetic iris contact lens:

Trial lens:

Base curve: 8.6 mm
Power: plano D
Overall diameter: 14.5mm
Color: complements brown
Spherocylinder overrefraction:
OS: −0.25 −3.00 × 175 (20/50)

Overkeratometry readings:
OS: 45.00 @ 15/47.00 @ 105; 2+ mire distortion

Interestingly, the overrefraction through the plano power diagnostic lens differed from the manifest refraction by approximately 1.00 D less minus power. This result may be due to (a) a significant reduction in glare from the opaque iris decreasing peripheral aberrations and providing more reliable refractive results, (b) the hydrogel lens may have provided a mild smoothing effect of the underlying irregular cornea, resulting in less minus correction required for equivalent or better visual acuity, and/or (c) a minus tear layer may have been created beneath the soft lens requiring less minus in the overrefraction.

As expected, persistent decreased vision remained with the soft lens alone; therefore, a GP lens piggyback fitting of the left eye was initiated. The following spherical GP trial contact lens was applied over the soft lens (OS):

Base curve: 46.25 D (7.30 mm)
Power: −4.75 D
Overall diameter: 9.4 mm
Optic zone diameter: 8.0 mm
Secondary curve radius: 8.30 mm
Peripheral curve radius: 11.50 mm @ 0.2-mm width
Spherocylinder overrefraction:
OS: +1.75 DS (20/25)
Final GP lens power required:
OS: −3.00 D

The final GP lens power is consistent with the patient's predicted spherical equivalent refraction through the soft lens and the induced tear lens power between the hydrogel and rigid lens, as the following calculations demonstrate:

Patient's spherical equivalent refraction (with plano soft lens in place): −1.75 D
Gas-permeable trial fit 1.25 D steeper than the flat keratometry reading; (+) tear lens is compensated with (−) power −1.25 D
Estimated final GP power: −3.00 D

The improved visual acuity obtained through the piggyback diagnostic lens system was most likely due to the significant reduction of irregular corneal astigmatism obtained with the GP contact lens, combined with reduction of peripheral glare and aberrations from the opaque iris soft contact lens. The GP lens moved in unison with the soft lens. High-molecular-weight fluorescein revealed mild central clearance and adequate peripheral edge clearance. Although there were no bubbles or impression rings from the GP over the hydrogel lens after 20 minutes of wear, the GP base curve was too steep, inducing adherence to the underlying hydrogel lens. In view of the significant improvement in vision with the GP/soft lens piggyback combination, the following piggyback lens system was prescribed:

1. Ciba Vision prosthetic soft contact lens:
Base curve: 8.6 mm; overall diameter: 14.5 mm; power: plano; color: complements brown with a black iris underprint and a 5-mm clear pupil.
2. Gas-permeable contact lens:
Base curve: 44.75 D (7.54 mm); overall diameter: 9.5 mm; optic zone diameter: 7.7 mm; power: −1.50 D; secondary curve radius: 9.50 mm; peripheral curve radius: 12.00 mm @ 0.3-mm width; material: Fluoroperm 92 (Dk = 92).

The prosthetic iris Ciba Vision soft contact lens was selected for the close color match to the patient's normal right eye. The Fluoroperm 92 GP contact lens was prescribed to obtain high oxygen transmissibility (Dk = 92), thereby reducing possible corneal edema secondary to piggyback lens wear. The base and peripheral curves of the GP lens were ordered flatter than the initial trial lens to achieve a more aligned fit and enhanced lens movement over the soft lens.

At the dispensing visit, visual acuity with the piggyback lens system was 20/30 with a plano spherocylinder overrefraction. The patient had been previously using a chemical soft contact lens care system, and he was instructed to continue with the same care system for both the soft and GP lenses. No specific solutions were dispensed for the GP lens due to potential incompatibility with the hydrogel lens and questionable patient compliance.

At the 2-week follow-up visit the patient reported a significant improvement in vision; however, he complained of continual glare. Biomicroscopy revealed approximately 2 mm movement of the GP lens with each blink; the soft lens moved approximately 0.5 mm with each blink. There was mild transillumination of the prosthetic iris, indicating that approximately 80% of the light was blocked by the double-printed opaque iris. The patient's complaint was attributed to excessive peripheral light transmission and it was recommended to reopaque the posterior side of the prosthetic iris soft lens with a solid black mask. Adventure in Colors (Golden, CO) was able to add an opaque black mask beneath the colored iris ring while preserving the clear 5-mm pupil.

Once the soft lens was tinted and redispensed, the piggyback system provided distance visual acuity of 20/25 − 2. There was less than 5% retroillumination visible through the reopaqued iris portion of the soft lens. The patient noted a tremendous improvement in clarity of his left image, with little to no glare, and was extremely pleased with the final piggyback system. The comparison of visual acuity with and without the GP/soft lens system documents that his visual problems were secondary to irregular corneal astigmatism and peripheral glare, which were corrected by a GP/prosthetic soft contact lens combination.

Summary

This case demonstrates the utility of GP lenses to correct irregular astigmatism secondary to corneal scars, as well as the value of specialty soft lenses in cases of unacceptable cosmesis due to severe ocular trauma. A piggyback lens system was the appropriate choice in this case where glare reduction and improved cosmesis were achieved with the opaque iris soft lens, and the crisp optics and tear lens "correction" of irregular astigmatism were provided by the GP lens. The greatest clinical concern for this patient was the possible development of corneal hypoxia. Significant central corneal clouding (acute) or neovascularization (chronic) can develop from contact lens–induced hypoxia. Fortunately, these complications did not develop for this patient. If signs or symptoms of hypoxia developed, one option would be to order a hyperpermeable GP material such as the Menicon Z (Dk = 163). However, the most significant barrier to oxygen transmission is the hydrogel lens, which has a Dk value of approximately 16. Therefore, if hypoxia did develop, discontinuation or a reduction in wearing time of the soft lens may have been required.

Important factors to consider when prescribing a prosthetic soft contact lens include: (a) selecting a tinting process/tinting laboratory, (b) selecting an iris diameter, (c) selecting a pupil diameter, (d) prescribing the hydrogel lens parameters, and (e) prescribing a lens care regimen. Standard hydrogel fitting techniques were used to achieve a lens fit that fully covered the cornea and moved approximately 1 mm with each blink. The iris diameter from Ciba Vision was a default 12.5-mm iris that was sufficiently large for this patient to provide a full block of peripheral light transmission, even with the allowance of slight lens movement. The pupil diameter (5.0 mm) was sufficient to minimize peripheral field constrictions.

The clinician should also always remember to also care for the "normal" eye in such cases, optimally by recommending use of safety spectacles instead of contact lenses for optimum protection.

REFERENCES

1. Edrington TB, Barr JT, Zadnik K, et al. Standardized rigid contact lens fitting protocol for keratoconus. *Optom Vis Sci* 1996;73: 369–375.
2. Korb DR, Finnemore VM, Herman JP. Apical changes and scarring in keratoconus as related to contact lens fitting techniques. *J Am Optom Assoc* 1982;53:199–205.
3. Krachmer JH, Feder RS, Belin MS. Keratoconus and related non-inflammatory corneal thinning disorders. *Surv Ophthalmol* 1984; 28:293–322.
4. Krachmer JH. Pellucid marginal corneal degeneration. *Arch Ophthalmol* 1978;96:1217–1221.
5. Brightbill, Frederick S, eds. *Corneal surgery: theory, technique, and tissue.* St. Louis: Mosby-Year Book, 1993.
6. Amoils SP, Deist MB, Gous P, et al. Iatrogenic keratectasia after laser in situ keratomileusis for less than -4.0 to -7.0 diopters of myopia. *J Cataract Refract Surg* 2000;26:967–977.
7. Seiler T, Quurke AW. Iatrogenic keratectasia after LASIK in a case of forme fruste keratoconus. *J Cataract Refract Surg* 1998;24: 1007–1009.
8. Szczotka LB, Aronsky M. Contact lenses after LASIK. *J Am Optom Assoc* 1998;69:775–784.

Index